APPLIED
BLOOD GROUP SEROLOGY

APPLIED
BLOOD GROUP SEROLOGY
Fourth Edition

Peter D. Issitt, PhD, FRCPath, FIBMS, FIBiol

Emeritus Professor of Pathology
Formerly Scientific Director
Blood Transfusion Service
Duke University Medical Center
Durham, North Carolina, USA

David J. Anstee, BSc, PhD, FRCPath

Director, Bristol Institute for Transfusion Sciences
Director, World Health Organization International
Blood Group Reference Laboratory
Honorary Professor of Transfusion Sciences
University of Bristol, Bristol, UK
and
Research and Development Coordinator
National Blood Service, England

Montgomery Scientific Publications
Durham, North Carolina, U.S.A

First Edition	**October 1970**
First Reprinting	December 1971
Second Reprinting	November 1972
Second Edition	**July 1975**
First Reprinting	July 1976
Second Reprinting	February 1977
Third Reprinting	August 1978
Fourth Reprinting	September 1979
Fifth Reprinting	June 1980
Sixth Reprinting	January 1981
Seventh Reprinting	May 1982
Third Edition	**October 1985**
First Reprinting	March 1986
Second Reprinting	October 1986
Third Reprinting	May 1987
Fourth Reprinting	May 1988
Fifth Reprinting	September 1989
Fourth Edition	**April 1998**

Library of Congress Catalog Card Number: 98-65364

ISBN 0-935643-05-2

Page layout in the U.S.A. by Clean Data, Inc., Durham, North Carolina

This fourth edition of Applied Blood Group Serology represents the culmination of three years of work in writing, revising, editing and proof reading the copy. The book differs in many respects from the third edition published in 1985. First and most significantly, this edition represents the combined efforts of two authors. In 1983 and 1984 when the third edition was being written, knowledge about the biochemistry, molecular structure and molecular genetics of the red cell blood groups was sparse enough that one blood group serologist felt competent to tackle the task of writing the book. The enormous explosion of information about the blood groups at the molecular level, that occurred between 1985 and 1995, when work on this edition began, left the sole author of the third edition ill-prepared to attempt the task of writing a comprehensive account of the current state of knowledge of our science. Fortunately, for that sole author of the third edition, a scientist who has personally made major contributions to the said explosion of information was willing to become a co-author. For the most part, the sections of this book that deal with the serology, practical applications in transfusion therapy and conventional genetics of the blood groups, were written by Peter Issitt. Those sections that deal with the immunological, biochemical and molecular aspects of the subject, were written by David Anstee. Naturally, since this is one book, about one subject, the red cell blood groups, those distinctions sometimes blurred and a section was written by one of us, when the other would have been expected to do so.

A second and obvious difference between the last edition and this one is that the third edition contained 30 chapters, this one contains 46. Often such expansion was a natural consequence of growth of knowledge about the blood groups. For example, in the third edition the Xg, Diego, Cartwright, Scianna, Dombrock and Colton blood group systems were all described in Chapter 16; the Gerbich and Cromer systems and some antigens now known to belong to the Dombrock system were included in a chapter on unrelated antigens of high incidence. In this edition each of those systems warrants, and is given, a chapter in its own right. Less obvious expansion involves the division of some major topics into more manageable pieces. In the third edition, a single chapter included descriptions of all known autoantibodies. In this edition the now considerably increased amount of information has resulted in the use of four separate chapters, one each on warm-reactive, cold-reactive and benign autoantibodies and one on antibodies produced as a result of drug therapy.

Third, the sequence of chapters in this book differs from that in previous editions. After topics such as terminology, immunology, serology, biochemistry and molecular genetics have been discussed, the blood group systems are arranged in a sequence based on certain characteristics that they share. To begin are chapters on the ABO, Hh, Lewis, Ii and P systems, in all of which the antigens are primarily carbohydrate in nature. Next, because of its importance in all aspects of blood grouping and transfusion comes the Rh system, it is immediately followed by the LW and Duffy systems because of their serological relationships with Rh. Then come chapters on the MN and Gerbich systems so that glycophorins A, B, C, D and E are described in adjacent chapters. This in spite of the admonition in Chapter 16 that if glycophorins C and D are so named, so too should be some other membrane-borne structures. The Diego, Kell, Kidd, Lutheran and Colton systems are described next, each involves a glycoprotein carrier for which a function (not necessarily on red cells) has been recognized. The Dombrock, Cartwright and Cromer systems are then described in sequential chapters because each represents a collection of antigens carried on a different protein attached to the red cell membrane via a phosphatidyl-inositol anchor. Next come chapters on the Xg, Scianna, Ch/Rg, Knops and Indian systems where there are fewer similarities between the systems. Antigens not currently assigned to systems follow in four chapters, then a number of antigens defined by cold-reactive autoantibodies are described. Each chapter on a blood group system begins with a lengthy introduction that covers salient points about that system for readers who require only an overview. Following the introduction, complete details about the system are given. After the blood group systems have been described there are chapters that illustrate use of the information previously given, at the practical level. These chapters, among them, discuss antibody detection and identification, compatibility testing, transfusion reactions, autoantibodies and hemolytic anemia, drug-induced antibodies, hemolytic disease of the newborn and polyagglutination. It is this series of chapters that give rise to use of the term, applied, in the title of the book.

As in previous editions, the length of the text, the number of tables and figures used and the number of references cited have increased. The third edition contained some 700,000 words, this one contains about 1.3 million. Some readers may recall that the first edition, published in 1970, had about 110,000 words. Thus the fourth edition, arriving 28 years later, is some 12 times the length of the first. One wonders, if the author had known what would come to pass, would he have written the first edition at all? The third edition included 9279 references, this one contains more than 13,500. Further, over 5000 of those references, that is, more than 37 percent, have been published since the third edition was released. This enormous number of new references again reflects the explosion of knowledge about the blood groups, mentioned above. As an example, among them, the chapters on the Gerbich, Diego, Colton, Dombrock, Cartwright, Cromer, Knops and Indian systems contain 1003 references; 572 (57%) of those papers had not been published when the third edition was written. In three chapters, ABO, Rh and HDN the number of references now exceeds 1000 per chapter. (The entire first edition of the book had 954.) A similar fate would have befallen a chapter on autoantibodies, the four replacement chapters described above contain, among them, 1564 citations. As the size of the book and its references grew, one author wondered if it should be sold with hernia insurance.

In this edition, we have included a number of tables that describe early information about certain subjects. No authors would ever write about the ABO system without describing the contributions of Landsteiner, nor about Rh without listing the work of Levine, Landsteiner, Wiener and Race. We have taken this approach a little further. In Chapter 12, table 12-8 depicts the results of early studies by Tippett and Sanger on the categories of D+ people who make alloimmune anti-D, table 12-9 shows later expanded data from those same investigators. In Chapter 15, table 15-13 shows Cleghorn's 1966 summation of the Miltenberger subsystem. Although later tables and figures (tables 12-10 and 12-11 and figures 12-7 and 12-8 for partial D, and table 15-14 for the formerly named Miltenberger series) give current information about these subjects, we believe that the earlier seminal studies that presaged contemporary knowledge and laid the very firm foundations on which that knowledge is built, should be remembered. Other examples will be found throughout the book. To do less than acknowledge such contributions would serve to dishonor those investigators on whose work our science is based.

Finally, the previous editions of this book have been graciously and generously received by members of our profession. We hope that this new edition will be of value.

Peter D. Issitt, Durham, NC, U.S.A.
David J. Anstee, Bristol, U.K.
January 1998

This is a book, written for blood bankers, about the red cell blood groups. It attempts to explain both theoretical and practical considerations from a level understandable to the newcomer to the field but at the same time progresses to information that, it is hoped, will encourage and enable the worker already competent to deal with all routine situations to attempt and to solve problems beyond the scope of his own previous experience. It further includes recently acquired information about the blood groups, in all their beautiful complexity, that although not strictly necessary for the daily running of the routine blood bank will serve as a source of reference for advanced workers dealing with the more exotic problems that make the study of the blood groups so fascinating and rewarding.

Because this book is about red cell blood groups, it does not attempt to deal with the administrative aspects of blood banking, the running of donor programs, blood component therapy nor with the groups of leukocytes or serum proteins. It does, however, concern itself closely with the physicochemistry of antigen-antibody reactions, methods employed in the blood bank, characteristics of red cell antigens and antibodies, compatibility testing, the detection and identification of red cell antibodies, autoantibodies, hemolytic disease of the newborn, and transfusion reactions for in each of these areas the blood groups themselves are intimately involved.

Finally, for the sake of clarity, no references are given in Chapter 1, the introduction to the subject. Each phase of blood group serology described in that Chapter is more fully described in the following Chapters and, in these, recognition is made of original work in the more than 900 references in this book.

Peter D. Issitt
Oxnard, California, May 1970

ACKNOWLEDGMENTS

We thank the many friends and colleagues, whose contributions are cited in the following chapters, who generously allowed us to list the results of studies in press or in progress and other unpublished observations.

Extra special thanks go to Linda Issitt for many reasons. First, she single-handedly convinced the senior author that this fourth edition should be written. Since he knew full well what was entailed, such persuasion was not easy, it took much time and perseverance. Second, having got the process started, Linda committed the complete text to word processor disks, entirely in her "spare" time and with many chapters, more than once as they were rewritten or revised. Third, once the contents of the disks had been formatted into page style, Linda proof read the entire book. There is no doubt whatever that without Linda, this book would not exist.

Sincere thanks also go to Sherrie Ayles who created most of the figures that appear herein. Review of those figures will provide testimony to her skills. Unlike the senior author, the junior author did not know in advance what was entailed in writing a book of this magnitude and would not have got through his part of the process without Sherrie's help, encouragement and fortitude.

We thank Chris Herndl, President of Clean Data, Inc., for sage advice about the composition, style and setting of the text and for keeping the production process on time on a preset schedule. Chris was more than ably abetted by Karen Haley and Amanda Albro who: converted the text from disks into page style; produced almost all the tables from hand written drafts; created some of the characters (such as $\overline{\overline{R}}^N$) that are unique unto the blood groups; recreated the figures retained from the third edition; and cheerfully and patiently made changes in what they had been told were final versions, when the authors changed their minds. We thank these two young ladies, the elegance of the final typescript reflects their considerable professional skills.

TABLE OF CONTENTS

6 | The Antiglobulin (Coombs) Test, Complement in Antigen-Antibody Reactions and in the Antiglobulin Test, the Alternative Pathway of Complement Activation, In Vivo Destruction of Incompatible Red Cells, Some Biological Consequences of Complement Activation in Man

7 | A General Introduction to Blood Group Antibodies, Red Cell Typing Reagents and the Use of Monoclonal Antibodies in Blood Group Serology

8 | The ABO and H Blood Group Systems

9 | The Lewis System

10 | The Ii Antigen Collection

11 | The P Blood Group System and the Antigens P, P^k and LKE

12 | The Rh Blood Group System

13 | The LW Blood Group System

14 | The Duffy Blood Group System

15 | The MN Blood Group System

16 | The Gerbich Blood Group System

17 | The Diego Blood Group System

18 | The Kell and Xk Blood Group Systems

19 | The Kidd Blood Group System

20 | The Lutheran Blood Group System

21 | The Colton Blood Group System

22 | The Dombrock Blood Group System

23 | The Cartwright Blood Group System

29 | The Indian Blood Group System and the Antigen AnWj

30 | Notes on the ISBT Collections of Antigens: the Antigens Cs^a and Cs^b; Er^a and Er^b; and Some Notes on HTLA Antibodies

31 | Well Characterized Independent Antigens of High Incidence

32 | Well Characterized Independent Antigens of Low Incidence

33 | Less Fully Investigated Antigens

34 | Antigens Defined by Cold-Reactive Autoantibodies

35 | Antibody Detection and Identification and Compatibility Testing

36 | Transfusion Reactions

37 | "Warm" Antibody-Induced Hemolytic Anemia (WAIHA)

38 | Cold Hemagglutinin Disease and Paroxysmal Cold Hemoglobinuria

39 | Autoantibodies that are Benign In Vivo

40 | Drug-Induced Antibodies

41 | Hemolytic Disease of the Newborn

42 | Polyagglutination

43 | Miscellaneous Conditions that may Affect Results in the Blood Transfusion Laboratory

44 | A Catalog of Antigens

1 | An Introduction to Immunohematology, Definition of a Blood Group System, Correct Use of Blood Group Terminology, The ISBT Terminology

Some of mankind's earliest records contain accounts of attempts to cure disease or prevent death, by transfusion. The difficulties faced by early proponents of the art proved insurmountable. Animal blood and substances other than blood (such as ale and wine) were frequently substituted as the transfusion fluid; blood was not always administered intravenously nor was anything known of coagulation or sterility. In 1628, Harvey advanced his theory of circulation of the blood in man, thus removing one major obstacle to transfusion. Although James Blundell, an English obstetrician, is generally credited as having performed the earliest transfusions with human blood in 1818 and 1819 (1,2), Schmidt (3) has pointed out that a transfusion, about which the outcome is not known, was given in Philadelphia in 1795 (4). Dr. Physick who performed that transfusion, apparently performed no others and both Schmidt (3) and Myhre (5), in an interesting account of Blundell's life and career, believe that credit for the experimental pioneering work in human transfusion, devolves on Blundell. Readers interested in the history of blood transfusion are referred to some other writings of Schmidt (6) and Myhre (7) and to a publication by Gottlieb (8) that reproduces numerous pictures of devices and equipment used in early (and some in later transfusions).

In 1900, Karl Landsteiner (9,10), by extending his own observation that the blood of one individual when mixed with the blood of another might cause visible clumping of the red cells, or hemolysis, discovered the existence of the ABO groups that are, to this day, the most important of the known human blood groups. The long history of unsuccessful attempts at blood transfusion, over a period of so many centuries, serves to make even more dramatic the tremendous growth in the amount of knowledge about the human blood groups that has taken place in the ninety-six years since Landsteiner's original discoveries. In that time, the original three blood groups have been extended so that today many hundreds of different red cell characters have been recognized.

Some of these advances, such as the discovery, in 1927, of the MN and P systems (11,12) have come from deliberate immunization of animals with human red cells and subsequent in vitro tests with the animal serum on still other human red cells. Others, such as the discovery of the Rh and/or LW system(s) in 1940 (13), have come from the immunization of one animal with red cells from a differ-ent, non-human species and subsequent tests of the serum from the immunized animal against human red cells.

Advances in technique provided still more opportunities for discovery. The use, in 1944, of the blocking antibody test (14,15), demonstrated the existence of a whole new group of antibodies that attach to red cells but cause no visible reaction: the so-called "incomplete" or "sensitizing" antibodies. Once their existence was known new methods were quickly devised to enable these antibodies to be demonstrated more easily. In 1945, bovine albumin was first used (16,17). The presence of this additive enabled some of these incomplete antibodies to cause agglutination of red cells. Later in the same year (18,19) the much more sensitive antiglobulin test, that detects immunglobulin (antibody) and/or complement that has bound to red cells following an antigen-antibody reaction was introduced. In 1947, it was shown (20) that the presence of certain proteolytic enzymes in the cell-serum mixture, or exposure of red cells to those enzymes, resulted in agglutination by otherwise "incomplete" antibodies. The introduction of these new methods resulted in a rapid accumulation of new data. To the already known ABO, MN, P and Rh systems were soon added the Lutheran system, discovered (21) in 1945 by means of the older direct agglutination method and a series of blood group systems, demonstrated mainly by the then new antiglobulin technique. The Kell and Lewis systems were discovered in 1946 (22,23), vast amounts of new data accumulated about the Rh system, the Duffy system was found in 1950 (24) and the Kidd system in 1951 (25).

Between 1951 and the mid 1970s, new discoveries were made at an exciting and at times breath-taking pace. To every one of the already described blood group systems was added enough new information to show that where, at first, there appeared to be a two antigen, two allele situation, a highly complex and sometimes confusing polymorphism of red cell antigens probably exists. Inter-relationships were found between the actions of blood group genes, sometimes within a system and sometimes between genes of independent systems. In addition, new systems were added to the "classic" nine independent blood group systems: ABO; MN; P; Rh; Lutheran; Kell; Lewis; Duffy and Kidd, known before 1951. Initially, serological studies were used to identify new systems. With the advent of new biochemical and molecular genetic methods, see below, it has become possible to be far more certain which systems are independent of all others. As described in the section dealing with the ISBT nomenclature, to the original nine systems listed above, can now be added the Diego; Cartwright; Xg; Scianna; Dombrock; Colton; LW; Chido/Rodgers; Hh; Kx; Gerbich; Cromer; Knops and Indian systems. In addition, an assortment of other antigens, some related to each other and some independent of all others, has now been recognized. In all this expansion there has been some consolidation. As a few examples, the rare antigens Go^a, Wiel (D^w), Be^a and Evans, each of which was at one time thought to be independent, are now all known to belong to the ever-expanding Rh system (26-29). The very common and very important antigen En^a, that at first (30,31), appeared to be the harbinger of a new blood group system, has now been recognized as a group of different antigens (32) carried on the glycoprotein structure on which some MN system antigens reside (33-40). The rare antigens Wb, Ls^a, An^a and Dh^a, all of which began their careers as rare antigens apparently not associated with any blood group system, have now all been admitted as fully fledged members of the Gerbich system (41-45). The three examples given illustrate the ways in which different types of study can provide information about the blood groups. The low incidence antigens Go^a, D^w, Be^a and Evans were shown to be part of the Rh system using serological methods in classical family studies. Control of production of each antigen was seen to involve a gene at the *Rh* locus. In the case of En^a, serological studies showed lack of expression of M and N on En(a-) red cells. Biochemical studies then showed that such red cells lack glycophorin A that carries M and N. Tests using untreated En(a+) red cells and those same cells treated with trypsin or ficin, together with recognition of the sites on glycophorin A that are subject to cleavage by those enzymes, lead to the recognition of the specificities anti-En^{a}TS, anti-En^{a}FS and anti-En^{a}FR (see also Chapter 15). Because the antigens Wb, Ls^a, An^a and Dh^a are all extremely rare and because Ge-negative red cells are equally uncommon, there was virtually no chance that classical family studies would ever have shown the place of the rare antigens in the Gerbich system. However, recognition of the fact that the high incidence Gerbich antigens (Ge2, Ge3 and Ge4) are carried on glycophorins C and D (46-48) and that alterations of those glycophorins (or the genes that encode them) are associated with presence of the rare antigens (41-45), allowed Wb, Ls^a, An^a and Dh^a to be taken out of limbo and into Gerbich.

In the mid 1970s new information about the blood group systems began to arrive from several different sources. Classic serology using tests based primarily on the hemagglutination reaction expanded many of the blood group systems, new antigens were found, details about those already known were added. In a few instances, characters found on red cells were seen (49) to be primarily leukocyte antigens. However, in the last 10 to 15 years more has been learned about the blood groups from biochemical and molecular genetic studies, than from traditional hemagglutination tests. A major contribution to these advances came with the demonstration by Kohler and Milstein (50) that monoclonal antibodies can be produced by cells maintained in continuous culture. Initially such antibodies were produced by fusing mouse B-cells, that carried the genetic information that imparted antibody specificity, with myeloma cells that secrete large amounts of immunoglobulin. Both mouse myeloma and human myeloma cell lines were used in the formation of antibody-secreting hybridomas. Because mice, when immunized, do not recognize some human red cell (or other) antigens, alternative methods for producing monoclonal antibodies were devised. Human B-cells from individuals already making blood group antibodies were transformed with Epstein-Barr virus (EBV) and were grown in tissue culture where they too secrete antibody. Early success in the production of anti-D by this method was reported (51-54) although it was also found (55) that the cultured cell lines tended to be unstable. Goosens et al. (56) and later others (57) developed methods to stabilize the cultured cell lines. Alternatively, the EBV-transformed B cells can be fused with human myeloma cells to form antibody-secreting hybridomas. Additional details about monoclonal antibodies and their use as blood typing reagents are given in Chapter 7. Once potent monoclonal antibodies to blood group antigens were available, it became somewhat easier for biochemists to isolate red cell antigen-bearing membrane components from intact red cells, red cell ghosts or solubilized red cell membranes. This, coupled with the development of improved techniques, such as sodium dodecyl sulphate, polyacrylamide gel electrophoresis (SDS-PAGE) (58) resulted in many advances in understanding the composition of antigen-bearing membrane structures. Further, once the partial amino acid sequences of these structures were determined it was possible to screen cDNA libraries to find genetic material encoding production of the antigen-bearing components. Thus instead of being limited to studying intact antigens on red cells via hemagglutination techniques, it became possible to work at the genetic level (59). In addition to working with cDNA (often isolated from reticulocytes) it is now possible to amplify genomic DNA using the polymerase chain reaction (PCR). Details about the principles of these methods are given in Chapters 4 and 5. In almost every chapter on the blood group systems, advances made possible by these biochemical and molecular genetic methods are documented.

Definition of a Blood Group System

With so many workers active in the field of human blood grouping, it might be thought that this section and the one that follows on the correct use of blood group nomenclature, would be unnecessary. Regrettably this is not the case. The high level of technical competence seen at the bench in so many blood banks, is often accompanied by a somewhat less impressive knowledge of the basic laws of inheritance and genetic concepts that govern immunohematology. For example, one of these authors has seen on a lecture schedule for medical technology students, a lecture titled "The ABH Blood Group System". A publication has appeared titled "Blood Group Systems: ABH and Lewis". While it is true (60) that the presence of at least one *H* gene is required for the *A* and *B* genes to be able to express themselves at the phenotypic level, the term ABH does not describe a blood group system. The ABO system genes *A*, *B* and *O* reside at one genetic locus, the *H* and *h* genes occupy a different locus and independent segregation of genes at the two loci has been demonstrated (60-62). Indeed, lack of an *H* gene (presumed presence of two *h* genes) does not even stop the *A* and *B* genes from functioning. As described more fully in Chapter 8, in persons genetically *hh*, who are therefore phenotypically O_h, an *A* or *B* gene, if present, still effects production of its specific transferase enzyme (63, 64). Because O_h red cells lack the H structure, *A* or *B*-specified transferase enzymes made, are unable to add immunodominant sugars to their usual site. Nevertheless, the well documented finding that genes at the *Hh* and *ABO* loci segregate independently, the *ABO* locus is on chromosome 9 (65,66) the *Hh* locus is on chromosome 19 (67) means, by definition, that ABO is one system and *Hh* is another. The error in the lecture and book titles could have been corrected simply by describing the ABO and H systems.

A blood group system includes those antigens that are produced by alleles at a single genetic locus or those produced by alleles at loci that are so closely linked that crossing-over between them either does not occur or is extremely rare. As simple examples, in the Kidd blood group system the antigens Jk[a] and Jk[b] are the products of the co-dominant alleles *Jk^a* and *Jk^b* (24,68). The third antigen in the system, Jk3, is made whenever a functional *Jk^a* or *Jk^b* gene is inherited. The only red cells that lack Jk3, and these are described phenotypically as Jk:-3, are those from individuals who have inherited two *Jk* genes (69). Family studies have shown, beyond reasonable doubt, that *Jk* is a silent allele at the *Jk^aJk^b* locus. That is to say, *Jk* effects no production of Jk[a], Jk[b] or Jk3. In the MN blood group system, the antigens M and N are the products of the alleles *M* and *N*, at a single genetic locus (11,12). The antigens S and s are the products of a different pair of alleles, *S* and *s*, at a closely linked locus (70-73). In other words, an individual with *M* and *S* on one chromosome and *N* and *s* on the other, will almost always pass *MS* or *Ns* to his/her offspring. Because crossing-over between the *MN* and *Ss* loci is so rare, in the example given it would result in the new chromosome alignments *Ms* and *NS*, the M, N, S and s antigens and the products of other alleles at the *MN* and *Ss* loci, are usually thought of as part of the same blood group system. Even so, some workers (28) refer to the system as the MNSs blood groups, because two loci are involved.

This seems as good a point as any to try to correct a misconception apparently held by many workers who should know much better. ALTERNATIVE GENES AT A SINGLE LOCUS ARE ALLELES. THE ANTIGENS PRODUCED BY ALLELES ARE ANTITHETICAL TO EACH OTHER. NO MATTER WHAT (even well known) TEXTBOOKS MAY SAY, BY DEFINITION, ANTIGENS *CANNOT* BE ALLELIC, *NOR CAN* GENES BE ANTITHETICAL.

There are many examples in the human blood groups where antigens display a phenotypic association that is not necessarily understood at the basic science level. Again to use a simple example, Rh_{null} red cells are LW(a-b-) (74-76). However, since the *Rh* and *LW* genes have been shown (77-80) to segregate independently (the *Rh* locus is on chromosome 1 (81, 82), the *LW* locus is on chromosome 19 (83)) it follows that the phenotypic association does not extend to the genetic level and that Rh and LW are separate blood group systems.

Antibodies that detect very common antigens, present on all except the null cells of a certain blood group system, likewise define antigens that at first can be said only to have a phenotypic association with the blood group system involved. For example, when anti-K11 was first found (84) it reacted with all red cells except those from individuals with two *K^o* genes. *K^o* is the silent allele at the *Kell* complex locus (85). While this finding strongly suggested that K11 might be a Kell system antigen, it did not prove that point. Because the *K^{11}* gene and those Kell system genes present in most individuals *(k, Kp^b, Js^b)* are all very common, trying to demonstrate linkage between *K^{11}* and the genes at the *Kell* complex locus, was a daunting proposition. However, it was later found (86) that the low incidence antigen Wk[a] (K17) is antithetical to K11 meaning that *Wk^a(K^{17})* and *K^{11}* must be alleles. *Wk^a* was shown (86, 87) always to travel with *k* and never with *K*, when passed by an individual genetically *KkWk^a*. Thus, since *Wk^a(K^{17})* had been shown to reside at the *Kell* complex locus, it followed that its allele, *K^{11}*, must reside there as well. Workers should always remember that failure of an antibody to react only with the null cells of a certain system provides a clue that the antibody may define an antigen of that system but does not prove that to be the case. Genetic evidence is required before any antigen is assigned to a blood group system.

Until the mid 1970s most assignments of antigens to established blood group systems had to be accomplished by traditional family studies. When pairs of antithetical antigens such as Di^a and Di^b, and Yt^a and Yt^b, in which one antigen was very common and the other very rare were encountered (88-91) finding informative families was next to impossible. In this particular example individuals phenotypically Di(a+b+), Yt(a+b+) would have to be found in whom transmission of Di^a, Di^b, Yt^a and Yt^b to their offspring could be clearly seen. If the genes of the Diego and Cartwright systems segregated independently, one family might show independence of the *Di* and *Yt* loci. If they did not segregate independently, several families may have had to be found in order to provide statistically significant evidence of linkage. In this particular example the difficulty caused by the low incidence of Di^a and Yt^b would be further compounded by the fact that Di^a is primarily a characteristic of persons of Mongolian extraction while Yt^b is primarily a characteristic of European Whites. Fortunately, use of the biochemical and molecular genetic technology described briefly above, has resolved some problems of this type as well. To continue the example, it is now known (92,93) that Di^a and Di^b represent a polymorphism of the major anion transport protein, band 3, of the red cell membrane. Production of band 3 is encoded from a locus on chromosome 17 (94,95). Yt^a and Yt^b, on the other hand, are known (96,97) to represent a polymorphism of red cell membrane associated acetylcholinesterase, a phosphatidylinositol-linked protein. The gene encoding production of acetylcholinesterase and hence the *Yt* locus, is on chromosome 7 (98-100). In other words, there is absolute proof that the Diego and Cartwright blood group systems are genetically independent of each other. This has been shown although, as far as these authors are aware, no individual phenotypically Di(a+b+), Yt(a+b+) has ever been found. In addition to advances made by studies on blood group genes at the molecular level, it is now often possible to use substitute markers. Zelinksi (101) has eloquently described the use of DNA restriction fragment length polymorphisms (RFLP) in conjunction with blood group genetics. Essentially such methods involve the detection of pieces of DNA that are variably cut by a large variety of bacterially produced endonucleases and are highly polymorphic in different individuals. Association of these DNA markers with various blood group system genes has enabled their use as substitutes for numerous blood group markers.

Correct Use of Blood Group Terminology

The rules that govern the use of various types of names for blood group genes, genotypes, antigens, phenotypes and antibodies are relatively straightforward. In spite of this, these names are regularly misused, particularly in the written form in reports, letters and to the chagrin of editors and reviewers, in manuscripts submitted for publication. This section will deal with the principles of the various nomenclature systems in use. For highly complex systems, such as Rh, where the terminology is more specialized, additional details are given in the appropriate chapters.

Gene and Antigen

In the majority of blood group systems the same term is used to describe the blood group gene and the antigen whose production it effects. Thus, the *M* gene encodes production of M antigen, the Jk^a gene encodes production of Jk^a antigen. In order to indicate whether gene or antigen is intended, two methods exist. In printed communications, gene symbols are set in italics, i.e. *M*, Jk^a, antigen symbols are set in regular type, i.e. M, Jk^a. In typed or handwritten communications, when italics are not available, gene symbols are underlined, i.e. <u>M</u>, <u>Jk</u>^{a}, antigen symbols continue in regular type without underlines.

Systems Using Single Letters

Typical examples are the ABO and P blood group systems. In the former, the antigens are A and B. The (common) genes are A^1, A^2, *B* and *O*. Note that A_1, A_2, B and O can also be used as phenotype names (as in group A_1, group A_2, etc.) as can A, i.e. group A, when a test for reactivity of the red cells with anti-A_1 has not been performed. As will be seen, in gene symbols the 1 and 2 are used as superscripts, in phenotype symbols as subscripts. In the P system the remaining antigen is P_1. It is now known that the P and P^k antigens are encoded by genes that are not located at the same locus as P^1 (see Chapter 11).

Systems Using Superscript Letters

Many blood group systems employ this type of terminology that is based on conventions introduced (102) for the Lewis and Lutheran systems. As examples, the Colton and Diego systems can be used. In the Colton system the antigen names are Co^a and Co^b. The genes that encode production of these antigens are, respectively, Co^a and Co^b (103,104). However, there is a third allele (105,106) in the Colton system the presence of which does not effect production of either Co^a or Co^b. This gene is called *Co*. Lack of a superscript letter indicates the silent nature of *Co*. If, at some time in the future, an antibody is found that detects a product of *Co*, the terminology will need revision. The *Co* gene could then be called *Co^c* (or more likely, with the current trend towards numbers, *Co^4*) and the antigen produced could be called Co^c (or Co4) see below, numerical terminology. Co4 and not Co3 would be used since the antibody made by individuals with red cells phenotypically Co(a-b-) has already been called anti-Co3.

The Diego system is less complex for no silent allele at the *Di^aDi^b* locus is known. In other words, the antigens are Di^a and Di^b the genes *Di^a* and *Di^b* (88,89,107). As can be seen, in antigen names the letters a and b are used as superscripts. As described later in this chapter, when phenotype designations are used, the rules are quite different.

Systems Using Numerical Terminology

Since the Scianna blood group system underwent a nomenclature change when permission to use the family name was obtained (108), it can conveniently be used as an example of this type of terminology. The antigens are Sc1 and Sc2 (formerly Sm and Bu^a respectively). The genes are *Sc^1* and *Sc^2* and, since a silent allele at the *Sc^1Sc^2* locus is known (109), *Sc*. Note that the antigen names do not employ colons. Sc1 and Sc2 are the antigens, Sc:1 , Sc:2 (and Sc:1,-2, Sc:-1,-2, etc.) are phenotype designations, as explained below. In antibody names, i.e. anti-Sc1, anti-Sc2, the colon is not used.

Combinations

Several blood group systems utilize combinations of more than one type of terminology. For example, in the Kell blood group system, K, k, Kp^a, Kp^b, Js^a, Js^b, K11 and K17 are antigens (among many others). Their production is controlled by the genes *K, k, Kp^a, Kp^b, Js^a, Js^b, K^{11} and K^{17}*, respectively.

Antigen versus Phenotype

This is the area where many blood bankers appear unaware of the rules and where mistakes are most often made. The antigen is the structure on the red cell membrane that is able to complex with its specific antibody. Further, the antigen can, after appropriate processing (see Chapter 2) elicit the production of an antibody when introduced into the circulation of some individuals whose red cells lack that antigen. A phenotype, on the other hand, is a description of which antigens are present on a given individual's red cells and simply indicates the

results of serological tests on those cells. Examples of how phenotype designations should be written will be given for each type of terminology described in the previous sections of this chapter.

In the ABO system the antigens, as stated, are A and B. However, the phenotypes (that are almost universally known as ABO blood groups) are A, A_1, A_2, B, O, AB, A_1B, A_2B, etc. As can be seen, all that the phenotypes do is to list which antigens are present (A or B) and, if the cells in question have been tested with anti-A_1, the result of that test (A_1 equals positive reaction, A_2 equals negative reaction of red cells that reacted strongly with anti-A). As can also be seen, negative reactions are indicated by lack of use of a term. In other words, group A_1 cells reacted with anti-A, anti-A_1 and anti-A,B (if used) but not with anti-B. Group O cells failed to react with anti-A, anti-B and, if used, anti-A,B and anti-A_1. The ABO terminology is different from others in that negative reactions are not reported but must be inferred. In other words, group A cells are called group A, not A+B-. Somewhat similarly, the phenotype designation group O, indicates the lack of A and B antigens but not the presence of an O antigen since the *O* gene is silent, that is it does not code for production of a serologically demonstrable character.

In the P blood group system, presence of the antigen can be expressed in one of two different ways in a phenotype designation. Red cells that carry the P_1 antigen (as revealed by a positive reaction when tested with anti-P_1) can be called P_1+ or simply P_1 (in the latter instance the antigen name and the phenotype are the same). When red cells are typed with a single antibody, such as anti-P_1, the phenotype designation should indicate only the result of that test and should not imply results of tests not performed. Red cells reactive with anti-P_1 can be called P_1+ or P_1. Red cells non-reactive with anti-P_1 but not tested with anti-P should be called P_1-. They should not (but unfortunately often are) be called P_2 for that phenotype designation implies the presence of the P antigen, for which no test has been performed.

Somewhat similarly, red cells found to be reactive with anti-M and non-reactive with anti-N are phenotypically M or M+ or M+N-. They are not MM (a term often incorrectly used to indicate the absence of N) for such a designation implies that the individual from whom the M+N- red cells came is genetically *MM*. Obviously, simple typing tests with anti-M and anti-N suggest MN system zygosity but fall short of proving it. Persons of the rare genotypes *MM^g, MEn, MM^k*, etc. (see Chapter 15) all have red cells that also type as M+N-. As can be seen from the examples given thus far, a phenotype is no more than a description of the results of serological tests.

For antigen names that use superscript letters, the terminology rules are quite different. Red cells typed with anti-Co^a are phenotypically Co(a+) or Co(a-) dependent on the result of the test. Those typed with anti-Co^b are Co(b+) or Co(b-). Those typed with both anti-bodies fall in to one of the phenotype designations Co(a+b-), Co(a+b+), Co(a-b+) and Co(a-b-). The phenotype designation must never imply results of tests not performed. Thus, red cells non-reactive with anti-Co^a must be called Co(a-) not Co(a-b+). They can be called Co(a-b+) only after they have been tested and shown to give a positive reaction with anti-Co^b. It can be added that the rules as applied to Co^a, Co(a+) and Co(a-) also apply to other antigens such as Jk^a, Jk^b, Fy^a, Fy^b, Kp^a, Kp^b, etc., that use this type of terminology.

In the numerical terminology, the antigen names use the code letters for the blood group system, i.e. Sc for Scianna, K for Kell, Rh for Rh, etc., and unadorned numbers. Thus in the Scianna blood group system the antigens are Sc1, Sc2 and Sc3. When a phenotype is to be written, the code letters are followed by a colon, i.e. Sc: then the results of the typing studies. When an antigen is present no symbol other than its number is used, i.e. Sc:1 (the cells gave a positive reaction when tested with anti-Sc1). When the antigen is absent (cells non-reactive with anti-Sc1) the number is preceded by a minus sign, i.e. Sc:-1. When two or more typing sera have been used, the results are separated by a comma, i.e. Sc:-1,2 or Sc:1,-2,3 etc. Again, the phenotype must describe only tests actually performed. Since the phenotype Sc:-1,-2,-3 is so rare, almost all red cells that fail to react with anti-Sc1 will react with anti-Sc2 and with anti-Sc3 (if it is available). However, red cells found to be non-reactive with anti-Sc1 are phenotypically Sc:-1 only. They must not be called Sc:-1,2 (or Sc:-1,2,3) until tested with anti-Sc2 and/or anti-Sc3. As indicated, if red cells are found to be non-reactive with anti-Sc1 and reactive with anti-Sc3, but anti-Sc2 is not available, the possible phenotypes (dependent on the results of the test with anti-Sc3) are Sc:-1,3 and Sc:-1,-3. Nothing can be said about Sc2

unless a test with anti-Sc2 has been performed.

An exception to the accepted way of reporting phenotypes occurs when a table is used to list the results of typing tests on a number of different blood samples. On such an occasion it is acceptable to list antigen names across the top of the table and identifying symbols for the blood samples on one side. The table can be completed by using + and 0 symbols to indicate presence or absence of the antigens. An example of this type of reporting method is given in table 1-1.

Lists

When a list of antigens is to be written, the terminology will vary dependent on the context. For example, when a single patient's red cells are being described the statement that "the patient's red cells lacked the antigens C, D, E; K, Kp^a, Js^a; Fy^a; Jk^b" would be correct. As can be seen, the antigens missing from the patient's cells are listed by system, with a comma between each antigen in the same system and a semi-colon between systems. To list a patient's phenotype, a related but slightly different, rule applies. Thus, "the patient's red cells were group A; D+ C+ E- c+ e+; M+ N- S+ s+; K -k+ Kp(a-b+) Js(a-b+); Fy(a+b-); Jk(a+b+); etc. As can be seen the antigens of a given system are still contained within semi-colons but since positive and negative signs are now used, no comma between the antigens is necessary. It is also correct, but aesthetically less pleasing, to omit the spaces after each positive or negative sign, see the MN system in the next example. The numerical terminology differs in that commas but no spaces are used. The example used above would become, group A; Rh:1,2,-3,4,5; M+N-S+s+ (the numerical terminology is seldom used for the MN system); K:-1,2,-3,4,-6,7; Fy:1,-2; Jk:1,2. To list antigens on different red cell samples, semi-colons would be used since each statement (antigen) refers to a different cell

TABLE 1-1 Acceptable Method for Listing Phenotypes in Table Form

Samples*	Antigens												
	C	D	E	c	e	M	N	S	P$_1$	Fy^a	Fy^b	Jk^a	Jk^b
I-1	+	+	+	+	+	+	0	+	+	+	+	+	0
I-2	0	0	0	+	+	+	+	0	+	+	+	+	+
II-1	+	+	0	+	+	+	+	+	+	+	0	+	0
II-2	0	+	+	+	+	+	0	+	+	+	+	+	0
II-3	+	+	0	+	+	+	0	0	0	0	+	+	0
II-4	0	+	+	+	+	+	+	0	0	0	+	+	+

*All samples tested were s+, U+, K-, k+

sample. Thus "the patient's serum was shown to be reactive with red cells lacking the antigens: hr^S; Hr^S; hr^B; Hr^B; Rh29; Kp^b; Js^b; Ge2; Ge3; Yt^a; Lan; etc.

Phenotype and Genotype

There are two considerations here that are of paramount importance. First, red cells can be phenotyped they CANNOT be genotyped. Second, unless a family study has been performed with completely conclusive results, a genotype is ALWAYS a probable interpretation of a phenotype. There are two major reasons why red cells cannot be genotyped. First, serological tests reveal the presence or absence of antigens not genes. Second, even if the first reason did not apply, red cells do not carry genes (their precursor cells do). Since red cells cannot be genotyped and because most of the time blood from an individual and not a complete family has been phenotyped, it follows that on most occasions a genotype will be an interpretation as to which genes the individual probably carries in order to have red cells of the observed phenotype. Most of the time there is nothing wrong with making such an interpretation so long as it is realized that is what it is and that it will occasionally be incorrect. As examples, almost all persons with red cells of the phenotype Jk(a+b-) will be genetically *Jk^{a}Jk^a* because the other genotype *Jk^{a}Jk*, that results in the production of phenotypically Jk(a+b-) red cells, is exceedingly rare (see Chapter 19). Most persons with red cells that are phenotypically M+ N- will be genetically *MM* since the other genotypes giving rise to the M+ N- phenotype (*MM^g*, *MEn, MM^k*, etc.) are also very rare. However, there are some occasions on which the interpretation of a phenotype as a single genotype should not be made. In Blacks, the *Fy* gene (that is located at the *Fy^{a}Fy^b* locus but that does not code for production of Fy^a or Fy^b, see Chapter 14) is common (110). As a result, the phenotype Fy(a+b-) will, in Blacks, represent the genotype *Fy^{a}Fy* more often than the genotype *Fy^{a}Fy^a*. Since tests with anti-Fy4 (also see Chapter 14) will not always reveal the presence of an *Fy* gene in Blacks (111) interpretation of phenotypes as single genotypes in such individuals is hazardous. A more complete explanation of the gene that is here called *Fy*, is given in Chapter 14. Briefly, although that gene behaves as *Fy* in that it does not encode a serologically demonstrable product, it is in fact most often an *Fy^b* gene in which a mutation has caused a defective promoter region (139).

As described in more detail in other chapters in this book there are some serological, biochemical and molecular genetic methods that can be used better to determine a genotype from an observed phenotype. As an example, red cells from an individual genetically *MM*

can usually be shown to carry more M antigen (double dose) than those, say from in individual genetically *MM^g* (single dose) in carefully controlled titration studies. Much better than manual titrations are dosage studies performed on the flow cytometer (112,113). In the Rh system, use of antibodies directed against the antigens f(ce), rh$_i$(Ce), cE and CE (see Chapter 12) will sometimes reveal the chromosomal alignment of *C, c, D, E* and *e* genes that must be present to explain an observed phenotype. As an example at the biochemical level, techniques such as SDS-PAGE (see Chapter 4) may reveal the presence of a single gene-specified amount of glycophorin B thus strongly suggesting (if not proving) that an individual with S- s+ red cells is genetically *sS^U* and not *ss* (114, for a definition of *S^U* see Chapter 15). The ability, via cDNA cloning or genomic DNA amplification, to determine which genes are actually present may appear as a fool-proof way of determining a genotype. Indeed, successful cloning and characterization of the ABO system genes (115-117) has provided, for the first time, a method of distinguishing between persons genetically *AA* and *AO* (118-121, see Chapter 8 for additional information). However, even such direct methods can sometimes be misleading. In the Rh system (see Chapter 12) there are already some known instances (122-126) where presence or absence of a gene is not absolutely correlated with expression of antigen at the phenotypic level (some *r'r* individuals have portions of, or a whole *D* gene). Such instances are likely to be rare but investigators must be aware that they exist. The differences do NOT represent false positives or negatives since the tests used are designed to detect DNA and in that respect the test results are correct. The differences arise because genes, when present, are not always expressed at the phenotypic level. That observation should come as no surprise to blood bankers who have known for a long time that O$_h$ (Bombay) individuals have normal, functional *ABO* genes (60,63,64) and that *X^{o}rX^{o}r* Rh$_{null}$ individuals have normal *Rh* genes (127-128).

Readers of the third edition of this book who have good memories may note that the suggested one dollar contribution to a Hawaiian beach bum existence for misuse of genotype for phenotype, has been discarded. First, nobody ever paid and second, the author who suggested it is now too old even to contemplate such a lifestyle. In one institution we did try a "swear-box" system of a dollar fine for each verbal misuse of terminology. The system was vetoed when, at the end of the first week, the medical director found that he owed more than he had earned!

Common Errors

It would be virtually impossible, in a book of this

size to list all the transgressions against the correct use of blood group terminology that these authors have had the misfortune to see. As outlined above, at both the antigen and phenotypic level the rules for the use of single letter, superscript and numerical terminology are relatively straightforward. An extraordinary feature of common errors is that often the terms are harder to create than the correct ones. Compassion requires that we leave unreferenced a paper that used the terms Jk^a and JK^b throughout. Symbols such as K1+, K:1+, K+1, K:+1 are harder to write than the correct phenotypic term K:1. One of our favorites is K$^+$ that we think is intended to mean K+ or K:1 but actually means potassium ions. We are never sure if K(+) means K+ with weak expression of K or K+ from an author who did not know that the + should not have been in parentheses; K+^{w} always tells us that the K antigen that is present is weakly expressed. Table 1-2 lists examples of correct and incorrect terms in the various nomenclature systems. It should be remembered that the rules outlined (involving both correct and incorrect symbols) can be extrapolated to other blood group systems (129) that use the same type of terminology. Table 1-3, that is by no means all inclusive, lists examples of the correct use of each type of terminology.

Antibodies

The most common mistake made in writing antibody names is to omit the hyphen, e.g. anti A and anti D instead of anti-A and anti-D. Since anti is a prefix it cannot stand alone. The name of the antibody must include the name of the antigen it defines (A and D in the examples). Thus anti-A and anti-D are each single words and are incorrectly written if the hyphen is omitted. In writing a list of antibodies it is permissible to use only the first as a full name, providing the hyphens are used for other specificities. For example "the serum contained anti-D, -E, -Fy^a, -Jk^a and -S". It is often grammatically tidier to rephrase the sentence "the serum contained antibodies to the D, E, Fy^a, Jk^a and S antigens".

The most common mistake in verbal descriptions of antibodies is to omit the anti entirely. Statements such as "this serum contains Fy^a (or worse, Duffy^a, or still worse, Duffy)" do not correctly describe the situation since Fy^a is an antigen and is not found in soluble form in serum.

TABLE 1-2 Examples of Correct and Incorrect Terminology

Term describes	Correct	Incorrect
Phenotypes	ARh+, BRh-	A+, B- (B-negative means negative for B antigen)
Phenotype	P$_1$+, P$_1$-	P$_1^+$, P$_1^-$, P$_1^{(+)}$, P$_1^{(-)}$
Phenotype	M+N- or M	M(+), MM (infers unproved genotype)
Antigen	K	Kell (name of sytem)
Antibody	Anti-K	Anti-Kell (still name of system)
Phenotypes	K:1, K:-1	K1+, K:1+, K(1), K:(1), K1-, K:1-, K1-negative
Phenotype	K-k+Kp(a+b+)	K$^-$, k$^+$, Kp^a+Kp^b+ K-k+Kp^a+Kp^b+
Antigens	Rh1, Rh2	Rh:1, Rh:2 (no colon in antigen names)
Phenotype	Rh:1,-2,3,4,-5	Rh:+1,-2,+3,+4,-5 Rh:1+,2-,-3+4+5- Rh1,-2,3,4,-5
Antibody	Anti-Rh32	Anti Rh32, Anti-Rh^{32}, Anti-$\overline{\overline{R}}$^{N} (See Chapter 12)
Phenotype	Le(a+)	Le^a+, Lea(+), Lea+, Le^a+, Lewis^a+, Lewis^a-positive
Phenotype	Lu(a+b+)	Lu^{a+b+}, Lu^a+Lu^b+, Lu(a+)(b+), Lu^a+Lu^b+, Lua+b+
Antibody	Anti-Fy3	Anti-Fy^3, Anti-Duffy3
Phenotype	Fy(a+b-)	Fy^{a+b-}, Fy$^{(a+b-)}$, Fy$^{a(+)b(-)}$, Fy^a-posFy^b-neg
Antigens	Jk^a, Jk^b	JK^a, JK^b
Phenotype	At(a+), At(a-)	At^a(a+), At^a(a-)

TABLE 1-3 Some Examples of Gene, Antigen and Phenotype Terms

System	Genes	Antigens	Phenotypes
ABO	$A\ A^1\ A^2\ B$	A A$_1$ A$_2$ B	A A$_1$ A$_2$ B
MN	$M\ N\ S\ s\ Ny^a$	M N S s Ny^a	M+N+S-s+Ny(a+)
P	p^1	P$_1$	P$_1$+ P$_1$-
Lewis	$Le\ le$	Le^a Le^b	Le(a+) Le(a-b+)
Duffy	$Fy^a\ Fy^b\ Fy^5$	Fy^a Fy^b Fy5	Fy(a+b+) Fy:5
Lutheran	$Lu^a\ Lu^b\ Lu$	Lu^a Lu^b	Lu(a-b-) Lu:-3
Rh	$D\ C^w\ Go^a$	D C^w Go^a	D+ C^w- Go(a+)
Rh	$R^1\ R^8\ R^{30}$	Rh1 Rh8 Rh30	Rh:1,-8,30
Kell	$K\ k\ Kp^a$	K k Kp^a	K-k+Kp(a+)
Kell	$K^1\ K^2\ K^3$	K1 K2 K3	K:-1,2,3
Scianna	$Sc^1\ Sc^2\ Sc$	Sc1 Sc2	Sc:-1,-2,-3
Colton	$Co^a\ Co^b$	Co^a Co^b Co3	Co(a-b-) Co:-3

On rare occasions an antibody may be misnamed by implication that it detects a gene, not an antigen. In the Rh blood group system (see Chapter 12) the rare genes $\bar{\bar{R}}^N$ and R^{oHar} encode production of the low incidence antigens Rh32 and Rh33 respectively. Some workers, who should know better, talk about anti-$\bar{\bar{R}}^N$ and anti-R^{oHar}. Since $\bar{\bar{R}}^N$ and R^{oHar} are genes and since antibodies define antigens, the terms are obviously nonsensical.

Some Other Common Errors

Although not relating strictly to blood group antigen names, there are a number of other errors that creep (sometimes gallop) into the immunohematologist's vocabulary. The word titer is a noun; the verb is to titrate. Thus, an antibody can be titrated; it cannot be titered. The titer is correctly expressed as the reciprocal of the serum dilution; it is incorrect to use the serum dilution as a synonym for titer. For example, if a serum dilution of 1 in 64 is the endpoint of the titration, the titer is 64; it is not 1 in 64. A dilution of 1 in 64 should not be written as 1:64 since that term describes a ratio, that is 1 part to 64 parts or a dilution of 1 in 65. While the difference between 1 in 64 and 1 in 65 is not often important, the term 1:2 creates a more serious error. 1:2 implies 1 part to 2 parts or a dilution of 1 in 3; 1 in 2 implies equal parts, clearly there is a 50% variance between the two.

The word data is plural. Thus the commonly used "the data is" and "the data shows" are incorrect and should be "the data are" and "the data show". A single piece of information is a datum.

The terms homozygous and heterozygous refer to genes not antigens. Thus red cells cannot correctly be described by either of those terms. Statements such as "homozygous Jk^a red cells" are incorrect, red cells of the type being described can be said to be "from a *Jk^a* homozygote". The use of the immediate spin compatibility test (the correct term for the slang "crossmatch") and the introduction of antibody-screening cells from three instead of two donors has led to a plethora of statements about the use of homozygous (for Jk^a, Jk^b, Fy^a, Fy^b, etc.) red cells when, all the time, the cells come from (presumed) homozygous donors.

The ISBT Terminology

When computers first became available, it was natural that blood groupers would use them to store information. By 1980 there was concern that since no standard system existed, individual workers were devising their own terminologies thus eliminating a major benefit of the use of computers, namely the capability of electronic transfer and exchange of information. In response to these concerns, Dr. B.P.L. Moore, the then President of the International Society of Blood Transfusion (ISBT), initiated formation of a Working Party on Terminology for Red Cell Surface Antigens. The charge to this Working Party was to devise a uniform nomenclature that would be both eye and machine readable and in keeping with the genetic basis of the blood groups. It is important to note that in its very first report (130) a statement appeared that "the ISBT Working Party is not trying to change the nomenclature of the blood groups. Numbers assigned to specificities are proposed as standard alternatives to current alphabetical names in those circumstances where numbers are necessary, as in some computer systems." In other words, since its inception, the Working Party has sought to provide an additional terminology, suitable for use in electronic data processing equipment, not a replacement. This point has not always been understood and attempts have sometimes been made to dictate use of the new system to the exclusion of traditional terms.

In the early 1980s many computers lacked the sophistication of their modern counterparts. Partly because of this and partly to keep the terminology easy to use, the ISBT Working Party elected to use only on line capital letters and Arabic numerals (e.g. ABO, RH, KEL, etc. systems; 001001, 001002, etc. for system and antigen codes). New antigens named after the terminology was introduced would have names using from 3 to 6 on line capital letters (e.g. NFLD, BOW, JONES, etc.).

In addition to assigning names and numbers to antigens, the Working Party has insisted on absolute evidence of genetic independence before recognizing a blood group system. Sometimes such evidence has come from traditional family studies showing independent segregation of the genes of one blood group system from the genes of all others. At other times biochemical evidence has been used to show that certain blood group antigens are carried on the same, or different, red cell membrane components. Most recently direct evidence from molecular genetic studies has been used, often with great help from substitute DNA markers and restriction fragment length polymorphisms (101), to prove genetic linkage or independence. Regular reports and updates of the Working Party's decisions have been published (131-137). As of this writing (April 1995) the Working Party has recognized the 23 blood group systems listed in table 1-4. Each system is given a number and an alphabetical symbol (001, ABO; 002, MNS, etc.). Each antigen within the system is then also given a number (001 for A, 002 for B, etc.). Thus in the full computer-intended code, the A antigen is 001001, the B antigen is 001002, etc. Sinistral zeros may be omitted when convenient so that A would be 1.1 and B 1.2, etc. In the Rh system (004) the first three antigens are D, 001; C, 002; E, 003. Thus in full computer-talk, D, C and E are 004001, 004002 and 004003 respectively. The system symbol and the antigen number (minus sinistral zeros) may also be used, thus RH1, RH2 and RH3 in the example used. Whenever a system already had (even partial) numerical terms (Rh, Lutheran, Kell, etc.) the same sequence was used, thus RH1, RH2 and RH3 in the ISBT terminology are Rh1, Rh2 and Rh3 in the numerical terminology. Since, like the journal TRANSFUSION(138), the chapters of this

book will use conventional rather than ISBT terms, table 1-4 is not fully comprehensive. For example, numbers up to RH51, MNS38 and KEL24 have been assigned to antigens. Table 1-4 records numbers for systems but not the antigens therein. In each of the chapters on blood group systems in this book, ISBT terms for the antigens are listed in an introductory table. For those readers with fingers already poised on computer keyboards, the most recent compilation of numbers assigned is given in reference 137. Since it is a convenient place to list them, table 1-4 includes the chromosomal locations of the blood group system genes. References to the many outstanding studies that generated such information are given in appropriate chapters of this book. After the 207 antigens in the 23 systems listed in table 1-4 had been assigned numbers (some of which are now obsolete since the defining reagents are no longer available or the antigen has been transferred to a different system) there were naturally antigens left over. This because in many instances antigens not part of any of the 23 systems have been recognized. In some instances these additional antigens were put into Collections. A Collection is a group of antigens that display clear phenotypic association to each other, but where there is insufficient evidence that the antigens of the collection comprise a blood group system genetically independent of all others. Table 1-5 lists the Collections that existed as of April 1995. Two other classifications are used. The 700 series comprises antigens of low incidence not yet known to be part of any recognized system; the 901 series lists high incidence antigens of similar, as yet apparently independent status. Brief details of the 700 and 901 series are also given in table 1-5, again the Collection, 700 and 901 series terms are listed in later chapters of this book.

Finally, since the ISBT Working Party has dealt with polymorphic characters and has required evidence of the discreet nature of an antigen before assigning a number, there any many red cell surface markers that do not have an ISBT term. Antigens such as IA, IB, IH (see Chapter 10), En^{a}TS, En^{a}FS, En^{a}FR (see Chapter 15), the Pr series, Sa, Gd, etc. (see Chapter 34) and many others, do not have (and may never have) ISBT numbers. Clearly those antigens and the antibodies that define them must be (and are) described in a book of this type.

References

1. Blundell J. Med Chir Trans 1818;9:56
2. Blundell J. Med Chir Trans 1819;10:295
3. Schmidt PJ. Transfusion 1995;35:4
4. Anon. Phila J Med Physic Sci 1825;9:207
5. Myhre BA. Transfusion 1995;35:74
6. Schmidt PJ. New Eng J Med 1968;279:1319
7. Myhre BA. Transfusion 1990;30:358

TABLE 1-4 Blood Group Systems Recognized by the ISBT Working Party

System Name Conventional	System Name ISBT	System Symbol Conventional	System Symbol ISBT	Chromosomal Location
ABO	001	ABO	ABO	9q34.1-q34.2
MN	002	MN	MNS	4q28-q31
P	003	P	P1	22q11.2-qter
Rh	004	Rh	RH	1p36.2-p34
Lutheran	005	Lu	LU	19q12-q13
Kell	006	K	KEL	7q33
Lewis	007	Le	LE	19p13.3
Duffy	008	Fy	FY	1q22-q23
Kidd	009	Jk	JK	18q11-q12
Diego	010	Di	DI	17q12-q21
Cartwright	011	Yt	YT	7q22
Xg	012	Xg	XG	Xp22.32
Scianna	013	Sc	SC	1p36.2-p22.1
Dombrock	014	Do	DO	12p13.2-p12.1
Colton	015	Co	CO	7p14
LW	016	LW	LW	19p13.2-cen
Chido/Rodgers	017	Ch/Rg	CH/RG	6p21.3
Hh	018	H	H	19q13
Kx	019	Kx	XK	Xp21.1
Gerbich	020	Ge	GE	2q14-q21
Cromer	021	Cromer	CROM	1q32
Knops	022	Kn	KN	1q32
Indian	023	In	IN	11p13

TABLE 1-5 Collections and Series in the ISBT Terminology

Conventional Name	ISBT Number	Collection Symbol	Antigens included (Conventional Symbols)
Cost/Stirling	205	COST	Cs^a, Cs^b
I	207	I	I, i
Er	208	ER	Er^a, Er^b
Previously P	209	GLOB	P, P^k, Luke
H-associated	210	Not named	Le^c (Type 1 chain)*
			Le^d (Type 1 H)*

ISBT 700 series - As of April 1995, 32 low incidence antigens

ISBT 901 series - As of April 1995, 12 high incidence antigens

* See Chapter 9

8. Gottlieb AM. A Pictorial History of Blood Practices and Transfusion. Scottsdale, AZ:Arcane, 1992
9. Landsteiner K. Zbl Bakt 1900;27:357
10. Landsteiner K. Wien Klin Wschr 1901;14:1132
11. Landsteiner K, Levine P. Proc Soc Exp Biol NY 1927;24:600
12. Landsteiner K, Levine P. Proc Soc Exp Biol NY 1927;24:941
13. Landsteiner K, Wiener AS. Proc Soc Exp Biol NY 1940;43:223
14. Race RR. Nature 1944;153:771
15. Wiener AS. Proc Soc Exp Biol NY 1944;56:173
16. Cameron JW, Diamond LK. J Clin Invest 1945;24:793
17. Diamond LK, Denton RL. J Lab Clin Med 1945;30:821
18. Coombs RRA, Mourant AE, Race RR. Lancet 1945;2:15
19. Coombs RRA, Mourant AE, Race RR. Brit J Exp Path 1945;26:255
20. Morton JA, Pickles MM. Nature 1947;159:779
21. Callender S, Race RR, Paykoc ZV. Brit Med J 1945;2:83
22. Coombs RRA, Mourant AE, Race RR. Lancet 1946;1:264
23. Mourant AE. Nature 1946;158:237
24. Cutbush M, Mollison PL, Parkin DM. Nature 1950;165:188
25. Allen FH Jr, Diamond LK, Niedziela B. Nature 1951;167:482.
26. Lewis M, Chown B, Kaita H, et al. Transfusion 1967;7:440
27. Chown B, Lewis M, Kaita H, et al. Transfusion 1964;4;169
28. Race RR, Sanger R. Blood Groups in Man, 6th Ed, Oxford:Blackwell, 1975
29. Contreras M, Stebbing B, Blessing M, et al. Vox Sang 1978;34:208
30. Darnborough J, Dunsford I, Wallace JA. Vox Sang 1969;17:241
31. Furuhjelm U, Myllyla G, Nevanlinna HR, et al. Vox Sang 1969;17:256
32. Issitt PD, Tippett P, Daniels GL. Transfusion 1981;21:473
33. Anstee DJ, Barker DM, Judson PA, et al. Br J Haematol 1977;35:309
34. Dahr W, Uhlenbruck G, Leikola J, et al. J Immunogenet 1976;3:329
35. Dahr W, Uhlenbruck G, Wagstaff W, et al. J Immunogenet 1976;3:383
36. Gahmberg CG, Myllyla G, Leikola J, et al. J Biol Chem 1976;251:6108
37. Tanner MJA, Anstee DJ. Biochem J 1976;153:271
38. Tanner MJA, Jenkins RE, Anstee DJ, et al. Biochem J 1976;155:701
39. Wasniowska K, Drzeniek Z, Lisowska E. Biochem Biophys Res Comm 1977;76:385
40. Dahr W, Uhlenbruck G, Janssen E, et al. Hum Genet 1977;35:335
41. Macdonald EB, Gerns LM. Vox Sang 1986;50:112
42. Reid ME, Shaw M-A, Rowe G, et al. Biochem J 1985;232:289
43. Macdonald EB, Condon J, Ford D, et al. Vox Sang 1990;58:300
44. Daniels G, King M-J, Avent ND, et al. Blood 1993;82:3198
45. King MJ, Avent ND, Mallinson G, et al. Vox Sang 1992;63:56
46. Anstee DJ, Ridgwell K, Tanner MJA, et al. Biochem J 1984;221:97
47. Colin Y, Rahuel C, London J, et al. J Biol Chem 1986;261:229
48. Cartron JP. In: Blood Cell Biochemistry, Vol 1, Plenum: New York, 1990:299
49. Seaman MJ, Benson R, Jones MN, et al. Br J Haematol 1967;13:464
50. Kohler G, Milstein C. Nature 1975;256:495
51. Kosimies S. Scand J Immunol 1980;11:73
52. Boylston AW, Gardner B, Anderson RL, et al. Scand J Immunol 1980;12:355
53. Crawford DH, Barlow MJ, Harrison JF, et al. Lancet 1983;1:386
54. Rouger P, Goosens D, Champomier F, et al. Rev Franc Transf Immunhematol 1985;28:671
55. Melamed MD, Gordon J, Ley SJ, et al. Eur J Immunol 1985;15:742
56. Goosens D, Champomier F, Rouger P, et al. J Immunol Meth 1987;101:193
57. Kumpel BM, Leader KA, Merry AH, et al. Eur J Immunol 1989;19:2283
58. Laemmli UK, Nature 1970;227:680
59. Maniatis T, Fritsch EF, Sambrook J. Molecular cloning. A laboratory manual. New York:Cold Spring Harbor, 1982
60. Levine P, Robinson E, Celano M, et al. Blood 1955;10:1100
61. Aloysia M, Gelb AG, Fudenberg H, et al. Transfusion 1961;1:212
62. Lanset S, Ropartz C, Rousseau PY, et al. Transfusion (Paris) 1966;9:255
63. Schenkel-Brunner H, Chester MA, Watkins WM. Eur J Biochem 1972;30:269
64. Race C, Watkins WM. FEBS Lett 1972;27:125
65. Robson EB, Cook PJL, Buckton KE. Ann Hum Genet 1977;41:53
66. Lewis M, Kaita H, Giblett ER, et al. Cytogenet Cell Genet 1978;22:452
67. Ball SP, Tongue N, Gibaud A, et al. Ann Hum Genet 1991;55(pt3):225
68. Plaut G, Ikin EW, Mourant AE, et al. Nature 1953;171:431
69. Pinkerton FJ, Mermod LE, Liles BA, et al. Vox Sang 1959;4:155
70. Walsh RJ, Montgomery C. Nature 1947;160:504
71. Levine P, Kuhmichel AB, Wigod M, et al. Proc Soc Exp Biol NY 1951;78:218
72. Sanger R, Race RR. Nature 1947;160:505
73. Sanger R, Race RR, Walsh RJ, et al. Heredity 1948;2:131
74. Levine P, Celano MJ, Falkowski F, et al. Nature 1964;204:892
75. Ishimori T, Hasekura H. Proc Jap Acad 1966;42:658
76. Levine P, Celano MJ, Falkowski F, et al. Transfusion 1965;5:492
77. Tippett P. Serological Study of the Inheritance of Unusual Rh and Other Blood Group Phenotypes. Ph.D. Thesis, Univ London, 1963
78. deVeber LL, Clark GW, Hunking M, et al. Transfusion 1971;11:33 and 389
79. Swanson JL, Azar M, Miller J, et al. Transfusion 1974;14:470
80. White JC, Rolih SD, Wilkinson SL, et al. Transfusion 1975;15:368
81. Marsh WL, Chaganti RSK, Gardner FH, et al. Science 1974;183:966
82. Chérif-Zahar B, Mattei MG, Le Van Kim C, et al. Hum Genet 1991;86:398
83. Sistonen P. Ann Hum Genet 1984;48:239
84. Guévin RM, Taliano V, Waldmann O. Vox Sang 1976;31(Suppl 1):96
85. Chown B, Lewis M, Kaita H. Nature 1957;180;711
86. Strange JJ, Kenworthy RJ, Webb AJ, et al. Vox Sang 1974;27:81
87. Sabo B. McCreary J, Gellerman M, et al. Vox Sang 1975;29:450
88. Layrisse M, Arends T, Dominguez SR. Acta Med Venezuela 1955;3:132
89. Thompson PR, Childers DM, Hatcher DE. Vox Sang 1967;13:314

90. Eaton BR, Morton JA, Pickles MM, et al. Br J Haematol 1956;7:333
91. Giles CM, Metaxas MN. Nature 1964;202:1122
92. Spring FA, Bruce LJ, Anstee DJ, et al. Biochem J 1992;288:713
93. Bruce LJ, Anstee DJ, Spring FA, et al. J Biol Chem 1994;269:16155
94. Zelinski T, Coghlan G, White L, et al. Genomics 1993;17;665
95. Solomon E, Ledbetter DM. Cytogenet Cell Genet 1991;58:686
96. Spring FA, Gardner B, Anstee DJ. Blood 1992;80:2136
97. Bartels CF, Zelinski T, Lockridge O. Am J Hum Genet 1993;52:928
98. Li Y, Camp S, Rachinsky TL, et al. J Biol Chem 1991;266:23083
99. Zelinski T, White L, Coghlan G, et al. Genomics 1991;11:165
100. Getman DK, Eubanks JH, Camp S, et al. Am J Hum Genet 1992;51:170
101. Zelinski T. Transfusion 1991;31:762
102. Andresen PH, Callender ST, Fisher RA, et al. Nature 1949;163:580
103. Heisto H, van der Hart M, Madsen G, et al. Vox Sang 1967;12:18
104. Giles CM, Darnborough J, Aspinall P, et al. Br J Haematol 1970;19:267
105. Rogers MJ, Styles PA, Wright J. (abstract). Transfusion 1974;14:508
106. Moulds JJ, Dykes D, Polesky HF. (abstract). Transfusion 1974;14:508
107. Levine, P, Robinson EA, Layrisse M, et al. Nature 1956;177:40
108. Lewis M, Kaita H, Chown B. Vox Sang 1974;27:261
109. Nason SG, Vengelen-Tyler V, Cohen N, et al. Transfusion 1980;20:531
110. Sanger R, Race RR, Jack JA. Br J Haematol 1955;1:370
111. Behzad O, Lee CL, Gavin J, et al. Vox Sang 1973;24:337
112. Oien L, Nance S, Arndt P, et al. Transfusion 1988;28:541
113. Nance ST. In: Progress in Immunohematology, Arlington, VA: Am Assoc Blood Banks. 1988:1
114. Dahr W, Weber W, Kordowicz M. In: Biomathematical Evidence of Paternity, Springer-Verlag, 1981:131
115. Yamamoto F, Clausen H, White T, et al. Nature 1990;345:229
116. Yamamoto F, Marken J, Tsuji T, et al. J Biol Chem 1990;265:1146
117. Yamamoto F, Hakomori S. J Biol Chem 1990;265:19257
118. Lee JC, Chang JG. J Foren Sci 1992;37:1269
119. Chang JG, Lee LS, Chen PH, et al. Blood 1992;79:2176
120. Ugozzoli L, Wallace RB. Genomics 1992;12:670
121. Yamamoto F, McNeill PD, Yamamoto M, et al. Vox Sang 1993;64:175
122. Carritt B, Blunt T, Avent N, et al. Ann Hum Genet 1993;57:273
123. Chérif-Zahar B, Raynal V, Le Van Kim C, et al. Blood 1993;82:656
124. Cartron J-P. Blood Rev 1994;8:199
125. Hyland CA, Wolter LC, Saul A. Blood 1994;84:321
126. Chérif-Zahar B, Raynal V, D'Ambrosio AM, et al. Blood 1994;84:4354
127. Levine P, Celano MJ, Falkowski F, et al. Nature 1964;204:892
128. Levine P, Celano MJ, Falkowski F, et al. Transfusion 1965;5:492
129. Issitt PD, Crookston M. Transfusion 1984;24:2
130. Allen FH Jr, Anstee DJ, Bird GWG, et al. Vox Sang 1982;42:164
131. Allen FH Jr. ISBT Newsletter No. 18, April 1983
132. Lewis M, Allen FH Jr, Anstee DJ, et al. Vox Sang 1985;49:71
133. Lewis M. ISBT Newsletter No. 34, April 1987
134. Lewis M, Anstee DJ, Bird GWG, et al. Vox Sang 1990;58:152
135. Lewis M, Anstee DJ, Bird GWG, et al. Vox Sang 1991;61:158
136. Daniels GL, Moulds JJ, Anstee DJ, et al. Vox Sang 1993;65:77
137. Daniels GL, Anstee DJ, Cartron J-P, et al. Vox Sang 1995;69:265
138. Issitt PD, Moulds JJ. Transfusion 1992;32:677
139. Tournamille C, Colin Y, Cartron J-P, et al. Nature Genetics 1995;10:224

2 | The Immune Response, Production of Antibodies, Antigen-Antibody Reactions

Introduction - Immunology Grew out of Bacteriology

The branch of science known as immunology arose out of a desperate need to understand and combat the ravages of infectious diseases. In the eighteenth century smallpox was rife. However, those who survived smallpox did not succumb to the disease again, they were immune. The word immune derives from the Latin *immunis*-not serving. Freedom from obligation to serve (presumably in battle) meant freedom from danger hence those that are immune to a disease are free from the danger the disease provides. Clearly, if immunity could be achieved without having to endure or risk the disease itself then its threat could be subverted. "It was common practice in the East for people to infect themselves deliberately from a sufferer who had smallpox in a mild form, in order to avoid getting it badly - a practice that found its way into Europe in the eighteenth century" (1). The first to apply this principle to generate a general method for protection from the disease was Edward Jenner, a physician who lived in Berkeley, Gloucestershire, England only a short drive from Bristol, the home of one of the authors. Jenner noticed that cowpox was a very similar disease to smallpox and, in 1796, showed that a person inoculated with cowpox gets a very mild disease which confers immunity to smallpox. The virus which causes cowpox is named *Vaccinia* from the Latin word for a cow and the process by which immunity was conferred to smallpox by inoculation with cowpox became known as vaccination.

By the late nineteenth century rapid progress was being made in understanding the nature of micro-organisms which cause disease. Chick et al. (2) describe a historic meeting held in August 1881 at King's College, London and attended by Louis Pasteur and Joseph Lister, at which the German physician, Robert Koch demonstrated techniques for isolating and culturing bacteria in the laboratory - the first demonstrably pure culture of a bacterium. "Before the end of the nineteenth century the agents responsible for fourteen different diseases had been identified, including the germs of tuberculosis, tetanus, typhoid and diphtheria" (2).

Research into the prevention of disease by vaccination using mild or attenuated strains of the relevant micro-organism continued most notably with the work of Pasteur on rabies, but how was immunity conferred? The answer to this question came from the work in Paris, of Roux and Yersin, who showed in 1888 that the diphtheria bacillus produced a soluble factor (toxin) which was responsible for the disease. Two years later von Behring and Kitasato, working in Berlin, showed that a similar toxin produced by tetanus bacilli when injected in low doses into rabbits and mice, conferred immunity to subsequent challenges with tetanus bacilli. Furthermore, these workers showed that a factor in the serum (anti-toxin) of these immunized animals could neutralize tetanus toxin (but not toxins from other types of bacteria) in a test tube (2). For toxin read antigen and for anti-toxin read antibody and the basis of immunology is established.

It soon became apparent that antibodies could be made to the surface of the bacteria themselves. Mixing the serum of an immunized individual with a suspension of the bacteria to which they had been immunized caused clumping (agglutination) or lysis of the bacteria. Furthermore, the exquisite specificity of antibodies for the antigen to which they had been exposed meant that in vitro tests of bacterial agglutination, lysis or precipitation (in the case of soluble antigen) could be used in a diagnostic way to identify the particular strains of bacilli causing disease (3). Landsteiner applied the same methodology and found that by mixing the red cells and serum of different individuals agglutination and/or lysis could be observed and immunohematology was born (4). Almost a century later basically the same methodology is applied worldwide to ensure the compatibility of blood for transfusion (see Chapter 3). The progress that has taken place in the intervening period and which forms the basis of this book, has served to expand the body of knowledge concerning the diversity of structures at the red cell surface and thereby improve the safety of blood transfusion. Progress has also been made in the provision of diagnostic antibodies for blood typing and in the improvement and/or automation of the methods used for blood typing and the detection of antibodies in patients' sera. The fundamental principles which underpin this work were elucidated by bacteriologists more than a century ago.

Vaccination confers immunity so that man will survive exposure to a disease at some time in the future. In order to treat a patient who already has the disease the practice developed of producing anti-toxin in animals and then treating patients with the serum of the immunized animal. Chick et al. (2) noted that one of the first persons to be treated in this way was a child with diphtheria given horse anti-diphtheria toxin on Christmas night, 1891 by a Dr. Geissler in Berlin. The practice of treating all wound cases with horse anti-tetanus toxin reduced the incidence of tetanus from 16 per thousand in 1914 to 2 per thousand in subsequent years of World War I (1). Antibodies have been used to prevent or cure disease for more than a century. For most of that time little was known about the structure of antibodies. An understanding of structure had to wait for the development of methodologies for protein purification and analysis in the 1950's and 1960's (5).

Lymphocytes Play a Central Role in Immunity

As the preceding section explains, the existence of antibodies and their value in the treatment of infectious diseases was appreciated a century ago. Where and how the antibodies were made remained a mystery for another 50 years. In 1931, Wells et al. (1) wrote "Where these substances (antibodies) are produced is at present not clear. There is some evidence that that versatile organ, the liver, plays a considerable part in their manufacture". In 1946, Wintrobe (6) wrote "the lymphocytes ......seem to be involved in some way in the healing process, for they are generally increased during convalescence from infections". Wintrobe goes on to quote a paper by Harris et al. (7) who showed that antibodies to typhoid antigen or to sheep red cells were produced in highest titer by lymphocytes present in "the efferent lymph draining the injected area".

During the 1960's it became clear that lymphocytes are a heterogeneous group of cells and that a broad distinction can be made between B cells and T cells. B cells are able to synthesize and secrete antibody. In man B cells develop in fetal liver and subsequently the bone marrow. The central role of B cells in antibody production was in large part deduced from studies on birds. In birds B cells are produced by a gut-associated organ known as the Bursa of Fabricius. If this organ is removed at the time of hatching then the birds are unable to make antibodies (8).

The cycle of events that involves recognition of foreign material (antigen), stimulation of lymphocytes to produce antibody and removal/destruction of foreign material by antibody is usually referred to as humoral immunity. Humoral means pertaining to or preceding from the humours. The humours (humour literally means to be moist, from the Latin *humere*) were, in early medicine, the four bodily fluids (blood, phlegm, yellow bile and black bile) which were considered to be the source of all diseases. Antibodies are found in blood and in other body fluids hence humoral immunity.

Not all immunity is conferred by antibodies and it is useful to distinguish between humoral (antibody-mediated) immunity and cell-mediated immunity. Humoral immunity is generally ineffective against viral infections because the virus is within the body's cells and tissues. A different defense mechanism has evolved to deal with this problem. Fragments of foreign (viral) proteins synthesized within the cell are transported to the cell surface where they are recognized and immune effector cells (cytotoxic T lymphocytes, CTLs) are stimulated to destroy the infected cells.

T cells are made in the thymus. If the thymus is removed from chickens they can make antibodies, albeit less efficiently than normal chickens, but are unable to effect cell-mediated immunity (8). Cell-mediated immunity is effected by a class of T cells known as cytotoxic T cells but there are other types of T cell. In particular, a class of T cells known as helper T cells are required for mounting a humoral immune response and this explains why thymectomized animals not only lack cell-mediated immunity but also have impaired humoral immunity. Proof that cell-mediated immunity is a vital part of mans' defense against viral assault has been obtained relatively recently from the work of Zinkernagel and Doherty (9). There are about 2×10^{12} lymphocytes in the human body making the immune system comparable in mass to the liver or the brain (10).

The foregoing discussion has considered the development of an understanding of immunological processes from the point of view of fighting infectious diseases. There are a number of pathological complications that may arise when something goes wrong with immune processes. The success of mechanisms which seek to destroy invading microbes depends upon their ability to recognize differences between the microbes and the hosts' own cells and tissues, that is, the ability to distinguish 'self' from 'non-self'. It is, of course, in the microbes' interest to evolve in such a way as to make it difficult for the host to distinguish self from non-self. The most successful microbes colonize their host without killing it and they frequently achieve this by acquiring surface structures which are similar to those of the host. If the host should mount an immune response to self then humoral and/or cell-mediated damage to host cells and tissues occurs and an autoimmune disease results.

Polymorphism Ensures Survival of the Species

Man's humoral and cell-mediated immune mechanisms are not the first line of defense against microbial assault. The commonest routes of microbial infection are through the respiratory tract and mucosal surfaces of the gut. The organisms seek to colonize the respiratory and/or mucosal surfaces by binding to receptors on cell surfaces. In order to survive man must be able to generate diversity in the structures at cell surfaces wherever those surfaces are exposed to microbes. Such diversity (polymorphism) is vital to the survival of the species because through this mechanism some individuals will avoid colonization by a micro-organism (because they lack the appropriate receptor) and survive without the need for immune mechanisms. The level of structural diversity among proteins which are found in locations regularly exposed to microbes is far greater than the level of structural diversity found in proteins not so exposed, like intracellular proteins. Murphy (11) compared the sequences of 615 human proteins with the corresponding rodent (mouse or rat) homologs. For 79% of all the proteins in the database the mean divergence (human sequence from rodent sequence) was in the range 1-12%. In contrast, among the 75 proteins known to be host defense ligands and receptors the divergence was 35%.

The large number of inherited blood group antigens that form the subject of this book are one consequence of the need to generate diversity at cell surfaces. Numerous blood group antigens are known to provide receptors for micro-organisms and the reader will find many references to this property throughout the book. Many of the blood group antigens which are defined by carbohydrate sequence like A, B and H are not confined to red cells but are widely distributed at mucosal surfaces (see Chapter 8). Perhaps one of the best examples is the Le^b antigen which provides a receptor for the bacterium *Helicobacter pylori* which is thought to be the causative agent of gastric ulcers and gastric carcinoma (12, and Chapter 9). Inheritance of the Fy(a-b-) phenotype is demonstrably a selective advantage because red cells of this phenotype are not invaded by the malarial parasite *Plasmodium vivax* (13, and Chapter 14). Clearly, absence of the microbial receptor is the best way to avoid infectious disease.

If the microbe binds to a host receptor and the host can shed the receptor and with it the microbe then this is also a highly satisfactory defense system. The constant production of mucus by the respiratory tract and the gastrointestinal tract provides a very effective way of removing potentially harmful microbes. If the host has the appropriate receptor for the microbe and the microbe evades the mucosal barriers then an immune system is needed.

Genetic mechanisms for the generation of diversity are not only relevant to the first phase of protection from microbes outlined in the preceding paragraph. Once the microbe has infected the host, the ability of the host to mount a successful immune response to the infection is also under genetic control. The genetic variability is exhibited primarily through the Major Histocompatibilty Complex (MHC). The function of the MHC will be discussed in more detail later in this chapter but in order to explain the relevance of these genes to the overall scheme of defense mechanisms to infectious diseases, it is necessary to make some preliminary comments here. Two types of molecules are the major products of genes in the MHC relevant to this discussion. They are known as class I and class II molecules respectively. Class I molecules are found at the surface of nearly all nucleated cells and their function is to present foreign antigen (made for example by a virus infecting the cell) at the surface of the cell so that the infected cell becomes a target for cytotoxic T lymphocytes and the infected cell can be destroyed (cell-mediated immunity). Class II molecules are relevant to mounting a humoral response. They are confined to cells which function by taking up antigen derived from extracellular foreign proteins [B lymphocytes and macrophages and other antigen-presenting cells (APC's)] which with the assistance of helper T lymphocytes, eliminate pathogens either by the production of antibody to foreign antigen (by B lymphocytes) or phagocytosis and destruction of the pathogen (by activated macrophages). The range of class I and class II molecules that an individual can produce is dependent on the genes that an individual inherits and this in turn determines the number of different foreign proteins that can be presented to elicit antibody production, phagocytosis or cytotoxic T cell activity. Thus it may seem that the more class I and class II genes the better. This is true, in part. The number and type of class I and class II genes varies greatly in different racial groups. Some populations have many fewer than others. The relatively restricted number of genes found among the indigenous peoples of America has been directly related to an increased susceptibility to viral infections and used to explain why approximately 56 million died as a result of European exploration of the New World (14). However, the number of genes is likely to be limited by the constraints within the system imposed by the need to avoid raising an immune response to self. This because each time a new MHC molecule is added the T cells which recognize self peptides in the context of the new MHC molecule must be eliminated. "The number of MHC molecules we express may represent a balance between the advantages of presenting a wide diversity of foreign peptides to T cells against the disadvantages of restricting the T cell repertoire" (10).

The mechanisms described above, antibody-mediated immunity, cell-mediated immunity and the genetic diversity which underpins it has evolved over millions of years to protect the individual from "non-self". In the light of this information, it is not surprising that blood transfusion and organ transplantation create complex problems!

The following sections focus on aspects of the immune response which are particularly relevant to the use of blood group serology in the practice of blood transfusion.

The Structure of Antibodies (10,23)

The same basic structural unit gives rise to all antibody molecules. It comprises two different polypeptide chains denoted heavy and light chains. Light chains are common to all antibody molecules and can be of two types, kappa (κ) and lambda (λ). A single antibody molecule always contains either κ or λ light chains never both. There are five different types of heavy chain denoted, μ, γ, α, δ, ε and it is the type of heavy chain that determines the class of the antibody molecule (IgM, IgG, IgA, IgD, IgE respectively). Four different subclasses of IgG (IgG1, 2, 3, 4) and two of IgA (IgA1, 2) are recognized.

The basic structural unit of all the classes and subclasses comprises two heavy chains held together by a variable number of disulphide bonds. Each heavy chain has one light chain bound to it by disulphide bonds (see figure 2-1). The terms heavy and light chain simply refer to the relative sizes of the two polypeptides. The heavy chain is larger (usually about 440 amino acids) than the light chain (usually about 220 amino acids). Major contributions to an understanding of the structure of antibody molecules were made by RR Porter working at St Mary's Hospital Medical School in London (15). Porter showed that IgG could be digested with papain to yield three fragments of approximately equal size. Two of these fragments were identical and able to bind antigen and these were named Fab (fragment containing antibody binding site). The third fragment could be crystallized easily from IgG of some species and was named Fc (fragment crystalline). These experiments together with evidence that heavy and light chains could be separated from one another by reduction with thiol reagents and were therefore held together by disulphide bonds allowed the basic unit structure of antibody molecules to be demonstrated (see figure 2-2). Pepsin cleaves IgG in a different way. The two Fab fragments remain linked (F(ab')₂) and the rest of the molecule is degraded into small peptides (see figure 2-3). F(ab')₂ fragments are bivalent and therefore able to cross-link antigens while Fab fragments are monovalent and cannot. In addition to the interchain disulphide bonds there are intrachain disulphide links which form globular domains (see figure 2-4).

In the intervening years since these pioneering experiments were carried out an enormous amount of information has accumulated concerning the structure and function of antibody molecules. The first antibody class to be synthesized is IgM. It is synthesized as a surface bound form on B lymphocytes and comprises two heavy (μ) and two light chains and it is this surface immunoglobulin which binds foreign antigen and triggers a primary immune response (see next section). Surface bound IgD of the same specificity is also found on these cells but its function is unclear.

IgM is also the first antibody class to be secreted into the plasma in a primary response. The secreted form of IgM is a pentamer of Mr 900,000 with 10 antigen binding sites and comprises about 10% of the immunoglobulin found in plasma. It also contains an additional polypeptide known as the J (joining) chain (see figure 2-5) which is required for the polymerization of the basic antibody units. As discussed below and in more detail in Chapter 6, IgM is particularly efficient at binding the first component of complement (C1q) thereby activating the complement cascade and effecting lysis of foreign cells. Electron micrographs of IgM molecules have shown that most of them are symmetrical with a diameter of 30-31nm, with occasional molecules having a diameter of 39nm (16). Following binding to antigen the Fab arms of IgM molecules are frequently bent at 90° to the central Fc region (16). This may serve to expose sites for C1q binding.

The major component of the immunoglobulin fraction of plasma is IgG which is found as a monomer Mr 150,000 and comprises about 75% of the total plasma immunoglobulin. IgG is produced in large quantities during secondary immune responses. There are four subclasses of IgG which differ in the nature of their respective heavy chains. The heavy chains of IgG3 are linked by 11 disulphide bonds, those of IgG2 by 4. IgG1 and

FIGURE 2-1 Basic Structural Unit of Immunoglobulin

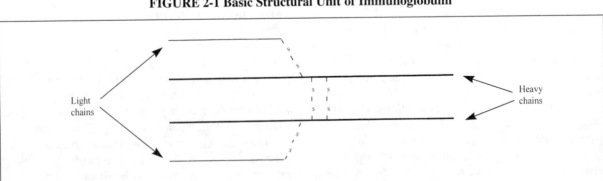

FIGURE 2-2 Papain Cleavage of an IgG Molecule to Create Fab and Fc Fragments

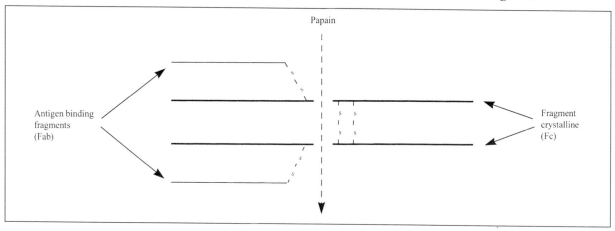

FIGURE 2-3 Pepsin Cleavage of an IgG Molecule to Create F(ab′)₂ Fragment

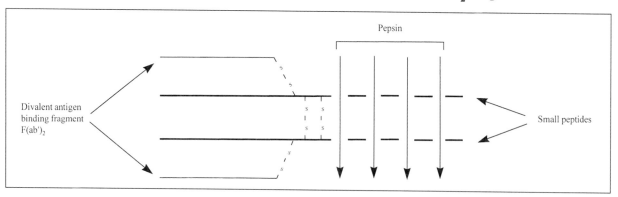

FIGURE 2-4 The Domain Structure of an IgG Molecule

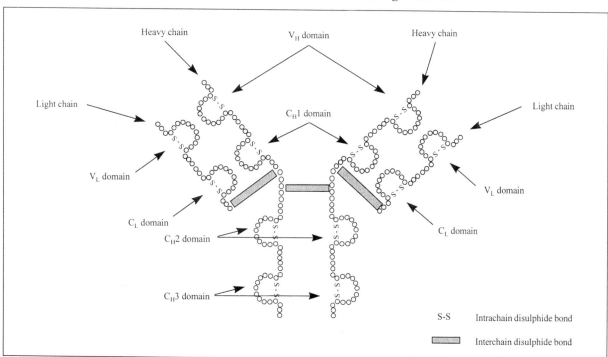

FIGURE 2-5 The Classes of Immunoglobulin Molecules (drawn from reference 10)

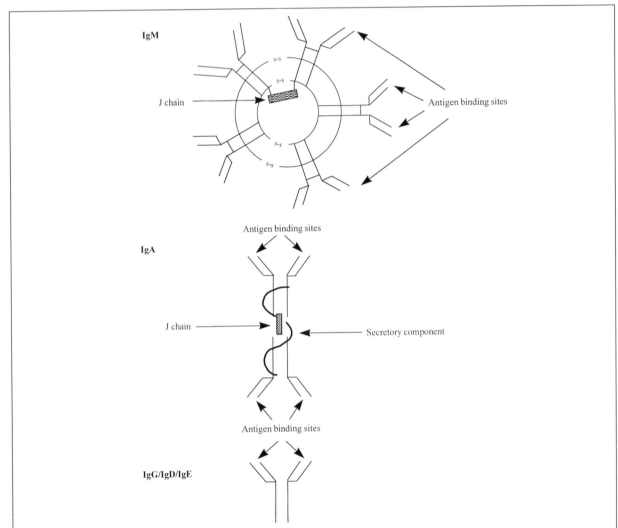

IgG4 each have two (17,18). The predominant subclass in human serum is IgG1 (65-77% of total IgG) compared with IgG2 (11-23%), IgG3 (8-9%) and IgG4 (3-4%). IgG1 and IgG3 can bind C1q, IgG2 binds it less well and IgG4 probably not at all. IgG3 and IgG1 are readily recognized by macrophages, IgG2 less well and IgG4 probably not at all. All four subclasses can cross the placenta (19). Red cell alloantibodies are predominantly IgG1 and/or IgG3. IgG3 differs markedly from the other subclasses in having a much longer hinge region (distance between Fab and Fc portions) which gives it greater flexibility than the other subclasses (see figure 2-6 (20)). Structural studies have shown that the maximum distance between the two antigen binding sites on an IgG molecule is about 14nm (21).

IgA comprises about 15% of human serum immunoglobulin but it is the major immunoglobulin class in secretions. The secretory form of IgA is a dimer linked by a small J (joining) piece and secretory component (see figure 2-5). Monomeric IgA is found in plasma. There are two subclasses of IgA, IgA1 and IgA2. IgA1 comprises about 80-90% of total IgA.

IgD and IgE are minor antibody classes in terms of abundance and together account for less than 1% of the immunoglobulin found in human serum.

All immunoglobulin molecules are glycosylated usually with several N-glycans. The IgA1 class is unusual in that it has O-glycans (22). Some properties of IgG, IgM and IgA are summarized in table 2-1.

The Genes that Encode Antibody Molecules

In the previous section the fact that all antibody molecules are composed of a basic unit comprising two heavy chains and two light chains was discussed. Both

FIGURE 2-6 Comparison of the Structures of IgG1 and IgG3

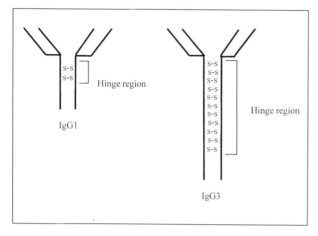

TABLE 2-1 Some Properties of IgG, IgM and IgA

	IgG	IgM	IgA
Type of heavy chain	γ	μ	α
Type of light chain	κ or λ	κ or λ	κ or λ
J chain	No	Yes	Yes
Secretory component	No	No	Yes
Carbohydrate content (%)	3	12	7.5
Molecular weight of 4 chain (2H, 2L) monomer	150,000	180,000	170,000
Molecular weight of heavy chain	53,000	70,000	64,000
Molecular weight of light chain	23,000	23,000	23,000
Molecular weight of J chain		20,000	20,000
Molecular weight of secretory component			60,000

the heavy chain and the light chain contain regions of amino acid sequence hypervariability that carry the information necessary for antigen binding (V_H and V_L respectively) and a region of amino acid sequence which is fairly constant (C_H and C_L) and which is necessary for effector functions of antibody molecules like binding the complement component C1q and interaction with Fc receptors. The regions of hypervariability are mostly confined to three small sections in each of the V_H and V_L regions known as complementary-determining regions or CDR's. This section will consider the way in which different sets of genes are utilized to create antibodies of different immunoglobulin classes and how the diverse array of antigen-binding structures is selected from a large number of different genes.

The human heavy chain loci are found on three chromosomes at 14q32.3, 15q11.2 and 16p11.2 (24). The locus at 14q32.3 comprises approximately 95 (51 functional) V_H (Variable) genes. Downstream of the V_H genes are about 30 D (Diversity) segments, 6 functional J_H (Joining) segments and 9 functional constant region genes (C_H). The C_H genes are in the order μ, δ, $\gamma1$, $\gamma2$, $\gamma3$, $\gamma4$, ε, $\alpha1$ and $\alpha2$, see figure 2-7 (23). The V_H gene loci at 15q11.2 and 16p11.2 have a further 24 V_H genes and D segment genes are also found at 15q11.2 but these genes do not appear to be functional because of the lack of J and C genes at these loci (24).

There are two light chain loci κ and λ. The κ locus is located on chromosome 2 it contains about 76 V_κ genes and pseudogenes. Downstream of the V_κ genes are 5 J_κ segments and a single C_κ gene (24). The λ locus is on chromosome 22 and contains 52 V_λ genes (about half are pseudogenes). Commonly there is a downstream J_λ segment and 7 C_λ genes of which 4 are functional (24).

Heavy and light chain genes for a given antibody are generated by combinatorial rearrangement of V_H, D and J_H segments (Heavy chain genes) and V_L and J_L segments (Light chain genes). The J_H and J_L segments are spliced to constant region genes (C_H and C_L respectively) following transcription of RNA (23, see figure 2-7). Wu and Kabat (25) compared the amino acid sequences of different heavy and light chains and noted three regions of hypervariability in sequence. These hypervariable regions correspond to regions of the V_H and V_L sequences which are in direct contact with antigen and therefore define the specificity of any given antibody. Two of the three hypervariable regions are encoded by the V_H gene product and the third is encoded in the region corresponding to the junction of V_H, D and J_H segments. A similar arrangement accounts for the three hypervariable regions encoded by the V_L and J_L segments which encode the light chain.

By the selection of different combinations of V, D and J genes it is clear that there is enormous potential for generating diversity in antibody structures and thereby, specificity for different antigens. Selection from the different C genes determines the effector functions of the antigen binding VDJ segment and the class/subclass of the resultant antibody molecule.

When the nucleotide sequences of V_H genes are compared it can been seen that they can be classified into seven families denoted V_H1-V_H7 with different members of the same family being at least 80% homologous at the nucleotide sequence level (23). When the different V_H gene families are compared with each other three groups, or clans, of similarity can be discerned. Clan I contains V_H1, V_H5 and V_H7, clan II contains V_H2, V_H4 and V_H6, clan III contains only V_H3. V_H3 has the largest number of V_H gene segments followed by V_H1 and V_H4 (23).

In addition to the structural diversity allowed by the selection of different V, D and J gene segments, antibody

FIGURE 2-7 Generation of IgG Heavy Chain by Combinational Rearrangement of V_H, D and J_H Gene Segments followed by Transcription and RNA Splicing of a Cγ Gene

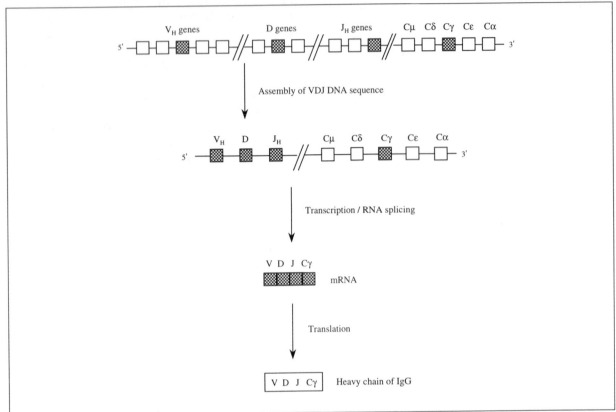

molecules can also undergo a process of affinity maturation (26). Affinity maturation results from point mutations in heavy and light chain variable region coding segments. This process takes place in memory B cells and explains why the antibody produced in a secondary response generally has a higher affinity than antibody produced as a primary response. Not all mutations will result in an increase of antibody affinity but those that do will be preferentially selected because the increased affinity of antigen binding to the surface Ig receptor will increase the signal for B cell proliferation. The effects of affinity maturation can be assessed at the level of protein sequence by comparing the sequences of different monoclonal antibodies with the germ line sequences from which the V, D and J segments were derived. The germ line sequences are those of V_H families 1 to 7, and D and J segments in individuals who have not been exposed to the particular antigen of interest. A human monoclonal anti-D can be taken as an example. Bye et al. (27) determined the nucleotide sequence of the V genes of 14 different human monoclonal anti-D (4 IgM and 10 IgG) derived from 7 different donors. The four IgM appeared to be derived from two germ line gene segments and were not extensively mutated (average 8.9 point muta-

tions/V gene segment). In fact, 10 of the 14 V_H appeared to be derived from one or two V_H germ line segments. These results suggest that the V_H gene response to D is restricted. The V_H genes utilized by the IgG anti-D had a higher number of point mutations (average 19.0 point mutations/V gene) than found in the IgM and consistent with this the IgG had higher affinity for D antigen than IgM. The four antibodies of highest affinity had an average of 25.5 point mutations/V gene.

Studies on pathological cold autoagglutinins of anti-I and anti-i specificity have shown that they are restricted in V_H gene usage to a single gene (V_H4.21) (28). Jefferies et al. (29) provide evidence that natural cold autoagglutinins may preferentially utilize the V_H3 gene. These authors speculate that different stimuli give rise to different V_H gene usage and that while microbes with I antigen might stimulate natural cold autoagglutinins other mechanisms may operate for pathological antibodies.

Knowledge of the particular V, D, J segments used to generate a given antibody specificity and the point mutations which lead to high affinity are of considerable value in molecular modeling of antigen binding sites and can also provide the basis for attempts to generate high affinity antibodies using recombinant DNA technology. Point mutations can be inserted into an appropriate germ line sequence by site directed mutagenesis (see Chapter 5). The mutated sequence can be inserted into a vector containing the appropriate C region gene and the whole gene can be expressed in a suitable cell line so that antibody of the desired specificity is obtained without the need to immunize with antigen.

How Antigen Stimulates the Synthesis of Antibodies

As mentioned briefly in the introduction to this chapter, antibodies are made by B lymphocytes which are produced in fetal liver and bone marrow but this process also requires helper T cells. A third cell type known as an antigen-presenting cell (APC) is also required.

The problem of how the body is able to produce antibody specific for each of the bewildering variety of foreign antigens to which it is exposed was addressed by Sir Macfarlane Burnet in the late 1950's (30). Burnet considered that lymphocytes are not produced in response to antigen but that the body contains millions of lymphocytes which are each "pre-programmed" to respond to a particular antigen structure. When foreign antigen is introduced into an animal a process of selection takes place which identifies the particular B cell able to produce antibody of the desired specificity. Once the required B cell has been found then a signal is transmitted to the cell which causes it to proliferate and produce a clone of B cells able to synthesize the required antibody. Burnet described this process as "The clonal selection theory of acquired immunity" (30).

This theory requires that foreign antigen is recognized when it enters the body and is in some way brought into contact with ("presented to") the relevant B cell and that when the B cell is in contact with antigen, a transmembrane signal causes the B cell to proliferate. Such a process must be extremely specific for antigen and demands that there should be antigen-specific receptor molecules on all B cells. In practice, antigens are complex structures able to stimulate several different B cells because different parts of the antigen (different epitopes) are recognized by different B cells. In other words, several clones of antibody secreting cells are produced, each secreting antibody specific for a different part (different epitope) of the antigen. The serum of the immunized animal will contain a mixture of these antibodies and since the mixture of antibodies is the product of several B cell clones it is known as a polyclonal response. If a complex structure like a bacterium or whole red cell is recognized as foreign then a mixture of antibodies to different epitopes on a large number of different antigens is obtained. Monoclonal antibody technology which is discussed in a later section allows individual B cell clones to be isolated and grown in culture so that antibody to a single epitope is obtained.

The process by which antigen stimulates B cells is complicated and not fully understood (10,31). The first step is recognition and endocytosis of foreign antigen by antigen-presenting cells (APCs) leading to the presentation of peptide derived from the foreign antigen on the surface of the APC by class II MHC molecules (APCs can be loosely defined as those cell types that express MHC class II molecules). MHC class II molecules, unlike class I molecules, have a very restricted distribution being found on certain bone marrow-derived cells (dendritic cells in lymphoid organs, Langerhans cells in skin as well as B cells and macrophages). The APC ingests foreign antigen by endocytosis and delivers it to endosomes where limited proteolysis of antigen occurs. MHC class II molecules are transported from the Golgi apparatus to the antigen-containing endosomes by a carrier protein (denoted invariant chain). The invariant chain is then proteolyzed and peptide derived from antigen becomes bound to the class II molecule. The complex containing class II molecule and antigen-derived peptide is then transported to the surface of the APC and the residual material not transported is degraded in lysosomes.

The second step involves recognition of the antigen-class II complex at the surface of the APC by helper T cells. Helper T cells bind to the antigen-class II complex via the T cell receptor (see figure 2-8) and this interaction induces a transmembrane signal in the helper T cell which activates a tyrosine kinase. Binding to the T cell receptor alone is not sufficient to activate the helper T cell, other interactions between the APC and the T cell are required and these may include interaction between a molecule known as B7 on the APC and CD28 on the helper T cell and several other interactions which promote cell-cell adhesion.

Once the helper T cell has been activated it synthesizes the receptor for the growth factor IL-2 on its surface and at the same time secretes IL-2 so that it can signal its own proliferation.

APCs other than B cells function in a general way by ingesting foreign antigen wherever it enters the body and presenting that antigen to helper T cells. Helper T cells then proliferate and help the appropriate B cell to make antibody. The process by which helper T cells stimulate B cells to make antibody is as follows: B cells express on their surface membrane-bound immunoglobulin (B cell receptor) whose specificity defines the type of antigen that can trigger the proliferation of the cell. When the foreign antigen is bound by the B cell receptor, the antigen-receptor complex is internalized by endocytosis and processed antigen is presented together with MHC class II molecule at the B cell surface in a manner analogous to

FIGURE 2-8 Cellular Mechanisms Involved in the Production of Antibodies

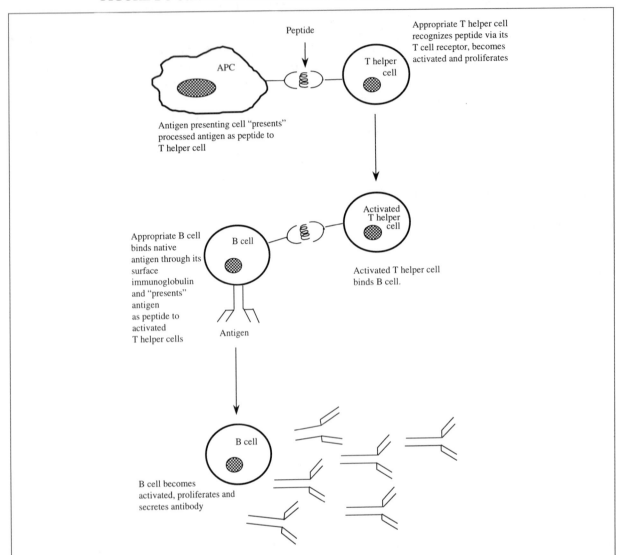

that described above for other APCs. The antigen-specific helper T cells which were activated by APCs other than B cells then bind to the antigen-class II complex on the B cell The antigen-specific interaction between helper T cell and B cell will cause the B cell to proliferate and secrete antibody specific for antigen provided other interactions also take place between the two cells. Binding to CD40 on the B cell by a molecule which specifically recognizes CD40 on the helper T cell is one such essential accessory interaction (see figure 2-8).

The reader may be thinking that this process is rather complicated and wonder why antigen cannot bind to the appropriate B cell and stimulate it to proliferate and secrete antibody without the need for other APCs or helper T cells. The process of natural selection ensures that the most effective method of immune surveillance is utilized and so there should be good reasons for doing it the complicated way. It is possible to generate antibody without involving helper T cells. So-called T cell independent responses are well documented and usually involve large polysaccharide antigens but the antibody produced is usually of the IgM class and of low affinity. Another possibility would be for B cells to act as APCs and stimulate helper T cell proliferation directly without involving other types of APC. This process may well happen when an organism is exposed to the same antigen on a second occasion when B cells which responded to the first antigen challenge (memory B cells) are circulating in larger numbers than before any antigen exposure. It seems likely that the requirement for a range of cell types in different tissues which are capable of presenting antigen is a reflection of the need to ensure that foreign antigen is detected wherever it enters the body and as soon as possible.

In order for the process of antibody synthesis in response to antigen to work it is essential that lymphocytes are mobile. This mobility ensures that lymphocytes come into contact with foreign antigen and with each other. B and T lymphocytes circulate around the blood stream, through lymphoid tissues and back to the blood continuously.

A model of MHC class II protein is given in figure 2-9. The protein consists of two polypeptide chains (an α chain of 34kDa and a β chain of 28kDa). Each polypeptide has a single membrane spanning domain and a short cytoplasmic domain. The extracellular regions of both polypeptides comprise two domains one, that nearest the membrane, is like an immunoglobulin domain. The N-terminal domains of both polypeptides associate together to form a groove which binds foreign antigen as peptide and presents it to helper T cells. The amino acid sequences of the α and β chains are highly variable (polymorphic) in the regions that define the peptide binding groove (32). There are three main loci giving rise to class II molecules (HLA-DP, DQ and DR) located on the short arm of chromosome 6 in man.

The T cell receptor (TcR) is a heterodimer composed of two polypeptide chains (α, β) each of 40-50kDa. The α and β genes are located on chromosome 14q11.2 and 7q35 respectively (33,34). Each polypeptide has two extracellular immunoglobulin-like domains (see figure 2-10). The Ig-like domains at the extreme N-termini are extremely polymorphic and homologous to the variable domains of antibody molecules. Although TcR genes contain fewer variable region genes than the genes giving rise to antibody molecules there is considerable potential for the production of different TcR through the differential use of D and J gene segments. It is this region of the TcR which recognizes antigen presented by MHC class II molecules on APCs. The TcR is non-covalently associated with a multi-subunit protein (CD3). CD3 comprises three chains (γ, δ, ε) encoded by genes at chromosome 11q23. CD3γ has an Mr of 25-28kDa and has two potential sites for N-glycosylation, CD3δ has an Mr of 20kDa and two potential N-glycosylation sites, CD3ε also has an Mr of 20kDa but lacks N-glycosylation sites. Also associated with the TcR/CD3 complex are polypeptides (ζ, η) encoded by a gene at chromosome

FIGURE 2-9 MHC Class II Protein

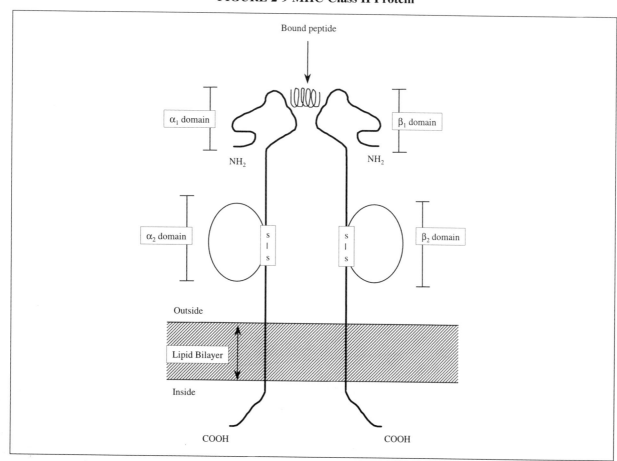

1q22-25. CD3 is essential for the activation of T cells when antigen/class II is recognized by the TcR. This process of helper T cell activation is complex and involves CD4 and other accessory protein interactions in addition to CD3 (35).

The response on first exposure to antigen is called a primary response. If an animal is exposed to the same antigen on a second occasion it will mount a secondary response. Antibody production in the secondary response differs from that in the primary response in that antibody is produced more quickly, the antibody may be of a different class and of higher affinity (see below for further discussion). This is because the immune system has remembered its previous exposure to antigen. Immunological memory is thought to work because when an animal is exposed to antigen for the first time some of the helper T cells and antigen-specific B cells become activated and produce a primary immune response while others are stimulated to become memory cells, that is they proliferate in response to antigen but do not participate in the actual immune response (36). Cells that are activated and participate in an immune response die within a few days whereas memory cells remain in the circulation for

years. This ability to remember exposure to a foreign antigen explains why vaccination works.

The Functions of Antibodies

The primary physiological function of antibodies is to effect the destruction of "non-self". Recognition of antigen is only one aspect of this process. When antibody binds to antigen on a foreign cell it does so through the Fab portions of the molecule. The Fc portion of the antibody molecule is then oriented to the outer surface of the cell where it may facilitate the binding of components of complement which ultimately lead to the assembly of the membrane attack complex (MAC) on the surface of the foreign cell and the destruction of that cell by lysis (37). Antibody molecules of the IgM class are particularly efficient at activating complement but other antibody classes are also able to carry out this function. The main requirement for complement fixation is that there should be two Fc domains sufficiently close together to allow cross linking by C1q. The large pentameric IgM molecule is particularly suited for this purpose (see Chapter 6

FIGURE 2-10 T Cell Receptor

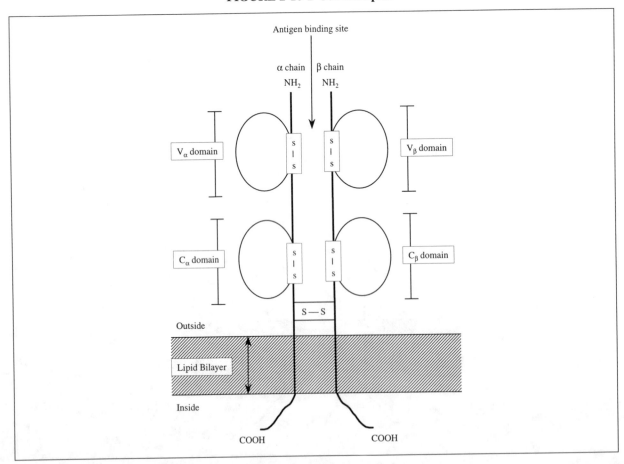

for a more detailed discussion of the importance of complement in immunohematology).

Another mechanism for antibody-mediated destruction of foreign cells involves the interaction of the Fc portion of the antibody molecule with receptor molecules (Fc receptors) on the surface of other cells (38,39, see Chapter 6 for a more detailed discussion). Binding of IgG-coated cells to Fc receptors on macrophages and neutrophils may lead to ingestion and destruction (phagocytosis) while binding to Fc receptors on a subset of lymphocytes (natural killer, NK cells) may effect lysis by triggering the release of perforin (antibody-dependent cellular cytoxicity, ADCC). Perforin (pore-forming protein) is homologous to the complement component C9 and polymerizes in the target plasma membrane to form transmembrane channels. Perforin is stored in secretory vesicles together with serine proteases and other proteins which may induce death of the target cells by entering the cell through the channels created by perforin (40). Another type of Fc receptor is found on placenta and this is responsible for the transport of IgG from mother to fetus, a process whereby the fetus acquires passive immunity from the mother to protect it from microbial assault in the first few months after birth while its own immune system is developing. The Fc receptor for placental transfer of IgG has been cloned (41) and the crystal structure of the rat homologue determined (42,43). The structure of the placental Fc receptor (FcRn) is unique among Fc receptors in having structural similarity with MHC class I molecules (see below for discussion of the structure of class I molecules and see also figure 2-11). However the peptide binding groove in FcRn is altered in comparison with class I molecules. FcRn does not bind Fc of immunoglobulin via this altered groove however but through interactions along the length of its extracellular domain.

Antibodies of the IgA class mainly function at the mucosal surfaces of the respiratory and gastro-intestinal tracts and in other secreted body fluids (tears, saliva, milk) in areas that are exposed to microbial assault. They therefore provide additional protection to that given by mucus (see also introduction to this section). IgA is transported across epithelial cells to the secreted body fluids by a specialized Fc receptor protein (poly-Ig receptor). Dimeric IgA containing a J chain and a secretory component is transported to the lumen of secretory organelles by receptor-mediated endocytosis (44). Nevertheless, IgA in secretions is not essential for the viability of twentieth century man because total deficiency of IgA is not uncommon, occurring in about 1 in 500 apparently healthy adults. However, IgA deficient individuals may have a greater propensity for autoimmune, infectious and less commonly, malignant diseases (45). Individuals who have a total IgA deficiency may make

anti-IgA when given blood components and this may lead to severe anaphylactic transfusion reactions (46 and see Chapter 36). The presence of this transfusion risk has led many blood centers to maintain a small panel of IgA-deficient donors (45). Sandler et al. (45) found that 4 of 44 IgA-deficient blood donors and 14 of 44 IgA-deficient patients also had deficiency of IgG2. They cite evidence that combined deficiency of IgA and IgG2 is often associated with recurrent pulmonary, sinus, ear or gastrointestinal infections. These authors propose that donors selected for IgA deficiency should have their serum tested for IgG2 and if found to be deficient in this immunoglobulin, should be evaluated for a history of recurrent bacterial infections and counseled accordingly.

IgD is rarely secreted, instead it remains bound to the B lymphocyte that synthesized it. Its function is unknown. Secreted IgE binds to another type of Fc receptor (FcεR1) on the surface of mast cells in tissues and basophils in blood. When antigen binds to this cell-bound IgE it signals the cell to secrete a number of molecules, notably histamine, which cause dilation and increased permeability of blood vessels, and cytokines and other chemical messengers. These changes are thought to help leukocytes, antibodies and complement components to enter the sites of inflammation. The release of these factors is also associated with allergic reactions such as those experienced by sufferers of asthma and hay fever (10). Roitt (23) argues that infectious agents penetrating the IgA defenses would meet and be bound by IgE on mast cells and that this would trigger the release of chemicals leading to vasodilation thereby facilitating an influx of IgG and complement and effecting the recruitment of granulocytes to combat the infectious agents. Activated mast cells are known to release factors that recruit eosinophils that are able to damage antibody coated parasites (helminths) (23).

Cell-Mediated Immunity

Antibody-mediated immunity is not very successful against viral infections because the viruses infect cells and "hide" within them. A different pathway of antigen recognition and killing of foreign material is required. This pathway involves MHC class I molecules and not the class II molecules which are utilized to generate the antibody response discussed earlier.

MHC class I molecules comprise two non-covalently linked polypeptides. The larger polypeptide (α chain) has an Mr of 45,000. It is a type I membrane protein of approximately 340 amino acids with a single transmembrane domain, a cytoplasmic domain of approximately 30 residues and an extracellular region comprising three distinct domains denoted α1, α2, and α3. The smaller non-glycosylated polypeptide (β_2 microglobulin) has approximately 100 amino acids (Mr 12,000) and is non-covalently linked to the extracellular domain of the α chain (see figure 2-11). The MHC class I locus is on chromosome 6 while that for β_2 microglobulin is on chromosome 15 (10,23).

The structure of class I molecules has been determined (47). The conformation of the class I molecule is very dependent upon the presence of β_2 microglobulin which interacts with each of the α domains. The $\alpha3$ domain and β_2 microglobulin have structures which are homologous to those found in immunoglobulins. The $\alpha1$ and $\alpha2$ domains have a quite different structure and fold together to create a groove which binds peptides. The $\alpha1$ and $\alpha2$ domains form the peptide binding groove from the sequence at their N-termini. Each domain has an N-terminal portion which forms a four stranded antiparallel β sheet followed by an α helical domain. The two domains align so that the 8 strands of β sheet form the floor of the peptide-binding groove and the two α-helical domains form the sides of the groove (see figure 2-11).

The products of the major class I loci (HLA-A, B and C) are expressed on the surface of most nucleated cells and function by presenting processed antigen as peptide to CD8 positive (cytotoxic) T lymphocytes (48). These loci carry the most polymorphic genes in man. Serological typing defines 27 HLA-A alleles, 59 HLA-B alleles and 10 HLA-C alleles (49) but this technique gives a gross underestimate of the underlying polymorphism revealed by nucleotide sequencing (49 and see Chapter 44).

Class I molecules present antigen (peptide) to the T cell receptor on cytotoxic T cells. The structure of the T cell receptor was described in an earlier section (see also figure 2-10). Cytotoxic T cells kill cells which are making foreign antigen and since viruses can infect any cell in the body it is not surprising that class I molecules which present foreign antigen to cytotoxic T cells are found on most nucleated cells. When class I molecules on an infected cell present peptide which is recognized by cytotoxic T cells, the initial interaction must be strengthened by the binding of CD8 on the T cell to the $\alpha3$ domain of the class I molecule. CD8 is a member of the immunoglobulin superfamily. It has an extracellular Ig domain, a single transmembrane domain and a cytoplasmic domain which is associated with a tyrosine-specific protein kinase (*Lck* protein). When CD8 binds the class I molecule the tyrosine kinase is activated to phosphorylate other proteins and

FIGURE 2-11 MHC Class I Protein

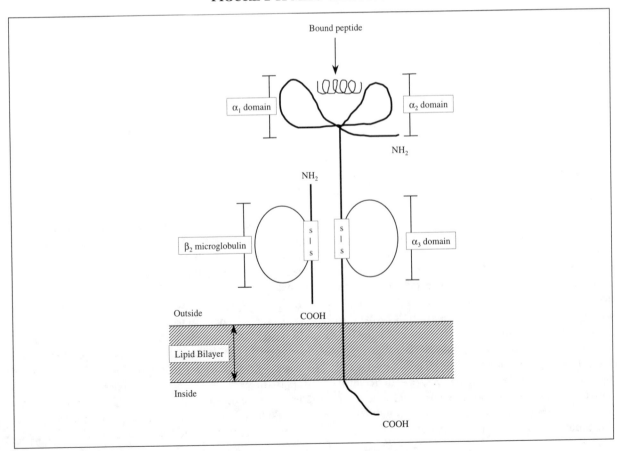

initiate the activation of the bound T cells to kill the infected cell by release of perforin, a molecule homologous to complement component C9 (10). The pathway for cell-mediated immunity is therefore quite different from that of humoral immunity where extracellular foreign antigens are removed by the combined forces of APC, helper T cells and B cells (see above).

The presentation of virally-derived peptide on MHC class I molecules at the surface of the infected cell is mediated by specialized transport proteins in the membrane of the endoplasmic reticulum (ER). After a cell is infected, viral proteins synthesized inside the cell are degraded by proteases in specialized structures known as proteasomes and the peptides that result are transported across the ER membrane where they bind to class I molecules. The peptide-class I complex is transported to the cell surface via the Golgi apparatus. Viral peptide in the context of the class I molecule is then recognized by the appropriate cytotoxic T cell. The transport proteins in the ER are known as TAP (transporters associated with antigen processing) proteins and are members of a family of ATP-dependent transporter proteins. Peptide binding to TAP is ATP independent but ATP hydrolysis is required for peptide translocation (50,51).

Cell-mediated immunity is of profound importance in organ transplantation. The same process that functions to eliminate virally infected cells also destroys a transplanted organ. It appears that endogenous peptide presented by a foreign class I molecule is recognized as non-self (10).

In immunohematology the focus has been much more on the effects of antibody-mediated immunity and the importance of cell-mediated immunity in transfusion has not received so much attention. A transfusion is, of course, a kind of transplant and certainly any transfusion which contains donor lymphocytes is a potential source of immunological problems.

Normally when lymphocytes are transfused they are recognized as foreign and eliminated by the recipient's immune system. If the transfused cells are not eliminated they proliferate and may cause graft-versus-host disease (GVHD). Transfusion associated GVHD is associated with transfusion to severely immunosuppressed recipients but can also occur with viable T lymphocytes from a donor who is homozygous for HLA antigens for which the recipient is heterozygous. The donated T lymphocytes are not recognized as foreign because they do not express antigens which are absent in the recipient. This latter problem is associated with fresh blood transfusions from donors who are related to the recipient. These problems can be overcome by irradiation of the blood before transfusion, this inhibits the proliferation of donor lymphocytes (52).

Autoimmunity

The success of the immune system in protecting man from microbial assault depends on its ability to distinguish 'self' from 'non-self'. There is a very thin line between recognition of all foreign antigens and recognition of 'self'. Successful microbes will evolve so that their surface proteins are similar to those of their host and occasionally the system fails and antibodies or cytotoxic T cells which react with 'self' antigens are produced and an autoimmune disease results. The first disease proved to be autoimmune in origin was autoimmune thyroiditis. Doniach and Roitt in the UK and Witebsky and Rose in the USA discovered autoantibodies to thyroglobulin in 1957 (53,54).

Tolerance to 'self' is thought to be acquired through T cell selection in the thymus. T cells which bind strongly to 'self' peptide in the context of 'self' MHC molecules are eliminated in the thymus while those that react only weakly survive and provide helper T cells and cytotoxic T cells for the normal immune response. Since this process of T cell selection operates on both helper and cytotoxic T cells both the humoral and cell-mediated immune responses of the host are protected from the risk of autoimmunity.

The risk of developing an autoimmune disease increases with age. Sir Macfarlane Burnet (30) considered that autoantibodies arise as a consequence of random somatic mutations in antibody genes generating new patterns of reactivity with 'self' antigens rather than with microbial antigens. As discussed above, somatic mutation in antibody (variable region) genes is the normal way in which affinity maturation of antibodies is achieved during a secondary immune response. Burnet (30) also considered the possibility that viral infection might interfere in some way with the normal mechanism for eliminating autoreactive clones and cites infectious mononucleosis as an example of this. Autoantibodies arising as a consequence of such a viral infection usually cause a transient hemolytic anemia suggesting that the change induced in the normal mechanism for eliminating auto-reactive clones is dependent on the continued presence of virus in the clones concerned (30). Burnet's hypotheses have stood the test of time (55). A more detailed discussion of the roles of random somatic mutation and viral infection in the generation of auto-reactive red cell antibodies will be found in Chapters 37 and 38.

Production of Antibodies: Polyclonal Antibodies

Nearly all human blood group antibodies found in patients' sera are polyclonal in nature. That is, they are the products of several B cell clones and contain a mixture of antibodies recognizing different epitopes on the same antigen. Monoclonal blood group antibodies in patients' sera are seen from time to time, particularly in patients with myeloma where a clone of B cells has proliferated. In these cases the cold agglutinin anti-I is sometimes found (see Chapter 38). The occurrence of monoclonal antibodies produced in large quantities by patients with myeloma provided material which allowed the first studies of the amino acid sequence of antibodies. Certain myeloma patients secrete light chains ("Bence-Jones proteins") in their urine and so light chains were studied first. It was soon found that the sequence of the N-terminal half of the light chain varies from one protein to another but the C-terminal end was common to all and it was through this work that the concept of variable and constant regions arose (56).

Polyclonal antisera are relatively easy to obtain by the deliberate immunization of laboratory animals commonly rabbits, goats or sheep. The production of antibodies by immunization of rabbits with human red cells led to the discovery of the P and the MN blood group systems (4). Where a soluble antigen is concerned it is common practice to homogenize a solution of the antigen in adjuvant (usually Freund's Complete Adjuvant) (FCA) and to inject 50-200µg of antigen via either the subcutaneous or intramuscular route. Second and subsequent injections are given at intervals of a month to generate a secondary immune response. Second and subsequent injections are usually given in Freund's Incomplete Adjuvant (FCA contains killed tubercle bacilli which may cause hypersensitivity reactions if used repeatedly). Freund's adjuvant is essentially a water-in-oil emulsion. When a solution of antigen is homogenized in FCA a thick white "treacle" results. When the treacle is injected into the laboratory animal it releases antigen slowly over a long period as it is gradually degraded. This prolonged release of antigen is thought to be one of the main reasons why this procedure is so successful for stimulating an immune response. Intact cells are highly immunogenic and do not need adjuvants and can be injected intravenously. Detailed methods for the production of polyclonal antisera are to be found in Goding (57). Antiglobulin reagents were prepared in this way until the development of monoclonal antibody technology provided the opportunity to make monoclonal anti-IgG and monoclonal anti-C3d (see Chapter 6). As discussed in that chapter, anti-IgG for use as an antiglobulin reagent is often still prepared by immunization of animals, anti-C3 is more often a monoclonal antibody produced in a hybridoma.

The reader should not assume that monoclonal antibody technology has rendered the production of polyclonal antibodies obsolete. It is a great deal cheaper and easier to raise a polyclonal antibody than to produce a monoclonal antibody and there are circumstances where a polyclonal antibody is preferred. One such circumstance concerns the production of antibodies to peptides and in particular to synthetic peptides. Methods for the automated synthesis of peptides have improved markedly in recent years and because protein sequences are largely obtained by deduction from cDNA sequences (nucleotide sequencing is much easier than protein sequencing) it is common practice to prepare synthetic peptides corresponding to a portion (usually N- or C-terminus) of the deduced protein sequence and to raise antibodies to the peptides. These antibodies can then be used to prove that a cDNA sequence does indeed encode the amino acid sequence of the protein that the researchers thought they were studying! An example of this approach will be found in Chapter 25 where polyclonal anti-peptide sera were used to show that a gene denoted *PBDX* encoded proteins which expressed the Xg^a blood group antigen (58). Another common use of polyclonal antisera to synthetic peptides concerns the determination of the topology of a membrane protein. For example, when cDNA corresponding to the Rh blood group polypeptides was first obtained, two different structures were proposed for the predicted protein. One group predicted a protein with its N-terminus on the cytoplasmic side of the red cell membrane and its C-terminus on the extracellular face (59) while another predicted both N- and C-termini on the cytoplasmic side (60). That the latter model was correct was proved by the use of polyclonal antisera raised to synthetic peptides corresponding to the N- and C-termini of the predicted protein. It was demonstrated that neither antiserum would react with intact red cells but both reacted with red cell ghosts which are leaky to antibody molecules (61).

Polyclonal sera are particularly valuable when peptides are used as antigen because the peptides can exist in a wide variety of structures in solution and even if less than 1% of the antibody response is to the peptide in a conformation that is found in the native protein then the antiserum is useful. Production of monoclonal antibodies to synthetic peptides, that then react with native protein is not impossible (see 58) but can be very time consuming. In one study three synthetic peptides corresponding to the whole cytoplasmic domain of glycophorin C were used as antigens for the preparation of polyclonal and monoclonal antibodies. Whereas polyclonal antibodies reactive with the native protein were obtained with all peptides, only that containing the extreme C-terminus yielded a monoclonal antibody (62,63).

The message of this section is that if very large quantities of antibody of a particular specificity are needed, the investment in monoclonal antibody technology will probably be justified, if not, it may be better to try to produce a polyclonal antibody.

Production of Antibodies: Rodent Monoclonal Antibodies

A major advance in the use of antibodies for diagnosis and therapy was heralded by the introduction of monoclonal antibody technology in 1975. Kohler and Milstein (64) reported the successful production of antibodies in vitro by the culture of individual clones of antibody-producing cells. In essence, antibody-producing B lymphocytes obtained from the spleen of an immunized mouse were fused with a B cell tumor line (myeloma) grown in culture and hybrid cells (hybridomas) were obtained which had the growth characteristics of the tumor cell line and the antibody-secreting characteristics of the splenic lymphocytes. In this way immortal cell lines secreting antibody of a defined specificity could be obtained - a revolution in biological sciences had begun!

In practice, the successful utilization of this technology required some special tricks. The splenic lymphocytes and tumor cells can be fused by the addition of polyethylene glycol but this process is not very efficient and unfused splenic lymphocytes and tumor cells remain. Unfused splenic lymphocytes do not survive in in vitro culture for much more than 48 hours but the unfused tumor cells rapidly overgrow the hybridomas. It is therefore essential to grow the cells in a culture medium which allows the hybridomas to flourish but does not support the growth of unfused tumor cells. This is achieved by selecting a tumor cell with a metabolic disorder which affects DNA synthesis.

The main biosynthetic pathway for guanosine monophosphate, one of the four components essential for DNA synthesis (see Chapter 5) can be completely inhibited by the addition of aminopterin. In the presence of aminopterin the normal cell can continue to synthesize guanosine monophosphate and hence DNA by alternative pathways known as 'salvage' pathways. These 'salvage' pathways utilize an enzyme known as hypoxanthine guanine phosphoribosyl transferase (HGPRT) to convert the nucleotide metabolites guanine and hypoxanthine to guanosine monophosphate. The essential trick which allows hybridoma cells to flourish while unfused myeloma cells die, is the use of a myeloma cell which lacks HGPRT suspended in a culture medium containing aminopterin. The hybridoma cells will contain HGPRT because the gene will be derived from the rodent spleen cells and so provided hypoxanthine is present in the culture medium the hybridoma cells will be able to synthesis guanosine monophosphate by the salvage pathway. Another salvage pathway involves the enzyme thymidine. In summary, the fusion mixture containing unfused spleen cells, unfused HGPRT deficient myeloma cells and hybridomas is cultured in a medium containing hypoxanthine, aminopterin and thymidine (HAT medium). The unfused spleen cells

die, the HGPRT deficient cells die and HGPRT containing hybridomas flourish (57,65).

A further complication is the need for the selected tumor cell to have a defect in antibody synthesis. If the tumor cell line used as a fusion partner itself makes antibody then the hybridoma may make antibody molecules which utilize heavy and light chains derived not from the splenic lymphocyte but from the tumor cell itself. In this case mixed antibodies will result with, for example, heavy chains derived from the splenic lymphocyte and light chains from the tumor cell. The first experiments utilized a tumor cell (NS-1) which was deficient in heavy chain synthesis but not in light chain synthesis and monoclonal anti-blood group A were obtained which contained light chains derived from the tumor cell (66). Later studies utilized tumor cell lines devoid of indigenous heavy or light chains so that the monoclonal antibodies originated from the splenic lymphocytes alone.

Once the splenic lymphocytes have been fused with tumor cells to form hybridomas it is essential to clone the individual hybridomas in order to derive a stable hybridoma secreting the monoclonal antibody of choice. The culture of the fusion mixture in HAT medium will ensure that unfused splenic lymphocytes and unfused tumor cells die but it will not have any effect on hybridomas which are not secreting antibody and these hybridomas, if left in the culture, will tend to overgrow those secreting antibody because they are not committing a large proportion of available metabolic energy to antibody synthesis. Furthermore, fusion of splenic lymphocytes and tumor cells creates hybrid cells which are often tetraploid and these cells may be unstable in culture.

Cloning individual hybridomas is usually done by limiting dilution (the hybridoma mixture is distributed into the wells of microplates at a concentration of one cell per well). In early experiments clones were obtained by plating the mixtures of hybridomas on soft agar and then picking individual colonies for subsequent liquid culture. The culture supernatant from each well is tested for the presence of the desired antibody and cells from the wells secreting the desired antibody are recloned again by limiting dilution until a stable hybridoma secreting the desired antibody is obtained.

When a hybridoma secreting the desired antibody is obtained (this may require numerous fusion experiments) it is often necessary to evaluate its properties from the point of view of large scale antibody production. If the antibody is required for research purposes it may be possible to obtain enough from small scale cultures (1-5 liters) but if the antibody is required for diagnostic or therapeutic use then the hybridomas must be sufficiently robust to survive large scale culture conditions. It does not follow automatically that a hybridoma which appears to have the required properties in terms of antibody specificity and level of antibody production in the research laboratory will be able to sustain those properties in large scale culture. Many promising cell lines fall by the wayside at this stage. Large scale culture involves either the use of fermenters or hollow fibers. Both methods require the careful and continuous monitoring of temperature, gases and nutrients in the culture vessel.

Fermenters, as the name suggests, are vessels designed for other purposes which can be adapted for hybridomas. The process is essentially one of large scale (up to 1,000 liters) liquid culture. Hybridomas regularly secrete 50-100 ug of antibody/ml of culture medium and so hundreds of grams of antibody can be obtained from the largest fermenters. Hollow fibre technology is very different. In this method the hybridomas are allowed to grow on the inside of hollow fibres while medium and nutrients are pumped through the fibres. Antibody is collected from the spent medium and replaced by fresh medium over a period of several months. The process is less like making beer and more like milking a cow. A hybridoma that grows well in fermentation culture will not necessarily grow well in hollow fibre culture. This is not unexpected because the technologies are obviously very different. Fermentation culture requires cells to grow in suspension with relatively little cell:cell contact, hollow fibre technology demands that the cells like living close together.

Even when a hybridoma has been produced which grows well in large scale culture and secretes antibody of the desired specificity in acceptable quantities there are still a number of pitfalls of which to be wary. How stable is the antibody when it is in solution? The antibody isolated and purified from large scale culture may, over time, disintegrate or aggregate when suspended in the medium chosen for use of the product in diagnosis or therapy. Most important of all, the cell line may change its characteristics over time in continuous culture. To ensure that this hard won cell line is not lost it is essential to create a master cell bank in which numerous vials of the original clone are stored in liquid nitrogen. At regular intervals, vials from this bank should be thawed, cultured, the cell line recloned and vials again stored in the master cell bank.

The foregoing discussion has concentrated on monoclonal antibodies made in a mouse system. It should be noted that a similar system is available in the rat (66). Most monoclonal antibodies utilized in immunohematology are of mouse origin but there are some studies describing rat anti-human red cell monoclonal antibodies. Rat monoclonal anti-C3g has been used as a component of antiglobulin reagent (67) and a series of rat monoclonal antibodies were raised against human red cells by Smythe (68,69). Perhaps not surprisingly, the range and specificity of antibodies produced in rats appears

very similar to those made in mice (68) although, to the authors' knowledge anti-In[b] has been made in rats (70) but not in mice.

In almost every chapter about a blood group system in this book the reader will find reference to monoclonal antibodies. These antibodies have had a major impact on the understanding of the structure of blood group antigens and the molecules which carry those antigens. Monoclonal antibodies raised to intact red cells have been used to identify blood group-active molecules by immunoprecipitation and immunoblotting techniques, to purify blood group-active molecules by immunoaffinity methods and to study the structure and function of blood group-active molecules by epitope mapping and inhibition assays (see Chapter 4 for further discussion).

Monoclonal antibodies are now almost universally used as diagnostic reagents for ABO typing. Determining the ABO type of a patient or donor is the most important task an immunohematologist ever undertakes since a mistake could result in the death of a patient. This risk is directly related to the fact that antibodies to the A and B antigens, unlike other blood group antibodies, occur naturally, that is, without stimulation by transfusion or pregnancy. It is thought that the original immune stimulation comes from bacteria in the gut which have A and/or B antigen on their surface (71 and see also Chapter 8). These "natural" antibodies (anti-A in group B individuals, anti-B in group A individuals, anti-A and anti-B in group O individuals) were used for decades as reagents with which to type donors and patients of unknown ABO type in just the same way as Landsteiner had done. However, the potency of such natural antibodies varies considerably from one individual to another and quite a lot of work is involved in screening donors to find those with the most potent antibodies for use as reagents. A widely used alternative before the 1980's was to hyperimmunize volunteers with purified A or B antigen to boost the existing polyclonal antibody. ABO typing reagents made in this way are excellent. Nevertheless when it became clear that monoclonal antibody technology could be used to obtain mouse hybridomas secreting anti-A and anti-B in in vitro culture (72,73) it was only a matter of time before this became the method of choice for reagent manufacturers. In the early days there was a little confusion over whether or not anti-B could be made in the mouse because mouse red cells have a B-like antigen (74) but this was more to do with a lack of familiarity with early literature than any fundamental immunological problem since it had been shown by several workers between the 1930s and the 1950s that the B-like antigens of animal red cells, including mouse, are not the same as human B and are not a barrier to making anti-human B (75,76).

It will come as no surprise to the reader that the replacement of polyclonal anti-A and anti-B with monoclonal anti-A and anti-B was not without problems. Some monoclonal anti-A's and B's react with epitopes that are not relevant to the selection of compatible blood for transfusion (see discussion of B(A) and A(B) phenotypes and acquired B phenotype in Chapter 8). The solution has been to prepare reagents which are mixtures of two or more monoclonal antibodies so that the final product mimics the properties of the best polyclonal reagents and any unwanted reactivities are eliminated. This pick 'n mix approach may appear to have more in common with cookery than science but it recognizes the practical requirements for these reagents and once an acceptable formulation has been found the composition can be precisely defined so that each batch of a given reagent is identical to all others - a precision not possible with polyclonal reagents.

Rodent monoclonal antibodies of some other blood group specificities have been made and some of these are of a quality that permits their use as reagents for blood typing (anti-M, -N (77,78); -P_1 (79); -Le^a, -Le^b (80,81)). The fact that rodent monoclonal antibodies of these specificities can be made and that others, to antigens such as c, C, D, e, E, K, Fy^a, etc., cannot, is of no surprise. It merely reflects the observations of others who tried to raise polyclonal reagents of these specificities many years previously. Rabbit anti-M, -N (4,82,83); anti-P_1 (4, 82,83); goat anti-Le^a, anti-Le^b (84-86) but not anti-Rh, -K or -Fy^a, were made. Why rodents do not make these other specificities is a question yet to be answered but it may be related to the presence of a different repertoire of V_H genes (see earlier section on antibody genes and reference 27).

Production of Antibodies: Human Monoclonal Antibodies

As discussed in the previous section, certain antibody specificities cannot be made in rodents. There are a number of ways of trying to produce monoclonal antibodies of such specificities. The most direct approach would be to take human B lymphocytes from an individual who is already making antibody of the desired specificity and to grow these cells in culture. Unfortunately, this does not work, the cells die in laboratory culture. Human B cells can however be immortalized using Epstein-Barr virus (EBV). Some of the earliest studies in this field were carried out with B lymphocytes derived from individuals making anti-D (87,88). Since numerous volunteers were being immunized to produce high titer anti-D for use in the prevention of immunization to D (see Chapters 12 and 41) B cells making anti-D were

readily available for such experiments. These early studies demonstrated that EBV-transformed lymphocytes secreting anti-D could be maintained in in vitro for several months but that the cell lines were not immortal. While some workers persisted in their attempts to obtain stable clones of EBV-lymphoblastoid cells which secreted human monoclonal antibody, others looked for alternative ways to stabilize the cell lines. Some attempted to produce human lymphoblastoid cell lines which were stable in vitro and could act as the fusion partner for antibody-secreting B cells (89,90). Others fused human B cells with the same mouse tumor cell lines used to make mouse monoclonal antibodies and created man:mouse heterohybridomas. Early fears that such heterohybridomas would be unstable in culture proved to be unfounded. One of the first groups to use this approach did so to produce an anti-A (91). Yet more complex fusion strategies were designed in which human B cells were fused with mouse-human heterohybridomas (92). In the event, two approaches proved to be robust. In 1983, Dorothy Crawford working at University College, London was the first to clone a stable anti-D secreting line from EBV transformed human lymphocytes (93) while at Babraham, near Cambridge, Nevin Hughes-Jones and his colleagues generated several cloned heterohybridomas which secreted anti-D (94).

The potential use of human monoclonal anti-D for prophylaxis in D-negative pregnancies and for blood typing was quickly realized and numerous laboratories sought to capitalize on these early successes. However, just as described for the rodent monoclonal antibodies in the previous section, it does not follow that a cell line generated in the research laboratory will have characteristics which are robust enough to take it through to large scale culture and then to prophylactic or diagnostic use and it takes time to generate suitable cell lines.

The first successful clinical trial (in male volunteers) of human monoclonal anti-D for prevention of immunization to D was reported in 1995 (95). In this case the IgG antibodies were obtained from cloned EBV-lymphoblastoid cell lines. The technique which has been most useful for producing blood typing reagents has been the production of heterohybridomas using human B cells obtained from donors whose immune response has been recently boosted. In this case IgM is the preferred antibody class (96,145,146).

Production of Antibodies: Humanized Rodent Monoclonal Antibodies

While rodent monoclonal antibodies are of great value in research and for use in diagnosis, considerable disadvantages accompany their use in vivo. The antibodies elicit an immune response in the recipient. Anti-rodent immunoglobulin can cause the rapid removal of the injected antibody, the blocking of antibody function (anti-idiotype) and hypersensitivity reactions.

For these reasons such antibodies can only be used on a few occasions in the same patient before efficacy is compromised and adverse reactions occur. There is, of course, nothing to stop the use of such antibodies for therapeutic processes which involve ex vivo exposure to antibody. A rat anti-CAMPATH-1 (CDw52) of the IgM class has been used with great success for the ex vivo depletion of T lymphocytes from bone marrow before allogeneic bone marrow transplantation in order to reduce the severity of graft versus host disease in the transplant recipients (97,98). Another monoclonal anti-CAMPATH-1 of the IgG class has been used in vivo and has been shown to reduce the tumor burden of patients with lymphoma (providing of course that the lymphomas express the CDw52 antigen). Because of the limitations imposed by the immune response to rodent immunoglobulin which is elicited in the recipient, efforts have been made to use recombinant DNA technology to "humanize" the rodent antibody. It might be thought that it would be easier to generate an entirely human anti-CAMPATH-1 using EBV-transformation of B lymphocytes derived from an individual making anti-CAMPATH-1 in a manner analogous to that described in the previous section for anti-D. However, such an approach is far from straightforward. EBV transformation of donor lymphocytes is really only an option if the target antigen is polymorphic in man and if volunteers lacking the antigen can be immunized so that lymphocytes actively secreting the desired antibody can be obtained shortly after the immunizing dose has been given. Attempts to derive human monoclonal antibodies from the lymphocytes of patients with autoantibodies have been largely unsuccessful.

The process of "humanizing" rodent monoclonal antibodies has been described by Winter and Harris (99). In the first experiments appropriate V_H and V_L genes were amplified from mRNA derived from the cell line producing the monoclonal antibody of desired specificity, using PCR. The rodent V_H gene was then inserted into a vector encoding the constant domains of human antibody (C_H1-hinge-C_H2-C_H3) and the rodent V_L gene inserted into a second vector encoding the C_L domain of human light chain. The two vectors were then co-expressed in a suitable mammalian cell line and cells secreting chimeric antibody of the desired specificity selected.

A more sophisticated approach involves inserting the CDR regions of the rodent monoclonal antibody into human antibody framework. As described above, most of the information critical for antigen binding is located in the sequence of the CDRs and so it is theoretically possible to create an antibody which is comprised mostly of

human antibody sequence and yet has antigen binding characteristics which are identical with those of the rodent antibody from which the CDRs were derived (100). In practice, other parts of the antibodies' V_H and V_L domains may influence antigen binding and it may be necessary to change additional residues outside the CDRs to obtain antibody of the desired specificity. This was the experience when anti-CAMPATH-1 was humanized and computer modeling of the rat and human V_H-CDR1 loop was used to identify a critical residue which, when mutated, restored the desired specificity of the engineered antibody (101). The antigen binding characteristics of such antibodies can sometimes be improved by changing the light chain (light chain shuffling) (102) or by random mutation (103).

Apart from minimizing problems with the recipient's immune response to rodent antibody "humanizing" such antibodies has the additional advantage of improving effector functions like complement binding and Fc receptor interactions. If a particular effector function is required a suitable human constant region sequence can be incorporated into the final product, selection for example of an IgG3 subclass rather than IgG1.

The final product still contains rodent CDR and so an anti-idiotype response which inhibits its activity is possible but this is also a potential problem with monoclonal antibodies which are entirely human in origin when they are given repeatedly over a long time. CDR-grafted anti-CDw52 has been used in clinical trials. Two patients with non-Hodgkin's lymphoma were given escalating doses (1-20 mg/day) for up to 43 days without mounting an antibody response, the treatment reduced the tumor mass and achieved clinical remission (104). When the antibody was used for a single course of therapy in patients with rheumatoid arthritis no antibody response was observed but further treatment did effect such a response (105).

Production of Antibodies: Making Human Antibodies Using Phage Display Technology

The use of bacteriophage as a novel expression vector was first described by Smith (106) who showed that small peptides could be displayed on the surface of filamentous phage by fusing them to the minor coat protein pIII. Phage expressing the peptides could be enriched by selecting with monoclonal antibodies which were specific for the peptides.

Bacteriophages are viruses that infect bacteria. Phages bind to the surface of a bacterium and inject their DNA into it. The DNA circularizes and either integrates into the host genome and remains dormant (a latent infection) or replicates to synthesize new phage which are released through lysis of the bacterial host cell and can infect further bacteria. The natural biology of the replication of phage in bacteria has been adapted for the expression of antigen binding fragments (107). One methodology which has been widely used involves the expression of single chain Fv fragments (scFv). An scFv comprises the V_H and V_L domains of an antibody molecule artificially joined by a flexible polypeptide spacer (108,109, see figure 2-12). DNA coding for the scFv is inserted into a vector containing the gene for the phage coat protein pIII (the vector is called a phagemid because it is a plasmid with a phage origin of replication) and transfected into *E. coli*. The phagemid is packaged into phage (helper phage) infecting the *E. coli* and this results in the appearance of the scFv at the surface of newly synthesized phage particles. Another methodology allows the display of Fab fragments. In this case one chain is fused to pIII and the other is secreted into the periplasm (110-112). The two chains associate and are expressed as Fab fragments on the phage surface protein pIII.

This system of "phage display" has been adapted to develop a method for generating libraries of scFv or Fab fragments which can be screened against an antigen of interest. Winter et al. (107) draw a parallel between the normal processes of the immune system and the phage display system. In a normal immune response a small number of B cells are selected from about 10^{12} cells through the binding of antigen. Once selected, the B cells proliferate and secrete antibody. In the phage display system a large number of V_H and V_L genes are amplified by the polymerase chain reaction and then randomly recombined with a flexible polypeptide linker and cloned into a vector containing the phage pIII gene. Mixtures of phage displaying different scFv are screened with antigen (usually by panning with antigen bound to microplates). Phage expressing scFv of the desired specificity are then enriched by several rounds of antigen selection. Libraries of more than 10^{10} specificities have been prepared from both germ line genes (non-immune libraries) as well as from the antibody genes of individuals who are immune to the antigen of interest. Libraries prepared from the antibody genes of immune individuals would be expected to yield scFv of higher affinity than those from non-immune ("naive") libraries because the genes have already undergone somatic mutation.

Nevertheless, somatic mutation can occur in the phage display system during successive rounds of selection with antigen and so affinity maturation is possible.

Once the phage population displaying scFv of the desired specificity has been cloned it is desirable to obtain the scFv in soluble form rather than linked to phage protein (here the analogy with the normal primary immune response is again helpful viz. the switch from expression of surface bound IgM on the B cell to secretion of IgM having the same specificity). The option of expressing the scFv on the surface of phage or secreting it into the culture medium can be engineered into the phagemid vector which carries the antibody genes. An amber codon (a stop codon which can be selectively suppressed) is inserted between the antibody genes and the pIII gene in the phagemid vector (see figure 2-13). If phage is grown in bacterial strains which suppress the amber codon the scFv will be displayed on the phage. If phage is grown in non-suppresser bacterial strains then the amber stop codon will disrupt synthesis of the scFv-pIII protein and the scFv will be secreted as soluble antibody fragments. The phagemid vector is designed so that the secreted scFv has a small peptide "tag" attached (see figure 2-13). Monoclonal anti-"tag" can then be used to purify the scFv and to enable the use of the scFv in immunological assays. Antibody fragments can be obtained from large scale culture in fermenters at concentrations above 500mg/l (113).

It is anticipated that phage display technology will be of considerable value for the construction of novel diagnostic and therapeutic agents. The desired antigen-binding domain can be isolated as described above and then cloned into a vector containing the DNA necessary to encode the remainder of the antibody molecule to create 'designer' monoclonal antibodies. The scFv and Fab fragments generated by this technology are likely to have limited therapeutic value in vivo because of their very short half-life in the circulation. There are however, some clear advantages from the use of scFv. In particular, scFv are much smaller than antibodies and can therefore penetrate tissues more easily and are less likely to be immunogenic. These properties have been exploited in the use of a scFv with high affinity for carcinoembryonic antigen (CEA). Begent et al. (114) used ^{123}I labeled scFv anti-CEA to locate tumor deposits in patients with CEA-producing cancers.

FIGURE 2-12 Structure of a Single Chain Fv (scFv) Fragment

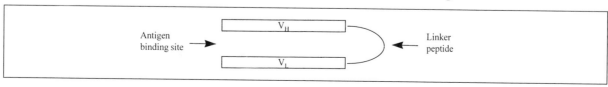

Several scFv and Fab fragments with blood group specificity have been isolated (specificities for the B, D, E, I and Kp[b] antigens (115-117)). IgM murine monoclonal antibodies to the "tag" decapeptide denoted myc were used to convert scFv (two anti-B and one anti-D) into direct agglutinins for use as blood typing reagents (118). Provided the ratios of IgM anti-myc and scFv are optimized they can be mixed and used as a single reagent (119).

Production of Antibodies: Making Human Antibodies in Transgenic Mice

In the preceding sections various strategies for making monoclonal antibodies for diagnostic and therapeutic use have been discussed. It has been pointed out that existing technologies have delivered a range of rodent and human antibodies that are suitable for blood typing and that human monoclonal anti-D can protect against immunization to D. It could be argued that the requirements of blood group serologists have been largely satisfied but there are still some blood group antibodies which are not available as monoclonal reagents (e.g. anti-Fy[a]) and there will always be a place for a better reagent or for a novel technology that allows for even greater reliability and convenience of testing. However, the primary drive for improvements in antibody production technology is the prospect of using antibodies for therapy in a vast array of diseases. Nevertheless, improvements in blood banking are likely to come by applying new technologies as and when they occur.

The advantages of monoclonal antibody technology are obvious. A potentially unlimited supply of a protein of known sequence makes the monoclonal antibody as reliable a product as a designer drug. For therapeutic use human antibodies are required but the existing technology is difficult and limited. "Humanizing" rodent antibodies is a powerful approach but also has its limitations. If the antibody genes of a mouse could be replaced by the complete human antibody gene repertoire then it should be possible to immunize the mouse to make human antibodies of the desired specificity and then to isolate the B lymphocytes which are secreting the desired antibody and use them to make a hybridoma secreting human monoclonal antibody, i.e., problem solved! However, to transfer the entire human antibody gene repertoire into a mouse is not a trivial undertaking. The human heavy chain locus, located on chromosome 14, is 1.5Mb in size. The human kappa light chain locus is located on chromosome 2 and spans 3Mb. The human lambda light chain locus is on chromosome 22 and spans 1.5Mb (120). Three experimental approaches have been used, miniloci, yeast artificial chromosomes (YACs) and bacteriophage P1 vectors.

In miniloci, several V_H gene segments have been placed artificially close to J and D gene segments together with relevant regulatory sequences in a construct of about 30kb. Constructs comprising V_H genes, D and J segments and C_μ or C_δ have been cloned on YACs of up to 300kb. Bacteriophage P1 vectors can carry about 90kb of inserted DNA and use *E. coli* as a host. In order to

FIGURE 2-13 Generation of Single Chain Fv Fragments by Phage Display

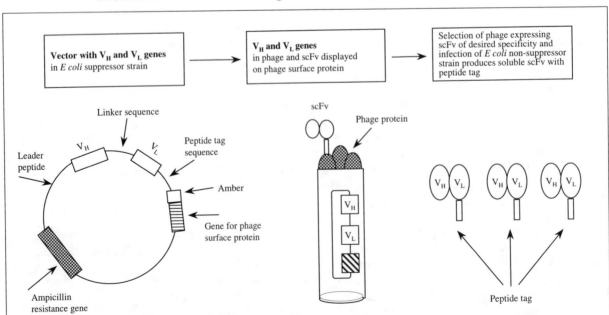

replace mouse genes with human genes, DNA can be injected directly into mouse eggs to effect random integration of the human DNA into the mouse genome and the resulting transgenic mice can then be crossed with mice which have deletions in their own antibody genes. Bruggeman and Neuberger (120) suggest that rather than relying on random integration of human DNA it may be possible to direct DNA to the mouse antibody gene loci and thereby directly substitute human antibody genes for mouse antibody genes.

Mice carrying transgenic miniloci or YAC-based transloci produce human antibody to a variety of antigens as judged both by serum antibody titer and by the derivation of hybridomas. Human monoclonal antibodies to tetanus toxoid (121) and human CD4 (122) have been produced in this way. The human anti-human CD4 is particularly interesting since it follows from these experiments that it might be possible to generate hybridomas secreting human monoclonal anti-D from suitable transgenic mice. Since numerous different monoclonal anti-D have been cloned and sequenced there is a lot of information about V_H, D and J gene usage in monoclonal anti-D (27) and so a suitable minigene should be relatively easy to design. This experiment might be interesting for another reason since it would address the question as to why mice do not make anti-D. Is it simply because they lack a suitable V_H gene repertoire or is there some other reason?

Antigen:Antibody Interactions

The interaction between an antigen and its corresponding antibody is reversible and analogous to that between an enzyme and its substrate. This reversible reaction is usually represented as:

$$Ag + Ab = AgAb$$

since there will be an equilibrium between free antigen (Ag), free antibody (Ab) and the complex of antigen and antibody (AgAb). The relative amounts of bound versus unbound antigen and antibody will depend on the strength of the interaction between Ag and Ab (binding affinity) and the concentrations of Ag and Ab in the mixture. The binding affinity or affinity constant (K) is obtained from the formula:

$$K = \frac{(AgAb)}{(Ag)(Ab)} \quad \text{-equation 1}$$

where (AgAb) is the concentration of bound and (Ag) and (Ab) the concentration of unbound elements. Clearly the higher the affinity the greater the amount of bound complex. The affinity constant is a measure of the sum of a variety of weak non-covalent interactions between antigen and antibody including, hydrogen bonds, ionic bonds, van der Waals forces and hydrophobic bonds (123).

Antibody molecules are bivalent or multivalent not monovalent (see figure 2-5). Immunohematologists usually observe the interaction of antibody with antigen under circumstances where more than one antigen binding site on the antibody is complexed with antigen - in a direct agglutination test for example. Under these circumstances the affinity constant of the antibody:antigen interaction is much greater than that observed for Fab:antigen interactions. This explains why secretory IgM is an effective weapon against microbial infection in a primary immune response. The individual Fab fragments of IgM molecules have very low affinity for antigen but multiple interactions with antigen by this pentameric molecule have a high functional affinity (avidity).

Measurement of antibody affinity can be achieved by a variety of methods. Different concentrations of radioiodinated antibody or Fab are incubated with a constant amount of antigen (e.g. a known number of red cells) and after allowing sufficient time for equilibration, the unbound antibody is separated from the bound antibody and the concentration of each determined from their respective specific activities (radioactive counts/min/mg antibody or Fab protein). The amount of antibody or Fab bound at saturation can be used to determine the number of antigen sites (assuming 1:1 binding in the case of Fab) and the affinity constant can be determined from knowledge of the concentration of antigen required to fill half the available antibody or Fab sites since when half the sites are filled, the concentration of bound antibody = concentration of free antibody and it follows from equation-1 above that K = 1/(Ag). Most polyclonal antisera contain antibodies with a wide range of affinities (equilibrium constants ranging from 10^6 to 10^9 liters/mole) (124).

The binding affinity of an antibody or Fab is affected by the composition of the solution in which antibody/Fab and antigen are suspended (ionic strength and pH) and by the temperature at which the reaction is carried out (123). The binding of polyclonal antibodies to their antigen is usually stable over a wide range of pH (4-9), (57). Although there may be discernible optima with individual sera, Hughes-Jones et al. (125) found that the equilibrium constant for polyclonal anti-D was highest between pH 6.5 and 7 but there was little change in reactivity between pH 5.5 and 8.5. Some examples of monoclonal anti-M and N are extremely dependent on pH (77). Many, but not all, blood group antibodies have a higher rate of association with antigen under conditions of low ionic strength (126,127). Antibodies to the A, B and H antigens are an exception (128).

Goding (57) notes that some monoclonal antibodies to a given cell surface antigen take longer than others to reach equilibrium binding to the antigens with saturation being reached in as little as 15 or as long as 90 minutes.

This, he suggests, may be related to the need for an antigen to be in a particular (transient) confirmation before antibody can bind. Differences like this are not so apparent with polyclonal antisera because such sera represent a mixture of antibodies and the behavior of the antiserum is likely to be dominated by a small fraction of antibody molecules with very high affinity. The precise nature of the interaction between antigen and antibody has been elucidated for several different antigens and antibodies by X-ray crystallographic studies of crystals containing antigen complexed with antibody (129-131).

The best studied of these interactions is that between a Fab fragment from a monoclonal antibody to hen egg white lysozyme (anti-HEL) and the lysozyme itself (129,130). Analysis of the structure of this complex revealed that the Fab is in a fully extended conformation in the complex and that its quaternary structure is no different from the structure of Fab fragments which are not complexed to antibody. This shows that, at least in this case, binding of antigen to Fab does not result in a significant conformational change in the antibody molecule. Inspection of the points of contact between Fab and lysozyme revealed that 16 amino acids in the lysozyme are in contact with 17 amino acids in the Fab. Ten of the residues in the Fab are in the heavy chain and 7 in the light chain. The residues involved in lysozyme are not in a continuous sequence but distributed in different regions of the protein. The epitope recognized by Fab anti-HEL is therefore a conformational epitope. Alzari et al. (129) comment that all the 3-dimensional structures of antigen-antibody complexes studied so far have revealed conformational epitopes and conclude that "therefore most antibodies directed against native protein molecules probably recognize non-continuous determinants". Alzari et al. (129) also comment that "the overall picture of the antigen-antibody interface in the Fab-lysozyme complex is that of two irregular, rather flat surfaces with protuberances and depressions that fit into the complementary features of the other".

Agglutination

The agglutination test is the essential tool by which compatible blood for transfusion is selected. The test is easy to perform but those who are not content simply to observe the beauty of agglutinated red cells and wish to understand how it happens will find the literature full of controversy (132,133). Essentially, the bivalent (IgG) and multivalent (IgM) antibody molecules crosslink red cells. IgM is a large molecule with a maximum distance of 30 nM between antigen binding sites. IgG is smaller with a maximum distance of 14 nM between antigen binding sites (21). Studies of the structure of blood group-active

molecules at the red cell surface (discussed in Chapter 4) have led to a model where some antigens are located at a distance from the lipid bilayer while others are located at the surface of the bilayer (see figure 2-14).

Clearly for crosslinking of red cells to take place, the antibody must be able to bind with antigens on each of two red cells. For IgM those antigens may be a maximum of 30 nM apart while for IgG the maximum distance is 14 nM. It is possible to calculate the position of an antigen relative to the bilayer from a consideration of the structure of the molecule that carries the antigen but in order to compare the position of antigens with the ability of antibodies to those antigens to agglutinate red cells it is necessary to know the distance between two red cells in isotonic solution. This problem was addressed by van Oss and Absolom (134). The distance between two cells is a balance between forces which tend to repel and those which attract. Repulsive forces are attributable to the surface negative charge of the red cell which is largely the result of its high content of sialic acid residues (predominantly found on glycophorins). This can be measured by cell electrophoresis and has been referred to as zeta potential (135). Intercellular attraction is induced by van der Waals forces. The problem of calculating the distance between two red cells in solution is compounded by the fact that red cells are not spheres but biconcave discs. Nevertheless van Oss and Absolom (134) calculated that the distance between the cell surfaces of two red cells in isotonic solution was a minimum of 7.9 nM if the red cell is a sphere or 10.3 nM if the flat sides of the biconcave disc are facing one another. It is now well established that IgM anti-D can directly agglutinate red cells in saline suspension and that the D antigen is known to be located on a hydrophobic polypeptide which extends very little above the lipid bilayer. It follows from this that the distance between the lipid bilayers of two red cells in saline suspension is unlikely to exceed 30 nM. It is also known that IgG anti-D does not agglutinate red cells directly so that the distance between the lipid bilayers of two red cells is unlikely to be as little as 14 nM. In contrast, IgG anti-A, IgG anti-B and IgG anti-M are potent agglutinins (136,137). A and B antigens are located on oligosaccharide structures on a wide variety of membrane proteins and glycolipids but the M antigen is confined to the extreme N-terminus of glycophorin A (Chapter 15). The M antigen (and at least some A and B antigens) must therefore be above the surface of the lipid bilayer relative to D antigen. These considerations led van Oss and Absolom (134) to conclude that the position of an antigen relative to the bilayer governs whether or not an IgG antibody, specific for that antigen can agglutinate red cells. These conclusions remain valid now that the structure of the red cell membrane and the nature of the antigen is known in greater detail (see figure 2-14).

FIGURE 2-14 Some Antibodies of the IgG Class are Direct Agglutinins (anti-M) Others are Not (anti-D) Because they Cannot Form a Bridge Between Two Red Cells in Suspension

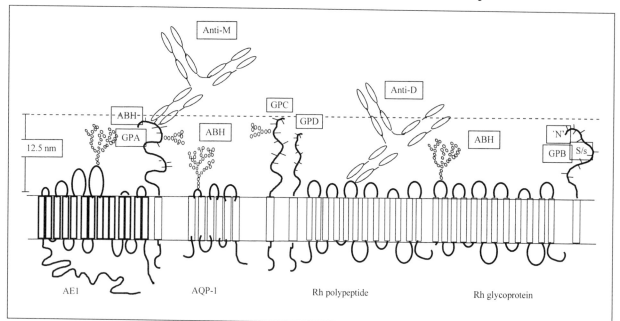

Detection of non-agglutinating IgG is achieved using the antiglobulin test whereby an anti-IgG crosslinks (predominantly through the Fc region) IgG molecules bound to different cells, see Chapter 6. Various ways of increasing the sensitivity of the antiglobulin test are also discussed in that Chapter.

The above considerations yield a fairly simple explanation of agglutination. There are however a number of other variables which can influence the agglutination reaction and problems of interpretation arising from these variables have unfortunately served to complicate this simple picture.

One of these variables is the number of antigen sites on a red cell. It has been argued that the number of antigen sites (rather than their position relative to the bilayer) determines whether or not an IgG antibody can agglutinate red cells. There are in excess of 2×10^6 A, B and H sites compared with about 30,000 D sites on most red cells, but since selected IgG anti-D will agglutinate D-- cells, that have 100-200,000 D sites (138) the inference was drawn that site number was the relevant factor. That this is not a valid conclusion is readily apparent from studies using monoclonal antibodies to CD44 which carries the Indian blood group antigens (see Chapter 29). There are about 10,000 molecules of CD44/red cell (139) but monoclonal anti-CD44 are usually direct agglutinins (140). It seems likely that the selected IgG anti-D that agglutinate D-- red cells contain aggregated IgG or an IgM component since none of the many monoclonal IgG anti-D that have been studied in three international work-

shops are able to agglutinate D-- cells (Kumpel B, personal communication). It seems more likely that the number of antigen sites determine the number of possible crosslinks between cells and thereby the strength of agglutination observed.

Another area of past controversy concerns the effect of treating red cells with sialidase or proteases and the ability of IgG antibodies to agglutinate such treated red cells (133). It has been noted that when the surface negative charge of a red cell is reduced to the same extent by sialidase treatment and protease treatment, the protease treated cells are more agglutinable by anti-D than are the sialidase-treated cells. Thus surface charge cannot be the only factor which determines agglutinability (141). Stratton et al. (141) argue that this difference relates to a greater decrease in steric hindrance (accessibility to D antigen sites). This argument hinges to a large extent on what happens to glycophorins when they are stripped of sialic acid since glycophorin A and B together contribute about 85% of the surface sialic acid (142). It has been argued that sialidase-treatment of glycophorins would cause the proteins to fold or contract (143) but more recent evidence suggests that the polypeptides would remain rigid because the main interaction which affects rigidity is between N-acetylgalactosamine and the adjacent peptide chain (144). These results suggest that the residual desialylated glycophorin molecules may indeed form a barrier to the accessibility of some D antigen sites thereby reducing the potential number of crosslinking sites and so the strength of agglutination. Protease treatment, in contrast, removes the entire glycosylated region of these proteins as released glycopeptides. Both sialidase-treated red cells and protease-treated red cells are closer together in saline suspension than are untreated red cells, sufficiently close in fact, to allow bridging of the treated cells by IgG (143).

Water molecules cluster around polar molecules and so the surface of the red cell contains bound water (a hydration shell). It is possible that the agglutination enchancing effects of bovine serum albumin and other potentiating molecules may be mediated through the binding of water molecules thereby reducing the hydration shell and potentiating ionic interactions between charged groups on the antigen and antibody (133). Depletion of the hydration shell by sialidase or protease treatment may also be a factor in the enhanced agglutinability of these cells.

References

1. Wells HG, Huxley J, Wells GP. The Science of Life. London:Cassell, 1931:630
2. Chick H, Hume M, Macfarlane M. War on Disease. London:Deutsch, 1971:19
3. Heidelberger M. Lectures in Immunochemistry. New York:Academic, 1956
4. Landsteiner K. The Specificity of Serological Reactions. Boston:Harvard Univ Press, 1946
5. Porter RR. Essays Biochem 1967;3:1
6. Wintrobe MM. Clinical Haematology. London:Himpton, 1946:157
7. Harris TN, Grimm E, Mertens E, et al. J Exp Med 1945;81:73
8. Cooper MD, Petersen RDA, South MA, et al. J Exp Med 1966;123:75
9. Zinkernagel RM, Doherty PC. Adv Immunol 1979; 27: 51
10. Alberts B, Bray D, Lewis J, et al. Molecular Biology of the Cell, 3rd Ed. New York:Garland, 1994:1250
11. Murphy PM. Cell 1993;72:823
12. Boren T, Falk P, Roth KA, et al. Science 1993;262:1892
13. Miller LH, Mason SJ, Clyde DF, et al. New Eng J Med 1976;295:302
14. Black FL. Science 1992;258:1739
15. Porter RR. Nature 1958;182:670
16. Feinstein A, Munn EA, Richardson NE. Ann NY Acad Sci 1971;190:104
17. Nisonoff A, Hopper JE, Spring SB. The Antibody Molecule. New York:Academic, 1975
18. Michaelson TE, Frangione B, Franklin EC. J Biol Chem 1977;252:883
19. Morell A, Skvaril F, Loghem E van, et al. Vox Sang 1971;21:481
20. Gregory L, Davies KG, Sheth B, et al. Mol Immunol 1987;24:821
21. Sarma VR, Silverton EW, Davies DR, et al. J Biol Chem 1971;246:3753
22. Kerr MA. Biochem J 1990;271:285
23. Roitt I. Essential Immunology 7th Ed. Oxford:Blackwell, 1991
24. Cook GP, Tomlinson IM. Immunol Today 1995;16:237
25. Wu TT, Kabat EA. J Exp Med 1970;132:211
26. Tonegawa S. Nature 1983;302:575
27. Bye JM, Carter C, Cui Y, et al. J Clin Invest 1992;90:2481
28. Pascual V, Victor K, Spellerberg M, et al. J Immunol 1992;149:2337
29. Jefferies LC, Carchidi CM, Silberstein LE J Clin Invest 1993;92:2821
30. Burnet M. The Clonal Selection Theory of Acquired Immunity. London:Cambridge Univ Press, 1959
31. Cresswell P. Ann Rev Immunol 1994;12:259
32. Brown JH, Jardetzky TS, Gorga JC, et al. Nature 1993;364:33
33. Barclay AN, Birkeland ML, Brown MH, et al. The Leucocyte Antigen Facts Book. London:Academic, 1993:106
34. Davies MM. Ann Rev Biochem 1990;59:475
35. Bierer BE, Sleckman BP, Ratnofsky SE, et al. Ann Rev Immunol 1989;7:579
36. Zinkernagel RM, Bachmann MF, Kundig TM, et al. Ann Rev Immunol 1996;14:333
37. Reid KB. Essays Biochem 1986;22:27
38. van der Winkel JGJ, Capel PJA. Immunol Today 1993;14:215
39. Indik ZK, Park J-G, Hunter S, et al. Blood 1995;86:4389
40. Podack ER, Hengartner H, Lichtenheld MG. Ann Rev Immunol 1991;9:129
41. Story CM, Mikulska JE, Simister NE. J Exp Med 1994;180:2377
42. Burmeister WP, Gastinel LN, Simister NE. Nature 1994;372:336
43. Burmeister WP, Huber AH, Bjorkman PJ. Nature 1994;372:379
44. Ravetch JV. Cell 1994;78:553
45. Sandler SG, Trimble J, Mallory DM. Transfusion 1996;36:256
46. Vyas GN, Perkins HA, Fudenberg HH. Lancet 1968;2:312
47. Bjorkman PJ, Saper MA, Samraoui B, et al. Nature 1987;329:506
48. Monaco JJ. Immunol Today 1993;13:173
49. Bodmer JG, Marsh SGE, Albert ED, et al. Tissue Antigens 1992;39:161
50. Howard JC. Curr Opin Immunol 1995;7:69
51. Lehner PJ, Cresswell P. Curr Opin Immunol 1996;8:59
52. Novotny VMJ, Brand A. In: Modern Transfusion Medicine. Ann Arbor:CRC Press, 1995:107
53. Doniach D, Roitt IM. J Clin Endocrinol Metab 1957;17:1293
54. Witebsky E, Rose NR, Terplan K, et al. J Am Med Assoc 1957;164:1439
55. Adams D. Immunol Today 1996;17:300
56. Hilschmann N, Craig LC. Proc Nat Acad Sci USA 1965;53:1403
57. Goding J. Monoclonal Antibodies: Principles and Practice, 2nd Ed. London:Academic, 1986
58. Ellis NA, Tippett P, Petty A, et al. Nature Genet 1994;8:285
59. Chérif-Zahar B, Bloy C, Le Van Kim C, et al. Proc Nat Acad Sci USA 1990;87:6242
60. Avent ND, Ridgwell K, Tanner MJA, et al. Biochem J 1990;271:821
61. Avent ND, Butcher SK, Liu W, et al. J Biol Chem 1992;267:15134
62. Hemming NJ, Anstee DJ, Mawby WJ, et al. Biochem J 1994;299:191
63. King M-J, Holmes CH, Mushens RE, et al. Br J Haematol 1995;89:440
64. Kohler G, Milstein C. Nature 1975;256:495
65. Littlefield JW. Science 1964;145:709
66. Voak D, Lowe AD, Lennox E. Biotest Bull 1983;1:291
67. Lachmann PJ, Oldroyd RG, Milstein C, et al. Immunology 1980;41:503
68. Smyth JS. MPhil Thesis. Univ West England, 1994

69. Smythe JS, Spring FA, Gardner B, et al. Blood 1995;85:2929
70. Stoll M, Dalchau R, Schmidt RE. In: Leucocyte Typing IV. Oxford:Oxford Univ Press, 1989:619
71. Springer GF, Horton MR, Forbes M. J Exp Med 1959;110:221
72. Voak D, Sacks SS, Alderson T, et al. Vox Sang 1980;39:134
73. Sacks S, Lennox ES. Vox Sang 1981;40:99
74. Friedenreich V, With S. Z Immunforsch 1933;78:152
75. Owen RD. J Immunol 1954;73:29
76. Joysey VC. Br Med Bull 1959;15:158
77. Fraser RH, Munro AC, Williamson AR, et al. J Immunogenet 1982;9:303
78. Bigbee WL, Vanderlaan M, Fong SSN, et al. Mol Immunol 1983;20:1353
79. Bailly P, Chevaleyre J, Sondag D, et al. Mol Immunol 1987;24:171
80. Fraser RH, Allen EK, Inglis G, et al. Exp Clin Immunogenet 1984;1:145
81. Cowles JW, Cox MT, McMican A, et al. Vox Sang 1987;52:83
82. Landsteiner K, Levine P. Proc Soc Exp Med NY 1927;24:941
83. Landsteiner K, Levine P. J Exp Med 1928;48:731
84. Graham HA, Hirsch HF, Davies DM. Human Blood Groups. Basel:Karger, 1977:257
85. Marcus DM, Bastani AM, Rosenfield RE, et al. Transfusion 1967;7:277
86. Zopf DA, Ginsburg A, Ginsburg V. J Immunol 1975;115:1525
87. Boylston AW, Gardner B, Anderson RL, et al. Scand J Immunol 1980;12:355
88. Koskimies S. Scand J Immunol 1980;11:73
89. Croce CM, Linnenbach A, Hall A, et al. Nature 1980;288:488
90. Edwards PAW, Smith CM, Neville AM, et al. Eur J Immunol 1982;12:641
91. Nowinski R, Berglund C, Lane J, et al. Science 1980;210:537
92. Bron D, Feinberg MB, Teng NNH, et al. Proc Nat Acad Sci USA 1984;81:3214
93. Crawford DH, Barlow MJ, Harrison JF, et al. Lancet 1983;1:386
94. Thompson KM, Hough DW, Maddison PJ, et al. J Immunol Meth 1986;94:7
95. Kumpel BM, Goodrick MK, Pamphilon DH. Blood 1995;86:1701
96. Scott ML, Voak D. In: Immunobiology of Transfusion Medicine. New York:Marcel Dekker, 1994:365
97. Hale G. Transfusion Med 1993;3:1
98. Hale G, Phillips JM. Biochem Soc Trans 1995;23:1057
99. Winter G, Harris WJ. Immunol Today 1993;14:243
100. Jones PT, Dear PH, Foote J, et al. Nature 1986;321:522
101. Reichmann L, Clarke M, Waldmann H, et al. Nature 1988;332:323
102. Marks JD, Griffiths AD, Malmqvist M, et al. Biotechnology 1992;10:779
103. Hawkins RE, Russell SJ, Winter G. J Mol Biol 1992;226:889
104. Hale G, Dyer MJS, Clark MR, et al. Lancet 1988;2:1394
105. Isaacs JD, Watts RA, Hazelman BL, et al. Lancet 1992;340:748
106. Smith GP. Science 1985;228:315
107. Winter G, Griffiths AD, Hawkins RE, et al. Ann Rev Immunol 1994;12:433
108. Huston JS, Levinson D, Mudgett HM, et al. Proc Nat Acad Sci USA 1988;85:5879
109. Bird RE, Hardman KD, Jacobson JW, et al. Science 1988;242:423
110. McCafferty J, Griffiths AD, Winter G, et al. Nature 1990;348:552
111. Hoogenboom HR, Griffiths AD, Johnson KS, et al. Nucleic Acids Res 1991;19:4133
112. Garrard LJ, Yang M, O'Connell MP, et al. Biotechnology 1991;9:1373
113. Carter P, Kelley RF, Rodrigues ML, et al. Biotechnology 1992;10:163
114. Begent RHJ, Verhaar MJ, Chester K, et al. Nature Med 1996;2:979
115. Marks JD, Ouwehand WH, Bye JM, et al., Biotechnology 1993;11:1145
116. Siegel DL, Silberstein LE. Blood 1994;83:2334
117. Czerwinski M, Siegel DL, Moore PF, et al. Transfusion 1995;35:137
118. Hughes-Jones NC, Gorick BD, Bye JM, et al. Br J Haematol 1994;88:180
119. Scott ML, Mushens RE, Guest AR, et al. (abstract). Vox Sang 1996;70(Suppl 2):48
120. Bruggemann M, Neuberger MS. Immunol Today 1996;17:391
121. Green LL, Hardy MC, Maynard-Currie CE, et al. Nature Genet 1994;7:13
122. Lonberg N, Taylor LD, Harding FA, et al. Nature 1994;368:856
123. Hughes-Jones NC. Br Med Bull 1963;19:171
124. Mason D, Williams AF. Biochem J 1980;187:1
125. Hughes-Jones NC, Gardner B, Telford R. Immunology 1964;7:72
126. Hughes-Jones NC, Polley MJ, Telford R, et al. Vox Sang 1964;9:385
127. Elliot M, Bossom E, Dupuy ME, et al. Vox Sang 1964;9:396
128. Messeter L, Brodin T, Chester MA, et al. Vox Sang 1984;46:185
129. Alzari PM, Lascombe M-B, Poljak RJ. Ann Rev Immunol 1988;6:555
130. Amit AG, Marinzza RA, Phillips SEV, et al. Science 1986;233:747
131. Stanfield RL, Fieser TM, Lerner RA, et al. Science 1990;248:712
132. van Oss CJ, Absolom DR, Neumann AW. Prog Clin Biol Res 1980;43:157
133. Steane EA, Greenwalt TJ. Prog Clin Biol Res 1980;43:171
134. van Oss CJ, Absolom DR. Vox Sang 1983;44:183
135. Pollack W, Hager HJ, Reckel R, et al. Transfusion 1965;5:158
136. Mollison PL. Blood Transfusion in Clinical Medicine, 7th Ed. Oxford:Blackwell, 1983:256
137. Smith ML, Beck ML. Transfusion 1979;19:472
138. Hughes-Jones NC, Gardner B, Lincoln PJ. Vox Sang 1971;21:210
139. Anstee DJ, Gardner B, Spring FA, et al. Immunology 1991;74:197
140. Anstee DJ, Gardner B. (abstract). Transf Med 1991;1 (Suppl 2):59
141. Stratton F, Rawlinson VI, Gunson HH, et al. Vox Sang 1973;24:273
142. Anstee DJ. Prog Clin Biol Res 1980;43:67
143. van Oss CJ, Absolom DR. Vox Sang 1984;47:250
144. Jentoft N. Trends Biochem Sci 1990;15:291
145. Thompson K, Barden G, Sutherland J, et al. Immunology 1990;71:323
146. Thompson K, Barden G, Sutherland J, et al. Transf Med 1991;1:91

3 | Principles of Serological Methods

In the three previous editions of this book details of some serological methods were given. The chapters involved were never intended to be fully comprehensive, rather the methods described were those that the author had found useful and reliable. The need for a chapter giving detailed methods has now passed. The same company that publishes this book has published two editions (1988 and 1994) of W. John Judd's *METHODS IN IMMUNOHEMATOLOGY*. That book should be regarded as a companion publication to this one and since it gives step by step procedures for over 150 serological methods, those details need not be repeated here. Instead, this chapter will discuss some principles of serological methods. As in the previous editions many methods will be discussed as separate entities. In actual practice, of course, methods are usually combined. As examples, while the principles of low ionic strength tests and those that use polyethylene glycol (PEG) and Polybrene are described individually, each of them is usually combined with an indirect antiglobulin test, in practice. Principles of biochemical methods are outlined in Chapter 4 together with a description of red cell membrane structure. The principles, use and interpretation of molecular genetic studies are described in Chapter 5. The antiglobulin test and complement, together with in vivo red cell destruction are discussed in Chapter 6.

Sensitivity and Relevance

In any discussion of serological methods, it is inevitable that comparisons of sensitivity between various methods will be made. Since the objective of many immunohematological tests is to prevent the transfusion of red cells that will not survive normally in vivo, it is often assumed that the more sensitive the method, the better. One often hears comments to the effect that the (new) method detects more antibodies so it MUST be better. This is not necessarily the case. If a method detects antibodies that are clinically meaningless, transfusion of the patient may be delayed while a search for "compatible" blood is mounted and large amounts of time and money may be spent in the search. Included in this Chapter are references to some reports that document the existence of antibodies that, based on their specificity, would be expected to be clinically significant. These antibodies, in fact, neither cleared antigen-positive red cells in vivo, nor increased in strength after the patient received antigen-positive blood. That is to say, there was no immediate or delayed transfusion reaction, nor any secondary immune response. It is clear that clinical significance of an antibody cannot be forecast based on specificity alone. While most Rh and Kell system antibodies are clinically-significant, some are not. This whole topic of trying to determine the likelihood of in vivo red cell clearance based on the results of in vitro tests, is discussed in detail in Chapters 6 and 35. However, it was felt necessary to place an admonition here, before the various methods were described, to remind readers that in vitro test sensitivity does not always correlate with in vivo clinical relevance.

Controls

Previous discussions of serological tests usually included a statement to the effect that all such tests must be controlled. Time and experience have modified thinking in this area. For example, most workers now agree that use of an autocontrol in antibody screening tests is not necessary since most such tests will be negative and the autocontrol will contribute no useful information. In such tests, IATs are individually controlled with IgG-coated (Coombs control) red cells. When the antibody screening test is positive and a panel study is performed an autocontrol is usually included to help distinguish allo from autoantibodies. Thus perhaps the correct statement now is that control tests must be included when their results are necessary to verify correct interpretation of the test. In tests using antisera of known specificity both positive and negative controls should be included. Whenever possible the positive control should be one in which the antigen involved is present in single dose. Thus in typing tests using anti-Jk^a, the negative control would be Jk(a-b+) red cells, the positive control should be Jk(a+b+) and not Jk(a+b-) cells. Correct results in the control tests will thus demonstrate the ability of the anti-Jk^a in use to detect the weakest expression of Jk^a likely to be encountered in routine tests.

Direct Agglutination Methods

These methods are ones in which red cells suspended in saline are tested with antibodies that can cause direct agglutination or ones in which known phenotype red cells are used to test serum for the presence of such antibodies. The methods can be used in a variety of ways.

1. Immediate Spin Tests

In these tests the red cells and serum are mixed and the tubes are centrifuged immediately or within a few minutes of addition of the cells to the serum. The tests are used predominantly in ABO reverse typing and in immediate spin (IS) compatibility tests in patients in whom no atypical antibodies have been found and in whom the compatibility test is designed only to detect major side ABO incompatibility (see Chapter 35). Although potent examples of some cold-reactive alloantibodies, such as anti-P$_1$ and anti-Le^a, will react by this method, its prime justification for use is for ABO system antibodies. Both IgM and IgG anti-A and anti-B will react in immediate spin tests.

2. Room Temperature Tests

The only difference between IS and room temperature direct agglutination tests is that in the latter an incubation period is used between adding the red cells to the serum and centrifugation. Once used as a standard procedure in compatibility testing, this method has now largely been abandoned for that purpose since antibodies detected only by this method are clinically benign. The method is now used primarily in phenotyping studies using agglutinating antibodies such as those directed against M, N, P$_1$, Le^a, Le^b, etc.

3. Tests at 37°C

These tests are somewhat more relevant than those incubated at room temperature since there is a greater likelihood that an agglutinin active at 37°C will be clinically significant. However, two points should be considered. First, antibodies that agglutinate red cells at 37°C but are not demonstrable in the antiglobulin test are rare. While some workers (1) contend that a 37°C reading for agglutination is necessary in antibody screening and compatibility tests and that recently formed IgM antibodies that portend the development of IgG antibodies of the same specificity can be detected in the test, others have eliminated the 37°C reading without adverse consequences. For example, in one of our services (2) we use PEG as a routine additive (3) and wash the test cells for IAT immediately the incubation period is complete. We believe that the difference between the observations of Judd et al. (1) and our own (2) relate directly to the antigen-antibody reaction enhancement method used. Judd et al. (1) used LISS and found a significant number of 37°C+/IAT-negative alloantibodies. In direct contrast, while using PEG we find a number of IgM antibodies

apparently reactive by IAT, although we read our tests with a heavy chain specific anti-IgG. We believe that at 37°C the IgM antibodies we detect cause agglutination of the red cells and that the agglutination is not dispersed during the washing steps that precede the IAT reading. Thus IgM agglutinins active at 37°C appear to be detected by IAT although, in fact, the agglutination has been "carried-through" and is not mediated by the anti-IgG (see the addendum).

Second, tests at 37°C are sometimes used as an aid in determining the clinical significance of an antibody (4-6). If such tests are to be used, it is important that they be performed strictly at 37°C. In tests set up at room temperature, then transferred to 37°C, antigen-antibody complexes may form before the contents of the tube reach 37°C and may not dissociate once that temperature is reached. The antibody may then appear to be active at 37°C when it does not actually have that capability.

4. Prewarmed Tests

As discussed in the previous section, antibody activity at 37°C should not be gauged from tests not maintained at 37°C. Instead, the test cells and serum should be warmed separately to 37°C before being mixed, using warm pipettes. Centrifugation before reading should also be at 37°C via the use of a heated centrifuge or centrifuge buckets filled with warm water. After centrifugation the tubes should be kept at 37°C and read one at a time. While the agglutination reaction at 37°C only seldom needs to be considered in assessing an antibody's potential activity in vivo, prewarmed tests are often set up, then converted to IAT for that purpose. The prewarmed test used in that manner has recently been criticized (7) and defended (8). There is no doubt that if a technologist has made a preconceived judgment that an antibody detected in routine tests is a "nuisance cold-agglutinin" prewarmed tests can be read in such a manner that the antibody is not detected. However, this is a failure of the technologist, not the test. If the test is used correctly and read properly, alloimmune and autoimmune antibodies truly reactive at 37°C will be detected.

It follows, of course, that if the antibody to be tested by the prewarmed technique was first detected in a test using a potentiator (e.g. LISS, PEG) that potentiator be used (by being warmed separately to 37°C) in the prewarmed test. If an antibody first detected in a LISS or PEG method is tested in a saline system at 37°C, failure to obtain a positive reaction may be due to the use of a less sensitive method and not to the fact that the antibody is inactive at 37°C. It seems probable that failure to remember this principle accounts for many of the so-called "failures" of the prewarmed method, in which antibodies of potential clinical significance have gone undetected.

5. Tests at 4°C

Clearly if tests at room temperature detect clinically insignificant antibodies, those performed at lower temperatures will detect even more examples. Nevertheless, there are occasions on which agglutination tests at 4°C can be useful. These include but are not limited to: the detection of weak ABO agglutinins in reverse typing (see Chapter 8 for the use of controls); the titration of cold-agglutinins in patients with cold hemagglutinin disease (see Chapter 38); and the use of weak antibodies in phenotyping studies when no better reagents are available.

Use of Reducing Agents

On occasion it is necessary to prevent agglutination by IgM antibodies. For example, antibody-screening tests on the serum of a patient with severe cold hemagglutinin disease, for the presence of IgG alloantibodies, may be difficult when the IgM autoagglutinin reacts with all red cells. The serum containing the IgM antibody can be mixed with a sulphydryl compound such as 2-mercaptoethanol (2-ME) or dithiothreitol (DTT) so that some of the disulphide bonds that connect the basic antibody structural units to the J chain (see Chapter 2) and some that join other chains in the molecule are cleaved. The pentameric IgM molecules will be reduced to the monomeric form and most often will lose their ability to agglutinate red cells. Although DTT is somewhat better than 2-ME at maintaining reduction, more resistant to oxidation in air and lacks the awful smell of 2-ME, it may be less efficient than 2-ME in its actions (9). A point not often remembered is that reduction cleavage by 2-ME and DTT is more efficient at 37°C than at room tem-

perature (9). Serum that has been treated with 2-ME may be used without dialysis (10) in agglutination studies but false positive reactions may be seen at IAT (9). It must also be remembered that 2-ME and DTT are anticomplementary and that treated sera must be dialyzed free of the reducing agent, then used in tests to which fresh serum has been added, if detection of cell bound complement is part of the aim of the test.

As discussed further in Chapter 41, tests with 2-ME or DTT can occasionally prove useful in forecasting the possibility of hemolytic disease of the newborn.

Inhibition of Agglutination

Agglutination by specific antibodies can sometimes be inhibited by the addition of material that contains the antigen involved in soluble form. Such inhibition of hemagglutination may be useful in identification of one antibody in the presence of another (one inhibited, one still active), in the confirmation of antibody specificity and in determination of the secretor status. Table 3-1 lists some sources of material suitable for use in inhibition studies.

Potentiators of the Hemagglutination Reaction and Enhancement of Antibody Uptake by Red Cells

Since the agglutination of red cells in a saline system is not a very sensitive method of antibody detection or of demonstrating antigen-antibody reactions in phenotyping studies, many methods to increase the sensitivity of in vitro test methods have been developed. In some instances relatively strong IgG antibodies that do not agglutinate red cells in a saline system can be prompted to behave as agglutinins in the more sensitive tests. More often, the test modifications increase the amount of anti-

TABLE 3-1 Some Materials Useful in Antibody Inhibition

Source and rbc phenotype where appropriate	Antigens present
Saliva from ABH secretors of corresponding phenotype	A,B,H (see also Le^a and Le^b)
Saliva from Le(a+b-) donors Saliva and plasma from Le(a-b+) donotrs	Le^a Le^a Le^b (see also A,B,H)
Hyadatid cyst fluid Pigeon egg white Earthworms (night crawlers)	P$_1$
Human milk	I (Seldom sufficient amounts to effect total antibody inhibition)
Serum and plasma from Ch+, Rg+ donors	Ch Rg
Urine from Sd(a+) donors and guinea pigs	Sd^a

body that binds to red cells and/or increase the rate of antibody association. Such changes considerably enhance the detection of such antibodies in the antiglobulin test.

1. Bovine Albumin

In 1945, it was shown (11,12) that the addition of bovine albumin to a test system caused some otherwise non-agglutinating antibodies to behave as agglutinins. As discussed in Chapter 2, the addition of bovine albumin does not enhance the first stage of the hemagglutination reaction (antibody uptake) (13). Exactly how it affects the second stage (crosslinking) is still controversial (14-24). The least sensitive methods of using bovine albumin are the simple addition of the material at the start of the test and the use of albumin-suspended red cells. The albumin replacement and albumin layering techniques (25,26) are more sensitive but are seldom used (at least in the USA) since faster and easier methods of in vitro test enhancement are now available.

2. Tests at Low Ionic Strength

It has been known since 1964 that lowering the ionic strength of the test medium greatly enhances the rate at which antibodies bind to red cells (27,28). Indeed, early studies (27) showed that the rate of uptake of anti-D by D+ red cells was increased one thousand fold at an ionic strength of 0.03I, compared to normal ionic strength. However, it proved difficult to use this observation at the level of routine blood banking. At very low ionic strength, immunoglobulins aggregate and activate complement. Both the aggregated immunoglobulins and complement bind to red cells so that positive antiglobulin tests are seen even in the absence of a specific blood group antigen-antibody reaction (28,29). Many of these difficulties were overcome in 1974 when Löw and Messeter (30) reported that if a test system in which the final ionic strength is 0.09I is used, sensitivity is retained and few unwanted (non-specific) positives are seen. The starting ionicity of the medium in which the red cells are suspended is 0.03I, the 0.09I level is reached when an equal volume of serum is added to the red cells in low ionic strength solution (LISS). Other workers (31-37) confirmed the sensitivity and speed of LISS tests. Because the final ionic strength is critical, it is important always to use the correct volumes of LISS and serum (and red cell suspensions if a LISS additive is used). That is to say, unlike tests at normal ionic strength, increasing the serum:cell ratio decreases instead of increases sensitivity of the test. When cells are suspended in LISS the amount of serum specified in the method must be used. When cells in nor-

mal ionic strength saline are mixed with serum and then a LISS reagent is added to bring the whole mixture to 0.09I, specified volumes of all reagents must be used. Use of an additional amount of serum increases the ionicity above 0.09I and reduces sensitivity of the method. Use of additional LISS reagent reduces the ionicity below 0.09I and results in non-specific positive reactions.

When LISS techniques were first used at the routine level, a number of reports (36,38-40) appeared describing the non-detection or difficulty in detection of anti-K. Merry at al. (41,42) studied this situation and made two findings. First, when a LISS method is used anti-K binds to K+ red cells more slowly than anti-D binds to D+ cells. Second, when red cells are coated (under low ionic strength conditions) with equal amounts of IgG anti-D and IgG anti-K, those coated with anti-D are better agglutinated by anti-IgG in antiglobulin tests. This may mean that the steric presentation of the IgG Fc pieces to anti-IgG differs between anti-D and anti-K. However, in a very large study, Dankbar et al. (43) tested 195 examples of anti-K by saline-IAT and by LISS-IAT. They showed that 189 of the antibodies reacted by both methods, two reacted by saline to IAT but not by LISS to IAT, while four reacted by LISS-IAT but not by saline-IAT. As the authors (43) pointed out, there is no single serological method that will detect all antibodies. Their data certainly seemed to show that LISS-IAT is as reliable as other methods for the detection of anti-K. Indeed, since 1986 when this study was reported, the use of methods based on low ionic strength (that include PEG and Polybrene methods, see below) has become widespread. As far as we are aware, there has been no increase in the number of transfusion reactions caused by anti-K that were not detected in routine tests.

Many workers who use tests based on low ionic strength claim to do so because of the increase in sensitivity of such tests over those performed at normal ionic strength. In fact this is not strictly accurate. Using the then newly introduced enzyme-linked antiglobulin test (ELAT)(44), Leikola and Perkins (13) measured the uptake of IgG antibodies by red cells at normal and reduced ionic strength. With anti-D, anti-Fy^a and anti-Jk^a approximately the same amount of IgG was bound in 10 minutes at low ionic strength as was bound in 60 minutes at normal ionic strength. After 10 minutes incubation in LISS, no appreciable increase in binding occurred. In other words, antibody binding at low ionic strength is much faster than at normal ionic strength but the total amount of antibody eventually bound is not appreciably different. In the same study (13) it was shown that the rate of binding of IgG anti-A, anti-Le^b and anti-IgG to IgG-coated red cells was not increased at low ionic strength. When papain-treated red cells were used, no increase in the rate of binding of anti-D at low ionic strength occurred. It was this study that also showed that albumin does not enhance the first stage of the hemagglutination reaction, i.e. antibody-uptake.

3. Tests using Polybrene

Polybrene is hexadimethrine bromide, a quaternary ammonium polymer. The principle of the manual test in which it is used (45) is that antibody uptake occurs at low ionic strength in the first stage, Polybrene is added in the second stage to prompt red cell aggregation then, in the third stage, the non-specific aggregation is dispersed with sodium citrate solution. If antibody-binding occurred in the first stage, specific antibody cross-linking occurs in the second and unlike the Polybrene-induced non-specific aggregation, is not dispersed in the third stage. Since the amount of low ionic strength medium used in the first stage is large, the antibody-uptake (first stage) of the test is completed in one minute. If agglutination is not seen at the end of the third stage, the test may be continued to an antiglobulin test reading. Initial reports on the Polybrene-IAT method specified that the tests should be read with anti-IgG since the anti-C3 component in a polyspecific antiglobulin reagent caused unwanted and clinically irrelevant positive reactions. While anti-IgG seems eminently suitable for use in the test, many workers have now used broad spectrum antiglobulin reagents to read the tests without experiencing excessive difficulties.

After the test was introduced, a number of reports appeared that either described the use of the Polybrene method in a routine setting (43-48) or documented the existence of antibodies detectable by this method but not by others (49-51). In our study (52) on 10,000 samples that had no antibodies demonstrable by LISS-IAT, in which we found 36 antibodies reactive with ficin-treated red cells (see below), we showed that of the 31 available for testing in Polybrene, 11 reacted. With regard to the detection of antibodies by some sensitive methods, that are not detected by others, readers are reminded of the admonition about sensitivity and relevance that appears earlier in this Chapter. Perhaps not surprisingly, since antibody uptake is potentiated in a low ionic strength milieu, the Polybrene-IAT method has been said not always to be efficient in the detection of anti-K (48,53).

4. Tests Using Polyethylene Glycol (PEG)

In 1987, Nance and Garratty (54) described the use of polyethylene glycol (PEG) as a potentiator of blood group antigen-antibody reactions. PEG is a water-soluble linear polymer of ethylene glycol that affects the anti-body-uptake stage of the hemagglutination reaction. When the polymers are added to the test system, steric exclusion of water molecules in the diluent (55, see also Chapter 2) occurs so that antigens and antibody molecules come into close proximity; the rate and amount of red cell-antibody collisions and hence antibody binding, increase. In the test, PEG is added to the serum-cell mixtures that, after a suitable incubation period, are washed and read with antiglobulin serum. The PEG-IAT is similar to the Polybrene-IAT in that reading with anti-IgG is recommended, the methods differ in that no reading for agglutination before the IAT is used in the PEG method. The low ionic strength feature of the PEG method is achieved when a volume of PEG greater than the volume of serum used is added to the test.

After introduction of the PEG method, a number of studies (56-59) confirmed its suitability as a routine method for antibody detection and identification. In our study (52) on the 36 enzyme-active, LISS-IAT-negative antibodies, 33 were available for testing by PEG-IAT, 12 of them reacted. Thus from our study, the PEG and Polybrene methods looked very similar in sensitivity (12 of 33 (36.4%) detected in PEG, 11 of 31 (35.5%) detected in Polybrene, the different methods detected different antibodies). Similar conclusions were reached by others (60) although in the initial report PEG-IAT appeared more sensitive than Polybrene-IAT (54). As far as we have been able to determine no difficulties in detecting anti-K using the PEG method have been reported.

In July of 1991 the PEG-IAT procedure was adopted as the routine method in the Transfusion Service of the Duke University Medical Center. Since we perform some 40,000 to 42,000 antibody screening and identification tests and transfuse between 35,000 and 40,000 units of red blood cells each year, we gain a great deal of experience with any new technique, very quickly. A number of points gleaned from this experience are worth documenting. First, when the procedure was introduced some difficulties accrued because the cell-serum-PEG mixtures were not adequately mixed when the tests were first set up (20% PEG is quite viscous). Based on a suggestion from Ron Roy (61) in St. John, New Brunswick, we ran parallel tests with a 20% PEG solution (as specified (54) in the original method) and a 15% solution. As Roy (61) had found, we saw no loss of sensitivity and found the tests easier to set up. Second, the use of PEG in antibody screening enabled us to abandon direct antiglobulin tests on new samples from recently transfused (within the last 15 days) patients. Earlier, Combs and Telen (62) had shown that in this setting PEG detected antibodies in eluates that were not demonstrable in serum, using a LISS-IAT method. However, when we ran parallel tests on eluates and sera from these patients using PEG in all studies, we found no antibodies in the eluates that were not also demonstrable in the posttrans-fusion sera. Thus our routine became to screen the sera by PEG-IAT and to eliminate DATs in these patients. In the last four years we have seen no evidence that we have missed an antibody formed in a recently transfused patient. Third, we have experienced some difficulties after reading PEG-IATs in that the antibody-coated (Coombs control) cells were not agglutinated. This is particularly prone to occur in patients with abnormal serum protein levels. The solution used at present is to set up the tests again then hand wash them. We are currently investigating the use of cell washers from different manufacturers to see if one (or some) of them injects wash saline with sufficient force, thoroughly to mix (and thus remove) the viscous PEG-serum mixture. It is of note that in spite of the extra work involved in repeating antibody screening tests when the control cells failed to react, there were very few complaints from the technologists. It seems they accepted the extra work as a worthwhile trade-off for not having to check to see which patients had recently been transfused, then perform DATs on all such samples and eluates on some.

5. Tests Using Proteolytic Enzymes

In 1947, Morton and Pickles (63) showed that two enzyme solutions, one extracted from cultures of *Vibrio cholera* and the other, trypsin from hog's stomach, could be used to enhance some agglutination reactions. Addition of enzyme to the cell-serum mixture, or pretreatment of the red cells with the enzyme, resulted in agglutination of those red cells by some antibodies that otherwise bound to but did not agglutinate the cells. Since that time a number of other proteinases (enzymes that specifically cleave proteins) have been found to be somewhat more useful, namely: papain from papayas (64); ficin from figs (65); bromelin from pineapples (66); and pronase from *Streptomyces griseus* culture supernatants (67). Comparative studies (68,69) have shown very clearly that pretreatment of red cells with the enzyme results in a much more sensitive method than simple addition of enzyme to the tests. Enzyme methods are very sensitive for the detection of some antibodies, for example those of the Rh system, but must be used as adjunct and replacement procedures in serological studies, since some antigens (see below) are no longer detectable on properly enzyme-treated red cells.

There are multiple effects of treating red cells with proteinases that contribute to the sensitivity of test systems using such cells. First, the enzymes cleave and release portions of a series of glycoproteins from the red cell membrane. Since most of these glycoproteins carry N-acetyl-neuraminic acid (NeuAc) that is the major con-tributor to the red cell membrane's negative charge, that charge and hence the zeta potential (see Chapter 2) is reduced when red cells are treated with proteinases. Second, the same glycoproteins that carry NeuNAc attract water and comprise the major mechanism of hydration of the red cell membrane. Once portions of the glycoproteins are removed, different red cells are obliged to share water molecules and thus approach each other more closely. Again as discussed in Chapter 2, this change also enhances agglutination by enabling small (IgG) antibody molecules to span the gap between the cells. Third and perhaps just as important as the two physicochemical changes described above, cleavage of portions of membrane glycoproteins allows some antibody molecules better access to their antigens. For example, red cells carry in the order of 1×10^6 copies of glycophorin A (70-72) the glycoprotein that carries M, N and some other MN system antigens. These copies extend out from the red cell membrane and must surely block the approach of some antibodies, such as those of the Rh system, that define antigens situated at or very close to the outer leaflet of the membrane (73-77). When red cells are treated with a proteinase, large portions of the million copies of glycophorin A are removed. Thus it would be expected that the steric presentation of Rh antigens to their antibodies would result in easier access of those antibodies to the antigens. Such a suggestion correlates well with the finding that many Rh system antibodies react better with enzyme-treated red cells than by any other method (52, and see below).

The sites at which various enzymes cleave proteins are listed in table 3-2, the information in that table is extracted from a review by Rolih (78) that should be consulted for references to reports of the original findings on enzyme substrate specificities. From looking at the multiple cleavage sites listed in table 3-2 it may initially appear that every protein structure on the red cell membrane should be cleaved when red cells are proteinase-treated. As most workers will be aware, this is not the case. The reason is that an enzyme is able to cleave a protein only when the appropriate site is accessible to the enzyme. The way in which proteins bearing blood group antigens are folded, in situ, often results in the potential cleavage site being protected from the enzyme's actions. A classic example is the fact that the S and s antigens are not affected when intact red cells are treated with trypsin (79). Once glycophorin B, the red cell membrane component that carries S and s (80,81) is isolated from the red cell membrane, it has a number of sites now accessible to trypsin (72,82,83). Availability of enzyme cleavage sites is reflected by the sensitivity or resistance of various red cell antigens to different proteinases. Table 3-3 includes data culled from references 63-67, 79 and 84-117 and lists which antigens are denatured (or removed)

TABLE 3-2 Sites at Which Some Proteinases Effect Cleavage (from 78)

Enzyme	Substrate
Trypsin	Arginine, Lysine
Ficin	Arginine, Lysine, Glutamine, Tyrosine, Glycine, Asparagine, Leucine, Valine
Papain	Alpha-amino substituted Arginine, Lysine, Glutamine, Tyrosine, Glycine, Histidine
Bromelin	Arginine, Lysine, Tyrosine, Glycine, Serine, Phenylalanine
Pronase	Tyrosine, Glycine, Leucine, Valine, Alanine, Isoleucine, Tryptophan, Phenylalanine

by which enzymes. It should be remembered that the data in table 3-3 come from direct tests (adsorption and elution studies were not always performed) and relate to the treatment of intact red cells. For the sake of convenience, the actions of aminoethylisothiouronium bromide (AET) that are discussed below, are also listed in table 3-3. References to those observations are 118-126.

As documented in the footnotes to table 3-3, different studies on the enzyme sensitivity of red cell antigens have sometimes reached different conclusions. There are a variety of reasons for this, some of which are technical in nature. First, strength of the enzyme solution used will directly affect the results. For many years for immunohematological studies, enzyme solutions were prepared on a weight/volume basis. Since not all lots of dry enzyme powder have the same amount of enzyme activity per given weight, comparative studies using like-percentage enzyme solutions sometimes, in fact, used preparations that contained different units of enzyme activity. This problem can be overcome by performing assays on enzyme solutions to standardize their level of activity (127-133). Second, the pH and ionic strength of the enzyme solution and the time and temperature used for the treatment of red cells, will all affect the degree of modification of the cells (134-136). Any time that an enzyme preparation is used to treat red cells it is incumbent on the user to ensure that the optimal conditions for the enzyme's function are used. Failure to do so may well result in different to expected modification of the red cells.

As will be apparent from what has been written in this section thus far, the use of proteinase-treated red cells provides a very sensitive method for the detection of some blood group antibodies. Both the sensitivity of the methods and the fact that certain blood group antigens are denatured by proteinase treatment of red cells, can be used to considerable advantage in antibody identification, see Chapter 35. However, enzyme tests are not suitable for routine antibody screening. First, because some antigens are destroyed, some antibodies will not be detected. Second, because enzyme-treated red cells react with clinically benign autoantibodies that are not detected by other methods, routine use of such cells results in far too many investigations that are of no benefit to the patients. In our study (52) on 10,000 samples, we found 216 (2.16%) that contained benign autoantibodies and another 77 (0.77%) that contained antibodies too weak to identify, that may well have been additional examples of benign autoantibodies. In other words, if enzyme-treated red cells are used in routine antibody screening, it can be anticipated that three of every 100 samples tested will have to be fully investigated (including autoadsorption tests) without any useful information being generated. Third, our study (52) also showed that some specific antibodies that react by enzyme but not by LISS-IAT methods are also clinically benign. In all we found 19 patients with Rh antibodies who, among them, had received 32 units of antigen-positive blood before the "enzyme-only" antibody was detected in the retrospective study. Among those 19 patients one had a delayed transfusion reaction, the other 18 had neither a transfusion reaction nor a secondary immune response following transfusion of the antigen-positive blood. The claim made earlier that enzyme-treated red cells provide the most sensitive method for the detection of Rh antibodies may be disputed by some advocates of the Polybrene and PEG methods. However, of the 29 "enzyme-positive, LISS-IAT-negative" Rh antibodies we found, 16 were non-reactive in Polybrene and 16 (not all the same antibodies) were non-reactive in PEG. As already discussed, the fact that enzyme techniques detected more antibodies does not, automatically, make them "better". Indeed, in our 10,000 patients, detection of 35 of the 36 antibodies was of no benefit to the patient concerned. From all this it can be concluded that the true value of enzyme techniques is in specialized situations such as when the patient has formed multiple antibodies, some of which are defying identification (see Chapter 35), when the patient has experienced a clinical reaction to transfusion and other test methods have been non-informative, or when investigational studies for weak antigen expression are being conducted. When enzyme treated red cells are used and the most sensitive system possible is required, the final reading can be by IAT. However, careful control of the antiglobulin reagent used is essential since some reagents will agglutinate enzyme-treated red cells that are not coated with antibody.

It has been claimed (137) that the routine use of enzyme-treated red cells in prenatal serology is justified since such tests detect (particularly Rh) antibodies that might cause hemolytic disease of the newborn, earlier in pregnancy than would otherwise be the case. However,

TABLE 3-3 Antigen Reactivity on Proteinase and AET Treated Red Cells

Antigens	T	F	P	B	C	AET
M, N	0	0	0	0	0	+
S, s	+	0[1]	0[1]			+
En^{a}TS	0	0	0			+
En^{a}FS	+	0	0			+
En^{a}FR	+	+	+			+
Fy^a , Fy^b, Fy6		0	0	0	0	+
Fy3, Fy4		+	+	+	+	+
Xg^a	0	0	0			+
Lu^a, Lu^b	V	V	V			0
Lu-H.I.[2]	0	0	V[3]		0	0
K	See footnote 4					0
Yt^a, Yt^b	+	V	V	V	0	0
LW^a, LW^b, see [5]	+		+		W	0
Ch, Rg	0	0	0	0	0	+
Ge2	0		0		W	+
Ge3	0		+		+	+
Ge4	0		0		+	+
In^a, In^b	0	0	0	0	0	0
Cromer System[6]	+		+		0	W
JMH	0	0	0	0	0	0

T = Trypsin; F = Ficin; P = Papain; B = Bromelin; C = Chymotrypsin
O = Antigen no longer demonstrable. However, very potent antibodies may still react weakly with vestige of antigen remaining
+ = Antigen unchanged
W = Antigen expression weakened
V = Variable results reported in the literature, i.e. some report antigen denaturation, others report antigen unchanged
Blank spaces = No definitive information

1. Must use proteinases under optimal conditions to cleave S and s
2. Lu-H.I = High incidence Lutheran system antigens, e.g. Lu3, Lu4, Lu5, etc.
3. Lu3, Lu4, Lu5, Lu6, Lu12, Lu13 said to survive papain treatment, Lu8 said to be denatured, Lu17 variable results
4. Sequential treatment with trypsin then chymotrypsin denatures K, k and Kp^b and either weakens or denatures other Kell system antigens. All antigens of the system denatured by AET
5. Some but not all workers have found that pronase denatures LW system antigens
6. Includes Cr^a, Tc^a, Dr^a, Es^a, IFC, WES^b and UMC

this claim has been vigorously disputed (138-140). First, we have never seen a case of clinical HDN caused by an "enzyme-only" antibody present at term. Second, when such antibodies were present, most infants had a negative DAT at birth. Third, if an antibody is going to cause clinical HDN it will be detectable, well before the end of pregnancy, by far less sensitive methods. In other words, presence of an "enzyme-only" antibody does not mandate clinical intervention in the pregnancy meaning that early knowledge of maternal immunization is of no benefit to the mother or the fetus.

The Gel Test

In 1990, Lapierre et al. (141) introduced a rather different test for immunohematological studies. In this method very small volumes of cells and serum are mixed in a reservoir at the top of a narrow microtube that contains any one of a number of dextran gels (Sephadex G100, Sephadex G200, Sephacryl S2000, all from Pharmacia Fine Chemicals, Uppsala, Sweden). The microtubes with the integral reservoirs are supplied in card form (DiaMed, AG, Switzerland). After a suitable incubation period the cards containing the tests are spun in a centrifuge in which the axis of the tube is strictly in line with the direction of the centrifugal force. The red cells but not the medium in which they are suspended, enter the gel column. Agglutinated red cells are trapped at the top of the gel, unagglutinated red cells form a pellet at the bottom of the microtube.

The system can be modified for different types of tests. For simple agglutination studies, e.g. ABO typing, a neutral gel is used, the antibody and red cells are allowed to react in the reservoir before centrifugation. This version of the test can be modified in a number of ways. As examples, the test cells can be suspended in a low ionic strength medium, or an enzyme solution can be added to the cells and serum before incubation begins. For antigen typing studies, the antibody can be incorporated in to the gel (141,148). The red cells can be suspended in LISS or an enzyme can be added. As the cells are centrifuged through the gel plus antibody, those that are antigen positive will be agglutinated and trapped in the upper portion of the gel, those that are antigen negative will form a pellet in the bottom of the microtube. For many of the antigen typing tests the antibody in the gel has been calibrated to react with enzyme-treated cells, clearly if the commercially prepared cards are used, the manufacturer's directions must be followed. For the indirect antiglobulin test, the cells, serum and/or LISS and/or enzyme are incubated in the reservoir. This time the gel contains antiglobulin reagent (in the original report (141) it was stated that many polyvalent antiglobulin reagents are unsuitable, presumably few problems are encountered if anti-IgG is used). Because, during centrifugation, the red cells but not the suspending fluid pass through the gel, the red cells do not have to be washed before coming into contact with the antiglobulin reagent. For the direct antiglobulin test, the patient's red cells are simply centrifuged through the gel.

Naturally when a test as different as the gel test is introduced, numerous workers conduct (and attempt to publish) evaluation and comparison studies. We have been told (but have not verified) that over 400 publications about the gel test have already appeared. Many of these must surely have been abstracts, some that we have seen make the statement already decried in this chapter that "it detects more antibodies so it must be better". As stated, if the additional antibodies detected are clinically relevant there is some merit in the conclusion; a simple increase in the number of antibodies found does not automatically mean that the test is better. Among the reports we have seen, some (141-144) have found the gel-IAT to be more sensitive than other methods while others (145-147) have found it marginally, but perhaps not significantly, less sensitive. Pinkerton et al. (147) made the highly pertinent observation that comparative studies will

result in different conclusions being drawn, based on the specifics of the method to which the gel test is compared. In their own study in which the gel-IAT appeared slightly less sensitive than a saline-IAT, they report that in their saline-IAT method they used a 120:1 to 200:1 ratio of serum to red cells. This is considerably higher than that used by others that is often in the range of 40:1. Not surprisingly, these authors (147) report that the use of albumin or LISS has not provided added sensitivity over the saline-IAT method as performed in their service.

Aside from considerations of sensitivity and relevance, the gel test system offers some advantages over other systems. First, it is easy to use and can be performed by persons with little training or theoretical knowledge about the blood groups. Second, since no cell washing before IATs is required, time is saved and the chance of aerosol contamination from infected samples is reduced. Third, the test cards can be kept (for at least 24 hours) after the tests are completed and can be reviewed by senior staff at a later time. Fourth, copies of the completed cards can be made on xerographic equipment (an enterprising, off-site reference laboratory could copy the actual results then FAX them to the submitting laboratory within minutes of completing of the tests) for permanent records. Fifth, because no washing is required, low affinity allo and autoantibodies may be better detected by the gel test than by other methods. Sixth, the gel test clearly lends itself to automation in both operating and reading features. Against these advantages must be weighed the facts that under normal working conditions the gel test detects some clinically irrelevant antibodies such as those directed against M, N, P_1, Le^b, etc. Second, if purchased in kit form the test is almost certain to cost more per test than conventional tube methods. It will be interesting to see if blood bank managers and directors are prepared to lower their operating costs by replacing skilled technologists with less highly trained persons (with considerably lower salaries) to a degree that will offset the presumed higher costs incurred by routine use of gel tests.

Solid Phase Testing

An alternative method to hemagglutination studies involves a system in which a known antibody or known antigens are immobilized on a solid matrix (149-153). The unknown sample is then applied to the immobilized reactant and the test is read by adherence.

Originally, for red cell ABO typing, monoclonal or affinity-purified anti-A and anti-B were bound to the test plates by simple adsorption of antibody (150) or via the use of poly-D-lysine (151). Antibody binding was considerably facilitated if the plates were first coated with A or B-containing saliva, as appropriate (154). For the test, red cells were added to the plate that was allowed to stand briefly and was then centrifuged. In a positive reaction the cells spread over the surface of the well since they adhered to the immobilized antibody. In a negative reaction there was no adherence and the cells formed a small button in the center of the well when the plates were centrifuged. Originally, for reverse typing, A and B cells were immobilized in the wells and were then hemolyzed by the addition of water. The hemoglobin was washed away leaving colorless immobilized A and B antigens attached to the matrix. The unknown serum was then added. If anti-A and/or anti-B were present they bound to the immobilized antigens on the plate. Excess serum was removed then A and B indicator cells, that were often enzyme-treated, were added to detect any anti-A or anti-B bound from the unknown serum.

For D typing a somewhat similar system was used. First, the wells were coated with affinity-purified anti-human IgG. Anti-D that had been isolated from other antibodies present in the starting serum by adsorption-elution, was then added and was immobilized by the anti-IgG. When the test cells were added positive and negative reactions were differentiated by the spread or button pattern described above.

Studies using these original methods generated some excellent results (155-159). For example, in ABO typing tests on more than 2000 samples, the results showed 99.6% concordance with those from conventional tests (158). The results of the solid phase tests were read in an automated system (see below) and the few discrepancies encountered were easily resolved by visual examination of the solid phase plates. In the same study it was shown that some samples that would have been classed as D^u from the results of conventional tests, were directly detected as D+ in the solid phase tests.

Some recent advances in development of the solid phase technology have made the system even more reliable. First, it was found (160) that chemical coupling of red cells to the matrix provided a more robust system than the use of passively adsorbed antibodies or the use of poly-D-lysine. This was an important advance since the test plates are often prepared commercially and then used in routine blood bank situations where they may not always be subjected to the same tender loving care afforded them in a research and development environment. Second, it was shown that the antibodies used in ABO and D typing can be better immobilized by attaching them to dried red cells already coupled to the plate, than by attaching the antibodies themselves to the plate. Thus in the methods described by Sinor (160) ABO and D typing plates are prepared by immobilizing A_1, B and D+ red cells to chemically modified U-bottom stripwells. The cells are then exposed to the appropriate antibody

and the sensitized red cell monolayers are then dried. The unknown test cells are added to the prepared plates and the tests are read as described above.

For reverse ABO typing and antibody screening tests, similar modifications are now used (160). A_1, B and group O screening cell monolayers are prepared and dried. The test serum is added and if antibodies to any of the immobilized antigens are present, they attach to the monolayer. The tests are read by the addition of group A_1B red cells that are coated with anti-IgG. If the unknown serum contained anti-A or anti-B, that (or those) antibodies will now be bound to the monolayer of dried A_1 and B cells and will, in turn, bind the A_1B indicator cells, a positive reaction will result. If the unknown serum contained an IgG antibody directed against an antigen on the dried monolayer of antibody screening cells, that IgG antibody will bind the indicator cells because they are coated with anti-IgG. Again, a positive reaction will be seen. It has been reported (160-164) that the solid phase antibody screening method is at least as sensitive as other currently used methods. Again, there is little information on the clinical significance of antibodies detected only by the solid phase method.

Clearly solid phase tests are highly suited for automated reading by passing a light beam through the well at a point at which it will not be interrupted by the button of cells in a negative test, but will be dispersed by the layer of red cells spread across the well in a positive test.

Because this section has dealt with the principles of solid phase tests that are likely to be readily available to readers, it has not included descriptions of a number of tests that are performed in tubes but read by a solid phase method or those that use substrate hydrolysis in the final reading for quantitative assays (165-167). A solid phase dipstick test for ABO red cell typing has also been described (168).

A Method Using Electrode Sensors

Following many physicochemical reactions, including the complexing of an antibody with its antigen, there is a change in charge at the site of the interaction. If a suitably sensitive sensor is in contact with one (or both) of the reactants, the change in charge can be measured within seconds (169-175). By setting predetermined levels of change to differentiate between a positive and a negative reaction, sensor readings in millivolt or microvolt amounts can be scanned through a logic table and can be interpreted. Moulds (176) has described how this principle might be applied in blood grouping tests including, presumably, antibody-screening and compatibility tests where two unknowns are used. A huge advantage of such technology, in addition to its speed, is that it would measure antibody uptake and would not be subject to all the variables involved in reading hemagglutination tests. Clearly, such technology would have to be automated with preset changes being interpreted as indicating a positive reaction or no reaction. From the description of the technology by Moulds (176) it is clear that it holds much promise but equally clear that many obstacles remain to be resolved before practical application of the method becomes a reality.

Flow Cytometry

Since relatively few blood banks can afford, or have access to a flow cytometer, only brief details will be given here. However, there is no doubt that flow cytometric studies have already contributed significantly in the field of immunohematology or that they can be expected to continue to do so at an ever increasing rate. In a flow cytometer, cells in suspension pass through a laser-beam light source in single file. As they pass the beam they cause light to scatter. If labeled with a fluorescent dye, attached to an antibody in many instances, the emitted light is a different color than the laser light. The selected color light can then be measured at a preselected wavelength and the amount converted to an electrical signal by light sensing devices. If more than one fluorescent dye is used, simultaneous measurements of more than one parameter can be made. In relatively short periods of time sufficient events occur that highly accurate results are generated. For example, in the detection of fetal cells in the maternal circulation, a very large number of cells can be examined so that even if the detection of fetal cells is a rare event, sufficient numbers will be seen for the size of the fetal-maternal hemorrhage accurately to be estimated. If the flow cytometer is equipped with a cell sorter, different populations of cells can be separated and collected for further analysis. Some applications of the flow cytometer in immunohematology are listed (with references) in table 3-4. Of particular interest to blood groupers are the extraordinary results obtained in antigen dosage studies designed to determine zygosity in the red cell donors. The results of these studies have clearly demonstrated that manual titration studies that were used before the flow cytometer became available, can sometimes give quite misleading results (199).

Readers wishing to learn more about flow cytometry are referred to the excellent reviews of Nance (202), Garratty (211) and Freedman and Lazarus (181).

Automated Blood Grouping

Because so many tests in the blood bank rely on the hemagglutination reaction as the end point and because automated reading of such reactions has proved difficult, the blood bank is perhaps the last of the clinical laboratories to convert to automated systems. However, over the years progress has been made and automated testing systems are gradually being introduced.

The greatest successes in the use of automated systems in immunohematology have come from the introduction of machines that perform mass typing tests on samples from blood donors. The Technicon Autogrouper reads tests via an optical density system, correlates results with bar code labels on the samples and feeds data into a computer where the results are interpreted. The Kontron Groupamatic system is available in three sizes

TABLE 3-4 Some Applications of Flow Cytometry in Immunohematology

Application	References
1. Detection and quantitation of cell-bound proteins, particularly IgG, and particularly in patients with autoimmune disorders	177-181
2. Quantitation of antigen sites	182-192
3. Detection of variant red cell membrane components and calculation of mutation rates	193-198
4. Measurement of antigen dose and zygosity studies	199-202
5. Detection of minor cell populations	
a) Investigation of transfusion reactions	203-205
b) Chimeric state after bone marrow transplantation	206
c) In vivo red cell survival studies	184, 207-211
d) Detection and quantitation of maternal-fetal hemorrhage	212-218
e) Detection and quantitation of maternal-fetal hemorrhage (in mice)	219
6. Detection or non-detection of "red cell" antigens on other cells	220

that handle 340, 180 or 240, and 55 samples an hour, respectively. The samples are tested in individual cups, again the system is fully automated to identify samples, interpret tests and print out results. The Olympus ProGroup systems are also fully automated, tests are performed in microtiter trays and read in a manner similar to that described above for solid phase tests. The Olympus machines are supplied in different sizes so that the user may select a machine most suitable for the volume of samples to be handled. Other systems that use microtiter trays include the Dynatech 220 Blood Grouping System, the Kontron Micro Groupamatic and the IBG Inverness System. The systems vary somewhat in their degree of automation, their reading system and their integral computers or interface capabilities.

Most of the automated systems can be adjusted in terms of sensitivity. This has resulted in most of them being able to perform D typing in such a way that the indirect antiglobulin test for the D^u phenotype is not necessary. That is to say, sensitivity of D typing can be adjusted so that samples that might appear to be of the D^u phenotype in manual tests, are typed as D+ in the automated systems. Most of the automated systems will also perform antibody screening tests. It is a mistake to make these tests too sensitive when processing donor samples (221, 222), particularly since the passive transfer of most antibodies from donor to patient is not a significant problem in transfusion.

Automation in the hospital transfusion service lags somewhat behind automation in donor processing centers. This often reflects the reluctance of some workers to perform testing in batches although such testing can be successfully instituted in large and/or centralized testing services (223). In addition to some of the systems mentioned above that can be used in a hospital transfusion service, other applicable systems are the Gamma Biologicals Micro V System (224) and the same company's Standardized Test System-Microtear. Virtually all the solid phase test systems mentioned in the earlier section are available from Immucor. The Biotest SolidScreen system is only partially automated. Readers wishing to obtain additional details about automated test systems should read Whitrow and Ross (225) and should certainly spend a considerable amount of time at the trade show at meetings of the American Association of Blood Banks or the British Blood Transfusion Society. Presumably, by the time this book is published, considerable advances in the development of automated systems will have been made.

Tests in Microtiter Trays, Capillary Tubes and Using Applicator Sticks

As already mentioned, many solid phase and auto-

mated methods use microtiter trays. Manual tests can also be performed in such trays, the major advantage of their use is that they are very economical in the use of reagents. The tests can be performed in V (226, 227) or U (228-231) bottomed well trays. When V bottomed well trays are used, a very light cell suspension (1/32 of 1%, that looks to the naked eye like saline) is used and reading is accomplished by inclining the trays at the end of the test (following incubation and centrifugation or following washing and the addition of antiglobulin serum). Negative tests are seen as a stream of cells running from the bottom of the well. Positive tests usually involve one clump of cells that may or may not fall out of the bottom of the V well. In U bottom well trays that have become somewhat more popular, heavier cell suspensions are used and results are read by viewing the settling patterns or by looking for agglutination following gentle agitation. In both types of tray, economy in the use of serum is possible since much higher than normal dilutions of typing sera can satisfactorily be used. For example, using V bottomed trays, we (232) typed 1000 samples for Hu and He, using less than 2 ml of each antibody.

Another method that is highly economical in the use of reagents involves the use of capillary tubes (233-240). In this method, serum is allowed to run into about one third of the length of a small capillary tube, an approximately equal volume of a heavy cell suspension (20-30%) or a much smaller volume of packed cells is allowed to run into the same capillary with no air space between the serum and cells. The capillary tube is then sealed and inclined at an angle of 60° so that the cells run through the serum. Results are read at any time up to 15 minutes following inclination of the tubes. The tubes are inverted for the cells to run through the serum again if necessary. Positive tests show beads of agglutinated cells down the length of the capillary while negatives appear as thin unbroken lines of cells down the center of the tube. The method uses only about 0.005 ml of serum per test (239-241) and can be modified for use with albumin, enzymes or antiglobulin serum (239-243). Another advantage of the method is that in the hands of experts, such as the workers in Winnipeg (244-247) the method is semi-quantitative. In addition to being read for positive or negative, the length of time required for development of a visible positive test can be recorded. With regularly used typing reagents or in comparative studies, a longer than normal time required for the test to become positive is often an indication that the antigen involved is present in a weaker than normal form. As a single example, the depression of D on Tar+ (Rh:40) red cells was not seen in tube tests using commercially prepared anti-D. It was noticed from the results of capillary tests using single donor anti-D with which the investigators were very familiar (246,247). Similarly, samples with increased levels of antigens can sometimes be identified because of the rapid development of agglutination.

Since both tests in microtiter plates and in capillary tubes use very small amounts of serum, they are particularly suited for use with antibodies in short supply and with expensive reagents. While the microtiter method is well worthwhile if large numbers of samples are to be typed at the same time, the capillary method, that requires some expertise and is better suited to workers with deft fingers than to those who tend to be clumsy, is perhaps more applicable for small numbers of occasional tests.

A rapid and useful test method is to put one or two drops of typing serum in a tube and to transfer cells directly from a clotted or unclotted sample by means of wooden applicator sticks. Enough cells should be transferred to make a final concentration, in the serum, equivalent to one drop of a 2-5% suspension but such is the excellence of most commercially available reagents that considerable latitude in the strength of the cell suspension will not prevent correct results from being obtained. Stick tests are usually spun and read after very brief incubation times (3-5 minutes). Negative results can be confirmed by allowing longer incubation after initial readings. Tests of this sort are of particular value in screening large numbers of bloods to find those that are, for example, c-negative or e-negative. While commercially-obtained human polyclonal Rh typing reagents work well in stick tests, it is possible that some monoclonal antibodies may not be as well suited for use by this method. This is because some monoclonal antibodies are more dependent on a correct pH in the test system than their human polyclonal counterparts. It is at least theoretically possible that the addition of unwashed cells plus the small amount of plasma or serum carried over, could produce an unfavorable pH in the test system.

Quantitation of Antibodies

The most common method used in a routine laboratory to estimate the strength of an antibody is to perform a titration. In this procedure, dilutions (usually doubling) of the serum are made and are then tested against appropriate red cells by a suitable method. The procedure has a number of drawbacks. First, unless considerable care is taken, serum carry-over occurs when the dilutions are made. Second, even if the dilutions are made in an accurate manner, different binding constants of antibodies of similar specificity in one serum, profoundly affect the results. Hughes-Jones (248) has shown that if two antibodies are present in the same quantity in a serum but with one having a ten times higher binding constant than the other, that antibody will react to a titer ten times greater than the other. At the routine practical level this

disadvantage may not be too serious since the object of the exercise is often to measure the maximum strength of any antibody present. Third, manual titrations are invariably read in a subjective manner, like other hemagglutination tests where the main objective is to distinguish between positive and negative.

For studies in which more exact antibody quantitation is required, more elegant methods have been devised. These include direct labeling of antibody with a radioisotope (249-252), measurement of bound antibody with a radiolabeled anti-IgG (252-254), use of the Technicon AutoAnalyzer (255-260) and immunoprecipitation (261). By using the AutoAnalyzer, antibody can be measured in terms of nanograms per ml (261,262), the whole system and hence the accuracy of the results can be validated by the use of reference standards (263,264). The enzyme-linked antiglobulin test (13, also see Chapter 6) can also be used for the quantitation of immunoglobulins or complement bound to red cells (265-267). However, for routine use in many blood banks and red cell reference laboratories, time and equipment constraints dictate that manual titrations will often be used. It must again be stressed that in order for useful data to be generated, impeccable technique and attention to detail are essential to exclude laboratory variables.

Titration End Point and Titer Scores

The titer of an antibody is correctly expressed as the reciprocal of the highest dilution of the antibody giving a 1+ reaction. Thus an antibody that gives greater than 1+ reactions at dilutions up to 1 in 8, a 1+ reaction a dilution of 1 in 16 and weaker than 1+, then negative reactions at dilutions of 1 in 32 and greater, has a titer of 16 (not 1 in 16, that is a dilution; not 1:16, that is a ratio). As can be seen, reactions weaker than 1+ are ignored in determining the end point. Since there are now so many serological methods available, it is necessary to specify the method used in determining the titer.

An additional useful way of reporting titration results is to assign a numerical value to each positive reaction in the titration, the value being based on the strength of agglutination in each tube. In the original description (268) of this scoring system a 3 plus reaction scored 10, a 2 plus 8, a 1 plus 5, a (+) 3 and a weak reaction 2. In most laboratories in the U.S.A., the strongest grade of agglutination is recorded as 4 plus and this reaction can be assigned a score of 12. To determine the titration score of an antibody the scores assigned to each positive reaction are totaled. Titration scores are useful in comparative titrations using one antibody and different red cell samples and in comparing the reactions of different antibodies with the same cell sample. Titration scores measure not only the strength (titer) of an antibody but also its avidity. For example, an antibody with a titer of 256 will have a lower score if it reacts to a strength of 1+ at all dilutions while another antibody, with the same titer of 256, will give a much higher score if high concentrations of that antibody give 4 and 3+ reactions. Often, differences in strengths of antigens on red cells and differences in antibody activity can be more easily seen from titer scores than from titers. The scoring system that one of us (PDI) has used for many years is reproduced in table 3-5, it is almost identical to that described by Marsh (269) that has been adapted by many workers for individual readings. That is to say instead of the 4+ (strongest) to 1+ (weakest) reaction scale, many workers now use a 12 (strongest) to 2 (weakest) scale of reactions.

TABLE 3-5 Scoring System for use with Agglutination Reactions

Strength of Reaction	"Synonomous" Reading	Score Value
4	"Complete"	12
3½	4^W or 3^S	11
3		10
2½	3^W or 2^S	9
2		8
1½	2^W or 1^S	6
1		5
½	1^W or ± or (1)	3
Trace		2
0	Negative	0

Reading Titration Studies

In order to prevent over-reading and falsely high end points, some workers routinely read titrations from the greatest serum dilution (1 in 1024 or 1 in 512) back to the tubes containing the highest amount of serum (1 in 2 and 1 in 1). This effectively prevents carry-over of subjective reading just as use of separate pipettes prevents serum carry-over.

Workers who do not believe that it is difficult to perform titrations in an accurate and reproducible manner should try the following exercise. Set up the titration in the normal way then have a co-worker code the tubes so that they are totally out of sequence of serum dilutions. Now try to read the titration and put the tubes back into the correct sequence of serum dilutions, before the code is broken!

Adsorption

An antibody can be removed from serum by adsorp-

tion on to red cells. The serum containing the antibody is mixed with cells that carry the antigen against which the antibody is directed. By allowing the antigen-antibody complexes to form and then removing the red cells all antibody activity can be removed from a serum. Practical applications are mentioned in many chapters of this book. Briefly, adsorption techniques are of value in:

1. Separation of antibodies in sera containing several specificities.
2. Confirmation of antibody specificity.
3. Preparation of human polyclonal typing reagents.
4. Confirmation of the presence or absence of weak antigens on red cells.

Because the aim of an adsorption method is sometimes totally to remove antibody activity from a serum, a much higher cell:serum ratio is required than in agglutination tests. A good practical proportion is one volume of packed cells for each volume of serum to be adsorbed.

A question is often asked about the use of the words adsorption and absorption. Some workers believe that the antibody is absorbed on to red cells and that the serum from which the antibody has been removed can be described as having been adsorbed. However, sentence construction often results in either word apparently being correct or both being incorrect (depending on whether one believes the glass is half full or half empty). Accordingly, one of us (PDI) took the sage advice of Dr. Richard Rosenfield who, as editior of TRANSFUSION used adsorption exclusively, and now pretends that absorption does not exist.

Elution

Once an antibody has attached to red cells, either in vivo or in vitro, or to any other solid matrix, it can be recovered by a process called elution. The recovered antibody, in whatever fluid has been used to recover it, is called an eluate. Antibody elution is a valuable serological tool and can be applied to:

1. Identification of antibodies in sera containing mixtures of specificities.
2. Confirmation of antibody specificity.
3. Preparation of a typing reagent. If the only available example of an antibody is from a group O individual and group A cells are to be typed, the antibody can be adsorbed on to group O antigen-positive red cells and an eluate containing the required antibody but no anti-A, can be made.
4. Confirmation of the presence of weak antigens on red cell samples.

5. Identification of antibodies causing hemolytic disease of the newborn.
6. Identification of antibodies that have caused transfusion reactions.
7. Investigation of antibodies in patients with acquired hemolytic anemia.
8. Purification of antibodies to be used in biochemical studies. (e.g., immunoblotting - see Chapter 4).

Elution of an antibody requires that antigen-antibody complexes be disrupted so that intact, dissociated antibody molecules are obtained. Many methods that result in the elution of antibodies from red cells, hemolyze the red cells in the process.

A huge number of different elution methods have been devised. Judd (270) gives detailed instructions regarding 16 different methods. Generally speaking they can be divided into four major groups. First, those that effect the release from red cells of cold-reactive antibodies, or antibodies reactive across a broad range of temperatures. These techniques are particularly useful for the recovery of antibodies from the red cells of infants suffering from ABO HDN. Second, are elution methods that seem best suited for the recovery of warm-reactive, non-agglutinating IgG antibodies that are either alloimmune or autoimmune in nature. Third, are the elution procedures that free the antibody-coated red cells of much of the bound immunoglobulin but leave many of the cells intact for use in autoadsorption procedures. Fourth are methods, mentioned in Chapter 4, that cause the release of antibodies from a solid matrix, such as a staph protein A column, that are used in antibody purification procedures.

Since, as mentioned, full details of many elution methods have been summarized by Judd (270,271), this section will comment only on the practical suitability of various methods and some basic principles that apply. The heat elution (272) and freeze-thaw methods (273,274) are particularly useful for the recovery of cold-reactive antibodies from red cells. Thus they are of value in investigating cases of ABO HDN. In the heat elution method the increase of temperature reverses the exothermic reaction involved in the formation of antigen-antibody complexes and effects the release of bound antibody. In the freeze-thaw methods the formation of ice crystals alters both intra and extracellular osmolarity so that eventually the red cells shrink and hemolyze, releasing antibody as the complimentary of fit between antigen and antibody is lost. Sonication methods (275-277) are also said to be useful in this setting. The microwave method probably works similarly to the heat method, as described above. Ultrasound causes alterations of pressure within fluids, gas bubbles are formed and eventually implode. The shock waves created appear to cause antibody molecules to dissociate from their antigens.

Methods that use organic solvents such as ether (278-280), chloroform (281,282), xylene (283-286), or methylene chloride (287) are very useful for the recovery of IgG warm-reactive allo and autoantibodies from the red cells. There are probably several mechanisms involved that result in the efficiency of these elution methods. First, organic solvents probably disrupt the lipid bilayer of the cell membrane. Second, they probably alter the tertiary structure of antibody molecules and third, they reverse some of the attraction forces that hold antigens and antibodies together. Although elution methods that use organic solvents are highly efficient, they have fallen into disfavor in some laboratories since the solvents may be flammable and/or toxic and/or carcinogenic. Fortunately, there are other elution methods that are also efficient and well suited to routine use. A widely used technique is a modification (288) of an earlier-introduced (289) acid-digitonin method. At the acid pH at which this method is used, antigen and antibody both apparently become negatively charged and are thus forced apart by repulsive charges. There are a number of other methods (290-293) that similarly use an acid pH system to disrupt antigen-antibody bonding and include one (294) that is designed for the recovery of antibody from placental tissue, a valuable but frequently overlooked source of a large amount of antibody.

At least in the USA, it is common for workers to make eluates using commercially prepared kits. Some of these kits are extremely efficient and in spite of their cost may be cheaper to use in routine situations since their purchase obviates the technologist time required to prepare reagents to use with original methods. Sometimes the principle of the elution method involved when a complete kit is used, is known, there are often proprietary changes made from the published descriptions that have been found, by the manufacturer, to increase the efficiency of the method.

A number of comparative studies on the efficiency of different elution methods have been published (295-302) not all of them reached the same conclusions as to which methods were best. One of us (PDI) was gratified to see that the ether method, that he used almost all the time until ether was essentially banned from the clinical laboratory, was not bettered consistently by any other method.

Elution procedures described thus far have been primarily those designed to recover usable antibody from red cells. Consequently destruction of the red cells during the elution procedure is of no significant disadvantage although it often results in a hemoglobin-stained eluate. When autoadsorption studies are necessary on the serum of patients with a positive DAT, in order that any alloantibodies simultaneously present can be detected and identified (see Chapter 37), elution is undertaken with a somewhat different objective. That is to say, the aim is to remove sufficient (not necessarily all) antibody from the red cells that they can be used in autoadsorption of the patient's serum. Obviously, the aim is best accomplished by having intact red cells at the end of the elution step. Perhaps the first method introduced for this purpose was the brief heat technique in which the cells are heated for a sufficient time that some autoantibody elutes, while some red cells survive intact (303). This method was superseded by others that remove more autoantibody and cause less red cell hemolysis. Edwards et al. (304) described the use of chloroquine disphosphate that, it is believed, neutralizes charged groups on amino acids that determine the tertiary structure of antibody molecules and hence causes antibody dissociation without red cell destruction. Branch and Petz (305) described the use of ZZAP, a mixture of activated papain and dithiothreitol that degrades red cell bound IgG again without destruction of the red cells. Unlike chloroquine disphosphate, ZZAP treatment of red cells destroys all antigens of the Kell system and those sensitive to proteinases (see table 3-3). Hanfland (306) described a method in which IgG coated red cells are subjected to discontinuous, combined density and pH gradient centrifugation. While the Hanfland (306) method may remove more autoantibody than either chloroquine disphosphate or ZZAP treatment of red cells, it is somewhat fussy in its requirements. Measured volumes, chilled pipettes and tubes, angle racks, etc., are required. The method resisted our (307) attempts to turn it into the type of "slop-bucket" technique with which blood bankers are familiar. Each deviation from the impeccable technique of Peter Hanfland, who is a biochemist with finely developed impeccable technique, reduced the efficiency of the method.

Thus, most workers wishing to remove autoantibodies from red cells so that the cells can be used for autoadsorption, rely on the chloroquine diphosphate (304) or ZZAP (305) method. Use of these techniques is discussed again in Chapter 37. As mentioned, elution of antibodies from affinity columns and the like, is discussed in Chapter 4.

Treatment of Red Cells with 2-Aminoethylisothiouronium Bromide (AET)

For the sake of convenience, table 3-3 listed those red cells antigens that are denatured when red cells are treated with AET. At an alkaline pH, the condition in which it is used to treat red cells, AET is rapidly converted to 2-mercaptoethyl guanidine, a sulphydryl compound (308,309). Both AET and ZZAP treatment destroy all Kell system antigens (Kx remains but is not a Kell system antigen, see Chapter 18) meaning that "artificial

K_o red cells" can be prepared to use in antibody identification studies. While such cells are extremely useful it must be remembered that unlike the natural (genetic) K_o cells, AET and ZZAP-treated red cells lack certain other high incidence blood group antigens (119-126 and see table 3-3). This does not detract from the use of AET-treated cells when working with Kell system allo or autoantibodies.

Separation of Two Cell Populations in a Single Patient

Sometimes, after a patient has been transfused and when the pretransfusion blood sample has been used, it becomes necessary to separate the patient's cells from those that were transfused. Such an exercise permits determination of the patient's phenotype. Somewhat similarly, it is sometimes useful to estimate the percentage of transfused red cells in a mixture of cells to gain an idea as to how well the transfused cells are surviving. On other occasions, such as when natural chimerism or artificial chimerism following a bone marrow transplant is suspected, it is useful to be able to demonstrate two distinct red cell populations. Most methods for the separation (or demonstration) of a two cell population rely on differences in blood group antigen composition between the two. The simplest, though perhaps least efficient method is differential agglutination. If, for example, the patient's red cells are M+ N- and the transfused cells are M+ N+, anti-N can be used to try to agglutinate the transfused cells and leave the patient's cells unagglutinated. Conversely, an attempt can be made to agglutinate the patient's cells and estimate the survival of the transfused cells from the number left unagglutinated. In the example given different antibodies would be required since the patient's and transfused cells are M+. The decision as to whether the patient's or the transfused cells will be the target of the agglutinating antibody used will depend on what is known about the phenotypes of the two populations, the availability of suitable agglutinating antibodies and the reason that separation is required i.e. to phenotype the patient's cells or to determine the survival of the transfused cells. There are a number of methods that have been described for the separation of two cell populations by simple agglutination (310-314), in antiglobulin tests (315), in agglutination tests on radiolabeled red cells (316), in the AutoAnalyzer (317-319) and on a tea plate (320).

As would be expected, as immunohematological techniques have been refined, so have methods for the detection of mixed cell populations. From what has been written above, it will be clear that the flow cytometer is ideally suited for this purpose (184, 203-219). For workers with access to antibodies but not to a flow cytometer, accurate modern methods are still available. For example, in a suspected chimera with a believed minor population of C+ E+ K+ cells in her major C- E- K- population, we (321) incubated the cells with IgG anti-C, anti-E or anti-K then passed them over a staph protein A column. The cells coated with IgG were retained in the column and were later recovered by elution, while the non-antibody coated cells passed through the column. Not only was excellent separation of the two populations accomplished, it could be seen to be happening as the top of the column changed color as the IgG-coated red cells were bound.

Using differential agglutination methods and some non-antibody based methods described below it is unlikely that complete separation of the two populations of red cells will be accomplished. Thus when the unagglutinated cells are used in phenotyping studies, the reactions of the majority of the cells must be read. Reactions of a small percentage of the cells (i.e. small agglutinates in a sea of unagglutinated cells) may represent unseparated cells of the other cell population and their presence may have to be ignored.

When it is not known how (or if) the patient's and the transfused cells differ in terms of antigens that they carry, a different approach can be used. Following transfusion, most of the young cells in the patient's circulation will be his own, having been recently released from the marrow providing, of course, that the patient is making blood. Stephens (322) showed that young red cells are less dense than old ones and several techniques for the separation of young and old cells, based on this difference, have been described (323-332,412).

Some of the density gradient separation methods referenced above are relatively complex. For blood typing studies, simpler methods sometimes prove suitable. If red cells are mixed with phthalate esters of different densities and then centrifuged in microhematocrit tubes, the esters effect separation of cells of different densities (333). Others (334,335) have found that similar separation can be obtained simply by hard centrifugation of red cells in capillary tubes, without use of phthalate esters. Brown (336) described a unique method for use with sickle cell patients. Since red cells from patients with hemoglobin S or SC disease are resistant to lysis by hypotonic saline while those from donors with hemoglobin A or Hb S trait are not, the mixed population sample is washed with 0.3% saline until gross hemolysis stops. The remaining red cells, that must be washed with 0.9% saline to restore tonicity, are those of the SSD or SCD patient.

Even better methods exist for the separation of reticulocytes. In one (337), affinity chromatography is used and it is reported that 25 to 35% of the cells separated are reticulocytes. In another (411) a monoclonal antibody to transferrin was used in conjunction with immunomagnetic beads. It was reported that 98 to 100% pure preparations of reticulocytes could be obtained (see also Chapter 43).

Forecasts of In Vivo Red Cell Survival

In spite of, and sometimes because of their sensitivity, in vitro blood bank tests do not always accurately forecast what will happen to red cells in vivo. That is to say, sensitivity does not always correlate exactly with clinical significance. Because of this, blood for transfusion is often selected with a safety margin in the patient's favor. When antibodies in say the Rh, Kell, Duffy and Kidd systems are found, antigen-negative blood is selected for transfusion, first because finding such units is not particularly difficult and second, because some antibodies in those systems have caused accelerated clearance of antigen-positive red cells. There is little doubt that some of the antibodies honored by the transfusion of antigen-negative blood would not cause in vivo red cell destruction, however, there is at present no quick, easy or reliable in vitro method to distinguish between clinically significant and benign antibodies. While the situation is relatively easy to handle when there is a reasonable incidence of the required antigen-negative phenotype, it is much more of a problem when the antibody involved is directed against an antigen of very high incidence. If the antibody is clinically significant, mass screening tests or use of one of the rare donor files may be necessary to provide suitable blood for the patient. If the antibody would not destroy antigen-positive red cells in vivo, or would destroy them at so slow a rate as to cause no clinical problems, more harm than good will be done by undertaking searches for antigen-negative blood. Delays in necessary surgery, non-transfusion in a clinical situation in which additional oxygen carrying capability is needed and the psychological trauma involved when the patient believes that no blood is available, must be avoided whenever possible by recognizing that serologically incompatible blood can safely be transfused. Sometimes the specificity of the antibody will be such that the decision to use antigen-positive blood can be made. As examples, antibodies to Ch, Rg, McC[a], Cs[a], etc. do not cause any, or any significant, in vivo destruction. On other occasions, antibodies to Yt[a] and the high incidence Ge antigens are good examples, the specificity will be such that it will be known that some examples of those antibodies are clinically significant while others are benign. On such occasions some attempt must often be made to forecast how the antibody will behave in vivo.

The most reliable way to forecast antibody behavior in this situation is to perform an in vivo red cell survival study. A small aliquot, usually about 1 ml, of antigen-positive red cells is labeled with a radioisotope, most often ^{51}Cr, and is injected into the patient. Unless very rapid and substantial red cell destruction is anticipated, a sample is drawn from the patient 3 minutes after the labeled red cells were injected and the isotope level is measured. This level is taken to represent 100% survival since at 3 minutes, near total mixing of the injected dose with the patient's red cells should have occurred and the lag period between injection and red cell destruction is such that marked clearance should not have occurred. If appreciable rapid destruction is anticipated different procedures must be used (338) including, perhaps, comparison of survival of the antigen-positive and the patient's own red cells via use of a double label. If the 3 minute sample is to be taken to represent 100% survival of the test dose, further samples are drawn say at 10 minutes and at 1 and 24 hours after injection of the labeled red cells. Red cell survival is estimated from measurements of remaining radioactivity. Levels of radioactivity in the plasma as well as in the red cells must be measured, particularly in the 10 and 60 minute samples in case intravascular hemolysis, with release of radioactivity in to the plasma has occurred. Normal red cell survival as measured by this method is such that 97% of the test dose should be present in the patient's circulation, 24 hours after injection (338-341). In the original descriptions of this method for use in forecasting in vivo survival of serologically incompatible red cells it was stated (339,342) that if greater than 70% of the test dose was present 1 hour after injection, blood of that phenotype could be transfused with little risk of a catastrophic transfusion reaction. This was intended as a guide in emergency situations where no compatible blood was available and transfusion was essential. Unfortunately, some workers have taken the 70% survival figure at 1 hour to indicate satisfactory in vivo survival. This is most certainly not the case. Survival of 70% of the cells at 24 hours indicates accelerated in vivo red cell clearance, the figure is intended only to permit transfusion in a dire emergency when no alternative exists. A survival of greater than 70% of the test dose at 24 hours may indicate that while accelerated in vivo clearance will occur, the amount may be such that transfusion may be safer than withholding blood (343,344).

It has been suggested (338,341) that when survival is less than 97% at 1 hour, further samples be taken to determine if substantial red cell destruction is likely. By extending survival studies over a period of days a T_{50}Cr can be calculated, usually by extrapolation of the rate of destruction measured over a number of days. The T_{50}Cr is the length of time that it takes for the radioactivity of the test dose to fall to half of its original value, it is commonly called the T_{50} or half-life of the test dose. Because of minor variations in both techniques and patients, a normal T_{50} range is 25 to 37 days (most often 27-32 days). In a patient in whom initial survival is normal or near normal but in whom the T_{50} is say 14 days, transfusion may be better than a delay while "compatible" blood is found. As discussed in more detail in Chapter 35, the object of transfusion is often to get a patient through surgery or to replace blood lost following trauma. In both instances, once the acute phase (surgery or correction of injury) has passed, the patient will make blood to correct his anemia. Thus transfused red cells may well serve the purpose for which they are intended, even if they survive only say, 7 days, in the patient.

While it is undoubtedly the "gold standard" for forecasting the in vivo survival of serologically "incompatible" red cells, the ^{51}Cr method is not without its drawbacks. First, it is not an easy method to perform (338-341,345,346), it is even harder to do it well. Second, unless considerable care is taken, the red cells may be damaged during the labeling step and their consequent accelerated clearance may be due to mechanical damage, not antibody activity in the patient. Third, estimates of red cell clearance based on tests with a small dose of red cells may not always accurately reflect what will happen when a whole unit is transfused (347,348). Fourth, specialized equipment is needed and the patient must be on site.

As mentioned in the section on flow cytometry, red cell survival studies can also be performed using that equipment (207-211). An advantage to use of the flow cytometer for this purpose is that samples from the patient can be collected and stored, then all shipped off site at one time. When this was done (210) no loss of accuracy occurred, the results were the same as those from a ^{51}Cr study performed simultaneously. A disadvantage of using the flow cytometer is that, in current methods, 10 ml of the test cells must be injected to obtain accurate estimates of survival.

The Monocyte Monolayer Assay

Because many transfusion services do not have the necessary facilities to perform ^{51}Cr survival studies and do not have access to a flow cytometer, alternative methods have been devised to attempt to forecast in vivo red cell survival from in vitro tests. One such test is the monocyte monolayer assay (MMA). The test is based on the findings that in vivo, IgG-coated red cells are bound and eventually destroyed by macrophages in various organs (349-362). Thus in vitro, tissue derived macrophages (363-366) or peripheral blood monocytes (330,367-390) have been used in monolayer assays to simulate what might occur in vivo. The reason that monocytes can be used is that they are the precursors of tissue bound macrophages (391,392). Monocytes are released from the bone marrow and circulate in the blood for a few days before taking up residence, many in the spleen and the liver, as macrophages of the reticuloendothelial system. Thus monocytes are immature macrophages. They do not have as many active Fc receptor sites as macrophages and may carry no, or relatively few activated receptor sites for complement. Nevertheless, they are sufficiently developed for use in the MMA.

In the test, peripheral blood leukocytes are separated from whole blood using a ficol-hypaque method (393). Aliquots of the leukocyte preparation are then placed in the wells of tissue culture slides. The slides are incubated, in some test systems in 5% CO_2, in others in air. During the incubation, monocytes but not other leukocytes (with the exception of a few large lymphocytes) adhere to the glass of the tissue culture slide. At the end of the incubation, the remaining contents of the tissue culture wells are discarded, leaving a monolayer of monocytes attached to the slide. While the monocyte monolayers are being prepared, the antibody whose clinical significance is in question is incubated, in separate tubes, with antigen-positive and, if available, antigen-negative red cells as a control, in about the same ratio as that used in performing IATs. Many workers add fresh whole serum to the antibody-red cell mixtures for the incubation stage. The red cells are then washed, again as for the IAT, and added to the prepared monocyte monolayers. Another incubation follows, again in CO_2 or air dependent on the method in use, then the dividers on the tissue culture slide are removed, the slides are rinsed in saline and allowed to dry in air, usually overnight. The slides are stained and examined microscopically. Various different reading methods are used. Some workers count the number of monocytes that have phagocytosed red cells, others count the number of red cells phagocytosed, while still others count for both phagocytosis and adherence of red cells to the monocytes. It is extremely important that a large number of monocytes are counted, 600 is a suitable number (379) unless there is obvious and marked (i.e. greater than 20%) phagocytosis and/or adherence.

It is also extremely important that each laboratory performing the MMA establish its own figures for positive and negative results. The techniques are sufficiently variable and reading methods sufficiently different, that no one number representing significant phagocytosis and/or adherence can be given for all variations of the method. When the test is first set up, a series of antibodies known to have caused in vivo red cell destruction and a series of antibodies known to have allowed normal in vivo survival of antigen-positive red cells should be used to establish positive and negative cut-offs. Ideally some of those sera will then be available to use as positive and negative controls each time the MMA is performed.

Particularly useful in establishing positive and negative values, are sera from patients who have suffered a delayed transfusion reaction (378). The pretransfusion serum can be expected to give a negative result as no red cell destruction occurred at the time of transfusion. The serum collected at the time of the delayed reaction should give a positive result if antibody-induced red cell clearance was, in fact, occurring. When the MMA is performed in air and read for phagocytosis and adherence, a positive value may well be in the region of 3 to 6% (379). When the test is performed in CO_2 and read only for phagocytosis, a figure of 1% may correlate with clinical significance of an antibody (378). Most workers have found, by experience, that there is a gray (a.k.a. grey) area between positive and negative values in to which an occasional clinically-significant and an occasional benign antibody will fall.

There are two probable reasons why such low numbers in the MMA correlate with clinical significance of an antibody. First, as explained above, monocytes are immature macrophages. Once tissue-bound they apparently develop more active Fc binding sites. Second, as discussed in Chapter 6, phagocytosis is a minority action of macrophages. More red cell destruction occurs when biconcave red cells are converted to spherocytes by macrophage action, than occurs by phagocytosis.

If the MMA is set up and controlled in a careful and consistent manner, its results correlate well with clinical significance or insignificance of the antibodies tested. In a number of studies (377-379,383,387,389,394-396) good correlation between the results of MMA and ^{51}Cr in vivo cell survival studies have been seen, but the MMA results are not infallible (377). Workers planning to use the MMA (or other cellular assays) to forecast in vivo red cell survival in immunized patients, should also read the section headed "Macrophage Variation" in Chapter 6. Since there is considerable variation of macrophage and monocyte activity in different normal individuals and in the same individual over time, pools of monocytes from healthy donors should be used to reduce this variable (383,413).

The MMA does not seem to be a quantitative test. In our study on sera that had caused immediate or delayed transfusion reactions (378) we saw vastly different degrees of in vivo red cell destruction by antibodies that gave the same level of positive results in the MMA. Another point deserves consideration. When the MMA is negative, antigen-positive blood is often transfused (387) so that correlation between a negative MMA and an antibody that is benign in vivo is seen. However, when the MMA is positive and ^{51}Cr survival studies cannot be performed, antigen-positive blood is seldom transfused. Thus the correlation between a positive MMA and clinical significance of an antibody is less firmly established.

In spite of the shortcomings of the MMA it is still a highly valuable tool in transfusion medicine as currently practiced. Although the test is somewhat labor intensive, it requires no sophisticated or expensive equipment. Further, it can be performed off site using a single sample of serum from the patient involved.

It is important to remember that antibody characteristics, including subclass composition, can change following the transfusion of antigen-positive red cells. Thus, if the MMA indicates that antigen-positive blood can safely be transfused and if such transfusions are successful, then further transfusions are required, the MMA should be repeated with a posttransfusion serum sample from the patient. In other words, a negative MMA does not indicate that the patient can receive antigen-positive blood with impunity, for ever. In this respect the MMA is no different from a compatibility test in that a current sample of the patient's serum must be tested.

Other Cellular Assays

There are a number of other assays that use mononuclear phagocytic cells and similar principles to the MMA. Since these tests have been used primarily in attempts to forecast the clinical severity of HDN, the significance of the results obtained is discussed in Chapter 41. The principles of the tests are discussed briefly, below. In the rosette assay (358,397) peripheral blood monocytes or other Fc receptor-bearing cells are mixed with antibody-coated red cells, centrifuged slowly, incubated at room temperature, resuspended gently, then examined for rosette formation. The test is used more often for investigation of Fc receptors on effector cells (398,399) than for determining clinical significance of antibodies.

The antibody-dependent cellular cytotoxicity (ADCC) assay measures the lysis of antibody-coated red cells by monocytes (400) or lymphocytes (362,401,402). The monocyte driven test is usually called ADCC(M) while the K-cell driven test is called ADCC(L). Red cells are labeled with ^{51}Cr, coated with antibody, then incubated with monocytes or lymphocytes (K-cells). The test is read by measuring the release of ^{51}Cr from the lysed red cells.

The chemiluminescence test (CLT) relies on the fact that during erythrophagocytosis and following activation of the respiratory burst, monocytes produce oxygen radicals that react with luminol. The product of this reaction is generation of light that can be measured in a luminometer (403,404). The test is fast and objective, it does not require counting cells with a microscope. However, the test is said (395) to be less sensitive than the MMA.

Readers interested in learning more about the rosette test, ADCC assay and CLT are referred to the excellent reviews of Garratty (394) and Zupanska (395). The role of IgG subclassing studies in the determination of clinical significance or lack thereof, of an antibody, is discussed in Chapters 2 and 6.

Miscellaneous Notes and Other Methods

The use of a dry button of red cells from which most of the wash saline has been decanted, for hemagglutination tests results in two advantages. First, no dilution of subsequently added antibody occurs. As mentioned above, Pinkerton et al. (143) have shown that if the serum:cell ratio is sufficiently high, a system with no additives may be as sensitive as any of the newly devised methods. Second, preparation of a (relatively) dry button of cells results in the test cells being washed before use. Some caution in the overly liberal use of cell buttons is perhaps necessary since some commercially prepared additives (low ionic solutions, etc.) are formulated to achieve the correct test conditions when the equivalent of one drop of saline is included in the test mixture. When in doubt, follow the manufacturer's instructions.

Antibody Salvage Method

When a serum of particular value is being used, some of it can be recovered after completion of the tests (405). Those tests giving negative reactions are centrifuged hard and supernatant serum is carefully pipetted off and pooled for re-use. In this way a small quantity of a rare serum can be used repeatedly, especially if the antigen it detects is of low incidence. It must be remembered that some dilution will have occurred and when the salvaged serum is re-used proportionally more must be used for each test. If cell buttons are used the dilution factor will be small; if cell suspensions are used the dilution factor will be higher. Obviously, positive controls with the salvaged serum are essential in order to show that dilution to non-reactivity has not occurred.

This modification can, obviously, be applied to other tests, such as the antiglobulin method where the cell-serum mixtures are spun and the serum saved before washing starts. The serum cannot be pooled until after the tests are read and it is known which were negative. Salvage of serum from albumin and one stage enzyme tests is more difficult because the serum is mixed with the additive when recovered, but it can be applied to tests using red cells pre-treated with enzymes. Serum should be harvested only from negative tests. The temptation to recover serum from weakly positive tests must be resisted because although not much agglutination may have taken place, there may have been a considerable amount of antibody adsorbed from the serum.

Plasma Recalification

Plasmapheresis is a convenient and practical way of obtaining large volumes of plasma from individuals with usable antibodies. In some but not all instances, the antibody present may react better if the plasma is converted into serum. Blood collected into ACD or CPD has been prevented from clotting by the action of the citrate, that chelates the calcium that is present in the blood and is essential for coagulation. Such plasma can be converted into serum by the addition of an excess of calcium. This, in effect, completes the coagulation cycle by converting fibrinogen to fibrin (all the factors necessary for coagulation with the exception of calcium being present in fresh plasma). A fibrin clot forms (in the absence of red cells that play no part in the coagulation cycle) and retracts, leaving serum instead of plasma. With some samples of plasma it may be necessary to add thrombin as well as calcium. A method is given by Judd (270).

Addition of Preservative to Serum

The most commonly used preservative in blood typing serum is sodium azide that has a bacteriostatic effect and at the concentration used does not interfere with serological reactions. After plasma has been recalcified to serum, sodium azide to a final concentration of 0.1% should be added. A convenient way of accomplishing this is to prepare a 10% solution of sodium azide in distilled water then to add 1ml of this for each 100ml of serum. Reagents containing sodium azide should not be discarded into sinks with copper or lead pipes. The azide complexes with copper or lead to form a potentially explosive compound. When the plumber arrives to clear a clog and hits the copper (azide) pipe accidentally with a wrench (spanner in England) or deliberately with a hammer, the pipe may explode.

Methods for Preserving Small Quantities of Red Cells in the Frozen State

Red cells used in blood grouping tests are normally used while fresh but the majority of red cell antigens survive fairly well for three weeks at 4°C. Cells may be stored frozen for long periods of time but before being frozen their aqueous content must be replaced by glycerol to prevent the formation of intracellular ice crystals that would otherwise cause hemolysis.

The best method for the long term preservation of red cell samples is to freeze them as droplets in liquid nitrogen (406). This is accomplished using expensive and specially designed equipment or by devising a parallel system employing what materials are available or can be purchased at the local five and dime store (407). There is little point in describing the freezing method in detail here. Workers who already have the specially designed equipment will not need to be told how to use it. Workers who are in the process of setting up droplet cell freezing in liquid nitrogen will need to obtain practical guidance from those already expert in the manipulation of tea-strainers, sieves, polystyrene boxes with holes cut in them and the like! Thawing cells frozen as droplets in liquid nitrogen is extremely easy. Enough droplets for the number of tests planned are simply placed in physiological saline prewarmed to 37°C. The cells are washed two or three times in saline and are then ready for use. The huge advantage of this method is that tiny volumes of cells can be recovered from the frozen state (loss by hemolysis during the washing steps is minimal) so that excess amounts need not be thawed and one five ml sample of frozen cells will last almost indefinitely. Cells frozen as droplets in liquid nitrogen seem to metabolize so slowly that there seems no danger that their red cell antigens will ever deteriorate. Certainly, samples that have been frozen for more than 30 years behave as normal red cells once thawed.

For those workers not fortunate enough to have liquid nitrogen freezers available alternative (but less satisfactory) methods exist. Red cells can be protected with glycerol, stored in mechanical freezers, and recovered from the frozen state for use in serological tests (26,270,332,408-410).

Reading Methods for In Vitro Tests

Now that most routine tests are carried through to an antiglobulin reading the question of how to read them does not often arise. They are usually read macroscopically in order that the cells and serum are left in the tube for progression of the test. A few cells may, of course, be removed and examined microscopically at any stage if this type of reading is required. However, one of us (PDI) has believed for years that routine use of the microscope in the blood bank creates far more problems than it solves. Almost any cell suspension, including those in which washed cells have never been exposed to antibody, if examined carefully enough under the microscope will be found to contain a few small clumps of red cells. Thus, while reading aids such as mirrors or hand lenses are acceptable, routine use of the microscope is not condoned. This reasoning also applies to the reading of antiglobulin tests. Again if agglutination cannot be seen with the naked eye, a hand lens, a convex mirror, or the type of microscope in which the contents of the tube are viewed while still inside the tube by placing the tube itself on the microscope stage, IT IS NOT THERE. Were it not for special tests, such as those in which mixed-field reactions may have occurred or when a small percentage of fetal cells might be present in a maternal sample, the microscope should be banned from the blood bank.

Enzyme tests for agglutination or following conversion to antiglobulin reading, should NEVER be read microscopically.

Commercially Prepared Reagents and Monoclonal Antibodies

While it can be stated here that these reagents should always be used in accordance with the manufacturers' directions, they are discussed in more detail in Chapter 7.

References

1. Judd WJ, Steiner EA, Oberman HA, et al. Transfusion 1992;32:304
2. Issitt PD, Combs MR. Unpublished observations 1992
3. Nance SJ, Garratty G. Am J Clin Pathol 1987;87:633
4. Garratty G. In: Immune Destruction of Red Blood Cells, Arlington, VA: Am Assoc Blood Banks, 1989:109
5. Garratty G. Gerentology 1991;37:68
6. Mollison PL, Engelfriet CP, Contreras M. Blood Transfusion in Clinical Medicine, 9th Ed. Oxford:Blackwell 1993
7. Judd WJ. Transfusion 1995;35:271
8. Mallory DM. Transfusion 1995;35:268
9. Freedman J, Masters CA, Newlands M, et al. Vox Sang 1976;30:231
10. Reesink HW, van der Hart M, van Loghem JJ. Vox Sang 1972;22:397
11. Cameron JW, Diamond LK. J Clin Invest 1945;24:793
12. Diamond LK, Denton RL. J Lab Clin Med 1945;30:821
13. Leikola J, Perkins HA. Transfusion 1980;20:224
14. Brooks DE, Millar JS, Seaman GVF, et al. J Cell Physiol 1967;69:155
15. Leikola J, Pasanen VJ. Int Arch Allerg 1970;39:352
16. Pollack W, Reckel RP. In: Human Blood Groups, Basel:Karger, 1977:17
17. Brooks DE. In: Human Blood Groups, Basel:Karger, 1977:27
18. Steane EA, Greenwalt TJ. In: Human Blood Groups, Basel:Karger 1977:36
19. Greenwalt TJ, Steane EA. Br J Haematol 1973;25:207
20. Steane EA. In: Antigen-Antibody Reactions Revisited, Washington, D.C.:Am Assoc Blood Banks, 1982:67
21. van Oss CJ, Good RJ. J Prot Chem 1988;7:179
22. van Oss CJ, Good RJ. J Disper Sci Tech 1988;9:355
23. van Oss CJ, Good RJ. J Disper Sci Tech 1991;12:273
24. van Oss CJ. In: Immunobiology of Transfusion Medicine, New York:Marcel Dekker 1994;327.
25. Case J. Vox Sang 1959;4:403
26. Moore BPL, Humphreys P, Lovett-Moseley C. Serological

and Immunological Methods, 7th Ed. Toronto: Canad Red Cross Soc, 1972
27. Hughes-Jones NC, Polley MJ, Telford R, et al. Vox Sang 1964;9:385
28. Elliot M, Blossom E, Dupuy ME, et al. Vox Sang 1964;9:396
29. Mollison PL, Polley MJ. Nature 1964;203:535
30. Löw B, Messeter L. Vox Sang 1974;26:53
31. Moore HC, Mollison PL. Transfusion 1976;16:291
32. Langley JW, McMahan M, Smith N. Am J Clin Pathol 1980;73:99
33. Wicker B, Wallas CH. Transfusion 1976;18:469
34. Rock G, Baxter A, Charron M, et al. Transfusion 1978;18:228
35. Garratty G, Petz LD, Webb M, et al. Clin Res 1978;26:347
36. Lown JAG, Barr AL, Davis RE. J Clin Pathol 1979;32:1019
37. Fitzsimmons JM, Morel PA. Transfusion 1979;19:81
38. Voak D. Biotest Bull 1981;1:24
39. Molthan L, Strohm PL. Am J Clin Pathol 1981;75:629
40. Molthan L. Canad J Med Tech 1981;43:176
41. Merry AH, Thomson EE, Rawlinson VI, et al. Vox Sang 1984;47:73
42. Merry AH, Thomson EE, Lagar J, et al. Vox Sang 1984;47:125
43. Dankbar DT, Blake BE, Pierce SR, et al. (abstract). Transfusion 1986;26:549
44. Leikola J, Perkins HA. Transfusion 1980;20:138
45. Lalezari P, Jiang AF. Transfusion 1980;20:206
46. Fisher GA. Transfusion 1983;23:152
47. Steane EA, Steane SM, Montgomery SR, et al. Transfusion 1985;25:540
48. Mintz PD, Anderson G. Transfusion 1987;27:134
49. Snyder EL, Spivak M, Novodoff D, et al. Transfusion 1978;18:79
50. Garratty G, Vengelen-Tyler V, Postoway N, et al. (abstract). Transfusion 1982;22:429
51. Maynard BA, Smith DS, Farrar RP, et al. Transfusion 1988;28:302
52. Issitt PD, Combs MR, Bredehoeft SJ, et al. Transfusion 1993;33:284
53. Letendre PL, Williams MA, Ferguson DJ. Transfusion 1987;27:138
54. Nance SJ, Garratty G. Am J Clin Pathol 1987;633
55. Laurent TC. Biochem J 1963;89:253
56. Wenz B, Apuzzo J. Transfusion 1989;29:218
57. Slater JL, Griswold DJ, Wojtyniak LS, et al. Transfusion 1989;29:686
58. De Man AJM, Overbeeke MAM. Vox Sang 1990;58:207
59. Wenz B, Apuzzo J, Shah DP. Transfusion 1990;30:318
60. Knight R. Unpublished observations cited in Mollison PL, Engelfriet CP, Contreras M. Blood Transfusion in Clinical Medicine, 9th Ed. Oxford:Blackwell, 1993:347
61. Roy RB. Personal communication 1991
62. Combs MR, Telen MJ. (abstract). Transfusion 1989;29(suppl 7S):58S
63. Morton JA, Pickles MM. Nature 1947;159:779
64. Löw B. Vox Sang 1955;5:94
65. Haber G, Rosenfield RE. In: PH Andreson, papers in dedication of his 60th birthday. Copenhagen:Munksgaard, 1957
66. Pirofsky B, Mangum MEJ. Proc Soc Exp Biol NY 1959;101:49
67. Judson PA, Anstee DJ. Med Lab Sci 1977;34:1
68. Kissmeyer-Nielsen F. Sangre 1964;9:221
69. Dybkjaer E. Proc 10th Cong ISBT, Stockholm, 1964
70. Anstee DJ, Mawby WJ, Tanner MJ. In: Membranes and Transport, a Critical Review. New York:Plenum, 1982
71. Dahr W. In: Recent Advances in Blood Group Biochemistry.

Arlington, VA:Am Assoc Blood Banks, 1986:23
72. Blanchard D, Dahr W. In: Immunobiology of Transfusion Medicine. New York:Marcel Dekker, 1994:37
73. Le Van Kim C, Mouro I, Cherif-Zahar B, et al. Proc Nat Acad Sci USA 1992;89:10925
74. Anstee DJ, Tanner MJA. Bailliere's Clin Haematol 1993;6:401
75. Arce M, Thompson ES, Wagner S, et al. Blood 1993;82:651
76. Cherif-Zahar B, Le Van Kim C, Rouillac C, et al. Genomics 1994;19:68
77. Cartron JP. Blood Rev 1994;8:199
78. Rolih SD. Immunohematology 1986;2:105
79. Issitt PD, Jerez GC. Transfusion 1966;6:155
80. Dahr W, Geilen W, Beyreuther K, et al. Hoppe-Seyler's Z Physiol Chem 1980;361:145
81. Dahr W, Beyreuther K, Steinbach H, et al. Hoppe-Seyler's Z Physiol Chem 1980;361:895
82. Dahr W, Uhlenbruck G. Hoppe-Seyler's Z Physiol Chem 1978;359:835
83. Blanchard D. Transf Med Rev 1990;4:170
84. Unger LJ, Katz J. J Lab Clin Med 1951;38:188
85. Morton JA. Br J Haematol 1962;8:134
86. Pavone BG, Billman R, Bryant J, et al. Transfusion 1981;21:25
87. Issitt PD, Daniels GL, Tippett P. (Letter). Transfusion 1981;21:473
88. Marsh WL, Jenkins WJ. Vox Sang 1968;15:177
89. Roelcke D. Vox Sang 1969;16:76
90. Roelcke D, Uhlenbruck G. Z Med Mikrobiol Immunol 1969;155:156
91. Roelcke D, Anstee DJ, Jungfer H, et al. Vox Sang 1971;20:218
92. Middleton JI. Canad J Med Tech 1972;34:41
93. Crookson MC. In: Transfusion with Crossmatch Incompatible Blood. Washington, D.C.:Am Assoc Blood Banks, 1975:17
94. Longster G, Giles CM. Vox Sang 1976;30:175
95. James J, Stiles P, Boyce F, et al. Vox Sang 1976;30:214
96. Rolih SD. In: High Titer Low Avidity Antibodies. Washington, D.C.:Am Assoc Blood Banks, 1979:1
97. Wright J. In: High Titer Low Avidity Antibodies. Washington, D.C.:Am Assoc Blood Banks 1979:13
98. Moulds MK. In: High Titer Low Avidity Antibodies. Washington, D.C.:Am Assoc Blood Banks 1979:33
99. Judd WJ. Personal communication 1982, cited in the 3rd Edition of this book
100. Mäkelä O, Cantell K. Ann Med Exp Fenn 1958;36:366
101. Springer GF, Ansell NJ. Proc Nat Acad Sci USA 1958;44:182
102. Habibi B, Tippett P, Lebesnerais M, et al. Vox Sang 1979;36:367
103. Romanowska E. Vox Sang 1964;9:578
104. Springer GF, Huprikar SV. Haematologica 1972;6:81
105. Springer GF, Tegtmeyer H, Huprikar SV. Vox Sang 1972;22:325
106. Bird GWG, Wingham J. Vox Sang 1970;18:240
107. Lomas CG, Tippett P. Med Lab Sci 1985;42:88
108. Albrey JA, Vincent EER, Hutchinson J, et al. Vox Sang 1971;20:29
109. Nichols ME, Rubinstein P, Barnwell J, et al. J Exp Med 1987;166:776
110. Mohammed MT, O'Day T, Sugasawara E. Transfusion 1986;26:120
111. Giles CM. Vox Sang 1960;5:467
112. Garratty G. Unpublished observations cited in Mollison PL, Engelfriet CP, Contreras M. Blood Transfusion in Clinical Medicine, 9th Ed. Oxford:Blackwell 1993:327

113. Poole J, Giles CM. Vox Sang 1982;43:220
114. Giles CM. Vox Sang 1982;42:256
115. Rouger PH, Dosda F, Girard M, et al. Rev Franc Transf Immunohematol 1982;25:45
116. Vengelen-Tyler V, Morel P. (abstract). Transfusion 1979;19:650
117. Daniels GL. Immunohematology 1992;8:53
118. Advani H, Zamor J, Judd WJ, et al. Br J Haematol 1982;51:107
119. Moulds JJ, Moulds MK. Transfusion 1983;23:274
120. Levene C, Harel N. Transfusion 1984;24:541
121. Moulds JJ, Moulds MK, Patriquin P. (Letter). Transfusion 1986;26:305
122. Levene C, Karniel Y, Sela R. Transfusion 1987;27:505
123. Marsh WL, DiNapoli J, Øyen R, et al. Transfusion 1985;25:364
124. Marsh WL, DiNapoli J, Øyen R, et al. (Letter). Transfusion 1986;26:305
125. Telen MJ, Eisenbarth GS, Haynes BF. J Clin Invest 1983;71:1878
126. Parsons SF, Mallinson G, Judson PA, et al. Transfusion 1987;27:61
127. Lambert R, Edwards J, Anstee DJ. Med Lab Sci 1978;35:233
128. Phillips PK, Prior D, Dawes B. J Clin Pathol 1984;37:329
129. Mazda T, Ogasawara K, Nakata K, et al. Vox Sang 1987;52:63
130. Scott ML, Whitton CM. Transfusion 1988;28:24
131. Ogasawara K, Mazda T. Vox Sang 1989;57:72
132. Scott ML, Voak D, Phillips PK, et al. Vox Sang 1994;67:89
133. Mazda T, Makino K, Yabe R, et al. Transf Med 1995;5:43
134. Scott ML, Johnson CA, Phillips PK. Vox Sang 1987;52:223
135. Scott ML, Voak D, Downie DM. Med Lab Sci 1988;45:7
136. Campbell E, Scott ML. Med Lab Sci 1991;48:52
137. Garner SF, Devenish A, Barber H, et al. (Letter). Vox Sang 1991;61:219
138. Judd WJ, Steiner EA, Nugent CE. (Letter). Vox Sang 1992;63:293
139. van Dijk BA. (Letter). Transfusion 1993;33:960
140. Issitt PD. (Letter). Transfusion 1993;33:960
141. Lapierre Y, Rigal D, Adam J, et al. Transfusion 1990;30:109
142. Bromilow IM, Adams KE, Hope J, et al. Transf Med 1991;1:159
143. deFigueiredo M, Lima M, Morais S, et al. Transf Med 1992;2:115
144. Lillevang ST, Georgsen J, Kristensen T. Vox Sang 1994;66:210
145. Phillips PK, Whitton CM, Lavin F. Transf Med 1992;2:111
146. Voak D. (Editorial) Transf Med 1992;2:177
147. Pinkerton PH, Ward J, Chan R, et al. Transf Med 1993;3:201
148. Tills D, Bushrod J, Ward DJ, et al. Immunohematology 1991;7:94
149. Fagraeus A, Espmark A, Jonsson J. Immunology 1965;9:161
150. Catt K, Tregear GW. Science 1967;158:1570
151. Rosenfield RE, Kochwa S, Kaczera Z. (abstract). Proc 15th Cong ISBT;1976:27
152. Mage MG, McHugh LL, Rothstein TL. J Immunol Meth 1977;14:47
153. Wysocki IJ, Sato VI. Proc Nat Acad Sci USA 1978;75:2844
154. Beck ML, Sinor LT, Rachel JM, et al. Med Lab Sci 1985;42:86
155. Beck ML, Rachel JM, Sinor LT, et al. Med Lab Sci 1984;41:374
156. Plapp FV, Sinor LT, Rachel JM, et al. Am J Clin Pathol 1984;82:719
157. Plapp FV, Rachel JM, Beck ML, et al. Lab Manag 1984;22:39

158. Rachel JM, Sinor LT, Beck ML, et al. Transfusion 1985;25:21
159. Rachel JM, Sinor LT, Beck ML, et al. Transfusion 1985;25:24
160. Sinor LT. Transf Med Rev 1992;6:26
161. Rolih SD, Moheng MC, Farlow SJ, et al. (abstract). Transfusion 1988;28:40S
162. Rolih SD, Sinor LT. (abstract). Transfusion 1989;29:19S
163. Wilson SM, Fosdick M. (abstract). Transfusion 1994;34:19S
164. Senko DF, Hahn LF, Wood K, et al. (abstract). Transfusion 1994;34:19S
165. Scott ML. Transf Med Rev 1991;5:60
166. Moore HH, Conradie JD. (Letter). Transfusion 1982;22:540
167. Scott ML, Guest AR, King MJ, et al. Rev Franc Transf Immunohematol 1987;30:515
168. Plapp FV, Rachel JM, Sinor LT. Lancet 1986;1:1465
169. Shearan P, Fernandez-Alvarez JM, Smyth MR. J Pharm Biomed Analy 1990;8:555
170. Fernandez-Alvarez JM, Smyth MR, O'Kennedy R. Talantia 1991;38:391
171. Buckley E, Fernandez-Alvarez JM, Smyth MR, et al. Electroanalysis 1991;3:43
172. John R, Spencer M, Wallace GG, et al. Analytica Chimica Alta 1991;249:381
173. Wang J, Dempsey E, Ozsoz M, et al. Analyst 1991;116:997
174. Hua C, Walsh S, Smyth RM, et al. Electroanalysis 1992;4:107
175. Konig B, Gratzel M. Analytica Chimica Acta 1993;276:329
176. Moulds J. Lab Med 1994;25:82
177. van der Meulen FW, de Bruin HG, Goosen PCM, et al. Br J Haematol 1980;46:47
178. de Bruin HG, van der Meulen FW, Aaig C. Flow Cytom 1980;4:233
179. de Bruin HG, de Leur-Ebeling I, Aaig C. Vox Sang 1983;45:373
180. Nance SJ, Garratty G. J Immunol Meth 1987;101:127
181. Freedman J, Lazarus AH. Transf Med Rev 1995;9:87
182. van Bockstaele DR, Berneman ZN, Muylle L, et al. Vox Sang 1986;51:40
183. Kornprobst M, Rouger PH, Goosens D, et al. J Clin Pathol 1986;39:1039
184. McHugh TM, Reid ME, Stites DP, et al. Vox Sang 1987;53:231
185. Arndt P, Garratty G. (abstract). Transfusion 1987;27:514
186. Reid ME, Anstee DJ, Jansen RH, et al. Br J Haematol 1987;67:467
187. Hasekura H, Ota M, Ito S, et al. Transfusion 1990;30:236
188. Berneman ZA, van Bockstaele DR, Uyttenbrook WM. Vox Sang 1991;61:265
189. Sharon R, Fibach E. Cytometry 1991;12:545
190. Lublin DM, Thompson ES, Green AM, et al. J Clin Invest 1991;87:1945
191. Nicholson G, Lawrence A, Ala FA, et al. Transf Med 1991;1:87
192. Murai J, Naka K, Shimojo N, et al. Clin Chim Acta 1994;266:21
193. Langlois RG, Bigbee WL, Jensen RH. Hum Genet 1986;74:353
194. Langlois RG, Bigbee WL, Kyoizumi S, et al. Science 1987;236:445
195. Kyoizumi S, Nakamura N, Hakoda M, et al. Cancer Res 1989;49:581
196. Langlois RG, Bigbee WL, Jensen RH, et al. Proc Nat Acad Sci 1989;86:670
197. Bigbee WL, Langlois RG, Swift M, et al. Am J Hum Genet 1989;44:402
198. Bigbee WL, Wyrobek AJ, Langlois RG, et al. Mutat Res 1990;240:165
199. Oien L, Nance S, Garratty G. (abstract). Transfusion 1985;25:474
200. Nelson J, Choy C, Vengelen-Tyler V, et al. Immunohematology 1985;2:38
201. Valinksy JE, Ralph H, Øyen R, et al. (abstract). Blood 1988;71(Suppl):273a
202. Nance SJ. In: Progress in Immunohematology, Arlington, VA:Am Assoc Blood Banks, 1988:1
203. Postoway N, Nance S, O'Neill P, et al. (abstract). Transfusion 1985;25:453
204. Valinsky JE, Marsh WL, Bianco C. (abstract). Transfusion 1985;25:478
205. Crabill H, Davey R, AuBuchon J, et al. (abstract). Transfusion 1985;25:474
206. Gerritsen WR, Jagiello CA, Bourhis J-H. Bone Marrow Transpl 1994;13:441
207. Read EJ, Crabill HE, Davey RJ. (abstract). Transfusion 1985;25:451
208. Nance S, Gonzales B, Postoway N. (abstract). Transfusion 1985;25:482
209. DiNapoli J, Gingras A, Diggs E, et al. (abstract). Transfusion 1986;26:545
210. Issitt PD, Valinksy JE, Marsh WL, et al. Transfusion 1990;30:258
211. Garratty G. Bailliere's Clin Haematol 1990;3:267
212. Medearis AL, Hensleigh PA, Parks DR, et al. Am J Obstet Gynecol 1984;148:290
213. Cupp JE, Leary JF, Cernichiari E, et al. Cytometry 1984;5:138
214. Nance S, Nelson J, O'Neill P, et al. (abstract). Transfusion 1986;26:571
215. Nance S, Nelson J, Garratty G. (abstract). Transfusion 1988;28:(Suppl 6S):9S
216. Nance S, Nelson JM, Arndt PA, et al. Am J Clin Pathol 1989;91:288
217. Bayliss KM, Kueck BD, Johnston ST, et al. Transfusion 1991;31:303
218. Nelson M, Popp H, Korky K, et al. Immunohematology 1994;10:55
219. Shimamura M, Ohta S, Suzuki R, et al. Blood 1994;83:926
220. Dunstan RA. Br J Haematol 1986;62:301
221. Perrault R, Högman C. Vox Sang 1971;20:356
222. Morehead RT, Anderson K, Grunewald S, et al. Transfusion 1974;14:586
223. Triulzi DJ, Portman WH, Mango PD, et al. Transf Med Rev 1995;6:123
224. Kutt SM, Larison PJ, Lewis CA. Am Clin Prod Rev 1988;7:8
225. Whitrow W, Ross DW. Bailliere's Clin Haematol 1990;3:255
226. Wegmann T, Smithies O. Transfusion 1966;6:67
227. Wegmann TG, Smithies O. Transfusion 1968;8:47
228. Crawford MN, Gottman FE, Gottman CA. Transfusion 1970;10:258
229. Myers M, Reynolds A. In: Micromethods in Blood Group Serology. Arlington, VA:Am Assoc Blood Banks, 1984:3
230. Dixon MR. In: Micromethods in Blood Group Serology, Arlington, VA:Am Assoc Blood Banks, 1984:37
231. Knight RV, Poole G. The Use of Microplates in Blood Group Serology. Manchester:Br Blood Transf Soc, 1987
232. Issitt PD, Haber JM, Allen FH Jr. Vox Sang 1968;15:1
233. Ponsold A. Munch Med Wschr 1933;41:1594
234. Ponsold A. Dtsch Zschr Gerichtl Med 1939;31:415
235. Ponsold A. Munch Med Wschr 1941;11:305
236. Chown B. Am J Clin Pathol Tech Suppl 1944;14:144
237. Chown B, Lewis M. Canad Med Assoc J 1946;55:66
238. Chown B, Lewis M. J Clin Pathol 1951;4:464

239. Chown B, Lewis M. Am J Phys Anthropol 1957;15:149
240. Lewis M, Kaita H, Chown B. J Lab Clin Med 1958;52:163
241. Hardman JT, Pierce SR, Crawford MN, et al. Transfusion 1981;21:330
242. Crawford MN, Gottman FE, Rogers LC. Vox Sang 1976;30:144
243. Crawford MN. Transfusion 1978;18:598
244. Chown B, Lewis M, Kaita H. Vox Sang 1971;21:126
245. Chown B, Lewis M, Kaita H, et al. Am J Hum Genet 1972;24:623
246. Lewis M, Kaita H, Allderdice PW, et al. Am J Hum Genet 1979;31:630
247. Humphreys J, Stout TD, Kaita H, et al. Vox Sang 1980;39:277
248. Hughes-Jones NC. Immunology 1967;12:565
249. Masouredis SP. J Clin Invest 1959;38:279
250. Hughes-Jones NC, Gardner B. Biochem J 1962;83:404
251. Hughes-Jones NC, Gardner B, Telford R. Biochem J 1962;85:466
252. Hughes-Jones NC, Stevenson M. Vox Sang 1968;14:401
253. Holburn AM, Cleghorn TE, Hughes-Jones NC. Vox Sang 1970;19:162
254. Hughes-Jones NC, Ellis M, Ivona J, et al. Vox Sang 1971;21:135
255. Rosenfield RE, Szymanski IO, Kochwa S. Cold Spring Harbor Symp Quant Biol 1964;29:427
256. Moore BPL. Canad Med Assoc J 1969;100:381
257. Judd WJ, Jenkins WJ. J Clin Pathol 1970;23:801
258. Sturgeon P, Kaye B. Vox Sang 1970;19:14
259. Berkman EM, Nusbacher J, Kochwa S, et al. Transfusion 1971;11:317
260. Moore BPL, Fernandez L. Scand J Haematol 1972;9:492
261. Hughes-Jones NC, Gardner B. Vox Sang 1973;24:317
262. Perrault R, Hogman C. Vox Sang 1971;20:340
263. Gunson HH, Bowell PJ, Kirkwood TBL. J Clin Pathol 1980;33:249
264. Phillips PK. Br J Haematol 1987;65:57
265. Postoway N, Nance SJ, Garratty G. Med Lab Sci 1985;42:11
266. Kiruba R, Han P. Transfusion 1988;28:519
267. Sokol RJ, Hewitt S, Booker DJ, et al. J Immunol Meth 1988;106:31
268. Race RR, Sanger R. Blood Groups in Man, 1st Ed. Oxford:Blackwell 1950
269. Marsh WL. Transfusion 1972;12:352
270. Judd WJ. Methods in Immunohematology, 2nd Ed. Durham:Montgomery, 1994:75
271. Judd WJ. In: A Seminar on Antigen-Antibody Reactions Revisited. Arlington, VA:Am Assoc Blood Banks, 1982:175
272. Landsteiner K, Miller CP. J Exp Med 1925;42:853
273. Weiner W. Br J Haematol 1957;3:276
274. Feng CS, Kirkley KC, Eicher CA, et al. Transfusion 1985;25:433
275. Bird GWG, Wingham J. Acta Haematol 1972;47:344
276. Jimerfield CA. Am J Med Technol 1977;43:187
277. Meier TJ, Wilkinson SL, Utz G. (abstract). Transfusion 1983;23:411
278. Vos GH, Kelsall GA. Br J Haematol 1956;2:342
279. Vos GH. Vox Sang 1960;5:472
280. Rubin HJ. J Clin Pathol 1963;16:70
281. Branch DR, Hian ALS, Petz LD. Vox Sang 1982;42:46
282. Massuet L, Martin C, Ribera A, et al. Transfusion 1982;22:359
283. Chan-Shu SA, Blair O. Transfusion 1979;19:182
284. Bueno R, Garratty G, Postoway N. Transfusion 1981;21:157
285. Deisting B, Douglas D, Ellisor S. (abstract). Transfusion 1986;26:549

286. Garratty G, O'Neill P. (Letter). Transfusion 1986;26:487
287. Ellisor SS, Papenfus L, Sugasawara E, et al. (abstract). Transfusion 1982;22:409
288. Jenkins DE, Moore WH. Transfusion 1977;17:110
289. Kochwa S, Rosenfield RE. J Immunol 1964;92:682
290. Rekvig OP, Hannestad K. Vox Sang 1977;33:280
291. Araszkiew P, Huff SR, Szymanski IO. Transfusion 1983;23:72
292. Louie J, Jiang A, Zaroulis C. (abstract). Transfusion 1986;26:550
293. Burich MA, AuBuchon JP, Anderson HJ. (Letter). Transfusion 1986;26:116
294. Moulds JJ, Mallory D, Zodin V. (abstract). Transfusion 1978;18:388
295. Cousins CR, Schanfield MS. (abstract). Transfusion 1978;18:631
296. Ellisor SS, Reid ME, Marks M. (abstract). Transfusion 1979;19:654
297. Steane SM, Steane EA, Reyes VG. (abstract). Transfusion 1982;22:430
298. Wilson MJ, Hare V, Peloquin KP. (abstract). Transfusion 1982;22:430
299. Gibble JW, Salmon JL, Ness PM. Transfusion 1983;23:300
300. Panzer S, Salama A, Bodeker RH, et al. Vox Sang 1984;46:330
301. McKelvey JK, Edwards JM. Lab Med 1984;15:44
302. South SF, Rea AE, Tregellas WM. Transfusion 1986;26:167
303. Morel PA, Bergren MO, Frank BA. (abstract) 1978;18:388
304. Edwards JM, Moulds JJ, Judd WJ. Transfusion 1982;22:59
305. Branch DR, Petz LD. Am J Clin Pathol 1982;78:161
306. Hanfland P. Vox Sang 1982;43:310
307. Issitt PD, Wren MR. Unpublished observations 1986-1988
308. Doherty DG, Shapira R, Burnett WT Jr. J Am Chem Soc 1957;79:5667
309. Marsh WL, DiNapoli J, Øyen R, et al. Transfusion 1985;25:364
310. Wiener AS, Peters HR. Ann Intern Med 1940;13:2306
311. Dacie JV, Mollison PL. Lancet 1943;1:550
312. Young LE, Platzer RF, Rafferty JA. J Lab Clin Med 1947;32:489
313. Booth PB, Plaut G, James JD, et al. Br Med J 1957;1:1456
314. Mayer K, D'Amaro J. Scand J Haematol 1964;1:331
315. Jones AR, Silver S. Blood 1958;13:763
316. Mollison PL. Blood Transfusion in Clinical Medicine, 6th Ed. Oxford:Blackwell, 1979
317. Szymanski IO, Valeri CR, McCallum LE, et al. Transfusion 1968;8:65
318. Szymanski IO, Valeri CR. Transfusion 1968;8:74
319. Szymanski IO, Valeri CR, Almond DV, et al. Br J Haematol 1967;13:Suppl 50
320. Renton PH, Hancock JA. Vox Sang 1964;9:187
321. Issitt PD, Combs MR, Sammons TD, et al. (abstract). Transfusion 1992;32 (Suppl 8S):55S
322. Stephens JG. J Physiol 1940;99:30
323. Constandoulakis M, Kay HEM. J Clin Pathol 1959;12:311
324. Rigas DA, Koler RD. J Lab Clin Med 1961;58:242
325. Renton PH, Hancock JA. Vox Sang 1964;9:183
326. O'Connell DJ, Caruso CJ, Sass MD. Clin Chem 1965;11:771
327. Rennie CM, Thompson S, Parker AC, et al. Clinica Chimica Acta 1979;98:119
328. Vettore L, DeMatteis DC, Zampini P. Am J Hematol 1980;8:291
329. Branch DR, Sy Siok Hian AL, Carlson F, et al. Am J Clin Pathol 1983;80:453
330. Branch DR, Gallagher MT, Mison AP, et al. Br J Haematol 1984;56:19

331. Vincenzi FF, Hinds TR. Blood Cells 1988;14:139
332. Lutz HU, Stammler P, Fasler S, et al. Biochim Biophys Acta 1992;1116:1
333. Wallas CH, Tanley PC, Gorrell LP. Transfusion 1980;20:332
334. Reid ME, Toy P. Am J Clin Pathol 1983;79:364
335. Mougey R. In: Micromethods in Blood Group Serology. Arlington, VA:Am Assoc Blood Banks, 1984:19
336. Brown DJ. Transfusion 1988;28:21
337. Light ND, Tanner MA. Anal Biochem 1978;87:263
338. Mollison PL, Engelfriet CP, Contreras M. Blood Transfusion in Clinical Medicine, 9th Ed. Oxford:Blackwell 1993
339. International Committee for Standardization in Haematology. Br J Haematol 1971;21:241
340. International Committee for Standardization in Haematology. Br J Haematol 1980;45:659
341. Mollison PL. In: A Seminar on Immune-Mediated Red Cell Destruction. Washington, D.C.:Am Assoc Blood Banks, 1981:45
342. Mollison PL. Haematologia 1972;6:139
343. Davey RJ, Rosen SL, Gustafson ML, et al. Blood 1979;54(Suppl 1):121
344. Davey RJ, Simpkins SS. Transfusion 1981;21:702
345. Garby L, Mollison PL. Br J Haematol 1971;20:527
346. Bentley SA, Glass HI, Lewis SM, et al. Br J Haematol 1974;26:179
347. Chaplin H Jr. Blood 1959;14:24
348. Mollison PL, Johnson CA, Prior DM. Vox Sang 1978;35:149
349. Archer GT. Mod Med Aust 1964;10:55
350. Archer GT. Vox Sang 1965;10:590
351. LoBuglio AF, Cotran RS, Jandl JH, et al. Science 1967;158:1582
352. Huber H, Polley MJ, Linscott WD, et al. Science 1968;162:1281
353. Huber H, Fudenberg HH. Int Arch Allergy App Immunol 1968;34:18
354. Abramson N, Schur PH. Blood 1972;40:500
355. Holm G, Engwall E, Hammarstrom S, et al. Scand J Immunol 1974;3:173
356. von dem Borne AEG KR, Beckers D, Engelfriet CP. Br J Haematol 1977;36:485
357. Kay NE, Douglas SD. Blood 1977;50:889
358. van der Meulen FW, van der Hart M, Fleer A. Br J Haematol 1978;38:541
359. Alexander MD, Andrews JA, Leslie RGQ, et al. Immunology 1978;35:115
360. Kurlander RJ, Rosse WF, Logue GL. J Clin Invest 1978;61:1309
361. Kurlander RJ, Rosse WF. Blood 1979;54:1131
362. Randazzo B, Hirschberg T, Hirschberg H. Scand J Immunol 1979;9:351
363. Schanfield MS, Schoeppner SL, Stevens JO. In: Immunobiology of the Erythrocyte, New York:AR Liss, 1980:305
364. Schanfield MS, Stevens JO, Bauman D. Transfusion 1981;21:571
365. Schanfield MS. In: Immune Hemolytic Anemias, New York:Churchill Livingstone, 1985:135
366. Herron R, Clark M, Young D, et al. Clin Lab Haematol 1986;8:199
367. Ohta S, Shimizu K. Acta Haematol 1974;51:270
368. Hunt JS, Beck ML,Hardman JT, et al. Am J Clin Pathol 1980;74:259
369. Hunt JS, Beck ML, Wood GW. Transfusion 1981;21:735
370. Brojer E, Zupanska B, Michalewska B. Haematologia 1982;15:135
371. Hunt JS, Beck ML, Tegtmeier G, et al. Transfusion 1982;22:355
372. Nance S, Garratty G. (abstract). Transfusion 1982;22:410
373. Gallagher MT, Branch DR, Mison A, et al. Exp Hematol 1983;11:82
374. Nance S, Nelson J, O'Neill P, et al. (abstract). Transfusion 1984;24:415
375. Douglas R, Rowthorne NV, Schneider JV. Transfusion 1985;25:535
376. Garratty G, Nance S, O'Neill P. (abstract). Transfusion 1985;25:474
377. Schoeppner-Esty S, Chin J, Mallory D. (abstract). Blood 1986;68(suppl 1):302a
378. Wren MR, Issitt PD. (abstract). Transfusion 1986;26:548
379. Garratty G, Nance S, O'Neill P. (abstract). Transfusion 1986;26:570
380. Branch DR, Gallagher MT. (Letter). Br J Haematol 1986;62:783
381. Zupanska B, Brojer, Thomson EE. Vox Sang 1987;52:212
382. Zupanska B, Thompson E, Brojer E, et al. Vox Sang 1987;53:96
383. Nance SJ, Arndt P, Garratty G. Transfusion 1987;27:449
384. Wiener E, Garner SF. Clin Lab Haematol 1987;9:399
385. Nance SJ, Arndt PA, Garratty G. (Letter). Transfusion 1988;28:398
386. Issitt PD, Gutgsell NS, Hervis L. (Letter). Transfusion 1988;28:399
387. Gutgsell NS, Issitt LA, Issitt PD. (abstract). Transfusion 1988;28(suppl 6S):32S
388. Nance SJ, Nelson JM, Horenstein J, et al. Am J Clin Pathol 1989;92:89
389. Zupanska B, Brojer E, McIntosh Y, et al. Vox Sang 1990;58:276
390. Bromilow IM, Duguid JKM. Br J Haematol 1991;78:588
391. Cline MJ, Lehrer RI. Blood 1968;32:432
392. Furth RV, Cohn ZA, Hirsch JG, et al. Bull WHO 1972;46:845
393. Boyum A. Scand J Clin Lab Invest 1968;21(suppl 97):77
394. Garratty G. Transf Med Rev 1990;4:297
395. Zupanska B. In: Immunobiology of Transfusion Medicine, New York:Marcel Dekker, 1994:465
396. Mudad R, Rao N, Issitt PD, et al. Transfusion, 1995;35:925
397. Zupanska B, Brojer E, Maslanka K, et al. Vox Sang 1985;49:67
398. Zupanska B, Maslanka K, van Loghem E. Vox Sang 1982;43:243
399. Merry AH, Brojer E, Zupanska B, et al. Vox Sang 1989;56:48
400. Ouwehand WH, Mallens TEJM, Huiskes E, et al. In: The Activity of IgG1 and IgG3 Antibodies in Immune Mediated Destruction of Red Cells. Doctoral Thesis, Amsterdam:Rodopi University 1984:87
401. Urbaniak SJ. Br J Haematol 1979;42:315
402. Urbaniak SJ, Greiss MA, Crawford RJ, et al. Vox Sang 1984;40:323
403. Hadley AG, Kumpel BM, Merry AH. Clin Lab Haematol 1988;10:377
404. Downing I, Templeton JG, Mitchell R, et al. J Biolumin Chemilumin 1990;5:243
405. Allen FH Jr. Personal communication 1964, cited in previous editions of this book
406. Rowe AW, Allen FH Jr. (abstract). Transfusion 1965;5:379
407. Reid ME, Ellisor SS. Transfusion 1974;14:75
408. Yagnow R, Shannon S, Weiland D. Red Cell Free Press 1978;3:8
409. Issitt PD, Applied Blood Group Serology, 3rd Ed. Miami:Montgomery 1985:65

410. Weiner W. Lancet 1961;1:1264

411. Brun A, Gaudernack G, Sandberg S. Blood 1990;76:2397

412. Sorette MP, Shiffer K, Clark MR. Blood 1992;80:249

413. Munn LR, Chaplin H Jr. Vox Sang 1977;33:129

4 | Structure of the Red Cell Membrane and Biochemical Methods for the Analysis of Blood Group Antigens

The human red cell membrane is one of the best characterized human plasma membranes. The reasons for this are fairly obvious. Red cells are readily available in large quantities and since they lack a nucleus and other intracellular organelles, the isolation of pure plasma membranes is technically simple.

The usual method for the isolation of red cell membranes involves hypotonic lysis in 5 mM sodium phosphate buffer on ice (1). Red cells subjected to hypotonic lysis under these conditions retain their biconcave shape and are often referred to as "ghosts" because they look like transparent red cells under a phase contrast microscope. The fact that red cells can be washed free of hemoglobin and other intracellular components without affecting the shape of the red cell is significant because it means that the shape of the red cell is entirely defined by the components which are found in the plasma membrane. The preparation of red cell "ghosts" should be distinguished from the preparation of red cell "stroma". When red cells are exposed to more severe conditions of lysis like suspension in distilled water or detergents, the membrane preparation recovered after washing to remove hemoglobin and other proteins comprises membrane fragments which do not retain the normal red cell shape. These membrane fragments are often referred to as "stroma".

The earliest studies of red cell membrane components concentrated on major protein components which could be solubilized in aqueous solutions. The glycoprotein which carries MN blood group antigens (now known as glycophorin A) is very hydrophilic because of its high sialic acid content and can be solubilized with salt solutions. Glycophorin A is one of the major proteins in red cell "ghosts" comprising approximately one million molecules / red cell (see Chapter 15 for a detailed discussion). Several different groups reported studies on glycophorin A-rich material in the late 1950's and early 1960's (2-5). When, in the early 1970's, detergents were used for the purification of membrane proteins it became clear that these glycophorin A extracts contained minor glycophorins (subsequently denoted B, C and D) in addition to glycophorin A (6,7). The structure of the N-terminal portion of glycophorin A released by trypsin-treatment of red cells was reported by Winzler in 1969 (8).

A second major membrane protein (spectrin) was extracted from red cell "ghosts" with 1 mM EDTA/5 mM Tris HCl pH 7.5. This long filamentous molecule could be visualized in the electron microscope (9). Subsequent studies described in a later section of this chapter established the fundamental importance of spectrin in maintaining the flexibility and deformability of the red cell membrane.

A third component of the red cell membrane which yielded to analysis between the 1940's and 1960's was lipid (10,11). Plasma membranes are essentially a phospholipid bilayer containing proteins, glycoproteins and glycolipids. The basic structure of all plasma membranes, the lipid bilayer, was elucidated by Davson and Danielli (12). Some ABH and Lewis active glycolipids were isolated in low yield from red cells and their structures elucidated in the 1960's (13,14) but most of the fundamental work which led to the elucidation of the structure of these antigens was derived from the analysis of alternative sources of these antigens, particularly glycoproteins purified from ovarian cyst fluids (15-17, and see Chapter 8 for a more detailed discussion of this work).

The major breakthrough which allowed the detailed characterization of the proteins of the red cell membrane was the application of SDS-PAGE to the study of plasma membranes (18). Individual polypeptide chains could be separated from one another by electrophoresis and when used in conjunction with methods for labeling protein on intact red cells and red cell ghosts it was possible to draw a model of the red cell membrane showing that some polypeptides were located on the extracellular surface of the plasma membrane, some on the cytoplasmic surface and some were accessible on both surfaces and hence transmembrane proteins. Blood group antigens were particularly useful in this context because they represent specific markers for proteins with extracellular domains. Monoclonal antibody technology (discussed in Chapter 2) was also particularly useful because it could be used to generate antibodies to proteins in the red cell membrane which were not necessarily marked by blood group antigens or readily labeled and also because large quantities of antibody available from in vitro culture could be used to purify membrane proteins by immunoaffinity methods.

In a similar way, the application of labeling methods specific for carbohydrate would be used to determine that all the carbohydrate of the red cell membrane is located on the extracellular face of the membrane.

By the mid 1980's the broad organization of the red cell membrane was established but the detailed structures of the individual protein components were poorly understood. It was clear that the extracellular face of the membrane comprised numerous glycoproteins and glycolipids, that all the carbohydrate was on the extracellular face and that most proteins with extracellular domains were transmembrane proteins. It was also clear that a substantial number of red cell membrane proteins (including spectrin discussed above) were located on the cytoplasmic face where they interacted to form the red cell skeleton. It also became clear during the mid 1980s that proteins could be 'anchored' in plasma membranes not only by transmembrane protein sequences but also by covalent attachment of lipid to protein. A whole new family of membrane proteins (GPI-family) was described (19,20). Several of these GPI-linked proteins are found on the red cell and as described elsewhere in this chapter, the synthesis of these molecules is defective in paroxysmal nocturnal hemoglobinuria (PNH, 21,22).

Structure of the Red Cell Membrane: Some General Principles

The major function of the red cell membrane is to provide a container for hemoglobin. The encapsulation of proteins with a high affinity for O_2 inside a membrane represented a major step in evolution. Crustaceans and annelids contain O_2-binding proteins in solution but osmotic problems limit the concentrations of such proteins and hence the total capacity for O_2. Much larger concentrations of Hb can be maintained within membranes allowing for the efficient delivery of O_2 to tissues and thus for higher metabolic activity and larger organisms (23).

The membrane must be able to regulate the exchange of O_2 and HCO_3 - between the intracellular Hb and external tissues and retain a minimal metabolism for its own self maintenance. In essence then, the human red blood cell is a remarkable example of economy in design, bereft of the baggage of intracellular organelles (nucleus, mitochondria, endoplasmic reticulum, Golgi apparatus). This exquisite corpuscle circulates in the vasculature and squeezes through capillaries for 120 days before it runs out of energy and is sequestered in the spleen. The red cell membrane must therefore be flexible and deformable while at the same time allowing the transport processes essential for the viability of the organism.

The red cell membrane, in common with all plasma membranes, comprises a lipid bilayer with numerous associated proteins. Several proteins and a small proportion of the lipids are glycosylated and this glycosylation is on the outer (extracellular) face of the membrane giving the red cell a surface carbohydrate 'coat' known as the glycocalyx. Underlying the lipid bilayer is a highly specialized network of peripheral proteins known as the red cell skeleton. The proteins of the skeleton determine the durability and flexibility of the red cell thereby allowing it to traverse capillaries (3μ) less than half the diameter of the red cell (7μ). A model of these various elements of the membrane is shown in figure 4-1. The gross composition of the red cell membrane is lipid 43%, protein 49% and carbohydrate 5-10% (24).

Lipids

The lipid bilayer provides the basic structure of plasma membranes. The main lipid components are phospholipids. Phospholipids are asymmetric molecules. One

FIGURE 4-1 The Red Cell Membrane: Glycocalyx, Lipid Bilayer and Skeleton

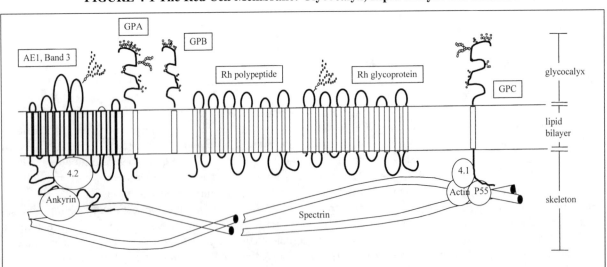

end is hydrophilic and the other hydrophobic. The hydrophobic 'tail' comprises two fatty acid chains one saturated and the other unsaturated. The double bonds in unsaturated fatty acids produce a kink in the structure (see figure 4-2). When phospholipids of the type found in plasma membranes are mixed with water they orient themselves to avoid contact of the hydrophobic fatty acid tails with water and form bilayers with the polar head groups oriented towards the water molecules (see figure 4-2). There are four major phospholipids in mammalian plasma membranes, phosphatidyl ethanolamine (PE), phosphatidyl serine (PS), phosphatidylcholine (PC) and sphingomyelin (SM). PS differs from the other phospholipids in that it has a net negative charge. Phospholipid molecules are very mobile within their respective half of the bilayer but exchange of phospholipid molecules from one half of the bilayer to the other ("flip-flop") does not occur with any significant frequency in lipid bilayers ("flip-flop occurs less than once a month"). "An average lipid molecule diffuses the length of a large bacterial cell (ca 2 μ) in about one second" (25). Most eukaryotic plasma membranes contain a considerable content of cholesterol. Cholesterol aligns itself with the phospholipids (see figure 4-2) and in so doing decreases the mobility of the phospholipid molecules and makes the membrane less permeable (25).

This lipid asymmetry is maintained by an enzyme known as a flippase. This is an ATP dependent transport system which translocates PS and to a lesser extent PE from the outer to the inner bilayer. The half lives for PS and PE are about 5 and 60 minutes respectively at 37°C (26). There may also be floppase which is able to transport PC, PS and PE to the outer bilayer (27). Neither the flippase nor the floppase has been isolated. There was a suggestion that the flippase might be a property of Rh proteins however Rh$_{null}$ red cells have normal flippase activity (28). Since phospholipid asymmetry is altered in Rh$_{null}$ cells (30) flippase may in some way be associated with the Rh proteins. Phospholipid asymmetry is also lost in sickle cells and in red cells from diabetics (29). The reader is referred to Lux and Palek (29) for a more detailed review of phospholipid asymmetry.

The lipid of the red cell membrane is mainly phospholipid (70%) and cholesterol (25%) with a small content of glycolipid (5%). Globoside, the P antigen, accounts for over 70% of all the glycolipids (29). The four major phospholipids SM, PS, PE and PC are asymmetrically distributed in the bilayer with 80% of the PE and 100% of the PS found on the inner half of the bilayer and 75% of the PC and 80% of the SM in the outer half (31).

Proteins

A general distinction is usually made between

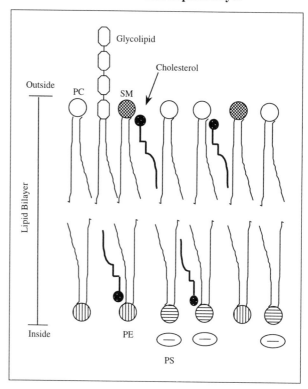

FIGURE 4-2 The Lipid Bilayer

peripheral and integral membrane proteins (32). Peripheral proteins are those which can be solubilized without the use of detergents while integral proteins require detergent solubilization because they have significant regions of hydrophobic amino acids which interact directly with lipids in the bilayer.

Integral membrane protein structures found in the red cell fall into three broad types: those that have a single membrane spanning domain (a single stretch of predominantly hydrophobic amino acids comprising 15-25 residues); those that have multiple membrane spanning domains; and those that are inserted into the bilayer through covalently linked lipid. Membrane spanning domains are thought to span the membrane as a single α-helix. This assumption is derived from X-ray crystallographic analysis of bacteriorhodopsin (33,34). There are many red cell membrane proteins which have a single membrane spanning domain and most of these are ordered with their amino-terminus on the outside of the cell and the carboxy-terminus on the inside (type I, for examples see models of the glycophorins, Chapters 15, 16), Indian blood group glycoprotein (Chapter 29) LW (Chapter 13) and Lutheran (Chapter 20). The Kell blood group glycoprotein also has a single membrane spanning domain but its orientation is unusual in that the amino-terminus is intracellular and the carboxy-terminus extracellular (type II, Chapter 18).

Membrane proteins with multiple membrane spanning domains often have a transport function. The number of membrane spanning domains in different proteins varies considerably for example, the Rh associated protein CD47 has 5 (Chapter 12) the Colton blood group glycoprotein has 6 (Chapter 22), the Duffy glycoprotein has 7 (Chapter 14), the Rh proteins have 12 (Chapter 12) and the Diego protein (band 3) may have 14 (Chapter 17). Proteins of this structural type usually have both the amino terminus and the carboxy-terminus intracellular.

The third type of integral membrane protein results from post translational processing. The carboxy-terminus of the translated protein is replaced with a lipid glycosylphosphoinositol, (GPI)-tail. Several red cell membrane proteins including some blood group-active molecules are known to have a structure of this type, Cromer (Chapter 24), Cartwright (Chapter 23), CD58, CD59 and there is some evidence that the Dombrock protein is also a GPI-linked molecule (Chapter 21).

Single and multiple membrane spanning proteins may have covalently linked fatty acids which are inserted into the cytoplasmic leaflet of the bilayer further increasing the hydrophobicity of the proteins. This fatty acylation (palmitoylation) is well established for the Rh polypeptides (35,36, see also Chapter 12) and may well occur in other blood group proteins like CD44 which carries the Indian system antigens (37, Chapter 29).

Most of the peripheral proteins are found on the cytoplasmic face of the membrane and comprise the red cell skeleton. It seems appropriate to point out here that some peripheral proteins are linked to the lipid bilayer through protein:protein interactions involving integral membrane proteins and that these interactions may be further stabilized by fatty acids covalently linked to the peripheral protein which insert into the cytoplasmic leaflet of the bilayer (reviewed by Schmidt (38)). The two major links between red cell skeletal proteins and the membrane involve ankyrin and p55 respectively, and both these proteins are fatty acylated (39,40) (see a later section of this chapter for a more detailed discussion of the red cell skeleton).

The mechanisms by which integral membrane proteins are inserted into a lipid bilayer has been extensively reviewed (41-43). An excellent summary is also provided by Alberts et al. (25) pages 582-591. It is well established that proteins which are secreted from cells have a hydrophobic sequence of 20-25 amino acids at the amino terminus of the protein which directs the polypeptide to the endoplasmic reticulum (ER) where the hydrophobic sequence is thought to be recognized and bound by a translocator protein. The translocator has a hydrophilic channel through which the polypeptide chain can pass to the lumen of the ER. The signal sequence is then cleaved by a "signal peptidase" on the lumen side of the ER and the protein is secreted. In several of the

Chapters in this book reference is made to such a cleavable signal sequence. If the protein is a membrane protein rather than a secreted protein the polypeptide chain will contain internal sequences of 20-25 hydrophobic amino acids which form transmembrane domains. In the simplest model, illustrated by glycophorin A, the polypeptide has a cleavable signal sequence and a single transmembrane domain. When the transmembrane domain comes into contact with the translocator protein this stops the process of secretion and the protein moves into the lipid bilayer.

A cleavable signal sequence is not an essential prerequisite for the synthesis of a membrane protein. Hydrophobic sequences within the polypeptide chain can themselves act as signal sequences. That is, an internal hydrophobic sequence can initiate binding to the translocator protein and also form a transmembrane domain in the final protein. When an internal signal sequence is used it is possible for the protein to be oriented with its amino terminus in the lumen of the ER and subsequently on the extracellular face of the plasma membrane (type I) or with its carboxy terminus in the lumen of the ER and hence the extracellular face of the plasma membrane (type II). The orientation depends on the distribution of charged amino acid residues on either side of the hydrophobic transmembrane domain (44). Glycophorin C (Chapter 16) is an example of a type I protein which lacks a cleavable signal sequence and uses the single transmembrane domain as an internal signal sequence. Membrane proteins oriented in this way typically have a cluster of basically charged amino acids (arginine, lysine) on the C-terminal side of the transmembrane domain and glycophorin C is no exception. In contrast, the Kell protein has a cluster of basically charged residues on the N-terminal side of its single transmembrane domain. This causes the polypeptide chain to orient itself with its carboxy terminal segment in the lumen of the ER and so the Kell protein is a type II glycoprotein (see Chapter 18).

Integral membrane proteins with multiple transmembrane domains are oriented in the membrane in an analogous manner with the binding of internal hydrophobic sequences to the translocator protein determining the folding of the protein.

The biosynthesis of the third major class of membrane proteins involves replacement of a carboxy terminal transmembrane sequence of 15-20 hydrophobic amino acids with a glycosylphosphatidylinositol (GPI) anchor. The first evidence that integral membrane proteins could be anchored by other than polypeptide came from the work of Low and Finean (19) who showed that alkaline phosphatase could be released from membranes by a bacterial enzyme denoted phosphatidylinositol-specific phospholipase C (PIPLC). This enzyme cleaves the bond between phosphate and glycerol found in phospho-inositol. Subsequent studies on similar proteins in try-panosomes (45) the glycoprotein Thy-1 from rat brain (46) and human red cell acetylcholinesterase (47) estab-lished the structure of this GPI membrane anchor (see figure 4-3). The biosynthesis of GP anchors has been reviewed by Stevens (20). GPI anchored proteins are of considerable interest in immunohematology because several blood group-active proteins are anchored in the red cell membrane in this way and because defective synthesis of the GPI anchor is responsible for the disease paroxysmal nocturnal hemoglobinuria (PNH, 48). The defect in PNH is caused by a failure to attach N-acetyl-glucosamine to the phosphoinositol membrane anchor and results from a diverse array of mutations, Rosse and Ware (22) quote 84 mutations in 72 patients with PNH,

in the gene (*PIG-A*) which encodes the enzyme neces-sary for this step in the biosynthetic pathway (reviewed in references 21,22).

Table 4-1 lists the amino acids used in the assembly of proteins and the one and three letter codes used to describe them.

Carbohydrate

Almost all the carbohydrate of the red cell mem-brane is on the outside. (One exception is protein 4.1 which has a single O-linked N-acetylglucosamine residue attached to 20-40% of the molecules, 49). The carbohydrate is found covalently linked to lipids or to proteins. The carbohydrate of most glycolipids is linked

FIGURE 4-3 Structure of a Glycosyl-phosphatidylinositol (GPI) Anchor

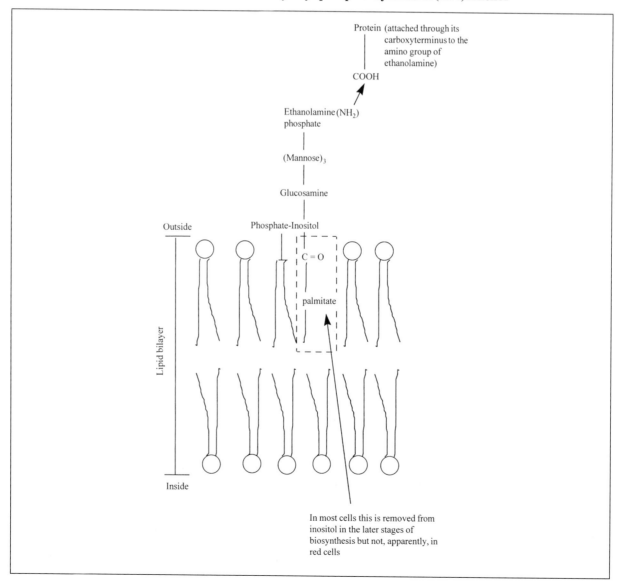

Protein (attached through its carboxyterminus to the amino group of ethanolamine)

COOH

Ethanolamine (NH₂) phosphate

(Mannose)₃

Glucosamine

Phosphate-Inositol

Outside

C = O

palmitate

Lipid bilayer

Inside

In most cells this is removed from inositol in the later stages of biosynthesis but not, apparently, in red cells

TABLE 4-1 Amino Acids and Their Symbols

One Letter Code	Abbreviation	Amino Acid	One Letter Code	Abbreviation	Amino Acid
A	Ala	Alanine	M	Met	Methionine
C	Cys	Cysteine	N	Asn	Asparagine
D	Asp	Aspartic acid	P	Pro	Proline
E	Glu	Glutamic acid	Q	Gln	Glutamine
F	Phe	Phenylalanine	R	Arg	Arginine
G	Gly	Glycine	S	Ser	Serine
H	His	Histidine	T	Thr	Threonine
I	Ile	Isoleucine	V	Val	Valine
K	Lys	Lysine	W	Trp	Tryptophan
L	Leu	Leucine	Y	Tyr	Tyrosine

B = Asx = Asparagine or Aspartic acid

Z = Glx = Glycine or Glutamic acid

X when used in a sequence = any amino acid that does not alter the character (e.g., glycosylation) of the sequence

through D-glucose to ceramide although small amounts linked through D-galactose are also found. The most abundant glycolipid in red cells is globoside which carries the P antigen and is discussed in detail in Chapter 11 (11). Carbohydrate covalently attached to protein is either attached through N-glycosidic links involving N-acetyl-D-glucosamine and asparagine (N-glycans) or O-glycosidic links through N-acetyl-D-galactosamine and either serine or threonine (O-glycans).

Whether or not a protein can be N-glycosylated is governed by the presence or absence of a tripeptide signal motif. The consensus sequence of the signal motif is asparagine-X-serine or threonine where X can be any amino acid except proline (50). The presence of such a signal motif does not guarantee that the protein will be glycosylated at that asparagine. N-glycosylation is only found on regions of membrane proteins that are on the extracellular face of the membrane. N-glycosylation consensus motifs found in regions of the protein which are predicted to be exposed on the cytoplasmic face are not glycosylated. Not all N-glycosylation signal sequence motifs found on predicted extracellular domains are utilized but N-glycosylation never occurs in the absence of a signal motif (51). Predicted structures for blood group-active proteins described in other Chapters of this book are usually obtained from cDNA sequences. The primary amino acid sequence can be predicted from the cDNA sequence and scanned for N-glycosylation signal motifs. It is important to realize that structures drawn from cDNA sequences show possible rather than actual N-glycan sites. Additional information is needed to show that a predicted N-glycan site is actually utilized.

The pattern of O-glycosylation of serine or threo-nine residues in a protein is much harder to predict than N-glycosylation because there is no simple signal motif. Extensive O-glycosylation is a feature of specialized secreted and membrane bound glycoproteins often referred to as mucin-type proteins. The ovarian cyst glycoproteins which yielded the structures of ABH and Lewis antigens are mucins (see Chapters 8 and 9). Glycophorin A is the archetypal membrane bound mucin glycoprotein (see Chapter 15). Hansen et al. (52) compared the sequences of 48 O-glycosylated proteins with a total of 264 O-glycosylation sites in an attempt to define common features predictive of O-glycosylation. These authors found that the glycosylation signal for threonine differs from that for serine. When threonine is O-glycosylated proline is frequently found at positions -1 and +3 (i.e. Pro-Thr-X-X-Pro). X could be any other amino acid but cysteine, tryptophan, methionine, aspartic acid or asparagine are rarely found juxtaposed to the O-glycosylated residue. However, optimal prediction of glycosylated threonine residues required that the nature of the eight amino acids on either side of the threonine be considered. Prediction of the glycosylation of a serine residue was optimal if seven amino acids on either side were considered. In the case of serine glycosylation, proline at position -1 and +3 was, as for threonine, of predictive value but there was also an increased frequency of proline, threonine and serine at positions -9, -8 and +1. It is interesting to note that proline appears to facilitate O-glycosylation while inhibiting N-glycosylation (52). Other factors to be taken into consideration are that O-glycosylation sites are frequently clustered. (Hansen et al. (52) found that more than 25% of O-glycan sites have another O-glycan site next to them) and that if, as has been suggested (53) O-glycosylation occurs after N-glycosylation and after protein folding only serine and threonine residues at the surface of the protein will be available for O-glycosylation.

N-glycans on red cell proteins range in size from Mr 3,000 e.g., that found on glycophorin A (54) to Mr 11,000, e.g. that found on band 3, Diego blood group protein (55) and may be simple biantennary structures (that for GPA illustrated in figure 4-4) or complex multibranched structures (that for Diego illustrated in figure 4-4).

The biosynthesis of N-glycans has been studied in detail (56). In brief, a complex oligosaccharide (N-acetyl glucosamine$_2$-mannose$_9$-glucose$_3$) is added to asparagine through the use of dolichol containing glycolipids. This structure is usually processed down by α-glucosidases and α-mannosidases to give a trimannoside core before addition of repeating N-acetyl lactosaminyl units by the action of glycosyltransferases. The number of repeating N-acetyl lactosaminyl units determines the overall size of the final N-glycan. Finally, other monosaccharides, commonly L-fucose, N-acetyl-neuraminic acid (sialic acid), D-galactose and N-acetylgalactosamine, are added to complete the structure. Some proteins have mannose-rich N-glycans (high mannose) reflecting termination of biosynthesis at an intermediate stage (56) but such high mannose structures have not yet

been described in the red cell membrane. Several blood group antigens are defined by N-glycans (A, B, H, I, i, Sd^a, Tk - see appropriate Chapters).

O-glycans are usually much simpler than N-glycans and in the human red cell the commonest structure is a tetrasaccharide comprising N-acetyl galactosamine covalently linked to serine or threonine on the polypeptide. D-galactose is linked to the N-acetylgalactosamine and two sialic acid residues complete the structure; one linked to the D-galactose and one to the N-acetylgalactosamine (see figure 4-5). Small amounts of di and trisaccharide structures may also be found in normal cells (57). The major source of O-glycans on the human red cell are the glycophorins but at least two other molecules (those that carry the Cromer and Indian antigens) also have a substantial O-glycan content. The Cad antigen is defined by O-glycans containing an additional residue (N-acetyl galactosamine (58), Chapter 42).

The functions of the numerous N and O-glycans at the surface of the red cell appear to be diverse. Glycosylation of proteins in general may serve to protect the polypeptide chain from proteolytic digestion and to confer the correct folding during translation and intracellular processing (59). At the cell surface the N-glycans extend out from the lipid bilayer to form the glycocalyx which acts as a barrier to cell fusion. Viitala and Jarnefelt (60) estimated that about half the total carbohydrate mass

FIGURE 4-4 Structure of the N-glycans Found on Glycophorin A (GPA) and Band 3 (Diego blood group glycoprotein)

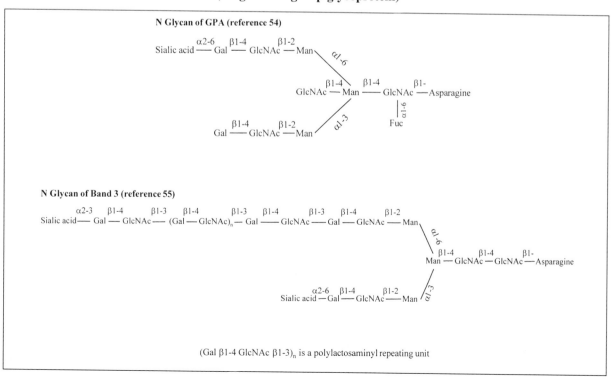

(Gal β1-4 GlcNAc β1-3)$_n$ is a polylactosaminyl repeating unit

FIGURE 4-5 Structure of the Predominant O-glycan on Glycophorin A

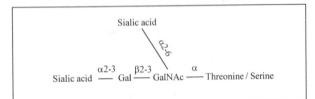

of the red cell surface is formed by poly-N-acetyl lactosamine chains. This calculation was based on the assumption that band 3 and band 4.5 (glucose transporter) which each have one polylactosaminyl (N-glycan) and polylactosaminyl glycolipids comprise $2\text{-}4 \times 10^6$ copies/cell. It is likely that the Rh glycoprotein and to a lesser extent the Colton glycoprotein (CHIP, Aquaporin 1) also contribute significantly to this question but given the approximate nature of the calculation the overall conclusion that polylactosaminyl chains contribute a major portion of the total carbohydrate mass at the red cell surface remains valid. Viitala and Jarnefelt (60) also suggested that the polylactosaminyl N-glycans, if extended, would reach 8 to 12.5 nm from the lipid bilayer. In the same paper these authors made the rather surprising assumption that glycophorin A is a globular protein, a conclusion which led them to suggest that the carbohydrate of GPA extends about 5 nm from the lipid bilayer. This conclusion must be seen as highly unlikely. Mucin-like glycoproteins such as GPA have a large number of O-glycans along the length of the peptide chain which confer an extended rather than a globular structure. The extended, stiff structure appears attributable to steric interactions between the peptide-linked GalNAc residues and adjacent amino acids in the peptide core (61). The elongation of the oligosaccharide chains by addition of other sugars appears to have little additional effect on the rigidity of the molecule, an observation which suggests that glycophorins on Tn red cells remain in an extended structure (see Chapter 42).

Assuming an extended structure, Jentoft (61) suggests an average length of 2.5Å per amino acid residue in an O-glycan-rich region of protein and argues that the conformation of glycosylated sequences containing up to 50 amino acid residues would approach that of a rigid rod. GPA has 72 amino acids in its extracellular domain and O-glycans are found within the first 50 residues (62, see also Chapter 15) suggesting that the molecule could extend up to 15 nm from the lipid bilayer. These considerations led to a model of the red cell membrane in which the glycocalyx is dominated by polylactosaminyl N-glycans and the mucin-like structures of the glycophorins (see figure 4-1).

Proteins exported from the endoplasmic reticulum are glycosylated in the Golgi apparatus. Proteins are glycosylated in an orderly sequence as they pass through the dif-

ferent compartments of the Golgi by a series of glycosyltransferase enzymes that utilize sugar nucleotides present in the lumen of the Golgi. The glycosylated protein is transported from the Golgi to the plasma membrane in membrane vesicles which fuse with the plasma membrane and expose the glycosylated protein on the extracellular face (25). The sequential addition of sugars as the molecule passes through the Golgi explains why sugars like fucose and sialic acid are always found at the ends of oligosaccharide chains, the relevant transferases are in the last compartment of the Golgi before transport of the protein to the plasma membrane. Glycosyltransferases are themselves usually N-glycosylated and this appears to be necessary to maintain the stability of the enzyme. A mutant ß-1,4-N-acetylgalactosaminyl transferase lacking all N-glycosylation sites had only 10% of the enzyme activity of the wild type enzyme (63). A number of glycosyltransferases are the products of blood group genes (A, B, H, Le^a, Le^b, Sd^a/Cad, P^1, P, P^k) and these are considered in detail in the relevant Chapters.

Structure of the Red Cell Membrane

As discussed in the preceding section, the red cell membrane can be thought of as comprising three layers, an outer carbohydrate-rich layer (glycocalyx), a lipid bilayer containing numerous transmembrane proteins, and an inner network of proteins which comprise the red cell skeleton.

The Glycocalyx and the Plasma Membrane

The blood group antigens which form the central theme of this book are located in the glycocalyx or at the extracellular face of integral membrane proteins embedded in the lipid bilayer. Very few proteins or glycoproteins which are accessible at the outer surface of the red cell apparently lack blood group antigens. Blood group antigens mark 24 such proteins while seven are not yet marked in this way (see table 4-2). It is of course, quite possible that blood group antigens which are presently unassigned to membrane molecules (see Chapters 31 and 32) will subsequently be shown to be located on one or other of the seven unmarked proteins. For example, the Rh glycoprotein may carry the Duclos antigen (see Chapters 12 and 31). It is also possible that antigens which have not yet been assigned to membrane molecules will identify new membrane molecules not listed in table 4-2. Irrespective of these qualifying remarks it is quite clear that most of the molecules at the surface of the red cell are capable of eliciting an immune response in the context of transfusion or pregnancy. Since the structure of the blood group-active molecules is considered in detail in other Chapters, the discussion here will focus more on those proteins not yet marked by antigens, which are not described in detail elsewhere in this book. The Rh glyco-protein and CD47 are described in Chapter 12. The glu-cose transporter (GLUT-1), the nucleoside transporter, the cell adhesion molecule CD58 (LFA-3) and the comple-ment regulatory molecules CD59 and C8 binding protein are described below.

The glycocalyx of the red cell membrane extends about 10 to 12.5nm from the surface of the lipid bilayer. The major constituents of the glycocalyx are the polylac-tosaminyl glycans found on the most abundant transport proteins, band 3 (10^6 molecules/cell) and GLUT-1 (500,000 molecules/cell) and the numerous O-glycans found on glycophorin A (10^6 molecules/cell) and gly-cophorin B (250,000 molecules/cell). Polylactosaminyl glycans carried on glycolipids are also thought to be of significance (500,000 molecules/cell) (60). This extensive surface carbohydrate layer is thought to provide a barrier to membrane fusion and to protect the red cell from micro-bial invasion (61).

The position of antigens in the glycocalyx is of con-siderable relevance to blood group serology since antigens located at the surface of the glycocalyx can be crosslinked by antibodies of the IgG class while those at the surface of the lipid bilayer cannot. Thus IgG anti-A, anti-B, anti-M and anti-N can agglutinate red cells while IgG anti-D can-not (see figure 2-14 in Chapter 2). The explanation for this difference is simply related to the distance between red cells in suspension. Obviously A, B, M and N antigens will be closer than D antigens on two adjacent red cells in suspension and so more easily crosslinked by IgG (see discussion of agglutination in Chapter 2).

Certain red cell membrane molecules extend out from the lipid bilayer above the glycocalyx (see figure 4-6). Molecules which have such a structure are likely to have functions which involve interaction between the red cell and its environs. Such functions may be impor-tant during the production of red cells, that is, in the process of erythropoiesis or in the function of the mature red cell during its circulation in the blood stream. Molecules like CD44, which carries the Indian blood group antigens (see Chapter 29), seem to have a role in the development of hemopoietic cells through interaction with extracellular matrix proteins, particu-larly hyaluronic acid, and on the mature red cell the hyaluronic binding domain of CD44 would be predict-ed to be presented above the glycocalyx (see figure 4-6). In this case a mucin-like domain (O-glycan-rich) analogous to the extracellular domains of glycophorins serves to present the hyaluronic-binding domain above the glycocalyx. The Lutheran blood group glycoprotein may also bind a component of the extracellular matrix in some tissues (laminin) (221). In this case the N-ter-minal domain of the protein is also predicted to be above the glycocalyx but presentation of the domain is achieved not through a mucin-like O-glycan-rich domain but through multiple Ig superfamily domains (see Chapter 20). Even more striking examples of the presentation of receptor binding domains above the gly-cocalyx are provided by red cell membrane molecules involved with the regulation of complement. The regu-latory component CD55 which carries Cromer blood group antigens (see Chapter 24) has four N-terminal globular domains (SCRs) which function by inhibiting the activation of C3 convertase and thus preventing autologous lysis of red cells when complement is acti-

TABLE 4-2 Most of the Known Red Cell Surface Proteins are Marked by Blood Group Antigens

Known Proteins Marked by Blood Group antigens		Known Proteins not Marked by Blood Group Antigens
Band 3 (AE1, Diego blood group)	Sc	CD47
Aquaporin 1 (CHIP, Colton blood group)	JMH	CD58
Urea Transporter (Jk)	Ok^a	Rh glycoprotein
Fy	Xk	GLUT-1
Rh polypeptide	CR1 (Kn blood group)	CD59
Lu	CD44 (In blood group)	Nucleoside Transporter
Xg	GPC/D (Gerbich blood group)	C8 binding protein
CD99	Do	
CD55 (Decay Accelerating Factor, Cromer blood group)		
Acetylcholinesterase (Yt)		
GPA/GPB (MNS blood group)		

FIGURE 4-6 Models of Minor Blood Group-active Proteins at the Red Cell Surface

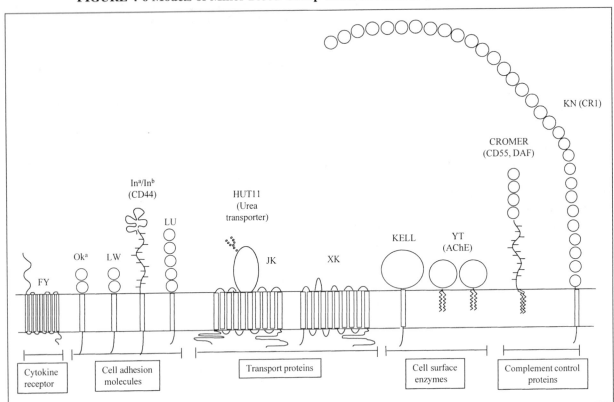

vated. These functional domains are presented above the glycocalyx by a mucin-like O-glycan-rich domain. The regulatory component CR1 which carries the Knops blood group antigens (see Chapter 28) is an extraordinarily long filamentous molecule which when fully extended would present its N terminus at a distance of 100nm from the lipid bilayer. CR1 functions on the red cell by binding C3b in the context of immune complexes. The immune complexes are subsequently removed in the liver and spleen. Presentation of the N-terminal domain of CR1 above the glycocalyx is achieved not by use of an O-glycan-rich domain but by multiple repeats of small globular domains (short concensus repeats or SCRs). This alternative strategy is likely to produce a much more flexible molecule than the rather rigid mucin-like structure.

It should not be assumed that all receptor binding proteins protrude above the glycocalyx. The well characterized adhesion molecule CD58 (LFA-3) contains two Ig family domains and would be predicted to extend with its N-terminus 7nm above the lipid bilayer (222). The LW blood group glycoprotein (see Chapter 13) would be predicted to have a similar size. It may be that molecules of this type are involved in the second stage of adhesive interactions between cells. There is evidence that this is so in the case of CD58 and the LW analog ICAM-2

(63,64). Initial long range low affinity interactions between cells involving L-selectin/Le^x are followed by LFA1/ICAM-2 interaction and subsequent intracellular signaling through 7-membrane spanning GDP binding proteins (64). CD58 is found on nearly all hemopoietic cells. It has a molecular weight of 60-70kDa on SDS-PAGE. This reduces to 26kDa after treatment with peptidyl N-glycanase to remove N-glycans. In red cells CD58 is found only as a GPI-linked protein but in most cells and tissues where it is expressed, an alternatively spliced form with a transmembrane domain and carboxy-terminal peptide is also found (65). Rosetting of activated T lymphocytes by red cells is due to CD2 on the lymphocytes binding to CD58 on the red cells (66).

A similar, second stage role is carried out by CD59. In this case the function relates to regulation of complement-mediated red cell lysis rather than adhesive interactions. As discussed above, CD55 functions by inhibiting the activation of C3 convertase. CD59 functions by inhibiting the assembly of the membrane attack complex (MAC, see Chapter 6). MAC assembly is the final step in complement-mediated hemolysis and results in the generation of a hole in the red cell membrane. CD59 plays a vital role in preventing destruction of autologous red cells when complement is activated by foreign antigen. The importance of CD59 is clearly demonstrated by the clinical features of an individual with an inherited absence of the protein (67). CD59 is a GPI-linked protein which along with all GPI-linked red cell proteins, is deficient from the surface of the red cells of patients with PNH (21,22). Studies of a young Japanese male with PNH-like symptoms revealed that he had normal expression of other GPI-linked proteins and a complete deficiency of CD59. The severe hemolysis in this patient and by inference in PNH patients can therefore be related to CD59 (67). The structure of CD59 is known in detail and its three-dimensional structure has been reported (68). It is a small protein of 128 amino acids, including a 25 amino acid N-terminal signal peptide. The molecular weight predicted from the amino acid sequence is 11.5kDa. On SDS-PAGE, the protein runs with an Mr of 18-29,000 reflecting the presence of a large N-glycan (69). The residues critical for inhibition of MAC (amino acid 27-38) have been located by inhibition studies using synthetic peptides (70). CD59 may also function as an adhesion molecule because cells transfected with CD2 bind purified CD59 and vice versa (71). Another, less well characterized complement regulatory component found on the red cell is the C8 binding protein (syn. HRF60) (72,73).

The red cell surface also contains the GPI-linked enzyme acetylcholinesterase which carries the Cartwright blood group antigens (see Chapter 23) and the Kell protein which has a structure which suggests an enzymatic function. The Kell protein has a large extracellular disulphide-bonded domain whose structure is not yet clearly defined but it is possible that the active site of the enzyme is located at or near the surface of the glycocalyx (see Chapter 18 for further discussion).

The surface of the bilayer itself is the province of various transport proteins. Several of these are marked by blood group antigens and are discussed in detail elsewhere in this book (anion transporter, Chapter 17; urea transporter, Chapter 19; water transporter, Chapter 22). The proteins involved in expression of the Rh antigens (Chapter 12) and the Kx antigen (Chapter 18) also have structures which suggest that they function as transporter proteins although this has not been proved. Other transporter proteins not yet known to express blood group antigens are the glucose transporter, the nucleoside transporter and the Ca^{++}-ATPase. The predicted structure of the glucose transporter (syn. GLUT1, band 4.5) is shown in figure 4-7. The glucose transporter has 12 membrane spanning domains with a single complex N-glycan on the first extra cellular loop (74). The protein transports glucose across the membrane to facilitate glycolysis and thereby maintain the basal metabolism of the cell. The structure of the other minor transporters is not yet known in detail. The multiple membrane spanning domains of GLUT-1 (see figure 4-7) are typical of the transporter

FIGURE 4-7 Structure of the Red Cell Glucose Transporter (GLUT-1) (reference 74)

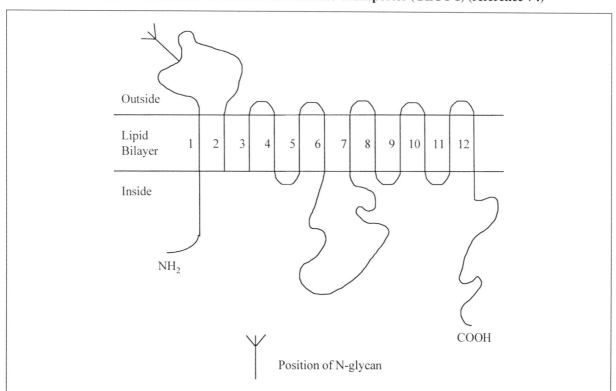

proteins. They frequently, but not always (see Rh polypeptides and Kx polypeptide) have a large N-glycan. The extracellular loops vary considerably in size. The N-glycans of GLUT-1, band 3, the water transporter (CHIP 28, Aquaporin 1) and the Rh glycoprotein are known to have blood group ABH activity and it would be expected that the N-glycans present on other transport proteins would be similarly blood group active. The anion transport function of the anion transporter, band 3, is important for maintaining ionic homeostasis by transporting Cl⁻ and HCO₃⁻ ions (75). The other transporters may serve more to maintain the metabolism of the red cell. In addition to the transporter proteins, the red cell membrane contains a chemokine receptor (Duffy glycoprotein, see Chapter 14). Chemokine receptors on cells are normally involved in transmembrane signaling through interaction with G-proteins (64). In the case of the Duffy protein however, there is some doubt whether signaling occurs (see Chapter 14). Chemokines bind to the N-terminal extracellular domain of the Duffy protein. This domain would not be expected to extend above the glycocalyx but since chemokines are small molecules and the glycocalyx is a barrier to large molecules, this structure does not pose any functional constraints. The most abundant glycolipid in the red cell membrane is a small molecule which expresses the P blood group antigen (globoside, see Chapter 11). Globoside is present in about 14 x 10⁶ copies/red cell (76). It is of interest that the so-called Donath Landsteiner antibodies, which have anti-P specificity, are of the IgG class and yet efficiently effect complement-mediated hemolysis suggesting that there are regions of the red cell membrane which are not covered by the glycocalyx and that the P lipid is found in these regions. Freeze-fracture electron microscope studies of the red cell membrane have shown the presence of intramembranous particles in the red cell membrane which are likely to represent protein "islands" (77). These "islands" certainly contain band 3 because they are altered in band 3 deficient mice and cattle (78-80).

The red cell membrane contains at least one membrane protein that although deeply embedded in the lipid bilayer does not appear to be accessible on the outer membrane surface. This protein is known as stomatin (syn. band 7.2b). Its cDNA encodes a protein of 288 amino acids (81,82). Stomatin deficiency is found in rare disorders known variously as hereditary stomatocytosis (syn. hereditary hydrocytosis) and hereditary xerocytosis depending on whether there is an excess or a deficiency of intracellular water respectively (83). Nucleotide sequencing of stomatin cDNA in these patients has not revealed any abnormality suggesting that the primary defect in these patients may affect another protein which associates with stomatin in the red cell membrane (83).

The Red Cell Skeleton

The preceding discussion has considered the role of the glycocalyx of the red cell, the functions of some molecules that extend above it, and the role of membrane proteins that are for the most part embedded in the lipid bilayer, several of which carry out essential transport functions which maintain the red cells' metabolism, and band 3 which carries out Cl⁻ and HCO₃⁻ exchange. The third element of the red cell membrane is a network of proteins which underlie the bilayer and which are collectively known as the red cell skeleton. The term red cell skeleton is generally used for the insoluble residue that remains after red cell ghosts are extracted with Triton X-100. This material comprises about 55-60% of the membrane protein and includes a number of different proteins including spectrin, actin, ankyrin, protein 4.1 and protein 4.2 (syn. pallidin), protein 4.9 (syn. dematin), p55, adducin, tropomyosin, tropomodulin and myosin (29). This network of interacting proteins gives the red cell membrane the strength and stability that it needs to survive the 120 day circulation in the body. It also imparts a large degree of flexibility and deformability to the membrane which allows red cells to pass through narrow blood capillaries. The mechanical strength and deformability of the red cell derives primarily from the unique structure of spectrin (84). Spectrin consists of two structurally similar subunits (α and ß) each present at about 200,000 copies/red cell (32). The α chain comprises 2429 amino acids (ca 280kDa, (85)) and the ß chain 2137 amino acids (ca 246kDa (86)). Both subunits consist of a repeating 106 amino acid motif which folds into triple stranded α-helical segments (87). Alpha spectrin has 20 such repeats while ß spectrin has 17. The two chains are aligned side by side in an anti-parallel arrangement with respect to their N and C terminal ends to form heterodimers (88). Each heterodimer is then arranged in a "head to head" configuration to produce tetramers and higher order oligomers (89). The free "tails" of the tetramers bind to actin filaments. This interaction is facilitated by the binding of several other proteins (protein 4.1 to ß spectrin, and the binding of several actin-associated proteins, adducin, dematin, tropomyosin, tropomodulin and myosin). The point at which spectrin, actin, protein 4.1 and the other proteins associate is known as the junctional complex. Under the electron microscope spectrin is seen as a long thread-like molecule which extends up to 100nM (89,90).

The skeletal network is linked to the red cell membrane by at least two sets of protein:protein interactions. One interaction involves ankyrin, pallidin, spectrin and band 3. The other involves protein 4.1, spectrin, p55 and glycophorins C/D.

Ankyrin links spectrin to the membrane through its association with the N-terminal cytoplasmic domain of band 3 (91) (see figure 4-1.) Ankyrin (syn. band 2.1) comprises a series of polypeptides generated by alternative splicing of mRNA (92,93). It is a large pyramid-shaped protein (8.3 x 10nM) of 206kDa (94). The molecule comprises three domains. An 89kDa N-terminal domain of 24 consecutive 33 amino acid repeats (92,93) the last 12 of which form the band 3 binding site (91,94,95), a central globular domain of 62kDa (spectrin binding domain) and a 55kDa C-terminal domain which contains a sequence that regulates spectrin and band 3 binding (96). It is in the C-terminal region that the alternatively spliced products are generated.

Band 3 (syn. AE-1) is discussed in detail in Chapter 17. For the purposes of this discussion it is relevant to note that the protein exists in the red cell membrane as a mixture of dimers, tetramers and higher oligomers (97,98). In vivo there are about ten times more copies of band 3 than ankyrin and ankyrin appears to bind predominantly to band 3 tetramers (98).

Pallidin (syn. band 4.2) can bind to both ankyrin and band 3 and it has been proposed that pallidin serves to stabilize the ankyrin:band 3 interaction. Pallidin is a 77kDa protein (reviewed in 99) which has been cloned and sequenced from a human reticulocyte cDNA library (100,101). The protein comprises 691 amino acids and is derived from a gene of about 20Kb comprising 13 exons (103). Pallidin has significant sequence homology with transglutaminase but lacks transglutaminase activity (99-102). The absence of pallidin from the membranes of band 3 deficient mice (78,79) clearly establishes that the two proteins interact in vivo.

The interaction between protein 4.1, spectrin, p55 and glycophorin C/D has only recently been clearly established. Protein 4.1 is a globular protein (5.7nm in diameter) which has a molecular weight of 66kDa (reviewed in 29,103). In the mature red cell, protein 4.1 exists in two predominant forms denoted 4.1a and 4.1b. Protein 4.1b is derived from 4.1a by deamidation of Asn502. The extent of this conversion is a good indication of the age of a red cell (104). Careful chymotrypsin digestion of protein 4.1 reveals four major fragments of 30kDa, 16kDa, 10kDa and 22/24kDa (105). The 10kDa domain is the spectrin binding domain (106,107) and the 30kDa domain contains the binding sites for glycophorin C/D and p55 (see below and figure 4-1). Protein 4.1 contains an O-linked N-acetyl glucosamine residue in the 22/24kDa domain (49). The function of this is unknown. The protein 4.1 gene is complex. It is more than 90Kb long and contains at least 23 exons which are subject to extensive alternative splicing (108-110). The first evidence that protein 4.1 interacts with GPC/D came from studies of protein 4.1 deficient red cells. Mueller and Morrison (111) observed that GPC (called glycoconnection in the paper) was present in normal red cell skeleton preparations but absent from skeletons prepared from protein 4.1 deficient cells. Subsequent studies showed that protein 4.1 is more readily extracted from GPC/D deficient red cells (syn. Leach phenotype cells, see Chapter 16) than from normal red cells (112). Another protein, p55, was implicated in this interaction when it was found that p55 is absent from both protein 4.1 deficient red cells and Leach phenotype red cells (113).

Direct evidence for protein 4.1, p55, GPC/D interactions was obtained using the purified proteins in various association assays (114-117). Protein 4.1 binds directly to GPC/D at a site on GPC/D close to the lipid bilayer. Protein 4.1 also binds to p55 and p55 binds to the extreme C terminal region of GPC/D (see figure 4-1).

Inherited Abnormalities Involving the Red Cell Skeleton

The importance of the proteins of the red cell skeleton in maintaining the shape and stability of the red cell membrane is clearly illustrated by studies carried out on the red cell membranes of individuals with abnormally shaped red cells.

Hereditary Spherocytosis (HS)

Patients with HS have fragile spherical red cells which are trapped in the spleen. Spherical red cells arise as a consequence of the loss of microvesicles from the cell surfaces. The molecular basis of HS is heterogeneous and so the degree of red cell destruction in the spleen and hence the severity of anemia associated with the disease varies considerably between patients (reviewed in 29). Severe anemia resulting from HS is usually corrected by splenectomy. The majority of HS patients inherit their disease in an autosomal dominant manner but the rarer, most severe cases are usually recessively inherited (118,119). Analysis of red cell membrane proteins in patients with HS usually identifies a defect which affects the interaction between spectrin, ankyrin, pallidin and band 3. Most HS patients have some deficiency of spectrin and in the rare (<2% of all HS patients) recessively inherited forms of disease the level of spectrin can be reduced to as little as 20-40% of normal (29). In fact, most HS patients are deficient in ankyrin as well as spectrin. Sauvides et al. (120) report that spectrin and ankyrin were both reduced in 75-80% of HS cases. It appears that the primary defect in most of these cases resides in the ankyrin gene and several different ankyrin mutations have now been identified (121).

In a study of 46 HS patients, Eber et al. (121) found 12 ankyrin mutations and five band 3 mutations. These authors concluded that ankyrin mutations are a major cause of dominant and recessive HS and that causative band 3 mutations are less common (20% of cases). They also suggested that most other HS cases result from ß-spectrin mutations (29,122). Jarolim et al. (123) found 18 different band 3 mutations in 38 of 166 families (23% of cases) with HS. Other minor (<10% of cases) causes are defects in α-spectrin (124) and pallidin (99). Pallidin deficiency is relatively common in Japan (99, 125) but rare elsewhere (126). Pallidin deficiency has been found in patients with mutations in the N-terminal cytoplasmic domain of band 3 (band 3 Montefiore (127) and band 3 Tuscaloosa (128)) suggesting that pallidin is bound to band 3 through interaction with this domain. The binding site for band 3 on pallidin has been defined as V63RRGQPFTIILYF using synthetic peptides (129). It would be expected that red cells from patients with HS resulting from mutations which cause band 3 deficiency would have reduced levels of Wr^b and Di^b antigens but this does not seem to have been reported (see Chapter 17 for further discussion).

Hereditary Elliptocytosis (HE)

HE is a relatively common disorder in which elliptocytic red cells are seen in the peripheral blood. About 1% of natives in equatorial Africa have HE as a result of mutations in α-spectrin. This high frequency has been attributed to selective pressure exerted by malaria (130). In individuals of European origin HE is 15 to 25 times less common. 60% of cases in Europeans are due to α-spectrin mutations and 40% to defects in protein 4.1 (29). Most of the spectrin mutations found in association with HE occur where the spectrin molecules associate "head to head" to form tetramers (29,83 and see figure 4-1). HE may be asymptomatic but where it is associated with hemolysis this is frequently due to the co-inheritance of an α-spectrin mutation with the α^{LELY} spectrin allele (131). Severe forms of HE may be classified as hereditary pyropoikilocytosis (HPP). HPP red cells but not HE red cells are partially deficient in spectrin. This partial spectrin deficiency is thought to explain the large number of spherocytes relative to elliptocytes found in some cases (29,132).

HE also results from the heterozygous or homozygous absence of protein 4.1. Heterozygous 4.1 deficiency is a mild condition (133). Homozygous 4.1 deficiency results in a severe hemolytic anemia which can be controlled by splenectomy (134-136). Red cells from individuals who are homozygous for 4.1 deficiency fragment more rapidly than normal cells when subject-ed to moderate shear stress (137). This fragility can be corrected by reconstituting 4.1 deficient membranes with a 62 amino acid 4.1 peptide containing the 21 residue spectrin binding domain (107).

Protein 4.1 deficient red cells also lack p55 (113) and have a reduced content of glycophorins C and D (138). The relationship between GPC, GPD, protein 4.1 and p55 has been discussed in the previous section of this chapter. For the sake of completeness it should be noted here that inherited deficiency of GPC/D (Leach phenotype) is associated with a mild elliptocytosis (139). The Leach phenotype is discussed in detail in Chapter 16. The elliptocytosis in these cells appears to be related to a partial deficiency (about 20%) of protein 4.1 (113) rather than absence of GPC/D because the mechanical fragility of Leach phenotype membranes can be restored by addition of the spectrin binding domain of protein 4.1 (107).

South East Asian Ovalocytosis (SAO)

South East Asian Ovalocytosis is a relatively common dominantly inherited condition in Melanesia and Malaya (140,141) where it may reach frequencies of 5 to 25% in certain native tribes (29). When peripheral blood smears are examined under the light microscope most of the red cells are like elliptocytes but with a more oval shape than HE. A few cells look like stomatocytes and for this reason the condition is sometimes known as stomatocytic elliptocytosis.

The condition appears to confer some resistance to malaria in these populations where malaria is endemic. The frequency of SAO increases with age in these populations, an observation that clearly suggests that the condition has some survival advantage (142). Studies carried out in vitro have suggested that SAO cells are resistant to invasion by *Plasmodium knowlesi* as well as *Plasmodium falciparum* (143). Since these parasites use different receptors on red cells (144,145) these results suggest that a general property of the SAO membrane is conferring resistance rather than absence of a specific receptor. In fact, this resistance to invasion by malaria parasites is not absolute. When parasites are cultured in fresh SAO cells invasion can take place (146). Analysis of the mechanical stability of SAO cells revealed that the membrane is 10 to 20 times more rigid than the normal red cell membrane (147,148).

The SAO phenotype has been shown to result from a mutation in one band 3 allele. The amino acid sequence of SAO band 3 deduced from the cDNA sequence reveals that SAO band 3 has a deletion of nine amino acids corresponding to part of the first transmembrane domain of normal band 3 (residues 400-408, (149-152)). SAO band 3 also contains another mutation (Lys 56 → Glu) corresponding to the band 3 Memphis variant which is common in many populations of the world and occurs in the absence of ovalocytosis (see Chapter 17 for further discussion of band 3 Memphis).

SAO cells therefore contain one normal band 3 protein and one mutant band 3 protein lacking nine amino acids. SAO cells exhibit only about half the anion transport activity of normal red cells suggesting that the mutant protein does not have transport activity (153), a conclusion supported by the demonstration that SAO band 3 when expressed in *Xenopus* oocytes is inserted into the plasma membrane of the oocytes but does not transport anions (154). It appears that the organization of the membrane domain of SAO band 3 is completely disrupted in SAO red cells. SAO band 3 lacks the polylactosaminyl oligosaccharide normally found on the fourth extracellular loop of band 3 (155) and it also lacks epitopes on the third extracellular loop of normal band 3 recognized by monoclonal antibodies (156). Such a distortion of the membrane domain is consistent with the weak reactivity of SAO cells with anti-Wr[b] and anti-Di[b] first described by Booth et al. (157, see Chapter 17 for further discussion).

Band 3 in normal red cells associates to form dimers and tetramers in the membrane with the tetramers preferentially interacting through ankyrin with the underlying red cell skeleton. Band 3 in SAO cells has a higher proportion of tetramers (50%) than normal red cells (33% (155)). Electron microscopy of SAO cell membranes shows that the increased oligomerization of SAO band 3 corresponds with the presence of linear strands of intramembraneous particles (157,223). The mutation in SAO band 3 clearly has a major affect on the organization of the red cell membrane in these cells and it seems likely that these changes are not restricted to band 3 but also affect other red cell membrane proteins which may exhibit some functional interdependence with band 3, for example, GPA, GPB, Rh polypeptides and the Rh glycoproteins (158). The weakened reactivity of SAO cells for Rh (D, C, e) and MNS (En[a], S, s, U) antigens observed by Booth et al. (224) may be a reflection of such interdependence and since Booth et al. (224) also noted weakening of Jk[a], Jk[b], Xg[a] and Sc1 it is tempting to suggest that the molecules which carry these antigens are also affected because of an altered association with band 3.

To take this speculation even further it is of note that Booth et al. (224) observed weakening of antigens denoted I[T] and I[F]. Since the I-active N-glycan found on band 3 is absent in SAO cells (155) it may be that this result reflects the dramatic reduction of I antigens sites on band 3 SAO cells. Since band 3 is the major red cell protein, absence of the N-glycan on SAO band 3 would reduce I antigen sites (and also ABH sites) by 500,000 / red cell. The studies of Booth et al. (224) provide an excellent example of how red cell serology, in skilled hands, can lead to new insights of broad biological significance.

General Methods for the Analysis of Red Cell Membrane Components: Lipid Analysis

The first step in the isolation and characterization of membrane lipids usually involves extraction of membranes with organic solvents, commonly butanol or chloroform/methanol in various ratios. When red cell membranes are extracted with n-butanol/water (or lysis buffer) most of the lipids partition into the butanol phase while protein constituents partition into the water phase. If n-butanol/high salt (mM phosphate) is used the upper lipid rich butanol phase is separated from the low aqueous phase by an interface of insoluble protein. In this case the high salt phase is a rich source of glycophorins and further purification of glycophorins is easily achieved from this material (7,159). Glycolipids are usually extracted using chloroform:methanol (2:1 v/v) after Folch et al. (160). The residue remaining after this procedure is further extracted with chloroform:methanol (1:2 v/v) containing 5% water to obtain polyglycosyl ceramides and more polar glycolipids like the sialic-acid containing gangliosides (161,162).

The aqueous phase from the initial extraction procedure is usually concentrated on a rotary evaporator and further purification of its individual constituents achieved by a suitable chromatographic step. Acidic-glycolipids can be separated from neutral glycolipids using anion exchange chromatography (e.g. DEAE-Sepherase A-25). Purification of minor lipid constituents can be extremely arduous (see Chapter 11 on the P system) but preparative thin layer chromatography (TLC) on silica gel plates is an extremely useful tool for this purpose (162).

Preliminary identification of individual lipids is usually achieved using TLC by reference to the mobility of standards of known structure. If the lipid of interest is a glycolipid with antigenic activity then it can be identified by overlaying the relevant antibody on the TLC plate and assaying for specifically bound antibody using a suitable detection system (163). This method has been particularly useful for the analysis of blood group glycolipids, see for example Henry et al. (164).

Structural analysis of the purified glycolipid is also difficult. It is possible to determine the sequence and anomeric configuration of sugars by sequential treatment with exo-glycosidases but this is laborious and requires quite large amounts of material (100μg, 162). Fast atom bombardment mass spectrometry is now the method of choice for analysis of glycolipids (162).

General Methods for the Analysis of Red Cell Membrane Components: Protein Analysis

As discussed in the introduction to this Chapter, early studies on red cell membranes were largely confined to proteins that were readily solubilized in aqueous solutions and present in large amounts (glycophorin A, spectrin). A major technical breakthrough came with the introduction of an ionic detergent, sodium dodecyl sulphate (SDS), to solubilize membrane proteins (18). When proteins are heated at 100°C for 2-5 minutes in the presence of SDS they unfold and bind SDS. SDS displaces lipid bound to integral membrane proteins and binds itself to the hydrophobic regions exposed. This results in a mixture of solubilized membrane proteins which are negatively charged because of bound SDS. The effect of SDS on a suspension of red cell membranes (ghosts) is instant and impressive. The cloudy suspension becomes transparent. When this mixture of solubilized negatively charged proteins is subjected to electrophoresis in a matrix which separates proteins according to molecular size (polyacrylamide gel) and the resultant gel stained with a protein stain, a ladder of stained bands is revealed (see figure 4-8). Under these conditions the electrophoretic mobility of a protein band is inversely proportional to the logarithm of its molecular weight meaning that the apparent molecular weight of an unknown protein band can be determined from a standard curve constructed from the mobility of a mixture of proteins of known molecular weight subjected to electrophoresis under identical conditions (165). A few red cell membrane proteins, mainly glycophorins, do not take up protein stains very well and these can be revealed using the periodic acid Schiffs base stain which stains sialic acid-rich proteins (16, figure 4-8). SDS-PAGE has been a major technical development leading to the elucidation of the structure of red cell membrane proteins.

When SDS-PAGE was introduced for the study of red cell membrane proteins the nature of the protein staining bands revealed was largely unknown and so the convention of numbering protein staining bands from the top (origin) of the SDS-gel was adopted (32). This convention is still in use although many of the bands originally defined by numbers now have other more descriptive names. The numbers, names, apparent molecular weight and abundance of each of the major proteins revealed by protein staining of SDS-gels is given in table 4-3. The glycophorins were not numbered in this way because they are not readily apparent on protein stained gels. Several different nomenclatures were developed for these proteins (166, table 4-4). Naming the glycophorin bands on SDS-gels is complicated because GPA and GPB form homo and heterodimers which are stable in SDS and so these two proteins are revealed as 5 different bands (GPA dimer, GPA monomer, GPB dimer, GPB monomer and GPA/GPB heterodimer) on single dimension SDS-gels stained with PAS stain (see Chapter 15 for further discussion). The best resolution of glycophorin bands in a single dimension gel is achieved using the discontinuous buffer system of Laemmli (167). In this method a short "stacking" gel is placed on top of the "separating" gel. The stacking gel is of a low acrylamide concentration (commonly 3% (w/v) acrylamide). The purpose of the stacking gel is not to separate proteins

FIGURE 4-8 Analysis of Red Cell Membrane Proteins using SDS-PAGE

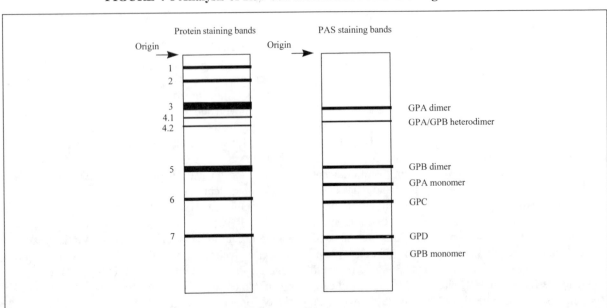

according to molecular size but to concentrate the solubilized proteins at the interface between the "stacking" and "separating" gels. This concentrating effect eliminates problems associated with the volume of sample applied to the gel (if a separating gel is used alone the greater the volume of sample applied the less effective the separation of components in the sample).

The concentration effect is achieved by the use of different buffers in the stacking gel (Tris-HCl pH 6.8), the separating gel (Tris-HCl pH 8.8) and the electrode chamber (Tris-glycine pH 8.3). On application of current, a moving boundary is created in the stacking gel with chloride ions at its leading edge and glycinate at its trailing edge. Protein-SDS complexes have a mobility less than the fully ionized chloride ions but greater than the uncharged glycinate ions and so the proteins are "stacked" and enter the separating gel as a very narrow band. When the protein enters the separating gel the pH rises from 6.8 to 8.8, the glycinate ions become negatively charged and migrate faster than the proteins (168). The acrylamide concentration of the separating gel can be varied according to the size range of the particular proteins of interest, concentrations of between 5 and 15% are commonly selected.

SDS-PAGE may be carried out under reducing or non-reducing conditions. The terms reducing and non-reducing simply refer to whether or not the protein sample has been boiled in the presence of a thiol reagent (commonly 2-mercaptoethanol or dithiothreitol). Reducing agents break inter- and intrachain disulphide bonds in proteins and so gels run under reducing conditions separate individual polypeptide chains rather than individual proteins. If a protein comprises two polypeptide chains of different molecular weights linked by interchain disulphide bonds two bands will be stained under reducing conditions and only one (of higher molecular weight) under non-reducing conditions. An example of this is provided by the Kell protein which is linked by disulphide bonding to the Kx protein (169,170, see also Chapter 18). Polypeptide chains whose folding is defined by intrachain disulphide bonds may give different apparent molecular weights when examined under reducing or non-reducing conditions. This may be related to the fact that under non-reducing conditions the protein is not completely unfolded and therefore binds less SDS than under reducing conditions. An example of this is provided by the Duffy glycoprotein (171, see also Chapter 14).

Stained polyacrylamide gels subjected to electrophoresis in one dimension give an oversimplified picture of the complexity of the red cell membrane. Different polypeptides may have similar apparent molecular weights and so run in the same place on a single dimension gel. What appears to be one protein band may actually comprise several. In addition, proteins present in very small amounts may not be visualized at the level of sensitivity of conventional protein stains. The problem of multiple bands running in the same place can be addressed by the technique of two-dimensional SDS-PAGE. In this technique SDS-PAGE provides the second dimension and is preceded by separation of proteins according to charge rather than size. Commonly the membranes are solubilized in a non-ionic detergent and individual proteins separated according to their isoelectric point in a tube gel (172,173). This gel is then placed at the origin of a polyacrylamide slab gel containing SDS and electrophoresis is carried out at right angles to the direction of current used in the original gel. When this

TABLE 4-3 Major Protein-staining Bands of the Red Cell Membrane

Number	Name	Apparent Molecular Weight	Abundance Copies/Cell
Band 1	Spectrin α chain	240,000	2×10^5
Band 2	Spectrin β chain	215,000	2×10^5
Band 2.1	Ankyrin	210,000	10^5
Band 3	Anion Transporter (AE1)	90,000	10^6
Band 4.1		78,000	2×10^5
Band 4.2	Pallidin	72,000	2×10^5
Band 4.5	Glucose Transporter (GLUT1)	50,000	5×10^5
Band 5	Actin	43,000	4×10^5
Band 6	Glyceraldehyde 3-phosphate dehydrogenase	35,000	5×10^5
Band 7	Stomatin	29,000	2×10^5

TABLE 4-4 Major PAS-staining Bands of the Red Cell Membrane (from reference 166)

	Alternative Names			Apparent Molecular Weight
GPA dimer	PAS-1	α_2	MN glycoprotein dimer	
GPA/GPB heterodimer	PAS-4	$\alpha\delta$		
GPB dimer		δ_2	Ss glycoprotein dimer	
GPA monomer	PAS-2	α	MN glycoprotein	37,000
GPC	PAS-2′	β	D-sialoglycoprotein, glycoconnectin	35,000
GPD		γ	E-sialoglycoprotein	27,000
GPB monomer	PAS-3	δ	Ss glycoprotein monomer	24,000

technique is used for the red cell membrane more than 200 protein-staining spots are observed (174). This technique although providing high resolution has several drawbacks, apart from being technically quite difficult to perform. Glycoproteins tend to run as diffuse rather than discrete spots presumably because of heterogeneity in glycosylation and since most blood group proteins are glycosylated, additional treatment with glycosidases is often needed to give clear results. Nevertheless, the technique has been used with considerable success for the identification of mutant forms of spectrin (175), increased sensitivity of detection can be obtained with radioactive labels and subsequent autoradiography of the two-dimensional gel.

Methods for Labeling Membrane Proteins

SDS-PAGE separates membrane proteins according to their size but does not provide any information concerning the position of those proteins in the membrane. Is the protein on the outer surface of the cell membrane, the cytoplasmic surface or does it traverse the membrane? Various labeling methods can be employed to answer these questions. One of the most useful is lactoperoxidase-catalyzed radioiodination (176). Lactoperoxidase (LPO) is a relatively large protein (Mr 77,500) which does not penetrate plasma membranes. Thus when intact red cells are incubated with LPO ^{125}I and hydrogen peroxidase, only tyrosine residues accessible on the outside of the cell will be labeled. Red cell "ghosts" are permeable to LPO so that the same experiment carried out on "ghosts" will label accessible tyrosine residues on both the outer and cytoplasmic surfaces of the membrane.

SDS-PAGE of membranes derived from LPO labeled intact red cells and LPO labeled red cell "ghosts" followed by autoradiography of the gels will therefore provide information concerning the organization of protein in the membrane because it will distinguish proteins confined to the inside or outside of the membrane and those which traverse the membrane. Autoradiography involves exposing the acrylamide gel to X-ray film and developing the film to identify radioactive bands. The developed film can then be overlaid on the protein stained gel so that the radioactive bands can be correlated with individual protein stained bands. It is usually convenient to dry the protein stained gel under vacuum before autoradiography. The sensitivity of detection of ^{125}I-labeled bands can be greatly increased by the use of an intensifying screen causing the release of multiple photons which expose the film (177).

Carbohydrate can also be labeled. Particularly useful for studies of red cell membranes is the periodate/NaB³H₄ method (178). Sialic acid is readily oxidized by periodate so that this method provides a good way of labeling glycophorins on red cells. Alternatively, galactose residues may be labeled using galactose oxidase/NaB³H₄ (179). SDS-PAGE of membranes derived from labeled cells or ghosts is visualized by fluorography. Fluorography rather than autoradiography is used for the detection of ³H because the energy of this isotope is too low to emerge from the gel or penetrate the X-ray film. For ³H it is necessary to soak the gel in a fluor such as 1M sodium salicylate before drying. The fluor, or scintillant, captures the radiation extremely efficiently and converts it into photons which can leave the gel and expose X-ray film. Fluorography is only effective at -70°C (180, also see Goding, 168, for details concerning methodology).

The Use of Antibodies to Identify Membrane Proteins

One of the most attractive ways of approaching the characterization of a red cell membrane protein is to exploit the availability of an antibody to it. In the case of blood group-active proteins it may be possible to utilize existing polyclonal antibodies of human or animal origin. Human polyclonal anti-D, -c, -E and -Fy^a were used by Moore et al. (181) to identify the proteins carrying Rh and Fy^a antigens, respectively, using immune precipitation (see Chapters 12 and 14 for a detailed discussion). In this method intact red cells with appropriate antigens are usually labeled with radioactive iodine or tritium using either the lactoperoxidase or periodate/NaB^{3}H$_4$ methods (described in the previous section) and then incubated with the appropriate antiserum to produce "sensitized cells". A non-ionic detergent (commonly Triton X-100) is then added to the washed sensitized cells in order to solubilize the membrane proteins. The assumption is made that the detergent will not denature the antibody or its antigen and that the antigen-antibody complex will be solubilized as a complete unit. It is then necessary to isolate the antigen-antibody complex from the mixture of detergent-solubilized membrane components. This can be achieved using protein A or protein G since these proteins bind specifically to the Fc portion of antibodies. If the protein A or protein G is itself covalently coupled to a particle like sepharose beads (a polymer of D-galactose) then the protein A or protein G beads when mixed with the Triton solubilized components will specifically bind only the antigen-antibody complex and that complex can be removed from the mixture of proteins simply by centrifugation and recovery of the beads. The antigen-antibody complexes can then be solubilized in SDS, a process which separates antigen from antibody and analyzed by SDS-PAGE. If the antibody:antigen complex is solubilized under reducing conditions and the resulting gel is stained with a protein stain, bands corresponding to the heavy and light chains of the antibody and a band(s) corresponding to the reactive antigen will be observed (provided that the antigen does not have the same Mr as either the heavy or light chain). If the antigen has been labeled (e.g. with ^{125}I or ^{3}H) it can be revealed by exposing the gel to X-ray film using autoradiography or fluorography as appropriate. Immune precipitation has been used extensively with both human polyclonal blood group antibodies and monoclonal antibodies, to identify blood group-active proteins on human red cells and the reader will find numerous examples in the chapters of this book dealing with the blood group systems.

An alternative and simpler method for identifying blood group-active red cell membrane proteins is immune blotting (syn. Western blotting, 182). In this technique the components of red cell membranes of appropriate blood group phenotype are separated by SDS-PAGE. The separated components are then electrophorectically transferred to nitrocellulose paper or another suitable matrix. If all the proteins have transferred from the gel to the paper (some of the higher molecular weight components may not transfer as well as

other components) it can be used to detect antigenically active components. Before this can be done it is necessary to mix the paper with a suitable protein solution (5% w/v bovine milk powder is very suitable) to coat all areas of the paper which are not occupied by membrane protein. Antibody (polyclonal or monoclonal) can then be incubated with the paper (better results are usually obtained if polyclonal blood group antibodies are prepared for use as eluates rather than crude serum). After appropriate washes bound antibody can be detected with an enzyme-antiglobulin conjugate (usually alkaline phosphatase or horseradish peroxidase) or if preferred by ^{125}I protein A. The position of the antigen can be visualized by adding enzyme substrate, the product of enzymatic activity is insoluble and colored and marks the position of antigen, or by autoradiography. This extremely useful technique has a major caveat. It will only work if the antigen of interest is not denatured by the process of SDS-PAGE. This is a disadvantage that does not apply to immune precipitation but because immune blotting is less laborious than immune precipitation it is common practice, when trying to identify a previously unidentified antigenically active protein, to begin with immune blotting and if this fails to try immune precipitation. When one considers that the process of SDS-PAGE separates and unfolds polypeptide chains it is quite surprising how successful immunoblotting has been for the identification of blood group-active proteins. Several blood group-active proteins were identified for the first time using this method, (Indian antigens Chapter 29, Cromer antigens Chapter 24, Lutheran antigens Chapter 20, Sc antigens Chapter 26 and Dombrock antigens Chapter 22, to name but a few). It should be said, however, that it is usually necessary to carry out immunoblotting under non-reducing conditions to achieve success. This is because many of the blood group proteins have intrachain disulphide bonds which maintain their structure and the antigens are not detectable if these bonds are broken (see Chapters on Indian, Cromer and Lutheran for examples).

Purification of Membrane Proteins

Although purification of membrane proteins can be achieved by conventional protein fractionation procedures which rely on separation on the basis of charge or size (see for example 183) these methods are laborious and particularly difficult to apply to proteins which represent only a small percentage of the total membrane protein. The commonest approach is to utilize a monoclonal antibody specific for the protein of interest. As described in Chapter 2, monoclonal antibodies are available in virtually unlimited quantities and so constraints on availability that might apply to polyclonal blood group antibodies do not apply.

One approach is to purify red cell membrane proteins by large scale immune precipitation. This method was used to purify the Rh polypeptides (and the Rh glycoproteins which coprecipitate with the polypeptides) in sufficient quantity to allow partial amino acid sequence analysis (184-186). In one experiment human monoclonal anti-D (1.5 liters of culture supernatant) was used to obtain approximately 7nmol of D polypeptide from 500ml of whole blood (185). Preparative immune precipitates were run on SDS-PAGE and the desired polypeptides localized by autoradiography utilizing a similar analytical immune precipitate from ^{125}I-labeled red cells run on the same gel. The Rh polypeptide could then be excised from the wet gel and recovered by a process known as electroelution (187). In essence, the excised gel is placed in a tube with an acrylamide plug and a dialysis sac bound to one end and subjected to electrophoresis until the protein passes out of the gel and into the dialysis sac.

This approach is suited for the purification of extremely hydrophobic proteins like the Rh proteins which are difficult to separate from other associated membrane proteins. However, many membrane proteins are not so difficult to handle and their purification can be achieved by a simple form of immunoaffinity chromatography. Monoclonal antibody of the desired specificity is purified and bound through its Fc portion to a solid phase using protein A which has been covalently coupled to sepharose beads. The long term stability of the antibody/protein A interaction can be improved by covalently crosslinking the antibody to protein A (188,189). Membrane proteins solublized in a suitable non-ionic detergent and after high speed centrifugation to remove soluble material, are applied to the antibody column in a suitable buffer (usually between pH 7 and pH 8). After application of the membrane proteins the column is washed extensively to remove "non-specifically bound" proteins and then the protein of interest is eluted from the column usually at acid pH (2.5 to 4). The eluate can be collected into a buffer which will restore the pH to neutral to minimize the exposure of the protein of interest to acidic conditions. If elution under acid conditions is unsuccessful high pH (5mm diethylamine, pH 11.5) may be successful. This approach has been used to purify several blood group-active proteins from red cells including LW (190,191), Lutheran (192) and Kell (170). Further purification of the eluted material can be achieved by subjecting it to SDS-PAGE and elution from the gel.

Amino Acid Sequence Analysis of Proteins

In order to determine the amino acid sequence of a protein the usual procedure is to obtain a partial amino acid sequence which is suitable for the design of a synthetic oligonucleotide which can be used to screen cDNA libraries (see Chapter 5 for further discussion of this procedure). The first step is usually to try to obtain the sequence of amino acids at the amino-terminus of the protein but sometimes the amino terminus is blocked and cannot be sequenced. This was the case with Kell protein (193). The Kell protein does not have a cleavable signal sequence. There is an initiator methionine which is likely to be posttranslationally cleaved exposing glutamic acid at the amino terminus. Glutamic acid is easily deaminated to form pyroglutamic acid which blocks the process of amino acid sequence analysis. In this case it becomes necessary to isolate peptides from the purified protein so that amino acid sequence of an internal piece of the protein can be obtained and a suitable oligonucleotide synthesized from this. Trypsin which cleaves polypeptide chains at lysine or arginine is a commonly used enzyme for this purpose. When the protein has been digested with a suitable protease the peptides are separated by SDS-PAGE, electrophoretically transferred to a suitable solid phase, visualized with a protein stain, and the stained bands excised and used for sequence analysis. Amino acid sequence analysis is a repetitive process in which the free amino group of each amino acid (starting with the amino terminal residue of the protein or peptide) is reacted with phenylisothiocyanate (Edman reagent) to produce a phenylthiocarbamyl peptide and then treated with a weak acid to produce the phenylthiohydantoin (PTH) of the N-terminal amino acid. The nature of the PTH amino acids is determined as they are released by the position at which they elute from a chromatographic column (194). Each of the 23 amino acids has a characteristic elution point which allows the sequence to be determined. This whole process is automated and sufficient sequence for the design of an oligonucleotide probe can be obtained from very small quantities of protein or peptide overnight. However, to determine the complete amino acid sequence of a large protein is a lengthy process even with automated sequencing because it is necessary to sequence a series of overlapping peptides to be able to assemble a complete sequence. Nowadays this is rarely done because the sequence can be deduced from cDNA. This approach does have some disadvantages however. When protein sequences are predicted from cDNA sequences the possible sites of glycosylation can be predicted but not proved. Comparison of the cDNA sequence and the actual amino acid sequence does demonstrate the actual sites of N-glycosylation because asparagine when it is glycosylated is recorded as aspartic acid on an amino acid sequence. Such discrepancies (asparagine predicted by cDNA sequence and aspartic acid obtained by amino acid sequence) have allowed definite conclusions about some possible sites of N-glycosylation in the Rh associated protein CD47 (195 and see Chapter 12) and the LW glycoprotein (191 and see Chapter 13).

Determining the Structure of Proteins

The 3-dimensional structures of relatively few membrane proteins have been elucidated. This is in large part because of the difficulty in obtaining sufficient purified membrane protein for X-ray crystallography. The archetypal membrane protein for which the crystal structure has been determined is bacteriorhodopsin (33,34). The human red cell membrane proteins CD59 (68) and the Colton blood group glycoprotein (CHIP, Aquaporin-1, 196, 197 and see Chapter 22) have been studied at this level but most of the structures for membrane proteins described in this book are predicted not actual. These predictions are based on comparisons with homologous proteins found on other cells and tissues for which more detailed structural information is available.

The first steps in trying to predict the structure of a blood group-active membrane protein whose primary amino acid sequence has been deduced from cDNA sequence will include a search of international protein sequence and DNA sequence databases to see if the protein has already been described under another name in another cell or tissue (this is not an uncommon occurrence, see CD47 (Chapter 12) and Ok^a antigen (Chapter 31)). If the sequence describes a novel protein there will frequently be other proteins in the database which have regions of homology with it which provide clues regarding the structure of the protein and its probable function. Proteins which show significant sequence homology are grouped in superfamilies (198). Two superfamilies which are well represented by blood group-active proteins on the human red cell membrane are the immunoglobulin superfamily (IgSF) and the complement control protein (CCP) superfamily. The Ig superfamily is the largest superfamily of cell surface proteins and approximately 40% of leukocyte membrane polypeptides contain IgSF domains. An IgSF domain comprises about 100 amino acids and is folded through characteristic disulphide bonds. Comparison of the protein sequence of a novel candidate IgSF member with known IgSF members is achieved by alignment according to the position of the cysteine residues which are critical for disulphide bonding and hence the folding of the domains. IgSF domains may have homology with variable domains of antibody molecules (V-set) or constant domains (C-set).

The CCP superfamily is represented by the Cromer (syn. DAF, CD55) and Knops (syn. CR1, CD35) blood group-active proteins. The CCP domain is commonly called a short consensus repeat (SCR). SCRs comprise about 60 amino acids and their folding is defined by conserved cysteines which form disulphide bonds (199).

The Duffy blood group glycoprotein is a member of the chemokine receptor family (200) while the Kell protein is a member of a small subfamily of membrane bound metalloproteinases (201).

A second step in attempting to understand the structure of a novel membrane protein is to examine the predicted amino acid sequence for regions rich in hydrophobic amino acids which could form transmembrane domains. This is normally achieved by a hydropathy plot (202) which essentially scans segments of the polypeptide chain (usually 10 amino acids at a time) for hydrophobicity and hydrophilicity. This is a quick and useful method of predicting the orientation of a membrane protein in the bilayer and provides a model around which to design experiments to confirm or disprove the predicted structure.

General Methods for the Analysis of Red Cell Membrane Components: Carbohydrate Analysis

The analysis of carbohydrate structures on membrane glycolipids and glycoproteins is complex and difficult. The same glycoprotein may have both N-glycans and O-glycans, it may have several N-glycans and/or many O-glycans. There is commonly heterogeneity in the structure of N- and O-glycans on a given molecule and individual molecules of the same protein may have differences in their carbohydrate content. Several of these points are illustrated by glycophorin A. It has a single N-glycan (54) and several, maybe 16 O-glycans (203). Most of the O-glycans are tetrasaccharides but some trisaccharides are found (57) and also some pentasaccharides (204). Individual GPA molecules on the same red cell appear to have different glycosylation patterns because only a proportion (ca 40%) of GPA is susceptible to digestion with chymotrypsin, the resistant portion appears to be due to additional O glycosylation on this fraction of the molecules (205,206).

Similar heterogeneity of polylactosaminyl N glycans is also observed. For example, the N-glycan of band 3 differs in structure depending on whether or not the I antigen or i antigen is expressed (55,207) but red cells from adults react with both anti-I and anti-i (Chapter 10) indicating heterogeneity of carbohydrate structure within band 3 molecules. The large polylactosamyl glycolipids show a similar heterogeneity of structure. The structure of smaller glycolipids can be more precisely defined.

Given the complex nature of the problem it is not

surprising that the glycosylation patterns of most red cell membrane glycoproteins and glycolipids are known in general rather than in precise terms.

It is relatively easy to establish that a red cell membrane protein is glycosylated. The first clue is often the fact that the protein gives a diffuse band when studied using SDS-PAGE. The diffuse nature of the band indicates heterogeneity of glycosylation. Confirmation of glycosylation can then be achieved by the use of exo or endoglycosidases. Exoglycosidases release terminal sugars from oligosaccharides whereas endoglycosidases cut glycosidic bonds within the oligosaccharide itself (reviewed in 208). The most widely used enzymes for this purpose are sialidase (syn. neuraminidase, receptor destroying enzyme) and peptidyl N-glycanase. Sialidases are available from a variety of microbial sources and most of them cleave sialic acid from glycoproteins, irrespective of the nature of the linkage to other sugar residues in the oligosaccharide (209). If the protein band of interest is sharpened after sialidase treatment and, more significantly, if it shows a shift in apparent molecular weight, this suggests a significant content of O-glycans. The presence of O-glycans can be confirmed by the use of an endo-glycosidase sometimes called O-glycanase which cleaves the N-acetylgalactosamine-serine/threonine linkage (210). O-glycanase is rather expensive and a cheaper alternative available in most blood grouping laboratories is to look at the mobility of the protein of interest in membranes derived from Tn red cells. Tn syndrome results from a deficiency of the ß-galactosyltransferase required for O-glycan synthesis so that a proportion of the O-glycans present on those cells comprise N-acetylgalactosamine alone or an oligosaccharide of sialic acid and N-acetyl galactosamine (see Chapter 42). Proteins with a significant content of O-glycans show a marked shift in apparent molecular weight in membranes from Tn positive red cells (see Spring et al. 211 for example).

Peptidyl-N-glycanase hydrolyzes the N-acetylglucosamine-asparagine bond which links N-glycans to proteins. The enzyme is obtained from cultures of *Flavobacterium meningosepticum* (212). These cultures also contain a second enzyme endo ß-N acetyl glucosaminidase F (Endo F). Proteins treated with this enzyme show a marked shift in apparent molecular weight and sharpening of the band on SDS-PAGE if they contain N-glycans. For example, treatment of the Duffy glycoprotein on red cells with an enzyme preparation containing Endo F and peptidyl N glycanase results in a dramatic shift of a very diffuse band of Mr 40,000 to 70,000 to a sharp band of 28 kDa (213).

Another endoglycosidase which is of particular value in blood group research is endo-ß-galactosidase. This enzyme can be found in *Streptococcus pneumoniae*,

Escherichia freundii and *Bacteriodes fragilis*. The enzyme cleaves internal ß-galactoside linkages and so is particularly useful for the study of polylactosaminyl structures. Band 3 which has a large polylactosaminyl N-glycan is noticeable sharpened when examined on SDS-PAGE after endo ß-galactosidase treatment (213). This enzyme is responsible for the exposure of the Tk antigen in vivo and can be used to make Tk red cells in vitro. Tk antigen is defined by the appearance of terminal N-acetyl glucosamine residues after exposure to the enzyme (214,215 and Chapter 42).

Other glycosidases are not commonly used on intact red cells although there has been some interest in the use of α-galactosidase and α-N-acetyl galactosaminidase to cleave B and A antigens respectively from red cells of appropriate blood group thereby converting them into O cells for transfusion purposes (216). The ability of coffee bean α-galactosidase to change B cells to O cells has been known for a long time (217). This enzyme is now widely available and it works well. Attempts to find a source of α-N-acetyl galactosaminidase that is similarly robust have not been so successful.

The determination of the complete structure of an oligosaccharide requires that it be isolated in pure form. Methods for the purification of glycoproteins and glycolipids have been discussed in the preceding sections. O-glycans can be released from glycoproteins by treatment with alkali. Montreuil et al. (208) suggest 0.05 - 0.1M NaOH or KOH at 4-45°C for 0.5 - 6 days. $NaBH_4$ (0.8 - 2M) is included in the reaction mixture in order to minimize damage or alteration of the released glycans.

The sequential use of exoglycosidases can be a useful approach to the determination of an oligosaccharide structure particularly for determining the anomeric linkage (α or ß) of one sugar to another.

N-glycans are usually released by hydrazinolysis. Hydrazine cleaves N-glycosidase linkages and deacetylates the released glycans. Re-acetylation is achieved using acetic anhydride with the glycan material dissolved in saturated $NaHCO_3$. Finally the glycan is stabilized by reduction with $NaBH_4$ (208).

For proteins which contain both O- and N-glycans, O-glycans are released by alkali treatment and then hydrazinolysis is performed to release N-glycans.

The above procedures may produce a complex mixture of oligosaccharides which require further purification before structural analysis can be undertaken. Conventional biochemical approaches of separation by size (gel filtration) or charge (ion-exchange chromatography) can be used and the judicious use of lectin affinity columns is also of value. Lectins have been used widely in blood group serology and it is well known that the ability of a lectin to agglutinate red cells is frequently inhibited by the addition of the appropriate monosaccharide. Indeed inhibition of ABH-active lectins by monosaccharides together with the use of exoglycosidases was of considerable value in the elucidation of the nature of ABH antigens (218). It is now clear that lectins are not simply reacting with monosaccharides but bind with very different affinities to different complex oligosaccharides. This property can be exploited to purify complex mixtures of oligosaccharides. The oligosaccharide mixture is applied to a lectin-sepharose column and different oligosaccharide fractions eluted by application of gradually increasing concentrations of a suitable inhibitory mono or oligosaccharide (208).

One of the most powerful methods for determining the structure of oligosaccharides utilizes fast atom bombardment mass spectrometry (FABMS). The power of this approach is demonstrated by the work of Fukuda and Dell on the oligosaccharides of band 3 (55,207) and GPA (204).

References

1. Dodge JT, Mitchell C, Hanahan DJ. Arch Biochem Biophys 1965;100:119
2. Baranowski T, Lisowska E, Morawiecki A, et al. Arch Immunol i Terapii Dosw 1959;7:15
3. Klenk E, Uhlenbruck G. Hoppe-Seyler's Z Physiol Chem 1960;319:151
4. Kathan RH, Winzler RJ, Johnson CA. J Exp Med 1961;37:37
5. Springer GF, Nagai Y, Tegtmeyer H. Biochemistry 1966;5:3254
6. Hamaguchi H, Cleve H. Biochim Biophys Acta 1972;278:271
7. Anstee DJ, Tanner MJA. Vox Sang 1975;29:378
8. Winzler RJ. In: Red Cell Membrane: Structure and Function. Philadelphia:Lippincott, 1969:157
9. Marchesi VT, Steers E, Tillack TW, et al. In: Red Cell Membrane: Structure and Function. Philadelphia:Lippincott 1969:117
10. Parpart AK, Dzieman AJ. Cold Spr Harb Symp Quant Biol 1940;8:17
11. Sweeley CC, Dawson G. In: Red Cell Membrane: Structure and Function. Philadelphia:Lippincott, 1969:172
12. Davson H, Danielli JF. The Permeability of Natural Membranes. New York:Cambridge,1952
13. Hakomori SI, Strycharz GD. Biochemistry 1968;7:1279
14. Koscielak J. Biochim Biophys Acta 1963;78:313
15. Kabat EA. Blood Group Substances. New York:Academic 1956
16. Morgan WTJ. Proc Roy Soc Series B 1960;151:308
17. Watkins WM. Science 1966;152:172
18. Fairbanks G, Steck TL, Wallach DFH. Biochemistry 1971;10:2606
19. Low MG, Finean JB. Biochem J 1977;167:281
20. Stevens VL. Biochem J 1995;310:361
21. Kinoshita T, Inoue N, Takeda J. Adv Immunol 1995;60:57
22. Rosse WF, Ware RE. Blood 1995;86:3277
23. Lux SE. Sem Hematol 1979;16:21
24. Rosenberg SA, Guidotti G. J Biol Chem 1968;243:1985
25. Alberts B, Bray D, Lewis J, et al. Molecular Biology of the Cell, 3rd Ed. New York:Garland, 1994:480
26. Morrot G, Herve P, Zachowski A, et al. Biochemistry 1989;28:3456
27. Connor J, Pak CH, Zwaal RFA, et al. J Biol Chem 1992;267:19412
28. Schroit AJ, Bloy C, Connor J, et al. Biochemistry 1990;29:10303
29. Lux SE, Palek J. In: Blood: Principles and Practice in Hematology. Philadelphia:Lippincott, 1995:1701
30. Kuypers FM, van Linde-Sibenius-Trip B, Roelfson B, et al. Biochem J 1984;221:931
31. Bretscher MS. Science 1973;181:622
32. Steck TL. J Cell Biol 1974;62:1
33. Henderson R, Unwin PNT. Nature 1975;257:28
34. Deisenhofer J, Epp O, Miki K, et al. Nature 1985;318:618
35. de Vetten MP, Agre P. J Biol Chem 1988;263:18193
36. Hartel-Schenk S, Agre P. J Biol Chem 1992;267:5569
37. Idzerda RL, Carter WG, Nottenburg C. Proc Nat Acad Sci USA 1989;86:4659
38. Schmidt MFG. Biochim Biophys Acta 1989;988:411
39. Staufenbiel M, Lazarides E. Proc Nat Acad Sci USA 1986;83:318
40. Ruff P, Speicher DW, Husain-Chishti A. Proc Nat Acad Sci USA 1991;88:6595
41. Singer SJ. Ann Rev Cell Biol 1990;6:247
42. Singer SJ, Yaffe MP. Trends Biochem Sci 1990;15:369
43. High S, Dobberstein B. Curr Opin Cell Biol 1992;4:581
44. Hartmann E, Rapoport TA, Lodish HF. Proc Nat Acad Sci USA 1989;86:5786
45. Ferguson MA, Homans SW, Dwek RA, et al. Science 1988;239:753
46. Homans SW, Ferguson MAJ, Dwek RA, et al. Nature 1988;333:269
47. Roberts WL, Santikarn S, Reinhold VN, et al. J Biol Chem 1988;263:18776
48. Bessler M, Mason PJ, Hillmen P, et al. EMBO J 1994;13:110
49. Inaba M, Maede Y. J Biol Chem 1989;264:18149
50. Bause A. Biochem J 1983:209:331
51. Opdenakker G, Rudd RM, Ponting CP, et al. FASEB J 1993;7:1330
52. Hansen JE, Lund O, Engelbrecht J, et al. Biochem J 1995;308:801
53. Carraway K, Hull S. Glycobiology 1991;1:131
54. Yoshima H, Furthmayr H, Kobata A. J Biol Chem 1980;255:9713
55. Fukuda M, Dell A, Oates JE, et al. J Biol Chem 1984;259:8260
56. Kornfeld R, Kornfeld S. Ann Rev Biochem 1985;54:631
57. Lisowska E, Duk M, Dahr W. Carbohyd Res 1980;79:103
58. Blanchard D, Cartron J-P, Fournet B, et al. J Biol Chem 1983;258:7691
59. Wickner WT, Lodish HF. Science 1985;230:400
60. Viitala J, Jarnefelt J. Trends Biochem Sci 1985;10:392
61. Jentoft N. Trends Biochem Sci 1990;15:291
62. Dahr W. In: Recent Advances in Blood Group Biochemistry. Arlington, VA:Am Assoc Blood Banks, 1986:23
63. Haraguchi M, Yamashiro S, Furukawa K, et al. Biochem J 1995;312:273
64. Springer TA. Cell 1994;76:301
65. Klickstein LB, Springer TA. In: Leucocyte Typing vol V, Oxford:Oxford Univ Press 1995;2:1475
66. Springer TA, Dustin ML, Kishimoto TK, et al. Ann Rev Immunol 1987;5:223
67. Yamashina M, Ueda E, Kinoshita T, et al. New Eng J Med 1990;323:1184
68. Kieffer B, Driscoll PC, Campbell ID, et al. Biochemistry 1994;33:4471

69. Klickstein LB, Springer TA. In: Leucocyte Typing vol V, Oxford:Oxford Univ Press 1995;2:1476

70. Nakano Y, Tozaki T, Kikuta N, et al. Mol Immunol 1995;32:241

71. Hahn WC, Menu E, Bothwell ALM, et al. Science 1992;256:1805

72. Schonermark S, Rauterberg EW, Shin ML, et al. J Immunol 1986;136:1772

73. Zalman LS, Wood LM, Müller-Eberhard HJ. Proc Nat Acad Sci USA 1986;83:6975

74. Mueckler M, Caruso C, Baldwin SA, et al. Science 1985;229:941

75. Tanner MJA. Sem Hematol 1993;30:34

76. Fletcher KS, Brewer EG, Schwarting GA. J Biol Chem 1979;254:11196

77. Weinstein RS. In: Red Cell Membrane: Structure and Function. Philadelphia:Lippincott, 1969:36

78. Southgate CD, Chishti AH, Mitchell B, et al. Nature Genet 1996;14:227

79. Peters LL, Shivdasani RA, Liu SC, et al. Cell 1996;86:917

80. Inaba M, Yawata A, Koshino I, et al. J Clin Invest 1996;97:1804

81. Heibl-Dirschmeid C, Entler B, Glotzmann C, et al. Biochim Biophys Acta 1991;1090:123

82. Stewart GW, Hepworth-Jones BE, Keen JN, et al. Blood 1992;79:1593

83. Delaunay J. In: Blood Cell Biochemistry, vol 6. New York:Plenum, 1995:1

84. Chasis J, Mohandas N. J Cell Biol 1986;103:343

85. Sahr KE, Laurila P, Kotula L, et al. J Biol Chem 1990;265:4434

86. Winkelmann JC, Chang J-G, Tse WT, et al. J Biol Chem 1990;265:11827

87. Speicher DW, Marchesi VT. Nature 1984;311:177

88. Speicher DW, Morrow JS, Knowles WJ, et al. J Biol Chem 1982:257:9093

89. Liu S-C, Windisch P, Kim S, et al. Cell 1984;37:587

90. Shotton DM, Burke BE, Branton D. J Mol Biol 1979;131:303

91. Davis LH, Otto E, Bennett V. J Biol Chem 1991;266:11163

92. Lambert S, Yu H, Prchal JT, et al. Proc Nat Acad Sci USA 1990;87:1730

93. Lux SE, John KM, Bennett V. Nature 1990;344:36

94. Davis LH, Bennett V. J Biol Chem 1990;265:10589

95. Michaely P, Bennett V. J Biol Chem 1993;268:22703

96. Hall TG, Bennett V. J Biol Chem 1987;262:10537

97. Jennings ML. Ann Rev Biophys Chem 1989;18:397

98. Casey JR, Reithmeier RAF. J Biol Chem 1991;266:15726

99. Yawata Y. Biochim Biophys Acta 1994;1204:131

100. Korsgren C, Lawler J, Lambert S, et al. Proc Nat Acad Sci USA 1990;87:613

101. Sung LA, Chien S, Chang L-S, et al. Proc Nat Acad Sci USA 1990;87:955

102. Korsgren C, Cohen CM. Proc Nat Acad Sci USA 1991;88:4840

103. Conboy JG. Sem Hematol 1993;30:58

104. Inaba M, Guptka KC, Kuwabara M, et al. Blood 1992;79:3355

105. Leto TL, Marchesi VT. J Biol Chem 1984;259:4603

106. Correas I, Speicher DW, Marchesi VT. J Biol Chem 1986;261:13362

107. Discher D, Parra M, Conboy JG, et al. (abstract). Blood 1993; 82:(suppl 1) 4a

108. Huang J-P, Tang C, Kou G, et al. J Biol Chem 1993;268:3758

109. Conboy JG, Chan JY, Chasis JA, et al. J Biol Chem 1991;266:8273

110. Conboy JG, Chan JY, Mohandas N, et al. Proc Nat Acad Sci USA 1988;85:9062

111. Mueller TJ, Morrison M. In: Erythrocyte Membranes 2: Recent Clinical and Experimental Advances. New York:Liss, 1981:95

112. Pinder JC, Chung A, Reid ME, et al. Blood 1993;82:3482

113. Alloisio N, Dalla Venezia N, Rana A, et al. Blood 1993;82:1323

114. Hemming NJ, Anstee DJ, Mawby WJ, et al. Biochem J 1994;299:191

115. Hemming NJ, Anstee DJ, Staricoff MA, et al. J Biol Chem 1995;270:5360

116. Marfatia SM, Lue RA, Branton D, et al. J Biol Chem 1994;269:8631

117. Marfatia SM, Lue RA, Branton D, et al. J Biol Chem 1995;270:715

118. Agre P, Orringer EP, Bennett V. New Eng J Med 1982;306:1155

119. Agre P, Casella JF, Zinkham WH, et al. Nature 1985;314:380

120. Savvides P, Shalev O, John KM, et al. Blood 1993;82:2953

121. Eber SW, Gonzalez JM, Lux ML, et al. Nature Genet 1996;13:214

122. Hassoun H, Vassiliadis JN, Murray J, et al. (abstract). Blood 1995;86 (Suppl 1):467a

123. Jarolim P, Murray JL, Rubin HL, et al. Blood 1996;88:4366

124. Wichterle H, Palek J, Hanspal M, et al. (abstract). Blood 1995;86 (Suppl 1):468a

125. Takaoka Y, Ideguchi H, Matsuda M, et al. Br J Haematol 1994;88:527

126. Hayette S, Morle L, Bozon M, et al. Br J Haematol 1995;89:762

127. Rybicki AC, Qiu JJH, Musto S, et al. Blood 1993;81:2155

128. Jarolim P, Palek J, Rubin HL, et al. Blood 1992;80:523

129. Rybicki AC, Musto S, Schwartz RS. Biochem J 1995;309:677

130. Lecomte MC, Dhermy D, Gautero HY, et al. CR Acad Sci Paris 1988;306:43

131. Wilmotte R, Marechal J, Morle L, et al. J Clin Invest 1993;91:2091

132. Hanspal M, Hanspal JS, Sahr KE, et al. Blood 1993;82:1652

133. Alloisio N, Morle L, Dorleac E, et al. Blood 1985;65:46

134. Tchernia G, Mohandas N, Shohet SB. J Clin Invest 1981;68:454

135. Conboy JG, Mohandas N, Tchernia G, et al. New Eng J Med 1986;315:680

136. Dalla Venezia N, Gilsanz F, Alloisio N, et al. J Clin Invest 1992;90:1713

137. Mohandas N, Chasis JA. Sem Hematol 1993;30:171

138. Alloisio N, Morle L, Bachir D, et al. Biochim Biophys Acta 1985;816:57

139. Anstee DJ, Parsons SF, Ridgwell K, et al. Biochem J 1984;218:615

140. Lie-Injo LE. Nature 1965;208:1329

141. Amato D, Booth PB. Papua New Guinea Med J 1977;20:26

142. Foo LC, Rekhra JV, Chiang GL, et al. Am J Trop Med Hyg 1992;47:271

143. Hadley T, Saul A, Lamont G, et al. J Clin Invest 1983;71:780

144. Miller LH, Mason SJ, Clyde DF, et al. New Eng J Med 1976;295:302

145. Sim BKL, Chitnis C, Wasniowska K, et al. Science 1994;264:1941

146. Dluzewski AR, Nash GB, Wilson RJM, et al. Mol Biochem Parasitol 1992;55:1

147. Mohandas N, Lie-Injo LE, Friedman M, et al. Blood 1984;63:1385

148. Saul A, Lamont G, Sawyer WH, et al. Papua New Guinea J

Cell Biol 1984;98:1348

149. Jarolim P, Palek J, Amato D, et al. Proc Nat Acad Sci USA 1991;88:11022
150. Tanner MJA, Bruce L, Martin PG, et al. Blood 1991;78:2785
151. Mohandas N, Winardi R, Knowles D, et al. J Clin Invest 1992;89:686
152. Schofield AE, Tanner MJA, Pinder JC, et al. J Mol Biol 1992;223:949
153. Schofield AE, Reardon DM, Tanner MJA. Nature 1992;355:836
154. Groves JD, Ring SM, Schofield AE, et al. FEBS Lett 1993;330:186
155. Sarabia VE, Casey JR, Reithmeier RAF. J Biol Chem 1993;268:10676
156. Smythe J, Spring FA, Gardner BG, et al. Blood 1995;85:2929
157. Liu S-C, Palek J, Scott J, et al. Blood 1995;86:349
158. Anstee DJ, Hemming NJ, Tanner MJA. In: Transfusion Immunology and Medicine. New York:Marcel Dekker, 1995:187
159. Anstee DJ, Tanner MJA. Eur J Biochem 1974;45:31
160. Folch J, Lees M, Sloane Stanley GH. J Biol Chem 1957;226:497
161. Susuki K. J Neurochem 1965;12:629
162. Morrison IM. In: Carbohydrate Analysis: A Practical Approach. Oxford:IRL Press, 1986:205
163. Hagashi H, Sugii T, Kato S. Biochim Biophys Acta 1988;963:333
164. Henry SM, Oriol R, Samuelsson BE. Glycocon J 1994;11:593
165. Weber K, Osborne M. J Biol Chem 1969;244:4406
166. Anstee DJ, Tanner MJA. Br J Haematol 1986;64:211
167. Laemmli UK. Nature 1970;227:680
168. Goding JW. Monoclonal Antibodies: Principles and Practice, 2nd Ed. London:Academic, 1986
169. Redman CM, Marsh WL, Mueller KA, et al. Transfusion 1984;24:176
170. Khamlichi S, Bailly P, Blanchard D, et al. Eur J Biochem 1995;228:931
171. Mallinson G, Soo KS, Schall TJ, et al. Br J Haematol 1995;90:823
172. O'Farrell PH. J Biol Chem 1975;250:4007
173. O'Farrell PZ, Goodman HM, O'Farrell PH. Cell 1977;12:1133
174. Harell D, Robinson M. Arch Biochem Biophys 1979;193:158
175. Gallagher PG, Forget BG. Sem Hematol 1993;30:4
176. Marchalonis JJ, Cone RE, Santer V. Biochem J 1971;124:921
177. Laskey RA. Meth Enzymol 1980;65:363
178. Gahmberg CG, Andersson LC. J Biol Chem 1977;252:5888
179. Gahmberg CG, Hakomori S. J Biol Chem 1973;248:4311
180. Bonner WM, Laskey RA. Eur J Biochem 1974;46:83
181. Moore S, Woodrow CF, McClelland DBL. Nature 1982;295:529
182. Burnette WN. Anals Biochem 1981;112:195
183. Saboori AM, Smith BL, Agre P. Proc Natl Acad Sci USA 1988;85:4042
184. Avent ND, Ridgwell K, Mawby WJ, et al. Biochem J 1988;256:1043
185. Avent ND, Ridgwell K, Tanner MJA, et al. Biochem J 1990;271:821
186. Bloy C, Blanchard D, Dahr W, et al. Blood 1988;72:661
187. Hunkapiller MW, Lujan E, Ostrander F, et al. Meth Enzymol 1983;91:227
188. Gersten DM, Marchalonis JJ. J Immunol Meth 1978;24:305

189. Schneider C, Newman RA, Sutherland DR, et al. J Biol Chem 1982;257:10766
190. Bailly P, Hermand P, Callebaut I, et al. Proc Nat Acad Sci USA 1994;90:5306
191. Mallinson G. PhD Thesis, Univ West England, 1995
192. Parsons SF, Mallinson G, Holmes CH, et al. Proc Nat Acad Sci USA 1995;92:5496
193. Redman C, Marsh WL. In: Protein Blood Group Antigens of the Human Red Cell. Baltimore:Johns Hopkins Univ Press, 1992:53
194. Koningsberg W, Hill RJ. J Biol Chem 1962;237:2547
195. Mawby WJ, Holmes CH, Anstee DJ, et al. Biochem J 1994;304:525
196. Mitra AK, van Hoek AN, Weiner MC, et al. Nat Struct Biol 1995;2:726
197. Walz T, Typke D, Smith BL, et al. Nature Struct Biol 1995;2:730
198. Barclay AN, Birkeland ML, Brown MH, et al. The Leucocyte Antigen Facts Book. London:Academic, 1993:38
199. Bodian DL, Jones EY, Harlos K, et al. Structure 1994;2:755
200. Murphy PM. Ann Rev Immunol 1994;12:593
201. Rawlins ND, Barrett AJ. Biochem J 1995;290:205
202. Kyte J, Doolittle RF. J Mol Biol 1982;157:105
203. Pisano A, Redmond J, Williams K, et al. Glycobiology 1993;3:429
204. Fukuda M, Laufenberger M, Sasaki H, et al. J Biol Chem 1987;262:11952
205. Gardner B, Parsons SF, Merry AH, et al. Immunology 1989;68:283
206. Dahr W, Mueller T, Moulds J, et al. Hoppe-Seyler's Z Biol Chem 1985;366:41
207. Fukuda M, Dell A, Fukuda MN. J Biol Chem 1984;259:4782
208. Montreuil J, Bouquelet S, Debray H, et al. In: Carbohydrate Analysis; A Practical Approach. Oxford:IRL Press, 1986:143
209. Corfield T. Glycobiology 1992;2:509
210. Sutherland DR, Abdullah KM, Cyopick P, et al. J Immunol 1992;148:1458
211. Spring FA, Judson PA, Daniels GL, et al. Immunology 1987;62:307
212. Plummer TH, Elder JH, Alexander S, et al. J Biol Chem 1984;259:10700
213. Tanner MJA, Anstee DJ, Mallinson G, et al. Carbohyd Res 1988;178:203
214. Inglis G, Bird GWG, Mitchell AAB, et al. J Clin Pathol 1975;28:964
215. Doinel C, Andreu G, Cartron J-P, et al. Vox Sang 1980;38:94
216. Goldstein JG, Sivigliar R, Hurst L, et al. Science 1982;215:168
217. Zarnitz ME, Kabat EA. J Am Chem Soc 1960;82:3953
218. Morgan WTJ, Watkins WM. Br Med Bull 1959;15:109
219. van Schravendijk MR, Handunnetti SM, Barnwell JW, et al. Blood 1992;80:2105
220. Handunnetti SM, van Schravendijk MR, Hasler T, et al. Blood 1992;80:2097
221. Udani M, Jefferson S, Daymont C, et al. (abstract). Blood 1996;88(Suppl 1):6a
222. Springer TA. Nature 1990;346:425
223. Che A, Cherry RJ, Bannister LH, et al. J Cell Sci 1993;105:655
224. Booth PB, Serjeantson S, Woodfield DG, et al. Vox Sang 1977;32:99

5 | Molecular Biology and Application of the Methods of Molecular Biology to the Study of Human Blood Groups

That certain individual characteristics are inherited has been noted for centuries. "Hippocrates knew that baldness begets baldness and squinting, squinting" (1). In the Origin of Species, first published in 1859, Darwin (2) commented that "The number and diversity of inheritable deviations of structure both those of slight and those of considerable physiological importance, is endless". However, the mechanism by which inherited characteristics are passed from one generation to another was unclear at that time. In 1865, shortly after the publication of The Origin of Species, Mendel presented his studies on "Experiments in Plant Hybridization" to the National Science Society in Brünn (now Brno), Moravia (1). Mendel's observations on plants led him to conclude that there is a unit of inheritance (now known as a gene) and that this unit is passed from one generation to another according to two simple rules. The first rule is that alternative forms of any given gene segregate into different gametic cells (sperm or eggs). The second rule is that different genes are inherited independently of one another. Mendel also invented the terms dominant and recessive to distinguish genes whose characteristics are expressed in each generation (dominant) from those which are sometimes latent (recessive).

Mendel's observations did not really influence the development of genetics until the beginning of the twentieth century when other scientists verified his work. The next crucial step was the realization that the units of inheritance were transmitted from one cell to another by chromosomes (3). The chromosomes present in the nucleus of a cell are revealed during the process of cell division known as mitosis (from the Greek for thread). "As soon as mitosis had been accurately described, it was pointed out that if the chromosomes were the bearers of something essential for life, and if this something existed in the form of units strung along the chromosome-like beads along a string, then this longitudinal splitting would ensure that each daughter-cell inherited a complete set of these essential somethings" (4). Human somatic cells contain 46 (23 different pairs) chromosomes (44 autosomes and two sex chromosomes (5,6)). Before the cells divide by mitosis the number of chromosomes doubles so that each of the daughter-cells will have the same number of chromosome pairs as the parent cell. Cells with 23 pairs of chromosomes are known as diploid. During sexual reproduction a different process takes place (meiosis) which results in the gametes (sperm cells or ova) having only one set of 23 chromosomes. Cells with only one set of 23 chromosomes are known as haploid. When the gametes fuse at fertilization a diploid cell is formed in which one set of chromosomes is derived from the sperm and the other from the egg. Since chromosome pairs segregate during gamete formation it follows that segregation of the units of inheritance (genes) described by Mendel can be explained if the genes are carried on chromosomes. Another crucial observation was that the different chromosome pairs segregate independently of each other, that is every gamete does not have an identical set of 23 chromosomes. This explains Mendel's second rule that different genes are inherited independently of one another. Much of the experimental work which led to these conclusions was based on studies of breeding experiments with the fruit fly Drosophila.

"It (Drosophila) makes peculiarly convenient material because it breeds every ten days, it produces several hundred offspring in each generation, it is so small that the whole of one of these generations can be successfully reared in a pint milk bottle. Like the fruits of paradise, it is in season all the year round. Thus a graduate student in the two years allotted for his higher degree can work out a problem covering seventy generations, equal to decades in the selection of rabbits, centuries in the case of cattle, and millennia of human reproduction" (4).

Studies on Drosophila notably in the laboratory of Thomas Hunt Morgan (7,8) in the United States also established the phenomena of crossing-over (syn. recombination) and linkage. Crossing-over occurs when maternal and paternal chromosomes become intertwined during meiosis, so that genetic material can pass from one to the other. If two genes are on the same chromosome they will tend to be inherited together and they are said to be linked. The frequency of crossover involving two genes on the same chromosome is a measure of the distance between them. This formed the basis of a method by which the location of a gene on a chromosome (its locus) could be mapped (reviewed in 9,10).

When it became clear that the structure of genes could be altered (mutation) for example by exposure to radiation (see for example reference 11) this provided an explanation for the inheritable deviation of structure observed by Darwin. The processes of inheritance and natural selection were thereby defined by the structure of genes which were located on chromosomes.

In order to understand these processes at the molecular level it was necessary to study the chemical composition of chromosomes. When it was shown that deoxyribonucleic (DNA) acid is only found in the nucleus (12) and that the amount of DNA in gametic cells is half that in somatic (diploid) cells (13) it became clear that the secret of inheritance might be revealed in the structure of DNA. The elucidation of the structure of DNA by Watson and Crick in 1953 (14) gave birth to molecular biology and molecular genetics.

In his book, Science and the Quiet Art (1), Sir David Weatherall quotes Francis Crick as saying that the term molecular biology is unfortunate because it has two meanings. "In the broad sense, it covers an explanation for any biological phenomena in terms of atoms and molecules. However, as it is usually used, it encompasses the structure and interactions of the building blocks of living things, particularly proteins and nucleic acids, and studies of gene structure, replication, and expression". It is the latter definition which forms the subject of this chapter. The structures of all the molecules of life are controlled by individual genes and so an understanding of the structure of genes should lead to an understanding of how they work in health and disease, this aspect is sometimes referred to as molecular genetics.

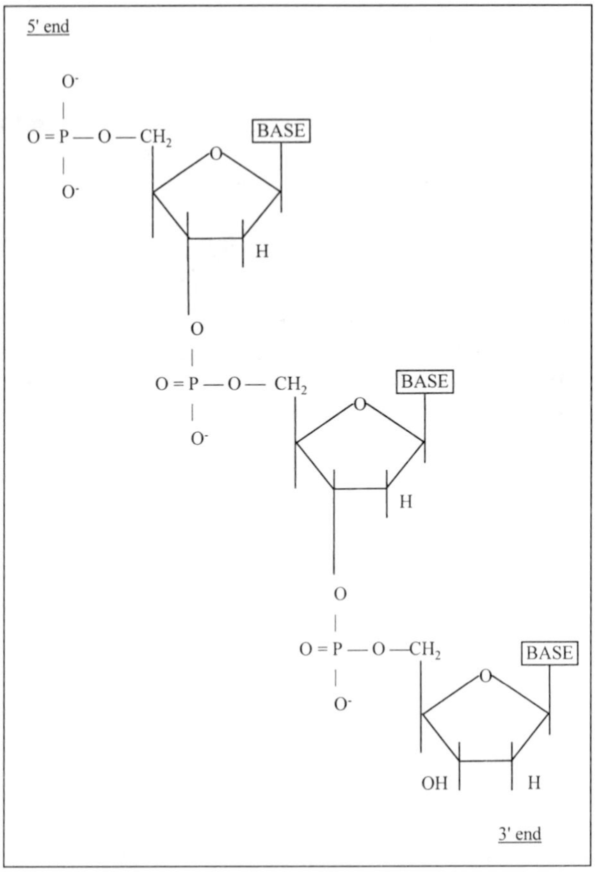

The Structure of DNA

DNA is composed of four chemical bases adenine (A), cytosine (C), guanine (G), and thymine (T). The bases are covalently linked to deoxyribose (sugar) forming nucleosides and each nucleoside is linked to another by phosphoester bonds (see figure 5-1). A phosphorylated nucleoside is referred to as a nucleotide. The carbon atoms of sugars are numbered, deoxyribose is a 5 carbon sugar. The bases are covalently attached to carbon 1 and the phosphoester linkages covalently link carbon 5 of one deoxyribose molecule to carbon 3 of another. In this way a chain of nucleotides can be assembled. The deoxyribose molecules at each end of the chain will have a free carbon 5 (5′ end) and a free carbon 3 (3′ end) respectively. The chain of nucleotide sugars is usually written as a series of letters each letter representing the particular base present, for example 5′ ACCCGCGGTAA 3′. The DNA molecule itself is a polymer comprising two nucleotide chains which form a double helix. The two nucleotide chains are antiparallel, that is the 5′ end of one chain is opposite the 3′ end of the other chain and vice versa (see figure 5-2). The bases are arranged on the inside of the double helix and are paired by hydrogen bonding, G with C and A with T (see figure 5-2).

FIGURE 5-1 The Structure of Nucleotide Chains which Comprise DNA

Since the double helix consists of two chains with sequences that are complementary, if the chains separate another complementary strand can be synthesized for each of the separated chains so that two molecules of identical sequence are produced. This explains how the genetic information contained within the DNA sequence is passed from one cell to another during mitosis. The process of DNA replication requires an enzyme called DNA polymerase. New DNA strands are generated by sequential addition of deoxyribose nucleotides to the 3′ end. The accuracy of replication is controlled through the specificity of base pairing (G with C and A with T) and mistakes are fewer than one in 10^9 nucleotides (15).

The Genetic Code (how genes encode proteins)

The DNA sequence contains the information necessary to make proteins. Proteins are assembled by the sequential addition of amino acids to a developing polypeptide chain. A sequence of bases in DNA which encodes the information necessary to make a protein (a

FIGURE 5-2 The Double Helix of DNA (two anti-parallel nucleotide chains with bases arranged on the inside of a double helix)

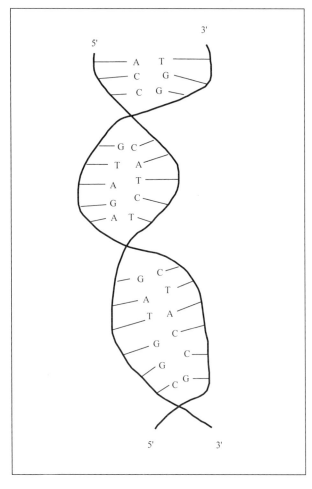

gene) is first transcribed into another type of nucleic acid known as ribonucleic acid or RNA. RNA, like DNA, is composed of a chain of nucleotides but the sugar component of these nucleotides is ribose not deoxyribose and the base thymine (T) found in DNA is replaced by uracil (U). RNA is single stranded and is transcribed from the DNA sequence which corresponds to its gene. It is released from the DNA. This mRNA (messenger RNA) contains a coded message from the DNA which can be translated into the sequence of a protein. The mechanisms of translation are quite complicated and involve other types of RNA (tRNA, rRNA) and numerous proteins (more than 50) forming a complex known as a ribosome (see reference 15 for more details). The mRNA sequence can be translated into protein because certain triplet sequences of bases encode particular amino acids (the genetic code). Since there are four bases there are 4^3 or 64 possible triplets (codons). There are only 20 different amino acids but several different codons can give rise to the same amino acid (degeneracy in the code, see figure 5-3). Three codons do not give rise to

amino acids at all but act as stop signals and define the point at which translation of the mRNA stops.

Not only does the translation machinery need to know when to stop it also needs to know where to start. Since each amino acid is encoded by a sequence of three bases any sequence of bases could give rise to three different proteins depending upon where the start occurs in the sequence, that is there are three possible reading frames. The cell has a mechanism to ensure that translation of a given mRNA always begins in the same place, at an initiator codon. Translation beginning at an initiator codon will result in an "open reading frame" and synthesis of the correct polypeptide sequence. The initiator codon is the base sequence AUG which encodes the amino acid methionine. A messenger RNA contains many AUG codons (proteins frequently contain several methionine residues) and so a special mechanism is required to ensure that the correct AUG (start codon) is selected. Eukaryotic mRNAs are modified after transcription. At the 5' end 7-methyl guanosine is added through a triphosphate linkage and at the 3' end a run of about 200 adenine residues is added (poly A tail). The addition of 7-methyl guanosine is referred to as a "cap" structure. A small ribosomal subunit binds to the mRNA at the capsite and scans the mRNA until it locates the first AUG site when protein synthesis begins. Protein synthesis is effected by specific (transfer) tRNA molecules which recognize a particular codon sequence. Each tRNA molecule has a particular amino acid attached to it by covalent linkage (see figure 5-4). The first tRNA (initiator tRNA) always carries methionine. Once the initiator tRNA has located the initiator AUG a large ribosomal subunit binds to the smaller one already present and protein synthesis begins. Protein synthesis proceeds by the sequential binding of tRNA molecules which recognize the codon corresponding to the amino acid carried. Once the amino acid is covalently linked to the developing polypeptide chain the tRNA is released and the next tRNA can be formed to attach the next amino acid and so on. Protein synthesis is terminated at a stop codon and the completed protein is either released into the cytoplasm or if it is either a membrane protein or a secreted protein it is inserted into the membrane of the endoplasmic reticulum (ER) (see Chapter 4 for further discussion of the assembly of membrane proteins). Usually only one initiator codon is used and so a single polypeptide chain is synthesized. However, there are examples of the use of more than one initiator AUG. Translation from a second initiator codon 3' or "downstream" of the first initiator is often referred to as a "leaky initiation" and this is the mechanism which gives rise to two Gerbich active proteins, glycophorins C and D, from a single gene (the *GYPC* gene, see Chapter 16). The occurrence of leaky initiation can be explained by inspection of the nucleotide sequence around AUG sites. Comparison of hundreds of mRNA sequences revealed

FIGURE 5-3 The Genetic Code

First Position (5' end)	Second Position				Third Position (3' end)
	U	C	A	G	
U	Phe	Ser	Tyr	Cys	U
	Phe	Ser	Tyr	Cys	C
	Leu	Ser	Stop	Stop	A
	Leu	Ser	Stop	Trp	G
C	Leu	Pro	His	Arg	U
	Leu	Pro	His	Arg	C
	Leu	Pro	Glu	Arg	A
	Leu	Pro	Glu	Arg	G
A	Ile	Thr	Asn	Ser	U
	Ile	Thr	Asn	Ser	C
	Ile	Thr	Lys	Arg	A
	Met	Thr	Lys	Arg	G
G	Val	Ala	Asp	Gly	U
	Val	Ala	Asp	Gly	C
	Val	Ala	Glu	Gly	A
	Val	Ala	Glu	Gly	G

that the sequence A/GNNAUGG is optimal for initiation (where N is any nucleotide (16)). If this optimal sequence is not present at the first AUG, translation may skip the first AUG and start at a downstream AUG which does have the optimal sequence.

The Structure of Genes

As a general rule, eukaryotic genes contain some regions of DNA sequence which are not translated into protein sequence. These regions are known as introns. Those regions of DNA sequence which are translated into protein sequence are referred to as exons. Thus, at the DNA (genomic) level eukaryotic genes usually comprise several exons interspersed with introns (see figure 5-5). Exceptions to this rule do occur but they are rare. When the blood group gene which gives rise to antigens of the Duffy blood group system was first described it appeared that the polypeptide it encoded was the product of a contiguous (intron-less gene). However, subsequent studies by Iwamoto et al. (17) revealed the presence of an additional small exon at the 5' end of the gene (see Chapter 14 for further discussion). Most members of the fucosyltransferase gene family, including the *H*, *Se* and *Le* gene products are derived from intron-less genes (see Chapters 8 and 9).

The realization during the 1970's, that eukaryotic

genes contain introns came as something of a surprise. At that time work on the structure of genes had been established from studies of bacteria. Bacterial genes do not contain introns and it had been assumed that genes in eukaryotes would be organized in the same way as in prokaryotes. "It was naturally assumed that this bacterial gene structure was universal. It followed that if the gene structure was the same, then the mechanisms of regulation were probably very similar, and thus what was true of a bacterium would be true of an elephant" (18).

Among the first genes to be shown to be split (i.e., contain intervening sequences or introns) were the globin genes (19) and the immunoglobulin genes (20). It is now clear that the average cellular gene contains approximately eight introns (18).

If eukaryotic genes are comprised of exons and introns and the protein products of these genes are encoded by the DNA sequence of exons alone, the obvious questions which arise are: how are the intronic sequences ignored and why are they there?

Intronic sequences are not present in mRNA and so are not translated into protein. When a gene is transcribed the first RNA product contains sequences which correspond to intronic sequences as well as exonic sequences. This RNA product (pre-mRNA or heterogeneous nuclear (hn) RNA) is typically four to ten times larger than the mRNA (18). The sequences corresponding to introns are removed (spliced out) to produce the mRNA which will

FIGURE 5-4 Translation of mRNA (drawn from reference 15)

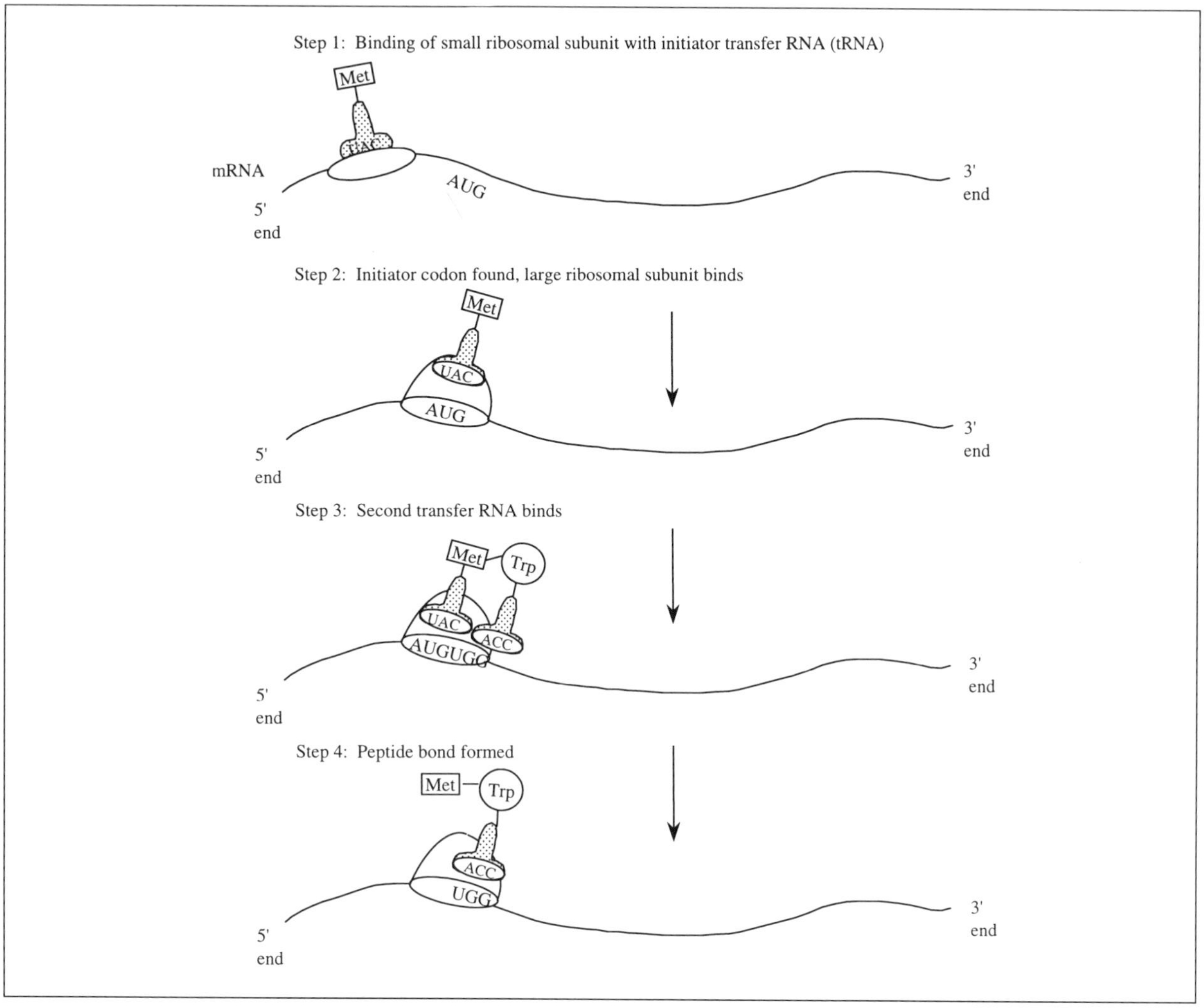

Step 1: Binding of small ribosomal subunit with initiator transfer RNA (tRNA)

Met

mRNA

AUG

5' end

3' end

Step 2: Initiator codon found, large ribosomal subunit binds

Met

UAC

AUG

5' end

3' end

Step 3: Second transfer RNA binds

Met   Trp

UAC   ACC

AUGUGG

5' end

3' end

Step 4: Peptide bond formed

Met — Trp

ACC

UGG

5' end

3' end

be translated into protein. The actual sequences of introns present in eukaryotic genes are not usually considered to have important functions, although evidence is emerging that in some genes they may be important for regulating gene expression. What is clear is that the presence of introns certainly provides much greater flexibility to the process of protein synthesis because it enables different protein variants to be produced from a single gene by a process of differential splicing in which alternative exons are spliced into or out of the mRNA. Differential or alternative splicing allows different protein products of the same gene to be expressed in different tissues and thereby provides a powerful mechanism for generating proteins which can function in the different cellular environments of multicellular organisms. Alternative splicing also provides a powerful mechanism for generating diversity in protein structures which are concerned with the protection of multicellular organisms from microbial assault. The supreme example of such diversity is provid-

ed by the genes which give rise to antibody molecules (discussed in Chapter 2). Alternative splicing is the genetic mechanism which underlies the creation of many blood group antigens and the reader will meet this term on numerous occasions in the chapters describing the blood group systems.

RNA Splicing

When pre-mRNA is transcribed in the nucleus by an enzyme RNA polymerase II, the 5' end is capped by addition of 7-methyl guanosine and a poly A tail is added at the 3' end. Termination of pre-mRNA synthesis is achieved by cleavage of the developing chain and addition of the poly A tail (by poly A polymerase). Cleavage of the developing chain is signaled by the sequence AAUAAA located 10-30 nucleotides upstream of the cleavage site and a less well defined nucleotide sequence

FIGURE 5-5 Transcription and RNA Splicing of Eukaryotic Genes

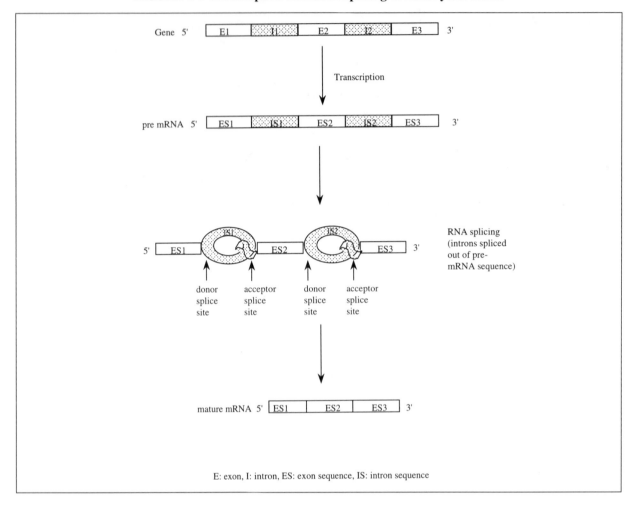

E: exon, I: intron, ES: exon sequence, IS: intron sequence

downstream of the cleavage site (15). The poly A tail (usually 100-200 residues of adenylic acid) is thought to aid transport of the pre-mRNA from nucleus to cytoplasm. Poly A tails are found on pre-mRNA and mRNA but not tRNA or rRNA.

RNA splicing occurs in the nucleus and RNA is transported to the cytoplasm only when splicing is complete. RNA splicing depends on conserved nucleotide sequences which are found at the 5′ end (donor splice site) and 3′ end (acceptor splice site) of intron sequences. The 5′ consensus splice sites comprise C/AAG of the preceding exon sequence and GUA/GAGU at the 5′ end of the intron. The 3′ consensus splice site comprises (U/C)n N, C/U, AG at the 3′ end of the intron and G/A of the next exon (the underlined residues 5′ GU and 3′ AG are the most conserved). Splicing occurs in RNA-protein complexes known as spliceosomes which are almost as large as ribosomes. An A within the intron (branch point) close to the 3′ poly (UC) sequence is also critical for splicing. This complex process (reviewed in reference 18) requires a series of small nuclear ribonucleoproteins (snRNPs known as "snurps") and results in the release of intronic RNA in which the 5′ end of the intron is joined to the branch point forming a circle of RNA with a tail which corresponds to the 3′ end of the intron. This structure is referred to as a lariat because that is what it looks like (see figure 5-5). The lariat RNA is rapidly degraded in the nucleus. This mechanism of splicing involves interactions between 5′ and 3′ splice sites across an intron. The average vertebrate gene consists of multiple small exons (average 137 nucleotides) separated by much larger introns (21). Some introns can be extremely long (for example intron 1 of the gene that encodes glycophorin A, see Chapter 15). Berget (22) quotes figures on the order of 100 kilobases for a single intron. The occurrence of very large introns has led researchers to focus on exon recognition rather than intron recognition and to consider pairing between splice sites across an exon rather than pairing across an intron (22). Intron recognition may be appropriate in some situations but not for a gene with small exons and large introns.

In this latter mechanism the first and last exons require special mechanisms for their recognition. Evidence that the cap and nuclear proteins that bind the cap are essential for in vitro splicing of simple one-intron pre-mRNAs (23) suggests that the cap is essential for recognition and removal of the first intron. Last exons begin with a 3' splice site and end with a poly A site and mutations in the poly A site inhibit the in vitro removal of proximal but not distal introns. It appears that splicing factors and polyadenylation factors are required (22). Although the complex mechanisms involved in RNA splicing are not fully understood it is obvious that mutations in splice sites could have dramatic effects. The process of splicing must be very precise to ensure that the mRNA corresponding to a given gene always gives rise to a polypeptide of the same sequence. Berget (22) cites a database search in the summer of 1994 by Nakai and Sakamoto (24) which revealed over 100 splice site mutations. The mutations gave rise to four types of abnormalities: exon skipping, activation of a cryptic splice site, creation of a pseudo-exon within an intron, and intron retention. These abnormalities represented 51, 32, 11 and 6% of the mutations, respectively.

Several blood group phenotypes appear to result from mutations in splice sites and the reader is referred to Chapter 15 (the MN system) in particular, for examples, from the work carried out by Huang and Blumenfeld at the Albert Einstein College of Medicine in New York (25). A nucleotide mutation which created a cryptic splice site was considered to provide an explanation for the very low level expression of CD55 in the Dr(a-) phenotype (26 and see Chapter 24).

Regulation of Gene Expression

Thus far the way in which a gene can be transcribed (into mRNA) and then translated into protein has been described. This process requires that the mRNA has a beginning (initiator codon) and an end (termination codon) and usually involves the removal of intronic sequences from the primary RNA transcript. Clearly the level of expression of each gene must be regulated since the products of all the genes in the genome are not expressed at the same level in every cell. The ability to regulate gene expression is crucial to the development of multicellular organisms since it directs the process by which a single fertilized egg becomes a multicellular organism comprising many specialized tissues.

Some genes encode proteins which are required for functions which nearly all cells need. Genes of this type are often referred to as "housekeeping" genes. Other genes are expressed in a restricted number of cells and tissues because they have a specialized function not required by all cells. In extreme cases the product of a particular gene or set of genes is only expressed in a single cell type. The process of erythropoiesis ultimately gives rise to a highly specialized end stage cell, the red blood cell. The red blood cell is not really a cell in the strict sense of the word since it lacks a nucleus and is therefore incapable of protein synthesis. During the process of erythropoiesis, particularly the later stages, a number of genes are "switched on" and encode proteins found exclusively or almost exclusively in erythroid cells. A classical example of tissue specific regulation is provided by the globin genes. Hemoglobin is found only in erythroid cells where its function of O_2 transport is fundamental to the viability of higher organisms. Several blood group-active proteins found in the red cell membrane also have a very restricted distribution. Available evidence suggests that the Rh polypeptides, Rh glycoproteins and Kell proteins are probably found only in red cells (see Chapters 12 and 18), while the anion transport protein band 3, glycophorin A, the urea transporter and the water transporter are restricted to erythroid cells and certain cells in the kidney (see Chapters 15,17,19,22). Other red cell membrane proteins, like glycophorin C/D have a wider, but still restricted distribution while CD44, CD59 and CD47 are almost ubiquitous and their respective genes fall into the category of "housekeeping" genes, that is these genes encode proteins which all cells need irrespective of any specialized functions (see Chapters 16, 4, 29 and 12, respectively). A more detailed discussion of the tissue distribution of the products of blood group genes will be found in the chapters describing blood group systems.

Every cell (bar the red cell) has a nucleus containing chromosomes which carry all the genes needed to make a multicellular organism but these genes are selectively expressed. How does the control of gene expression work? It is clear from earlier sections of this chapter that the process by which the information contained within a gene is converted to proteins is complicated and that there are numerous stages where regulatory factors could operate (at the level of the gene itself, i.e. at transcription or during the process of RNA splicing or translation).

For most genes it appears that the critical controls apply at the level of transcription. Certain DNA sequences, usually upstream of a gene, act as receptors for specialized DNA binding proteins (transcription factors) which control the expression of that gene. Hundreds of DNA binding proteins have been identified. The binding of such proteins to DNA is highly specific and of high affinity. DNA binding proteins are usually dimers (hetero or homo-dimers) a feature which greatly increases the affinity of protein-DNA interactions. Given the mind boggling problems of regulating all the genes in the genome to produce an organism with all its organs and tissues in working order and in the right place, it is not surprising to discover that many different types of DNA binding proteins have evolved.

Most DNA-binding proteins bind through regions of α-helix, although some are two stranded ß sheets. The first DNA-binding protein described binds DNA through a "helix-turn-helix" motif. The two helices are connected by a short stretch of amino acids (the turn) and are held at a fixed angle through interactions between the helices. One helix (recognition helix) binds DNA. Another family of DNA-binding proteins uses one or more molecules of zinc to form its structure. The amino acids which bind zinc (often Cys-Cys-His-His) are called "zinc finger" motifs. A third family of DNA-binding proteins contain so called "leucine zipper" motifs. The leucine zipper describes a method of forming dimers between two DNA binding proteins. Two α-helices, one from each monomer bind together through a short region of hydrophobic amino acids (usually leucine) in each helix. Beyond the hydrophobic interaction the two helices separate to form a Y-shaped structure which binds the DNA. Yet another type of DNA binding motif is known as "helix-loop-helix". Dimers formed with this motif have structures very similar to dimers formed via leucine zippers. This summary of the structure of DNA proteins is derived from the excellent book by Alberts et al. (15). The reader is referred to this book for a more detailed discussion.

Most eukaryotic genes are transcribed by RNA polymerase II (Pol II). Transcription by Pol II requires the binding of transcription factors upstream of the initiator site. The first step in this sequence involves binding to the nucleotide sequence TATA which is usually located about 25 nucleotides upstream of the initiator site. The sequential binding of transcription factors recruit Pol II and when Pol II is phosphorylated it is released from the complex of transcription factors and transcription begins. The region around the TATA site where the general transcription factors and Pol II bind is known as the promoter. Activation of transcription is also influenced by other DNA binding proteins which recognize different nucleotide motifs. Such nucleotide motifs may be located 5′ or 3′ of the gene and even within large introns. In some cases the motifs are a long way from the gene itself and it is thought that transcription factors bound at these distant sites come into close contact with the factors bound at the promotor because of looping out of the intervening DNA. Proteins regulating transcription are not all activators, some are required to stop the process (repressors). The combined effects of many transcriptional factors are required for the regulation of gene expression in any given tissue. In erythropoiesis one transcription factor (GATA-1) plays a key role.

Regulation of Erythropoiesis

All blood cells are produced from pluripotent progenitor cells (hemopoietic stem cells). These pluripotent stem cells can be maintained in a dormant (non-dividing) state, they can undergo cell division to produce identical progeny (self-renewal) and they can produce multipotent precursor cells. As their name suggests multipotent precursor cells have more limited developmental potential than pluripotent stem cells. These multipotent precursor cells give rise to single cell lineages which result in end stage cells (red cells, granulocytes, monocytes, lymphocytes). The process by which these end-stage cells are generated is essentially a process by which the developmental potential of a progenitor cell is progressively restricted (pluripotent → multipotent → single lineage). In the mammalian embryo the site of hemopoiesis is in blood islands in the yolk sac. As the embryo develops hemopoiesis occurs in fetal liver and then in bone marrow.

The process of hemopoiesis is complex but can be considered as containing essentially three "levels" of activity. At the first level a soluble growth factor binds to a growth factor receptor on the progenitor cell and triggers a transmembrane signal. At the second level the transmembrane signal causes activation of intracellular signaling pathways. At the third level these intracellular signaling pathways cause activation or repression of the DNA binding proteins (transcription factors) which control gene expression. For example, activation of a growth factor receptor gene results in the expression of novel protein at the cell surface and allows the cell to be influenced by binding of a growth factor which it was previously unable to bind. A new sequence of intracellular signaling events is stimulated and new genes are activated and so the cycle of events continues until end stage cells are produced. Developing erythroblasts express the erythropoietin receptor (EpoR). Erythropoietin (EPO) is a hormone produced by the kidney in response to anemia and hypoxia. EPO interacts with EpoR on developing erythroblasts causing intracellular signaling which results in proliferation of the cells and differentiation along the erythroid lineage (reviewed in 27). Activation of the *EpoR* gene results from the binding of the transcription factor GATA-1 to the promotor of the *EpoR* gene (28). Studies with transgenic mice lacking the *EPO* gene or the *EpoR* gene have shown that EPO and EpoR are crucial in vivo for the production of circulatory red cells but are not required for the generation of committed erythroid progenitor cells (29). Binding of EPO to EpoR results in a transmembrane signal causing the activation of a protein tyrosine kinase (JAK2) which binds to the cytoplasmic domain of EpoR and phosphorylates both itself and a critical site (tyrosine 429) in the cytoplasmic domain of EpoR. This phosphorylation event is associated with proliferation and differentiation of erythroid cells. The process of proliferation and differentiation is stopped by the binding of a phosphorylase (SH-PTP1). These findings (30) explain why mutations in the cytoplasmic domain of EpoR which result in loss of Tyr 429 are associated with a rare benign familial erythrocytosis which in heterozygotes results in high hemoglobin concentration and increased oxygen carrying capacity (31).

GATA-1 is essential for the development of red cells. The name GATA-1 derives from the specificity of the protein. It binds specifically as a monomer to a consensus nucleotide sequence (T/A)GATA(A/G). This consensus sequence is found upstream of all globin genes and other erythroid genes that have been examined. GATA-1 is a member of the family of zinc finger proteins described in an earlier section. It has two zinc binding regions (Cys-X-X-Cys) separated by 29 amino acids but only one of these zinc fingers (the second, most carboxy terminal region) is necessary for specific DNA binding (32,33). The binding of a 66 residue fragment of chicken GATA-1 which contains the DNA binding site (residues 158-223) to a 16bp double-stranded oligonucleotide containing the consensus sequence AGATAA has been studied and its 3-dimensional structure determined using nuclear magnetic resonance spectroscopy (34). Omichimski et al. (34) describe the overall structure of the complex as "analogous to that of a right hand holding a rope, with the rope representing the DNA, the palm and fingers of the hand the core of the protein, and the thumb the carboxy tail".

The crucial importance of GATA-1 to erythroid development is clearly demonstrated by studies of transgenic mice in which the *GATA-1* gene is absent (knockout mice). Knockout mice can be produced using embryonic stem cells (ESC) derived from the inner cell mass of early mouse embryos. ESC can be maintained in culture and a particular gene of interest can be disrupted by homologous recombination in ESCs to create a heterozygous mutation in which one chromosome lacks a functional gene (35).

If the knockout ESCs are injected into the blastocytes of a wild type host embryo it is possible through breeding to produce mice that are homozygous for the non-functional gene, that is "knockout mice". This process is possible because ESCs contribute to germ line cells (sperm and eggs) and so the defective gene is transmitted from one generation to another. It is also possible to produce ESCs that are homozygous for the gene knockout in culture before injection into blastocytes or to culture the mutant ESCs in vitro. The latter option has been used to great effect in the study of genes critical for hemopoiesis (36). The experiments carried out show that *GATA-1* gene-deficiency results in a complete block of erythropoiesis. This block occurs after the proerythroblast stage, that is, it prevents the terminal stage of erythroid maturation. There are at least 5 other GATA binding proteins and there is evidence that several of these play a role in hemopoiesis (37). The relationship between appearance of GATA-1 and EpoR can be demonstrated in vitro using hemopoietic stem cells cultured in the presence of EPO and low levels of IL-3 and GM-CSF (38).

The discussion here has concentrated on GATA-1, which is of particular interest to blood group serologists, because mutation of the GATA-1 binding site upstream of the blood group *Duffy (FY)* gene of hemopoietic cells explains the tissue-specific absence of Duffy (FY) proteins from the red cells of Africans with the Fy(a-b-) phenotype (39, see Chapter 14 for further discussion). It should be appreciated, however, that numerous other transcription factors and intracellular signaling molecules are involved in erythropoiesis (see references 36,40,41).

Transgenic Mice and Blood Group Null Phenotypes

The production of "knockout" mice by the procedure illustrated in the previous section with respect to GATA-1 is a very powerful method for obtaining information about the functional significance of a particular gene product. However, the technique has not been used widely to study the function of blood group-active proteins on red cells. The reader will find references to band 3 knockout mice in Chapter 4 and Chapter 17, to knockout mice lacking the Ok^a blood group glycoprotein in Chapter 31 and to knockout mice lacking the Rh associated protein CD47 in Chapter 12. There are however, many examples of human "knockouts" of blood group genes (blood group null phenotypes) where a defect in the gene itself (rather than an erythroid-specific regulatory defect as described for the Fy(a-b-) phenotype in the previous section) is responsible for the phenotype. Those null phenotypes which result from defects at the level of the blood group gene itself provide information about the functional importance of blood group proteins not only in the red cell but in all tissues where the gene is normally expressed.

The fact that these human null phenotypes have been found at all is a clear indication that most blood group proteins are not essential for the viability of man (63). Indeed it is only in relatively few cases (McLeod syndrome Chapter 18, Rh$_{null}$ syndrome Chapter 12) that there is any associated pathology. It follows from this that the proteins which carry the antigens of blood group systems which lack a known null phenotype are likely to have more critical functions. The generation of knockouts of the analogous genes in mice may therefore prove to be a fruitful avenue of research, for example, the human blood group phenotype Di(a-b-) is unknown and band 3 knockout mice have a severe form of hereditary spherocytosis (42,43, see also Chapter 17).

Genetic Mechanisms for the Generation of Diversity

Evolution depends on mechanisms which introduce change in existing genes and create new genes. By a process of natural selection, species can retain advantageous changes and survive. At the simplest level changes in gene structure result from point mutations which change one nucleotide (i.e. one nucleotide is substituted for another). A single nucleotide substitution does not necessarily alter the amino acid sequence of the protein corresponding to the gene because degeneracy in the genetic code (see earlier in this chapter) means that several different codons encode the same amino acid. Nucleotide changes which do not result in an altered amino acid sequence are called silent mutations. A nucleotide substitution which changes an amino acid is called a mis-sense mutation. This is a very common mechanism responsible for the creation of blood group antigens and numerous examples will be found in the chapters of this book which are concerned with blood group systems. It is also possible for a nucleotide substitution to change a codon which encodes an amino acid in to a stop codon (non-sense mutation). The effect of introducing a stop codon depends to some extent on where the stop codon occurs but can have a major affect on the expression of a membrane protein.

If a single nucleotide is deleted or inserted into the gene during the process of DNA or RNA synthesis this will alter the reading frame of the mRNA with the result that it is translated as a completely different amino acid sequence after the point of the insertion/deletion. Such events are called frameshift mutations. Sometimes the nucleotide insertion/deletion creates a stop codon at the site of the mutation. In other cases the amino acid sequence of the protein is changed and translation of the protein is terminated because a premature stop codon is created downstream of the site of the mutation.

A very powerful mechanism for generating novel proteins follows as a consequence of eukaryotic genes being composed of exons and introns. A pre-mRNA can often be spliced in different ways to create several different but related proteins from the same gene. This process, known as alternative splicing, can result in the addition or omission of different exons to create a whole series of different proteins adapted for function in different tissues. Good examples of alternative splicing are

provided by the glycoprotein CD44 which carries Indian blood group antigens (see Chapter 29).

A mutation in a consensus nucleotide sequence required for RNA splicing may knock out or reduce the efficiency of that splice site so that the nucleotide sequence normally removed remains in the translated protein. A mutation may also create a new splice site which affects the sequence of the resulting protein product. A nucleotide substitution in glycophorin A associated with the ERIK antigen alters a 5' splice site at the end of exon 3 and results in four different transcripts instead of one (44 and see Chapter 15).

Novel proteins can be created by crossover events during misalignment of genes at meiosis. Such intragenic crossover events appear to explain the occurrence of glycophorin C/D variant genes with deleted exon 2, deleted exon 3, duplicated exon 2 and duplicated exon 3 (see Chapter 16).

By far the most powerful mechanism for generating structural diversity is that of gene duplication. The way in which gene duplication occurs is poorly understood. It may be related to errors in the process of DNA repair. Once tandem duplication has occurred there are opportunities for further gene duplication by unequal crossing over between genes at meiosis so that a whole series of genes, each of which can mutate independently, can arise and a family of related genes is created. Among the blood group genes the variations consequent on unequal crossing over are illustrated by the genes giving rise to MN system antigens. In the late 1970s it became apparent that some glycophorin molecules were hybrid molecules comprising portions of glycophorin A sequence and a portion of glycophorin B sequence and unequal crossing over at meiosis was proposed to explain their origin (reviewed in 45, see also Chapter 15 for more detailed discussion).

Another mechanism which can generate diversity in tandemly repeated genes is called gene conversion. Gene conversion, like unequal crossing over, usually occurs during meiosis but in this case a portion of the DNA sequence of a gene on one chromosome misaligns with the corresponding gene on the other chromosome. The mismatch between the misaligned DNA sequences is repaired by the normal DNA repair process so that either the paternal strand acquires the DNA sequence of the maternal strand or vice versa. Such gene conversion events usually involve a small section of DNA and only a small part of the gene is changed (15). The mechanism is therefore quite different from crossing over which creates hybrid proteins. Gene conversion events are thought to explain a number of glycophorin variants in the MN system (Chapter 15) and the origin of partial D antigens in the Rh system (Chapter 12). Tandemly arranged genes are found in the Rh and MN systems but not in any of the other blood group systems. The greater opportunities for genetic variation, that crossover and gene conversion involving tandemly arranged genes provides, are reflected by the presence of far more blood group antigens in these systems than in any others.

It is remarkable that the greatest level of structural variation on the red cell should involve major surface proteins (GPA, GPB) and Rh polypeptides. This fact raises the question as to the nature of the selective pressure which is driving this level of polymorphism. It has been argued for many years that selection is driven by infectious disease (Haldane 1949 cited in 46) and this argument has been developed more recently by Howard (46). In the case of red cells, the major selective pressure must surely be malaria, an argument discussed by Miller (47) and considered in more detail with respect to glycophorin variants in Chapter 15. While there is experimental evidence in support of a role for GPA in invasion of red cells by *Plasmodium falciparum* (48) evidence for an involvement of Rh polypeptides is lacking.

Application of the Methods of Molecular Biology to the Study of Human Blood Groups

DNA was first isolated by Friedrick Miescher in 1868 in the laboratory of Hoppe-Seyler in Tubingen. Miescher isolated nuclei from pus cells obtained from discarded surgical bandages and showed that they contained an unusual phosphorus-containing compound he called "nuclein" (49). More than 100 years passed before methods were developed which allowed the isolation and sequence analysis of the genes contained within this DNA. A crucial step in this process was the discovery of bacterial enzymes known as restriction endonucleases. When viruses that infect bacteria (bacteriophage) are transferred from growth in one bacterial host to another the efficiency of phage growth is impaired, frequently several thousand fold. This is because bacterial restriction endonucleases degrade the phage DNA and thereby protect the bacterium. The bacterium's own DNA is not degraded because it is protected by methylation of its bases (A or C). Restriction enzymes have, as their name suggests, restricted specificity and cut DNA very specifically. Base sequences of 4-8 nucleotides are usually recognized. More than 100 different restriction endonucleases have been identified and most are available in purified form from commercial sources, for use in recombinant technology today. Without this pioneering work on bacteria the modern revolution in molecular medicine would not have occurred. Restriction enzymes from bacteria can be used to cut mammalian DNA into pieces. The pieces of DNA can then be separated and isolated by gel elec-

trophoresis. Polyacrylamide gel electrophoresis (PAGE) can be used to separate small pieces of DNA (< 500 nucleotides) but for large fragments agarose (1-2%) gel electrophoresis is used. The separated pieces of DNA can be visualized by staining with the dye ethidium bromide which fluoresces under ultraviolet light when bound to DNA. Alternatively, ^{32}P can be incorporated into phosphate groups in the DNA and the bands detected by autoradiography.

The size of the DNA fragments is determined by reference to fragments of known molecular weight which are run in neighboring tracks on the gel. The reader who refers to Chapter 4 will note that the electrophoretic methods for separation of membrane polypeptides are similar to those for DNA although in the case of DNA, addition of the detergent SDS is not required because the nucleotides already carry a negative charge (phosphate).

Restriction enzymes allow DNA to be cut into manageable pieces which can be separated and isolated by electrophoresis. The next requirement is to determine the nucleotide sequence of the DNA pieces. Methods for rapid sequencing of DNA were developed in the late 1970s (50,51). The method developed by Sanger et al. (50) forms the basis of automated DNA sequencing procedures used today. The method utilizes the enzyme DNA polymerase, the enzyme which is required for DNA synthesis from its deoxyribonucleotide precursor. An exact copy of a single-stranded DNA sequence can be obtained by incubating the single-stranded DNA with DNA polymerase and deoxyribonucleoside triphosphate precursors (dATP, dCTP, dGTP, dTTP). A small oligonucleotide sequencing primer is required which corresponds to the 5′ end of the strand to be synthesized and hybridizes to the 3′ end of the strand to be sequenced. If one of the deoxyribonucleotide triphosphate precursors is radiolabeled with ^{32}P the newly synthesized DNA will be labeled. The critical step which allows the sequence of the new strand to be determined is the inclusion in the reaction mixture of a small amount of dideoxy ribonucleoside triphosphate (ddATP, ddCTP, ddGTP or ddTTP in four different DNA synthesis reactions). When the dideoxy ribonucleoside triphosphates are incorporated into the new DNA chain the addition of further nucleotides is prevented, that is, the dideoxy ribonucleoside triphosphates act as inhibitors of chain synthesis. Provided the deoxynucleotide precursors are in excess a series of DNA fragments is produced, the smallest of which comprises the primer plus a single dideoxynucleotide and the largest corresponding to 300 or 400 deoxynucletides terminated by a dideoxynucleotide. The composition of the four reaction mixtures is analyzed by electrophoresis in four parallel lanes of a polyacrylamide gel. An autoradiograph of the gel or "ladder" of bands the smallest (at the bottom of the gel) corresponding to the 5′ end of the newly synthesized sequence (primer sequence + 1 dideoxynucleotide) is made. By reading the gel from the bottom up, the DNA sequence of the new strand can be determined.

Modern automated DNA sequencers allow the determination of a complete DNA sequence using only one lane of a polyacrylamide gel. This is achieved by labeling each dideoxy ribonucleotide triphosphate with a different fluorochrome. This means that four times as many sequences can be obtained from a single gel and each sequence can be read automatically by detection of the different fluorescence signals.

DNA Cloning

Restriction enzymes and DNA sequencing methods provide the basic tools but how are the genes that encode blood group-active proteins found, among the three thousand million nucleotides of a human genome? There are different ways of approaching this problem but they all involve DNA cloning. The term "DNA cloning" describes a method by which a single fragment of human DNA can be replicated in a bacterial cell. A clone is a stock of individuals derived asexually from one individual. Each individual in the clone has an identical genetic constitution to all the others. Bacteria reproduce asexually very rapidly and within the bacterial cell circles of double stranded DNA, known as plasmids, occur naturally. One way of DNA cloning is to use restriction enzymes to cut human DNA and to insert the human DNA pieces into plasmids (the plasmid DNA is cut with the same restriction enzyme so that the human DNA pieces will "fit" into the plasmid). This process by which human DNA is "recombined" with bacterial DNA gave rise to the term recombinant DNA technology. The plasmid is known as a vector (Latin vector, meaning carrier). Plasmids are easily isolated from bacteria since they are much smaller than chromosomal DNA. The recombinant plasmid can be put back into bacterial cells simply by making the bacterial cell wall transiently permeable. The different pieces of human DNA insert into different plasmids. The process of transfection is not 100% efficient and so it is usual to engineer into the plasmid a gene which can be used to select bacterial cells containing plasmids (commonly a gene that confers resistance to a particular antibiotic). The transfected bacterial cells are then cultured and those bacterial colonies which grow in the presence of antibiotic contain plasmids and hence human DNA fragments or clones. The set of bacterial clones containing different DNA fragments is known as a DNA "library".

There are two kinds of DNA library. If total DNA from the cell of interest is used to make the library it is known as a genomic DNA library. A genomic library contains large segments of DNA which do not encode proteins. It will also contain intronic sequences which do not encode proteins. Because genomic DNA libraries contain large amounts of DNA sequence which are not directly involved in encoding protein it is often more convenient to begin the search for a gene using a cDNA library. In an earlier section of this chapter the process by which a gene is transcribed to pre-mRNA and then to mRNA which is translated into protein was discussed. It would clearly be attractive to search the mRNA population of a cell for a gene of interest. It is possible to purify total mRNA from a cell by exploiting the fact that mRNA differs from other cellular RNAs by virtue of its poly A "tail" (see earlier section for a discussion). Since A pairs with T, mRNA can be purified by binding and elution from a poly T column (usually referred to as an oligo dT column). The process by which DNA gave rise to RNA can be reversed using a viral enzyme known as reverse transcriptase. In the presence of reverse transcriptase a DNA copy of the purified mRNA can be made (complementary DNA or cDNA). This cDNA is not the same as the genomic DNA sequence which gave rise to the mRNA because it lacks intronic sequences. The single stranded cDNA is converted to double stranded DNA using DNA polymerase and a cDNA "library" can be generated using the same methods described above to generate a genomic DNA library.

Although bacterial plasmids are the most commonly used they are not the only vectors available for recombinant DNA technology. Viral DNA can also be used as a vector and the reader will find reference to this in Chapter 2 since bacteriophage vectors have been used extensively genetically to engineer novel antibody molecules.

Genomic DNA libraries contain all the genes present in an organism but cDNA libraries reflect mRNA synthesis so that if a cDNA library is to be used to find a gene which gives rise to a red cell surface protein, it is necessary to use a library which has been prepared from a cell tissue which is known to express that protein. Commonly, but not exclusively, reticulocyte cDNA libraries and bone marrow libraries have been used to search for red cell genes. Successful use of cDNA libraries depends to some extent on the level of mRNA expression of the protein of interest in the cell used to make the library. For example, hemoglobin is such a major protein in the red cell that globin gene transcripts represent a high percentage of the total mRNA in reticulocytes and are easily found in a reticulocyte cDNA library. In contrast, the Lutheran glycoprotein is of low abundance on the red cell. Attempts to isolate Lutheran cDNA from a reticulocyte cDNA library were unsuccessful and it was eventually isolated from a placental cDNA library (52). This experience highlights the value of determining the tissue distribution of a protein of interest because the cell in which a protein is first described may not necessarily be the cell in which it is expressed at the highest levels.

Finding Genes in cDNA Libraries

As discussed in Chapter 4, the usual way of hunting for a gene is to obtain partial amino acid sequence of the protein of interest and to synthesize an oligonucleotide or mixture of oligonucleotides which can be used to probe a suitable cDNA library. Since there is substantial redundancy in the genetic code (see earlier section) some amino acids can be encoded by several different codons. Obviously, it is preferable to find a stretch of amino acid sequence in the protein of interest where this level of degeneracy is at a minimum in order to maximize the chances of finding a bacterial clone with the desired cDNA. Amino acids like tryptophan (codon UGG) and methionine (codon AUG) have only a single codon and so selection of protein sequences containing these residues is highly desirable. Phenylalanine, tyrosine, cysteine, histidine, glutamine, asparagine, lysine, aspartic acid and glutamic acid, each have two codons and are therefore better than the other amino acids. The synthetic oligonucleotide probe (usually about 30 nucleotides) is labeled (traditionally with ^{32}P although non-radioactive labels are also available) and used to screen the library. A typical screening protocol involves plating the cDNA libraries to generate large numbers of bacterial clones, placing a filter paper on each petri dish to obtain an aliquot of each clone on the paper (marking the paper and petri dish so that each desired clone can be identified again later), lysing the bacteria and denaturing the DNA contained within with alkali (the DNA remains bound to the paper), incubating the paper with labeled oligonucleotide probe and exposing the paper to autoradiography. If the procedure is successful, one or more bacterial colonies will give positive signals and these can be picked from the original petri dish, recloned and expanded. The next step is to see if the selected clones contain cDNA corresponding to the protein of interest. This can be achieved by a variety of methods but the most direct involves recovery of the plasmid vector and sequencing of the human DNA insert, to see if the protein sequence encoded by the cDNA corresponds to the protein sequence of the peptide or peptides obtained from the purified protein itself.

Sometimes amino acid sequence is not available for the protein of interest and researchers are tempted to use another type of cDNA library known as an expression library. The vectors used for expression libraries are designed so that they include a gene regulatory sequence (promoter) which allows the bacterium to synthesize mRNA and protein corresponding to the human cDNA sequence in the plasmid. The bacterial clones can then be screened for protein with antibody or some other unique probe for the protein of interest. This approach is not to be undertaken by the faint hearted. Fairbairn and Tanner (53) used a murine monoclonal anti-glycophorin A (BRIC 127) to search for glycophorin A clones in human fetal liver expression library and isolated strongly positive cDNA clones which turned out to encode not glycophorin A but a cytoplasmic enzyme, paroxysmal 3-oxoacyl-CoA thiolase. Comparison of the sequence of this enzyme with that of glycophorin A showed that residues 208-218 of the enzyme were homologous to residues 28-38 of glycophorin A and furnished evidence that both proteins contained the epitope for BRIC 127. A major problem with bacterial expression systems is that posttranslational modifications (for example glycosylation) of human proteins expressed in bacteria are not the same as those in eukaryotic cells. Since almost all blood group-active proteins are glycosylated this is obviously a major drawback. The alternative is expression in a mammalian cell and several systems are available for this. One of these involves expression in the oocyte of the amphibian *Xenopus*. A painstaking study involving injection and expression of cDNA in *Xenopus* oocytes and then screening the oocytes for urea transport led to the cDNA cloning of the first mammalian urea transporter (54). The sequence of this rabbit urea transporter was then used to isolate the human urea transporter and show that it carried the Kidd blood group system antigens (see Chapter 19). Expression cloning in mammalian cell lines has proved to be a successful route for identifying glycosyltransferase genes (see Chapters 8, 9 and 10).

Determining the Structure of Genes from Genomic DNA: Use of Cosmids

A cDNA clone identifies the portions of the gene which are ultimately incorporated into the gene product, a protein. It does not describe the structure of the gene itself which contains introns and regulatory sequences that determine in which tissue it will be expressed, when and how much. Genomic DNA libraries produced in bacterial plasmids like those described in the previous section are limited with respect to the length of human DNA that can be accommodated in the plasmid. Special vectors called cosmids which are derived from bacteriophage can accommodate about 30,000 base pairs. Cosmids have the potential to contain the whole gene for a protein of interest including introns and both 5′ and 3′ flanking (regulatory) sequences.

One approach to determining the structure of a gene of interest is to use cDNA to screen a cosmid genomic DNA library in an analogous manner to that described for cDNA cloning in the previous section. Having found suitable genomic clones a restriction map of the human DNA clone can be constructed by digesting the cosmid DNA with restriction enzymes of different specificities and determining the sizes of the fragments produced by electrophoresis. The restriction fragments which contain exons corresponding to the gene of interest can be identified by hybridization of the double stranded genomic DNA with cDNA, a technique known as Southern blotting. Genomic DNA fragments are separated by electrophoresis and then transferred to a nylon paper. This transfer is achieved simply by exposing one side of the gel to a suitable buffer, placing the nylon paper on the other side of the gel and a stack of paper towels on top of the nylon paper so that buffer is drawn through the gel towards the paper towels. The DNA fragments are drawn out of the gel and bound to the nylon paper. DNA fragments bound to the nylon are denatured by treatment with alkali or heat treatment so that the double stranded molecules unfold, are exposed to labeled cDNA and hybridization between the cDNA and the complementary genomic DNA strand is achieved by renaturation at 65°C. Suitable fragments hybridizing to the cDNA probe can be isolated and sequenced and if fragments of overlapping sequence are obtained the location of introns and regulatory sequences can be determined.

Determining the Structure of Genes from Genomic DNA: PCR

The "classical" method of determining gene struc- ture described above has to a large extent been superseded by the development of the polymerase chain reaction (PCR) and the easy availability of synthetic oligonucleotides. The PCR was described and refined during the latter half of the 1980s (55). PCR can be used if part of the nucleotide sequence of a gene is known. Two synthetic oligonucleotide primers are prepared, one complementary to each strand of the DNA molecule of interest. One binds to the 5' end of the region of interest and the other to the 3' end on the other strand (see figure 5-6). These primers serve to initiate synthesis of a copy of each DNA strand in the presence of DNA polymerase after the two strands of the target DNA have been separated by heat treatment. Most DNA polymerases are denatured by repeated and prolonged exposure to high temperatures and so the chain reaction of heat treatment, DNA synthesis, heat treatment, DNA synthesis is limited. There are however some bacteria which live at high temperatures and these "thermophilic" bacteria have DNA polymerases which are not denatured by heat. The DNA polymerase from one of these bacteria (*Thermophilus aquatica*) is called Taq polymerase. The inclusion of Taq polymerase in a reaction mixture containing double stranded DNA, complementary primers and the four deoxyribonucleoside triphosphates allows a chain reaction to take place over numerous cycles of heat (circa 90°C) and cool (circa 40°C) where heat separates the strands and cool allows hybridization of the oligonucleotide primers and Taq polymerase effects synthesis of DNA. Most amplifications are for about 30 cycles (each cycle takes about 5 minutes) and a single species of DNA

FIGURE 5-6 The Polymerase Chain Reaction (PCR)

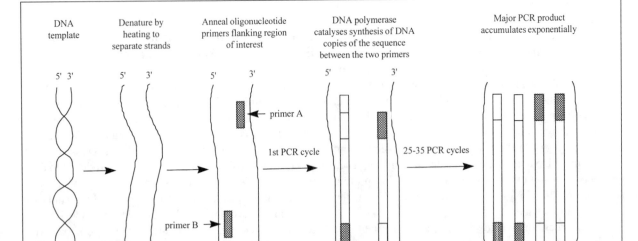

results which corresponds to the region between the two primers originally selected. By selecting pairs of primers from different regions of a cDNA sequence and performing the PCR with genomic DNA it is possible to determine the sequence of all the introns in a gene (see for example reference 56). If the gene contains one or more very large introns such an analysis is not so easy to perform. Obviously, determination of the 5′ and 3′ regions of the gene by PCR is not so straightforward because suitable primer sequences are not present in the cDNA.

Chromosome "Walking" and Positional DNA Cloning

It is possible to identify a gene of interest without knowing the nature of its protein product. This is achieved by linkage analysis, that is from the knowledge that the gene of interest is close to a known gene or a particular genetic marker (restriction fragment length polymorphisms) (RFLP) (9,10).

When a gene of interest is close to a known gene for which DNA probes are available it is possible to 'walk' along the chromosome to find the gene. Cloning of the gene giving rise to the Xg[a] blood group antigen was achieved by chromosome walking over 75Kb from the *CD99* (*MIC 2*) gene (57, see Chapter 25 for a more detailed discussion). Chromosome walking involves the use of large genomic clones. The process starts with a genomic clone which hybridizes to the known gene close to the unknown gene of interest. A probe is made from the end of this clone (say 3′ end) and this is used to screen a genomic DNA library for other positive clones which have the probe sequence at their 5′ end. A probe is made to the 3′ end of this new clone and the process repeated until the unknown gene is found. In this way a set of overlapping clones is generated which cover the area which includes the gene of interest. In the case of Xg[a], the gene was found by using genomic sequences from the set of overlapping clones to screen a bone marrow cDNA library.

The *XK* gene was found by positional cloning (58). The *XK* gene was known from studies of patients with McLeod syndrome to map between the gene which is dysfunctional in chronic granulomatous disease (CGD) and the gene which is dysfunctional in Duchenne's muscular dystrophy (DMD, 59). Ho et al. (58) obtained a set of overlapping genomic clones which spanned the CGD and DMD genes. Because of the large distance between the two genes yeast artificial chromosomes (YACs) were used. Chromosomes replicate during mitosis. For replication to take place certain critical regions of the chromosome must be present. In the case of yeast chromosomes their critical regions are very small and so recombinant DNA molecules can be prepared which contain the yeast critical sequence but in the context of very large human DNA sequences (Ω 10^6 nucleotide pairs) are much larger than cosmids. These recombinant DNA sequences can replicate in yeast cells and are known as yeast artificial chromosomes or YACs. YACs which contained the *XK* gene were found by utilizing hybridization experiments with DNA from patients with McLeod syndrome. One patient in particular had a very large deletion and this allowed the identification of the gene because of abnormal hybridization patterns on Southern blots. See Chapter 18 for a more detailed discussion.

Studying the Regulation of Genes

The usual method of elucidating the regulatory sequences which control transcription of a gene is to employ a "reporter" gene. A reporter gene is a gene selected because its protein product is easy to detect (usually an enzyme). The most commonly employed reporter genes are the genes for the bacterial enzymes ß-galactosidase and chloramphenicol acetyltransferase (CAT). Putative regulatory sequences from the gene of interest are inserted in a vector containing the reporter gene and the expression of the protein product of the reporter gene is assayed after transfection of the construct in a suitable cell line simply by assaying for the bacterial enzyme. Regulatory sequences are not confined to the promoter sequences in the 5′ non-coding region of a gene but may be several kilobases away. The various regulatory sequences act in combination. Regulatory sequences controlling the ß-globin gene locus are the most extensively studied (60).

Transcription factors involved in the regulation of genes are usually studied using a "gel shift" assay. In a "gel shift" assay a short DNA sequence containing a putative regulatory sequence is radiolabeled and incubated with a cell extract. If the extract contains a DNA-binding protein which recognizes nucleotide sequences within the target DNA sequence, the DNA binding protein will be detected because the mobility of the target DNA will be retarded when the mixture is subjected to electrophoresis. If there is more than one DNA binding protein capable of binding the target DNA in the cell extract then more than one retarded band will be found on electrophoresis. Once the DNA binding protein has been detected it can be purified from the cell extract using conventional protein purification procedures using the "gel shift" assay to monitor purification.

Determining the Chromosomal Location of a Gene Using Molecular Methods

One of the most powerful molecular methods for determining the chromosomal location of a gene is fluorescence in situ hybridization (FISH, 61). In this method the target DNA (a chromosomal spread from the cell of interest) and suitable DNA probe (frequently a cDNA) are denatured then hybridized. The position of the cDNA probe on a particular chromosome is then determined by fluorescence microscopy. The DNA probe may itself be directly labeled with fluorochrome or more commonly it is labeled with biotin and detected indirectly with a fluorescence probe. Alternatively radiolabeled DNA probes can be used and chromosomal location determined by autoradiography.

If FISH is performed using chromosomal spreads from cells undergoing mitosis at the metaphase stage the location of the gene to a particular region of a chromosome can be achieved. This is because at metaphase the chromosomes are maximally condensed and therefore maximally separated from one another before separation of the sister chromatids at anaphase and subsequent cell division. The condensed nature of the chromosome at metaphase does however limit the precision with which a gene can be located. By examining chromosomes very early in mitosis it is possible to study the order of genes that are very close on the same chromosome. In this case different fluorescences are used to label each DNA probe. Techniques are also available which allow examination of genes on chromosomes in cells at interphase. The cells are lysed and the long strands of uncondensed DNA are released. Under these conditions it is possible to distinguish fluorescence signals from probes which are a few kilobases apart (62).

References

1. Weatherall D. Science and the Quiet Art. Oxford:Oxford Univ Press, 1995:229
2. Darwin C. On the Origin of Species. New York:Ward, Lock:1901,20
3. Sutton WSS. Biol Bull 1903;4:231
4. Wells HG, Huxley J, Wells GP. The Science of Life. London:Cassell 1931;282
5. Ford CE, Hamerton JL. Nature 1956;178:1020
6. Tijo JK, Levan A. Hereditas 1956;42:1
7. Morgan TH. Science 1910;32:120
8. Morgan TH. Science 1911;34:384
9. Lewis M. In: Molecular and Functional Aspects of Blood Group Antigens. Bethesda:Am Assoc Blood Banks, 1995:127
10. Zelinski T. In: Molecular and Functional Aspects of Blood Group Antigens. Bethesda:Am Assoc Blood Banks, 1995:41
11. Langlois RG, Bigbee WL, Kyoizumi S, et al. Science 1987;236:445
12. Feulgen R, Behrens M, Mahdihassan S, et al. Z Physiol Chem 1937;246:203
13. Mirsky AE, Ris H. Nature 1949;163:666
14. Watson JD, Crick FHC. Nature 1953;171:737
15. Alberts B, Bray D, Lewis J, et al. Molecular Biology of the Cell, 3rd Ed. NewYork:Garland, 1994
16. Kozek M. J Mol Biol 1987;196:947
17. Iwamato S, Li J, Omi T, et al. Blood 1996;87:378
18. Sharp PA. Cell 1994;77:805
19. Jeffreys AJ, Flavell RA. Cell 1977;12:1097
20. Tonegawa S, Maxam AM, Tizard R, et al. Proc Nat Acad Sci USA 1978;75:1485
21. Hawkins JD. Nucleic Acids Res 1988;16:9893
22. Berget SM. J Biol Chem 1995;270:2411
23. Izaurralde E, Lewis J, McGuigan C, et al. Cell 1994;78:657
24. Nakai K, Sakamoto H. Gene 1994;141:171
25. Huang C-H, Johe KK, Seifter S, et al. Baillières Clin Haematol 1991;4:821
26. Lublin DM, Mallinson G, Poole J, et al. Blood 1994;84:1276
27. Youssoufian H, Longmore G, Neumann D, et al. Blood 1993;81:2223
28. Zon LI, Youssoufian H, Mather C, et al. Proc Nat Acad Sci USA 1991;88:10638
29. Wu H, Liu X, Jaenisch R, et al. Cell 1995;83:59
30. Klingmuller U, Lorenz K, Cantley LC, et al. Cell 1995;80:729
31. de la Chapelle A, Traskelin A-L, Juvonen E. Proc Nat Acad Sci USA 1993;90:4495
32. Martin DIK, Orkin SH. Genes Dev 1990;4:1886
33. Yang H-Y, Evans T. Mol Cell Biol 1992;12:4562
34. Omichinski JG, Clore GM, Schaad O, et al. Science 1993;261:438
35. Capechi MR. Science 1989;244:1288
36. Weiss MJ, Orkin SH. Exp Haematol 1995;23:99
37. Simmon MC. Nature Genetics 1995;11:9
38. Labbaye C, Valtieri M, Barberi T, et al. J Clin Invest 1995;95:2346
39. Tourmaville C, Colin Y, Cartron J-P, et al. Nature Genetics 1995;10:224
40. Condorelli G, Vitelli L, Valtieri M, et al. Blood 1995;86:164
41. Orkin SH. J Biol Chem 1995;270:4955
42. Peters LL, Shivdasani RA, Liu S-C, et al. Cell 1996;86:917
43. Southgate CD, Chishti AH, Mitchell B, et al. Nature Genet 1996;14:227
44. Huang C-H, Reid ME, Daniels GL, et al. J Biol Chem 1993;268:25902
45. Anstee DJ, Mawby WJ, Tanner MJA. In: Membranes and Transport: A Critical Review. New York:Plenum, 1982, vol 2:427
46. Howard JC. Nature 1991;352:565
47 Miller LH. Proc Nat Acad Sci USA 1994;91:2415
48. Sim BKL, Chitnis CE, Wasniowska K, et al. Science 1994;264:1941
49. Adams RLP, Burdon RH, Campbell AM, et al. In: The Biochemistry of Nucleic Acids. London: Chapman and Hall 1981:1
50. Sanger F, Nickless S, Coulson AR. Proc Nat Acad Sci USA 1977;74:5463
51. Maxam AM, Gilbert W. Proc Nat Acad Sci USA 1977;74:560
52. Parson SF, Mallinson G, Holmes CH, et al. Proc Nat Acad Sci USA 1995;92:5496
53. Fairbairn LJ, Tanner MJA. Nucleic Acids Res 1989;17:3588
54. You G, Smith CP, Kanai Y, et al. Nature 1993;365:844
55. Saiki RK, Gelfand DH, Stoffel S, et al. Science 1988;239:487
56. Parsons SF, Mallinson G, Daniels GL, et al. Blood 1997;89:4219
57. Ellis NA, Ye T-Z, Patton S, et al. Nature Genet 1994;6:394

58. Ho M, Chelly J, Carter N, et al. Cell 1994;77:869
59. Bertelson CJ, Pogo AO, Chaduri A, et al. Am J Hum Genet 1988;423:703
60. Crossley M, Orkin SH. Curr Opin Genet Dev 1993;3:232

61. Trask BJ. Trends Genet 1991;7:149
62. Parra I, Windle B. Nature Genetics 1993;5:17
63. Issitt PD. Transf Med Rev 1993;7:139

6 | The Antiglobulin (Coombs) Test, Complement in Antigen-Antibody Reactions and in the Antiglobulin Test, the Alternative Pathway of Complement Activation, In Vivo Destruction of Incompatible Red Cells, Some Biological Consequences of Complement Activation in Man

In 1945, Coombs, Mourant, and Race (1,2) described the use of anti-human globulin serum for the detection of red cell-bound non-agglutinating antibodies. Coming at that time in the progress of blood grouping, the discovery must rank as almost as important as the discovery of the ABO blood groups. The antiglobulin (Coombs) test was rapidly applied, by the authors describing it and by other prominent workers and soon proved responsible for a variety of important discoveries about blood groups, antibody-induced hemolytic anemia and hemolytic disease of the newborn. It was not until several years after his publications had appeared that Dr. Coombs found that the principle of the test had been applied by Moreschi (3) in 1908.

Since its rediscovery, the test has been in regular use in laboratories throughout the world and is probably still the most useful single tool at the disposal of the blood bank serologist. In 1957, Dacie et al. (4) showed that antibodies present in antiglobulin sera, that had been known up to that time as anti-non-gamma, were in fact directed against certain of the components of complement. Thus it was realized that anti-human globulin serum can detect not only non-agglutinating antibody molecules but also molecules of complement that have become attached to red cells following in vivo or in vitro antigen-antibody reactions.

Principle of the Antiglobulin Test and Monoclonal Antiglobulin Reagents

The principle of the test is straightforward. Originally, human serum (or purified components from human serum) were injected into animals, most often rabbits or goats. The proteins in the human serum acted as foreign antigens and the animals underwent immune responses the products of which were an assortment of anti-human-globulins. Once suitable levels of antibodies were being produced the animals were bled. Unwanted antibodies such as anti-species, anti-A and anti-B were removed by adsorption, or the animal serum was used at a dilution at which those antibodies did not interfere. The

useful antibodies in animal serum antiglobulin reagents are IgG (but see below with regard to monoclonal antiglobulins) but react with their antigens, human IgG or complement, that are attached to red cells, in a manner that promotes rapid agglutination of the protein-coated red cells (see below). An early problem with the production of anti-human globulin reagents by this method was that sometimes traces of the unwanted antibodies, mentioned above, remained active in the finished reagent and interfered in the test by causing weak positive reactions that were not due to antibody or complement binding to the test cells. This was not much of a problem with anti-IgG, the titer of which was invariably much higher than that of the unwanted agglutinins. It was far more of a problem in producing reagents containing adequate amounts of anti-complement, the strength of which in the raw animal serum, was sometimes not much greater than that of the unwanted agglutinins.

These problems have been in part overcome by the production of monoclonal anti-human-globulin reagents. Indeed, some of the first useful (in blood banking) monoclonal antibodies produced were directed against the third component of human complement, C3 (5-7 and see below). Monoclonal antiglobulins do not, of course, contain unwanted contaminating antibodies that must be removed by adsorption or by-passed by dilution. Thus it is now possible to make broad spectrum (anti-IgG plus anti-C3) antiglobulin reagents that contain suitable levels of anti-C3, without any danger that contaminating antibodies will interfere in the final reaction. The use of selected IgM monoclonal anti-C3 has further advanced the production of potent anti-complement reagents that are free of contaminants (8-10). Production of monoclonal anti-IgG has lagged somewhat behind production of monoclonal anti-C3. Some reagents have appeared but many broad spectrum reagents commercially available as of this writing (May 1995) contain monoclonal anti-C3 and polyclonal anti-IgG. It is possible that because of the epitope specificity of monoclonal antibodies (see Chapter 7) it may prove necessary to make pools of monoclonal anti-IgG for routine use, in order that all important epitopes of IgG are recognized. An early attempt to do this, with existing monoclonal anti-IgG, resulted in production of a reagent that was not as good as animal polyclonal anti-IgG pools (11). However, better clones have been identified (12) and pressure to reduce the use of animals in the production of biological reagents may provide an incentive for the development of high quality monoclonal anti-IgG reagents (13). At least one early example of a single clone derived monoclonal anti-IgG, that was known not to recognize IgG4, failed to detect one example of an eluted autoantibody made of IgG3 and IgG4 (14).

Because the IgG agglutinins in antiglobulin sera cause rapid agglutination of IgG-coated red cells the tests should be read by immediate spin methods. With some animal source reagents, the complement-anti-complement reaction develops more slowly so that the tests should be spun and read again after being left at room temperature for five minutes. However, this reading for the optimal detection of cell-bound complement should be in addition to and should not replace the immediate reading. The reason for this is that IgG-anti-IgG complexes dissociate fairly rapidly so that maximal strength positive reactions of that portion of the test are seen in tests spun immediately after the addition of anti-human-globulin serum. Reading tests only once, following a five minute incubation after addition of the antiglobulin serum, would result in some IgG-anti-IgG reactions being missed.

To use antiglobulin serum once it has been prepared, red cells are incubated with an incomplete antibody directed against an antigen that they carry. After a suitable incubation time the antibody becomes attached to the red cells but no agglutination occurs because the antibody is of the non-agglutinating type. The cells are then washed in order that the free globulin molecules in the cell-serum mixture, that are not attached to the cells, will be removed and will not neutralize the antiglobulin serum when it is added. Because the cells are now coated with human globulin (antibody) the anti-human globulin (Coombs serum) causes agglutination to occur. The complex formed comprises red cell-plus-antibody globulin-plus-Coombs serum-plus-antibody globulin-plus red cells (see figure 6-1).

Application of the Antiglobulin Test

It is easy to see that this test can be applied on a variety of different occasions in the blood bank.

1. Known antiserum and unknown cells (red cell typing).
2. Known phenotype red cells and unknown serum (antibody detection and identification).

3. Unknown cells and unknown serum (compatibility testing).
4. Direct tests on the red cells of individuals possibly suffering from hemolytic anemia, hemolytic disease of the newborn or a transfusion reaction, in any of which antigen-antibody complexes may have formed in vivo.

If an antigen-antibody reaction takes place (or has already taken place in the case of direct tests) antibody globulin will be attached to the red cell surface and a positive antiglobulin test will result. If no antigen-antibody complexes are formed the antiglobulin serum, when added, will find no antigen present and the antiglobulin test will be negative.

Control for Negative Antiglobulin Tests

There are a number of factors that can result in a false negative antiglobulin test. These include but are not limited to: failure to add the antiglobulin reagent; contamination (neutralization) of the antiglobulin reagent before it is used; and failure to wash the test cells adequately before the test is read. Thus an essential control for all negative tests is to show that the antiglobulin reagent was active during the test. One drop of a 5% suspension of red cells coated with an incomplete antibody is added to each negative test, after the test has been read. The tubes are then centrifuged and read again. A positive result indicates that the antiglobulin reagent was active and that the negative result of the original test is valid. A negative result in the control test indicates that the antiglobulin reagent was not active and that the original test is not valid. In other words, a negative reaction could have been seen although the test cells were coated with antibody. Since, on most occasions, antiglobulin neutralization is an all or nothing phenomenon, indicator cells coated with IgG can be used. There is no need to use complement-coated red cells in this control procedure.

Incubation Times in Solutions at Normal Ionic Strength and Indirect Antiglobulin Tests

When red cells and serum are first mixed and the serum contains an antibody directed against an antigen present on the red cells, the uptake of antibody by the red cells begins immediately. With strong enough antibodies, immunoglobulin can be shown to have bound to the red cells within seconds of addition. However, in indirect antiglobulin tests where the strength of the antibody is not known, time must be allowed for sufficient numbers

FIGURE 6-1 The Principle of the Anti-IgG Antiglobulin Test

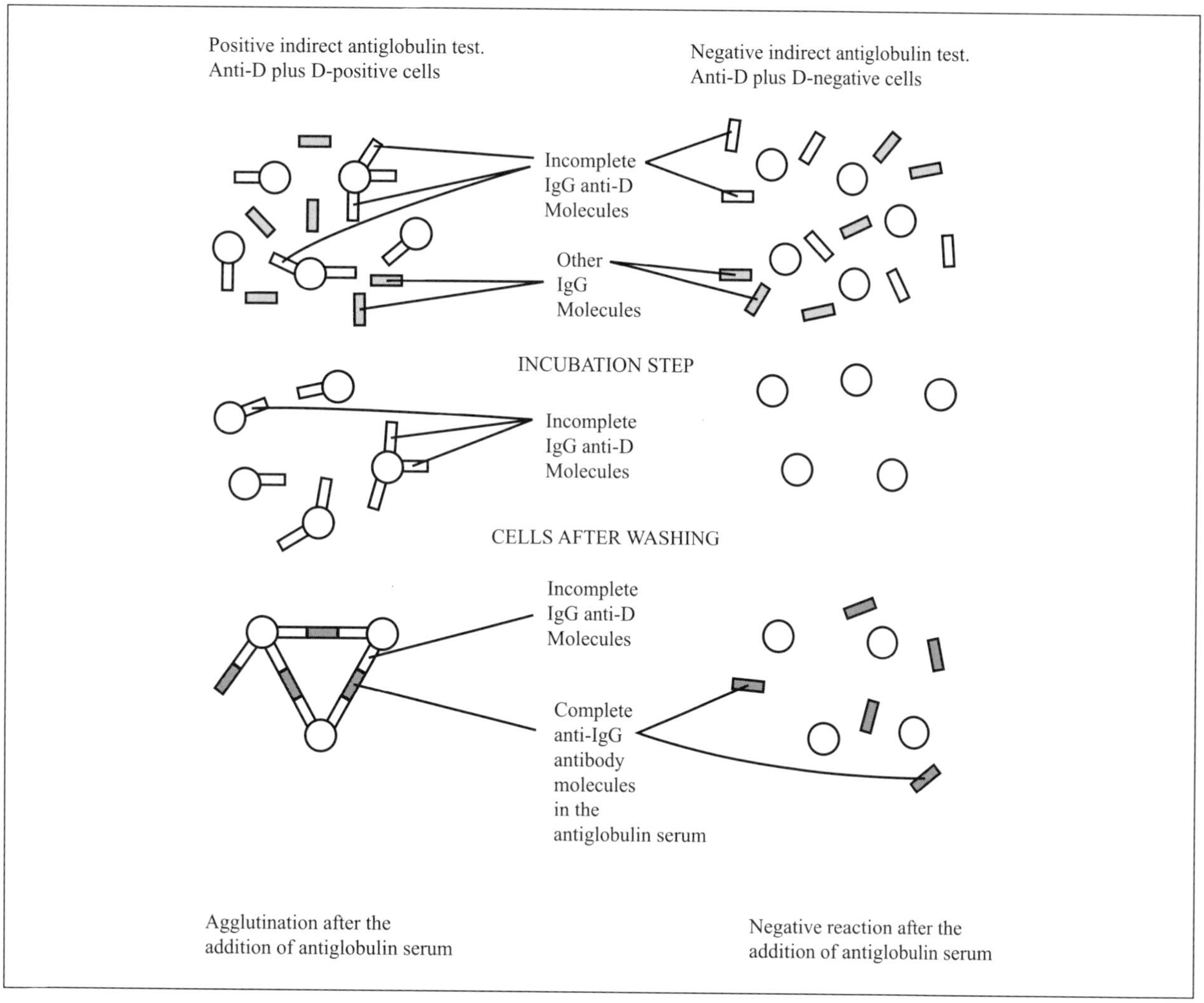

Positive indirect antiglobulin test. Anti-D plus D-positive cells

Negative indirect antiglobulin test. Anti-D plus D-negative cells

Incomplete IgG anti-D Molecules

Other IgG Molecules

INCUBATION STEP

Incomplete IgG anti-D Molecules

CELLS AFTER WASHING

Incomplete IgG anti-D Molecules

Complete anti-IgG antibody molecules in the antiglobulin serum

Agglutination after the addition of antiglobulin serum

Negative reaction after the addition of antiglobulin serum

of antibody molecules to attach to red cells for subsequent detection with antiglobulin serum. Various workers have tried to estimate the minimum number of IgG molecules necessary per red cell for detection of the antibody with a potent anti-IgG serum. Although no absolute agreement has been reached the number appears to be in the order of 100-200 molecules, dependent partly on the type of IgG involved and partly on the potency of the anti-IgG serum being used (15-22). The purpose of the incubation period, in indirect antiglobulin tests, is to allow sufficient antibody uptake by the cells for subsequent detection with antiglobulin serum. Many factors must be considered. When antigen and antibody are first mixed the rate of antibody association is high and the rate of dissociation low. After some time a point of equilibrium is reached with association and dissociation rates being about equal. After prolonged incubation less antibody may be detectable on the red cells although it is not clear whether this is because dissociation rates overtake association rates or because antigen and/or antibody

molecules undergo degenerative changes that render complexing less efficient, (23) see figure 6-2. Ideally, all indirect antiglobulin tests would be read at the time the equilibrium point is reached. This would provide the advantage of reading all tests when maximal amounts of antibody had bound, in minimal times. Thus the weakest antibodies detectable would be found and would give the strongest possible reactions. Indirect antiglobulin tests would also be read with minimum incubation times. Unfortunately, it is not possible exactly to apply this theory in practical situations. As can be seen in figure 6-2, no actual times of incubation are given. Although most antibodies follow the curve shown in that figure, they do not all do so at the same rate. When tests using saline or albumin are considered, a few antibodies reach the equilibrium point after 10-15 minutes, some not until 30 minutes and a few not until a full hour of incubation. Some antibodies will also reach the point where dissociation overtakes association fairly rapidly. Thus a few antibodies will show stronger reactions after 30 minutes than

FIGURE 6-2 To Show Levels of Antibody Bound to Red Cells During Incubation Period

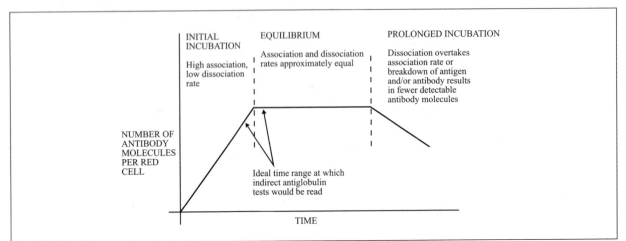

after 60 minutes incubation. In typing tests this presents no problem since the same antibody is used repeatedly and a suitable incubation time can easily be determined. In the detection and identification of unknown antibodies and in compatibility tests, an arbitrary time must be used that will allow the maximum number of antibodies to be detected. Most workers use an incubation period between 15 and 60 minutes. Many workers, by experience, have found incubation times of 30 to 45 minutes both practical and reliable although there are, as mentioned, a few antibodies that require a full hour's incubation before they will give reliable results. It should be emphasized that the incubation period is largely dependent on the serum:cell ratio of the test. The incubation times suggested here are for tests in normal ionic strength media, using one button, or one drop of a 2-5% saline suspension of cells, with two to four drops of serum, with or without the addition of albumin. Nowadays, of course, relatively few workers use tests at normal ionic strength so that the section below, on tests at low ionic strength most often applies. French (24), in a series of tests with antibodies of different specificities, found that most antibodies can be shown to have attached to red cells in sufficient quantity after 15 minutes incubation for detection with antiglobulin serum. Most workers, from practical experience, have adopted this incubation time as the absolute minimum in emergency situations when using this type of test.

Incubation Times In Low Ionic Strength Solutions and Indirect Antiglobulin Tests

As discussed in detail in Chapters 2 and 3, when red cells and serum are mixed in a solution with a starting ionic strength of 0.03I, the uptake of antibody by red cells occurs at a much more rapid rate than is the case at normal ionic strength. It is probable that antibody uptake by the cells follows a similar pattern to that shown in figure 6-2, but the time scale is markedly condensed. As a result, incubation times can be considerably reduced before the performance of indirect antiglobulin tests for antibody screening and identification and in compatibility tests, when a low ionic strength system is used. In fairly large scale studies Löw and Messeter (25) used five minutes, Moore and Mollison (26) 10 minutes and Wicker and Wallas (27), 15 minutes, incubation at 37°C. Since all these studies showed efficient antibody detection and identification it seems reasonable to conclude that routine tests incubated for 10 to 15 minutes in low ionic strength solutions are at least equivalent to those using saline and/or albumin that are incubated for 30 to 60 minutes and that in emergencies, tests incubated for five minutes in low ionic strength solutions are at least as good as those incubated for 15 minutes in saline and/or albumin. As described in Chapter 3, the manual polybrene test of Lalezari and Jiang (28) uses a one minute incubation time in a low ionic strength medium, the PEG test of Nance and Garratty (29) uses 15 minutes. Perhaps this is as good a place as any to point out that no single test exists (and probably never will) that will detect every weak blood group antibody likely to be encountered. In the very practical situation that is present day blood banking, workers must decide which test, or battery of tests, is most likely to yield the most meaningful results, most of the time. Again as discussed in some detail in Chapter 3, the main advantage of using low ionic strength test systems is the reduction in time needed for completion of the tests rather than an absolute increase in sensitivity.

As also mentioned in Chapter 3, use of a low ionic strength test system in which the starting ionic strength is less than 0.03*I* results in non-antibody-mediated uptake of complement by red cells. At ionic strengths below 0.03*I* immunoglobulins aggregate. Aggregated immunoglobulins cause the classical and perhaps also the alternative pathway of complement activation to begin. Since broad spectrum antiglobulin reagents contain anti-C3, positive antiglobulin tests will be seen in the absence of antigen-antibody reactions. Although tests in low ionic strength saline and those that use Polybrene or PEG do not result in many positive reactions due to the detection of non-antigen-antibody-mediated complement activation, many workers prefer to use anti-IgG to read those tests. It seems that most (perhaps all) antibodies detected via the C3-anti-C3 reaction in normal ionic strength tests, can be detected with anti-IgG in Polybrene and PEG, and perhaps in LISS, tests.

Cell Washing Before the Addition of Antiglobulin Serum

Because of the specificity of the antibodies in antiglobulin serum, it is vital that cells to be tested for the presence of antibody globulin or complement on their surface, be very thoroughly washed following incubation in serum. There are many globulin and complement molecules in human serum, most of which do not bind to red cells. If some of these unattached globulin or complement molecules are still present when the antiglobulin serum is added, they will combine with the antibody molecules in the antiglobulin serum and neutralize them. Negative reactions may then be obtained in spite of the fact that large numbers of antibody or complement molecules have bound to the test cells. The washing of cells before the addition of antiglobulin serum actually constitutes a series of dilutions in which the remaining unbound proteins (from the original serum) are diluted in successive lots of wash saline that are discarded once the red cells have been centrifuged. Since the normal IgG level of serum is between 1 and 1.5g/100 ml it can be calculated that serum used in antiglobulin tests will contain up to 15,000mg IgG/ml. It is known that as little as 2mg IgG/ml remaining at the end of the wash cycle can cause neutralization of antiglobulin serum when it is added. These figures indicate levels of IgG/ml. It does not matter that less than 1 ml of serum is used, or that less than 1 ml of cell-saline mixture is left at the end of the wash cycle, since it is the level of remaining IgG that is being considered. Most blood bank workers use 10 x 75 mm or 12 x 75 mm tubes to perform antiglobulin tests. If the cell button is well decanted between washings, three washes with 3 ml of physiological saline are sufficient to reduce the non-bound IgG below the required level. However, if this system is used and care is not taken to remove all (or

almost all) the wash saline, false negative tests can result due to antiglobulin serum neutralization. This point is illustrated in table 6-1. In 10 x 75 mm tubes 2 ml of saline is used and in 12 x 75 tubes, 3 ml. If the cells are well decanted between each wash the remaining serum-saline mixture can be measured as being as little as 0.01 ml. Each time 2 ml of saline is added a 1 in 200 dilution of the remaining IgG will occur. If 3 ml of saline is used the dilution will be 1 in 300. If the cells are poorly decanted and 0.1 ml of serum-saline mixture is left the dilution factor will be 1 in 20 in a 2 ml wash and 1 in 30 in a 3 ml wash. Table 6-1 also includes calculations based on leaving 0.05 ml serum-saline mixture in the tubes. As can be seen, bad technique can result in insufficient IgG being removed. This point is especially critical when tests are performed by newcomers to the field of immunohematology or by students. Senior staff should take care to ensure that these less experienced workers understand WHY it is necessary to be so scrupu-

TABLE 6-1 Cell Washing Before the Addition of Antiglobulin Serum Expressed in Terms of Remaining Non-Bound IgG

	0.1 ml Serum/Saline left on cells		0.05 ml Serum/Saline left on cells		0.01 ml Serum/Saline left on cells	
Saline Wash Volume	2ml	3ml	2ml	3ml	2ml	3ml
µg IgG/ml remaining*						
After 1 wash	750	500	375	250	75	50
After 2 washes	37.5	16.66	9.375	4.16	0.375	0.166
After 3 washes	1.875	0.55	0.234	0.07	0.0018	0.0005

*Starting level 15,000 µg IgG/ml

lously careful in the washing of cells before the addition of antiglobulin serum. It has long been the practice of most workers to ensure that following the last wash before the addition of antiglobulin serum, the cell buttons be decanted to almost total dryness. The object of this exercise has been to prevent dilution of the antiglobulin serum when it is added. However, as can be seen from what is written above and from table 6-1, decants after the first and second washes are equally critical. The introduction of automated equipment for cell washing has generally improved the performance of the test by improving the efficacy of the wash procedure. The machines can be adjusted so that the decant cycle leaves an almost totally dry button of red cells. Since the machines are automated this occurs not only before the addition of antiglobulin serum, but also after the first and second washes. It should be stressed that although the automated systems enable an efficient wash cycle to be achieved when properly adjusted, regular examination of the system's performance is vital to ensure that machine settings do not alter and that the efficiency of the system is maintained. It should also be stressed that by being aware of the need for an efficient wash cycle and by constantly practicing impeccable technique, workers can achieve performances as good as those of well adjusted machines, by manual washing methods. However, such efficiency in wash procedures is more easily repeatable on a continual basis if automated equipment is used.

Having included the above comments about manual cell washing before the addition of antiglobulin serum, these authors have realized that this book will be read by some blood bankers who have never used a manual system! These youngsters are encouraged to ask their older colleagues what antiglobulin testing involved in the bad old days!

The Combining Sites of Antiglobulin Molecules

As has been explained in Chapter 2, the combining site of an antibody is situated in the Fab portion of the molecule. In this respect (and indeed in most others) antibody molecules in antiglobulin serum are no different to other antibody molecules. The antigens, against which anti-IgG is directed, are carried on the Fc portions of the IgG blood group antibody molecules. Earlier in this chapter, in figure 6-1, molecules of non-agglutinating anti-D and molecules of anti-IgG in antiglobulin serum were depicted as neat little blocks, conveniently shaded according to specificity. It is stressed that figure 6-1 is highly diagrammatic and is used strictly to illustrate a principle. The actual combination between anti-D and red cells and anti-IgG and IgG (anti-D) are more accurately depicted in figure 6-3. However, for the sake of clarity only two red cells, two molecules of anti-D and one molecule of anti-IgG are used in that diagram. In the actual agglutination of antibody-coated red cells by antiglobulin serum, many hundred of molecules of both anti-D and anti-IgG are involved.

Figure 6-3 treats the Fc pieces of IgG and anti-IgG as single entities. In fact there are subtle differences in the Fc pieces associated with the IgG subclasses (see Chapter 2) and the Gm groups. When polyspecific antiglobulin reagents made in animals are used, differences in structure of Fc pieces of blood group antibody molecules appear to play no role in the IgG-anti-IgG reaction. Antiglobulin reagents containing appropriate

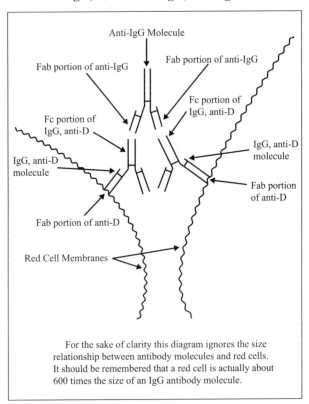

FIGURE 6-3 To Illustrate the Combining Sites of IgG, Anti-D and IgG, Anti-IgG

For the sake of clarity this diagram ignores the size relationship between antibody molecules and red cells. It should be remembered that a red cell is actually about 600 times the size of an IgG antibody molecule.

levels of anti-IgG will agglutinate red cells coated with IgG of any subclass. As already discussed in the section dealing with the principle of the antiglobulin test, the same may not hold true for monoclonal anti-IgG.

As illustrated in figure 6-3, the anti-IgG in antiglobulin serum is, itself, IgG. Chaplin (30) studied IgM anti-IgG made by immunized animals early in their response to the injection of human globulins. Although these antibodies were shown to bring about the agglutination of antibody-coated red cells, they were not particularly potent nor were they very stable on storage. It was concluded that it rather difficult to obtain these IgM antiglobulins and that their use does not involve advantage over the use of the later formed, more stable, IgG antiglobulins. Whether these conclusions will hold for monoclonal anti-IgG is not yet known. As already mentioned monoclonal IgM anti-C3 has been used in the production of antiglobulin reagents (8-10).

Degree of Agglutination Effected by Anti-IgG as it Relates to the Number of IgG Molecules Bound to Each Red Cell

Earlier in this chapter it was mentioned that in order for a (direct or indirect) antiglobulin test to give a visibly positive reaction, there must be an average of between 100 and 200 molecules of IgG bound to each red cell. With this number of molecules bound, the strength of the reaction is usually about 1+. However, different ways of measuring the amount of IgG per cell, yield different figures. In spite of this, the ratio of number of antibody molecules bound to the strength of the visible reaction, remains relatively well in balance. When Petz and Garratty (21) measured the amount of anti-D bound to the test cells, using a complement fixing antibody consumption test (17), their findings, expressed as number of IgG molecules per cell compared to degree of agglutination by anti-IgG were: <25 to 120, negative; 200, 1+; 300-500, 2+; >500, 3+ or 4+. Weakly positive reactions (less than 1+) were seen when between 120 and 200 molecules of IgG anti-D, were bound per red cell. Hughes-Jones et al. (16) investigated the same situation by measuring the degree of saturation of D antigen sites on red cells and the strength of reaction in IATs that detected the bound IgG anti-D. Their results, that used the degree of antigen site saturation to calculate the number of anti-D molecules bound and strength of IATs were: 2.6% saturation, 500 molecules, 1+ reaction; 5% saturation, 950 molecules, 2+ reaction; 9% saturation, 1700 molecules, 3+ reaction. Once the antiglobulin test reaches its maximum strength reaction, there can be no correlation between number of molecules bound and degree of agglutination. In the Petz and Garratty study (21), 500-700 molecules of IgG per red cell produced maximum strength (4+) reactions, in the Hughes-Jones et al. study (16) red cell IgG levels between 5,700 and 16,500 molecules per cell gave 4+ reactions. In other words, once the antiglobulin test reaches a strength of 4+ it does not provide much of a guide as to how much antibody (above a certain level) is bound to the red cells. The above findings are summarized in table 6-2. As discussed in detail in Chapter 37, a titration antiglobulin test or one using enzyme-linked or radiolabeled anti-IgG, can be of value in following the clinical response to therapy of patients with warm antibody-induced autoimmune hemolytic anemia.

Necessary Components of Antiglobulin Serum-Part 1, Anti-IgG

As described in Chapter 2, human IgG molecules vary considerably in terms of IgG subclass and within the subclasses, in terms of markers, such as the Gm groups, that they carry (31-33). Further, it is known that while many blood group antibodies are IgG1 and IgG3 in nature, IgG2 and IgG4 forms also exist (34-48). Natvig (49) has shown that a non-agglutinating, IgG, anti-D, produced by one individual, varied in its Gm composition over a period of time. In spite of this, it seems that the anti-IgG components in broad spectrum antiglobulin reagents that are

TABLE 6-2 Strength of Reaction of Anti-IgG in IATs as Correlated with Number of Molecules of IgG Anti-D Bound to D+ Red Cells

Number IgG Molecules per red cell*	Strength of IAT	
	From Petz and Garratty (21)	From Hughes-Jones et al. (16)
Up to 120	0	
120 to 200	+^{W}	
200	1+	
300 to 500	2+	1+
More than 500	3+,4+	
950		2+
1700		3+
More than 5000		4+

*For differences in methods used to calculate the number of IgG molecules per red cell, see text

heavy chain specific and are usually described simply as anti-IgG, react with determinants that are common to all gamma heavy chains. This does not mean that all anti-IgG (in polyspecific or monospecific reagents) are the same, nor that they are equally efficient in the detection of cell-bound IgG antibodies of different specificities. As described below, there are some differences among commercially available antiglobulin reagents. However, it does not seem that these differences relate directly to the IgG subclass and subtype within the subclass, of which the blood group antibodies are made.

Since the actions of anti-IgG can be described so briefly and since the actions of the anti-complement specificities that are also present in broad spectrum reagents take so long to describe (50-52), it should be stressed here that anti-IgG is, by far, the most important component in an antiglobulin reagent. Other than direct antiglobulin tests performed on the red cells of individuals with cold hemagglutinin disease (CHD), those of a small minority of patients with warm antibody-induced hemolytic anemia (WAIHA) and those sera of a tiny minority of patients who have formed blood group alloantibodies, the IgG-anti-IgG reaction predominates in cases in which antiglobulin tests are positive. Indeed, as already mentioned, in many currently used methods for antibody detection and identification and compatibility testing, anti-IgG can be substituted for broad spectrum antiglobulin serum.

Anti-light Chain Specificities in Antiglobulin Serum

When animals are immunized with human IgG most

of the antibodies they produce are directed against the gamma heavy chains of the IgG molecules. The result, as described above, is that the anti-IgG in antiglobulin serum combines with the Fc portion of non-agglutinating antibodies bound to red cells. However, the light chains of antibody molecules are also immunogenic in animals. The result is that sera from immunized animals may contain anti-kappa and anti-lambda in addition to anti-IgG and anti-complement. In most antiglobulin tests the participation of anti-light chain components is minimal and does little more than make figures such as 6-3 somewhat less than the whole story.

When monospecific antiglobulin reagents are considered, the presence of anti-light chain specificities must be taken more seriously (53). For example, an anti-IgG serum that contains anti-kappa may give a positive result when tested against red cells coated with an IgM antibody with light chains of the kappa type. Since the object of the test was to determine if the cells were coated with IgM or IgG it is obvious that a misleading result may be obtained. As has been fully explained in Chapter 2, IgG, IgM and IgA antibodies are found with similar kappa or lambda light chains. When an anti-immunoglobulin (i.e. directed against IgG, IgM or IgA) is being used to determine the immunoglobulin class of an antibody, one known to be heavy chain specific should be used. That designation indicates that only antibodies to the specified heavy chain (gamma, mu or alpha) are present. Many anti-IgG that are not labeled as heavy chain specific, in fact, lack other antibodies (anti-kappa, anti-lambda, etc.). However, those reagents may not have been tested for other specificities, the term heavy chain specific is used when tests have actually demonstrated the absence of other antibodies.

Complement

Complement is a normal constituent of human and animal serum that serves as one of the primary effectors of the immune system. In other words, once antigen-antibody reactions have occurred, the complement system is often mobilized to complete the task of destroying the invading organisms or cells. In what has become a classic definition, Müller-Eberhard (54) has described complement as "a multimolecular, self-assembling biological system that constitutes the primary humoral mediator of antigen-antibody reactions". The classical pathway of complement activation involves participation by eleven proteins each of which has been isolated and characterized (55). Some details about these components are given in table 6-3. The alternative pathway uses some of the same components as the classical pathway and three others that are not directly involved in classical activation

(56). Some details about those components are given in table 6-4. In addition, as described in more detail in a later section, there are a number of important proteins that act as regulators of the complement activation systems (57,58). Since this chapter will deal with complement primarily from the view of its role in immunohematology, readers wishing to learn more about other biological effects of the system are referred to a number of outstanding reviews (59-61). The role of complement in immunohematology has also been the subject of some excellent recent reviews (57,62,63). Again for those readers seeking more information about the biology of complement, the information in tables 6-3 and 6-4 was culled from references 21, 54 and 64-89.

Complement activation is important to the immunohematologist in a number of areas. First, some blood group antibodies activate large amounts of complement and act as hemolysins in vitro and/or in vivo. Second, many others activate complement at a slower rate so that red cells become coated with amounts of C3 that are insufficient to activate the terminal attack sequence (see below) meaning that these antibodies do not act as hemolysins. However, the activation of complement to the C3 stage is itself important in two respects. First, red cells coated with IgG and C3 are usually cleared more efficiently via the extravascular clearance mechanism (again see below) than those coated with IgG alone. Second, in the antiglobulin test, if a reagent containing anti-C3 is used, complement activation to the C3 stage will result in a positive direct or indirect antiglobulin test. As mentioned several times, this latter consideration is somewhat less important now than in the past since many currently used antibody detection and identification methods allow recognition of the antibody via the IgG-anti-IgG reaction of the antiglobulin test. The importance of anti-C3 in reagents used to perform direct antiglobulin tests has not diminished.

Many complement components deteriorate when serum is stored. Garratty (90) showed that around 60% of the starting level of complement in serum is necessary for reliable demonstration of complement activation by an antibody. In sera stored at -55°C or -90°C, more than 90% of the complement was still viable after 3 months of storage. More than 60% of the complement usually remained viable in sera stored for 2 months at -20°C or 2 weeks at 4°C. At higher temperatures complement was far less stable. At room temperature only about 40% of the complement was viable after 48 hours, almost none survived 72 hours storage. At 37°C only 30% was viable after 24 hours. Many anticoagulants act by chelating calcium that is essential for complement activation as well as for coagulation. Thus ACD or CPD plasma or that from samples collected with high levels of heparin, that is also anticomplementary, cannot be used to demon-

TABLE 6-3 Components of the Classical Activation Pathway and Terminal Attack Sequence of Complement

Protein	MW (kD)	Serum Conc µg/ml*1	Chromosome*2	Biological Activity (for interactions see text)
Clq	400	80-250	1*3	Antibody binding
Clr	85	50-100	12*4	Serine protease
Cls	85	50-80	12*4	Serine protease
C4	204	450-600	6*5	Component of C3 convertase
C2	95	20-25	6*5	Component of C3 convertase
C3	195	1300	19	C5 convertase
C5	190	70-85	9	Initiates terminal attack sequence
C6	120	50-65	5*6	Terminal attack
C7	120	50-55	5*6	Terminal attack
C8	150	50-55	1,9*7	Terminal attack
C9	71	50-60	5	Terminal attack

*1 Ranges represent figures given in different publications
*2 Shows chromosome on which encoding genes are carried
*3 A and B chain genes, chromosome 1; C chain gene not assigned
*4 Genes closely linked on chromosome 12
*5 Genes part of major histocompatibility locus on chromosome 6
*6 Genes closely linked on chromosome 5
*7 Alpha and beta chain genes, chromosome 1; gamma chain gene, chromosome 9

strate complement activation. These considerations are important in immunohematology tests designed to detect a C3-anti-C3 reaction in the antiglobulin test.

Terminology for Complement

The proteins involved in the classical activation pathway are described with a capital C followed by the number of the component involved, e.g. C1, C2, C4, etc. This terminology (19) replaces the old system that used C' and subscript numbers, e.g. C'_{14}. An unadorned term, e.g. C4 indicates the native protein, lower case letters, e.g. C4a, C4b, C3c, C3g, etc., indicate activated, functional or cleavage products. For many components the letter a, e.g. C3a indicates a cleaved product that plays no further role in the activation sequence, but often has a biological function. The letter b, e.g. C3b indicates the portion of the molecule that participates in continuation of the activation sequence. C2a and C2b were an exception to this rule in that C2a was used to describe the portion of C2 that complexes with C4b to activate C3. However, recently the C2 terminology has been used differently (92-94) and C2b has been used to describe the portion of C2 that complexes with C4b. This adapted terminology for C2b will be used in this chapter. The enzymatically active forms of complement are written with a bar over the symbol, e.g. $\overline{C4b2b}$.

The proteins associated with the alternative pathway are described with capital letters, e.g. factor B, factor D.

TABLE 6-4 Components of the Alternative Pathway of Complement Activation

Protein	MW (kD)	Serum Conc. µg/ml*1	Chromosome*2	Biological Activity (for interactions see text)
B	93	150-225	6*3	Serine protease
D	25	1-2	not known	Serine protease
P	150	25	X	Stabilizes $\overline{C3bBb}$
C3	195	1300	19	See text

*1 Ranges represent figures given in different publications
*2 Shows chromosome on which encoding genes are carried
*3 Gene part of major histocompatibility locus on chromosome 6

Again split products are designated with lower case letters, e.g. Ba, Bb. Terms for the inhibitors and regulators of complement activation are given in a later section.

The Classical Pathway Activation Sequence

The classical pathway of complement activation can be initiated by Fc pieces of antibody molecules bound to red cells. Two Fc pieces are required to activate the C1q portion of C1. This means that a single IgM molecule (that has five Fc pieces) can begin the sequence but that two IgG molecules (each of which has one Fc piece) working in tandem are required. It has been calculated (95) that in order to have two Fc pieces in close enough proximity for C1q to be bound, red cells must bind in the order of 1000 IgG molecules. Clq is composed of 18 disulphide-linked chains, arranged in six subunits (96,97) and has a MW of 400kD. The globular-like subunits extend from a central unit and are believed to bind to sites in the C_H2 domains of antibody Fc regions. Once bound, C1q undergoes a conformation change to expose a serine enzymatic site. This change results in $\overline{C1q}$ being able to activate the next component of the C1 trimolecular complex, C1r. This protein is a single chain proenzyme and once activated by $\overline{C1q}$ has serine protease activity. In the activation step C1r is cleaved into a heavy chain of 57kD and a light chain of 28kD (89). The esterase activity of the $\overline{C1r}$ light chain then cleaves C1s, activating a light chain serine protease $\overline{C1s}$ (98). Each molecule of $\overline{C1q}$ complexes with two $\overline{C1r}$ and two $\overline{C1s}$ molecules. The entire activated C1 complex is dependent on the presence of available calcium ions for its integrity.

The $\overline{C1qrs}$ complex then activates the next two components of the classical pathway, C4 and C2. The component C4 has a MW of 204kD and comprises three chains alpha, beta and gamma with MW of 93, 78 and 33kD respectively. $\overline{C1s}$ cleaves the alpha chain and releases a small component, C4a, with a MW of 9kD. While it plays no further role in the activation sequence, released C4a is an anaphylatoxin. The larger $\overline{C4b}$ piece of activated C4 is able to bind either to the red cell membrane close to the AgAbC1 site, via ester or amide bonds, or directly to the Fc piece of the antibody molecule that initiated complement activation, via a thioester bond. Bound $\overline{C4b}$ acts to protect $\overline{C1}$ from its inactivators (100). The activation and binding of $\overline{C4b}$ represents one of several amplification steps in the classical activation pathway. Each $\overline{C1s}$ molecule activates many molecules of C4 but not all of them form an active site on the red cell. Once activated at the $\overline{C1s}$ site, $\overline{C4b}$ must bind to the red cell membrane or the antibody Fc piece to form an active site. The decay time of $\overline{C4b}$ is short with the result that many molecules become inactive, i.e. C4bi, before binding to the red cell membrane or to an antibody molecule. Once $\overline{C4b}$ is bound it is able to bind C2 that is in turn cleaved by $\overline{C1s}$; the presence of magnesium ions is necessary for this interaction. C2 is a single chain molecule with a MW of 95kD. When cleaved by $\overline{C1s}$, C2a with a MW of 30kd is released (67), $\overline{C2b}$ remains bound to the $\overline{C4b}$ to form the complex $\overline{C4b2b}$ in which the active enzymatic site on $\overline{C2b}$ activates C3 (101). The $\overline{C4b2b}$ complex is labile, with a half-life of about one minute. Readers confused because what was for years called $\overline{C4b2a}$, is here called $\overline{C4b2b}$ are referred to the earlier section on terminology for complement. The Ch and Rg antigens that are carried on C4 (370-372) are described in Chapter 27.

The component involved next in the activation sequence, C3, is the most important and the most complex of the complement proteins. In its native state C3 is composed of an alpha chain of 120kD and a beta chain of 75kD, the chains are linked by disulphide bonds. C3 is present in serum at a level of about 1300mg/ml, the next most abundant complement protein is C4, present at a level between 450 and 600mg/ml. When C3 is activated by $\overline{C4b2b}$ a 9kD fragment of the alpha chain, C3a, is released. While C3a plays no further role in complement activation it is a powerful and important anaphylatoxin. The larger portion of activated C3, $\overline{C3b}$, continues the activation sequence. One $\overline{C4b2b}$ complex can activate hundreds of molecules of C3, thus providing a major amplification step in the pathway. However, C3b carries an identical active site to that on $\overline{C4b}$, and is highly labile. Activated $\overline{C3b}$ has a life span of approximately 60μ seconds, during which time it can travel some 40 nanameters (102). Thus although hundreds of $\overline{C3b}$ molecules are generated most of them are converted to the inactive form, iC3b, before they are able to bind to activated C4 and C2 to form the complex $\overline{C4b2b3b}$ that continues complement activation by acting as C5 convertase.

These observations explain why so many blood group antibodies activate complement to the C3 stage but do not go on, by activation of the terminal attack sequence, to act as hemolysins. In order for sufficient quantities of C5 convertase to be generated to continue the activation sequence, huge amounts of $\overline{C3b}$ must be generated very rapidly. The role of number of antibody molecules and antigen site density in this consideration are discussed in the section on intravascular red cell destruction. If a blood group antigen-antibody reaction occurs that, in spite of the amplification steps, generates the production of too little $\overline{C3b}$, or generates production of those molecules too slowly, complement activation stops at the $\overline{C3b}$ stage. However, the presence of C3 on the red cells augments their in vivo clearance if they are also coated with IgG (see below) and can be detected in the antiglobulin test.

When C3 is activated and C3a is released, the $\overline{C3b}$ molecule undergoes a rearrangement of shape. Among others things, this results in the exposure of a thioester site in the C3d region of the alpha chain that can effect binding of $\overline{C3b}$ to the red cell membrane (82,103). Red cell membrane bound $\overline{C3b}$ is then subject to additional modifications. Further cleavage of the alpha chain by factor I with factors H and CR1 as cofactors (see below) converts $\overline{C3b}$ to iC3b (see above) by the release of the 3kD fragment, C3f (104). Membrane bound iC3b can then be further degraded, at a different site, by factor I (previously called C3bINA) that releases C3c, a 145kD fragment and leaves C3dg a 41kD protein, membrane bound (105). When C3dg coated red cells are treated with trypsin (or biologically similar enzymes) as was frequently done in the blood bank to prepare red cells for the evaluation of anti-C3-containing antiglobulin reagents (106-111) C3g is removed and the 30kD C3d fragment remains membrane bound. In contrast, the red cells of patients with cold hemagglutinin disease, that were also used in such studies when available, are coated with C3dg. Presumably in the in vitro method of preparing C3d-coated red cells using long-term incubation with human serum rather than trypsin (52), C3dg was left intact.

As already mentioned, if sufficient amounts of C5 convertase are generated during the classical pathway of complement activation, the terminal attack sequence (C5-C9) is mobilized and red cell hemolysis (or lysis of invading bacteria, etc.) results. However, before describing the terminal attack sequence, it is convenient next to consider the alternative pathway of complement activation that begins at the C3 activation stage and, therefore, interacts with the classical pathway.

The Alternative Pathway of Complement Activation

Between 1954 and 1959, a number of reports by Pillemer and his associates were published (112-115) that purported to show that complement can sometimes be activated in situations in which no antigen-antibody reaction has taken place. Since a naturally-occurring serum protein, that was named properdin, seemed to be involved in an interaction with the substance initiating complement activation, the pathway became known as the properdin system. In retrospect it does not seem surprising that complement can be activated other than following an antigen-antibody reaction. Activated complement components play a number of important biological roles in host defense. Thus, again in retrospect, one might expect that complement activation would some-

times be required when no antibody against a foreign antigen is present. In spite of this, as knowledge about the classical pathway of complement activation and its initiation by antigen-antibody complexes accumulated, the concept of non-antibody-induced complement activation was disputed (116). More recently it has been shown (56,77,117-129) that C3 can indeed be activated in a pathway that does not use C1, C4 or C2. It has become apparent that the old properdin system has been rediscovered. Ironically, it is now known that properdin itself plays a relatively minor role as a stabilizing protein and the system is now called the alternative pathway of complement activation.

In the pathway, any one of a wide variety of substances can initiate complement activation. The list of activators includes but is by no means limited to, aggregates of IgA, and perhaps of IgG, bacterial and fungal membrane polysaccharides, bacterial endotoxins, cobra venom and some assorted substances such as inulin and trypsin. In the initial phase of the reaction there is autoactivation of the thioester bond of C3 to form $\overline{C3b}$. These activated $\overline{C3b}$ molecules (see section below on regulators and inhibitors of complement activation) are unstable in plasma but are able to bind to one of the activators of the alternative pathway, as listed above. The activated $\overline{C3b}$ complexes with factor B of the alternative pathway. Factor B, a 93kD protein is then cleaved by factor D of the alternative pathway, a 25kD serine protease. Cleavage of factor B in the $\overline{C3bB}$ complex results in the release of Ba a 30kD fragment that is a chemotactic agent. The larger portion of factor B, Bb, a 63kD serine protease, remains bound to C3 in the complex $\overline{C3bBb}$. This molecule has the same activity as $\overline{C4b2b}$ of the classical pathway. Thus additional molecules of C3 are activated in a positive feed back mechanism. As can be seen, once C3 is activated in the classical or the alternative pathway, the two pathways work in conjunction in the activation of additional C3 molecules. The role of properdin, factor P of the alternative pathway, a three subunit protein with a MW of around 150kD, is to bind to the C3 convertase that has been generated, to form the complex $\overline{C3bBbP}$. The binding of factor P in this manner, stabilizes the complex but $\overline{C3bBb}$ is still able to act as a C3 convertase in the absence of bound factor P.

Importance of the Alternative Pathway

As mentioned above, C3 is converted to $\overline{C3b}$ under normal physiological conditions. Both water molecules and proteolytic enzymes in plasma can activate the C3 thioester bond to generate activated $\overline{C3b}$. This means essentially that the alternative pathway is always "switched on" albeit slowly and at a low level of activation. When no external activator is present, as in normal healthy individuals, the activated $\overline{C3b}$ is rapidly converted to iC3b by factors H and I (see below). When an external activator, such as polysaccharide structures on the membranes of invading bacteria, is introduced, as in a bacterial infection, the already mobilized alternative pathway is amplified, as described in the previous section, with the result that an instant defense mechanism is generated. Clearly, even in the absence of antibody against the invading bacteria, activated components of the complement system can be deposited on the bacteria. If sufficient $\overline{C3bBbP}$ becomes attached to the organisms, C5 can be activated and the terminal attack sequence can be mobilized to destroy the bacteria. Because the alternative pathway is always activated, control mechanisms (described below) are required to prevent harmful levels of complement activation and autolysis under normal physiological conditions.

The Terminal Attack Sequence of Complement Activation

If sufficient quantities of $\overline{C4b2b3b}$ are generated in the classical pathway, or $\overline{C3bBbP}$ in the alternative pathway, that they are able to act before significant inactivation occurs, the terminal attack sequence (also known as the membrane attack complex or MAC) is mobilized, Both $\overline{C4b2b3b}$ and $\overline{C3bBbP}$ act as a C5 convertase enzyme. C5, a 190kD, two chain protein is cleaved and C5a, an 11kD anaphylatoxin, is released. The larger portion of activated C5, $\overline{C5b}$, binds to the membrane. The activation of C5 is the last enzymatic step in the complement activation sequence. Once attached to the membrane, $\overline{C5b}$ is able to bind C6 and C7, both single chain proteins of 120kD (78,79). When bound, C6 and C7 expose hydrophobic groups and the trimolecular complex C5b67 is inserted into the phospholipid bilayer that is the red cell membrane (79). C8, a three chain, 150kD protein then binds to the C5b67 complex and is also partially inserted into the membrane (80). Once assembled in the membrane the C5b678 complex effects the binding of C9 molecules (81). The C9 component is single chain protein unit with a molecular weight of 71kD. Each C5b678 complex is able to bind multiple C9 molecules (as many as 16) and the resultant structures are in fact pores or holes (130) in the membrane that allow water and solutes to enter or leave the red cell (131). Both sodium ions and water enter the cell in excess amounts and hemolysis results. Figure 6-4 is a schematic diagram to depict the classical and alternative pathways of complement activation, the interaction between the two, the positive feedback mechanism of the alternative pathway and the terminal attack sequence.

Regulators of Complement Activation

Because the complement activation systems are so important in host defense mechanisms, a certain degree of complement activation occurs at all times. In order to prevent the activated complement from causing destruction of autologous (red and other) cells, a counter system, to the activation mechanisms, exists. This comprises a series of fluid phase and cell-bound proteins that serve to regulate the level of autologous complement activation. Some details about the regulatory proteins are given in table 6-5.

C1-INH is a 110kD single chain glycoprotein that is a serine protease inhibitor. It can bind weakly to $\overline{C1r}$ in the $\overline{C1q1r_21s_2}$ complex but has a greater inhibitory effect on activated $\overline{C1}$ by binding to and inhibiting the active enzyme sites of $\overline{C1r}$ and $\overline{C1s}$ (58,70-72,132-134).

C4bp (C4-binding protein) is a 500kD protein that has two regulatory effects on C4 when that molecule is part of the C3-convertase enzyme. First, C4bp increases the rate of dissociation of the $\overline{C4b2b}$ complex. Second, in the presence of C4bp, $\overline{C4b}$ is subject to proteolysis by factor I (see below) that was originally called (58,128,135-138) C3b-inhibitor, or C3b-INA and acts similarly on $\overline{C4b}$ and $\overline{C3b}$.

Factor H is a 150kD protein that also has several regulatory functions. In the classical activation pathway factor H accelerates the rate of dissociation of $\overline{C4b2b}$ thus allowing increased proteolytic cleavage of $\overline{C4b}$ by factor I. In the alternative pathway, factor H competes with factor B for the active binding site on $\overline{C3b}$. Since $\overline{C3bBb}$ is the major activating enzyme for C3 in the alternative pathway, it follows that successful competition by factor H, in forming the complex C3bH, will reduce the number of $\overline{C3bBb}$ complexes and thus reduce the rate at which newly activated $\overline{C3b}$ is generated (139-140).

Factor I is a two chain 80kD protein that can cleave both $\overline{C4b}$ and $\overline{C3b}$ in the presence of cofactor H. Originally called C3b-INA or beta-1-H protein (105,128,135-138), this enzyme has long been recognized as an important regulatory protein. It cleaves C3f from the alpha chain of $\overline{C3b}$ and thus creates iC3b (104). Factor I can then further cleave iC3b to release C3c and leave C3dg membrane-bound. Clearly, since factor I acts directly on C3 and thus regulates the level of that component that remains in the activated form, it is important in regulation of both the classical and alternative activation pathways (141,142). The importance of the release of C3c is discussed again in the sections on extravascular destruction of complement coated red cells and the use of anti-C3 in antiglobulin tests.

Protein S or vitronectin is an 83kD component that is present in high levels, circa 500mg/ml in serum. In its regulatory role, it binds fluid phase C5b-C7 (57,78).

FIGURE 6-4 Complement Activation

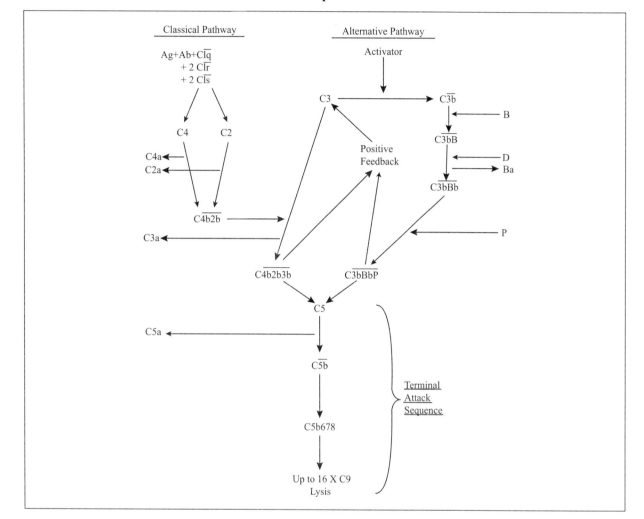

Protein S has also been shown (143) to augment the functional activity of monocyte receptors for IgG and C3.

In addition to the circulating plasma proteins described above, there are a number of cell-bound molecules that serve to regulate complement activation. Many of these are attached to red cells via a phosphatidylinositol (PI) anchor. In paroxysmal nocturnal hemoglobinuria (PNH) the PI anchor is defective and lack of some of the regulatory proteins results in the greatly increased susceptibility of PNH cells to complement-induced lysis (144-151). Red cell hemolysis in PNH sometimes occurs following normal autoactivation of the alternative pathway and lack of regulation of the components activated.

The glycoprotein CD55 or decay accelerating factor (DAF) is PI-linked to red cells and has a MW of 70kD. Its regulatory function is to inhibit formation and accelerate decay of both C3 and C5 convertases so that it is regulatory in both the classical and alternative pathways (152-154). Although PNH red cells are deficient in DAF, absence of that protein does not seem to represent a major defect leading to their sensitivity to activated complement. Red cells of the Inab phenotype of the Cromer blood group system are totally devoid of DAF. However, they display only a limited increase in sensitivity to complement-induced lysis. Indeed, the alteration in sensitivity cannot be detected by some test methods (155-157). The antigens of the Cromer blood group system, all of which reside on DAF (158-160) are described in Chapter 24.

Membrane cofactor protein (MCP) or CD46 has a MW of 53 to 66kD and is structurally similar to DAF. However, unlike DAF, MCP does not accelerate the decay of C3 and C5 convertases. Instead it serves as a cofactor for factor I cleavage of $C\overline{3b}$ and to a lesser degree $C\overline{4b}$ (161,162).

The protein CD59 that is also known as protectin, homologous restriction factor 20 (HCF20), P18, MAC-inhibitory factor (MACIF) and membrane inhibitor of reactive lysis (MIRL) serves to regulate the terminal attack sequence. This 18-20kD protein apparently binds

TABLE 6-5 Regulators of Complement Activation

Protein	MW (kD)	Serum Conc. µg/ml*1	Chromosome*2	Biological Activity (for interactions see text)
C1-INH	110	180-200	11	Serine protease inhibitor
C4bp	500	250	1*3	Accelerates decay of C$\overline{4b2b}$ and acts as cofactor for factor I
H	150	450-500	1*3	Accelerates decay of C$\overline{4b2b}$ and C$\overline{3bBb}$
I	80	35	4	Cleaves C3b at two different sites
S	83	500-600	not known	Binds fluid phase C5b-7
Sp-40,40	75	50	not known	Binds fluid phase C5b-7
CR1	160-250	cell bound	1*3	Binds C3b and allows factor I to act. See also Table 6-6
DAF	70	cell bound	1*3	Accelerates decay of C3 and C5
MCP	53-66	cell bound	1*3	Cofactor for factor I cleavage of C3, C4 and perhaps C5
MIRL	20	cell bound	11	Binds to C5b-6 and C8, inhibits terminal attack sequence
C8bp	65	cell bound	not known	Binds to C8, inhibits terminal attack sequence

For possible role of glycophorin A, see text.
*1 Ranges represent figures given in different publications
*2 Shows chromosome on which encoding genes are carried
*3 In regulators of complement activation (RCA) cluster on chromosome 1

to C5b-6 and thus inhibits the binding of C7 and C8 (57,58,148,157,163) or binds to C8 and prevents the insertion of C9 (164,165,170).

A protein known variously as C8-binding protein (C8bp), homologous restriction factor (HRF) and MAC inhibitory protein (MIP) also serves to regulate the terminal attack sequence. This 65kD protein binds C8 and this inhibits the interaction of C8 (and eventually C9) with C5b67 (166-169).

It is currently believed that it is lack of the PI-linked regulatory proteins that control the terminal attack sequence of complement, that results in the extreme sensitivity of PNH III red cells to complement-induced hemolysis.

It has been claimed (171-174) that glycophorin A is a complement regulatory protein. Under certain conditions glycophorin A will apparently bind C3 (171,172). In other reports (173,174) the glycoprotein was said to inhibit lysis by blocking the formation of C5b-7. Indeed, in one report (174) glycophorin A was called membrane inhibitor of reactive lysis, type II. (MIRL II). Glycophorin A is not PI-linked, instead it is an integral membrane protein with extracellular, transmembrane and cytoplasmic domains (175,176), the last of those regions probably being attached to the cytoskeleton of the red cell via protein 4.1 (177). It seems that if glycophorin A is a complement regulatory protein, its function can be performed by other components in its

absence. As far as we are aware, no increased susceptibility to complement-induced lysis has been noted with En(a-) or S- s- U- red cells, or those from M^k homozygotes, that lack glycophorin A, glycophorin B and both glycophorins, respectively. Thus if glycophorin A is involved in complement regulation its role may be no greater than that of DAF, as already mentioned the absence of DAF in the Inab phenotype does not substantially increase the sensitivity of the red cells to complement-induced lysis (155-157). Glycophorin A is present on red cells in very large amounts, i.e. 1×10^6 copies per red cell. Thus another possibility seems to be that an otherwise unrecognized complement regulatory protein may be co-precipitated with glycophorin A and then not recognized in the abundance of glycophorin A obtained. As readers will know, glycophorin A carries MN system antigens, accordingly its structure is discussed in detail in Chapter 15.

Complement Receptors

Many different cells carry receptors for the cleaved and activated complement components, some details are given in table 6-6, additional information will be found in references 57, 63, 101 and 178 to 181.

Complement receptor 1 (CR1, CD35) that is also known as the immune adherence or C3b/C4b receptor, is a glycoprotein that binds both $\overline{C3b}$ and C3 but has a 1000-fold higher affinity for the former than for latter. Thus the uptake of $\overline{C3b}$ by CR1, in the presence of a second signal that is usually IgG, may promote phagocytosis (182). CR1 is also involved in the breakdown of C3. Once $\overline{C3b}$ is bound to CR1 it is subject to the actions of factor I, that are described above, and is converted to iC3b (183). CR1 also participates in the clearance of immune complexes from the circulation. $\overline{C3b}$ binds to immune complexes and is then protected from cleavage

TABLE 6-6 Complement Receptors

Receptor	MW (kD)	Present on
Clq	65	Platelets, monocytes, macrophages, B-cells, endothelial cells
C3a	not known	Mast cells, monocytes, macrophages, neutrophils, basophils, T-cells, platelets
C5a	45	Mast cells, monocytes, macrophages, neutrophils
CR1	160-250	Red cells, monocytes, neutrophils, B-cells
CR2	140	B-cells, epithelial cells
CR3	245	Monocytes, macrophages, neutrophils, natural killer cells, epithelial cells
CR4	245	Monocytes, macrophages, neutrophils, natural killer cells

by factors H and I (again see above). The unaltered $\overline{C3b}$ attached to the immune complexes is then bound by red cell surface CR1 molecules and those red cells are recognized by tissue-bound macrophages, predominantly those in the liver (184-187). See also the section below, on extravascular destruction of red cells coated with IgG and C3. The role of CR1 as the site of the Knops system antigens Kn[a], Kn[b], McC[a], Sl[a] and Yk[a] (188,189) is described in Chapter 28.

Complement receptor 2 (CR2, CD21) is a 140kD glycoprotein that binds C3dg and C3d, after C3g has been cleaved. Presumably with such binding capabilities it plays no role in the immune destruction of red cells. On B-cells, CR2 is the binding site of Epstein-Barr virus (190).

Complement receptor 3 (CR3, CD18) is a two chain molecule of about 245kD. It is found on phagocytic and some other cells (see table 6-6) and is the receptor for iC3b. Like CR1, CR3 requires a second signal (e.g. IgG) in order to bind iC3b-coated red cells. CR3 on leukocytes is involved in antibody-dependent cell cytotoxicity (ADCC) and natural killer (NK) cell cytotoxicity. The protein is a member of the integrin family of adhesion

proteins (179,181,191).

Complement receptor 4 (CR4) is also a two chain, 245kD molecule. It is closely related to CR3 and binds iC3b and, with much lower affinity, C3dg. CR4 is the predominant complement receptor expressed by macrophages (191).

As can be seen from table 6-6, of the four complement receptors just discussed, only CR1 is present on red cells. All CR play important roles in the immune response, phagocytosis and the inflammatory response, clearly only brief mention of some of those functions has been made above. In terms of red cell clearance, those CR that bind to C3b and iC3b are important in vivo. For example, in cold hemagglutinin disease, the patient's red cells may be coated with as many as 20,000 C3dg molecules per cell but are not cleared by macrophages (192,193). For additional details about the other important biological roles of the CR molecules readers are again referred to references 57, 63, 101, 178-182 and 191.

As will be apparent by now, many of the proteins discussed in the last several sections are known by more than one name. Table 6-7 is an attempt to list the various synonyms used.

Variation in Ability of Blood Group Antibodies to Initiate Complement Activation via the Classical Pathway

If given the opportunity, many blood group antibodies will activate complement once they have bound to red cells. As explained above, most with that ability cause activation to the C3 stage, only a few activate enough C3 and at a sufficient rate, for the terminal attack sequence to be mobilized. The dogma regarding complement activation is that IgM antibodies are more efficient in this respect than are those made of IgG. The explanation, of course, is that each pentameric IgM molecule has five Fc pieces, two of which are required for activation of C1q (see above) while each IgG molecule has only one Fc region. Indeed, it has been shown (194-196) that a single IgM molecule can initiate complement activation. For an IgG antibody to bind C1q, two different molecules must work in tandem. This in turn means that they must bind to antigens in close proximity, complement activation by IgG is most efficient when two antibody molecules bind to epitopes on the same antigen (197). The requirement for two IgG Fc pieces for activation of C1q also means that complement activation will be more likely if there are large numbers of antigen sites on the red cell membrane and/or if they are situated in clusters, than if there is a paucity of antigen sites that are spread out on the membrane. While the dogma regarding IgM, IgG and

TABLE 6-7 Some Names used for Complement Proteins, Regulators and Receptors

In this Chapter	Synonyms
C$\overline{4b2b}$	C$\overline{4b2a}$ (older literature), C3 convertase of classical pathway
C$\overline{3bBb}$	C3 convertase of alternative pathway, C5 convertase
C$\overline{3bBbP}$	Stabilized C3 convertase of alternative pathway, C5 convertase
C$\overline{4b2b3b}$	C5 convertase of classical pathway
P	Properdin
Terminal attack sequence	Membrane attack complex or MAC
I	C3b-INA, C3-inhibitor, beta-1-H protein
Protein S	Vitronectin
DAF	CD55, Decay accelerating factor
MCP	CD46, Membrance cofactor protein
MIRL	CD59, Membrane inhibitor of reactive lysis, Protectin, P18, Homologous restriction factor 20 (HRF20), Membrane attack complex inhibitory factor (MACIF)
C8bp	MAC-inhibitory protein (MIP), Homologous restriction factor (HCF)
CR1	CD35
CR2	CD21
CR3	CD11b, CD18
CR4	CD11c, CD18
CR5	Not yet fully characterized. Believed to be on neutrophils and platelets

complement is quite true when blood group antibodies are tested in vitro, many blood bankers overlook the fact that IgM blood group antibodies seldom get the chance to behave similarly in vivo. This is because many IgM blood group antibodies are cold-reactive and simply do not bind to red cells in vivo. Obviously, if an IgM antibody can bind to red cells only at temperatures below, say 22 to 24°C, it may activate complement in room temperature tests in vitro, but will not bind to even antigen-positive red cells in vivo, so will not initiate complement binding. If in vitro tests are performed at or near 37°C (room temperature should be abandoned, see Chapter 35) it will be found that complement activation by blood group antibodies is associated with IgG molecules far more often than with those that are IgM.

A major consideration regarding complement activation by IgG antibodies involves subclass composition of the antibody. In activating complement, IgG3 is the most efficient, IgG1 efficient, IgG2 less efficient while IgG4 may not activate complement at all (198-200). However, for blood group antibodies this consideration applies with relative infrequence since most such antibodies are IgG3 or IgG1, or a mixture of those two subclasses (37-42,44,45,47,48,201,202).

As readers will know, some examples of antibodies in the Kell, Kidd, Duffy, etc., blood group systems, activate complement. In marked contrast, only very rare examples of Rh antibodies have that ability (203-205) in spite of the fact that most of them are made of IgG1 and/or IgG3 (35,202,206-209). For many years it was believed that these apparently divergent findings could be explained by the paucity of Rh antigens on the red cell membrane. It was assumed that even when large numbers of IgG Rh antibody molecules had bound to each red cell, the location of the antigens was such that no two antibody Fc pieces were close enough together for binding of C1q to occur (210). Experiments performed by Rosse (211) appeared at first to support such a concept. It was shown that when cDe red cells were coated with anti-D, no complement activation occurred. However, when the same cells were coated with anti-D, anti-c and anti-e, a limited amount of C1q binding (as demonstrated by the C1q transfer test) did seem to take place. It was assumed that Fc pieces from some molecules bound to D sites, some bound to c sites and some bound to e sites, were in close enough proximity to enable C1q to be bound. However, other workers were unable, at first, to duplicate these findings. Further, Freedman et al. (212) convincingly demonstrated that the uptake of complement by cDE/cDE red cells exposed to anti-c, anti-D and anti-E was not Rh antibody-mediated. Indeed, when the same three antibodies were incubated with cde/cde red cells, the same degree of complement activation apparently occurred (incubation of the cde/cde cells with anti-c alone did not result in any measurable complement activation). Thus it seems that the combined effects of potent Rh antibodies in causing small amounts of complement to be activated may not be antigen-antibody reaction-mediated. Perhaps, in such mixtures, there are enough aggregates of IgG present that complement activation begins without antibody binding specifically to antigen. Most recently the original observation of Rosse (211) appears to have been confirmed. Hughes-Jones and Ghosh (213) showed that if sufficient quantities of IgG anti-D are bound per red cell, C1q can be shown also to have been bound. However, when purified C1 is added to the test, C1r and C1s are not cleaved (214). Mollison et al. (215) suggest that the difference between IgG anti-K and IgG anti-D, in terms of complement activation, may relate to the fact that more than one anti-K molecule can bind to the K antigen whereas the D antigen site may be so small (216) that only a single molecule of anti-D can bind. In the study of Freedman et al. (212) it was found that complement was not activated when anti-D was allowed to bind to D--/D-- red cells. As far as we are aware, there have been no further studies on an observation made by Hidalgo et al. (236). Those workers reported that some Rh antibodies would activate complement when allowed to bind to red cell ghosts. Complement activation was said to occur only when very potent antibodies were used and was enhanced by papain-treatment of the ghosts, and use of red cells carrying a double dose of antigen against which the antibody was directed.

Another argument against the concept that IgG1 and IgG3 Rh antibodies fail to bind complement because the antigens with which they complex are widely separated on the red cell membrane, was advanced from experimental evidence (217-221) that suggested that after Rh antigens have complexed with their antibodies, they are capable of lateral movement through the red cell membrane and are thus able to cluster. If this was so, it followed that the Fc pieces of different IgG molecules should be close enough to initiate complement activation. It should be added that although the experimental evidence seemed to indicate the mobility of Rh antigens through the plane of the red cell membrane, Masouredis (221) was careful to point out that unusual experimental conditions were being used. He cautioned that perhaps in intact red cells, where different conditions prevail, antigen movement might not occur. That caution now seems to have been well justified for additional studies (222-225) have suggested that in intact red cells from adults, the complexing of antigen with antibody does not result in antigen movement and clustering.

Rosenfield (226) has offered a different explanation as to why Rh antibodies do not activate complement. He has suggested that Rh antigens protrude far enough above the red cell membrane that, even if C1 activation occurs at the Rh-anti-Rh antigen-antibody complexing site, the complement activation sequence cannot continue. It is known that once activated, some C4 and C2 molecules bind directly to membrane surfaces. It is also known that these components, once activated, decay quickly if they do not bind to a membrane (54). Rosenfield suggests that the distance between the C4 activation site ($\overline{C1}$) and the red cell membrane, is too great for activated C4 to reach the membrane before decay occurs. In support of this contention Rosenfield cites the observations of Douglas (227) and of Davis et al. (228), who believe that the distance of ferritin-labeled, red cell-bound, IgG anti-Rh, from the visualized lipid surface is in excess of 10 nanameters. Similarly, the observations of Sela (229) and of Rimon and Sela (230) suggest that when antibodies complex with antigens carried on long chains agglutination is enhanced, but that immune lysis occurs only when antibodies complex with antigens borne on short chains. Recent data (231-235) that seem to indicate that most Rh antigens are embedded in or located very close to the red cell membrane, tend to make this theory less tenable than was previously the case.

One of us (PDI) who has neither the benefit of supportive evidence, nor the ability to perform experiments that would test the hypothesis, has often wondered if yet a different explanation applies. It is believed that when IgG antibody molecules complex with their antigen, the molecules undergo a change in shape. Perhaps when anti-Fy^a or anti-Jk^a complex with Fy(a+) or Jk(a+) red cells, the shape change of the antibody molecule is such that the complement activation sites in the C_H2 domains are exposed. Perhaps the shape of the Rh antigen is such that when Rh antibodies bind to red cells they are simply unable to undergo the required shape change that results in exposure of the complement activation site. Although this last idea seems theoretically plausible it is not yet supported by experiment evidence. It would also have to contend with the fact that in IgM molecules the complement activation site is in the C_H3 region (215).

Finally, in discussing the failure of the overwhelming majority of IgG1 and IgG3 Rh antibodies to activate complement, it should be pointed out that IgM Rh antibodies also lack that ability. Although this is an established fact (215) it throws no light on the problem of explaining lack of complement activation by Rh antibodies. Paucity of Rh antigens on the red cell membrane, failure of the antibody to attach two Fab pieces to epitopes on the same antigen, distance of the antigens from the membrane surface, or shape of the antigens in preventing a required configurational change in a bound antibody molecule, would all equally well explain the lack of complement activation by IgM and IgG Rh antibodies.

The finding that some examples of IgG antibodies directed against the antigens K, S, Fy^a, and Fy^b and many IgG antibodies directed against the antigens Jk^a and Jk^b fix complement, adds further complexity to the situation. There is little doubt (237-249) that there are fewer of these antigens on red cells than there are Rh antigens. It is sometimes assumed that these observations simply mean that Duffy, Kidd and other antigen sites occur in clusters on the red cell membrane, while Rh antigen sites are randomly distributed. However, as far as these authors are aware, there is no good supportive evidence for this assumption. It is, of course, possible that these antigens are sterically arranged or large enough, such that more than one IgG molecule can bind, via different epitopes, to the same antigen.

The concept that antibodies that complex with antigens some distance from the red cell membrane are relatively inefficient in causing activated complement to become bound to the red cell membrane, may, at first, sound like a contradiction. This, because anti-A and anti-B often act as hemolysins although the A and B immunodominant sugars are thought of as being situated at the end of long glycosphingolipid chains extending from the membrane. However, Rosenfield (226) makes a number of pertinent statements. First, in view of the number of A and B antigens on red cells, anti-A and anti-B might be regarded as relatively inefficient hemolysins. Perhaps IgM anti-A and anti-B molecules, because of their size, cannot get close to the red cell membrane. Perhaps these antibodies act as agglutinins by complexing with A and B antigens carried on long glycosphingolipids and thus distal to the membrane. Some A and B antigens are known (250) to be carried on short chains. Perhaps the smaller IgG anti-A and anti-B molecules are able to approach these antigens and perhaps it is those molecules that activate complement and cause hemolysis. In support of this concept Rosenfield (226) points out that the most efficient blood group hemolysin known is the auto-anti-P that causes PCH (251-254). This autoantibody is IgG in nature and reacts with globoside that cannot extend more than 2.5 nanameters from the red cell membrane (255-260). The shortest ABH glycosphingolipid is a little longer than globoside (226). It is also known (256,733) that globoside is the most abundant red cell lipid and it has been estimated (734) that each red cell carries in the order of 14×10^6 copies of the P antigen.

In Vitro Hemolysins

One of the most fascinating aspects in the consideration of the actions of the components of complement is the speed with which they act. As can be seen, the description of the actions of the complement components from E+A+C1q through C9 (where E = erythrocyte and A = antibody) is of necessity long because of the nature of the interactions. In the blood bank, most workers have seen the speed with which group O sera from some patients can bring about total lysis of A and B cells. No matter how quickly this occurs in vitro (and in vivo if the wrong ABO group blood is transfused) all the steps described above, starting with the combination of the cells with the anti-A,B and proceeding through the C142356789 sequence have occurred. Anti-A and anti-B are the most commonly encountered in vitro hemolysins. If ABO reverse typing tests are performed with A_1 and B red cells suspended in saline, many group O sera will act as hemolysins. Because hemolysis is sometimes not as readily recognized as a positive test as strong agglutination, some manufacturers add EDTA to the suspending media in the preparation of red cells for ABO serum

grouping. As mentioned above, EDTA chelates calcium ions so that in its presence the trimolecular $\overline{C1}qrs$ complex does not form and complement activation does not proceed beyond the $\overline{C1q}$ stage. Sera that contain potent ABO system hemolysins will agglutinate but not hemolyze red cells in the presence of EDTA. The concept of "dangerous" group O donors, i.e. those with high titered anti-A,B hemolysins present, is discussed in Chapter 8.

In vitro alloimmune hemolysins with specificities outside the ABO system are rare. Anti-P+P$_1$+P^k (a.k.a. anti-Tj^a, see Chapter 11) and anti-Vel (see Chapter 31) sometimes act as hemolysins in vitro and in vivo. Anti-Le^a, for reasons discussed in Chapter 9, sometimes acts as a hemolysin in vitro but seldom behaves similarly in vivo.

Complement in the Antiglobulin Test

Before the introduction of some now routinely used tests, such as those using LISS, Polybrene, PEG, etc., the detection of activated complement via the indirect antiglobulin test (IAT) was important. Two major considerations applied. First, some IgM antibodies activated complement but were otherwise difficult to detect if they did not act as direct agglutinins. Second, a few IgG antibodies (notably some in the Kidd system) bound to red cells and activated complement, but were difficult to detect via the IgG-anti-IgG portion of the IAT. Because, as described, the classical pathway of complement activation involves several amplification steps, presence of these antibodies was easier to demonstrate via the C3-anti-C3 portion of the test (21,51,261-276). In one of the cases reported (270) a patient suffered a number of transfusion reactions when given blood that appeared compatible in tests using commercially prepared antiglobulin reagents. No antibody could be detected. When compatibility tests were performed using a potent home made anti-C3, non-reactive units could be transfused with no untoward effects, however, the specificity of the antibody activating the C3 was never established. In titration studies on 140 IgG complement binding antibodies it was shown (272) that 90 of them gave stronger reactions when the IATs were read with an antiglobulin reagent containing anti-IgG and anti-C3 than when read with an anti-IgG of comparable strength to that in the broad spectrum reagent. Thus while rare, some IgG antibodies detected only via the C3-anti-C3 reaction of the IAT were clinically important.

As mentioned earlier, use of different in vitro methods has greatly reduced, or perhaps even eliminated, the chance that an antibody of this type will be missed in an IAT if a reagent containing anti-C3 is not used. As mentioned in Chapter 3, one of us (PDI) has noticed that some antibodies that act as agglutinins at 37°C and which we presume include some that are IgM, are detected in our PEG method although those tests are not read following 37°C incubation, before being washed for the IAT. It appears that once the agglutination has taken place in PEG, it survives washing and is still present when the IATs are read with anti-IgG. With some of these antibodies we have shown that agglutination is still seen if saline instead of anti-IgG is added before the tests are read. For those IgG antibodies previously detected via the C3-anti-C3 reaction, it seems that the IgG bound in the newer test methods can be detected with anti-IgG. However, it should be remembered that this conclusion is based on assumption, not fact. We are not aware of any study that has taken known examples of IgG antibodies detectable only via the C3-anti-C3 reaction in a test at normal ionic strength and tested them via LISS, Polybrene or PEG methods using anti-IgG (but see the addedum).

The points made above, that suggest that the presence of anti-C3 in antiglobulin reagents is not as important as was the case in the fairly recent past, apply to indirect antiglobulin tests. There is no doubt that for direct antiglobulin tests, anti-C3 is still necessary (see below).

Necessary Components of Antiglobulin Serum, Part II, Anti-Complement

Over the years there has been considerable disagreement as to which antibodies to complement components are necessary in broad spectrum antiglobulin reagents, or indeed whether any are necessary at all. Rather than repeat the entire history of this disagreement and reasons used to support various points of view, condensed considerations of the more critical points are provided below. In many discussions of this topic, the term "false positive" is used. In fact, many times the positive reactions represent the detection of low levels of C3 and C4 on red cells by anti-C3 and anti-C4, respectively. While these reactions are unwanted and clinically irrelevant, they are not "false positives" since they represent specific antigen-antibody (C3-anti-C3, etc.) reactions. In the statements below, the term unwanted positive is used for these reactions.

1. All normal red cells carry low levels of C3 and C4 that gradually increase during in vitro storage of the cells (277-287). Thus antiglobulin reagents with unacceptably high levels of anti-C3 and/or anti-C4 will give unwanted positive reactions.
2. Since no case is known in which the presence of red cell bound C4, in the absence of C3, was clinically relevant (273), there is no need to have anti-

C4 in reagents that contain appropriate levels of anti-C3.
3. Anti-C4, if present, is more likely than anti-C3 to given unwanted positive reactions, as in 1 above (288).
4. In striving to achieve adequate levels of anti-C3, using polyclonal rabbit (or goat) antibodies, some manufacturers produced antiglobulin reagents that contained reactive levels of other unwanted antibodies (anti-species, anti-A, anti-B, etc.)(52,271,289). This phenomenon was often blamed on "too much anti-complement" but in fact represented the presence of contaminating antibodies.
5. Almost all workers used the same polyspecific antiglobulin reagent for direct and indirect antiglobulin tests. Since there is no doubt (see below) that anti-C3 is essential when DATs are performed, presence of that antibody was required.

Now that the activation and binding of C3 to red cells is better understood it is easier to consider which anti-C3 specificities are required in antiglobulin reagents. As described in the sections above dealing with complement activation and the regulation thereof, when native C3 is activated by $\overline{C4b2b}$ or $\overline{C3bBb}$, C3a is cleaved and $\overline{C3b}$ binds to the membrane. Bound $\overline{C3b}$ can be detected by anti-C3c or anti-C3d since epitopes on both those fragments are exposed on $\overline{C3b}$. However, the conversion of $\overline{C3b}$ to iC3b by the actions of factors I and H in the fluid phase, or I and CR1 on the membrane, exposes another antigen, this one on C3g. The conversion of C3 to iC3b is so rapid, that anti-C3g will also agglutinate $\overline{C3b}$ coated red cells (7,290). The conversion of $\overline{C3b}$ to iC3b does not prevent agglutination of the coated cells by anti-C3c or anti-C3d. The next regulatory step involving bound iC3b involves factor I-mediated cleavage of that molecule, C3c is released meaning that the red cells will now be agglutinated by anti-C3d and anti-C3g but not by anti-C3c. The release of C3c is time dependent and in most indirect antiglobulin tests, some C3c molecules will still be bound when the tests are read (10). However, if longer than normal incubation times are used (293), or if weak antibodies have caused the uptake of only low levels of $\overline{C3b}$, anti-C3c may give a negative reaction although the red cells are C3-coated, i.e. C3d and C3g still present (8,10,291,292). While anti-C3c is less prone to unwanted positive reactions caused by the small amounts of C3 on normal red cells, i.e. present predominantly in the form of C3d, its use in a broad spectrum (or anti-C3) reagent must be bolstered by the presence of anti-C3d or anti-C3g for the reasons just given (10). Since C3d accumulates on red cells stored at 4°C or incubated in fresh serum, more rapidly than C3g, the ideal partner for anti-C3c in an antiglobulin reagent would be anti-C3g. However, if a suitably potent anti-C3g is not available, anti-C3d must be used. Although antibodies to C3c , C3d and C3g can now be blended at optimal concentrations, a few unwanted positives (i.e. higher than usual levels of C3 bound) are still seen. There is one monoclonal with anti-C3d that can be blended with anti-IgG to make a satisfactory broad spectrum reagent without the use of anti-C3c (9). There are now also a variety of methods that can be used to measure the amount of the various anti-C3 specificities in antiglobulin reagents and to determine their epitope specificities (110,294-299).

There has never been any dispute about the need for anti-C3 in reagents to be used to perform direct antiglobulin tests. The almost universal practice is first to test the red cells with a polyspecific reagent containing anti-IgG and anti-C3. If this test is negative, further testing is not performed unless there are unusual clinical findings. If the test with the broad spectrum reagent is positive, the cells are then tested with separate anti-IgG and anti-C3 reagents. In patients with WAIHA or CHD and those with benign or drug-induced antibodies (see Chapters 37 to 40) any one of three patterns may be seen. The red cells may be coated with IgG alone, with IgG and C3, or with C3 alone. The anti-C3 specificities required are anti-C3g and/or anti-C3d, the C3c originally attached to the patient's red cells may be long gone before the sample is collected and tested. The occasional need for anti-IgA in the broad spectrum reagent is discussed below.

As can be seen, much is now known about the requirements for anti-C3 in antiglobulin reagents. Although great improvements over the reagents available 20 years ago (50-52,270,271,288,289,300-302) have been made, some problems remain. No doubt by the time this chapter appears in print the problems will have been further resolved, perhaps by the use of IgM monoclonal antibodies to IgG and C3. The currently accepted types of antibodies required in a broad spectrum antiglobulin reagent are shown in table 6-8.

Anti-IgM in Antiglobulin Reagents

From what has been written thus far, it does not seem that the presence of anti-IgM in a broad spectrum reagent would be of any great advantage. Most IgM antibodies agglutinate red cells or cause complement to be bound so that presence of the antibody can be detected via the C3-anti-C3 reaction. Polley et al. (262) showed that it was much easier to detect the bound C3 than it was to detect the antibody with anti-IgM. However, there is one report of non-complement binding IgM autoantibodies (303) so that the presence of anti-IgM in the reagent might occasionally be of value.

Anti-IgA in Antiglobulin Reagents

IgA blood group antibodies are not common and when found are usually present in the same sera as IgG and/or IgM antibodies of identical specificity (21,215,304-309). Thus anti-IgA will not regularly play an important role in antiglobulin tests. However, a few examples of non-agglutinating IgA autoantibodies have been reported (21,304,310-315) in patients in whom no IgG or IgM antibodies could be found. It is possible (see also Chapter 37) that the red cells of patients with hemolytic anemia, that appear to be coated only with IgA, also carry sub-detectable levels of IgG. Indeed, Petz and Garratty (21) and Wolf et al. (316) have reported cases in which, in conventional tests, the patients' cells reacted with anti-IgA but not with anti-IgG or anti-complement but that were, in more sensitive tests, shown to be coated with low levels of other proteins as well. At present there is some dispute as to how or if red cells coated only with IgA are destroyed in vivo. First, IgA antibodies do not activate complement. Second, although it has been reported (317-319) that some macrophages carry IgA receptors, the finding has not been confirmed by others (215). However, IgA-coated red cells may be bound by neutrophils (317,318) and, in vitro, are cytotoxically damaged by monocytes (313).

TABLE 6-8 Antibodies Currently Regarded as Minimum Requirements in a Broad Spectrum Antiglobulin Reagent

Antibody	Comments
Anti-IgG	Capable of detecting red cell-bound IgG1, IgG2 and IgG3. Detection of IgG1 and IgG3 required in antibody-screening and identification, compatibility and direct antiglobulin tests. Detection of IgG2 required in cases of ABO HDN (see Chapter 41). The ability to detect red cell bound IgG4 may not be essential.
Anti-C3	For use in compatibility testing in normal ionic strength systems, anti-C3c may be required. For direct antiglobulin tests the presence of anti-C3g is desirable. However, blends of anti-C3c plus anti-C3d or anti-C3c plus anti-C3g, or even potent anti-C3d (monoclonal source) may suffice for both direct and indirect antiglobulin tests.

The only way that non-agglutinating IgA antibodies can be detected on red cells that are not also coated with IgG or complement, is if the antiglobulin reagent in use contains anti-IgA. Since the incidence of IgA-only autoantibodies causative of antibody-induced hemolytic anemia is so low, it would be unreasonable to demand that all broad spectrum antiglobulin reagents contain anti-IgA. Instead, workers can have on hand some anti-IgA (that prepared for precipitation studies is satisfactory if suitably diluted, see below) and can use it to perform a direct antiglobulin test on the red cells of those rare patients who present with the clinical signs and symptoms of autoimmune hemolytic anemia, but in whom standard serological tests are negative. In those few cases of autoimmune hemolytic anemia with only IgA detectable in the direct antiglobulin test, that have been reported, it has been noticeable that some broad spectrum antiglobulin reagents would detect the cell-bound IgA while others would not. Thus, in the absence of an available monospecific anti-IgA (or more likely, in the absence of materials with which to control it) workers can perform the direct antiglobulin test with the products of different manufacturers. Based on the reported experiences it seems likely that at least one such reagent would yield a positive result.

It must be remembered that the presence of anti-IgA in broad spectrum antiglobulin reagents, made from the sera of immunized animals, often represents chance. That is to say the animal makes the antibody that gets into the finished reagent when anti-IgG and ant-C3 are blended. Once antiglobulin reagents are entirely monoclonal antibody-based, anti-IgA will be present only if deliberately added from a clone distinct from those producing epitope specific anti-IgG and anti-C3.

Use of Immunoprecipitating Antiglobulins

Because specific anti-IgM and anti-IgA are not widely available for use in hemagglutination methods, immunohematologists have sometimes had to use reagents prepared for use in immunoprecipitation studies. Such reagents will usually agglutinate IgM or IgA coated red cells since the hemagglutination test requires less antibody than the immunoprecipitation reaction. However, a danger is that the immunoprecipitating reagent will contain contaminating antibodies (such as anti-IgG) at too low a level to interfere in immunoprecipitation, but at a sufficient level to react in the hemagglutination reaction. Clearly, if this occurs an incorrect interpretation of a positive test may be made. Most workers have found that the immunoprecipitating reagents can be used at dilutions between 1 in 5 and 1 in 15. However, it then becomes necessary to prepare IgM or IgA coated

red cells for use as a positive control. Preparation of IgM-coated red cells is relatively straightforward since an IgM antibody can be used at a dilution at which it does not cause agglutination, in the first stage of the EDTA-2 stage test (261). Preparation of IgA coated cells is more difficult, a method using chromic chloride (320) to effect passive coupling of IgA and red cells, is given by Judd (321).

Anti-transferrin in Antiglobulin Reagents

The protein transferrin is a beta globulin. When rabbits are immunized to produce antiglobulins they may also form anti-transferrin (322). Jandl (333) and Sutherland et al. (186) found a close relationship between reticulocyte counts and positive direct antiglobulin tests and postulated that, on at least some occasions, the reaction was due to anti-transferrin and transferrin rich reticulocytes. However, Mollison et al. (215) point out that the bond between iron-free transferrin and reticulocytes is weak and that the transferrin is likely to dissociate in the washing stage before the addition of antiglobulin serum. It is of course to be expected that many patients with high reticulocyte counts will have positive direct antiglobulin tests due to autoantibodies bound to their red cells. One of the consequences of a hemolytic process is that red cells are needed by the body so that the patient should undergo a reticulocyte response.

Modifications to the Antiglobulin Test

The antiglobulin test is sufficiently versatile that workers who understand the underlying principles can modify the test for a variety of purposes. Details of many modifications were given in the previous editions of this book, some of them have now been replaced by newer techniques and are now primarily of historical interest. For the sake of completeness and to illustrate the utility of the antiglobulin reaction, brief details are given below.
1. Gamma globulin neutralization test. Purified IgG was added to a broad spectrum reagent that could then be used to demonstrate the presence or absence of complement on red cells. No longer needed since pure anti-IgG (H chain specific) and anti-C3 are readily available.
2. Antiglobulin consumption test. Essentially an adsorption of anti-IgG with red cells thought possibly to be coated with a low level of IgG that was insufficient to promote agglutination by anti-IgG in the standard (usually direct) test. The basis of the "Gilliland" test used to detect low levels of IgG on the red cells of patients with "warm" antibody-induced hemolytic anemia and a nega-

tive DAT (335,336). Now largely replaced by sensitive antiglobulin methods that use anti-IgG coupled to an enzyme (EIA) (337-340) or a radiolabel (RIA) (341-344) or better still (if one is available) by use of a flow cytometer (345-348).

3. Rescue of stored, complement-binding antibodies. When the stored serum contains altered complement that prevents the uptake of C3 that can be detected with anti-C3, either of two remedies can be tried. The addition of fresh serum to the stored serum results in competition between active and altered C1q for the antibody Fc pieces. In the EDTA two stage test Ag+Ab+C1q occurs in the first stage and C1r to C3 activation in the second (261). Little used now since methods such as those using PEG and Polybrene will often allow detection of IgG.

4. Antiglobulin titration to measure responses to treatment in patients with WAIHA, see Chapter 37. Seldom used now since the quantitative methods mentioned in 2, above, are better.

Having written that some modifications to the antiglobulin test devised and used by his colleagues are now primarily of historical interest, the elder of these authors can only apologize by pointing out that he is older than some of those colleagues.

Evaluation of Antiglobulin Reagents

When antiglobulin reagents are made wholly by blending selected monoclonal antibodies, whose activity levels can be measured by non-serological methods, it may become unnecessary for the blood banker to evaluate the purchased reagents. That time has not yet arrived. Accordingly for those workers who wish to compare antiglobulin reagents from different manufacturers, or who wish to evaluate home-made reagents, this section is retained from the previous edition of this book.

The preparation of a good broad spectrum antiglobulin reagent is a skilled task. It is virtually impossible to obtain a suitable reagent from one, or even a small number of animals. In order to obtain sufficient quantities of all the anti-IgG and anti-complement components optimally reactive at the same dilution, a pool of many raw sera from immunized animals must be made and suitably diluted. Because of the difficulties involved and the time required, many blood bankers now rely on commercially-prepared reagents.

Antiglobulin sera, as sold, are already diluted to the point where the antibodies present react optimally. Accordingly, any commercially obtained reagent should *NOT* be further diluted. In addition to the fact that further antibody dilution must be avoided, it must be realized that these sera are supplied in a carefully prepared diluent. Dilution of an antiglobulin serum with an equal vol-

ume of saline may destroy the environment in which that reagent was designed to react.

The correct way to evaluate batches of antiglobulin reagents is to test them against red cells coated with decreasing amounts of many different antibodies. It is the antibodies that should be diluted so that the ability of the antiglobulin reagents to detect smaller and smaller numbers of antibody and complement molecules bound to red cells is tested.

In order to test an antiglobulin reagent for its ability to detect membrane-bound IgG, the reagent should be tested against dilutions of a variety of different blood group antibodies. Studies using non-agglutinating Rh antibodies will seldom reveal significant differences between antiglobulin reagents. It seems that almost any anti-IgG is able to detect red cell-bound Rh antibodies with relative ease. More marked differences are often seen when IgG antibodies with specificities such as those against the Fy^a, Fy^b, Jk^a, Jk^b, Do^a, Xg^a, etc. antigens are used. One point that must be remembered is that many IgG antibodies, especially those in the Duffy and Kidd systems, fix complement. In order that the evaluation tests really detect the IgG antibody and not a mixture of the IgG antibody and complement, it is important that such sera be prevented from fixing complement. This can be accomplished by adding EDTA to the sera in a final concentration of 4 mg per 1 ml of serum. The evaluation of antiglobulin reagents for anti-IgG content is easy, providing different IgG antibodies are available. Titration of the antibodies will reveal more differences in antiglobulin reagents than will simple tests with undiluted antibodies. As pointed out in several published reports of evaluation studies (50,271,289,301) some examples of Duffy and Kidd system antibodies are particularly discriminating in this respect.

Evaluation of antiglobulin reagents for their anti-complement content is more complex but is still well within the capability of the blood banker. As described in an earlier section, anti-C3c is useful in indirect antiglobulin tests since it will react with cell-bound iC3b before that protein is further cleaved. Anti-C3d and anti-C3g are useful in indirect antiglobulin tests and at least one of them must be present in a reagent used for direct antiglobulin tests. This because by the time the sample is tested in a DAT, all (or most) C3c may have been cleaved, leaving C3dg cell-bound. Of the two specificities, anti-C3g may be more desirable than anti-C3d since the latter is more likely to give unwanted positive reactions by detecting the C3d present on normal red cells (10,215). The presence of anti-C4 (either as anti-C4b or anti-C4d) is undesirable. First, there is no known case in which the presence of C4 on red cells, in the absence of C3, represented a clinically relevant situation in vivo or in vitro (21). Second, because of the already described amplification step, red cells coated to the C1423 stage, carry far more C3 than C4. Thus, lower levels of anti-C3 than anti-C4 will effect positive tests in clinically relevant situations. Third, because of the situation described, reagents containing enough anti-C4 to cause agglutination of C1423-coated red cells, will often also agglutinate normal red cells coated to the C14 stage, i.e. unwanted positives.

Thus evaluation tests for anti-complement in antiglobulin reagents would ideally use red cells coated with C3 but not C4. Unfortunately, this ideal is difficult to attain in practice. The easiest methods to coat red cells with complement involve the use of sucrose solutions of low ionic strength. However, if care is not taken, reagents containing anti-C4 but little anti-C3 will appear satisfactory from the results of the evaluation studies.

The original "sugar-water" test (349) (i.e. a sucrose solution to which red cells and serum or whole blood was added) is now known (288) to result in the uptake of both C3 and C4 by red cells. The test can be modified (106,273) by the addition of EDTA to the sucrose solution. Since EDTA chelates magnesium ions that are necessary for the C42 complex to form, less C3 is activated (probably none via the classical pathway) and red cells coated to the C4 stage can be prepared. Thus by the use of the two methods, one set of red cells coated with C1423 and one set coated with C14 can be prepared. If the antiglobulin serum under test reacts with the C1423-coated red cells but not with the C14-coated cells, it can be said, with some confidence, to contain anti-C3. However, if the antiglobulin reagent reacts with both sets of cells, showing that it contains some anti-C4, the investigator will not know if anti-C3 is present as well.

The test has been further modified (108,110) by adding EDTA, varying the sucrose content, coating the red cells at 0-1°C and adding an excess of magnesium chloride, to prepare red cells coated with much higher levels of C3 than C4. However, some C4 may still become membrane bound so that in the absence of a pure anti-C4 to measure C4 uptake, it is difficult to be certain that the cells, as prepared, are detecting only anti-C3 in the evaluation study.

A more satisfactory way to test antiglobulin reagents for their anti-C3 content is to use the EDTA two-stage method. Lewis system antibodies used by this method are especially suitable since they are almost always IgM and always bind complement (215). Many Lewis system antibodies act as saline agglutinins but at dilutions at which they will not agglutinate red cells, most of them will still cause complement to be bound to the cells. In several large studies on different antiglobulin sera, Issitt et al. (52,271,289,301) utilized this fact. Each time a Lewis system antibody was used, a saline control was included. This consisted of a titration, treated in exactly

the same manner as those read with antiglobulin serum, that had two drops of saline instead of antiglobulin reagent, added at the reading stage. Any agglutination observed in the saline control was then subtracted from the degree of agglutination found in the antiglobulin tests. The difference, of course, represented the complement-anti-complement reaction. By using old stored Lewis system antibodies it is often possible to work in a system in which the saline agglutinating activity of the antibody has totally disappeared and in which positive reactions are only obtained with antiglobulin serum. Some diluents used in the preparation of antiglobulin reagents contain additives to enhance the positive reactions of the antiglobulin serum. Thus there is a small danger that when saline is used in place of antiglobulin serum, in the agglutination control just described, it will not provide a strictly comparable control. Some agglutination by the Lewis system antibody, enhanced by the additives in the antiglobulin serum diluent, may be interpreted as being due to a C3-anti-C3 reaction. This problem can be circumvented by using the antiglobulin reagent diluent in place of saline for reading the control titration. If commercially-prepared reagents are being studied and the diluents used in their manufacture are not available, neutralized antiglobulin serum can be used. Sufficient drops of serum are added to a vial of antiglobulin reagent so that the reagent will not longer agglutinate antibody-coated red cells. That neutralized reagent is then used as the diluent control.

By using the EDTA two-stage procedure it is possible to prepare red cells coated with appreciable amounts of C3b, C3d and C3g and relatively small amounts of C4b and C4d. Not only does this method allow full amplification from the $\overline{C4b2b}$ to the $\overline{C4b2b3b}$ stage to occur, it provides an evaluation system that closely resembles the situation in which the antiglobulin reagent will actually be used, once the evaluation studies are completed.

No matter which method is used to prepare the C3b-coated red cells (with or without C4b), further treatment can be used to cleave some of the complement components bound. First, the iC3b can be cleaved by long time incubation of the C3b-coated red cells in human serum. We used this method in many evaluation studies to convert cell-bound iC3b to C3d (52,271,289). We incubated the cells in fresh human serum for periods of 2 to 24 hours, with intermittent or constant agitation, to allow the C3b-INA (factor I) to cleave the bound iC3b. In the 24 hour incubation method, sodium azide to a final concentration of 0.1% was added to prevent bacterial growth. Others used trypsin in place of the fresh human serum and believed that iC3b was converted to C3d in some 15 to 30 minutes (283). Although for many years it was believed that both human serum and trypsin effected the same iC3b to C3d conversion, we always felt (52,289) that when the two methods were used in parallel, subsequent tests revealed some differences. It is now known (8,10,111,290,295,353,354) that when human serum is used iC3b is cleaved, C3c is released, and C3dg remains membrane bound. When trypsin is used in place of human serum, iC3b is cleaved, C3c and C3g are released and only C3d remains membrane-bound. As already mentioned, anti-C3g may be a more useful antibody than anti-C3d meaning that the serum-based cleavage of iC3b results in a better evaluation system than the trypsin-based method. For years, many workers told us that the two methods resulted in the same product, for years we felt our serum system to be better, we were right but we had no idea why!

Yet another method of testing antiglobulin reagents for the presence of anti-C3d and anti-C3g is to use red cells from a patient with cold hemagglutinin disease, or warm antibody hemolytic anemia where only complement is present on the red cells. However, the ability to prepare cells in vitro is of great advantage since red cells from appropriate patients are not always available when needed. Further, such cells cannot be stored in the frozen state, when the patients are available, since degradation of cell-bound C3 occurs during storage.

Finally, in the evaluation of antiglobulin reagents, some tests should be included to ensure that the reagents do not contain unwanted agglutinins. There are several different methods of determining the presence or absence of these antibodies. Issitt et al. (289) used unwashed A, B and O cells, suspended in their own serum in agglutination tests at RT and 4°C. Use of unwashed, serum-suspended cells ensured that the antiglobulins would be neutralized and that any agglutination observed could be attributed to unwanted antibodies. Use of A, B and O cells ensured that anti-A, anti-B, anti-H and anti-species, all of which can be present in animal sera, would be detected. Of course, if autologous serum is used, controls must be included to show that autoagglutinins are not present in the serum. When antiglobulin reagents are made, various methods including adsorption, dilution and heating (215,266,350,351) are used to free the reagents of these unwanted agglutinins. In the preparation of anti-IgG reagents this becomes a simple procedure since the level of anti-IgG is usually high and that of unwanted agglutinins low. As mentioned above, in the preparation of anti-complement reagents the difference between required and unwanted antibody titers is not nearly so marked. The result is that in an attempt to increase anti-complement levels it is very easy to increase levels of unwanted antibodies to dangerous levels. Again, this problem does not exist when monoclonal anti-C3 reagents are used.

Moore et al. (352) point out that in any antiglobulin

reagent evaluation study, the methods by which the reagent is to be used must be examined. Thus if the reagent is to be used in tests on enzyme-treated red cells it must be shown not to agglutinate non-antibody and non-complement-coated, enzyme-treated red cells. If the reagent is to be used in capillary tube tests it must be shown not to give unwanted positives by that method. These considerations are of importance since lower levels of contaminating agglutinins will cause unwanted positives by these methods than will cause such positives in conventional tube methods.

Mechanisms of Immune Red Cell Destruction

This section, on in vivo red cell destruction, has been included in this chapter because the same mechanisms that allow detection of antibodies in the antiglobulin test are involved in the in vivo destruction of red cells. Alloantibodies and autoantibodies destroy incompatible red cells by the same mechanism. Following transfusion, an alloantibody in the patient's blood, directed against an antigen on the donor's cells, binds to those cells and may cause red cell destruction. In antibody-induced hemolytic anemia the patient forms an antibody directed against an antigen on his own cells. Thereafter the ways in which these antibodies cause cell destruction are the same.

There are two major mechanisms of in vivo red cell destruction. One is intravascular destruction in which red cells are actually destroyed in the blood stream with consequent release of hemoglobin into the plasma. The second type is extravascular destruction in which intact red cells are removed from circulation by cells of the reticulo-endothelial system. This type of red cell removal results in hyperbilirubinemia but little release of hemoglobin into the plasma (215,355). The cells responsible for the removal of intact red cells are part of the reticuloendothelial (R-E) system but are situated primarily in the liver and spleen. These two organs are not, themselves, part of the R-E system but act as sites for the functions of the R-E system cells involved.

Intravascular Red Cell Destruction

Antibody-mediated intravascular red cell destruction is caused by exactly the same mechanism that causes red cell hemolysis in vitro, namely the sequential binding of the complement components C1 through C9 following the formation of antigen-antibody complexes. Most of the factors, described in detail earlier in this chapter, that influence the ability of antibody molecules to bind complement in vitro can be applied to the actions of antibodies in vivo. Thus, in the presence of a potent, complement binding antibody and large numbers of closely situated red cell antigens, intravascular hemolysis can occur. Antibodies that are readily hemolytic in vitro will often cause intravascular hemolysis in vivo. Thus, this type of cell destruction is usually seen following the transfusion of major-side ABO incompatible blood. As discussed above, both IgM and IgG ABO system antibodies activate complement. Further, both bind to red cells at 37°C. As mentioned, IgG ABO system antibodies may play a major role in intravascular lysis, that does not mean that IgM antibodies of the system do not act similarly. A second requirement for intravascular hemolysis to occur (in addition to the presence of potent complement-binding antibodies) is that large numbers of closely situated antigen sites be present on the red cells. Certainly the ABO system fulfills this criterion as well. From the results of direct measurements of the number of antibody molecules that bind to red cells it was suggested (356-358) that A and B sites number between 8×10^5 and 1.2×10^6 per red cell. However, Mollison et al. (215) point out that this assumes that each antibody molecule binds to one antigen. In fact there is evidence (359-362) that each molecule of anti-A and anti-B attaches to two antigens so that the number of A and B sites may be double those given above. In reviewing current knowledge about red cell membrane-borne glycoproteins and glycolipids, Anstee (248) pointed out that A and B are carried on many such structures. They are known (363) to be on the major anion transporter, protein band 3, that is present on red cells in 1×10^6 copies (364). They are known (365) to be carried on band 4.5, the glucose transport protein, that is present on red cells in 5×10^5 copies (366). A and B are also carried on poly-N-acetyl lactosaminyl glycolipids that occur in some 5×10^5 copies per red cell (367) and on other glycoproteins (such as the Rh-associated glycoproteins, circa $1 - 2 \times 10^5$ copies per red cell (368)) and glycolipids that occur in less profusion on the membrane. Anstee (248) concluded that these findings indicate that A and B cells carry more than 2 million copies of their antigens per cell, a figure that agrees well with the figures obtained in direct antibody binding measurements if those figures are doubled because of the antibodies' monogamous bivalency as first described by Klinman and Karush (369).

Other antibodies such as anti-P+P_1+P^k (anti-Tj[a]); anti-Vel; and potent examples of anti-Le[a]; all of which can cause in vitro hemolysis, can also cause intravascular destruction. However, the correlation between in vitro hemolysis and intravascular destruction is by no means absolute. For example, more Lewis system antibodies cause in vitro hemolysis than cause intravascular red cell destruction. The various reasons for this are considered more fully later in this chapter.

Recognition of the fact that intravascular hemolysis has occurred is not difficult. The resultant transfusion reaction is immediate, severe and sometime fatal (see Chapters 8 and 36). In cases where ABO incompatible blood has been transfused, intravascular hemolysis should always be considered as a very real possibility even if the ABO agglutinins of the patient are not acting as hemolysins in vitro. Mollison et al. (215) have pointed out that the majority of ABO antibodies can act as hemolysins in vitro if other than usual tests are used. For example, an increase of the serum:cell ratio or prolonged incubation times in in vitro tests will often result in hemolysis, where routine tests with the same antibodies did not. It should also be remembered that some commercial companies add EDTA to the A and B cells sold for use in reverse typing so that (for reasons already described) complement binding in the in vitro tests stops at the EAC1q point and potent hemolysins present as agglutinins.

Extravascular Red Cell Destruction

This type of in vivo red cell destruction occurs when red cells are coated with: IgG but no complement; immunoglobulin and complement bound to the C3 stage where insufficient quantities of the terminal attack components bind to cause intravascular lysis; and to a relatively limited degree when red cells are coated with complement to the C3 stage but do not have immunoglobulins simultaneously attached. In all three situations, the abnormal protein (IgG or C3) coating acts a signal to macrophages of the reticulo-endothelial system. The coated cells are bound by these macrophages, via specific receptor sites and may eventually be destroyed. More details about the specific receptor sites on tissue-bound macrophages, are given in the following sections.

Once macrophage trapping of IgG or C3-coated cells has occurred, it seems that the macrophages attempt to remove the abnormal protein from the red cell membrane. If the macrophage activities result in phagocytosis, or fragmentation of the cells, obviously red cell destruction within organs of the body (see below) has occurred. Often, it seems that the macrophage succeeds in removing the IgG or the C3 but at the same time removes a piece of the red cell membrane. Thus the red cell now has the same mean cell volume but has a reduced membrane surface area. In other words, the red cell has been converted from a biconcave disc to a spherocyte (373). As explained below, even if spherocytes are released in to the circulation, they are subject to trapping in the sinusoids in subsequent passages through the spleen. The spherocytes seen in the blood films of patients

FIGURE 6-5 The Passage or Non-Passage of Red Cells Through Microcapillaries

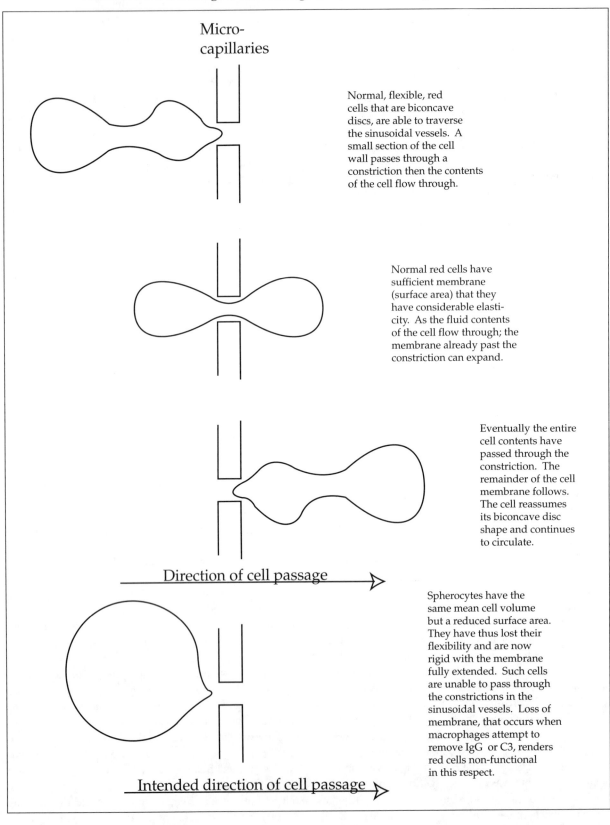

Micro-
capillaries

Normal, flexible, red
cells that are biconcave
discs, are able to traverse
the sinusoidal vessels. A
small section of the cell
wall passes through a
constriction then the contents
of the cell flow through.

Normal red cells have
sufficient membrane
(surface area) that they
have considerable elasti-
city. As the fluid contents
of the cell flow through; the
membrane already past the
constriction can expand.

Eventually the entire
cell contents have
passed through the
constriction. The
remainder of the cell
membrane follows.
The cell reassumes
its biconcave disc
shape and continues
to circulate.

Direction of cell passage

Spherocytes have the
same mean cell volume
but a reduced surface area.
They have thus lost their
flexibility and are now
rigid with the membrane
fully extended. Such cells
are unable to pass through
the constrictions in the
sinusoidal vessels. Loss of
membrane, that occurs when
macrophages attempt to
remove IgG or C3, renders
red cells non-functional
in this respect.

Intended direction of cell passage

with "warm" antibody-induced hemolytic anemia (see also Chapter 37), those who have suffered antibody-mediated transfusion reactions, and those infants suffering from (particularly ABO) HDN (see also Chapter 41) are red cells that were coated with IgG (and to a lesser degree with C3) that have become altered by macrophage-mediated removal of some red cell membrane.

As most workers well know, the biconcave shape of a normal red cell represents a deliberate functional design. The excess membrane (surface area) of the red cell allows the cell considerable flexibility and elasticity. As illustrated in figure 6-5, normal red cells with their excess of membrane surface, are able successfully to traverse constrictions such as those in the sinusoidal circulation of the spleen and the liver. Spherocytes on the other hand (whether they are malformed red cells, as in patients with hereditary spherocytosis, or are formed following macrophage action, as described above) become trapped in the sinusoids and eventually suffer metabolic starvation and death (374-377).

Extravascular Destruction of IgG-Coated Red Cells

Red cells coated with IgG alone, are removed from circulation predominantly by the spleen. Macrophages located within that organ carry receptors (see below) that bind the Fc pieces of IgG molecules attached to red cells (373,378-413). The red cells then suffer the consequences described in the previous section.

This ability of macrophages to fix IgG-coated red cells can be demonstrated in vitro. Macrophages begin life in the bone marrow, are released into the circulation in the form of monocytes and after circulating for a few days, become tissue bound macrophages (388). If monocytes from peripheral blood are isolated, they can be shown to bind to IgG-coated red cells, in rosette formations, in in vitro experiments (382,383,385,386). Further, the ability of the monocytes to form rosettes with IgG-coated red cells can be inhibited by adding IgG, whole Fc pieces from IgG molecules, or C_H3 portions of the Fc pieces of IgG molecules, to the test system (384,390,396,397).

Mollison et al. (215) report that splenic sequestration of IgG-coated red cells can result in the removal of up to 400ml of red cells per day and Arend and Mannik (393) have calculated that each macrophage has as many as 1×10^6 IgG receptors on its surface. Since it has been shown that IgG molecules (or IgG Fc pieces, or C_H3 portions of the IgG Fc piece) inhibit the ability of macrophages to bind to IgG-coated red cells, presumably because free IgG can itself bind to the macrophage receptors, it may be wondered how IgG-coated red cells

are removed from circulation via the mechanism described. It might be thought that in the presence of serum IgG the macrophage receptors would bind free IgG molecules and would not be able to bring about the removal of IgG-coated red cells. In answer to this question, it has been pointed out (383,396,398) that there is considerable concentration of red cells within the spleen. In other words, within the spleen, where the concentration of red cells is such that the hematocrit is 75 to 80% there are fewer free (unbound, serum) molecules of IgG to bind the macrophage Fc receptors. Thus as red cells pass through the sinusoids of the spleen the chance that they will encounter macrophages with available Fc receptors is much greater than would be the case in an organ where the hematocrit is the same as in peripheral blood. Further, the unique architecture of the spleen increases the chance that an IgG-coated red cell will encounter a macrophage with available receptors. Small arteries in the spleen branch at right angles to the larger ones. Since red cells tend to travel in the center of the stream of blood passing through those arteries, plasma, containing the unbound IgG gets skimmed from the edges of the vessels thus further decreasing the chance that macrophage receptors will be occupied with free IgG molecules when the IgG-coated red cell arrives (377,414,415). Although this concept has been questioned (416), the finding that in some disease states (though not necessarily with IgG-coated red cells) macrophage sequestration of IgG-coated particles can be blocked by the injection of IVIG, so that very high levels of free IgG are attained, seems to support the idea (417-432,729). Further, Kelton et al. (433) have demonstrated a direct correlation between the concentration of IgG in the serum and Fc-dependent reticuloendothelial cell function.

In the clearance of red cells coated with IgG but no complement, the spleen is the major site of red cell removal. Mollison et al. (215) report that when red cells are coated with 20 to 30mg of Rh antibody per red cell and then labeled and injected into volunteers, they are cleared by the spleen, with a half life of about 20 minutes. This shows that some 90% of the red cells are cleared during their first passage through the spleen. When red cells coated with the same amount of the same antibody are injected into an individual who has had a splenectomy (because of accidental injury to the spleen) the labeled cells are removed by the liver, with a half life of about 5 hours (434). Similarly, in patients with warm antibody-induced hemolytic anemia, splenectomy often alleviates the anemia (caused by the splenic removal of IgG-coated red cells) although the red cells can sometimes be shown to be coated with rather similar amounts of IgG, before and following the splenectomy. It is known that while the liver is a much larger organ than the spleen and that while it contains macrophages with IgG Fc receptors, hemoconcentration is not nearly as great in the hepatic as in the splenic circulation. It has been calculated (434) that on a weight basis, the spleen is about 100 times more efficient than the liver in the removal of IgG-coated red cells. Nevertheless, in patients with warm antibody-induced hemolytic anemia, in whom splenectomy has been performed, the level of autoantibody bound per red cell eventually reaches a high enough point that significant hepatic red cell sequestration and destruction occurs, if autoantibody production is not reduced by the use of immunosuppressive agents such as steroids (see Chapter 37). It should be pointed out that the above considerations apply to red cells coated only with IgG. When red cells are coated with IgG and C3 (see below) their in vivo clearance may be much more rapid and hepatic sequestration will play a far more significant role (215,435-445).

Thus far this discussion has been in somewhat general terms and has not considered differences in the rates of in vivo clearance, or indeed whether such clearance will occur at all, that might be correlated with the IgG subclass of the antibody involved. In fact, the IgG subclass of the antibody is of considerable importance in determining the in vivo fate of antibody-coated red cells. The group of investigators in Amsterdam showed (395,396,398,446-453) that when autoantibodies were considered, those that were IgG3 nearly always brought about marked in vivo red cell destruction. Those that were IgG1 varied in that about half of them caused hemolytic anemia while the other half were clinically benign. As described below, in vitro experiments have also shown that Fc receptors on macrophages bind IgG3 more efficiently than they bind IgG1. However, the situation is not as cut and dried (or should that be cut and spherocytosed) as those observations might indicate. First, Garratty and colleagues (202,455,456) have demonstrated IgG3 as the only immunoglobulin on the DAT-positive red cells of some blood donors, patients and neonates in whom there was no obvious hemolytic anemia. Second, in patients with a positive DAT with IgG but no complement on the red cells, the most common findings are that the cells are coated with both IgG3 and IgG1 or IgG1 alone. Observations on patients (with or without hemolytic anemia) who present with only IgG3 on the red cells have been made on a relatively small group of individuals (202,452). When the antibody is wholly IgG2, in vivo red cell destruction does not usually occur although exceptions have been seen (454,455). As far as we are aware, no case of WAIHA caused by an IgG4 autoantibody has been reported. However, this situation may change. As described in the next section, some Fc receptors on macrophages have now been shown to bind IgG4, albeit with considerable less affinity than that displayed for IgG3 and IgG1.

The difference between IgG3 and IgG1 in terms of macrophage binding has also been seen in in vitro studies. Rosetting assays and cytotoxicity tests showed higher values when IgG3-coated red cells were tested than when IgG1-coated red cells were used (403-406,449,452,457-459). IgG3 myeloma proteins were shown to be more efficient than those composed of IgG1 in inhibiting the reaction between monocytes and IgG-coated red cells (37,386,400). IgG2 and IgG4 myeloma proteins did not inhibit these reactions at all (452). In a series of in vitro studies using adherence or phagocytosis as the end point it was found that anywhere between 3 and 10 times as much IgG1 as IgG3 per red cell was needed to obtain the same degree of reactivity (403-406,457-459). The actual numbers of IgG molecules per cell vary in these different reports since different test systems were used, the ratios suggest the 3 to 1 to 10 to 1 numbers cited.

Somewhat similar observations have been made from studies on patients with a positive DAT due to an IgG autoantibody, some of whom had hemolytic anemia and some of whom did not. In two reports (451,452) it was suggested that as few as 100 molecules of IgG3 per red cell could effect in vivo red cell clearance (perhaps explaining some cases of DAT-negative, WAIHA in which enough IgG3 is bound to initiate in vivo red cell destruction, but too little for detection in the "standard" DAT, see also Chapter 37). In contrast, in a different study (22) it was reported that circa 1000 molecules of IgG1 per red cell were necessary for in vivo clearance to occur. While these numbers are useful and while they show a difference between the activities of IgG3 and IgG1, they should not be taken as absolutes. First, they take no account of the variable ability of the reticuloendothelial system in different individuals. Clearly one patient may have an RES that will clear red cells coated with 1000 molecules of IgG1 per red cell. Another patient may have an RES that will require 1200 or more molecules per cell to effect the same degree of in vivo red cell destruction. Second, the number of molecules per cell reported will be highly dependent on the method used to measure the bound IgG. It is not inconceivable that levels of 100 molecules per cell measured by one method represents the same amount of antibody binding as 500 molecules per cell measured by a different method. Third, the observations cited above that presence of IgG3 alone has been associated with some DAT-positive conditions in which there was no obvious in vivo red cell destruction, should be remembered. Since those cases involved positive DATs, it can be assumed that more than 100 molecules of IgG3 per red cell were bound (21).

When it was first found that about half of all individuals with autoantibodies made of IgG1 on their red cells had hemolytic anemia while the other half were hematologically normal, it was suspected that IgG1 antibodies might vary in some way that was not recognizable by the in vitro tests currently available. It seemed possible that then unrecognized factors might determine the pathological or benign characteristics of the autoantibodies involved. Once it had been reported (22,451,452) that levels of 900 or less IgG1 molecules per red cell are associated with normal in vivo red cell survival while levels of 1200 or more IgG1 molecules per red cell are associated with accelerated rates of in vivo red cell destruction, most workers assumed that the differences in IgG1 autoantibody behavior are purely quantitative. Indeed, the laboratory data currently available tend to lend considerable support to such a hypothesis. However, as Garratty (202) has pointed out, the question is still not entirely resolved. First, while there is no direct evidence for qualitative differences between IgG1 autoantibodies, there is no evidence against it, either. Second, as already mentioned, quantitative differences between the amount of IgG1 that becomes red cell-bound do not provide unequivocal evidence that they are the sole explanation of the differences. Third, it is still possible that differences in RES function among different individuals are at least as important as the quantitative differences described.

A considerable amount of work in this area has also been done by studying the red cells and sera of patients who had formed autoantibodies as the result of treatment with the anti-hypertensive drug alpha-methyldopa (aldomet). Before alternative drugs were available, large numbers of persons were treated with aldomet. It was found (460-465) that some 10 to 36% of such patients developed a positive DAT and that autoantibody production was dose dependent. In patients receiving 2g or more of the drug per day, the incidence of autoantibody formation was three to five times greater than in patients receiving 1g per day, or less (462). In spite of the fact that some 10 to 36% of patients made autoantibodies, only about 0.8% of all treated patients developed hemolytic anemia (465) although virtually all the autoantibodies made were IgG1 (441,452). Two quite different explanations emerged to posit the low incidence of hemolytic anemia in this group of autoimmunized individuals. Meulen et al. (448) reported that in nine patients suffering in vivo hemolysis due to aldomet-induced autoantibodies, the level of red cell-bound IgG1 was higher than in six similarly treated patients who had positive DATs but no in vivo hemolysis. Lalezari et al. (466) reported that in those patients with hemolysis, IgM autoantibodies of the same specificity as the IgG autoantibodies were simultaneously present, those patients in whom no hemolysis occurred had only IgG autoantibodies. The

IgM autoantibodies were said to fix complement and were incriminated as the antibodies causing the hemolysis. These findings must be interpreted with some caution. The complement bound to the red cells was detected only via the Polybrene-IAT method (28,466). The near universal experience of others has been that when DATs, IATs and tests on eluates made from the red cells of these patients are performed by conventional methods, only IgG non-complement binding autoantibodies can be found (21,308,460-465,467-469). In the aldomet-induced situation, the answer may now never be obtained. In the late 1960s aldomet was one of relatively few highly efficient antihypertensive drugs so was widely used in spite of its propensity to stimulate autoantibody formation. In the years since then many equally efficient antihypertensives, that do not cause autoimmunization, have been developed. Today, clinicians who continue to prescribe aldomet are well aware of its dose-dependent feature in causing autoantibodies to be made so that if the patient's blood pressure cannot be controlled on a dose of 1g or less of aldomet per day, an alternative drug is invariably substituted. Development of a positive DAT in patients receiving up to 1g of aldomet per day is around 10%, accelerated in vivo red cell destruction in those patients is rare. A possible effect of aldomet in reducing macrophage efficiency is discussed in Chapter 40.

Rather less work has been completed on the role of different IgG subclass alloantibodies in effecting different amounts of in vivo red cell clearance, than has been performed with autoantibodies. However, there seem to be no reasons to suppose that macrophage preference for IgG3-coated cells, their ability to sequester IgG1-coated cells if enough antibody is bound and their paucity of high affinity receptors for IgG2 and IgG4, would be any different for allo than for autoantibodies. It has been shown that a number of alloantibodies generally regarded as being of clinical significance, are IgG3 and/or IgG1 in nature. For example, Natvig and Kunkel (34) studied 100 Rh antibodies and found them all to be of subclasses IgG1 and/or IgG3. Abramson and Schur (37) found that: 10 Rh antibodies were IgG1 and/or IgG3, although some had IgG2 components; 3 anti-K and one anti-Kp[b] were IgG1 while a second anti-Kp[b] was IgG3; two anti-S were IgG3 although one of them might have contained an IgG2 component; and one anti-Jk[a] was IgG2. Frame et al. (36) found that: 41 Rh antibodies were IgG1 and/or IgG3, although four of them contained an IgG4 component; while eleven examples of anti-K and one each of anti-Fy[a] and anti-Jk[a] were IgG1 and/or IgG3. Hardman and Beck (44) attempted IgG subclassing studies on 204 red cell blood group alloantibodies and found that 150 of them could be classified with the reagents available. While many of the antibodies were shown to be mixtures of different IgG subclasses, the correlation between expected clinical significance (based on specificity) and IgG3 and IgG1 subclasses, generally held. More recent studies (201,207-209,470,471) have also documented the clinical significance of a number of IgG3 and IgG1 alloantibodies by means of in vivo cell survival studies or red cell destruction in HDN. However, perhaps not too much weight should be placed on these observations since most blood group alloantibodies are made of IgG3 and/or IgG1 anyway. Presumably some weak alloantibodies, detected only by highly sensitive methods (472) are also IgG3 and/or IgG1 although they are usually too weak to allow tests to determine that fact. Some of those antibodies (i.e. some in the Rh system) have been shown to be totally benign in vivo (472). In still other studies (43,45,46) it has been shown that at least some IgG2 and IgG4 blood group alloantibodies are clinically significant.

In spite of what has been written it should be remembered that when the antibody is IgG3 or IgG1, the amount of antibody that binds to the red cells is critical in terms of the rate at which red cells will be destroyed (215,434,436,473-475). In a classic experiment demonstrating this point, Mollison et al. (475) coated D+ red cells with 12 different amounts (ranging from 1.6 to 74mg) of purified IgG prepared from a serum containing anti-D. The IgG-coated red cells were labeled and used in in vivo cell survival studies. There was very close correlation between the amount of anti-D bound and the rate of red cell clearance.

Cell Bound Receptors for IgG

When the binding of IgG Fc to receptors on macrophages, monocytes and other cells was first recognized it was thought that a single receptor existed. That receptor was thought to bind IgG3 and IgG1, with later evidence for a higher affinity for the former than the latter, but not IgG2, IgG4 or IgA. As work has progressed it has become apparent that there are a series of receptors and that some of them may bind IgG2 and/or IgG4 and/or IgA, albeit with lower affinity than for IgG3 and IgG1.

Currently, IgG Fc receptors are divided into three classes, all three are present on macrophages. There is emerging evidence (413) that this classification is an oversimplification and that additional heterogeneity exists. However, in considering the in vivo clearance of IgG-coated red cells it is still convenient to describe the actions of the three broad categories of receptors. All three are members of the Ig supergene family and their production is encoded from a locus on the long arm of chromosome 1 (476).

FcγRI (Fc gamma receptor I) or CD64 is a glyco-protein of 70kD that is expressed predominantly on macrophages and monocytes. It binds human IgG1, IgG3 and IgG4 but not IgG2 (399) and has a high affinity for monomeric IgG (399,402). There is a polymorphism of FcγRI, at least three forms exist (477).

FcγRII (Fc gamma receptor II) or CD32 is a highly polymorphic 40kD integral membrane glycoprotein. At least three genes encode slightly different FcγRII that apparently exists in at least seven different forms (476,478). These slightly different versions of FcγRII are present on different cells and have different binding affinities for IgG Fc. Two versions of FcγRII are present on (at least) monocytes, macrophages and neutrophils, a third is present on (at least) monocytes, macrophages and lymphocytes (478). Other cells that carry at least one form of FcγRII include platelets but the receptor is not found on red cells, T-cells or NK (natural killer) cells (412). It was at first thought (479) that FcγRII bound IgG1 and IgG3 but had little affinity for IgG2 or IgG4. A later study (480) showed that the receptor binds IgG2 as well as it binds IgG1 but has only low affinity for IgG4. The differences seen in these studies presumably resulted from the polymorphic natue of FcγRII as described above. FcγRII has a low binding affinity for monomeric IgG (481) thus suggesting that in vivo the receptor binds only immune complexes or cells coated with large numbers of IgG molecules. The activity of FcγRII is enhanced by proteolytic enzymes (482) which may mean that receptor activity in vivo increases at the site of local inflammation or during macrophage activation when proteases are released.

FcγRIII (Fc gamma receptor III) or CD16 is also a polymorphic glycoprotein. Posttranslation glycosylation changes result in the receptor having a MW of 50-70 kD on neutrophils (483) and 45-65kD on macrophages (484). FcγRIII is also present on NK (natural killer) cells, eosinophils, trophoblasts and a subpopulation of monocytes (485). FcγRIII has a relatively low affinity for monomeric IgG, it binds IgG1 and IgG3 to about the same degree but does not bind IgG2 or IgG4 (486,487). The FcγRIII receptor on macrophages and NK cells is a transmembrane protein whereas the receptor on neutrophils is a phosphatidylinositol (PI)-linked protein (488,489). The two forms of the receptor are encoded by allelic genes. Although it has been shown that FcγRIII on macrophages can mediate phagocytosis, it is not clear whether the neutrophil-borne receptor can act similarly (411,490,491). There is also some dispute as to whether the macrophage FcγRIII receptor can cause direct cell lysis (410,484).

The FcγRIII on neutrophils carries the antigens of the neutrophil specific antigen system NA1-NA2. The difference between NA1 and NA2 has been established at the molecular level (492,493) and involves amino acid substitutions that result in two additional glycosylation sites on NA2 compared to NA1 (494). On macrophages and NK cells, the FcγRIII molecule is always of the NA2 type. Some features of the Fcγ receptors are summarized in table 6-9.

Mode of Action of Fc Receptors

Fc receptors bind IgG by attaching to the antibody molecule's C_H3 region although portions of the C_H2 region may sometimes also be involved (495). Lack of flexibility in the hinge region of IgG2 and IgG4 molecules, may account, in part, for the difficulty receptors have in binding molecules of those subclasses (see above). Because the affinity of many receptors for monomeric IgG is low, most are best able to bind red cells or immune complexes that carry multiple copies of the antibody. This feature also contributes to the ability of the receptors to bind antibody-coated cells in the presence of free (monomeric) serum IgG. The Fc receptors on many cells are able to move laterally in the plane of the cell membrane after they have bound IgG. Congregation of many receptors at a single site results in multiple binding, affinity activity thus increases. Once the receptors have bound IgG (with red cells attached) they migrate to membrane pits and stimulate the assembly of clathrin that leads to their internalization by the cell (494). In some instances the receptor is detached from the (usually monomeric) IgG molecule and returns to function again at the cell surface, on other occasions the receptor is degraded with the multiple IgG molecules after phagocytosis has occurred (497-499). On average, monocytes carry in the order of 2×10^4 high affinity

receptors, once tissue bound these cells (now macrophages) carry some 2×10^5 low affinity and the same 2×10^4 high affinity receptors (500).

Extravascular Destruction of Red Cells Coated with IgG and C3

As described above (see table 6-6) in addition to Fcγ receptors, macrophages carry receptors for certain components of complement (384,501-506). Unlike Fcγ receptors, the complement receptors do not bind native molecules present in plasma, but recognize complement components that have been cleaved during the complement activation cascade. This means that when red cells coated with complement (predominantly C3, see below) encounter macrophages carrying appropriate receptors they can be bound by those macrophages regardless of the amount of plasma (complement) present at the site of contact. As a result, red cells coated with IgG and C3 are sequestered in the liver (as well as in the spleen where Fcγ receptors are active) where the hematocrit is roughly equal to that of circulating blood. However, again as described below, red cells coated with C3 in the absence of IgG are subject to somewhat limited in vivo sequestration and destruction. Thus it seems that the action of C3 receptors on macrophages is primarily to augment the clearance of IgG-coated red cells. Mollison et al. (475,507) showed that red cells coated with a certain amount of anti-Fy^a and with complement were cleared from circulation with a half-life of about 2 minutes. In contrast, when red cells coated with a similar amount, in terms of mg/ml of antibody, of non-complement binding anti-D were used, their in vivo half life was around 75

TABLE 6-9 Simplified Features of Fcγ Receptors*

Receptor and carrier protein	Cell lines on which receptor is predominantly expressed	Functional characteristics
FcγRI CD64	Macrophages and monocytes	Binds IgG1, IgG3 and IgG4. Has high affinity for monomeric IgG and is primary receptor for IgG-coated red cells. Polymophic, exists in at least 3 forms.
FcγRII	In various forms on macrophages, monocytes, neutrophils, lymphocytes and platelets	Binds IgG1, IgG2, IgG3 but has poor affinity for IgG4. Low affinity for monomeric IgG of any type and binds predominantly immune complexes. Encoded by 3 different genes, polymorphic, exists in at least 7 forms. Different forms carried by different cell lines.
FcγRIII	In various forms on macrophages, neutrophils, natural killer (NK) cells, eosinophils, trophoblasts and a subpopulation of monocytes.	Binds IgG1 and IgG3 but not IgG2 or IgG4. Low affinity for monomeric IgG. Macrophage borne receptor can mediate phagocytosis, neutrophil-borne receptor may not possess that ability. Dispute as to whether receptor can mediate direct cell lysis. At least 2 genes encode different forms of the receptor.

*This table presents an oversimplified view of Fcγ receptor structure and function. For additional details, see text.

minutes. Somewhat similarly, Schreiber and Frank (439,440) showed that when red cells were coated with a complement binding IgG antibody then injected into guinea-pigs, some of which were normal and some of which were genetically deficient in terms of production of some of the complement components, the red cells survived for the shortest period of time in the animals that had intact complement systems.

These data are currently interpreted, together with those that show that red cells coated with C3 but no IgG are poorly cleared, to indicate that the C3 receptors serve to trap and immobilize red cells. In other words, if red cells coated with IgG but no C3 encounter macrophages on which the Fcγ receptors are blocked with free (plasma) IgG, they will not be bound by the macrophages. If red cells coated with IgG and C3 encounter macrophages on which the Fcγ are blocked, they can be bound by the C3 receptors on those or nearby macrophages since, as stated, the C3 receptors are not blocked by the native (non-activated) C3 in plasma. The binding of free IgG to Fcγ receptors is a reversible event. Eventually the free IgG will spontaneously elute and the Fcγ receptors will become available to bind the Fc of the IgG molecules on the IgG and C3 coated red cells (183,503,506,508-513).

As mentioned earlier in this chapter, there are a number of different complement receptors that are present on a variety of cells and bind different components of activated complement, or the same components but with markedly different affinities. In terms of extravascular clearance of complement coated red cells, some of these receptors are much more important than others. The CR1 molecule binds C3b and C3. As explained above (table 6-4), its role in binding C3 is a regulatory one, rather than one that promotes phagocytosis. When CR1 binds C3b, phagocytosis may follow (182), however since red cell bound C3b is rapidly converted to iC3b (that is recognized predominantly by CR3 and CR4, see below) CR1 does not play a major role in the in vivo clearance of complement coated red cells. While CR1 is able to bind iC3b it does so with a very much lower affinity than that with which it binds C3b. CR1 is able to bind C3b only in the presence of a second signal that is, of course, almost always IgG in the situation described here. The presence of IgG on C3b-coated red cells (or other particles) causes increased expression of CR1 on the membrane of the macrophage, the mechanism involves mobilization and capping of intracellular receptors (508,514-518). Although red cells carry CR1 molecules and because of their numbers compared to other cells carry the majority of the body's supply of such receptors, they do not participate directly in extravascular red cell clearance. Instead the red cell CR1 molecules serve to enable the red cells to act as scavengers in the clearance of immune complexes from circulation. The

immune complexes are bound to red cells via a C3b-CR1 interaction and are transported to the liver where the immune complexes are removed by CR3 molecules, for clearance. The red cells that transported the immune complexes may then be released and may return to the circulation (185,519).

The CR2 molecule binds C3dg and with lower affinity, C3d. It appears to play no role in intravascular red cell clearance.

The CR3 and CR4 molecules are the predominant receptors involved in the clearance of complement coated red cells via the extravascular mechanism. CR3 is present on monocytes, neutrophils and large granular lymphocytes, it binds predominantly iC3b. Like CR1, CR3 requires a second signal, such as IgG, in order to be able to bind iC3b coated red cells. As mentioned above, CR3 is involved in ADCC(M), ADCC(L) and NK cytotoxicity (179,181,520,521). The closely related CR4 molecule is found predominantly on tissue macrophages (191). It binds iC3b and, with considerably lower affinity, C3dg. Again, like CR1 and CR3, CR4 requires a second signal in order to be able to bind iC3b. As will be apparent from what is written above, the prime mediator of clearance of complement coated red cells is iC3b. As stated both CR2 and CR4 are able to bind C3dg and/or C3d coated red cells, albeit with low affinity. However, it does not seem that the binding of C3dg or C3d coated red cells results in erythrophagocytosis. First, CR2 is present on B-cells and epithelial cells but not on macrophages. Second CR4 has only low affinity for C3dg. It was at one time suggested (522-524) that very low levels of serologically undetectable C3d, on red cells that appear from the results of in vitro tests to be coated only with IgG, might augment the clearance of those cells. As far as these authors are aware no further proof for that supposition has been obtained although there is now no doubt that C3d receptors exist (190,522,525-529) a point that was earlier disputed (438-440,442,504,505,530).

Extravascular Destruction of Red Cells Coated with Complement Components but with No Immunoglobulin

Long before complement regulation was understood and the functions of complement receptors were characterized, Lewis et al. (531) showed that the in vivo clearance of red cells coated with C3 but no immunoglobulin is limited and rather inefficient. These investigators coated red cells with C3 via a method that does not use an antibody, labeled the red cells with an isotope, then injected them into volunteers. The cells were quickly sequestered with counts over the liver. However, within two to four hours after their injection, more than 50% of the small test dose of cells were back in circulation. Although the reason for reappearance of the red cells in circulation was not fully understood at the time, the observation was confirmed by others (437,438). Now, of course, it is relatively easy to explain what happened. At the time of their injection the red cells would have carried C3b and/or iC3b and would have been bound by the CR3 and CR4 and to a lesser extent by the CR1 molecules, on macrophages in the liver. In the absence of the second signal (IgG) on the red cells, hepatic sequestration but little phagocytosis would have occurred. Even after they have bound to red cells and to macrophage receptors, C3b and iC3b are still subject to cleavage regulation. Thus although all the C3 coated red cells were initially sequestered in the liver, any intact C3b on the cells would have been converted to iC3b by factor I in the presence of cofactor H and then the cell bound iC3b would have been further degraded by factor I, to leave only C3dg membrane-bound. (See also the earlier section on regulation of complement activation.) Since the macrophage receptors bind to C3c the conversion of iC3b to C3dg would have resulted in C3c being left attached to the macrophages and the C3dg-coated cells being released into the circulation. Red cells coated with C3dg or C3d function normally and, for reasons given in the previous section, are not subject to significant macrophage binding or phagocytosis.

The contemporary explanation of that 1960 experiment, essentially explains why red cells coated with C3 but no immunoglobulin are not destroyed at any significant rate in vivo. In cold hemagglutinin disease (see Chapter 38) an IgM autoantibody binds to the patient's red cells when the patient is exposed to cold temperatures and activates complement (most efficiently as the blood temperature returns to 37°C). Some intravascular hemolysis may occur if enough C3 becomes cell-bound to activate the C5-C9 terminal attack sequence. Those red cells not destroyed intravascularly are coated initially with iC3b in the absence of immunoglobulin (the IgM autoantibody most often spontaneously elutes at normal body temperature), the iC3b is then converted (as above) to C3dg then C3d. Little further red cell clearance occurs. Ross (532) has shown that red cells coated with as many as 20,000 molecules of C3dg per red cell, are not cleared from the circulation by tissue bound macrophages. Although they preceded the basic science explanation, there are other reports of limited (or no) in vivo destruction of red cells coated with C3 in the absence of immunoglobulin (438,504,505,533,730).

As mentioned earlier, some Lewis system antibodies are capable of causing rather limited intravascular hemolysis. The amount of intravascular destruction that occurs is often limited by the weakness of the antibodies and by some or all of the factors listed below. Since most Lewis antibodies are IgM in composition and since there are apparently no macrophages with receptors for that

immunoglobulin, those red cells that escape intravascular destruction when a Lewis-anti-Lewis reaction occurs in vivo (that is relatively rare since many Lewis antibodies are cold-reactive and cannot complex with red cells in vivo) are subject to the slow and limited removal of C3-coated red cells as described in this section. It should also be remembered that Lewis system antibodies are subject to some considerations that do not apply to other antibodies. Since the Lewis antigens are plasma (or soluble) antigens they adsorb onto red cells passively (534-538). Thus, when Le(a+b-) red cells are transfused to an Le(a-b-) person whose serum contains anti-Le^a several events may occur. First, if the anti-Le^a is powerful and has a wide thermal range some intravascular cell destruction may occur. Second, if the anti-Le^a binds complement rather slowly, red cells coated to the C3b stage may be subject to the actions of factors I and H and not be destroyed at all. Third, the Le^a substance present with the red cells may neutralize the anti-Le^a before very much (or any) red cell destruction has occurred. Fourth, even in the absence of much free plasma Le^a substance, the Le^a substance present on the red cells may elute from the cells and cause antibody neutralization, again before very much (or any) red cell destruction has occurred. Almost any combination of the four points above is possible. It should also be remembered that total inhibition (neutralization) of Lewis antibodies by deliberate means is possible (539-541). Most of these considerations about Lewis antibodies apply to anti-Le^a or anti-Le^a plus anti-Le^b. Anti-Le^b, when present alone, is nearly always a cold-reactive, clinically-insignificant antibody.

Cytokine Generation During In Vivo Red Cell Destruction

In the section below describing macrophage variation as it relates to in vivo red cell destruction, brief mention is made of the activities of various cytokines. In fact, it is now appreciated that many of the clinical sequalae that follow in vivo red cell destruction result directly from the generation of cytokines and other effector molecules. These effects are discussed in detail in Chapter 36 (Transfusion Reactions) where a series of tables list: effector molecules generated and physiological consequences; cytokines generated and the effects they promote; the interrelationships between in vivo red cell destruction and disseminated intravascular coagulation (DIC); and differences in cytokine generation that follow intravascular and extravascular red cell destruction.

In Vivo Clearance of IgM-coated Red Cells

The in vivo clearance of red cells by IgM antibodies

must be considered in a number of different ways. First, some IgM antibodies, such as anti-A and anti-B, are able to bind to red cells at 37°C and activate sufficient amounts of complement that intravascular hemolysis can occur. Second, IgM antibodies that can bind to red cells at 37°C and can cause the activation of smaller amounts of complement can effect the slow and limited clearance of red cells described in the previous section. Third, IgM non-complement binding antibodies may or may not effect in vivo red cell destruction, the question has not yet been fully resolved. It is generally agreed that no macrophage receptors for IgM exist. Thus if IgM non-complement binding antibodies effect in vivo red cell destruction at all, they may do so via a mechanism in which agglutinated red cells become mechanically trapped in the sinusoidal circulation. Early reports (436,542) suggested that examples of IgM anti-M, anti-D and anti-c had caused in vivo red cell destruction. However, in a retrospective analysis of these studies, Mollison (444) stated that the anti-M studied may have activated complement and that the anti-D may have contained a small IgG component. The in vivo clearance of c+ red cells by the IgM anti-c remained unexplained. In that case (436), labeled c+ red cells were sequestered in the liver suggesting that the anti-c had activated complement. However, no complement activation could be demonstrated in in vitro tests. Another series of findings still in search of an explanation involves the cases of warm antibody-induced hemolytic anemia apparently caused by non-complement binding IgM autoantibodies (303).

In Vivo Clearance of IgA-coated Red Cells

As mentioned in an earlier section, it is not clear how IgA-coated red cells are removed from circulation in vivo. There seems to be general agreement that IgA antibodies do not activate complement. There is less agreement as to the existence of macrophage-bound receptors for IgA. While some workers (317-319,543,544) claim to have identified such receptors the findings do not yet seem to have been generally accepted. There is also a claim (319) that peripheral blood monocytes carry receptors for IgA. It has also been demonstrated (543) that monocyte-mediated anti-menigococcal activity can be generated by the purified IgA component of serum from patients convalescing from C-meningococcal disease. This observation was taken to mean that macrophages (monocytes) can recognize IgA. In those rare patients in whom IgA autoantibodies seem to be causative of warm antibody-induced hemolytic anemia (21,304,310-315) spherocytes are seen in the blood films and splenic sequestration of labeled autoantibody-coated red cells occurs. While these findings might appear to suggest that splenic macrophages

with receptors for IgA exist, it must be remembered that in at least two cases (21,316) in which the autoantibodies appeared in conventional tests to be exclusively IgA in nature, more sensitive than usual tests revealed the presence of, at least, IgG on the red cells as well. In other words, the in vivo cell clearance may have been a function of the sub-routine-antiglobulin-test-detectable IgG autoantibodies and the serum and cell-bound IgA antibodies may have been red herrings.

In Vivo Clearance of Agglutinated Red Cells

Ironically, since the agglutination reaction is by far the most commonly used tool of the blood banker, less is known about the in vivo destruction of agglutinated red cells than about the removal of those coated with IgG and/or complement. Erythrophagocytosis may play a role in the removal of agglutinated red cells (215,507,545-547). The spleen and liver can, somewhat simply, be thought of as filters that trap agglutinates of red cells (215,547-550). It must also be remembered that red cells agglutinated by IgG antibodies, or by any antibody that causes complement activation, will be subject to the actions of macrophages with IgG and C3 receptors, as already described. As also mentioned above, it is possible (215) that agglutinated red cells trapped in the sinusoidal circulation of the liver or spleen, or any other organ for that matter, might suffer metabolic starvation and death.

One point, that is perhaps surprising to the blood banker since agglutination is so often significant in in vitro tests, is that agglutination itself does not cause irreversible damage to red cells. Loutit and Mollison (551) and Jandl et al. (552) have clearly shown that agglutinated cells, when injected into volunteers, are not always destroyed. If the agglutination is reversible in vivo, the previously agglutinated red cells may be capable of normal survival.

Macrophage Variation

Much (perhaps too much) has been written in this chapter about variables that affect the amount and rate of in vivo red cell destruction. Those parameters described so far, i.e. antibody class and subclass, antibody quantity, antibody specificity and thermal range, complement components activated in terms of type and amount, etc., lend themselves to measurement by in vitro tests (202,215). However, a major variable that is much more difficult to measure involves variation in activity of the reticuloendothelial system in different individuals. It would not be expected that all macrophages would be created equal nor that all individuals would have similar numbers of Fcγ and complement receptors on their cells. Indeed Munn and Chaplin (522) used an MMA in which readings were accomplished by measuring the monocyte binding of ^{51}Cr-labeled red cells coated with IgG anti-D, to demonstrate this point. They found considerable variation in the activity of monocytes from 10 healthy individuals, then studied monocytes collected at different times from two of them. Over a four month period, variation was seen in the activity of monocytes from a single donor, viral infection resulted in monocyte activity that was more than 10 times greater than the normal mean. Thus the amount of in vivo red cell destruction caused by similar specificity and similar quantities of antibodies in different subjects should be expected to vary over a considerable "normal" range. Within the limits of such variation, table 6-10 presents what might be expected, on average, in terms of in vivo clearance of antibody and/or complement coated red cells.

In some disease states the activity of the reticuloendothelial system is at least partially suppressed, in others it is, sometimes markedly, enhanced. As examples, in patients with systemic lupus erythematosus, red cells heavily coated with anti-D and labeled with ^{51}Cr were shown to survive in vivo for longer periods than in normal healthy individuals. Frank et al. (553) postulated that in these patients DNA-anti-DNA immune complexes were blocking macrophage Fcγ receptors. As mentioned earlier, although many patients treated with alpha-methyldopa (aldomet) form autoantibodies and have strongly positive DATs, relatively few of them suffer accelerated rates of in vivo red cell destruction. Kelton (554) performed studies similar to those described above and concluded that lack of in vivo red cell destruction is related to impairment of the reticuloendothelial system in these patients and not to characteristics of the autoantibodies made.

In contrast to suppression of the reticuloendothelial system there is evidence that in some diseases, e.g. "warm" antibody-induced hemolytic anemia, sarcoidosis, tuberculosis, Crohn's disease, solid tumors, etc.

TABLE 6-10 Correlation of Red Cell-Bound Proteins and Rate of in Vivo Red Cell Clearance by Macrophages

Red cell coating	Amount of macrophage-induced in vivo red destruction
IgG plus C3b	Maximal
IgG3	Much
IgG1	Less
C3b (alone)	Least
C3d (alone)	Probably none

macrophages become hyperactive (21, 335, 336, 393, 522, 547, 555-560). It is very clearly established that in patients with "warm" antibody-induced hemolytic anemia in whom the hemolysis is being controlled with corticosteroid therapy, concomitant infection can result in an exacerbation of the hemolysis (21, 336, 522, 547, 555, 559). Increases in the rate of hemolysis in patients with autoantibodies have also been seen following vaccination and immunization (21,547,555). Fries and Frank (336) showed that the increase in macrophage activity in patients with "warm" antibody-induced hemolytic anemia represents an increase in the number of Fc receptors expressed on the surface of the macrophages. They and others (561-563) have shown that one of the ways in which corticosteroids act to control the hemolytic process in these patients is to control the increased expression of Fc receptors on macrophages and other cells.

It is now well established that many of the changes in activity of the reticuloendothelial system are cytokine driven. As will be appreciated from the list of pathological conditions given above, many of them result in the generation of cytokines. As simple examples, in hemolytic anemia red cell destruction occurs, such destruction has been shown (580-588,595) to result in the release of many different cytokines. In the host defense against malignant tumors, cytokines play a number of important roles (589-594) often by enhancing reticuloendothelial system function to enhance tumor rejection. To list a few of the more fully investigated effects: interferon gamma stimulates an increase in the number of FcγI receptors expressed at the cell surface, causes an increase in activity of FcγII receptors without increasing their numbers and promotes increased ADCC activity (410,596-599). Somewhat similarly, IL-6 causes increased ADCC and FcγI activity, without increasing the number of receptors expressed (600). The T-cell cytokines cause an increase in the biological activity of CR1, chemotatic agents cause an increase in the expression of CR3 (514,601). As already discussed, bacterial and viral infections cause an increase in the activity of the reticuloendothelial system, probably in large part via stimulation of cytokine release, indeed the mechanism may be the initiating factor in both childhood autoimmune thrombocytopenia and childhood "warm" antibody-induced hemolytic anemia (602,603). As discussed in more detail in Chapter 37, at least as far as WAIHA is concerned, the secondary infection-induced disease in children (which is the most common form) is much more likely to be cured in total than the chronic form (603).

Rather less is known about macrophage variation in terms of individuals who make easily detectable red cell autoantibodies (i.e. DAT strongly positive) but who do not develop hemolytic anemia (21, 308, 564-566, 731,

732) and those who have clinical hemolytic anemia but so little autoantibody on their red cells that it cannot be detected in conventionally performed DATs (17, 18, 21, 30, 304, 567). In other words, it is not known if the former group are spared in vivo red cell destruction because they have relatively inefficient macrophages and if the latter group have hemolytic anemia because they have a hyperactive reticuloendothelial system. One point against the concept that the individuals with autoantibodies but no hemolytic anemia have defective macrophages is that those individuals do not present with histories of recurrent infections as might be expected if their macrophages had seriously impaired function in vivo.

K-Cell Lysis

When incompatible red cells are cleared from circulation via the intravascular route, free hemoglobin is almost always seen in the patient's plasma. When extravascular clearance is involved, the rate of red cell destruction is usually slow enough that hemoglobinemia is not seen. However, on some occasions free hemoglobin is found in the plasma when an IgG non-complement binding antibody has effected the red cell destruction (568-579). Many workers believe that the hemoglobinemia represents overload of the reticuloendothelial system with a consequent release of unbound hemoglobin into the plasma. However, it is also possible that the free plasma hemoglobin is from red cells destroyed in the circulation without participation of the terminal attack sequence of the complement cycle.

It has been shown that in vitro, monocytes and some large lymphocytes can destroy antibody-coated red cells following cell-cell contact. Monocytes can lyse anti-D coated red cells (524,605) the mechanism involves the the release of lysosomal enzymes by the monocytes after cell-cell contact (397). IgG3 is a much better potentiator of this reaction than IgG1 that, when present on red cells in low levels, may not prompt lysis by monocytes (452,606,607) at all. The large lymphocytes that are active in a similar reaction are natural killer (NK) cells, hereafter referred to simply as K-cells. Following cell-cell contact, K-cells release perforins (that are somewhat like the components of the terminal attack sequence of complement) that can produce holes in the red cell membrane (131). Human polyclonal anti-D that are IgG1 or contain such a component, seem best to stimulate K-cell lysis in vitro and use of the ADCC(M) and ADCC(L) tests to forecast the severity of HDN due to anti-Rh have been said to be more reliable than some other cellular assays for that purpose (608-613). In contrast, only a minority of monoclonal IgG1

and fewer monoclonal IgG3 antibodies prompted K-cell lysis (614,615). The direct lysis of red cells by monocytes and K-cells is the basis of the ADCC(M) and ADCC(L) tests described briefly in Chapter 3. While these mechanisms are generally called ADCC, Garratty (604) has pointed out that such a term applies equally well to the actions of tissue-bound macrophages in destroying IgG or IgG plus C3-coated red cells. Accordingly, since we (almost) always do what George tells us, the term K-cell lysis is preferred here.

In studies (608-611) on K-cell lysis of red cells coated with IgG Rh antibodies, it has been shown that the activity of the K cells is not inhibited by free (serum) IgG although it may be blocked by aggregates of that immunoglobulin. Yust et al. (616,617) claimed that in patients undergoing in vivo red cell destruction caused by antibodies against penicillin, simultaneous extravascular removal and K-cell lysis may occur. As far as we are aware that claim has not been investigated further. Since it had been reported (618-625) that IgM, in addition to IgG antibodies, could induce K-cell lysis, Wiedermann et al. (626) ran a series of experiments. They used three pure IgM antibodies and found that none of them would induce K-cell lysis. They suggested that in previous studies in which IgM antibodies appeared to be active in this respect, the IgM preparations also contained aggregates of IgG that are known to prompt K-cell lysis. As they pointed out, if IgM antibodies are purified by a method that isolates molecules of appropriate size, IgG aggregates in the starting solution may well separate with the IgM molecules if they have a similar molecular size.

While there can be no dispute that both monocytes and K-cells can lyse antibody-coated red cells in vitro, it is less clear what role these mechanisms play in the destruction of red cells in vivo. For example, if IgG-coated red cells are labeled with ^{51}Cr and are then injected into a human, the radioactivity is all found over the spleen. Apparently the IgG-coated red cells are sequestered by splenic macrophages via the mechanism described earlier in this chapter, a finding that appears to leave no room for partial red cell destruction in the circulation by K-cells or circulating monocytes. Perhaps the situation in which a small quantity of antibody-coated red cells is injected does not fully reflect what occurs when larger volumes of red cells are destroyed in vivo. Perhaps with a small test dose the splenic macrophages compete successfully with K-cells and circulating monocytes. Perhaps when a whole unit of incompatible blood is transfused or when an autoantibody is destroying the patient's own cells, K-cell lysis and lysis by circulating monocytes play some role in the in vivo red cell destruction. Thus although the hemoglobinemia mentioned at the start of this section may represent direct red cell lysis by K-cells and monocytes in circulation, that point does not yet seem to have been proved.

There seems little doubt (627-629) that K-cell lysis is important in host defense against tumors and in combating viral infections. Further, it may be significant in transplantation immunology. As discussed in the earlier sections, various lymphocytes (and other cells) carry Fcγ and complement receptors, presumably to equip them for their role in cellular immunity.

Some Other Consequences of Complement Activation (see also table 6-11)

As mentioned several times in this chapter, the activation of complement via the classical or alternative pathway results in the generation of components with important biological functions, not all such components participate in the fixation of complement to the red cell membrane. Thus complement activation, in addition to causing red cell clearance, plays a role in the inflammatory response, the phagocytosis of bacteria, virus killing and initiation of the coagulation system. While a full description of these mechanisms is beyond the scope of this book, listed below are brief descriptions of some of the additional activities of activated complement components. Many of the activities described are initiated when complement components bind to the specific receptors. Those receptors and the cells on which they are present are listed in table 6-6.

1. Anaphylatoxins

When cleaved from C3 and C5 respectively, C3a and C5a act as anaphylatoxins. These small molecular weight proteins (C3a 9kD, C5a 11kD) cause smooth muscle contraction and the release of histamine from mast cells and platelets (630). The released histamine causes increased vascular permeability, that is, it causes dilation of capillary blood vessels allowing a larger supply of blood that contains leukocytes to reach the site of injury or infection (630-634). While anaphylatoxins are obviously important in the body's total defense mechanism, the activation of large amounts of complement and the release of huge quantities of C3a and C5a can have an adverse effect. Following an ABO incompatible blood transfusion, large amounts of complement are activated and the symptoms of flushing, headache, chest pain and fever are largely caused by C3a and C5a-mediated histamine release. C5a is more than 200 times more potent than C3a in causing anaphylactic reactions (63). While C3a and C5a have long been incriminated as causing hypersensitivity-type reactions, it is now clear that

leukotrienes are also involved (635). These substances are potent bronchoconstrictors. During cardiopulmonary bypass, plasma levels of C3a increase, plasma levels of C5a do not. During the post bypass period, granulocytopenia may be seen suggesting that C5-activated granulocytes may be trapped in the pulmonary circulation. Complement activation during cardiopulmonary bypass occurs when blood comes into contact with plastic surfaces and during oxygenation of the blood. The use of heparin and protamine during bypass surgery may also contribute to complement activation (178,179,636-640). Some perfluorocarbon blood substitutes (641) and some biomedical polymers (642) also activate complement, the latter observation is important in the selection of materials used in the manufacture of plastic blood bags and leukocyte filters.

2. Kinins and Chemotaxis

C3a and C5a, perhaps by their ability to interact with plasmin, effect generation of at least the kinins, bradykinin and kallikrein (643,644). C3a, C5a and the trimolecular complex C567 are chemotactic, that is they attract granulocytes and monocytes (macrophages) to the site of an infection (632,645). C5a is apparently the most active chemotactic agent in attracting granulocytes (631,634), it acts directly on the endothelial cells of capillaries to cause vasodilution and thus increased permeability (215).

3. Immune Adherence

Antigen-antibody-complement complexes are capable of binding to surfaces other than those on which the original antigen-antibody reaction took place. For example, bacteria coated with antibody and complement may bind to red cells or leukocytes (646,647). The immune adherence (IA) reaction is largely dependent on the presence of C3 receptors on the membrane of the cell to which the antigen-antibody-complement complex binds and it has been shown (648) that more than 100 molecules of C3 per cell are necessary for weak reactions to be seen in a system using sheep red cells. While some cells carry receptors for C4 it seems (649) that in the order of more than 3000 C4 molecules per cell are necessary for IA to occur. The role of red cells in binding immune complexes via their CR1 molecule and subsequent clearance of those immune complexes (185,519) is described above in the section dealing with extravascular destruction of red cells coated with IgG and C3.

Petz and Garratty (21) point out that macrophage sequestration of complement-coated cells may be the in vivo equivalent to in vitro immune adherence. Further, since B cells carry receptors for C3b and for C4b it follows that IA may play a role in the early stages of the immune response.

4. Innocent Bystanders (Reactive Lysis)

The term innocent bystanders is used to describe cells that have played no part in the original antigen-antibody reaction but that have become coated with the activated components of complement C567 (651-653). The term reactive lysis is commonly used to describe cell destruction by this mechanism. In terms of red cell hemolysis it is supposed that following formation of an immune complex (antigen-antibody complex) that does not involve any antigen on the red cells, complement is activated and the C567 complex is transferred (655) on to nearby red cells (innocent bystanders) that can then bind C8 and C9 and undergo intravascular lysis. This mechanism was first described (654) in patients with paroxysmal nocturnal hemoglobinuria (PNH) in whom the red cells are susceptible to lysis by very small amounts of complement because those red cells lack complement inhibitory proteins (see below). The phenomenon may also occur in patients with SLE (see above), hemolytic anemia, drug-induced hemolysis and in malarial and protozoal infections (651-653,656,657).

Reactive lysis may also occur following hemolytic transfusion reactions. For example, a group O patient, transfused in error with a quantity of group A blood will destroy the A cells infused. The A-anti-A reaction will activate complement and some of the activated components may attach to the patient's own group O cells. By this mechanism red cell destruction in excess of the amount of incompatible blood actually transfused may occur (658-660). The phenomenon has also been associated with the passenger lymphocyte syndrome following ABO incompatible bone marrow transplants (661).

In terms of red cell destruction, reactive lysis is an unwanted event. In other circumstances the phenomenon plays a role in host defense. For example, complement activation may occur at the site of an injury. Invading bacteria may then become coated with activated complement even though no antibody against those bacteria was present. The bacteria will then be more susceptible to phagocytosis (662).

5. Coagulation

For many years it was believed that the disseminated intravascular coagulation (DIC) that is often seen following intravascular hemolysis, e.g. following major-

side ABO incompatible transfusion, was initiated by interactions between activated complement components and proteins of the coagulation cycle. The interactions were poorly understood. The lysosomal enzyme that cleaves C5 was reported to be able to activate Hageman factor (663,664). Red cell stroma were believed also to be able to initiate the complement cascade (665,666). Activators of the alternative pathway were shown to decrease the clotting time in rabbits but not in man (667,668). Reports (669,670) that plasmin can activate C1 and C3 were thought, perhaps to indicate the existence of a positive feed-back mechanism. More recently it has become appreciated that the generation and release of certain cytokines following ABO antibody-induced hemolysis (580,581,584,586-588) has a profound effect on the coagulation system. As examples, tumor necrosis factor (TNF) can act directly to activate the common coagulation pathway (671,672), it also degrades cell surface thrombomodulin (673). Both interleukin-1 (IL-1) and TNF change the hemostatic properties of endothelial cell surfaces (that are now known to play important roles in coagulation) and effect an increase in tissue factor and a decrease in thrombomodulin (674,675). The net effect of these changes is to alter the activity of protein C that acts as an anticoagulant by proteolytic cleavage of factors V and VIII. Thus while the activation of complement during intravascular red cell destruction is involved with disturbances in the coagulation cycles, its effects seem less direct than was originally believed (585, see also Chapter 36).

Complement Deficiency (see also table 6-11)

It is somewhat ironic, in view of the wide range of biological systems in which complement is involved, that individuals who have genetic deficiencies leading to lack or markedly reduced production of a particular component are often not particularly ill. Genetic deficiencies of most of the components have been documented (70-73,676-681) sometimes the deficiency does not result in any clinical abnormality. In individuals with a genetic lack of C1, C4 or C2, complement activation can still proceed via the alternative pathway that does not use those components.

Systemic lupus erythematosus (SLE) or an SLE-like syndrome have been associated with deficiencies of C1r, C1s, C4, C2, C5, C8 and C1-inhibitor in different individuals (682). However, as mentioned above, other persons with similar deficiencies have been free of disease. The strongest association between complement deficiency and disease appears to involve SLE in patients deficient in C4. From a review of many reports (683-690) Moulds (691) noted that of 18 published cases of total C4 deficiency, 14 of the patients had SLE. In Whites the *C4A* null gene is most often associated with the HLA-A1, B8, DR3 phenotype, in Blacks it is associated with that phenotype and with the HLA-B44 and DR2 haplotypes. The *C4A* null gene has also been associated with other autoimmune diseases including Graves' disease, systemic sclerosis, rheumatoid arthritis, Sjogren's syndrome, juvenile dermatomyositis, IgA nephrophathy and subacute sclerosing panencephalities (692-695). The *C4B* null gene has been associated with IgA nephropathy, rheumatoid arthritis (696-698) and lack of C4B protein in children results in increased susceptibility to bacterial meningitis (699). Presence of the *C4B* null gene in HIV infected individuals may be associated with the progression of ARC to AIDS (700,701). Further discussion of these associations and the association of C4 allotypes with disease will be found in Chapter 27.

Deficiencies in Complement Regulation (see also table 6-11)

As might be expected, since the autologous activation of complement is an ongoing and dynamic event, individuals with genetic deficiencies of production of complement regulatory proteins sometimes suffer more serious clinical problems than those who do not make certain complement components (70-73,702-707).

In hereditary angioneurotic edema (HAE) a C1-esterase inhibitor (C1-INH) is produced at a level far below that of healthy individuals (132,702). Normally, this inhibitor acts not only on C1-esterase but also on several enzymes activated during the coagulation cascade. In acute attacks of HAE the available C1-INH is used so that as complement activation continues vascular permeability (due to the effects of C3a and C5a) increases and considerable tissue edema results (75). This situation can become life-threatening (132,702) if the edema is in an area such as the throat, that restricts breathing. However, the simple infusion of plasma containing C1-INH effects a speedy and dramatic reversal of the symptoms. The severity of a severe acute attack of HAE illustrates the biological importance of complement component regulatory proteins in normal individuals.

Two patients have been described (704,708) in whose plasma there was no C3b INA (now more often called factor I, see earlier in this chapter). The patients had low levels of C3 and of factor B and it was felt that lack of C3b INA represented consumption of that protein following constant activation of the alternative pathway and utilization of the C3b INA. The patients presented with frequent infections and the activated C̄3b became red cell bound so that the DAT when performed with a reagent containing anti-C3 was positive. The positive

DAT was not associated with an accelerated rate of in vivo red cell clearance (see earlier in this chapter for a discussion of the relatively poor macrophage clearance of red cells coated with C3 in the absence of immunoglobulin).

As described earlier, decay accelerating factor (DAF) is a phosphatidyl-inositol linked red cell membrane protein that acts to inhibit formation and accelerate decay of both C3 and C5 convertases. Lack of DAF from PNH red cells (that have a defective P-I anchor) was at first thought to explain their exquisite sensitivity to complement-induced hemolysis. However, the finding (155-157) that red cells of the Inab phenotype, that are devoid of DAF, have only a limited increase in susceptibility to complement-induced lysis, showed that the role of DAF can presumably be performed by other proteins present on Inab red cells.

In contrast to the lack of DAF, lack of CD59, the membrane inhibitor of reactive lysis (147,151,167), seems severely to compromise red cells. It is currently believed that absence of this PI-linked regulatory protein, that inhibits the binding of C7 and C8 to the membrane (57,58,148,157,163) and/or binds to C8 to prevent the attachment of C9 (164,164,170) represents the major defect that imparts sensitivity to complement-induced lysis to PNH (actually PNH III) red cells.

Complement Utilization

In some disease states such as SLE, acute glomerulonephritis, bacterial endocarditis and some in which large numbers of immune complexes are formed, complement activation may proceed at a rate greater than synthesis of complement components, resulting in reduced levels of some of the components in the patients' plasma. In cold hemagglutinin disease (see Chapter 38) acute episodes of red cell destruction involve complement-mediated intravascular hemolysis of the red cells. If enough intravascular hemolysis occurs (with all the components of complement from C1 to C9 involved) depletion of the supply of one or more of the components may become the limiting factor in the hemolytic process. For this reason, blood bankers are sometimes asked to supply washed cells for transfusion to these patients. Use of such cells avoids the infusion of complement components present in the donor's plasma. However, limitation of antibody or restriction of the antibody's thermal range are much more often the limiting factors than is complement depletion by utilization. Accordingly, it used to be recommended that complement assays be performed to demonstrate depletion before washed cells were issued. However, it is now considerably easier to wash donor red cells than it is to perform complement assays.

TABLE 6-11 Some Non-Immunohematological Considerations about Complement

1. Some consequences of complement activation
   a) Generation of anaphylatoxins that cause smooth muscle contraction, release of histamine and increased vascular permeability
   b) Generation of the kinins, bradykinin and kallikrein
   c) Chemotaxis, attract granulocytes and macrophages to the site of injury
   d) Immune adherance leading to clearance of immune complexes and possible participation in generation of an immune response
   e) Reactive lysis, clearance of cells that played no role in the initiation of complement activation
   f) Interaction with components of the coagulation cascade

2. Diseases that may sometimes be associated with complement deficiency
   a) Systemic lupus erythematosus (SLE)
   b) SLE-like syndromes
   c) Graves' disease
   d) Rheumatoid arthritis
   e) Sjogren's syndrome
   f) Juvenile dermatomyositis
   g) Subacute sclerosing panencephalites
   h) IgA nephropathy
   i) Susceptibility to bacterial meningitis

3. Diseases associated with deficiencies of complement regulation
   a) Hereditary angioneurotic edema
   b) Paroxysmal nocturnal hemoglobinuria
   c) Susceptibility to bacterial infections
   d) Possibly a protein-losing enteropathy

In patients with liver disease there may be a reduced amount of complement components present because of impaired synthesis of the proteins. In inflammatory conditions such as rheumatoid arthritis, ulcerative colitis, gout, etc., there may be increased levels of complement in the plasma.

The In Vivo Clearance of Senescent Red Cells

It is perhaps fitting that in a chapter in which so much has been written about red cell clearance in vivo, the last section should deal with the clearance of such cells at the end of their normal life span. In spite of the optimistic title of this section there is, as yet, no complete agreement as to how aged red cells are removed from the circulation. Originally it was believed that red cell simply died as the activity of various membrane associated enzymes diminished and/or was lost (323-326). While there is no doubt that some enzymes, such as hexokinase, are present in much higher quantities in reticulocytes than in mature red cells while others, such as pyruvate kinase, gradually decrease in levels as red cells age, there is no proof that these changes actually cause cell death (327-329). Beutler (327,328) has pointed out that the questions about relationship of red cell age to levels of enzyme activity are not likely to be completely answered until such time as a better method for the isolation of pure suspensions of old red cells is developed, than exists at present.

One incontrovertible finding is that red cells shed pieces of their membranes as they age and that vesicles comprised of shed membrane particles can be isolated and studied (330-332,715-718). This phenomenon occurs both in vivo (717) and in vitro (716) and loss of portions of the membrane results in the conversion of red cells from their discoid to a spherocyte-like shape (332). However, this finding could represent loss of portions of the membrane that carry enzymes, or loss of membrane structures that expose de novo antigens on the membrane surface, that would be compatible with the alternative theories of senescent red cell clearance discussed below.

In 1975, Kay (719) reported discovery of what was called the senescent cell antigen (SCA). Since then, Kay and her colleagues have performed a huge number of studies on this structure, for full details see a recent review (720) that includes references to 32 publications by these workers. To summarize, briefly, it is claimed that as red cells age, physiological changes result in cleavage of protein band 3 and that the SCA is thus exposed or created by a new orientation of the protein. Further, it is claimed that all normal sera contain natural IgG antibodies to SCA, that the oldest red cells in circulation with the maximum number of exposed copies of SCA bind that IgG and are then sequestered and destroyed by macrophage recognition of the red cell bound IgG, as described in the section above on extravascular clearance of IgG-coated red cells. While the studies on isolation of the IgG anti-SCA, its binding to the oldest population of red cells and the molecular biological studies on band 3 and SCA appear convincing, the findings are not always in complete agreement with those of others.

Some workers (721,728) have produced evidence that they interpret as indicating binding of IgG to clusters of band 3 that are formed by denaturation of hemoglobin in older red cells. This concept and that of Kay (720) are not mutually exclusive. However, Galili et al. (722,723) claimed that the IgG antibody that binds to aged red cells and causes them to be subject to macrophage-mediated phagocytosis, had anti-alpha-galactosyl residue specificity. It was claimed that as sialic acid was removed from aging red cells (a proved event (715,724)) the alpha-galactosyl residues became exposed. This conclusion was disputed by Kay et al. (725) who, among other findings, reported that their anti-SCA was inhibited by non-glycosylated synthetic peptides.

The concepts that senescent red cells are cleared by phagocytosis because they are coated with IgG autoantibody (whatever its specificity) may explain the finding that normal red cells carry some IgG on their surface. In various studies (17,18,21,726,727) it has been shown that normal red cells carry (on average) some 30 to 40 molecules of IgG per cell. Clearly that number is too small (see earlier section) to promote in vivo phagocytosis. However, the 30 to 40 molecules per cell estimates were made using whole red cell populations. Since some 1% of an individual's red cells are cleared per day, the average of 30 to 40 molecules per cell might represent none on young cells and far more than 30 to 40 on old cells (i.e. perhaps 300 to 400 molecules per cell on the oldest 1% of cells). Perhaps the flow cytometer will prove useful in determining if the IgG on normal red cells is evenly distributed among many cells, or concentrated on a few.

Attractive as theories about the removal of senescent red cells by IgG autoantibody coating may be (some workers believe that some cases of WAIHA may represent over production of this physiological autoantibody), there are still some unanswered questions. To mention just a few, first, it has not yet been completely proved that the IgG bound represents autoantibody and not simply cytophilic IgG adsorbed non-specifically from the plasma. Second, since aged red cells have not yet been isolated in pure form (except by the so-called physiological autoantibodies that may be selecting a population of cells different from those 100 to 120 days old) it cannot be said for sure that they have increased levels of IgG bound and/or reduced levels of certain enzymes. Third, prolonged red cell life is not seen in individuals from whom the spleen has been removed following injury, as might be expected if phagocytosis of red cells coated with (relatively low levels of) IgG was the sole mechanism of senescent cell removal. Suffice it here to say that obviously much remains to be learned about what is clearly a normal physiological event.

References

1. Coombs RRA, Mourant AE, Race RR. Lancet 1945;2:15
2. Coombs RRA, Mourant AE, Race RR. Br J Exp Path 1945;26:255
3. Moreschi C. Zbl Bakt 1908;46:49
4. Dacie JV, Crookston JH, Christenson WN. Br J Haematol 1957;3:77
5. Lachmann PJ, Oldroyd RG, Milstein C, et al. Immunology 1980;41:503
6. Barker JM. Transfusion 1982;22:507
7. Lachmann PJ, Voak D, Oldroyd RG, et al. Vox Sang 1983;45:367
8. Voak D, Downie DM, Moore BPL, et al. Biotest Bull 1986;1:7
9. Holt PDJ, Donaldson C, Judson PA, et al. Transfusion 1985;25:267
10. Engelfriet CP, Voak D. Vox Sang 1987;53:241
11. Downie DM, Voak D, Jarvis J, et al. Biotest Bull 1983;4:348
12. Voak D, Nilsson U. J Immunogenet 1990;17:331
13. Scott ML, Voak D. In: Immunobiology of Transfusion Medicine, New York:Marcel Dekker, 1994;365
14. Kugele F, Wilkerson P, Carney M. (abstract). Transfusion 1993;33(suppl 9S):29S
15. Dupuy ME, Elliot M, Masouredis SP. Vox Sang 1964;9:40
16. Hughes-Jones NC, Polley MJ, Telford R, et al. Vox Sang 1964;9:385
17. Gilliland BC, Baxter E, Evans RS. New Eng J Med 1971;285:252
18. Gilliland BC, Evans RS. In: Recent Advances in Immunohematology, Washington, D.C.:Am Assoc Blood Banks, 1973:31
19. Romano EL, Hughes-Jones NC, Mollison PL. Br Med J 1973;1:524
20. Burkhardt D, Rosenfield RE, Hsu TCS, et al. Vox Sang 1974;26:289
21. Petz LD, Garratty G. Acquired Immune Hemolytic Anemias. New York:Churchill Livingstone 1980:307
22. Stratton F, Rawlinson VI, Merry AH, et al. Clin Lab Haematol 1983;5:17
23. Steane EA. In: A Seminar on Antigen-Antibody Reactions Revisited. Arlington, VA:Am Assoc Blood Banks, 1982:67
24. French EE. Lancet 1968;1:664
25. Löw B, Messeter L. Vox Sang 1974;26:53
26. Moore HC, Mollison PL. Transfusion 1976;16:291
27. Wicker B, Wallas CH. Transfusion 1976;16:469
28. Lalezari P, Jiang AF. Transfusion 1980;20:206
29. Nance SJ, Garratty G. Am J Clin Pathol 1987;87:633
30. Chaplin H Jr. Prog Hematol 1973;8:25
31. Grey HM, Kunkel HG. J Exp Med 1964;120:253
32. Terry WD, Fahey JL. Science 1964;146:400
33. Steinberg AG, Cook CE. The Distribution of the Human Immunoglobulin Allotypes. Oxford: Oxford Univ Press, 1981
34. Natvig JB, Kunkel HG. Nature 1967;215:68
35. Natvig JB, Kunkel HG. Ser Hematol 1968;1:66
36. Frame M, Mollison PL, Terry WD. Nature 1970;255:641
37. Abramson H, Schur PH. Blood 1972;40:500
38. Schur PH. Prog Clin Immunol 1972;1:71
39. Morrell A, Skvaril F, Rufener JL. Vox Sang 1973;24:323
40. Devey ME, Voak D. Immunology 1974;27:1073
41. Hunt JS, Beck ML, Hardman JT, et al. Am J Clin Pathol 1980;74:259
42. Pierce SR, Hardman JT, Hunt JS, et al. (abstract). Transfusion 1980;20:627
43. Tregellas WM, Pierce SR, Hardman JT, et al. (abstract). Transfusion 1980;20:628
44. Hardman JT, Beck ML. Transfusion 1981;21:343
45. Szymanski IO, Huff SR, Delsignore R. Transfusion 1982;22:90
46. Vengelen-Tyler V, Morel P. Transfusion 1983;23:114
47. Devenish A, Burslem MF, Morris R, et al. Transfusion 1986;26:426
48. Anderson G, Gray LS, Mintz PD. Am J Clin Pathol 1991;95:87
49. Natvig JB. Acta Path Microbiol Scand 1965;65:467
50. Issitt PD. Adv Immunohematol 1977; Vol 4:No 4
51. Issitt PD. Adv Immunohematol 1977; Vol 4:No 5
52. Issitt PD. Adv Immunohematol 1977; Vol 4:No 6

53. Shore SL, Phillips DJ, Reimer CB. Immunochemistry 1971;8:562
54. Müller-Eberhard HJ. Ann Rev Biochem 1975;44:697
55. Vroon DH, Shulz DR, Zarco RM. Immunochemistry 1970;7:43
56. Pangburn MK. Fed Proc 1983;42:139
57. Devine DV. Transf Med Rev 1991;5:123
58. Parker CJ. In: Current Topics in Microbiology and Immunology. Heidelberg:Springer Verlag 1992;178:184
59. Müller-Eberhard HJ. Springer Sem Immunopathol 1983;6:2
60. Frank MM, Fries LF. In: Fundamental Immunology, 2nd Ed. New York:Raven, 1989:679
61. Morgan BP. Complement. Clinical Aspects and Relevance to Disease. London:Academic Press, 1990
62. Garratty G. CRC Crit Rev Clin Lab Sci 1985;20:25
63. Freedman J, Semple JW. In: Immunobiology of Transfusion Medicine. New York:Marcel Dekker 1994:403
64. Mayer MM. Experimental Immunochemistry.Springfield:Thomas, 1961
65. Müller-Eberhard HJ. Textbook of Immunopathology. New York:Grune and Stratton, 1968
66. Müller-Eberhard HJ. In: Adv Immunol 1968, Vol 8
67. Müller-Eberhard HJ. Ann Rev Biochem 1969;38:389
68. Rapp HJ, Borsos T. Molecular Basis of Complement Action.New York:Appleton-Century-Crofts, 1970
69. Schultz DR. Monographs in Allergy. Basel:Karger, 1971, Vol 6
70. Ruddy S, Gigli I, Austen KF. New Eng J Med 1972;287:489
71. Ruddy S, Gigli I, Austen KF. New Eng J Med 1972;287:545
72. Ruddy S, Gigli I, Austen KF. New Eng J Med 1972;287:592
73. Ruddy S, Gigli I, Austen KF. New Eng J Med 1972;287:642
74. Mayer MM. Proc Nat Acad Sci USA 1972;69:2954
75. Brown DL. Br J Haematol 1975;30:377
76. Frank MM, Atkinson JP. Complement in Clinical Medicine. Chicago:Year Book Pub,1975
77. Cuman B, Sandberg-Tragardh L, Peterson PA. Biochemistry 1977;16:5368
78. Podack ER, Kolb WP, Müller-Eberhard HJ. J Immunol 1978;120:1841
79. Podack ER, Kolb WP, Esser AF, et al. J Immunol 1979;123:1071
80. Steckel EW, York RG, Monahan JB, et al. J Biol Chem 1980;255:11997
81. Biesecker G, Müller-Eberhard HJ. J Immunol 1980;124:1291
82. Isenman DE, Cooper NR. Mol Immunol 1981;18:331
83. Petz LD, Swisher SN. Clinical Practice of Blood Transfusion. New York:Churchill Livingstone, 1981:45
84. Discipio RG, Gagnon J. Mol Immunol 1982;19:1425
85. Steckel EW, Welbaum BE, Sodetz JM. J Biol Chem 1983;258:4318
86. Silversmith RE, Nelsestuen GL. Biochemistry 1986;25:841
87. Müller-Eberhard HJ. Ann Rev Immunol 1986;4:503
88. Podack ER. J Cell Biochem 1986;30:133
89. Schonermark S, Filsinger S, Berger B, et al. Immunology 1988;63:585
90. Garratty G. Am J Clin Pathol 1970;54:531
91. Bulletin of the World Health Organization 1968;31:935
92. Roitt AM, Brostoff J, Male DK. Immunology. Toronto:Mosby, 1985:7
93. Coleman RM, Lombard MF, Sicard RE, et al. Fundamental Immunology.Dubuque:Wm C Brown, 1989:209
94. Letendre P. (Letter). Transfusion 1990;30:478
95. Müller-Eberhard HJ, Nilsson UR, Dalmasso AP, et al. Arch Pathol 1966;82:205
96. Svehag SE, Manheim L. Bloth B. Nature New Biol 1972;238:117
97. Shelton E, Yonemasu K, Stroud RM. Proc Nat Acad Sci USA 1972;69:65
98. Schumaker VN, Zavodsky P, Poon PH. Ann Rev Immunol 1987;5:21
99. Colomb MJ, Arloud GL,Villiers CL. Complement 1984;1:69
100. Tenner AJ, Frank MM. J Immunol 1986;137:625
101 .Hughes-Jones NC. In: Immunobiology of the Complement System. London:Academic Press, 1986
102. Sim RB, Twose TW, Paterson DS, et al. Biochem J 1981;193:115
103. Tack BF, Harrison RA, Janatova J. Proc Nat Acad Sci USA 1980;77:5764
104. Law SK, Levine RP. Proc Nat Acad Sci USA 1977;74:2701
105. Harrison RA, Lachmann PJ. Mol Immunol 1980;17:9
106. Jenkins DE Jr, Moore WH, Luthringer DG, et al. Transfusion 1975;15:402
107. Freedman J, Mollison PL. Vox Sang 1976;31:241
108. Fruitstone MJ. (Letter). Transfusion 1978;18:125
109. Carlo JR, Ruddy S, Studer EJ, et al. J Immunol 1979;123:523
110. Chaplin H Jr, Freedman J, Massey A, et al. Transfusion 1980;20:256
111. Engelfriet CP, Overbeeke MAM, Voak D. In: Progress in Transfusion Medicine Vol 2. Edinburgh:Churchill:Livingstone, 1987
112. Pillemer L, Blum L, Lepow IH, et al. Science 1954;120:279
113. Pillemer L. Ann NY Acad Sci 1956;66:233
114. Pensky J, Wurz L, Pillemer L. Z Immun Forsch 1959;118:329
115. Blum L, Pillemer L, Lepow IH. Z Immun Forsch 1959;118:349
116. Nelson RA. J Exp Med 1958;108:515
117. Schur PH, Becker EL. J Exp Med 1963;118:891
118. Gewurz H, Shin HS, Mergenhagen SE. J Exp Med 1968;128:1049
119. Ellman L, Green I, Frank MM. Science 1970;170:74
120. Marcus RL, Shin HS, Mayer MM. Proc Nat Acad Sci USA 1971;68:1351
121. Frank MM, May J, Gaither T, et al. J Exp Med 1971;134:176
122. Götze O, Müller-Eberhard HJ. J Exp Med 1971;134:91
123. Sandberg AL, Oliveira B, Osler AG. J Immunol 1971;106:282
124. Lepow IH, Rosen FS. New Eng J Med 1972;286:942
125. Naff GB. New Eng J Med 1972;287:716
126. Goldlust MB, Shin HS, Hammer CH, et al. J Immunol 1974;113:998
127. Schreiber RD, Pangburn MK, Lesavre PH, et al. Proc Nat Acad Sci USA 1978;75:3948
128. Pangburn MK, Schreiber RD, Müller-Eberhard HJ. J Exp Med 1977;146:257
129. Pangburn MK, Müller-Eberhard HJ. Springer Sem Immunopathol 1984;7:163
130. Rosse WF, Dourmashkin R, Humphrey JH. J Exp Med 1966;123:969
131. Podack ER. In: Immunobiology of the Complement System. London:Academic Press, 1986
132. Donaldson VH, Evans RR. Am J Med 1963;35:37
133. Rothfield N, Ross HA, Minta JO, et al. New Eng J Med 1972;287:681
134. Alper CA. New Eng J Med 1973;288:109
135. Tamura N, Nelson RA. J Immunol 1967;99:582
136. Lachmann PJ, Müller-Eberhard HJ. J Immunol 1968;100:691
137. Ruddy S, Austen K. J Immunol 1969;102:533
138. Ruddy S, Austen K. J Immunol 1971;107:742
139. Conrad DH, Carlo JR, Ruddy S. J Exp Med 1978;147:1792
140. Weiler JM, Daha MR, Austen KF, et al. Proc Nat Acad Sci USA 1976;73:3268

141. Fearon DT. Proc Nat Acad Sci USA 1979;76:5867
142. Lambris JD, Dobson NJ, Ross GD. J Exp Med 1980;152:1625
143. Parker CJ, Frame RN, Elstad MR. Blood 1988;71:86
144. Rosse WF, Dacie JV. J Clin Invest 1966;45:736
145. Parker CJ, Baker PJ, Rosse WF. J Clin Invest 1982;69:337
146. Parker CJ, Wiedmer T, Sims PJ, et al. J Clin Invest 1985;75:2074
147. Holguin MH, Wilcox LA, Bernshaw NJ, et al. J Clin Invest 1989;84:1387
148. Holguin MH, Fredrick LR, Bernshaw NJ, et al. J Clin Invest 1989;84:7
149. Parker CJ, Stone OL, Bernshaw NJ. J Immunol 1989;142:208
150. Rosse WF. Blood 1990;75:1595
151. Yamashina M, Ueda E, Kinoshita T, et al. New Eng J Med 1990;323:1185
152. Nicholson-Weller A, Burge J, Fearon DT, et al. J Immunol 1982;129:184
153. Medof ME, Kinoshita T, Nussenzweig V. J Exp Med 1984;160:1558
154. Nicholson-Weller A. In: Current Topics in Microbiology and Immunology. Heidelberg:Springer Verlag 1992;178:7
155. Telen MJ, Green AM. Blood 1989;74:437
156. Merry AH, Rawlinson VI, Uchikawa M, et al. Br J Haematol 1989;73:248
157. Holguin MH, Martin CB, Bernshaw NJ, et al. J Immunol 1992;148:498
158. Spring FA, Judson PA, Daniels GL, et al. Immunology 1987;62:307
159. Telen MJ, Hall SE, Green AM, et al. J Exp Med 1988;167:1993
160. Telen MJ. In: Blood Groups: Chido/Rodgers, Knops/McCoy/York and Cromer.Bethesda, MD:Am Assoc Blood Banks, 1992:45
161. Seya T, Turner J, Atkinson JP. J Exp Med 1986;163:837
162. Liszewski MK, Atkinson JP. In: Current Topics in Microbiology and Immunology. Heidelberg:Springer-Verlag, 1992;178:45
163. Holguin MH, Wilcox LA, Bernshaw NJ, et al. Blood 1990;75:284
164. Meri S, Morgan BP, Davies A, et al. Immunology 1990;71:1
165. Rollins SA, Zhao J, Ninomiya H, et al. J Immunol 1991;146:2345
166. Zalman LS, Wood LM, Müller-Eberhard HJ.Proc Nat Acad Sci USA 1986;82:7711
167. Schonermark S, Rauterberg EW, Shin ML, et al. J Immunol 1986;136:1772
168. Hansch GM, Weller PF, Nicholson-Weller A. Blood 1988;72:1089
169. Sugita Y, Nakano Y, Tomita M. J Biochem 1988;104:663
170. Sugita Y, Takashi T, Oda E, et al. J Biochem 1989;106:555
171. Okada N, Yasuda T, Tsumita H, et al. Biochem Biophys Res Comm 1982;108:770
172. Okada H, Tanaka H. Mol Immunol 1983;20:1233
173. Brauch H, Roelcke D, Rother U. Immunobiology 1983;165:115
174. Tomita A, Radike E, Parker CJ. J Immunol 1993;151:3308
175. Anstee DJ.Sem Hematol 1981;18:13
176. Dahr W. In: Recent Advances in Blood Group Biochemistry.Arlington, VA:Am Assoc Blood Banks, 1986:27
177. Anderson RA, Lovrien RE. Nature 1984;307:665
178. Berger M, Gaither TA, Frank MM. Clin Immunol Rev 1983;1:471
179. Schreiber AD. Springer Sem Immunopathol 1984;7:221
180. Ross GD, Medof ME. Adv Immunol 1985;37:217
181. Sim RB, Malhotra V, Day AJ, et al. Immunol Lett

182. Unkeless JC, Wright SD. In: Inflammation: Basic Principles and Clinical Correlates. New York:Raven 1988:343
183. Ehlenberger AG, Nussenzweig V. J Exp Med 1977;145:357
184. Medorf ME, Iida K, Mold C, et al. J Exp Med 1982;156:1739
185. Cornacoff JB, Hebert LA, Smead WL, et al. J Clin Invest 1983;71:236
186. Ng YC, Schifferli JA, Walport MJ. Clin Exp Immunol 1988;71:481
187. Walport MJ, Lachmann PJ. Arthritis Rheum 1988;31:153
188. Moulds JM, Nickells MW, Moulds JJ, et al. J Exp Med 1991;173:1159
189. Rao N, Ferguson DJ, Lee SF, et al. J Immunol 1991;146:3501
190. Cooper NR, Moore MD, Nemerow GR. Ann Rev Immunol 1988;6:85
191. Ross GD. Curr Opinion in Immunol 1989;2:50
192. Ross CR, Yount WJ, Walport MJ, et al. J Immunol 1985;135:2005
193. Ross GD. In: Immunobiology of the Complement System. New York:Academic Press, 1986
194. Borsos T, Rapp HL. Science 1965;150:505
195. Ishizaka T, Ishizaka K, Borsos T, et al. J Immunol 1966;97:716
196. Humphrey JH, Dourmashkin RR. Adv Immunol 1969;11:75
197. Hughes-Jones NC, Gorick BD, Miller NGA, et al. Eur J Immunol 1984;14:974
198. Ishizaka K, Ishizaka T, Lee EH, et al. J Immunol 1965;95:197
199. Müller-Eberhard HJ, Hadding U, Calcott MA. In: Immunopathology 5th International Symposium. Basel:Schwabe, 1967:179
200. Augener W, Grey HM, Cooper NR, et al. Immunochemistry 1971;8:1011
201. Michaelsen TE, Kornstad L. Clin Exp Immunol 1987;67:637
202. Garratty G. In: Immune Destruction of Red Blood Cells. Arlington, VA:Am Assoc Blood Banks, 1989:109
203. Waller M, Lawler D. Vox Sang 1962;7:591
204. Ayland J, Horton MA, Tippett PA, et al. Vox Sang 1978;34:40
205. Kline WE, Sullivan CM, Pope M, et al. Vox Sang 1982;43:335
206. Frankowska K, Gorska B. Arch Immunol Therap Exp 1978;26:1095
207. Parinaud J, Blanc C, Grandjean H, et al. Am J Obstet Gynecol 1985;151:1111
208. Mattila PS, Seppala IJT, Eklund J, et al. Vox Sang 1985;48:350
209. Shaw DR, Conley ME, Knox FJ, et al. Transfusion 1988;28:127
210. Mollison PL. Br J Haematol 1970;18:249
211. Rosse WF. J Clin Invest 1968;45:2430
212. Freedman J, Massey A, Chaplin H, et al. Br J Haematol 1980;45:309
213. Hughes-Jones NC, Ghosh S. FEBS Lett 1981;128:318
214. Hughes-Jones NC. Unpublished observations cited by Mollison, PL, Engelfriet CP, Contreras M. In: Blood Transfusion in Clinical Medicine, 9th Ed. Oxford:Blackwell, 1993:224
215. Mollison PL, Engelfriet CP, Contreras M. Blood Transfusion in Clinical Medicine, 9th Ed. Oxford:Blackwell, 1993
216. Lomas C, Tippett P, Thompson KM, et al. Vox Sang 1989;57:261
217. Nicholson GL, Masouredis SP, Singer SJ. Proc Nat Acad Sci USA 1971;68:1416
218. Singer SJ, Nicholson GL. Science 1972;175:720
219. Romano EL, Stolinsky C, Hughes-Jones NC. Br J Haematol 1975;30:507

1986;14:183

220. Victoria EJ, Muchmore E, Sudora E, et al. J Clin Invest 1975;56:292

221. Masouredis SP. In: Membrane Structure and Function of Human Blood Cells.Washington, D.C.:Am Assoc Blood Banks, 1976:37

222. Elsaeter A, Branton D. J Cell Biol 1974;63:1018

223. Peters R, Peters J, Tews KH, et al. Biochem Biophys Acta 1974;367:282

224. Schekman R, Singer SJ. Proc Nat Acad Sci USA 1976;73:4075

225. Furcht LT, Jensen NJ, Palm S. (abstract). Transfusion 1978;28:644

226. Rosenfield RE. In: A Seminar on Performance Evaluation. Washington, D.C.; Am Assoc Blood Banks, 1976:93

227. Douglas SD. Unpublished observations 1976 cited by Rosenfield RE. In: A Seminar on Performance Evaluation. Washington, D.C.; Am Assoc Blood Banks, 1976

228. Davis WC, Douglas SD, Petz LD, et al. J Immunol 1968;101:621

229. Sela M. Unpublished observations 1976 cited by Rosenfield RE. In: A Seminar on Performance Evaluation. Washington, D.C.; Am Assoc Blood Banks, 1976

230. Rimon A, Sela M. Biochem Biophys Acta 1966;124:408

231. Cartron J-P. Blood Rev 1994;8:199

232. Colin Y, Bailly P, Cartron J-P. Vox Sang 1994;67(Suppl S3):67

233. Anstee DJ, Mallinson G. Vox Sang 1994;67 (Suppl S3):1

234. Anstee DJ, Tanner MJA. Bailliere's Clin Hematol 1993;6:401

235. Cartron J-P, Agre P. Sem Hematol 1993;30:193

236. Hidalgo C, Romano CL, Linares J, et al. Transfusion 1979;19:250

237. Edgington TS. J Immunol 1971;106:673

238. Masouredis SP. J Clin Invest 1960;39:1450

239. Rochna E, Hughes-Jones NC. Vox Sang 1965;10:675

240. Masouredis SP, Dupuy ME, Elliot M. J Clin Invest 1967;46:681

241. Hughes-Jones NC, Gardner B. Vox Sang 1971;21:154

242. Hughes-Jones NC, Gardner B, Lincoln P. Vox Sang 1971;21:210

243. Masouredis SP, Sudora E, Mahon L, et al. Blood 1980;56:969

244. Merry AH, Thomson EE, Anstee DJ, et al. Immunology 1984;51:793

245. Merry AH, Hodson C, Thomson EE, et al. Biochem J 1986;233:93

246. Merry AH, Gardner B, Parsons SF, et al. Vox Sang 1987;53:57

247. Anstee DJ, Spring FA. Transf Med Rev 1989;3:13

248. Anstee DJ. Vox Sang 1990;58:1

249. Anstee DJ. J Immunogenet 1990;17:219

250. Watkins WM. Proc Roy Soc Lond B 1978;202:31

251. Levine P, Celano MJ, Falkowski F. Transfusion 1963;3:278

252. Knapp T. Can J Med Tech 1964;26:172

253. Kortekangas AE, Kaarsalo E, Melartin L, et al. Vox Sang 1965;10:385

254. Worlledge SM, Rousso C. Vox Sang 1965;10:293

255. Fraser BS, Malette MF. Immunochemistry 1974;11:581

256. Naiki M, Marcus DM. Biochem Biophys Res Comm 1974;60:1105

257. Marcus DM, Naiki M, Kundu SK. Proc Nat Acad Sci USA 1976;73:3263

258. Marcus DM, Kundu SK, Suzuki A. Sem Hematol 1981;18:63

259. Marcus DM. Immunol Ser 1989;43:701

260. Spitalnik PF, Spitalnik SL. Transf Med Rev 1995;9:110

261. Polley MJ, Mollison PL. Transfusion 1961;1:9

262. Polley MJ, Mollison PL, Soothill JF. Br J Haematol 1962;8:149

263. Adinolfi M, Polley MJ, Hunter DA, et al. Immunology 1962;2:566

264. Stratton F, Gunson HH, Rawlinson VI. Transfusion 1962;2:135

265. Stratton F, Smith DS, Rawlinson VI.Clin Exp Immunol 1968;3:81

266. Stratton F, Smith DS, Rawlinson VI. J Clin Pathol 1968;21:708

267. Holburn AJ. Immunology 1973;24:1019

268. Petz LD, Garratty G. Prog Clin Immunol 1974;2:175

269. Stratton F. Wadley Med Bull 1975;5:182

270. Sherwood GK, Haynes BF, Rosse WF. Transfusion 1976;16:417

271. Issitt PD, Smith TR. In: A Seminar on Performance Evaluation. Washington, D.C.:Am Assoc Blood Banks, 1976:25

272. Wright MS, Issitt PD.Transfusion 1979;19:688

273. Garratty G, Petz LD. (Letter). Transfusion 1975;15:397

274. Howard JE, Winn LC, Gottlieb CE, et al. Transfusion 1982;22:269

275. Nasongkla M, Hummert J, Chaplin H Jr. Transfusion 1982;22:273

276. Howell P, Giles CM. Vox Sang 1983;45:129

277. Fischer JT, Petz LD, Garratty G. Blood 1974;44:359

278. Graham H, Davies DM Jr, Tigner JA, et al. Transfusion 1976;16:530

279. Rosenfield RE, Jagathambal.Transfusion 1978;18:517

280. Tilley CA, Romans DG, Crookston MC. Nature 1978;276:613

281. Freedman J, Massey A. Vox Sang 1979;37:1

282. Freedman J, Massey A. J Clin Pathol 1980;37:977

283. Chaplin H, Nasongkla M, Monroe MC. Br J Haematol 1981;48:69

284. Freedman J, Barefoot C. Transfusion 1982;22:511

285. Merry AH, Thomas EE, Rawlinson VI, et al. Clin Lab Haematol 1983;5:387

286. Giles CM. Exp Clin Immunogenet 1988;5:99

287. Giles CM, Davies KA,Walport MJ. Transfusion 1991;31:223

288. Garratty G, Petz LD. Transfusion 1976;16:297

289. Issitt PD, Issitt CH, Wilkinson SL. Transfusion 1974;14:103

290. Lachmann P, Pangburn HK, Oldroyd RS. J Exp Med 1982;156:205

291. Stratton F, Rawlinson VI. J Clin Pathol 1974;27:359

292. Chaplin H, Monroe MC, Lachmann PJ. Clin Exp Immunol 1984;51:639

293. Holburn AM, Prior DM. Clin Lab Haematol 1987;9:33

294. Chaplin H Jr, Coleman ME, Monroe MC. Blood 1983;62:965

295. Chaplin H, Hoffman NL. Transfusion 1982;22:6

296. Holburn AM. In: Immune Hemolytic Anemias NewYork: Churchill Livingstone,1985:231

297. Chaplin H Jr, Monroe MC. Vox Sang 1986;50:42

298. Chaplin H Jr, Monroe MC. Vox Sang 1986;50:87

299. Dobbie D, Brazier DM, Gardner B, et al. Transfusion 1987;27:453

300. Garratty G, Petz LD. Transfusion 1971;11:79

301. Issitt PD, Issitt CH, Wilkinson SL. Transfusion 1974;14:93

302. Petz LD, Garratty G. Transfusion 1978;18:257

303. Salama A, Mueller-Eckhardt C. Br J Haematol 1987;65:67

304. Worlledge SM, Blajchman MA. Br J Haematol 1972;23 Suppl:61

305. Adinolfi A, Mollison PL, Polley MJ, et al. J Exp Med 1966;123:951

306. MacKenzie MR. Vox Sang 1970;19:451

307. Vos GH, Petz LD, Fudenberg HH. J Immunol 1971;106:1172

308. Issitt PD, Pavone BG, Goldfinger D, et al. Br J Haematol

1976;34:5

309. Lubenko A. Unpublished observations cited in: Mollison PL, Engelfriet CP, Contreras M. Blood Transfusion in Clinical Medicine, 9th Ed. Oxford:Blackwell 1993:266

310. Stratton F, Rawlinson VI, Chapman SA, et al. Transfusion 1972;12:157

311. Wagner O, Haltia K, Rasauen JA, et al. Ann Clin Res 1971;3:76

312. Sturgeon P, Smith LE, Chun HMT, et al. Transfusion 1979;19:324

313. Clark DA, Dessypris EN, Jenkins DE, et al. Blood 1984;64:1000

314. Reusser P, Osterwalder B, Burri H, et al. Acta Haematol 1987;77:53

315. Göttsche B, Salama A, Mueller-Eckhardt C. Vox Sang 1990;58:211

316. Wolf CFW, Wolf DJ, Peterson P, et al. Transfusion 1982;22:238

317. Lum LG, Muchmore AV, Keren D, et al. J Immunol 1979;122:65

318. Lum LG, Muchmore AV, O'Connor N, et al. J Immunol 1979;123:714

319. Fanger MW, Shen L, Pugh J, et al. Proc Nat Acad Sci USA 1980;77:3640

320. Gold ER, Fudenberg HH. J Immunol 1967;99:859

321. Judd WJ. Methods in Immunohematology, 2nd Ed. Durham, N.C.:Montgomery, 1994

322. Nelken D. Vox Sang 1961;6:348

323. Allison AC, Burn GP. Br J Haematol 1955;1:291

324. Löhr GW, Waller HD. Klin Wochenschr 1959;37:833

325. Brewer GJ, Powell RD. Nature 1963;199:704

326. Chapman RG, Schaumburg L. Br J Haematol 1967;13:665

327. Beutler E. Blood Cells 1988;14:1

328. Beutler E. Blood Cells 1988;14:69

329. Suzuki T, Dale GL. Proc Nat Acad Sci USA 1988;85:1647

330. Lutz HU, Liu S-C, Palek J. J Cell Biol 1977;73:548

331. Seaman GVF, Knox RJ, Nordt FJ, et al. Blood 1977;50:1001

332. Rumsby MG, Trotter J, Allan D, et al. Biochem Soc Trans 1977;5:126

333. Jandl JH. J Lab Clin Med 1960;55:662

334. Sutherland DA, Eisentraut AM, McCall MS. Br J Haematol 1963;9:68

335. Gallagher MT, Branch DR, Mison A, et al. Exp Hematol 1983;11:82

336. Fries LF, Frank MM. J Immunol 1983;131:1240

337. Leikola J, Perkins HA. Transfusion 1980;20:138

338. Leikola J, Perkins HA. Transfusion 1980;20:224

339. Postoway N, Nance SJ, Garratty G. Med Lab Sci 1985;42:11

340. Wilson L, Wren MR, Issitt PD. Med Lab Sci 1985;42:20

341. Costea N, Schwartz R, Constantoulakis, et al. Blood 1962;20:214

342. Rochna E, Hughes-Jones NC. Vox Sang 1965;10:675

343. McConahey PJ, Dixon FJ. Int Arch Allgy 1966;29:185

344. Jenkins DE Jr, Moore WH, Hawiger A. Transfusion 1977;17:16

345. de Bruin HG, van der Meulen FW, Aaig C. Flow Cytom 1980;4:233

346. de Bruin HG, de Leur-Ebeling I, Aaig C. Vox Sang 1983;45:373

347. Nance SJ, Garratty G. J Immunol Meth 1987;101:127

348. Nance SJ. In: Progress in Immunohematology. Arlington, VA:Am Assoc Blood Banks, 1988:1

349. Mollison PL, Polley MJ. Nature 1964;203:535

350. Hunter DA, Thomas AR. J Clin Pathol 1957;10:245

351. Rawson AJ, Abelson NM. Vox Sang 1964;9:79

352. Moore BPL, Humphreys P, Lovett-Moseley CA. Serological and Immunological Methods, 7th Ed. Toronto:Canad Red Cross Soc, 1972

353. Voak D, Lachmann PJ, Downie DM, et al. Biotest Bull 1983;4:339

354. Currie MS, Rustagi PK, Wojcieszak R, et al. Blood 1988;71:786

355. Fairley NH. Br Med J 1940;2:213

356. Greenbury CL, Moore DH, Nunn LAC. Immunology 1963;6:421

357. Economidou J, Hughes-Jones NC, Gardner B. Vox Sang 1967;12:321

358. Cartron J-P, Gerbal A, Hughes-Jones NC, et al. Immunology 1974;27:723

359. Greenbury CL, Moore DH, Nunn LAC. Immunology 1965;8:240

360. Economidou J, Hughes-Jones NC, Gardner B. Immunology 1967;13:227

361. Romans DG, Tilley CA, Dorrington KJ.Molec Immunol 1979;16:859

362. Romans DG, Tilley CA, Dorrington KJ. J Immunol 1980;124:2807

363. Tanner MJA, Martin PG, High S. Biochem J 1988;256:703

364. Steck TL. J Cell Biol 1974;62:1

365. Mueckler M, Caruso C, Baldwin SA, et al. Science 1985;229:941

366. Allard W-J, Lienhard GE. J Biol Chem 1985;160:8868

367. Koscielak J, Miller-Podruza H, Kranze R, et al. Eur J Biochem 1976;71:9

368. Moore SJ, Green G. Biochem J 1987;244:735

369. Klinman NR, Karush F. Immunochemistry 1967;4:387

370. Middleton J, Crookston MC, Falk JA, et al. Tissue Antigens 1974;4:366

371. O'Neill GJ, Yang SY, Tegoli J, et al. Nature 1978;273:668

372. Tilley CA, Romans DG, Crookston MC. Nature 1978;273:713

373. Brown DL, Nelson DA. Br J Haematol 1973;24:301

374. Weed RI. Am J Med 1970;49:147

375. Cooper RA. J Clin Invest 1972;51:16

376. Mohandas N, de Boisfleury A. Blood Cells 1977;3:187

377. Weiss L, Geduldig U, Weidanz WP. Am J Anat 1986;176:251

378. Abt AF. Am J Child 1931;42:1364

379. Vaughan RB, Boyden SV. Immunology 1964;7:118

380. Archer GT. Mod Med Austral 1964;7:55

381. Archer GT. Vox Sang 1965;10:590

382. Lo Buglio AF, Cotran RS, Jandl JH. Science 1967;158:1582

383. Huber H, Fudenberg HH. Int Arch Allgy Appl Immunol 1968;34:18

384. Huber H, Polley M, Linscott W, et al. Science 1968;162:1281

385. Abramson N, Lo Buglio AF, Jandl JH, et al. J Exp Med 1970;132:1191

386. Abramson N, Gelfand EW, Jandl JH, et al. J Exp Med 1970;132:1207

387. Huber H, Douglas SD, Nusbacher J, et al. Nature 1971;229:420

388. van Furth R, Cohn ZA, Hirsch JG, et al. Bull WHO 1972;46:845

389. Hay FC, Torrigiani G, Roitt IM. Eur J Immunol 1972;2:257

390. Yasmeen D, Ellerson JR, Dorrington KJ, et al. J Immunol 1973;110:1706

391. Brown DL. Ser Haematologica 1974;3:348

392. Holm G, Engwall E, Hammarstrom S, et al. Scand J Immunol 1974;3:173

393. Arend WP, Mannick M. In: Mononuclear Phagocytes in Immunity, Infection and Pathology. Oxford:Blackwell, 1975

394. Logue G, Rosse WF. Sem Hematol 1976;13:277

395. Borne von dem AEG Kr, Beckers D, Engelfriet CP. Br J Haematol 1977;36:485

396. Fleer A, Meulen van der FW, Linthout E, et al. Br J Haematol 1978;39:425

397. Fleer A, Schaik van MLJ, Borne von dem AEG Kr, et al. Scand J Immunol 1978;8:515

398. Meulen van der FM, Hart van der M, Fleer A, et al. Br J Haematol 1978;38:541

399. Anderson CL, Abraham GN. J Immunol 1980;125:2735

400. Alexander MD. Arch Allgy Appl Immunol 1980;62:99

401. Fries LF, Hall RP, Lawley TJ, et al. J Immunol 1982;129:1041

402. Kurlander RJ, Batker J. J Clin Invest 1982;69:1

403. Douglas R, Rowthorne NV, Schneider JV. Transfusion 1985;25:535

404. Zupanska B, Brojer E, Maslanka R, et al. Vox Sang 1985;49:67

405. Zupanska B, Thomson EE, Merry AH. Vox Sang 1986;50:97

406. Zupanska B, Thompson E, Brojer E, et al. Vox Sang 1987;53:96

407. Duncan AR, Woof JM, Partridge LJ, et al. Nature 1988;332:563

408. Williams AF, Barclay AN. Ann Rev Immunol 1988;6:381

409. Unkless JC. J Clin Invest 1989;83:355

410. Fanger MW, Shen L, Graziano RF, et al. Immunol Today 1989;10:92

411. Anderson CL, Shen L, Eicher DM, et al. J Exp Med 1990;171:1333

412. Ravetch JV, Anderson CL. In: Fc Receptors and the Action of Antibodies. Washington, D.C.:Am Soc Microbiol, 1990:211

413. Winkel van de JGJ, Anderson CL. J Leuk Biol 1991;49:511

414. Weiss L. Am J Anat 1963;113:51

415. Horsewood P, Kelton JG. In: Immunobiology of Transfusion Medicine. New York:Marcel Dekker, 1994:435

416. Scornick JC, Salinas MC, Drewinko B. J Immunol 1975;115:901

417. Fehr J, Hofmann V, Kappelar V. New Eng J Med 1982;306:1254

418. Bussel JB, Kimberly RP, Inman RD. Blood 1983;62:480

419. Bussel J, Lalezari P, Hilgartner M, et al. Blood 1983;62:398

420. Kekomaki R, Elfeinbein G, Gardner R, et al. Am J Med 1984;76:199

421. Bierling P, Cordonnier C, Rodet M, et al. Scand J Haematol 1984;33:215

422. Junghans RP, Ahn YS. Am J Med 1984;76:204

423. Becton DL, Kinney TR, Schaffee S, et al. Pediatrics 1984;74:1120

424. Schiffer CA, Hogge DE, Aisner J, et al. Blood 1984;64:937

425. Knupp C, Chamberlain JK, Raab SO. Blood 1985;65:776

426. Bussel JB, Goldman A, Imbach P, et al. J Pediat 1985;106:886

427. Imbach P, Berchtold W, Hirt A, et al. Lancet 1985;2:464

428. Atrah HI, Sheehan T, Gribben J, et al. Scand J Haemotol 1986;36:160

429. Neppert J, Clemens M, Muller-Eckhardt C. Blut 1986;52:67

430. Ziegler ZR, Shadduck RK, Rosenfeld CS, et al. Blood 1987;70:1433

431. Lee EJ, Norris D, Schiffer CA. Transfusion 1987;27:245

432. Kickler T, Braine HG, Piantadose S, et al. Blood 1990;75:313

433. Kelton JG, Singer J, Rodger C, et al. Blood 1985;66:490

434. Crome P, Mollison PL. Br J Haematol 1964;10:137

435. Mollison PL, Hughes-Jones NC. Vox Sang 1958;3:243

436. Cutbush M, Mollison PL. Br J Haematol 1958;4:115

437. Mollison PL. In: Complement. London:Churchill, 1965:323

438. Brown DL. Lachmann PJ, Dacie JV. Clin Exp Immunol 1970;7:401

439. Schreiber AD, Frank MM. J Clin Invest 1972;51:575

440. Schreiber AD, Frank MM. J Clin Invest 1972;51:583

441. Fischer JT, Petz LD, Garratty G, et al. Blood 1974;44:359

442. Atkinson JP, Frank MM. J Clin Invest 1974;54:339

443. Jaffe CJ, Atkinson JP, Frank MM. J Clin Invest 1976;58:942

444. Mollison PL. Transfusion 1986;26:43

445. Gaither T, Vargas I, Inada S, et al. Immunology 1987;62:405

446. Engelfriet CP, Pondman KW, Wolters G, et al. Clin Exp Immunol 1970;6:721

447. Loghem van JJ, Meulen van der FW, Fleer A, et al. In: Human Blood Groups, Basel:Karger 1977:75

448. Borne von dem AEG Kr, Engelfriet CP. Br J Haematol 1977;36:467

449. Meulen van der FW, Hart van der M, Fleer A, et al. Br J Haematol 1978;38:541

450. Fleer A, Roos D, Borne von dem AEG Kr. Blood 1979;54:407

451. Meulen van der FW, de Bruin HG, Goosens PCM, et al. Br J Haematol 1980;46:47

452. Engelfriet CP, Borne von dem AEG Kr, Meulen van der FW, et al. In: A Seminar on Immune-Mediated Cell Destruction, Washington, D.C.:Am Assoc Blood Banks, 1981:93

453. Engelfriet CP, Beckers TAP, Veer vant MB, et al. In: Recent Advances in Haematology. Budapest:Akademia Kiado, 1982

454. Dacie JV. Arch Int Med 1975;135:1293

455. Nance S, Bourdo S, Garratty G. (abstract). Transfusion 1983;23:413

456. Nance S, Nelson J, O'Neill P, et al. (abstract). Transfusion 1984;24:415

457. Thompson KM, Hough DW, Maddison PJ, et al. J Immunol Meth 1986;94:7

458. Armstrong SS, Wiener E, Garner SF, et al. Br J Haematol 1987;66:257

459. Wiener E, Atwal A, Thompson KM, et al. Immunology 1987;62:401

460. Carstairs KC, Breckenridge A, Dollery CT, et al. Lancet 1966;2:133

461. Worlledge SM, Carstairs KC, Dacie JV. Lancet 1966;2:135

462. Worlledge SM. Sem Hematol 1969;6:181

463. Dacie JV, Worlledge SM. Prog Hematol 1969;6:82

464. Worlledge SM. Br J Haematol 1969;16:5

465. Worlledge SM. Sem Hematol 1973;10:327

466. Lalezari P, Louie JE, Fadlallah N. Blood 1982;59:61

467. Garratty G, Petz LD. Am J Med 1975;58:398

468. Petz LD, Fudenberg HH. Prog Hematol 1975;9:185

469. Petz LD, Garratty G. Clin Haematol 1975;4:181

470. Taslimi MM, Sibai BM, Mason JM, et al. Am J Obstet Gynecol 1986;154:1327

471. Issitt PD, Valinsky JE, Marsh WL, et al. Transfusion 1990;30:258

472. Issitt PD, Combs MR, Bredehoeft SJ, et al. Transfusion 1993;33:284

473. Mollison PL. Br Med J 1959;2:1035

474. Mollison PL. Br Med J 1959;2:1123

475. Mollison PL, Crome P, Hughes-Jones NC, et al. Br J Haematol 1965;11:461

476. Qiu WQ, Bruin de D, Brownstein BH, et al. Science 1990;248:732

477. Allen JM, Seed B. Science 1989;243:378

478. Brooks DG, Qiu WQ, Luster A-D, et al. J Exp Med 1989;170:1369

479. Rosenfeld SI, Anderson CL. In: Platelet Immunology. Philadelphia:Lippincott, 1989:337

480. Warmerdam PAM, Winkel van der JGJ, Vlug A, et al. J Immunol 1991;147:1338

481. Karas SP, Rosse WF, Kurlander RJ. Blood 1982;60:1277

482. Winkel van der JGJ, Ommen van R, Huizinga TWJ, et al. J

Immunol 1989;143:571

483. Fleit HB, Wright SD, Unkeless JC. Proc Nat Acad Sci USA 1982;79:3275
484. Klaasen RJL, Ouwehand WH, Huizinga TWJ, et al. J Immunol 1990;144:599
485. Passlick B, Flieger D, Ziegler-Heitbrock HWL. Blood 1989;74:2527
486. Simmons D, Seed B. Nature 1988;323:568
487. Huizinga TWJ, Kent M, Nuijens JH, et al. J Immunol 1989;142:2359
488. Selvaraj P, Rosse WF, Silker R, et al. Nature 1988;333:565
489. Huizinga TWJ, Schoot van der CE, Jost C, et al. Nature 1988;333:667
490. Clarkson SB, Ory PA. J Exp Med 1988;167:408
491. Salmon JE, Kapur S, Kimberly RP. J Exp Med 1987;166:1798
492. Ravetch JV, Perussia B. J Exp Med 1989;170:481
493. Ory PA, Clark MR, Kwoh EE, et al. J Clin Invest 1989;84:1688
494. Huizinga TWJ, Kleijer M, Roos D, et al. In: Leukocyte Typing IV. New York:Oxford Univ Press, 1989:582
495. Ramasamy R, Secher DS, Adetugbo K. Nature 1975;253:656
496. Takemura R, Stenberg PE, Bainton DF, et al. J Cell Biol 1986;102:55
497. Mellman I, Plutner H, Ukkonen P. J Cell Biol 1984;98:1163
498. Ukkonen P, Lewis V, Marsh M, et al. J Exp Med 1986;163:952
499. Mellman I, Plutner H. J Cell Biol 1984;98:1170
500. Rosse WF. Clinical Immunohematology. Boston:Blackwell, 1990:107
501. Lay WH, Nussenzweig V. J Exp Med 1968;128:991
502. Cooper RA, Shattil SJ. New Eng J Med 1971;285:1514
503. Mantovani B, Rabinovitch M, Nussenzweig V. J Exp Med 1972;135:780
504. Griffin FM Jr, Bianco C, Silverstein SC. J Exp Med 1975;141:1269
505. Bianco C, Griffen FM Jr, Silverstein SC. J Exp Med 1975;141:1278
506. Ehlenberger AG, Nussenzweig V. In: Clinical Evaluation of Immune Function in Man. New York:Grune and Stratton, 1976
507. Mollison PL. Blood Transfusion in Clinical Medicine, 6th Ed. Oxford:Blackwell, 1979
508. Jack RM, Fearon DT. J Immunol 1984;132:3028
509. Panzer S, Niessner H, Lechner K, et al. Scand J Haematol 1986;37:97
510. Lutz H, Bussolino F, Flepp R, et al. Proc Natl Acad Sci USA 1987;84:7368
511. Tenner AJ, Robinson SL, Borchelt J, et al. J Biol Chem 1989;264:13923
512. Newman SL, Mikus LK, Tucci MA. J Immunol 1991;146:967
513. Waytes AT, Malbran A, Bobak DA, et al. J Immunol 1991;146:2694
514. Griffin JA, Griffin FM. J Exp Med 1979;150:653
515. Pommier CG, Inada S, Fries LF, et al. J Exp Med 1983;157:1844
516. Wright SD, Craigmyle LS, Silverstein SC. J Exp Med 1983;158:1338
517. Changelian PS, Jack RM, Collins LA, et al. J Immunol 1985;134:1851
518. Jack RM, Ezzel RM, Hartwiz J, et al. J Immunol 1986;137:3996
519. Wong WW. J Invest Dermatol 1990;6:64S
520. Rothlein R, Springer TA. J Immunol 1985;135:2668
521. Ramos OF, Kai C, Yefenof E, et al. J Immunol 1988;140:1239
522. Munn LR, Chaplin H Jr. Vox Sang 1977;33:129

523. Atkinson JP, Frank MM. Prog Hematol 1977;10:211
524. Kurlander RJ, Rosse WF, Logue GL. J Clin Invest 1978;61:1309
525. Ross GD, Polley MJ, Rabellino EM, et al. J Exp Med 1973;138:798
526. Ross GD, Polley MJ. J Exp Med 1975;141:1163
527. Reynolds HY, Atkinson JP, Newball HH, et al. J Immunol 1975;114:1813
528. Ehlenberger AG, Nussenzweig V. Fed Proc 1975;34:854
529. Wellek B, Hahn HH, Opferkuch W. J Immunol 1975;114:1643
530. Bianco C. In: Comprehensive Immunology. New York:Plenum, 1977
531. Lewis SM, Dacie JV, Szur L. Br J Haematol 1960;6:154
532. Ross GD. In: Immunobiology of the Complement System. New York:Academic Press, 1986
533. Griffin FM Jr, Griffin JA, Leider JE, et al. J Exp Med 1975;142:1263
534. Grubb R. Acta Path Microbiol Scand 1951;28;61
535. Sneath JS, Sneath PHA. Nature 1955;176:172
536. Cutbush M, Giblett ER, Mollison PL. Br J Haematol 1956;2:210
537. Tilley CA, Crookston MC, Brown BL, et al. Vox Sang 1975;28:25
538. Cooper RA. New Eng J Med 1977;297:371
539. Mollison PL, Polley MJ, Crome P. Lancet 1963;1:909
540. Hossaini AA. Am J Clin Pathol 1972;57:489
541. Pelosi MA, Bauer JL, Langer A, et al. Obstet Gynecol 1974;4:590
542. Holburn AM, Frame M, Hughes-Jones NC, et al. Immunology 1971;20:681
543. Lowell GH, Smith LF, McLeod G. J Exp Med 1980;152:452
544. Gauldie J, Richards C, Lamontagne L. Mol Immunol 1983;20:1029
545. Zinkham WH, Diamond LK. Blood 1952;7:592
546. Bonnin JA, Schwartz L. Blood 1954;9:773
547. Pirofsky B. In: Autoimmunization and the Autoimmune Hemolytic Anemias. Baltimore:Williams and Wilkins, 1969
548. Jandl JH, Simmons RL, Castle WB. Blood 1961;18:133
549. Jandl JH. Lab Clin Med 1960;55:663
550. Romano EL, Mollison PL. Br J Haematol 1975;29:121
551. Loutit JJ, Mollison PL. J Path Bact 1946;58:711
552. Jandl JH, Jones AR, Castle WB. J Clin Invest 1957;36:1428
553. Frank MM, Hamburger MI, Lawley TJ, et al. New Eng J Med 1979;300:518
554. Kelton JG. New Eng J Med 1985;313:596
555. Rosse WF. Prog Hematol 1973;8:51
556. Arend WP, Mannik M. J Immunol 1973;110:1455
557. MacKenzie MR. (abstract). Clin Res 1975;23:132A
558. Kay NE, Douglas SD. Blood 1977;50:889
559. Rhodes J. Nature 1977;265:253
560. Issitt PD. Prog Clin Pathol 1978;7:137
561. Rinehart JJ, Balcerzak SP, Sargone AL, et al. J Clin Invest 1974;54:1337
562. Friedman D, Nettl F, Schreiber AD. J Clin Invest 1985;75:162
563. Petroni KG, Shen L, Guyre PM. J Immunol 1988;140:3467
564. Weiner W, Vos GH. Blood 1963;22:206
565. Weiner W. Biblio Haematol 1966;25:35
566. Allan J, Garratty G. (abstract). Book of Abstracts, 16th Cong ISBT, 1980:150
567. Evans RS, Weiser RS. Arch Int Med 1957;100:371
568. Wiener AS, Peters HR. Ann Int Med 1940;13:2306
569. Wiener AS. Arch Pathol 1941;32:227
570. Vogel P, Rosenthal N, Levine P. Am J Clin Pathol 1943;13:1
571. Swisher SN, Young LE. Trans Assoc Am Phys 1954;67:124

572. Roy RB, Lotto WN. Transfusion 1962;2:342
573. Croucher BEE, Crookston MC, Crookston JH. Vox Sang 1967;12:32
574. Meltz DJ, Bertles JF, David DS, et al. Lancet 1971;2:1348
575. Rothman IK, Alter HJ, Strewler GJ. Transfusion 1976;16:357
576. Pickles MM, Jones MN, Egan J, et al. Vox Sang 1978;35:32
577. Halima D, Postoway N, Brunt D, et al. (abstract). Transfusion 1982;22:405
578. Baldwin ML, Barrasso C, Ness PM, et al. Transfusion 1983;23:40
579. Harrison CR, Hayes TC, Trow LL, et al. Vox Sang 1986;51:96
580. Davenport RD, Strieter RM, Standiford TJ, et al. Blood 1990;76:2439
581. Davenport RD, Strieter RM, Kunkel SL. Br J Haematol 1991;78:540
582. Hoffman M. Vox Sang 1991;60:184
583. Butler J, Parker D, Pillai R, et al. Br J Haematol 1991;79:525
584. Davenport RD, Burdick M, Moore SA, et al. Transfusion 1993;33:19
585. Capon SM, Goldfinger D. In: Alloimmunity: 1993 and Beyond. Bethesda:Am Assoc Blood Banks, 1993;141
586. Davenport RD, Burdick M, Strieter RM, et al. Transfusion 1994;34:16
587. Davenport RD, Burdick MD, Strieter RM, et al. Transfusion 1994;34:297
588. Davenport RD, Polak TJ, Kunkel SL. Transfusion 1994;34:943
589. Durum SK, Schmidt JA, Oppenheim JJ. Ann Rev Immunol 1985;3:263
590. Ruddle NH. Immunol Today 1987;8:129
591. Ulich TR, del Castillo J, Keys M, et al. J Immunol 1987;139:3406
592. Butler LD, Layman NK, Cain RL, et al. Clin Immunol Immunopathol 1989;53:400
593. Caussy D, Sauder DN. Transf Med Rev 1989;3:194
594. Nathan C, Sporn M. J Cell Biol 1991;113:981
595. Davenport RD, Kunkel SL. Transf Med Rev 1994;8:157
596. Guyre PM, Morganelli M, Miller R. J Clin Invest 1983;72:393
597. Shen L, Guyre PM, Fanger MW. J Immunol 1987;139:534
598. Mannel DN, Falk W. Cell Immunol 1983;79:396
599. Perussia B, Dayton ET, Lazarus R, et al. J Exp Med 1983;158:1092
600. Erbe DV, Collins JE, Shen L, et al. Mol Immunol 1990;27:57
601. Miller LJ, Bainton DF, Borregaard N, et al. J Clin Invest 1987;80:535
602. McClure PD. Pediatrics 1975;55:68
603. Habibi B, Homberg J-C, Schaison G, et al. Am J Med 1974;56:61
604. Garratty G. Personal communication 1981, cited in the 3rd Edition of this book
605. Handwerger BS, Kay NW, Douglas SD. Vox Sang 1978;34:276
606. Engelfriet CP, Ouwehand WH. Balliere's Clin Haematol 1990;3:321
607. Wiener E, Joliffe VM, Scott HCF, et al. Immunology 1988;65:159
608. Urbaniak SJ. Br J Haematol 1976;33:409
609. Urbaniak SJ. Br J Haematol 1979;42:303
610. Urbaniak SJ. Br J Haematol 1979;42:315
611. Urbaniak SJ, Greiss MA. Br J Haematol 1980;46:447
612. Urbaniak SJ, Greiss MA, Crawford RJ, et al. Vox Sang 1984;46:323
613. Mollison PL reporting studies from nine collaborating laboratories. Vox Sang 1991;60:225
614. Kumpel BM, Leader KA, Merry AH, et al. Eur J Immunol 1989;19:2283
615. Kumpel BM, Wiener E, Urbaniak SJ, et al. Br J Haematol 1989;71:415
616. Yust I, Goldsher N. Br J Haematol 1981;47:443
617. Yust I, Frisch B, Goldsher N. Am J Hematol 1982;13:53
618. Lamon EW, Skurzak HM, Andersson B, et al. J Immunol 1975;114:1171
619. Lamon EW, Whitten HD, Skurzak HM, et al. J Immunol 1975;115:1288
620. Blair PB, Lane MA, Mar P. J Immunol 1976;116:606
621. Fuson EW, Lamon EW. J Immunol 1977;118:1907
622. Wahlin P, Perlmann H, Perlmann P. J Exp Med 1976;144:1375
623. Fuson EW, Whitten HD, Ayers RD, et al. J Immunol 1978;120:1726
624. Andersson B, Skoglund AC, Rosen A. J Immunol 1979;123:1976
625. Lamon EW, Shaw MW, Goodson S, et al. J Exp Med 1977;145:302
626. Wiederman G, Rumpold H, Stemberg H, et al. J Clin Exp Immunol 1981;2:39
627. Perlmann P, Holm G. Adv Immunol 1969;11:117
628. Pearson GR. Top Microbiol Immunol 1978;80:65
629. Perlmann P, Cerottini SC. In: The Antigens, Vol 5. New York:Academic Press 1979:173
630. Johnson AR, Hugli TE, Müller-Eberhard HJ. Immunology 1975;28:1067
631. Bokish VA, Müller-Eberhard HJ, Cochrane CG. J Exp Med 1969;129:1109
632. Ward PA, Cochrane CG, Müller-Eberhard HJ. J Exp Med 1965;122:327
633. Lepow IH, Willms-Kretschmer K, Patrick RA. Am J Pathol 1970;61:13
634. Snyderman R, Phillips JK, Morgenhagen SE. J Exp Med 1971;134:1131
635. Dahlen SE, Bjork J, Hedqvist P, et al. Proc Nat Acad Sci USA 1981;78:3887
636. Rent R, Ertel N, Eisenstein R, et al. J Immunol 1975;114:120
637. Chenoweth DE. (Letter). New Eng J Med 1981;305:51
638. Chenoweth DE, Cooper SW, Hugli TE, et al. New Eng J Med 1981;304:497
639. White JV. (Letter). New Eng J Med 1981;305:51
640. Wurzner R, Schuff-Werner P, Franzke A, et al. Eur J Clin Invest 1991;21:288
641. Hong F, Shastri KA, Logue GL, et al. Transfusion 1991;31:642
642. Janatova J, Cheung AK, Parker CJ. Complement Inflamm 1991;8:61
643. Kaplan AP, Austen KF. J Immunol 1970;105:802
644. Kaplan AP, Austen KF. J Exp Med 1971;133:696
645. Ward PA, Offen CD, Montgomery JR. Fed Proc 1971;30:1721
646. Nelson RA Jr. Science 1953;118:733
647. Nelson RA Jr. Proc Roy Soc Med 1956;49:55
648. Nishioka K, Linscott WD. J Exp Med 1963;118:767
649. Cooper NR. Science 1969;165:396
650. Dukor P, Hartmann KU. Cell Immunol 1973;7:349
651. Lachmann PJ, Thompson RA. J Exp Med 1970;131:643
652. Thompson RA, Rowe DS. Immunology 1968;14:745
653. Thompson RA, Lachmann PJ. J Exp Med 1970;131:629
654. Yachnin S, Ruthenberg JM. J Clin Invest 1965;44:518
655. Götze O, Müller-Eberhard HJ. J Exp Med 1970;132:898
656. Salama A, Bahkdi S, Mueller-Eckhardt C. Transfusion 1987;27:49
657. Woodruff AW, Ansdell VE, Pettitt LE. Lancet 1979;1:1055
658. Salama A, Mueller-Eckhardt C. Transfusion 1984;24:188

659. Salama A, Mueller-Eckhardt C. Transfusion 1985;25:528
660. Ness PM, Shirey RS, Thomas SK, et al. Transfusion 1990;30:688
661. Petz LD. In: Clinical and Basic Science Aspects of Immunohematology. Arlington, VA:Am Assoc Blood Banks, 1991:73
662. Gigli I, Nelson RA Jr. Exp Cell Res 1968;51:45
663. Perlmann P, Perlmann H, Müller-Eberhard HJ, et al. Science 1969;163:937
664. Ratnoff OD. Hosp Prac 1971;6:119
665. Rabiner SE, Friedman LH. Br J Haematol 1968;14;105
666. Birndorf NI, Lopas H. (abstract). Clin Res 1970;18:398
667. Zimmerman TS, Müller-Eberhard HJ. J Exp Med 1971;134:1601
668. Heusinkveld RS, Leddy JP, Klemperer MR, et al. J Clin Invest 1974;53:554
669. Ratnoff OD, Naff GB. J Exp Med 1967;125:337
670. Taylor FB Jr, Ward PA. J Exp Med 1967;126:149
671. Poll van der T, Buller HR, Ten CH, et al. New Eng J Med 1990;322:1622
672. Conkling PR, Greenburg CS, Weinberg JB. Blood 1988;72:128
673. Moore KL, Esmon CT, Esmon NL. Blood 1989;73:159
674. Nawroth PP, Handley DA, Esmon CT, et al. Proc Nat Acad Sci USA 1986;83:3460
675. Nawroth PP, Stern DM. J Exp Med 1986;163:740
676. Klemperer MR, Austen KF, Rosen FS. J Immunol 1967;98:72
677. Alper CA, Propp PP, Klemperer MR. J Clin Invest 1969;48:553
678. Klemperer MR. J Immunol 1969;102:168
679. Kohler PF, Müller-Eberhard HJ. Science 1969;163:474
680. Miller ME, Nilsson UR. New Eng J Med 1970;282:354
681. Ruddy S, Austen KF. Prog Med Genet 1970;7:69
682. Kohler PF. Ann Int Med 1975;82:420
683. Fielder AHL, Walport MJ, Batchelor JR, et al. Br Med J 1983;286:425
684. Hauptmann G, Goetz J, Uring-Lambert B, et al. Prog Allergy 1986;39:239
685. Kemp ME, Atkinson JP, Skanes VM, et al. Arthritis Rheum 1987;30:1015
686. Dunckley H, Gatenby PA, Hawkins B, et al. J Immunogenet 1987;14:209
687. Goldstein R, Arnett FC, McLean RH, et al. Arthritis Rheum 1988;31:736
688. Wilson WA, Perez MC, Michalski JP, et al. J Rheumatol 1988;15:1768
689. Kumar A, Kumar P, Schur PH. Clin Immunol Immunopathol 1991;60:55
690. deMessias IJT, Reis A, Brenden M, et al. Comp Inflamm 1991;8:288
691. Moulds JM. In: Blood Groups: Ch/Rg, Knops/McCoy/York and Cromer. Bethesda:Am Assoc Blood Banks 1992:13
692. Rittner C, Meier EMM, Stradman B, et al. Immunogenet 1984;20:407
693. Robb SA, Fielder AHL, Saunders CEL. Hum Immunol 1988;22:31
694. Wyatt RJ, Julian BA, Woodford SY, et al. Clin Nephrol 1991;36:1
695. Ratanachaiyavong S, Demaine AG, Campbell RD, et al. Clin Exp Immunol 1991;84:48
696. Thomson W, Sanders PA, Davis M, et al. Arthritis Rheum 1988;31:984
697. Welch TR, Beischel LS, Choi EM. Hum Immunol 1989;26:353
698. Hillarby MC, Strachan T, Grennan DM. Ann Rheum Dis 1990;49:763
699. Rowe PC, McLean RH, Wood RA, et al. J Infect Dis 1989;160:448
700. Cameron PU, Cobain TJ, Zhang WJ, et al. Br Med J 1988;296;1627
701. Plum G, Siebel E, Bendick C, et al. Vox Sang 1990;59(Suppl 1):15
702. Donaldson VH, Evans RR. Pediatrics 1966;37:10174
703. Alper CA, Abramson N, Johnston RB. New Eng J Med 1970;282:349
704. Abramson N, Alper CA, Lachmann PJ, et al. J Immunol 1971;107:19
705. Rothfield N, Ross HA, Minta JO, et al. New Eng J Med 1972;287:681
706. Lachmann PJ. In Ciba Foundation Symposium. Amsterdam: Knight, 1972:194
707. Alper CA. New Eng J Med 1973;288:109
708. Thompson RA, Lachmann PJ. Clin Exp Immunol 1977;27:23
709. Groux H, Huet S, Aubrit F, et al. J Immunol 1989;142;3013
710. Stefanova I, Hilgert I, Kristofova H, et al. Mol Immunol 1989;26:153
711. Davies A, Simmons DL, Hale G, et al. J Exp Med 1989;170:637
712. Sawada R, Ohashi K, Okano K, et al. Nucl Acids Res 1989;17:6728
713. Sawada R, Ohashi K, Anaguchi H, et al. DNA Cell Biol 1990;9:213
714. Taguchi R, Funahashi Y, Ikezawa H, et al. FEBS Lett 1990;261:142
715. Greenwalt TJ, Lau FO. Br J Haematol 1978;39:545
716. Greenwalt TJ, Bryan DJ, Dumaswala UJ. Vox Sang 1984;47:261
717. Dumaswala UJ, Greenwalt TJ. Transfusion 1984;24:490
718. Greenwalt TJ, Zehner-Sostok C, Dumaswala UJ. Vox Sang 1990;58:90
719. Kay MMB. Proc Nat Acad Sci USA1975;72:3521
720. Kay MMB. In: Immunobiology of Transfusion Medicine. New York:Marcel Dekker, 1994:173
721. Low PS, Waugh SM, Zinke K, et al. Science 1985;227:531
722. Galili U, Rachmilewicz EA, Peleg, et al. J Exp Med 1984;160:1519
723. Galili U, Flechner I, Knyszynski A, et al. Br J Haematol 1986;62:317
724. Greenwalt TJ, Flory LL, Steane EA. Br J Haematol 1970;19:701
725. Kay MMB, Bosman GJCGM. Exp Hematol 1985;13:1103
726. Merry AH, Thomson EE, Rawlinson VI, et al. Clin Lab Haematol 1982;4:393
727. Jeje MO, Blajchman MA, Steeves K, et al. Transfusion 1984;24:473
728. Schluter K, Drenkhahn D. Proc Nat Acad Sci USA 1986;83:6137
729. Imbach P, Barandun S, d'Apuzzo V, et al. Lancet 1981;1:1228
730. Rosse WF, de Boisfleury A, Bessis M. Blood Cells 1975;1:345
731. Darnborough J. Br Med J 1958;2:1451
732. Stratton F, Tovey G. Br Med J 1959;1:115
733. Naiki M, Marcus DM. Biochemstry 1975;14:4837
734. Schwarting GA, Marcus DM, Metaxas M. Vox Sang 1977;32:257

7 | A General Introduction to Blood Group Antibodies, Red Cell Typing Reagents and the Use of Monoclonal Antibodies in Blood Group Serology

From what has been written in earlier chapters it will be obvious that no absolute generalizations can be made about antibodies to red cell blood group antigens. Throughout the chapters of this book that deal with blood group systems, an early table lists the major features of antibodies of the system under discussion. Rather than include lists of explanations with each of those tables, this section describes their interpretation. The headings that are used are listed below together with the most usual interpretations of the findings listed.

1. Antibody specificity
   Interpretation: obvious
2. Positive reactions seen in vitro
   a) Sal. (agglutination in a saline system)
   b) LISS (low ionic strength solutions, i.e. LISS, Polybrene®, PEG)
   c) AHG (anti-human globulin, Coombs, almost always IAT)
   d) Enz (tests with enzyme pretreated red cells)
   Interpretation: The most usual optimal test systems are shown. The LISS and Enz columns *include* tests performed by that method then converted to IAT readings. Blank spaces in these columns often mean that the antibody will react by that method (with the common exception of Sal.) but will give stronger reactions or will be more easily detected by the method(s) marked.
3. Usual immunoglobulin
   a) IgG
   b) IgM
   Interpretation The most commonly encountered form is shown. Examples of antibodies made of the other immunoglobulin will be found, but less frequently. Since IgA red cell blood group antibodies are rare, footnotes are used to indicate when they might be seen in a particular system.
4. Ability to bind complement
   Interpretation: Shown only if sufficient examples of the antibody have been studied for this characteristic.
5. Ability to cause in vitro hemolysis
   Interpretation: Refers to tests on untreated red cells using human serum as the source of complement. It has been shown (1) that the use of complement from other species (e.g. rabbits) results in more

antibodies being lytic in vitro than when human complement is used. Similarly, more antibodies will hemolyze enzyme pretreated red cells than will hemolyze untreated cells (2).
6. Implicated in
   a) Transfusion reactions
   Interpretation: Some antibodies, such as anti-En^a (3,4) and anti-Co3 (5) would presumably cause transfusion reactions. That they have not done so is sometimes simply because no one with the antibody has been transfused with antigen-positive blood. In some cases in vivo ^{51}Cr survival studies have shown that accelerated clearance of antigen-positive red cells occurs. Such antibodies are marked Prob (for probable) indicating that they would probably cause a transfusion reaction if given that opportunity.
   b) Hemolytic disease of the newborn
   Interpretation: Some attempt is made to indicate the most probable severity (i.e. severe, moderate, mild) of HDN caused by those antibodies that have already caused the disease. Others are marked Prob (for probable) indicating that an IgG form of the antibody could be expected to cause the disease if an infant with the antigen was born to a mother with the antibody.
7. Usual form of stimulation
   a) Red cells
   b) Other than red cells
   Interpretation: To replace the commonly used terms "immune" and "naturally-occurring" respectively. While the term "immune" antibody seems appropriate (i.e. antibody-maker previously exposed to the antigen on foreign red cells), the term "naturally-occurring" does not. We believe that in order to mount an antibody response, the immune system must "see" the antigen. Thus it follows that in non-transfused, never pregnant individuals, the antigen was introduced via a non-red-cell carrier. It is known that antigens such as A and B are ubiquitous in nature, being present on bacteria, pollen, corn-flakes, etc. Anti-A and anti-B are apparently made when antigen-negative persons are exposed to structures that closely resemble the A and B antigens that are present on other than red cells. Other so-called "naturally-occurring" anti-

bodies such as anti-E and anti-C^w may be directed against non-red cell antigens but may have the ability to cross-react with some structures on red cells (see also Chapter 35). As in the descriptions of other characteristics of the antibodies, exceptions will be seen.

8. Percentage of White population positive
    Interpretation: Some incidences given as 100% indicate that the only negatives are likely to be other persons with the antibody (e.g. Bombay bloods are the only H-negative red cells). Other incidences of 100% indicate that no White has ever been found to lack the antigen (e.g. Js^b) except in "deletion" instances (in this case K$_o$) (6), but in these cases bloods from Blacks may be found to lack the antigen. A given high incidence below 100% indicates that negative donors will be found if enough random bloods are screened (e.g. Lu(b-), Kp(b-)). There is too little information in the literature for accurate figures to be given for the incidence of many antigens in Blacks. Where accurate figures are available they are included in the text of each chapter.

9. ISBT antigen name
    Interpretation: The "shorthand" symbol from the ISBT terminology (7,8) that uses letters for the blood group system and sequential numbers for antigens within that system.

10. ISBT computer code
    Interpretation: The six digit number indicating blood group system (first three digits) and antigen (last three digits) as the system was originally intended to permit storage of data in electronic processing equipment (9).
    General Comments: Throughout the chapters that follow, the tables described above attempt to indicate what is most likely. Thus terms such as rare, few, most; possible, probable; some, many, all; mild, moderate, severe; are used. It must be remembered that exceptions will be seen in many categories. For example, in Chapter 12, anti-D is shown as an IgG antibody, reacting in antiglobulin and enzyme tests. It is further shown as red cell-stimulated, an immune antibody. These are the characteristics of thousands of examples of anti-D and it can be expected that many more like them will be found. However, as explained in Chapter 2, if a patient in the process of forming anti-D is bled at the opportune time, IgM anti-D may be present. Anti-D has even been reported (10-15) as a non-red-cell-stimulated antibody. Similarly, anti-K is nearly always a red cell immune antibody but cases of anti-K in individuals who have never been transfused, pregnant or injected with blood, have been

reported (16-22). In some instances involving non-red cell stimulated anti-D (15) and anti-K (22) the introduction of antigen-positive red cells neither resulted in their accelerated clearance nor prompted a secondary immune response. Similar findings were made (23) on a series of anti-E several of which were apparently non-red cell stimulated i.e. present in the sera of never-transfused males. It is findings such as these that prompt the suggestion that at least some "naturally-occurring" antibodies are really directed against other than red cell antigens and have the ability to cross-react with blood group antigens. It is presumed that the antigen that provoked the initial immune response would have to be reintroduced to prompt a secondary response. In the case of anti-K, at least one example appears to have been provoked by a strain of *E. coli* causing enteritis in an infant (18), several others have been seen in individuals with bacterial (notably tuberculosis or intestinal) infections (17,19,21). Further, Wong et al. (24) have shown that some strains of *Camphylobacter jejuni* and *Camphylobacter coli*, both of which cause gastrointestinal infections, carry structures that bind anti-K.

Since exceptions to the statements in the tables are comparatively rare, any antibody that violates several of them should be reexamined. In such circumstances, it is possible that the specificity ascribed the antibody is not the correct one. Another possibility is the presence, in the same serum, of a second antibody whose coexistence has to that point not been suspected. In this instance it may be the second antibody that is responsible for the unexpected characteristics. A classic case of this sort was the second discovered example of anti-Xg^a. When this antibody was found (25) relatively few cells had been typed for Xg^a. The anti-C, that was also present in the serum, appeared to be binding complement (a very rare event). It was not until the anti-Xg^a was identified that it was shown that when tested against C+ and C-, Xg(a+) cells it was the anti-Xg^a and not the anti-C that was binding complement.

Red Cell Typing Reagents

These reagents fall in to two major categories. First, those that are purchased from commercial companies and second, those that are not available from such sources so comprise previously identified antibodies from individual patients, characterized in one's own laboratory or that of a generous colleague. Commercially available reagents come in a number of varieties that are described below. There is no point in discussing home-identified sera that are used for typing, clearly workers using them will be aware of their characteristics.

Until fairly recently, commercially supplied reagents were made using polyclonal human antibodies as the starting material. As monoclonal antibodies with blood group specificity (see below) have become available, the use of human polyclonal material has been discouraged. First, the use of in vitro produced monoclonal reagents removes the (admittedly miniscule) possibility that the reagent will contain an infectious agent. Second and of more significance, introduction of monoclonal-based reagents obviates the need to hyperimmunize humans (and thus risk transmission of an infectious agent) to produce reagent grade antibodies. Thus by the time this book is published, reagents made from human polyclonal antibodies may be rarities. That is not to say that monoclonal reagents are always superior to the long used human-based reagents. Indeed, as discussed below, use of monoclonal blood group antibodies in immunohematology has introduced a number of problems not previously encountered by blood bankers.

Commercially supplied reagent antisera may be pools made from a number of individual sera containing antibodies of the same specificity or, particularly when the raw material is in short supply and few potent examples of a specificity are available, may be from one individual donor. Often the user is not aware if the reagent he is using is a pool of sera or an individual antibody. However, if knowledge of that difference is important, most manufacturers will supply the necessary information on request. One point that is now more appreciated than was previously the case, is that several manufacturers may make a reagent using serum from the same donor. In other words if a red cell sample is typed for say, C, using anti-C from four different companies, it may not have been tested with four different anti-C. Indeed it is possible that the sample has been typed four times with the same anti-C because of the situation described. Again, when the user is in doubt, most companies will supply the relevant information.

Directions for Use

Undoubtably the most important point that can be made about commercially supplied reagent antisera is that they be used exactly as the manufacturer instructs in the directions for use circular that accompanies the reagent. The reagents have been extensively tested before issue and the methods recommended are those that have been found to give the most reliable results. These reagents are licensed to be specifically reactive by the test methods described and are not necessarily specific by other methods. A slide and rapid tube reagent may, for

example, contain other antibodies that react by the antiglobulin method. There is a simple explanation for this fact. Not enough pure sera are available for all reagents to be specific by all methods. The demand for typing reagents probably could not be met if only pure sera (by all methods) had to be used. FDA regulations do not require that all reagents be specific by all methods.

Some sera are totally specific by any method and if so a statement to this effect will appear in the directions for use circular. In cases of doubt, the manufacturer should be consulted. He is usually completely aware of what antibodies are present in each serum and has no reason not to divulge this information when it is requested.

Slide and Rapid Tube Reagents

These reagents are not usually complete agglutinins by nature, although they do react by agglutinating red cells suspended in saline. They are often made from potent incomplete antibodies, with a purification step sometimes being included in the manufacturing process, that are resuspended in a synthetic medium that includes a variety of potentiators of the hemagglutination reaction. For this reason, controls using the potentiating medium without antibody are necessary to avoid false positive interpretations when red cells already coated with immunoglobulins (i.e. DAT+) are typed (26). Some of these reagents contain albumin and the manufacturers usually recommend that they be stored at 2 - 8°C but not frozen.

Chemically-Modified Reagents

When IgG, non-agglutinating antibodies are subjected to mild reduction by sulphydryl compounds some of them develop the ability to agglutinate saline suspended red cells (27-30). Once treated with the sulphydryl compound the antibody molecules are stabilized by treatment with an alkylating agent such as iodoacetamide (2). Not all IgG antibodies are equal in terms of susceptibility to conversion to agglutinins. It was shown (30) that the change is brought about by reduction cleavage of the inter-heavy-chain disulphide bonds in the hinge region of the IgG molecule (see Chapter 2). After reduction of these bonds the two Fab pieces of the IgG molecule are able to stretch further apart, or at very least, acquire more flexibility. The two halves of the reduced molecules are held together by strong non-covalent bonds in the C_H3 domains. Since the number of inter-heavy-chain disulphide bonds varies by IgG subclass, i.e. two in IgG1, four in IgG2, eleven in IgG3 and two in IgG4 (31,32), it might be expected that the production of IgG agglutinins by reduction cleavage would be more successful with antibodies of some subclasses than with those of others. However, this point did not seem to be proved with human polyclonal antibodies perhaps because it is difficult to determine how many molecules of each subclass are present. Using monoclonal anti-D, Scott et al. (33) showed that reduced IgG3 molecules were more potent agglutinins than were reduced IgG1 molecules. This finding presumably relates to the much larger hinge region in IgG3 than in IgG1 (34, see also Chapter 2) so that after reduction cleavage the antigen binding sites on IgG3 are farther apart than those on any other reduced IgG molecules.

Chemically reduced, commercially-prepared typing sera were introduced as dual purpose reagents. First, they were intended for use in the same situations that slide and rapid tube reagents are used. Second, because they lack (or have low levels) of potentiators they can be used safely to type DAT-positive red cells that may give false positive reactions in tests with slide and rapid tube reagents. In spite of these advantages and the claims that diluent (potentiator without antibody) controls are not required, not all workers have adopted chemically reduced reagents for routine use. First, some workers have found that these reagents are often less avid than their slide and rapid tube equivalents. Second, there is sometimes a price differential with the chemically reduced reagents being more expensive than the slide and rapid tube reagents. Third, it has been claimed but apparently not well documented in the literature, that false positives can occur when these reagents are used to type heavily coated (with IgG) red cells.

Affinity Purified Reagents

If a serum containing an IgG blood group antibody is passed over a column with an immunoadsorbant constructed so that only the antibody will bind, then the bound antibody is recovered by elution from the column, the antibody will be largely free of other serum immunoglobulins and proteins (35,36). Such purified blood group antibodies can then be used to coat red cells (as in the incubation step in the indirect antiglobulin test) and the tests can be read with anti-IgG without washing the red cells after the incubation step. The cells need not be washed since in a positive test virtually all the IgG molecules present will be bound to the red cells, while in a negative test too few free IgG molecules will be present to neutralize the anti-IgG. For those workers still concerned that some neutralization of anti-IgG may occur, it can be pointed out that non-bound IgG will be present with the red cells, only in a negative test anyway.

The Use of Monoclonal Antibodies in Blood Group Serology

The 1975 report of Köhler and Milstein (37) that described the in vitro production of unlimited quantities of monoclonal antibodies (MAb) of predetermined specificity, generated enormous excitement in almost every branch of science. Twenty years later it is clear that the high expectations for this new technology were amply justified. Since the principles of MAb production and the various improvements over the initial methods have been described in Chapter 2, this section will be primarily concerned with descriptions of the use of MAb as typing reagents.

Initially many MAb were made in mouse-mouse hybridomas or human-mouse heterohybridomas. The antibodies were made of mouse IgG so required the use of anti-mouse IgG for optimal detection. Later human-human hybridomas or supernatants from EBV-transformed human B-cell lines grown in tissue culture were used so that the more readily available anti-human IgG could be used. Most recently emphasis has been placed on the transformation and immortalization of human B-cells that are synthesizing IgM antibody of the required specificity. Thus it does not seem inconceivable that in the foreseeable future, most or all red cell phenotyping will be done using antibodies that react by immediate spin methods in tests using saline suspended red cells. While this will make phenotyping tests quick and easy it seems, to some of us, that is will also take away much of the fun.

Advantages of Monoclonal Antibody-Based Reagents

Two major sets of advantages of MAbs involve specificity and availability. As described earlier, when a human is immunized to a blood group antigen by transfusion, pregnancy or deliberate injection, or when a reagent antiserum is made following immunization of a laboratory animal, the immune system of the individual or animal produces a series of different antibodies. While these antibodies may have apparently the same specificity, each is the product of a different clone and the antibodies may vary in binding constant, affinity, and portion of the antigen (epitopes) against which they are directed. In contrast, a MAb produced in a clone of identical cells, comprises molecules of identical structure, specificity and binding constant. An advantage of the single epitope specificity of a MAb is that if correctly used it will not give unexpected or unwanted positive reactions due to the presence of another antibody. For example, a polyclonal anti-A reagent made from human serum may have been in use for many years without any problems having been encountered. Then suddenly that reagent may agglutinate an other-than-group A sample because the red cells involved carry a low incidence blood group antigen and the anti-A happens to have been made from plasma that contains a previously undetected antibody to that antigen. Since there are so many different low incidence blood group antigens, even the most extensive tests performed by the reagent manufacturer cannot be guaranteed to have excluded presence of all such possible antibodies. When a MAb is produced by subculture of a single antibody-secreting cell that is making anti-A, the possibility that another antibody may be present is excluded. However, as discussed below, the single epitope specificity of a MAb is not always an advantage in blood group serology.

Ironically, a second advantage of MAbs in terms of specificity is that some of them can be used as screening reagents although they may not have exact specificity for the antigen in question. For example, MAbs that react with almost all e+ red cells and are non-reactive with almost all e- samples have been described (38,39). Similarly, MAbs with a specificity very close to anti-M are known (40-42). If extensive tests with red cells of rare phenotypes are performed, it can be seen that these antibodies do not have exactly the same specificity as human anti-e and anti-M, respectively. However, by using the antibodies under controlled test conditions (pH, temperature, time of incubation, etc.) they can be made to perform very similarly to human anti-e and anti-M. Clearly since human polyclonal anti-e is in short supply and is often not very avid when found, the MAb can be used in mass screening and the 2 percent of non-reactive samples can be confirmed as being e-negative with a human reagent (or the patient's serum). Having suggested that some MAb that do not have the exact specificity required can be used as screening reagents, it should be added that new MAb are being made by so many workers and at such a pace, that use of the "near-specificity" ones may not be necessary since others, with more exact specificity will be made.

In terms of availability, MAbs have some very clear advantages over human source reagents. First, once a suitable clone has been produced, those cells can be propagated and used to produce an unlimited supply of antibody. Obviously, human source reagents must be made from antibody-containing plasma as it becomes available; some human antibodies such as those directed against C, e, Jk^b, and Fy^b are chronically in short supply in terms of antibodies potent enough for reagent production. The production of MAb-based reagents is not devoid of problems. The antibody-secreting cells may die during subculture or mutation may occur so that the required antibody is no longer made. To guard against

these possibilities, most workers making MAbs keep aliquots of useful clones frozen so that a fresh culture can be made if problems occur during production.

A second advantage in terms of availability relates to consistency of the reagents made. With human source material, potency and avidity of the finished product will sometimes vary based on the quality of the starting material available. With a MAb-based reagent, identical antibody molecules will be present in each lot made; further, a relatively simple assay can be used to ensure that each new lot is identical to its predecessors in terms of antibody content.

A third and related advantage pertains to the production of reagents for which human source material is in short supply. If one person already immunized, say to the Rh antigen e is found, lymphocytes from a peripheral blood sample from that person can be used to develop a clone of cells making anti-e. Once developed, subcultures of that clone can be used continually to make the antibody, a far cry from collection of plasma from a donor who may or may not continue to produce a usable antibody and may or may not continue to be available to donate.

Disadvantages of Monoclonal Antibody-Based Reagents

Even at the time that production of MAb was described, experienced workers predicted that the introduction of these antibodies would not provide a panacea for all the ills of blood group antigen typing. Indeed it was anticipated that some new problems would be encountered. It is highly probable that all human red cell blood group antigens are comprised of a series of epitopes. If all red cells positive for a given antigen carry all the epitopes, use of a MAb directed against any one of those epitopes would yield results identical to those obtained with human source reagents. However, it is known for sure with some antigens and is probably true of the majority of (or all) others, that all antigen-positive cells do not carry every epitope of the antigen. Thus if 99% of antigen-positive red cells carry the epitope recognized by the MAb, but 1% lack that epitope (but carry others) typing tests with the MAb will fail to identify an occasional antigen-positive sample. As a single example, MAb to D have allowed the recognition of numerous epitopes of D (43-59) and have advanced our understanding of that antigen but, at the same time, the single epitope specificity of the MAb has resulted in no single MAb to D reacting with all D+ samples. Since MAb-based blood typing reagents will often be used to screen for antigen-negative units for an immunized patient, occasional units may fail to react with the MAb, yet will be incompatible if the patient's polyclonal antibody includes molecules directed against the epitope in question (a situation with a very high probability). This problem is not too difficult to overcome. It is often possible to blend two or more MAb or to add some human polyclonal antibody to the reagent, so that its reactions exactly mirror those of antibodies in patients. While it may seem ironic to go to all the trouble of producing single epitope specific MAb, then to mix them for use as typing regents, it should be remembered that in this instance the MAbs are being used to select blood for a patient whose immune system has recognized multiple epitopes of a red cell blood group antigen. In other words, a new wheel should not be invented if it will not fit the vehicle for which it is intended. An entirely different perspective on the single epitope specificity of a MAb applies at the research level. If a series of MAbs can be used to characterize different epitopes of what had previously been recognized as a single blood group antigen, progress in understanding that antigen at the serological, biochemical, structural, genetic and immunological levels can be expected to follow.

A second disadvantage in using MAbs is that with their restricted specificity for a single epitope, some of them may cross-react with closely related epitopes on more than one antigen. While such a problem might well be resolved by using the MAb at a dilution at which it would give visible positive reactions only with red cells carrying the antigen that the antibody was intended to detect, it might also mean that the MAb was not suitable for use in adsorption-elution studies. That is to say, false positive reactions might be seen if antigen-negative red cells carrying a closely related epitope were used. It has been known for some time that the combining site of an antibody is able to bind structurally similar epitopes, (60,61) indeed the higher the affinity of an antibody, the greater the chance that it will cross-react (62). That is not to say that all MAb have high affinity and will be involved in problems of this nature. Mollison et al. (2) point out that while all molecules in a MAb have the same binding affinity and while polyclonal antibodies contain molecules with varying affinities, the affinities of most MAb are within the range seen in polyclonal antibodies.

Some problems with cross-reactivity have already been described. Thorpe (63) used a series of monoclonal anti-D in immunostaining and immunoprecipitation methods and reported that three of them bound to leukocytes and various tissue cells of D+ and D- persons and to tissue cells of various animals. These conclusions were in direct contrast to a very large body of evidence that Rh antigens are present only on red cells and some of their precursors (for details see Chapter 12). Eventually the same investigator (64) showed that one of the reactive anti-D was binding to the intermediate fila-

ment protein vimentin (65) and not to D, on the leukocytes and tissue cells. Somewhat similarly, two monoclonal anti-A that appeared highly specific for A in tests with red cells bound, in immunochemical studies, to muscle and nerve cells and to lymphocytes of group O and group B individuals (66). Adsorption studies showed the presence of a single antibody, again cross-reactivity of the MAb with structurally similar epitopes seemed to be the explanation.

A third possible problem that can be encountered in the use of MAb relates to the way in which the MAb is produced. When antibody-secreting cells are grown in tissue culture and the supernatant fluid is used as a source of the antibody, the immunoglobulin concentration is often in the order of 0.05 mg/ml. If the hybrid, antibody-producing cells are injected into a mouse and if the mouse then develops a liquid-secreting tumor, the ascitic fluid from that tumor may have a protein concentration as high as 5 mg/ml of which 90% is antibody. That is to say, the antibody concentration may be close to 100 fold greater in ascitic fluid than in culture supernatant. If the culture supernatant and the ascitic fluid are then used undiluted in serological tests, they may appear to have different specificities. Usually this apparent difference relates to antibody strength and not specificity. Blood bankers are well aware that weakened expressions of some antigens can result in red cells being seen to be antigen-positive when a potent antibody is used although the same cells may fail to react (visibly) when a weaker example of an antibody of the same specificity is used. While this explanation usually accounts for apparent differences in specificity between the same MAb in ascitic fluid and a culture supernatant, it should be remembered that ascitic fluids sometimes also contain an antibody (e.g. "natural" anti-A) of the host animal (66,67). As already mentioned, "true" specificity of a MAb (as seen in tests on ascitic fluid) does not necessarily exclude the use of diluted MAb as a typing reagent. Since the injection of antibody-secreting cells into a laboratory animal has the potential to result in a 100-fold increase in antibody level (ascitic fluid versus culture supernatant) it may appear that all MAbs should be made by such a method. However, there is no guarantee that the injected animal will develop a liquid-secreting tumor; if a solid tumor forms instead, antibody may not be secreted at all.

A fourth potential problem with MAb is that they may be sufficiently potent as to detect a trace amount of antigen on red cells that is not detectable using human source polyclonal reagents. The B(A) phenotype is discussed in detail in Chapter 8, it will be mentioned briefly here, for illustrative purposes. Using one particular MAb to A in routine ABO typing it was found that between 1 in 100 and 1 in 1000 bloods previously typed as group B, were reactive with the monoclonal anti-A (68,69). It was already known that the *A* and *B* gene-specified trans-ferases have overlapping specificities (70-72) and the explanation of the finding was that persons with high levels of *B* gene-specified transferase are able to add a small amount of N-acetyl-galactosamine (the A immunodominant sugar) and a lot of D-galactose (the B immunodominant sugar) to their red cells (69,73). The small amount of A antigen on their red cells was detected by the monoclonal anti-A in question, but not by polyclonal-based reagents. The important points about these observations are first that the persons involved (i.e. with the B(A) phenotype) are group B, for all practical purposes. That is, they have B on their red cells and anti-A in their serum. As donors their red cells can be safely transfused to group B patients, as patients they must receive group B not group AB blood. In other words for clinical purposes the trace amount of A detected by the monoclonal anti-A on red cells of the B(A) phenotype, is better not detected than found. Also involving the ABO system, one monoclonal anti-B reacted with red cells with acquired B antigens so strongly that no differentiation between acquired B and genetically inherited B could initially be seen (74-77). At least one fatal case in which a group A individual with an acquired B antigen was typed as group AB and transfused with AB blood, has occurred (78). Problems such as those involving the detection of some A antigen on B(A) red cells, and detection of acquired B on group A_1 red cells, tend to be associated with MAb made in particular clones. In other words, not all monoclonal anti-A and anti-B cause these problems. Since the monoclonal products of various clones, particularly those such as anti-A, anti-B and anti-D that will be widely used, are often carefully characterized with descriptions of their characteristics published,

it is to be earnestly hoped that FDA regulations will be promulgated that require reagent manufacturers to identify the clones whose products have been used to prepare the monoclonal-based reagents or that, in the absence of a regulatory requirement, manufacturers will supply this information voluntarily. By knowing from which clones the MAbs originated and by knowing the characteristics of the products of those clones, the user may well be able to anticipate and thus avoid potential problems.

Two final potential problems with MAb in blood group serology are that some of them fail to cause cross-linking (agglutination) of red cells while others are pH, time or temperature dependent. The first of these problems can sometimes be overcome by supplying the MAb in a milieu in which it will act as an agglutinin. The second may be resolved by using the MAb in a suitably adjusted test system. The advantages and disadvantages of using MAb in blood group serology, are summarized in table 7-1.

Having discussed potential pitfalls in the use of MAbs at some length, it must now be added that the practical blood banker who purchases a MAb-based reagent for routine use, should not be overly concerned about them save for knowing the source (originating clone) of the MAb. That is to say, by the time the reagent reaches the blood bank from a commercial supplier, the potential problems outlined above should already have been identified and addressed. However, as can be seen, some MAb have more fastidious requirements than their polyclonal counterparts meaning that it is even more important that the user follow the manufacturer's directions for use.

As will be noticed, relatively few of the hundreds of monoclonal antibodies to blood group antigens produced

TABLE 7-1 Some Advantages and Disadvantages of Using MAb in Blood Group Serology

	Advantages		Disadvantages
1.	Single epitope specificity may reveal new information about blood group antigens	1.	Single epitope specificity may be too restrictive for typing purposes. Blends of MAb often resolve this problem
2.	Unwanted positive reactions due to the presence of contaminating antibodies such as anti-T, Anti-Tn, anti-Wrᵃ, etc. will not occur	2.	Some MAb may "cross-react," i.e. define shared epitopes on different antigens
3.	Rare antibodies can sometimes be made using immortalized human B cells	3.	Use of culture supernatant or ascitic fluid may result in apparent differences in specificity
4.	Unlimited quantities of antibodies can be made	4.	Potent MAb may detect trace amounts of antigen that would be better left undetected
5.	Standardized reagents with no lot to lot variation in terms of antibody content and reactivity can be made	5.	Some MAb may fail to agglutinate red cells
6.	Highly reliable typing reagents can sometimes be made even when the MAb has a slightly different specificity	6.	Some MAb may be technique, i.e. pH, temperature, time, dependent
		7.	Due to points 2, 3, and 4 above, some MAb may not be entirely suitable for use in adorption-elution tests

thus far (79-83) have been mentioned in this chapter. They are described, together with references to their production, in the blood group system chapters of this book. It will rapidly become apparent that many (perhaps most) of the recent advances in understanding the serology, immunology, biochemistry, molecular biology and genetics of the blood group systems would not have occurred had monoclonal antibodies not been available. The excitement generated by the original report of Köhler and Milstein (37) persists and should be expected to increase.

References

1. Mollison PL, Thomas AR. Vox Sang 1959;4:185
2. Mollison PL, Engelfriet CP, Contreras M. Blood Transfusion in Clinical Medicine, 9th Ed. Oxford:Blackwell, 1993
3. Darnborough J, Dunsford I, Wallace JA. Vox Sang 1969;17:241
4. Furuhjelm U, Myllylä G, Nevanlinna HR, et al. Vox Sang 1969;17:256
5. Rogers MJ, Stiles PA, Wright J. (abstract). Transfusion 1974;14:508
6. Stroup M, MacIlroy M, Walker R, et al. Transfusion 1965;5:309
7. Lewis M, Anstee DJ, Bird GWG, et al. Vox Sang 1990;58:152
8. Daniels GL, Anstee DJ, Cartron J-P, et al. Vox Sang 1995;69:265
9. Allen FH Jr, Anstee DJ, Bird GWG, et al. Vox Sang 1982;42:164
10. Wiener AS. In: Studies in Pediatrics and Medical History. New York:Froben, 1949
11. Allen FH Jr, Newell JL. New Eng J Med 1958;259:236
12. Perrault RA, Högman CF. Acta Univ Uppsaliensis 1972:No 120
13. Nordhagen R, Kornstad L. (abstract). Book of Abstracts, 18th Cong ISBT, 1984:218
14. Lee D, Remnant M, Stratton F. Clin Lab Haematol 1984;6:33
15. Contreras M, De Silva M, Teesdale P, et al. Br J Haematol 1987;65:475
16. Morgan P, Bossom EL. Transfusion 1963;5:397
17. Tegoli J, Sausais L, Issitt PD. Vox Sang 1967;12:305
18. Marsh WL, Nichols ME, Øyen R, et al. Transfusion 1978;18:149
19. Kanel GC, Davis I, Bowman JE. Transfusion 1978;18:472
20. O'Brien M, King G, Dube VE, et al. Transfusion 1979;19:558
21. Clark A, Monaghan WP, Martin CA. Am J Med Technol 1981;47:983
22. Judd WJ, Walter WJ, Steiner EA. Transfusion 1981;21:184
23. Issitt PD, Combs MR, Bredehoeft SJ, et al. Transfusion 1993;33:284
24. Wong KH, Shelton SK, Feeley JC. J Clin Microbiol 1985;22:134
25. Cook IA, Polley MJ, Mollison PL. Lancet 1963;1:857
26. White WD, Issitt CH, McGuire D. Transfusion 1974;14:67
27. Chan PCY, Deutsch HF. J Immunol 1960;85:37
28. Pirofsky B, Cordova M de la S. Nature 1963;197:392
29. Mandy WJ, Fudenberg HH, Lewis FB. J Clin Invest 1965;44:1352
30. Romans DG, Tilley CA, Crookston MC, et al. Proc Nat Acad Sci USA 1977;74:2531
31. Nisonoff A, Hopper JE, Springs SB. The Antibody Molecule. New York:Academic Press, 1975
32. Michaelson TE, Frangione B, Franklin EC. J Biol Chem 1977;252:883
33. Scott ML, Guest AR, Anstee DJ. (abstract). Transfusion 1989;29(Suppl 7S):57S
34. Roitt I, Brostoff J, Male D. Immunology, 2nd Ed. London:Gower, 1989
35. Product Insert. Gamma ID series, anti-Fy^a and anti-Fy^b. Houston:Gamma Biologicals, 1982
36. Product Insert. Gamma ID series, Kell system antibodies. Houston:Gamma Biologicals, 1983
37. Köhler G, Milstein C. Nature 1975;256:495
38. Bourel D, Lecointre M, Genetet N, et al. Vox Sang 1987;52:85
39. Fraser RH, Inglis G, Allan JC, et al. Transfusion 1990;30:226
40. Fraser RH, Inglis G, Mackie A, et al. Transfusion 1985;25:261
41. Nichols ME, Rosenfield RE, Rubinstein P. Vox Sang 1985;49:138
42. Jaskiewicz E, Moulds JJ, Kraemer K, et al. Transfusion 1990;30:230
43. Tippett P. In Blood Group Systems: Rh. Arlington,VA:Am Assoc Blood Banks, 1987:25
44. Gorick BD, Thompson KM, Melamed MD, et al. Vox Sang 1988;55:165
45. Lomas C, Tippett P, Thompson KM, et al. Vox Sang 1989;57:261
46. Leader KA, Kumpel BM, Poole GD, et al. Vox Sang 1990;58:106
47. Hughes-Jones NC, Gorick BD, Brown D. Immunol Lett 1991;27:101
48. Lomas C, McColl K, Tippett P. Transf Med 1993;3:67
49. Lomas C, Tippett P, Mannessier L. (Letter). Transfusion 1993;33:535
50. Mouro I, Le Van Kim C, Rouillac C, et al. Blood 1994;83:1129
51. Colin Y, Bailly P, Cartron J-P. Vox Sang 1994;67 (Suppl S3):67
52. Lomas C, Grassman W, Ford D, et al. Transfusion 1994;34:612
53. Cartron J-P. Blood Rev 1994;8:199
54. van Rhenen DJ, Thijssen PMHJ, Overbeeke MAM. Vox Sang 1994;66:133
55. Scott ML, Voak D, Jones J, et al. (abstract). Transf Med 1994;4 (Suppl 1):45
56. Rouillac C, Le Van Kim C, Blancher A, et al. Br J Haematol 1995;89:424
57. Rouillac C, Le Van Kim C, Beolet M, et al. Am J Haematol 1995;49:87
58. Rouillac C, Colin Y, Hughes-Jones NC, et al. Blood 1995;85:2937
59. Tippett P, Lomas-Francis C, Wallace M. Vox Sang 1996;70:123
60. Talmage DW. Science 1959;129:1463
61. Richards FF, Konigsberg WH, Rosenstein RW, et al. Science 1975;187:130
62. Steiner LA, Eisen HM. J Exp Med 1967;126:1185
63. Thorpe SJ. Br J Haematol 1989;73:527
64. Thorpe SJ. Br J Haematol 1990;76:116
65. Steinert PM, Roop DR. Ann Rev Biochem 1988;57:593
66. Le Pendu J. In: Monoclonal Antibodies Against Human Red Blood Cell and Related Antigens. Paris:Librairie Arnette, 1987;193
67. Shaw MA. Med Lab Sci 1986;43:194

68. Beck ML, Hardman JT, Kowalski M, et al. In: Monoclonal Antibodies Against Human Red Blood Cell and Related Antigens. Paris:Librairie Arnette, 1987;224

69. Beck ML, Yates AD, Hardman J, et al. Am J Clin Pathol 1989;92:625

70. Yates AD, Watkins WM. Biochem Biophys Res Comm 1982;109:958

71. Yates AD, Greenwell P, Watkins WM. Biochem Soc Transact 1983;11:300

72. Yates AD, Feeney J, Donald ASR, et al. Carbohydr Res 1984;130:251

73. Beck ML, Yates AD, Hardman JT, et al. (abstract). Transfusion 1987;27:535

74. Beck ML, Kowalski MA, Kirkegaard J, et al. (Letter). Immunohematology 1992;8:22

75. Beck ML, Korth J, Judd WJ. (abstract). Transfusion 1992;32 (Suppl 8S): 17S

76. Beck ML, Kirkegaard J, Korth J, et al. (Letter). Transfusion 1993;33:623

77. Kirkegaard J, Beck ML. (abstract). Transfusion 1993;33 (Suppl 9S):63S

78. Garratty G, Arndt P, Co S, et al. (abstract). Transfusion 1993;33 (Suppl 9S):47S

79. Issitt PD. Transfusion 1989;29:58

80. Voak D. (Editorial). Transfusion 1989;29:191

81. Issitt PD. Murex Biologicals Scientific Publication Series, No 6, 1991

82. Lemieux R, Bazin R. Transf Med Rev 1993;7:25

83. Scott ML, Voak D. In: Immunobiology of Transfusion Medicine. New York:Marcel Dekker, 1994:365

8 | The ABO and H Blood Group Systems

Importance of the ABO System

The ABO system, discovered in 1900 by Landsteiner (1,2) is without doubt the most important of the blood group systems as far as the transfusion of blood is concerned. Generally, blood should not be transfused if it carries an ABO antigen that the recipient lacks. Transfusion accidents producing the most serious results (death on some occasions) are, by far, most often caused by ABO incompatibility involving transfusion of the wrong ABO group blood. Fortunately, it is comparatively easy to determine the ABO groups of blood donors and recipients. As described in more detail later in this chapter, tests for red cell antigens using potent ABO typing sera and tests on the plasma or serum of the blood samples for the presence of reciprocal ABO agglutinins, provide a system in which each sample is, in effect, typed twice. If the results of the tests are carefully checked to be sure that they correlate, laboratory errors in ABO typing should be virtually eliminated. As a result, serious transfusion accidents due to mistakes in determining the ABO group of a donor or a recipient are extremely rare. A number of individuals (3-6) reviewed all cases of transfusion-associated fatalities reported to the Bureau of Biologics from 1976-1978. Of the 70 deaths reported it appeared that 42 involved immune destruction of transfused red cells. Of those 42 cases, 38 involved the transfusion of ABO major side (i.e. recipient antibody directed against donor antigen) incompatible blood. In a further analysis, Honig and Bove (3) noted that in only four of the 38 cases was a serological error in the blood bank responsible for issue of the incompatible unit. However, clerical errors in the blood bank (samples or records transposed, incorrect unit released) accounted for another nine fatal reactions. In 24 cases the error resulted from a mislabeled sample or requisition form (7 cases) or involved transfusion of blood to the wrong patient (17 cases). In the remaining case (as in some of the non-ABO-related cases) the error could not be identified for sure. More recent reviews of reports of transfusion-associated fatalities made to the Center for Biologics Evaluation and Research (CBER, formerly the Bureau of Biologics) of the United States Food and Drug Administration (FDA) have been published by Edinger (7) and Sazama (8). The first of these reports covers a 7 year period and the second a 10 year period from 1976, both include the data reviewed in the earlier (3-6) publications. Sazama (8) noted that in 10 years 355 deaths had been reported but excluded 99 of them from her review since they were unrelated to transfusion or involved hepatitis or acquired immune deficiency syndrome. Of the remaining 256 cases, 158 were said to involve acute hemolysis, of those 158 cases, 131 involved the transfusion of ABO incompatible blood. Of the 158 cases involving acute hemolysis, 13 resulted from a mislabeled sample or requisition form, 20 from serological errors in the blood bank, 25 when the samples or records were confused in the blood bank or when the wrong unit was issued and 77 when blood was transfused to the wrong patient. In the remaining 23 cases the error was unclear or could not be determined. Thus the most common single cause of a transfusion-related death continues to be transfusion of blood to the wrong patient. Among errors leading to the 77 transfusions given to the wrong patient, 51 were made by nurses alone, 15 by physicians alone and 11 by both a nurse and a physician. As Schmidt (4) had noted earlier, a scenario that was repeated (8) involved the anesthesiologist in the operating room when one patient's surgery had been completed, surgery on the next patient had begun, but blood intended for the first patient was held in the operating room and transfused to the second patient.

Although close to half of all the transfusion-related deaths involving acute hemolysis resulted when blood was given to the wrong patient, there is no room for complacency in the blood bank. First, at least 20 deaths (12.7%) occurred following a serological error, at least another 25 (15.8%) occurred when samples or records were muddled or the wrong unit was issued. These numbers may be higher since in 23 of the 158 cases, cause of the error could not be established.

There are two important points that should be considered when data such as those given above are reviewed. First, it is commonly accepted that there is underreporting of transfusion accidents. In some instances the connection between death and the transfusion is not recognized. Probably more common, it is supposed that some reports are not made to the CBER because many persons involved in transfusion medicine are unaware of the legal requirement that such events be reported. As Sazama (8) stated, figures obtained and used in reviews such as hers are the best available but the true numbers are "generally unknown and probably unknowable".

Second and perhaps compensating for underreporting to some degree, there is no doubt that some of the deaths reported were not caused by the transfusion of incompatible blood. For example, in reviewing deaths supposedly caused by delayed hemolysis, Sazama (8) notes that one is attributed to anti-Ch and another to an HTLA. While one need not dispute that an anti-Ch and an HTLA were present, nor that the patients died, experienced workers are likely to conclude that those situations were true, true and unrelated.

To put the above figures in perspective it is commonly believed that in the 10 year period in which 355 deaths were reported, some 100 million units of red cells were transfused to some 28 to 30 million patients. Although such figures show that error rates as percentages are small, it should be remembered that the errors are also preventable by adherence to correct serological, clerical and management techniques and systems. It is clear that there is a real need for transfusion services to establish a foolproof system to ensure that all units of blood transfused are given to the patients for whom they are intended. Further, the system must include a mechanism that prevents mislabeling or misidentification of samples submitted to the service for compatibility testing. It is ironic that over the years, huge amounts of energy and an untold sum of money have been expended in the development of methods for the detection of weak antibodies in the sera of potential recipients of blood transfusions. While it is true that some of these antibodies, if not detected before transfusion, can bring about reduced survival of the transfused red cells, they do not usually cause reactions as serious as those that occur when ABO incompatible blood is transfused. Antibodies other than those in the ABO system seldom cause fatal transfusion reactions (see Chapter 36). Accordingly, it would seem prudent for blood bankers to direct a large portion of their current efforts (and money) to the establishment of a system designed to eliminate ABO incompatible transfusions that, at their worst, may kill the patient. In concluding this sermon it should be mentioned that fatal transfusion reactions caused by ABO antibodies always involve major side incompatibility. The passive transfer of donor ABO antibodies to patients (minor side incompatibility, as in the transfusion of platelet concentrates containing plasma from ABO mismatched donors, see below) seldom causes real difficulties and often causes no difficulties at all.

The reasons that major side ABO incompatible transfusions often result in severe transfusion reactions are several. First, antibodies against the A or B antigens that an individual lacks, are almost always present. Thus, virtually all group A persons will have anti-B in their plasma, virtually all those who are group B will have anti-A and virtually all those who are group O will have anti-A,B. Second, these antibodies will often be of high titer and/or avidity even in individuals who have never been exposed to foreign red cells. Third, although ABO typing is invariably performed at room temperature,

almost all ABO system antibodies are capable of binding to red cells carrying the appropriate ABO system antigens, at 37°C. (Anti-A_1 in A_2 and A_2B individuals is usually a notable exception.) Thus, anti-A, anti-B and anti-A,B (in the plasma of group B, A and O persons respectively) are not cold-reactive antibodies that can be ignored in transfusion therapy. Fourth, both IgM and IgG forms of anti-A, anti-B and anti-A,B are invariably capable of activating complement. This fact, coupled with the fifth consideration, namely that the A and B antigens are present in very large amounts (circa two million or more copies per red cell (9) and see section on intravascular hemolysis in Chapter 6 for derivation of this number) means that when major side ABO incompatible blood is transfused, all the conditions necessary for acute intravascular hemolysis (see Chapter 6) exist.

Because many patients who receive blood transfusions are already seriously ill, it is difficult to determine the smallest volume of ABO incompatible blood that has caused the death of a patient. In other words, as in any transfusion-associated death, it is difficult to determine the contribution of the incompatible transfusion in relation to the contribution of the patient's disease. Mollison (10) reports that of some 50 individuals injected with quantities between 0.2 and 1.0 ml of ABO incompatible red cells, only one displayed any clinical symptoms of a transfusion reaction. Jandl et al. (11,12) gave injections of 10 ml of washed incompatible red cells and observed transient reactions in some but by no means all the recipients. When reactions to small amounts of ABO incompatible red cells are encountered, anti-A or anti-B hemolysins can invariably be demonstrated in the individual's pretransfusion (preinjection) serum (10-12). If the reviews of reports to the FDA (3-8) and individual reports of fatal transfusion reactions (13-18) are studied, it appears that death following the transfusion of less than 125 ml of red cells is unusual. In the reports submitted to the CBER and reviewed by Sazama (8) it was stated that one patient supposedly suffered a fatal reaction after receiving 30 ml of red cells and three others succumbed after receiving some 60 ml. In the other 120 patients who died, in whom the amount of blood given was reported: 8 had received half a unit; 74 had received one unit; 22 had received 2 units; and 16 had received 3 units. In considering the report of death following a small volume of incompatible red cells it should be remembered that both Sazama (8) and we (above) have questioned the absolute accuracy of the reports. Nevertheless, the fact that the incidence of a fatal outcome from the transfusion of ABO major side incompatible blood is directly proportional to the amount of blood transfused means that the requirement that the patient be monitored for the first 10 to 20 minutes of the transfusion, is critical. If the signs and symptoms of a severe transfusion reaction (see Chapter 36) are seen and the transfusion is stopped before 100 ml or so of blood has been infused, the patient stands a good chance of surviving the episode.

Major Side ABO Incompatible Transfusions and Mild Reactions

In spite of what has been written above, about the serious consequences that can result when ABO incompatible blood is transfused, there are a number of reports in the literature (19-24) about transfusion accidents of this type that were not associated with severe transfusion reactions. In most of these it was found that the patient's ABO antibodies were of relatively low titer and were not readily hemolytic in in vitro tests at the time of the transfusion. Although, in some cases the transfusion of ABO incompatible blood caused the ABO antibodies to increase in strength so that the transfused red cells were later cleared, the weakness of the antibodies at the time of transfusion prevented immediate intravascular hemolysis of all the incompatible cells. As a result, the signs and symptoms usually associated with ABO incompatible transfusions were not seen. The immune response that follows the transfusion of major side ABO incompatible blood is described below.

Incidence of Major Side ABO Incompatible Transfusions

It is, of course, very difficult to determine how often blood incompatible with a patient's ABO antibody is transfused. Wallace (21) reported that in the 1950s he had studied data from transfusions of more than 60,000 units of blood to some 20,000 patients. In six cases ABO incompatible blood was transfused (twice due to mislabeled samples from the patient, twice due to laboratory errors and twice due to transfusion to the wrong patient). Thus in this study one transfused unit in 10,000 was ABO incompatible, 1 in 3300 patients received ABO incompatible blood. Mayer (25) reported 27 ABO hemolytic reactions in close to half a million transfusions for an incidence of about 1 unit in 18,000 transfused or once in every 6,000 patients. At the Mayo Clinic where the transfusion service staff have total control of all aspects of transfusion, from the collection of samples from the patients through the administration of units outside the operating rooms and monitoring of transfusions in the operating rooms (26), only one of 268,000 units of blood, given over a 10 year period, was ABO incompatible (18). If the calculation (22) that 10% of major side ABO incompatible transfusions are fatal is accepted, it can be calculated, from the review of Sazama (8) that 1310 units of some 100 million transfused were ABO incompatible (i.e. 131 deaths from ABO incompatible transfusions). This gives an incidence of 1 transfusion in 76,000 and leads to the suspicion (based on the observations of Wallace (21) and Mayer (25)) that there is underreporting to the CBER. Given the excellence of the service reporting 1 unit in every 18,000 as ABO incompatible (25), one suspects that the national average is probably higher than that, i.e. perhaps closer to the 1 in 10,000 observed by Wallace (21).

Deliberate Transfusions with Major Side ABO Incompatible Blood

In view of all the terrible consequences that can result from major side ABO incompatible transfusions, many blood bankers are surprised to learn that some workers transfuse such blood deliberately. In allogeneic bone marrow transplantation, success can be achieved even when the donor marrow is ABO incompatible with the recipient, i.e. marrow donor group A, recipient group O (28-34,44). In such ABO incompatible situations engraftment may take longer than when the donor and recipient are ABO identical (35-38,45) and persistence of recipient anti-A and/or anti-B may result in destruction of some red cells produced by the donor marrow (36,39). This problem may be more noticeable in patients treated with cyclosporine to prevent GVHD than in those who do not receive that drug (35-38). Another more immediate problem is that when the donor marrow has been frozen (particularly when dimethyl sulphoxide (DMSO) is used) it must be infused very rapidly, i.e. within 5 to 10 minutes after being thawed since in the liquid form DMSO is toxic to marrow cells. Marrow harvests are invariable heavily contaminated with red blood cells with the result that when ABO incompatible marrow preparations are infused rapidly, acute intravascular hemolytic transfusion reactions are seen. One solution to this problem is to remove as many red cells as possible from the marrow preparation using sedimentation with or without a sedimenting agent such as hydroxyethyl starch (35,41-43,46). Alternatively a cell separator may be used (40).

The methods described above are designed to remove ABO incompatible red cells from the marrow preparations before those preparations are infused. An alternative approach, that was common in early work on marrow transplantation, is to try to remove or reduce the level of the ABO antibodies of the patient. Plasma exchange was often used but suffers from a number of disadvantages (28-31,47,48). First, because such large volumes of plasma must be exchanged the procedure is protracted and is performed at a time, immediately before transplantation, when the patient is undergoing intensive chemotherapy and/or radiation treatment. Second, even when intensive plasma exchange is used, e.g. equivalent to eleven or more plasma volume exchanges (29,34) ABO antibodies are not always sufficiently reduced in strength that large numbers of ABO incompatible red cells can safely be infused. Third, if large amounts of donor ABO type plasma are used, the risk of disease transmission exists. Fourth, if fluids such as albumin solutions are used for the exchange, to avoid the risk of disease transmission, rapid equilibration of the IgG level occurs from the extravascular compartment so that reduction of ABO antibody levels is only transient. Fifth, particularly in children, vascular access may be difficult.

To overcome some of these problems, plasma exchange was sometimes followed by the infusion of soluble A and/or B substances (49) or the transfusion of donor ABO type blood (28-30,38,50-52). The idea was to use plasma exchange to reduce the level of ABO antibodies to the point at which they would cause relatively mild transfusion reactions, then adsorb the remaining antibodies in vivo by the transfusion of incompatible red cells. Although methods to remove red cells from the marrow preparations are probably more in vogue than those that effect in vivo antibody adsorption, the latter have not been abandoned.

Tichelli et al. (53) selected patients with low levels of ABO antibodies and transfused them with ABO incompatible blood, without first performing plasma exchange, to effect in vivo antibody adsorption. Most recently Nussbaumer et al. (54) began their study similarly, then extended it to all patients, regardless of the initial starting levels of the ABO antibodies. Even when ABO agglutinin levels were as high as 64 and IAT active antibodies had titers of 1024, two units of ABO incompatible blood were transfused. The transfusions were on days -2 and -1 before transplantation, were performed in the intensive care unit, each unit was given over an 8 hour period, the patients were hyperhydrated (3000 ml per meter^2 per day) with equal volumes of normal saline and 5% glucose from day -6 to day -1 and sodium bicarbonate was given to keep the urine pH above 7.0. The units of red cells were leukodepleted, washed and irradiated (15Gy). It was reported that the patients suffered mild nausea and chills at the beginning of the transfusions and passed dark urine after the transfusions. One patient with impaired renal function before transfusion suffered reversible renal failure and it was recommended that the procedure not be used for patients with preexisting renal impairment. It was further reported that other than the mild reactions described above, none of 12 patients treated in this manner suffered untoward reactions during the transfusion of red cells or the subsequent

marrow transfusions. It was claimed that this protocol has the advantages of: not requiring plasma exchange that results in the removal of immunoglobulins in addition to anti-A and anti-B and in the removal of coagulation factors; not introducing significant risk of transmitting disease (two units of leukoreduced, washed red cells but no plasma is used); avoiding the manipulation of the marrow preparation to remove red cells, that introduces a risk of loss or damage to stem cells (40,55,56).

When the ABO Chapters of the first three editions of this book were written the authors had no idea that in the fourth edition the deliberate transfusion of 2 units of ABO incompatible blood to a patient with an ABO antibody with an IAT of 1024, *for the patient's benefit,* would be described!

Passive Transfer of ABO System Antibodies

In spite of the very real danger that exists when red cells carrying an antigen against which the patient has an ABO system antibody, are transfused, the passive transfer of ABO agglutinins directed against an A or B antigen on the recipient's red cells (minor side incompatibility) only occasionally causes serious consequences. There are three principle reasons why this is so. First, when the donor plasma is infused rapid dilution of the antibodies by the patient's plasma occurs. This is the case even in anemic patients where the red cell mass may be low but where the total blood volume is likely to be normal. Second, when a major side incompatible unit is transfused there is a whole body full of antibodies (the patient's) and a limited number of red cells (the donor's) so that each red cell is likely to have multiple antibody molecules bound. In minor side incompatibility, the number of antibody molecules present (the donor's) are distributed among a body full of red cells (the patient's) so that each red cell may bind only a few antibody molecules. On most occasions the number of antibody molecules bound per cell is too low for macrophage recognition of IgG coated cells or for appreciable amounts of complement to be activated (for both considerations, see also Chapter 6). Third, in addition to the ABO antigens present on the patient's red cells, there will be like-specificity blood group substance free in the plasma (57-62) so that some antibody inhibition will occur. As a simple example, if a unit of group O plasma is transfused to a group A patient, the anti-A,B in the donor plasma will be diluted by the patient's own plasma. At the same time some of the donor's antibody will be neutralized by the A substance in the patient's plasma. The soluble A and B substances in plasma are almost certainly different (and additive to) the A and B antigens found in units of stored red cells where microvesicles released from such cells during storage (63,64) carry some antigens from the red cells from which they were formed (65,66).

In spite of the protective factors listed above, there are some reports (23,67-71) that describe destruction of the patient's own red cells by antibodies in the donor plasma. Most of these involved the infusion of plasma from a group O donor to a group A patient. When transfusions with minor side incompatible whole blood were relatively frequent, efforts were made to identify "dangerous" group O donors. That is, those with levels of anti-A,B such that their blood was suitable only for group O recipients. Several different test methods to identify dangerous group O donors were used. Mollison (22) showed that if the donor serum, when diluted 1 in 4, failed to hemolyze A₁ or B cells, there was little danger that it would cause appreciable red cell destruction in a group A or B recipient. This test was not particularly applicable to routine use since it involved the addition of fresh serum (as a source of complement) to each test. Others considered group O donors as "safe" if their sera did not agglutinate A₁ or B cells at a dilution of 1 in 50, different workers set the cut-off point as non-agglutination by the donor serum at a dilution of 1 in 100. Still others considered the group O donors as "safe" if their serum failed to hemolyze A₁ and B cells in reverse grouping tests incubated at 37°C. While there is little doubt that each of these methods identified dangerous group O donors, it is probable that they also eliminated many group O units that could have been transfused to group A or B recipients with impunity. As described below, current blood banking practices have virtually eliminated the need for tests to detect dangerous group O donors. While occasional anecdotal reports of this problem are still heard, a cost benefit ratio would be unlikely to suggest continuation of tests for "dangerous" O donors. In considering the passive transfer of ABO system antibodies it is convenient to consider separately, the use of red cell products, plasma, platelet concentrates, cryoprecipitate and factor VIII concentrates.

Passive Transfer of ABO Antibodies in Red Cell Transfusions

Most workers now agree that group O packed cells can be transfused to patients of any ABO type without it being necessary to measure anti-A,B levels in the group O donors. It is felt that the small amounts of plasma left on the packed red cells are unlikely to effect very much (if any) destruction of non-group O recipient red cells. Use of red cells from which most of the plasma has been removed and replaced with a synthetic additive is likely to make red cell destruction by passively transferred anti-A and/or anti-B an even less common event. It is possi-

ble that the danger was not as great as theoretically conceived even when group O whole blood was used. Ebert and Emerson (69) transfused a series of group A, B and AB patients with group O blood as a routine. They noted frank evidence of red cell destruction in only 1% of the recipients but did feel that asymptomatic accelerated rates of red cell destruction occurred in some others.

Because infants and children have smaller blood volumes than adults, less passively transferred antibody may bring about in vivo lysis meaning that ABO minor side incompatible transfusion should be avoided. For example, it is sometimes necessary to prepare blood for an exchange transfusion for an infant in whom it is believed that HDN will be severe, before birth of the infant and before its ABO type is known. Group O packed or washed cells can be used. If the physician who will perform the exchange transfusion does not wish to use packed cells because of their viscosity and the mechanical difficulties that ensue, the group O cells can be resuspended in group AB plasma.

Passive Transfer of ABO Antibodies in Plasma Transfusions

Since transfusions with fresh frozen, cryoprecipitate extracted and banked plasma involve the infusion of relatively large volumes of plasma, it is advisable (and easy to accomplish) to use ABO type specific plasma for such transfusions. Indeed, there are reports (72,73) of destruction of the patient's red cells in hemophiliacs given minor side incompatible fresh frozen plasma.

Passive Transfer of ABO Antibodies in Platelet Transfusions

When platelets are stored at room temperature, those from each donor may be suspended in as much as 50 to 65 ml of plasma. Thus when eight platelet concentrates are pooled, the plasma volume may be as high as 400 to 500 ml. Because such pools may contain appreciable amounts of antibody it seems prudent to use platelets from ABO matched donors whenever possible. In fact, a better reason for using ABO major side compatible platelets is that such transfusions are more effective in increasing the patient's platelet level, than are platelets from ABO incompatible donors (74-78). Because platelet transfusion demands seldom match platelet concentrate inventories it is sometimes necessary to use ABO mismatched platelets. Two considerations apply. If the platelets carry A and/or B antigens to which the patient has the antibody, the platelet increment will be reduced. If the plasma in which the platelets are suspended contains anti-A and/or anti-B and the patient is A, B or AB the platelet increment will be better but some hemolysis of the recipient's red cells may occur. Most authorities recommend the use of minor side incompatible over major side incompatible platelets when the choice must be made. In spite of the infusion of large volumes of minor side incompatible plasma with the platelets, serious difficulties are not commonly encountered. The patient may develop a positive DAT and anti-A and/or anti-B may be recovered from the patient's red cells by elution. Appreciable in vivo red cell destruction is a much less frequently encountered event. If necessary the platelet concentrate can be volume reduced, i.e. centrifuged to isolate the platelets, some plasma removed, then the platelets resuspended, immediately before issue. Removal of some plasma from both pools of platelet concentrates from individual donors and from single donor platelets collected by pheresis can be used. Such removal should be done as close to the time of transfusion as possible to prevent damage to the platelets, although demonstration of suitable resuspension of the platelets is essential before they are issued. It should also be remembered that whatever centrifugation method is used before plasma removal, some loss of platelets (i.e. circa 15%) is inevitable (79,80). Volume reduction of even ABO identical platelets is indicated for some patients, particularly children, to prevent volume overload.

In 1977 a case was described (81) in which a patient of phenotype $A_{int}B$ (see later in this chapter for a description of the A_{int} phenotype) was transfused with 10 units of platelets from group O donors. When subsequently transfused with A_1B red cells, the patient had a transfusion reaction that was described by the investigators as being due to anti-A_1. What the patient really had, of course, was a transfusion reaction due to anti-A. The antibody remaining in the patient's plasma was not anti-A_1, but anti-A,B passively transferred in the plasma from the 10 group O donors, that was now present in a dilution that allowed it to react (visibly) with A_1 but not with A_{int} or A_2 red cells. No doubt, if the patient had been of phenotype A_1B instead of $A_{int}B$ the antibody would have caused destruction of some of the patient's cells as well. The difference between A_1 and A_2 and the specificity of the antibody most conveniently described as anti-A_1 are discussed in more detail later in this chapter.

Passive Transfer of ABO Antibodies in Cryoprecipitate and Factor VIII Concentrates

This is perhaps the area in which the passive transfer of ABO antibodies causes a problem most frequently.

Since cryoprecipitate or factor VIII concentrate must usually be administered over an extended period of time, and since the concentration methods used to prepare the factor VIII product also concentrate IgG, the amount of ABO antibody in the recipient's plasma may gradually accumulate and eventually reach a level at which it causes destruction of some of the recipient's red cells. Cases where this has occurred, when factor VIII concentrate was used, have been reported (82-84) and one of us has seen a similar situation in two other group A hemophiliacs (85). In one of them it occurred on four separate occasions separated by several years. Since it is the IgG immune form of anti-A and anti-B that causes the problem (22) the DAT on the patient's red cells is invariably positive and anti-A (or anti-B or both) can be shown to be present in eluates made from the patient's red cells. The fact that this occurred several times in one group A hemophiliac but never in other similarly treated patients, caused us to speculate that the phenomenon is most likely to be seen in a patient who is unfortunate enough to have both hemophilia and a high A antigen site density on his red cells.

Passive Transfer of ABO Antibodies in Intravenous Immune Globulin Preparations

Based on what has been written above, it should come as no surprise that intravenous immune globulin preparations (IVIG) contain a whole variety of antibodies. Indeed the whole purpose of IVIG is that it supply required IgG antibodies or IgG molecules that the patient lacks. Clearly as the result of methods used to concentrate IVIG, anti-A and anti-B will be among the immunoglobulins present in potent form. In spite of this there are relatively few reports in the literature about deleterious effects following the passive transfer of anti-A and/or anti-B in IVIG (86). Perhaps the paucity of reports simply reflects the fact that clinicians using IVIG expect to see anti-A and/or anti-B mediated hemolysis in some of their patients so do not report such an event when it occurs. In a recent case in which we (87) studied a group O child who had been transplanted with her brother's group B marrow, hemolysis of the group B red cells produced by the engrafted marrow was clearly occurring. However, since the child was receiving IVIG, HLA matched platelets from primarily group O donors and group O red cells because anti-B was still demonstrable in her serum, it was difficult to determine which source anti-B was causing the red cell destruction. Since the fraternal marrow had engrafted, HLA matched platelet transfusions were discontinued, washed group O red cells were transfused and IVIG administration was tapered then stopped. Eventually anti-B disappeared from the patient's plasma and hemolysis of the group B red cells stopped.

Solution to the Problem

The passive transfer of ABO antibodies can be prevented by the use of ABO type specific (or minor side compatible) plasma. When platelet concentrates containing minor side incompatible plasma, or cryoprecipitate, or factor VIII concentrates must be used, the patient's course can be followed with serial DATs. As long as the DAT remains negative and there is no evidence of in vivo hemolysis, changes in therapy are not required. Once the DAT becomes positive, or if there are signs that indicate that a hemolytic process has begun, further transfusions of platelet concentrates or cryoprecipitate should be with ABO minor side compatible components, within the confines mentioned above regarding avoidance of transfusing ABO major side incompatible platelets. Since ABO specific transfusion cannot be accomplished with factor VIII concentrates it may be necessary to replace treatment with that product with minor side compatible cryoprecipitate.

If sufficient levels of free ABO antibodies are present in the patient's serum that compatibility tests are positive with red cells of the patient's own ABO type and if red cell transfusions are indicated, it becomes necessary to use packed or washed group O red cells. A similar situation may arise in patients given group O blood in an emergency, before their own ABO types were determined. Once such group O blood has been transfused it becomes difficult to know when a switch to blood of the patient's own type can be made. A good rule of thumb seems to be to rely on the compatibility test. In other words, if group A red cells appear to be compatible in in vitro tests, with a current serum sample from a group A patient known to have received group O blood, it is probable that the A cells will survive normally in vivo.

ABO Minor Side Incompatibility following Bone Marrow Transplantation

An ABO minor side incompatibility problem that cannot be solved by the measures outlined in the previous paragraph involves the production of anti-A and/or anti-B by immunologically competent cells transferred to the recipient at the time of marrow transplantation. The antibodies produced then complex with and destroy the recipient's own red cells and any transfused cells that were of the patient's ABO type. This type of hemolysis is typically delayed and is seen one to two weeks after the marrow is transplanted, presumably at a time when the transplanted antibody-producing cells are producing sufficient levels of antibody to cause red cell destruction. The term passenger lymphocyte syndrome is used to describe this situation. Hemolysis caused by anti-A and/or anti-B in this setting may begin abruptly, may be severe (intravascular hemolysis has been reported) and necessitate either additional red cell transfusions or plasma exchange in severe cases (88,89). A similar phenomenon involving both ABO (90-94,154) and other system antibodies (94-101) has been reported following solid organ transplants. In a number of the reports on ABO antibody production following organ transplantation, the antibody has been described as anti-A_1. If the transplanted organ was from a group O donor, the antibody must have been anti-A not anti-A_1. Certainly the level of antibody made may have been such that the antibody agglutinated A_1 but not A_2 red cells so appeared to have anti-A_1 specificity. However, that feature is a function of antibody strength and A antigen site density of A_1 and A_2 red cells. Immunocytes from a group O donor make anti-A (and anti-B) not anti-A_1. The quantitative difference between the A_1 and A_2 phenotypes is discussed again, later in this chapter. It should also be remembered that the passenger lymphocytes involved were already primed to make antibody before they were taken out of the donor and transplanted in the recipient. In the donor, of course, the antibodies made were alloimmune in nature. In the recipient, until total engraftment has occurred, the antibodies will appear to be autoimmune.

As in the case of immune hemolysis of red cells from the transplanted marrow in ABO major side incompatible transplants (36), hemolysis due to minor side incompatibility in which transplanted immunocytes produce the antibody, appears to be related to the use of cyclosporine. In one series (88), five patients with red cell hemolysis associated with the passenger lymphocyte syndrome were receiving cyclosporine, in the same institution among 13 patients who received minor side incompatible bone marrow transplants but who received methotrexate instead of cyclosporine, no donor-derived antibody caused hemolysis. In a large series of patients receiving ABO unmatched kidneys, 2 of 34 patients on cyclosporine but none of 108 on azathioprine, experienced minor side antibody-induced hemolysis (102).

Petz (27) and Gajewski et al. (103) have pointed out that when the passenger lymphocyte syndrome results in the production of minor side ABO incompatible antibodies (i.e. directed against the recipients' red cells) far more red cell destruction may occur than can be explained by destruction of the recipients' red cells alone. In three patients studied in detail (27) in whom transfusion involved the use of group O washed red cells (to avoid introduction of red cells incompatible with the donor

ABO antibodies and to avoid the passive transfer of additional amounts of ABO antibodies) it was clear that a large proportion of the group O red cells were also destroyed. It was concluded that destruction of the group O red cells occurred via the "innocent bystander" (reactive lysis, see Chapter 6) mechanism. In two of the three patients renal dialysis was required when the hemolysis caused renal failure. Again the hemolysis in these patients was associated with the use of cyclosporine. In an attempt to prevent severe hemolysis via the reactive lysis mechanism, four patients scheduled to receive ABO minor side incompatible transplants from unrelated donors and scheduled to receive cyclosporine to prevent GVHD, were given 8 unit exchange transfusions with group O red cells before receiving their transplants. Hemolysis due to donor-derived antibodies was not prevented but was less than in those patients not treated by pretransplant exchange transfusions. Further, in three of the four patients, the degree of red cell destruction could be explained by destruction of the patient's remaining ABO incompatible (with the donor-derived ABO) antibodies (27). Petz (27) reports that in addition to the exaggerated immune response to ABO blood group antigens by donor-derived immunocytes in patients receiving cyclosporine, the events are more severe in patients receiving transplants from unrelated donors, than in those receiving transplants from siblings.

Triulzi et al. (996) documented their findings in 41 consecutive patients who had received a liver transplant. Nine of the 41 received a total of 10 ABO-unmatched livers. Five of those nine patients developed donor derived antibodies and hemolysis In all five patients the liver donor was group O and the patient was group A. Indeed, just as with ABO HDN (see Chapter 41) most problems of this type seem to result from the production of anti-A and anti-B by group O individuals or transplanted immunocytes (94,997-1002). However, we (1003) have recently encountered one case in which a group AB recipient experienced hemolysis caused by donor-derived anti-A from the group B liver donor's cells. The problem is sufficiently common and severe following liver transplantation that Triulzi et al. (996) recommended the transfusion of donor ABO type red cells during and after surgery.

Benign ABO System Antibodies

As will be apparent from what has been written in this chapter thus far, ABO antibodies are of great importance in transfusion therapy most of the time. In spite of this, there are some ABO system and ABO system-related antibodies that are benign in vivo. Between 1 and 8% of persons of the phenotype A_2 and between 22 and 35% of per-

sons of the phenotype A_2B (or more in some populations) present with anti-A_1 in the serum (104-108, see below for details about the A_1 and A_2 phenotypes). Most of the time anti-A_1 is a cold-reactive antibody that will not complex with red cells at 37°C. Like other cold-reactive antibodies with this limited thermal range (see Chapter 35) these anti-A_1 are incapable of destroying antigen-positive (in this case A_1) red cells in vivo. Accordingly, there is no need to select A_2 or A_2B blood for transfusion to these patients. On very rare occasions an example of anti-A_1 may be found that is active at 37°C and that may be capable of destroying (often limited numbers of) A_1 red cells in vivo (109-113). There are several important points to be made about the observation that anti-A_1 can sometimes be a clinically-significant antibody. First, when the incidence of anti-A_1 (see above) is compared to the number of reports of that antibody causing in vivo red cell clearance, it becomes abundantly clear that clinically-significant forms of anti-A_1 are extraordinarily rare. Indeed, if one calculates the number of patients with anti-A_1 who must have been encountered since the first report of in vivo red cell destruction by that antibody was made, and if one couples this with the assumption that 50% of all patients with that antibody who have been transfused were given A_1 blood, it appears that only one example of anti-A_1 in about 125,000 examples found, is capable of destroying A_1 red cells in vivo. Obviously, most blood bankers will spend their entire careers without encountering a clinically-significant example of anti-A_1. Second, when patients with cold-reactive anti-A_1 are transfused with A_1 blood, very few of them (109,110,112,114,115) mount an immune response that results in an increase in strength or a widening in thermal amplitude, of their antibody. As with the overwhelming majority of patients with cold-reactive antibodies, the introduction of red cells carrying the antigen to which the antibody is directed, almost always fails to cause any alteration in the immune response in the patient (23,116). Third, if red cell survival studies using small amounts (circa 1.0 ml) of ^{51}Cr-labeled A_1 red cells are performed in patients with anti-A_1 (some of the antibodies in the patients studied were weakly reactive at 37°C) limited destruction of a small amount of the test dose (say 20% of the 1 ml of labeled red cells) with normal survival of the remainder, almost always means that survival of a whole unit of cells, if transfused, would be expected to be normal (22,23,117-123). A detailed study (124) illustrated this point very clearly. The patient had anti-A_1 that, in in vitro studies, agglutinated red cells up to 32°C and caused some complement activation at 37°C. When a test dose of 0.55 ml of ^{51}Cr-labeled A_1 cells was injected, 65% of the cells were destroyed within 30 minutes of the injection. When a test dose of 18.9 ml of labeled A_1 cells was injected about 45% of the cells were destroyed within 30 minutes. When a whole unit of A_1 blood was transfused, 90% of the cells were present in the patient's circulation 24 hours after the transfusion. In other words, in spite of accelerated clearance of the small dose test samples, survival of the A_1 cells was essentially normal when a whole unit was transfused. Further, this example of anti-A_1 was unusual in that it caused complement activation. Most antibodies of this specificity lack that ability. Fourth, in vitro tests with anti-A_1 can, like tests with any cold-reactive antibody, be extremely misleading if not performed with considerable care. For example, if antibody screening or compatibility tests are read by immediate spin and/or following incubation at room temperature and then incubated at 37°C, positive reactions after the 37°C incubation do NOT indicate that the antibody is active at 37°C. Instead, a test in which the red cells and serum are separately warmed to 37°C before being mixed and in which these tests are read at 37°C, is essential to determine whether an example of anti-A_1 (or any other antibody) is truly active at 37°C. As already indicated, when this test is used it is found that the overwhelming majority of examples of anti-A_1 are not active at 37°C and accordingly, are of no consequence in transfusion therapy.

As mentioned above, we believe that those reports that describe red cell destruction by anti-A_1, made by passenger lymphocytes following transplantation from a group O donor (90,93,125), those that describe red cell destruction by anti-A_1 following the transfusion of platelets from group O donors (81) and those that describe destruction of red cells by anti-A_1 following the transfusion of whole blood or plasma from group O donors, misinterpret the true situation. Again, we believe that the antibody involved is actually anti-A (126-129) that looks like anti-A_1 because it agglutinates A_1 but not A_2 red cells. We believe that in each instance, adsorption of the antibody with A_2 red cells would have revealed its anti-A specificity.

Similar observations regarding lack of clinical significance have been made about other ABO system or related antibodies. Anti-H as made by A_1, B and A_1B individuals is invariably benign in vivo. The only examples of clinically-significant anti-H of which we are aware, were made by H-negative (O_h or Bombay, see later in this Chapter) individuals. The example described by Davey et al. (130) rapidly cleared H-positive cells in a ^{51}Cr survival study, the example described by Moores et al. (131) caused hemolytic disease of the newborn. Again, the difference in clinical significance of these antibodies relates directly to their thermal range. Anti-H as made by A_1, B and A_1B individuals is almost always optimally reactive at low temperatures. Anti-H made by O_h persons can be as active at 37°C as at room temperature or 4°C.

Antibodies that react only with red cells from individuals who have I or i on their red cells and certain functional ABO or P system genes (antibodies to IH, IB, IA,

iH, IP_1, etc.) are described in detail in Chapters 10 and 11. Suffice it here to say that these antibodies too are almost always active only at temperatures below 37°C so are clinically insignificant. As discussed in detail in previous editions of this book, the overwhelming majority of patients with anti-A_1, anti-IH, etc., do not need to be transfused with antigen negative blood. They can safely be transfused with blood that has not been phenotyped but which has been shown to be serologically-compatible in tests using a prewarmed method.

Predominantly Benign ABO System Autoantibodies

Most of the ABO system autoantibodies that have been reported in the literature (132-153,252-256) can be classified as being one of two types. The first type is a cold-reactive benign autoantibody, the reactions of which may interfere in ABO grouping or antibody screening tests but whose clinical relevance is nil. The second type is an autoantibody capable of causing some in vivo destruction of the patient's red cells because of its wider than normal thermal range. These antibodies, although of some clinical importance, have not often caused severe disease. As described in Chapter 38, cold antibody-induced hemolytic anemia (cold hemagglutinin disease or CHD) is often a relatively mild disorder because the autoantibody can bind to the patient's cells (and hence cause in vivo red cell destruction) only when the patient's body temperature falls below normal. With both types of autoantibody mentioned above, the specificity has often but not always been different from ordinary anti-A and anti-B and autoantibodies directed against the IH, IA, IB, iH, etc., determinants (see also Chapter 10) have been identified. A recent review (256) has listed the serological features and clinical relevance or lack thereof of many of the ABO autoantibodies described in the reports listed above.

Although they did not initially appear to be autoantibodies, this is a convenient place to record that some anti-A have been found in A_1 persons and some anti-B in A_1B persons (22,132,155). The antibodies failed to agglutinate the antibody-maker's red cells but did react with other A or B cells respectively. In one of the cases (155) the anti-B was adsorbed by the subject's A_1B red cells although it would not agglutinate them. In the other cases incomplete adsorption occurred (132) or details of autoadsorption studies were not included. One auto-anti-A reactive only in the presence of borate (156) and one reactive only in the presence of chloramphenicol (157) have been described. The presence of anti-B in the sera of individuals whose red cells acquire a B antigen is discussed in a later section of this chapter.

Pathological ABO System Autoantibodies

Some ABO system autoantibodies have behaved quite differently. In a case reported by Szymanski et al. (158) an A_1 patient developed auto-anti-A (anti-IA specificity was excluded) that was capable of binding to and causing intravascular destruction of the patient's red cells at normal body temperature. The antibody caused severe, acute autoimmune hemolytic anemia from which the patient died. Somewhat similar cases were reported by Parker et al. (159), Kuipers et al. (257) and one perhaps similar by McGinniss (258). In the last case the auto-anti-A was recognized retrospectively when a blood sample was sent to a reference laboratory after the patient had died. Obviously an autoantibody directed against A or B, that is capable of causing intravascular red cell destruction at normal body temperature will cause a very serious form of hemolytic anemia. It is indeed fortunate that autoantibodies of this type seem be exceedingly rare. Autoantibodies of this type are discussed again in Chapter 37 in the sections dealing with in vivo red cell destruction in hemolytic anemia and in the description of hemolytic anemia caused by ABO system antibodies.

Routine ABO Grouping

Because of the presence of the expected ABO agglutinins whenever an antigen is absent, ABO typing can be performed on both cells and serum. Further, because of the immense importance of the system in transfusion it is essential that all patients and donors have cell and serum typings determined in order to reduce the possibility of errors. Satisfactory results can be obtained by slide or tube methods. Commercially-prepared or laboratory-made reagents using human sera as the source material are entirely suitable. Extracts of snails have proved a rich source of anti-A (160-175) while anti-B has been made from plants, seeds and fish (176-188). In manual tests the typing reagents should give unequivocal and strong reactions by immediate spin methods or on tiles. In automated blood typing machines some of the non-human-source reagents have proved particularly useful. First, in such machines a longer period of time is often available for the reactions to develop. Second, some such systems use enzyme (often bromelin) treated red cells that react very well with some of the non-human-source reagents (172). Perhaps by the time this book is published most or all routine ABO typing will be performed using monoclonal antibody based reagents that are discussed in more detail below.

In reverse typing tests using the sera of patients and donors, some reactions will develop rather slowly because of low levels of ABO system antibodies in a few sera. Some workers believe that tube tests are better than tile tests for reverse grouping procedures, for this reason. In reverse typing tests that are designed to detect hemolysins as well as agglutinins, care must be taken not to use red cells suspended in a medium that contains EDTA. That chemical will, of course, block complement activation (see Chapter 6) so that even potent hemolysins will present as agglutinins.

Table 8-1 illustrates the expected results when ABO typing is performed at a basic level. The reactions of anti-A,B (group O serum) are shown in that table, at least in part for historical reasons. As discussed below, when anti-A from group B persons is used as a typing reagent, it may fail to react with the red cells of some subgroups of A that carry low numbers of copies of the A antigen. Such red cells are usually agglutinated by potent anti-A,B made in group O individuals. Thus when human anti-A was used for routine typing, some workers elected also to use human anti-A,B to ensure that all weak subgroups of A were recognized. Now that monoclonal antibody-based anti-A is used it can be engineered to react with red cells of all A subgroups. Thus most workers agree that if monoclonal anti-A is used as the routine typing reagent, typing tests with anti-A,B are not necessary. While some workers use A_1 and A_2 cells in reverse typing tests to obtain an early indication of the presence of anti-A_1 in the sera of A_2 and A_2B individuals, most do not. The majority view is that anti-A_1 as a typing reagent and A_1 and A_2 red cells in reverse typing should be excluded from routine tests and used only in investigating those cases in which the serum of a group A person agglutinates group A red cells. Reactions with anti-A_1 as a typing reagent and the expected reactions of A_1 and A_2 cells in reverse typing are shown in a later table. The ISBT terminology for the ABO and H systems is listed in table 8-2.

Monoclonal Anti-A and Anti-B as Typing Reagents

Fairly soon after Köhler and Milstein (189) described the production of monoclonal antibodies in an in vitro system, an example of anti-A was made (190). Naturally since anti-A and anti-B are in such widespread use worldwide, many other workers set out to produce these antibodies. Many, including some with anti-A,B specificity were made and a large body of literature (191-207) now exists to document the production and characteristics of these antibodies. As would be expected, monoclonal ABO typing reagents share the same major advantages of other monoclonal antibody-based reagents, i.e. available in unlimited quantities, standard-

TABLE 8-1 Expected Results in Routine ABO Typing Tests

Unknown Cells Against			Unknown Serum Against				
Anti-A	Anti-B	Anti-A,B	A Cells	B Cells	O Cells	ABO Group	ABO Antibodies in Serum
0	0	0	+	+	0	0	Anti-A and Anti-B
+	0	+	0	+	0	A	Anti-B
0	+	+	+	0	0	B	Anti-A
+	+	+	0	0	0	AB	None

ized in terms of antibody content from lot to lot, lack of unwanted antibodies to rare and cryptantigens, etc., that are listed in table 7-1 of Chapter 7. However, monoclonal-based ABO typing reagents have some of the disadvantages listed in that table as well. It has been shown (203,204) that some monoclonal antibodies are more suitable than others for use as typing reagents. For example, some monoclonal anti-A react avidly and strongly with A_1 and A_2 red cells. Others agglutinate red cells that carry low levels of A antigen, such as those of phenotype A_x (see later in this chapter), as well as they agglutinate A_1 and A_2 cells. A single monoclonal anti-A seldom has both features. Thus to make a good anti-A typing reagent with the features described, it is often necessary to blend the products of two or more clones (206). Similarly, for reasons discussed in Chapter 7, some monoclonal anti-A and anti-B are not suitable for use in adsorption-elution studies (208).

Lubenko (277), Lubenko et al. (278,279) and Oehlert (280) have reported that some monoclonal anti-B and anti-A,B fail to agglutinate A_1B_{weak} and B_{weak} red cells. Since some donors of those phenotypes have low levels of anti-B in the serum, they can be mistakenly typed as group A and group O, respectively, if the B-anti-B reaction is not detected. The significance of transfusing A_1B_{weak} and B_{weak} red cells to group A and group O persons, respectively, is not known. Lubenko and Redman (279) make a highly sensible plea that when

monoclonal-based typing reagents are sold, the package insert contain information as to which clone (or clones in blended reagents) was (were) used in their production. Clearly such information would be of great value to workers using the reagents since details of reactivity of antibodies from various clones is often available in reports from International Workshops on Monoclonal Antibodies (e.g. 278).

In addition to suffering some of the disadvantages of monoclonal antibodies discussed in Chapter 7, some MAb directed against A and B have been seen to have problems unique unto themselves. As discussed in more detail later in this chapter, some monoclonal anti-A detect a trace amount of A antigen on cells of the so-called B(A) phenotype (209,210). One particular monoclonal anti-B reacts with A_1 red cells that have an acquired B antigen in a manner that suggests that the cells are of phenotype AB (211-213). A phenotype called A(B) in analogy to B(A), recognized by certain monoclonal anti-B has also been reported (214,215).

As mentioned in Chapter 7, it would be hoped that by the time monoclonal-based anti-A, anti-B and anti-A,B reach the routine blood banker, the problems described above would have been recognized and reserved. However, the existence of difficulties such as those mentioned and presumably others not yet uncovered, would suggest that exactly following the manufacturer's directions for use may be even more important

TABLE 8-2 Conventional and ISBT Terminology for the ABO and H Systems

System (Conventional Name)	ISBT System Symbol	ISBT System Number	Antigen (Conventional Name)	ISBT Antigen Number	ISBT Full Code Number
ABO	ABO	001	A	001	001001
			B	002	001002
			A,B	003	001003
			A_1	004	001004
Hh	H	018	H	001	018001

with monoclonal-based typing reagents than with human source reagents.

Origin of ABO Antibodies

There has long been considerable debate regarding the origin of "naturally-occurring" ABO system antibodies. One group of workers believe that these and other "naturally-occurring" antibodies are produced without exposure to antigen. Indeed early workers suggested that the production of anti-A and anti-B was controlled by genes linked to the genes that control production of ABO antigens. While this gene linkage now seems unlikely, the findings (see Chapter 2) that immunocompetent T and B cells carry immunoglobulins on their surface, show that a genetic mechanism is involved in the production of immunoglobulin molecules with antibody specificity. Other workers have suggested that anti-A and anti-B are stimulated by substances that are ubiquitous in nature (216-219). For example, bacteria have been shown to contain substances that are chemically very similar to human A and B antigens and therefore may stimulate the production of anti-A or anti-B (220-223). Springer et al. (221) demonstrated that White Leghorn chicks raised in a germ free environment did not make anti-B agglutinins, while chicks raised under normal conditions had significant titers of anti-B and further, chicks that were fed *E. coli* O$_{86}$ formed potent anti-B agglutinins. Øyen et al. (224) took advantage of the fact that *E. coli* O$_{86}$:B7 organisms carry A and B antigens and used suspensions of killed bacteria to adsorb anti-B and (somewhat less effectively) anti-A, from sera that contained antibodies to high frequency blood group antigens, when suitable antigen-negative A and B red cells were not available. Obviously, this technique has considerable potential in rendering valuable antisera suitable for use for typing red cells of all ABO groups. Rodgers et al. (225) attached lipopolysaccharide from *E. coli* O$_{86}$ to red cells, then used those cells to study various B lectins.

Conger et al. (226) used A-type and B-type terminal trisaccharides in an ELISA method (227) in in vitro studies, to examine the abilities of B cells of persons of different ABO groups to make anti-A, anti-B and anti-A,B. They found that 9% of clones from group O persons made antibody that, from serological studies, would be considered to be inseparable anti-A,B. Fewer B cells from group A and group B persons were able to make anti-B and anti-A, respectively, although autoreactive antibodies not detectable by conventional methods were seen. It was suggested that auto-anti-A and auto-anti-B are not seen in conventional tests either because a highly purified antigen is necessary for their detection or because the epitopes with which they complexed in the ELISA method are not present on red cells. It was also considered possible that, in vivo, T cells suppress the activation of self-reactive B cells (228) or that cell surface-associated self-antigens effectively mediate autoreactive B-cell clonal deletion (229).

Development of ABO Antibodies

Newborn infants are not capable of synthesizing appreciable amounts of IgG and are able to make only limited quantities of IgM. The majority of anti-A and anti-B present in cord serum is IgG and is passively acquired from the mother (230). IgM anti-A and anti-B synthesized by the fetus can be demonstrated in occasional cord sera (231-233). Anti-A and anti-B that have been synthesized by the infant can usually be demonstrated 3 to 6 months after birth (234-236). Anti-A and anti-B titers are at their highest at 5 to 10 years of age and have been said to be higher in girls than in boys (237). Blood bankers are sometimes asked to perform titration studies on the anti-A and anti-B in a patient's serum to see if "normal" amounts of these antibodies are being made. This request is sometimes made when immunodeficiency or abnormal globulin synthesis is suspected, in the patient. The titration values are difficult to interpret, the "normal ranges" of titers of anti-A and anti-B are in the order of 8 to 2048 and 8 to 256, respectively (23). However, some normal healthy individuals have titers higher than those listed. Lack of expected ABO agglutinins may be more informative (see below). One of us (PDI) remembers one terrifying case in which determination of ABO titer levels was requested "to confirm immune deficiency" in a child. The child was group AB, we are not sure that we ever convinced the physician that absence of anti-A and anti-B in the child was expected and that there are much better laboratory tests to aid in the diagnosis of immune deficiency (even in 1970 when this case was studied). For many years it has been believed that with advancing age, the levels of anti-A and anti-B synthesized gradually decline. Recently that supposition has been challenged (238,239), the authors of the studies in which no such decline could be demonstrated pointed out that the supposition is based primarily on a single study performed in 1929 (240). In spite of the recent studies, many workers will continue to believe that in at least some older individuals, ABO antibody levels are lower than in younger persons. Indeed, there are some additional reports (241,242,251) that suggest that the IgM but not the IgG levels of anti-A and anti-B decline in persons aged 65 or older. Further, many practical blood bankers will know that in reverse ABO typing it is not unusual to have to incubate tests at low temperatures in order to detect the ABO agglutinins of elderly patients. As mentioned below, such tests must be carefully controlled. Most workers will also be aware of at least anecdotal reports of relatively mild reactions in elderly patients accidentally transfused with major side ABO incompatible blood. In at least some such occurrences of which we are aware, lack of serious consequences seemed to be associated with low levels of anti-A and/or anti-B in the pretransfusion serum sample. As Mollison et al. (23) point out, the most important factor determining severity of an ABO incompatible transfusion reaction is the level of the causative ABO antibody in the patient's serum at the time of the transfusion.

As mentioned earlier, some workers (243,244) believe that a genetic control mechanism determines the levels of ABO agglutinins that will be made, while others (245) were unable to find supporting evidence for such claims. Vos and Vos (246) produced evidence that the amounts of ABH substances in saliva (see later in this chapter) affect the immune response to A, B and H-like determinants on bacteria and other exogenous material. Some workers (247,248) have not been able to confirm these findings. The characteristics of ABO antibodies are given in table 8-3 and in line with common convention (23), the IgM forms of the antibodies are called natural and the IgG forms called immune. As a later section of this chapter will show, this division is certainly an over simplification, albeit a convenient one since the importance of the antibodies is, on some occasions (such as when they cause ABO HDN) different.

For reasons that are not entirely clear, but which may result from some sort of genetic control of the immune response to A and B, group A and group B persons seem to make more IgM and less IgG anti-B and anti-A, respectively, than group O persons (259). This is particularly noticeable following known immunogenic exposure such as when vaccinations are given and following deliberate immunization with purified A and B substances. The effects of this are seen in ABO hemolytic disease of the newborn where only IgG antibodies cross the placenta. Almost all cases of ABO HDN severe enough to warrant some form of treatment occur in infants born to group O mothers (see Chapter 41 for a discussion of the ABO groups of affected infants in different ethnic groups). The finding that when immunized, group O persons tend to make more IgG than IgM anti-A,B while group A and group B people tend to make more IgM than IgG, anti-B and anti-A, has sometimes been taken to indicate that most or all anti-A,B are IgG while most or all anti-A and anti-B are IgM. This is certainly not the case.

TABLE 8-3 Usual Characteristics of ABO and H System Antibodies

Antibody Specificity	Positive Reactions in In Vitro Tests[*1]				Usual Immunoglobulin[*2]		Ability to Bind Complement		Ability to Cause In Vitro Lysis		Implicated in		Usual Form of Stimulation		% of White Population Positive
	Sal	LISS	AHG	Enz	IgG	IgM	Yes	No	Yes	No	Transfusion Reaction	HDN	Red Cells	Other	
Anti-A (Natural)	X				Some	Most	X		X		X			X	44
Anti-A (Immune)	X	X	X	X	Some	Some	X		X		X	X	X	X	44
Anti-B (Natural)	X				Some	Most	X		X		X			X	14
Anti-B (Immune)	X	X	X	X	Some	Some	X		X		X	X	X	X	14
Anti-A,B (Natural)	X				Some	Some	X		X		X			X	58
Anti-A,B (Immune)	X	X	X	X	Most	Some	X		X		X	X	X	X	58
Anti-A$_1$	X					Most	Rare	Most	Rare	Most	Rare	No		X	37
Anti-H (in Bombay)	X	X	X	X	Some	Some	X		X		Prob[*3]	X		X	100

[*1] Test systems yielding maximal strength reactions are shown. In fact, almost all ABO system antibodies shown, with the exception of anti-A$_1$, react by all methods.

[*2] ABO system antibodies often include an IgA component (23).

[*3] Has caused accelerated clearance of H+ (group O) red cells in a ^{51}Cr cell survival study (130).

Use of IgG or IgM to make antibody is a relative tendency associated with the ABO type of the antibody-maker. When 38 donors (8 group O, 16 group B, 14 group A) donors were immunized with purified blood group substances, 37 of them showed increases in IgG ABO antibody levels, the 38th was lost to follow-up (296).

Levels of ABO System Antibodies in Individuals in Different Populations

In Whites, titers of anti-A are often higher than those of anti-B, in one study (240) anti-B levels in group A and group O people were found to be comparable. In another (261) anti-B was found to be higher in group O than in group A persons. Grundbacher (244) reported that in Blacks, anti-A and anti-B levels are generally higher than in Whites and anti-B levels often equal those of anti-A. In studying Nigerian blood donors, Worlledge et al. (262) found that anti-A agglutinin levels often exceed those of anti-B but that hemolysins were more common among the anti-B. Redman et al. (263) addressed the question of variation of ABO antibody levels in persons of different ethnic backgrounds by studying antibody levels in Asian, White and Black blood donors, all of whom were living in the north London area of England. Although the highest levels of IgG anti-A and anti-B were found in Black female donors, the differences in the groups studied were not statistically significant. The authors (263) suggested that previously reported differences, seen when tests were performed on individuals living in different parts of the world, were the result of environmental rather than hereditary factors. There is already evidence that infections with intestinal and other parasites, some of which carry A and B-like antigens, result in the stimulation of high levels of anti-A and/or anti-B (264-269). Another finding in support of the concept that external environmental factors play a large role in the stimulation of ABO antibody levels was that of Toy et al. (270). These workers showed that among nearly 10,000 infants born in San Francisco during a six-year period, there was no difference in the incidence of clinical ABO HDN among those born to Asian, Black, Hispanic and White mothers.

Absence of Expected ABO Antibodies

As mentioned above, sera from newborn infants may not contain the expected ABO antibodies. Sometimes the expected or even the unexpected (based on ABO group) agglutinins may be present but as has been stated, these are in most instances maternal IgG antibodies that have entered the infant's circulation via the placenta. As discussed above there is (debatable) evidence that ABO agglutinins decrease in strength as individuals grow older. Thus in elderly patients the agglutinins may be difficult to detect and tests at 4°C may be necessary to demonstrate their presence. If this is done, a control of the patient's own cells and serum is essential to prove that ABO agglutinins and not cold-reacting autoagglutinins are being detected.

Anti-A and anti-B may be absent or present in only low levels in patients with hypogammaglobulinemia. The antibodies are absent from the plasma of boys with the X-linked Wiskott-Aldrich syndrome. In this condition the patient is unable to make antibodies to polysaccharide antigens but may be able to respond (by producing antibodies) to protein antigens (271-274).

As would be expected, in chimeras who receive a graft of blood forming tissue from a twin, in utero, no antibodies are made against the subject's own antigens or those on cells produced by the engrafted tissue. Thus in a chimera with a major population of group O and a minor population of group A red cells, anti-B but no anti-A will be present in the plasma. This observation applies to blood group systems other than ABO, individuals do not make antibodies to antigens to which they were exposed in utero (275,276).

In very rare instances anti-A or anti-B may be absent from sera in which they would be expected, although the individuals involved are not hypogammaglobulinemic nor, as far as can be determined, suffering from any other pathological condition. Dobson and Ikin (281) estimated that only one healthy donor in 10,000 would be found to lack expected ABO agglutinins from the plasma. Two such cases had been seen (282,283) before Springer et al. (284) described a very extensively studied case in which a woman had A and H, but not B on her red cells and no anti-B in her serum. Heroic efforts were made to try to find B antigen on the individual's cells but even highly sensitive serological and immunochemical tests failed to do so. The woman's red cells also failed to elicit the production of anti-B when injected into animals. The woman herself failed to form anti-B after being injected with B substance. The investigators in this case (284) concluded that lack of anti-B formation by the group A_1 subject might represent absence of suitable B lymphocytes, a situation thought most likely to be the result of somatic mutation since other members of the family made anti-B or anti-A,B dependent on their ABO types. Alternatively, it was suggested that the woman might be homozygous for rare recessive genes that somehow prevented an immune response to B substances. A group O individual whose serum lacked anti-A,B has also been reported (285).

Anti-A,B (Group O) Serum

As mentioned briefly above, anti-A,B (group O) serum, when used as a typing reagent, has the ability to agglutinate red cells belonging to some of the subclasses of A, such as A_x (286), that are not agglutinated by anti-A. The serum must be obtained from selected group O individuals (i.e. those with high titered, avid anti-A,B in their serum). Anti-A,B possesses serological reactivity not found in mixtures of anti-A from group B and anti-B from group A individuals. This applies even if the antibodies in the mixture are of as high a titer as those in the group O serum.

Eluates prepared from group A or B red cells that have been incubated with anti-A,B may react not only with cells of the same ABO group as the adsorbing cells but also with cells of the opposite ABO group. Thus an eluate prepared from group A red cells that have been incubated with anti-A,B will react strongly with A cells and may react with group B cells (287). Some workers report that this phenomenon occurs only with anti-A,B (from group O persons) (288,289) while others have been able to demonstrate the same findings with mixtures of anti-A and anti-B (290,291). Rosenfield et al. (230,292,293) demonstrated that anti-A,B crosses the placenta more frequently than do anti-A or anti-B, the relative differences in production of immune IgG anti-A,B and IgM anti-A and anti-B have been discussed above. Some group O sera contain separable anti-A and anti-B but only small amounts of cross-reacting anti-A,B (294); the level of the cross-reacting antibody increases when group O individuals are immunized (295,296) this applies when either purified A or B substance is used as the immunogen (296).

A number of different suggestions have been made to explain the presence of cross-reacting anti-A,B in group O sera and the ability of such sera to agglutinate red cells such as those of phenotype A_x that are not agglutinated by similar strength anti-A from group B donors. These suggestions are briefly described below.

1. In addition to containing anti-A and anti-B, group O serum is said to contain a third antibody: anti-C. Group A, B and AB red cells are thought to possess not only the A and/or B determinants, but also the C antigen (57,297-301). However, Jones and Kaneb (302) demonstrated that if group A red cells were incubated with anti-A (group B serum), their reaction with anti-A,B could be blocked. These results argue against the existence of a separate antigen, C.

2. Some workers have suggested that some antibody molecules may have both anti-A and anti-B specificity (288,289,303). In light of what is known about immunoglobulin production and structure (see Chapter 2) this theory seems somewhat doubtful.

3. Matuhasi and Ogata (290,291,304,305) suggested that anti-A,B might be a simple mixture of anti-A and anti-B. They postulated that presence of the "wrong" antibody in eluates was due to the non-specific binding of antibody to antigen-antibody complexes. While this theory does explain "wrong antibody eluates" it does not attempt to account for other observed results, such as the fact that anti-A,B reacts with A_x cells while anti-A does not. Further, it has now been shown (306) that the non-specific uptake of antibody by red cells is no different from the non-specific binding of IgG to those red cells, that was recognized many years ago (307-312). There is no evidence (306) that antibody-coated red cells bind more IgG non-specifically, than do those that have no antibody bound.

4. Owen (313) and Kabat (218) suggested that anti-A,B is an antibody that recognizes a structure common to the A and B determinants. Certainly this seems to be the best of the explanations advanced. The theory receives strong support from biochemical studies on the A and B antigens. The results of these studies have shown that the immunodominant sugars determining A and B specificity are N-acetyl-D-galactosamine and D-galactose, respectively. Structurally these two sugars are similar; in fact the only difference is the substituent at the number 2 carbon position. Thus an antibody that reacts with a portion of one of these two molecules, that does not include the carbon number 2 group in its combining site, would appear to be capable of reacting with the same region of the other molecule. Again this theory is supported by observations on monoclonal antibodies. If anti-A,B was merely "cross-reacting" anti-A plus anti-B, or a mixture of anti-A and anti-B, one would not expect a monoclonal antibody with anti-A,B specificity to exist. The fact that several such antibodies have been found (196,199,205 and others described at ISBT Workshops on monoclonal antibodies, e.g. 314) shows that A and B must share at least one (probably several) epitope(s) that are recognized by monoclonal anti-A,B. Oriol et al. (205) have shown that such an epitope can be located terminally or at an internal portion of the antigen.

It seems that monoclonal antibody-based reagents that serve as anti-A,B come in two varieties. Some are single MAb or blends of MAb that have anti-A,B specificity. Others are mixtures of potent monoclonal anti-A and anti-B. In many publications the first type are called anti-A,B and the second type anti-A+B. However, it is not clear that this distinction will always be made for commercially available reagents. As mentioned earlier in this chapter, if a monoclonal-based anti-A reagent known to agglutinate the red cells of subgroups of A such as A_x is used, there is no need to use anti-A,B in routine typing tests. If anti-A,B is used alone, to reconfirm that group O units from a transfusion service's supplier do not include any mislabeled A or B units, almost any anti-A,B or anti-A+B is likely to be satisfactory. However, for critical investigatory studies it may be more important to know whether the reagent is anti-A,B or anti-A+B. The anti-A+B reagents were introduced at a time when there was a paucity of good monoclonal anti-A,B. Perhaps by the time this book is published enough clones making potent anti-A,B will have been developed that anti-A+B will no longer be offered as a reagent.

Inheritance of the ABO Blood Groups

The exact structure of the ABO blood group genes is now known. A later section of this chapter describes the structure of *A, B* and *O* at the molecular level. Thus for the first time reliable methods exist by which *AA* and *AO*, and *BB* and *BO* individuals can be differentiated. In spite of this advanced knowledge it is convenient still to consider inheritance in the ABO system as it can be recognized from the results of simple, routine serological tests. Again as explained in later sections of this chapter, there are rare exceptions to the usual rules of ABO inheritance. However, in the overwhelming majority of cases inheritance is straightforward.

Three allelic genes *A, B* and *O* in the various possible combinations of two, account for the four recognized ABO groups: A, B, AB and O. The ways in which these genes control the production of the ABO antigens was first recognized by Bernstein (315,316) in 1924. His explanation, to which only minor changes have been necessary, is now known to be correct. Bernstein showed that each individual inherits two *ABO* genes, one from each parent and that genes then determine which ABO antigens will be present on that individual's red cells. The presence of A or B antigen on the red cells can be recognized by serological tests with the appropriate antiserum so that the presence of the gene that controls its production can be deduced. The presence of an *O* gene can be deduced only in the absence of both the *A* and *B* genes when no A or B antigen is present on the red cells. The *O* gene produces no detectable antigen and is therefore regarded as silent (see later for the exact explanation of lack of activity of *O*). This means that the ABO typing of an individual sometimes reveals exactly which genes are present, or a genotype, while in other instances only one gene product can be recognized and thus only a phenotype is determined. Individuals who type as group AB

and have, therefore, both the A and B antigens on their red cells, must have one *A* and one *B* gene present. (See later in this chapter for rare exceptions.) Those who type as group O must have two *O* genes present (since both the *A* and the *B* genes cause the production of serologically recognizable antigens, neither of which is present on group O red cells. Again see later in this chapter for very rare exceptions). In these two instances, ABO grouping has revealed a genotype, *AB* and *OO* respectively. Typings that show persons to be group A or group B reveal only a phenotype, since the product of only one of the two genes present has been recognized. Persons of phenotype A can be of genotype *AA* or *AO*, while those of phenotype B can be genotypically *BB* or *BO*. There is no serological method of determining the presence or absence of an *O* gene when the individual has an *A* or *B* gene present. Family studies may reveal the identity of the second gene in an A or B individual. As an example, if the mating of one A and one B parent produces a group O child, it has been shown that the second gene present in each parent, must be *O* since the child has inherited one *O* gene from each parent. The mating can thus be rewritten as *AO* X *BO* producing an *OO* child.

Based on these very straightforward principles, the genetic control of the inheritance of the ABO groups shown in table 8-4 can be determined. It is but a simple (albeit lengthy) exercise to extend table 8-4 to include the other known alleles at the ABO locus, such as A^1, A^2, A^3, A^x, A^m, etc. While it might seem logical next to explain anomalies of inheritance of the ABO groups, it is in fact necessary to discuss the synthesis and structure of the ABO and some related antigens. Again the molecular genetics and biochemistry are described in later sections of this chapter. In the sections that follow this one, basic information is provided that allows interpretation of serological test results.

Genetic Control of A, B and H Antigen Production (Basic Concepts)

As discussed in some detail in Chapter 5, genes encode the production of proteins. As mentioned briefly earlier and as discussed in more detail later in this chapter, the immunodominant structures of the H, A and B antigens are carbohydrate. Therefore it follows that the H, A and B antigens are not the direct gene products of *H, A* and *B*. Nevertheless, as the section on the normal inheritance of the ABO blood groups clearly shows, inheritance of the appropriate ABO system gene or genes nearly always results in the presence of the corresponding antigen or antigens on the red cells. The explanation of the gap between protein synthesis under control of the genes and the carbohydrate nature of the antigens is rel-

TABLE 8-4 ABO Groups of the Offspring of Different ABO Matings (Normal Inheritance)

Mating Phenotypes	Mating Genotypes	Offspring Possible Phenotypes (and Genotypes)
A x A	*AA* x *AA*	A(*AA*)
	AA x *AO*	A (*AA* or *AO*)
	AO x *AO*	A (*AA* or *AO*) or O (*OO*)
B x B	*BB* x *BB*	B (*BB*)
	BB x *BO*	B (*BB* or *BO*)
	BO x *BO*	B (*BB* or *BO*) or O (*OO*)
AB x AB	*AB* x *AB*	AB (*AB*) or A (*AA*) or B (*BB*)
O x O	*OO* x *OO*	O (*OO*)
A x B	*AA* x *BB*	AB (*AB*)
	AO x *BB*	AB (*AB*) or B (*BO*)
	AA x *BO*	AB (*AB*) or A (*AO*)
	AO x *BO*	AB (*AB*) or A(*AO*) or B (*BO*) or O (*OO*)
A x O	*AA* x *OO*	A (*AO*)
	AO x *OO*	A (*AO*) or O (*OO*)
A x AB	*AA* x *AB*	AB (*AB*) or A (*AA*)
	AO x *AB*	AB (*AB*) or A (*AA* or *AO*) or B (*BO*)
B x O	*BB* x *OO*	B (*BO*)
	BO x *OO*	B (*BO*) or O (*OO*)
B x AB	*BB* x *AB*	AB (*AB*) or B (*BB*)
	BO x *AB*	AB (*AB*) or B (*BB* or *BO*) or A (*AO*)
AB x O	*AB* x *OO*	A (*AO*) or B (*BO*)

atively easy to explain. It is well established (317-352) that *H*, *A* and *B* each encode production of an enzyme that is protein in nature. The enzymes act as transferases. That is to say, each catalyzes the transfer of a sugar molecule from a donor substrate to a predetermined precursor substance. These enzyme actions were first recognized from studies on soluble substances that include H, A and B (317-320); it is now clear that similar enzyme activities result in the addition of carbohydrate moieties to some glycoproteins and glycolipids of the red cell membrane and account for red cell-borne as well as secreted H, A and B antigens.

Again in brief (the subject is explained more fully in a later section in this chapter on the biochemical structure of the H, A and B antigens and in Chapter 9 on the structure of the Lewis antigens) the *H* and *Se* (*Secretor*, see below) genes each encode production of fucosyl transferase enzymes that effect the addition of L-fucose to a series of precursor structures known as the type 1, 2, 3 and 4 chains. Once L-fucose has been added, the *A* and *B* gene-specified products can act to add sugars to the chains that now carry H. The *A* gene encodes production

of a galactosaminyl transferase that effects the addition of N-acetylgalactosamine to the preformed H-bearing chains. The *B* gene encodes production of a galactosyl transferase that effects the addition of D-galactose to the same H-bearing structures. Thus the immunodominant carbohydrate of the H antigen is L-fucose; of the A antigen, N-acetylgalactosamine; and of the B antigen, D-galactose. As described in the section on the B(A) phenotype, there is some overlap in specificity of the *A* and *B* gene-specified transferases and each can add a small amount of the opposite immunodominant carbohydrate to preformed H structures. Of the four precursor chains mentioned above: type 1 is the predominant carrier of secreted H, A and B (353); type 2 carries most of the red cell glycoprotein-associated H, A and B (331,353,354); type 3 chains are found in mucins isolated from substances such as the gastric mucosa or ovarian cyst fluid and may not be present on red cells (355-357) although reports of "A-associated" type 3 chains in red cell membrane glycolipids have appeared (356,357); and type 4 chains are believed to be components of red cell membrane glycolipids (343,358). It is believed that the *H* gene-specified fucosyl transferase adds L-fucose to type 2 and type 4 chains (340,359) to form red cell membrane-associated type 2H and type 4H, while the *Se* gene-specified enzyme adds L-fucose to type 1 and type 3 chains (340,357) to form type 1H and type 3H, as found in secretions.

Even at this simple level of explanation a number of additional points need to be made. First, in the absence of L-fucose (the immundominant structure of H) A and B sugars cannot be added. In other words, if an individual does not inherit a functional *H* gene, the A and B immunodominant sugars cannot be added at the red cell level because no type 2 or type 4H has been made. This is the basis of the explanation of the Bombay or O_h phenotype. Such individuals inherit two *h* genes, *h* being the silent allele of *H*, so make no red cell membrane associated *H*. Although any *A* and/or *B* gene that they inherit is functional (see below, the *A* and/or *B* gene-specified transferase(s) is (are) made) no A or B antigen can be constructed.

Second, in individuals who inherit two *se* genes, *se* being the silent allele of *Se*, no type 1 or type 3H is made. Again, any *A* or *B* gene-specified transferase made will be unable to add its immunodominant sugar to type 1 and type 3 chains so that these individuals will have no H, A or B in their secretions (non-secretors, see below). The *sese* genotype is much more common than the *hh* genotype meaning that non-secretors of ABH are much more common than O_h (Bombay) individuals. As will be seen, the concept that the *H* gene-specified transferase operates on type 2 and type 4 chains, while the *Se* gene-specified transferase operates on type 1 and type 3 chains, explains why persons who initially appear to be of the Bombay phenotype can present with no H, A or B in their saliva (*hh, sese*) or with H-negative red cells but H (and/or A and/or B) in their saliva (*hh, Se*).

Third, in spite of the dependence of A and B antigen assembly on the presence of H at the biochemical level, the *Hh* and *Sese* genes are not part of the ABO system. Independence of the *ABO* and *Sese* loci was apparent right from the time that the ability of some individuals to secrete ABH substances was recognized (58,360-363). Independence of the *ABO* and *Hh* loci was originally demonstrated in a number of families in which there were O_h members (364-366).

Fourth, as mentioned above, inheritance of two *h* genes does not block function of any *A* or *B* genes simultaneously inherited. In other words, the *A* and *B* gene-specified transferase enzymes are still produced and can be detected (367,368) dependent, of course, on the inheritance of an *A* or *B* (or both) gene but, because of lack of H (L-fucose) on the type 2 and type 4 precursor chains, cannot add galactosamine or galactose (respectively) to those chains on red cells.

Fifth, the *O* gene is silent. That is to say in the presence of two *O* genes (phenotype O, genotype *OO*, see table 8-4) no further addition of carbohydrate to H-bearing structures occurs. As described below, it is now known that there are several different forms of the *O* gene.

Chromosomal Locations of the *ABO*, *Hh* and *Sese* Loci

It has been known for some time that the *ABO* locus is linked to the *Np* and *AK* loci (369-381). A rare dominant gene at the *Np* locus causes nail-patella syndrome or hereditary onychoosteodysplasia, a condition in which the finger nails have an unusual convex shape. Genes at the *AK* locus are responsible for a polymorphism of the enzyme adenylate kinase. The *ABO*, *Np* and *AK* loci are now known (382-385) to be located on chromosome number nine.

Both the *Hh* and *Sese* loci are located on chromosome 19 (386-390), indeed it is entirely possible that one arose by duplication of the other (386). However, recent studies (see a later section in this chapter on the biochemistry of H, A and B) and review of reports in the literature on families with *hh* members who apparently had differing *Sese* genotypes (391-393) suggest that while genes at the two loci may show some linkage, that linkage is not absolute indicating that two distinct loci exist (386,394,446). Clearly, both the *Hh* and *Sese* loci are genetically independent of the *ABO* locus on chromosome 9.

Development of the ABO Antigens

Like the antibodies of the system, the ABO antigens are not fully developed in newborn infants (395-397) even though some antigens can be detected on the red cells of the embryo as early as five weeks after conception (398). Red cells from group A and group B cord bloods react less strongly with anti-A and anti-B than do cells from adults. In addition, many group A infants, at birth, type as A_2 (399) but can be shown by the time they are six to 18 months old to be type A_1. Bird (400) showed that the red cells of newborn infants who have inherited an A^1 gene are more likely to react with *Dolichos biflorus* lectin than with human-source anti-A_1; others (401) found that the red cells of genetically A^2 infants reacted better with anti-A,B than with anti-A. While Haddad (402) believed that the H antigen was weaker on cord red cells than on those from adults, one of us (137,403-405) felt that H was fairly well developed on cord cells while the determinant defined by anti-IH was present in an amount considerably less than on the red cells of adults. Economidou et al. (406) found that the cord cells of A_1 infants have fewer A sites than do those of A_1 adults but Tilley et al. (407) showed that the level of A^1-specified transferase enzyme is in fact higher in cord blood serum from A^1 infants than in the sera of A^1 (non-pregnant) adults. In pregnancy, the level of A^1-specified transferase enzyme in the serum drops to less than half the amount present in the sera of non-pregnant A^1 adults (407,408). Many blood bankers will be aware of the marked reduction of production of Lewis system antigens during pregnancy. Indeed, the weakening of Le^b in particular, is far more dramatic than the reduction of A and B. It is sometimes assumed that the mechanisms responsible for reduced production of antigens in the two systems are the same. In fact they are quite different. In the ABO system, reduced levels of antigens represent reduced production of *A* and/or *B* gene-specified transferases. There is no similar reduction in the production of *Le* gene-specified transferase in pregnancy, instead, the reduced level of red cell antigen expression represents partition of the Lewis antigen-bearing glycolipids between red cells and plasma lipoproteins. In pregnancy the plasma lipoproteins increase dramatically in amount and bind a high proportion of the Lewis system antigen-bearing structures (409).

Romans et al. (410) addressed the relatively weak reactivity of many cord blood samples with anti-A and anti-B. They suggested that one of the reasons that makes the detection of IgG anti-A and anti-B on cord cells difficult is the fact that many of the molecules are attached to the cells via only one of their two antigen-binding sites. When an antibody molecule is able to attach both combining sites to antigen, a condition termed monogamous bivalency (411), the rate of dissociation of the antibody is considerably less than when only one antibody-binding site attaches (412,413). The inability of IgG anti-A and anti-B to bind both antigen combining sites to antigens on cord blood red cells relates directly to the state of development of the A and B antigens on those cells. As described in more detail later in this chapter, the H, A and B immunodominant sugars are attached to red cell membrane-borne glycoproteins and glycolipids. On the red cells of adults many of these glycoproteins and glycolipids are complex branched structures that place different copies of the same antigen in close proximity to each other (414-420). Others are straight chain structures on which the antigens are distal to others. On the red cells of newborn infants almost all the ABH-bearing structures are of the straight chain variety. Thus the antigens are fewer in number (406,421-424) and those that are present are arranged in a different spatial configuration than those on the red cells of adults. The enzyme responsible for converting the straight chain structures to the branched form is a beta 1→6 glucosaminyl trans-

ferase that is made in only low levels in newborns. The level of synthesis of the enzyme gradually increases and reaches the same level as seen in adults between six and 18 months of age (422-427,432). It is this same branching of the ABH bearing structures that results in the change from the i to the I phenotype during the first 18 months of life (425-427). Blood bankers often talk about the conversion of i to I during this period but, as discussed in more detail in Chapter 10, the true situation is probably that as chain branching occurs and the structure recognized by anti-I develops, access of anti-i to its antigen is sterically impeded.

These considerations regarding the stage of development of A and B antigens on cord blood red cells help to explain a phenomenon that most blood bankers with a reasonable amount of experience will have noticed. When a direct antiglobulin test is performed on the red cells of a newborn infant suffering from ABO HDN, it often yields only a weakly positive reaction. However, if an eluate is made from those cells and is then tested against red cells from adults of the appropriate ABO group, strongly positive indirect antiglobulin tests are invariably seen. It seems that because of the relatively low numbers of A or B antigen sites on the cord blood cells, their spatial distribution on straight chain glycoproteins and glycolipids and the inability of the IgG molecules to attach via both combining sites because of the arrangement of the A and B antigens, not all the maternal ABO antibody molecules that cross the placenta can bind to the infant's red cells. Further, those that do bind have a relatively high rate of dissociation. However, when the antibody molecules are recovered by elution, from a much larger number of cord cells than are tested in a DAT and are then tested against the red cells of adults, a different situation exists. The antibody molecules now find far more copies of their antigens on the cells, the antigens are present in several copies on branched chains allowing monogamous bivalency to occur and the rate of antibody dissociation is markedly reduced. Accordingly, many IgG antibody molecules are cell-bound when the anti-IgG is added and strongly positive indirect antiglobulin tests result. Romans et al. (410) pointed out that there is a very strong natural selection against the early branching of glycoprotein and glycolipid red cell membrane-borne chains that carry H, A and B. The paucity of A and B antigens and the positioning of the ones that are present in such a way that monogamous bivalency is severely restricted, act as a defense against hemolytic disease of the newborn even when large amounts of maternal antibody enter the fetal circulation. The very same situation acts as a defense mechanism against severe ABO HDN in a second way. When DATs are performed on the red cells of infants with clinical ABO HDN it is found that the test with anti-

IgG may be positive but the test with anti-C3 is negative (23,260). However, if the causative antibody is recovered by elution, mixed with fresh serum as a source of complement and allowed to bind to appropriate ABO group red cells from adults, both IgG and C3 are detectable in IATs. Clearly, the IgG ABO antibodies involved can activate complement, they are prevented from doing so in the infants in large part by the paucity of ABO antigen sites and the distance between those sites (see Chapter 6 for a discussion of complement activation by IgG molecules and the need for Fc contributions from two different antibody molecules). Clearly if intravascular lysis occurred in infants with red cells ABO incompatible with the maternal antibodies, a high rate of fetal loss would be seen. In other words, paucity of A and B sites on the red cells of the fetus and their location on straight chain structures prevents serious and frequent ABO HDN by limiting the amount of IgG that can bind, by effecting poor association of those molecules that do bind, and by preventing complement activation.

Although Brouwers et al. (260) and Vescio and Castro (464) found that the DAT was positive with anti-IgG and negative with anti-C3 in several hundred newborns with maternal IgG anti-A and/or anti-B bound to their red cells, Pujol et al. (465) later claimed that 2 of 46 infants in their study had IgG and C3 on their red cells at the time of birth. While Pujol (466) defended the supposition that it was the ABO antibodies that had activated the complement, Garratty (467) pointed out that a few infants, whose red cells are not ABO incompatible with the maternal antibodies, are seen to have some C3 on their red cells at birth.

Having credited the paucity and spatial arrangement of A and B antigens on cord red blood cells as the major defense mechanism against severe ABO HDN, it should be added that there are additional factors involved. First, much of the maternal IgG that crosses the placental is IgG2 (468) that, as described in Chapter 2, is far less efficient at activating complement than IgG3 or IgG1. Second, the levels of complement components present in newborns are less than those present in adults (469). Third, some A or B substances in the infants' plasma and on tissue cells probably serve partially to neutralize maternal antibodies.

As mentioned earlier in this chapter, Economidou et al. (406) estimated the number of A and B sites on the red cells of adults and newborn infants of various different ABO phenotypes. In part for historical reasons their findings, that are in good general agreement with those of others (428-431) are reproduced in table 8-5. However, as discussed in Chapter 6 (section on Intravascular Red Cell Destruction) the calculations leading to data such as those shown in table 8-5 were all based on the premise that each antibody molecule

counted in the studies, had bound to one red cell antigen. With the monogamous bivalency concept described above borne in mind (23,410) it can be concluded that the estimates, that were based on the number of antibody molecules that bound, underestimated the actual number of antigen sites by a factor of 50%. As discussed in Chapter 6, one of us (9) has calculated the number of copies per red cell of the many membrane structures known to carry ABH antigens (at least: protein band 3; band 4.5, the glucose transport protein; poly-N-acetyl lactosaminyl glycolipids; the Rh glycoproteins; and some minor glycolipids; for references see Chapter 6) and has concluded that, at least on the red cells of adults, the figures given in table 8-5 represent only half of the antigens actually present. These new figures are also shown in table 8-5. It is not clear if the numbers of antigens on cord red blood cells should be doubled (they are not in table 8-5). The reasons for this hesitation will be clear from what has been written above. While there is reason to believe that on the red cells of adults each molecule of anti-A and anti-B may bind to two antigens, on cord blood red cells each antibody molecule might bind to a single antigen. This possibility would, of course, make the difference in ABO antigen site density on the red cells of adults and those of newborn infants even greater than has previously been supposed.

The genotypes *AA*, *AO*, and *BB* and *BO* cannot be differentiated from tests that measure the number of antigen sites per red cell. As described in more detail below, A^1A^1 individuals produce more *A*-specified transferase than do people who are genetically A^1O, but enough enzyme is made by A^1O heterozygotes that the same number of copies of A can be added to their red cells as to the red cells of persons homozygous for A^1. Also as mentioned below, the A^1A^1 and A^1O (and *BB* and *BO*) phenotypes can now be differentiated at the molecular level by demonstrating the presence of an *O* gene.

The Bombay and Other H-deficient Phenotypes

In 1952, Bhende et al. (433) described a new phenotype in the ABO system. The red cells of the individuals concerned were not agglutinated by anti-A, anti-B, anti-A,B or by anti-H. The individuals' sera contained anti-A, anti-B and anti-H. At first it was thought that the Bombay or O_h phenotype, as it has become known, might represent the existence of an additional allele at the *ABO* locus. However, Ceppellini et al. (434) and Watkins and Morgan (435) suggested that the phenotype might involve the presence of suppressor genes at a locus independent of *ABO*. When a family in which persons of the Bombay phenotype were present was studied, Levine et al. (364)

TABLE 8-5 Number of A and B Antigens per Red Cell as Measured by Economidou et al. (8) and as Calculated by Anstee (9)*

Red Cell Source	Measured (8)	Calculated (9)
A_1 Adult	810,000 to 1,170,000	>2,000,000
A_1 Cord	250,000 to 370,000	
A_2 Adult	240,000 to 290,000	
A_2 Cord	140,000	
A_1B Adult	460,000 to 850,000 A 310,000 to 560,000 B	
A_1B Cord	220,000 A	
A_2B Adult	120,000 A	
B Adult	610,000 to 830,000	>2,000,000

* For details of monogamous bivalency and the difference between the measured and calculated numbers, see text.

showed that the genetic background of phenotype does indeed involve genes that are not residents of the *ABO* locus. Figure 8-1 reproduces some of the findings in the family studied by Levine et al. (364). As can be seen, the mother in the second generation of that family has red cells that are non-reactive with anti-A, anti-B and anti-A,B. However, she has passed a *B* gene to her daughter (where it is partnered by *A¹* from the child's father) and in the daughter the *B* gene is functional. That is, the daughter's red cells react with anti-B as well as with anti-A and anti-A_1. It was supposed that in normal individuals an additional gene (called *X* by Levine et al. (364)) was necessary in order for an *A* or *B* gene present to be able to function, in terms of controlling production of serologically recognizable A or B antigen. In Bombay individuals, it was supposed that *X* was not present and that its allele *x* (present in the homozygous form in Bombay individuals) prevented the production of A and/or B. As the biochemical structure of the H, A and B antigens was elaborated, only minor modifications to these concepts were necessary. As already discussed, the *A* and *B*-specified transferases can add the immunodominant sugars of A and B only to a structure that carries H (that is, a precursor to which the *H* gene-specified transferase has added L-fucose). Thus, it became clear that the *X* and *H* genes are the same thing. The *x* gene was renamed *h*; individuals of the Bombay phenotype were recognized as being genetically *hh*; and the phenotype became known as O_h. It follows that *h* does not effect production of an enzyme that allows the addition of a carbohydrate moiety to the precursor chain. As additional examples of the O_h phenotype were studied, the independent segregation of *H* and *h* from genes at the *ABO* locus, first demonstrated by Levine et al. (364) was confirmed (365,366). From the family study depicted in figure 8-1 it is apparent that individuals of the O_h phenotype can carry *ABO* system genes. While these genes do not effect the production of A or B antigen on the red cells of the O_h individual they can be passed by the O_h person to his or her offspring. Providing that the child inherits *H* from the other parent, the A or B gene from the O_h individual can then be expressed in the child. The terms O_h^{A1}, O_h^{A2}, O_h^{B}, O_h^{O}, etc. indicate the *ABO* gene carried by the O_h individual if such a determination can be made from a family study. In those instances where no family study is possible, or when one is done but is non-informative (i.e. O_h X A, producing an A child) the term O_h is used unadorned. Since the early examples of the O_h phenotype were studied, other examples have been found and many of them (365,366,436-452) have been described in print. The examples just referenced were found in people from the Indian subcontinent and in Whites. The phenotype has also been found in a Sudanese said to be of Arab and African Black extraction (453); a Japanese (454); a Thai-Muslim (455); an American Black (456) and in peoples of Indian extraction living in South Africa (457).

That it is incorrect to say that the genotype *hh* suppresses the action of *A* and/or *B* became clear when it was demonstrated (367,368) that the sera of O_h individuals contain transferase enzymes specified by the *A* or *B* genes that those individuals carry. In other words, in O_h individuals the *A* and/or *B* gene(s) present is(are) functional and code for production of a galactosaminyl or a galactosyl transferase respectively, just as in people who are phenotypically A or B. Lack of demonstrable A or B antigen on O_h red cells is a function of lack of a suitable acceptor site, not lack of *A* or *B* gene action. As expected, the *H* gene-specified fucosyl transferase is not present in the sera of O_h persons (367,368). Thus the correct way to describe the genetic situation in O_h persons is that lack of

FIGURE 8-1 The Family with O$_h$ Members Studied by Levine et al. (364)

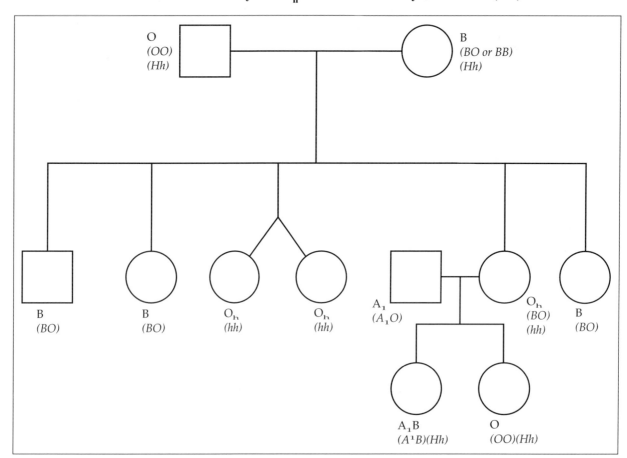

an *H* gene results in the absence of acceptor sites to which functional *A* and/or *B* gene-specified transferases would attach the immunodominant sugar of A or B.

As more examples of red cells deficient in H were studied it became clear that they are not all identical. By definition, O$_h$ red cells are non-reactive with anti-H, anti-A and anti-B in agglutination and antiglobulin tests. In the classical Bombay phenotype (now sometimes called Bombay, Indian or O$_h$, Indian) no H, A or B is secreted. As described below, several different H-deficient phenotypes that do not fit these criteria have been described and many of them have been lumped together under the designation para-Bombays.

Even before the genetic differences giving rise to the various H-deficient phenotypes were recognized, some serological heterogeneity among O$_h$ samples had been seen. For example, when adsorption-elution methods were used, some examples (364,366,449) could be shown to carry trace amounts of H, A or B, while in others (458,459) even the use of highly potent antibodies still resulted in negative adsorption-elution tests. Moores et al. (459) and later Bhatia (1061) suggested that these findings might mean that additional alleles existed at the

Hh locus. It did not seem unreasonable to suppose that one form of *h* might effect no production of the usual fucosyl transferase and hence no H, while another might encode a small amount (or a defective version) of the enzyme and allow production of a small amount of H that then became converted to A or B if *A* or *B* was present. Such a suggestion was not invalidated by the two locus theory of Oriol et al. (386) that is described below, see also table 8-6. Wagner and Flegel (1043) have now produced evidence at the DNA level that any one of at least seven different changes in the *H* gene can result in a gene that behaves as *h* or a very similar gene. Studies are currently in progress (1064) to determine whether there is any correlation between the various forms of *h* and the production of no or a very low level of H on the red cells.

Another claim that predated the explanation of the H-deficient phenotypes presented below was that presence of an *O*, *A* or *B* gene in an O$_h$ individual might be indicated by the level of antibody in the individual's serum. That is, it was suggested (449) that in an O$_h^A$ individual the amount of anti-A might be less than the amount of anti-H and anti-B, in an O$_h^B$ individual the amount of anti-B might less than the amount of anti-A and anti-H, and so forth. We (459) tested this hypothesis by running blind titrations on the sera of O_h individuals in whom family studies had revealed which *ABO* genes were carried. The results of our titrations did not correlate in any way with the ABO genotypes of the individuals studied.

As described in detail in Chapters 12 and 18, red blood cells of the Rh_{null} and McLeod phenotypes do not enjoy normal in vivo survival. Persons with red cells of either of those phenotypes suffer an often well compensated form of red cell deficiency hemolytic anemia. In 1973, Levine et al. (460) pointed out that individuals of the O_h phenotype are not similarly afflicted. This was taken as evidence that the Rh antigens are essential for red cell membrane integrity while those of the ABO system are not. One of us has pointed out elsewhere (461) that this comparison between Rh_{null} and O_h red cells may not be entirely valid. Rh_{null} cells seem to be totally lacking in Rh protein. There is no reason to suppose that O_h red cells lack any more than terminal carbohydrates normally attached to red cell membrane-borne glycoproteins and glycolipids. In other words, if the structures to which the terminal carbohydates are attached play a functional role in red cell membrane integrity, it would not be surprising that their functional role is still accomplished in the absence of the immunodominant terminal carbohydrates of H, A and B. There is now actual evidence from red cell survival studies that O_h red cells survive normally in the circulation of the O_h individual (462,463).

The Para-Bombay and other H-deficient Phenotypes

As bloods with phenotypes similar to but not identical with those of the O_h phenotype were studied, the term para-Bombay was introduced to describe them. Unfortunately, through no fault of the investigators since the different genetic backgrounds had not been recognized, the term was applied to a heterogeneous set of phenotypes. It is now known (483) that some H-deficient bloods arise because of the inheritance of *hh* with *sese* while others represent the genotype *hh, Se*. A more complete explanation of the H-deficient, secretor phenotype (representing the *hh, Se* genotype) is given below in the section on the two locus theory.

The terms A_h and B_h (470-489) were used to describe phenotypes in which the red cells carried traces of A or B but no detectable H and came from individuals whose saliva lacked H, A and B. Terms such as O_m^h, O_{Hm}, A_m^h, O_{Hm}^A, B_m^h and O_{Hm}^B have been used (366,391,393,490,491,493-501) to describe phenotypes in which there was either no H, A or B, or only trace amounts of those antigens (dependent on which *ABO*

genes had been inherited) on the red cells, but normal or near normal amounts of H, H and A, or H and B (again dependent on the *ABO* genes inherited) in the saliva. Again it must be stessed that at the serological level both categories are heterogeneous. In some cases anti-H from different sources gave variable (weak or negative) reactions; adsorption-elution tests sometimes suggested presence of small amounts and sometimes total absence of H. In addition to the heterogeneity of the samples, some of these variations no doubt reflected differences in source and strength of the reagents and the methods by which they were used.

H-deficient Phenotypes and the Three Locus Theory

In order to explain all the serological findings mentioned in the previous two sections, a three locus theory was developed. It was supposed that various combinations of genes at the *Hh*, *Sese* and *Zz* loci gave rise to the various phenotypes. For example, since all the early studied examples of the O_h (Indian) phenotype involved absence of H, A and B from the red cells and the secretions it was assumed that at least one *H* gene was necessary in order that an *Se* gene present could function. That is to say that since in the Indian and related populations, *Se* is considerably more common than *se*, it could not be supposed that all *h* homozygotes were also homozygous for *se*. Thus the theory held that in the genotype *hh, Se*, the *Se* gene was unable to function since no *H* was present.

The *Zz* genes were invoked to explain the lack of A on the red cells in say O_{Hm}^A individuals who had red cells that lacked H and A but who secreted both H and A substance. Thus the theory held that in the genotype *A, H, Se, zz*, the *H, Se* and *A* genes were able to function at the secretory cell level but that in the absence of *Z* (i.e. the *zz* genotype) no H or A could be made at the red cell level.

The theory was somewhat cumbersome and supposed that both *Se* and *Z* were regulatory genes that controlled *H*. For example it was assumed that in a normal individual of genotype *A, H, Se, Z*, the *Se* gene allowed *H* to act at the secretory cell level, while *Z* allowed *H* to act in the synthesis of red cell-borne H. *A*, of course, then acted on preformed H on both red cells and in the secretions, i.e. group A, secretor of H and A. In an individual genetically *A, H, sese, Z*, lack of *Se* prevented *H* from acting at the secretory cell level while presence of *Z* allowed *H* to act at the red cell level which in turn allowed *A* to act, i.e. group A, non-secretor. The *Zz* locus had to be invoked to explain a phenotype in which H and A were present in the saliva but absent from the red cells, i.e. *A, H, Se, zz* with *Se* allowing *H* to act in secretory cells but *zz* preventing synthesis of H and subsequently A, on the red cells.

Because we favor the two locus theory of Oriol et al. (386) that is described below, a full explanation of the Bombay and para-Bombay phenotypes based on the three locus theory will not be given. Readers interested in seeing how all the findings were explained are referred to two publications (994,995) in which it is still used.

The H-deficient Réunion and H-deficient Secretor Phenotypes

In 1982 and 1983 Gerard et al. (485) and LePendu et al. (486) reported a higher incidence of H-deficient phenotypes on the small island of Réunion, in the Indian Ocean off the east cost of Africa, than seen anywhere else in the world. In the Indian population of Réunion the H-deficient phenotype represented the classic O_h Indian phenotype in that the red cells and secretions were devoid of A, B and H. In the White (European extraction) population of Réunion, the phenotypes were O_h, A_h, B_h and AB_h (see above) showing that the supposed O_h phenotype in the European population represented the inheritance of the same *h* alleles as the A_h and B_h individuals, in the absence of inheritance of *A* or *B*. To differentiate this form of O_h from the O_h phenotype described above, the terms O_h Réunion and O_h Indian are now used. Red cells of the two phenotypes can be distinguished at the serological level. The anti-H lectin *Ulex europaeus* will agglutinate papain-treated O_h Réunion but not O_h Indian cells. The most potent anti-H made by persons of the O_h Indian phenotype will react with red cells of the O_h Réunion phenotype (486). Like the O_h Indian phenotype, the O_h Réunion phenotype occurs in non-secretors of A, B and H. Since the terms A_h and B_h can be used to describe para-Bombays and the Réunion phenotype, it follows that much more useful terms are para-Bombay non-secretors and para-Bombay secretors with the secretion relating to A, B and/or H. It is probable that para-Bombay non-secretors (and O_h Indian phenotype) individuals draw attention to themselves by making potent anti-H. Since the para-Bombay secretors have H in the secretions they do not make potent anti-H. No doubt this is one explanation as to why more O_h Indian and para-Bombay non-secretors than para-Bombay secretors have been described in the literature in spite of the fact that *Se* is more common than *se* in all populations involved.

It is noteworthy that the O_h Indian phenotype is seen at its highest level in individuals either native to the Indian subcontinent (particularly the area around Bombay, 365,366,436-452) or in their direct descendants, such as an enclave of persons of Indian extraction living in Natal (457). The O_h Réunion phenotype is seen (i.e.

including A_h and B_h non-secretors) among European Whites but with a much higher incidence in Whites living in Réunion. Since Réunion island is a French possession off the coast of Madagascar, in the Indian Ocean, it would seem that a deficiency of H in the general geographic area around the Indian Ocean must originally have conveyed some form of selective advantage. If so, the advantage involved is not likely ever to be recognized.

H-deficient Phenotypes and the Two Locus Theory

Armed with the data generated by studies on O_h Indian, O_h Réunion and para-Bombay individuals and their families, Oriol et al. (386) considered the possibility that rather than being a regulatory gene, *Se* might encode a product. It was supposed that *H* encodes a fucosyl transferase that adds L-fucose to type 2 and type 4 precursor chains and is thus responsible for the presence of H and eventually, if *A* and/or *B* is present, for A and/or B on red cells. It was further supposed that *Se* encodes a similar fucosyl transferase that adds L-fucose to type 1 and type 3 precursor chains and is thus responsible for the presence of H and eventually, if *A* and/or *B* is present, for A and/or B in the secretions. The theory is highly attractive in that it is economical in the use of genes and loci, it obviates the need to suppose that a third locus (*Zz*) exists and, as discussed below, accommodates all the observed serological findings.

Studies on fucosyl transferases isolated from human tissues and at the molecular level on the genes that encode their production, have lent considerable support to the two locus theory. First, type 1 and type 2 disaccharides are different (505) suggesting that transferases adding L-fucose to each would need to have slightly different substrate specificities. Second, a fucosyl transferase isolated from an individual genetically *hh, Se*, had different characteristics from one isolated from an individual genetically *H, sese* (341,487,488). Third, other studies (351,506-514) along similar lines have all supported the concept that the *H* and *Se* gene-specified fucosyl transferases are different.

Dramatic as the progress described above has been, the answers are not yet all in. In addition to the fucosyl transferases encoded by *H* and *Se*, humans produce at least four others. In the geneticists' language the *H* gene is *FUT 1*, the *Se* gene is *FUT 2* (502,507, 1069, *FUT* for fucosyl transferase). *FUT 1* (*H*) and *FUT 2* (*Se*) are closely linked on the long arm of chromosome 19, it seems entirely probable that one arose by duplication of the other. *FUT 3* will be familiar to blood bankers, it is what we call *Le* (see Chapter 9). *FUT 3* (*Le*) and *FUT 6* are closely linked on the short arm of chromosome

19. *FUT 6* is also involved in the synthesis of Lewis system determinants but will be less familiar than *Le* (*FUT 3*) to blood bankers since the structures eventually produced are tissue bound (again see Chapter 9). *FUT 4* has been mapped to chromosome 11q21 and encodes a monomorphic myeloid enzyme. *FUT 5* has been cloned and sequenced, the function of its product has not yet been determined. Of the six *FUT* genes, all except *FUT 4* are genetically polymorphic. Again blood bankers will recognize some of these polymorphisms, i.e. *FUT 1*, H and h (and others, see below); *FUT 2*, *Se* and *se* (again others, see below); and *FUT 3*, *Le* and *le*. Readers wishing to learn more about *FUT 3* and *FUT 6* are referred to Chapter 9, those wishing to learn more about all these genes at the molecular level and about *FUT 4* and *FUT 5* are directed to references 351, 508 to 521 and 1070 to 1076.

The O$_h$ Indian, O$_h$ Réunion and Para-Bombay Phenotypes and the Two Locus Theory: A Summation

As mentioned earlier, the two locus theory of Oriol et al. (386) will accommodate all the findings involving phenotypes in which H is deficient. Table 8-6 provides such explanations. While the table is based on the proposal of Oriol et al. (386) we have added some conjectures of our own. Thus readers who find fault with some of the explanations given should consult Oriol et al.

(386) in the original, the portions to which they object may be our additions, not those of the original authors. For the sake of completeness the table begins with two common genotypes. The combination of at least one *H* and one *Se* gene (together with whichever *ABO* gene is inherited) results in the production of H (then A or B) on the red cells (*H* then *A* or *B* gene action) and in the secretions (*Se* then *A* or *B* gene action). The phenotype is that of a normal ABH secretor.

The combination of at least one *H* with two *se* genes (together with whichever *ABO* gene is inherited) results in the production of H (then A or B) on the red cells (*H* then *A* or *B* gene action) but no H, A or B in the secretions (no *Se* is present). The phenotype is that of a normal ABH non-secretor.

The next three combinations represent the *hh, sese* genotype (i.e. H-deficient, non-secretors). In the first, *hh* results in no production of H on the red cells, *sese* results in no production of H in the secretions. The result is the classic O$_h$ Indian type of Bombay blood in which the red cells will not adsorb or yield on elution, anti-H, anti-A or anti-B. In the second genotype of this subsection it is supposed that a different form of *h* gene is present, that allows production of a small amount of H on the red cells. If *A* or *B* is present the small amount of H is converted to A or B, if neither *A* nor *B* is present the small amount of H remains. The phenotype is almost identical to the classic O$_h$ Indian type of Bombay blood but the red cells will adsorb and yield on elution anti-H, anti-A, or anti-B, dependent on whether *O, A* or *B* has been inher-

TABLE 8-6 ABH Substances on Red Cells and in the Saliva in Common and in H-deficient Phenotypes

Phenotype	Genes	ABH Substances on Red Cells	ABH Substances in Saliva
Common ABH Secretor	*H, Se, (ABO)*	H (A and/or B)	H (A and/or B)
Common ABH Non-secretor	*H, sese, (ABO)*	H (A and/or B)	None
O$_h$ Indian type *1	*hh*[2], *sese, (ABO)*	None	None
O$_h$ Indian Type Variant	*hh*[2], *sese, (ABO)*	Trace of H, A and/or B[3]	None
O$_h$ Réunion Type, A$_h$ and B$_h$	*hh*[2], *sese (ABO)*	Trace of H, A and /or B [4]	None
H-deficient Secretor with two O genes[5]	*hh, Se, OO*	Trace of H [6]	H [7]
H-deficient Secretor with *A* and/or *B*[8]	*hh, Se, A or B*	Trace of A or B [6]	H, A or B [7]

[1] Red cells do not absorb anti-A, anti-B or anti-H.
[2] Assumes the existence of variants of *h* that effect no, a trace, or a little more synthesis of H (see text).
[3] Detectable only in adsorption-elution studies.
[4] Small amounts of antigens detectable in direct agglutination tests.
[5] Previously called O$_{Hm}$, O$_m^h$, etc.
[6] Detection or non-detection of H and/or A and/or B dependent on amount of uptake of antigen bearing glycolipids from the plasma, by red cells. Antigen-bearing structures made in secretory tissues because of presence of *Se* (see text, two locus model).
[7] In normal or near normal amounts.
[8] Previously called O$_{Hm}^A$, A$_m^h$, O$_{Hm}^B$, B$_m^h$, etc.

ited. Lack of *Se* in the genotype *sese* results in no H, A or B being present in the secretions. In the third genotype in this subsection it is supposed that yet a different form of *h* is present. This variant of *h* supposedly allows production of more H than in the previous genotype. If *A* or *B* is present the available H is converted to A or B. The resulting phenotype is A_h or B_h with the small amounts of A or B detectable in direct tests. The red cells are H-negative because all the available H has been converted to A or B, no H, A or B is present in the secretions since there is no *Se* in the *sese* genotype. In all three phenotypes resulting from the genotypes in this subsection the red cells are H-negative in direct agglutination tests (H never made or fully converted) so that the individuals can make anti-H. As will be apparent from what is written above, the second and/or third genotypes could represent the O_h Réunion phenotype.

The final two combinations represent the *hh, Se* genotypes. In the first, the genotype *hh, Se, OO* results in no synthesis of H on the red cells because no *H* gene-specified fucosyl transferase is present to add L-fucose to the type 2 or type 4 precursor chains. H is present in the secretions (in normal amounts) because the *Se* gene-specified fucosyl transferase adds L-fucose to the type 1 and type 3 precursor chains. The phenotypes resulting from this genotype are heterogeneous. It is known that some glycolipids are incorporated from the plasma into the red cell membrane (503,504). While type 3H is found primarily in mucins (355-357) some may be demonstrable on red cells (356,357). Thus if enough H-bearing glycolipids are incorporated into the membrane, the red cells may type as weakly H-positive. If fewer glycolipids are incorporated, the red cells may appear to be H-negative. In the second genotype in this subsection *hh* and *Se* are accompanied by *A* or *B*. Exactly the same reasoning as given above applies, except that in the *hh, Se, A* or *B* genotypes the red cells may incorporate glycolipids carrying A or B instead of H. If sufficient conversion of the available plasma glycolipid-borne H to A or B occurs, the red cells may type as H-negative or as H very weakly positive. Because *Se* is present, H, that is then partially converted to A or B, is found in the secretions with A or B. It is likely that these two genotypes explain all the previously named para-Bombay (e.g. $O_m^h A_m^h$, H_m, H_z, etc.) phenotypes in which secretion of H and/or A and/or B, is seen. Because of the presence of large amounts of H in the secretions, these individuals seem not to make anti-H.

If the two gene concept is correct, it is theoretically possible that sibs, one with the O_h Indian and the other with the H-deficient secretor phenotype, could exist. The mating could be *Hh, Sese* X *Hh, sese* producing *hh, sese* (O_h Indian) and *hh, Sese* (H-deficient secretor) offspring. Clearly such an event would be extremely rare. First, *h* itself is very rare. Second the

possibility of the event would be directly related to the tightness of linkage between the *Hh* and *Sese* loci. In spite of the expected rarity, one family has been described (446) in which there was recombination between the two loci, in another (393) recombination may well have occurred

The above sections describing the interpretations listed above and shown in table 8-6 are written in a dogmatic fashion. This because it seems to us that the two locus theory best explains the O_h Indian, O_h Réunion and para-Bombay (H-deficient secretor) phenotypes. However, some points should be borne in mind. First, although different forms of *h* have been recognized at the DNA level (1043) it is not yet known if they differ at the functional level (i.e. do some of them encode low levels of fucosyl transferase?). However, postulating differently functioning alleles at the *Hh* locus is more economical and thus probably more likely, than postulating a whole additional locus, *Zz*. Second, as mentioned several times, some of the variation in the phenotypes described may have resulted from technical differences. The reports reviewed have been generated over a long time period and have often described work using different reagents. It remains possible that some of the subtle differences that we have been at pains to explain may have resulted from technical rather than genetic variation. Third, while as discussed there is abundant evidence that *H* and *Se* encode different fucosyl transferases, it is possible that each can act to a limited degree on the other's substrate. Thus while the *H* gene-specified enzyme is described as adding L-fucose to type 2 and type 4 precursor chains, it may have limited specificity for type 1 and type 3 chains. Similarly, while the *Se* gene-specified transferase may prefer type 1 and type 3 chains, it may be able to add small amounts of L-fucose to type 2 and type 4 chains. Such cross-specificity might perhaps explain some of the weak expressions of antigens described above.

The H-deficient H_m Phenotype

Table 8-6 does not include one family in which the H-deficient phenotype, called H_m, was inherited as a dominant characteristic (393). Rather than considering this phenotype here, we would liken it to the dominant suppressor of A and B that is described in a later section of this chapter. The H_m phenotype was characterized (393) by markedly depressed H (and A or B) on red cells, normal H (and A or B) in saliva and plasma, and absence of anti-H from the serum (anti-A and/or anti-B were present dependent on the ABO phenotype). In addition to being unusual because of the dominant inheritance pattern, H_m

was unusual in that fucosyl transferases were present.

Secretion of ABH Substances

Setting aside all the complexities described above, which is appropriate since over 99.9% of random individuals have a functional *H* gene so have no impediment to their synthesis of H, A and B; hemagglutination inhibition tests show that the saliva of about 80% of people contains H, H and A, or H and B substance dependent, of course, on the ABO group. Secretion of these substances is controlled by a pair of alleles *Se* and *se*, that segregate independently of genes at the *ABO* and *Hh* loci (58,360-363). The same substances as found in the saliva are present in other secreted body fluids such as the tears and semen of secretors. *Se* is dominant over *se* so that persons heterozygous or homozygous for *Se* are secretors. Individuals who are homozygous for *se* do not secrete H, A or B, regardless of the presence of *H*, *A* and *B* genes. Table 8-7 lists the expected ABH substances in secretions. As described in detail in the next chapter, there is considerable interplay between the *Hh*, *ABO*, *Sese* and *Lele* (*Lewis*) genes although four separate loci are involved. As described below, the detection of some A or B substance in the saliva of a secretor can be a useful confirmatory test when establishing a phenotype that involves a subgroup of A or B. Tests for the secretor status are usually performed by using saliva in attempts to inhibit anti-A, anti-B or anti-H at single, predetermined dilutions (reference 522, page 379). In aberrant secretors (399) the titration method (reference 522, page 383) is more sensitive and should be used. Use of the titration method may reveal the presence of very small amounts of specific substances in the saliva of non-secretors (399). For a possible explanation of this finding see the section above on para-Bombays regarding the specificities of the *H* and *Se* gene-specified fucosyl transferases. Because it has a direct effect on the Lewis phenotype of an indivicual, the *Se^w* (w for weak) gene (1065-1067) is described in Chapter 9. Just as different mutations of *H* result in *h* (1043), at least two mutations of *Se* leading to *se* have been documented (1068).

ABO Typing Discrepancies Due to High Levels of Soluble ABH Substances

On rare occasions (523-528) the level of A or B substance in an individual's plasma may be so high that it interferes with ABO typing. Treacy et al. (528) described four patients, three with advanced carcinoma of the GI tract and one with an intestinal obstruction, whose plasma contained so much A or B substance that it inhibited the anti-A or anti-B used when typing studies on whole blood were attempted. In ABO grouping tests using washed red cells from the patients, the correct ABO groups could be determined without difficulty.

TABLE 8-7 Expected ABH Substances in Saliva

ABO Group	Substance		
Secretors	A	B	H
A	much	none	some
B	none	much	some
O	none	none	much
AB	much	much	less
Non-Secretors			
A, B, O and AB	none*	none*	none*

* The sensitive titration method may show the presence of small amounts of specific substances in the saliva of non-secretors (399).

Transfusion and the O_h Phenotype

As discussed above and again below, anti-H made by an A_1 or B individual is invariably a cold-reactive agglutinin of no clinical-significance (the same can be said for anti-IH). While the anti-H made by O_h individuals is almost always more potent and is usually active at 37°C, one of us (PDI) had often wondered if an O_h individual could be transfused (in an emergency situation when no O_h donor blood was available) with group O red cells. Fortunately the question was never more than an academic exercise. It seems that the answer is a resounding no! Davey et al. (130) labeled a small sample of group O cells with ^{51}Cr and injected them in to an O_h individual. The T1/2 of the group O cells was six minutes and only 2% of them were present 24 hours after the injection. Obviously, O_h individuals should be strongly encouraged to have their blood frozen for autotransfusion. The above statement was going to read O_h individuals should be strongly encouraged to become blood donors but that comment, of course, applies to people who are O, A, B or AB as well! A related question as to what should be done when no compatible blood is available (including blood for an O_h individual) and it is certain that the patient will die if not transfused, is discussed in Chapter 35 (as a preview, transfuse, do not let the patient die). Another report that documents the clinical significance of anti-H as made by a Bombay individual is that of Moores et al. (131) who described HDN in two group O infants born to an O_h mother. Interestingly, in both affected infants the DAT at birth was weakly positive with anti-C3 but negative with anti-IgG.

Transfusion in Other H-deficient Phenotypes

As might be expected, the requirement that H-negative blood be transfused is dictated by the presence of anti-H, reactive at 37°C, in the patient's serum. In those individuals in whom the presence of H substance in the plasma and saliva prevents the formation of anti-H and in those who make only cold-reactive anti-IH, transfusion with group O blood appears to produce satisfactory and maintained increases in hemoglobin concentrations.

Anti-H

Although it was not fully appreciated at the time, the specificity of the anti-H used to study O_h and para-Bombay bloods contributed significantly to the sometimes discrepant findings. Based on the two locus theory (386) described in detail above, it is not surprising to learn (489) that the anti-H made by an individual genetically *hh, sese* (classical Bombay) recognizes both type 1H (saliva) and type 2H (red cells) while that made by an individual genetically *hh, Se*, recognizes predominantly type 2H. A large number of lectins including those made from the seeds of: *Ulex europaeus* (530-533); *Lotus tetragonolobus* (534,535); *Laburnum alpinum* (23,394); *Galactia filiformis* (536); *Galactia tenuiflora* (537); *Cytisus sessilifolius* (394); *Cerastium tomeatosum* (394); and *Cystius glabrescens* (394); have anti-H (or anti-IH) specificity. Similar reactivity can be found in extracts from *Streptomyces species* (538) and in some sera from the eels *Anguilla anguilla* (539). Care is apparently necessary in using eel sera since some contain anti-H, some anti-IH and some anti-I (the red cell phenotypes of the eels were not determined).

It would be highly satisfactory to be able to construct a table showing the reactivities of the various lectins and other reagents listed above with types 1, 2, 3 and 4H. Unfortunately, if information on the fine specificities of these anti-H reagents is known, it does not appear to be in the published literature. What can be said is that the *Ulex europaeus* lectin, that is the most commonly used plant anti-H, reacts best with type 2H but has some specificity for type 1H (535). The *Lotus tetragonolobus* lectin has marked affinity for L-fucose-alpha 1-6 GlcNac structures (540). The lectin from *Galactia tenuiflora* seeds reacts predominantly with the type 2H trisaccharide but has some cross-reactivity with

type 3H and type 4H trisaccharides (537). In tissue staining studies the *Ulex europaeus* lectin was shown to label surface epithelial cells of the stomach where the H was known to be produced by the actions of the *Se* gene, whereas the *Galactia tenuiflora* lectin labeled those cells regardless of the secretor status of the tissue donor (537).

The Subgroups of A: A_1 and A_2

In 1911, von Dungern and Hirszfeld (541) showed that not all group A bloods are identical in terms of their A antigen. These observations led to the division of group A bloods into the subgroups now known as A_1 and A_2. Group AB bloods can be similarly divided into subgroups A_1B and A_2B. Of group A bloods, about 78% are A_1 and about 22% are A_2, similar proportions apply among AB bloods (542). Although, as discussed below, the difference between A_1 and A_2 is primarily quantitative, meaning that A_1 and A_2 cells carry different amounts of the same antigen, the serological differentiation between bloods of subgroups A_1 and A_2 is relatively easy.

First, if anti-A from a group B person is adsorbed with A_2 cells, a typing serum can be prepared that will agglutinate A_1 but not A_2 cells. For many years this finding was interpreted as indicating that the anti-A from group B persons contained two components, anti-A and anti-A_1. A_1 cells were said to carry A and A_1, while A_2 cells were thought to carry A without A_1. Thus, the adsorbed anti-A_1 from group B persons were regarded as the component left when the A+, A_1-, group A_2 cells, had adsorbed the anti-A. In light of antigen site density measurement on A_1 and A_2 cells, a different explanation now seems much more likely. The anti-A in group B serum behaves like a single antibody. In the raw state (i.e. unabsorbed) this antibody can agglutinate A_1 cells that carry about two million copies of the A antigen and A_2 cells that carry about 500,000 copies of the antigen. When the anti-A is adsorbed with A_2 cells, its strength (i.e. number of antibody molecules left unadsorbed) is reduced. At a certain strength, the antibody will retain its ability to agglutinate red cells carrying a large number of copies of the antigen, that is A_1 cells, but not those that carry a smaller number of copies, that is A_2 cells. There does not seem to be any good evidence that adsorption with the A_2 cells removes a population of antibody molecules that specifically or preferentially agglutinate A_2 cells. This concept about the nature of anti-A in group B serum and a quantitative difference between A_1 and A_2 is supported by a serological finding. As long ago as 1924, it was shown (543) that the anti-A_1 typing reagent, made by adsorbing group B serum with A_2 cells, could be adsorbed to exhaustion if additional A_2 cells were used further to adsorb the reagent, after it had apparent anti-A_1

specificity. In other words, A_2 cells carry the antigen (A) against which the antibody (anti-A, agglutinating A_1 but not A_2 cells) is directed. The failure of anti-A_1 to agglutinate A_2 cells relates not to its specificity but to the restricted number of copies of the antigen that it defines, on A_2 cells. This concept also explains the statements made in the section on the passive transfer of ABO system antibodies. Patients who experience hemolysis of their own A_1 cells after receiving plasma from group O or B donors, have anti-A, not anti-A_1 in their serum. The antibody may look like anti-A_1 since it is of a strength that agglutinates A_1 (high A antigen site density) but not A_2 cells (lower A antigen site density), nevertheless it is anti-A not anti-A_1 (81). Further to this conclusion, anti-A or anti-A,B in group O serum might be expected to destroy group A red cells, anti-A_1 that is usually a cold-reactive, benign antibody, would not. Data provided by Lopez et al. (544) on A antigen levels on red cells of various A subgroups and the adsorption of anti-A (from group B sera) are entirely consistent with the above conclusions.

Second, people of phenotypes A_2 and A_2B often present with anti-A_1 in their sera and those antibodies can be used in typing tests to differentiate between A_1 and A_2 red cells. If such reagents are used it must be remembered that the sera of A_2 individuals that contain anti-A_1 also contain anti-B. Thus potent examples of these antibodies can be used to differentiate between A_1 and A_2, but not between A_1B and A_2B cells. Estimates of the frequency of anti-A_1 in sera vary between 1 and 8% of A_2 bloods and 22 and 35% of A_2B samples (104-106). Since anti-A_1 in this setting is almost always a cold-reactive antibody, the frequency with which it is found will depend on the nature of the tests performed and the temperature at which they are incubated. Juel (106) has claimed that if sensitive enough procedures are used and if the serum:cell ratio is high enough, anti-A_1 can be detected in all sera from A_2 persons. The fact that A_2 persons make anti-A_1, that apparently fails to react with their own red cells, was for many years taken as evidence that there must be a qualitative difference between A_1 and A_2. Again, the explanation relates to the number of copies of the antigen. A_2 people who form anti-A_1 are actually group A people who have made a weak auto-anti-A. The reason that the antibody appears to be alloimmune and not autoimmune in nature is that there is a sufficient number of copies of the antigen defined on A_1 cells that the antibody can agglutinate those cells. A_2 cells, including those of the antibody-maker, carry fewer copies of the antigen, so are not agglutinated. The presence of a benign, cold-reactive autoagglutinin (anti-A_1) in so many A_2 individuals should not come as a surprise. As discussed in Chapter 10, all people with I+ red cells have cold-reactive, benign anti-I in their sera. As discussed in Chapter 15, people with M+ N- red cells who

form anti-N, have made a cold-reactive, benign autoantibody if their red cells are S+ or s+. The N antigen missing from their MN SGP is present as an exact copy on their Ss SGP. Again, insufficient copies of the antigen are present for this type of anti-N to agglutinate M+ N-, S or s+ red cells. Those cells can be shown to adsorb anti-N.

The third and probably the most practical way to differentiate between A_1 and A_2 red cells is by the use of the lectin from *Dolichos biflorus* seeds (400). The raw lectin has anti-A and not anti-A_1 specificity, some lots of undiluted lectin agglutinate A_2 cells, albeit less strongly than A_1 cells. However, it is easy to find a dilution at which the lectin will agglutinate A_1 but not A_2 cells. *Dolichos* lectins sold as anti-A_1 typing reagents are already suitably diluted. As should by now be obvious, the ability of diluted *Dolichos* lectin to agglutinate A_1 but not A_2 cells is related to the number of copies of the A antigen on those cells. The *Dolichos* lectin is not totally specific for A_1 since it also agglutinates some group O or group B cells that carry the antigens Cad or super Sd^a and some that are polyagglutinable via certain other mechanisms (see Chapter 42). However, such cells are rare enough that their existence does not significantly reduce the usefulness of the *Dolichos* lectin as an anti-A_1 reagent.

The reactions of A_1, A_2, A_1B and A_2B red cells in straightforward typing tests are listed in table 8-8. Again it will be stressed that the anti-A_1 found so frequently in the sera of A_2 and A_2B people is almost never a clinically-significant antibody and that A_2 or A_2B blood need not be selected for transfusion to those individuals.

Having written this strongly worded section on the quantitative difference between A_1 and A_2, this author (PDI) is prepared to admit that at the biochemical level, qualitative differences between the two phenotypes do exist. However, he does not accept that such differences, that are described in the next section of this chapter, contribute significantly to the serological findings described above. Instead he believes that the serology of A_1 and A_2 represents almost, if not entirely, the fact that A_1 red cells carry a lot of A antigen, while A_2 red cells carry a lot less.

A_1 and A_2: How Much of the Difference is Quantitative and How Much Qualitative?

As stated in the previous section, the differences seen in serological tests between red cells that are said to be phenotypically A_1 and those said to be phenotypically A_2, can essentially all be explained by the fact that A_1 cells carry some 2 million and A_2 cells some 500,000 to 600,000 copies of the same antigen. Indeed, the distinction between A_1 and A_2 is made from the results of agglutination tests, the positive or negative reactions of which

TABLE 8-8 Subdivision of A and AB Phenotypes using Anti-A$_1$

Unknown Cells Against				Unknown Serum Against				
Anti-A	Anti-A$_1$	Anti-B	Anti-A,B	A$_1$ Cells	A$_2$ Cells	B Cells	O Cells	Interpretation
+	+	0	+	0	0	+	0	A$_1$
+	0	0	+	0	0	+	0	A$_2$
+	0	0	+	+	0	+	0	A$_2$ with anti-A$_1$ in the serum
+	+	+	+	0	0	0	0	A$_1$B
+	0	+	+	0	0	0	0	A$_2$B
+	0	+	+	+	0	0	0	A$_2$B with anti-A$_1$ in the serum

are directly related to antigen site density. Those who question that statement should remember that while A$_2$ cells are not agglutinated by anti-A$_1$, they will adsorb it.

The fact that the antigen on A$_1$ and A$_2$ red cells is the same, does not mean that the A^1 and A^2 genes are the same. Indeed, the inheritance of the A$_1$, A$_2$, A$_1$B and A$_2$B phenotypes shows clearly that A^1 and A^2 are alleles at the *ABO* locus. Straightforward inheritance of the alleles occurs. Individuals of genotype A^1A^2 are phenotypically A$_1$, presence of their A^2 gene can be deduced when it is seen in a parent or child in whom it is paired with *O*, *B*, another A^2 or a gene whose presence results in the production of even less A (e.g. A^3, see below). Both A^1 and A^2 encode an alpha-N-acetylgalactosaminyl transferase that transfers the A immunodominant carbohydrate from a donor substrate to preformed H (408,492,529). The A^1 and A^2 gene-specified transferases differ considerably in the kinetics of their reactions. These differences, that involve Km values, pH optima and pI values, result in the A^1 gene-specified transferase being much more efficient than the A^2 gene-specified transferase, in adding the A immunodominant sugar to H-bearing chains (492,529). In reviewing these observations, Watkins (331,546) comments that the difference in isoelectric points (pI) of the A^2 gene-specified transferase in cyst fluid and serum, indicates secondary modifications to the enzyme rather than coded amino acid sequence differences in assembly of the protein. Thus the difference between A^1 and A^2 at the genetic level results in a quantitative difference between A$_1$ and A$_2$ at the serological level.

In spite of the above mentioned findings there is now some evidence for a qualitative difference between A$_1$ and A$_2$ at the biochemical level. Originally it was suggested (333,547) that in the A$_1$ phenotype, galactosamine is added to type 1 and type 2 precursor chains while in the A$_2$ phenotype only type 2 chains carry that sugar. Other investigators (325,408) were not able to confirm that observation. Another suggestion (548,549) was that the pattern of attachment of galactosamine on A$_1$ and A$_2$

cells differed, suggesting that the acceptor sites for the A^1 and A^2 gene-specified transferases might be different. In many other studies (414, 417, 422-424,550-558) it was found that the same branched structures on A$_1$ and A$_2$ cells carry A antigenic determinants and that variation involved primarily the number of copies of A that became attached.

Most recently it has been suggested that the major difference at the biochemical level, between A$_1$ and A$_2$, involves lipid-linked type 3 chains. It has been suggested (345,356,359,559) that in the A$_1$ phenotype type 3H (and possibly type 4H) chains have galactosamine added by the A^1 gene-specified transferase, whereas the A^2 gene-specified enzyme is less efficient in this activity. Thus A$_1$ red cells are said to have repetitive A determinants on type 3 (and perhaps type 4) chains, a feature not seen in A$_2$ cells. The type 3 (and perhaps type 4) chains on A$_2$ cells carry H, thus in part explaining the higher level of H on A$_2$ than on A$_1$ cells (see below).

As described below, there are many subgroups of A in addition to A$_1$ and A$_2$. In most instances the serological findings suggest that these subgroups represent the presence of additional alleles at the *ABO* locus. As described above, the transferase enzymes encoded by A^1 and A^2 have been studied in some detail but it is still not yet absolutely clear how they account for the differences between A$_1$ and A$_2$. Even less is known about the products of apparent additional alleles such as A^3, A^x, et al. (571).

The Reciprocal Relationship of H to A and B

For reasons that will become apparent in the descriptions of red cells of various subgroups of A and B, it is necessary next to consider the reciprocal relationship of H to A and B. As described earlier, the A and B immunodominant sugars are added to type 1, 2, 3 and 4 H-bearing chains. Thus, most of the time, as the amount of A and B on red cells increases the amount of serologically detectable H decreases. Since A_1 and B cells have large numbers of copies of the immunodominant sugars added and since the level of H detectable on those cells in serological tests is small, it appears that the A and B structures limit access of anti-H to its determinant. In other words, while the original amount of H antigen is still present, it is now blocked by the added sugars of A and B. This concept receives considerable support from tests on A_2 and O red cells. On A_2 cells, the amount of A is much less than on A_1 cells and the A_2 cells react more strongly with anti-H than do A_1 and B cells. It is felt that in A_2, where fewer copies of the A immunodominant sugar are added than in A_1 cells, more H is left uncovered and available to its antibody. The covering of H sites is so dramatic that some A_1 and B people make anti-H that does not react with their own red cells. People of the A_2 phenotype virtually never make anti-H. As described in an earlier section, the anti-H and anti-IH (see also Chapter 10) made in group A_1 and B individuals is almost always a clinically benign, cold-reactive antibody. Anti-IH seems to be made by A_1, B or A_1B secretors of ABH.

The concept that H is covered on A_1 and B cells is also supported by observations that cells of the subgroups of A lower than A_2, have levels of H that are roughly similar to those on O cells. Since the *O* gene is silent, none of the H structures are covered by other carbohydrates. As expected, group O cells react more strongly with anti-H than do A_2 cells. Group O people do not make anti-H. (The anti-H in O_h individuals represents an alloantibody made by persons with no readily demonstrable H on their red cells.)

The concept that H-bearing structures are necessary for the addition of A and B immunodominant carbohydrates is also supported by some other observations. Group O cells have been converted into A and B cells in vitro, by use of the *A* and *B* gene-specified transferases and suitable donor substrates (560,561). O_h cells could not be similarly converted (561). Further, Romano et al. (562) used: group O cells from adults and cord bloods; group B serum (containing the *B* gene-specified transferase); and UDP-galactose. It was found that some 200,000 B sites per cell were added to the group O cells from adults, but only 40,000 to 70,000 to the group O cells from newborn infants (see also, the earlier section dealing with branched acceptor chains on the red cells of adults and lack (or lower numbers) of similar chains on the cells of newborn infants (410)).

The reciprocal relationship between H and A and B that is seen both on red cells and in secretions is the rule in the overwhelming majority of individuals. However, there are some notable, albeit very rare, exceptions. First, as already discussed, some of the para-Bombay bloods have expressions of A or B without H. Table 8-6 lists the

A, B and H found on red cells and in secretions in some of those phenotypes. Second, there is a subgroup of A called A_{int} (see a later section) in which the reciprocal H to A relationship is markedly disturbed.

Additional Subgroups of A

Although much less frequent than A_1 and A_2, there are many other subgroups of A that, other than A_{int}, involve the presence of less A and more H antigen than on A_2 cells. The classification of weak subgroups of A is based on: the reactivity of red cells with anti-A, anti-A,B, anti-H and anti-A_1 (*Dolichos biflorus*); the presence or absence of anti-A_1 in the serum; and the secretion of A and H substance by secretors. The serological characteristics of the subgroups of A are given in table 8-9.

Genetically controlled subgroups of A result from the inheritance of rare alleles at the *ABO* locus. However, serological findings that closely resemble those seen when subgroups of A are encountered may be the result of: genes at other loci (modifying genes) that alter the expression of normal *ABO* genes; mixtures of blood; changes in antigen strength due to disease; and acquired A antigens.

Some investigators (394,563,568,588) have reported that in individual persons of a low (in terms of detectable A antigen) subgroup of A, the red cells vary greatly in the number of copies of A that they carry. That is to say, in one given individual: some of the red cells will carry enough A that those cells can be agglutinated by anti-A; others will carry A that can be detected only by methods such as those that use fluorescent antibodies; while still others will carry so few copies of A that the antigen can be detected only by adsorption/elution techniques. It is not thought that different populations of red cells arising from different genetic control are involved, rather it is felt that the variation of A antigen numbers represents limitation in the amount of *A* gene-specified transferase available. The supposition that all red cells of a person of a low subgroup of A carry some A antigen, albeit sometimes at a level too low for detection by earlier used methods, seems to be supported by the finding that some monoclonal anti-A will agglutinate the red cells of some subgroups strongly, see below, particularly the section on the subgroup A_x.

As will be seen, the various subgroups of A have been given different names that tend to imply that each is a distinct entity. This is not the case. The elegant quantitative and thermodynamic studies conducted by Salmon and his colleagues in Paris (429,563,565-567 and see reference 563 for many additional papers published in French and not referenced here) have shown that the distribution and characteristics of A antigen,

TABLE 8-9 Serological Characteristics of Some of the Subgroups of A

Name of Subgroup	Reactions with				Substance(s) in Saliva if Secretor
	Anti-A	Anti-A,B	Anti-A₁*	Anti-H	
A_{int}	++++	++++	++	+++	A and H
A_3	++ mixed field	++ mixed field	0	++++	A and H
A_x	O/+ʷ	+/++	0	++++	H
A_m	+ʷ	+ʷ	0	++++	A and H
A_{end}	+ʷ(1%)**	+ʷ(1%)**	0	++++	H
A_{el}	0	0	0	++++	H
A_{bantu}	+/++(5%)** mixed field	+/++(5%)** mixed field	0	++++	H
A_{pae}	O/+ʷ	O/+ʷ	0	++++	H
A_{lae}	0	0	+++	++++	H
A_{finn}	+ʷ	+ʷ	0	++++	H

*   *Dolichos biflorus*
**   Figures represent the approximate percentage of red cells invoved in the agglutinates.

from the weakest subgroup, A_{end}, to the strongest, A_3, comprise a continual curve. The multitude of names applied to the subgroups by others, refer to serological characteristics and sometimes rather miniscule or meaningless differences that allow bloods from unrelated individuals to be called by the same name. Similar findings regarding the antigenic continuum in A subgroups have been made by others (568-70).

The Subgroup A_{int}

The term A_{int} (for $A_{intermediate}$) was originally introduced to describe red cells that are intermediate between A_1 and A_2 in terms of their reactions with anti-A and anti-A_1 (458,572,573). However, A_{int} cells react more strongly with anti-H than do A_2 cells, an observation cited by Brain (573,574) as indicative of genetic control of H antigen production that is independent of the effects of the *ABO* genes. Published responses to a question about A_{int} terminology revealed some minor differences of opinion about definition of the subgroup (574-580). The question about the A_{int} terminology arose because of a report by Sathe and Bhatia (581) of a phenotype in which the red cells reacted strongly with anti-A_1 and considerably better than most A_1 samples with anti-H. It was agreed (574-580) that such cells should not be called A_{int} and a better term would be A_{1H}↑. Such terminology fits well with the term $A_{int↓}$, introduced by Voak et al. (582) to describe bloods that would be clas-

sified as A_{int} by their reactions with anti-A, but had much less H than is characteristic of the A_{int} subclass. The A_{int} subclass as originally defined, is relatively common among Blacks (583,584).

The Subgroup A_3

The subgroup A_3 was first described in 1936 by Friedenreich (585) and was said to represent inheritance of a gene, A^3, that resides at the *ABO* locus. A_3 bloods give a highly unusual agglutination pattern with anti-A and anti-A,B of small agglutinates in a sea of unagglutinated cells. Gammelgaard (586) and Dunsford (587) found occasional anti-A,B sera that would agglutinate all the red cells of an A^3O individual.

Using labeled anti-A, Reed (588) demonstrated marked cell-to-cell variability in the fluorescence of agglutinated A_3 cells. This variation was thought to reflect differences in A antigen content of individual A_3 red cells. As mentioned above, variation in antigen content on the red cells of a given individual is thought to represent a fairly consistent pattern among the subgroups of A. Cohen and Zuelzer (568) using the same technique, demonstrated only weak fluorescence of occasional A_3 cells with the majority of cells being nonfluorescent. The apparent discrepancy of these reports may be due to the fact that Reed (588) examined only agglutinated A_3 cells whereas Cohen and Zuelzer (568) examined both agglutinated and unagglutinated cells.

Reed (588) further demonstrated that anti-A could be eluted from both agglutinated and unagglutinated A_3 red cells. Cotterman (589), on the other hand, was able to elute anti-A only from agglutinated A_3 red cells (589). Again, this result would appear to represent lack of sensitivity of some tests available in 1958. As already mentioned, tests with monoclonal anti-A strongly suggest that all A subgroup red cells carry some A antigen. Cotterman (590,591) has suggested that A_3 bloods may be a mixture of A_2 and O red cells. However, the inheritance of A^3 makes this suggestion unlikely unless the A^3 gene is actually an *AO cis* gene, somewhat like the *AB cis* genes described later in this chapter. Even then, the *A* and *O* of the *AO* hybrid would have to have separate functional and non-functional ability to allow for production of a mixture of A and O cells. Oguchi et al. (592) used affinity chromatography to separate A_3 cells carrying A antigen from those not agglutinated by anti-A. Although they found low site density of A on A_3 cells, they found no evidence to suggest that the A antigen of those cells was qualitatively different from the A of A_1 cells.

Gammelgaard (586) found no anti-A_1 in the sera of 58 A_3 individuals but Dunsford (587) found the antibody in the serum of 2 of 11 A_3 persons studied. Gammelgaard (586) estimated the frequency of A_3 as 1 in 1000 group A persons. The saliva of A_3 secretors contains A and H substance.

The Subgroup A_x

The subgroup A_x was first described by Fischer and Hahn (286) in 1935. A_x red cells efficiently adsorb and yield on elution, anti-A, although they are not often agglutinated by it. However, A_x red cells are clearly agglutinated by anti-A,B. Alter and Rosenfield (593) claimed that eluates from A_x red cells that had been incubated with anti-A would agglutinate A_x cells. They postulated that the adsorption procedure "selected" those anti-A molecules with the greatest degree of fit for the A_x antigen. We (594) were not able to duplicate these findings and concluded that the A_x phenotype represents presence of very low levels of A and not A_x antigen. Lopez et al. (595) found that the ability of different examples of anti-A and anti-A,B to agglutinate red cells of low subgroups of A, was directly related to the association constants of those antibodies for the A antigen. The serum from A_x individuals usually contains anti-A_1 (587,596) and will on occasion also agglutinate A_2 cells (597). According to Salmon (598) the frequency of A_x is 1 in 40,000. The saliva of A_x secretors contains H but no detectable A substance.

The A_x phenotype, rare as it is, has contributed significantly, although not necessarily in an appropriate manner, to routine red cell phenotyping. First, it was the reactivity of A_x red cells with most anti-A,B, when those cells fail to react with anti-A, that was largely responsible for the introduction of anti-A,B (i.e. group O serum) as a routine typing reagent. Hundreds of millions of ABO typing tests with anti-A,B must have been performed, in large part so that A_x donors would not be "missed". As mentioned above, the sera of some A_x persons contains anti-A that agglutinates A_1 and A_2 red cells (597). Thus even if A_1 and A_2 red cells are used in routine reverse ABO typing (not a recommended technique) but anti-A,B is not used in forward typing, some A_x samples will pass as unremarkable group O. Ironically, the strenuous efforts and appreciable sums of money expended to ensure that no group A_x unit was labeled as group O, may not have been necessary. As described below, the only transfusion reaction reported when A_x red cells were transfused to a group O individual, involved exceptional circumstances. Since the A_x phenotype has presumably existed since the time that blood transfusion in man was first used and since the routine use of anti-A,B came much later, one can speculate that other A_x units have been transfused to group O patients, who did not notice that anything was wrong.

The second contribution of A_x to routine ABO grouping is that it has become a sort of unofficial gold standard for the evaluation of monoclonal-based anti-A typing reagents (190,191,198,199,599). That is to say, if the MAb-based reagent will agglutinate A_x red cells, the use of anti-A,B in routine typing can be discontinued. Logical as this decision may be, it is not without disadvantages. As described in detail below, it was a monoclonal anti-A used because it strongly agglutinated A_x red cells that uncovered the problems associated with detection of the B(A) phenotype.

In most families the A_x phenotype appears to result from the inheritance of an allele, A^x, at the *ABO* locus (586,600-608). In others the inheritance is not straightforward and the A_x phenotype appears as if it might result from the presence of modifying genes (608-610).

The Subgroup A_m (Includes A_y)

The A_m phenotype was first described by Gammelgaard (586) in 1942 and was called A_x. However, the term A_x had already been used so that the phenotype was renamed A_m (611). A_m red cells are not, or are only very weakly, agglutinated by anti-A or anti-A,B, but they are capable of adsorbing and yielding on elution, anti-A. The serum of A_m individuals does not usually contain anti-A or anti-A_1. Saliva from A_m secretors contains A and H substances.

The phenotype A_m can result from inheritance of a gene, A^m, an allele at the *ABO* locus (611-616). In other families it appears that the A_m phenotype results from the inheritance of two rare recessive genes, y, that are not at the *ABO* locus. It has been assumed that at least one common gene, Y, is necessary for normal expression of the A antigen on red cells. Absence of a Y gene (yy) results in decreased expression of the A antigen on the red cells but does not usually affect the secretion of A substance, nor the expression of the B antigen on red cells (617). Darnborough et al. (618) reported a case of the A_m phenotype in which they believed that the yy genes not only caused reduction of red cell A antigen but also a reduction in the amount of A substance in the saliva. Ducos et al. (619) have described another family in which the A_m phenotype provides additional evidence for existence of the modifier yy genes. In some reports (618,619,1063) the subgroup of A that results from the inheritance of two y genes, has been called A_y. The subgroups A_m and A_y may (arguably) be differentiated at the serological level. A_m red cells appear, from the results of adsorption-elution studies, to carry more A than do A_y cells. Secretors of the A_m phenotype have more A and less H in their saliva than do secretors of the A_y phenotype. Many workers believe that the mode of inheritance, i.e. A^m (*ABO* locus) versus genes not at the *ABO* locus, provides a more reliable way of classifying A_m and A_y, respectively. From the serological findings reported in persons thought to be genetically yy, it would not be too surprising eventually to learn that these individuals can be explained, at the genetic level, by the two locus (*Hh* and *Sese*) model described above. Other examples of the A_m and A_mB phenotype have been reported, but family studies did not disclose their genetic background (620,621).

The Subgroup A_{end}

The phenotype A_{end} was first described by Weiner et al. (622) and was named by Sturgeon et al. (623). A_{end} red cells give extremely weak reactions with anti-A and anti-A,B. The saliva of A_{end} secretors contains H but not A substance. The serum of A_{end} individuals does not contain anti-A or anti-A_1 active at room temperature. Family studies show the A_{end} phenotype to be the result of inheritance of an allele at the *ABO* locus (622,624). Other reports of examples of the A_{end} phenotype are: Moore et al. (625) and Jakobowicz et al. (626).

The Subgroup A_{el}

Reed and Moore (627) first described the A_{el} phenotype. A_{el} red cells are not agglutinated by anti-A or anti-A,B, but eluates prepared from A_{el} red cells that have been exposed to anti-A or anti-A,B have anti-A specificity. The term A_{el} was suggested to indicate that A specificity can only be demonstrated via an eluate made following exposure of the A_{el} cells to anti-A. The saliva of A_{el} secretors contains H but not A substance. The serum of A_{el} individuals may contain anti-A_1. The phenotype is thought to result from inheritance of an allele, A^{el}, at the *ABO* locus (627-629).

The Subgroup A_{bantu}

The subgroup A_{bantu} that represents approximately 4% of Bantu group A bloods, was first described by Brain (573). A_{bantu} red cells react weakly with anti-A and anti-A,B. The saliva of A_{bantu} secretors contains H but not A. The serum of 33 A_{bantu} individuals tested contained anti-A_1 (573). A population study (630) revealed: that the A_{bantu} phenotype is present in 38 South African populations; that it probably originated in the Khoikhoi peoples; and that it was only recently acquired by Blacks as they moved south. This would explain lack of the A_{bantu} phenotype in West African Blacks and in their descendants in the Americas. The same study (630) clearly established that the phenotype is controlled by a variant gene, A^{bantu}, that resides at the *ABO* locus.

The Subgroup A_{lae}

Schuh et al. (631) described the subgroup A_{lae} in nine members of a French family. A_{lae} red cells are not agglutinated by anti-A or anti-A,B but will adsorb and yield on elution, anti-A. A_{lae} red cells are agglutinated by anti-A_1 lectin prepared from the seeds of *Dolichos biflorus*. The name A_{lae} represents the above characteristics: the subscript l indicates the reactivity with the lectin *Dolichos biflorus* and the subscript ae denotes the ability of the cells to adsorb and yield on elution, anti-A. The serum from A_{lae} individuals reacts with A_1, A_2 and B red cells and saliva of secretors contains H but no A substance. The A_{lae} phenotype appears to be the result of inheritance of an allele at the *ABO* locus.

The serological characteristics of A_{lae} red cells bear a remarkable resemblance to those of group O, Cad positive red cells (see Chapter 42). However, adsorption of *Dolichos biflorus* lectin with A_{lae} red cells abolishes the lectin's reactivity with A_1 red cells while adsorption of the lectin with Cad-positive red cells does not remove its reactivity for A_1 cells.

The Subgroup A$_{finn}$

The subgroup A$_{finn}$ that occurs in approximately 1 in 6000 Finnish blood donors was first described (632) in 1973. A corrected version of another 1973 report, giving additional details, appeared later in the same year (633). The reaction of A$_{finn}$ red cells with anti-A and anti-A,B can only be seen microscopically. It was reported that there were 2-10 agglutinates per low-power field, with each agglutinate consisting of 4-6 red cells. Saliva of A$_{finn}$ secretors contains H but no A substance. Anti-A$_1$ has been demonstrated in the sera of all A$_{finn}$ persons studied. It seems that the only difference between the subgroups A$_{end}$ and A$_{finn}$ is that the former lack anti-A$_1$ from their sera, while the latter have that antibody. One of us (PDI) remains unconvinced that a new name was justified when this phenotype was found.

The Subgroup A$_{pae}$

This subgroup was described (1062) in 1987. The p in the subscript indicates that the red cells are agglutinated by *Helix pomatia* anti-A without the need for enzyme-treatment of the cells. The ae indicates that the red cells adsorb and yield on elution selected examples of anti-A. The subgroup was seen in members of three unrelated White families and genetic control from the *ABO* locus seemed likely. Had the authors chosen to call A$_{pae}$ a form of A$_x$, it is doubtful that many would have argued.

Practical Importance of the Detection of Bloods of Low Subgroups of A

Failure to detect a weak A antigen usually results in the blood being typed as group O. If the blood is from a potential recipient of transfusion this is of little significance since group O blood can be given to these people with no ill-effects. Indeed, as described, many of them have anti-A in the serum that will agglutinate A$_1$ and A$_2$ red cells. In other words, even when abbreviated compatibility tests are used (see Chapter 35) only group O units will appear compatible. If the blood is from a donor the typing may create a few more (primarily in vitro) problems. That is, if the red cells fail to react with anti-A, anti-B, and anti-A,B while the serum agglutinates A$_1$ and B cells and sometimes A$_2$ cells if they are used, the unit will be labeled as group O. If it is then tested for compatibility with a group O patient, using a full IAT compatibility test, the unit will likely appear to be incompatible. The problem is likely to be resolved in vitro, before the unit is issued. If an abbreviated compatibility test is performed, using only an immediate spin

test, or if a computer issue system is used with the unit already entered as being group O, it may well be issued (and transfused) to a group O patient. A transfusion reaction is possible (634) but is by no means guaranteed. Many blood bankers will be familiar with cases in which the donor's weak A subgroup was not recognized until a repeat donation of blood was tested, meaning that previous units were probably issued as group O. In follow-up studies it is extraordinarily difficult to obtain any evidence that the subgroup units caused any untoward reactions when given to group O patients. Mollison (22) points out that red cells carrying very low levels of A are relatively unsusceptible to damage by ABO antibodies. It may be that the very rare combination of a donor unit with a very weak (and undetected) A antigen and a patient with a very potent anti-A (the one mentioned earlier (634) had an anti-A titer of 1000 before transfusion) is necessary for a noticeable reaction to occur.

The adsorption and elution method used to detect very weak A antigens has been described by Judd (522). Readers of the last edition of this book may remember the expressed hope that the terms A$_{end}$ and A$_{finn}$ really indicated the end and finish of the proliferation of names for phenotypes that are extraordinarily difficult to differentiate at the practical level. Those who have read the above sections carefully will appreciate that the hope was almost realized. As far as we have been able to determine, the only new name applied to a subgroup of A since 1985, is A$_{pae}$, as listed above. Most of the references in the section on the subgroups of A are those cited in the third edition of this book. The proliferation of names for these subgroups (where it is sometimes easier to see the difference in the name than that in the serology) must surely be close to completion. Most monoclonal-based anti-A typing reagents will type most samples of an A subgroup phenotype, as group A. The remaining problem likely to be encountered is the presence of anti-A in the sera of some of these people, that will have to be recognized for what it is, in spite of the presence of A antigen on their red cells.

Subgroups of A in Persons of Group AB

Some care is necessary in the interpretation of subgroups of A in persons of group AB. The phenotype A$_2$B is sometimes, mistakenly called A$_3$B because of the weakening of the A antigen in the presence of B. One reliable way of typing such persons is to carry out family studies in the hopes that the products of the same *A* gene will be found in a family member who lacks the *B* gene. When this occurs it can frequently be shown that the amount of A antigen produced is much greater than in the AB member and is, in fact, normal for an A$_2$ subject. The simple explanation for this phenomenon is that in genetically A^2B individuals, the B gene-specified transferase competes successfully with A^2 gene-specified enzyme, for available H sites to which immunodominant sugars can be attached. It has been shown that in the genotype A^1B, the A^1 and B gene-specified transferases are about equal in terms of efficiency in adding immunodominant sugars to H-bearing chains (but see below). In the genotype A^2B (or A^3B, A^xB, etc.) the B gene-specified transferase is more efficient than the A^2 (or A^3, A^x, etc.) specified transferase. As a result, more of the H-bearing structures receive a galactose residue (B), than receive a galactosamine residue (A). In the genotype A^2O, where there is no B gene-specified transferase to compete with the one for which A^2 codes, more A is added to H. Thus, A_2 red cells carry more A sites than do those that are A_2B.

In spite of the statement made above that the A^1 gene-specified transferase usually equals the B gene-specified transferase in its ability to add an immunodominant carbohydrate to H, exceptions are seen. Frederick et al. (635) described two cases in which paternity was apparently excluded when an A_2B male was alleged to have fathered an A_1 child. In both cases, transferase enzyme studies showed that the alleged fathers were genetically A^1B in spite of their phenotypic A_2B red cell expression. Other examples of genetically A^1B individuals presenting with an A_2B phenotype have been reported (636-638).

Anomalies of Inheritance of the ABO Groups

1. The *Yy* genes

Throughout the remainder of this chapter, various situations that can lead to anomalies in the inheritance of the ABO groups will be described. Rather than group them together, they will be discussed near other pertinent sections. In a section above, dealing with the A_m subgroup, it was pointed out that an additional gene, Y, is apparently necessary for the expression of A on the red cell surface, to be manifest by the A gene (617-619). In individuals believed to be genetically yy, an A^1 or A^2 gene present may be represented by the A_m and not the A_1 or A_2 phenotype. Thus it follows that the mating A^1B, Yy by O, Yy, can result in a child of the A_m phenotype. In fact, the child is genetically A^1O, yy, with y in double dose preventing the full expression of the A^1 gene at the phenotypic (red cell) level. Similarly the mating A_m X O can produce an A_1 child if the mating is actually A^1O, yy X O, YY producing A^1O, Yy. There are

several families reported in the literature in which A^1 is apparently transmitted by an individual of a weak A subgroup or in which A^1 or A^2 when passed to a child fails to effect the appearance of the A_1 or A_2 phenotype. Genes such as Yy provide one explanation for such anomalies of inheritance.

As mentioned in the section on the A_m subgroup, it may eventually be necessary to reconsider even the existence of Y and y, if A_m can be explained by alleles at the Hh and/or $Sese$ loci.

The Subgroups of B

The subgroups of B are rarer than the subgroups of A. Unfortunately in many instances the terminology used to describe the subgroups of B is inconsistent. As with the subgroups of A, the French workers have shown (563,639-642 and again see reference 563 for many additional papers in French, not listed here) that while any subgroup of B may be consistent within a single family, the subgroups form an antigenic continuum when viewed as a whole. These same workers (643) have proposed a terminology for the subgroups of B that is based on the percentage of cells of the sample agglutinated by a standard human immune anti-B, when the number of cells not agglutinated is determined in a cell counter. The findings (643) were that three major subgroups, B_{60}, B_{20} and B_0 exist. That is, in the B_{60} subgroup, 60% of the cells were agglutinated by the immune anti-B, in the B_{20} subgroup 20% and in the B_0 subgroup, none. Obviously the B antigen on red cells of the B_0 subgroup had to be detected by more sensitive tests, such as adsorption-elution studies. There is no doubt that the approach of the French workers is the most logical in terms of the collection and collation of data about the subgroups of B. Unfortunately, most of the rest of us have to manage without their cell counting equipment and standard immune anti-B and more importantly, without their very considerable skills in performing the tests. Accordingly, there is still a need for a system of naming bloods of the rare subgroups of B, based on the results of tests that can be performed in most blood banks. As in the second and third editions of this book, one of us (PDI) has concluded that terms such as B_3, B_x and B_m have been used with so little consistency as to be no longer of any real value. A major problem is that terms such as B_3, B_x and B_m imply analogies to A_3, A_x and A_m that are sometimes impossible to see. Again as in the second and third editions, the classification of Race and Sanger (644) that divides the subgroups of B into three (somewhat heterogeneous) categories will be reproduced, see also table 8-10.

Subgroups of B: Category 1

The red cells of persons with subgroups of B in this group are weakly agglutinated by anti-B and anti-A,B. Anti-B is present in the serum. The saliva of secretors contains B and H substances: examples have been described by Battagline et al. (645), Bennett et al. (646), Boorman and Zeitlin (647), Mäkelä and Mäkelä (648), Ruoslahti et al. (649) and Babcock et al. (650). Marsh et al. (501) have reported a blood phenotypically similar to these, that they called B_m^H, that appeared to be due to a suppressor gene because the *B* gene appeared to function normally in other family members.

Subgroups of B: Category 2

Red cells from bloods belonging to this group are weakly agglutinated by anti-B and anti-A,B. Anti-B is not present in the serum. Saliva from secretors contains B and H substances. Examples have been reported by many workers (652-661). In one of these cases (661) a unit of blood from one of six family members with the subgroup of B had been transfused to a group O patient with no ill-effects.

Subgroups of B: Category 3

Red cells from individuals belonging to this group are not, or only weakly agglutinated by anti-B and anti-A,B. Saliva from secretors contains H but no, or markedly decreased amounts of, B substance. Anti-B is not present in the serum. Many examples have been reported (662-667).

Other Terms Used to Describe Some Subgroups of B

Although, as already stated, we believe that the category 1, 2 and 3 classification could be used to accom-modate all serological findings for the subgroups of B, other terms have been introduced in various publications. The term B_4 was used (755) to describe a phenotype reported but not named previously (756,789). In one of those publications (756) the phenotype was said to be analogous to A_x. Mak et al. (790) described B_v, a subgroup of B with an incidence of 1 in 12,330 among Chinese donors in Hong Kong. A subgroup intermediate between B_1 and B_2 was called (792) B_{int}. Other samples with weak B antigens have been described (795,796) no doubt still others have escaped our literature search. Since, as mentioned, the categories for the subgroups of B were known (644) to contain heterogeneous examples when first introduced, it seems that the samples described above could have been assigned to one of the categories, if necessary on a "nearest neighbor" basis. Readers may wish to try the exercise of listing the serological findings in the cases described in this section, then assigning the samples to one of the three categories.

Anomalies of Inheritance of the ABO Groups

2. The Subgroups of B

Although not yet clearly documented, it is entirely possible that genes analogous to those proposed as *Yy* exist and control the expression of B on the red cell membrane. Thus it would come as no great surprise to learn that a normal *B* gene had been transmitted to a child, in whom it functioned in terms of full expression of B antigen on the red cells, from a parent who had red cells of one of the B subgroup phenotypes. Similarly, it would not be surprising to see an apparently normal *B* gene transmitted from a parent to a child, in whom it effected a B subgroup phenotype. As previously, unusual alleles at the *Hh* or *Sese* loci could conceivably result in a variant that had some of the characteristics of a subgroup of B and some of a phenotype such as B_h (see sec-

TABLE 8-10 Subgroups of B, The Categories of Race and Sanger (644)

Classification	Synonyms used by others	Reactions of red cells	Serum contains	Saliva of secretors contains
Category 1	B_v	Weakly agglutinated by anti-B and anti-A,B	Anti-B (and anti-A)	Some type of B and H
Category 2	B_m, B_w, B_x	Weakly agglutinated by anti-B and anti-A,B	No anti-B (Anti-A)	B and H
Category 3	B_3, B_x[*1]	Weakly agglutinatied by anti-A,B and a few anti-B. Adsorb and yield on elution, anti-B	No anti-B (Anti-A)	H (Some examples dubious B)

[*1]   Race and Sanger (644) point out that the synonyms are not suitable since the subgroup is not analagous to A_3 or A_x. For other names that have been used, see text.

tion on Bombay and other H-deficient phenotypes).

Anomalies of Inheritance of the ABO Groups

3. Variants of *H* and *h*

As will be apparent from the previous sections on the Bombay and other H-deficient phenotypes, the existence of recessive genes, that when present in double dose can modify the expression of A and B on the red cells, will result in unusual inheritance of an ABO group. For example, an individual with two variant genes at the *Hh* locus that permit the production of only a small amount of H, may carry an A^1 gene, but may have red cells of the phenotype A_h. If that individual passes the A^1 gene to a child and that child inherits a normal *H* gene from the other parent, the child will have red cells of the A_1 phenotype.

The B(A) Phenotype

Between 1986 and 1989, Beck and his colleagues (209,210,668,669) studied an ABO system phenotype, the existence of which was revealed by the use of one particular monoclonal anti-A. It was found that one group B sample in about 100, previously typed as straightforward group B, would react visibly with a monoclonal antibody-based anti-A typing reagent. The reagent was a blend of two monoclonal anti-A, one selected for its rapid avid reactions with A_1 and A_2 cells and the other (BS 63), for its ability strongly to agglutinate A_x red cells. It was shown that the monoclonal anti-A able to agglutinate A_x red cells in immediate spin tests, was the one that agglutinated the samples previously typed as group B. The reaction was shown to be A-anti-A specific. First, it could be inhibited by the addition of saliva containing A substance. Second, a single adsorption with A_1 cells removed all reactivity for A and B cells. It was further found that if group B red cells were treated with proteases, a higher percentage of them would react with the monoclonal anti-A. No enzyme-treated group O cells would react.

The explanation of the B(A) phenotype, as it was called, was provided when Beck and his colleagues collaborated with Yates et al. who had previously shown that the *A* and *B* gene-specified transferases have overlapping specificities (335,338,670). That is to say, the *A* gene-specified transferase adds large amounts of N-acetyl-galactosamine to preformed H structures, but also has some ability to add D-galactose to a few H structures. Similarly, the *B* gene-specified transferase adds large amounts of D-galactose to preformed H, but also has some ability to add N-acetyl-galactosamine to other H structures. Beck et al. (210) produced clear evidence that those group B individuals on whose red cells some A antigen could be detected (i.e. the B(A) phenotype), were those with levels of *B* gene-specified transferase enzyme at the top of a variable distribution curve. Clearly, the A antigen on B(A) red cells is best not detected. First, B(A) individuals have anti-A in their serum, like other group B persons, and must be transfused with B, not AB, red cells. Second, the red cells of B(A) donors can be, and have been, transfused to group B patients without any signs of accelerated rates of in vivo red cell destruction.

Two groups (673,674) have pointed out that care is necessary to differentiate between bloods of the B(A) phenotype and those of individuals who have a variant form of A and normal or near normal B.

The A(B) Phenotype

After Beck et al. documented and explained the B(A) phenotype (209,210) an allegedly analogous phenomenon, A(B), was reported (215,671) in which some group A red cells reacted with a particular monoclonal anti-B (BS 85). It was assumed that the B antigen detected on the A cells represented cross-reactivity of the *A* gene-specified transferase in transferring some D-galactose to preformed H. However, unlike persons of B(A) phenotype, in whom high levels of *B* gene-specified transferase could be demonstrated, those of the A(B) phenotype could not be shown to have elevated levels of *A* gene-specified transferase (215). In view of this and in view of the fact (see below) that another monoclonal anti-B (ES 4) is particularly efficient at detecting red cells that acquire a B antigen, some doubt must remain that the A(B) phenotype represents a direct analogy to B(A). Given the incidence of acquired B detected by some MAb, that showed that the situation is far more common than had been supposed and the lack of high levels of *A* gene-specified transferase in persons said to have the A(B) phenotype, it seems possible that some, perhaps many, of them could have represented group A persons with an acquired B antigen. In both circumstances, A(B) and acquired B, genetically A^1 and A^2 individuals were involved.

Whether the overlapping specificities of the *A* and *B* gene-specified transferases explain a finding reported by Deryugina and Chertkov (214) is not clear. Those workers found that 8 of 9 monoclonal anti-B would agglutinate A but not O red cells, when PEG was used as a potentiator in the tests. PEG did not cause a monoclonal anti-A to agglutinate B cells.

The Acquired B Antigen, Deacetylation of A Type

In 1959, Cameron et al. (675) described seven patients whose group A$_1$ red cells had acquired a B antigen in vivo. Since then, numerous similar cases have been reported (498,672,676-698). Many of these have been in patients with carcinoma, particularly of the colon or rectum and many others have been in patients with infections, notably involving massive growth of organisms in the gut. Much less frequently, the acquisition of a B-like antigen in a healthy individual has been reported (688,699). In tests on blood samples in which a B antigen has been acquired in vivo it has been shown that: the red cells react with most anti-B but give weaker reactions than do those of genetically group B people; the sera contain a form of anti-B that fails to react with autologous cells or with those of other individuals with an acquired B antigen; eluates made from red cells that have acquired the B antigen do not usually contain anti-B. It has been reported that anti-B from group A$_2$ bloods may be better at detecting the acquired B antigen than is anti-B from A$_1$ bloods (680). Clearly, the unsuspected presence of an acquired B antigen can result in an ABO typing discrepancy. Judd (522,700) showed that such a problem can be resolved quickly. If ordinary anti-B from a group A donor is acidified to pH 6.0 it no longer reacts with red cells that carry an acquired B although it will still agglutinate group B cells from persons with a *B* gene. With some minor modifications, this method for resolving the typing problem can be applied when monoclonal anti-B, some of which detect many examples of acquired B (see below) are used.

The finding that a B antigen could be acquired by people whose red cells are phenotypically A$_1$, but not usually by those whose cells are phenotypically A$_2$ and not at all by those whose cells are phenotypically group O, remained a puzzle for some time. The explanation of this finding became apparent from a series of elegant experiments reported by Gerbal et al. (498,690,691). These workers showed that deacetylation of the A$_1$ antigen by bacterial enzymes results in a change of structure of that antigen so that it can bind anti-B. Acetylation of the acquired B antigen resulted in the loss of B activity and the reappearance of A$_1$ that had been deacetylated in vivo. Since the difference between A and B involves only a substitution of the number two carbon atom of the terminal immunodominant monosaccharide, the change from A$_1$ to B by deacetylation can be explained. This structural change also explains why, as the B character is acquired, the level of detectable A antigen drops proportionally and why, as the acquired B structure is reacetylated and B activity is lost, there is a proportional return of A activity. Marsh (699) described the transfusion of A$_1$ red cells to one individual with an acquired B antigen and the transfusion of O cells to another. Forty-eight hours later the transfused and the patients' cells were separated by differential agglutination. The transfused A$_1$ cells had acquired a B antigen, the transfused O cells had not. This finding is, of course, in complete accord with the mechanism of deacetylation of A, as demonstrated by Gerbal et al. (498,690,691). Thus it follows that this form of acquired B antigen can develop only in individuals who have A antigen on their red cells, on which the bacterial enzymes can act. The larger number of A sites on A$_1$ than on A$_2$ red cells explains why acquired B antigens are most often found in group A$_1$ individuals. After Stayboldt et al. (1004) described the conversion of group A$_1$ red cells, to cells with an acquired B antigen using serum from a patient with acquired B, Herron and Smith (1005) reported that in the previous 15 years they had tested sera from 10 persons with acquired B for similar activity. One of the 10 sera converted A$_1$ cells to a form in which they would react with antibodies specific for acquired B, described earlier by the same authors (1006). Presumably the sera able to effect conversion contain a deacetylase enzyme. Herron and Smith (1005) reported that the active serum they had found was still able to transform A$_1$ cells to the acquired B state after 4 years storage at -20°C.

Further observations on the deacetylation mechanism that is responsible for this form of acquired B, were provided when monoclonal antibodies specific for the acquired B structure were produced (701,702). Others are not totally specific but still display a very marked preference for the acquired B structure. Okubo et al. (702) used two totally acquired-B-specific MAb in agglutination studies and in thin layer chromatography immunostaining of glycolipids extracted from red cells. Group A$_1$, A$_1$B, A$_2$, A$_3$, cis A$_2$B$_3$ (see below) and A$_{mos}$ (also see below) red cells were treated with a deacetylase enzyme from *Clostridium tertium*. Once treated, all reacted with both MAb, further, the strength of the reaction was largely proportional to the amount of A on the different red cells that were treated. Again in all cases, reacetylation of the samples with acetic anhydride resulted in their becoming non-reactive with the two MAb. No production of acquired B (i.e. no reactivity with either MAb) could be accomplished by treating group O or group B cells with the *Clostridium tertium* derived enzyme. The two MAb were non-reactive with untreated T, Tn, Th and Tk polyagglutinable red cells (see Chapter 42).

Another interesting aspect of the acquired B phenomenon is why these patients have, in their serum, an anti-B that reacts with all normal group B red cells yet does not react with their own red cells although those cells react with most normal anti-B. Marsh et al. (677) and Garratty et al. (689) demonstrated that adsorption of anti-B with red cells that have acquired a B antigen will not remove all activity for normal B antigens. Group B secretor saliva inhibits the reaction between anti-B and red cells with an acquired B antigen while group A and group O secretor salivas cause no inhibition (689). These findings suggest that a subpopulation of anti-B molecules may have the ability to complex with the acquired B antigens, while other anti-B molecules may lack that ability. Such a suggestion certainly seems to be supported by the finding (described above) that monoclonal antibodies specific for acquired B, that do not react with normal group B cells, have been produced (701,702). The possibility that different populations of anti-B molecules might exist led to the suggestion that only those patients whose anti-B already lacks the specific anti-B fraction are capable of acquiring a B antigen. However, now that the deacetylation mechanism has been shown to be the cause of this type of acquired B antigen, a different explanation seems much more likely. It seems probable that the responsible enzyme, once present, would cause deacetylation of the soluble A substance present in the individual's plasma, as well as that on the red cells. Thus, it is not difficult to imagine that once a B-like antigen has been acquired in the plasma as well as on the red cells, those anti-B molecules in the serum, capable of combining with the acquired B antigen, would simply be neutralized.

As mentioned several times above, the introduction of a monoclonal anti-B as a routine ABO typing reagent resulted in a sudden and rather dramatic increase in the number of cases of acquired B recognized. In one large service that used to see one or two cases of acquired B each year, five new cases were found in eight months after a monoclonal-based anti-B, containing the product of clone ES 4, was put into use (211). Other similar reports followed (212,704-706,710), one 92 year-old group A patient was mistyped as group AB because of the presence of acquired B, was transfused with group AB blood and died 10 days later (213). It was shown (704,710) that if the anti-B based on ES 4 was used in a test system at pH 6.0, it did not agglutinate red cells with acquired B. However, it was also pointed out (212) that since different manufacturers using ES 4 use different buffering systems, anywhere from 0.1 to 0.3 ml of 0.2N HCl per 1 ml of anti-B was required to adjust the pH of their anti-B containing ES 4 to 6.0 (±0.1) when this situation was recognized. While adjustment of pH may resolve the problem with the acquired B phenotype, it may introduce a new problem. When unwashed red cells from some patients with cold reactive agglutinins are tested in a system at pH 6, agglutination of the patient's red cells by the patient's autoantibody, not by the anti-B,

is potentiated (see also Chapter 34). Thus a positive reaction may be attributed to anti-B although, in fact, the patient is group O or group A.

Beck et al. (212) showed that the agglutination of red cells with an acquired B antigen by a monoclonal antibody, such as one containing the product of the ES 4 clone, could be rapidly dispersed by the addition of one drop of 0.1M (0.1 mol/L) galactosamine in 0.85% sodium chloride solution at pH 7.5 to 8. Removal of the supernatant anti-B before addition of the galactosamine solution facilitated dispersal of the agglutination. The reaction between the anti-B and normal group B cells was not dispersed by the addition of the galactosamine solution. As expected, when DNA from subjects with the acquired B phenotype was studied, no B gene was present (1078).

The Acquired B Antigen, "Passenger Antigen" Type

While the deacetylation of A, in the A$_1$ or A$_1$B (696) phenotype accounts for most examples of the acquired B phenotype, another mechanism by which red cells can acquire B, exists. Several groups of workers (564,651,678,703,707) have obtained evidence that some types of bacteria produce lipopolysaccharides that include B-like structures. Thus, the passive adsorption of these materials by red cells can result in those cells acquiring a B-like antigen without any reduction of A in the case of A$_1$ and A$_2$ cells. Unlike the deacetylation mechanism, the transfer of "passenger B antigen" can result in O cells acquiring B. However, it seems that this mechanism has resulted in the acquisition of B in vitro, but never in vivo (708).

Acquired B Antigens and Polyagglutination

It has been known for some time that red cells that have acquired a B antigen may be polyagglutinable (498,651,687,690,691,712-715). Further, since the deacetylase that effects the change that results in the acquired B phenotype is almost always bacterially-produced, it is not surprising to find that other enzymes produced by the same bacteria, or by others concurrently infecting the host, cause a variety of different forms of polyagglutination. Thus the acquired B phenotype may be accompanied by T or Tk-activation, or both, or by another form that is more closely related to the deacetylation phenomenon than are T and Tk (701,711,715). Although the various types of polyagglutination are discussed in detail in Chapter 42, it can be mentioned here that the T and Tk-activation as seen in cases of acquired

B, are not reversible by reacetylation of the acquired B, to A. That is to say, red cells that have an acquired B antigen and are agglutinated by *Arachis hypogea* (anti-T) and/or *Griffonia simplicifolia II* (anti-Tk) lectin, remain agglutinable by the lectin or lectins after in vitro reacetylation has resulted in the acquired B antigen no longer being detectable. In direct contrast, the form of polyagglutination associated with acquired B that is detected by an antibody in AB serum (498,690,691) is reversed when the acquired B antigen is reacetylated (701,711). Not surprisingly the antibody that causes this type of polyagglutination is inhibited by galactosamine.

Although much less fully investigated, there is some evidence (708,715,716) that the passenger type acquisition of B may sometimes be associated with polyagglutination. Presumably the adsorption of bacterial lipopolysaccharides on to the red cell membrane, could result in agglutination of those red cells by human antibodies directed against bacterial antigens.

Acquired A-like Antigens

Berman et al. (717) seem to have been the first to point out that Tn-activated red cells behave as if they have acquired an A antigen, an observation later confirmed by others (718,719). The reason that group O or group B, Tn-activated cells react with some anti-A reagents is that like A, the immunodominant sugar of Tn is N-acetyl-galactosamine (718,720,721). The nature of this determinant, that is present in incompletely formed side chains attached to the MN and Ss sialoglycoproteins, is discussed in more detail in Chapters 15 and 42. Somewhat similarly, the immunodominant carbohydrate of Sd[a] (Chapter 31)(722-725) and Cad (Chapter 42)(726-729) is N-acetyl-galactosamine (722-729). Accordingly, red cells with a high expression of Sd[a] ("Super-Sid") and Cad-polyagglutinable red cells, will sometimes behave in serological studies as if they have an acquired A antigen (730).

Anomalies of Inheritance of the ABO Groups

4. The *AB cis* genes

There are now many well investigated and well documented cases (332,731-752) in which the *A* and *B* genes seem to have been inherited on a single chromosome. The type of inheritance pattern seen is illustrated in figure 8-2. Although as described later in this chapter there

are now known to be a number of different genetic backgrounds that lead to this situation, it is convenient here to describe all the causative genes as *AB cis*, that is A and B produced by the same gene on one chromosome.

Many of the phenotypes resulting from the presence of an *AB cis* gene have been described as A_2B_3, etc. That is, the amount of A antigen produced is often typical of the amount seen in the A_2 phenotype, the amount of B made is often very much less. In contrast, one of the French *AB cis* genes was clearly A^1B although the B antigen produced was weaker than normal (394). In most individuals with an *AB cis* gene, the B antigen produced is abnormal enough that an allo-anti-B is present in the individual's serum. Thus there are several clues that suggest that an investigation for the *cis AB* situation is in order. First, as described below, inheritance of the ABO groups may be seen to be abnormal. Second, the A and/or B antigens on the red cells may be weaker than expected in an AB blood. Third, in spite of the fact that the red cells of the person react with anti-B, the individual may have anti-B in the serum.

Many of the individuals carrying an *AB cis* gene were first noticed because of an anomaly of inheritance of the ABO groups. For example, the mating AB X O producing an AB child cannot be explained in terms of the usual inheritance patterns seen within the system. (See table 8-3. Most of the time the mating will be *AB X OO,* producing *AO* (phenotype A) or *BO* (phenotype B) children.) However, if the mating is *AB/O X OO*, the AB child (genetically *AB/O*) can be explained. Similarly, the mating AB X O is not expected to produce an O child, unless the AB parent is genetically *AB/O*.

Although the structure of the various *AB cis* genes is described in detail below, it can be mentioned here that unequal crossing over between *A* and *B* with subsequent gene fusion (749,751) and point mutation resulting in a new gene (750,752) have both been seen to explain the *AB cis* phenomenon. The two can sometimes

FIGURE 8-2 To Show Inheritance of the Rare *AB CIS* Gene

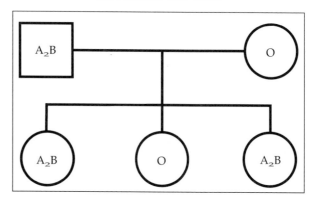

be differentiated by determination as to whether one or two transferases are made.

Situations in Which Phenotypes Similar to Those Caused by *AB cis* Are Seen

The *AB cis* gene is itself rare. There are some even less common situations in which it at first appears that a *cis AB* gene may be present but in which careful investigations provide a different explanation of the serological findings. Watkins (753) described an $A_{weak}B$ phenotype in which a *B* gene-specified transferase enzyme was so efficient (velocity of the reaction five to ten times greater than normal) that it added galactose to most of the H-bearing receptors before the slower acting A^2 gene-specified transferase could add galactosamine. Thus, although the individual was genetically A^2B, the $A_{weak}B$ phenotype resulted. Lopez et al. (754) used quantitative and thermodynamic studies to conclude that the A_1B_x phenotype present in a family was not the result of the presence of an *AB cis* gene but instead represented a situation perhaps like that described by Watkins (753). Now that it is known that some *AB cis* genes make separable transferases that add the immunodominant sugars of A and B, while others make a single enzyme with both functions, cases such as those described by Lopez et al. (754) may stand reevaluation.

Anomalies of Inheritance of the ABO Groups

5. Other Unexpected Findings

As will by now be apparent, there are a variety of situations that can result in an unexpected ABO phenotype in a child. The mating A_h X O, producing an A_1 child, sometimes means that the A_h parent carries an A^1 gene that is suppressed in the parent by alleles at the *Hh* or *Yy* loci, but not in the child who gets one *H* and one *Y* from the O parent. The mating AB X O producing AB or O children can be explained if the AB parent is genetically *AB/O*. There remain other instances of anomalous inheritance for which a complete or a convincing explanation is not yet available. In a number of families (608,610,754,757) A_x has been transmitted by an A_2B parent. That the explanation is not simply A^2B/A^x X *OO* is clear from the finding that more than once the A_2B X O matings have produced phenotypically A_x and B children. Somewhat similarly, A_x children have been born of two group O parents in at least three families (758-760).

Other not yet fully explained patterns of inheritance of the ABO groups have been reported (491,761,762).

Inherited Mosaicism Affecting the ABO Blood Groups

When group A and B red cells are agglutinated by anti-A and anti-B respectively, some cells always remain unagglutinated (763,764). In the case of B cells, at least, it has been shown (765) that the unagglutinated cells carry B antigen. A different situation was described in 1975 when Marsh et al. (766) reported that some individuals (who were not chimeras) had two populations of red cells that differed in terms of ABO phenotype. In those persons with some A and some O cells, it was shown that the cells not agglutinated by anti-A, did not carry the A antigen. From a study on the blood of members of two families and three unrelated individuals, in whom the phenomenon was seen, it was concluded that the dual population of cells was determined at the genetic level and that alleles at the *ABO* locus were responsible. The ABO mos phenotypes as they were called (mos being short for mosaic) were punctiliously transmitted to different generations within the families. It was argued that control as to whether the cell population would be group A or group O, for example, was determined at the somatic cell level although it was not clear why only a portion of the somatic cells were affected.

Anomalies of Inheritance of the ABO Groups

6. A Dominant Suppressor of *A* and *B*

In 1973, Rubinstein et al. (767) reported a family in which there was a dominant suppressor of *A* and *B*. The propositus had red cells that typed as group O but his serum lacked anti-A. A and H substances were present in his saliva and a family study showed that he was genetically A^1O. His mother, who was group O and who had donated the dominant suppressor, had married twice and her second husband was group B. A half brother had group O cells, had no anti-B in his serum, yet secreted B and H substances in his saliva. Apparently he was genetically *BO* for his father and one of his sibs had red cells with a normal expression of B. The family pedigree is shown in figure 8-3. As seems often to be the case, the dominant suppressor caused marked but not total suppression of antigen expression. While the red cells of the two men typed as group O, those of the propositus would adsorb and yield on elution, a small amount of anti-A. Those of his half brother would adsorb and yield on elution, a small amount of anti-B. A family studied earlier (768) had suggested that a dominant suppressor of *A* and *B* might exist but the ABO phenotypes of the members of that family did not demonstrate the point beyond doubt.

Transferase Enzymes

As will be apparent from much of what has been written in this chapter, the detection and measurement of *H*, *A* and *B* gene-specified transferase enzymes in sera is often a key in the investigation of complex situations in the ABO system. Further, transferase production can now be studied in parallel with the molecular structure of normal and variant *ABO* system genes. As described later in this chapter, findings such as those that show that *AB cis* genes are not all the same have even more exciting counterparts. As a single example, there are at least three different genes whose presence in the homozygous state leads to group O. While most routine blood bankers will not have many occasions on which they wish to study transferase enzyme production and, in those complex cases in which such information might contribute new knowledge, are likely to enlist the help of expert bio-

chemists, a simple method to demonstrate presence or absence of *B* gene-specified transferase has been published (769) full are details are given by Judd (522); variation in reagents used would enable detection of the *A* gene-specified enzyme.

As discussed in Chapter 41, hemolytic disease of the newborn caused by ABO system antibodies occurs and on relatively infrequent occasions is severe enough that exchange or simple transfusion of the infant is required. The personal experience of many workers and anecdotal evidence suggest that clinically significant disease most often occurs in group A infants born to group O White mothers and group A or B infants born to group O Black mothers. However, this anecdotal evidence has been hard to confirm in various populations studied (23). The unproved but widely held beliefs about the settings in which severe ABO HDN most often occurs are often explained by the suggestions that in Whites some *A* genes are highly efficient, while in Blacks some *A* and more *B* genes are highly efficient and produce high levels of transferases. Again, these suggestions are based more on serological studies that show strong A antigens on the red cells of some Whites, and strong B antigens on the red cells of some Blacks, than on actual transferase assays. However, that some "super" *B* genes do exist is clear from the studies of

FIGURE 8-3 The Family with a Dominant Suppressor of A and B Studied by Rubinstein et al. (767)

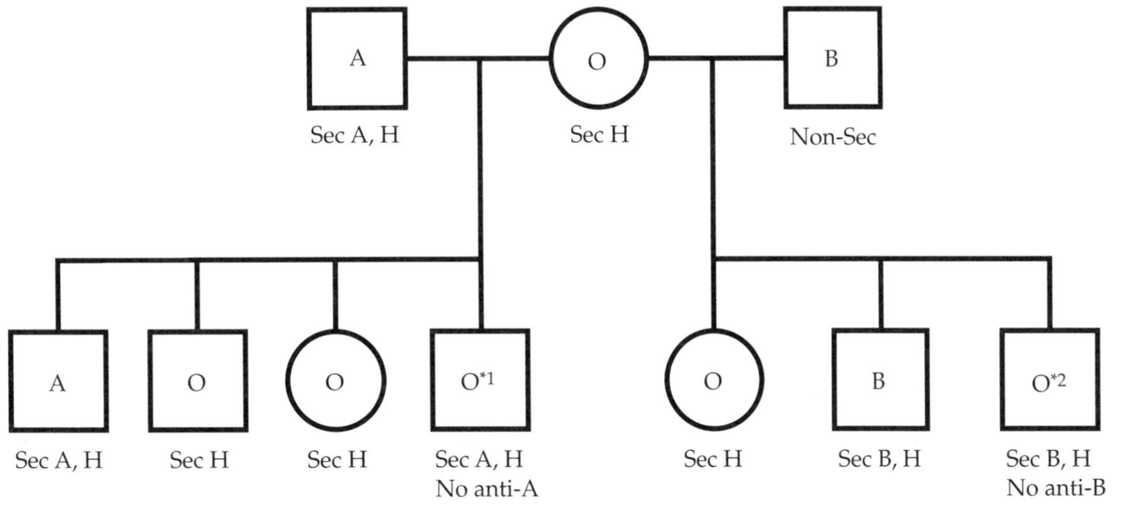

Sec = Substances secreted

*1   Red cells typed as O, would adsorb anti-A and yield that antibody on elution, A and H substance in the saliva, no anti-A in the serum

*2   Red cells typed as O, would adsorb anti-B and yield that antibody on elution, B and H substances in the saliva, no anti-B in the serum

Palatnik and Schull in Brazil (90) and those of Yoshida et al. (793) on individuals living in Hiroshima and Nagaski in Japan.

Cellular Acquisition of H, A and B from Plasma

While most of the H, A and B antigenic material on red cells is synthesized by red cell precursors, some is acquired from the plasma. As described briefly earlier and in more detail later in this chapter, some precursor chains to which H, A and B immunodominant sugars are added, are synthesized in secretory tissues. Glycosphingolipids present in the plasma and carrying H and/or A and/or B can then be inserted into red cell membranes.

Many years ago, Renton and Hancock (770) showed that group O cells transfused into a group A individual, acquired A antigens. They found that these cells were agglutinated by anti-A,B but not by anti-A. Tilley et al. (503) extended these observations and showed that acquired (from the plasma) glycolipid-borne A and B antigens could be detected with anti-A,B but not anti-A, anti-B or with *Dolichos biflorus* (anti-A or anti-A$_1$) lectin. The presumption of Crookston and Tilley (504,771) was that anti-A,B (group O serum) contains antibody molecules that react with antigens on type 1 and type 2 chains whereas anti-A (group B serum), anti-B (group A serum) and the *Dolichos* anti-A$_1$ lectin, react predominantly or exclusively with antigens on type 2 chains. Somewhat similarly, O$_h$ red cells exposed to the glycosphingolipid fraction of the plasma from an O, Le(a-b-) secretor were agglutinated by anti-type 1H but not by anti-H from O$_h$ donors or by *Ulex europaeus* anti-H lectin (772). Again it was presumed (504) that the anti-H made by most O$_h$ persons and the *Ulex* anti-H lectin have predominantly anti-type 2H specificity.

Lymphocytes and platelets acquire H, A and B from the plasma via the same mechanism. That is, the insertion of preformed glycosphingolipids into the membrane. It is currently believed (773-775) that little, if any, H, A or B is synthesized during lymphocyte development. Instead, it is felt that all the lymphocyte membrane-borne H, A and B antigens are acquired from the plasma. Antibodies present in HLA typing sera, that react with the antigens that lymphocytes have acquired from the plasma, can cause positive and confusing results in lymphocytotoxicity tests (776-782).

The H, A and B antigens on platelets are apparently derived from two sources. First, if platelets are suspended in plasma containing A and/or B substance, they rapidly acquire A and/or B antigens (783-785). Second, there is good evidence (76-78,786-788,791) that H, A and B are also synthesized on the platelet

membrane. Platelets from group A$_2$ donors carry less A antigen than do those from A$_1$ donors (791). As first shown by Aster (74) in 1965, transfusions using major side ABO incompatible platelets result in smaller increments of the platelet count (74,77,78) and more rapid in vivo clearance of the transfused platelets (76).

The ABO System and Disease

Over the years there have been a huge number of reports that describe the incidence of the ABO groups in various different disease states and the effects of certain clinical conditions on expression of the ABO phenotypes. Some of these associations have been well characterized and can be considered proved. Others have been suggested by some groups of workers but disputed by others. Still more associations may apply only to small, relatively inbred populations. A clear indication of the amount of work conducted in this area is given by the number of publications on the subject. In some excellent reviews, Garratty (269,794) and others (267,797,798) have listed hundreds of publications about the subject. Clearly, a fully comprehensive review of these numerous publications is beyond the scope of this book. The associations between the ABO system and disease that are discussed briefly below are either ones that are well established or ones that the authors feel will be of particular interest to readers of this book. Workers seeking additional information are referred to the reviews cited above. Table 8-11 summarizes some of the well established associations.

Depression of A, B and H Antigens in Leukemia and in Other Disorders

Since the first description (799) of weakening of the A antigen in a patient with leukemia, a large number of reports (800-838) describing similar situations have appeared. It has been shown that like A, red cell B and H levels can be depressed although in a few cases as the level of A or B decreased, the level of H detectable on the red cells was seen to increase. This presumably represents the uncovering of remaining H as A or B is lost since, as described below, transferase level measurements have suggested that the *H* gene-specified transferase may be more markedly affected than those encoded by *A* and *B*. Somewhat similar findings have been made in patients with Hodgkin's disease, lymphomas, or refractory anemia associated with abnormal red cell enzymes (822,830,839,840). In some cases the blood appears to be a mixture of A and O red cells; in others it appears to be a mixture of A$_1$ and weak A red cells; and in still others all the red cells appear to have weak A antigens. Hoogstraten et al. (807) described a case of an A_1 individual with leukemia whose red cells became unagglutinable by anti-A but were strongly agglutinated by anti-H. The subscript g has been suggested (794,801,841), as in A_g to indicate an antigen weakened by the leukemic process but this term has not been widely used.

Salmon et al. (808) transfused A_1 red cells to 3 patients with leukemia whose A antigens were depressed. The A antigens on the transfused red cells were not altered thus showing that the weak antigens on the patients' cells represent a defect in synthesis and are not caused by an external agent, such as the deacetylase enzyme that weakens A in persons with the acquired B phenotype (see earlier in this chapter). A case described by Gold et al. (801) and by Tovey (842) suggested the possibility that, in some cases at least, antigen depression is related to the course of the disease for a return to more normal levels of antigen production accompanied a clinical remission. Starling and Fernbach (824) performed serial studies on 30 group A children with acute leukemia over a one year period. The red cells of 11 of the 30 children demonstrated depression of A antigen strength. Significant differences were noted in the occurrence of A antigen depression and different forms of chemotherapy. No correlation was noted between status of disease and A antigen depression.

In a number of cases (829,834,835,838,840) depression of expression of A, B or H was seen before the patient developed leukemia. That is to say, it was seen during a preleukemic syndrome and in some cases augured later development of leukemia. As Garratty (269) points out, it is of considerable interest that depression of ABH antigens on red cells sometimes predicts leukemia, just as loss of ABH antigens from tissue cells sometimes predicts malignant metastases (see also below).

As would be expected, in a number of the reported cases, quantitative measurements of H, A and B gene-specified transferase enzymes have been made. Salmon (840) reported that in two group A leukemics with depressed expression of A, the level of A gene-specified transferase was markedly less than in healthy family members who had inherited the same A gene. Kuhns et al. (833) found that while the H gene-specified transferase level was often decreased in leukemic patients, the level of A gene-specified enzyme was often unchanged. In those patients in whom the A gene-specified enzyme was decreased, a remission in the disease was accompanied by a return to more normal levels of A gene-specified product. Koscielak et al. (836) pointed out that platelets are a rich source of at least one form of fucosyltransferase and that the presence of such cells in some of the samples analyzed might explain some of the discrepancies noted. Crookston (797) noted that the locus for A and B is on the long arm of chromosome 9 and that in chronic myelogenous leukemia there is often a reciprocal translocation between a portion of the long arm of chromosome 9 and a portion of the long arm of chromosome 22. However, the depression of A or B is seen more frequently in acute myelogenous leukemia than in the chronic form, in the acute disease translocations between chromosomes 8 and 21 are more common than those between chromosomes 9 and 22.

As many workers will know, weakening of A and B is also seen in some elderly patients who do not have leukemia. Salmon et al. (839,840) have produced evidence that in disease, multiple modifications occur. They have shown, concurrent with depressed red cell antigen

Table 8-11 Established Associations Between the ABO Groups and Disease, as Summarized by Garratty (269), largely from Vogel and Druger (849) Vogel (850) and Berger et al. (955)

Statistically more common in group A than in group O:

Carcinoma of the salivary glands, ovaries, stomach, uterus, cervix, colon and rectum. Pernicious anemia, rheumatic disease, cholecystitis and cholelithiasis. Smallpox, leprosy (lepromatous form). Increased levels of coagulation factors VIII, vWF, V and IX (see text for relationship to thromboembolitic disease).

Statistically more common in group O than in group A:

Duodenal ulcer, gastric ulcer, bleeding ulcer (see text for role of secretor status and levels of coagulation factors). Bubonic plague, cholera, leprosy (tuberculoid form), tuberculosis, mumps.

Statistically more common in group B than in other groups:

Gonorrhoea, *Streptococcus pneumoniae* and *Escherichia coli* infections.

Statistically more common in ABH non-secretors than in secretors:

Infections with *Neisseria meningitidis*, *Haemophilus influenzae*, *Candida albicans*. Ulceration and bleeding diathesis (see text).

levels, reduced amounts of red cell enzymes and of immunoglobulin markers in some of the cases. Salmon (840) has contrasted this situation to the depression of red cell antigen levels sometimes seen in the elderly. In those cases it is believed that depression of a single clone of cells and hence only one marker, is involved. This view of multiple modification in disease is supported by the earlier observation of Renton et al. (810) who studied a leukemic patient of the A_1B phenotype. At one point in the patient's disease, the circulation contained separable AB, A, B and O red cells; clearly many different cell lines were modified in that patient.

Many of the observed changes have been seen in patients with leukemia and have affected the expression of H, A and B on red cells. The case described by Tegoli et al. (843) was different. First, there was marked depression of the amount of A substance secreted with very little alteration of A on the red cells. Second, the patient had osteogenic sarcoma and not leukemia.

ABO System, Cancer and Other Diseases of the Gastrointestinal Tract

There is no doubt that persons of different ABO groups have different susceptibilities to some diseases of the GI tract. Group A individuals have about a 20% greater chance than do group O people of developing carcinoma of the stomach (844). While it was originally thought (845,846) that group O persons had a 20% greater chance than group A people of developing a duodenal or gastric (primarily duodenal) ulcer it is now appreciated (847,848) that the increased chance involves development of a bleeding ulcer (see also the section below on ABO groups and coagulation). Although early reports of association between ABO groups and cancer of the stomach and duodenal ulcer were disputed by some workers, Garratty (269) points out that the validity of the findings is now beyond doubt. For example, over 150 sets of patients, involving more than 50,000 individuals have been studied all over the world and in each series an A:O ratio of circa 1.2:1 for cancer of the stomach has been seen. Somewhat similarly, other malignancies involve an increased risk for group A persons. Carcinoma of the colon and rectum show an A:O ratio of 1.11:1 based on 17 series that included 7435 patients (849,850). Carcinoma of the ovary, uterus and cervix show A:O ratios of 1.28:1, 1.15:1 and 1.33:1 respectively based on 17 series of 2326 patients, 14 series of 2598 patients and 19 series of 11,927 patients, also respectively (849,850). Based on smaller numbers, that is 2 series of 285 patients, the A:O ratio in patients with salivary tumors was 1.64:1 (849,850). As discussed below, the malignant cells of group O and group B people not infre-

quently express an A or A-like antigen. Thus it has been suggested (863) that the immune system of a group A (or AB) individual may be less capable of rejecting cancerous cells than those of group O and group B people who, of course, have already made anti-A.

It should be pointed out that real as these relative susceptibilities to disease are, they confer no selective advantage in terms of propagation of the various *ABO* genes. The diseases mentioned above most often develop well after the individuals' reproductive years. Thus although more group A than group O individuals may die of carcinoma of the stomach, they will have passed on their *A* genes to their offspring well before the disease develops. Thus cancer of the stomach selects against the A phenotype but not the *A* gene. In this respect these disease susceptibilities are quite different from the selective advantages enjoyed say, by persons of the Fy(a-b-) phenotype who live in parts of the world where certain forms of malaria are endemic. As discussed in detail in Chapter 14, individuals with Fy(a+) and/or Fy(b+) red cells who live in those areas are much more susceptible to certain forms of malaria than are those with Fy(a-b-) red cells. Since malaria kills many individuals before their reproductive years, there is very strong selection against Fy^a and Fy^b and in favor of the gene(s) that encode neither of those antigens.

It contrast to the susceptibility to cancer of the stomach, as mentioned above group O individuals have a greater susceptibility to duodenal and gastric ulcers and to bleeding ulcers than do people who are group A. The O:A ratios for the three conditions are 1.35:1, 1.17:1 and 1.46:1, respectively. Many routine blood bankers will recognize these findings as contributing factors to the shortages of group O blood that seem to occur much more frequently than do shortages of group A. The ABH secretor status (controlled by the *Sese* genes, see earlier in this chapter) also contributes (851). The highest incidence of patients with a duodenal ulcer is among group O nonsecretors, the next highest in group A and B non-secretors, the next in group O secretors and the lowest in group A and B secretors. Associations between other diseases and the ABO groups are reviewed in comprehensive detail by Garratty (269).

Loss of ABH Antigens from Malignant Cells

A number of early studies (852-855) provided evidence that the epithelial cells of various tissues that carry ABH antigens, may not express those markers when malignancy develops in the tissue. Davidsohn et al. (856-862) confirmed these findings and used a modification of the mixed cell agglutination test to stain tissue sections and demonstrate absence of expected antigens. It was found that antigen loss was correlated with development of metastases and the test was used for the diagnosis of early cancer and in assessing the degree of progression of known cancer. Many subsequent studies (863-867) confirmed these observations and it has been suggested (868) that loss of antigen expression in cancerous cells may represent alterations in glycosyltransferase production and/or alterations of the sites to which A, B and H immunodominant sugars are usually added. As described in the next section, antigen loss does not always occur, in some cases different than expected antigens are present. Exposure of the cryptantigens T and Tn on malignant cells is discussed in Chapter 42.

Presence of "Illegitimate" ABH Antigens on Malignant Cells

An "illegitimate" antigen, as described here, is one that is detectable on malignant tumor cells but not on the red cells or normal tissues of the host. That is to say, an antigen produced by an individual who lacks the gene that encodes production of that antigen. A very large body of literature exists (869-878) in which this phenomenon is described, since antigens related to the Lewis system are often involved, this subject is considered further and appropriate references are cited in the next chapter. In terms of the ABO system, the most common but certainly not an exclusive finding, is that the malignant cells of group O and group B persons carry an A or an A-like antigen. Thus it has been suggested (421) that in oncogenesis the step-by-step development of precursor to antigen bearing chains is disrupted. In some instances an expected antigen is not made, or is made in less than the expected amount, in others a transferase acts differently to usual and adds an unexpected immunodominant structure. It is not difficult to envisage that both alteration from usual structure of the carbohydrate-bearing chains and abnormal production or action of transferase enzymes could contribute to the general situation. In support of such ideas it has been pointed out (670) that the *A* and *B* gene-specified transferases have overlapping specificities so that addition of the unexpected immunodominant carbohydrate might be explained during abnormal chain synthesis, as in malignant cells (670).

ABO System and Coagulation

There are two major effects demonstrable when the ABO groups and coagulation are considered. First, group O individuals tend to bleed more often than do persons of other groups; second, the incidence of thromboembolic disease is higher in group A than in other

ABO group individuals.

As already mentioned, the incidence of gastrointestinal hemorrhage among individuals with duodenal and gastric ulcers is higher in group O than in group A people (847,848). This tendency to hemorrhage is markedly influenced by the presence or absence of the *Se* gene with the group at highest risk being group O non-secretors. Indeed, duodenal ulcers are 50% more likely in *sese* individuals than in those with one or two *Se* genes. Such is the influence of the *Se* gene that duodenal ulceration is more likely in A and B non-secretors than in O secretors. The groups at lowest risk are A and B secretors.

As mentioned above, there is an increased incidence of thromboembolic disease in individuals who are group A compared to persons of other ABO groups. The studies (891-903) on disease incidence included coagulation abnormalities among women taking oral contraceptives, similar abnormalities in pregnant women and among those who had delivered children, and patients with coronary thrombosis. Mourant et al. (900) and Garratty (269) pointed out that if the results from the admittedly small number of patients studied were extrapolated, it could be calculated that among one million group O women using oral contraceptives for 20 years, some 211 deaths from coronary thrombosis due to the medication, could be expected. Among one million group A women using oral contraceptives for the same period, the fatality incidence from the medication could be expected to be about 680. Similar findings about the incidence thromboembolic diseases were reported in the other papers cited above and from some more recent studies (904,905).

As attempts have been made to explain these differences in bleeding and clotting that are associated with the ABO groups, some other differences have been noted. In adults of Western European ethnic extraction, group A individuals have higher average serum cholesterol levels than persons of other ABO groups (906-913). This finding did not seem to apply in Asians (914-916), African-Americans (917) or newborns and young children (916,917). However, from a study on 656 White and Black adolescent children that was adjusted for other variables, Fox et al. (918) concluded that in Whites, cholesterol levels are higher in group A than in group O individuals, while in Blacks the levels might be higher in group B than in group O persons. Clearly these differences have the potential to affect the incidence of thromboembolic disease in persons of different ABO groups.

The levels of serum alkaline phosphatase also differ in persons of different ABO groups (919-923). On starch-gel electrophoresis, human alkaline phosphatase can be separated into a fast moving component thought to be derived from liver or bone, and a slower moving component thought to be derived from the small intestine. The slower moving component is present in group A secretors and a small number of non-secretors, in only about 10 to 15% of the amount found in group O and group B secretors. Although the exact function of alkaline phosphatases is not known it is suspected (924-927) that they may be involved in the active transport of substances across cell membranes and/or fat handling in the intestine. Thus a role for variation in alkaline phosphatase levels associated with ABO groups has not yet been excluded as a contributory factor in the incidence of thromboembolic disease in persons of various ABO groups.

One other set of findings that may well relate to the increased tendency of group O people to bleed and the increased tendency of group A people to form thromboemboli involves levels of coagulation factors made. In a number of studies it has been shown that the average levels of factor VIII (879-884), von Willebrand factor and factors V and IX (883,885-890) are higher in group A than in group O individuals.

ABO System and Worldwide Epidemics

Although it is difficult to be certain so long after the events, there are some rather convincing arguments that can be made to suggest that people of certain ABO groups may have been more susceptible than others to some very widespread diseases. *Yersinia pestis*, the causative organism of bubonic plague is said (928) to carry an H-like antigen. Thus group O people, who cannot form anti-H, may have been more susceptible to this disease than non-group O persons. The smallpox virus carries an A-like antigen (928) so that group O and group B people may have had more resistance to smallpox than people of group A and group AB, whose sera do not contain anti-A. Population studies completed long after the plague and smallpox epidemics tend to support these ideas. For example, the *O* gene is now very common in areas that were not the sites of plague epidemics and has a much lower incidence in areas such as Mongolia, Turkey and North Africa (929,930) where the plague is known to have killed huge numbers of people. Similarly, the low incidence of the *A* gene in areas such as Asia and Africa (929,930) and isolates such as Iceland (938) where smallpox was widespread, suggests a selection against people with the *A* gene who could not make anti-A. In Mongolia, China, India and parts of Russia where both plague and smallpox epidemics were widespread there is now an increased incidence of the *B* gene compared to other parts of the world (929,930). Obviously, the worldwide differences in incidence of the ABO groups cannot be explained solely by plague and smallpox epidemics. Other widespread infectious disease may

well have played a role in the selective advantage or disadvantage of certain ABO groups and less lethal epidemics (such as those that involved *Shigella* and *Salmonella* infections where the organisms may carry (931-934) appreciable quantities of a B-like substance) may have contributed. Nevertheless, the suggestions of Mourant (929,930) that infectious diseases, caused by bacteria and viruses that carry ABH-like antigens, may be a primary factor in the now existing world-wide distribution of the ABO groups (and perhaps even a reason for development of the ABO polymorphism) are highly attractive to many. However, such suggestions have not gone unchallenged (935-937).

It can be assumed that all readers of this book will be glad that there have been no recent worldwide epidemics of bubonic plague, smallpox, or the like. One of us is even more pleased. Lack of any recent epidemic has allowed reproduction of the above section of the 3rd edition of this book, without major change. As such it represents a minority of sections in this edition!

ABO Groups and Other Bacterial Infections

The concept that some ABO phenotypes may convey increased susceptibility or increased resistance to certain bacterial infections is highly controversial. In theory at least, there are two major ways in which the ABO groups might be involved. First, if the bacterium carries an ABH or ABH-like antigen on its surface, individuals with an ABO antibody to that antigen might have increased resistance to infection while those who have the antigen on their red cells so cannot make the protective antibody, might be more susceptible. Second, if the bacterium uses one of the ABH antigens, or an epitope within one of those antigens to bind to cells, individuals with the antigen might be more susceptible to infection while those without it might be more resistant. The controversy revolves around the supposed evidence that either of these mechanisms is operative and, if so, to what degree. As later chapters of this book illustrate, antigens of other blood group systems are sometimes considered in similar ways although in some cases the evidence is rather more clear-cut.

While this section is by no means a catalog of all the alleged associations that have been reported, it lists some of the more commonly discussed ones and gives some pertinent references. Already mentioned is the possible protection against *Salmonella* and *Shigella* infections provided by anti-B in group O and group A persons (931-934). Anti-B has also been said to retard the growth of *E. coli* O_{86} (931) in the absence of complement and kill the organism when complement is present (939). Similarly enteric infections by other organisms sometimes seem to be more common in persons of groups O and A than in those of groups B and AB (934,941) although other studies (942,943) did not produce similar findings. Lack of anti-B also seems (944-949) to confer increased susceptibility to infection with *Neisseria gonorrhoeae*. It is possible that some of the increased incidences of resistance or susceptibility reported in the literature relate to some ethnic groups but not others; such a possibility may explain some of the discrepancies reported. There seems little doubt that group O persons are more susceptible to cholera than are persons of other ABO groups, such an association has been seen in several studies (950-954). Readers interested in obtaining more information on bacterial infections and ABO groups are directed to references 269 and 955.

ABO System and AIDS

Although there is no clear-cut association between the ABO groups and the acquired immune deficiency syndrome (AIDS), a number of interesting observations have been reported. Adachi et al. (991) found that T cells from patients infected with human immunodeficiency virus (HIV) expressed the Le[y] antigen (see Chapter 9) while those from non-infected persons did not. Arendrup et al. (992) showed that anti-A neutralized HIV from lymphocytes of group A, but not from those of group O or group B patients. It was suggested that HIV may carry the ABH determinant of the host, whose T cells are infected. The whole topic of glycoepitopes in the immunogenesis and pathogenesis of AIDS and the possible use of anti-carbohydrate therapy has been reviewed by Glinsky (993).

ABO System and Heat Shock

There is some evidence (970) that the H, A and B determinants carried on glycoproteins may play a role in the resistance of cells to damage by heat and that this function may be independent of heat shock protein synthesis. Presumably the wide distribution of H, A and B on tissue cells could be important in this regard.

ABO System and Other Disease Associations

The associations between the ABO system and disease, discussed above, all have the merit of some sort of scientific explanation or involve studies large enough that the mathematical probabilities of association are reasonably high. There are many others that probably represent chance observations, apply only in small inbred populations, are not supported by scientific findings, or involve studies too small to permit valid conclusions. Some of the more amusing examples are mentioned briefly in the section of this chapter on other findings.

Chemical Changes of Red Cell ABO Group

In 1980, Lenny and Goldstein (956) reported that they had removed the B antigen from intact gibbon red cells using an alpha-galactosidase enzyme obtained from green coffee beans. The cells had in effect been transformed from group B to group O by in vitro modification. Further, in both in vitro and in vivo studies (some of the transformed red cells were labeled with ^{51}Cr and transfused to a gibbon) the transformed cells seemed to have undergone no change other than removal of the B antigen. Since the A and B antigens of gibbon red cells are thought to be identical in structure to those on the red cells of humans, these experiments were the first to raise the possibility that the ABO group of a unit of donor blood might be changed after the unit had been collected. The following year it was reported (957) that similar conversion of group B cells from a human donor had been achieved. The converted cells had lost only their B and P$_1$ determinants (both of which are structurally dependent on the presence of terminal alpha-linked galactose) and appeared from all the in vitro studies performed, to be essentially normal group O red cells. In cell survival studies, 1 ml aliquots of the transformed red cells were labeled with ^{51}Cr and were injected into a group O and a group A volunteer and the group B donor from whom the cells were obtained. In all three individuals, in vivo survival of the transformed cells was normal (957,958). In 1982, it was shown (959) that the transformed group O cells can, like any others, be metabolically rejuvenated. Following these early successes in enzymatic conversion of group B cells to group O, the New York workers have performed a series of studies (960-964) in which gradually increasing amounts of transformed cells have been transfused to group A and group O recipients. It has been convincingly demonstrated that transfusion of as many as three units of the transformed cells results in: no reaction or development of abnormalities at the time of transfusion; normal in vivo survival and function of the transformed red cells; no significant increase in anti-B levels in the group O and group A recipients; and no development of antibodies directed against the transformed red cells. This last observation shows that either no cryptantigens are exposed during the enzymatic conversion or that if such antigens are exposed they are apparently not immunogenic.

Clearly the ability to convert group B to group O red cells for transfusion raises the exciting possibility that inventory control could be simplified by increasing the number of group O units available. Since excesses of group B donor blood are much less common than excesses of group A units, the conversion of group A to group O would be even more exciting. However, it has been suggested (965) that because of the presence of repeating type 3 chain epitopes on group A_1 red cells (356) the conversion of group A to group O may be more difficult than the conversion of group B to group O. Questions regarding long-term safety and use of transformed red cells in patients with high levels of ABO antibodies are being answered by the studies in New York (962-964), the question of cost-effectiveness of the procedure remains. Natural alpha-galactosidase purified from green coffee beans is relatively expensive. However, in their most recent report, Lenny et al. (964) describe the use of the specific enzyme synthesized using recombinant DNA technology. If, as may be anticipated, cost of production of the enzyme can be dramatically reduced, the whole procedure may become more practically applicable.

While routine application of the method may not yet be cost effective, it can be envisioned that on rare occasions it might still be applied. If, for example, red cells of the McLeod phenotype were needed for a patient who had formed anti-Kx (with which even K_o cells are incompatible, see Chapter 18) and there was a major side ABO incompatibility between the patient and the only available donors, the enzymatic conversion mechanism might be used. Similarly, as described in Chapter 11, the immunodominant sugars of some of the very common antigens in the P blood group system include galactose. Thus it might prove possible to make a unit of blood with an ultra rare P system phenotype, from a random donor unit.

The ABO System, Some Irreverent Observations

By popular demand some less practical observations about the ABO system are reproduced here from the third edition of this book. It does seem that transfusion medicine has become more serious in the last decade, there are few additions for this section.

Some early reports on the association of the ABO groups and various conditions, as cited by Prokop and Uhlenbruck (966), stated that group A people have the worst hangovers, group B people defecate most, while group O people have the best teeth. One cannot help but feel for those group AB individuals with awful hangovers, G-I hurry and bad teeth! According to Woods et al. (967) one species of mosquito bites group O people more often than it bites those who are group A. Strange as that observation may sound, it may eventually have to be moved into the scientific section of this chapter. We have

been told that since the sweat of A, B and O secretors contains different carbohydrates, sensitive chemical methods may differentiate between them. Perhaps there is a lesson to be learned from the mosquitoes. In 1973, it was reported (968) that group A_2 people have higher IQs than persons of other phenotypes. Another report (983) claimed that the group A phenotype is more common among persons of higher socioeconomic groups. Following one of those reports (983) almost everyone including an anesthesiologist in Brooklyn, New York (984) and a cellular geneticist in Chile (985) who could do a blood group (and who was presumably not group A) wrote (969,984-987) to dispute the findings. Ironically, one of us would have accepted the suggestion without any supporting data. Fortunately, Karl Landsteiner who was group O was unaware of either of the last two alleged associations.

Among other disorders at different times described as being associated with the ABO groups, obsessive-compulsive neurosis has been said (971) to be associated with group A, the alleged association was disputed (972). Somewhat similarly, there are alleged associations between the ABO groups and schizophrenia (973-975), bipolar and unipolar disorders (975-977), neurosis (974,978) and alcoholism (979,980). Readers wishing to determine their relative risks of the above are referred to the original publications. Those who become concerned that their lives are doomed because of their unfortunate inheritance of a particular *ABO* gene are referred to references 935,937 and 981 that dispute the validity of most of the conclusions.

The ABO groups apparently extend into the animal kingdom. As mentioned earlier in this chapter, it seems that death caused by a major-side ABO incompatible transfusion is very rare if less than 120 ml of blood is transfused. In contrast, death of a cat who received only 4 ml of major-side incompatible blood has been reported (982). Even given the size of a cat, one would suspect that other major contributory factors must have been involved!

Two reports published in 1982 (988,989) describe four plasma proteins and the ABO groups of house sparrows that invaded Costa Rica in 1974 and 1975 and were well established there by 1981. Blood bankers may find these reports difficult to accept at face value since the Rh types of sparrows were also described. Most of us will have difficulty in accepting that sparrows (even in Costa Rica) have Rh antigens.

The Structure of the A, B and H Antigens: The First 90 Years

It took 90 years from the discovery of the A and B antigens to elucidate the nature of the genes which give rise to them. How this was achieved is a fascinating story worthy of a book in its own right. The story is a paradigm of progress in the biological sciences in the twentieth century. Once the antigens had been described and their clinical importance appreciated the challenge was to determine their structure. "The task of the immunochemist in the field of human blood groups is to isolate and characterize the substances which possess the specific blood-group properties and to elucidate the chemical structures in these materials which are responsible for their complete serological independence." (1046).

Isolation of A and B antigens from red cells proved difficult. A and B antigens on red cells are not water-soluble and although some progress was made using ethanol extraction it soon became clear that water-soluble A and B antigens were available in large quantities from other tissues and that these were the most promising sources of material for structural studies. Kabat (218) notes that "the most definitive studies on the distribution of blood group substances in human tissues were carried out by Freidenreich and Hartmann (1047) and by Hartmann (1048)". Freidenreich and Hartmann (1047) took 5g of a wide range of human organs, ground the tissues in a mortar with 25ml of water, placed the extract in a boiling water bath for 10 minutes, centrifuged, evaporated the extract to dryness then redissolved the dried residue in 2.5ml saline. The saline extracts were then tested for A and B antigen activity by hemagglutination inhibition. These studies and those of others showed that the largest quantities of antigenically active material could be obtained from secretory tissues like stomach and salivary gland. Subsequent studies demonstrated that the best sources of antigenically active material were pseudomucinous ovarian cyst fluids (1049) and meconium (1050). Kabat (218) notes that the presence of blood group substances in ovarian cyst fluids and in meconium was first recorded in the English literature by Yosida in 1928. These discoveries led to a substantial amount of work aimed at the purification and characterization of A, B and H-active substances (blood group substances) from a variety of sources (human ovarian cyst fluid, human meconium, horse, cow and pig stomachs). For a detailed review of these early studies the reader is referred to the excellent monograph by Kabat (218).

The isolation of blood group substances from these various sources was usually achieved by freeze-drying the fluid or water-soluble tissue extract and then extracting the dried material with cold 90% phenol. The phenol-insoluble residue contains most of the antigenic activity. Further purification could be achieved by high-speed centrifugation and/or fractionation with organic solvents like ethanol. The resulting blood group substances are extremely large mucins (often referred to as mucopolysaccharides in the early literature) which con-

tain circa 85% carbohydrate and 15% protein. The carbohydrate comprises four sugars, L-fucose, D-galactose, N-acetyl D-glucosamine and N-acetyl D-galactosamine. The carbohydrate is covalently linked to the polypeptide through N-acetyl D-galactosamine residues and serine or threonine on the polypeptide chain (O-glycosylation). Numerous O-glycans are attached to the polypeptide chain forming the "test tube brush" structure typical of the glycosylated regions of mucins. In the late 1940s and early 1950s it became clear that the A, B and H antigens were likely to be defined by carbohydrate structures in the blood group substances. Mild acid hydrolysis of blood group substances caused the loss of blood group activity with the concomitant release of sugars (1046). Of particular interest was the observation that mild acid hydrolysis caused a marked increase in the reactivity of the remaining mucin with antibodies to the type XIV pneumoccocal bacterium (1051). Pioneering studies on the structure of bacterial cell wall polysaccharides demonstrated that differences in antigen structure between different strains of pneumococcal bacteria were due to differences in the structures of bacterial cell wall polysaccharides. These studies on the relationship between carbohydrate structure and antigen structure in bacteria greatly influenced studies on the structure of A, B and H antigens and the interested reader is encouraged to read the account of this early work given by Heidelberger (1052).

The breakthrough which ultimately led to the elucidation of the molecular basis of A, B and H antigens came in 1952 when Watkins and Morgan (1053) working in London showed that the ability of eel anti-H serum to agglutinate red cells of group O could be inhibited by a single monosaccharide, L-fucose (1053). Subsequent studies showed that the ability of lectins with anti-A specificity to agglutinate red cells of group A could be specifically inhibited by N-acetyl D-galactosamine (1054) and that the B antigen is defined by D-galactose (1055). These results were soon confirmed by the use of exoglycosidases from *Trichomonas foetus* and *Clostridium welchii*. It was shown that enzymes derived from these organisms were capable of destroying A, B and H activity and that this property could be inhibited by N-acetyl D-galactosamine, D-galactose and L-fucose respectively (1056). Subsequent studies on the structure of oligosaccharides released from blood group substances established the structure of A, B and H antigens in exquisite detail (321,324, and see figure 8-4).

Once the structure of the A, B and H antigens was known attention turned to the process by which the antigens are synthesized. Carbohydrate structures are assembled by the sequential addition of monosaccharides. This process takes place in the Golgi apparatus. Proteins synthesized in the endoplasmic reticulum pass through the various functional compartments of the Golgi en route to the plasma membrane or to secretion from the cell. Monosaccharides in the form of nucleotide sugars are present in the lumen of the Golgi and enzymes (glycosyl transferases) catalyze the addition of monosaccharide to the developing chain of sugars (see also Chapter 4). There are a large number of different glycosyl transferases in mammalian cells and each has a very precise specificity for nucleotide sugar and substrate. The presence of these various transferases in different tissues allows for a great variety of carbohydrate structures to be formed and tissue-specific regulation of their expression allows for different carbohydrate structures to be formed on the same polypeptide in different tissues. The process of glycosylation therefore provides the potential for enormous structural diversity at cell surfaces.

In 1959, Watkins and Morgan (318) proposed that the H-active blood group substance found in individuals of blood group O was converted into blood group A or blood group B by the action of glycosyltransferases which added $\alpha1\rightarrow3$-N-acetylgalactosamine or $\alpha1\rightarrow3$-galactose to H antigens. Experimental support for this hypothesis came from a variety of sources during the 1960s. Transfer of N-acetylgalactosamine to H substance with a homogenate of pig gastric mucosa from a group A pig but not with a comparable preparation from a group O pig was described by Tuppy and Staudenbauer in 1966 (1057). Subsequent studies with preparations from human maxillary glands (1058), gastric mucosa (1007), colonic mucosa (1008), colonic cancer (1008), milk (1009) and plasma (1010) confirmed these findings. In 1968, Race et al. (1011) identified the galactosyltransferase required for synthesis of B antigen.

During the 1970s several groups undertook the very difficult task of purifying the A, B and H transferases. The fortuitous discovery that blood group A transferases were absorbed onto certain batches of sepharose 4B (a polymer of galactose) and could be eluted from this matrix by the nucleotide sugar UDP provided an affinity chromatography step which allowed a 50,000-fold purification of the enzyme and made protein sequence studies a realistic possibility (1012,1013). Nevertheless, it was not until 1990 that sufficient protein sequence information was obtained to allow the search for, and identification of, the *A* transferase gene. Clausen et al. (347) purified the A transferase from lung tissue by a process of detergent solubilization (with Triton X-100), affinity chromatography on sepharose 4B and cation exchange chromatography. Starting with 5Kg of human lung tissue (approximately 3 lungs) 54μg of purified A transferase were obtained representing a 630,000-fold purification.

FIGURE 8-4 Structure of A, B and H Antigens

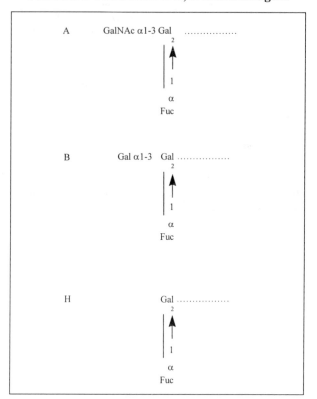

Cloning the *A* Transferase Gene

Yamamoto et al. (348) used protein sequence information obtained for human lung A transferase by Clausen et al. (347) to isolate a full length cDNA clone corresponding to the A transferase. A cDNA library was prepared from human stomach cancer cell line (MKN45) known to contain high levels of A antigen and high A transferase activity. Redundant oligonucleotide probes were used in a PCR to amplify a 98bp cDNA fragment and this fragment was used to screen the cDNA library. One clone was found which contained the entire coding sequence of the putative A transferase and contained nucleotide sequences which corresponded to the sequence of peptides obtained from the purified enzyme. The cDNA encoded a protein predicted to have a molecular weight of 41kD with a short N-terminal domain, a single transmembrane domain and a large C-terminal domain containing a signal motif for N-glycosylation. The protein is a type II transmembrane protein with its N-terminus in the cytosol and C-terminus in the lumen of the Golgi (see figure 8-5). This structure is commonly found in glycosyltransferases, the active site of these enzymes is located in the large C-terminal domain. Southern blot analysis indicated that the A transferase is encoded by a single gene. Northern blotting revealed that RNA transcripts of this gene were not confined to cell lines expressing blood group A or AB but were also present in cell lines expressing blood group B and O. These results indicated that the B transferase has a very similar structure to the A transferase and that the absence of A and B antigens in individuals of group O is not due to the absence of a gene but the inability to produce a functional enzyme.

Molecular Basis of the A and B Antigens

Yamamoto et al. (349) used the A transferase cDNA probe described in the previous section to investigate the molecular basis of A and B antigens. Four cDNA libraries were constructed from four different human colon adenocarcinoma cell lines. Three of the patients from which these lines were derived were of known blood group (O, AB and B). The A transferase cDNA probe was used to screen each of these cDNA libraries and hybridizing clones were isolated and sequenced. Inspection of the sequences allowed the following conclusions to be drawn. Seven nucleotide substitutions (four of which changed amino acids at residues 176, 235, 266, 268) were found in cDNAs isolated from cells of group B when compared with the A transferase sequence (see figure 8-6). All the predicted O allelic cDNA clones had a sequence which differed from that of the A transferase at only one position, a single nucleotide deletion (nt258) in the coding region resulting in a frameshift and this was presumed to result in an inactive transferase. These observations were verified on genomic DNA from 14 individuals of known ABO phenotype.

The importance of the four amino acid sequence differences between the A_1 enzyme (Arg176, Gly235, Leu266, Gly268) and the B enzyme (Gly176, Ser235, Met266, Ala268) was investigated by Yamamoto and Hakomori (350). These authors constructed chimeric proteins with B-enzyme-specific amino acids in an A enzyme and vice versa. The normal A_1 enzyme was denoted AAAA to indicate that each of the four amino acids at positions 176, 235, 266 and 268 were of the A enzyme type and by analogy the normal B enzyme was denoted BBBB. When chimeric proteins of type BAAA, ABAA, BBAA, AAAB and BAAB were expressed in a suitable cell line the cells became A antigen positive. When chimeric proteins of type ABBB, BABB, or AABB were expressed the cells became B antigen positive. Chimeric proteins of type AABA, ABBA, BABA and BBBA produced cells expressing both A and B antigens while ABAB and BBAB produced both A and weak B antigens. These results imply that the amino acids at the third position (residue 266) and the fourth position (residue 268) are crucial in defining the specificity of the A_1-enzyme and the B-enzyme. These studies also show

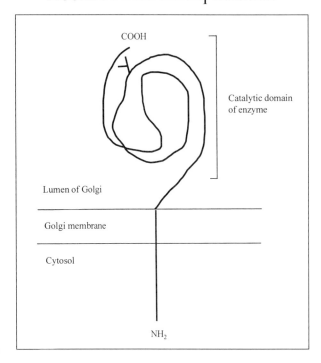

FIGURE 8-5 Model of the A_1 Transferase

that the residue at position 176 is of little importance. B antigen can be produced as well as A antigen when the A specific residue is third and the B-specific residue is fourth indicating that the fourth residue is important for B-enzyme activity. These studies also indicate that the residue at the second position (residue 235) can also influence substrate specificity.

The role of the amino acid at position 268 was further defined by Yamamoto and McNeill (1014). These authors introduced a series of mutations into codon 268 of the A and B transferases to create a panel of mutant enzymes in which every possible amino acid substitution at codon 268 was present. They then examined the effect of each amino acid substitution on the nucleotide sugar donor substrate specificity and the enzymatic activity of the A and B transferases that resulted. The results showed that if the glycine 268 found in wild type A transferase is substituted by alanine, serine or cysteine the expressed mutant enzymes have both A and B transferase activity. Weak A activity was detected if histidine or phenylalanine was at residue 268 while asparagine or threonine at this position gave rise to weak B activity. All other amino acid substitutions had neither A nor B activity and were therefore artificially generated *O* alleles. If the alanine 268 found in wild type B transferase is replaced with glycine which occupies this position in the A transferase the mutant enzyme expresses both A and B transferase activity. These experiments clearly establish the critical role of residue 268 in determining the activity and nucleotide sugar specificity of the A and B transferases.

FIGURE 8-6 Genetic Basis of *A¹*, *B*, *O* and Some Variant Alleles
(see text for discussion of variant allelles *O¹* and *O³*)

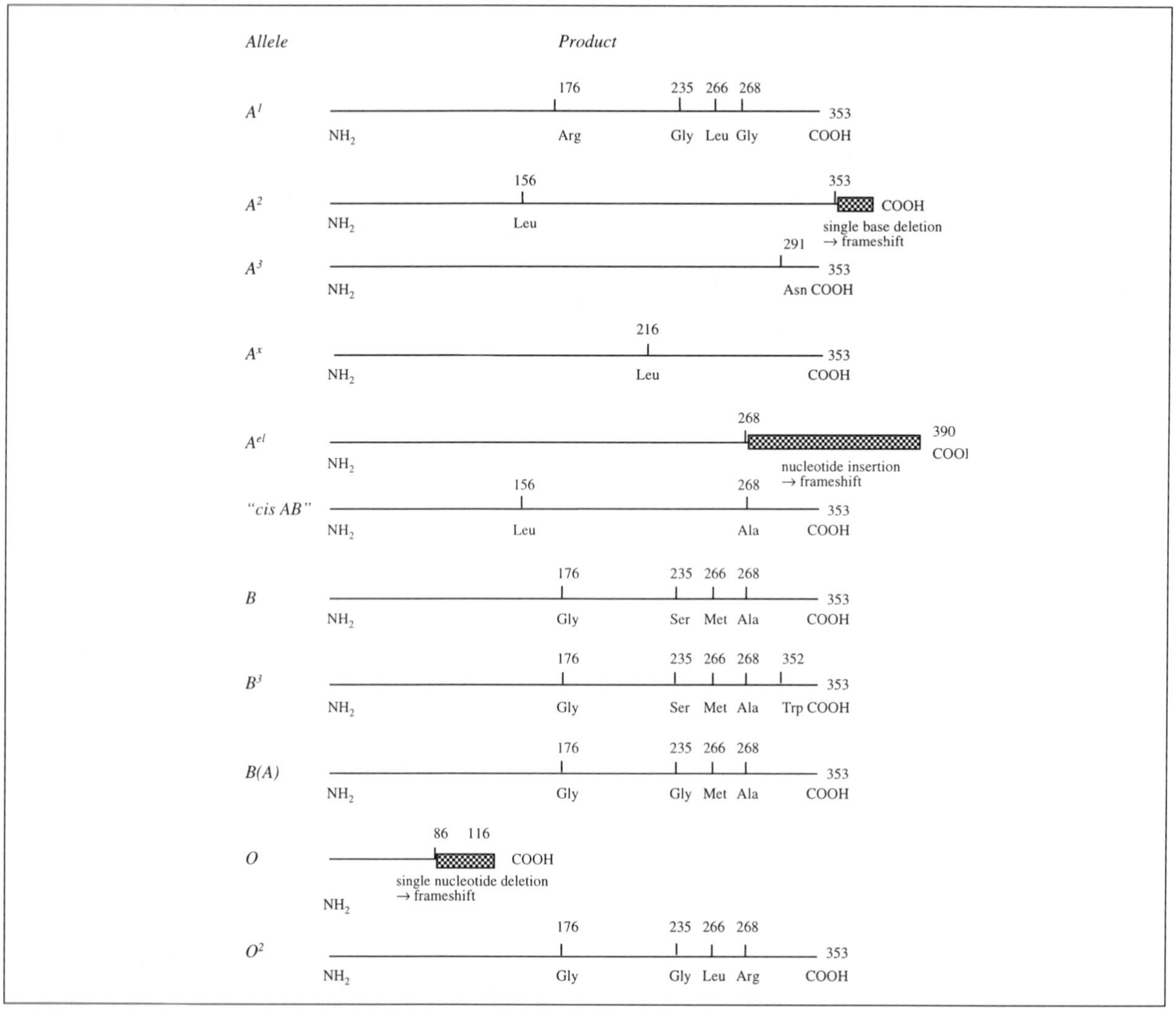

Structure of the Transferase Gene Responsible for A, B and O Phenotypes

As described above, different allelic forms of a single gene give rise to the A, B and O phenotypes. The first allelic form of this gene to be cloned was that which gives rise to A antigen (termed A-transferase in this chapter). The *ABO* locus on chromosome 9q34 therefore comprises a single gene. The *ABO* locus is sometimes described as the human histo-blood group locus (345). The prefix histo- is used to convey that A and B antigens are expressed in a wide variety of tissues and not simply confined to blood cells. In 1995, two groups described the structure of the single gene at the *ABO* locus (1015,1016). Yamamoto et al. (1015) screened genomic DNA libraries derived from human leukocytes and human placenta with the A transferase cDNA probe. They obtained five genomic clones which spanned a region of more than 30kb and contained the entire *ABO* gene.

The coding region of the human *ABO* gene spans over 18kb and comprises 7 exons (see figure 8-7). The region of the gene encoding the transmembrane domain of the enzyme is mostly in exon 2 with its last four amino acids in exon 3. The first five exons are small, comprising 28, 70, 57, 48, and 36 nucleotides respectively. Most of the coding sequence for the C-terminal catalytic domain is contained within exons 6 (135 nucleotides) and the largest exon, exon 7 (688 nucleotides). The single nucleotide deletion found in most *O* alleles is found in exon 6 as is the first of the seven nucleotide substitutions that distinguish the *A* and *B* alleles. Exon 7 contains the other six nucleotide substitutions that distinguish *A* and *B* alleles. Bennett et al. (1016) used fluorescence in situ hybridization (FISH) to confirm the chromosomal location of the *ABO* locus at 9q34. The last two coding exons of the *ABO* gene are homologous to the last two coding exons of the murine α1,3 galactosyltransferase gene (1017,1018). A number of alternatively spliced products of the *ABO* gene have been isolated and there is evidence that transcripts with different exon usage are found in different organs. However, it is not clear whether these alternatively spliced transcripts are translated and if translated, enzymically active (1016,1017). These questions are reminiscent of problems of interpreting the physiological significance of alternatively spliced transcripts in the Rh system (see Chapter 12).

Variant A and B Antigens Result from Mutations in the Transferase Gene

Once cDNA encoding the A transferase had been obtained and the molecular bases of B and O phenotypes determined it was a comparatively simple task to explore the nature of this gene in individuals whose red cells expressed unusual A and/or B antigens.

A_2 Phenotype

The transferase gene in 8 individuals expressing the A_2 phenotype was found to have a single base substitution at nt467 which changed Pro156 to Leu and a single base deletion within the codon corresponding to the last amino acid (residue 353) of the predicted protein corresponding to the original cloned A transferase (see figure 8-6) (1019). The single base deletion results in a frameshift which deletes the carboxy-terminal proline residue and adds 21 amino acids to the C terminus generating a predicted protein of 374 amino acids compared with 353 in the original A transferase reported. The original A transferase sequence (348, presumed A_1 transferase) was used to construct a cDNA with the additional 21 amino acids found in the transferase from the A_2 individuals but without the Pro156→Leu change. When

this was transfected into HeLa cells a weak A transferase activity with properties similar to that reported previously for A_2 transferase was found. The single base substitution Pro156→Leu was found to have little effect on enzyme activity (350). Pro→Leu is a significant change to the amino acid sequence of the protein and such a change is frequently associated with antigenicity in cell surface proteins (many examples will be found in this book). The fact that this change does not affect the enzymic activity of this protein suggests that it occurs outside the active site of the enzyme.

The occurrence of two different mutations in the A^2 gene only one of which influences enzymic activity seems unlikely to be the only genetic background of this phenotype since it would require two separate genetic events to create. Individuals with the A_1 phenotype having Pro156→Leu and individuals with the A_2 phenotype having only the additional 21 amino acids at the C-terminus must surely exist. The analogy of M^c in the MNS system comes to mind (see Chapter 15). Leucine at 156 was found in one A^1 allele from a human stomach cancer cell line MKN45 (1019).

There is a substantial literature documenting differences between A_1 and A_2 and the structural basis for the difference between these phenotypes has been a subject of controversy. There is clear evidence that the difference is quantitative because A_1 cells have more A antigen sites than A_2 cells (406). There is clear evidence that the difference is qualitative because individuals of phenotype A_2 sometimes make anti-A_1 (287). The molecular studies outlined above demonstrate that the A_2 phenotype results from a mutation in the A^1 transferase gene and in this respect provide the possibility of a structural explanation for well documented differences in the enzymic activity of transferases obtained from individuals of the A_1 and A_2 phenotypes. The enzyme from A_1 individuals has a pH optimum of 5.6 whereas that from A_2 individuals has a pH optimum between 7 and 8 (492). The enzymes differ in their isoelectric points and although both are active in the presence of Mn^{++} only the A_1 enzyme is active in the presence of Mg^{++} (492). These molecular

FIGURE 8-7 Structure of the *ABO* Gene (references 1015, 1016)

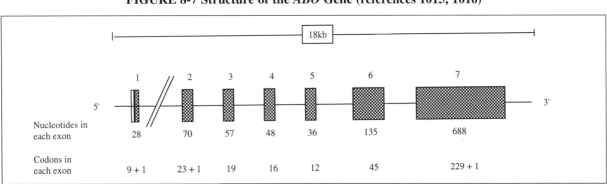

results do not, however, directly address the controversy regarding qualitative/quantitative differences in the A_1 and A_2 antigens. Structural studies have shown the occurrence of A-active structures on A_1 red cells that are not found on A_2 red cells (357,359). These A active structures (denoted type 3A and type 4A) arise because the A_1 transferase can utilize substrates that the A_2 transferase cannot. The type 3A structure can be created on existing A antigens by the following steps: galactose is added to the N-acetylgalactosamine residue of an existing A antigen in the linkage ß1→3, addition of fucose to this galactose in the linkage α1→2 creates an H antigen (type 3 H) and this structure can then be converted into A antigen by addition of N-acetylgalactosamine in an α1→3 linkage. The type 4A structure is created by addition of GalNAcα1→3(Fucα1→2) Galß1→3 to the major red cell membrane glycolipid globoside which carries P antigen (see Chapter 11). The answer to the question what is the difference between A_1 and A_2 therefore appears to be that the phenotypes differ both quantitatively and qualitatively. The A_1 enzyme is more efficient at transferring GalNAc to available H antigen sites under physiological conditions and so there are quantitatively more A antigen sites on A_1 red cells but the A_1 transferase also has a slightly different substrate specificity which allows it to add GalNAc to substrates (type 3H, type 4H) which the A_2 enzyme cannot utilize and thus create qualitative differences because some of the A antigens on A_1 red cells are of a type not present on A_2 red cells.

The A_3 Phenotype

Yamomoto et al. (1020) used the PCR to amplify the last two coding exons (exons 6 and 7) of the A transferase from genomic DNA obtained from two individuals with the A_3 phenotype and two with the A_3B phenotype. Exons 6 and 7 encode most of the C-terminal domain of the enzyme and 91% of the soluble form of the transferase (see figure 8-7). The two individuals with the A_3B phenotype had a single base substitution at nt871 which converted Asp291→Asn in the predicted protein sequence of the enzyme (see figure 8-6). DNA from the two individuals with the A_3 phenotype did not show any nucleotide sequence differences when compared with the A_1 transferase in the last two exons. These authors conclude that the results demonstrate heterogeneity in the molecular mechanisms giving rise to the A_3 phenotype and note that this conclusion is consistent with studies of the properties of A transferases in this phenotype which also indicate heterogeneity (571,1021). Interpretation of these studies must be tempered with the knowledge that not all the coding sequence of the enzyme was examined. Nevertheless the

substitution of Asp291 with Asn represents a major change from an acidic to an uncharged residue and would not be inconsistent with disruption of the active site of the enzyme and thereby weak transferase activity. This could be studied by transfection of the mutant enzyme. The authors speculate that their failure to detect sequence changes in the other two A^3 alleles may reflect a weakening of A antigen as a result of factors unrelated to the transferase gene since A and B antigens are known to be transiently weakened in disease. Clearly, there are several different possibilities which could account for these results including general or tissue-specific defects in the regulation of the transferase gene and these will require further study.

The A_X Phenotype

The nucleotide sequence of the last two exons of the A transferase gene was determined for the corresponding gene of one individual with the A_X phenotype (1022). One nucleotide substitution was found at nucleotide 646 which would have the effect of changing amino acid Phe216 to Ile. Whether this change of one nonpolar amino acid for another is sufficient to account for the gross reduction in A transferase activity found in this phenotype will require study of the enzymic activity of the mutant enzyme after transfection.

The A_{el} Phenotype

The A^{el} allele correlates with an A transferase sequence with a nucleotide insertion which changes the amino acid sequence of the predicted protein product immediately after the critical Gly268 and extends the polypeptide by 37 amino acids compared to the A_1 transferase and a further 16 amino acids compared to the A_2 transferase (1059). The occurrence of this mutated sequence in the A^{el} allele suggests that the translated protein has weak A-enzyme activity but this has not been formally proved by expression studies at the time of this writing.

The B_3 Phenotype

The last two coding exons of the B allele of the A_1 transferase gene cloned by Yamamoto et al. (348) were amplified and sequenced from two individuals with the B_3 phenotype and one with the A_1B_3 phenotype (1020). The B^3 allele in the individual with phenotype A_1B_3 had a nucleotide substitution at nt1054 resulting an amino acid substitution Arg352→Trp almost at the C-terminus of the protein. Substitution of the very basically charged arginine by a non-polar tryptophan residue in this region of the protein may account for the weak α-galactosyl transferase activity in this individual but transfection studies will be required to establish this unequivocally. No nucleotide sequence differences were found in the last two exons of the B^3 allele of the other two individuals studied. Elucidation of the genetic mechanism(s) giving rise to this phenotype in these two individuals is likely to require analysis of the complete transferase gene and its regulatory sequences.

The B(A) Phenotype

Nucleotide sequence analysis of the last two exons of the *B* allele of the A transferase gene from an individual with the B(A) phenotype revealed two nucleotide substitutions (T657C and A703G) not associated with the common *B* allele (1022). The substitution A703G changed the amino acid sequence of the predicted protein from Ser235 to Gly. Both of these nucleotide substitutions are found in the A_1 transferase. Individuals exhibiting the B(A) phenotype have small amounts of A antigen in addition to normal levels of B antigen. These results suggest that Ser235Gly mutation may alter the specificity of the B enzyme for nucleotide sugars thereby allowing synthesis of some A antigen. Direct evidence that this residue affects the specificity of A and B transferases was obtained from expression studies in HeLa cells using manufactured chimeric A_1-B transferase constructs (350).

The "cis-AB" Phenotype

Nucleotide sequence analysis of the last two exons of A transferase gene in two individuals with *cis-AB* alleles revealed that the *cis-AB* alleles in both individuals were identical to A^1 alleles except for two nucleotide substitutions (752). The first substitution Pro156→Leu is identical to that found in the A_2 phenotype (see above). The second substitution changes Gly268→Ala. Alanine is found at residue 268 in the normal *B* allele (see figure 8-6) and this is known to be a critical residue in defining the nucleotide sugar specificity of the B transferase (350,1014). These results suggest that the *cis-AB* allele in these two Japanese individuals produces a transferase which is capable of catalyzing the synthesis of both A and B antigens. Formal proof of this interpretation will require expression of the *cis-AB* sequence in a suitable cell line and the demonstration of this dual catalytic activity.

Subsequent studies by Fukumori et al. (1023) on 27 cis-AB samples from Japanese donors have shown that all of them have a chimeric allele consisting of a mixture of the nucleotide sequences present in normal *A* and *B* alleles. All samples had A transferase-specific nucleotides at nt526, 703 and 796 and a B-specific nucleotide at nt803 (amino acid 268). These authors further showed that examples of cis-AB with phenotypes A_2B_3, A_1B_3 and A_2B had genotypes that were *cis-AB/O*, *cis-AB/A* and *cis-AB/B* respectively. In the terminology used by Yamamoto and Hakomori (350) for their chimeric enzyme constructs these cis-AB enzymes would be of the type AAAB. In their original paper Yamamoto and Hakomori (350) reported that AAAB constructs produced only A antigen but it was later recorded that weak B activity was found in one of three different experiments (752). The occurrence of weak B activity would be consistent with serological studies of the cis-AB phenotype.

Variant *O* Alleles

The initial study of the molecular basis of blood group O found that the phenotype results from a single base pair deletion in the A^1 transferase gene within codon 87 (denoted O^1 allele). This deletion caused a translational frameshift thereby producing a truncated protein of 116 amino acids with a completely different amino acid sequence beyond residue 86 (348). This truncated protein is presumed to be inactive with respect to glycosyltransferase activity since it would lack the large enzymically-active cytoplasmic domain (see figures 8-5 and 8-6).

A different molecular mechanism associated with the O phenotype was found by Yamamoto et al. (1024) during the study of DNA from an individual with a weak B phenotype (1024). The weak *B* allele (denoted B^{60}) had a nucleotide sequence in the last two exons of the transferase gene that was indistinguishable from the normal *B* allele but the other allele, presumed *O*, was found to have two nucleotide substitutions which change amino acids found in the A_1 transferase, Arg176Gly which is also found in the normal B enzyme, and Gly268Arg which is unique to this allele. As described above, the amino acid at position 176 does not appear to be important for activity of the A or B enzyme but the nature of the residue at 268 is critical (350,1014). Replacement of glycine (A-enzyme) or alanine (B-enzyme), both small nonpolar residues, with arginine, an amino acid with a large and very basic side chain, would be expected to have a profound affect on the activity of the translated protein. When this sequence was expressed in HeLa cells no A or B antigen could be detected on the cells suggesting that the translated protein is either completely inactive or active at a very low level below the detection threshold of the assay system. This result was of particular interest because of earlier studies which had suggested that a polyclonal antibody raised to the A_1 transferase could bind "cross-reactive" material in the plasma of individuals of group O (1025). This result, which could not be repeated by others using a different polyclonal anti-A_1 transferase (1026) could be explained if some group O alleles produce an inactive transferase which shares substantial sequence homology with the A_1 transferase. The unusual O allele described by Yamamoto et al. (1024) clearly fulfills these criteria. This O allele has been denoted O^2.

In the initial study which described the molecular basis of A, B and O, a variant O^1 allele was found in a human colon adenocarcinoma cell line COLO 205 which had, in addition to the nucleotide deletion in codon 87 which creates the truncated protein product, nine other mutations in comparison with the A_1 transferase sequence (349). These 10 mutations are distributed throughout the gene occurring in exon 3 (one mutation), exon 4 (2 mutations), exon 5 (one mutation), exon 6 (two mutations), and exon 7 (four mutations). The same unusual O allele, at least with respect to mutations in exon 6 and exon 7, was found in a donor with the B(A) phenotype (1022). Olsson and Chester (1027) used an ABO genotyping method based on amplification of the last two exons (exons 6 and 7) of the transferase gene using the PCR (1028) and RFLP analysis of the PCR products to examine DNA from 150 blood samples obtained from Swedish blood donors. These authors detected 180 O^1 alleles and 10 O^2 alleles. Of the 180 O^1 alleles, 105 gave a single nucleotide deletion at nt261 (nucleotide 258 in the original paper because of a deletion of three bases in the original A allele sequenced, 347,349). The remaining 75 alleles were identical to the variant O^1 allele described by Yamamoto (349) and described above. These results suggest that the variant O^1 allele is much more common than formerly thought and accounts for approximately 40% of the O alleles found in Swedish blood donors. In another study of 300 Danish blood donors the frequency of the O^2 allele was found to be 4% (1029). A study of 30 Indians from two Amazonian tribes (Yanomami and Arara) found that all were of the O^1 allelic type and none of the O^2 allelic type (1030).

Yet another O allele (O^3) has been described (1060). The group O propositus had an O^1 allele and a novel allele (O^3). Initial analysis of DNA from the propositus using RFLP-PCR indicated the genotype A^2/O^1 because one allele had the deletion of nucleotide 1060 characteristic of A^2 but sequence analysis of exons 6 and 7 revealed the same nucleotide insertion at nt798-804 that is found in the A^{el} allele (1023). These results suggest that the O^3 allele has resulted from the same mutation that creates the A^{el} allele occurring on a A^2 allele. The translated protein derived from this allele is apparently

enzymatically inactive because the phenotype of the propositus is group O.

ABO Typing from DNA

A cursory glance at the sections discussing mutations at the *ABO* locus which precede this section will be sufficient to convince the reader that ABO typing from DNA is unlikely to replace agglutination as the routine method for typing donors and patients. Clinical transfusion is concerned with obviating the risks inherent in transfusion and, ipso facto, phenotype not genotype. Clearly, many different mutations give rise to different ABO phenotypes and more significantly, in the context of routine typing, many different mutations can give rise to the same phenotype (see for example, the discussion of O variants in the preceding section and 1028,1031-1033,1060). ABO typing from DNA may have a role in forensic and paternity testing but even here the usage is likely to be limited given that DNA fingerprinting is a much more powerful technique for discriminating between people (1034).

Various DNA-based methods for determining ABO type have been reported and all use the PCR. Some workers have used PCR to amplify the region of the *ABO* gene which encompasses known polymorphic sites and then used restriction enzymes which will selectively cleave the PCR product depending upon which polymorphism is present. When the digested PCR products are separated by agarose gel electrophoresis the antigen type can be inferred from the size of fragments observed (349,1028,1032,1035). Other workers have used allele-specific primers in a multiplex PCR (1033,1036, 1037,1077).

Molecular Basis of H Antigen

The H antigen is produced by the action of an $\alpha1\rightarrow2$ fucosyltransferase gene (*FUT1*) which catalyses the transfer of L-fucose from GDP-L-fucose to either type 1 (Galß1$\rightarrow$3GlcNac-) or type 2 (Galß1$\rightarrow$4GlcNAc-) acceptors. The huge problems inherent in trying to purify mammalian glycosyltransferases led John Lowe's group in Ann Arbor, Michigan (346) to try expression cloning as a route to obtaining a cDNA corresponding to the H transferase. Fragments of human genomic DNA (approximately 100kb in size) were transfected into a mouse cell line which was deficient in the H transferase and lacked H antigen on its surface. The rare cells which expressed H antigen were collected via their ability to adhere to plastic dishes coated with anti-H (346). Southern blot analysis of the H-positive mouse transfectant revealed two human DNA restriction fragments. The largest of these fragments was shown to encode the H transferase when expressed in an H transferase-deficient cell line (506). A 1.2kb *Hin*fI restriction fragment derived from this fragment was used to screen a cDNA library, when the largest cDNA was transfected into COS-1 cells the cell expressed H transferase activity de novo (507). The cDNA predicted a protein of 365 amino acids with a calculated molecular weight of 41,249. Hydropathy analysis of the predicted protein sequence indicated a type II transmembrane protein similar to that of the A transferase described above with a short N-terminal domain of 8 residues, a single membrane spanning domain of 17 residues and a large C-terminal domain of 340 amino acids containing two signal motifs for N-glycosylation. Although the overall topology of this enzyme was similar to that of other cloned glycosyltransferases it demonstrated no significant sequence homology with these other transferases (507). Larsen et al. (507) prepared a chimeric protein comprising the C-terminal 333 amino acids of the H-transferase and the secreted form of the IgG-binding domain of *Staphylococcus aureus* protein A and showed that the secreted chimeric protein retained H-transferase activity. The H-transferase gene is small (less than 9kb) and its coding region is contained within a single exon of 1.1kb (1038). The H-transferase gene, *FUT1* has been localized to chromosome 19q13.3 using fluorescence in situ hybridization (FISH,1039).

Molecular Basis of the Bombay and Para-Bombay Phenotypes

Kelly et al. (513) studied the H-transferase gene of an individual with the Bombay phenotype and found six single base pair differences between the normal and *Bombay* allele. Each of these mutations was created in the "wild-type" transferase sequence and expressed in COS-1 cells which lack H-transferase activity. Only one of these base pair differences was found to be significant and this change converted codon Tyr316 to a termination codon and would therefore be predicted to yield a truncated (lacking the last 50 amino acids of the "wild-type" enzyme) and enzymatically inactive product. Transfection studies showed that this mutant was indeed enzymatically inactive and furthermore that correction of the Tyr316→ter mutation in the *Bombay* allele to the "wild-type" tyrosine fully restored enyme activity (1038). The H-deficient donor was homozygous for this mutation (see figure 8-8).

Studies of the H-transferase gene in a para-Bombay individual previously described by Solomon et al. (490) revealed one allele with a missense mutation converting Leu164 to His and the other allele with a mutation con-

verting codon Gln276 to a termination codon which would cause a truncated enzyme lacking the last 90 amino acids. Gene transfer studies showed that each of these mutations results in an inactive enzyme (513). These studies provided strong evidence for the existence of another α(1→2)fucosyltransferase gene distinct from the H-transferase because this individual had normal levels of H antigen in her secretions. Oriol et al. (386) proposed that the *Secretor* gene encodes a second α(1→2)fucosyltransferase, a hypothesis consistent with the observations of Kelly et al. (513) on this para-Bombay donor and subsequently proved to be correct (see earlier section on H-deficient phenotypes and the two locus theory and Chapter 9).

Wang et al. (1040) describe studies of the *FUT1* gene in a para-Bombay individual in which two further enzyme-inactivating mutations were found. Two single nucleotide mutations resulted the conversion of Tyr154 to His and Glu348 to Lys in the same *FUT1* allele. Transfection of this mutant allele in COS-7 cells showed that it does not produce an active fucosyltransferase. In order to assess the individual effect of each amino acid change on enzyme activity chimeric constructs involving the wild type *FUT1* allele and the mutant allele were prepared. The chimeric construct containing His154 but not Lys348 when transfected into COS-7 cells produced 1% of the fucosyltransferase activity of the wild type construct. The chimeric construct containing Lys348 but not His154 produced 9.3% of the fucosyltransferase activity of the wild type construct. H antigen on the surface of COS-7 cells could be demonstrated by immunofluorescence when the chimeric constructs were expressed but not when the double mutant was expressed. These results show that both mutations have a dramatic effect on enzyme activity and that the combined effect of the mutations is to produce a totally inactive enzyme.

Fernandez-Mateos et al. (1041) identified an enzyme inactivating mutation (Leu242Arg) in the *FUT1* gene found in natives of the Réunion island whose ancestors came from the South West Coast of India. This represents the first mutation found in Indian individuals of the Bombay phenotype and these authors argue that it may correspond to the original Bombay phenotype described in 1952 (433).

Costache et al. (1042) review the catalogue of known mutations in fucosyltransferase genes including those described by Yu et al. (1044), Wagner and Flegel (1043), and Johnson et al. (1045) and record more than 20 different mutations in the *FUT1* gene (see figure 8-8). Two of these are missense mutations which result in only partial inactivation of the enzyme, a further 14 missense mutations are enzyme inactivating, 4 are nucleotide deletions which change the reading frame and 3 are mutations which introduce a stop codon. The mutations extend

FIGURE 8-8 Inactivating Mutations in the *H* Gene (*FUT1*) (data from references 1041, 1042)

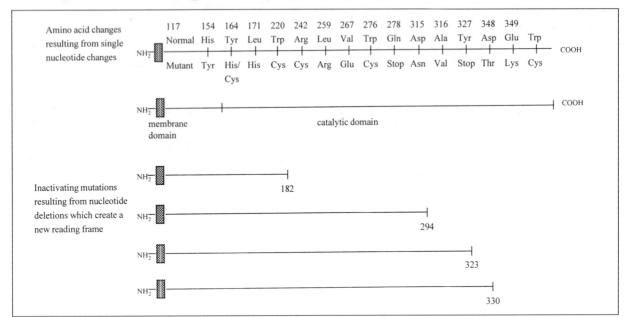

along the whole length of the C-terminal catalytic domain of the enzyme.

Molecular Basis of the H-deficient Réunion Phenotype

The H-deficient Réunion phenotype is found in individuals of French ancestry living in the mountains of Réunion island. Individuals expressing this phenotype have a very weak expression of ABH antigens on their red cells and in their saliva and weak anti-H in their plasma. When the *FUT1* gene of an individual of this phenotype was sequenced a single nucleotide missense mutation was found which converted amino acid His117 to Tyr (1041) (see figure 8-8). Expression studies confirmed that this mutation caused the weakened H antigen activity in these individuals.

References

1. Landsteiner K. Zbl Bakt 1900;27:357
2. Landsteiner K. Wien Klin Wschr 1901;14:1132
3. Honig CL, Bove JR. Transfusion 1980;20:653
4. Schmidt PJ. J Fl Med Assoc 1980;67:151
5. Mhyre BA. J Am Med Assoc 1980;244:1333
6. Camp FR, Monoghan WP. Am J Foren Med Pathol 1981;2:143
7. Edinger SE. Med Lab Obs 1985;April:41
8. Sazama K. Transfusion 1990;30:583
9. Anstee DJ. Vox Sang 1990;58:1
10. Mollison PL. Blood Transfusion in Clinical Medicine 3rd Ed. Oxford:Blackwell 1961:497
11. Jandl JH, Tomlinson AS. J Clin Invest 1958;37:1202
12. Jandl JH, Kaplan ME. J Clin Invest 1960;39:1145
13. Muirhead EE. Surg Gynecol Obstet 1951;92:734
14. Binder LS, Ginsberg V, Harmel MH. Surg Gynecol Obstet 1959;108:19
15. Bluemle LW Jr. Trans Am Clin Climat Assoc 1962;74:201
16. Stuckey MA, Osoba D, Thomas JW. Canad Med Assoc J 1964;90:739
17. Yunis EJ, Ziegler N, Benson S. J Am Med Assoc 1964;189:907
18. Pineda AA, Brzica SM Jr, Taswell HF. Mayo Clin Proc 1978;53:378
19. Akeroyd JH, O'Brien WA. Vox Sang 1958;3:330
20. Buchholz DH, Bove JR. Transfusion 1975;15:557
21. Wallace J. Blood Transfusion for Clinicians. Edinburgh:Churchill Livingtone, 1977
22. Mollison PL. Blood Transfusion in Clinical Medicine 6th Ed. Oxford:Blackwell, 1979
23. Mollison PL, Engelfriet CP, Contreras M. Blood Transfusion in Clinical Medicine 9th Ed. Oxford:Blackwell, 1993
24. Rydberg L, Breimer ME, Samuelsson BE. Transfusion 1988;28:483
25. Mayer K. In: Safety in Transfusion Practices. Skokie, IL. Coll Am Pathol, 1982
26. Taswell HF, Pineda AA, Moore SB. In: A Seminar on Immune Mediated Cell Destruction. Washington, D.C.:Am Assoc Blood Banks, 1981;71
27. Petz LD. In: Clinical and Basic Science Aspects of Immunohematology. Arlington, VA:Am Assoc Blood Banks, 1991;73
28. Gale RP, Feig S, Ho W, et al. Blood 1977;50:185
29. Buckner CD, Clift RA, Sanders JE, et al. Transplantation 1978;26:233
30. Hershko C, Gale RP, Ho W, et al. Br J Haematol 1980;44:65
31. Curtis JE, Messner HA. Canad Med Assoc J 1982;126:649
32. Bensinger WI, Buckner CD, Thomas ED, et al. Transplantation 1982;33:427
33. Petz LD. In: Red Cell Antigens and Antibodies. Arlington,

VA:Am Assoc Blood Banks, 1986:195

34. Petz LD. Transf Med Rev 1987;1:85
35. Braine HG, Sensenbrener LL, Wright SK, et al. Blood 1982;60:420
36. Sniecinski IJ, Oien L, Petz LD, et al. Transplantation 1988;45:530
37. Barge AJ, Johnson G, Witherspoon R, et al. Blood 1989;74:1477
38. Gmur J, Burger J, Schaffner A, et al. Blood 1990;75:290
39. Sniecinski IJ, Petz LD, Oien L, et al. Transplant Proc 1987;19:4609
40. Blacklock HA, Prentice H, Evans JPM, et al. Lancet 1982;2:1061
41. Dinsmore RE, Reich LM, Kapoor N, et al. Br J Haematol 1983;54:441
42. Ho WG, Champlin RE, Feig SA, et al. Br J Haematol 1984;57:155
43. Sniecinski I, Henry S, Ritchey B, et al. J Clin Apheresis 1985;2:231
44. Storb R, Thomas ED. Immunol Rev 1983;71:77
45. Hows JM, Chipping PM, Palmer S, et al. Br J Haematol 1983;53:145
46. Warkentin PI, Hilden JM, Kersey JH, et al. Vox Sang 1985;48:89
47. Bensinger WI, Baker DA, Buckner CD, et al. New Eng J Med 1981;304:160
48. Lasky LC, Warkentin PI, Kersey JH, et al. Transfusion 1983;23:277
49. Bleyer WA, Blaese RM, Bujak JS, et al. Blood 1975;45:171
50. Berkman EM, Caplan S, Kim CS. Transfusion 1978;18:504
51. Bensinger WI, Buckner CD, Clift AR, et al. J Clin Apheresis 1987;3:174
52. Slavc I, Urban C, Schwinger W, et al. Wien Klin Woch 1992;104:93
53. Tichelli A, Gratwohl A, Wenger R, et al. Transplant Proc 1987;19:4632
54. Nussbaumer W, Schwaighofer H, Gratwohl A, et al. Transfusion 1995;35:592
55. Wagner A, Hocker P, Gerhartl K. In: Therapeutic Plasmapheresis (XII). Utrecht:VSP BV, 1993:333
56. Areman EM, Cullis H, Spitzer T, et al. Transfusion 1991;31:724
57. Moss WL. Bull Johns Hopkins Hosp 1910;21:63
58. Schiff F. Klin Wschr 1924;3:679
59. Aubert EF, Boorman KE, Dodd BF. J Pathol Bact 1942;54:89
60. Hostrup H. Vox Sang 1963;8:557
61. Denborough MA, Dowling JH, Doig AG. Br J Haematol 1969;16:103
62. Holburn AM, Masters CA. Br J Haematol 1974;28:157
63. Allan D, Billah MM, Finean JB, et al. Nature 1976;261:58
64. Lutz HU. J Supramolec Struct 1978;8:375
65. Cole WF, Rumsby MG, Longster GH, et al. Biochem Soc Trans 1978;6:1375 65
66. Oreskovic RT, Dumaswala UJ, Greenwalt TJ. Transfusion 1992;32:848
67. Wiener AS, Moloney WC. Am J Clin Pathol 1943;13:74
68. Gasser C. Helv Pediat Acta 1945;1:38
69. Ebert RV, Emerson CP. J Clin Invest 1946;25:627
70. Stevens AR Jr, Finch CA. Am J Clin Pathol 1954;24:612
71. Inwood MJ, Zuliani B. Ann Intern Med 1978;89:515
72. Keidan SE, Lohoar E, Mainwaring D. Lancet 1966;1:179
73. Delmas-Marsalet Y, Parquet-Gernez A, Bauters F, et al. Rev Franc Transf 1969;12:351
74. Aster RH. Blood 1965;26:732
75. Duquesnoy RJ, Anderson AJ, Tomasulo PA, et al. Blood

1979;54:595
76. Brand A, Sintnicolaas K, Claas FHJ, et al. Transfusion 1986;26:463
77. Heal JM, Blumberg N, Masel D. Blood 1987;70:23
78. Lee EJ, Schiffer CA. Transfusion 1989;29:384
79. Simon TL, Sierra ER. Transfusion 1984;24:173
80. Moroff G, Friedman A, Robkin-Kline L, et al. Transfusion 1984;24:144
81. Zoes C, Dube VE, Miller JH, et al. Transfusion 1977;17:29
82. Rosati LA, Barnes B, Oberman HA, et al. Transfusion 1970;10:139
83. Tamagnini GP, Dormandy KM, Ellis D, et al. (Letter). Lancet 1975;2:188
84. Hach-Wunderle V, Texidor D, Zumpe P, et al. Infusionstherapie 1989;16:100
85. Issitt PD, Issitt CH, Glueck H. Unpublished observations 1976-1981, cited in the second edition of this book
86. Kim HC, Park C, Cowan JH, et al. Am J Pediat Hematol Oncol 1988;10:69
87. Issitt PD, Combs MR, Laughlin M. Unpublished observations, 1995
88. Hows J, Beddow K, Gordon-Smith E, et al. Blood 1986;67:177
89. Hazelhurst GR, Brenner MK, Wimperis JZ, et al. Scand J Haematol 1986;37:1
90. Bracey AW, Van Buren C. Transfusion 1986;26:282
91. Bracey AW. Vox Sang 1987;53:181
92. Solheim BG, Albrechtsen DA, Berg KJ, et al. Transplant Proc 1987;19:4236
93. Brecher ME, Moore SB, Reisner RK, et al. Am J Clin Pathol 1989;91:232
94. Ramsey G. Transfusion 1991;31:76
95. Herron R, Clark M, Tate D, et al. Vox Sang 1986;51:226
96. Ramsey G, Israel L, Lindsay GD, et al. Transplantation 1986;41:67
97. Ahmed KY, Nunn G, Brazier DM, et al. Transplantation 1987;43:163
98. Swanson JL, Sastamoinen RM, Steeper TA, et al. Vox Sang 1987;52:75
99. Solheim BG, Albrechtsen D, Egeland T, et al. Transplant Proc 1987;19:4520
100. Albrechtsen D, Solheim BG, Flatmark A, et al. Transplant Proc 1988;20(Suppl 3):959
101. Hjelle B, Donegan E, Cruz J, et al. Transfusion 1988;28:496
102. Povlsen JV, Rasmussen A, Hansen HE, et al. Nephrol Dial Transplant 1990;5:148
103. Gajewski JL, Petz LD, Calhoun L, et al. (abstract). Blood 1990;76(Supl 1):398a 103
104. Taylor GL, Race RR, Prior AM, et al. J Pathol Bact 1942;54:514
105. Speiser P, Schwartz J, Lewkins D. Klin Med 1951;6:105
106. Juel E. Acta Pathol Microbiol Scand 1959;46:91
107. Speiser P. Acta Genet Med (Roma) 1956;3:192
108. Lenkiewicz B, Sarul B. Arch Immunol Ther Exp 1971;19:643
109. Boorman KE, Dodd BE, Loutit JF, et al. Br Med J 1946;1:751
110. Salmon C, Schwartzenberg L, Andre R. Sangre 1959;30:223
111. Kliman AP, Schmidt PJ, Hoye RC, et al. Transfusion 1961;1:40
112. Jakobowicz R, Simmons RT, Carew JP. Vox Sang 1961;6:320
113. Lundberg WB, McGinniss MH. Transfusion 1975;15:1
114. Northoff H, Wölpl A, Sugg U, et al. Blut 1986;52:317
115. Domen RE, Calero A, Keehn WH. Lab Med 1988;19:739
116. Stratton F. In: Modern Trends in Blood Diseases, London:Butterworth, 1955
117. Mollison PL, Cutbush M. Lancet 1955;1:1290

118. Cutbush M, Mollison PL. Br J Haematol 1958;4:115
119. Mollison PL. Br Med J 1959;2:1035
120. Mollison PL. Br Med J 1959;2:1123
121. Mollison PL. Br Med Bull 1959;15:92
122. Mollison PL. Acta Hematol 1959;10:495
123. Issitt PD. In: Clinically Significant and Insignificant Antibodies. Washington, D.C.:Am Assoc Blood Banks, 1979:13
124. Mollison PL, Johnson CA, Prior DM. Vox Sang 1978;35:149
125. Haas RJ, Rieber P, Helmig M, et al. Blut 1986;53:401
126. Ervin DM, Young LE. Blood 1950;5:61
127. Grove-Rasmussen M, Shaw RS, Marceau E. Am J Clin Pathol 1953;23:828
128. Mangal AK, Growe GH, Sinclair M, et al. Transfusion 1984;24:201
129. Salamon DJ, Ramsey G, Nusbacher J, et al. Vox Sang 1985;48:309
130. Davey RJ, Tourault MA, Holland PV. Transfusion 1978;18:738
131. Moores PP, Smart E, Garbriel B. (Letter). Transfusion 1994;34:1015
132. Seyfried H, Walewska I, Giles CM. Vox Sang 1963;8:273
133. Rosenfield RE, Schroeder R, Ballard R, et al. Vox Sang 1964;9:415
134. Salmon C, Homberg J, Liberge G, et al. Rev Franc Clin Biol 1965;5:552
135. Schmidt PJ, McGinniss MH. Vox Sang 1965;10:109
136. Yokoyama M. Nature 1965;208:411
137. Tegoli J, Harris JP, Issitt PD, et al. Vox Sang 1967;13:144
138. Drachmann O. Vox Sang 1968;14:185
139. Voak D, Lodge TW, Hopkins J, et al. Vox Sang 1968;15:353
140. Rochant H, Tonthat H, Eitevant MF, et al. Vox Sang 1972;22:45
141. Bird GWG, Wingham J. Vox Sang 1972;22:364
142. Banopoulos H, Lopez M, Homberg JC, et al. Rev Franc Transf 1975;18:47
143. Lopez M, Banopoulos H, Liberge G, et al. Vox Sang 1975;28:371
144. Morel P, Garratty G, Willbanks E. Vox Sang 1975;29:231
145. Finke M, Sachs V, Vollert B, et al. Blut 1976;32:371
146. Bird GWG, Wingham J. Vox Sang 1977;32:280
147. Lopez M, Sachs V, Badet J, et al. Vox Sang 1978;34:18
148. Wright J, Lim FC, Freedman J. Vox Sang 1980;39:222
149. Rogers VB, Reid ME, Ellisor SS, et al. Transfusion 1981;21:92
150. Castella A, Labarge BP, Lanenstein KJ, et al. Transfusion 1983;23:339
151. Atichartakarn V, Chiewsilp P, Ratanasirivanich P, et al. Vox Sang 1985;49:301
152. Uchikawa H, Tohyama H. Transfusion 1986;26:240
153. McClelland WM, Bradley A, Morris TCM, et al. Vox Sang 1981;41:231
154. Bird GWG, Wingham J. J Immunol Comm 1980;9:155
155. Ehnholm C, Mäkelä O. Vox Sang 1970;18:414
156. Strange CA, Cross J. Vox Sang 1981;41:235
157. Hegarty JS, Dolphin E, Leonard WR. (abstract). Transfusion 1982;22:411
158. Szymanski IO, Roberts PL, Rosenfield RE. New Eng J Med 1976;294:995
159. Parker AC, Willis G, Urbaniak SJ, et al. Br Med J 1978;1:26
160. Prokop O, Rackwitz A, Schlesinger D. J Foren Med 1965;12:108
161. Prokop O, Schlesinger D, Rackwitz A. Z Immun Forsch 1965;129:402
162. Boyd WC, Brown RA. Nature 1965;208:593
163. Boyd WC, Brown R, Boyd LG. J Immunol 1966;96:301
164. Prokop O, Uhlenbruck G, Köhler W. Vox Sang 1968;14:321
165. Hammarstrom S, Kabat EA. Biochemistry 1969;8:2696
166. Uhlenbruck G, Sprenger I, Leseney AM, et al. Vox Sang 1970;19:488
167. Ishiyama I, Dietz W, Uhlenbruck G. Comp Biochem Physiol 1973;44:529
168. Cann GB. Med Lab Sci 1974;31:11
169. Cann GB. Med Lab Sci 1975;32:69
170. Dahr W, Uhlenbruck G, Bird GWG. Vox Sang 1975;28:133
171. Myers RJ, Med Lab Sci 1976;33:331
172. Salmon C, Cartron J-P. In: Handbook Series in Clinical Laboratory Science. Cleveland:CRC Press, 1977, Section D:71
173. Beck ML, Poehler C, Webb D, et al. (abstract). Transfusion 1979;19:658
174. Beck ML, Miles CD, Moheng MC. (abstract). Transfusion 1981;21:609
175. Brasssel J, Beck M, Hendricks E, et al. (abstract). Transfusion 1981;21:609
176. Mäkelä O, Mäkelä P, Kruppe M. Z Immun Forsch 1959;117:220
177. Chattoraj A, Boyd WC. J Immunol 1965;96:898
178. Prokop O, Schlesinger G, Geserick G. Z Immun Forsch 1967;132:491
179. Baldo BA, Boettcher B. Immunology 1970;19:569
180. Pardoe GI, Uhlenbruck G, Anstee DJ, et al. Z Immun Forsch 1970;139:468
181. Todd GM. Vox Sang 1971;21:451
182. Anstee DJ, Holt PDJ, Pardoe GI. Vox Sang 1973;25:347
183. Hayes CE, Goldstein IJ. J Biol Chem 1974;249:1904
184. Judd WJ, Steiner EA, Freidman BA, et al. Vox Sang 1976;30:261
185. Rodgers DJ, Blunden G, Evans PR. Med Lab Sci 1977;34:193
186. Downie DM, Madlin DF, Voak D. Med Lab Sci 1977;34:319
187. Judd WJ, Murphy LA, Goldstein IJ, et al. Transfusion 1978;18:274
188. Rodgers DJ. Med Lab Sci 1978;35:239
189. Köhler G, Milstein C. Nature 1975;256:495
190. Barstable EJ, Bodmer WF, Brown G, et al. Cell 1978;14:9
191. Voak D, Sachs S, Alderson T, et al. Vox Sang 1980;39:13
192. Sachs S, Lennox E. Vox Sang 1981;40:99
193. Voak D, Lennox E, Sachs S, et al. Med Lab Sci 1982;39:109
194. Munro AC, Inglis G, Blue A, et al. Med Lab Sci 1982;39:123
195. Voak D, Lennox E. Biotest Bull 1983;4:281
196. Voak D, Lowe AD, Lennox E. Biotest Bull 1983;4:291
197. Salmon C, Rouger PH, Doinel C, et al. Biotest Bull 1983;4:300
198. Lowe AD, Lennox E, Voak D. Vox Sang 1984;46:29
199. Messeter L, Brodin T, Chester MA, et al. Vox Sang 1984;46:185
200. Moore S, Chirnside A, Micklem LR, et al. Vox Sang 1984;47:427
201. Scott ML, Guest AR, King M-J, et al. Rev Fr Transf Immunohematol 1987;30:443
202. Scott ML, Guest AR, King M-J, et al. Rev Fr Transf Immunohematol 1987;30:515
203. Gane P, Vellayoudom J, Mollicone R, et al. Vox Sang 1987;53:117
204. Rouger P, Anstee D. Vox Sang 1988;55:57
205. Oriol R, Samuelsson BE, Messeter L. J Immunogenet 1990;17:279
206. Voak D. Bailliere's Clin Haematol 1990;3:219
207. Judson PA, Smythe JS. Transf Med 1991;1:97
208. Zelinksi KR. (abstract). Book of Abstracts, 19th Cong ISBT,

1986:502

209. Beck ML, Hardman JT, Kowalski M, et al. In: Monoclonal Antibodies Against Human Red Cells and Related Antigens. Paris:Librarie Arnette, 1987:224

210. Beck ML, Yates AD, Hardman JT, et al. Am J Clin Pathol 1989;92:625

211. Beck ML, Kowalski MA, Kirkegaard J, et al. (Letter). Immunohematology 1992;8:22

212. Beck ML, Kirkegaard J, Korth J, et al. (Letter). Transfusion 1993;33:623

213. Garratty G, Arndt P, Co S, et al. (abstract). Transfusion 1993;33(Suppl 9S):47S

214. Deryugina EI, Chertkov JL. (Letter). Transfusion 1990;30:766

215. Voak D, Sonneborn H, Yates A. Transf Med 1992;2:119

216. DuPont M. Arch Int Med Exp 1934;9:33

217. Wiener AS. J Immunol 1951;66:287

218. Kabat EA. Blood Group Substances. New York:Academic Press, 1956

219. Springer GF, Horton RE. J Clin Invest 1969;48:1280

220. Springer GF. J Immunol 1956;76:399

221. Springer GF, Horton RE, Forbes M. J Exp Med 1959;110:221

222. Springer GF, Williamson P, Readler BL. Ann NY Acad Sci 1962;97:104

223. Springer GF, Schuster R. Vox Sang 1964;9:589

224. Øyen R, Colledge KI, Marsh WL, et al. Transfusion 1972;12:98

225. Rodgers DJ, Topliss J, Blunden G. Med Lab Sci 1979;36:79

226. Conger JD, Chan MM, DePalma L. Transfusion 1993;33:200

227. Buchs JP, Nydegger UE. J Immunol Meth 1989;118:37

228. Miller RD, Calkins CE. J Immunol 1988;140:3779

229. Hartley SB, Crosbie J, Brink R, et al. Nature 1991;353:765

230. Kochwa S, Rosenfield RE, Tallal L, et al. J Clin Invest 1961;40:874

231. Thomaidis T, Fouskaris G, Matsaniotis N. Am J Dis Childh 1967;113:654

232. Chattoraj A, Gilbert R Jr, Josephson AM. Transfusion 1968;8:368

233. Toivanen P, Hirvonen T. Scand J Haematol 1969;6:42

234. Morville P. Acta Path Microbiol Scand 1929;6:39

235. Yliruokanen A. Ann Med Exp Biol Fenn 1948;26:Suppl 6

236. Fong SW, Qaqundah BY, Taylor WF. Transfusion 1974;14:551

237. Grundbacher FJ. Z Immun Forsch 1967;134:317

238. Rieben R, Buchs JP, Flückiger E, et al. Transfusion 1991;31:607

239. Auf der Maur C, Hodel M, Nydegger UE, et al. Transfusion 1993;33:915

240. Thomsen O, Kettel K. Z Immun Forsch 1929;63:67

241. Somers H, Kuhns WJ. Proc Soc Exp Biol Med 1972;141:1104

242. Baumgarten A, Kruchok AH, Weirich F. Vox Sang 1976;30:253

243. Carlinfanti E. J Immunol 1948;59:1

244. Grundbacher FJ. Transfusion 1976;16:48

245. Nijenhuis LE, Bratlie K. Vox Sang 1962;7:236

246. Vos GH, Vos D. Afr J Clin Exp Immunol 1980;1:103

247. Shaw DH, Stone WH. Proc 6th Cong Eur Soc Haematol, 1957:724

248. Mayeda K. Am J Med Technol 1966;32:187

249. Vetter O. Z Ges Inn Med 1966;21:466

250. Tovey LAD, Taverner JM, Longster GH. Vox Sang 1970;19:64

251. Grundbacher FJ, Shreffler DC. Z Immun Forsch 1970;141:20

252. Doinel C, Ropars C, Salmon C. Vox Sang 1974;27:515

253. Dodds AJ, Klarkowski D, Cooper D, et al. Am J Clin Pathol 1979;71:473

254. McGinniss MH, Binder RA, Kales AN, et al. Immunohematology 1987;3:20

255. Govoni M, Turbiani C, Menini C, et al. Vox Sang 1991;61:75

256. Sokol RJ, Booker DJ, Stamps R, et al. Haematologia 1995;26:121

257. Kuipers EJ, van Imhoff GW, Hazenberg CAM, et al. Br J Haematol 1991;78:283

258. McGinniss MH. (Letter). Immunohematology 1987;3:23

259. Rawson AJ, Abelson NM. J Immunol 1960;85:640

260. Brouwers HAA, Overbeeke MAM, Huiskes E, et al. Br J Haematol 1988;68:363

261. Ichikawa Y. Jpn J Med Sci Biol 1959;12:1

262. Worlledge S, Ogiemudia SE, Thomas CO, et al. Ann Trop Med Parasitol 1974;68:249

263. Redman M, Malde R, Contreras M. Vox Sang 1990;59:89

264. Rose HM. Proc Soc Exp Biol Med 1945;58:93

265. Heiner DC, Kevy SV. New Eng J Med 1956;254:629

266. Shrand J. Lancet 1964;1:1357

267. Bird GWG. In: Blood Group Antigens and Disease. Arlington, VA:Am Assoc Blood Banks 1983:1

268. Kulkarni AG, Ibazebe R, Fleming AF. Vox Sang 1985;48:39

269. Garratty G. In: Immunobiology of Transfusion Medicine. New York:Marcel Dekker 1994;201

270. Toy PTCY, Reid ME, Papenfus L, et al. Vox Sang 1988;54:181

271. Krivit WE, Good RA. Am J Dis Childh 1959;97:137

272. Blaese RM, Brown RS, Strober W, et al. Lancet 1968;1:1056

273. Cooper MD, Chase HP, Lowman JT, et al. Am J Med 1968;44:499

274. Miescher PA, Müller-Eberhard HJ. Sem Immunopathol. Berlin:Springer Verlag 1978:Vol 1

275. Owen RD. Science 1945;102:400

276. Burnet FM, Fenner F. The Production of Antibodies. Melbourne: Macmillan, 1949

277. Lubenko A. In: Monoclonal Antibodies against Human Red Blood Cells and Related Antigens. Paris:Librairie Arnette, 1987:161

278. Lubenko A, Redman M, Contreras M. Rev Fr Transf Immunohematol 1987;30:503

279. Lubenko A, Redman M. (Letter). Vox Sang 1989;57:275

280. Oehlert P. (Letter). Vox Sang 1989;56:133

281. Dobson A, Ikin EW. J Path Bact 1946;58:221

282. Weisert O, Heier AW. Vox Sang 1961;6:692

283. Campbell JS. Unpublished observations 1958 cited by Race RR, Sanger R. Blood Groups in Man 6th Ed. Oxford:Blackwell, 1975

284. Springer GF, Tegtmeyer H. Vox Sang 1974;26:247

285. Ogata H, Hasegawa S. Transfusion 1977;17:651

286. Fisher W, Hahn F. Z Immun Forsch 1935;84:177

287. Landsteiner K, Witt D. J Immunol 1926;11:221

288. Dodd BE. Br J Exp Pathol 1952;33:1

289. Bird GWG. Br J Exp Pathol 1953;34:131

290. Ogata T, Matuhasi T. Proc 8th Cong ISBT. Basel:Karger, 1962:208

291. Ogata T, Matuhasi T. Proc 9th Cong ISBT. Basel:Karger 1964;528

292. Rosenfield RE. Blood 1955;10:17

293. Rosenfield RE, Ohno G. Rev Hematol 1955;10:231

294. Yokoyama M, Fudenberg HH. J Immunol 1964;92:966

295. Dodd BE, Lincoln PJ, Boorman KE. Immunology 1967;12:39

296. Contreras M, Armitage SE, Hewitt PE. Vox Sang 1984;47:224

297. Koeckert HL. J Immunol 1920;5:529

298. Matsunaga E. Proc Imp Acad Jpn 1950;26:59

299. Wiener AS. Ann Eugen 1953;18:1

300. Wiener AS, Samwick AA, Morrison H, et al. Exp Med Surg

1953;11:276

301. Unger LJ, Wiener AS. J Lab Clin Med 1954;44:387
302. Jones AR, Kaneb L. Blood 1960;13:395
303. Harley D. Br J Exp Pathol 1936;17:35
304. Matuhasi T. Proc 15th Gen Assem Jpn Med Cong 1959;4;80
305. Matuhasi T, Kumazawa H, Usui M. J Jpn Soc Blood Transf 1960;6:295
306. Bove JR, Holburn AM, Mollison PL. Immunology 1973;25:793
307. Boursnell JC, Coombs RRA, Rizk V. Biochem J 1953;55:745
308. Masouredis SP. J Clin Invest 1959;38:279
309. Hughes-Jones NC, Gardner B. Biochem J 1962;83:404
310. Pirofsky B, Cordova MS, Imel TL. Vox Sang 1962;7:334
311. Masouredis SP. Transfusion 1964;4:69
312. Gergely J, Arky I, Medgyesi GA. Vox Sang 1967;12:252
313. Owen RD. J Immunol 1954;73:29
314. Messeter L, Johnson U. J Immunogenet 1990;17:213
315. Bernstein F. Klin Wschr 1924;3:1495
316. Bernstein F. Z Indukt Abstamm u Vereb 1925;37:237
317. Morgan WTJ, Watkins WM. Nature 1956;177:521
318. Watkins WM, Morgan WTJ, Vox Sang 1959;4:97
319. Watkins WM. In: Biochemistry of Human Genetics, London:Churchill, 1959:217
320. Ceppellini R. In: Biochemistry of Human Genetics. London:Churchill, 1959:242
321. Morgan WTJ. Proc Roy Soc, Series B, 1960;151:308
322. Watkins WM. Science 1966;152:172
323. Morgan WTJ, Watkins WM. Br Med Bull 1969;25:30
324. Kabat EA. In: Blood and Tissue Antigens. New York:Academic Press, 1970:187
325. Watkins WM. In: Blood and Tissue Antigens. New York:Academic Press, 1970:200
326. Morgan WTJ. In: British Biochemistry Past and Present. London:Academic Press, 1970:99
327. Sawicka T. FEBS Lett 1971;16:346
328. Watkins WM. Ann Rep Lister Inst Prev Med 1972:12
329. Ginsburg V. Adv Enzymol 1972;36:131
330. Watkins WM. Ref Fr Transf Immunohematol 1979;22:35
331. Watkins WM. Adv Hum Genet 1980;10:1
332. Watkins WM, Greenwell P, Yates AD. Immunol Comm 1981;10:83
333. Kabat EA. Am J Clin Pathol 1982;78:281
334. Cook GA, Greenwell P, Watkins WM. Biochem Soc Trans 1982;10:446
335. Yates AD, Watkins WM. Biochem Biophys Res Comm 1982;109:958
336. Abe K, Levery SB, Hakomori S. J Immunol 1984;132:1951
337. Kumazaki T, Yoshida A. Proc Nat Acad Sci USA 1984;81:4193
338. Yates AD, Feeney J, Donald ASR, et al. Carbohyd Res 1984;130:251
339. Betteridge A, Watkins WM. Glycocon J 1985;2:61
340. Betteridge A, Watkins WM. Biochem Soc Trans 1985;13:1126
341. Le Pendu J, Cartron J-P, Lemieux RU, et al. Am J Hum Genet 1985;37:749
342. Clausen H, Levery SB, Nudelman E, et al. Biochemistry 1986;25:7075
343. Greenwell P, Edwards YH, Williams J, et al. Biochem Soc Trans 1987;15:601
344. Weinstein J, Lee EU, McEntee K, et al. J Biol Chem 1987;262:17735
345. Clausen H, Hakomori SI. Vox Sang 1989;56:1
346. Ernst LK, Rajan VP, Larsen RD, et al. J Biol Chem 1989;264:3436
347. Clausen H, White T, Takio K, et al. J Biol Chem

1990;265:1139

348. Yamamoto F, Marken J, Tsuji T, et al. J Biol Chem 1990;265:1146
349. Yamamoto F, Clausen H, White T, et al. Nature 1990;345:229
350. Yamamoto F, Hakomori S. J Biol Chem 1990;265:19257
351. Mollicone R, Gibaud D, Francois A, et al. Eur J Biochem 1990;191:169
352. Oriol R. J Immunogenet 1990;17:235
353. Oriol R, Le Pendu J, Mollicone R. Vox Sang 1986;51:161
354. Laine RA, Rush JH. Adv Exp Med Biol 1988;228:331
355. Sadler JE. In: Biology of Carbohydrates, Vol 2. New York:Wiley, 1984:199
356. Clausen H, Levery SB, Nudelman E, et al. Proc Nat Acad Sci 1985;82:1199
357. Le Pendu J, Lambert F, Samuelsson BE, et al. Glycoconjugate J 1986;3:255
358. Kannagi R, Levery SB, Hakomori S. FEBS Lett 1984;175:397
359. Clausen H, Holmes E, Hakomori S. J Biol Chem 1985;261:1388
360. Moss WL. Folia Serol 1910;5:267
361. Lehrs H. Z Immun Forsch 1930;66:175
362. Putkonen T. Acta Soc Med Fenn 1930;A14,No12
363. Schiff F, Sasaki H. Klin Woch 1932;11:1426
364. Levine P, Robinson E, Celano M, et al. Blood 1955;10:1100
365. Aloysia M, Gelb AG, Fudenberg H, et al. Transfusion 1961;1:212
366. Lanset S, Ropartz C, Rousseau Y, et al. Transfusion (Paris) 1966;9:255
367. Schenkel-Brunner H, Chester MA, Watkins WM. Eur J Biochem 1972;30:269
368. Race C, Watkins WM. FEBS Lett 1972;27:125
369. Renwick JH, Lawler SD. Ann Hum Genet 1955;19:312
370. Jameson RJ, Lawler SD, Renwick JH. Ann Hum Genet 1956;20:348
371. Renwick JH. Ann Hum Genet 1956;21:159
372. Lawler SD, Renwick JH, Wildervanck LS. Ann Hum Genet 1957;21:410
373. Lawler SD, Renwick JH, Hauge M, et al. Ann Hum Genet 1958;22:342
374. Renwick JH, Izatt MM. Ann Hum Genet 1965;28:369
375. Sharma JC. Ann Hum Genet 1966;30:193
376. Rapley SE, Robson EB, Harris H, et al. Ann Hum Genet 1968;31:237
377. Weitkamp LR, Sing CF, Shreffler DG, et al. Am J Hum Genet 1969;21:600
378. Schleutermann DA, Bias WB, Murdoch JL, et al. Am J Hum Genet 1969;21:606
379. Willie B, Ritter H. Humangenetik 1969;7:263
380. Wendt GG, Ritter H, Zilch I, et al. Humangenetik 1971;13:347
381. Sobel RS, Tiger A, Gerald PS. Am J Hum Genet 1971;23:146
382. Ferguson-Smith M, Aitken D, Turleau C, et al. Hum Genet 1976;34:35
383. Westerveld A, Jongsma A, Meera Khan P, et al. Proc Nat Acad Sci USA 1976;73:895
384. Robson EB, Cook PJL, Buckton KE. Ann Hum Genet 1977;41:53
385. Lewis M, Kaita H, Giblett ER, et al. Cytogenet Cell Genet 1978;22:452
386. Oriol R, Danilovs J, Hawkins BR. Am J Hum Genet 1981;33:421
387. Westerveld A, Naylor S. Cytogenet Cell Genet 1984;37:156
388. Donis-Keller H, Green P, Helms C, et al. Cell 1987;51:319
389. Le Beau MM, Ryan D, Pericak-Vance MA. Cytogenet Cell Genet 1989;51:338

390. Ball SP, Tengue N, Gibald A, et al. Ann Hum Genet 1991;55:225

391. Hrubisko M, Laluha J, Mergancova O, et al. Vox Sang 1970;19:113

392. Hrubisko M. Rev Fr Transf Immunohematol 1972;15:157

393. Salmon C, Rouger P, Rodier L, et al. Blood Transf Immunohematol 1980;23:251

394. Salmon C, Cartron J-P, Rouger P. In: The Human Blood Groups. New York:Masson, 1984

395. Witebsky E, Engasser LM. J Immunol 1949;61:171

396. Crawford H, Cutbush M, Mollison PL. Blood 1953;8:620

397. Grundbacher FJ. Nature 1964;204:192

398. Kemp T. Acta Path Microbiol Scand 1930;7:146

399. Wiener AS. In: Blood Groups and Transfusion 3rd Ed. Springfield:Thomas 1943

400. Bird GWG. Lancet 1952;170:674

401. Constantoulakis M, Kay HEM, Giles GM, et al. Br J Haematol 1963;9:63

402. Haddad SA. Canad J Med Tech 1974;36:373

403. Issitt PD. In: A Seminar on the ABO Blood Group System. Chicago:Am Assoc Blood Banks, 1966:33

404. Issitt PD. J Med Lab Technol 1967;24:90

405. Issitt PD, J Med Lab Technol 1968;25:1

406. Economidou J, Hughes-Jones NC, Gardner B. Vox Sang 1967;12:321

407. Tilley CA, Crookston MC, Crookston JH, et al. Vox Sang 1978;34:8

408. Schachter H, Michaels MA, Crookston MC, et al. Biochem Biophys Res Comm 1971;45:1011

409. Hammer L, Mansson S, Rohr T, et al. Vox Sang 1981;40:27

410. Romans DG, Tilley CA, Dorrington KJ. J Immunol 1980;124:2807

411. Klinman NR, Karush F. Immunochemistry 1967;4:387

412. Hornick CL, Karush F. Immunochemistry 1972;9:325

413. Crothers DM, Metzger H. Immunochemistry 1972;9:341

414. Koscielak J, Miller-Podraza H, Krauze R, et al. Eur J Biochem 1976;71:9

415. Hakomori S, Watanabe K, Laine RA. Pure Appl Chem 1977;49:1215

416. Dejter-Juszynski M, Harpaz N, Flowers HM, et al. Eur J Biochem 1978;83:363

417. Gardas A. Eur J Biochem 1978;89:471

418. Takasaki S, Yamashita K, Kobtata A. J Biol Chem 1978;253:6086

419. Jarnefelt J, Rush J, Li Y-T, et al. J Biol Chem 1978;253:8006

420. Krusius T, Finne J, Rauvala H. Eur J Biochem 1978;92:289

421. Watanabe K, Hakomori S. J Exp Med 1976;14:644

422. Fukuda M, Fukuda MN, Hakomori S. J Biol Chem 1979;254:3700

423. Fukuda M, Fukuda MN, Hakomori S. J Biol Chem 1979;254:5458

424. Koscielak J, Zdebska E, Wilczynska Z, et al. Eur J Biochem 1979;96:331

425. Watanabe K, Laine RA, Hakomori S. Biochemistry 1975;14:2725

426. Feizi T, Childs RA, Watanabe K, et al. J Exp Med 1979;149:175

427. Watanabe K, Hakomori S, Childs RA, et al. J Biol Chem 1979;254:3221

428. Greenbury CL, Moore DH, Nunn LAC. Immunology 1963;6:421

429. Cartron J-P, Gerbal A, Hughes-Jones NC, et al. Immunology 1974;27:723

430. Filitti-Wurmser S, Jacquot-Armand Y, Aubel-Lesure G, et al. Ann Eugen 1954;18:183

431. Williams MA, Voak D. Br J Haematol 1972;23:427

432. Hakomori S. Sem Hematol 1981;18:39

433. Bhende YM, Deshpande DK, Bhatia HM, et al. Lancet 1952;1:903

434. Ceppellini R, Nasso S, Tecilazich F. In: La Malattia Emolitica del Neonata. Milan: Belfanti, 1952:204

435. Watkins WM, Morgan WTJ. Vox Sang (Old Series) 1955;5:1

436. Simmons RT, D'Sena GWL. J Ind Med Assoc 1955;24:325

437. Bhatia HM, Sanghvi LD, Bhide YG, et al. J Ind Med Assoc 1955;24:545

438. Parkin DM. Br J Haematol 1956;2:106 438

439. Roy MN, Dutta S, Mitra PC, et al. J Ind Med Assoc 1957;29:224

440. Pettenkofer JH, Luboldt W, Lawonn H, et al. Z Immun Forsch 1960;120:288

441. Hakim SA, Vyas GN, Sanghvi LD, et al. Transfusion 1961;1:218

442. Jakobowicz R, Whittingham S, Simmons RT. Med J Austral 1961;2:868

443. Aust CH, Hocker ND, Keller ZG, et al. Am J Clin Pathol 1962;37:579

444. Giles CM, Mourant AE, Atabuddin A-H. Vox Sang 1963;8:269

445. Gandini E, Sacchi R, Reali G, et al. Vox Sang 1968;15:142

446. Yunis EJ, Svardal JM, Bridges RA. Blood 1969;33:124

447. Pretty HM, Taliano V, Fiset D, et al. Vox Sang 1969;16:179

448. Prodanov P, Hrubisko M, Beranova G, et al. Rev Fr Hematol 1970;10:31

449. Dzierzkowa-Borodej W, Meinhard W, Nestorowicz S, et al. Arch Immunol Ther Exp 1972;20:841

450. Bryant JG, Lloyd B, Davis J, et al. (abstract). Transfusion 1974;14:506

451. Bhatia HM, Sathe MS. Vox Sang 1974;27:524

452. Sathe M, Bhatia HM. Vox Sang 1976;30:312

453. Abu Sin AYH, Abdelrazig H, Ayoub M, et al. Vox Sang 1976;31:48

454. Iseki S, Takizawa H, Takizawa H. Proc Jpn Acad 1970;46:803

455. Sringarm S, Sombatpanich B, Chandanayingyong D. Vox Sang 1977;33:364

456. Beattie KM, Saeed SM. (Letter). Transfusion 1976;16:290

457. Moores PP. PhD Thesis, Univ Natal, 1980

458. Race RR, Sanger R. Blood Groups in Man 5th Ed. Oxford:Blackwell, 1968

459. Moores PP, Issitt PD, Pavone BG, et al. Transfusion 1975;15:237

460. Levine P, Tripodi D, Struck J Jr, et al. Vox Sang 1973;24:417

461. Issitt PD. In: Serology and Genetics of the Rhesus Blood Group System. Cincinnati: Montgomery, 1979

462. Bhatia HM, Sathe M, Gandhi S, et al. Vox Sang 1974;26:252

463. Poschmann A, Fischer K, Seidl S, et al. Vox Sang 1974;27:338

464. Vescio LAC, Castro RA. Vox Sang 1990;58:231

465. Pujol M, Ribera A, Abella E, et al. Vox Sang 1991;61:76

466. Pujol M. (Letter). Vox Sang 1992;63:240

467. Garratty G. (Letter). Vox Sang 1992;63:240

468. Brouwers HHA, Overbeeke MAM, Gemke RJBJ, et al. Br J Haematol 1987;66:267

469. Edwards MS, Buffone GJ, Fuselier PA, et al. Pediatr Res 1983;17:685

470. Levine P, Uhlir M, White J. Vox Sang 1961;6:561

471. Bhatia HM. Vox Sang 1962;7:485

472. Bhtia HM. Ind J Med Res 1966;54:345

473. Molthan L. (abstract). Transfusion 1967;7:384

474. Voak D, Stapleton RR, Bowley CC. Vox Sang 1968;14:18

475. Beranova G, Prodanov P, Hrubisko M, et al. Vox Sang

1969;16:449

476. Gerard G, Guimbretiere J, Guimbretiere L. Rev Fr Transf 1970;13:267

477. Liberge G, Salmon C, Gerbal A, et al. Rev Fr Transf 1970;13:357

478. Rodier L, Lopez M, Liberge G, et al. Biomedicine 1974;21:312

479. Mulet C, Cartron J-P, Badet J, et al. FEBS Lett 1977;84:74

480. Prodanov P, Drazhev G. Vox Sang 1978;34:162

481. Mulet C, Cartron J-P, Lopez M, et al. FEBS Lett 1978;90:233

482. Mulet C, Cartron J-P, Schenkel-Brunner H, et al. Vox Sang 1979;37:272

483. Salmon C, Cartron J-P, Rouger P, et al. Blood Transf Immunohematol 1980;23:233

484. Le Pendu J, Lemieux RU, Lambert F, et al. Am J Hum Genet 1982;34:402

485. Gerard G, Vitrac D, Le Pendu J, et al. Am J Hum Genet 1982;34:937

486. Le Pendu J, Gerard G, Vitrac D, et al. Am J Hum Genet 1983;35:484

487. Le Pendu J, Clamagirand C, Cartron J-P, et al. Am J Hum Genet 1983;35:497

488. Le Pendu J, Oriol R, Juszczak G, et al. Vox Sang 1983;44:360

489. Le Pendu J. Lambert F, Gerard G, et al. Vox Sang 1986;50:223

490. Solomon JM, Waggoner R, Leyshon WC. Blood 1965;25:470

491. Jakobowicz R, Simmons RT, Graydon JJ, et al. Vox Sang 1965;10:552

492. Schachter H, Michaels MA, Tilley CA, et al. Proc Nat Acad Sci USA 1973;70:220

493. Lewi S. Transfusion (Paris) 1967;10:335

494. Kitahama M, Yamaguchi H, Okubo Y, et al. Vox Sang 1967;12:354

495. Bhatia HM, Solomon JM. Vox Sang 1967;12:457

496. Kogure T, Tohyama H, Iseki S. J Jpn Soc Blood Transf 1968;15:161

497. Fawcett KJ, Eckstein EG, Innella F, et al. Vox Sang 1970;19:547

498. Gerbal A, Liberge AGG, Lopez M, et al. Rev Fr Transf 1970;13:61

499. Sringarm S, Chupungart C, Giles GM. Vox Sang 1972;23:537

500. Yamaguchi H, Okubo Y, Tanaka M. Proc Jpn Acad 1972;48:629

501. Marsh WL, Ferrari M, Nichols ME, et al. Vox Sang 1973;25:341

502. Shows TB, McAlpine PJ, Bouchieux C, et al. Cytogenet Cell Genet 1987;46:11

503. Tilley CA, Crookson MC, Brown BL, et al. Vox Sang 1975;28:25

504. Crookston MC, Tilley CA. In: Blood Groups and Other Red Cell Surface Markers in Health and Disease. New York:Masson 1982:111

505. Lemieux RU, Le Pendu J, Hindsgaul O. Jpn J Antibiot 1979;32(Suppl):21

506. Rajan VP, Larsen RD, Ajmera S, et al. J Biol Chem 1989;264:11158

507. Larsen RD, Ernst LK, Nair RP, et al. Proc Nat Acad Sci USA 1990;87:6674

508. Sarnesto A, Köhlin T, Thurin J, et al. J Biol Chem 1990;265:15067

509. Oriol R, Mollicone R, Masri R, et al. (abstract). Glycoconjugate J 1991;8:147

510. Oriol R, Mollicone R, Couillin P, et al. APMIS 1992;100:28

511. Sarnesto A, Köhlin T, Hindsgaul O. J Biol Chem 1992;267:2745

512. Couillin P, Mollicone R, Grisard MC, et al. Cytogenet Cell Genet 1991;56:108

513. Kelly RJ, Ernst LK, Larsen RD, et al. Proc Nat Acad Sci USA 1994;91:5843

514. Mollicone R, Candelier JJ, Reguigne I, et al. Transf Clin Biol 1994;2:91

515. Mollicone R, Candelier JJ, Mennesson B, et al. Carbohyd Res 1992;228:265

516. Koszdin KL, Bowen BR. Biophys Biochem Res Comm 1992;187:152

517. Weston BW, Nair RP, Larsen RD, et al. J Biol Chem 1992;267:4152

518. Weston BW, Smith PL, Kelly RJ, et al. J Biol Chem 1992;267:24575

519. Easton EW, Schiphorst WECM, van Drunen E, et al. Blood 1993;81:2978

520. Reguigne I, James MR, Richard III CW, et al. Cytogenet Cell Genet 1994;66:104

521. Mollicone R, Reguigne I, Fletcher A, et al. J Biol Chem, in press 1995

522. Judd WJ. Methods in Immunohematology, 2nd Ed. Durham:Montgomery, 1994 52

523. Freda V. Am J Obstet Gynecol 1958;76:407

524. Barber M, Dunsford I. Br Med J 1959;1:607

525. Freiesleben E, Kissmeyer-Nielsen F, Christensen KJ, et al. Vox Sang 1961;6:304

526. Hatton J, Walsh RJ. Vox Sang 1961;6:568

527. Hostrup H. Acta Pathol 1963;59;407

528. Treacy M, Geiger J, Goss MF. Transfusion 1967;7:443

529. Topping MD, Watkins WM. Biochem Biophys Res Comm 1975;64:89

530. Matsumoto I, Osawa T. Biochim Biophys Acta 1969;194:180

531. Horejsi V, Kocourek J. Biochim Biophys Acta 1974;336:329

532. Pereira MEA, Kisailus EC, Gruezo F, et al. Arch Biochem Biophys 1978;185:108

533. Solomon JM. Transfusion 1964;4:3

534. Kalb AJ. Biochim Biophys Acta 1968;168:532

535. Pereira MEA, Kabat EA. Biochemistry 1974;13:3184

536. Ranadive KJ, Bhatia HM. Ind J Med Res 1967;55:369

537. Le Pendu J, Gerard G, Lambert F, et al. Glycoconjugate J 1986;3:203

538. Kameyama T, Oishi K, Aida K. Biochim Biophys Acta 1979;587:407

539. Chessin LN, McGinniss MH. Vox Sang 1968;14:194

540. Debray H, Decout D, Strecker G, et al. Eur J Biochem 1981;117:41

541. von Dungern E, Hirszfeld L. Z Immun Forsch 1911;8:526

542. Ikin EW, Prior AM, Race RR, et al. Ann Eugen Lond 1939;9:409

543. Lattes L, Cavazutti A. J Immunol 1924;9:407

544. Lopez M, Benali J, Cartron J-P, et al. Vox Sang 1980;39:271

545. Issitt PD, Jackson VA. Vox Sang 1968;15:152

546. Watkins WM. In: Human Blood Groups Basel:Karger, 1977:134

547. Moreno C, Lundblad A, Kabat EA. J Exp Med 1971;134:439

548. Hakomori S, Watanabe K, Laine RA. In: Human Blood Groups. Basel:Karger, 1977:150

549. Fujii H, Yoshida A. Proc Nat Acad Sci USA 1980;77:2951

550. Hakomori SI, Steller K, Watanabe K. Biochem Biophys Res Comm 1972;49:1061

551. Gardas A. Eur J Biochem 1976;68:177

552. Fukuda MN, Matsumura G. J Biol Chem 1976;251:6218

553. Finne J. Eur J Biochem 1980;104:181

554. Schenkel-Brunner H. Eur J Biochem 1980;104:529

555. Finne J, Krusius T, Rauvala H, et al. Blood Transf

Immunohematol 1980;23:545
556. Donald ASR. Eur J Biochem 1981;120:243
557. Schenkel-Brunner H. Eur J Biochem 1982;122:511
558. Fukuda MN, Hakomori SI. J Biol Chem 1982;257:446
559. Breimer ME, Samuelsson BE. Transplantation 1986;42:88
560. Schenkel-Brunner H, Tuppy H. Eur J Biochem 1970;17:218
561. Race C, Watkins CM. Vox Sang 1972;23:385
562. Romano EL, Mollison PL, Linares J. Vox Sang 1978;34:14
563. Salmon C, Lopez M, Cartron J-P, et al. Transfusion 1976;16:580
564. Springer GF, Ansell J. Fed Proc 1960;19:70
565. Cartron J-P, Gerbal A, Badet J, et al. Vox Sang 1975;28:347
566. Lopez M, Habibi B, Lemeud J, et al. Vox Sang 1975;28:57
567. Cartron J-P, Reyes F, Gourdin MF, et al. Immunology 1977;32:233
568. Cohen F, Zuelzer WW. Transfusion 1965;5:223
569. Reyes F, Gourdin MF, Lejonc JL, et al. Br J Haematol 1976;34:613
570. Bakacs T, Totpal J, Ringwald G, et al. J Clin Lab Immunol 1988;25:53
571. Cartron J-P, Badet J, Mulet C, et al. J Immunogenet 1978;5:107
572. Bird GWG. PhD Thesis, Univ Lond 1958
573. Brain P. Vox Sang 1966;11:686
574. Brain P. (Letter). Vox Sang 1974;26:383
575. Bhatia HM. (Letter). Vox Sang 1974;26:383
576. Bird GWG. (Letter). Vox Sang 1974;26:383
577. Levine P. (Letter). Vox Sang 1974;26:383
578. Race RR, Sanger R. (Letter). Vox Sang 1974;26:384
579. Voak D. (Letter). Vox Sang 1974;26:384
580. Davey MG. (Editorial). Vox Sang 1974;26:384
581. Sathe M, Bhatia HM. Vox Sang 1974;26:374
582. Voak D, Lodge TW, Stapleton RR, et al. Vox Sang 1970;19:73
583. Wiener AS. Am J Hum Genet 1950;2:177
584. Bird GWG. Vox Sang 1964;9:629
585. Friedenreich V. Z Immun Forsch 1936;89:409
586. Gammelgaard A. In: Hospital Mennesket. Copenhagen:Arnold, 1942
587. Dunsford I. Proc 7th Cong ISBT. Basel:Karger, 1959:685
588. Reed TE. Transfusion 1964;4:457
589. Cotterman CW. Unpublished observations 1958, cited in Reed TE. Transfusion 1964;4:457
590. Cotterman CW. Proc 1st Int Cong Hum Genet 1956:94
591. Cotterman CW. J Cell Comp Physiol 1958;52(Suppl 1):69
592. Oguchi Y, Kawaguchi T, Suzuta O, et al. Vox Sang 1978;34:32
593. Alter AA, Rosenfield RE. Blood 1964;23:605
594. Issitt PD, Sanders CW, Jackson VA. Unpublished observations, 1965
595. Lopez M, Benali J, Bony V, et al. Vox Sang 1979;37:281
596. Andre R, Salmon C. Rev Hematol 1957;12:668
597. Issitt PD. Applied Blood Group Serology, 1st Ed. Oxnard CA:Spectra,1970
598. Salmon C. DSc Thesis, Univ Paris, 1960
599. Scott ML, Voak D. In: Immunobiology of Transfusion Medicine. New York:Marcel Dekker, 1994:365
600. Johnsson B, Fast K. Acta Path Microbiol Scand 1948;25:649
601. Dunsford I, Aspinall P. Ann Eugen 1952;17:30
602. Estola A, Elo J. Ann Med Exp Fenn 1952;30:79
603. Grove-Rasmussen M, Soutter L, Levine P. Am J Clin Pathol 1952;22:1157
604. Fine M, Eyquem A, Thebault J. Ann Inst Pasteur 1956;91:892
605. Ellis FR, Cawley LP. Proc 6th Cong ISBT. Basel:Karger, 1958:135
606. Glover SM, Walford RL. Am J Clin Pathol 1958;30:539

607. Vos GH. Vox Sang 1964;9:160
608. Salmon C, Salmon D, Reviron J. Nouv Rev Fr Hematol 1965;5:275
609. Cahan A, Jack JA, Scudder J, et al. Vox Sang 1957;2:8
610. Fisher N, Cahan A. Vox Sang 1962;7:484
611. Wiener AS, Gordon EB. Br J Haematol 1956;2:305
612. Kindler M. Blut 1958;4:373
613. Salmon C, Borin P, Andre R. Rev Hematol 1958;13:529
614. Salmon C, Reviron J, Liberge G. Nouv Rev Fr Hematol 1958;4:359
615. Hrubisko M, Calkovska Z, Mergancova O, et al. Blut 1966;13:1
616. Hrubisko M, Calkovska Z, Mergancova O, et al. Blut 1966;13:7
617. Weiner W, Lewis HBM, Moores P, et al. Vox Sang 1957;2:25
618. Darnborough J, Voak D, Pepper RM. Vox Sang 1973;24:216
619. Ducos J, Marty Y, Ruffie J. Vox Sang 1975;28:456
620. Junqueira PC, Garangau FM, Wishart PJ. Vox Sang 1957;2:386
621. Dodd BE, Gilbey BE. Vox Sang 1957;2:390
622. Weiner W, Sanger R, Race RR. Proc 7th Cong ISBT. Basel:Karger, 1959:721
623. Sturgeon P, Moore BPL, Weiner W. Vox Sang 1964;9:214
624. Moore BPL, Newstead PH, Marson A. Vox Sang 1961;6:624
625. Moore BPL, Newstead PH, Johnson J. Vox Sang 1961;6:151
626. Jakobowicz R, Noades JE, Simmons RT. Med J Austral 1963;1:657
627. Reed TE, Moore BPL. Vox Sang 1964;9:363
628. Solomon JM, Sturgeon P. Vox Sang 1964;9:476
629. Lanset S, Liberge G, Gerbal A, et al. Nouv Rev Fr Hematol 1970;10:389
630. Jenkins T. Vox Sang 1974;26:537
631. Schuh V, Vyas GN, Fudenberg HH. Am J Hum Genet 1972;24:11
632. Nevanlinna HR, Pirkola A. Vox Sang 1973;24:404
633. Mohn JR, Cunningham RK, Pirkola A, et al. Vox Sang 1973;25:193
634. Schmidt PJ, Nancarrow JF, Morrison EG, et al. J Lab Clin Med 1959;54:38
635. Frederick J, Hunter J, Greenwell P, et al. Transfusion 1985;25:30
636. Perkins HA, Morel PA. Am J Clin Pathol 1980;73:263
637. Singh G, Janoson B, McClung M, et al. Am J Clin Pathol 1981;75:271
638. Yoshida A. Am J Hum Genet 1983;35:1117
639. Badet J, Ropars C, Cartron J-P, et al. Biomedicine 1974;21:230
640. Lopez M, Bouguerra A, Lemeud J, et al. Vox Sang 1974;27:243
641. Salmon C, Liberge G, Gerbal A, et al. Biomedicine 1974;21:465
642. Badet J, Ropars C, Cartron J-P, et al. Vox Sang 1976;30:105
643. Lopez M, Lemeud J, Gerbal A, et al. Nouv Rev Fr Hematol 1973;13:107
644. Race RR, Sanger R. Blood Groups in Man 6th Ed. Oxford:Blackwell, 1975
645. Battaglini P, Melis C, Bridonneau C. Transfusion (Paris) 1967;10:121
646. Bennett MH, Brumley A, Giles CM, et al. Vox Sang 1962;7:579
647. Boorman KE, Zeitlin RA. Vox Sang 1964;9:278
648. Mäkelä O, Mäkelä P. Ann Med Exp Fenn 1955;33:33
649. Ruoslahti E, Enholm C, Mäkelä O. Vox Sang 1967;13:511
650. Babcock L, Tregellas WM, McCormick SB, et al. (abstract). Transfusion 1982;22:421

651. Marsh WL. Vox Sang 1960;5:387
652. Dunsford I, Stacey SM, Yokoyama M. Nature 1956;178:1167
653. Yokoyama M, Stacey SM, Dunsford I. Vox Sang 1957;2:348
654. Levine P, Celano MJ, Griset T. Proc 6th Cong ISBT. Basel:Karger, 1958:132
655. Yokoyama M, Barber M, Dunsford I. Juntendo Med J 1959;5:273
656. Liotta I, Russo G, Gandini E. Vox Sang 1961;6:698
657. Kout M, Totin P. Vox Sang 1963;8:741
658. Furukawa K, Iseki S. Proc 1st AsianCong Blood Transf, 1963:183
659. Yamaguchi H, Okubo Y, Hazama F, et al. Proc Imp Acad Jpn 1964;40:357
660. Ikemoto S, Kuniyuki M, Furuhata T. Proc Imp Jpn Acad 1964;40:362
661. Boose GM, Issitt CH, Issitt PD. Transfusion 1978;18:570
662. Moullec J, Sutton F, Burganda M. Rev Hematol 1955;10:574
663. Vyas GN, Bhatia HM, Sanghvi LD. Vox Sang 1960;5:509
664. Sussman LN, Pretshold H, Lacher MJ. Blood 1960;16:1788
665. Alter AA, Rosenfield RE. Blood 1964;23:600
666. Bhatia HM, Undevia JV, Sanghvi LD. Vox Sang 1965;10:506
667. Wiener AS, Cioffi AF. Am J Clin Pathol 1972;58:693
668. Beck ML, Hardman JT, Henry R. (abstract). Transfusion 1986;26:572
669. Beck ML, Yates AD, Hardman JT, et al. (abstract). Transfusion 1987;27:535
670. Yates AD, Greenwell P, Watkins WM. Biochem Soc Transact 1983;11:300
671. Sonneborn HH, Voak D. (abstract). Cong Int Soc Hematol, Milan, 1988
672. Levene C, Levene NA, Buskila D, et al. Transf Med Rev 1988;2:176
673. Lau P, Serarat S, Beatty J, et al. Transfusion 1990;30:142
674. Beck ML, Korth J, Kirkegaard J, et al. (Letter). Transfusion 1993;33:624
675. Cameron C, Graham F, Dunsford I, et al. Br Med J 1959;2:29
676. Giles CM, Mourant AE, Parkin D, et al. Br Med J 1959;2:32
677. Marsh WL, Jenkins WJ, Walther WW. Br Med J 1959;2:63
678. Stratton F, Renton PH. Br Med J 1959;2:244
679. Andersen J. Acta Path Microbiol Scand 1960;48:280
680. Andersen J. Acta Path Microbiol Scand 1960;48:289
681. Claflin AJ, Zinneman HH. Am J Clin Pathol 1963;39:355
682. Jouvenceaux A, Betuel H, Paillet H, et al. Transfusion (Paris) 1964;7:713
683. Majsky A. Neoplasma 1965;12:617
684. Burns W, Friend W, Scudder J. Surg Gynec Obstet 1965;120:757
685. Marantz C, Dimmette RM. Transfusion 1969;9:160
686. Beck ML, Dixon J, Oberman HA. J Med Lab Technol 1970;27:528
687. Beck ML, Walker RH, Oberman HA. J Med Lab Technol 1971;11:296
688. Lanset S, Ropartz C. Vox Sang 1971;20:82
689. Garratty G, Willbanks E, Petz LD. Vox Sang 1971;21:45
690. Gerbal A, Maslet C, Salmon C. Vox Sang 1975;28:398
691. Gerbal A, Ropars C, Gerbal R, et al. Vox Sang 1976;31:64
692. Campbell B, Palmer RN. Transfusion 1980;20:467
693. Chang MS. Lab Med 1981;12:506
694. O'Leary M. Diagnostic Med 1982;5:41
695. Beck ML. In: Blood Group Antigens and Disease. Arlington, VA:Am Assoc Blood Banks, 1983:45
696. Kikuchi M, Endo N, Seno T, et al. Jpn J Transf Med 1984;30:134
697. Yamaguchi H. Jpn J Med Technol 1985;34:3
698. Anstall HB. In: Blood Group Systems: ABH and Lewis.

Arlington, VA:Am Assoc Blood Banks, 1986:135
699. Marsh WL. (Letter). Transfusion 1970;10:41
700. Judd WJ. Unpublished observations 1980, cited in the Addendum of the 3rd Edition of this book
701. Janvier D, Veaux S, Reviron M, et al. Vox Sang 1990;59:92
702. Okubo Y, Seno T, Tanaka M, et al. (Letter). Transfusion 1994;34:456
703. Andersen J. Nature 1961;190;730
704. Beck ML, Korth J, Judd WJ. (abstract). Transfusion 1992;32(Suppl 8S):17S
705. Pedreira PP, Noto TA. (abstract). Transfusion 1992;32(Suppl 8S):17S
706. Judd WJ, Annesley T, Kirkegaard J, et al. (abstract). Transfusion 1992;32(Suppl 8S):18S
707. Springer GF, Horton RE. J Gen Physiol 1964;47:1229
708. Bird GWG. In: Handbook Series in Clinical Laboratory Science, D, Blood Banking. Cleveland:CRC Press, 1977;1:443
709. Case J. (Letter). Transfusion 1993;33:964
710. Kirkegaard J, Beck M. (abstract). Transfusion 1993;33(Suppl 9S):63S
711. Janvier D, Reviron M, Reviron J. (abstract). Transfusion 1983;23:412
712. Beck ML, Myers M, Moulds JJ. Transfusion 1976;16:527
713. Judd WJ, Beck ML, Hicklin BL, et al. Vox Sang 1977;33:246
714. Judd WJ, McGuire-Mallory D, Anderson KM, et al. Transfusion 1979;19:293
715. Judd WJ. In: Polyagglutination. Washington, D.C.:Am Assoc Blood Banks, 1980:23
716. Issitt PD. In: A Seminar on Problems Encountered in Pretransfusion Tests. Washington, D.C.:Am Assoc Blood Banks, 1972:81
717. Berman HJ, Smarto J, Issitt CH, et al. Transfusion 1972;12:35
718. Dahr W, Uhlenbruck G, Bird GWG. Vox Sang 1974;27:29
719. Jiji RM, Jahn EFW, Bilenki LA. (abstract). Transfusion 1973;13:359
720. Dahr W, Uhlenbruck G, Gunson HH, et al. Vox Sang 1975;28:249
721. Dahr W, Uhlenbruck G, Gunson HH. Vox Sang 1975;29:36
722. Soh CPC, Morgan WTJ, Watkins WM, et al. Biochem Biophys Res Comm 1980;93:1132
723. Donald ASR, Yates AD, Soh CPC, et al. Biochem Biophys Res Comm 1983;115:625
724. Donald ASR, Yates AD, Soh CPC, et al. Biochem Soc Trans 1984;12:596
725. Donald ASR, Soh CPC, Yates AD, et al. Biochem Soc Trans 1987;15:606
726. Blanchard D, Cartron J-P, Fournet B, et al. J Biol Chem 1983;258:7691
727. Duffy FA, Marshall RD. Biochem Soc Trans 1985;13:1128
728. Catelani G, Marra A, Paquet F, et al. Carbohydr Res 1986;155:131
729. Marra A, Sinay P. Gazz Chim Ital 1987;117:563
730. Issitt PD. In: Blood Groups P, I, Sd^a and Pr. Arlington, VA:Am Assoc Blood Banks, 1991:53
731. Kossovitch N. Rev Antropol 1929;39:374
732. Haselhorst G, Lauer A. Z Konstit 1930;15:205
733. Haselhorst G, Lauer A. Z Konstit 1931;16:227
734. Moullec J, LeChevrel P. Nature 1959;183:1733
735. Moullec J, LeChevrel P. Transfusion (Paris) 1959;2:47
736. Seyfried H, Walewska I, Werblinska B. Vox Sang 1964;9:268
737. Yamaguchi H, Okubo Y, Hazama F. Proc Imp Acad Jpn 1965;41:316
738. Yamaguchi H, Okubo Y, Hazama F. Proc Imp Acad Jpn 1966;42:517

739. Reviron J, Jacquet A, Delarue F, et al. Nouv Rev Fr Hematol 1967;7:425

740. Madsen G, Heisto H. Vox Sang 1968;14:211

741. Bouguerra-Jacquet A, Reviron J, Salmon D, et al. Nouv Rev Fr Hematol 1969;9:329

742. Yamaguchi H, Okubo Y, Tanaka M. Jpn J Hum Genet 1970;15:198

743. Yamaguchi H. Jpn J Hum Genet 1973;18:1

744. Kogure T. Vox Sang 1975;29:51

745. Pacuszka T, Koscielak J, Seyfried H, et al. Vox Sang 1975;29:292

746. Salmon C, Lopez M, Liberge G, et al. Rev Fr Transf Immunohematol 1975;18:11

747. Hummel K, Badet J, Bauermeister W, et al. Vox Sang 1977;33:290

748. Valdes MD, Zoes C, Froker A. Vox Sang 1978;35:176

749. Yoshida A, Yamaguchi H, Okubo Y. Am J Hum Genet 1980;32:332

750. Yoshida A, Yamaguchi H, Okubo Y. Am J Hum Genet 1980;32:645

751. Sabo BH, Bush M, German J, et al. J Immunogenet 1978;5:87

752. Yamamoto F, McNeill PD, Kominato Y, et al. Vox Sang 1993;64:120

753. Watkins WM. In: Blood Group Serology '82. A symposium held at Reading University, April 1982. Abstracts published by IBMS, London

754. Lopez M, Danielescu M, Liberge G, et al. Vox Sang 1975;29:459

755. Wheeler DA, Nelson JM, Shulman IA, et al. Blood 1984;63:711

756. Yamaguchi H, Okubo Y, Tanaka M. Proc Jpn Acad 1970;46:446

757. Ducos J, Marty Y, Ruffie J. Vox Sang 1975;29:390

758. Loghem JJ van, Hart M van der. Vox Sang (Old Series) 1954;4;69

759. Beckers T, Loghem JJ van, Dunsford I. Vox Sang (Old Series) 1955;5:145

760. McGuire D, Webster G, Mougey R, et al. (abstract). Book of Abstracts, 25th Ann Mtg AABB,13th Cong ISBT. 1972:45

761. Prokop O, Simon A, Rackwitz A. Dtsch Z Ges Gerichtl Med 1960;50:448

762. Badet J, Lopez M, Habibi B, et al. J Immunogenet 1982;9:169

763. Solomon JM, Gibbs MB, Bowdler AJ. Vox Sang 1965;10:54

764. Solomon JM, Gibbs MB, Bowdler AJ. Vox Sang 1965;10:133

765. Winkelstein JA, Mollison PL. Vox Sang 1965;10:614

766. Marsh WL, Nichols ME, Øyen R, et al. Transfusion 1975;15:589

767. Rubinstein P, Allen FH Jr, Rosenfield RE. Vox Sang 1973;25:377

768. Rosenfield RE. In: Hartford Found Conf on Blood Groups. New York:Bellevue Assoc, 1967:47

769. Valko DA, Rolih SD, Moulds JJ, et al. (abstract). Transfusion 1981;21:624 769

770. Renton PH, Hancock JA. Vox Sang 1962;7:33

771. Crookston MC, Tilley CA. In: Human Blood Groups. Basel:Karger, 1977:246

772. Tilley CA, Graham HA. Unpublished observations 1976, cited by Crookston MC, Tilley CA. In: Blood Groups and Other Red Cell Surface Markers in Health and Disease. New York:Masson, 1982

773. Mayr WR, Pausch V. J Immunogenet 1976;3:367

774. Rachkewich RA, Crookston MC, Tilley CA, et al. J Immunogenet 1978;5:25

775. Oriol R, Danilovs J, Lemieux R. Hum Immunol 1980;3:195

776. Dorf ME, Eguro SY, Cabrera G, et al. Vox Sang 1972;22:447

777. Jeannet M, Bodmer JG, Bodmer WF, et al. In: Histocompatibility Testing. Copenhagen:Munksgaard, 1972:493

778. Jeannet M, Schapira M, Magnin C. Schweiz Med Woch 1974;104:152

779. Mayr WF, Mayr D. J Immunogenet 1974;1:43

780. Marcelli-Barge A, Poirier JC, Benajam A, et al. Vox Sang 1976;30:81

781. Park MS, Oriol R, Nakata S, et al. Transpl Proc 1979;11:1947

782. Pullen S, Hersey P. Clin Exp Immunol 1980;39:403

783. Kelton JG, Aker S, Hamid C, et al. (abstract). Transfusion 1980;20:625

784. Kools A, Collins J, Aster RH. (abstract). Transfusion 1981;21:615

785. Kelton JG, Hamid C, Aker S, et al. Blood 1982;59:980

786. Dunstan RA, Simpson MB. Br J Haematol 1985;61:603

787. Dunstan RA, Simspon MB, Knowles RW, et al. Blood 1985;65:615

788. Dunstan RA. Br J Haematol 1986;62:587

789. Zelinski SK, Litsenberger B, Aster RH. Vox Sang 1974;26:189

790. Mak KH, Voak D, Chu RW, et al. Transf Med 1992;2:129

791. Skogen B, Rossebo Hansen B, Husebekk A, et al. Transfusion 1988;28:456

792. Zhang GL, Wang Y, Zheng J, et al. Immunohematology 1993;9:11

793. Yoshida A, Dave V, Hamilton HB. Am J Hum Genet 1988;43:422

794. Garratty G. In: Cellular Antigens and Disease. Washington, D.C.:Am Assoc Blood Banks, 1977:1

795. Simmons A, Twaitt J. Transfusion 1975;15:359

796. Heier HE, Kornstad L, Namork E, et al. Immunohematology 1992;8:94

797. Crookson MC. In: Blood Group Antigens and Disease. Arlington, VA:Am Assoc Blood Banks, 1983:67

798. Reid ME, Bird GWG. Transf Med Rev 1990;4:47

799. Loghem JJ van, Dorfmeier H, Hart M van der. Vox Sang 1957;2:16

800. Salmon C, Dreyfus B, Andre R. Rev Hematol 1958;13:148

801. Gold ER, Tovey GH, Benney WE, et al. Nature 1959;181:62

802. Salmon C. Rev Hematol 1959;14:205

803. Salmon C, Andre R, Dreyfus B. Rev Fr Etud Clin Biol 1959;4:468

804. Bhatia HM, Sanghvi LD. Ind J Med Sci 1960;14:534

805. Gandini E, Ceppellini R. Att A G I 1960:5:283

806. Salmon C, Bernard J. Rev Fr Etud Clin Biol 1960;5:912

807. Hoogstraten B, Rosenfield RE, Wasserman LR. Transfusion 1961;1:32

808. Salmon C, Andre R, Philippon J. Rev Fr Etud Clin Biol 1961;8:792

809. Tovey GH, Lockyer JW, Tierney RBH. Vox Sang 1961;6:628

810. Renton PH, Stratton F, Gunson HH, et al. Br Med J 1962;1:294

811. Hart M van der, Veer M van der, Loghem JJ van. Vox Sang 1962;7:449

812. Richards AG. Lancet 1962;2:178

813. Salmon C, Salmon D. Nouv Rev Fr Hematol 1963;3:653

814. Gold ER, Hollander L. Blut 1963;9:188

815. Gold ER. Sangre 1964;9:131

816. McGinniss MH, Kirkham WR, Schmidt PJ. Transfusion 1964;4:310

817. Salmon C, Debray J, Lemaire A. Nouv Rev Fr Hematol 1964;4:425

818. Bernard J, Bessis M, Bussard A, et al. Nouv Rev Fr Hematol 1965;5:291

819. Shirley R, Desai RG. J Med Genet 1965;2:189
820. Undevia JV, Bhatia H, Sharma RS, et al. Ind J Med Res 1966;54:1145
821. Ayres M, Salzano FM, Ludwig OK. J Med Genet 1966;3:180
822. Salmon C. Ser Hematol 1969;11:3
823. Kassulke JT, Halgren HM, Yunis EJ. Am J Pathol 1969;56:333
824. Starling KA, Fernbach DJ. Transfusion 1970;10:3
825. Rivat L, Ropartz C, Lebreton JP, et al. Nouv Rev Fr Hematol 1970;10:371
826. Kahn A, Vroclans M, Hakim J, et al. (Letter). Lancet 1971;2:933
827. Kahn A, Boivin P, Vroclans M, et al. Nouv Rev Fr Hematol 1972;12:609
828. Bird GWG, Wingham J, Chester GH, et al. Br J Haematol 1976;33:295
829. Rochant H, Tonthat H, Henri A, et al. Blood Cells 1976;2:237
830. Saichua S, Chiewsilp P. Vox Sang 1978;35:154
831. Kollins J, Holland PV, McGinniss MH. Cancer 1978;42:2248
832. Kollins J, Allgood JW, Burghardt DC, et al. Transfusion 1980;20:574
833. Kuhns WJ, Oliver RTD, Watkins WM, et al. Cancer Res 1980;40:268
834. Yoshida A, Kumazaki T, Dave V, et al. Blood 1985;66:990
835. Lopez M, Bonnet-Gajdos M, Reviron M, et al. Br J Haematol 1986;63:535
836. Koscielak J, Pacuszka T, Miller-Podraza H, et al. Biochem Soc Transact 1987;15:603
837. Atkinson JB, Tanley PC, Wallas CH. Transfusion 1987;27:45
838. Benson K. Immunohematology 1991;7:89
839. Dreyfus B, Sultan C, Rochant H, et al. Br J Haematol 1969;16:303
840. Salmon C. Blood Cells 1976;2:211
841. Beattie KM. In: Problems Encountered in Pretransfusion Tests. Washington, D.C.:Am Assoc Blood Banks, 1972;129
842. Tovey GH. Proc 7th Cong Eur Soc Haematol 1959:1167
843. Tegoli J, Sanders CW, Harris JP, et al. Vox Sang 1967;13:285
844. Aird I, Bentall HH, Roberts JAF. Br Med J 1953;1:799
845. Aird I, Bentall HH, Mehigan JA, et al. Br Med J 1954;2:315
846. Clark CA, Cowan WK, Edwards JW, et al. Br Med J 1955;2:643
847. Langman MJS, Doll R. Gut 1965;6:270
848. Merikas G, Christakopoulos P, Petropoulos E. Am J Disgest Dis 1966;11:790
849. Vogel F, Druger J. Blut 1968;16:351
850. Vogel F. Am J Hum Genet 1970;22:464
851. Clark CA, Edwards JW, Haddock DRW, et al. Br Med J 1956;2:725
852. Oh-Huti K. Tohoku J Exp Med 1949;51:297
853. Masamune H, Yosizawa Z, Masukawa A. Tohoku J Exp Med 1953:58:381
854. Kawasaki H. Tohoku J Exp Med 1958;68:119
855. Kay HEM, Wallace DM. J Nat Cancer Inst 1961;26:1349
856. Davidsohn I, Kovarik S, Lee CL. Arch Pathol 1966;81:381
857. Kovarik S, Davidsohn I, Stejskal R. Arch Pathol 1968;86:12
858. Davidsohn I, Kovarik S, Ni LY. Arch Pathol 1969;87:306
859. Davidsohn I, Ni LY, Stejskal R. Cancer Res 1971;31:1244
860. Davidsohn I, Ni LY, Stejskal R. Arch Pathol 1971;92:456
861. Davidsohn I, Stejskal R. Haematologia 1972;6:177
862. Davidsohn I. Am J Clin Pathol 1972;57:715
863. Hakomori S. Prog Biochem Pharmacol 1975;10:167
864. Hakomori S. Am J Clin Pathol 1984;82:635
865. Coon JS, Weinstein RS. Hum Pathol 1986;17:1089
866. Lloyd KO. Am J Clin Pathol 1987;87:129
867. Hakomori S. Adv Cancer Res 1989;52:257

868. Singhai A, Hakomori S. BioEssays 1990;12:223
869. Hakkinen I. J Nat Cancer Inst 1970;44:1183
870. Yokata M, Warner G, Hakomori S. Cancer Res 1981;41:4185
871. Hattori H, Uemura K, Taketomi T. Biochim Biophys Acta 1981;666:361
872. Hakomori S. Cancer Res 1985;45:2405
873. Feizi T. Cancer Surv 1985;4:425
874. Clausen H, Hakomori S, Graem N, et al. J Immunol 1986;136:326
875. Hakomori S, Clausen H, Levery SB. Biochem Soc Trans 1987;15:593
876. Uemura K, Hattori H, Ono K, et al. Jpn J Exp Med 1989;59:239
877. Hakomori S. Curr Opin Immunol 1991;3:646
878. Liotta LA. Sci Am 1992;266:54
879. Preston AE, Barr A. Br J Haematol 1964;10:238
880. Jeremic M, Weisert O, Gedde-Dahl TW. Scand J Clin Lab Invest 1976;36:461
881. McCallum CJ, Peake IR, Newcombe RG, et al. Thromb Hemostas 1983;50:757
882. Mohanty D, Ghosh K, Marwaha N, et al. Thromb Hemostas 1984;51:414
883. Ørstavik KH, Magnus P, Reisner H, et al. Am J Hum Genet 1985;37:89
884. McLelland DS, Knight SR, Aronstam A. Med Lab Sci 1988;45:131
885. Fagerhol M, Abildgaard U, Kornstad L. Lancet 1971;2:664
886. Korsnan-Bengsten K, Wilhelmsen L, Nilson LA, et al. Thromb Res 1972;1:549
887. Gedde-Dahl TW, Jeremic M, Weisert O. Scand J Clin Lab Invest 1975;35:25
888. Stormorken H, Erikssen J. Thromb Hemostas 1977;38:874
889. Mazurier C, Samor B, Mannessier L, et al. Blood Transf Immunohematol 1981;24:3
890. Gill JC, Endres-Brooks J, Bauer PJ, et al. Blood 1987;69:1691
891. Bronte-Stewart B, Botha MC, Krut LH. Br Med J 1962;1:1646
892. Denborough MA. Br Med J 1962;2:927
893. Dick W, Scheider W, Brockmuller K, et al. Thromb Diath Haemorrh 1963;9:472
894. Allan TM, Dawson AA. Br Heart J 1968;30:377
895. Jick H, Slone D, Westerhold B, et al. Lancet 19691:539
896. Nefzger MD, Hrubee Z, Chalmers TC. Lancet 1969;1:887
897. Havlik RJ, Feinleib M, Garrison RJ, et al. Lancet 1969;2:269
898. Talbot S, Wakley EJ, Ryrie D, et al. Lancet 1970;1:1257
899. Kingsbury KJ. Lancet 1971;1:199
900. Mourant AE, Kopec AC, Domaniewska-Sobczak K. Lancet 1971;1:223
901. Medalie JH, Levene C, Papier C, et al. New Eng J Med 1971;285:1348
902. Weiss NA. Am J Hum Genet 1972;24:65
903. Morris T, Bouhoutsos J. Br J Surg 1973;60:89
904. George VT, Elston RC, Amos CI, et al. Genet Epidemiol 1987;4:267
905. Whincup PH, Cook DG, Phillips AN, et al. Br Med J 1990;300:1679
906. Oliver MF, Geizerova H, Cumming RA, et al. Lancet 1969;2:605
907. Langman MJS, Elwood PC, Foote J, et al. Lancet 1969;2:607
908. Flat G. Humangenetik 1970;10:318
909. Beckman L, Olivecrona T, Hernell O. Hum Hered 1970;20:569
910. Morton NE. J Med Genet 1976;13:81
911. Garrison RJ, Havlik RJ, Harris RB, et al. Atherosclerosis

1976;25:311

912. Sing CF, Orr JD. Am J Hum Genet 1976;28:453
913. Polychronopoulou A, Georgiadis E, Kalandidi A, et al. Hum Biol 1977;49:605
914. Srivastava BK, Sinha AS. J Ind Med Assoc 1966;47:261
915. Banergee B, Saha N. Lancet 1969;2:961
916. Saha N, Banergee B. Lancet 1971;1:969
917. Hames CG, Greenberg BG. Am J Public Health 1961;51:374
918. Fox MH, Webber LS, Srinivasan SR, et al. Hum Biol 1981;53:411
919. Arfors KE, Beckman L, Lundin L. Acta Genet 1963;13:89
920. Arfors KE, Beckman L, Lundin LG. Acta Genet 1963;13:366
921. Beckman L. Acta Genet 1964;14:286
922. Bamford KF, Harris H, Luffman JE, et al. Lancet 1965;1:530
923. Schreffler DC. Am J Hum Genet 1965;17:71
924. Langman MJS, Leuthold E, Robson EB, et al. Nature 1966;212:41
925. Inglis NI, Krant MJ, Fishman WH. Proc Soc Exp Biol Med 1967;124:699
926. Kleerekoper M, Horne M, Cornish CJ, et al. Clin Sci 1970;38:339
927. Kaplan MM. New Eng J Med 1972;286:200
928. Voegl F, Pettenkofer HJ, Helmbold W. Acta Genet Statis Med 1960;10:267
929. Mourant AE. The Distribution of the Human Blood Groups. Oxford:Blackwell, 1954
930. Mourant AE, Kopec AC, Domaniewska-Sobczak K. The Distribution of the Human Blood Groups and Other Biochemical Polymorphisms 2nd Ed. London:Oxford Univ Press, 1976
931. Springer GF, Ansell N, Brandes W, et al. Proc 6th Cong ISBT. Basel:Karger 1958:190
932. Springer GF. In: Blood and Tissue Antigens, New York:Academic Press 1970:265
933. Springer GF. Prog Allgy 1971;15:9
934. Robinson MG, Folchin D, Halpern C. Am J Hum Genet 1971;23:135
935. Wiener AS. J Foren Med 1960;7:166
936. Springer GF, Wiener AS. Nature 1962;193:444
937. Wiener AS. Am J Hum Genet 1970;22:476
938. Adalsteinsson S. Ann Hum Genet 1985;49:275
939. Muschel LH, Osawa E. Proc Soc Exp Biol Med 1959;101:614 939
940. Moody MP, Young VM, Faber JE. Proc Conf Am Soc Microbiol. Antimicrobiol Agents Chemother 1969:424
941. Wittels EG, Lichtman HC. Transfusion 1986;26:533
942. Sachs V. (Letter). Transfusion 1987;27:504
943. van Loon FPL, Clemens JD, Sack DA, et al. J Infec Dis 1991;163:1243
944. Foster MT, Labrum AH. J Infec Dis 1976;133:329
945. Miler JJ, Novotney P, Walker PD, et al. Infect Immunol 1977;15:713
946. Kinane DF, Blackwell CC, Winstanley FP, et al. Br J Vener Dis 1983;59:44
947. Blackwell CC, Kowolik M, Winstanley FP, et al. J Clin Lab Immunol 1983;10:173
948. Kinane DF, Blackwell CC, Weir DM, et al. J Clin Lab Immunol 1983;12:83
949. Mandrell RE, Griffiss JM, Macher BA. J Exp Med 1988;168:107
950. Chaudhuri A. Lancet 1977;2:404
951. Barua D, Paquio AS. Ann Hum Biol 1977;4:489
952. Levine MM, Nalin DR, Rennels MB, et al. Ann Hum Biol 1979;6:359
953. Glass RI, Holmgren J, Haley CE, et al. Am J Epidemiol

1985;121:791

954. Clemens JD, Sack DA, Harris JR, et al. J Infec Dis 1989;159:770
955. Berger SA, Young NA, Edberg SC. Eur J Clin Microbiol Infec Dis 1989;8:681
956. Lenny L, Goldstein J. (abstract). Transfusion 1980;20:618
957. Goldstein J, Siviglia G, Hurst R, et al. (abstract). Transfusion 1981;21:602
958. Goldstein J, Siviglia G, Hurst R, et al. Science 1982;215:168
959. Lenny L, Goldstein J, Rowe AW. (abstract). Transfusion 1982;22:420
960. Goldstein J. In: Recent Advances in Haematology, Immunology and Blood Transfusion. Budapest:Hungarian Acad Sci, 1983:89
961. Goldstein J. In: The Red Cell, Sixth Ann Arbor Conf. New York:Liss, 1984:139
962. Goldstein J. Transf Med Rev 1989;3:206
963. Lenny LL, Hurst R, Goldstein J, et al. Blood 1991;77:1383
964. Lenny LL, Hurst R, Zhu A, et al. Transfusion 1995;35:899
965. Lubenko A. (Editorial). Transfusion 1991;31:577
966. Prokop O, Uhlenbruck G. Human Blood and Serum Groups. London:Maclaren, 1969;690
967. Woods CS, Hattison GA, Dore C, et al. Nature 1972;239:165
968. Gilson JB, Harrison CA, Clarke VA, et al. Nature 1973;246:498
969. Golding J, Hicks P, Butler NR. Nature 1984;309:396
970. Menoret A, Otry C, Labarriere N, et al. J Cell Sci 1995;108:1691
971. Rinieris PM, Stefanis CN, Rabavilas AD, et al. Acta Psychiat Scand 1978;57:377
972. McKeon JP, McColl D. Acta Psychiat Scand 1982;65:74
973. Irvine DG, Miyashita H. Canad Med Assoc J 1965;92:551
974. Masters AB. Br J Psychiat 1967;113:1309
975. Mendlewicz J, Massart-Guiot T, Wilmotte J, et al. Dis Nerv System 1974;35:39
976. Parker JB, Theile A, Speilberger CD. J Ment Sci 1961;103:773 976
977. Shapiro RW, Rafaelson OJ, Ryder LP, et al. Am J Psychiat 1977;134:2197
978. Beckman L, Cedergren B, Perris C, et al. Hum Hered 1978;28:48 978
979. Camps FE, Dodd BE, Lincoln PJ. Br Med J 1969;4:457
980. Swinson RP, Madden JS. Quart J Stud Alcohol 1973;34:64
981. Wiener AS. Lancet 1962;1:813
982. Auer L, Bell K, Coates S. J Am Vet Med Assoc 1982;180:729
983. Beardmore JA, Karimi-Booshehri F. Nature 1983;303:522
984. Hartung J. Nature 1984;309:398
985. Valenzuela CY. Nature 1984;309:398
986. Mascie-Taylor CGN, McManus IC. Nature 1984;309:395
987. Hawkins JD. Nature 1984;309:397
988. Reynolds J, Stiles FG. Rev Biol Trop 1982;30:65
989. Reynolds J. Rev Biol Trop 1982;30:73
990. Palatnik M, Schull WJ. Am J Hum Genet 1986;38:390
991. Adachi M, Hayami M, Kishiwagi N, et al. J Exp Med 1988;167:323
992. Arendrup M, Hansen J-ES, Clausen H, et al. AIDS 1991;5:441
993. Glinsky GV. Med Hypoth 1992;39:212
994. Harmening Pittiglio D. In: Blood Group Systems: ABH and Lewis. Arlington, VA:Am Assoc Blood Banks 1986;44
995. Harmening DM. Modern Blood Banking and Transfusion Practices, 3rd Ed. Philadelphia:Davis, 1994:101
996. Triulzi DJ, Shirey RS, Ness PM, et al. Transfusion 1992;32:829
997. Ramsey G, Nusbacher J, Starzl TE, et al. New Eng J Med

1984;311:1167

998. Gordon RW, Iwatsuki S, Esquivel CO, et al. Transplant Proc 1987;19:4575

999. Jenkins RL, Georgi BA, Gallik-Karlson CA, et al. Transplant Proc 1987;19:4580

1000. Angstadt J, Jarrell B, Maddrey W, et al. Transplant Proc 1987;19:4595

1001. Shanwell A, Eleborg L, Blomqvist BI, et al. Transplant Proc 1989;21:3532

1002. Ramsey G, Cornell FW, Hahn LF, et al. Transfusion 1991;31:76

1003. Telen MJ, Issitt PD, Combs MR. Unpublished observations, 1995

1004. Stayboldt C, Rearden A. Lane TA. (abstract). Transfusion 1985;25:481

1005. Herron R, Smith DS. (Letter). Transfusion 1986;26:303

1006. Herron R, Young D, Clark M, et al. Transfusion 1982;22:525

1007. Tuppy H, Schenkel-Brunner H. Eur J Biochem 1969;10:152

1008. Stellner K, Watanabe K, Hakomori S. Biochemistry 1973;12:656

1009. Kobata A, Grollman EF, Ginsburg V. Biochim Biophys Acta 1968;32:272

1010. Kim YS, Perdomo J, Bella A, et al. Proc Nat Acad Sci USA 1971;68:1753

1011. Race C, Ziderman D, Watkins WM. Biochem J 1968;107:733

1012. Whitehead JS, Bella A, Kim YS. J Biol Chem 1968;107:733

1013. Nagai M, Dave V, Kaplan BE, et al. J Biol Chem 1978;253:377

1014. Yamamoto F, McNeil PD. J Biol Chem 1996;271:10515

1015. Yamamoto F, McNeil PD, Hakomori S. Glycobiology 1995;5:51

1016. Bennett EP, Steffensen R, Clausen H, et al. Biochem Biophys Res Comm 1995;206:318

1017. Joziasse DH. Glycobiology 1992;2:271

1018. Joziasse DH, Shaper NL, Kim D. et al. J Biol Chem 1992;267:5534

1019. Yamamoto F, McNeil PD, Hakomori S. Biochem Biophys Res Comm 1992;187:366

1020. Yamamoto F, McNeil PD, Yamamoto M, et al. Vox Sang 1993;64:116

1021. Nakamura I, Takizawa H, Nishinok K. Exp Clin Immunogenet 1989;6:143

1022. Yamamoto F, McNeil PD, Yamamoto M, et al. Vox Sang 1993;64:171

1023. Fukumori Y, Ohnoki K, Yoshimura K, et al. Transf Med 1996;6:337

1024. Yamamoto F, McNeil PD, Yamamoto M, et al. Vox Sang 1993;64:175

1025. Yoshida A, Yamaguchi YF, Dave V. Blood 1979;54:344

1026. Takizawa N, Iseki S. In: Glycoconjugates. Tokyo:Jpn Sci Soc Press, 1981:379

1027. Olsson ML, Chester MA. Vox Sang 1996;70:26

1028. Olsson ML, Chester MA. Vox Sang 1995;69:242

1029. Grunnet N, Steffensen R, Bennett EP, et al. Vox Sang 1994;67:210

1030. Franco RF, Simoes BP, Guerreiro JF, et al. Vox Sang 1994;67:299

1031. Dzik W. In: Molecular and Functional Aspects of Blood Group Antigens. Bethesda:Am Assoc Blood Banks, 1995:1

1032. Stroncek DF, Konz R, Clay ME, et al. Transfusion 1995;35:231

1033. Olsson ML, Chester MA. Transfusion 1996;36:309

1034. Jeffreys AJ. In: Human Genetics 1994: A Revolution in Full Swing. Bethesda:Am Assoc Blood Banks, 1994:97

1035. Chang JG, Lee LS, Chen PH, et al. (Letter). Blood 1992;79:2176

1036. Ugozzoli L, Wallace RB. Genomics 1992;12:670

1037. Crouse C, Vincek V. Biotechniques 1995;18:478

1038. Lowe JB. Blood Cell Biochemistry. New York:Plenum, 1995;75

1039. Rouquier S, Giorgi D, Bergmann A, et al. Cytogenet Cell Genet 1994;66:70

1040. Wang B, Koda Y, Soejima M, et al. Vox Sang 1997;72:31

1041. Fernandez-Mateos P, Cailleau A, Henry S, et al. Am J Hum Genet in press 1997

1042. Costache M, Cailleau A, Fernandez-Mateos P, et al. Transf Clin Biol in press 1997

1043. Wagner FF, Flegel WA. Transfusion 1997;37:284

1044. Yu LC, Yang YH, Broadberry RE, et al. Vox Sang 1997;72:36

1045. Johnson PH, Mak MK, Leong S, et al. (abstract). Vox Sang 1994;67 (Suppl 2):67

1046. Morgan WTJ, Watkins WM. Br Med Bull 1959;15:109

1047. Friedenreich V, Hartmann G. Z Immun Forsch 1938;92:141

1048. Hartmann G. In: Group Antigens in Human Organs. Copenhagen:Munksgaard, 1941

1049. Aminoff D, Morgan WTJ, Watkins WM. Biochem J 1950;46:426 1049

1050. Gordon RW, Iwatsuki S, Esquivel CO, et al. Transplant Proc 1987;19:4575

1051. Kabat EA, Baer H, Bezer AE, et al. J Exp Med 1948;87:295

1052. Heideberger M. In: Lectures in Immunochemistry. New York:Academic, 1956

1053. Watkins WM, Morgan WTJ. Nature 1952;169:852

1054. Morgan WTJ, Watkins WM. Br J Exp Path 1953;34:94

1055. Kabat EA, Leskowitz S. J Am Chem Soc 1955;77:5159

1056. Watkins WM, Morgan WTJ. Nature 1955;175:676

1057. Tuppy H, Staudenbauer Z. Nature 1966;210:316

1058. Hearn VM, Smith ZG, Watkins WM. Biochem J 1968;109:315

1059. Olsson ML, Thuresson B, Chester MA. Biochem Biophys Res Comm 1995;216:642

1060. Olsson ML, Chester MA. Vox Sang 1996;71:113

1061. Bhatia HM. In: Human Blood Groups. Basel:Karger, 1977:296

1062. Stamps R, Sokol RJ, Leach M, et al. Transfusion 1987;27:315

1063. Drozda EA, Dean JD. Transfusion 1985;25:280

1064. Flegel WA, Wagner FF, Issitt PD, et al. In progress, 1997

1065. Henry SM, Benny AG, Woodfield DG. Vox Sang 1990;58:61

1066. Henry SM, Oriol R, Samuelsson BE. Vox Sang 1995;69:166

1067. Henry SM, Mollicone R, Fernandez P, et al. Biochem Biophys Res Comm 1996;219:675

1068. Henry S, Mollicone R, Lowe JB, et al. Vox Sang 1996;70:21

1069. Ropers HH, Pericak-Vance MA, Siciliano MJ, et al. Cytogenet Cell Genet 1992;60:88

1070. Tetteroo PAT, de Heij HT, van der Hijnden DH, et al. J Biol Chem 1987;262:15984

1071. Paulson JC, Colley KJ. J Biol Chem 1989;264:17615

1072. Goelz SE, Hession C, Goff D, et al. Cell 1990;63:1349

1073. Lowe JB. Sem Cell Biol 1991;2:289

1074. Johnson PH, Donald ASR, Watkins WM. Glycoconjugate J 1993;10:152

1075. Lowe JB, Kukowska-Latallo JF, Nair RP, et al. J Biol Chem 1991;266:17467

1076. Kumar R, Potvin B, Muller WA, et al. J Biol Chem 1991;266:21777

1077. O'Keefe DS, Dobrovic A. Hum Mutat 1993;2:67

1078. Yip SP, Choy WL, Chan CW, et al. J Clin Pathol 1996;49:180

9 | The Lewis System

This chapter on the Lewis system has been placed immediately after the one on the ABO and H systems because genes at the *Lele* (*Lewis*) and *Sese* loci interact in the production of antigens of the system. Further, the amount of Lewis system antigens detectable on red cells is directly influenced by the *ABO* genes present.

Lewis Red Cell Phenotypes

Unlike most other blood group antigens, those of the Lewis system are not synthesized on red cells. Instead, they are present in the plasma and in body secretions, such as saliva. In plasma, the Lewis antigens are carried on oligosaccharide chains that are bound through D-glucose, to sphingolipids (1,2). In saliva, the Lewis antigens are carried on identical oligosaccharides that are bound through N-acetyl-D-galactosamine, to proteins (3). Obviously, once the Lewis antigen-bearing oligosaccharides have been attached, these structures are glycosphingolipids and glycoproteins, respectively. Once the Lewis antigen-bearing structures have been assembled in the plasma, the glycosphingolipids can be inserted (3) into the membranes of red cells, lymphocytes and platelets. All the Lewis antigens carried on red cells are derived from the plasma. Throughout most of this chapter, the descriptions given pertain to the assembly of Lewis determinants on type 1 chains in the plasma. However, it should be remembered that almost everything that is written about the development of Lewis substances in plasma, applies also to the development of those substances in saliva and other body secretions. In other words, the Lewis substances on type 1 chains are identical in the plasma and body secretions, only their carrier molecules differ. Because the plasma glycosphingolipids that carry

the Lewis substances are inserted into red cell membranes, those cells can be typed with Lewis system antibodies and various phenotypes can be recognized.

Discovery of the Lewis System

In 1946, Mourant (4) reported the discovery of anti-Le[a]. The antibody described reacted with red cells and was recognized as defining a new antigen. However, antibodies in chicken sera, found several years earlier in Japan (5-7) (papers in Japanese), were almost certainly anti-Le[a] for they caused formation of a precipitate when mixed with saliva from non-secretors of ABH substances. In 1948, Andresen (8) described the first example of anti-Le[b]. It is now known that Le[a] and Le[b] are not antithetical antigens produced under the control of allelic genes. Instead, as described in more detail later in this chapter, inheritance of the gene *Le* results in development of Le[a] in persons who are non-secretors of ABH substances and of Le[b] in persons who inherit at least one *Se* gene. The allele of *Le* is *le*, a silent gene and in persons genetically *lele*, neither Le[a] nor Le[b] is made. Thus, by using anti-Le[a] and anti-Le[b] to type red cells, the phenotypes listed in table 9-1 can be identified. The reactions of the antibodies originally called anti-Le[c] and anti-Le[d], the specificity of anti-Le[x], the rare phenotype Le(a+b+) and a different antibody also called anti-Le[x] (or anti-X) and one called anti-Le[y], are all described in later sections of this chapter.

Lewis Antigens from Plasma are Taken-up by Red Cells

In 1948, Grubb (9,10) and Brendemoen (11) each

TABLE 9-1 Lewis Phenotypes of Red Cells

Phenotype	Frequency	
	Whites[*1]	Blacks[*2]
Le(a+b-)	22%	19.5%
Le(a-b+)	72%	52%
Le(a-b-)	6%	28.5%
Le(a+b+)	Rare[*3]	Rare[*3]

* 1. Phenotype frequencies in Whites from references 10 and 117 to 120.
* 2. Phenotype frequencies from tests on the red cells of 883 American Black adults by Molthan (122). Others (26,117,123-125) have given phenotype frequencies for Le(a-b-) in Blacks that vary (dependent on the population studied) from 16 to 22%.
* 3. Rare in Whites and Blacks, more common in other populations, see text.

noticed that the saliva of individuals whose red cells typed as Le(a+) would inhibit anti-Le^a. It was Grubb who first suggested (12) that Lewis is a system of saliva and plasma antigens. In 1955, Sneath and Sneath (13) found that Le(a-b-) red cells could be transformed into Le(a+) or Le(b+) cells by incubation in appropriate plasma. This finding was confirmed by others (14) who also reported that saliva from individuals with Le(b+) red cells failed to effect the same transformation as could be achieved with plasma. Later it was shown (15) that red cells previously treated with tannic acid would take up Le^a from saliva. It is now appreciated that red cell uptake of Lewis substances from the plasma involves the insertion of glycosphingolipids into the membrane (1). In contrast, the uptake of Le^a from saliva, by tanned red cells, involves non-specific adsorption. Indeed, tanned red cells will adsorb almost any protein from a solution in which they are suspended. Mäkelä et al. (16) studied the transformation of Le(a-b-) red cells, incubated in plasma containing Le^a or Le^b substance and found no evidence to suggest that enzymes in the plasma were altering structures on the membrane. Like the earlier workers, they concluded that Le^a and Le^b reach the membrane by adsorption from the plasma. This conclusion was supported by some observations made in studies on the blood of chimeric twins (17-22). In informative pairs it was shown that both populations of red cells carried the Lewis substance present in the plasma, regardless of the genes present in the erythropoetic tissue. As a single example (17), one pair of twins comprised one who was group O and had the *Le*, *Se* and *H* genes. This twin made Le^b in the secretory cells and was a secretor of H substances. The other twin was group A and was genetically *sese*, that is a non-secretor of ABH substances. The O twin had received a graft from the A twin and had a mixed cell population of almost equal numbers of O and A cells. Both cell populations (that could be separated easily because of the difference in ABO group) were Le(a-b+). The A cells were from an ABH non-secretor so would have been Le(a+b-) if their Lewis antigens had been synthesized on the red cells. Instead, they were Le(a-b+) reflecting the Lewis phenotype of the plasma of the group O twin in which they were being made. Such cases show that all the red cell-borne Lewis antigens are derived from the plasma. In 1969, Marcus and Cass (1) showed that the mechanism by which red cells acquire Lewis antigens is by insertion of plasma glycosphingolipids into the cell membrane. A similar mechanism is operative in lymphocytes and as discussed later in this chapter, many cytotoxic antibodies directed against the acquired antigens have now been reported. Because their structure has not yet been described in this chapter, little will be said at this point about the antigens originally called Le^c and Le^d or about antigens such as A$_1$Le^b.

However, it can be mentioned that, like Le^a and Le^b, these antigens reach the red cell and lymphocytes membranes from the plasma, via the same mechanism.

Red cells that have acquired Le^a or Le^b from the plasma can lose those antigens if suspended in plasma from an Le(a-b-) person (23). As discussed in the later section of this chapter that deals with blood transfusion in persons who have Lewis system antibodies, the loss of antigens also occurs in vivo. For example, if Le(a-b+) blood is transfused into an Le(a-b-) individual, Le(b+) cells usually cannot be demonstrated in the patient's circulation some 7 to 10 days later. Lack of Le(b+) cells does not represent the destruction of transfused cells because other antigenic markers (M, N, etc.) can be used to show that the expected numbers of transfused cells are still present. Instead, lack of demonstrable Le^b antigen in the patient's blood represents loss of that antigen from the transfused cells, into the recipient's plasma (24).

Lewis Saliva and Plasma Phenotypes

The saliva of individuals whose red cells type as Le(a+b-) contains Le^a but not Le^b substance (9-11). The saliva of persons who have red cells that type as Le(a-b+) contains both Le^b and Le^a substance (10,13,14,25,26). The saliva of persons whose red cells type as Le(a-b-) usually contains neither Le^a nor Le^b substance.

In 1948, Grubb (9) reported that individuals who had red cells that typed as Le(a+) were non-secretors of ABH substances. Individuals whose red cells typed as Le(b+) were secretors of ABH substance. Individuals with red cells that typed as Le(a-b-) could be either secretors or non-secretors of ABH substances (see table 9-2). With very few exceptions (27,28) identical findings have been made in other studies.

It should be stressed that the presence of Lewis substances in the saliva is not dependent on the presence of an *Se* gene. Individuals who are genetically *SeSe* or *Sese* secrete ABH substances (dependent on which *ABO* gene(s) is(are) present). Individuals with an *Le* gene all secrete Le^a or Le^a and Le^b, while individuals genetically *lele* have what have previously been called Le^c or Le^d in their saliva. These findings are summarized in table 9-2.

As will be apparent from this and previous sections, the Lewis saliva and plasma (serum) phenotypes are identical. They differ from red cell phenotypes in that individuals whose red cells type as Le(a-b+) have both Le^a and Le^b in the saliva and plasma. The reason for this difference is quantitative. In an individual genetically *Le*, *Se*, sufficient quantities of Le^b are made in the plasma that the red cells bind enough of it to react with anti-Le^b. There is less Le^a substance present and although some of it does get on to red cells, too little is present for detec-

TABLE 9-2 Lewis Phenotypes and ABH Secretion

Red Cell Lewis Phenotype	ABH Secretor Status	Lewis Secretor Status
Le(a+b-)	ALL ABH non-secretors	ALL secretors of Le^a
Le(a-b+)	ALL ABH secretors	ALL secretors of Le^a and Le^b
Le(a-b-)	80% ABH secretors 20% ABH non-secretors	See section on the antigens originally called Le^c and Le^d

tion with many examples of anti-Le^a. Very potent examples of anti-Le^a will react with red cells typed as Le(a-b+) with other anti-Le^a and anti-Le^b reagents. Indeed, as discussed below, some antibodies that appear to have anti-Le^a plus anti-Le^b specificity, are actually examples of anti-Le^a capable of reacting with the small amounts of Le^a on the so-called Le(a-b+) red cells.

The trace amounts of Le^a or Le^b found in the plasma and saliva of a few individuals with Le(a-b-) red cells (327) may be representative of the fact that the term *le* describes more than one allele. This point is discussed in more detail in the section on the *Lele* genes and chromosome 19.

The Antigens Le^a and Le^b and the Phenotypes Le(a+b-), Le(a-b+) and Le(a-b-)

Although the biochemical structure of Le^a and Le^b is described in detail in a later section of this chapter, it is necessary here to include basic details about those antigens in order to explain the serology of the Lewis system. As mentioned several times, Le^a and Le^b are synthesized on type 1 precursor chains in the plasma and saliva and are taken up by red cells from the plasma (29-52). Figure 9-1 shows the structure of the relevant portion of the type 1 chain and, for reasons that will become apparent, the equivalent portion of the type 2 chain. The *Le* gene encodes a fucosyl transferase that adds L-fucose in alpha 1→4 linkage to the subterminal N-acetyl-D-glucosamine of the type 1 chain (figure 9-2). The *Le* gene-specified transferase cannot act similarly on the type 2 chain since that chain has galactose added in beta 1→4 linkage to the subterminal N-acetyl-D-glucosamine (figure 9-1) meaning that the acceptor site for the actions of the *Le* gene-specified transferase is blocked. The addition of L-fucose to the subterminal N-acetyl-D-galactosamine on the type 1 chain results in Le^a specificity (figure 9-2). In persons genetically *sese* no other addition to the type 1 chain occurs (63) with the result that ABH non-secretors, who have at least one *Le* gene, have red

cells that are Le(a+b-) (see table 9-2 and figure 9-2).

In persons who have at least one *Se* and one *Le* gene, the *Se* gene-specified fucosyl transferase adds L-fucose in alpha 1→2 linkage to the terminal galactose of the type 1 chain to form type 1 H. The *Le* gene-specified fucosyl transferase then adds L-fucose in alpha 1→4 linkage to the subterminal N-acetyl-D-glucosamine of the same chain (figure 9-2) the resultant structure is Le^b (38). Thus ABH secretors who have at least one *Le* gene have red cells that are Le(a-b+) (see table 9-2 and figure 9-2). Since the Le^b structure is made by *Se* individuals who have *Le*, some Le^a is made as well. Thus the saliva of individuals with Le(a-b+) red cells contains both Le^b and Le^a substance. Apparently too few Le^a-bearing type 1 chains are made in those individuals for their red cells to take up enough such structures for Le^a to be readily detected on the red cells. However, as mentioned above, trace amounts of Le^a are taken up by those red cells and they may give positive reactions when tested with very potent examples of anti-Le^a (see section below on anti-Le^a plus anti-Le^b).

The saliva of persons genetically *Se, Le* also contains H and if the individual inherits A or B, A or B substance as well. As described in detail in Chapter 8, the two gene theory about *Hh* and *Sese* proposes that H in the secretions is produced by the actions of the *Se* gene-specified transferase (54).

An additional point to be considered in this basic description of the actions of the *Le* and *Se* gene-specified fucosyl transferases is that if the *Le* specified enzyme acts first, by adding L-fucose to the subterminal N-acetyl-D-glucosamine, the presence of that residue may sterically block the addition of L-fucose to the terminal galactose by the *Se* gene-specified enzyme (53). In other words, the addition of L-fucose to the subterminal carbohydrate may act as a chain synthesis ending event. Thus in individuals with a particularly efficient *Le* gene-specified fucosyl transferase and/or a relatively inefficient *Se* gene-specified transferase, more type 1 chains bearing Le^a, that cannot subsequently be converted to Le^b, may be taken up by the red cells.

As will be seen from this discussion, the synthesis of Le^a and Le^b has been described in terms of the actions of *Le* and *Se*. As discussed in detail in Chapter 8, this is because we subscribe to the two gene theory of Oriol et al. (54). In other words, no role for the *H* gene-specified fucosyl transferase is invoked in the synthesis of Le^a and Le^b. In many of the papers cited (29-46) the older three gene theory was used to explain the serological and biochemical findings. That theory held that at least one *H* gene was necessary for *Se* to function at the secretory cell level. Now we believe that *H* and *Se* encode different fucosyl transferases (47-51, 55-62) and that the evidence shows that each can act alone as a structural gene.

FIGURE 9-1 Structure of the Precursor Chains

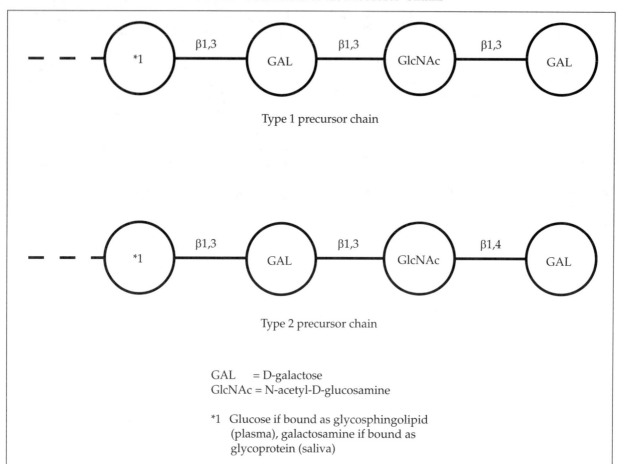

Type 1 precursor chain

Type 2 precursor chain

GAL   = D-galactose
GlcNAc = N-acetyl-D-glucosamine

*1   Glucose if bound as glycosphingolipid
     (plasma), galactosamine if bound as
     glycoprotein (saliva)

That is to say, neither regulates the other. It should be remembered that since the *H* gene-specified fucosyl transferase acts on type 2 precursor chains, H substance will be present on the red cells of persons genetically *H, sese*, including those who inherit *Le* and those who are genetically *lele* (i.e. have Le(a-b-) red cells).

As readers of the third edition of this book will realize, this section of the chapter has been changed to provide basic biochemical information that is needed to understand the serology of the system. This has resulted in many papers on this topic not being cited in this section. Readers wishing to compile a more complete set of original papers are referred to those publications referenced as 67-108, that list includes papers about Le[c] and Le[d] that are described in a later section.

The Phenotype Le(a+b+)

As described in the previous section, the red cell Lewis phenotypes of Whites of European extraction and of U.S. Blacks are Le(a+b-), Le(a-b+) and Le(a-b-). In these populations the Le(a+b+) phenotype is rare although, as discussed below, particularly potent examples of anti-Le[a] react with some apparently Le(a-b+) red cells.

The red cell phenotype Le(a+b+) is more common in other populations. It has been found in Japanese (64,65), Australian Aborigines (66,328) and Thais (28). Henry et al. (152) reported that the incidence of the Le(a+b+) phenotype varied from 10 to 40% in different Polynesian populations, Broadberry and Lin (153) found that between 22 and 25% of Chinese living in Taiwan were of that phenotype.

The Le(a+b+) red cell phenotype is believed to represent a situation described in the previous section. That is to say, if the *Le* gene-specified transferase adds L-fucose to the subterminal N-acetyl-D-glucosamine before the *Se* gene-specified transferase adds L-fucose to the terminal galactose, Le[a] cannot be converted to Le[b] (see figures 9-1 and 9-2). Since both Le[a] and Le[b]-bearing chains will be present in the plasma, they can be taken up by red cells that will then have the Le(a+b+) phenotype. Originally two different mechanisms could be invoked as possible explanations of the Le(a+b+) phenotype. First,

FIGURE 9-2 Action of the *Le* Gene-specified Transferase Enzyme

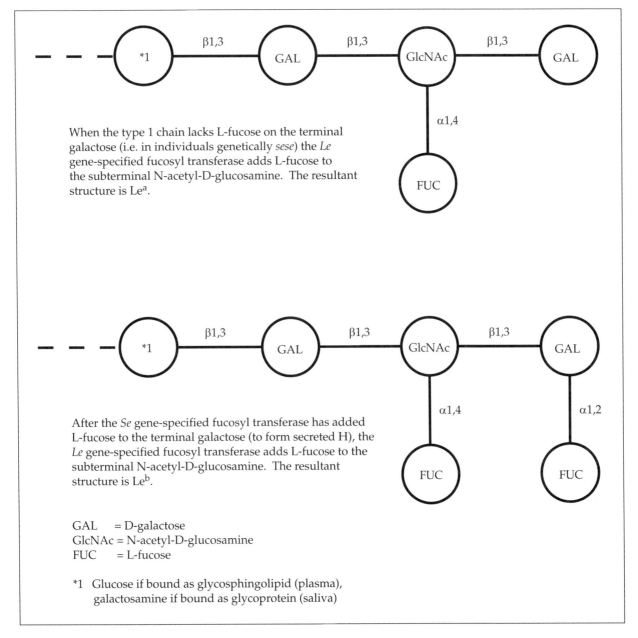

When the type 1 chain lacks L-fucose on the terminal galactose (i.e. in individuals genetically *sese*) the *Le* gene-specified fucosyl transferase adds L-fucose to the subterminal N-acetyl-D-glucosamine. The resultant structure is Le[a].

After the *Se* gene-specified fucosyl transferase has added L-fucose to the terminal galactose (to form secreted H), the *Le* gene-specified fucosyl transferase adds L-fucose to the subterminal N-acetyl-D-glucosamine. The resultant structure is Le[b].

GAL = D-galactose
GlcNAc = N-acetyl-D-glucosamine
FUC = L-fucose

*1 Glucose if bound as glycosphingolipid (plasma), galactosamine if bound as glycoprotein (saliva)

if an *Le* gene making a high level of fucosyl transferase was present it could be supposed that Le[a] might be made on many type 1 chains before the *Se* gene-specified transferase could act to add L-fucose to the terminal galactose residue. Alternatively, if the *Se* gene present encoded less than normal amounts of its transferase, or an enzyme that functioned less efficiently than the normal product, again the *Le* gene-specified transferase might convert enough type 1 structures to Le[a] (with those structures then not amenable to conversion to Le[b]) before the *Se* gene-specified product acted to add L-fucose to the terminal galactose. In either situation, competition between the *Le* and *Se* gene-specified transferases for available sites on type 1 chains, could result in the Le(a+b+) phenotype.

Henry et al. (152,329,330) studied the above situation at the serological level and concluded that the causative gene is an allele of *Se*, that they named *Se[w]*, and not a super-active form of *Le*. The workers in Taiwan (153-155) used the *Se[w]* explanation for the Le(a+b+) phenotype in their population. Later studies by Henry et al. (334,353) at the biochemical and DNA levels, confirmed the existence of *Se[w]*. As mentioned in Chapter 8, Henry et al. (348) also showed that two different mutations can lead to the *se* gene. One of these changes accounts for the *se* gene in Whites, both changes are seen among Polynesian non-secretors. While the roles of *Se*, two forms of *se*, and *Se*^{w} in aberrant secretors (331,332) is not known, the phenotypic findings suggest that genes at the *Sese* locus may be involved.

To these somewhat complicated considerations of the Le(a+b+) phenotype, it now seems that a third less involved explanation must be added for some examples of the phenotype, particularly in Whites of European and Blacks of African extraction. As discussed elsewhere in this chapter and as shown in figure 9-2, red cells that have adsorbed Le^b-bearing structures from the plasma and type as Le(a-b+) will always also have some structures recognized by anti-Le^a. While human polyclonal anti-Le^a and anti-Le^b may type such red cells as Le(a-b+) with only the very potent examples of anti-Le^a able to recognize the Le^a structure, the same may not be true of monoclonal anti-Le^a. In other words, when some monoclonal anti-Le^a are used, particularly in typing studies on the red cells of other than Oriental people, the trace amount of Le^a that has always been present, but not detected by human polyclonal anti-Le^a, may be recognized and the Le(a+b+) phenotype may result. Possible correlation between the newly detectable Le^a on the Le(a+b+) red cells of Whites and Blacks and presence of an allele similar to the *Se*^{w} gene of Orientals, has not yet been studied.

The Antigens Originally Called Le^c and Le^d

In 1957, Iseki et al. (109,110) immunized animals and raised an antibody that reacted with all Le(a-b-) red cells. It was assumed that this antibody must be defining a product of the *le* gene and the antibody was named anti-Le^c. Later (see below) the name anti-Le^c was applied to an antibody that reacts only with the Le(a-b-) red cells of non-secretors of ABH. Throughout the remainder of this chapter, the second meaning of anti-Le^c is intended when that term is used, that is, Le^c is the structure present in individuals who are genetically *lele*, *sese*. (In fact, see below, the current concept of Le^c is that it is unaltered type 1 precursor chain.) In 1965, Lodge et al. (111) tested a number of potent anti-Le^a, present in human sera and found one that contained a component that reacted with Le(a-b-) red cells.

In 1970, Potapov (112) immunized animals and raised an antibody that reacted only with the Le(a-b-) red cells of persons who were secretors of ABH substances. This antibody was named anti-Le^d and Potapov (112) forecast that an antibody reacting only with the Le(a-b-) red cells of ABH non-secretors, would also be found. In 1972, Gunson and Latham (113) identified

such an antibody that became known as anti-Le^c. One possibility at that time was that anti-Le^c and anti-Le^d were detecting structures somewhat analogous to Le^a and Le^b in that they were made by joint actions or non-actions of the *le*, *Se* and *se* genes. However, this possibility was effectively excluded by Graham et al. (114). If Le^a and Le^c were made, respectively, by *Le* and *le* in the absence of *Se*, and if Le^b and Le^d were made, respectively, by *Le* and *le* in the presence of *Se*, individuals heterozygous for *Le* and *le*, who were non-secretors of ABH, should have red cells of the phenotype Le(a+b-c+d-). Those who were genetically *Lele* and were secretors of ABH should have red cells of the phenotype Le(a-b+c-d+). In tests on the red cells of 98 adults, Graham et al. (114) found only one of the antigens Le^a, Le^b, Le^c and Le^d on each sample. The conclusion from this study was that Le^c and Le^d are made in the absence of *Le* without any action on the part of *le*. The authors (114) suggested that when *Le* is absent, but *Se* is active in the secretory cells, Le^d is made because it is the H determinant of type 1 chains. Further, they proposed that in individuals genetically *lele*, *sese*, where no addition to the type 1 chain occurs, the unconverted chain was what anti-Le^c recognized. As discussed in detail in the section below on the biochemical structure of the Lewis antigens, these proposals of Graham et al. (114) were exactly correct. Mollison (115) suggested that since the structure of what was originally called Le^d has now been recognized, the term Le^d should be abandoned (no *Lewis* gene action is involved in the synthesis of Le^d) in favor of the term "H type 1". Along similar lines Lodge (116) has suggested that Le^c become known as "precursor type 1". These concepts are illustrated diagramatically in figure 9-3. As would be expected, the antigens originally called Le^c and Le^d are taken up by red cells from the plasma (99).

In describing a series of Lewis antibodies made in goats, Potapov (172) used some terms that should be mentioned to aid readers who may encounter them. Anti-Le^s was used to describe a mixture of anti-Le^b and anti-Le^d. In other words, anti-Le^s detected the determinant present in secretors of ABH substances, that is Le^b when *Le* and *Se* are present and Le^d (type 1 H) when *lele* and *Se* are inherited. Anti-Le^{ns} was used to describe a mixture of anti-Le^a and anti-Le^c, or the antibody that defines the Lewis antigens of ABH non-secretors. In other words, anti-Le^{ns} defines Le^a made by persons genetically *Le*, *sese* and Le^c (type 1 precursor) as present in persons genetically *lele*, *sese*. Anti-Le^m was the name used to describe a goat serum with anti-Le^b plus anti-Le^c specificity. It was stressed (172) that the new symbols of divalent anti-Le sera did not imply the existence of corresponding antigens, Le^s, Le^{ns} and Le^m.

FIGURE 9-3 Structure of the Antigens Originally Called Le^c and Le^d

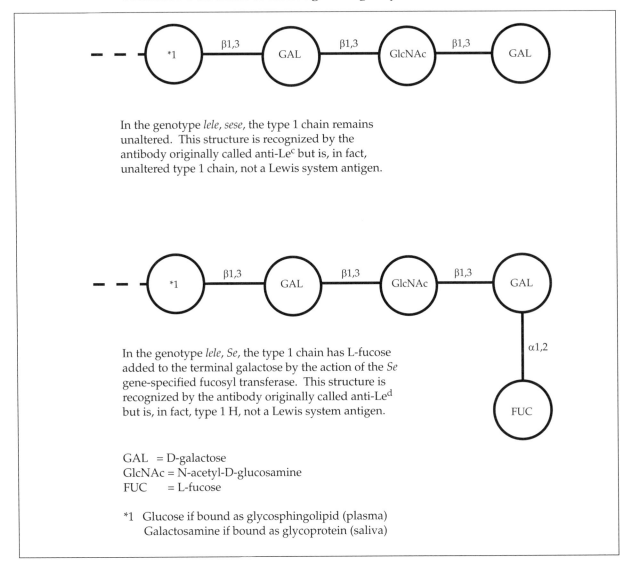

In the genotype *lele, sese*, the type 1 chain remains unaltered. This structure is recognized by the antibody originally called anti-Le^c but is, in fact, unaltered type 1 chain, not a Lewis system antigen.

In the genotype *lele, Se*, the type 1 chain has L-fucose added to the terminal galactose by the action of the *Se* gene-specified fucosyl transferase. This structure is recognized by the antibody originally called anti-Le^d but is, in fact, type 1 H, not a Lewis system antigen.

GAL   = D-galactose
GlcNAc = N-acetyl-D-glucosamine
FUC   = L-fucose

*1   Glucose if bound as glycosphingolipid (plasma)
     Galactosamine if bound as glycoprotein (saliva)

The Antigens A$_1$Le^b, BLe^b, A$_1$Le^d and BLe^d

In individuals who inherit at least one *Se* and one *Le* gene, the Le^b determinant is formed on type 1 chains (figure 9-2). Since the *Se* gene-specified fucosyl transferase adds L-fucose to the terminal galactose residue, H is formed. In individuals who inherit at least one *Se* gene, but two *lele* genes, Le^b is not made (no *Le* gene-specified transferase) but the *Se* gene-specified enzyme still adds L-fucose to the terminal galactose residue, so that H is made. Because H is present in both situations, the type 1 chain is a suitable acceptor for the addition of the immunodominant carbohydrates added by the *A* and *B* gene-specified transferases. As depicted in figure 9-4 the *A* gene-specified galactosaminyl transferase adds N-acetyl-D-galactosamine to the type 1 chain of *Le, Se* individuals and to the type 1 chain of *lele, Se* persons. The resultant antigens are called A$_1$Le^b and A$_1$Le^d, respectively. Similarly, because the type 1 chains each carry H, the *B* gene-specified galactosyl transferase adds D-galactose to form BLe^b in persons with Le^b and BLe^d in persons with type 1 H but no Le^b. The type 1 chains are then taken up by red cells on which the antigens can be detected. In other words, the red cells of all A and B secretors who have an *Le* gene will carry A$_1$Le^b or BLe^b, dependent on the inheritance of A^1 or *B*, while the red cells of all A and B secretors of the Le(a-b-) phenotype will carry A$_1$Le^d or BLe^d, again dependent on the inheritance of A^1 or *B* (figure 9-4)

A number of points are pertinent. First, the A$_1$Le^b, BLe^b, A$_1$Le^d and BLe^d determinants are defined by single antibodies directed against those antigens. In other words, anti-A$_1$Le^b is one antibody, not a separable mix-

FIGURE 9-4 To Show the Structures of A$_1$Le^b, BLe^b, A$_1$Le^d and BLe^d

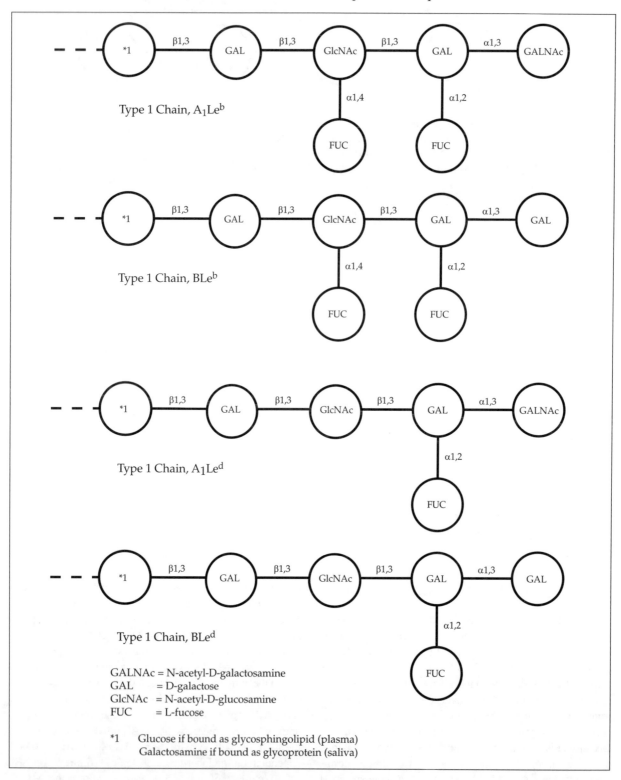

GALNAc = N-acetyl-D-galactosamine
GAL   = D-galactose
GlcNAc   = N-acetyl-D-glucosamine
FUC   = L-fucose

*1   Glucose if bound as glycosphingolipid (plasma)
         Galactosamine if bound as glycoprotein (saliva)

ture of anti-A$_1$ and anti-Le^b; the same applies to the antibodies that define BLe^b, A$_1$Le^d and BLe^d (2,18,19,126).

Second, it will be noticed that in discussing the determinants made when A is attached to Le^b or Le^d, the terms A$_1$Le^b and A$_1$Le^d are used. This probably represents the fact that an A^1 gene that produces a more efficient galactosaminyl transferase than does A^2, is necessary for large enough amounts of these antigens to be made in the plasma for enough to become attached to red cells or lymphocytes, for subsequent detection with the antibodies.

Third, there are no equivalent A and B-related antigens involving Le^a or Le^c. Individuals with Le(a+b-) red cells are genetically *Le, sese*, those who have Le(a-b-) red cells and are non-secretors of ABH, are genetically *lele, sese*. Since both groups of individuals lack *Se*, no H is made on their type 1 chains meaning that no addition of A or B immunodominant sugars can occur (63). These individuals have A and/or B on their red cells, dependent on which *ABO* gene(s) is(are) inherited because the overwhelming majority of them have *H* so make H substance on their type 2 chains. However, as discussed in Chapter 8, *H* is not operative in the secretory tissues while *Se* and *Le* are not operative at the level of antigen synthesis on red cells. Thus non-secretors of ABH have no equivalent antigens to A$_1$Le^b, BLe^b, A$_1$Le^d and BLe^d, regardless of whether their red cells are Le(a+b-) or Le(a-b-).

Table 9-3 summarizes the red cell and saliva phenotypes that result from the inheritance of various combinations of genes at the *Lele, Sese* and *ABO* loci; table 9-4 lists the ISBT terms for antigens in the Lewis system and for those originally called Le^c and Le^d. As will be seen, the Working Party has not assigned numbers to A$_1$Le^b, A$_1$Le^d, etc.

Development of the Lewis Antigens

At birth, an infant does not necessarily have red cells of the Lewis phenotype that will be present later in life.

Andresen (8) found that in agglutination tests, most cord red blood cells type as Le(a-b-). However, Cutbush et al. (127) showed that if the indirect antiglobulin test is used, many cord blood samples type as Le(a+). By pooling data from several studies (127-130) it can be seen that the Le(a+) phenotype has an incidence of: about 50% if White infants are typed at birth; between 80 and 90% if they are typed at around two months of age; about 45% if they are typed at one year of age; and about 22% (the incidence in adults) if they are typed when two or three years old. It seems clear that at birth, the *Se* gene-specified transferase is produced in low levels and the *Le* gene-specified transferase in higher amounts. Thus, the immunodominant Le^a specificity can be added to type 1 chains, before type 1 H is made. The Le(a+b-) phenotype results. At around 2 months of age, the *Le* gene-specified transferase must be made in levels approximating those in adults, to account for the very high incidence of the Le(a+) phenotype. Thereafter, it seems that the *Se* gene-specified transferase gradually increases in amount made so that by one year of age, half those children previously found to have Le(a+) red cells, have cells that are Le(a-b+). By two to three years of age the Le(a+b-) and Le(a-b+) phenotypes of children seem to reflect the genes that have they have inherited, that is *Le, sese* and *Le, Se* respectively. When *Se* gene-specified transferase production begins to approach the levels seen in adults, many Le(a+) red cells will still be present in the child's circulation. Accordingly, for a one to two month period, the child's red cells may type as Le(a+b+) (127,130).

Mäkelä and Mäkelä (14) demonstrated that the plasma of newborn infants would not transform Le(a-b-) red cells from adults into Le(a+), but that Le(a-b-) red cells from infants could be transformed into Le(a+) by incu-

TABLE 9-3 ABO and Lewis Substances on Red Cells and in Saliva of Individuals with Various Combinations of the *Lele, Sese* and *ABO* Genes

Genes Present				
Lewis	Secretor	ABO*1	Red Cell Phenotype	Substances in Saliva
LeLe or *Lele*	*SeSe* or *Sese*	*O*	O,Le(a-b+c-d-)	H,Le^a,Le^b
lele	*SeSe* or *Sese*	*O*	O,Le(a-b-c-d+)	Type 1 H (Le^d)
LeLe or *Lele*	*sese*	*O*	O,Le(a+b-c-d-)	Le^a
lele	*sese*	*O*	O,Le(a-b-c+d-)	Type 1 chain(Le^c)
LeLe or *Lele*	*SeSe* or *Sese*	A^1	A$_1$,Le(a-b+c-d-)	A,H,Le^a,Le^b,A$_1$Le^{b*2}
lele	*SeSe* or *Sese*	A^1	A$_1$,Le(a-b-c-d+)	A,Type 1 H (Le^d), A$_1$Le^d
LeLe or *Lele*	*sese*	A^1	A$_1$,Le(a+b-c-d-)	Le^a
lele	*sese*	A^1	A$_1$,Le(a-b-c+d-)	Type 1 chain(Le^c)

* 1   *O* and A^1 used as examples, obviously *B*, A^2 etc., can substitute with slightly different results

* 2   Less Lewis substances in group A than in group O

TABLE 9-4 Conventional and ISBT Terminology for the Lewis System and some Associated Antigens

System (Conventional Name)	ISBT System Symbol	ISBT System Number	Antigen (Conventional Name)	ISBT Antigen Number	ISBT Full Code Number
Lewis	LE	007	Le^a	001	007001
			Le^b	002	007002
			Le^ab*1	003	007003
Unnamed Collection*2	None	210	Le^c*3	001	210001
			Le^d*4	002	210002

* 1   The authors do not know if the antigen designated Le^ab is the same as the one called Le^x in this chapter
* 2   While these two antigens have been put in Collection 210 (for definition of a Collection see Chapter 1) no name or symbol has been assigned to that Collection
* 3   Le^c is unconverted type 1 chain (see text)
* 4   Le^d is type 1H (see text)

bation with plasma from an Le(a+) adult. These results support the theory that it is the low level of transferase activity and hence plasma antigens that results in the absence of some Lewis antigens from cord blood red cells. The experiments show that the red cells of infants have the ability to take up Lewis antigens if those antigens are present in the plasma.

The situation seems to be different in Orientals. In studies in Taiwan (154,155) it was found that Le^b develops before Le^a in infants. It was concluded that in these infants the *Se* gene is more active than *Le* at the time of birth. Thus it was assumed that in infants with *Le* and *Se*, the *Se* gene-specified transferase made type 1 H before the low level of *Le* gene-specified transferase could make Le^a (see above section for a description of the synthesis of Le^a and Le^b). This concept does not fit particularly well with the *Se^w* gene mentioned in the discussion of the Le(a+b+) phenotype. However, it is possible that levels of enzymes produced by *Se*, *Le*, and *Se^w*, are different in newborn infants and adults. A preliminary study (155) has suggested that neonatal hyperbilirubinemia, that is much more common in Taiwanese than in White infants, (156-159) may be associated with late development of Le^a. However, no role for the *Le* gene-specified transferase in the hyperbilirubinemia (that is not caused by antibody-mediated red cell destruction) is apparent.

Lewis System Antibodies

(See also table 9-5.)

Anti-Le^a

Anti-Le^a is a common antibody (129,131-134) and

examples will be found frequently in any service that tests blood samples from Black patients or donors. One reason for this is that almost all persons who form the antibody have red cells that are Le(a-b-) and that phenotype is considerably more frequent in Blacks than in Whites (see table 9-1). A second reason is that anti-Le^a occurs regularly in persons who have never been transfused or pregnant. In routine tests, examples of anti-Le^a most often react as if they are entirely IgM in nature (115,135,136). However, occasional examples of IgG anti-Le^a had been found (115,136) before Holburn (137) showed that sera that contain anti-Le^a, often contain both IgM and IgG components with that specificity. The IgM component seems usually to have a higher binding constant than the IgG form and it was suggested (137) that the IgG antibody might easily be overlooked in conventional tests, in the presence of IgM antibody. At least the IgM form of anti-Le^a is highly efficient in activating complement.

As mentioned above, almost all examples of anti-Le^a are formed by persons who have red cells of the Le(a-b-) phenotype. As explained earlier, individuals who have red cells of the Le(a-b+) phenotype have an *Le* gene and secrete both Le^a and Le^b in their saliva. Further, tests with potent examples of anti-Le^a show that the red cells of these people carry trace amounts of Le^a. In spite of this, at least two examples of anti-Le^a made by persons with Le(a-b+) red cells have been reported (138,151). One patient had carcinoma of the esophagus and although his saliva contained H, Le^a and Le^b, the amount of Le^b on his red cells was only half that on control Le(a-b+) cells. It was suggested (138) that perhaps his disease process (squamous cell carcinoma was diagnosed) had caused sufficient depletion of the Lewis antigen production that he was able to recognize Le^a as a for-

TABLE 9-5 Usual Characteristics of Lewis System Antibodies

Antibody Specificity	Positive Reactions in In Vitro Tests				Usual Immuno-globulin		Ability to Bind Complement		Ability to Cause In Vitro Lysis		Implicated In		Usual Form of Stimulation		% of White Population Positive
	Sal	LISS	AHG	Enz	IgG	IgM	Yes	No	Yes	No	Trans-fusion Reaction	HDN	Red Cells	Other	
Anti-Le^a	X	X	X	X	Tr	X	X		Some		Yes	No		X	22
Anti-Le^{bH}	X	X	X	X		X	X				No	No*5		X	*1
Anti-Le^{bL}	X	X	X	X		X	X		Few		No	No		X	72
Anti-Le^a+Le^b	X	X	X	X		X	X		Some*2		Yes	No		X	94
Anti-Le^{c*3}											No	No		X	1
Anti-Le^{d*4}											No	No		X	5

Tr = Trace
* 1   See text, reacts with group O, Le(a-b+) red cells
* 2   More likely to hemolyze Le(a+b-) than Le(a-b+) red cells
* 3   Anti-Le^c is anti-precusor chain 1, see text
* 4   Anti-Le^d is anti-type 1 H, see text
* 5   See text for a claim to the contrary.

eign antigen. The antibody was correctly described (138) as being autoimmune in nature because although it did not react with the patient's red cells, it was totally inhibited by his own saliva. Naturally, since it did not react with the patient's red cells, it did not cause any shortening of the in vivo life span of those cells.

The secretor status appears to affect the ability of individuals with Le(a-b-) red cells to make anti-Le^a. Miller et al. (26) noticed that anti-Le^a was usually made by *lele* individuals who also had *Se*. The reason for this is not clear. In the genotype *lele, Se* L-fucose is added to the terminal galactose residue of the type 1 chain. In the genotype *lele, sese* the type 1 chain is unaltered. Why the former and not the latter group of individuals are able to make an antibody that recognizes a structure that has L-fucose attached to the subterminal glucosamine residue, has not yet been explained.

The ABO group also affects the ability of individuals to make anti-Le^a. Several groups of workers (26,129,133,139-141) have noticed that anti-Le^a is more commonly made by group A, B and AB people than would be expected on a random basis. In one study (139) only 11% of people who had made anti-Le^a were group O, in another study (133) the figure was 30%. Walker et al. (141) found a somewhat different incidence. Approximately 41% of the people who had made anti-Le^a were group O but the figure for those who had made anti-Le^a plus anti-Le^b was lower, only 20% of those individuals were group O. It is perhaps easier to understand why group O secretors of ABH substances are in the minority among people who make anti-Le^a plus anti-Le^b

since those people have H in their secretions and H and Le^b are structurally similar.

While many examples of anti-Le^a are clinically-insignificant because they do not bind to Le(a+) red cells at 37°C, less frequent examples are active in vivo. A number of transfusion reactions caused by anti-Le^a have been documented (142-150). As discussed below, in the section on the clinical significance of Lewis system antibodies, there are a number of reasons why the in vivo destruction of Le(a+) cells in a patient with anti-Le^a may be rather limited. However, those examples of anti-Le^a that are active in vitro at 37°C, particularly those that present as in vitro hemolysis and those reactive in indirect antiglobulin tests, should not be ignored in the selection of blood. Again as discussed in more detail later, it is not necessary to select Le(a-b-) blood for transfusion to patients with anti-Le^a. The small amount of Le^a present on Le(a-b+) red cells can be ignored and units compatible with the patient's serum in in vitro tests performed at 37°C are perfectly suitable. As would be expected, since anti-Le^a is usually predominantly IgM in nature and since the Le^a antigen is not fully developed at birth, no case of HDN due to anti-Le^a has been reported. Spitalnik et al. (205) studied 13 mother-infant pairs in whom anti-Le^a was demonstrable by standard hemagglutination tests in the maternal serum. Although none of the cord sera contained similarly demonstrable anti-Le^a, 12 of them were found to contain some IgG anti-Le^a when a sensitive enzyme-linked immunosorbent assay (203) assay was used. The authors (205) concluded that IgG anti-Le^a does cross the placenta but does not cause HDN because of low levels of Le^a on fetal red cells. However, it seems likely that the very low levels of anti-Le^a in the cord serum (i.e. demonstrable only by the immunosorbent assay) must have contributed to the benign situation, particularly in view of the findings cited above (127-130) that many samples of cord blood red cells can be shown to be Le(a+) when the IAT is used.

Unlike anti-Le^b that are described in detail below, anti-Le^a react to about the same degree with Le(a+) red cells of any ABO group. This is not surprising since, as explained above, the immunodominant sugars of A and B cannot be added to type 1 chains that carry Le^a, since those chains lack H (i.e. made by individuals genetically *sese*).

Anti-Le^b

Anti-Le^b is often present as a weak antibody in the sera of individuals who have made potent anti-Le^a. It is also common on its own and is then most often made (10,26,160) by persons with Le(a-b-) red cells who are non-secretors of ABH substances. Persons who are genetically *lele*, *Se*, that is ABH secretors who have Le(a-b-) red cells, make type 1 H (Le^d) and that structure seems similar enough to Le^b (see figures 9-2 and 9-3) that they do not regularly make anti-Le^b.

Theoretically, persons with Le(a+b-) red cells should be able to make anti-Le^b for neither their plasma nor their saliva contains Le^b substance. A number of such antibodies made by these persons have been reported (25,161-163). While the production of anti-Le^b by persons with Le(a+b-) red cells appears to be a comparatively rare event it should be added that nowadays Lewis phenotypes are seldom determined on the red cells of persons who make anti-Le^b since they do not provide useful information.

Two different forms of anti-Le^b have been described (25,124,164,165). Anti-Le^{bH} reacts with group O and sometimes A$_2$, but not with group A$_1$ or B, Le(b+) red cells. Further, it is neutralized by saliva from ABH secretors with red cells of the phenotypes Le(a-b+) and Le(a-b-). In other words, anti-Le^{bH} can be neutralized by saliva that contains H, or H and Le^b. Clearly, anti-Le^{bH} has a specificity that recognizes predominantly the type 1 H on group O red cells when that structure is not blocked by the addition of an immunodominant sugar of A or B. However, the L-fucose residue added by the actions of the *Le* gene-specified transferase must also be involved in the determinant with which the antibody reacts since anti-Le^{bH} does not agglutinate red cells that are Le(a-b-) and come from ABH secretors (i.e. red cells that carry type 1 H (Le^d) but not Le^b).

Anti-Le^{bL} on the other hand, reacts with Le(a-b+) red cells regardless of their ABO type and is inhibited by saliva that contains H and Le^b but not by saliva that contains

H but no Le^b. It seems that anti-Le^{bL} requires the L-fucose residues added by the actions of *Le* and *Se* gene-specified transferases to type 1 chains in order to be able to complex with its determinant and further, is able still to complex after the A or B immunodominant sugar has been added to Le^b. Obviously, if group A, B or AB red cells are to be typed for Le^b, anti-Le^{bL} must be used. False negative typings will result if the tests are performed with anti-Le^{bH}. While the reactions of anti-Le^{bH} and anti-Le^{bL} are profoundly influenced by the addition of the A and/or B immunodominant carbohydrates to the Le^b-bearing type 1 chain, or by the exposed Le^b antigen on group O cells in which no further addition to the type 1 chain occurs, anti-Le^{bL} is different from anti-A$_1$Le^b and anti-BLe^b. Anti-Le^{bL} reacts with group O Le(a-b+) red cells, anti-A$_1$Le^b and anti-BLe^b react only with red cells carrying Le^b and the appropriate A or B determinant.

Like anti-Le^a, most examples of anti-Le^b appear to be predominantly IgM in composition and to be non-red cell stimulated, complement binding antibodies. There is one report in the literature (166) that describes a case of HDN said to have been caused by anti-Le^b. If this was so, it follows that IgG anti-Le^b must exist since IgM antibodies are not able to cross the placenta and cause HDN. The single report was challenged (167) and defended (168) after it appeared. Part of the challenge was based on the rarity of IgG anti-Le^b and the rest on the known poor development of Le^b on cord red blood cells (see an earlier section of this chapter). In writing about the single case reported (166), Mollison et al. (169) comment that there was no clinical or hematological evidence of a hemolytic process.

While a few examples of anti-Le^b are capable of causing in vitro hemolysis of Le(b+) red cells, such sera are rarer than examples of anti-Le^a that hemolyze Le(a+) cells. Although there is no doubt that occasional examples of anti-Le^b have caused in vivo destruction of Le(b+) red cells in ^{51}Cr survival studies (24,115), there is no well-documented report of anti-Le^b ever having caused a transfusion reaction in Whites or American Blacks (170). The situation may be different in some areas in Asia where Lewis antibodies are more potent (171). In the USA and Europe the overwhelming majority of examples of anti-Le^b are cold-reactive and, as discussed below, are of no clinical-significance. When an example of anti-Le^b reactive at 37°C is encountered, blood for transfusion can safely be selected by performing compatibility tests, with the patient's serum, at 37°C. There is no need to use Le(a-b-) blood or to type units and select those that are Le(b-).

The Incidence of Anti-Le^a and Anti-Le^b

The number of Lewis system antibodies found in any given service will be markedly influenced by the ethnic make-up of the population served. Most such antibodies are made in persons with Le(a-b-) red cells, a phenotype found in some 6% of Whites and between 20 to 30% of Blacks. Clearly Lewis antibodies will be expected three to four times more often in Blacks than in Whites. The in vitro antibody detection methods used will also influence the number of these antibodies found. If room temperature tests are performed, more Lewis system antibodies can be expected than if only tests at 37°C are used. Conversely, if methods such as PEG and Polybrene are used, some Lewis system antibodies active only in room temperature tests in saline will be detected at 37°C. Because of variation in test methods used, figures for the incidence of Lewis antibodies in older surveys will not be given. Instead it will be reported that in tests on 72,000 individuals in Paris, Salmon et al. (251) found 249 anti-Le[a], 49 anti-Le[x] (for a definition of that specificity see below) and 31 anti-Le[b], for an incidence of one Lewis antibody in every 218 patients. Of the 31 anti-Le[b], 29 were anti-Le[bH], two were anti-Le[bL]. In the Transfusion Service at Duke University Medical Center in the year 1994, we tested samples from approximately 40,000 patients. We found 167 anti-Le[a] and 39 anti-Le[b] for an incidence of Lewis antibodies the same as that seen in France.

Anti-Le[c]

As already described, this antibody reacts with the Le(a-b-c+d-) red cells of persons genetically *lele, sese*. In fact, the antibody complexes with the unaltered type 1 chains that those red cells have taken up from the plasma. Although anti-Le[c] has been made in a human (113) more potent examples of the antibody have been made by animal immunization (99,109,114,172). As far as this author is aware, no clinical significance for anti-Le[c] has ever been claimed.

Anti-Le[d]

As described earlier, this antibody reacts with the Le(a-b-c-d+) red cells of persons genetically *lele, Se*. In fact, the antibody defines the type 1 H that those red cells have taken up from the plasma. Like anti-Le[c], anti-Le[d] has been produced by immunization of animals (99,112, 114,172).

Anti-Le[a] plus Anti-Le[b]

As mentioned above, a number of individuals with red cells of the phenotype Le(a-b-) have antibody activity in the serum such that it appears that both anti-Le[a] and anti-Le[b] are present. There is no doubt that in some cases both antibodies have been made. For example, in at least one reported case (24), the anti-Le[b] was clearly demonstrable after the anti-Le[a] had been neutralized. There are no doubts either that on some occasions a potent example of anti-Le[a] can give reactions that are taken to indicate the presence of anti-Le[a] plus anti-Le[b]. The red cells of persons genetically *Le, Se* usually type as Le(a-b+). However, as explained, such individuals make both Le[a] and Le[b] in the plasma so that both antigens may be present on the red cells. Potent enough examples of anti-Le[a] may detect the trace amount of Le[a] on the supposed Le(a-b+) red cells. For those workers interested in making the serological distinction between a very potent anti-Le[a] and a true mixture of anti-Le[a] plus anti-Le[b], simple saliva inhibition studies can be used. If the antibody is anti-Le[a], its activity against Le(a+b-) and Le(a-b+) cells will be neutralized by the addition of saliva from an individual with Le(a+b-) red cells. If the antibodies are anti-Le[a] plus anti-Le[b], the addition of saliva from an Le(a+) individual will neutralize the activity of the serum against Le(a+b-) but not against Le(a-b+) cells. Saliva from an individual with Le(a-b+) red cells cannot be used in this differential inhibition since it contains both Le[a] and Le[b] substance. Much of the time making the differentiation just described is an academic exercise. If the patient with the antibody or antibodies requires transfusion, compatibility tests at 37°C, using the patient's serum, will select suitable Le(a-b-) units (or Le(a-b+) units if the antibody reacting with such cells is only active at temperatures below 37°C). However, if the patient requires a large number of units of blood and a decision is made to neutralize the Lewis antibodies in vivo (see below) it is worth knowing if plasma from an Le(a+) and from an Le(b+) donor must be transfused, or if total antibody inhibition can be expected from the infusion of plasma from just an Le(a+) donor. Obviously, the in vivo antibody neutralization pattern will be the same as the saliva inhibition pattern just described.

Like anti-Le[a] or anti-Le[b] when present alone, mixtures of anti-Le[a] and anti-Le[b] occur as non-red cell stimulated, complement binding antibodies. Some examples of anti-Le[a] plus anti-Le[b] as described in this section may be what has been called anti-Le[x] (see below). This may pertain particularly to those examples that can be totally inhibited by saliva that contains Le[a] but not Le[b].

Anti-A₁Le[b] and Anti-BLe[b]

As described earlier, the addition of the A or B immunodominant sugar to the Le[b] structure results in the formation of determinants defined by these antibodies.

Although it was not appreciated at the time, an antibody described by Seaman et al. (173) in 1968, was the first example of anti-A_1Le^b. The antibody was made by an individual with red cells of the phenotype A_1B Le(a-b-) and reacted with A_1 or A_1B Le(a-b+) red cells but not with those that were A_2 or O, Le(a-b+) nor with those that were A_1, A_1B, A_2 or O Le(a-b-). Neutralization studies showed that the only saliva samples that would inhibit the antibody were those of A_1 and A_1B, ABH secretors. Some time later (2,18) it was shown that glycosphingolipids carrying A_1Le^b and BLe^b are present in the plasma of persons genetically A^1, Le, Se, and B, Le, Se, respectively. These two antigens can be taken up by lymphocytes as well as by red cells (21,174,175). As far as we aware, neither anti-A_1Le^b nor anti-BLe^b has complicated the transfusion of red cells.

Anti-A_1Le^d and Anti-BLe^d

In 1958, Andersen (176) described an antibody made in an individual with red cells of the phenotype A_2, Le(a-b+), that reacted with group A_1, Le(a-b-) and less strongly with group A_2, Le(a-b-) cells, but only when those cells were from ABH secretors. The exact specificity of the Magard serum, as it was known for many years, remained unclear until the already described biochemical structure of A_1Le^d (type 1 A) was established. It is of considerable interest that Andersen (176) postulated that Se in the absence of Le caused an altered expression of A and that the Magard antibody was detecting that altered A. That idea was advanced in 1958; almost 20 years later (177) it became appreciated that the Magard serum was the first described example of anti-A_1Le^d, an antibody that defines type 1 A. Like A_1Le^b and BLe^b, A_1Le^d and BLe^d can be taken up by lymphocytes as well as by red cells (21,174,175). Again, neither anti-A_1Le^d nor anti-BLe^d seem to have complicated red cell transfusions.

Anti-ILe^{bH}

An antibody in the serum of an individual with A_1, Le(a-b-) red cells, that reacted with group O or group A_2, Le(a-b+) red cells only when those cells were I+, was described by Tegoli et al. (178). The antibody was inhibited by the saliva of persons with O or A_1, Le(a-b+), I+, and A_1, Le(a-b+), I-, i+ (see Chapter 10) red cells. It was not inhibited by saliva from persons with red cells of the O or O_h, Le(a+b-), I+ phenotypes. It was concluded that the antibody was defining an antigen made by individuals with functioning Le and Se genes in whom I was present on the red cells. At least one other example of anti-

ILe^{bH} has been described (179).

The Antigen Le^x and the Antibody that Defines It

In 1949, Andresen and Jordal (180) described an agglutinin at first called anti-X, that was later renamed anti-Le^x (129,132,181), that reacted with all red cells tested except those of the Le(a-b-) phenotype. The initial differentiation between anti-Le^x and other Lewis system antibodies was that anti-Le^x agglutinated 90% of cord blood red cell samples while those cells typed as Le(a-b-) with other Lewis system antibodies. Although Andresen (35,181) originally suggested that production of Le^x is dependent on the presence of an additional Lewis system gene, no evidence in support of that concept has emerged. Accordingly, Sturgeon and Arcilla (65) concluded that genetic control of production of Le^a, Le^b and Le^x rests with Le. At the serological level, the reactions of anti-Le^x can be explained by considering it as anti-Le^a and anti-Le^b in an inseparable form. That is to say, adsorption studies do not separate anti-Le^x into anti-Le^a and anti-Le^b although sera that contain anti-Le^x sometimes contain anti-Le^a and anti-Le^b as well (186).

The reactions of anti-Le^x with cord blood red cells can be in part explained by later findings that many cord blood samples will react with anti-Le^a if the indirect antiglobulin test is used (127 and see section above on development of Lewis antigens). While anti-Le^a is usually made by persons who are secretors of ABH substances and anti-Le^b by persons who are ABH non-secretors, anti-Le^x is most often but not invariably made by A, B or AB, Le(a-b-) persons who secrete ABH substances. Clearly if some individuals can make separable anti-Le^a and anti-Le^b while others can make those two antibodies and anti-Le^x, it follows that the rules regarding the secretor-non-secretor status of Lewis system antibody-makers are not inviolate.

Arcilla and Sturgeon (182-185) reported that amniotic fluids from fetuses genetically Le, sese contained high levels of Le^x that fell as Le^a appeared. However, such a conclusion would have to be dependent on the antibodies used and predetermination as to which would be called anti-Le^a and which anti-Le^x.

Anti-Le^x is efficiently inhibited by saliva that contains Le^a, weakly by saliva that contains Le^b and, surprisingly, partially by saliva from Le(a-b-) non-secretors (180,181). Inhibition by Le^b-containing saliva is more efficient than that effected by saliva from Le(a-b-) non-secretors.

The exact biochemical structure of Le^x is not yet known (52). Although the information that is available is discussed in more detail below in the section on biochemistry of the Lewis antigens, the serological reactions of anti-Le^x can be explained in large part by the simple statement that a series of elegant biochemical studies (52,182,187-190) have suggested that the determinant recognized by anti-Le^x is smaller than those recognized by anti-Le^a and anti-Le^b and is contained within both the Le^a and Le^b structures. No matter what the exact structure of Le^x, anti-Le^x can be regarded as inseparable anti-Le^a plus anti-Le^b, for practical transfusion purposes.

Monoclonal Lewis System Antibodies

A number of monoclonal antibodies suitable for determining Lewis phenotypes have been produced (189,191-193,244,250,293-295) some of them are available commercially. Like some human Lewis antibodies, some of the MAb have been found to be cytotoxic to white cells (see below). The later section on the X and Le^y tissue antigens describes findings made exclusively with monoclonal antibodies.

Lewis Antigens and Antibodies in Pregnancy

It has been known for some time (25,194,195) that red cell Lewis antigens are much weaker in pregnant than in non-pregnant women. Indeed, some women with red cells of the Le(a-b+) phenotype may lose Le^b altogether while pregnant and have red cells that type as Le(a-b-). The finding of Schachter et al. (196) that the serum level of the *A* gene-specified N-acetyl-galactosaminyl transferase is dramatically reduced in pregnancy, suggested that a similar explanation may apply to the reduction or loss of Lewis system antigens. However, on investigation, Hammer et al. (197) found that the situation is quite different. In pregnant and non-pregnant women, the level of Le^b-active glycolipid in the blood is nearly the same. The authors (197) found that in non-pregnant women two thirds of the Le^b-active glycolipid is reversibly bound to plasma lipoprotein and the rest is attached to red cells. In pregnancy the ratio of lipoprotein to red cell mass increases more than fourfold so that much more of the available Le^b-active glycolipid is attached to plasma lipoprotein and a smaller proportion is red cell-bound.

There seems little doubt that some pregnant women can form anti-Le^b while their red cell Le^b antigen level is depressed. The incidence of the antibody is higher in pregnant women than in others (133) and one of us (198) has seen a case in which a woman who was seven months pregnant had a very strong anti-Le^b in her serum but when bled, as a potential antibody donor three months after her child was delivered, had no antibody in her

serum and had Le(a-b+) red cells.

Workers who undertake prenatal serological studies, particularly for clinics whose patients include many who are Black, will not need to be told that anti-Le^b and to a lesser extent anti-Le^a, are very common in the sera of pregnant women. Since neither of these specificities causes HDN, a great deal of time, effort and money can be spent in detecting and identifying the antibodies with no practical benefit to the patient. The argument that antibody identification is necessary in case the mother requires transfusion at the time of delivery is fallacious. First, very few women need transfusion at delivery. Second, even in those who do, blood compatible in in vitro tests performed at 37°C is perfectly suitable for patients with anti-Le^a or anti-Le^b (or both) in the serum. The best solution to the overabundance of anti-Le^b in prenatal samples that we have heard is that devised by Steane (199). When his antibody identification service was about to collapse under the sheer volume of work involved in detecting and identifying anti-Le^b in the sera of pregnant women, the screening cells were changed. Those used in the revised system carried, between them, all antigens to which clinically-relevant antibodies might be directed but were all Le(a-b-)!

The In Vitro Inhibition of Lewis System Antibodies

There are several materials that have structures similar enough to the Lewis determinants that they will effect neutralization of Lewis system antibodies. The materials range from gum arabic (200) that neutralizes anti-Le^a, to commercially-prepared materials (201,234) to synthetic antigens (202) that can also be used in solid-phase antibody quantitation (203). While there is no doubt that these materials work, blood bankers should remember that saliva works just as well and if collected from staff members, is much less expensive (i.e. free!). A method for the treatment of saliva for use in antibody inhibition tests is given by Judd (204). Once prepared as described, the saliva can be stored frozen for many years without loss of activity. It has been said (200) that if red cells are added directly to saliva, hemolysis may occur. This problem is easily overcome by mixing the saliva with an equal volume of saline. One of us (PDI) has always found sufficient amounts of Le^a and Le^b substance in saliva that the 1 in 2 dilution in saline does not impair the ability of the saliva to inhibit antibodies.

The major use of these materials is to block activities in sera that contain Lewis system antibodies, so that other antibodies simultaneously present can be detected and identified (233). Accordingly, they are of most use with sera that react with Le(a+) and with Le(b+) cells, if sufficient numbers of Le(a-b-) samples are not available.

The Clinical Significance of Lewis System Antibodies

As has already been stated, some examples of anti-Le^a have caused transfusion reactions and a few examples of anti-Le^b have been shown to be capable of at least some in vivo destruction of small aliquots of Le(b+) red cells used in survival studies. However, there are also huge numbers of Lewis system antibodies that are totally incapable of destroying antigen-positive red cells in vivo. One of the main reasons that these antibodies (particularly examples of anti-Le^b) are benign in vivo is that they are unable to complex with red cells, carrying the antigens against which they are directed, at 37°C. Unfortunately, many routine blood bankers have assumed that since some Lewis system antibodies destroy antigen-positive red cells in vivo, all antibodies in the system must be honored when blood is selected for transfusion. In 1981, Waheed et al. (206) reported on a nationwide survey to determine transfusion practices when Lewis antibodies were present. Most distressingly, they found that almost 60% of the respondents believed that when the patient's serum contained anti-Le^a or anti-Le^b that was reacting as an agglutinin in tests at room temperature or below, but was not active at 37°C or by the indirect antiglobulin test, antigen-negative blood must be selected for transfusion. Selection of suitable units had to be made by use of appropriate typing sera, in the opinion of the respondents. Even worse, over 63% of respondents believed that if the patient had a history of having anti-Le^a or anti-Le^b, but currently had no demonstrable antibody in the serum, antigen-negative units must still be selected by use of typing reagents. Unfortunately, these responses clearly indicate that well over half the blood bankers who answered the survey have not read the literature for there is abundant evidence that random units, compatible with the patients' sera in in vitro tests at 37°C, survive normally in vivo. Many of the data in the literature have been there for a very long time (127,147,207-211) and have more recently been reviewed by several different authors (169,171,212-218). In each of the reviews cited, the authors dogmatically state that antibody-screening and compatibility tests at temperatures below 37°C (which is where a majority of Lewis system antibodies are found) are not necessary since antibodies detected only in tests below 37°C HAVE NO CLINICAL SIGNIFICANCE. In line with these statements neither the AABB standards (219) nor the AABB Technical Manual (220) require that room temperature antibody-screening or compatibility be performed. Indeed, like the other books cited the AABB

Technical Manual (220) recommends that these tests NOT be done.

The cost of screening units with anti-Le^a and anti-Le^b must be astronomical when considered at a national level. First, because the most commonly used reagents are those made in goats or in hybridomas and because the production methods are reasonably complex, the cost of the reagents is high. Second, labor costs constitute at least 60 to 80% of the operating costs of most transfusion services so that the time consumed by the unnecessary tests could profitably be used for important tasks. Clearly it is time that blood bankers realize that enough is known about Lewis system antibodies that many of them should be ignored in transfusion therapy.

Those who have utilized a modern approach to these antibodies have found, once again, that the earlier reports (127,147,207-211) of their benign nature in vivo are completely accurate. Waheed et al. (221) reported on the transfusion of blood to patients with anti-Le^a or anti-Le^b in the serum, when that blood was selected solely by compatibility tests with the patient's serum. Those Lewis antibodies that caused hemolysis in vitro were excluded from the study (we do not understand why, obviously such antibodies demonstrate incompatibility very clearly), all others were included. In all, 207 patients with anti-Le^a or anti-Le^b in the serum were studied. A total of 995 compatibility tests were performed, 875 of which yielded negative reactions. By using the incidence of the phenotypes Le(a+b-) and Le(a-b+) in the donor population in the area, it becomes possible to calculate that between 290 and 310 of the units found to be compatible, must have carried the Le^a or Le^b antigen against which the serum contained the antibody. Of the 207 patients for whom 875 compatible units were found, 33 received a total, among them, of 222 units (one sincerely hopes that the service has instituted a type and screen and maximum surgical blood order schedule since the study was completed!). Again, use of phenotype incidence permits the calculation that of the 222 units transfused, between 70 and 80 must have carried the Le^a or Le^b antigen against which the patient had the antibody. Of the 33 patients transfused, records were available for 28. No transfusion reactions were reported and in all 28 cases the hemoglobin and hematocrit levels increased as expected (based on the amount of blood transfused) and were maintained over the next few weeks. In other words, blood selected for patients with anti-Le^a or anti-Le^b, using the patients' sera as the sole means of selection, survives normally even when it is antigen-positive and causes neither immediate nor delayed transfusion reactions. Identical conclusions were reached by others (222-225) not all of whom collected such extensive data.

AuBuchon et al. (333) described three examples of anti-Le^x reactive at 37°C. In one patient an in vitro monocyte monolayer assay suggested that the antibody might be clinically significant and a ^{51}Cr red cell survival study using Le(a-b+) red cells showed accelerated clearance of those cells. The authors suggested that patients with anti-Le^x active at 37°C should be transfused with Le(a-b-) red cells. Since, as described earlier, anti-Le^x reacts with both Le(a+b-) and Le(a-b+) red cells, blood compatible with the patient's serum in compatibility tests performed at 37°C would still seem suitable.

Even on those rare occasions that Lewis antibodies cause the in vivo clearance of antigen-positive red cells, the amount of cell destruction may be limited. There are a number of reasons for this. First, when a two component curve is seen in a cell survival study (particularly when Le(b+) red cells are injected into a patient with anti-Le^b) a whole unit of blood will often survive normally. When 1 ml of antigen-positive red cells are injected and say 20% of the test dose is destroyed within the first hour but the other 80% survives normally or near normally, antibody limitation is often the explanation. In other words, if a much larger quantity of blood is given, still only about 20% of 1 ml (obviously an amount too small to matter or to be noticed if a unit is transfused) will be destroyed because there are insufficient antibody molecules to bring about the destruction of the rest of the cells. The question about increased antibody production following the introduction of antigen-positive red cells is addressed at the end of this section.

Second, since Lewis antigens are present in the plasma, neutralization of some of the patient's antibody will occur if antigen-positive blood is used. Obviously, whole blood contains more plasma than do packed red cells but the latter product still contains enough plasma that appreciable antibody neutralization can be expected. Often, antibody neutralization by the plasma Lewis substance will occur before any appreciable red cell destruction takes place.

Third, as already explained, red cells lose their Lewis antigens into plasma as readily as they acquire them (226). Thus, Le(a-b+) red cells transfused into an Le(a-b-) individual will quickly become Le(a-b-) themselves. The Lewis substances that come off the red cells also act to neutralize any Lewis antibody present.

Fourth, as stated, anti-Le^{bH} reacts with group O but not with group A, Le(a-b+) red cells. Thus, a group A patient who has made anti-Le^{bH} can be transfused with (in vitro compatible) group A, Le(a-b+) red cells and no in vivo antigen-antibody complexes will form.

Some workers use antigen-negative blood, for transfusion to patients with clinically-insignificant anti-Le^a or anti-Le^b in the plasma, because they believe that the infusion of antigen-positive red cells may cause increased levels of antibody to be produced, or may cause the antibody being made to broaden its thermal range. While there is some evidence that such events occur rarely, the experience of most workers has been that secondary immune responses to Le^a and Le^b are seen only in those patients in whom the antibodies were active at 37°C before transfusion or the injection of purified Lewis substances (24,227,228). The de novo appearance of anti-Le^a or anti-Le^b after transfusion is a sufficiently rare event (229) that it may have been coincidental and not transfusion-induced at all (true, true and perhaps unrelated). The best piece of evidence in support of the statements about the benign nature of Lewis antibodies may be that although many workers, for many years, have been using (often antigen-positive) serologically compatible blood for transfusion to patients with cold-reactive Lewis antibodies, there seems to be only one claim (230) that such a practice has resulted in a delayed transfusion reaction.

In short, this long section can be summarized with the statement that red cells that are compatible in in vitro tests at 37°C, with the serum of a patient who has made any antibody in the Lewis system, can be expected to survive normally in vivo. The clinical significance of Lewis system antibodies that are cytotoxic to lymphocytes is discussed below.

The In Vivo Neutralization of Lewis Antibodies

When a patient has anti-Le^a and anti-Le^b in the serum and when both have been shown capable of destroying antigen-positive red cells in vivo, the antibodies can be neutralized to permit the transfusion of antigen-positive red cells. The first case of this type was reported by Mollison et al. (24) when the alternative was to try to obtain many group B, Le(a-b-) units. Either purified Le^a or Le^b concentrates, or plasma from Le(a+) and/or Le(b+) donors can be used to effect antibody neutralization. In the case reported (24), the patient's antibodies were neutralized in vivo and many units of Le(a-b+) blood were transfused. Some days later, the anti-Le^a and anti-Le^b were again present in the patient's plasma, now in stronger forms (both had been clearly active at 37°C before being neutralized). The direct antiglobulin test became positive because many of the transfused Le(a-b+) cells were still in the patient's circulation, but before any in vivo cell destruction began, the transfused cells shed their Le^b antigen, became Le(a-b-) and the DAT became negative. This process of in vivo antibody neutralization to permit the use of antigen-positive blood has since been used by others (231,232). It is not yet known whether the fear of Andorka et al. (231), that the IgG anti-Le^a that formed after an initial course of in vivo antibody neutralization might be harder to neutralize on a second occasion, is justified. It may well be that plasma from an Le(a+) donor contains enough Le^a substance that an IgG anti-Le^a could still be neutralized.

While it may be tempting to transfuse plasma containing Le^a and/or Le^b to inhibit Lewis antibodies in vivo to permit the transfusion of antigen-positive blood, the procedure should probably not be undertaken lightly. First, as described in earlier sections of this chapter, many examples of anti-Le^a and, more frequently, anti-Le^b, do not cause in vivo red cell destruction. In other words, on many occasions the transfusion of antigen-positive blood will not result in any untoward events nor accelerated in vivo clearance of the antigen-positive red cells. Second, the in vivo neutralization of Lewis system antibodies presumably results in the formation of immune complexes in the patient's circulation. It is not yet known if such immune complex formation results in any long-term deleterious consequences. Third, as is true of any unnecessary transfusion, the risk of disease transmission is unjustifiably increased any time a non-essential blood product is transfused.

Cytotoxic Lewis System Antibodies and Renal Transplantation

Several of the plasma Lewis substances are taken up by lymphocytes via the same mechanism (1) by which they attach to red cells. Indeed, a number of authors (2,21,97,106,126,174,175,235-237) have reported that just as with red cells, all lymphocyte Lewis antigens are derived from the plasma. In spite of this, one series of experiments involving in vitro lymphocyte culture indicated that Lewis antigens are intrinsic to lymphocytes (252). Regardless of how Lewis antigens reach the lymphocyte membrane, there are no doubts that Lewis antibodies are often cytotoxic to such cells (21,126,175, 193,235,236,238-244).

The role of the Lewis system in renal transplantation has been vigorously debated. Oriol et al. (242) performed a retrospective analysis on the effects of Lewis incompatibility in renal transplant recipients. Because the kidney donors had not been typed, the analysis considered that recipients who had *Le* and/or *Se* (as determined by red cell typing and saliva secretion studies) had received a Lewis compatible kidney while recipients with Le(a-b-) red cells who were non-secretors of ABH substances were considered to have received a Lewis incompatible graft. It was felt that any significant differences would still be seen since 255 recipients were included so that the figures could be expected to overcome the fact that a small number of *lele*, *sese* recipients would have received a kidney from an *lele*, *sese* donor. The recipients were divided into four groups: Le and

HLA matched; Le matched, HLA mismatched; Le mismatched, HLA matched; and Le and HLA mismatched. From the mean survival times of the grafts is was concluded that both HLA and Lewis matching are significant in renal transplantation. Those recipients with an HLA and Lewis matched kidney had the best survival times, those with an HLA and Lewis mismatched kidney, the worst. The groups with an HLA matched, Lewis mismatched or an HLA mismatched, Lewis matched kidney showed about the same survival rate. Thus, it seemed to the investigators (242) that the effect of HLA and Lewis mismatching were separate and additive. A number of other studies (253-259) appeared to support a role for Lewis matching (i.e. *Le* recipients to receive kidneys from *Le* or *lele* donors, *lele* recipients only from *lele* donors) in kidney transplantation although different investigators did not agree on the significance of the event. The same workers who had reported that the Lewis antigens are intrinsic structures on lymphocytes (252) showed that the Lewis gene products induce lymphoproliferative responses in vivo (243). It should be stressed that the studies cited considered Lewis (and HLA) matching and not the presence of Lewis system antibodies, detected by conventional tests, in the patients. However, using the ELISA assay that they had developed earlier (203), Spitalnik et al. (260) did find Lewis system antibodies in some of the patients.

When Salmon et al. (251) reviewed renal allograft survival times in a large series of patients, they found no significant effect attributable to the presence or absence of *Le*. However, when the effects of HLA and Lewis matching were combined, the survival times were better than those in the series of patients who were matched for HLA alone. In contrast, Posner et al. (245) found no difference between Lewis matched and mismatched recipient when one year graft survival rates were reviewed.

The final answer regarding the role of Lewis matching in kidney transplantation may never be known. The introduction of cyclosporine as an immunosuppressant to prevent graft rejection has greatly reduced the importance of donor-recipient matching (261,262) and may have obviated the need for pretransplant transfusions to aid in the reduction of rejection rates (263).

Lewis Antigens on Platelets but not on Granulocytes or Monocytes

As would be expected, Lewis antigens are present on platelets (246). As described in Chapter 8, a large proportion of the A and B antigens on platelets are taken up from the plasma when type 1 glycosphingolipids are incorporated into platelet membranes (247,248). Thus it is not surprising that Lewis antigens are present on platelets since they are carried on the same type 1 chains as A and B. Unlike red cells and platelets, granulocytes and monocytes do not seem to take up Lewis antigens from the plasma (237,249).

Some Other Aspects of the Lewis System and Disease

Evans et al. (264) have suggested that the presence of Le^a substance in the urine may be a guide to response to treatment in patients with coeliac disease. The Le^a substance in the alimentary tract is a large molecule (265,266) that must be broken down by secretions from the ileal and jejunal mucosa before it can be excreted in the urine. The authors (264) believe that presence of dialysable Le^a substance in the urine may indicate return to normal ileal and jejunal secretion in treated patients and that its absence (or presence in very small amounts) may indicate a failure of the patient's disease to respond to treatment.

Lee et al. (267) noticed that of four patients with infectious mononucleosis complicated by antibody-induced hemolytic anemia (see Chapter 38), three had red cells that were phenotypically Le(a-b-) and that the fourth had cells that were Le(a+b-). Three of the four patients were shown to be non-secretors of ABH and the fourth was presumably a non-secretor since the red cells were Le(a+b-). It was suggested that perhaps in Le(a-b-) individuals, more i antigen is accessible to anti-i. It is known (268) that the ABO and Lewis structures described in this chapter are present on some chains that carry I and i. If Le(a-b-) cells have more i antigen available than do other cells, then perhaps lower levels of anti-i might cause hemolytic episodes. It is known that cord blood red cells, that usually type as Le(a-b-) or as Le(a+b-), carry large amounts of i.

Additional associations between the Lewis system and disease are discussed below in the section on the X and Le^y antigens.

The Lewis System and the Plant Kingdom

Although not widely used in routine blood group serology, the lectin BS-IV (GS-IV) made from the seeds of *Bandeiraea simplicifolia* (a.k.a. *Griffonia simplicifolia*) can be used as anti-Le^b (269). In fact, the lectin also has marked affinity for the type 2 chain based determinant Y (or Le^y, see below)(270,271).

In an earlier section some readily available substances that can be used to inhibit anti-Le^a and anti-Le^b sere described. Yamamoto (272) found that similar inhibition, particularly of anti-Le^a, can be achieved using extracts from the fruit or seeds of species of higher plants. Wang et al. (273) found that a substance that will inhibit anti-Le^a is present in Chinese medicinal herbs.

The Antigens X (a second Le^x) and Y or Le^y

A large number of monoclonal antibodies developed in the hope that they would recognize determinants on malignant tissue cells of different types have been shown to have Lewis antigen-related specificity (274-292). In some instances the MAb recognize antigens present on red cells and tissues, in other instances the antigens are confined to, sometimes malignant, tissue cells. Some of the determinants defined are present when *Le* is inherited and active, others are structures in which the *Le* determined character serves as a core or a base to which other structures are added.

An antigen originally known as CD-15 or SSEA-1 (for Stage Specific Embryonic Antigen) (274,296) was later called X (297) and later still (298) Le^x. This last designation was particularly unfortunate because the antigen is not the same as the Le^x antigen found on red cells, that is described in an earlier section of this chapter. Accordingly, in this section the antigen will be called X, not Le^x. X is a common character in human and animal tissues, it is present as both a basic structure and as a sialoyl derivative. The X antigen in plasma is encoded by a gene closely linked to *Le* on chromosome 19 (299,300) the myeloid type of X is encoded by a gene on chromosome 11 (301,202). The X antigen is involved in cell-cell adhesion (285,303-311) hence its importance in metastasis of human cancers. The X antigen is based on a type 2 chain core structure, it is not present on red cells.

The Y or Le^y antigen is also a common structure on human and animal tissue cells, its synthesis is controlled by the products of the *Se* and *Le* genes. Like X, Y is based on a type 2 chain structure and like Le^b requires the actions of both *Se* and *Le* for its synthesis. Thus X and Y can be regarded as type 2 isomers of Le^a and Le^b respectively (298). Again like X, most glycolipids carrying Y have been isolated from adenomas or adenocarcinomas of the GI tract and mammary glands (312-314). The Y antigen accumulates in various tumors and hence has at least the potential to serve as a stage specific marker. Y is also involved in cell-cell adhesion, it is not found on red cells although its close similarity to Le^b results in some monoclonal antibodies being able to complex with both Y (Le^y) and Le^b.

Clearly since they are not present on red cells, X and Y (Le^y) will be less familiar to blood bankers than the antigens described earlier in this chapter. Additional information on the structures of X, sialoyl X and Y (Le^y) are given in the section on biochemistry of the Lewis system, readers wishing to learn more about the important roles of these antigens in human malignancies are referred to the many papers cited in that section.

The *Lele* Genes and Chromosome 19

The *Lele* locus is located on the short arm of chromosome 19 (315-320) at position 19p13.3. Chromosome 19 is home to many blood group loci: *LW* is between 19p13.2 and the centromere (321); *Lu* (Lutheran), *Hh*, and *Sese* are on the long arm of chromosome 19 (60,300,316,322,323) with *Lu* at 19q12-q13; *Hh* at 19q13 and *Sese* very close to *Hh*. In addition, the loci *Pep D* (Peptidase D); *C3* (third component of human complement); *APOC2*, *D1957* and *D1959* are members of the chromosome 19 linkage group.

Le is one of a series of genes that encode production of fucosyl transferases. In the language of the geneticists *FUT1*, *FUT2*, *FUT3*, *FUT5* and *FUT6* (*FUT* for fucosyl transferase) are genes on chromosome 19 (324). To blood bankers *FUT1* is better known as *H*, *FUT2* as *Se* and *FUT3* as *Le*. Clearly, polymorphisms exist at the *FUT1*, *FUT2* and *FUT3* loci, to account for *Hh*, *Sese* and *Lele*, respectively. *FUT3* and *FUT6* may be involved in the production of X (see earlier, the tissue antigen known as Le^x, not the red cell antigen called by the same name). *FUT6* and *FUT2* may jointly control the synthesis of the tissue antigen, Le^y.

Throughout this chapter thus far, *le* has been described as a silent allele of *Le*, that is to say, in the genotype *lele* no *Le* gene-specified fucosyl transferase is made. In fact the symbol *le* describes a series of different genes. As explained in detail below, four different amino acid substitutions lead to the production of defective transferase (317-319,325,326). It is possible that one or more of these defective enzymes is involved in the production of low levels of Lewis substances sometimes seen (327) in the tissues and saliva of individuals with Le(a-b-) red cells.

Introduction to the Biochemistry of Lewis Antigens

The antigens of the Lewis system (Le^a and Le^b) are not synthesized by red cell progenitors in the bone marrow. They are antigens of the secretions which are acquired by red cells via a passive adsorption process (3,13). In this respect the Lewis antigens are unlike the antigens of all the other blood group systems except the Chido/Rodgers system (see Chapter 27). The realization that Lewis antigens are not red cell antigens in the strictest sense is fundamental to an understanding of their structure, biosynthesis and genetic basis. The description of the molecular basis of A, B and H antigens given in Chapter 8 alluded to the fact that there are two $\alpha(1\rightarrow2)$ fucosyltransferase genes, one of which encodes the H-transferase (*FUT1*) which is responsible for intrinsic H antigen on red cells and another which has historically been described as the product of the *Secretor* gene but is now known as *FUT2*. The $\alpha(1\rightarrow2)$ fucosyltransferase produced by the *FUT2* generates H antigen in secretions but not in red cells. The *Lewis* (*Le*) gene encodes yet another fucosyltransferase gene which has the ability to add L-fucose to suitable acceptor molecules in either the $\alpha(1\rightarrow3)$ or the $\alpha(1\rightarrow4)$ linkage.

The structure of the Le^a and Le^b antigens has been known for many years from structural studies of blood group substances derived, in the main, from ovarian cyst fluid (23) but the nature of the fucosyltransferases that synthesize these antigens has only been unraveled comparatively recently. Put simply, when the *Le* gene (*FUT3*), which encodes an }$\alpha(1,3/1,4)$ fucosyltransferase, catalyses the addition of L-fucose to acceptors which contain the terminal sequence Gal$\beta1\rightarrow$3GlcNAc (type 1 precursor chains) the fucose residue is added to carbon 4 of the GlcNAc residue and the structure recognized by anti-Le^a is formed (see figure 9-2). If the product of the *Secretor* gene (*FUT2*) is expressed it catalyses the addition of L-fucose to carbon 2 of the terminal Gal residue to create H antigen (see figure 9-2). If both *FUT2* and *FUT3* are expressed two fucose residues are added to the acceptor molecule and the Le^b antigen is formed (see figure 9-2). Since the H antigen can be converted to A or B antigen by the action of the product of the *ABO* gene, structures like ALe^b, BLe^b, as well as HLe^b can be also be synthesized. In the strictest sense the foregoing summary defines the totality of the Lewis blood group system-a single gene gives rise to an $\alpha(1,4)$ fucosyltransferase which can create Le^a antigen on type 1 precursor chains and Le^b antigen on H type 1 precursor chains.

Apparent complications have arisen because the type 1 precursor chain has been described by some as Le^c antigen and H type 1 precursor chain as Le^d antigen. Clearly Le^c and Le^d are not generated by the action of the Lewis gene (see figure 9-3) and so these names are inappropriate and, worse than that, are misleading.

Real complications have arisen because the *Le* gene product is "bigamous" rather than "monogamous", that is, it can fucosylate not only type 1 but also type 2 precursor chains. Fucosylation of type 2 precursor chains requires an $\alpha(1,3)$ fucosyltransferase activity. The *Le* gene (*FUT3*) product has both $\alpha(1,4)$ and $\alpha(1,3)$ fucosyltransferase activity and in this respect is unlike the other six human fucosyltransferases that have been studied in detail (with the possible exception of *FUT5*, the other six members have $\alpha(1,3)$ fucosyltransferase activity but do *not* have α(1,4) fucosyltransferase activity (see section on the family of α(1,3) fucosyltransferases later in this chapter). When the *Le* gene product fucosylates a type 2 precursor chain the antigen known as Le[x] is formed and in the case of H type 2 precursor chains the antigen Le[y] is formed (see figure 9-5). Similarly the action of the ABO transferase can produce ALe[y] and BLe[y]. The term Le[x] has also been used to mean Le[ab] (185) which is something completely different from Le[x] as defined above - mentioned in case it appeared that this subject was becoming easy to follow! A further complication arises because both type 1 and type 2 precursor chains can be sialylated by addition of a sialic acid residue in α(2,3) linkage to the non-reducing βGal of any type 1 or type 2 precursor chain. In this way sialyl-Le[a] and sialyl-Le[x] antigens are created (see figure 9-5). As will be apparent, what was called Le[x] in the section on the serology of the Lewis system is not the same as what is called Le[x] in this section on biochemistry of the system. The Le[x] of this section is the antigen called X in the serology section. A review of what is written in the serology and biochemistry sections will rapidly reveal the reason, a blood group serologist (PDI) and a biochemist (DJA) have different views of X/Le[x] at both the practical and the philosophical level.

All these complications are reviewed by Henry et al. (334). As far as transfusion practice is concerned only Le[a] and Le[b] are of major concern but in terms of biology, in general, the antigens Le[x] and sialyl-Le[x] are far more important (see section on fucosyltransferase family at the end of this chapter).

Having listened frequently to my co-author PDI (and several other blood group fanatics) describe the Rh blood group system at length, delighting in its apparent complexity, it was a refreshing experience to read "The Lewis system is perhaps the most complicated blood group system in humans. The type, amount and size of a particular antigen formed depends on the interaction of a range of products coded by alleles of at least three genetically independent loci; *Lewis*, *Secretor* and *ABO*." (335). The aforementioned blood group fanatics answer this comment by pointing out that all workers (including DJA, see above) acknowledge that Lewis is not really a blood group system at all, but a system of the secretions.

Cloning the *Lewis* Gene (*FUT3*)

The *Lewis* (*Le*) gene was cloned from experiments designed to find genes with α(1→3) fucosyltransferase activity. This may at first sight seem surprising since the Le[a] and Le[b] antigens are formed by the action of an α(1→4) fucosyltransferase acting on type 1 precursor chains (see figure 9-2) but various lines of evidence

FIGURE 9-5 Structure of Le[x], Le[y], Sialyl-Le[x] and Sialyl-Le[a]

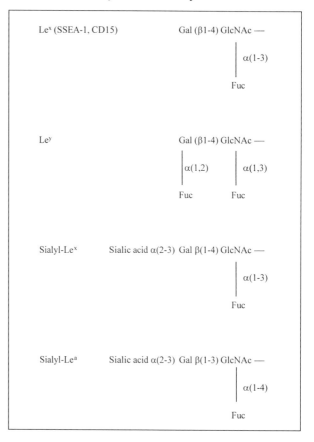

(reviewed in 336) suggested that the Lewis enzyme could also catalyze the transfer of fucose to carbon 3 of the GlcNAc of type 2 precursor chains to form the antigen known as Le[x] or SSEA-1 (stage-specific embryonic antigen) (see figure 9-5). A cDNA expression library prepared from a Lewis positive mammalian cell line (A431) was used to transfect COS-1 cells which lack any endogenous α(1→3) fucosyltransferase activity (COS-1 cells are known to express type 2 precursor chains). The transfected cells were then screened for the expression of the antigen SSEA-1 by plating them onto dishes coated with anti-SSEA-1 and looking for cells that adhered to the plate. The cloned α(1→3) fucosyltransferases could then be isolated from the SSEA-1 positive adherent cells. Using this experimental approach, Kukowska-Latallo et al. (315) isolated a full length cDNA with an open reading frame which predicted a protein of 361 amino acids with an N-terminal domain of 15 amino acids, a transmembrane domain of 19 amino acids and a large C-terminal domain of 327 amino acids. The C-terminal domain contained two signal motifs for N-glycosylation which were shown to be utilized in vitro. The overall structure of the predicted protein is that of a type 2 protein typical of glycosyltransferases. The protein encoded by this cDNA was shown to exhibit both $\alpha(1\rightarrow3)$ and $\alpha(1\rightarrow4)$ fucosyltransferase activity (315) and the enzymatic activity was shown to be located in the C-terminal 319 amino acids. The recombinant transferase was shown to be able to effect the synthesis of Le[a], Le[b], and Le[x] (SSEA-1) antigens as well as sialyl-Le[a] and sialyl-Le[x] structures (see figures 9-2 and 9-5) (315,337,338). These results all indicate that the cloned transferase is the product of the *Le* gene since they mirror results obtained with Lewis transferase purified from human milk (339) but clear and unambiguous evidence that this is indeed the case has come from studies of rare Lewis negative individuals (*le* genes) who have enzyme inactivating mutations in the *FUT3* gene (see next section).

Molecular Bases of the Lewis Negative and Lewis Weak (Le[w]) Phenotypes

Several mutations in the coding region of the *FUT3* gene have been associated with inactivation of the fucosyltransferase. Koda et al. (317) found two mutations in the *FUT3* gene of a Lewis negative Japanese. One mutation changed Leu20 to Arg and the other Gly170→Ser. Chimeric cDNAs were produced which expressed only one of these mutations and these were expressed in COS cells to see if both mutations inactivated the Lewis transferase. The results showed that Gly170 to Ser produced an inactive enzyme whereas Leu20 to Arg resulted in an active enzyme as judged by the expression of Le[b] antigen on the surface of the COS cells. Mollicone et al. (319) also found the Leu20 to Arg mutation (denoted L1 mutation by these authors) in several Indonesians who have Lewis negative red cells but express Lewis antigens in saliva. This is a particularly interesting mutation because it occurs in the transmembrane domain of the enzyme rather than in the catalytic C-terminal domain (see figure 9-6). Presumably the replacement of nonpolar leucine for the basically charged arginine affects the efficiency/stability of membrane insertion resulting in quantitatively less enzyme in the membrane of the Golgi and thereby weak Lewis antigen expression.

Mollicone et al. (319) also describe another mutation, Ile356→Lys (denoted L2 mutation) found in Lewis negative Indonesians. Homozygosity for this mutation was found in 18 of 19 Indonesians who were Lewis negative both on their red cells and in their saliva. Expression of the Ile356Lys mutant resulted in an inactive enzyme. The Ile356Lys mutation has also been found in Japan (320). The Leu20Arg mutation was found in a second Japanese study (325) and also in a Swedish study (340).

Two further mutations Trp68→Arg and Thr105→Met

found originally in Sweden have not been found on separate alleles (318,340). In order to determine the significance of each mutation with respect to enzyme activity Elmgren et al. (341) constructed chimeric proteins. *FUT3* constructs with the Trp68Arg mutation but lacking the Thr105Met mutation generated an enzyme with only 1% of the activity of the wild type enzyme whereas *FUT3* constructs having Thr105Met without Trp68Arg were indistinguishable from the wild type enzyme. These results show that it is the homozygous presence of Trp68Arg that gives rise to the Le(a-b-) phenotype in these individuals. Orntoft et al. (342) describe an additional mutation (C445A) in a Lewis negative cancer patient which created a methionine residue at position 146. It is not clear if this mutation occurs in normal healthy donors. Information relating to these various mutations is summarized in figure 9-6.

Plasma $\alpha(1,3)$-fucosyltransferase Gene (*FUT6*) Deficiency

Mollicone et al. (343) found that 9% of individuals on the island of Java do not express an $\alpha(1,3)$ fucosyltransferase normally found in plasma and that 95% of those individuals who lack the plasma enzyme had the Lewis negative blood group phenotype. The linkage between enzyme deficiency and Lewis phenotype suggested that the gene for the plasma enzyme might be located in the same cluster of genes on chromosome 19 that contains the Lewis transferase gene (*FUT3*) and that the plasma enzyme might be encoded by either *FUT5* or *FUT6*. Cloning and sequencing the *FUT5* and *FUT6* genes from an individual with deficiency of this plasma enzyme revealed mutations in both genes (compared to wild type). Three point mutations which changed codons in the *FUT5* gene were identified (Arg173Cys, Pro187Leu, Thr388Met). Expression studies indicated that this mutant enzyme had the same activity as the wild type enzyme and so the mutations in the *FUT5* gene could not explain the plasma fucosyltransferase deficiency. When the *FUT6* gene was studied four single base pair mutations were identified within the coding region of the gene and three of these changed amino acids (in comparison with wild type sequence). The mutations resulted in the following changes, Pro124Ser, Glu247Lys and Tyr315 to a stop codon. Expression studies demonstrated that the mutation Pro124Ser does not inactivate the enzyme but that the other two mutations are inactivating and therefore *FUT6* is responsible for the plasma enzyme in wild type individuals. The mutations Glu247Lys and Tyr315stop in *FUT6* also correlate with plasma enzyme deficiency in Polynesia and Sweden (344).

FIGURE 9-6 Mutations Affecting the Function of the Lewis Gene (*FUT3*) Product

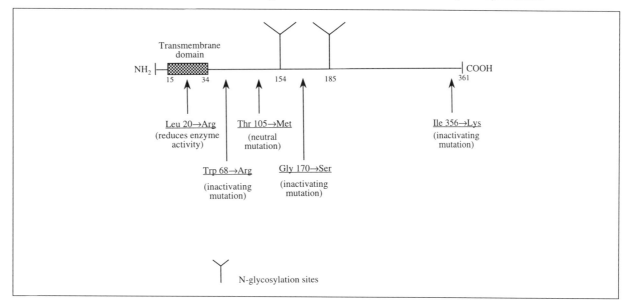

Cloning the Secretor Gene (*FUT2*) and the Molecular Basis of the Non-secretor Phenotype

In the work that resulted in the cloning of the H-transferase gene (*FUT1*) evidence was obtained for the existence of a second α(1→2) fucosyltransferase - that is, a cloned segment of the coding region of the H enzyme cross-hybridized with DNA fragments distinct from the *H* gene (345). Consequently, the H-transferase cDNA was used to screen chromosome 19 cosmid libraries to look for this second gene which was presumed to be the *Secretor* gene known to be located on chromosome 19 (346). One cosmid was found which contained two distinct segments which cross-hybridized with H-transferase cDNA and this was mapped to chromosome 19q13.3, the same site as *FUT1*. In order to map the relationship between *FUT1* and the candidate *Secretor* gene a series of overlapping cosmid clones (contig) was assembled. A five-cosmid contig spanning 100kb was assembled which contained *FUT1* and two candidate *Secretor* genes denoted *Sec1* and *Sec2*. *FUT1* and the *Sec2* locus were separated by approximately 35kb. In order to see if either *Sec1* or *Sec2* are transcribed, double-stranded cDNA prepared from human fetal brain mRNA was hybridized with biotinylated cosmid DNA and cosmids with bound cDNA selected with streptavidin-coated magnetic beads. A 500bp cDNA corresponding to *Sec2* was obtained which identified a 3.35kb transcript in colon, small intestine and lung but not in liver or kidney. The tissue distribution of the *Sec2* gene product mirrored that of the human *Secretor* gene product (346) suggesting that *Sec2* did indeed correspond to the *Secretor* gene. No transcripts corresponding to *Sec1* were obtained suggesting that it represents a pseudogene (346).

Sequence studies confirmed that *Sec1* is a pseudogene and that *Sec2* is the *Secretor* gene *FUT2* (347). The *Sec2* sequence predicts a protein of 332 amino acids and an isoform of 343 amino acids which has 11 additional N-terminal amino acids. Put another way, there are two 'in-frame' initiator codons (methionine). The first initiator methionine would yield a protein of 343 amino acids, the second would yield a protein of 332 amino acids. Two potential initiator codons account for the production of glycophorins C and D from a single gene (see Chapter 16). The N-terminal domain of the transferase is predicted to comprise either 3 or 14 amino acids depending on which isoform is translated, there is a hydrophobic transmembrane domain of 14 residues, and a large C-terminal domain of 315 amino acids which contains three potential N-glycosylation sites. The overall structure of the *Se* (*FUT 2*)-specified transferase therefore corresponds to a type 2 membrane spanning protein and is typical of glycosyltransferases in general. The Secretor transferase has substantial sequence homology with the H transferase in its C-terminal domain. Two of the N-glycosylation sites are in the same place and a sequence of 292 amino acids distal to Ala66 in the H transferase shows 68% homology with the Secretor transferase. Both the 'short' and 'long' isoforms of the enzyme have α(1→2) fucosyltransferase activity when expressed in COS-7 cells (347).

Approximately 20% of people are non-secretors of ABH substances (see earlier in this Chapter). Kelly et al. (347) found that 10 of 52 unselected people were homozygous for a mutation in the *Se* (*FUT 2*) gene which converted Trp143 to a termination codon and each of six individuals known to be non-secretors were found to be homozygous for the same mutation. This mutation produces a truncated protein lacking 189 amino acids at the C-terminus. Expression of the mutated protein in COS-7 cells confirmed that it is enzymatically inactive. The mutation Trp143→ter therefore seems to account for the blood group phenotype Le(a+b-) at least in Whites. Henry et al. (348) described a different mutation occurring in two Polynesians with the Le(a+b-) phenotype. In these cases Arg191 was mutated to a stop codon (see figure 9-7). This mutation would be predicted to result in a truncated protein lacking 141 amino acids from the C-terminal domain. Transfection of the mutated gene in COS-7 cells confirmed that it does produce an inactive enzyme (349). Two other nonsense mutations found in Japan and Taiwan resulted in Arg210STOP (350) and Trp283STOP (351) respectively. Koda et al. (350) described a *FUT2* deficient allele which is a fusion gene presumed to result from unequal crossover and comprising the 5′ region of the pseudogene (*Sec1*) and the 3′ region of *FUT2*.

Molecular Basis of the Partial-secretor Phenotype Le(a+b+)

The red cell phenotype Le(a+b+) is rare in Whites but is more common in other populations (Polynesians, Asians, Indonesians, Australian aborigines). The phenotype is associated with a partial-secretor type in which the secretions contain a level of ABH substance less than that found in White secretors (330). Examination of the

Secretor gene *FUT2* in Asians, Indonesians and Polynesians with this phenotype, has revealed a single base-pair mutation ntA385T which would change a single amino acid Ile129 to Phe in the resulting fucosyltransferase (349,352,353). Expression of this mutant gene in COS-7 cells revealed that it encodes an enzyme with the same apparent specificity as the "wild type" enzyme but with reduced fucosyltransferase activity (349). Comparative kinetic studies using phenyl-β-D-galactoside as acceptor revealed that the mutant transferase and the "wild-type" *FUT2* allele had a similar K_m but the V_{max} was five times lower for the mutant enzyme. Henry et al. (349) also review the occurrence of several other single nucleotide mutations in the *FUT2* gene only one of which changes an amino acid (Gly247 to Ser), in this case without apparent effect on fucosyltransferase activity.

The Family of α(1→3) fucosyltransferases

To summarize, there are five members of the α(1,3) fucosyltransferase family. Two members (*FUT4* and *FUT7*) have not yet been shown to exhibit polymorphism in man and both appear to have extremely important functions. Three members (*FUT3, FUT5, FUT6*) exhibit polymorphism and benign human null phenotypes are known for two of these (*FUT3, FUT6*). It would be interesting to know the consequences of a triple gene knockout which inactivated *FUT3, FUT5* and *FUT6* to see to what extent one enzyme in this cluster can compensate for the loss of another. Legault et al. (362) constructed a series of chimeric enzymes derived from *FUT3, FUT5* and *FUT6* and looked at the ability of each chimera to catalyze the synthesis of Le^x, sialyl Le^x, Le^a and sialyl

FIGURE 9-7 Mutations Affecting the Function of the Secretor Gene (*FUT2*) Product

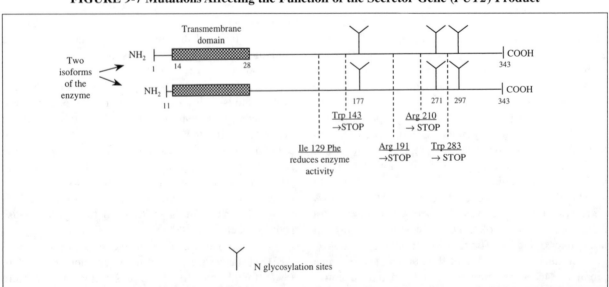

Le^a after transfection into a suitable cell line. The three wild type enzymes share approximately 85% amino acid sequence identity but whereas all three enzymes can fucosylate type 2 acceptors to produce Le^x and sialyl Le^x only the *FUT3* product can fucosylate type 1 acceptors to produce Le^a and sialyl Le^a. These authors concluded that the ability to fucosylate type 1 precursor chains was determined by about 11 amino acids in a region of the C-terminal catalytic domain of the enzyme proximal to the transmembrane domain. Xu et al. (363) came to similar conclusions. Since the *FUT3* product is the only wild type enzyme capable of generating Le^a and Le^b antigens it seems clear that these particular structures have far less importance in man than α-fucosylated structures created on a type 2 precursor chain (Le^x, Le^y, see figure 9-5). A preliminary general model for the three-dimensional structure of fucosyltransferases has been developed by analogy with the β-glucosyltransferase from bacterio-phage T4 whose crystal structure is known (364).

References

1. Marcus DM, Cass LE. Science 1969;164:553
2. Tilley CA, Crookston MC, Brown BL, et al. Vox Sang 1975;28:25
3. Watkins WM, Morgan WTJ. Vox Sang 1959;4:97
4. Mourant AE. Nature 1946;158:237
5. Ueyama R, Hanzaigaku-Zaschi 1939;13:51
6. Furuhata T, Ueyama R. Tokyo Izisinisi 1939;3120:271
7. Ueyama R. Jpn J Med Sci 1940;3:23
8. Andresen PH. Acta Path Microbiol Scand 1948;25:728
9. Grubb R. Nature 1948;162:933
10. Grubb R. Acta Path Microbiol Scand 1951;28:61
11. Brendemoen OJ. J Lab Clin Med 1949;34:538
12. Grubb R. Rev Hematol 1950;5:268
13. Sneath JS, Sneath PHA. Nature 1955;176:172
14. Mäkelä O, Mäkelä P. Ann Med Exp Fenn 1956;34:157
15. Levine P, Celano M. Vox Sang 1960;5:53
16. Mäkelä O, Mäkelä P, Kortekangas A. Ann Med Exp Fenn 1967;45:159
17. Nicholas JW, Jenkins WJ, Marsh WJ. Br Med J 1957;1:1458
18. Crookston MC, Tilley CA, Crookston JH. Lancet 1970;2:1110
19. Swanson J, Crookston MC, Yunis E, et al. Lancet 1971;1:396
20. Wrobel DM, McDonald I, Race C, et al. Vox Sang 1974;27:395
21. Mayr W, Pausch V. J Immunogenet 1976;3:367
22. Szymanski IO, Tilley CA, Crookston MC, et al. J Med Genet 1977;14:279
23. Watkins WM. In: Advances in Human Genetics, New York:Plenum 1980
24. Mollison PL, Polley MJ, Crome P. Lancet 1963;1:909
25. Brendemoen OJ. Acta Path Microbiol Scand 1952;31:579
26. Miller EB, Rosenfield RE, Vogel P, et al. Am J Phy Antrhopol 1954;12:427
27. Lewis M, Kaita H, Chown B. Am J Hum Genet 1957;9:274
28. Chandanayingyong D, Sasaki TT, Greenwalt TJ. Transfusion 1967;7:269
29. Anderson J. Vox Sang 1958;3:251
30. Morgan WTJ. In: Ciba Foundation Symposium on Biochemistry of Human Genetics. London:Churchill, 1959:194
31. Watkins WM. In: Ciba Foundation Symposium on Biochemistry of Human Genetics. London:Churchill, 1959:217
32. Ceppellini R. In: Ciba Foundation Symposium on Biochemistry of Human Genetics. London:Churchill, 1959:242
33. Ceppellini R. Folia Hered Pathol 1959;8:201
34. Morgan WTJ. Proc Roy Soc, Ser B 1960;151:308
35. Andresen PH. Am J Hum Genet 1961;13:396
36. Watkins WM. Proc 10th Cong ISBT. Basel:Karger, 1965:443
37. Watkins WM. Science 1966;152:172
38. Marr AMS, Donald ASR, Watkins WM, et al. Nature 1967;215:1345
39. Morgan WTJ, Watkins WM. Br Med Bull 1969;25:30
40. Ginsberg V. Adv Enzymol 1972;36:131
41. Kabat EA. In: Advances in Chemistry, Series 117. Washington,D.C.:Am Chem Soc, 1973:334
42. Watkins WM. Proc Roy Soc Lond (Biol) 1978;202:31
43. Watkins WM. Adv Hum Genet 1980;10:1
44. Watkins WM, Greenwell P, Yates AD. Immunol Comm 1981;10:83
45. Watkins WM, Yates AD, Greenwell P. Biochem Soc Transact 1981;9:186
46. Hanfland P, Graham H. Arch Biochem Biophys 1981;220:383
47. Johnson PH, Yates AD, Watkins WM. Biochem Biophys Res Comm 1981;100:1611
48. Prieels JP, Monnom D, Dolmans M, et al. J Biol Chem 1981;256:10456
49. Kukowaska-Latallo JF, Larsen RD, Nair RP, et al. Genes Dev 1990;4:1288
50. Lowe JB, Stoolman LM, Nair RP, et al. Cell 1990;63:475
51. Lowe JB. In: Immunobiology of Transfusion Medicine. New York:Marcel Dekker, 1994:3
52. Schenkel-Brunner H. Human Blood Groups. Vienna:Springer-Verlag, 1995:146
53. Kobata E, Grollman EF, Ginsberg V. Arch Biochem Biophys 1968;124:609
54. Oriol R, Danilovs J, Hawkins BR. Am J Hum Genet 1981;33:421
55. Kumazaki T, Yoshida A. Proc Nat Acad Sci USA 1984;81:4193
56. LePendu J, Cartron JP, Lemieux RU, et al. Am J Hum Genet 1985;37:749
57. Betteridge A, Watkins WM. Biochem Soc Transact 1986;13:1126
58. Ernst LK, Rajan JP, Larsen RD, et al. J Biol Chem 1989;264:3436
59. Sarnesto A, Kohlin T, Thurin J, et al. J Biol Chem 1990;265:15067
60. Larsen RD, Ernst LK, Nair RP, et al. Proc Nat Acad Sci USA 1990;87:6674
61. RajanVP, Larsen RD, Ajmera S, et al. J Biol Chem 1991;24:1158
62. Sarnesto A, Kohlin T, Hindsgaul O, et al. J Biol Chem 1992;267:2737
63. Annison EE, Morgan WTJ. Biochem J 1952;50:460
64. Lewis M, Kaita H, Chown B. Am J Hum Genet 1957;9:274
65. Sturgeon P, Arcilla MB. Vox Sang 1970;18:301
66. Boettcher B, Kenny R. Hum Hered 1971;21:334
67. Kabat EA, Bendich A, Bezer E. J Exp Med 1948;87:295
68. Grubb R, Morgan WTJ. Br J Exp Pathol 1949;30:198
69. Watkins WM, Morgan WTJ. Vox Sang (Old Series) 1955;5:1
70. Watkins WM, Morgan WTJ. Nature 1957;180:1038

71. Brown PC, Glynn LE, Holborow EJ. Vox Sang 1959;4:1
72. Morgan WTJ, Watkins WM. Br Med Bull 1959;15:109
73. Lodge TW, Usher A. Vox Sang 1962;7:329
74. Marcus DM, Grollman AP. J Immunol 1966;97:867
75. Lloyd KO, Kabat EA, Layug EJ. Biochemistry 1966;5:1489
76. Lloyd KO, Kabat EA, Rosenfield RE. Biochemistry 1966;5:1502
77. Marcus DM, Bastani A, Rosenfield RE, et al. Transfusion 1967;7:277
78. Lloyd KO, Kabat EA. Proc Nat Acad Sci 1968;61:1430
79. Lloyd KO, Kabat EA, Licerio E. Biochemistry 1968;7:2976
80. Grollman EF, Kobata A, Ginsberg V. J Clin Invest 1969;48:1489
81. Chester MA, Watkins WM. Biochem Biophys Res Comm 1969;34:835
82. Marcus DM. New Eng J Med 1969;280:994
83. Marcus DM. Ann NY Acad Sci 1970;169:161
84. Jarkovsky Z, Marcus DM, Grollman AP. Biochemistry 1970;9:1123
85. Vicari G, Kabat EA. Biochemistry 1970;9:3414
86. Lundblat A, Kabat EA. J Immunol 1971;106:1572
87. Rovis L, Anderson B, Kabat EA. Biochemistry 1973;12:5340
88. Rovis L, Kabat EA, Pereira MEA. Biochemistry 1973;12:5355
89. Savvas RS. Vox Sang 1975;29:280
90. Lemieux RU, Baker DA, Bundle DR. Canad J Biochem 1977;55:507
91. Crookston MC, Tilley CA. In: Human Blood Groups. Basel:Karger, 1977:246
92. Lemieux RU. Chem Soc Rev 1978;7:423
93. Prohaska R, Schenkel-Brunner H, Tuppy H. Eur J Biochem 1978;84:161
94. Hanfland P. Eur J Biochem 1978;87:161
95. Hanfland P, Kladetzky RG, Egli G. Chem Phys Lipids 1978;22:141
96. Yazawa S. Furukawa K. J Immunogenet 1980;7:137
97. Carton J-P, Mulet C, Bauvois B, et al. Blood Transf Immunohematol 1980;23:271
98. Oriol R. Blood Transf Immunohematol 1980;23:517
99. Hirsch HF, Graham HA. Transfusion 1980;20:474
100. Hanfland P, Graham HA. Arch Biochem Biophys 1981;210:383
101. Egge H, Hanfland P. Arch Biochem Biophys 1981;210:396
102. Dabrowski J, Hanfland P, Egge H, et al. Arch Biochem Biophys 1981;210:405
103. Oriol R, LePendu J, Sparkes RS, et al. Am J Hum Genet 1981;33:551
104. Ratcliffe RM, Baker DA, Lemieux RU. Carbohydr Res 1981;93:25
105. Lemieux RU, Baker DA, Weinstein WM, et al. Biochemistry 1981;20:199
106. Crookston MC, Tilley CA. In: Blood Groups and Other Red Cell Surface Markers in Health and Disease. New York:Masson, 1982:111
107. LePendu J, Lemieux RU, Oriol R. Vox Sang 1982;43:188
108. LePendu J, Lemieux RU, Lambert F, et al. Am J Hum Genet 1982;34:402
109. Iseki S, Masaki S, Shibasaki K. Proc Imp Acad Jpn 1957;33:492
110. Iseki S, Masaki S, Shibasaki K. Proc Imp Acad Jpn 1957;33:686
111. Lodge TW, Andersen J, Gold ER. Vox Sang 1965;10:73
112. Potapov MI. Probl Haemathol 1970;11:45 (In Russian, translated into English by Russian Language Studies Dept., Univ Cincinnati and into Lewis by Wilkinson SL).
113. Gunson HH, Latham V. Vox Sang 1972;22:344
114. Graham HA, Hirsch HF, Davies DM. In: Human Blood Groups. Basel:Karger, 1977:257
115. Mollison PL. Blood Transfusion in Clinical Medicine, 6th Ed. Oxford:Blackwell, 1979
116. Lodge TW. Biotest Bull 1982;3:196
117. Miller EB, Rosenfield RE, Vogel P. Am J Phys Anthropol 1951;9:115
118. Thompson JS. Unpublished observations, 1953 cited by Race RR, Sanger R. Blood Groups in Man, 2nd Ed. Oxford:Blackwell, 1954
119. Brendemoen OJ. Unpublished observations, 1953 cited by Race RR, Sanger R. Blood Groups in Man, 6th Ed. Oxford:Blackwell, 1975
120. Ikin EW. Unpublished observations, 1953 cited by Mourant AE. The Distribution of the Human Blood Groups. Oxford:Blackwell, 1954:438
121. Salmon C, Malassenet R. Rev Hematol 1953;8:183
122. Molthan L. Vox Sang 1980;39:327
123. Barnicot NA, Lawler SD. Am J Phys Anthropol 1953;11:83
124. Ceppellini R, Dunn LC, Innella F. Fol Hered Pathol 1959;8:261
125. Lawler SD, Marshall R, Roberts DF. Ann Hum Genet 1960;24:271
126. Park MS, Oriol R, Nakata S, et al. Transpl Proc 1979;11:1947
127. Cutbush M, Giblett ER, Mollison PL. Br J Haematol 1956;2:210
128. Jordal K, Lyndrup S. Acta Path Microbiol Scand 1952;31:476
129. Jordal K. Acta Path Microbiol Scand 1956;39:399
130. Lawler S, Marshall R. Vox Sang 1961;6:541
131. Kissmeyer-Nielsen F, Bastrup-Masden K, Stenderup A. Dan Med Bull 1955;2:202
132. Jordal K. Acta Path Micrbiol Scand 1958;42:269
133. Kissmeyer-Nielsen F. Scand J Haematol 1965;2:331
134. Issitt PD. In: Rhesus Problems in Clinical Practice. Groningen:Red Cross Blood Bank, 1979:58
135. Polley MJ, Mollison PL, Soothill JF. Br J Haematol 1962;8:149
136. Adinolfi M, Polley MJ, Hunter DA, et al. Immunology 1962;5:566
137. Holburn AM. Br J Haematol 1974;27:489
138. Judd WJ, Steiner EA, Friedman BA, et al. Transfusion 1978;18:436
139. Giblett ER. Unpublished observations, 1961 cited by Mollison PL. Blood Transfusion in Clinical Medicine, 6th Ed. Oxford:Blackwell, 1979
140. Mollison PL. Blood Transfusion in Clinical Medicine, 3rd Ed. Oxford:Blackwell, 1961
141. Walker RH, Griffin LD, Kashgarian M. Am J Clin Pathol 1969;51:13
142. Krieger VI, Simmons RT. Med J Austral 1949;1:85
143. Vries de SI, Smitskamp HS. Br Med J 1951;1:280
144. Brendemoen OJ, Aas K. Acta Med Scand 1952;141:458
145. Lauer A, Clauss J, Hoppe HH. Dtsch Med Wschr 1954;79:1869
146. Matson GA, Coe J, Swanson J. Blood 1955;10:1236
147. Mollison PL, Cutbush M. Lancet 1955;1:1290
148. Merrild-Hansen B, Munk-Andersen G. Vox Sang 1957;2:109
149. Peterson ET, Chisholm R. Proc 7th Cong ISBT. Basel:Karger,1958:59
150. Roy RB, Wesley RH, Fitzgerald JDL. Vox Sang 1960;5:545
151. Cowles JW, Spitalnik SL, Blumberg N. Vox Sang 1986;50:164
152. Henry SM, Simpson LA, Woodfield DG. Hum Hered 1988;38:111

153. Broadberry RE, Lin-Chu M. Hum Hered 1991;41:290
154. Lin M, Shieh SH. Vox Sang 1994;66:137
155. Lin M, Shieh SH, Hwang FY, et al. Vox Sang 1995;69:131
156. Lu TC, Lee TC, Chen CL. Acta Paediat Sin 1963;4:1
157. Brown WR, Boon WH. Pediatrics 1965;36:745
158. Chen CL. In: Medical Review. Taipei:Chinese Cultural and Scientific Series, 1980:27
159. Linn S, Schoenbaum SC, Monson RR, et al. Pediatrics 1985;75:770
160. Grubb R. Am J Phys Anthropol 1955;13:663
161. Garratty G, Kleinschmidt G. Vox Sang 1965;10:567
162. Granger A, Cjuiko C, Moreau L. Unpublished observations 1966, cited in Mollison PL. Blood Transfusion in Clinical Medicine, 6th Ed. Oxford:Blackwell, 1979
163. Kornstad L. Vox Sang 1969;16:124
164. Ceppellini R. Proc 6th Cong ISBT, Basel:Karger, 1955:207
165. Sneath JS, Sneath PHA. Br Med Bull 1959;15:154
166. Bharucha ZS, Joshi SR, Bhatia HM. Vox Sang 1981;41:36
167. Reid ME, Ellisor SS. (Letter). Vox Sang 1982;42:278
168. Bhatia HM. (Letter). Vox Sang 1982;42:278
169. Mollison PL, Englefriet CP, Contreras M. Blood Transfusion in Clinical Medicine, 9th Ed. Oxford:Blackwell, 1993
170. Garratty G. In: Clinically Significant and Insignificant Antibodies. Washington, D.C.:Am Assoc Blood Banks, 1979:39
171. Chandanayingyong D. Unpublished observations cited by Mollison PL, Englefriet CP, Contreras M. Blood Transfusion in Clinical Medicine, 9th Ed. Oxford:Blackwell, 1993:183
172. Potapov MI. Vox Sang 1976;30:211
173. Seaman MJ, Chalmers DJ, Franks D. Vox Sang 1968;15:25
174. Rachkewich RA, Crookston MC, Tilley CA, et al. J Immunogenet 1978;5:25
175. Oriol R, Danilovs J, Lemieux R, et al. Hum Immunol 1980;3:195
176. Andersen J. Vox Sang 1958;3:251
177. Hirsch HF, Graham HA, Davies DM Jr. (abstract). Transfusion 1975;15:521
178. Tegoli J, Cortez M, Jensen L, et al. Vox Sang 1971;21:397
179. Branch DR, Powers T. (Letter). Transfusion 1979;19:353
180. Andresen PH, Jordal K. Acta Path Microbiol Scand 1949;26:636
181. Andresen PH. Vox Sang 1972;23:262
182. Schenkel-Brunner H, Hanfland P. Vox Sang 1981;40:358
183. Arcilla MB, Sturgeon P. Pediat Res 1972;6:853
184. Arcilla MB, Sturgeon P. Vox Sang 1973;25:72
185. Arcilla MB, Sturgeon P. Vox Sang 1974;26:425
186. Andersen J. Acta Path Microbiol Scand 1960;48:374
187. Hanfland P, Kordowicz M, Peter-Katalinic J, et al. Arch Biochem Biophys 1986;246:655
188. Oriol R, LePendu, Mollicone R. Vox Sang 1986;51:161
189. Young WW, Johnson HS, Tamura Y, et al. J Biol Chem 1983;258:4890
190. Cagas P, Bush CA. Biopolymers 1990;30:1123
191. Brockhaus M, Magnani JL, Blaszczyk M, et al. J Biol Chem 1981;256:13223
192. Messeter L, Brodin T, Chester MA, et al. Vox Sang 1984;46:66
193. Mayr WR, Kemkes A, Kowalkski R, et al. Proceedings 2nd International Workshop on Monoclonal Antibodies Against Human Red Cells and Related Antigens. Lund, 1990:52
194. Camoens H, Sathe M, Joshi VB, et al. Ind J Med Sci 1971;25:313
195. Taylor PA, Rachkewich RA, Gare DJ, et al. Transplantation 1974;17:142
196. Schachter H, Michaels MA, Crookston MC, et al. Biochem

197. Hammer L, Mansson S, Rohr T, et al. Vox Sang 1981;40:27
198. Issitt PD. Unpublished observations, 1963
199. Steane EA. Unpublished observations, 1982 cited by Issitt PD. Br J Biomed Sci 1994;51:158
200. Wilson MJ, Fruitstone MJ. (abstract). Transfusion 1976;16:523
201. Marsh WL, Øyen R. Transfusion 1978;18:743
202. Spitalnik S, Cowles J, Cox MT, et al. Am J Clin Pathol 1983;80:63
203. Spitalnik S, Cowles J, Cox MT, et al. Vox Sang 1983;45:440
204. Judd WJ. Methods in Immunohematology, 2nd Ed. Durham:Montgomery, 1994
205. Spitalnik S, Cowles J, Cox MT, et al. Vox Sang 1985;48:235
206. Waheed A, Kennedy MS, Gerhan S. Transfusion 1981;21:542
207. Cutbush M, Mollison PL. Br J Haematol 1958;4:115
208. Mollison PL. Br Med J 1959;2:1035
209. Mollison PL. Br Med J 1959;2:1123
210. Mollison PL. Br Med Bull 1959;15:92
211. Mollison PL. Acta Hematol 1959;10:495
212. Giblett ER. Transfusion 1977;17:299
213. Issitt PD. In: Clinically Significant and Insignificant Antibodies. Washington, D.C.:Am Assoc Blood Banks, 1979:13
214. Issitt PD. In: Pathology-Anatomical and Clinical. Oxford:Pergamon, 1982:395
215. Petz LD. In: Clinical Practice of Transfusion Medicine, 2nd Ed. New York:Churchill: Livingstone, 1989:173
216. Rosse WF. Clinical Immunohematology: Basic Concepts and Clinical Applications. Boston:Blackwell, 1990
217. Greenwalt TJ. In: Principles of Transfusion Medicine. Baltimore:Williams and Wilkins, 1991:79
218. Shirey RS, Ness PM. In: Scientific Basis of Transfusion Medicine. Philadelphia:Saunders, 1994:507
219. Klein HG, Ed. Standards for Blood Banks and Transfusion Services, 16th Ed. Bethesda:Am Assoc Blood Banks, 1994
220. Walker RH, Ed. Technical Manual, 11th Ed. Bethesda:Am Assoc Blood Banks, 1993
221. Waheed A, Kennedy MS, Gerhan S, et al. Am J Clin Pathol 1981;76:294
222. Morel PA, Garratty G, Perkins HA. Am J Med Technol 1978;44:122
223. Owen IA, Blajchman MA, O'Hoski P, et al. Transfusion 1979;19:95
224. Perkins HA, Mallory D, Bergren M, et al. (Letter). Transfusion 1982;22:346
225. Orlin JB, Domm A, Vroon DH. (abstract). Transfusion 1982;22:421
226. Cooper RA. New Eng J Med 1977;297:371
227. Hossaini AA. Am J Clin Pathol 1972;56:3
228. Holburn AM. Immunology 1973;24:1019
229. Cheng MS, Lukomskyj L. Vox Sang 1989;57:155
230. Wier AB III, Woods LL, Chesney C, et al. Vox Sang 1987;53:105
231. Andorka DW, Arosomena A, Harris JL. Am J Clin Pathol 1974;62:47
232. Pelosi MA, Bauer JL, Lander A, et al. Obstet Gynecol 1974;4:590
233. Shulman IA, Nakayama R. Transfusion 1993;33:37
234. Obarski G, Edwards-Moulds JM. J Med Technol 1984;1:377
235. Dorf ME, Eguro SY, Cabrera G, et al. Vox Sang 1972;22:447
236. Marcelli-Barge A, Poirier JC, Benajam A, et al. Vox Sang 1972;30:81
237. Dunstan RA. Br J Haematol 1986;62:301
238. Jeannet M, Bodmer JG, Bodmer WF, et al. In:

Biophys Res Comm 1971;45:1011

Histocompatibility Testing 1972. Copenhagen:Munksgaard, 1973:493

239. Jeannet M, Schapira M, Magnin C. Sch Med Woch 1974;104:152

240. Mayr WF, Mayr D. J Immunogenet 1974;1:43

241. Oriol R, Baur MP, Danilovs J, et al. In: Histocompatibility Testing 1980. Los Angeles:UCLA Tissue Typing Laboratory, 1980

242. Oriol R, Cartron J-P, Yvart J, et al. Lancet 1978;1;574

243. Singal DP, Blajchman MA, Naipaul N, et al. Hum Immunol 1981;2:201

244. Nielsen LS, Eiberg H, Mohr J. Tissues Antigens 1983;21:177

245. Posner MP, McGeorge MB, Mendez-Picon G, et al. Transplantation 1986;41:474

246. Dunstan RA, Simpson MB, Knowles RW, et al. Blood 1985;65:615

247. Kools A, Collins J, Aster RH. Transfusion 1981;21:615

248. Kelton JG, Hamid C, Aker S, et al. Blood 1982;59:980

249. Dunstan RA, Simpson MB, Borowitz M. Br J Haematol 1985;60:651

250. Good AH, Yau O, Lamontagne LR, et al. Vox Sang 1992;62:180

251. Salmon C, Cartron J-P, Rouger P. The Human Blood Groups. New York:Masson, 1984

252. Singal DP, Blajchman MA, Naipaul N, et al. Transplt Proc 1981;13:1193

253. Oriol R, Cartron J, Yvart J, et al. Lancet 1978;1;574

254. Oriol R, Carton J-P, Cartron J, et al. Transplantation 1980;29:184

255. Oriol R, Opelz G, Chun C, et al. Transplantation 1980;29:397

256. Lenhard V, Roelcke D, Driekorn K, et al. Transplt Proc 1981;13:930

257. Cecka M. In: Clinical Kidney Transplants. Los Angeles:UCLA Tissue Typing Laboratory, 1985:179

258. Roy R, Terasaki PI, Chia D, et al. Transplt Proc 1987;19:4498

259. Terasaki PI, Chia D, Mickey MR. Transplt Proc 1988;20:21

260. Spitalnik S, Pfaff W, Cowles J, et al. Transplanation 1984;37:265

261. Kerman RH, Van Buren CT, Lewis RM, et al. Transplantation 1988;45:37

262. Opelz G, for the Collaborative Transplant Study. Transplt Proc 1988;20:1069

263. Anonymous, Editorial. Lancet 1988;1:567

264. Evans DAP, Donohoe WTA, Hewitt S, et al. Vox Sang 1982;43:177

265. Morgan WTJ. In: Lectures on the Scientific Basis of Medicine, Vol 4. London:Athlone, 1954:92

266. Smith EL, McKibbin JM, Karlsson K-A, et al J Biol Chem 1975;250:6059

267. Lee CH, Hagen MA, Chong BH, et al. Transfusion 1980;20:585

268. Feizi T, Kabat EA. J Exp Med 1972;135:1247

269. Shibata S, Goldstein IJ, Baker DA. J Biol Chem 1982;257:9324

270. Kaladas PM, Kabat EA, Shibata S, et al. Arch Biochem Biophys 1983;223:309

271. Spohr U, Hindsgaul O, Lemieux RU. Canad J Chem 1985;63:2644

272. Yamamoto S. J Immunogenet 1982;9:137

273. Wang XM, Terasaki PI, Loon J, et al. Vox Sang 1983;45:320

274. Solter D, Knowles BB. Proc Nat Acad Sci USA 1978;75:5565

275. Koprowski H, Brockhaus M, Blaszczyk M, et al. Lancet 1982;1:1332

276. Iwaki Y, Kasai M, Terasaki PI, et al. Cancer Res 1982;42:409

277. Brockhaus M, Magnani JL, Herlyn M, et al. Arch Biochem

Biophys 1982;217:647

278. Hansson GC, Karlsson KA, Larsen G, et al. J Biol Chem 1983;258:4091

279. Fredman P, Richert ND, Magnani JL, et al. J Biol Chem 1983;258:11206

280. Abe K, McKibbin JM, Hakomori SI. J Biol Chem 1983;258:11793

281. Blaineau C, LePendu J, Arnaud D, et al. EMBO J 1983;2:2217

282. Brown A, Feizi T, Gooi HC, et al. Biosci Rep 1983;3:163

283. Lloyd KO, Larson G, Strömberg N, et al. Immunogenetics 1983;17:537

284. Blaszczyk M, Hansson GC, Karlsson KA, et al. Arch Biochem Biophys 1984;233:161

285. Fukushi Y, Hakomori SI, Nudelman E, et al. J Biol Chem 1984;259:4681

286. Huang LC, Brockhaus M, Magnani JL, et al. Arch Biochem Biophys 1983;220:318

287. Fukushi Y, Nudelman E, Levery SB, et al. J Biol Chem 1984;259:10511

288. Fukushima K, Hirota M, Terasaki P, et al. Cancer Res 1984;44:5279

289. Gooi HC, Pickard JK, Hounsell EF, et al. Mol Immunol 1985;22:689

290. LePendu J, Fredman P, Richter ND, et al. Carbohydr Res 1985;141:347

291. Kaizu T, Levery SB, Nudelman E, et al. J Biol Chem 1986;261:11254

292. Steplewski Z, Blaszczyk-Thurin M, Lubeck M, et al. Hydridoma 1990;9:201

293. Clausen H, McKibbin JM, Hakomori S. Biochemistry 1985;24:6190

294. Lemieux RU, Hindsgaul O, Bird P. Carbohyr Res 1988;178:293

295. Fraser RH, Allan EK, Murphy MT, et al. (abstract). 2nd Int Workshop on Monoclonal Antibodies to Human Blood Group and Related Antigens, Lund, 1990

296. Gooi HC, Feizi T, Kapadia A, et al. Nature 1981;292:156

297. Hakomori SI, Kobata A. In: The Antigens, Vol 2. New York:Academic Press, 1974:79

298. Hakomori SI, Nudelman E, Levery SB, et al. Biochem Biophys Res Comm 1981;100:1578

299. Wu JT, Olson J, Walker K. J Clin Lab Anal 1992;6:151

300. Nishihara S, Nakazato M, Kudo T, et al. Biochem Biophys Res Comm 1993;190:42

301. Tetteroo PAT, De Heij HT, Eijnden van der DH, et al. J Biol Chem 1987;262:15984

302. Couillin P, Mollicone R, Grisard MC, et al. Cytogenet Cell Genet 1991;56:108

303. Hakomori SI, Nudelman E, Kannagi R, et al. Biochem Biophys Res Comm 1982;109:36

304. Kannagi R, Nudelman E, Levery SB, et al. J Biol Chem 1982;257:14865

305. Taki T, Takamatsu M, Myoga A, et al. J Biochem 1988;103:998

306. Eggens I, Fenderson B, Toyokuni T, et al. J Biol Chem 1989;264:9476

307. Brandley BK, Swiedler SJ, Robbins PW. Cell 1990;63:861

308. Hakomori SI. Histochem J 1992;24:771

309. Kerr MA, Stocks SC. Histochem J 1992;24:811

310. Takada A, Ohmori K, Yoneda T, et al. Cancer Res 1993;53:354

311. Hakomori SI, Nudelman E, Levery SB, et al. J Biol Chem 1984;259:4672

312. Levery SB, Nudelman ED, Anderson NH, et al. Carbohydr

Res 1986;151:311

313. Nudelman E, Levery SB, Kaizu T, et al. J Biol Chem 1986;261:11247

314. Blaszczyk-Thurin M, Thurin J, Hindsgaul O, et al. J Biol Chem 1987;262:372

315. Kukowska-Latallo JF, Larsen RD, Nair RP, et al. Gene Dev 1990;4:1288

316. Ball SP, Tongue N, Gibaud A, et al. Ann Hum Genet 1991;55:225

317. Koda Y, Kimura H, Makeda E. Blood 1993;82:2915

318. Elmgren A, Rydberg L, Larson G. Biochem Biophys Res Comm 1993;196:515

319. Mollicone R, Reguigne I, Kelly RJ, et al. J Biol Chem 1994;269:20987

320. Nishihara S, Narimatsu H, Iwaski H, et al. J Biol Chem 1994;269:29271

321. Bailly P, Hermand P, Callebaut I, et al. Proc Nat Acad Sci USA 1994;91:5306

322. Parsons SF, Mallinson G, Holmes CH, et al. Proc Nat Acad Sci USA 1995;92:5496

323. Rouquier S, Georgi D, Bergmann A, et al. Cytogenet Cell Genet 1994;66:70

324. Mollicone R, Candelier J-J, Reguigne I, et al. Transf Clin Biol 1994;2;91

325. Nishihara S, Yazawa S, Iwasaki H, et al. Biochem Biophys Res Comm 1993;196:624

326. Koda Y, Soejima M, Kimura H. Vox Sang 1994;67:327

327. Ørntoff TF, Holmes EH, Johnson P, et al. Blood 1991;77:1389

328. Vos GH, Comley P. Acta Genet Stat Med 1967;17:495

329. Henry SM, Simpson LA, Benny AG, et al. NZ J Med Lab Technol 1989;43:64

330. Henry SM, Benny AG, Woodfield DG. Vox Sang 1990;58:61

331. McNeil C, Trentleman EF, Kreutzer VO, et al. Am J Clin Pathol 1957;28:145

332. Clark CA, McConnell RB, Sheppard PM. Ann Hum Genet 1960;24:295

333. AuBuchon JP, Davey RJ, Anderson HJ, et al. (Letter). Transfusion 1986;26:302

334. Henry S, Oriol R, Samuelsson B. Vox Sang 1995;69:166

335. Henry S. Doctoral Thesis, Goteborg Univ 1995

336. Lowe JB. In: Blood Cell Biochemistry. Volume 6. New York:Plenum 1995;75

337. Lowe JB, Kukowska-Latallo JF, Nair RP, et al. J Biol Chem 1991;266:17467

338. Dumas DP, Ichikawa Y, Wong CH, et al. Bio Med Chem Lett 1991;1:425

339. Prieels JP, Monnom D, Dolmans M, et al. J Biol Chem 1981;256:10456

340. Elmgren A, Borjeson C, Svensson L, et al. Vox Sang 1996;70:97

341. Elmgren A, Mollicone R, Costache M. J Biol Chem in press 1997

342. Orntoft TF, Vestergaard EM, Holmes E. J Biol Chem 1996;271:32260

343. Mollicone R, Reguigne I, Fletcher A. J Biol Chem 1994;269:12662

344. Larson G, Borjeson C, Elmgren A, et al. Vox Sang 1996;71:233

345. Kelly RJ, Ernst LK, Larsen RD, et al. Proc Nat Acad Sci USA 1994;91:5843

346. Rouquier S, Lowe JB, Kelly RJ, et al. J Biol Chem 1995;270:4632

347. Kelly RJ, Rouquier S, Giorgi D, et al. J Biol Chem 1995;270:4640

348. Henry S, Mollicone R, Lowe JB, et al. Vox Sang 1996;70:21

349. Henry S, Mollicone R, Fernandez P, et al. Glycoconjugate J. in press 1997

350. Koda Y,Soejima M, Liu Y, et al. Am J Hum Genet 1996;59:343

351. Yu L-C, Broadberry RE, Yang YH, et al. Biochem Biophys Res Comm 1996;222:390

352. Yu L-C, Yang Y-H, Broadberry RE, et al. Biochem J 1995;312:329

353. Henry S, Mollicone R, Fernandez P, et al. Biochem Biophys Res Comm 1996;219:675

354. Reguigne-Arnould I, Coullin P, Mollicone R, et al. Cytogenet Cell Genet 1995;71:158

355. McCurley RS, Recinor A, Olsen AS, et al. Genomics 1995;26:142

356. Reguigne-Arnould I, Wolfe J, Hornigold N, et al. C R Acad Sci, Paris 1996;319:783

357. Costache M, Cailleau A, Fernandez-Mateos P, et al. Transfus Clin Biol in press 1997

358. Springer TA. Cell 1994;36:301

359. Maly P, Thall AD, Petryniak B, et al. Cell 1996;85:643

360. Phillips ML, Schwartz BR, Etzioni A, et al. J Clin Invest 1995;96:2898

361. Holmes EH, Xu Z, Sherwood AL, et al. J Biol Chem 1995;270:8145

362. Legault DJ, Kelly RJ, Natsuka Y, et al. J Biol Chem 1995;270:20987

363. Xu Z, Vo L, Macher BA. J Biol Chem 1996;271:8818

364. Breton C, Oriol R, Imberty A. Glycobiology 1996;6:7

10 | The Ii Antigen Collection

The Ii antigen collection is described following the ABO and Lewis systems because the I and i antigens have been shown to have a definite serological relationship to those of the ABO system. As the title of the chapter indicates, the Ii collection does not satisfy the criteria established by the ISBT working party (see Chapter 1) for designation as a blood group system. The antigens I and i can be defined serologically and a fair amount is known about their biochemical structure. However, genetic control of the production of I, i and related antigens is incompletely understood. It has not been established for sure that what could be regarded as *I* and *i* genes exist, nor is the serologically defined reciprocal relationship between I and i fully defined in terms of gene action (see a later section for evidence that I and i are not encoded by alleles). The (rather limited) ISBT terminology for the Ii collection is shown in table 10-1.

Unlike the Lewis system that comprises a series of plasma and saliva antigens, with the former being taken up by red cells, antigens of the Ii collection appear to be synthesized in large part on red cells, on the same glycoprotein chains that carry H, A and B. There is evidence (see below) that I and i are also present on the same plasma glycolipids that carry Le^a and Le^b but the uptake of those antigen-bearing chains by red cells does not seem to represent a major contribution to the I and i antigens of those cells.

The I and i Antigens on Red Cells

In 1956, Wiener et al. (1) while working with a panagglutinating autoantibody from a patient with CHD (cold hemagglutinin disease, the "cold" antibody-induced form of hemolytic anemia, see Chapter 38) found that five of 22,000 donor samples tested, were non-reactive. The antibody present was called anti-I and the antigen it detects, I. Those samples that were compatible were called I-negative or i. In 1960, Jenkins et al. (2) showed that 50 sera containing what had previously been known as the non-specific-cold-agglutinin had anti-I specificity when tested with a single adult i and many I-positive red cell samples. Later in the same year, Marsh and Jenkins (3) and in 1961, Marsh (4), reported the first two examples of anti-i and knowledge of the I system increased rapidly as a result. The presently known facts about the system are summarized in tables 10-2 and 10-3.

As shown in table 10-3 and as discussed in more detail in later sections of this chapter, the red cells of most newborn infants carry high levels of i and low levels of I (2,31). Marsh (4) used serial titrations to show that between birth and about 18 months of age, the i antigen levels gradually fall and the I antigen levels gradual-

TABLE 10-1 Conventional and ISBT Terminology for the Ii Collection

Conventional Name	ISBT Collection Symbol	ISBT Collection Number	Antigen (Conventional Name)	ISBT Antigen Number	ISBT Full Code Number
Ii	I	207	I	001	207001
			i	002	207002

TABLE 10-2 Characteristics of Some Ii Collection Antibodies

Antibody Specificity	Positive Reactions in In Vitro Tests				Usual Immunoglobulin		Ability to Bind Complement		Ability to Cause In Vitro Lysis		Implicated in		Usual Form of Stimulation		% of White Population Positive
	Sal	LISS	AHG	Enz	IgG	IgM	Yes	No	Yes	No	Transfusion Reaction	HDN	Red Cells	Other	
Anti-I	X	X		X	Few	Most	Most		Few	Most				X	100
Anti-i	X	X		X	Few	Most	Most		Few	Most				X	100
Anti-j	X			X		Most				Most				X	100
Anti-I^T	X					Most				Most				X	100
Anti-IA	X					Most				Most				X	44
Anti IB	X					Most				Most				X	14
Anti IH	X			X	Few	Most	Most		Few	Most				X	100

TABLE 10-3 Some Characteristics of Ii Collection Antigens

1. The amount of I antigen on the I+ red cells of different people is variable.

2. All I+ red cells carry some i antigen.

3. Two components of the I antigen, I^F and I^D have been described (5).

4. Rare adults have red cells that carry a high level of i and only a trace of I. Such cells are said to be of the adult i phenotype.

5. Adults with red cells of the i phenotype are very rare. The phenotpe has a probable incidence of less than 1 in 10,000.

6. Two slightly different i phenotypes i_1 and i_2 may exist.

7. Rare adults have red cells that carry reduced amounts of I, but more than is present on i cells and increased levels of i, but less than is present on i cells. Such cells are said to be of the I_{int} phenotype (4).

8. In most instances the I antigen is poorly developed on cord red blood cells. For practical purposes i_{cord} red cells can often be used as I-, i+.

9. In spite of 8, cord red blood cells carry a trace of I.

10. Between birth and about 18 months of age, the i antigen on an infant's red cells is gradually replaced by I(4).

11. The I and i antigen levels on red cells are altered in some disease states.

12. I substance is present in small quantities in most saliva samples and in even smaller quantities in all others (6).

13. Human milk contains larger quantities of I substance, than does saliva (7).

14. I and i substances are present in sera from adults and newborn infants (6,8,9).

15. When anti-I and anti-i are studied by hemagglutination inhibition and the I and i antigens are studied at the biochemical level, great heterogeneity is seen (10-30).

16. Antibodies exist that define antigens that seem to be comprised in part of I and in part of ABO, or in part of I and in part of P determinants.

17. For details about j, see text.

ly increase, in a reciprocal manner, in the blood of the overwhelming majority of infants. The appearance of I and the gradual reduction of i on the red cells of growing infants coincides with the appearance of hemoglobin A and the gradual reduction of production of hemoglobin F. In spite of this, there is no evidence that the two changes are related in any way other than the time at which they occur. In other words, the i antigen is not a marker on hemoglobin F molecules. In very rare instances, the change from production of i to I does not occur and the red cell phenotype i persists into adult life (1-4). For the

remainder of this chapter the term adult i is used to describe red cells of that phenotype.

Historically the i adult phenotype has been divided (4) into two forms, i_1 and i_2, with i_2 being said to carry a little more I and a little less i than does i_1. However, it now seems rather more likely that differences in the i adult phenotype of different individuals represents a continuum that is dependent on the number of branched oligosaccharide chains that are formed on the red cells (see below). In other words, variation in the small amounts of the beta 1→6 N-acetylglucosaminyl transferase synthesized by different individuals would be reflected at the phenotypic levels by slight differences in i and I levels of i adult red cells.

Testa et al. (32) claimed that as red cells age in vivo, the small amount of i that is present on all I+ red cells is gradually reduced. This phenomenon does not seem to have been further studied. In spite of the findings about the disappearance of i and the appearance of I during the first 18 months of life, as the description below of the biochemical nature of I and i will make clear, it seems highly unlikely that control of production of I and i rests with genes that can be thought of simply as *I* and *i*. Marsh et al. (33) suggested that the ability to convert i to I is controlled by a gene *Z* that is very common. Individuals who lacked *Z* (presumably *zz*) would have red cells of the adult i phenotype and the I_{int} phenotype (see Table 10-3) might represent the *Zz* genetic state. Studies of families (8,31,34-40) in which there were adults with red cells of the i phenotype have indicated that the phenotype represents an inherited situation. However, as discussed in detail in the section on the biochemistry of I and i, conversion of i to I is now known (30,41-45) to involve the actions of a transferase enzyme that acts to convert straight chain oligosaccharides into branched structures. Thus while the product of *Z* could perhaps be thought of as the transferase that adds N-acetylglucosamine in beta 1→6 linkage to galactose and thus effects branching of the chains (see below) the i adult phenotype seems to represent lack of, or low level synthesis of this enzyme.

There is almost absolute correlation between lack (or small numbers) of branched oligosaccharide chains on the red cells of embryos and fetuses and the high content of i (76-79) and the development of branched oligosaccharides and the appearance of I (12,19,20,77,79). In the adult i phenotype it has been shown (77-79) that branching of the oligosaccharide chains has not occurred or has occurred to only a limited degree.

Although biochemical studies have shown that the I and i antigens represent a complex series of structures on red cells and that different examples of anti-I and anti-i complex with different portions of these structures, the differences are not often apparent in straightforward serological studies. The reason for this is that almost all I+ red cells carry all the determinants recognized by the various specificity anti-I, while i cord and i adult cells almost always carry all the determinants recognized by anti-i. More differences are seen when the various substances described below are used in hemagglutination inhibition studies. Sialylated I, i and related antigens are described in Chapter 34.

Soluble I and i Antigens

A series of studies revealed that some examples of anti-I and anti-i could be (often partially) neutralized with saliva (6,33,46,47), colostrum (11), human milk (5,7,33,46), serum and plasma (6,8,9,47,48), amniotic fluid (49) and urine (49). While much of the work on the biochemical structure of I and i has been performed on these soluble antigens, there are occasional differences when the red cell and soluble substances from the same individual are studied. For example, Marsh et al. (33) found that the milk and saliva of a woman with the i adult red cell phenotype contained essentially the same amount of I as the milk and saliva of women with I+ red cells. Further, the milk from the woman with the i adult red cell phenotype did not inhibit anti-i any more efficiently than did the milk of a woman with I+ red cells.

Although not dealing with the inhibition of anti-I, a recent paper (281) on the composition of human milk, described the material as human breast milk. That same term has been used by other authors (282-284). We much prefer the term human milk (5,7,33,36) we do not know from whence else it might be obtained!

Location of the I and i Antigens

As mentioned above and as described in more detail in the section on biochemistry of the Ii collection, the I and i antigens on red cells are carried on the same glycoprotein and glycolipid chains that carry H, A and B and in the secretions on the same glycolipids that carry H, A, B, Le^a and Le^b. Using solubilized extracts from red cell membranes and the materials mentioned above that carry soluble I and i (11,13,14,50-65) it became apparent (66-68) that I and i are present on the chains in a position closer to the membrane than are the terminal carbohydrates of H, A and B. The I and i antigens are predominantly carbohydrate in nature (12,69-71). The series of determinants recognized by various specificities of anti-i involve, predominantly, an N-acetyl-glucosamine residue in beta 1→3 linkage to a galactose residue on straight chain glycoproteins and glycolipids. The series of determinants recognized by various specificities of

anti-I involve, predominantly, the same N-acetyl-glucosamine residue in beta 1→3 linkage to a galactose residue plus a second N-acetyl-glucosamine in beta 1→6 linkage to the same galactose residue, on branched chain glycoproteins and glycolipids. As the immunodominant sugars of H, A and B are added to the chains, access of anti-I and anti-i to their antigenic determinants may be blocked (72). This is demonstrable at the serological level as well. O$_h$ red cells, that never have the H, A or B immunodominant sugars added to their precursor chains, have been shown (73-75) to react more strongly than other cells, with anti-I.

Viewed at its most simple level, the above explanations correlate exactly with the serological findings. On cord red blood cells where few branched chains are present and on red cells of the adult i phenotype where little development of branched chains occurs, the structures with which different anti-i complex are readily accessible to the antibodies. Accordingly, those cells react strongly with anti-i and weakly with anti-I. As the branched chains start to form, access for anti-i becomes restricted and the structures with which different anti-I combine, gradually increase in numbers. This corresponds to the apparent loss of i and the development of I during the first 18 months of life (4). Once the infants' red cells carry branched structures that are the same as those on the red cells of adults, the I antigens are readily detectable but the i antigens are now somewhat inaccessible to anti-i. The red cells of almost all adults type as strongly I+ and can be shown to react only weakly with anti-i (2,31). Figure 10-1 is an oversimplified diagram of some red cell membrane-borne structures that carry I and i. From what has been written about the structure of i and I, it will now be clear why, unlike most blood group systems where negative phenotypes exist when an allele is not inherited (e.g. individuals genetically *OO* have no A or B on their red cells) there are no negative phenotypes in the Ii collection. As shown in table 10-3, all red cells of the I adult phenotype carry some i, all i cord and i adult red cells carry some I.

When diagrams such as figure 10-1 are constructed to depict the straight chains that carry i and the branched chains that carry I, it appears that the ABH and Ii determinants are some distance from each other. When the chains are present in situ on red cells or in fluids, it is likely that the natural folding of the chains brings the determinants into close proximity. As described below, there are a series of antibodies that recognize determinants comprised in part of Ii, in part of ABH, and sometimes in part of Le^b, antigens. As described in Chapter 11, some similar spatial arrangements involve antigens of the Ii collection, the P$_1$ system and the GLOB collection.

FIGURE 10-1 Simplified Diagrams to Show the Locations of I and i

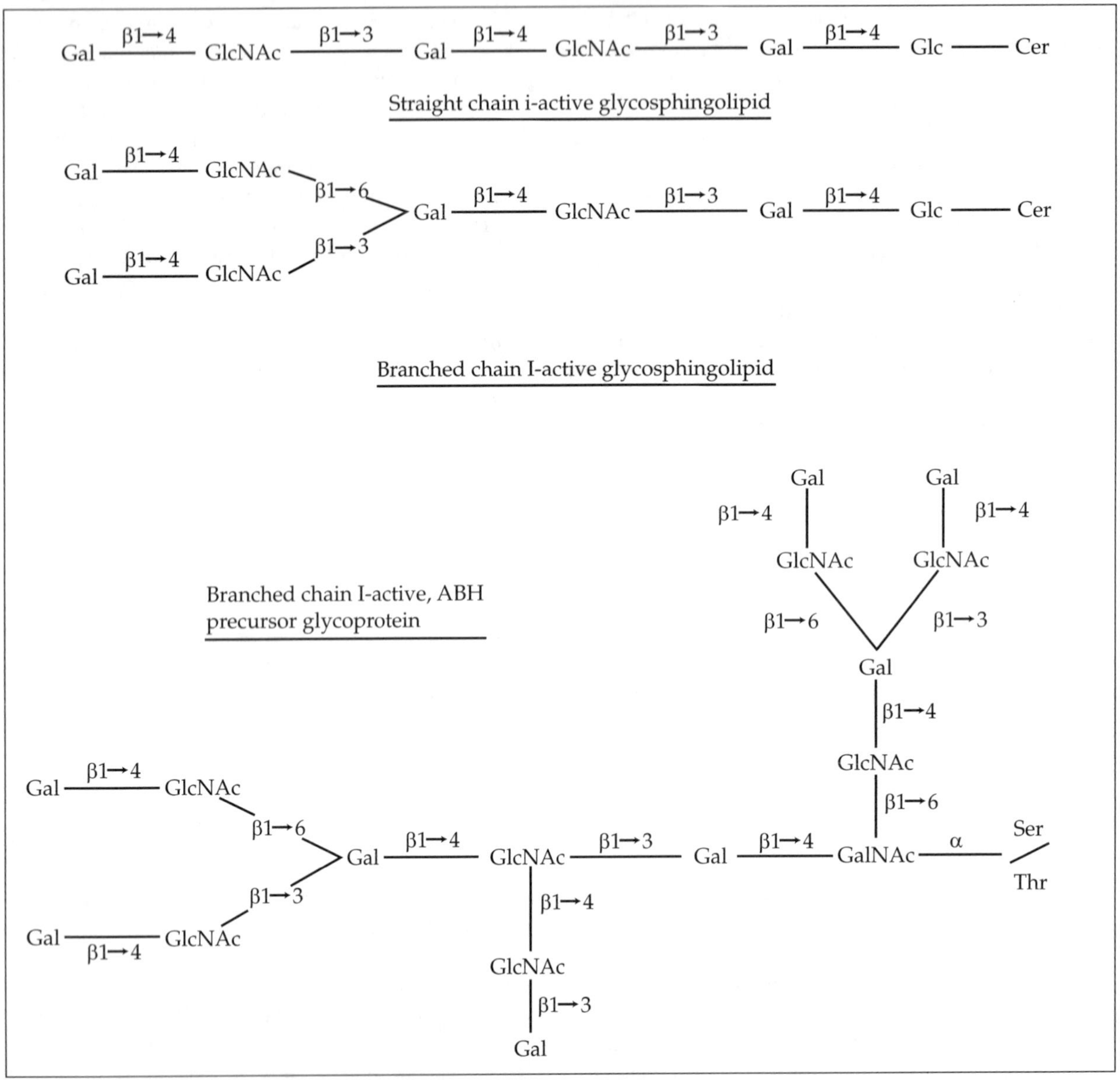

Gal —β1→4— GlcNAc —β1→3— Gal —β1→4— GlcNAc —β1→3— Gal —β1→4— Glc —— Cer

Straight chain i-active glycosphingolipid

Gal —β1→4— GlcNAc —β1→6↘
                            Gal —β1→4— GlcNAc —β1→3— Gal —β1→4— Glc —— Cer
Gal —β1→4— GlcNAc —β1→3↗

Branched chain I-active glycosphingolipid

Branched chain I-active, ABH precursor glycoprotein

Gal —β1→4— GlcNAc —β1→6↘
                            Gal —β1→4— GlcNAc —β1→3— Gal —β1→4— GalNAc —α— Ser/Thr
Gal —β1→4— GlcNAc —β1→3↗

(GlcNAc β1→4 below GlcNAc; GlcNAc β1→3 Gal)

(Upper right: Gal —β1→4— GlcNAc —β1→6↘ and Gal —β1→4— GlcNAc —β1→3↗ to Gal —β1→4— GlcNAc —β1→6— GalNAc)

Gal	= Galactose	Ser = Serine
GlcNAc	= Glucosamine	Thr = Threonine
Glc	= Glucose	β = Beta linkage
GalNAc	= Galactosamine	α = Alpha linkage
Cer	= Ceramide	

When the oligosaccharide is attached to a lipid, to form a glycolipid, linkage is via glucose, i.e. Glc-Cer. When it is attached to a protein, to form a glycoprotein, linkage is via galactosamine, i.e. GalNAc-Ser or Thr.

Based on diagrams kindly provided by W. John Judd

The Ii Collection at the Level of the Routine Blood Bank

Although only in the order of one person in 10,000 is of the i adult phenotype, the sera of all individuals con- tain anti-I (80). Often, tests at 4°C are necessary to demonstrate auto-anti-I and if blood samples are allowed to cool before the serum is harvested it may appear that no anti-I is present. This is because weak examples of auto-anti-I may be completely adsorbed by the patient's own I+ red cells. Sometimes, the auto-anti-I may be demonstrable in tests performed at room temperature. While such antibodies can cause problems in compatibility tests, the solution is simple. As discussed in several other places in this book, antibody-screening and compatibility tests at room temperature are not necessary, result in problems when clinically-insignificant cold-reactive antibodies are present and should not be performed. Rarely, a clinically-insignificant form of auto-anti-I may interfere in tests performed above room temperature. If the patient has no signs or symptoms of cold hemagglutinin disease (CHD), thus showing that the antibody is benign in vivo, again the solution is simple. Antibodies of this type can be removed from the patient's serum by autoadsorption. More potent than usual forms may require autoadsorptions using the patient's red cells previously treated with ficin, papain or bromelin (for methods, see Judd (81)). Examples of auto-anti-I that are causative of CHD may be very difficult to remove from serum by autoadsorption (82,83). Alternative methods for performing antibody-screening and compatibility tests in the presence of strongly reactive cold autoantibodies are discussed in Chapter 38. Benign cold agglutinins, including anti-I, seem to be produced at their highest levels in individuals between 11 and 25 years of age (84), thereafter the level of cold agglutinin produced decreases. There is some correlation between IgM levels and amount of cold agglutinin made in healthy individuals and a much stronger one when pathological cold autoantibodies are made (85-88), again see Chapter 38.

When anti-I is present in the serum of an individual of the i adult phenotype, it is traditional to use blood from i adult donors for transfusion. It is not clear to these authors, that such a procedure is always essential. While one example of anti-I made by an individual of the i adult phenotype was shown to be IgM in nature (89) and to fix complement at 37°C (90), in vivo red cell survival studies were not performed. In another case (91) in which an adult with red cells of the i phenotype had anti-I in the serum, random donor I+ red cells were cleared rapidly in vivo (99% cleared in 30 minutes in the first study, 92% cleared in 90 minutes in the second study, 10 months later, using the same I+ donor's red cells). However, the red cells of the patient's daughter, that typed as I+, were shown to survive in a nearly normal manner in the patient. It is by no means clear whether this case (91) represented an exception or the rule. The authors described their finding of rapid clearance of the I+ red cells as "so unexpected" that they looked for explanations other than red cell destruction by the anti-I, but found none. Along similar lines, one of us (PDI) has seen several individuals of the i adult phenotype in whom the anti-I present had no higher a titer, nor any wider a thermal range, than examples of anti-I

found in the sera of individuals with I+ red cells. Thus it seems that currently available data suggest that in i adults with anti-I in the serum, rarely i adult blood may be needed for transfusion but that need should not automatically be assumed. Instead the characteristics of the anti-I, particularly its thermal range, should be reviewed in each individual case.

There is one circumstance in which an individual with I+ red cells and benign auto-anti-I in the serum, may present with a serological picture that mimics an individual of the i adult phenotype. If the patient's serum contains an incomplete form of anti-I, the patient's red cells may be blocked to the actions of anti-I agglutinins and may type as I- (92). If this situation is suspected, the patient's cells should be collected and maintained at 37°C until they have been washed three times with saline warmed to 37-40°C. They can then be typed with agglutinating anti-I. The object is to prevent the incomplete anti-I in the patient's serum from binding to the red cells and blocking the I sites.

Other than cold hemagglutinin disease, some secondary "cold" autoantibody-induced hemolytic anemias or hemolytic episodes, and the one anti-I in the i adult patient described above, anti-I and anti-i have not been incriminated as causative of in vivo red cell destruction. Even in patients subjected to hypothermia during surgical procedures, no evidence of anti-I or anti-i-induced red cell destruction has been reported.

Anti-I

As already explained, the term anti-I describes a group of related but not identical specificity antibodies. However, in the blood bank, all such antibodies have certain characteristics in common and can be identified without difficulty. Because I+ red cells from adults vary in the amount of I antigen present (1,2,4), the antibody may give variable strength reactions with different samples. For reasons given above, cord blood red cells and those of the i adult phenotype (if available) will react to varying degrees with potent examples of anti-I and weakly or not at all with less potent anti-I. Weak examples of anti-I may not react with all I+ cells. They may react with those samples that carry the highest amount of I, experienced workers soon learn which red cells, on an antibody identification panel, carry large amounts of I. Similarly, some examples of anti-I may fail to agglutinate I+ red cells, but may combine with them and cause complement to be activated. Again, experienced workers soon learn which of the cell samples they use regularly, react only in indirect antiglobulin tests (with complement being detected on the red cells) with such examples of anti-I. Most anti-I can be identified without i adult red cells in the panel. It may be necessary to use several different cord samples because of variation in expression of the I antigen (93). Although most examples of anti-I react optimally at 4°C, as stated, incomplete forms do exist. If a serum fails to react in RT and 37°C saline tests but is weakly reactive with all red cells from adults by the antiglobulin test, anti-I may be suspected but is by no means proved, even if cord cells samples are non-reactive. Other high incidence antigens, such as Yt^a, are also poorly developed on cord cells so that other antibodies may give a similar reaction pattern. If the antibody is anti-I, the auto-control will usually be positive but confirmation tests can be performed. One such test is to carry out the already described autoadsorption with enzyme-treated cells; this should remove anti-I but leave other antibodies, such as anti-Yt^a, unadsorbed. Tests in saline at 4°C will enhance the reactions of anti-I but not those of clinically important antibodies. Incomplete anti-I is invariably accompanied by a complete antibody of the same specificity active at 4°C. Tests using enzyme-treated red cells enhance the reactions of anti-I so that positive reactions will often be seen in such tests at RT although the antibody is not active above 4°C in saline tests. Similarly, the use of LISS, PEG and Polybrene methods will sometimes result in the detection of anti-I at 37°C although that antibody may be reactive only at RT or 4°C in saline systems. Although most LISS, PEG and Polybrene tests converted to IAT are read with anti-IgG, some examples of anti-I may be detected in such tests. It is not entirely clear whether IgG anti-I is being detected or whether the agglutination seen in the IATs has "carried-through" the washing stage in the IATs.

Potent examples of anti-I may be more difficult to identify. Sometimes the anti-I is so strong that when undiluted serum is used, I adult, i cord and i adult red cells all react (the latter two because of the traces of I that they carry). In this situation titration studies can be of value. As illustrated in table 10-4 as the anti-I (or anti-i, see below) is diluted, its specificity becomes apparent.

Only rarely are inhibition studies using human milk of value in the identification of anti-I. In the paper describing the presence of I substance in milk, Marsh et al. (7) reported that of 13 examples of anti-I from patients with CHD, only one was totally inhibited and of the other 12, 11 still had a titer of 32 or more after addition of the milk. In tests on nine examples of benign auto-anti-I from persons with I+ red cells and two from persons of the adult i phenotype, again only one antibody was totally inhibited. Of the remaining 10, six were still active at dilutions between 1 in 4 and 1 in 64. In other words, inhibition of anti-I with human milk demonstrates the presence of I substance in that fluid, by partial and sometimes appreciable antibody neutralization but total antibody inhibition is rare. Clearly the objective of the experiments reported (7) was to advance knowledge of the biochemistry of I, not to identify a material for use in routine antibody identification studies.

Shirey et al. (94) described a benign, IgM, cold-active anti-I, the reactivity of which was greatly enhanced by the presence of thimerosal; Reviron et al. (230) described an example, the reactions of which were enhanced in the presence of sodium azide. The association of the Ii antigens with a number of drug-related antibodies is discussed below.

TABLE 10-4 Examples of Anti-I, Anti-i and Anti-j in Titration Studies

Cell Type and Antibody	Serum Dilutions												
	None	2	4	8	16	32	64	128	256	512	1024	2048	4096
ANTI-I													
Adult I	4+	4+	4+	4+	4+	4+	3+	3+	2+	2+	+	+	0
i cord	4+	4+	3+	2+	+	0	0	0	0	0	0	0	0
i Adult	4+	3+	2+	+	0	0	0	0	0	0	0	0	0
ANTI-i													
Adult I	4+	3+	2+	+	0	0	0	0	0	0	0	0	0
i cord	4+	4+	4+	4+	4+	4+	3+	3+	2+	2+	+	0	0
i Adult	4+	4+	4+	4+	4+	4+	3+	3+	2+	2+	+	+	0
ANTI-j													
Adult I	4+	4+	4+	3+	3+	3+	2+	2+	+	+	0	0	0
i cord	4+	4+	4+	3+	3+	3+	2+	2+	+	+	0	0	0
i Adult	4+	4+	4+	3+	3+	3+	2+	2+	+	+	0	0	0

Because anti-I can interfere in routine blood bank tests, it is sometimes necessary to remove the antibody from a serum, by adsorption. Autoadsorption in this circumstance has been described above. In 1980, it was reported (95) that formaldehyde-treated rabbit red blood cells could be used to adsorb anti-I. A commercial product made from rabbit red cell stroma became available and was widely used. However, it seems that the product should be used with some caution since there are reports (96-100) that alloantibodies to (at least) D, E and K (and some others that may not have been of clinical significance) may be partially or wholly adsorbed by rabbit red cells or stroma made therefrom. In contrast, one study (101) found no loss of alloantibody strength in sera adsorbed with rabbit red cell stroma. If antibodies to D, E, K, et al. can be adsorbed on to rabbit red cells or stroma, it might have to be presumed that the adsorption represents non-specific uptake of antibody by the cells. It would not be a comfortable thought to believe that rabbits have Rh and Kell system antigens on their red cells.

Anti-I and PPLO

Although anti-I made by patients with atypical pneumonia caused by *Mycoplasma pneumoniae* (often called the pleuropneumonia like organism or PPLO) are described in more detail in Chapter 38, they should be mentioned here. These antibodies are not uncommon following PPLO infections, they appear to represent transient increases in titer and thermal range of normal cold reactive anti-I. If these increases are sufficient in terms of antibody strength and widening of thermal amplitude, hemolytic anemia, that can be severe, may develop. Schmidt et al. (138-142) suggested that during PPLO-pneumonia, there is an alteration of expression of I antigen on the patient's red cells. The immune system no longer recognizes the altered I as a host or self antigen and anti-I directed against it, is made. This concept to explain the etiology of the situation was favored over one that suggested that the PPLO carried an I-like antigen because the autoantibodies made were not readily adsorbed by organisms, from the patients, grown in culture. However, biochemical studies (153,251-257,259) have shown that lipopolysaccharides prepared from PPLO are biochemically related to red cell I antigens. At the practical level, the hemolytic episodes that sometimes follow PPLO infections are self-limited because autoantibody production is transient. In other words, if the patient can be managed through the hemolytic episode (see Chapter 38) chronic cold agglutinin disease does not follow.

Anti-I^D^, Anti-I^F^ and Anti-I^S^

In 1971, Marsh et al. (5) reported studies that indicated that some of the heterogeneity of anti-I could be resolved at the serological level. These workers named the component of I that is present on cord cells, I^F, (F for fetal) and believed that the antigen did not change appreciably as I developed at the expense of i, during the first eighteen months of life (4). The I antigen that is not present on cord cells and that develops as i levels decrease, was called I^D (D for developed). In other words, cord cells were said to carry i and I^F, while the red cells of adults carry I^D, only a trace amount of i and about the same amount of I^F as is produced on cord cells. Marsh et al. (7) and Dzierzkowa-Borodej et al. (6) had already reported the presence of I substance in human milk when the terms I^F and I^D were introduced. In the new study (5) it was reported that anti-I^D can be inhibited by human milk while anti-I^F cannot.

Marsh et al. (5) found that the common, benign auto-anti-I that is present in the sera of all I+ individuals (80), usually had anti-I^D specificity. That is, the antibody reacted with red cells from adults but not with cord blood red cells. In contrast, the auto-anti-I causative of CHD was said usually to be a mixture of anti-I^D plus anti-I^F. Rarely, the causative autoantibody of CHD was said to have just anti-I^F specificity. One of us (102) has seen many examples of anti-I that violate this classification. First, examples of pathological cold autoantibodies that fail to react at all with cord blood red cells have been seen and second, some benign cold autoantibodies have been encountered that did react well with cord blood red cells.

In retrospect it seems that I^F probably represents structures on branched chains already present on an infant's red cells at the time of birth while I^D probably represents structures on the chains that undergo branching during the infant's first eighteen months of life.

The term I^S was applied (103) to the Ii collection determinant recognized by those anti-I that could be totally inhibited with the IgA component isolated from human milk or colostrum. Thus the term anti-I^S describes anti-I with certain characteristics, the I^S determinant is not a separate entity within the constellation of structures recognized by various specificity anti-I.

Anti-i

This is a fairly rare antibody that gives strong reactions with cord blood and i adult red cells and weaker reactions with I+ cells. Anti-i has been reported to occur in the serum of patients with reticuloses (3,4), infectious mononucleosis (104-116), alcoholic cirrhosis (117) and myeloid leukemia (118). While anti-i is relatively common in the sera of patients with infectious mononucleosis, that is 8% of 85 patients in one study (104), 68% of 38 patients in another (106) and a calculated incidence of 50% from a worldwide literature review (110), hemolytic anemia caused by the anti-i is rare, i.e. less than 1% of all cases (110). The reason for this seems to be that while the antibody is formed frequently, only a minority of examples are able to complex with red cells at 37°C. While most of the early reports of anti-i in patients with infectious mononucleosis described IgM anti-i, with those examples with a wide thermal amplitude able to cause a secondary hemolytic anemia, some different findings were reported. Capra et al. (109) and Goldberg and Barnett (120) implicated IgG anti-i as the cause of hemolytic episodes. Capra et al. (109) described cold reactive IgG anti-i in 45 of 50 patients with infectious mononucleosis and IgM anti-IgG in 36 of them. They postulated that the hemolytic episodes were caused when the IgM anti-IgG reacted with the IgG (anti-i) coated red cells. However, the study did not produce any evidence that either the IgG anti-i, or the IgM anti-IgG, could form complexes at 37°C. Indeed few of the anti-i reacted above 25°C while the anti-IgG reacted only at 4°C. In investigating this aspect further, Wilkinson et al. (112) conducted detailed studies on three patients with infectious mononucleosis and moderate to severe hemolytic anemia. One patient had an IgM, complement-binding anti-i active to 31°C. The other two patients had low titer, cold reactive IgM anti-i. Although both had anti-IgG in the serum, the hemolytic process could not be ascribed to those antibodies since the anti-i were IgM and did not react at 20°C. Wilkinson et al. (112) concluded that it is unlikely that a single explanation applies for all the hemolytic episodes associated with infectious mononucleosis. While the presence of high thermal range IgM anti-i explains some cases there are others, such as those described above, where different explanations must obtain. Petz and Garratty (83) point out that such a concept is supported by reports of acute hemolysis in infectious mononucleosis associated with a positive Donath-Landsteiner test (113,121) and a case associated with auto-anti-N (122).

Horwitz et al. (119) studied patients with heterophile antibody-positive infectious mononucleosis and heterophile antibody-negative mononucleosis syndromes and concluded that anti-i is usually made by patients infected with the Epstein-Barr virus. As mentioned in Chapter 9, there is a hint (115) that auto-anti-i causing a hemolytic episode following infectious mononucleosis may be more of a problem in people with red cells of the Le(a-b-) and Le(a+b-) phenotypes, than in those whose red cells are Le(a-b+).

Since the i antigen is present in such large (readily accessible) amounts on cord red blood cells and since IgG forms of anti-i are known to exist (109,123,124), it is not surprising that the antibody has been incriminated (125) as causative of HDN. In another case (126), an IgG anti-i crossed the placenta and although it could not be detected (with anti-IgG) on the infant's red blood cells, it had caused complement activation so that the DAT was positive. The infant did not suffer clinical HDN.

Like strong anti-I, potent examples of anti-i may react strongly with I, i, and cord cells when undiluted serum is used. As illustrated in table 10-4, titration studies may be necessary to identify such examples of the antibody. One example of anti-i that was not detected in immediate spin compatibility tests was blamed as the cause of a hemolytic transfusion reaction (249).

Anti-I^T

In 1966, Booth et al. (127) described an antibody, that they named anti-I^T, that was thought to be associated with I and i. Although there are now reasons, discussed at the end of this section, to doubt that anti-I^T defines an antigen in the Ii collection, the long historical association between anti-I^T and I and i, makes this an appropriate place to describe the specificity of the antibody. In the original study (127) it was found that anti-I^T reacted most strongly with i cord, well with adult I and least strongly with i adult red cells. From these findings, the authors (127) concluded that anti-I^T was defining a transitional antigen (the T in I^T), present during the change from i on the cells of newborn infants, to the adult I levels reached at eighteen months of age. As mentioned above, this interpretation has now been questioned. Anti-I^T was found frequently (but not exclusively) in two populations, Melanesians (127) and Venezuelans (128,129) in both of whom it was a benign, cold-reactive autoantibody.

In 1972, Garratty et al. (130) reported an IgG anti-I^T, optimally reactive at 37°C, in the serum of a White American patient with Hodgkin's disease. The antibody did not react with the patient's own red cells so appeared to be alloimmune in nature. A different picture emerged from a large study by some of the same investigators. In studies on the blood of 56 patients with Hodgkin's disease, six of whom had a positive DAT and in three of whom there was a hemolytic process, Garratty et al. (131) found three examples of IgG, warm-reactive auto-anti-I^T. The antibodies were present in the only three patients among the 56 with Hodgkin's disease, who had hemolytic anemia. In 70 other patients with hemolytic anemia, none of whom had Hodgkin's disease, no example of anti-I^T was found. In 1977, Freedman et al. (132)

described a case of autoimmune hemolytic anemia caused by an IgM form of anti-I^T that was active at 37°C. The patient did not appear to have Hodgkin's disease. Earlier, Schmidt et al. (133) had described a similar antibody that seemed to have caused a milder form of hemolytic anemia. In 1978, Hafleigh et al. (134) described three antiglobulin-reactive examples of anti-I^T in White patients, none of whom had Hodgkin's disease. Although all three antibodies were autoimmune in nature, none of the patients had any evidence of hemolytic anemia. Further, ^{51}Cr cell survival studies and transfusions with I^T+ red cells, did not provide evidence of in vivo cell clearance by the antibodies.

There is obviously more to the I^T story and the possible association of that antigen with disease than has been learned so far. First, Booth (135,136) has found that some Melanesians have red cells that have reduced levels of I^T, but normal levels of I and i and has questioned his own concept (127) that I^T may be a transitional form between i and I. Second, it has been suggested (128) that the cold-reactive examples of anti-I^T may have been produced transiently. Such transient production of Ii collection antibodies is known to occur follow infectious mononucleosis (104-116) and pleuropneumonia like (PPLO) infections (137-142) to name only two of many infectious diseases that could be listed. For anti- I^T, malarial infections have been suggested (143) as a cause, with little evidence save the geographical locations in which the antibodies are common. Third, Garratty et al. (130,131) tested red blood cells from fetuses and found that I^T is almost as well, or is as well developed in early fetal life as at birth. In addition to causing them to question the role of I^T as a transitional antigen between i and I, this finding caused them to wonder (131) about the role of anti-I^T in their patients with Hodgkin's disease. There is considerable evidence that the re-emergence of fetal antigens and the loss of other antigens may be associated with malignancies in man (144-149). Their (131) thoughtful discussion, only a small part of which can be repeated here, richly deserves to be read in the original.

Once more, like anti-I and anti-i, anti-I^T may react strongly with I, i and i cord red cells in tests with undiluted serum and may thus defy identification. Titration studies may be necessary for the antibody specificity to be recognized. To add yet one more complication, the example of anti-I^T described by Freedman et al. (132) had a marked prozone that the authors thought probably represented the presence of a high avidity blocking anti-I^T, as well as the agglutinin in the serum.

As indicated above, there is now considerable doubt about a close relationship of I^T to I and i. In reviewing a large number of papers about the serology and biochemistry of antigens recognized by pathological autoantibodies, that are not part of the Ii collection, one of us (150)

noticed that the serological and biochemical characteristics of the antigen Lud (151-153) are almost exactly those described for I^T. Since Lud appears to be a sialylated antigen carried on type 1 glycolipid chains, its identity with I^T would remove I^T from the Ii collection. As discussed in more detail in Chapter 34, the Lud antigen is denatured when red cells are treated with a sialidase, such as neuraminidase (151). The effects on I^T of such enzyme treatment of red cells, do not seem to have been reported.

Anti-I and Anti-i in the Same Serum

On rare occasions, sera contain both anti-I and anti-i (154) that can be separated by adsorption with carefully selected red cells (80). Sera containing the two antibodies may react to about the same dilution with I, i and i cord cells if the antibodies are of about the same strength. Such mixtures make antibody identification extremely difficult unless adsorption studies are undertaken. Marsh et al. (5) have pointed out that mixtures of what they have called anti-I^D and anti-I^F may also react equally with I , i and i cord cells in titration studies.

Anti-j

In 1994, Roelcke et al. (258) described two examples of a new antibody associated with the Ii collection. Anti-j was found in the sera of two patients with cold agglutinin disease. Serologically, the antibody reacted to equal titers with adult I, i cord and adult i red cells. However, adsorption studies and the finding that the antibodies were monotypic, with mu heavy and lambda light chains, showed that they were not simply mixtures of anti-I and anti-i. Association of anti-j with the Ii collection was demonstrated in a number of ways. First, the antibody reacted with both protease and sialidase-treated red cells. As described in Chapter 34, a number of cold-reactive autoantibodies that define antigens outside the Ii collection, recognize determinants that are denatured when red cells are treated with one, the other, or both of those enzymes (153). Both I and i are protease and sialidase resistant. Second, like anti-I and anti-i, the reactions of anti-j were enhanced in tests against the enzyme-treated red cells. Third, the reactions of anti-j were reduced or abolished in tests against red cells treated with endo-beta-galactosidase, an enzyme that removes I and i-bearing type 2 chains from red cells. Fourth, anti-j was inhibited by isolates containing straight chain, i-bearing, and by branched chain, I-bearing type 2 chains. It was concluded that anti-j defines an epitope present in both linear (straight chain) and branched chain type 2 structures.

As will be seen from table 10-1, as of this writing, the determinant recognized by anti-j has not yet been given an ISBT number. For the sake of completeness, the reactions of anti-j are shown in tables 10-2 and 10-4.

Monoclonal Antibodies that Detect Antigens of the Ii Collection

Many examples of human anti-I and anti-i are monoclonal in nature (see Chapter 38 for details about cold hemagglutinin disease). It has also proved to be relatively easy to produce monoclonal antibodies, via the hybridoma technology, that detect various components of I and i (20,23,25,27,155-157). Indeed, much of the work that has led to an understanding of the complex structures of I and i has been performed with such antibodies. Since human source anti-I and anti-i are relatively easy to obtain, the monoclonal antibodies have not been extensively used in red cell phenotyping studies. Accordingly, more complete descriptions of the specificities of these antibodies will be found below, in the section on biochemistry of the antigens.

Anti-I and Anti-i as Hemolysins

As will be seen, table 10-2 describes a few examples of anti-I, anti-i and anti-IH (see later in this chapter) as having the ability to cause hemolysis in vitro. In conventional tests, relatively few of these antibodies act as hemolysins. However, if tests are performed using serum that has been acidified to pH 6.5 to 6.8 (250) or if tests are performed using protease premodified red cells (80,82), more of the antibodies will act as hemolysins. While this characteristic is more common among pathological than among benign Ii antibodies (see Chapter 38), it is by no means exclusive to those that cause CHD. In tests against enzyme-treated red cells, high titered examples of anti-I from healthy individuals may cause hemolysis.

Red Cells With Unusual I and i Phenotypes

There have been a number of reports describing persons with red cells of unexpected I system phenotypes. In 1968, Jorgensen (159) described a patient who had Turner's syndrome, but no hematological abnormality, whose red cells lacked i but carried far less I antigen than is normal. In fact, the patient's cells reacted less strongly with anti-I than did cord blood red cells. In the same year an individual was reported (160) to have red cells that reacted normally with anti-I made by normal healthy I+ adults, but which failed to react with anti-I from patients with CHD. This finding did not fit with the later claimed

(5) difference in specificity between the two types of anti-I. The benign auto-anti-I was said to have anti-I^D specificity and the antibody causative of CHD was said usually to be anti-I^D plus anti-I^F. Thus, the individual described (160) could not have had I^D+, I^F- or I^D-, I^F+ red cells. In 1974, a 19 year-old prospective blood donor was said (161) to have red cells with markedly reduced levels of I^D and i, but normal levels of I^F. Joshi and Bhatia (162) tested blood samples from 5,864 healthy Indian blood donors and claimed that seven of them had red cells that were I-, i-, and carried only small amounts of I^T. Mougey et al. (163) described a family in which the propositus and his sister had red cells that typed as only weakly positive with many examples of anti-I and anti-i. The daughter of the propositus had red cells that carried a markedly reduced amount of I and although her cells carried more i than those of her father, they were still described as having less i than is expected in the adult i phenotype. In 1984, Joshi and Bhatia (164) described a large family in India in which 15 persons had markedly depressed red cell I and i antigens while another six had red cells showing less severe depression of those antigens. Again the term I-, i- was used to describe the phenotype in which marked depression of antigen presentation occurred.

In retrospect it seems highly probable that these unusual phenotypes were largely representations of the anti-I and anti-i used. As mentioned above and as described in more detail in the section on the biochemistry of I and i, the definitive antibodies recognize a complex series of structures with the result that great heterogeneity of antibodies is seen. Presumably, in the unusual phenotypes minor differences in antigen-bearing chain synthesis could lead to apparent major differences at the phenotypic level. In support of this idea, we have been told by a colleague that when the red cells of one of the individuals (160) described above were tested with a different battery of anti-I and anti-i, no abnormalities were seen. In none of the cited cases (160-164) were disturbances in expression of H, A or B, reported. Since I, i, H, A and B are carried on the same chains perhaps it can be concluded that those chains were present in the usual numbers and in something at least close to normal steric arrangement at their termini. It seems possible that alterations had occurred in the oligosaccharide regions that normally include I and i, that do not affect the ends of the chains, where H, A and B are located. For this reason, we much prefer the designation (163) I weak, i weak, over I-, i- for the phenotype.

Association of I and i With Other Blood Group Antigens

As has been mentioned several times in this chapter,

the membrane-associated chains that carry I and i, also carry antigenic determinants of several other blood group systems. Accordingly, it should come as no surprise that antibodies exist that complex with determinants that are comprised of portions of antigens of more than one blood group system. As a single example, the anti-IA described by Tippett et al. (31) in 1960, is not a mixture of anti-I and anti-A. Instead, it is an antibody that reacts with red cells that carry both the I and the A antigens. It does not react with group A, i adult, or with group O, I+, cells, as would a serum that contained anti-I and anti-A. Not surprisingly, a large number of antibodies with similar specificities have been reported. Rather than describe each specificity separately, table 10-5 lists the determinants that have been reported and gives references to many of the papers that have described them. As mentioned earlier, when diagrams such as that presented in figure 10-1 are drawn, it appears that determinants such as I, i H, A and B are some distance apart. Existence of the antibody specificities described in this section strongly suggests that in situ the chains are positioned (folded) in such a way that at least some I and some A, etc., antigens are in close proximity. Such steric orientation, that is not apparent from two dimensional diagrams such as figure 10-1, would be expected based on composition, charge, etc., of the chains involved. As shown in table 10-5, in addition to the Ii and ABH determinants, some in the Lewis (see Chapter 9) and the P (see Chapter 11) systems are also involved (248). As far as we are aware none of these antibodies has been clinically significant in transfusion therapy for patients who did not have cold hemagglutinin disease (see Chapter 38).

The I and i Antigens and Disease

The very considerable roles played by anti-I and less frequently by anti-i and anti-I^T as causative autoantibodies of cold hemagglutinin disease (cold antibody-induced hemolytic anemia) are described in detail in Chapter 38. The production of anti-I in patients with atypical pneumonia, caused by the pleuropneumonia-like-organism (PPLO) and of anti-i in patients with infectious mononucleosis have been mentioned above and, since in both instances the antibodies can cause secondary hemolytic anemia, are discussed again, also in Chapter 38.

In addition to the above very clear associations of the I and i antigens with disease, a number of others have been reported. In 1964, Giblett and Crookston (190) showed that the red cells of all of 17 patients with thalassemia major carried more i antigen than did the cells of healthy individuals. Similar findings were made in some but not all patients with hypoplastic anemia, acute leukemia and chronic hemolytic states. The amount of

TABLE 10-5 Antigens Dependent on the Presence of Determinants of more than one Blood Group System

Antigen	References *
IA	31,165-168
IB	169-172
IH	140,173-179
iH	165,173,180
IP_1	181
I^TP_1	182
iP_1	183
IP	184
ILe^{bH}	185,186
IBH	187,188
IAB	189

* Some of the earlier papers did not use terms such as anti-IH, anti-iH, etc., but the data presented clearly show the reactivity of the antibodies as being affected by ABO etc., type.

increase of i was not related to ABO group, degree of anemia or amount of fetal hemoglobin present. The authors (190) postulated that prolonged marrow stress might result in increased levels of i on red cells. The following year, Hillman and Giblett (191) conducted tests on a patient with hemochromatosis and huge iron stores. The patient was treated by repeated phlebotomy, that eventually caused anemia, to reduce the iron stores. It was shown that the appearance of i antigen on red cells released from the marrow was related to the maturation time of cells in the marrow. In other words, regardless of the degree of anemia, if red cells spent their full maturation time in the marrow, they were released into circulation carrying large amounts of I and very little i. If the marrow was stressed and red cells were released in less than the usual length of time (as shown by incorporation of a radio-label in the cells as they were formed) they emerged from the marrow carrying higher than normal levels of i. It does not seem unreasonable, now to suppose, that when first formed from erythroid precursor cells in the marrow, red cells have many straight chain oligosaccharides on their surface. Perhaps during the normal maturation time, branching of those chains occurs and the released cells then type as typical I+ red cells. If the time spent in the marrow by newly formed red cells is reduced, those cells may then be released before full branching has occurred with the result that more i than usual is detectable. However, it must be added that in virtually all cases where an increase in i on the red cells of a patient has been seen, the I level of those cells has either remained normal, or has also been increased (for a review see 192). Cooper et al. (193) found that the red cells of 13 of 15 patients with sideroblastic anemia and of 7 of 8 patients with megaloblastic anemia, had increased levels of I and i. They were unable to correlate the increase in levels of those antigens with decreased red cell marrow transit times and considered disordered erythropoeisis a more likely explanation. Somewhat similarly, Maniatis et al. (194) found increased levels of both I and i on the red cells of patients with sickle cell disease and some increases on the cells of patients with sickle cell trait. Berrebi and Levene (195) reported that the acanthocytic red cells of a patient with abetalipoproteinemia had i levels equal to those of cord red blood cells although their I content was not reduced.

In the above cited papers (190-194) and in others (196-199) that have demonstrated altered expressions of I and/or i in dyserythropoeisis, no correlation has been found between the level of hemoglobin F and the level of i antigen. In other words, as mentioned earlier, although the changes from i to I and from HbF to HbA production occur at about the same time in infants, there is no evidence at all that the i antigen and HbF are structurally related.

McGinniss et al. (138) reported that the red cells of 22 of 73 patients with leukemia failed to react with anti-I and further, that when clinical remissions were induced, the red cells of some of the patients typed as I+. Jenkins et al. (200) also described a leukemic patient with red cells that had depressed I and increased i, while another leukemic patient was found (201) to have altered I expression on the red cells that was associated with altered expression of the ABO and Rh antigens. In contrast, Ducos et al. (202) found no reduction of I antigen strength on the red cells of any of 56 patients with leukemia. Again, one might suspect that the fine specificities of the anti-I used in the various studies could account for these divergent findings.

Crookston et al. (203) found that the red cells of patients with hereditary erythroblastic multinuclearity with a positive acid serum lysis test (HEMPAS), carry higher than normal levels of i and are particularly susceptible to lysis by anti-I and anti-i. Although Worlledge (199) was not able to demonstrate increased levels of I on these cells there are several reports (204-207) that show that the increased susceptibility of HEMPAS red cells to lysis is due to their ability to bind more anti-I than do normal I+ red cells, so that more complement is activated. The mechanism by which lysis is induced by increased amounts of anti-I being bound (207) is different from the situation involving the red cells of patients with paroxysmal nocturnal hemoglobinuria. PNH is a red cell abnormality, not to be confused with PCH which is an antibody-induced hemolytic anemia. The red cells of persons with PNH bind the same amount of anti-I as do normal I+ cells but are susceptible to lysis by very small amounts of activated complement (207-217).

Several groups of workers (218-220) have reported an association between the i adult phenotype and congenital cataract. The early association that suggested genetic linkage between the two characters, was noticed in Oriental individuals. While the linkage did not seem to be as pronounced in Whites (221,246) some such families apparently showing the linkage, have been found (222,246).

The I Antigen and Drug-Induced Antibodies

There is now a fairly considerable body of evidence that the I antigen may act as a membrane receptor in some cases of drug-induced, antibody-mediated red cell destruction (223-229). The drugs involved have included dexchlorphenyramine maleate, rifampicin, nitrofurantoin, thiopental, fluorouracil (5-FU), nomifensine and its metabolities. In most instances the drug-antibody immune complexes would bind to I+ but not to i adult or i cord red cells. The antibodies to nomifensine and its metabolites were inhibited by soluble I antigen (227). These findings are described in more detail in Chapter 40.

The I and i Antigens on Leukocytes and Platelets

As would be expected from what has been written in this chapter thus far about the biochemical structures of I and i, the antigens are not confined to red cells. Anti-I and anti-i will agglutinate lymphocytes (231). Shumak et al. (232) found that lymphocytes from cord blood samples had decreased levels of I but that the i antigen was present in similar amounts on the lymphocytes of adults and newborn infants. Watkins and Shulman (233) demonstrated the presence of I and i on platelets. In view of the fact that I and i are present on lymphocytes and on other leukocytes, it is not surprising that I system antibodies that are lymphocytotoxic have been reported (234-241). Some of the antibodies also have the ability to kill granulocytes and monocytes when complement is available (238,239,242-244). The leukopenia and thrombocytopenia occasionally seen in patients with CHD may represent the destruction of white cells and platelets by the patient's autoantibody (245). More often, patients with CHD have normal leukocyte and platelet counts (83).

The level of i antigen on the lymphocytes of patients with chronic lymphocytic leukemia is markedly reduced and may be an early indicator of the disease since the amount of i is normal on the blast cells of patients with acute lymphoblastic leukemia and on the lymphocytes of some patients with lymphosarcoma (247).

The Molecular Basis of I and i

The first information regarding the structure of the I antigen was obtained by Marcus et al. in 1963 (10). These authors treated red cells with a mixture of exo-glycosidases (β-galactosidase and β-glucosaminidase) derived from cultures of *Clostridium tertium* and showed that the I antigen on the treated cells was weakened. These results therefore suggested that the I antigen was a carbohydrate structure containing galactose and N-acetylglucosamine. Studies of I antigen structure were hampered by the apparent absence of a water-soluble source of I substance until 1970 when it was realized that some anti-I could be inhibited by water soluble substances contained in human saliva (6) and human milk (7). The key observations which laid the foundation for an understanding of the structure of the I antigen came in a series of papers in the early 1970's from Ten Feizi working in Elvin Kabat's laboratory in New York. Feizi et al. (260) showed that 2 of 21 anti-I sera were inhibited by a partially purified blood group-like substance from human milk but more significantly one anti-I serum (anti-I, Ma) was strongly inhibited by a blood group substance (OG) isolated from ovarian cyst fluid, derived from a Nigerian, which lacked A, B, H, Le^a and Le^b activity. OG substance was considered to be a precursor substance in the pathways giving rise to A, B, H and Lewis antigens (261) and it could be shown that chemical degradation of ABH active substances from human ovarian cyst fluids and pig gastric mucin revealed I antigen activity and that I activity was also found in some blood group substances derived from cow stomach. These studies provided two important keys with which to unlock the structure of I. First, that I antigen is a precursor en route to ABH and Lewis and so its structure must be contained within that of the already well characterized blood group substances. Second, the availability of an inhibitable anti-I serum (Ma) would allow oligosaccharides of known structure derived from blood group substances to be tested for I activity. When such oligosaccharides were tested for their ability to inhibit the interaction between anti-I (Ma) and precursor blood group substance OG only one disaccharide inhibitor showed significant activity and this had the structure β-D-Galactose(1→4)-D-GlcNAc. The antibody was inhibited best by oligosaccharides with the structure β-D-Gal(1→4)β-D-GlcNAc(1→6)(12). Further studies on eleven anti-I and five anti-i revealed at least six types

of anti-I and four types of anti-i. The antigens recognized by all types of anti-I and anti-i were represented in varying amounts in the precursor blood group substance OG (262). I + P$_1$-active materials were also isolated from hydatid cyst fluid (see also Chapter 11) suggesting that this tapeworm derived glycoprotein had a similar structure to human and animal blood group substances (263).

The next advance in understanding the structure of Ii antigens came from studies of glycolipids derived from human and cow red cell membranes. A sialylated glycolipid (ganglioside) derived from bovine stroma was shown to have weak I activity with one anti-I (Step) but not with anti-I (Ma) and i antigen activity detected by several anti-i. If the sialic acid residue was removed from this ganglioside both the I antigen activity recognized by anti-I (Step) and the i antigen activity were significantly increased. The desialylated ganglioside goes by the unwieldy name of Lacto-N-*nor*-hexaosylceramide and has the structure shown in figure 10-1. The same structure is found in human red cell membranes and can be created from a blood group H-active glycolipid (H$_2$-glycolipid) by treatment with the exoglycosidase α-L-fucosidase whereupon I antigenic activity for anti-I (Step) and i antigenic activity is revealed de novo (264). These Ii activities can be removed by treatment with the exoglycosidase, β-D-galactosidase or removal of two N-acetyl groups from GlcNAc residues suggesting that the alternating sequence Galβ(1→4) GlcNAcβ (1→3)Galβ(1→4)GlcNAcβ(1→3)- defines the I antigen recognized by anti-I (Step) and the i antigen. These results when taken together with the earlier studies described above which defined the specificity of anti-I (Ma) led to the conclusion that the I antigen recognized by anti-I (Ma) can be created from the i antigen structure by addition of the Galβ(1→4)GlcNAcβ(1→6) sequence to Lacto N-*nor*-hexaosylceramide to create a branched structure (see figure 10-1). The results do not explain the reactivity of anti-I (Step). Subsequent studies confirmed the structure recognized by anti-I (Ma) as the branched oligosaccharide shown in figure 10-1 and further showed that anti-I (Step) reacts best with the Galβ(1→4)GlcNAcβ(1→3) structure in Lacto-N-*nor*-hexaosylceramide when it is part of the branched structure also recognized by anti-I (Ma), figure 10-1, (19,20).

Various studies carried out in the 1970's showed that I and i antigens could be expressed on both glycoproteins and glycolipids in the human red cell membrane and, where structural studies were carried out, I antigen-activity was exclusively associated with branched oligosaccharide structures of the type described above and in figure 10-1 (14,15,16,265-267,270). Childs et al. (268) showed that the I antigen is carried by the major anion transport protein of the red cell, band 3 and Fukuda et al.

(269) compared the structure of oligosaccharides from band 3 in adult red cells with those derived from band 3 in cord blood cells and with those from adult i cells. These studies showed that the oligosaccharride found on band 3 in adult cells differed from that found in cord cells and adult i cells in that it contained a branched structure consistent with expression of I antigen which was absent from band 3 on cord cells and adult i cells. Okada et al. (271) found the same for glycolipids derived from adult and cord red cells. All these results pointed to the creation of the branched structure as being the defining step in the synthesis of I antigen and lack of the glycosyltransferase which creates this branch as the cause of the adult i phenotype. A number of studies of glycosyltransferases involved in synthesis of Ii-active structures were carried out during the 1980's and these are reviewed by Roelcke (272). The gene encoding a β-1,6-N-acetylglucosaminyltransferase capable of generating the branched structure which carries I antigen activity was cloned by Bierhuizen et al. in 1993 (273).

Cloning the *I* Gene

A cDNA encoding a member of a β-1,6-N-acetylglucosaminyltransferase family was obtained by Bierhuizen et al. (273). These authors used an expression cloning strategy similar to that use by Kukowska-Latallo et al. (274) to clone the *Le* gene-specified transferase (see Chapter 9). Chinese hamster ovary cells (CHO cells) express the linear i antigen but not I antigen (275,276). Bierhuizen et al. (273) used a CHO cell line (CHO-Py.leu cells) which allowed transient expression cloning, utilizing vectors which have the polyoma virus replication origin. A cDNA expression library was constructed from mRNA derived from a cell line (PA-1 cells, a human teratocarcinoma cell line) known to express a large amount of I-active structures. The cDNA was then transfected into the CHO cell line and cells secreting I-active structures were selected by panning using anti-I. After several rounds of selection a plasmid was obtained which directed the expression of I antigen (detected by anti-I (Ma)). The plasmid contained a cDNA insert of 1807bp which predicted a protein of 400 amino acids with a molecular weight of 45,860. Hydropathy analysis indicated a type II membrane protein with a short N-terminal domain of 6 amino acids, a single transmembrane domain of 19 amino acids and a large C-terminal domain with 6 potential N-glycosylation sites which by analogy with other cloned glycosyltransferases would be expected to contain the catalytic site of the enzyme. Northern blotting studies carried out with the cDNA revealed a single RNA transcript of 4.4kb in PA-1 cells but no transcript in CHO-Py.leu cells as would be expected for an enzyme which effects I

antigen synthesis. The I enzyme (denoted IGnT for I acetylglucosaminyltransferase) showed substantial sequence homology in its C terminal domain with another β-1,6-N-acetylglucosaminyltransferase (denoted C2GnT). C2GnT catalyses the transfer of GlcNAcβ1→6 to Galβ1→3GalNAc but not to Galβ1→4GlcNAc (277). Determination of the chromosomal location of the genes giving rise to IGnT and C2GnT using in situ hybridization revealed that both are located on chromosome 9 at q21(273). The ABO transferase gene is located on chromosome 9 at q34 (see Chapter 8). Ropp et al. (280) describe another β-1,6-N-acetylglucosaminyltransferase isolated from bovine tracheal epithelium which has the substrate specificity of both IGnT and C2GnT and the additional ability to transfer GlcNAc to the 6 position of a GalNAc in the structure GlcNAcβ1→3GalNAc. Whether or not this third enzyme corresponds to an additional human gene related to those that encode IGnT and C2GnT located on chromosome 9q21 (see above) is not yet known. The enzyme IGnT certainly has the ability to generate I antigen but it would seem possible that a human analogue of the enzyme described by Ropp et al. (280) might also have this property. It would be desirable to study the gene encoding IGnT in individuals with the adult i phenotype (presumed to be genetically *ii*) to see if the expression of this genotype corresponds with mutations in the *IGnT* gene and whether or not there is any relationship between such mutations and the occurrence of congenital cataract (see earlier section). The search for similar mutations in the *H* gene (Chapter 8) and the *Le* and *Se* genes (Chapter 9) has been of great value in confirming that the products of these genes are the ones controlling blood group antigen expression. If the *IGnT* gene is confirmed as that which controls I antigen expression in red cells then there would seem to be no reason for denying system status to I since it would be in an analogous situation to H. The i antigen would not however, be part of the I system since it is not the product of the *IGnT* gene. Here again the analogy with A, B and H is valid. H antigen is a precursor of A and/or B antigen but it is not a product of the same gene as A and B and therefore ABO on the one hand and H on the other, are separate blood group systems.

The Structure of the *I* Gene

The genomic structure of the genes giving rise to IGnT and C2GnT was reported by Bierhuizen et al. (278). Genomic clones were isolated from a human placental genomic DNA library using a mixture of labeled cDNA for both *IGnT* and *C2GnT*. The human *C2GnT* gene was found to be composed of two exons. The first exon (326bp) contained a 5′ untranslated sequence. Exon

2 contained the rest of the 5' untranslated (143bp) and the entire coding sequence (1284bp) as well as the 3' untranslated sequence.

The human *IGnT* gene comprises 3 exons. Exon 1 (1629bp) contains the initiator codon at nt711 and encodes more than half the translation product. Exon 2 is small (93bp). Exon 3 (947bp) includes the rest of the coding sequence (188bp) and the 3' untranslated sequence. *C2GnT* and *IGnT* contain three regions of homology (> 60% identity) in their catalytic domains suggesting that they evolved from a common ancestral gene.

The Function of I Antigens

As discussed earlier it is well established that I antigen is developmentally regulated. The recent cloning of the mouse homologue of human *IGnT* has permitted a detailed study of the tissue distribution of I antigen in the mouse and opened the way for the production of "knock-out" mice lacking *IGnT* to study the functional significance of the enzyme (279). In the mouse, IGnT and I antigen appear in epithelial cells and dividing cells as well as cells exposed to the lumenal surface of tissues (279).

References

1. Wiener AS, Unger LJ, Cohen L, et al. Ann Intern Med 1956;44:221
2. Jenkins WJ, Marsh WL, Noades J, et al. Vox Sang 1960;5:97
3. Marsh WL, Jenkins WJ. Nature 1960;188:753
4. Marsh WL. Br J Haematol 1961;7:200
5. Marsh WL, Nichols ME, Reid ME. Vox Sang 1971;20:209
6. Dzierzkowa-Borodej W, Seyfried H, Nichols ME, et al. Vox Sang 1970;18:222
7. Marsh WL, Nichols ME, Allen FH Jr. Vox Sang 1970;18:149
8. Burnie K. Canad J Med Technol 1973;35:5
9. Cooper AG, Brown MC. Biochem Biophys Res Comm 1973;55:297
10. Marcus DM, Kabat EA, Rosenfield RE. J Exp Med 1963;118:175
11. Dzierzkowa-Borodej W, Lisowska E, Seyfried H. Life Sci 1970;9:111
12. Feizi T, Kabat EA, Vicari G, et al. J Immunol 1971;106:1578
13. Gardas A, Koscielak J. FEBS Lett 1974;42:101
14. Watanabe K, Laine RA, Hakomori SI. Biochemistry 1975;14:2725
15. Gardas A. Eur J Biochem 1976;68:185
16. Koscielak J, Miller-Podraza H, Krauze R, et al. Eur J Biochem 1976;71:9
17. Kabat EA, Liao J, Lemieux RU. Immunochemistry 1978;15:727
18. Wood E, Feizi T. FEBS Lett 1979;104:135
19. Watanabe K, Hakomori SI, Childs RA, et al. J Biol Chem 1979;254:3221
20. Feizi T, Childs RA, Watanabe K, et al. J Exp Med 1979;149:975
21. Kabat EA, Liao J, Burzynska MH, et al. Mol Immunol 1981;18:873
22. Hanfland P, Egge H, Dubrowski U, et al. Biochemistry 1981;20:5310
23. Gooi HC, Uemura K, Edwards PAW, et al. Carbohydr Res 1983;120:293
24. Lemieux RU, Wong TC, Liao J, et al. Mol Immunol 1984;21:751
25. Gooi HC, Veyrières A, Alias J, et al. Mol Immunol 1984;21:1099
26. Egge H, Kordowicz M, Peter-Katalinic J, et al. J Biol Chem 1985;260:4927
27. Dube VE, Kallio P, Tanaka M. Mol Immunol 1986;23:217
28. Tang PW, Scudder P, Mehmet H, et al. Eur J Biochem 1986;160:537
29. Feizi T, Hounsell EF, Alias J, et al. Carbohydr Res 1992;228:289
30. Gu J, Nishikawa A, Fujii S, et al. J Biol Chem 1992;267:2994
31. Tippett P, Noades J, Sanger R, et al. Vox Sang 1960;5:107
32. Testa U, Rochnant H, Henri A, et al. Blood Transf Immunohematol 1981;24:299
33. Marsh WL, Jensen L, Decary F, et al. Transfusion 1972;12:222
34. Claflin AJ. Transfusion 1963;3:216
35. Jakobowicz R, Simmon RT. Med J Austral 1964;1:194
36. Race RR, Sanger R. Blood Groups in Man, 5th Ed. Oxford:Blackwell, 1968
37. Yamaguchi H, Okubo Y, Tomita T, et al. Proc Jpn Acad 1970;46:889
38. Yamaguchi H, Okubo Y, Tanaka M. Proc Jpn Acad 1972;48:625
39. Dzierzkowa-Borodej W, Kazmierczak Z, Ziemniak J. Arch Immunol Ther Exp 1972;20:851
40. Signal T, Booth PB. Vox Sang 1976;30:391
41. Zielenski J, Koscielak J. FEBS Lett 1983;163:114
42. Eijnden van der DH, Winterwerp H, Smeeman P, et al. J Biol Chem 1983;258:3435
43. Basu M, Basu S. J Biol Chem 1984;259:12557
44. Piller F, Cartron J-P, Maranduba A, et al. J Biol Chem 1984;259:13385
45. Brockhausen I, Matta KL, Orr J, et al. Eur J Biochem 1986;157:463
46. Feizi T, Marsh WL. Vox Sang 1970;18:379
47. Rouger P, Juszczak G, Doinel C, et al. Transfusion 1980;20:536
48. Rouger P, Riveau D, Salmon C. Vox Sang 1979;37:78
49. Cooper AG. Nature 1970;227:508
50. Rosse WF, Lauf PK. Blood 1990;36:777
51. Zvilichovsky B, Gallop PM, Blumenfeld OO. Biochem Biophys Res Comm 1971;44:1234
52. Marchesi VT, Andrews EP. Science 1971;174:1247
53. Hamaguchi H, Cleve H. Biochim Biophys Acta 1972;278:271
54. Tanner MJA, Boxer DH. Biochem J 1972;129:333
55. Akiyama Y, Osawa Y. Hoppe Seylers Z Physiol Chem 1972;353:323
56. Lisowska E, Jeanloz RW. Carbohydr Res 1973;29:181
57. Roelcke D, Ebert W, Metz J, et al. Vox Sang 1973;21:352
58. Fukuda M, Osawa T. J Biol Chem 1973;248:5100
59. Liao T, Gallup PM, Blumenfeld OO. J Biol Chem 1973;248:8247
60. Anstee DJ, Tanner MJA. Biochem J 1974;138:381
61. Anstee DJ, Tanner MJA. Eur J Biochem 1974;45:31
62. Lisowska E, Dzierzkowa-Borodej W, Seyfried H, et al. Vox Sang 1975;28:122
63. Anstee DJ, Tanner MJA. Vox Sang 1975;29:378
64. Gardas A, Koscielak J. Vox Sang 1974;26:227

65. Wood E, Lecomte J, Childs RA, et al. Mol Immunol 1979;16:813

66. Koscielak J. In: Human Blood Groups. Basel:Karger, 1977:143

67. Hakomori S, Watanabe K, Laine RA. In: Human Blood Groups. Basel:Karger, 1977:150

68. Feizi T. In: Human Blood Groups. Basel:Karger, 1977:164

69. Feizi T, Kabat EA, Vicari G, et al. J Exp 1971;133:39

70. Feizi T, Kabat EA. J Exp Med 1972;135:247

71. Feizi T, Kabat EA. J Immunol 1974;112:145

72. Hakomori S. Sem Hematol 1981;18:39

73. Dzierzkowa-Borodej W, Meinhard W, Nestorowicz S, et al. Arch Immunol Ther Exp 1972;20:841

74. Lopez M, Gerbal A, Salmon C. Rev Fr Transf 1972;15:187

75. Moores PP, Issitt PD, Pavone BG, et al. Transfusion 1975;15:237

76. Watanabe K, Hakomori S. J Exp Med 1976;144:644

77. Fukuda M, Fukuda MN, Hakomori S. J Biol Chem 1979;254:3700

78. Fukuda M, Fukuda MN, Hakomori S. J Biol Chem 1979;254:5458

79. Koscielak J, Zdebska E, Wilcznska Z, et al. Eur J Biochem 1979;96:331

80. Issitt PD, Jackson VA. Vox Sang 1968;15:152

81. Judd WJ. Methods in Immunohematology, 2nd Ed. Durham:Montgomery, 1994

82. Petz LD, Garratty G. In: Laboratory Diagnosis in Immune Disorders. New York:Grune and Stratton, 1975:139

83. Petz LD, Garratty G. Acquired Immune Hemolytic Anemias. New York:Churchill Livingstone, 1980

84. Dube VE, Zuckerman L, Philipsborn HF Jr. Vox Sang 1978;34:71

85. Angevine CD, Andersen BR, Barnett EV. J Immunol 1966;96:578

86. Roelcke D, Ebert W, Feizi T. Immunology 1974;27:879

87. Dacie JV. Arch Int Med 1975;135:1293

88. Roelcke D. Ric Clin Lab 1977;7:11

89. Polley MJ, Mollison PL, Soothill JF. Br J Haematol 1962;8:149

90. Adinolfi M, Polley MJ, Hunter DA, et al. Immunology 1962;5:566

91. Chaplin H, Hunter VL, Malacek AC, et al. Transfusion 1986;26:57

92. Weiner W, Shinton NK, Gray IR. J Clin Pathol 1960;13:232

93. Mass D, Schubothe H. Vox Sang 1968;14:292

94. Shirey RS, Harris J, Moore L. (abstract). Transfusion 1979;19:642

95. Marks MR, Reid ME, Ellisor SS. (abstract). Transfusion 1980;20:629

96. Waligora SK, Edwards JM. Transfusion 1983;23:328

97. Edwards-Moulds J, Waligora SK. (Letter). Transfusion 1984;24:369

98. Strauss RA, Gasich L, Gloster ES. Lab Med 1985;16:551

99. Orsini LA, Haase JE, Poling SR, et al. (abstract). Transfusion 1985;25:452

100. Dzik WH, Yang R, Blank J. (Letter). Transfusion 1986;26:303

101. Weiland DL. (Letter). Transfusion 1984;24:369

102. Issitt PD. In: Progress in Clinical Pathology, Vol 7. New York:Grune and Stratton, 1978:137

103. Dzierzkowa-Borodej W, Seyfried H, Lisowska E. Vox Sang 1975;28:110

104. Jenkins WJ, Koster HG, Marsh WL, et al. Br J Haematol 1965;11:480

105. Calvo R, Stein W, Kochwa S, et al. J Clin Invest 1965;44:1033

106. Rosenfield RE, Schmidt PJ, Calvo RC, et al. Vox Sang 1965;10:631

107. Brafield AJ. Lancet 1966;1:982

108. Troxel DB, Innella F, Cohen RJ. Am J Clin Pathol 1966;46:625

109. Capra JD. Dowling P, Cook S, et al. Vox Sang 1969;16:10

110. Worlledge SM, Dacie JV. In: Infectious Mononucleosis. Oxford:Blackwell, 1969

111. Hossaini AA. Am J Clin Pathol 1970;53:198

112. Wilkinson LS, Petz LD, Garratty G. Br J Haematol 1973;25:715

113. Wishart MM, Davey MG. J Clin Pathol 1973;26:332

114. Woodruff RK, McPherson AJ. Austral N Z J Med 1976;6:569

115. Lee CH, Hagen MA, Chong BH, et al. Transfusion 1980;20:585

116. Gronemeyer P, Chaplin H, Ghazarian V, et al. Transfusion 1981;21:715

117. Rubin H, Solomon A. Vox Sang 1967;12:227

118. Loghem van JJ, Hart van der M, Veenhoven van RE, et al. Vox Sang 1962;7:214

119. Horwitz CA, Moulds J, Henle W, et al. Blood 1977;50:195

120. Goldberg LS, Barnett EV. Ann NY Acad Sci 1969;168:122

121. Ellis LB, Wollenman OJ, Stetson RP. Blood 1948;3:419

122. Bowman HS, Marsh WL, Schumacher HR, et al. Am J Clin Pathol 1974;61:465

123. MacKenzie MR, Creevy NC. Blood 1970;36:549

124. Mollison PL. Blood Transfusion in Clinical Medicine, 6th Ed. Oxford:Blackwell, 1979

125. Gerbal A, Lavallee R, Ropars C, et al. Nouv Rev Fr Hematol 1971;11:689

126. Branch DR. Transfusion 1979;19:348

127. Booth PB, Jenkins WJ, Marsh WL. Br J Haematol 1966;12:341

128. Layrisse Z, Layrisse M. Vox Sang 1968;14:369

129. Layrisse Z, Layrisse M. Vox Sang 1972;22:457

130. Garratty G, Hafleigh EF, Dalziel J, et al. Transfusion 1972;12:325

131. Garratty G, Petz LD, Wallerstein RO, et al. Transfusion 1974;14:226

132. Freedman J, Newlands M, Johnson CA. Vox Sang 1977;32:135

133. Schmidt PJ, McCurdy P, Havell T, et al. (abstract). Transfusion 1974;14:507

134. Hafleigh EB, Wells RF, Grumet FC. Transfusion 1978;18:592

135. Booth PB. Vox Sang 1972;22:64

136. Booth PB. Personal communication to and cited by Garratty G, Petz LD, Wallerstein RO, et al. Transfusion 1974;14:226

137. Channock RM, Mufson MA, Somerson NL, et al. Am Rev Resp Dis 1963;88(Suppl 2):218

138. McGinniss MH, Schmidt PJ, Carbone PP. Nature 1964;202:606

139. Schmidt PJ, Barile MF, McGinniss MH. Nature 1965;205:371

140. Schmidt PJ, McGinniss MH. Vox Sang 1965;10:109

141. Schmidt PJ, McGinniss MH. Nature 1967;214:1363

142. Smith CB, McGinniss MH, Schmidt PJ. J Immunol 1967;99:333

143. Curtain CC, Baumgarten A, Gorman J, et al. Br J Haematol 1965;11:471

144. Laurence DJR, Neville AM. Br J Cancer 1972;26:335

145. Simmons DAR, Perlmann D. Cancer Res 1973;33:313

146. Feizi T. Cancer Surv 1985;4:245

147. Nichols EJ, Kannagi R, Hakomori S, et al. J Immunol 1985;135:1911

148. Hakomori S. Cancer Res 1985;45:2405

149. Liotta LA. Sci Am 1992;266:54

150. Issitt PD. In: Blood Groups: P, I, Sd^a and Pr. Arlington, VA:Am Assoc Blood Banks, 1991:73
151. Roelcke D. Vox Sang 1981;41:316
152. Kajii E, Ikemoto S, Miura Y. Vox Sang 1988;54:248
153. Roelcke D. Transf Med Rev 1989;3:140
154. Jackson VA, Issitt PD, Francis BJ, et al. Vox Sang 1968;15:133
155. Feizi T. Nature 1985;314:53
156. Wasserman RL, Steane EA, Steane SM, et al. (abstract). Transfusion 1985;25:481
157. Hirohashi S, Clausen H, Nudelman E, et al. J Immunol 1986;136:4163
158. Messeter L, Johnson U. J Immunogenet 1990;17:213
159. Jorgensen JR. Vox Sang 1968;15:171
160. McGinnis MH, Grindon AJ. (abstract). Transfusion 1968;8:314
161. Dzierzkowa-Borodej W, Lisowska E, Leskiewicz A, et al. Vox Sang 1974;27:57
162. Joshi SR, Bhatia HM. Vox Sang 1979;36:34
163. Mougey R, Gaergen B, Troyer P, et al. (abstract). Transfusion 1978;18:643
164. Joshi SR, Bhatia HM. Vox Sang 1984;46:157
165. Gold ER. Vox Sang 1964;9:153
166. Yokoyama M. Nature 1965;206:411
167. Baumgarten A, Curtain CC, Golab T, et al. Br J Haematol 1968;15:567
168. Baumgarten A, Curtain CC. Vox Sang 1970;18:21
169. Tegoli J, Harris JP, Issitt PD, et al. Vox Sang 1967;13:144
170. Drachmann O. Vox Sang 1968;14:185
171. Voak D, Lodge TW, Hopkins J, et al. Vox Sang 1968;15:353
172. Morel P, Garratty G, Willbanks E. Vox Sang 1975;29:231
173. Rosenfield RE, Schroeder R, Ballard R, et al. Vox Sang 1964;9:415
174. Voak D. Scand J Haematol 1964;1:238
175. Salmon C, Homberg JC, Liberge G, et al. Rev Fr Etud Clin Biol 1965;5:552
176. Giblett ER, Hillman RS, Brooks LE. Vox Sang 1965;10:448
177. Lodge TW, Voak D. Vox Sang 1968;14:60
178. Dzierzkowa-Borodej W. Ann Immunol 1971;3:85
179. Ting A, Pun A, Dodds AJ, et al. Transfusion 1987;27:145
180. Pierce SR, Kowalski MA, Hardman JT, et al. (abstract). Book of Abstracts. ISBT/AABB Joint Cong 1990:79
181. Issitt PD, Tegoli J, Jackson VA, et al. Vox Sang 1968;14:1
182. Booth PB. Vox Sang 1970;19:85
183. McGinniss MH, Kaplan HS, Bowen AB, et al. Transfusion 1969;9:40
184. Allen FH Jr, Marsh WL, Jensen L, et al. Vox Sang 1974;27:442
185. Tegoli J, Cortez M, Jensen L, et al. Vox Sang 1971;21:397
186. Branch DR, Powers T. (Letter). Transfusion 1979;19:353
187. Baird JF, Hansel MJ, McCurdy PR. (abstract). Transfusion 1975;15:526
188. Cassidy K, Blajchman MA. (abstract). Transfusion 1975;15:526
189. Doinel C, Ropars C, Salmon C. Vox Sang 1974;27:515
190. Giblett ER, Crookston MC. Nature 1964;201:1138
191. Hillman RS, Giblett ER. J Clin Invest 1965;44:1730
192. Issitt PD. J Med Lab Technol 1968;25:1
193. Cooper AG, Hoffbrand AV, Worlledge SM. Br J Haematol 1968;15:381
194. Maniatis A, Frieman B, Bertles JF. Vox Sang 1977;33:29
195. Berrebi A, Levene C. Vox Sang 1976;30:396
196. Dacie JV, Lewis SM, Tills D. Br J Haematol 1960;6:362
197. Lewis SM, Dacie JV, Tills D. Br J Haematol 1961;7:64
198. Lewis SM. Br J Haematol 1962;8:322

199. Worlledge SM. In: Dyserythropoiesis. New York:Academic Press, 1977
200. Jenkins WJ, Marsh WL, Gold ER. Nature 1965;205:813
201. Walewska I, Zdziechowska H. Acta Haematol Pol 1970;1:263
202. Ducos J, Ruffie J, Colombies P, et al. Nature 1965;208:1329
203. Crookston JH, Crookston MC, Burnie KL, et al. Br J Haematol 1969;17:11
204. Crookston JH, Crookston MC, Rosse WF. (abstract). Blood 1969;34:844
205. Lewis SM, Garammaticos P, Dacie JV. Br J Haematol 1970;18:465
206. Crookston JH, Crookston MC. In: Blood Groups and Other Red Cell Surface Markers in Health and Disease. New York:Masson 1982:29
207. Rosse WF, Logue GL, Adams J. J Clin Invest 1974;53:31
208. Rosse WF, Dacie JV. J Clin Invest 1966;45:749
209. Jenkins DE Jr, Christenson WN, Engle RL Jr. J Clin Invest 1966;45:796
210. May JE, Rosse WF, Frank MM. New Eng J Med 1973;289:705
211. Rosse WF, Adams JP, Thorpe AM. Br J Haematol 1974;28:181
212. Jenkins DE Jr, Johnson RM, Hartman RC. Transfusion 1978;18:647
213. Packman CH, Rosenfeld SI, Jenkins DE Jr. J Clin Invest 1979;64:428
214. Rosse WF, Parker CJ. Clin Haematol 1986;14:105
215. Holguin MH, Wilcox LA, Bernshaw NJ, et al. J Clin Invest 1989;84:1387
216. Rosse WF. Clinical Immunohematology: Basic Concepts and Clinical Applications. Boston:Blackwell, 1990
217. Rosse WF. In: Clinical and Basic Science Aspects of Immunohematology. Arlington, VA:Am Assoc Blood Banks, 1991:13
218. Yamaguchi H, Okubo Y, Tomita M. Proc Jpn Acad 1972;48:625
219. Ogata H, Okubo Y, Akabane T. Transfusion 1979;19:166
220. Lin-Chu M, Broadberry RE, Okubo Y, et al. (Letter). Transfusion 1991;31:676
221. Marsh WL, DePalma H. Transfusion 1982;22:337
222. Macdonald EB, Douglas R, Harden P. Vox Sang 1983;44:322
223. Duran-Suarez JR, Martin-Vega C, Argelagues E, et al. Br J Haematol 1981;49:153
224. Duran-Suarez JR, Martin-Vega C, Argelagues E, et al. Vox Sang 1981;41:313
225. Habibi B, Basty R, Chodez S, et al. New Eng J Med 1985;312:353
226. Sandvei P, Nordhagen R, Michaelsen TE, et al. Br J Haematol 1987;65:357
227. Salama A, Mueller-Eckhardt C. Blood 1987;69:1006
228. Pereira A, Sanz C, Cervantes F, et al. Ann Hematol 1991;63:56
229. Habibi B, Bretagne Y. C R Acad Sci (series D) Paris 1991;296:693
230. Reviron M, Janvier D, Reviron J, et al. Vox Sang 1984;46:211
231. Lalezari P, Murphy GB. In: Histocompatibility Testing. Copenhagen:Munksgaard, 1967
232. Shumak KH, Rachkewich RA, Crookston MC, et al. Nature New Biol 1971;231:148
233. Watkins SP Jr, Shulman RN. Blood 1970;36:153
234. Shumak RH, Rachkewich RA, Crookston MC, et al. Clin Immunol Immunopathol 1975;4:241
235. Pruzanski W, Farid N, Keystone E, et al. Clin Immunol Immunopathol 1975;4:248
236. Crookston JH. Arch Int Med 1975;135:1314

237. Greally JF, Whelan CA, O'Connell L, et al. Acta Haematol 1977;57:206
238. Pruzanski W, Shumak KH. New Eng J Med 1977;297:538
239. Pruzanski W, Shumak KH. New Eng J Med 1977;297:583
240. Pruzanski W, Roelcke D, Armstrong M, et al. Clin Immunol Immunopathol 1980;15:631
241. Crisp D, Pruzanski W. Am J Med 1983;72:915
242. Pruzanski W, Farid N, Keystone E, et al. Clin Immunol Immunopathol 1975;4:277
243. Biberfeld G, Biberfeld P, Wigzell H. Scand J Immunol 1976;5:87
244. Pruzanski W, Delmage K. Clin Immunol Immunopathol 1977;7:130
245. Wintrobe MM, Lee GR, Boggs DR, et al. Clinical Hematology. Philadelphia:Lee and Febiger, 1981:936
246. Page PL, Langevin S, Petersen RA, et al. Am J Clin Pathol 1987;87:101
247. Shumak KH, Beldotti LE, Rachkewich RA. Br J Haematol 1979;41:399
248. Issitt PD. J Med Lab Technol 1967;24:90
249. Judd WJ, Steiner EA, Abruzzo LV, et al. Transfusion 1992;32:572
250. Dacie JV. The Haemolytic Anaemias, Part II, The Autoimmune Haemolytic Anaemais. New York:Grune and Stratton, 1963
251. Costea N, Yakulis VJ, Heller P. Proc Soc Exp Biol NY 1972;139:476
252. Lind K. Acta Path Micobiol Scand 1973;81:487
253. Janney FA, Lee LT, Howe C. Infect Immunol 1978;22:29
254. Feizi T. Med Biol 1980;58:123
255. Loomes LM, Uemura K, Childs RA, et al. Nature 1984;307:560
256. Loomes LM, Uemura K, Feizi T. Infec Immunol 1985;47:15
257. Konig AL, Kreft H, Hengge U, et al. Vox Sang 1988;55:176
258. Roelcke D, Kreft H, Hack H, et al. Vox Sang 1994;67:216
259. Roelkcke D, Kreft H, Northoff H, et al. Transfusion 1991;31:627
260. Feizi T, Kabat EA, Vicari G, et al. J Exp Med 1971;133:39
261. Vicari G, Kabat EA. Biochemistry 1970;9:3414
262. Feizi T, Kabat EA. J Exp Med 1972;135:1247
263. Feizi T, Kabat EA. J Immunol 1974;112:145
264. Niemann H, Watanabe K, Hakomori S. Biochem Biophys Res Comm 1978;81:1286
265. Ebert W, Roelcke D, Weicker H. Eur J Biochem 1975;53:505
266. Jarnefelt J, Rush J, Li Y-T, et al. J Biol Chem 1978;253:8006
267. Finne J, Krusius T, Rauvala H, et al. FEBS Lett 1978;89:111
268. Childs RA, Feizi T, Fukuda M, et al. Biochem J 1978;173:333
269. Fukuda M, Fukuda MN, Hakomori S. J Biol Chem 1979;254:3700
270. Feizi T, Childs RA, Hakomori S, et al. Biochem J 1978;173:245
271. Okada Y, Kannagi R, Levery SB, et al. J Immunol 1984;133:835
272. Roelcke D. In: Blood Cell Biochemistry. Volume 6. New York:Plenum 1995;117
273. Bierhuizen MFA, Mattei M-G, Fukuda M. Genes Dev 1993;7:468
274. Kukowska-Latallo JF, Larsen RD, Nair RP, et al. Genes Dev 1990;4:1288
275. Sasaki H, Bothner B, Dell A, et al. J Biol Chem 1987;262:12059
276. Smith DF, Larsen RD, Mattox S, et al. J Biol Chem 1990;265:6225
277. Bierhuizen MFA, Fukuda M. Proc Nat Acad Sci USA 1992;89:9326
278. Bierhuizen MFA, Maemura K, Kudo S, et al. Glycobiology 1995;5:417
279. Magnet AD, Fukuda M. Glycobiology 1997;7:285
280. Ropp PA, Little MR, Cheng PW. J Biol Chem 1991;266:23863
281. Wallace JMW, Ferguson SJ, Loane P, et al. Br J Biomed Sci 1997;54:85
282. Klagsbrun M, Neumann J, Tapper D. J Pediat Res 1979;26:417
283. Tapper D, Klagsbrun M, Neumann J. J Pediat Surg 1979;14:803
284. Narayanan I, Probosk K, Verma RF, et al. Lancet 1980;2:561

11 | The P Blood Group System and the Antigens P, Pᵏ and LKE

When the previous editions of this book were written it was believed that the antigens P_1, P and P^k, and perhaps Luke and p, were part of the same blood group system. It is now appreciated that although P_1, P and P^k, and probably Luke, derive from a common precursor, the genes that control their development are almost certainly not alleles and are, instead, located at independent loci. Accordingly, some changes in terminology have been suggested. In 1990, the ISBT working party on terminology for red cell surface antigens revised the P system to include just the antigen P_1 (1). The antigens P, P^k and LKE (for Luke) were placed in what, at that time, was an unnamed "collection". Antigens that display a phenotypic or other relationship to each other, when the genetic nature of the association is not known, are placed in collections pending an explanation of their genetic control. In 1991, the working party (2) assigned the name globoside, (shorthand symbol GLOBO) to the collection that houses P, P^k and LKE, because of the biochemical nature of these antigens. In 1996 (285) the term Globo was shortened to GLOB. The current ISBT terminology is shown in table 11-1. Because of the very close serological relationships between P_1, P, P^k and LKE, these antigens are considered in a single chapter here, they will be called the P blood groups, for ease of communication, although as said, genetic independence of the genes that control their synthesis is recognized.

This chapter follows those on the ABO and Lewis systems and the Ii antigen collection because antibodies showing phenotypic relationships between the four sets of antigens (ABO, Lewis, Ii and P blood groups) have been described. In spite of this the two or three (see below) P blood group loci are genetically independent of *Hh*, *ABO*, *Lele* and the genes that encode I and i.

The P_1 antigen (at that time called P) was discovered in 1927 when Landsteiner and Levine (3) immunized rabbits with human red cells and tested the anti-

body made by the animals against the red cells of other humans. Antibodies of the same specificity (i.e. anti-P_1) as that made by the rabbits were soon found in human serum (4). Unfortunately, common usage has resulted in the terms anti-P, P+ and P- sometimes still being used when anti-P_1, P_1+ and P_1- are intended. As discussed below, the antigen now called P is quite different from the P_1 antigen. In 1955, the P blood groups were expanded when Sanger (5) demonstrated a phenotypic association between Tjᵃ (described four years earlier by Levine et al. (6)) and the P blood groups. In 1959, Matson et al. (7) described the antigen, P^k, that although related to the P blood groups is not encoded from the *P¹* locus (8). In 1965, Tippett et al. (9) described Luke, another antigen with a phenotypic relationship to the P blood groups and in 1972, Engelfriet et al. (10) named another new antibody, anti-p. As described below, anti-p may define an antigen that has less of an association with the P blood groups than do those mentioned above. The pieces of the P blood groups, that is P_1, P, P^k, Luke and perhaps p, were in place, it remained for a satisfactory explanation to be provided to account for their serological, biochemical and genetic relationships to each other. Although a great deal of progress has been made (11) (see later sections of this chapter) some questions still remain unanswered, it seems likely that cloning of the genes involved will be necessary for the situation to be understood in full.

Unlike the biochemistry and genetics of the P blood groups, that are apparently as complex as those of any other blood group system, the P blood groups are relatively straightforward at the serological and clinical levels. Accordingly, the next several sections of this chapter will deal with those aspects, the complexities will be addressed again later in the chapter. While some of biochemistry and genetics must be understood to allow a full appreciation of the phenotypes and antibodies of the P

TABLE 11-1 Conventional and ISBT Terminology for the P System and the GLOB Collection

System/Collection (Conventional name)	ISBT Symbol	ISBT Number	Antigen (conventional name)	ISBT Antigen Number	ISBT Full Code Number
P	P1	003	P_1	001	003001
P (conventional) Collection 209 (ISBT)	GLOB	209	P	001	209001
			P^k	002	209002
			LKE	003	209003

295

blood groups, for the sake of easy reference tables 11-2 and 11-3 list some details about the antibodies and phenotypes, respectively, of the P blood groups. Again, more complete explanations of the data in tables 11-2 and 11-3 are given later in the chapter.

Anti-P$_1$

Tests with anti-P$_1$ divide red cells into two phenotypes, P$_1$+ and P$_1$-. Unfortunately, common practice often results in P$_1$- red cells being described as being of phenotype P$_2$. As discussed in more detail in a later section, red cells phenotypically P$_2$ are P$_1$- P+. A negative test result with anti-P$_1$ does not reveal the P status of the red cells tested. Since P is a common antigen, most P$_1$- red cells will be P+. However, unless a test with anti-P has been performed and a positive result obtained, P$_1$- red cells should be called P$_1$- and not P$_2$.

Anti-P$_1$ is a common antibody in the sera of patients and donors with red cells of the P$_1$- phenotype (12-15). Most examples of the antibody are IgM agglutinins that are only weakly reactive at low temperatures in in vitro tests. Most often the antibodies will not agglutinate P$_1$+ red cells at temperatures above 25 to 30°C. As the temperature at which in vitro tests are performed is reduced, the frequency with which anti-P$_1$ is found increases. Henningsen (12) showed that if prolonged incubation was used, in tests at low temperatures, anti-P$_1$ could be found in the sera of about two thirds of people with P$_1$- red cells. In tests using an automated antibody detection system (15), anti-P$_1$ was found in just over a quarter of the sera from 100 healthy donors with P$_1$- red cells. It seems entirely possible that if a high enough serum:cell ratio was used and if long enough incubation at a low enough temperature was included, anti-P$_1$ might be found in all sera from persons with P$_1$- cells. The above figures relate to weak examples of anti-P$_1$, found only in tests at reduced temperatures (such as those incubated at 4°C), in normal healthy individuals with no known exposure to the P$_1$ antigen. A rather different situation exists in persons with certain diseases or in those regularly exposed to substances that are chemically similar to, or identical with the P$_1$ antigen. In the following paragraphs, although the incidences of anti-P$_1$ may not appear appreciably higher, the antibodies are invariably much more avid. Although they often still only react at temperatures up to about 22°C, the antibodies described below, often give 3 and 4+ agglutination reactions, compared to the 1 and 2+ reactions of those described above.

In patients with hydatid cyst disease, those who are phenotypically P$_1$- may make potent anti-P$_1$. In different studies (15-18) the incidence of anti-P$_1$ production has been reported to vary from 8 to 100%. Presumably the antibody detection and identification methods used, again influenced the frequency with which the antibody

TABLE 11-2 Characteristics of P Blood Group Antibodies

Antibody Specificity	Positive Reactions in In Vitro Tests				Usual Immunoglobulin		Ability to Bind Complement		Ability to Cause In Vitro Lysis		Implicated in		Usual Form of Stimulation		% of White Population Positive
	Sal	LISS	AHG	Enz	IgG	IgM	Yes	No	Yes	No	Transfusion Reaction	HDN	Red Cells	Other	
Anti-P$_1$	X	X	Rare	X	Rare	X	Few		Rare		Rare	No		X	80
Anti-P^k	X					X					No	No		X	<1
Anti-Tj^a (anti-P+ P$_1$+P^k)	X				Few	Most	X		All		Yes	Yes		X	100
Anti-P	X				Some	X	X		X		Yes			X	100
Anti-IP$_1$	X					X					No	No		X	80
Anti-LKE	X		Some	Some	Some	Some	Some		Some			No		X	98

1 As shown above, anti-P$_1$ has been implicated as the rare cause of a transfusion reaction. The ability of the antibody to destroy P$_1$+ red cells in vivo, is dependent on activity at 37°C. In other words, the commonly-encountered, cold-reactive anti-P$_1$ does NOT cause transfusion reactions.

2 The anti-P shown is the antibody made by persons of the very rare P^k red cell phenotype. It is not the commonly encountered cold-reactive agglutinin that has anti-P$_1$ specificity.

TABLE 11-3 A Simplified View of P Blood Group Phenotypes

Red Cell Phenotype	Some Characteristics	Frequencies	
		Whites	Blacks
P_1	Cells react with anti-P_1 and anti P. Cells carry some P^k antigen but too little for detection in conventional tests.	80%	90-95%*
P_2	Cells react with anti-P but not with anti-P_1. The term P_2 is frequently misused to describe red cells that fail to react with anti-P_1. In fact, the term P_2 should not be used until the P_1- cells have been shown to be P+.	20%	5-10%*
P_1^k	Cells react with anti-P_1 and strongly with anti-P^k. Cells are non-reactive with anti-P.		Very Rare
P_2^k	Cells react strongly with anti-P^k but are non-reactive with anti-P_1 and anti-P.		Very Rare
p	Cells fail to react with anti-P_1, anti-P or anti-P^k. Previously known as Tj(a-)		Very Rare

* Insufficient figures published for more accurate frequencies to be calculated.

was found. As described later in this chapter, the discovery (16) that hydatid cyst fluid is a rich source of P_1 substance was utilized in the biochemical investigations that led to the elucidation of P blood group antigen structure. The incidence of anti-P_1 is even more dramatic in persons with phenotypically P_1- red cells who contract Fascioliasis (bovine liver fluke disease, also called acute hepatic distomiasis). From various studies (15,19-22) it seems that 100% of such persons make a potent anti-P_1.

The sport of breeding pigeons (most of those bred seem to be used for racing purposes (23)) also exposes phenotypically P_1- persons to materials that carry the P_1 structure and puts them at risk of making anti-P_1 (24-28). After the initial observation of the high incidence of anti-P_1 among pigeon fanciers was made (24) it was shown (25,26) that pigeon red cells, plasma and droppings, all contain P_1 substance. Similarly, it is now known (29,30) that the red cells, plasma, egg white (specifically the ovomucoid of the egg white) and droppings of the (presum-

ably related) turtledove also contain P_1 substance. Several groups of investigators (25,26,29-31) have successfully raised anti-P_1 in animals by using some of the above materials as immunogens. Some pigeon breeders suffer a bronchitis-like condition that seems to be allergic in origin and that is given the appropriate name, pigeon-breeders' disease. It has been shown (25,32) that the antibodies causative of this disease and the anti-P_1 often produced, have different specificities. It is suspected that the allergen involved in pigeon breeders' disease and P_1 substance are present in pigeon droppings and it is felt that P_1 gets there because of its presence in certain strains of avian gram negative bacteria (24,27,33).

P_1 substance has also been found in the common earthworm (nightcrawlers in the USA) *Lumbricus terrestris* (13,34,35). Indeed, it is possible to prepare extracts that will inhibit anti-P_1, in the blood bank, using earthworms as the starting material. From personal experience, one author (PDI) can warn workers with a keen olfactory sense not to undertake the exercise. Among the many examples of anti-P_1 that have been studied, one inhibitable by inosine, hypoxanthine, adenine and thymine was found (36).

As far as we are aware, the only report that suggests that heterogeneity might exist among examples of anti-P_1 is that of Norman et al. (37) who described an alloanti-P_1 in the serum of a pigeon-breeder whose red cells typed as P_1+ with other anti-P_1.

Cold-Reactive Anti-P₁ in Transfusion Therapy

Examples of anti-P_1 that do not react with red cells in in vitro tests at 37°C are of no consequence in transfusion therapy. Indeed there is abundant evidence that blood group antibodies that do not react with antigen-positive red cells at 30°C (38-44) or 37°C (45-49) in in vitro tests, do not bring about accelerated clearance of those red cells in vivo. The data cited above are substantiated by a common sense evaluation of current transfusion practice. First, as described in the previous section, cold-reactive anti-P_1 in the sera of P_1- persons are common. Second, as shown in table 11-3, over 80% of random donors (in the USA) will have P_1+ red cells. Third, currently used antibody-screening and immediate spin compatibility tests will fail to detect most examples of cold-reactive anti-P_1. Thus it follows that hundreds of thousands of persons with cold-reactive anti-P_1 in the serum must, by now, have been transfused with P_1+ red cells. In spite of this, reports of immediate or delayed transfusion reactions and secondary immune responses to P_1 following transfusion, are few in number (54,44,82). Cronin et al. (50) addressed the question as to the clinical significance of cold-reactive anti-P_1 directly. Among 56 patients with anti-P_1 in the serum, 19 received a total of 53 units of blood not typed for P_1; none of them suffered immediate or delayed transfusion reactions nor any other untoward effect. In other words, the most intelligent way to handle cold-reactive anti-P_1 in a transfusion service is, first, to use antibody-screening methods that will usually fail to detect the antibody. Second, on those occasions that anti-P_1 active in vitro only at temperatures below 37°C is encountered, blood compatible by immediate spin methods can be transfused with impunity. The considerable amounts of time and money expended in the detection and identification of cold-reactive anti-P_1, and in typing donor units to identify those that are P_1-, cannot be justified since they provide no additional benefit to the patients involved.

Some workers worry that the introduction of P_1+ red cells into the circulation of individuals who have cold-reactive anti-P_1, will cause an increase in the amount of anti-P_1 being made, or a widening in thermal range of the antibody. In fact, Mollison (51) found that the intravenous injection of P_1+ red cells in patients whose sera contain anti-P_1 active at 37°C, causes no increase in the titer of anti-P_1. Further, if such a practice caused any appreciable increase in the titer or thermal range of anti-P_1, delayed hemolytic transfusion reactions due to that antibody would be common since so many workers now use blood not typed for P_1 for the transfusions. In fact, delayed hemolytic transfusion reactions caused by anti-P_1 are rare. A few such reactions have been reported but when encountered were either mild in nature (52) or were of the type that could not be avoided (53-55). That is to say, the more severe delayed transfusion reactions due to this antibody did not occur in patients who had cold-reactive anti-P_1 demonstrable in the serum before transfusion. Instead, like other classic delayed transfusion reactions, they occurred in individuals in whom no serologically active antibodies were found when pre-transfusion antibody screening and compatibility tests were performed. It is of note that in describing perhaps the most severe case of a delayed transfusion reaction allegedly due to anti-P_1 ever claimed, Chandeysson et al. (55) pointed out that their policy was not to select P_1-blood for patients with anti-P_1 reactive at low temperatures. They comment in their paper that cases such as the one they are describing are so rare, that encountering this one has not caused them to modify their policy in any way. In considering this case of a severe delayed transfusion reaction it should be remembered that Mollison (83) has questioned whether the reaction was caused by anti-P_1 at all. It is also noteworthy that in what is perhaps the most comprehensive study ever performed on delayed transfusion reactions, Pineda et al. (56) did not find any caused by anti-P_1 among the 47 cases that they studied.

In extending the study to 171 cases (57,58) only two examples of anti-P_1 are mentioned and their roles in the delayed transfusion reactions were dubious at best. One was present in the serum of a patient who had also made anti-Jk^a and in the other in a serum that also contained anti-E, anti-K and anti-M.

As the above discussion clearly shows, there is overwhelming evidence first, that cold-reactive anti-P_1 does not cause the in vivo destruction of P_1+ red cells. Second, that blood compatible with the patient's serum in in vitro tests performed at 37°C survives normally in the presence of anti-P_1. Third, that the introduction of P_1+ red cells to the circulation of patients whose sera contain cold-reactive anti-P_1, does not usually cause an anamnestic antibody response. There is one report in the literature that is contrary to these findings. Strohm and Molthan (59) claimed that of five patients with anti-P_1 who were transfused with P_1+ blood, four suffered delayed transfusion reactions. Most workers will find it impossible to accept the evidence presented as supportive of this conclusion. First, clearance of the P_1+ red cells was said to be proved because P_1+ red cells were not detected in post-transfusion samples from the patients. However, it is known (60,61) that the P_1 antigen is fragile and difficult to detect as red cells age. Indeed, the detection of P_1+ red cells in the post-transfusion blood of P_1- patients who do not have anti-P_1 may be difficult or impossible. Second, it was claimed (59) that post-transfusion hemoglobin and hematocrit levels showed that the transfused red cells had been cleared. However, one of the patients was anemic as a result of chemotherapy and two had bleeding episodes before transfusion. The age of the units transfused was not given and it is possible that the post-transfusion hemoglobin and hematocrit levels were within expected increment levels, particularly in one patient who was not making blood and two who may have been losing it. Third, it is not clear whether the alleged 37°C reactions of the anti-P_1 were seen in tests transferred to 37°C from lower temperatures. This point is important since most workers (14,43,46-49) accept (see below) that anti-P_1 strongly active at 37°C can be of clinical significance. Fourth, the method used to measure IgM/IgG ratios in the anti-P_1 was naive. Titration of an antibody before and after treatment with 2-ME will not reveal respective IgM and IgG levels if two antibodies in the starting serum have the same titer, or if one of them is not an agglutinin. Finally, it should be pointed out that other findings totally divergent from the experience of other workers have been reported from the same laboratory. Molthan (62) reported a fatal outcome following intravascular destruction of transfused red cells by anti-Vw + Mi^a. However, the antibody was said to be mostly IgM and not to fix complement. By definition (14,63,64) intravascular hemolysis involves "rupture of red cells within the blood stream"; activation of the terminal attack sequence of complement is invariably involved. Even when challenged (66) the author (65) offered no explanation as to how an IgM non-complement binding antibody could cause intravascular lysis. Molthan et al. (67) and Molthan (68) have also claimed to have seen in vivo red cell destruction by antibodies directed against Ykᵃ, Csᵃ, McCᵃ and Knᵃ. The near universal experience of others (69-75) is that these antibodies are benign in vivo (see Chapters 28 and 30).

Thus it is clear that the report (59) that claims that cold-reactive anti-P₁ is a clinically-significant antibody comes from a laboratory in which findings and conclusions are frequently in direct contradiction to those of virtually all other workers. Readers who have ploughed through the long section above may wonder why so much space has been devoted to discrediting a single report. There are two major reasons. First, if a clinically-insignificant antibody is not recognized as such and handled by the transfusion of antigen-positive blood that will survive normally in vivo, delays in necessary transfusion or postponement of necessary surgery may result while searches for "compatible" blood are undertaken. Clearly, if antigen-negative blood is not required for supportive transfusion therapy, the patients' clinical outcome may be compromised by unnecessary delays. Second, in this age of cost containment in medical care, labor-intensive serological studies and expensive searches for antigen-negative blood are justified only when the transfusion of antigen-negative red cells is necessary for the patient's well being.

Anti-P₁ Reactive at 37°C and Transfusion Therapy

Having been at pains to document the clinical insignificance of cold-reactive anti-P₁, it must now be pointed out that very rare examples of the antibody are active at 37°C and are of clinical importance. Cutbush and Mollison (40) showed that anti-P₁ that act as agglutinins at 37°C may also fix complement so that they can be detected in the indirect antiglobulin test if a broad spectrum reagent is used, or may cause the hemolysis of ficin-treated P₁+ red cells. In the course of a long career in blood banking, one of us (PDI) has seen four examples of anti-P₁ that only weakly agglutinated P₁+ red cells, but that were strongly reactive by the indirect antiglobulin test. All four antibodies caused complement activation and bound to red cells in tests in which the serum and cells were prewarmed to 37°C before being mixed. In view of the poor abilities of these antibodies in agglutinating P₁+ red cells it is tempting to guess that

they may have been IgG in nature. However, Adinolphi et al. (76) investigated two examples and Polley et al. (77) one example, of anti-P₁ with similar characteristics and concluded that they were entirely IgM in composition. An IgG anti-P₁, active at 37°C and capable of causing complement activation, was described by DiNapoli et al. (54). The antibody apparently caused a delayed transfusion reaction. Thus, it seems that while the rare examples of antiglobulin-active, complement-binding anti-P₁ active at 37°C, that have been investigated have usually been IgM in nature, rarely, IgG forms may be encountered.

There is no doubt that those examples of anti-P₁ that fix complement at 37°C and that are clearly demonstrable in indirect antiglobulin tests, must be taken seriously when blood is issued for transfusion. Again, it is possible that in vitro tests with the patient's serum at 37°C provide the safest method for the selection of blood for transfusion. The reason this time is that anti-P₁ of this type often give stronger reactions with P₁+ red cells than do available typing sera. In considering anti-P₁ of this type it is important again to stress the correct use of prewarmed tests. If the antibody agglutinates red cells at temperatures below 37°C, positive reactions when the tests are read after incubation do not necessarily indicate that the antibody is active at 37°C. That is to say, agglutination that has occurred at lower temperatures may not disperse at 37°C so that the positive reactions may simply represent "carry-over" of agglutination. If the anti-P₁ is truly active at 37°C, tests set up by prewarming the test red cells and the serum to 37°C before they are mixed, will yield positive reactions (78). As mentioned above, detection of the positive reactions may be considerably enhanced by the use of indirect antiglobulin tests read with a reagent containing anti-complement.

Production of Anti-P₁ Following Transfusion

As already described, most examples of anti-P₁ are cold-reactive, IgM agglutinins found in the sera of individuals who have not been transfused. Thus it seems that most frequently these antibodies are of the non-red-cell stimulated variety (see Chapter 7). On rare occasions production of anti-P₁ following transfusion has been described (59,79-81). As already discussed, routine transfusion practices must result in huge numbers of patients with P₁- red cells, including many with cold-reactive anti-P₁ already present in the serum, being transfused with P₁+ blood. The paucity of reports describing immunization to P₁ by transfusion serves to emphasize that the phenomenon is a very rare exception to a very large rule.

Monoclonal Anti-P$_1$

A number of monoclonal antibodies directed against the P$_1$ antigen have been produced (84-88). Some of them have proved valuable in determination of the biochemical structures of the P blood group antigens (see later in this chapter). One of the monoclonal antibodies produced (86) behaved as if it had anti-P$_1$ and anti-P^k specificity. Since the antibody was monoclonal in nature, it follows that it must have been directed against an epitope shared by P$_1$ and P^k (see below). Other monoclonal antibodies against P blood group antigens are described below.

Development of the P$_1$ Antigen

The P$_1$ antigen appears to develop early in fetal life, then to be less well expressed as the fetus develops. Race and Sanger (89) showed that the red cells of a 12 week-old fetus were P$_1$+; Ikin et al. (90) found that the antigen is better developed on the red cells of 12 week-old than on those of 28 week-old fetuses. Henningsen (91) demonstrated that the antigen is not fully developed at birth and Heiken (92) suggested that P$_1$ antigen production may not reach its peak level for the first seven years of life. Issitt et al. (93) showed that some examples of apparent anti-P$_1$ have anti-IP$_1$ specificity. Obviously, if such antibodies are used to type cord blood red cells, some samples will fail to react although, as can be demonstrated by the use of anti-P$_1$, they are P$_1$+.

Variation in Strength of the P$_1$ Antigen

The amount of P$_1$ antigen on different P$_1$+ red cell samples varies considerably. This variation was first noticed by Landsteiner and Levine (3) and has subsequently been studied by others (12,91,94-97). The studies have all confirmed quantitative variation of the antigen, other than the one example of alloimmune anti-P$_1$ made by an individual with P$_1$+ red cells (37) that is mentioned above, no evidence of qualitative differences has emerged. Moharram's (94) family studies on P$_1$ antigenic strength suggested that the variable strength condition was inherited. Likewise Henningsen (12,98) thought that the amount of P$_1$ antigen produced is, like the presence of the P$_1$ antigen, genetically controlled but Fisher (9) found that Henningsen's data did not stand statistical analysis in this supposition.

As already mentioned, the P$_1$ antigen is not particularly stable (60,61) and difficulties are sometimes encountered in detecting the antigen on red cell samples that have been stored for a period of time. Most workers who use red cell samples to identify antibodies will have noticed for themselves that the P$_1$ antigen is often stronger on the red cells of Black donors than on those of Whites. Such is the variation of strength of the P$_1$ antigen on the red cells of different donors that many weak examples of anti-P$_1$ react visibly only with red cells on which the antigen is well expressed. The practice of some providers of panels of red cells for antibody identification, in indicating which samples have strong and which have weak expressions of P$_1$, is often of considerable value in the identification of weak anti-P$_1$.

The P$_1$ Antigen and the *In(Lu)* Gene

As described in detail in Chapter 20, there is a dominant gene called *In(Lu)* (195) that is not at the *Lutheran* (*Lu*) locus, that comes close to preventing *Lu^a* or *Lu^b* genes that are present, from being expressed at the phenotypic level. In 1974, Crawford et al. (196) reported that there was a significant excess of the phenotype P$_1$- among individuals who had inherited *In(Lu)*. Shortly thereafter an expected family, showing an apparent upset in the inheritance of P$_1$ was found (197). It became clear that an individual who inherits *In(Lu)* and *P^1*, that occupy genetically independent loci, can have red cells that type as P$_1$-.

The Phenotype p, the Antigen P and the Antibody Anti-P+P$_1$+P^k

In 1951, Levine et al. (6) described a red cell phenotype that they called Tj(a-). In 1955, Sanger (5) noticed that the Tj(a-) red cells of three unrelated persons studied by her, were P$_1$-. A literature review showed that the Tj(a-) red cells of three other unrelated persons and those of one Tj(a-) sib were also P$_1$-. Since the incidence of the P$_1$ antigen was known to be around 80%, the finding that all of six unrelated persons of the Tj(a-) phenotype had P$_1$- red cells, showed beyond doubt that Tj^a must be part of the P blood groups. As described below, Tj(a-) persons present with a potent antibody, that is often an in vitro hemolysin, in the serum. When Sanger (5) adsorbed this antibody, then known as anti-Tj^a, with P$_1$- red cells, anti-P$_1$ was left unadsorbed.

For reasons given below, the Tj(a-) phenotype is now most often called p. Although many examples of the phenotype have been reported (100-122) it is still extremely uncommon. Race and Sanger (123) calculated that in most populations the p phenotype has an incidence of around 1 in 5.8 million. Many of the examples studied were found in isolated communities or in populations in which higher than usual rates of inbreeding were known, or were thought to have occurred. In Japan, where the HLA types reveal that the population is genetically more homogeneous than most others (124,125,260-263) the p phenotype is somewhat more frequent (102,105-107,110,111,113-116). Cedergren (112) calculated that in the Vasterbatten area of Northern Sweden, the p phenotype frequency might be as high as 1 in 5000 to 1 in 7000. Somewhat similarly, clusters of p individuals have been found in a large Amish kindred in Northern Ohio (120) and in a cohort of persons of Spanish extraction living in Ecuador (122).

The antibody originally called anti-Tjᵃ was recognized, from the work of Sanger (5), as containing two specificities anti-P₁ and anti-P. As described below, it later became apparent that some antibodies made by p persons contain a third separable antibody, anti-Pᵏ as well. Anti-P was seen to detect a very common antigen, P, that is present on almost all P₁+ and P₁- red cells, but is lacking from p cells. As mentioned earlier, (see also table 11-3) red cells of the P₁ phenotype are P₁+ P+, those of the P₂ phenotype are P₁- P+. All persons with the p phenotype make anti-P₁ plus anti-P, about half of them also make separable anti-Pᵏ (see below). Obregon and McKeever (120) have shown that the antibody is not present at birth, in the sera of infants with p red cells, but that it develops early in life without exposure of the children to foreign red cells. Anti-P+P₁+Pᵏ often presents as a powerful in vitro hemolysin and may be IgM (76) or IgG (109) in nature. An anti-P+P₁+Pᵏ that was demonstrable in serological studies only after the serum in which it was present was concentrated to one fourth of its original volume, but that nevertheless destroyed P₁- P+ (P₂) red cells in vivo, has been reported (259).

More information about the p phenotype and about the antigens defined by anti-P and anti-Pᵏ, is given in the later sections of this chapter on the genetics and biochemistry of the P system.

Anti-P+P₁+Pᵏ and Cancer

The first reported (6) patient with anti-P+P₁+Pᵏ in the serum had adenocarcinoma of the stomach. She was injected with 25 ml of incompatible blood to determine whether or not the antibody needed to be avoided in transfusion therapy. This test showed that the antibody was indeed clinically-significant and further, resulted in it being produced in higher levels after injection of the incompatible red cells. Following a subtotal gastrectomy the patient lived another 22 years and died at age 88 with no clinical signs of metastatic cancer. The tumor cells were shown (126) to carry the P blood group antigens that the patient's red cells lacked, her anti-P+P₁+Pᵏ was alloimmune in nature. Levine (126-130) interpreted

these findings as showing that the tumor cells (the T in Tjᵃ stands for tumor (6)) carried an illegitimate antigen (Tjᵃ), for the patient lacked the encoding gene. Further, the anti-P+P₁+Pᵏ, present as a potent antibody following injection of the 25 ml of incompatible red cells, was credited with having acted as a cytotoxin in preventing the growth of metastatic cancer cells in the patient. The patient's sister, who was also of the p phenotype but in whom the titer of anti-Tjᵃ was not boosted by the injection of incompatible red cells, died of adenocarcinoma of the uterus in 1962 (136).

From other studies (137-145) there is evidence that cancer cells often carry illegitimate antigens, again ones for which the patient lacks the appropriate genes, some of which can be detected with blood group antibodies. As discussed in Chapter 8, the appearance on tumor cells of ABO antigens, for which the patients' lack the appropriate genes, is not particularly uncommon. Obviously, if these antigens can be recognized in time, the possibility that the carcinoma's growth can be stopped by local application of the appropriate antibody, exists. In this respect, the production of highly specific monoclonal antibodies in hybridomas could certainly play a major role in therapy, particularly if methods can be devised to transport those antibodies to the site of the cancer. The role of the Forsmann antigen, of which P antigen-bearing globoside is a precursor, in this setting, is discussed in detail by Garratty (145).

Anti-p

In 1972, Engelfriet et al. (10) described an antibody, made by a patient whose red cells typed as P₁+, that reacted preferentially with p red cells. The patient's serum contained warm-active and biphasic hemolysins and although activity against P₁+ and P₁- (P₂) red cells was initially demonstrated, the antibody clearly had a preference for p red cells. Antibody production in the patient was transient and may well have been initiated by an infection. Metaxas et al. (146) and Issitt et al. (147) have described antibodies with similar characteristics that had either a very similar or an identical specificity to the anti-p reported by Engelfriet et al. (10). Subsequent findings (148) suggested that the antigens recognized by what were called anti-p, may be sialylated forms of paragloboside and ceramide dihexoside (CDH) that are precursor substances on which the P blood group antigens are assembled (see below). Thus p may be closely related to the antigen Gd (149,150) that is described in detail in Chapter 34, although it seems (150) that anti-p and anti-Gd are not identical. It is now appreciated that all red cells carry the determinant recognized by anti-p in the quantitative sequence p>P₂>P₁.

The Antigen P^k

In 1959, Matson et al. (7) described a new antigen that revealed two new phenotypes within the P blood groups. In these phenotypes, P$_1$^{k} and P$_2$^{k}, the red cells carry the antigen P^k (that is detected by a separable component in some anti-P+P$_1$+P^k sera) but lack the very common antigen, P. In the P$_1$^{k} phenotype, P$_1$ and P^k are present but P is absent; in the P$_2$^{k} phenotype P^k is present, P$_1$ and P are absent. Persons phenotypically P$_1$^{k} and P$_2$^{k} can form anti-P, the antibody lacks the anti-P^k component found in the sera of persons phenotypically p; when made by an individual phenotypically P$_1$^{k}, it lacks anti-P^k and anti-P$_1$. Although the P^k phenotypes are rare, other examples have been described in the literature (8,114,115,132,135,159-161). Like the p phenotype, P^k is more common in Japan (114,115,135,157,159-161) than in other parts of the world.

For many years it was thought that the P^k phenotype must be controlled by a gene at a different locus than that at which P^1 and P^2 and p were thought to reside. Such assumptions were based in part on the results of family studies and in part on observations that the P$_1$, P$_2$, P$_1$^{k} and P$_2$^{k} phenotypes all existed. In other words, it seemed that most red cells of the P$_1$ phenotype lacked P^k, while others were P$_1$^{k} (i.e. positive for both antigens). It followed that if the P$_1$^{k} phenotype represented the inheritance of P^1 and P^k, then P^1 and P^k could not be alleles. Further, it initially appeared that only P$_1$^{k} and P$_2$^{k} red cells expressed the P^k antigen. Eventually, as described in the sections on biochemistry and genetics of the P blood groups, it became apparent (162) that P^k is not a low incidence antigen, as serological studies had suggested, but instead is present on the structure on which P is later assembled. Thus all red cells of the P$_1$ and P$_2$ phenotypes carry P^k, its presence is difficult to detect since anti-P^k cannot readily complex with P^k when continued synthesis has resulted in the conversion of P^k to P. This realization also explained why individuals phenotypically P$_1$ and P$_2$ do not make anti-P^k. They are, fact, positive for the P^k antigen although that antigen is largely covered by P on their red cells. Persons of the p phenotype make neither P^k nor P (nor P$_1$) on their red cells so are able to form anti-P+P$_1$+P^k. Individuals of the phenotypes P$_1$^{k} and P$_2$^{k} do not make P. Accordingly, the unconverted P^k antigen on their red cells is readily detectable in tests with anti-P^k. These findings are all more readily understood when the biosynthetic pathways leading to the production of P, P$_1$ and P^k are considered (see below).

Anti-P

As will be apparent from what has been written above, persons of the P^k phenotypes can make alloimmune anti-P but not anti-P^k. Those of the P$_1$^{k} phenotype cannot make alloimmune anti-P$_1$. When produced by individuals of the P^k phenotypes, anti-P is a potent antibody. It is probable that such immunized individuals will tolerate only transfusions with P-, (i.e. P$_1$^{k}, P$_2$^{k} or p) red cells. Just as all p persons found thus far have P system antibodies in the sera, all those of the P^k phenotypes have been seen to have anti-P. The anti-P produced will hemolyze P$_1$ and P$_2$ cells in vitro in the presence of complement, published reports have not provided any evidence for different amounts of P on red cells of the P$_1$ and P$_2$ phenotypes. This is not surprising, as illustrated in a later section of this chapter, the synthesis of P is independent of the synthesis of P$_1$. The anti-P component in the anti-P+P$_1$+P^k made by p individuals may be entirely IgM in nature (76) but as described below in the section on spontaneous abortion is not invariably so; the anti-P made by individuals of the P^k phenotypes are usually mixtures of IgM and IgG (109,135,163,164) and may contain IgA as well (165).

P Blood Group Antibodies and Spontaneous Abortion

From findings (107,118) that some women of the p phenotype had histories of spontaneous abortions and that their live-born children were of the P$_1$- phenotype, it was suggested (118,126-129) that the presence of anti-P+P$_1$+P^k might result in those women being unable or unlikely to carry fetuses that had inherited a P^1 gene from the father, to term. However, this theory was disputed and figures were presented (119,120) to show that at least the expected number of genetically P^1 infants had been born to p mothers. While there is evidence (121,123,130-133) that the presence of anti-P+P$_1$+P^k (and anti-P in P^k individuals, see below) may lead to spontaneous abortion two points are now better understood. First, while the spontaneous abortion rate in women with anti-P+P$_1$+P^k or anti-P in the serum is higher than in those who do not have those antibodies, it is by no means universal. That is, some women with these antibodies in the serum carry normal fetuses to term. Second, inheritance of P^1 from the father, does not put the fetus at increased risk.

Anti-P as made by women of the P^k phenotypes has also been incriminated (132,135) as a cause of early spontaneous abortion. Indeed, as discussed below, it may well be the anti-P component of the anti-P+P$_1$+P^k made by p women that is causative of the abortions.

Cantin and Lyonnaise (121) described a woman of the p phenotype who had anti-P+P$_1$+P^k in her serum and had three miscarriages. However, her twin sisters who were of the same red cell phenotype and who also had antibody in the serum, each delivered normal children following their first pregnancies. Both women who delivered normal infants had husbands with P_1+ red cells and one of the infants was of that phenotype. When the sera of the three women were fractionated, that of the one who had suffered miscarriages was found to contain IgM agglutinating activity and an IgG antiglobulin-active antibody reactive with P_1 and P_2 red cells. The serum of one sister who had delivered a normal child contained IgM agglutinating activity for P_1 and P_2 cells; the serum of the other contained that activity plus an IgG antiglobulin-active antibody that reacted with P_1 but not P_2 cells. The authors (121) suggested that IgG anti-P might be the antibody associated with risk of early abortion. Shirey et al. (132) described a woman, with red cells of the P_1^k phenotype, who had IgM and IgG anti-P in her serum, who had suffered fourteen first trimester miscarriages and who had not had a successful pregnancy. During the fifteenth pregnancy the woman was treated, from the fifth week of gestation, by plasma exchange. A one volume exchange was performed two or three times each week and the levels of IgM and IgG anti-P were reduced. At 33 weeks gestation a live child was delivered. The DAT on the infant's red cells was positive, anti-P was eluted from those cells but the child was not anemic and the highest bilirubin level reached was 8.6mg/100 ml. These findings also suggest that anti-P (when present alone or when (121) present in a serum containing anti-P+P_1+P^k) may be responsible for miscarriages in women of the p and P^k phenotypes. Yoshida et al. (135) used plasma removal and ex vivo antibody adsorption to reduce the level of anti-P in a pregnant woman of the P^k phenotype. Again the anti-P was IgG in nature and the woman had previously had four miscarriages. A total of 93 plasma adsorptions were performed before a live born infant, that did not require exchange transfusion, was delivered by Caesarian section. Other cases in which plasma removal was used with successful results have subsequently been described (133-135).

It seems that IgG anti-P is the most likely cause of spontaneous abortion in this setting. It has been shown (166) that tissue cells of the placenta carry higher levels of P (and P^k) than do the red cells of the fetus. Although evidence has been presented (161,163,167) that was interpreted as indicating a role for anti-P^k in these spontaneous abortions, it seems unlikely that anti-P^k alone can be responsible. The rationale for that statement is, of course, that such abortions have been seen in women of the P^k phenotype who had anti-P but not anti-P^k in the serum (132,135).

Vos et al. (168) and Vos (169-171) described a hemolysin directed against P_1 and P_2 red cells in the sera of women with a history of abortion. Unlike the situations described above, the women had red cells of the P_1 or P_2 phenotype and antibody production was transient. The hemolysin was found in women in Australia but not in women with similar obstetrical histories in other parts of the world (168,172). While exhaustive studies did not reveal one, it certainly seems possible that some unknown environmental factor was involved in stimulation of production of this transiently made antibody.

In concluding this section on the association between P blood group antibodies and spontaneous abortion, it will again be stressed that abortion is not the sole outcome of pregnancy in p and P^k women. In other cases infants with no (160,173,174) or only mild (107,118) HDN have been born to women with anti-P or anti-P+P_1+P^k in the serum. In the large Amish kindred in Northern Ohio (120), a total of 139 infants with P+ red cells (41 P_1+, 98 P_1-) were born to women with anti-P+P_1+P^k in the serum in an eleven and a half year period. Among those infants, at the time of birth, five had red cells that yielded anti-P+P_1+P^k on elution, none of the 139 required treatment for HDN (174).

Auto-anti-P and Paroxysmal Cold Hemoglobinuria

The disease paroxysmal cold hemoglobinuria (PCH) is caused by a usually powerful, IgG, biphasic hemolysin. As the body temperature of a patient with PCH falls, in vivo antigen-antibody complexes form because the biphasic hemolysin is an autoantibody. As the body temperature returns to normal, the preformed antigen-antibody complexes activate complement and an episode of intravascular red cell destruction results. While this mechanism is similar to that causative of cold hemagglutinin disease (CHD) a major difference is that in PCH the autoantibody is IgG while in CHD it is usually IgM (see Chapter 38). In part because of this difference and in part because of the location of the antigens defined by the autoantibodies, hemolytic episodes are almost always more severe in PCH than in CHD. After exposure to cold and before the body temperature returns to normal, some antibody elution occurs. Apparently the IgG autoantibody causative of PCH elutes less readily than does the IgM autoantibody causative of CHD. The net result is that once the body temperature reaches 37°C, where complement is most efficiently activated, more of the antigen-antibody complexes are still present in patients with PCH than in patients with CHD. As described below, autoantibodies causative of PCH complex with the P antigen. The close proximity of this antigen to the red cell membrane (11,151,175-180) allows much of the activated complement to attach to the membrane so that (often) considerable intravascular red cell hemolysis occurs.

For a very long time it was thought (181,182) that the biphasic hemolysin causative of PCH, that is also known as the Donath-Landsteiner antibody, was "nonspecific" for it had been found to hemolyze all red cells against which it was tested. In 1963, Levine et al. (183) showed that the antibody did not react with p red cells. Shortly thereafter, other workers (184-186) showed that the antibody does not react with P^k red cells either and is, in fact, auto-anti-P. As stated, auto-anti-P in PCH is always IgG and acts as a biphasic hemolysin. Dacie (187) has shown that if the antibody is denied an opportunity to activate complement, it will agglutinate red cells. A highly unusual auto-anti-P causative of PCH, was reported by Lindgren et al. (22). In addition to giving a positive D-L test, the antibody was reactive by indirect antiglobulin test in a system kept strictly at 37°C. Both IgG and C3 were detected on P+ red cells used in the 37°C IATs. We (264) described another atypical auto-anti-P that caused PCH. The antibody hemolyzed P+ red cells in tests using PEG, that were set up at room temperature, then immediately incubated at 37°C; that is, there was no incubation at a reduced temperature (265). We were able to test only one other auto-anti-P by the same method, it did not hemolyze P+ red cells but we had only stored, recalcified plasma to test.

There is some minor disagreement among workers regarding the exact definition of PCH. Some believe that the disease is always caused by IgG anti-P, presenting as a biphasic hemolysin. Others (192) believe that a positive D-L test is indicative of PCH regardless of the specificity of the causative antibody. Thus examples of anti-IH (188,189), anti-I (190) and anti-i (191) have been described as causing the disease. Those who believe that PCH is always caused by IgG, anti-P, prefer the term "Donath-Landsteiner hemolytic anemia" (193) to describe the clinically similar condition caused by an autoantibody other than anti-P (194). It is entirely possible that with other specificities, monophasic hemolysins may be involved. The occurrence of secondary PCH following infections, particularly in young children, is discussed in detail in Chapter 38.

Benign Auto-anti-P

In spite of the severity of many cases of PCH, benign examples of auto-anti-P have been found. In 1975, Judd (198) described a transiently produced auto-anti-P that would react in vitro only in a test system at pH 6.0 or lower. In 1982, Judd et al. (199) described two examples of auto-anti-P reactive in vitro only in tests at low ionic strength. In the cases mentioned above there was no evidence of antibody-induced red cell destruc-

tion, presumably because the autoantibodies did not bind to red cells in vivo. A similar LISS-dependent auto-anti-P was described by Cohen and Nelson (201) but in their case the patient had severe hemolytic anemia. The autoantibody was apparently IgM in nature and the D-L test in the patient was negative. In spite of the severe anemia, the authors were not able to demonstrate a cause-and-effect relationship for the auto-anti-P.

The Luke Antigen and Antibody

In 1965, Tippett et al. (9) described the Luke antibody. Based on the reactions of cell samples, three phenotypes: Luke-; Luke(w) (weak positive); and Luke+; were reported. The association between the Luke antibody and the P blood groups was that all p and P^k samples were Luke-. However, not all Luke- samples were p or P^k. Further, the Luke- and Luke(w) phenotypes were more common among P_1- than among P_1+ bloods. An additional finding was that people with red cells of the Luke- and Luke(w) phenotypes were more likely to carry A^1 than A^2, B or O. However, when the second human example and first monoclonal antibody with this specificity were studied, the same association with ABO was not seen. With the monoclonal antibody the Luke(w) phenotype was seen more frequently in persons with a *B* gene than in persons who lacked that gene (202,203); with the second human antibody no effect of ABO group was apparent (204).

The monoclonal antibody MC813-70 was shown to define a murine stage specific embryonic antigen (SSEA-4) (203) and to complex with the red cell antigen defined by the Luke antibody (204). Since it was now possible better to define the Luke antigen (the human antibodies were difficult to use with Luke(w) and Luke- red cells) it was renamed LKE. Since the second human anti-LKE was identified, three others have been encountered (205-207); two of them failed to cause HDN in the LKE+ infants born to women with anti-LKE in their serum (206,207).

As discussed in detail in the section on the biochemistry of the P blood groups, the LKE antigen is now known to be formed when two additional carbohydrate residues are added to the glycosphingolipid that carries P^k and P (203,204). This is reflected at the serological level by the finding (204) that P+, LKE- red cells express a stronger P^k antigen than do those that are P+, LKE+. In other words, when LKE is formed more P^k is covered and becomes less accessible to anti-P^k than when LKE is not made. It was also found (206) that P_1+, LKE- red cells react more strongly with anti-P^k than do P_1- (P_2), LKE- cells although P_1^k and P_2^k cells do not appear to differ in their P^k expression (7).

Anti-IP₁, Anti-IᵀP₁, Anti-iP₁, and Anti-IP

The serological reactions of anti-IP₁ (93), anti-IᵀP₁ (208), anti-iP₁ and anti-IP (210) have been mentioned in Chapter 10. All that is necessary here is to point out that the specificities of these antibodies and of some examples of the Luke antibody as described in the previous section, show that the red cell membrane-borne structures that carry the ABO and I system determinants, also carry those of the P blood groups.

Other Monoclonal Antibodies and the P Blood Groups

Some monoclonal anti-P₁ were mentioned earlier (84-88), the MAb directed against SSEA-4 and the LKE antigen was described in the previous section. In addition, a number of other monoclonal antibodies related to the P blood groups have been made. In many instances the specificity of these antibodies was revealed by inhibition studies using glycosphingolipid fractions known to carry precursor materials and/or Pᵏ, and/or P, and/or Forssman antigen and/or LKE; or related glycosphingolipid fractions known to carry precursor materials and/or P₁ and/or related structures (see section on biochemistry of the P blood groups). In most instances the MAb have also been shown to give the expected (based on inhibition studies) reactions with red cells of various P blood group phenotypes. At least three monoclonal anti-P have been reported (211-213). One them, MC631, (211) is directed against SSEA-3, an immediate precursor of both LKE and H type 4 (see Chapter 8). Another (212) acted as a hemolysin of red cells of phenotypes P₁ and P₂, it also reacted weakly with glycolipids exposed on protease-treated Pᵏ and p red cells. A third (213) had anti-P specificity in serological tests but was inhibited by the T antigen structure (85, and see Chapter 42).

A number of monoclonal anti-Pᵏ have also been produced (86,214,215). As mentioned above, one of several MAb to Pᵏ studied at an international workshop (86) reacted with P₁ and Pᵏ red cells. The MAb 38.13 (214) has considerable practical application since it reacts with Pᵏ red cells but defines a tissue antigen present on Burkitt lymphoma cells. Indeed several of the P blood group related monoclonal antibodies have proved useful in the study of malignant cells in tissues. This aspect and the role of these antibodies is establishing the biosynthetic pathways involved in the production of P blood group antigens are considered in detail, below.

Antibodies of the P Blood Groups in Salmon and Trout Roe and in Snake Serum

As described in the section on the biochemistry of the P system, an alpha-galactosyl-like determinant is common to the B, P₁ and Pᵏ antigens. Protectins from salmon and trout roe complex with such a structure so that antibody-like activity for these determinants is seen in extracts of these materials (216-223). Since the anti-B (and anti-A, see below) and the antibodies to the P blood group determinants are not separable, these materials are of use only in tests on group O red cells. Serum from the South African snake *Python sebae* contains anti-A and anti-B that react with untreated red cells and anti-P that reacts with protease-treated P+ red cells (224). Any reader prepared to collect python serum is cordially invited to write with additional comments.

A number of anti-P₁ have been produced by immunizing various animals with substances such as hydatid cyst fluid, ovomucoid of turtle dove egg white, etc. (see section on anti-P₁) (30,225-227). It seems that for success to be achieved in this venture, the substance containing the P₁ material must be coupled to a carrier or injected with an adjuvant (30,225). Again, the larger number of reports on the use of rabbits and goats, than those of snake serum, presumably represents differences in the ease of handling the antibody-producers. The P blood groups in man are obviously different to the P system in chickens for in those animals *P* genes are linked (233) to those that control recessive white (feathers not eggs), silkie feathering and naked neck!

Some Unusual P Blood Group Phenotypes

When the complexity of the P blood group biosynthetic pathways is considered (see below) it is not surprising that a total or partial block (often reduced or nonproduction of a necessary transferase) at almost any point, can result in an unusual P blood group phenotype.

In 1978, Kundu et al. (228) described a normal healthy individual whose red cells reacted less strongly than normal with several examples of anti-P+P₁+Pᵏ. Analysis of the glycosphingolipids of the red cells showed that they contained less than 25% of the normal amount of globoside (P) and only 30 to 40% of the normal amount of ceramide trihexoside (Pᵏ). The ganglioside content of the red cells was four times that of normal red cells and sialosylparagloboside was increased sixfold. The authors (228) concluded that their findings could be explained either in terms of the presence of an abnormal allele of *Pᵏ*, or by the presence of a gene at another locus affecting the action of *Pᵏ*.

In 1980, Kundu et al. (229) described another P system variant phenotype that had been mentioned briefly (230) in an earlier abstract. Initially it appeared that the phenotype was an example of P₁ᵏ, but analysis of the red cell glycosphingolipids showed that the cells carried half as much globoside (P) as do normal red cells, in addition to their high level of ceramide trihexoside (P^k). Previous studies (177) on red cells of the P^k phenotype had revealed an absence of globoside (P). The globoside on the red cells of the newly described individual (229) was not detectable in serological tests (the cells typed as P-) and the proposita's serum was shown to contain anti-P. As the genetic model described below shows, this case could have represented presence of an allele that affected incomplete or qualitatively different conversion of ceramide trihexoside (P^k) to globoside (P).

The P_1 Antigen and Parentage Studies

Because the P_1+ phenotype is common (table 11-3) and because the P_1 antigen is somewhat fragile (60,61), especially on traveled red cells, the P blood groups are not of great value in cases of disputed parentage. Some workers use P_1 typing primarily in a search for additional exclusions in cases with exclusions involving other markers or to increase the odds when calculating inclusion probabilities. In analyzing blood grouping results from 1000 cases of mother, child, putative father trios, Rasmuson and Hed (231) made the unexpected finding that among those cases in which the probability of paternity was high, the mating P_1 X P_1 was significantly more frequent than would be expected on a random basis. They then tried (232) to confirm this positive assortive mating for P_1 in typing tests on an additional series of parents but were unable to do so. In reviewing the world literature (for 15 references see 232) they found one series each in Germany, Norway and Sweden (their initial series (231) was the Swedish one) in which the P_1 X P_1 mating was significantly in excess of the expected number. However, when all the series were totaled, the excess of P_1 X P_1 mating that could still be seen, fell short of statistical significance. Thus the apparent attraction of P_1+ people for other P_1+ people, remains unexplained.

The P Blood Group System and Disease

As already discussed, the causative autoantibody of paroxysmal cold hemoglobinuria has anti-P specificity. Similarly, the concept of illegitimate antigens in cancer, that began with the P system has been described.

In 1973, Roland (234) reported the presence of a P_1-like antigen in some strains of gram-negative bacilli. In 1981, Lomberg et al. (235) presented data that they believed indicated that young girls who inherited the P^1 gene are more susceptible to urinary tract infections than are those who do not inherit the gene. They studied 28

girls, with a mean age of 9.5 years, each of whom had experienced at least one episode of acute pyelonephritis. The control group comprised 40 children, matched for age, who had no history of urinary tract infection. Among the 28 who had infections, 27 had P_1+ and one, P_1- red cells. Among the controls, 30 had P_1+ and 10, P_1- red cells. In a later study, the same investigators (236) reported that 35 of 36 girls (97%) with recurrent pyelonephritis, had P_1+ red cells compared to 63 of 84 (75%) healthy age-matched controls. To explain these findings, the authors (235,236) cited previous observations (237-241) that show that in order to cause an infection, the bacteria (most often *E. coli*) must ascend the urinary tract against the flow of urine and do so by adherance to uroepithelial cells. There is a body of evidence (242-244) that suggests that the bacteria adhere to glycolipids on the epithelial cells and Lomberg et al. (235,236) suggested that glycolipid chains that carry terminal D-galactose in alpha 1→4 linkage to a subterminal galactose, comprise the prime adhesion or recognition site for *E. Coli*. That combination (see below) represents the terminal end of both the P^k and P_1-bearing glycosphingolipids. Thus the theory is that in the presence of P_1-bearing glycosphingolipids on tissue cells of the urinary tract (236,243,245-256) (P^k is, of course, almost universally present) the *E. coli* organisms can bind and ascend the urinary tract more easily than in the absence of P_1-bearing glycosphingolipid. This concept is used to explain the higher rate of infections and pyelonephritis in P_1+ than in P_1- subjects. A similar role for some antigens of the Cromer blood group system is discussed in Chapter 24.

The Structure of the P_1 Antigen

The first studies on the biochemical nature of the P_1 antigen, like those on the A, B, H, Lewis and Ii antigens (Chapters 8,9,10) were not made on material purified from human red cells. In the case of P_1 the alternative source of antigen came from what is at first sight a rather unlikely source namely, hydatid cyst fluid. Hydatid cyst fluid is produced by the tapeworm *Echinococcus granulosus*, a very common parasite of farmyard animals and occasionally found in man. Cameron and Staveley (16) working in New Zealand noticed that patients with hydatid disease were much more likely to have anti-P_1 in their serum than patients with other diseases. This observation led them to show that hydatid cyst fluid is a potent inhibitor of hemagglutination caused by anti-P_1. Hydatid cysts are easily found in the liver and lungs of infected animals. In the late 1960s one of us (DJA) spent many Friday lunchtimes in a Bristol abbattoir collecting hydatid cyst fluid from the infected livers and lungs of sheep which came down from the Welsh mountains for slaughter. It is not a pleasant job but large quantities of fluid (several liters) are easily collected. Morgan and Watkins (266) applied the same methodology that had been used successfully to purify ABH and Lewis-active blood group substances from human ovarian cyst fluid to purify the P_1-active material from hydatid cyst fluid. They showed that it was a glycoprotein. Inhibition of agglutination of human P_1+ red cells by human and rabbit anti-P_1 could be demonstrated with the disaccharides Galα(1→3)Gal and Galα(1→4)Gal (226). The importance of α-linked D-galactose in the P_1 structure was confirmed in several subsequent studies of P_1 substance from hydatid cyst fluid (115, 219, 221, 267). Acid hydrolysis of the P_1 glycoprotein released a blood group P_1-active trisaccharide of structure αGal(1→4)βGal(1→4)GlcNAc (268).

While this work was in progress, Donald Marcus in New York was in the process of characterizing the P_1 antigen from red cells. In 1971, Marcus was able to report that the P_1 antigen is carried on a glycolipid in red cells although the glycolipid had not yet been purified to homogeneity (269). The reader should not underestimate the difficulty of this task. This author (DJA) recalls a letter from Donald Marcus received at the time in which he said that "no matter how many red cells we start with we still seem to finish up with less than a milligram of not quite pure P_1 glycolipid."

The endeavor was to prove worthwhile however, and in 1975, Naiki et al. (270) were able to report the structure of the human erythrocyte blood group P_1 glycolipid as Galα(1→4)Galβ(1→4)GlcNAcβ(1→3)Galβ(1→4)Glc-ceramide. The terminal trisaccharide structure of this lipid was exactly the same as that found for the glycoprotein in hydatid cyst fluid by Cory et al. (268).

Given that the structure of the P_1 glycolipid is formed by addition of galactose to a type 2 precursor sequence which can also be glycosylated to form ABH antigens, it would not be unreasonable to suppose that the P_1 glycosyltransferase competes with the A, B and H transferases for the same substrate. It would follow from this that since ABH antigens are widely expressed on red cell membrane glycoproteins (see Chapter 8) then P_1 antigen might also be found on glycoproteins as well as glycolipids in the red cell membrane. One publication (271) suggests that P_1 is associated with carbohydrate on band 3 (anion transporter, see Chapter 17 and band 4.5, glucose transporter, see Chapter 4). Another publication (272) disputes this and argues that P_1 is found only on glycolipids. This is an interesting point because it raises questions about the substrate specificity of glycosyltransferases. Most studies of glycosyltransferase specificity are carried out with model acceptor substrates because it is difficult to analyze the variety of natural

substrates available on a whole red cell but studies with model acceptors may not reveal subtelities that effect their specificity in nature. Recent studies on the specificity of the H-transferase alluded to in Chapter 8 show that this enzyme, when expressed in Chinese hamster ovary cells, preferentially fucosylates glycans containing polylactosamine and does not fucosylate O-glycans *or* glycolipids (273).

The Structure of the Pᵏ Antigen

The P_1-active glycoprotein from hydatid cyst fluid also inhibits agglutination caused by anti-P^k (7). Evidence that anti-P^k, like anti-P_1, recognizes α-linked D-galactose was first provided by Voak et al. (221) on the basis of hemagglutination inhibition experiments with simple sugars and loss of P^k antigen activity after treatment of P_1 substance with coffee bean α-galactosidase. Furukawa et al. (7) came to similar conclusions. The P_1-active trisaccharide isolated by Cory et al. (268) and the disaccharide αGal(1→4)Gal were also potent inhibitors of anti-P^k (274). Naiki and Marcus (176, 275) showed that P^k activity in the red cell membrane is carried on a previously described glycolipid known as ceramide trihexoside (CTH). CTH has the structure: Galα(1→4)Galβ(1→4)Glc-ceramide. The P_1 and P^k antigens are therefore identical with respect to the disaccharide sequence at the non-reducing end of the antigen. These results also explained the anti-α-galactosyl specificity of the lectin found in ova derived from the trout *Salmo trutta* (222) since purified P_1 glycolipid and CTH but not the P antigen (see next section) specifically inhibited hemagglutination caused by the lectin (275).

The Structure of the P Antigen

P antigen is easily detected in lipid extracts of red cell membranes (219, 276). Naiki and Marcus (176, 275) showed that this is because P antigen is expressed by a previously described lipid known as globoside I which is the most abundant glycolipid in the red cell membrane. Globoside I has the structure: GalNAcβ(1→3)Galα(1→4)Galβ(1→4)Glc-ceramide. Inspection of this structure reveals that the P^k antigen is the biosynthetic precursor of the P antigen (see figure 11-1). The number of molecules of P antigen/red cell are estimated at 14×10^6/cell (148).

The Biosynthesis of P_1, P and Pᵏ

The total amount of P antigen in P_1+ red cells and P_1- red cells is about the same but red cells of the P_1+

phenotype contain more P^k than do P$_1$- cells (about 1 molecule of P^k antigen (CTH) for every 8 molecules of P antigen (globoside)). P$_1$- cells contain about 1 molecule of P^k antigen to every 12 molecules of P antigen (245). The precursor of P^k, ceramide dihexoside (CDH) is present at levels more than twice that of P^k in P$_1$- cells but only half that of P^k in P$_1$+ red cells. These results led Fletcher et al. (245) to conclude that the same galactosyltransferase is able to convert CDH to CTH and to synthesize P$_1$ antigen from its precursor, paragloboside (figure 11-1, but see below).

These conclusions were supported by studies of the glycolipid composition of P^k and p red cells. Red cells of both phenotypes lack detectable globoside. P^k cells contain an abnormally large amount of CTH and p red cells have a marked increase in CDH (177,277). Red cells of p phenotype also have an increased content (3-5 fold increase) of two sialylated glycolipids (gangliosides) known as sialoparagloboside and G$_{M3}$ (see figure 11-1). Sialoparagloboside and related structures inhibit antibodies which react preferentially with red cells of phenotype p (148). There is evidence that at least some individuals with the P^k phenotype make small amounts of globoside suggesting that the P^k phenotype is not always the result of a totally inactive P-transferase (212).

An overall scheme for the biosynthesis of P$_1$, P and P^k is given in figure 11-1. Essentially there are two distinct pathways. Both pathways begin with CDH, one

leads to the synthesis of P^k and then to P, the other ultimately yields P$_1$. The pathway from CDH to P^k and P is assumed to result from the sequential action of two glycosyltransferases (an $\alpha(1\rightarrow4)$ galactosyltransferase (product of the *P^k* gene) and a $\beta(1\rightarrow3)$ N-acetylgalactosaminyl transferase (product of the *P* gene). A candidate for the *P^k* gene product has been reported in rat kidney, intestine, liver, human kidney and placenta (reviewed in 278). A candidate for the *P* gene product has been found in canine spleen, guinea pig kidney, human lung and lymphoblastoid cells (278). There has been some debate in the literature as to whether the galactosyltransferase responsible for P^k antigen is the same enzyme that gives rise to P$_1$. Bailly et al. (279) provide evidence that they are different enzymes.

Strategies for Cloning the Transferase Genes Giving Rise to the P$_1$, P and P^k Antigens

The transferase genes giving rise to these antigens have not been cloned at the time of writing. The problems of purifying glycosyltransferases in sufficient quantity to obtain protein sequence were discussed in Chapter 8 with respect to the blood group A transferase. Studies on the genes giving rise to the family of fucosyltransferases suggest a different strategy. Fucosyltransferases share a

FIGURE 11-1 Biosynthetic Relationships Between P^k, P$_1$ and P antigens

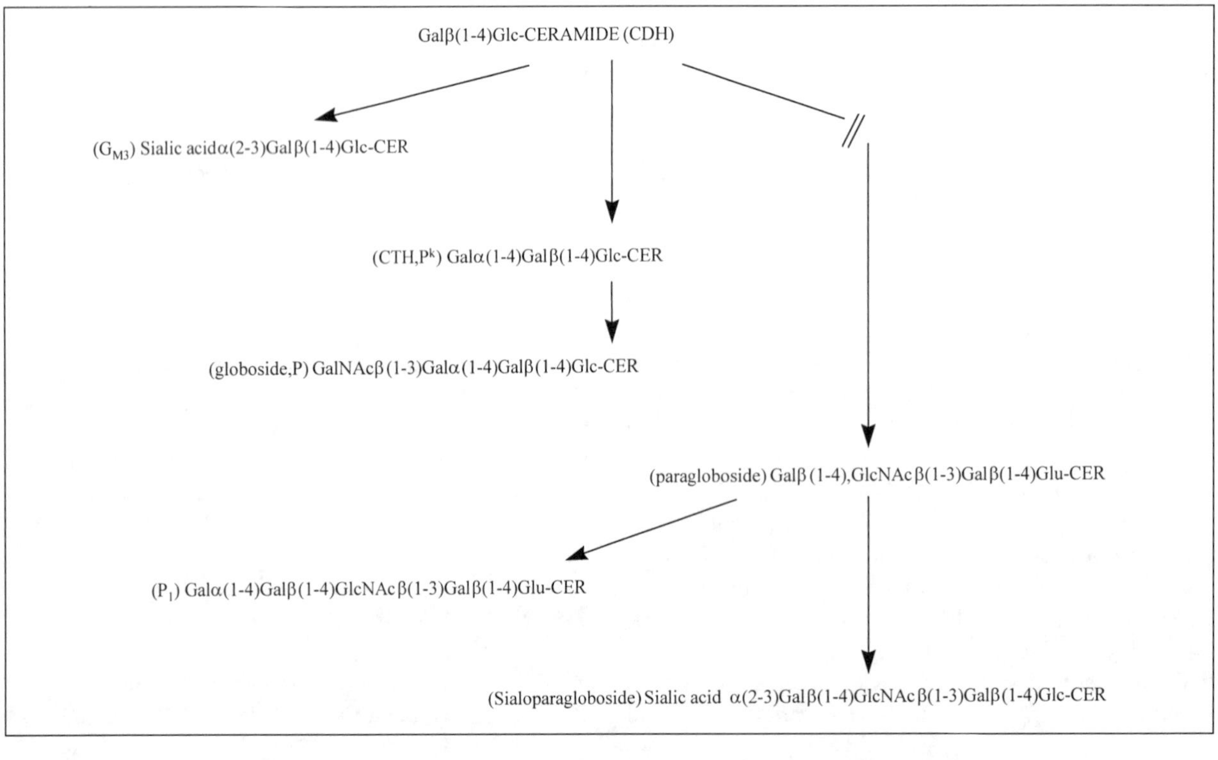

degree of sequence homology in their active site which has proved sufficient to allow the identification of a candidate α(1,3)fucosyltransferase gene in *Caenorhabditis elegans* (280). *C. elegans* is a nematode and is the first metazoan whose entire genome has been sequenced (281).

The P_1 antigen is known to be widely distributed in a wide variety of organisms including the nematode *Ascaris suum* (34) and the bacterium *Neisseria gonorrhoeae* (282). The P^k antigen is reported to be expressed on several different bacteria (*Neisseria gonorrhoeae, N. meningitidis, N. lactamica, Hemophilus influenzae, Branhamella catarrhalis,* 278,282). P_1 antigen is also found in earthworms (*Lumbricus terrestris,* 34), liver flukes (*Fasciola hepatica,* 15,19,21) and various parts of the pigeon (26,29) in addition to the tapeworm *Echinococcus granulosus* discussed in a previous section. These results clearly indicate that the αGal transferase(s) giving rise to P_1 and P^k are widespread and that it is likely that the sequence of the gene for one or more such enzymes is already known in *C. elegans*. The problem is finding it. If α-galactosyl transferases show a similar sequence homology around the active site to that shown by fucosyltransferases, one possibility would be to search the *C. elegans* database for homologies with the ABO-transferase and its murine homolog (283) and see if any sequences match a protein that would follow the general model of glycosyltransferase proteins. Failing this, it should be possible to clone the α-galactosyl transferase gene(s) using transfection cloning. This has been used successfully to identify the H-transferase (see Chapter 8). This method requires a cell line which itself fails to express the transferases it is desired to clone so that transfected cells obtaining the desired transferase gene can be detected by looking for surface expression of the antigen of interest (in this case P^k, P or P_1). Wiels et al. (284) describe Epstein-Barr virus (EBV) transformed B cell lines derived from individuals of phenotype p which could provide suitable cell lines for such a transfection cloning approach.

Structure of the Antigen LKE

Monoclonal antibodies reactive with embryonic antigens SSEA-3 and SSEA-4 react with red cells. These antigens are produced by the addition of galactose (β1→3) to the non-reducing end of globoside (P antigen) in the case of SSEA-3 and to both galactose and sialic acid (α2→3) in the case of SSEA-4 (see figure 11-2). Tippett et al. (203) tested monoclonal antibodies to these two antigens against Luke negative red cells and found that anti-SSEA-4 failed to react with these cells. Both anti-SSEA-3 and anti-SSEA-4 failed to react with red cells of phenotype p. Bruce et al. (206) reported that red cells that are negative for the Luke antigen (LKE-) have elevated expression of P^k antigen.

References

1. Lewis M, Anstee DJ, Bird GWG, et al. Vox Sang 1990;58:152
2. Lewis M, Anstee DJ, Bird GWG, et al. Vox Sang 1991;61:158
3. Landsteiner K, Levine P. Proc Soc Exp Biol NY 1927;24:941
4. Landsteiner K, Levine P. J Immunol 1930;18:87
5. Sanger R. Nature 1955;176:1163
6. Levine P, Bobbitt OB, Walker RK, et al. Proc Soc Exp Biol NY;1951;77:403
7. Matson GA, Swanson J, Noades J, et al. Am J Hum Genet 1959;11:26
8. Kortekangas AE, Kaarsalo E, Melartin L, et al. Vox Sang 1965;10:385
9. Tippett P, Sanger R, Race RR, et al. Vox Sang 1965;10:269
10. Engelfriet CP, Beckers D, von dem Borne AEG Kr, et al. Vox Sang 1972;23:176
11. Spitalnik PF, Spitalnick SL. Transf Med Rev 1995;9:110
12. Henningsen K. Acta Path Microbiol Scand 1949;26:769
13. Prokop O, Schlesinger D. Z Immun Forsch Exp Ther 1965;6:344
14. Mollison PL. Blood Transfusion in Clinical Medicine, 6th Ed. Oxford:Blackwell, 1979
15. Ben-Ismail R, Rouger P, Carme B, et al. Vox Sang 1980;38:165
16. Cameron GL, Stavely JM. Nature 1957;179:147

FIGURE 11-2 Biosynthetic Relationships Between P, Pᵏ and LKE Antigens

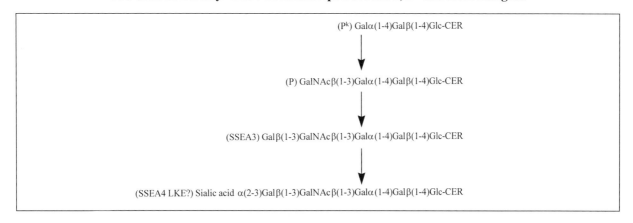

(P^k) Galα(1-4)Galβ(1-4)Glc-CER

(P) GalNAcβ(1-3)Galα(1-4)Galβ(1-4)Glc-CER

(SSEA3) Galβ(1-3)GalNAcβ(1-3)Galα(1-4)Galβ(1-4)Glc-CER

(SSEA4 LKE?) Sialic acid α(2-3)Galβ(1-3)GalNAcβ(1-3)Galα(1-4)Galβ(1-4)Glc-CER

17. DeTapia GM. Proc 9th Cong ISBT, Basel:Karger 1964:731
18. Raik A, Hunter E, Warner H. Med J Austral 1970;6:1055
19. Bevan A, Hammond W, Clark RL. Vox Sang 1970;18:188
20. Ben-Ismail R, Carme B, Gentilini M. Nouv Presse Med 1978;7:4300
21. Ben-Ismail R, Carme B, Gentilini M. Pathol Biol Paris 1979;26:487
22. Petit A, Duong TH, Bremond JL, et al. Rev Fr Transf Immunohematol 1981;24:197
23. Smythe R. Andy Capp Strikes Back. London:Mirror Syn, 1973
24. Roland F, Effler D. Chemosphere 1973;4:137
25. Brocteur J, Francois-Gerard C, Andre A, et al. Haematologia 1975;9:43
26. Radermecker M, Bruwier M, Francois C, et al. Clin Exp Immunol 1975;22:546
27. Roland F, Effler D, Redding R. Clin Exp Immunol 1977;29:95
28. Munro AC, Inglis G, Lynch PP, et al. Clin Allgy 1980;10:643
29. Francois-Gerard C, Gerday C, Beeley JG. Biochem J 1979;177:679
30. Francois-Gerard C, Brocteur J, Andre A. Vox Sang 1980;39:141
31. Inglis G, Watt AG, Munro AC. Med Lab Sci 1982;39:179
32. Radermecker MF, Bruwier MW. Chest 1977;72;546
33. Roland FP. Lancet 1981;1:946
34. Prokop O, Schlesinger D. Z Immun Allgy Forsch 1965;129:334
35. Prokop O, Schelsinger D. Acta Biol Med Germ 1965;15:180
36. Vengelen-Tyler V, Nason SG, Dugan M, et al. Transfusion 1981;21:224
37. Norman P, MacIntyre D, Poole J, et al. Vox Sang 1985;49:211
38. Mollison PL, Cutbush M. Lancet 1955;1:1290
39. Cutbush M, Giblett ER, Mollison PL. Br J Haematol 1956;2:210
40. Cutbush M, Mollison PL. Br J Haematol 1958;4:115
41. Mollison PL. Br Med J 1959;2:1035
42. Mollison PL. Br Med J 1959;2:1123
43. Mollison PL. Br Med Bull 1959;15:92
44. Mollison PL. Acta Hematol 1959;10:495
45. Giblett ER. Transfusion 1977;17:299
46. Morel PA, Garratty G, Perkins HA. Am J Med Technol 1978;44:122
47. Issitt PD. In: Clinically Significant and Insignificant Antibodies. Washington, D.C.:Am Assoc Blood Banks 1979:13
48. Garratty G. In: Clinically Significant and Insignificant Antibodies. Washington, D.C.:Am Assoc Blood Banks 1979:29
49. Issitt PD. In: Pathology-Anatomical and Clinical. Oxford:Pergamon 1982:395
50. Cronin CA, Pohl BA, Miller WV. Transfusion 1978;18:728
51. Mollison PL. Unpublished observations, cited in Mollison PL. Blood Transfusion in Clinical Medicine, 6th Ed. Oxford:Blackwell, 1979:281
52. Ahrons S, Kissmeyer-Nielsen F. Dan Med Bull 1968;15:259
53. Kissmeyer-Nielsen F, Kristoffersen K. Ugesk Laeger 1955;117:745
54. DiNapoli JB, Nichols ME, Marsh WL, et al. (abstract). Transfusion 1978;18:383
55. Chandeysson PL, Flye MW, Simpkins SM, et al. Transfusion 1981;21:77
56. Pineda AA, Brzica SM, Taswell HF. Mayo Clin Proc 1978;53:378
57. Moore SB, Taswell HF, Pineda AA, et al. Am J Clin Pathol 1980;74:94
58. Taswell HF, Pineda AA, Moore SB. In: A Seminar on Immune Mediated Red Cell Destruction. Washington, D.C.:Am Assoc Blood Banks, 1981:71
59. Strohm PL, Molthan L. Canad J Med Technol 1981;43:153
60. Crawford H, Cutbush M, Mollison PL. Vox Sang (Old Series) 1954;4:149
61. Linins I, McIntyre J, Moore BPL. Canad J Med Technol 1959;21:47
62. Molthan L. Vox Sang 1981;40:105
63. Fairley NH. Br Med J 1940;2:213
64. Anderson DR, Kelton JG. In: Immune Destruction of Red Blood Cells. Arlington, VA:Am Assoc Blood Banks, 1989:1
65. Molthan L. (Letter). Vox Sang 1982;42:55
66. Avoy DR. (Letter). Vox Sang 1982;42:54
67. Molthan L, Wick R, Gross BM. Blood Transf Immunohematol 1981;24:263
68. Mothan L. Blood Transf Immunohematol 1982;25:127
69. Wells RF, Korn G, Hafleigh B, et al. Transfusion 1976;16:427
70. Tilley CA, Crookston MC, Haddad SA, et al. Transfusion 1977;17:162
71. Shore GM, Steane EA. (abstract). Transfusion 1978;18:387
72. Ryden SE. (Letter). Transfusion 1981;21:130
73. Viggiano E, Ballas SK. (abstract). Transfusion 1981;21:603
74. Valko DA, Silberstein EB, Greenwalt TJ, et al. (abstract). Transfusion 1981;21:603
75. Grove W, Peters B, Ellisor SS, et al. (abstract). Transfusion 1981;21:607
76. Adinolphi M, Polley MJ, Hunter DA, et al. Immunology 1962;5:566
77. Polley MJ, Mollison PL, Soothill JF. Br J Haematol 1962;8:149
78. Garratty G, Arndt P, Marfoe R, et al. (abstract). Transfusion 1995;35(Suppl 10S):22S
79. Wiener AS, Unger LJ. Am J Clin Pathol 1944;14:616
80. Cheng MS. (Letter). Transfusion 1984;24:183
81. Cox MT, Roberts M, LaJoie J, et al. (Letter). Transfusion 1992;32:874
82. Moreau P. Rev Belg Sci Med 1945;16:258
83. Mollison PL. Blood Transfusion in Clinical Medicine, 7th ed. Oxford:Blackwell, 1983:317
84. Bailly P, Chevaleyre J, Sondag D, et al. Mol Immunol 1987;24:171
85. Rouger P, Anstee DJ, Salmon C. Rev Fr Transf Immunohematol 1987;30:627
86. Brodin NT, Dahmén J, Nilsson B, et al. Int J Cancer 1988;42:185
87. Chester MA, Johnson U, Lundblad A, et al. Proc 2nd Int Workshop on Monoclonal Antibodies Against Human Red Blood Cells and Related Antigens, 1990:86
88. Bouhours D, Bouhours JF, Willem C, et al. (abstract). Vox Sang 1994;67(Suppl 2):118
89. Race RR, Sanger R. Blood Groups in Man 3rd Ed. Oxford:Blackwell, 1958
90. Ikin EW, Kay HEM, Playfair JHL, et al. Nature 1961;192:883
91. Henningsen K. Acta Path Microbiol Scand 1949;26:639
92. Heiken A. Hereditas 1966;56:83
93. Issitt PD, Tegoli J, Jackson VA, et al. Vox Sang 1968;14:1
94. Moharram I. Lab Med Prog 1942;3;1
95. Cazal P, Mathieu M. Sangre 1950;2:717
96. Grosjean R. Sangre 1952;23:490
97. Spieser P, Weigel B. Z Clin Med 1952;7:54
98. Henningsen K. Rev Hematol 1950;5:276
99. Fisher R. Heredity 1953;7:81
100. Zoutendyk A, Levine P. Am J Clin Pathol 1952;22:630

101. Hirszfeld L, Grabowska M. Experienta 1952;8:355
102. Iseki S, Masaki S, Levine P. Nature 1954;173:1193
103. Levine P, Robinson EA, Pryer B, et al. Vox Sang (Old Series) 1954;4:143
104. Walsh RJ, Kooptzoff O. Austral J Exp Biol Med Sci 1954;32:387
105. Yasuda J, Yokoyama M. Proc 8th Cong ISBT. Basel:Karger 1960;IIa:20
106. Furukawa K. J Jpn Soc Blood Transf 1967;14:158
107. Hayashida Y, Watanabe A. J Jpn Legal Med 1968;22:10
108. Hornstein L, Pinkas-Schweitzer R. Israel J Med Sci 1969;5:114
109. Wurzel HA, Gottlieb AJ, Abelson NM. (abstract). Prog 24th Ann Mtg Am Assoc Blood Banks, 1971:103
110. Tomita K, Nakajima H. J Jpn Soc Blood Transf 1972;19:33
111. Kawase M. Proc 20th Cong Jpn Soc Blood Transf 1972
112. Cedergren B. Hereditas 1973;73:27
113. Miwa S, Matuhasi T, Yasuda J. Vox Sang 1974;26:565
114. Yamaguchi H, Okubo Y, Tanaka M, et al. J Jpn Soc Blood Transf 1974;20:33
115. Fukukawa K, Takizawa H, Takizawa H, et al. Jpn J Hum Genet 1974;19:137
116. Yokata T, Ohno K, Ito S, et al. J Jpn Soc Blood Transf 1974;20:31
117. Weiss DB. Levene C, Aboulafia Y, et al. Fertil Steril 1975;26:901
118. Levene C, Sela R, Rudolphson Y, et al. Transfusion 1977;17:569
119. Sanger R, Tippett P. (Letter). Transfusion 1979;19:222
120. Obregon E, McKeever BG. (abstract). Transfusion 1980;20:621
121. Cantin G, Lyonnais J. Transfusion 1983;23:350
122. Sweeney JD, Wenz B. Transfusion 1984;24:25
123. Race RR, Sanger R. Blood Groups in Man 6th Ed. Oxford:Blackwell, 1975
124. Otsuka S, Kunieda K, Kitamura F, et al. Transfusion 1991;31:260
125. Kimura A, Dong RP, Harada H, et al. Tissue Antigens 1992;40:5
126. Levine P. Ann NY Acad Sci 1976;277:428
127. Levine P. In: Onco-Developmental Gene Expression. New York:Academic Press, 1976:485
128. Levine P. In: Cancer Invasion and Metastasis. New York:Raven, 1977
129. Levine P. Transfusion 1977;17:573
130. Levine P. (Letter). Transfusion 1979;19:223
131. Levene C. (Letter). Transfusion 1979;19:224
132. Shirey RS, Ness PM, Kickler T, et al. Transfusion 1987;27:189
133. Shechter Y, Timor-Tritsch IE, Lewit N, et al. Vox Sang 1987;53:135
134. Cedergren B. Unpublished observations cited in Rydberg L, Cedergren B, Breimer ME, et al. Molec Immunol 1992;29:1273
135. Yoshida H, Ito K, Emi N, et al. Vox Sang 1984;47:216
136. Levine P. Semin Oncol 1978;5:25
137. Stellner K, Hakomori S, Warner G. Biochem Biophys Res Comm 1973;55:439
138. Springer GF, Desai PR, Scanlon EF. Cancer 1976;37:169
139. Hakomori S, Wang M, Young WW, et al. Proc Nat Acad Sci USA 1977;74:3026
140. Iwaki Y, Kasai M, Terasaki PI, et al. Cancer Res 1982;42:409
141. Lloyd KO. Am J Clin Pathol 1987;87:129
142. Hakomori S. Adv Cancer Res 1989;52:257
143. Hakomori S. Curr Opin Immunol 1991;3:646
144. Liotta LA. Sci Am 1992;266:54
145. Garratty G. In: Immunobiology of Transfusion Medicine. New York:Marcel Dekker, 1994:201
146. Metaxas MN, Metaxas-Bühler M, Tippett P. (abstract). Book of Abstracts, 14th Cong ISBT, 1975:95
147. Issitt CH, Duckett JB, Osborne BM, et al. Br J Haematol 1976;34:19
148. Schwarting GA, Marcus DM, Metaxas M. Vox Sang 1977;32:257
149. Roelcke D, Riesen W, Geisen HP, et al. Vox Sang 1977;33:304
150. Roelcke D, Riesen W, Geisen HP, et al. Vox Sang 1977;33:372
151. Marcus DM, Kundu SK, Suzuki A. Semin Hematol 1981;18:63
152. Kortekangas AE, Noades J, Tippett P, et al. Vox Sang 1959;4:337
153. Kortekangas AE, Kaarsalo E, Tippett P, et al. Acta Path Microbiol Scand 1962;154(Suppl):359
154. Stroup M, MacIlroy M, Suggs G, et al. (abstract). Transfusion 1964;4:314
155. Kaarsalo E. Unpublished observations, 1965 to 1967 cited by Race RR, Sanger R. Blood Groups in Man, 6th Ed. Oxford:Blackwell, 1975
156. Nevanlinna HR, Furuhjelm U. Unpublished observations, 1966 cited by Race RR, Sanger R. Blood Groups in Man 6th Ed. Oxford:Blackwell, 1975
157. Hayashida Y. J Jpn Soc Blood Transf 1968;15:181
158. Schneider W, Tippett P, Gooch A. Vox Sang 1969;16:67
159. Furukawa K. Jpn J Hum Genet 1975;20:32
160. Nakajima H, Yokata T. Vox Sang 1977;32:56
161. Kato M, Kubo S, Naiki M. J Immunogenet 1978;5:31
162. Fellous M, Gerbal A, Tessier C, et al. Vox Sang 1974;26:518
163. Lopez M, Cartron J, Cartron JP, et al. Clin Immunol Immunopathol 1983;28:296
164. Söderström T, Enskog A, Samuelsson BE, et al. J Immunol 1985;134:1
165. Hansson GC, Wazniowska K, Rock JA, et al. Arch Biochem Biophys 1988;260:168
166. Lindström K, von dem Borne AEG Kr, Breimer ME, et al. Glycocon J 1992;9:325
167. Cartron J, Cartron JP, Lopez M, et al. C R Acad Sci Paris Ser D 1979;288:1501
168. Vos GH, Celano MJ, Falkowski F, et al. Transfusion 1964;4:87
169. Vos GH. Transfusion 1965;5:327
170. Vos GH. Transfusion 1966;6:272
171. Vos GH. Transfusion 1967;7:40
172. Horvath E, Peisz L. Transfusion 1966;6:499
173. Yamaguchi H, Okubo Y, Tanaka M, et al. Proc Jpn Acad 1974;50:764
174. Sheehan J, Pochedley M, Toy E. (abstract). Book of Abstracts, Joint Cong ISBT/AABB, 1990:84
175. Fraser BA, Malette MF. Immunochemistry 1974;11:581
176. Naiki M, Marcus DM. Biochem Biophys Res Comm 1974;60:1105
177. Marcus DM, Naiki M, Kundu SK. Proc Nat Acad Sci USA 1976;73:3263
178. Rosenfield RE. In: A Seminar on Performance Evaluation. Washington, D.C.:Am Assoc Blood Banks, 1976:93
179. Heddle NM. Transf Med Rev 1989;3:219
180. Marcus DM. Immunol Ser 1989;43:701
181. Ehrlich P, Morgenroth J. Berlin Klin Wschr 1900;37:453
182. Donath J, Landsteiner K. Munch Med Wschr 1904;51:1590
183. Levine P, Celano MJ, Falkowski F. Transfusion 1963;3:278

184. Knapp T. Canad J Med Technol 1964;26:172
185. Hart van der M, Giessen van der M, Veer van der M, et al. Vox Sang 1964;9:36
186. Worlledge SM, Rousso C. Vox Sang 1965;10:293
187. Dacie JV. The Haemolytic Anaemias. II. The Autoimmune Haemolytic Anaemias. New York:Grune and Stratton, 1962
188. Weiner W, Gordon EG, Rowe D. Vox Sang 1964;9:684
189. Bell CA, Zwicker H. (abstract). Transfusion 1967;7:384
190. Bell CA, Zwicker H, Rosenbaum DL. Transfusion 1973;13:138
191. Shirey RS, Miller KP, Ness PM, et al. (abstract). Transfusion 1983;23:424
192. Rosse WF. Clinical Immunohematology: Basic Concepts and Clinical Applications. Boston:Blackwell, 1990
193. Wolach B, Heddle N, Barr RD, et al. Br J Haematol 1981;48:425
194. Judd WJ, Wilkinson SL, Issitt PD, et al. Transfusion 1986;26:423
195. Crawford MN, Greenwalt TJ, Sasaki T, et al. Transfusion 1961;1:228
196. Crawford MN, Tippett P, Sanger R. Vox Sang 1974;26:283
197. Contreras M, Tippett P. Vox Sang 1974;27:369
198. Judd WJ. Transfusion 1975;15:373
199. Judd WJ, Steiner EA, Capps RD. Transfusion 1982;22:185
200. Lindgren S, Zimmerman S, Gibbs F, et al. Transfusion 1985;25:142
201. Cohen DW, Nelson L. (Letter). Transfusion 1983;23:79
202. Kannagi R, Cochran NA, Ishigami F, et al. EMBO J 1983;2:2355
203. Tippett P, Andrews PW, Knowles BB, et al. Vox Sang 1986;51:53
204. Tippett P. In: Red Cell Antigens and Antibodies. Arlington, VA:Am Assoc Blood Banks, 1986:83
205. Boorman K. Unpublished observations cited by Daniels G. Human Blood Groups. Oxford:Blackwell, 1995
206. Bruce M, Watt A, Gabra GS, et al. Vox Sang 1988;55:237
207. Møller B, Jørgensen J. Transfusion 1988;28:88
208. Booth PB. Vox Sang 1970;19:85
209. McGinniss MH, Kaplan HS, Bowen AB, et al. Transfusion 1969;9:40
210. Allen FH Jr, Marsh WL, Jensen L, et al. Vox Sang 1974;27:442
211. Shevinsky LH, Knowles BB, Damjanov I, et al. Cell 1982;30:697
212. von dem Borne AEGKr, Bos MJE, Joustra-Maas N, et al. Br J Haematol 1986;63:35
213. Inglis G, Fraser RH, Mitchell AAB, et al. Vox Sang 1987;52:79
214. Nudelman E, Kannagi R, Hakomori S, et al. Science 1983;220:509
215. Kasai K, Galton J, Terasaki PI, et al. J Immunogenet 1985;12:213
216. Uhlenbruck G, Prokop O. Vox Sang 1967;12:465
217. Todd GM. Vox Sang 1971;21:451
218. Pardoe GI. Rev Inst Pasteur 1971;4:255
219. Anstee DJ. PhD Thesis, Univ Bristol 1972
220. Pardoe GI, Uhlenbruck G. Med Lab Technol 1972;29:351
221. Voak D, Anstee D, Pardoe G. Vox Sang 1973;25:263
222. Anstee DJ, Holt PDJ, Pardoe GI. Vox Sang 1973;25:347
223. Voak D, Todd GM, Pardoe GI. Vox Sang 1974;26:176
224. Lockyer WJ, Gold ER. Med Lab Sci 1977;34:303
225. Levine P, Celano M, Stavely JM. Vox Sang 1958;3:434
226. Watkins WM, Morgan WTJ. Proc 9th Cong ISBT. Basel:Karger 1962:230
227. Prokop O, Schlesinger D. Nature 1966;209:1255
228. Kundu SK, Steane SM, Bloom JEC, et al. Vox Sang 1978;35:160
229. Kundu SK, Evans A, Rizvi J, et al. J Immunogenet 1980;7:431
230. Rizvi J, Kundu SK, Glidden H, et al. (abstract). Transfusion 1979;19:662
231. Rasmuson M, Hed H. Hereditas 1981;94:105
232. Rasmuson M, Hed H. Hum Hered 1983;33:9
233. Bitgood JJ, Dochnahl J, Schlafly P, et al. Poultry Science 1984;63:592
234. Roland F. Ann Microbiol Inst Pasteur 1973;124A:175
235. Lombard H, Jordal U, Eden CS, et al. Lancet 1981;1:551
236. Lombard H, Hanson LA, Jacobsson B, et al. New Eng J Med 1983;308:1189
237. Svanborg EC, Hanson LA, Jordal U, et al. Lancet 1976;2:490
238. Fowler JE, Stamey TA. J Urol 1977;117:472
239. Källenius G, Winberg J. Lancet 1978;2:540
240. Svanborg EC, Jordal U. Infect Immun 1979;26:837
241. Svanborg EC, Hagberg L, Hanson LA, et al. In: Adhesion and Micro-Organism Pathogenicity. London:Pitman, 1980.
242. Svanborg EC, Leffler H. Scand J Infect Dis 1980;24(Suppl):144
243. Leffler H, Svanborg EC. FEMS Microbiol Lett 1980;8:127
244. Källenius G, Möllby R, Svenson SB, et al. FEMS Microbiol Lett 1980;7:297
245. Fletcher KD, Bremer EG, Schwarting GA, et al. J Biol Chem 1979;254:11196
246. Holmgren J, Elwing H, Fredman P, et al. Adv Exp Med Biol 1980;125:453
247. Väisänen V, Elo J, Tallgren LG, et al. Lancet 1981;2:1366
248. Källenius G, Svenson SB, Hultberg H, et al. Lancet 1981;2:1369
249. Momata K, Shimoda K, Naiki M. J Biochem 1982;92:2047
250. Korhonen TK, Väisänen V, Saxén H, et al. Infect Immun 1982;37:286
251. Sussman M, Parry SH, Rooke DM, et al. Lancet 1982;1:1352
252. Sobota AE. J Urol 1984;131:1013
253. Gander RM, Thomas VL, Forland M. J Infect Dis 1985;151:508
254. Schmidt DR, Sobota AE. Microbiosci 1988;55:173
255. Kaack MB, Roberts JA, Baskin G, et al. Infect Immun 1988;56:1
256. Anonymous, Editorial. Lancet 1988;2:1343
257. Zafriri D, Ofek I, Adar R, et al. Antimicrob Agents Chemotherap 1989;33:92
258. Ofek I, Goldhar J, Zafriri D, et al. New Eng J Med 1991;324:1599
259. Whitsett CF, Duffin LE, Heffner LT, et al. (abstract). Transfusion 1982;22:407
260. Rodey G. HLA Beyond Tears. Atlanta:De Novo, 1991
261. Ohto H, Yasuda H, Noguchi M, et al. Transfusion 1992;32:691
262. McMilan KD, Johnson RL. Transf Med Rev 1993;7:37
263. Takahashi K, Jiji T, Miyamoto M, et al. Lancet 1994;343:700
264. Combs MR, Issitt PD, Kirkland A. (abstract). Transfusion 1993;33(Suppl 9S):21S
265. Nance SJ, Garratty G. Am J Clin Pathol 1987;87:633
266. Morgan WTJ, Watkins WM. Proc 9th Congr ISBT Mexico City, Karger,Basel 1964:225
267. Russi S, Siracusano A, Vicari G. J Immunol 1974;112:1061
268. Cory HT, Yates AD, Donald ASR, et al. Biochem Biophys Res Comm 1974;61:1289
269. Marcus DM. Transfusion 1971;11:16
270. Naiki M, Fong J, Ledeen R, et al. Biochemistry 1975;14:4831
271. Haselberger CG, Schenkel-Brunner H. FEBS Lett

1982;149:126

272. Yang ZT, Bergstrom J, Karlsson K-A. J Biol Chem 1994;269:14620

273. Prieto PA, Larsen RD, Cho M, et al. J Biol Chem 1997;272:2089

274. Watkins WM, Morgan WTJ. J Immunogenet 1976;3:15

275. Naiki M, Marcus DM. Biochemistry 1975;14:4837

276. Anstee DJ, Tanner MJA. Biochem J 1974;138:381

277. Koscielak J, Miller-Podraza H, Krauze R, et al. FEBS Lett 1976;66:250

278. Bailly P, Bouhours J-F. Blood Cell Biochemistry. Volume 6. New York:Plenum 1995;299

279. Bailly P, Piller F, Gillard B, et al. Carbohydr Res

280. Costache M, Cailleau A, Fernandez-Mateos P, et al. Transf Clin Biol, in press 1997

281. Wilson R, Ainscough R, Anderson K, et al. Nature 1994;368:32

282. Mandrell RE. Infect Immun 1992;60:3017

283. Joziasse DH, Shaper NL, Kim D, et al. J Biol Chem 1992;267:5534

284. Wiels J, Taga S, Tetand C, et al. Glycoconjugate J 1996;13:529

285. Daniels GL, Anstee DJ, Cartron J-P, et al. Vox Sang 1996;71:246

1992;228:277

12 | The Rh Blood Group System

Well before the Rh system was discovered, a clinical condition called hydrops fetalis was known to exist (1). In the worst cases of this disease a severely edematous stillborn fetus was delivered. Liveborn infants with the disease frequently developed deep jaundice and kernicterus in the first few days of life and often died of the condition. Because of a wide variety of clinical symptoms in the patients it was not immediately appreciated that they resulted from a common cause. In 1921, von Gierke (2) suggested that the hydrops and kernicterus might be related. Although many of the affected infants were severely anemic they were found to have an excess of blood forming tissue and erythroblasts in the circulation. In 1932, Diamond et al. (3) correctly associated the edema, jaundice and kernicterus with hemolysis of red cells in these infants and named the condition erythroblastosis fetalis. At that time it was not known what caused the red cell hemolysis. In 1938, Darrow (4) suggested that fetal hemoglobin in the infant's red cells served as an immunogen in the mother and caused production of an antibody against it. Clearly, Darrow (4) had correctly theorized that an antigen-antibody reaction is the basis for the development of erythroblastosis fetalis (now more often called hemolytic disease of the newborn or HDN) but had not correctly identified the antigen-antibody reaction involved.

In 1939, Levine and Stetson (5) reported a fatal case of HDN and a transfusion reaction in the mother when she was given a unit of blood donated by her husband. Although an antibody was detected in the woman's serum and was believed to have caused the transfusion reaction, it was not named nor was it blamed as the cause of the HDN. The authors pointed out that the antibody reacted rather poorly and that inconsistent reactions were obtained. Further, the antibody was no longer demonstrable in the woman's serum some months after the transfusion reaction so that no definitive study could be performed. In retrospect, it can be seen that the authors were dealing with IgM anti-D that was not produced for very long. In 1939 no method existed to demonstrate the presence of IgG anti-D. Many years later a sample of serum from this lady, Mary Seno, was tested and was shown to contain potent IgG anti-D (6).

In 1940 and 1941, Landsteiner and Weiner (7,8) described the results of experiments in which they immunized guinea pigs and rabbits with red cells from rhesus monkeys. The antibody raised agglutinated the red cells of approximately 85% of random humans and was named anti-Rh. Those red cells agglutinated were said to be Rh+, those that were non-reactive were called Rh-. In 1941, Levine et al. (9) published a full report on the etiology of HDN. They correctly concluded that the severe anemia represented destruction of the infant's red cells by maternal antibody that had crossed the placenta. Moreover, in several of the cases that they studied, the antibody appeared to have the same specificity as the anti-Rh of Landsteiner and Wiener. In 1940, Wiener and Peters (10) had reported that the antibody, when present in humans, could cause hemolytic transfusion reactions. Although it now seems that the anti-Rh made in rabbits and ostensibly the same antibody made in humans, may have different specificities (the rabbit anti-Rh may have been anti-LW, see Chapter 13), there is no doubt that the combined reports of Levine and Stetson (5), Landsteiner and Wiener (7,8) and Levine et al. (9) represent the discovery of the Rh system. While it has been suggested (11-13) that a 1933 report by Buchbinder (14) may have described an Rh antibody, the paper does not describe clear differentiation between any such antibody and the species antibodies present in the animal sera studied.

The eventual realization that the rabbit anti-Rh and the human antibody, now known as anti-D, have different specificities, explained a number of early contradictory findings. For example, Fisk and Foord (15) reported that while cord blood red cells could be divided into Rh+ and Rh- using human antibodies, they all reacted with the rabbit anti-Rh. Murray and Clark (16) showed that the same anti-Rh specificity could be raised in animals using either Rh+ or Rh- red cells for the immunization. Further, these workers (16) showed that Rh- human red cells would adsorb the rabbit anti-Rh to exhaustion although they were not agglutinated by it. The explanations of these findings are described in Chapter 13.

It soon became apparent that the human anti-Rh defined one of many antigens that are part of the Rh system. The antibody was renamed anti-Rh$_0$ by one group of workers and anti-D by others. The enormous growth in knowledge about the system since then, has been accompanied by the introduction of three different terminologies to describe Rh antigens and genes and by innumerable theories that purported to explain how production of Rh antigens is controlled at the genetic level. At present, some 50 Rh antigens have been recognized. However, it is entirely possible that some of the named antigens are actually component parts of others. It is equally possible that some of the names oversimplify the situation because the same term is used to describe a group of similar, but not absolutely identical antigens.

Although full details and references to discovery of the antigens C, c, E and e are given below, it is necessary here at least to mention them in order that the following sections in this introduction can be understood. The antigens C (rh′) and E (rh″) are present most often on red cells that are D+. The antigens c (hr′) and e (hr″) are present on both D+ and D- red cells but most D- samples are C- c+ E- e+. At a practical working level, although rare exceptions are seen, C and c behave as one pair of antithetical antigens while E and e, behave as another pair.

While recent findings have provided some answers to long-held questions about the Rh system, it is necessary next to consider some historical aspects if, for no other reason, than to be able to appreciate the diversity of terms still used to describe Rh antigens and their antibodies. The early workers did not agree as to the probable nature of genetic control of Rh antigen production. Wiener and his colleagues (17-25) believed that a single gene at the *Rh* locus controls production of an agglutinogen. The agglutinogen was said to be comprised of a series of blood factors. The entire agglutinogen and each individual blood factor were believed capable of acting as immunogens. Rh antibodies were thought of as combining with one blood factor, a combination of blood factors, possibly a combination of portions of different blood factors (that by definition then became an alternative blood factor) or the whole agglutinogen. To express these concepts Wiener devised the Rh-Hr terminology. As an example, he believed that the gene *Rh⁰* encodes production of the agglutinogen Rh_o that is comprised (at least) of the blood factors Rh_o, hr′ and hr″. This theory easily accommodated later findings. For example, when it was found (26) that most bloods positive for hr″ also carry the blood factor hr^S, but that rare examples are hr″+ hr^S-, it was said that different *Rh* genes were encoding production of different agglutinogens. These, in turn, differed in the blood factors of which they were comprised. The term *Rh⁰* was retained to describe the gene that encodes production of an agglutinogen that includes hr″ and hr^S. The term *R̂h⁰* was introduced to describe the new gene that encodes production of an agglutinogen that includes hr″ but not hr^S.

While the work leading to Wiener's concepts was being done, similar discoveries were being made by Race and his colleagues (27-39). However, Fisher and Race (30,32) suggested that production of Rh antigens was controlled by three sets of alleles whose loci were so closely linked that crossing-over between them did not occur. This concept led to development of the CDE terminology to describe the genetics and serology of the system. The three loci were believed to carry the alleles *C* and *c*, *D* and *d*, and *E* and *e*, with later work demonstrating additional alleles at the loci. Many workers found the CDE terminology easier than the Rh-Hr

terms, for everyday use and it became widely applied. In spite of this, the terminology was at some difficulty in trying to accommodate later findings. To use the same example as described above, it was found that the gene complex *cDe* encodes (as its name implies) production of the antigens c, D and e. Most persons who inherit an *R⁰* gene (the shorthand name for *cDe*) have red cells that are e+ hr^S+. A few rare exceptions exist (26) in which c, D and e are not accompanied by hr^S. It then became rather awkward, using strictly *CDE* terms, to differentiate between an *R⁰* gene that encoded production of hr^S and one that did not. Over the years, the three closely linked loci model was modified to one that supposed that there were three subloci within a single genetic locus. Further, the evidence seemed to suggest that the sequence on the chromosome must be *DCE* rather than *CDE*. The term *d* became used merely to indicate the absence of *D*, no evidence for the existence of a *d* gene, or a d antigen ever emerged.

Ironically, in view of the debate they engendered, neither the one gene, nor the three gene theory proved to be totally correct. As described in detail later in this chapter, there is now direct evidence regarding the genetic control of production of the red cell membrane proteins that carry Rh antigens (40,41). In Rh+ persons, two genes, *RHD* and *RHCE* are involved. In most Rh-persons, at least in White populations and probably in others, *RHD* is deleted. Thus in Rh- persons only one gene, *RHCE*, is involved. *RHCE* is a term used to describe four common alleles, *RHCe*, *RHcE*, *RHce* and *RHCE*; most individuals with D- red cells are homozygous for *RHce*. *RHD* encodes production of a polypeptide that carries, at least, multiple epitopes of the D antigen (see below). The allele of *RHCE* present encodes production of a related polypeptide, with considerable homology to the D-bearing structure, that carries, at least, antigens of the Cc and Ee series (42). That the Rh antigens are encoded by two, not by one or three genes, was skillfully forecast by Tippett (43) well before direct evidence was available. In spite of the recent findings, information generated while the one gene and three gene theories were still in vogue, remains both viable and valuable. Indeed, for ease of communication, much of the rest of this chapter will use terms that were introduced when the previous theories prevailed.

From early studies on Rh it became apparent that the genes are inherited in sets. That is to say, a parent with C+ D+ E+ c+ e+ red cells who passes the genes making C, D and e to one child and those making c, D and E to another, is never likely to transmit a chromosome carrying genes that encode C and E or one that carries genes that encode c and e. If the most easily recognizable antigens, C, D, E, c and e are considered and if rare antigens such as C^w, C^x, E^w, etc. are excluded, it is clear that eight basic haplotypes exist with the system. These haplotypes were originally called *Rh* genes or *Rh* gene complexes but can be seen actually to be haplotypes, at least in Rh+ persons. For example what was called the *R¹* or *CDe* gene or gene complex can now be seen to be an *RHDRHCe* haplotype. Whether the term haplotype can be used when one of the two genes commonly involved is deleted (i.e. in D- persons) is debatable. Again for ease of communication, the term haplotype will be used here; that is most persons with D- C- E- c+ e+ red cells will be considered to be homozygotes for the haplotype *RHce*. Table 12-1 lists the eight most easily recognizable *Rh* haplotypes in CDE terms, indicates the shorthand symbols used in their description, lists the *RH* genes presumed to be present and the antigens made, and shows the frequency of each haplotype in three major population groups (44,45). As will be seen, table 12-1 and much of the text in this chapter, continue the tradition of using *d* to indicate the lack of a *D* gene, and d to indicate the lack of D antigen. This is done deliberately, to enhance communication although, as already mentioned, neither a *d* gene nor a d antigen exists.

By popular usage, the shorthand haplotype symbols *R¹*, *R²*, *r*, etc., have become acceptable as phenotype designations as well. The superscript numbers become lower case and regular type not italics is used. Thus, D+ C+ E- c- e+ red cells are often called R_1R_1 (they could also be R_1r'); D- C- E- c+ e+ cells are called rr, etc. Strictly speaking this convention is incorrect since *R¹*, *r*, etc. are haplotype symbols. However, for everyday use it is much easier to say (and write) R_1R_1, rr, etc., than D+ C+ E- c- e+ and D- C- E- c+ e+, etc. Traditionally, *Rh* haplotypes (and phenotypes) have been expressed in the

sequence CDE, for example *Cde*, *cde* (Cde, cde). In fact, the order on the chromosome is almost certainly DCE, for example *Dce*, *dce*. Currently the order *CDE* and *DCE* are both used and both are acceptable. Like many others, these authors write (and say) *Cde*, *(C)D(e)* etc., but *Dc-*, *D--*, *D••* etc., for the *Rh* deletion genes. No excuse other than habit is offered for this illogical application of the terminology.

By 1962, it was clear that the Rh system was far more complex than table 12-1 suggests. Twenty-five different Rh antigens had been recognized and a bewildering assortment of genes (now haplotypes) responsible for production of a few or many of those antigens was known to exist. It was apparent that use of either CDE or Rh-Hr terms sometimes made genetic implications that investigators did not wish to make. In an attempt to overcome these difficulties, Rosenfield et al. (46) introduced a new terminology. The new terms were intended to allow workers to report serological findings without necessarily including genetic interpretations. Each Rh antigen was given a number, D or Rh_o became Rh1, C or rh′ became Rh2, and so on. To illustrate one advantage of this terminology, the earlier example can be used. Since D became Rh1, c became Rh4, e became Rh5, and hr^S became Rh19, a blood typed as D+ c+ e+ hr^S+ would be described as Rh:1,4,5,19 while one typed as D+ c+ e+ hr^S- would be reported as Rh:1,4,5,-19. For workers wishing to describe haplotypes, the *R⁰* haplotype making e and hr^S would be $R^{1,4,5,19}$ while the $\hat{R}^o$ haplotype making e but not hr^S would be $R^{1,4,5,-19}$. To use the new terminology in an even simpler fashion, the haplotypes producing e and hr^S and e but not hr^S, could be described, respectively, as $R^{4,19}$ and $R^{4,-19}$. As can be seen, when an

TABLE 12-1 Eight *Rh* Haplotypes, Some of Their Products and Their Frequencies

Haplotype	Shorthand Symbol	Presumed Genes	Antigens Made	Phenotype Symbol	Frequency in		
					Whites	Blacks	Orientals
CDe	*R¹*	*RHDRHCe*	C, D and e	R_1	0.42	0.17	0.70
cDE	*R²*	*RHDRHcE*	c, D and E	R_2	0.14	0.11	0.21
cDe	*R⁰*	*RHDRHce*	c, D and e	R_0	0.04	0.44	0.03
CDE	*Rᶻ*	*RHDRHCE*	C, D and E	R_z	*1	*1	0.01
cde	*r*	*RHce*	c and e	r	0.37	0.26	0.03
Cde	*r′*	*RHCe*	C and e	r′	0.02	0.02*2	0.02
cdE	*r″*	*RHcE*	c and E	r″	0.01	*1	*1
CdE	*rʸ*	*RHCE*	C and E	rʸ	*1	*1	*1

* 1   Frequency less than 0.01
* 2   Includes *r′ˢ* (see text)
      Shorthand symbols are derived from Rh-Hr terms that are not given in full.
      Use of a capital *R* in shorthand symbols indicates presence of *D*, use of a lower case *r* indicates absence of *D*.

antigen is to be described, Rh and a number are used, e.g. Rh2. When a phenotype is to be reported, the term Rh is followed by a colon and a series of numbers, dependent on which serological tests have been performed. An unadorned number represents the presence of an antigen, a minus sign before the number indicates antigen absence, for example, Rh:1,4,5,-19. Haplotypes are written in a similar fashion. *R* indicates an *Rh* haplotype and superscript numbers indicate which antigens are and which are not made by the haplotype, e.g. $R^{1,4,5,-19}$. The new terminology was primarily intended for written communication. It was designed so that workers reporting new findings could describe not only what antigens were present on various red cell samples, but also which antisera had been used.

As mentioned above, use of the numerical terminology is also advantageous when blood samples have been typed with different antisera. As an example, listed below are the results of tests on three different samples.

Sample 1: D- C- E-
Sample 2: D- C- E- c+ e+
Sample 3: D- C- E- c+ e+ f+ G- C^G- Hr_o+ Rh:26.

To describe these three bloods in the CDE or Rh-Hr terms, the symbols rr, cde/cde, rh or rh/rh would have to used at the phenotypic level. Those terms all imply the absence of D(Rh_o), C(rh′) and E(rh″) and the presence of c(hr′) and e(hr″). With sample number 1, the absence of D, C and E has been demonstrated, the presence of c and e has not. For sample number 3, the CDE and Rh-Hr terms do not reveal that additional typings, beyond those for D, C, E, c and e, have been performed. Further, the terms cde/cde and rh/rh while describing phenotypes, both imply that two *r* or *rh* haplotypes are present in the individuals from whom the red cells were obtained. In fact, sample number one could be from an Rh_{null} individual (see later in this Chapter) while samples two and three could be from individuals with one *r* or *rh* haplotype, whose second haplotype did not make D, C, E, c or e (such as $\bar{\bar{r}}$, again see later). All these difficulties are resolved by use of the numerical terminology. The three blood samples would be described, phenotypically, as:

Sample 1: Rh:-1,-2,-3
Sample 2: Rh:-1,-2,-3,4,5
Sample 3: Rh:-1,-2,-3,4,5,6,-12,17,-21,26.

As can be seen, the exact results of serological tests are listed but no implications are made as to which *Rh* haplotypes are present to account for production of the antigens.

When the numerical terminology was introduced (46) the numbers Rh1 to Rh25 were allocated. Rh26 to Rh33 were assigned in 1972 (47), Rh34 in 1973 (48), Rh35 in 1975 (49,50), Rh36 to Rh39 in 1979 (51); Rh40 also in 1979 (52); Rh41 in 1981 (53); Rh42 in 1980 (54), Rh43 to Rh45 in 1985 (55); Rh46 to Rh48 in 1990 (56);

Rh49 in 1993 (57); Rh50 and Rh51 in 1995 (58) and Rh52 in 1996 (943). It is important to appreciate that the references given above are to the publications in which the Rh numbers were assigned, only a minority are to the papers reporting the actual discovery of the antigen. Table 12-2 gives references to the actual publications that described the discovery of the antigens (and in some instances also to the work that later showed that the antigen is part of the Rh system). As discussed in the section below that describes the ISBT terminology for Rh, two of the 52 antigens mentioned above have now been excluded from the Rh system while five others have been declared obsolete.

Another complexity of Rh that bears mention in this introductory section is that not all *Rh* haplotypes encode production of the same number of Rh antigens. As a simple example, the most common form of the R^1 (*CDe*) haplotype encodes production of (at least) D (that is itself composed of a large number of epitopes), C, e, rh_i, G, C^G, Hr_o, Hr, hr^S, Rh29, hr^B, Hr^B, Rh39, Rh41, Rh44, Rh46, Rh47 and Rh51, that is at least 18 antigens, or many more if each recognized epitope of D is considered an antigen (see below). In contrast, the *r″* (*cdE*) haplotype encodes production of E, c, Hr_o, Hr, Rh26, cE, Rh29, Hr^B, Rh39, Rh44, Rh46, Rh47 and Rh51, or 13 antigens. Of course, as mentioned briefly above and discussed in detail later in this chapter, the R^1 haplotype includes the genes *RHD* and *RHCe*, while the *r″* haplotype has only *RHcE*.

The *Rh* genes in each haplotype also control exactly how much of each antigen will be made. As discussed more fully later in this chapter, Rosenfield and his colleagues (59-65) have shown that the same *Rh* haplotype, in different members of the same family where the *Rh* haplotype on the paired chromosome causes no interference, encodes production of an exact quantity of each antigen made.

The ISBT Terminology

Since a numerical terminology for Rh already existed when the ISBT Working Party on Terminology for Red Cell Surface Antigens was formed, the terms were adopted en bloc by the working party. The Rh system (RH in ISBT terms) became system 004, the antigens were numbered 001 onwards. Thus in computer terms, D is 004001, C is 004002, and so forth to BARC which is 004052. As mentioned in earlier chapters, the ISBT terms all have shorthand equivalents. The only difference between the original numerical terminology (46) and the ISBT version (66) is that the former uses a lower case h, i.e. Rh, and the latter a capital H, i.e. RH, in the antigen designations. Several of the references cited above regarding the assignment of RH numbers are to publications from the Working Party, in which official recognition of new Rh antigens was made (55-58).

Since the Working Party requires that any antigen given a number within a system be shown to be encoded from the locus of the system, two antigens originally given Rh numbers have been excluded from the system. The antigen LW (later called LW^a, see Chapter 13) was originally called Rh25 (46). Since the *Rh* and *LW* loci are distinct (67), LW (actually LW^a) has become the first antigen of system 016, the LW system. The reason that this first antigen is called LW5 is given in Chapter 13. Somewhat similarly, the antigen Duclos (68) was seen to have a phenotypic association with Rh and was mistakenly assigned the number Rh38 (51). When evidence emerged (69) that the Duclos antigen is not encoded from the *Rh* locus, that antigen too was excluded from the system.

At the 1994 meeting, the ISBT Working Party noted that antibodies to define Rh^A (Rh13), Rh^B (Rh14), Rh^C (Rh15), Rh^D (Rh16) and E^T (Rh24) are no longer available. Accordingly the numbers for these antigens were declared obsolete. Even if new antibodies with ostensible specificities for those antigens are found, their identity with the original examples can never be proved. Once an ISBT number has been declared obsolete, it is never used again. Clearly use of a previously used number for a new and different antigen would cause confusion, Rh already has more than its share of that!

Terminology Used in the Rest of this Chapter

Having written at length on the various terminologies used for Rh, it is now incumbent on us as authors to justify the terms that we will use for the rest of this chapter. One guiding principle would seem to be, not to let logic interfere. Since the objective of this book is to communicate information we believe that the best terms to use are those that will be most familiar to readers. Thus, when CDE terms are widely used, we shall describe an antigen by its CDE name. Although one of us (70) has declared the Rh-Hr terminology officially dead, we will continue to use some Rh-Hr terms. In some cases, e.g. Hr, Hr$_o$, only numerical alternatives exist, in others, e.g. rh$_i$, the Rh-Hr term is more widely known than the CDE term Ce. When an antigen is best known by its numerical term we will use the number, choosing to use the Rosenfield et al. (46) small h over the ISBT capital H. For several of the numbered antigens the only alternative is to use the gene symbol, a practice that one of us (70) deplores. For example, a low incidence Rh antigen first seen to be encoded by the *Rh* haplotype $\bar{\bar{R}}^N$ is Rh32. It is

defined by anti-Rh32, not by anti-$\bar{\bar{R}}^N$. The folly of using the term anti-$\bar{\bar{R}}^N$ (as has been the practice in some publications) is now well illustrated by the finding that Rh32 is also present on red cells of the partial D phenotype DBT (71 and see a later section). In other words anti-$\bar{\bar{R}}^N$ (an antibody to a gene!) detects an antigen that is made by a gene that is not $\bar{\bar{R}}^N$. Even with the CDE, retained Rh-Hr and numerical terms available, alternatives are sometimes necessary. The antigens Go^a and Be^a are best known by those names. Both names were applied before the antigens were recognized as being part of the Rh system, so, naturally, do not indicate any relationship to Rh. When we use names such as Go^a, Be^a, Evans, Tar, Nou, Riv, etc., we will try, at least once to show the Rh numerical term in close proximity to the more familiar name.

The situation with the molecular genetics of Rh is a little more straightforward since most of the work in that area, described later in this chapter, has been completed since the terms *RHD* and *RHCE* (alleles *RHce*, *RHcE*, *RHce* and *RHCE*) were introduced. However, a variety of different names have been used to describe the protein structures encoded by the *Rh* genes and some related glycoproteins. Since that portion of the chapter will be many pages removed from this introductory section, the various synonyms used will be described in the section on the biochemistry of Rh.

With the numerous escape clauses in the previous paragraph in position, tables 12-2 and 12-3 can now be introduced. Table 12-2: lists the 45 Rh antigens still on active duty; gives their CDE, Rh-Hr, other and numerical names; shows their incidence in a White population; lists the year of discovery and gives references to their discovery for antigens seen immediately to be part of Rh, or to their discovery and later entry into the Rh system, in other cases. The ISBT terms are not listed, as already described the numerical terms can be converted to ISBT terms simply by changing Rh to RH. Table 12-3 lists the five antigens that were previously part of the Rh system but can no longer be recognized for lack of definitive antibodies. LW (LW^a) and Duclos are not included in table 12-3, both are alive and well and are living in other places in this book; LW (LW^a) in Chapter 13, Duclos in Chapter 31. Table 12-4 lists the most usual characteristics of antibodies that define Rh antigens.

The Rh System in Routine Work and the Immunogenicity of D

Though vastly complex, the Rh blood group system is used at its most basic level in almost every transfusion. The red cells of donors and patients are typed with anti-D. Those whose cells carry D are called Rh+, those whose cells lack the antigen are called Rh-. Later in this

TABLE 12-2 Antigens of the Rh Blood Group System

CDE	Rh-Hr	Other	Numerical	% Positive in Whites	Year Antigen Reported	References
D	Rh_o		Rh1	85	1939/40	5, 7
C	rh'		Rh2	70	1941	77
E	rh"		Rh3	30	1943	20, 28
c	hr'		Rh4	80	1941	9
e	hr"		Rh5	98	1945	78
ce or f	hr		Rh6	64	1953	79
CE			Rh22	<1	1961	80
Ce	rh_i		Rh7	70	1958	81
cE			Rh27	30	1961	82
C^w	rh^{w1}		Rh8	1	1946	83
C^x	rh^x		Rh9	<1	1954	84
E^w	rh^{w2}		Rh11	<1	1955	85
G	rh^G		Rh12	85	1958	86
C^G			Rh21	70	1961	87
V or ce^s	hr^v		Rh10	<1[*1]	1955	88
VS or e^s			Rh20	<1[*1]	1960	89
	Hr_o		Rh17	>99.9	1950	90, 91
	Hr or Hr^s		Rh18	>99.9	1960	26
	hr^s		Rh19	98	1960	26
	hr^H		Rh28	<1[*2]	1964	92
D^w			Rh23	<1	1962	93
c-like			Rh26	80	1964	94
			Rh29	>99.9	1967	95
D^{Cor}		Go^a	Rh30	<1[*2]	1958	96, 103
	hr^B		Rh31	98	1972	97
			Rh32	<1[*2]	1971	98, 99
			Rh33	<1[*3]	1971	100
	Hr^B		Rh34	>99.9	1972	97
			Rh35	<1[*3]	1971	101
		Be^a	Rh36	<1	1953	49, 102
		Evans	Rh37	<1	1968	49, 104
C-like[*4]			Rh39	>99.9	1979	51
		Tar	Rh40	<1	1975	52
Ce-like			Rh41	70	1980	53
Ce^S			Rh42	<1[*2]	1980	54
		Craw	Rh43	<1	1980	105
		Nou	Rh44	>99.9	1981	106
		Riv	Rh45	<1	1983	107
		Sec	Rh46	>99.9	1989	108
		Dav	Rh47	>99.9	1982	109, 110
		JAL	Rh48	<1	1990	111, 112
		STEM	Rh49	<1[*2]	1993	113

TABLE 12-2 Antigens of the Rh Blood Group System Continued

CDE	Rh-Hr	Other	Numerical	% Positive in Whites	Year antigen Reported	References
		FPTT	Rh50	<1	1988	114, 115
		MAR	Rh51	>99.9	1994	116
		BARC	Rh52	<1	1989	511, 943

* 1   The names ce^s and e^s may not be appropriate. V and VS are rare in Whites but are present in 20 to 25% of random Blacks.
* 2   Rare in Whites, more freqent in Blacks.
* 3   Rare but more frequent in Whites than in Blacks.
* 4   Anti-Rh39 has been found, thus far, only as an autoantibody.
    Blank spaces in terminology columns indicate that no equivalent term exists

TABLE 12-3 Former Antigens of the Rh Blood Group System

CDE	Rh-Hr	Obsolete Numerical	% Positive in Whites	Years Antigen Recognized	References
*1	Rh^A	Rh13	85	1957-1994*2	117
*1	Rh^B	Rh14	85	1959-1994*2	118
*1	Rh^C	Rh15	85	1959-1994*2	119
*1	Rh^D	Rh16	85	1959-1994*2	120
E^T		Rh24	30	1962-1994*2	121

* 1   Portions of the Rh_o mosaic. Similar but not correlated with the categories of partial D (122-124).
* 2   For obituaries see 58.
* 3   The LW (LW^a) antigen, formerly Rh25, is discussed in Chapter 13. The Duclos antigen, formerly Rh38, is discussed in Chapter 31.

TABLE 12-4 Characteristics of Some Rh System Antibodies

Antibody Specificity	Positive Reactions in In Vitro Tests				Usual Immuno-globulin		Ability to Bind Complement		Ability to Cause In Vitro Lysis		Implicated in		Usual Form of Stimulation		% of Caucasian Population Positive
	Sal	LISS	AHG	Enz	IgG	IgM	Yes	No	Yes	No	Trans-fusion Reaction	HDN	Red Cells	Other	
Anti-D		X	X	X	Most	Some		X		X	X	X	X	Rare	85
Anti-C		X	X	X	Most			X		X	X	X	X	Rare	70
Anti-E	X	X	X	X	Most	Some		X		X	X	X	X	Some	30
Anti-c		X	X	X	Most			X		X	X	X	X		80
Anti-e		X	X	X	Most			X		X	X	X	X		98
Anti-f		X	X	X	Most			X		X	X	Prob.	X		64
Anti-C^W	X	X	X	X	Most	Some		X		X	X	X	X	Some	1
Anti-G		X	X	X	Most			X		X	X	X	X		85
Anti-V		X	X	X	Most			X		X	X	X	X		<1
Anti-VS		X	X	X	Most			X		X	X	X	X		<1
Anti-Ce		X	X	X	Most			X		X	X	X	X		69
Anti-cE		X	X	X	Most			X		X	X	Prob.	X		30
Anti-CE		X	X	X	Most			X		X	X	Prob.	X		<1
Anti-Hr_o		X	X	X	Most			X		X	X	X	X		>99.9

chapter the more appropriate terms D+ and D- will replace Rh+ and Rh-. However, for this consideration of routine transfusion the more traditional terms of Rh+ and Rh- will be retained. Under ideal circumstances Rh-patients are transfused only with Rh- blood. Unlike the ABO system where major-side matching is necessary because of the virtual universal presence of alloantibodies, the use of Rh+ blood for Rh- recipients is avoided because of the very high immunogenicity of D. In other words, if an Rh- patient who has not made anti-D is transfused with Rh+ blood, it can be expected that the Rh+ red cells will survive normally. However, it can also be expected that 80% of Rh- patients transfused with one or more units of Rh+ blood will make anti-D (72-74,155,156). Since Rh+ red cells transfused to an Rh-individual survive normally if that individual has not previously been exposed to D, it may be asked why Rh+ blood is not used for the first series of transfusions and the switch to Rh- made when (and if) the recipient makes anti-D. The question is pertinent since some 85 to 87% of random donors are Rh+ and shortages of Rh-blood are not infrequent. There are three reasons to avoid the routine use of Rh+ blood for Rh- recipients. First, anti-D once made, can cause severe hemolytic disease of the newborn (HDN). Indeed, of infants requiring treatment for HDN, more than 90% are Rh+ and are born to Rh- women with anti-D in the serum (75). Further, the most severe form of HDN, that results in in utero death of the fetus, is almost always caused by anti-D (76). In cases of severe HDN and death of the fetus in utero, the anti-D is frequently accompanied by antibodies to C, E and/or G. Thus an Rh- woman immunized to D, by transfusion with Rh+ blood, is at risk of having children affected with HDN and at worst, of never being able to bear a live child. Since 85 to 87% of males are Rh+, the chances that the father of the Rh- woman's child and the child will be Rh+, are high. Second, although the first series of transfusions with Rh+ blood in an Rh- recipient can be expected to result in normal in vivo red cell survival, the chances are about 80% that Rh- blood will have to be used for subsequent transfusions. Accordingly, the use of Rh+ blood for Rh- recipients should be restricted to dire emergencies when no Rh- blood is available. Rh- patients must not be put at later risk of not being able to receive Rh+ blood, when no Rh- units are available, unless there is no alternative. Third, it is hard to be absolutely certain that an Rh- individual, with no anti-D demonstrable in the serum, has not previously been exposed to D. The use of Rh+ blood in an Rh- patient who has anti-D present in subdetectable levels, will invariably result in a delayed transfusion reaction. For example an Rh- woman who has borne Rh+ children many years before the current transfusion episodes, may have mounted a primary response

to D. Although anti-D may not be demonstrable in her serum, the transfusion of Rh+ blood may result in secondary immunization, an anamnestic response and a delayed transfusion reaction. Some classic cases of this type are described by Mollison et al. (74).

Platelet concentrates made from the blood of Rh+ donors can also stimulate the production of anti-D by Rh- recipients (125). There seems no doubt that it is the few red cells in the platelet concentrates that act as the immunogen. Although there have been claims (126,127) that platelets carry the D antigen, the preponderance of evidence (128-130) shows that this is not the case. Platelets from Rh+ donors transfused to Rh- individuals who already have anti-D, survive normally in vivo (131). Although the transfusion of platelets from Rh+ donors to Rh- patients who were receiving immunosuppressive drugs resulted in no cases of immunization to D in one series (132), other patients who made anti-D in spite of the immunosuppression have been described (133). Accordingly, when an Rh- female who may later bear children is transfused with platelets from an Rh+ donor, the use of Rh immune globulin (RhIG) to prevent immunization should be considered. Some physicians are reluctant to use intramuscular injections of RhIG in thrombocytopenic patients because of the risk that bleeding in to the tissues will occur. Clearly, when RhIG is to be used in this setting the product suitable for intravenous injection is preferable. For many years this presented a problem in the USA since no RhIG for intravenous injection was available. Happily this problem has now been resolved and the Canadian-made RhIG for intravenous use (134,473,474) is available.

Platelet concentrates that do not appear pink carry very few red cells, i.e. probably less than 0.5 ml, estimated average 0.37 (125). Nevertheless, repeated transfusions of platelets from Rh+ donors to Rh- patients who are not immunosuppressed results in a high rate of immunization to D. At Duke University Medical Center one of the major regimens for treating breast cancer is to collect bone marrow from the patient, attempt to kill the tumor by high dose chemotherapy or radiation, then reconstitute the patient's hematopoietic system via autologous bone marrow transplantaton. During the recovery period following marrow ablation, supportive transfusions are required. In part because of the supply and demand situation and in part because many of these patients require HLA-matched platelets, it is impossible to avoid giving platelets from Rh+ donors to Rh- patients. Immunization to D by the red cells in the platelet products is impressive; close to 100% of Rh- women treated in this manner make anti-D. Although production of anti-D by Rh- women who have delivered Rh+ infants can now be almost totally prevented (see Chapter 41), anti-D is still, by far, the most common antibody outside the ABO system, seen in our transfusion service. No attempts are made on a routine basis to prevent formation of anti-D in these patients, by the use of RhIG. Clearly because of the clinical condition being treated, the majority of patients are beyond child bearing age.

In terms of plasma transfusions, liquid plasma from Rh+ donors (that probably contained a few intact red cells) has been reported (135,136) to cause both primary immunization to D and a secondary response in an already immunized patient. Fresh frozen plasma does not seem to have been incriminated as a cause of primary immunization to D, but may rarely provoke a secondary response (135,137). There is one rather old note (138) that suggests that cryoprecipitate may contain enough material derived from D, to stimulate production of anti-D in an Rh- hemophiliac. If this occurs at all, it must be a very rare event.

One practical implication of the presence of enough red cell stroma in plasma derived from Rh+ donors to stimulate a secondary immune response to D, involves the use of plasma exchange to attempt to reduce the level of anti-D in pregnant women (137,139-146). First, in such procedures, plasma containing normal levels of IgG must be used as the replacement fluid. If a product (such as albumin) lacking IgG is used there will be a rebound effect in which rapid IgG synthesis (to bring the level in circulation back to normal) will occur in the patient and a large amount of anti-D will be included in the IgG made. Second, because the aim of the procedure is to reduce the level of circulating anti-D, plasma from Rh- donors should be used as the replacement fluid. If plasma from Rh+ donors is used, secondary immunization by the D-bearing stroma in the plasma may occur and the level of anti-D being made may increase rather than decline. Third, there is evidence from animal studies (147) that even when normal IgG levels are maintained in a plasma exchange, a rebound in antibody production may occur that will result in antibody being present in higher levels some days after the exchange than was the case before the procedure.

Although it appears logical to try to reduce the level of anti-D by plasma exchange, in a woman who has a history of severely affected infants and who is pregnant with an Rh+ fetus, the procedure is not one to be undertaken lightly. First, it may be necessary to replace large volumes of plasma at each procedure. Second, many plasma exchanges may be necessary, for example two or three times a week from fairly early in the pregnancy until the child is delivered. Third, the procedure is not always successful in terms of salvage of the fetus. Fourth, there has been at least one death of a pregnant woman perhaps caused by the repeated plasma exchange procedure. Bowman (148,149) has suggested that the treatment method should be reserved for women with a previous history of hydrops developing before 24 to 26 weeks of gestation and in whom the fetus is known to be D+. The intensive plasma exchange described above should then be started at 10 to 12 weeks gestation.

Because this section deals with immunization to D in situations involving the transfusion of red cells, platelets and plasma, other treatments and practices that result in anti-D being made are described in a later section. Immunization to D associated with pregnancy and the prevention of such immunization are discussed in Chapter 41.

Having discussed at length the contraindications for the use of Rh+ blood for Rh- patients, it will now be added that in certain circumstances the use of such blood is justified. When Rh- donor blood is not available, Rh+ blood will survive normally in an Rh- patient who has not already made anti-D. Thus, a non-immunized Rh- patient can be given Rh+ blood in a life-saving emergency situation. When Rh- blood is in short supply and a non-immunized (to D) Rh- patient requiring massive transfusion is encountered, it is better to begin such transfusions with Rh+ blood, than exhaust the supply of Rh- units and then switch to Rh+ blood. Much of the blood transfused during the situation that necessitated massive transfusion is likely to be lost by hemorrhage. If the patient did not already have anti-D, there is little point in switching to Rh- blood once the bleeding slows or is stopped. It is probable that the patient will make anti-D, such immunization is not likely to be prevented by the use of Rh- blood near the end of the emergency, nor is it likely that the patient will make anti-D quickly enough to have a delayed transfusion reaction. Somewhat similarly when Rh- blood is in short supply and an Rh- patient with anti-D is likely to require massive transfusion (i.e. replacing or approaching replacement of the patient's blood volume in a 24 hour period), it may be best to begin the transfusions with Rh+ blood. Again, much of the blood transfused initially will likely be lost by hemorrhage. However, this time there may be considerable advantage in finishing the transfusions (say the last six units transfused) with Rh- blood. By leaving the patient with primarily Rh- blood in circulation, at the end of the emergency, the degree of anemia caused by red cell destruction of the Rh+ blood (the patient already had anti-D) will be lessened.

When Rh- blood is in extremely short supply, Rh+ blood should be given to selected Rh- patients who do not have anti-D, in order that the Rh- units in hand are available for use in parous women, young girls and Rh- patients who have already made anti-D and are not candidates for massive transfusion. Those Rh- patients who will deliberately be given Rh+ blood can be selected on a rational basis. Obviously, the best choices are older males in whom it can be forecast that only one series of transfusions is likely. Equally obvious, any patient who will require a series of transfusions (such as those who experience repeated G-I hemorrhages, those with sickle cell disease, etc.) should not be immunized to D because of the already described possibility that urgent transfusions may later be required, when Rh- blood is not available. When Rh+ blood must be transfused to an Rh- patient, it is safer to select a male than a female beyond menopause. As discussed above, earlier pregnancies may have resulted in an Rh- woman being immunized to D and thus a prime candidate for a delayed transfusion reaction. The fact that older Rh-males who are likely to require only one series of transfusions can be given Rh+ blood with relative impunity, should not be used as an excuse to avoid strenuous attempts to obtain Rh- blood for their transfusions. For reasons already discussed, the decision to use Rh+ blood for an Rh- recipient is one that should never be made lightly.

Unlike the situation in which Rh+ blood must not routinely be given to an Rh- patient, there are no contraindications for the use of Rh- blood in non-immunized Rh+ patients. Regrettably there are still physicians who refuse to use Rh- blood unless the patient is Rh-. There is no scientific reason for such a refusal. While Rh- donor units are invariably c+ and e+, so are the majority of Rh+ units. Thus, Rh- blood is no more likely to stimulate the production of anti-c or anti-e than is Rh+ blood. In any case, as discussed later in this chapter, c and e are relatively poor immunogens and there is no need to match patient and donor for c or e (or C or E).

At one time it was felt that in order for blood to be considered Rh-, the red cells must be shown to be D- C- and E- with the test for D including sufficient sensitivity or an additional step that would detect weak D (formerly the D^u phenotype, see below). For reasons discussed in detail below, there is no justification for calling C+ D- or D- E+ donor blood anything other than Rh-. In the USA, negative tests for D and weak D qualify a unit of blood as Rh-.

While the division of a population into approximately 85% Rh+ and 15% Rh- is the norm in most parts of the USA and Europe, that is not the case throughout the world. For example, the frequency of *rr* in the Chinese is in the order of 1 in 1000 (44,150-152). It is strange for American and European blood bankers to have to think of the Rh- phenotype as being more unusual in some countries than, say the K+ k-, phenotype in their own. In Polynesians the *r* haplotype is apparently absent but some D- bloods are found since *r'*

exists in that population (44,153,154).

The Immunogenicity of D as it Relates to the Volume of Immunogen Introduced

As already mentioned, the D antigen is highly immunogenic in D- individuals and is the only Rh antigen for which the donor and patient need routinely be matched. Exceptions include those patients already immunized to one of the other Rh antigens and, in the opinion of some, patients such as those with sickle cell disease (SSD), who will receive multiple transfusions. Matching in SSD to prevent alloimmunization is sometimes done to prevent concomitant autoantibody production, that may have far more serious consequences than the alloimmunization (for a more complete discussion see Chapter 35). As mentioned earlier, among D-subjects transfused with one or more units of D+ blood, some 80% can be expected to make anti-D (72-74,155,156). When the amount of D+ blood introduced is smaller, the rate of immunization drops only slightly. Pollack (157) reported that 50% of D- individuals injected with 25ml of D+ red cells made anti-D. Davey et al. (158) found anti-D in 33% of D- recipients of 40ml of D+ red cells. When the immunizing dose is much smaller, a fair number of D- people still make anti-D. Mollison et al. (159) found anti-D in 15% of D- persons injected with 1ml of D+ red cells. Before the introduction of Rh immune globulin, a number of D- women who carried fetuses with D+ red cells became immunized to D when fetal red cells entered the maternal circulation. Usually, during the first D+ pregnancy, too few D+ red cells enter the maternal circulation for a primary response to D to occur. However, at the time of delivery, a larger amount of fetal cells is introduced so that a primary response to D may be initiated. Then, often in the second D+ pregnancy, the small amount of fetal cells that enter the maternal circulation is sufficient to serve as a secondary immunizing dose and serologically detectable anti-D is made. By pooling the numbers from several series (160-164) it can be seen that in D- women not treated with Rh immune globulin, between 15 and 22% eventually make anti-D. At first it seems that this figure may be lower than would be expected. In several series (165-168) repeated injections of small amounts (sometimes at little as 0.1ml per injection) of D+ red cells were given to D- volunteers. In most instances it was shown that this means of stimulating anti-D was as effective as the transfusion of a whole unit of Rh+ blood, namely close to 70% of the volunteers eventually made anti-D. Similarly, as described above, the very small amounts of D+ red cells in platelet concentrates are highly efficient in provoking production of anti-D in non-immunosuppressed D- patients. However, Mollison (169) calculated that, based on: the percentage of D-women who marry D+ men; the likelihood of each woman bearing two or more D+ children; and variation in size of fetal-maternal hemorrhages; the observed immunization rate was very close to what would be expected from the results of studies on the rate of immunization to D by deliberate (injection) means.

In both deliberate immunization experiments and in pregnancy, it has been noted by several workers (165,167,170,171) that individuals who form anti-D following few exposures to D+ cells (such as two small injections or following one D+ pregnancy) are the ones most likely to go on and make very potent antibodies. It has also been shown (172-177) that the ABO group of the fetus and mother affect the likelihood that anti-D will be made. In women who deliver infants with red cells that are ABO incompatible, D+ fetal red cells are cleared immediately they enter the maternal circulation, by the maternal ABO antibodies and thus provide a single immunizing dose. When the D+ fetal red cells are ABO compatible, they presumably circulate normally in the mother and probably provide a whole series of small immunizing doses as they are cleared at the end of their normal life-span. Vos (178) has suggested that the major difference related to ABO incompatibility does not involve the production or non-production of anti-D but that it does influence how soon and how much anti-D will be made.

In spite of the high immunogenicity of D, there are a number of D- individuals who do not make anti-D even after repeated exposures to the D antigen. The available evidence (summarized in Chapter 2 where responders and non-responders are described) suggests that some 8 to 10% of D- individuals are non-responders, that is they are unable to make anti-D. Also discussed in Chapter 2 and 41 are prevention of immunization to D by the use of Rh immune globulin and possible augmentation of the immune response to D. It will be mentioned here that the claims (179,476,477) that the immune response to D can be prevented or partially down regulated by oral administration of a preparation made from D+ red cells (i.e. a purported tolerizing dose of antigen) could not be confirmed by others (180-182) and are not generally accepted as true.

Other Situations Resulting in Immunization to D

As would be expected from the above descriptions of immune responses to D following the injection of very small quantities of red cells, anti-D production has also been seen in a number of situations in which red cells were introduced other than via transfusion. Both renal transplantation (135,183) and bone grafts (184,185) have been associated with production of anti-D in D- persons although attempts were made to remove red cells from the kidney and the bone grafts before they were transplanted or grafted. The reverse, that is production of anti-D by B cells carried in the transplant, is even more common (186-192). In one highly unusual case (186) transient anti-D production was seen in two D+ recipients of kidneys from the same immunized (to D) D- donor.

In the past, relatively small volumes of blood from one person, were injected into others in a practice known as heterohemotherapy (it was believed that immunity to disease could be passively transferred). Not surprisingly, cases of immunization to D and later, HDN, followed this practice (193,194). It might be expected that this type of immunization would no longer be seen since, for very good reasons, heterohemotherapy is no longer practiced by enlightened workers. Unfortunately, other similar forms have taken its place. There are documented cases (195-199) in which the use of syringes that have become contaminated with blood, for the injection of illegal drugs; "blood brotherhood" rituals; and the exchange of blood for "emotional gratification" purposes, have resulted in immunization to D and subsequently in HDN. During his term as Associate Editor for Correspondence for *Transfusion*, one of us received a number of submissions describing the production of anti-D in drug addicts who shared syringes that became contaminated with blood. Although, for the most part these letters were not accepted for publication, since they added nothing new to knowledge about the unfortunate practice that was already documented, they do serve to suggest that the event may be more common than is generally assumed.

HLA Antigens and The Immune Response to D

As discussed in Chapter 2, HLA antigens are intimately involved in antigen recognition and initiation of the immune response. Several groups of investigators have studied D- individuals who have formed anti-D, in search of an association between HLA and immune responsiveness to D. Murray et al. (925) reported an increased frequency of HLA-A3 in women immunized by pregnancy; Darke (926) described similar findings in women immunized by pregnancy but found no such association in males who made anti-D after deliberate exposure to D+ red cells. Differently, Brain and Hammond (927) reported an increased frequency of HLA-A1 in women immunized by pregnancy. In a later study, Darke et al. (928) described an increase of HLA-

DRw6 in the immunized males, but not in the females. Wojtulewicz-Kurkus et al. (929) also reported an increase of HLA-DRw6 in males immunized by transfusion while Raum et al. (940) suggested that immune responsiveness to D might be associated with HLA class III alleles. In contrast to the above findings, Hors et al. (930) and Petranyi et al. (931) studied a large number of deliberately immunized males while van Rood et al. (932) and Kruskall et al. (933) studied women immunized by pregnancy, without finding any association between HLA and the immune response to D. Of note in these studies that showed lack of any association, Petranyi et al. (931) studied high responders to D, while Kruskall et al. (33) typed their subjects for extended HLA haplotypes and linked markers (HLA-A, HLA-B, HLA-DR, and the complement components BF, C2, C4A and C4B). In a thoughtful discussion in their paper, Kruskall et al. (933) suggested ways in which studies of this type, particularly when limited numbers of subjects are available for study, can appear to indicate associations that do not actually exist. Support for their suggestion that type 1 statistical artifacts may have suggested associations was provided by Young et al. (941) who showed that immunoglobulin allotype frequencies were the same in individuals who had made anti-D, those known to be non-responders to D and the general population. Most recently, Hildén et al. (934) have described an excess of the *HLA-DQB1* allele among women producing the highest levels of anti-D. The study was, perforce, small, 13 of the women included had anti-D with a titer of 512 or higher. Clearly, in view of the other data cited in this section, additional studies will be required particularly since the authors (934) suggest that the presence of *HLA-DQB1* in a woman in whom anti-D is detected early in the pregnancy, might forecast severe HDN. Much of the work done in a search for an association between HLA and immune responsiveness to D, has focused on individuals who have made anti-D. Kruskall et al. (933) suggested that more information might be obtained by studying known non-responders to D. That is, D- individuals who have not made anti-D in spite of multiple exposures to the D antigen. Given the extreme polymorphism of HLA and the fact that 80% of D- individuals make anti-D if transfused with one unit of D+ blood, it seems that most HLA genotypes must allow recognition of D as foreign, in D- persons. Thirty-two non-responders were included in the study of Young et al. (941) that showed that immunoglobulin allotypes are no different in responders and non-responders to D.

What Makes D so Highly Immunogenic?

The question that heads this section has intrigued

blood group serologists for years. As documented above, 80% of D- persons transfused with one or more units of D+ blood, make anti-D. Some 20% of D- women who deliver D+ infants and are not protected with Rh immune globulin, make anti-D. In contrast, if the combined effects of transfusion and pregnancy are considered for all other Rh and non-Rh antigens (i.e. those of the Kell, Duffy, Kidd, etc., systems), the immunization rate probably does not exceed 3 to 5%. The high immunogenicity of D is now at least partially understood. As described in detail in later sections of the chapter, the *RH* genes encode production of non-glycosylated, fatty acid acylated polypeptides that are incorporated in to the red cell membrane. In 1991, Colin et al. (40) showed that in D+ persons two genes, *RHD* and *RHCE* encode products. In the overwhelming majority of White D- persons, *RHD* is deleted. *RHCE* is the name used for the gene whose alleles include *RHce*, *RHcE*, *RHce* and *RHCE*. Most persons with D- red cells are homozygous for *RHce*; those whose red cells lack D but carry C or E or both, have *RHCe*, *RHcE* and *RHCE*, respectively. The polypeptides encoded by the alleles of *RHCE* display very considerable homology. The polypeptide that carries C may differ from the one that carries c by four amino acids on the 416 amino acid protein (41). However, only one of those differences may be critical for the difference between C and c (202,203). The polypeptide that carries E differs from the one that carries e by a single amino acid change (41). In contrast, the polypeptide encoded by *RHD* differs from that encoded by *RHcE* by 36 amino acids (40,41,204-207). Thus when persons with C+ c- and C- c+ red cells are transfused with c+ and C+ red cells, respectively, the immune system of the recipient "sees" an Rh protein that differs from the host protein by only a few, or one, amino acids. When individuals with E+ e- and E- e+ red cells are exposed to e+ and E+ red cells, respectively, the immune system of the recipient "sees" an Rh protein that differs from the host protein by only a single amino acid. In marked contrast, when a person with D- red cells is exposed to D+ cells, the immune system of the recipient "sees" a protein for which there is no host counterpart (*RHD* deleted, no product made) and which differs by at least 36 amino acids from the nearest equivalent (the *RHce* encoded protein) of the recipient. Thus the immune response in D- persons, who are perhaps best described as D_{null}, becomes easier to understand. One worrying point about this concept is that antigens such as C, c, E, e, C^W and C^X involve changes of amino acids forecast (41,208) to be exofacial. Of the 36 amino acids in the D polypeptide that differ from those in the cE protein, only 9 or 10 are forecast to be exofacial (40,41,204-207). The difficulty of trying to reconcile this finding with the multiple epitopes of D already recognized (209-218) is discussed again in the section below on the partial D phenotypes.

Monoclonal Anti-D

The use of anti-D is clearly of very great importance in transfusion medicine. First, it is used as a routine reagent to type the red cells of patients and blood donors. Second, it is injected in a purified form (Rh immune globulin or RhIG) in D- women both during pregnancy and following delivery to prevent immunization to D. Thus great excitement was generated by the 1975 report of Köhler and Milstein (200) that described a method for the in vitro synthesis of monoclonal antibodies (MAb). It was hoped that high quality anti-D typing reagents could be made and that the shortage of raw material (human anti-D) used in the production of RhIG would be alleviated. The first of these goals has been achieved and monoclonal antibody-based anti-D typing reagents are already in widespread use. Considerable progress has also been made in testing MAb to D for their ability to clear D+ red cells in vivo, as a step towards using them in the production of RhIG.

In the original method for the production of MAb, spleen cells from immunized mice were fused with mouse myeloma cells. The lymphocytes from the spleens of the immunized animals provided instructions regarding antibody specificity, the myeloma cells synthesized the immunoglobulins. Unfortunately the mouse appears incapable of responding to D and no MAb to D was ever made by this method. In the early 1980s, a series of reports appeared describing the transformation of human antibody-producing lymphocytes with Epstein Barr virus (EBV). The EBV-transformed lymphoblastoid cells were then grown in tissue culture where they secreted antibody. By using lymphocytes from individuals already making anti-D, it became possible to produce both IgG and IgM MAb to D (219-222). Initially, some of the clones of antibody-producing cells were short lived (223) but the problem was overcome (221,224,225) and subsequently, numerous clones, many of which involved the fusion of EBV transformed lymphocytes with mouse myeloma cells to form heterohybridomas, making MAb to D have been produced. It has been reported (221,226) that the use of lymphocytes from immunized donors who have recently received booster doses of D+ red cells is most likely to lead to successful production of monoclonal anti-D. At least one IgA monoclonal anti-D has been made (227). In addition to the nine publications cited above, many others (228-242, 1069) have appeared and have described either new MAb to D or have presented the results of additional studies on those previously reported.

Like other MAb, those directed against D define a single epitope of the antigen. As discussed in detail in the section below on partial D, the D antigen is composed of multiple epitopes. Thus while the single epitope specificity of MAb to D is of tremendous advantage in work on partial D, it can be a liability in the use of these antibodies for routine typing. Most D+ red cells carry all the epitopes of D so react with all monoclonal anti-D. However, red cells with partial D lack one or more of the epitopes (again see below) so will fail to react with those MAb directed against the epitope(s) they lack. Early examples of monoclonal anti-D were seen often to fail to react with red cells of partial D, categories IV and/or VI. While the failure of a MAb typing reagent to react with the partial D antigen on a patient's red cells would be of no great moment (the patient would be transfused with D- red cells) it has the potential to be much more serious if it types the red cells of a donor as D-, when in fact those red cells carry some D antigen. To circumvent this problem different approaches were used. Some manufacturers blended monoclonal anti-D with human polyclonal antibody and required that if the direct agglutination test for D was negative, the test be converted to an indirect antiglobulin stage in which the reaction of the human polyclonal anti-D with weak D and/or category IV or VI red cells would be seen. Other manufacturers made blends of more than one MAb to D, as they became available, having shown that, between them, the constituents of the blend were capable of detecting all forms of weak and/or partial D. Now that more MAb to D are available, this latter approach has become the one of choice for most manufacturers.

When initial attempts to make MAb-based anti-D typing reagents were undertaken there were relatively few MAb available that reacted with category VI red cells. One suggestion was that two different anti-D reagents, one for use in typing donors and the other for use in typing patients, be made. The one for typing donors would be one selected because it reacted with category VI red cells. This because it is believed that such cells can provoke production of anti-D if transfused to a D- individual. The reagent for use in typing patients' samples would be formulated to be non-reactive with category VI red cells. Since persons with red cells of that category can form alloimmune anti-D against the epitopes of D that their red cells lack, it was argued that these patients would be best served by being typed as D- and then transfused with D- blood or given RhIG after a D+ pregnancy. While having some merit, this proposal was not very practical. First, it would result in rare individuals being called D+ as blood donors and D- as patients. The problems that the D^u phenotype has caused for so long would be reinvented! Second, the use of two different anti-D typing reagents would surely cause problems; the wrong one might be used or less well informed blood bankers might well refuse to purchase an anti-D deliberately formulated to miss one form of D+. It was even pointed out (201) that, theoretically at least, a patient donating blood for later autologous use might have the units typed as D+ then be told that the autologous units could not be given since they were the wrong Rh type, when the donor was typed as D- as a patient. Fortunately this idea was never put into practice, instead as more MAb to D became available, blends, often containing both IgM and IgG anti-D, that recognize all forms of partial D, were formulated as typing reagents.

Use of MAb-based anti-D typing reagents has created another problem similar to that involving partial D, category VI. The haplotype R^{oHar} (see later in this chapter for more details) encodes a form of D that is difficult to detect with most human polyclonal anti-D (100,243). When such reagents were the only ones available, individuals with R^{oHar} whose second haplotype did not encode D, were often typed as D- (244). They were transfused with D- blood and those who delivered D+ infants were protected with RhIG. Usually this was done without any knowledge that any form of D was present on the patient's red cells. As donors, $R^{oHar}r$ individuals were often called D-, (244) again because the weak D on their red cells went undetected. Many MAb to D react with the red cells of individuals genetically $R^{oHar}r$ as if a normal D is present (245). Thus now, these persons are called D+, are transfused with D+ blood and are not protected with RhIG. This, because the typing with MAb-based anti-D gives no indication that the D on their red cells is unusual. Unfortunately, $R^{oHar}r$ individuals can and do make anti-D (246,247) because their D is of the partial type (71,241,248). In terms of donors, no advantage is gained by recognition of the D on the red cells. As far as is known, no unit from an R^{oHar} donor has provoked production of anti-D in a D- recipient. It is difficult to imagine how this problem might be resolved. The use of two different anti-D typing reagents has already been decried in the section above. Presumably, individuals genetically $R^{oHar}r$ will now fall in to the same group as persons with partial D whose red cells typed as unremarkable D+, when human polyclonal anti-D were used to D type red cells.

As mentioned at the start of this section, the use of MAb to D in production of RhIG would alleviate the situation in which it becomes increasingly more difficult to obtain sufficient raw material to make the product. The more successful the program to prevent immunization to D by pregnancy, the fewer the source donors of human anti-D available. Considerable progress has been made (239,249-253) in studying the subclass composition of different monoclonal anti-D and their ability to bind to red cells and to mediate the effector functions of macrophages and monocytes, in in vitro models. Further

some in vivo studies have been completed (254,255) that demonstrated first, that three MAb to D cleared D+ red cells in vivo, while one other was shown to have a normal in vivo half life when injected in to D- volunteers. As far as we are aware, monoclonal anti-D has not yet been used to prevent immunization to D during or following pregnancy although it has been shown to be efficient in that respect in D- volunteers injected with D+ red cells (475). Perhaps by the time this book is published Rh immune globulin will, like most anti-D typing reagents now available, be monoclonal antibody-based.

Weak D (Formerly the D^u Phenotype)

In 1946, Stratton (256) described red cells that reacted with anti-D in what, at that time, was an atypical manner. Although it was at first thought that the red cells involved carried a new Rh antigen, it rapidly became apparent (36,257-260) that the antigen present was actually D, in a weakened form. Thus the term D^u, that Stratton (256) introduced, was seen to describe a phenotype, not an antigen. According to the original definition, red cells of the D^u phenotype fail to react in direct agglutination tests with IgM anti-D, but do react with IgG anti-D either in albumin enhanced tests (high grade D^u) or only by indirect antiglobulin test (low grade D^u). The original definition cannot be applied to the way D typing tests are now performed. First, the slide and rapid tube anti-D reagents that have been in use for many years, cause direct agglutination of red cells that would previously have been called high grade D^u. Second, many of the monoclonal antibody-based anti-D reagents described in the previous section, are formulated so that they will agglutinate most samples that would previously have been described as D^u of any type.

Over the years, it has become appreciated that the difference between the D+ and D^u phenotypes is quantitative, not qualitative. Accordingly, for the remainder of this section, red cells previously said to be of the D^u phenotype will be described by the more informative term (261-264) as having weak D. Studies (265,266) with both polyclonal and monoclonal anti-D have shown that D+ red cells of the R_1r and R_2R_2 phenotypes carry approximately 10,000 and 30,000 available D antigen sites per red cell, respectively. In contrast, on weak D red cells, the measured number of D antigen sites varied from 300 to 9000 per red cell (267-269). Presumably the finding that some weak D red cells carried 9000 D sites, i.e. the same or close to the number on some R_1r red cells, represented orientation of D on those red cells and/or epitope specificity of the anti-D used and/or differences in the method from that used to count D sites on R_1r red cells.

It is now appreciated that there are three major ways by which the weak D phenotype can arise. In some individuals, *RHC* on one chromosome affects the expression of *RHD* on the other, so that the weak D phenotype results (270,271). This *trans* position effect whereby a gene on one chromosome affects the expression of a gene on the paired autosome is discussed again later in this chapter. It should not be assumed that the *trans* position effect of *RHC* or *RHD* is inviolate. Some red cells from individuals genetically *r'R^o* (or *r'R^1*, etc.) have weak D, those of others with apparently the same genotype, express D normally. A second form of weak D (sometimes serologically indistinguishable from the first) represents the absence of some epitopes of D. This situation is discussed more fully below in the section describing partial D. However, it should not be assumed that the absence of one or more epitopes of D always results in the weak D phenotype. Indeed, the majority of red cells of the partial D phenotypes react with anti-D in a manner akin to red cells with all epitopes of D present (122-124). The least frequent type of weak D represents the inheritance of a gene, not influenced by its partner on the paired autosome, that encodes production of all epitopes of D but in less quantity than are present on D+ red cells.

Thus a working definition for the weak D phenotype that covers all three types but does not differentiate between them, is that the red cells involved react only weakly or fail to react at all in a routine D-typing test, but give a clearly positive reaction with anti-D when a more sensitive than usual method is used. The more sensitive method may be an IAT, a test with enzyme modified red cells, or any other test in which the antigen-antibody reaction is enhanced. However, to that working definition the caveat must be added that, such is the excellence of currently available anti-D typing reagents, the more sensitive method is now seldom needed to detect weak D. Red cells of the weak D phenotype always adsorb anti-D and yield that antibody on elution, there is no such specificity as anti-D^u.

Soon after its discovery, it was reported (260,272,273) that blood of the weak D phenotype (at that time called D^u) could provoke production of anti-D if transfused to a D- recipient. For this reason, most workers elected to use blood from donors with weak D as D+. Later, it was found that some recipients with weak D on their red cells could form anti-D if transfused with D+ blood (274-276). Thus the weak D phenotype came to be regarded as D- in patients, the opposite to what it was called in blood donors. The storm of confusion created has not yet subsided.

It is now appreciated that production of anti-D by persons with weak D on their red cells, who are transfused with D+ blood, is a very rare event. First, individu-

als with the *trans* position type of weak D cannot form alloimmune anti-D since their red cells carry all the epitopes of D. Second, the epitopes of D may be less immunogenic in persons with partial D than is D in D-individuals. Third, some red cells with weak D lack the Rh antigen G (see later) and there is doubt that partial D, G- blood has ever provoked production of anti-D (169). For these reasons, some workers now elect to type all patients for D and weak D (a test often incorrectly called the D^u test) and transfuse those with any representation of D on their red cells, with D+ blood. The rationale for this procedure was that it preserves the supply of D- blood by avoiding its use in patients with weak D on the red cells. While this is a laudable aim its execution may not be cost effective. Our experience has been that such is the excellence of currently available anti-D typing reagents that persons with weak D on the red cells are almost always recognized as D+ in the initial typing tests. Those whose red cells type as D- in initial tests, then are shown to have weak D by use of IAT with anti-D, are so few that routine searches for them are not justified.

As far as blood donors are concerned, virtually all workers agree that absence of weak D must be demonstrated before the donor blood is called D-. However, this may not indicate a need for an IAT with anti-D on red cells initially typing as D-. Many of the automated donor typing systems and many in which manual tests are still used, will detect weak D in the initial tests for D. It has been suggested (277) that absence of D as indicated by a direct test with potent currently available anti-D reagents used in a sensitive system, correlates with inability of the donor red cells to initiate primary immunization to D, in a D- recipient.

The controversy about weak D and whether patients and donors of that phenotype should be regarded as D-and D+, respectively, continues. A large prospective study would certainly be of value but it seems unlikely that such a study will ever be performed. It is not known how many patients with weak D make anti-D when given D+ blood. Better data are available about the immunogenicity of weak D in D- recipients. Schmidt et al. (278) transfused a total of 68 weak D units to 45 D- recipients none of whom made anti-D. The study has been criticized because 15 of the 45 recipients were receiving immunosuppressive drugs. However, it follows that if weak D was as immunogenic as D, 24 of the 30 (i.e. 80%) of the non-immunosuppressed patients would have been expected to make anti-D. As stated, none did. Another criticism of the study has been that insufficient follow-up was conducted to determine the true response to D. However, the paper (278) describes the production of anti-E by one recipient and anti-K by another. Given the low immunogenicity of E and K, compared to D, these findings certainly appear to indicate that sufficient follow-up was performed. Even if a large study showed that weak D blood only rarely causes production of anti-D, it is probable that some workers would continue to regard weak D donors as D+. Transfusion-induced anti-D, in a woman who later delivers a D+ child, constitutes enough evidence against the policy of regarding weak D donors as D- for some workers to remain loath to adopt the policy at all. While it is relatively easy to formulate a policy about blood donors with weak D on their red cells, it should be remembered that patients with D+ red cells, who lack one or more epitopes of D from their red cells and can form alloimmune anti-D, cannot be similarly recognized. As mentioned briefly above and as discussed in more detail in a later section on partial D, such individuals do not often present with weak D on their red cells. Indeed, the majority of them have red cells that give unremarkable positive reactions in typing tests with anti-D and their partial D status is recognized only when they present with alloimmune anti-D in the serum.

Workers who perform tests for the weak D phenotype will be well aware that on infrequent occasions interpretation of the result can be difficult. Much of the time the weak D phenotype is easy to recognize since the red cells give obvious positive reactions, i.e. 2+ to 4+, when typed with anti-D by IAT. However, occasional samples are found that react very weakly, i.e. 1+ or less in these tests. In the past, some of these reactions represented the presence of contaminating antibodies, such as anti-Bg (279,280) or other antibodies to low incidence antigens (281,282) in the anti-D. Adsorption-elution experiments with anti-D often, but not always (280) resolved the problem. It can be expected that problems created by unrecognized contaminating antibodies in the anti-D typing reagents will not occur when MAb-based reagents are used.

In summarizing this long section on weak D and the problems created in routine transfusion therapy it can be said that, at least in the opinion of these authors, tests with currently available anti-D typing reagents identify those donor units that carry sufficient D to be immunogenic in D- recipients, as D+. Others (283-288,348) apparently agree. It is noteworthy that when asked to write a commentary defending the test for weak D, the sole author (289) remarked to one of us (290) that she wished she had been allowed to include a statement to the effect that the views expressed were not necessarily those of the author. In short, if the red cells react visibly with anti-D, they are D+ (291), if they do not, they are D-. Since we believe that D- equates with Rh- (see section below on the use of r' and r'' blood) we do not agree with statements (292) that tests on donor blood beyond D (with sufficient sensitivity to detect weak D) are necessary.

The Phenotype D$_{el}$

As shown in table 12-1, the D- phenotype is rare in Oriental persons. Further, among those individuals with red cells that initially appear to be D-, some have a very weak form of the D antigen. Okubo et al. (293) showed that as many as 10% of samples from Japanese donors that were non-reactive in typing tests with anti-D, would adsorb anti-D and yield that antibody on elution. The phenotype was called D$_{el}$ and in a limited study it was shown that no individuals who had formed anti-D were of the D$_{el}$ phenotype. Ogasawara et al. (294) showed, in in vitro studies, that when D$_{el}$ red cells are coated with anti-D they are not phagocytosed by monocytes. Mak et al. (295) tested 172,222 Hong Kong Chinese donors and found that 99.71% were D+. Of those initially typing as D-, close to 30% had the D$_{el}$ phenotype. In several studies (293,295,296) it was noticed that a number of persons with D$_{el}$ red cells had an r' haplotype and it was suspected that C in *trans* to a gene making weak D might further have suppressed expression of D. Steers et al. (297) report that exons 2 and 5 of *RHD* (see below) have been detected in persons of the D$_{el}$ phenotype. It is not yet clear whether persons in other population groups with red cells phenotypically like D$_{el}$ (298,299) have the same genetic background.

The Antigens C, c, E and e

As can be seen from table 12-1, C and c and E and e normally occur as if they are produced by pairs of alleles. For most practical purposes in the routine blood bank, C and c; and E and e; behave as pairs of antithetical antigens. Each common *Rh* haplotype produces one of each while none produces both of either pair. In the light of what is now known about *Rh* genes at the molecular level, the alleles appear to be *RHCe*, *RHcE*, *RHce* and *RHCE*. Rare *Rh* alleles break the general rule cited above. For example, the *Dc-* haplotype produces neither E nor e nor any alternative antigen while the r'^{s} haplotype may produce some C and some c. Individuals who lack C, c, E or e may become immunized and form the corresponding antibody. With these four antigens, both transfusion and pregnancy are possible means of immunization but none of the antigens is even close to D in terms of immunogenicity. As mentioned, some 80% of D- individuals transfused with D+ blood form anti-D. It is difficult to determine the actual incidence of transfusion-induced immunization to C, c, E and e. While numerous studies have been published (300-316) the results are influenced by many factors. For example, the early studies used antibody detection methods that were far less sensitive than those used more recently, the apparent rates of immunization would be expected to increase as more sensitive in vitro methods were introduced. In some studies patients receiving few and those receiving many transfusions are considered together, in others they are reviewed separately. In some studies, random patients were included, in others many or most of the patients were receiving immunosuppressive therapy for the clinical condition that necessitated transfusion. Time intervals between transfusion and the last antibody detection tests vary widely in the different studies. Taking these and other variables into account, it seems that the total immunization rate to C, c, E and e following transfusion (i.e. non-red cell immune anti-E, see below, are excluded) is in the order of 1 to 3%. The immunization rates are higher in some, but certainly by no means all, groups of multiply transfused patients (317-327). The figures, when studied overall, show that other than perhaps in some selected groups of patients (see Chapter 35) the practice of matching non-immunized patients and donors for these antigens is not cost effective.

Immunization to C (in the absence of immunization to D) or to c, E or e by pregnancy probably occurs even less often than immunization by transfusion (75,328-330). It has been suggested (289,292) that if routine tests for weak D are discontinued (see above) the money, time and effort saved might be usefully applied to typing all females with child bearing potential for c and K and transfusing those lacking those antigens with antigen-negative blood. While this aim is laudable, anti-c and anti-K on occasion cause severe HDN, many workers do not believe that its application would be practical or cost-effective. Although c- and K- donors and their units from repeat donations can be readily identified via the donor center computer system, introduction of the plan would result in creation of a third inventory category. That is to D-, D+ c+ or D+ c-not typed, would be added a D+ c-classification of units. Further, routine typing of all females who have not yet reached menopause for c and provision of c- blood could delay emergency transfusions and/or scheduled surgery. While the cost of typing donors for c could be reduced by use of computerized records, the costs involved in typing patients, 80% of whom will be c+, would be high. Given the comparative rarity of severe HDN caused by anti-c, most workers believe that routine matching for c (and K) is not justified even in this group of patients.

When an antibody against C, c, E or e is found in a patient's serum, blood lacking that antigen is provided for transfusion most of the time. As discussed below and as shown in table 12-4, many Rh system antibodies are capable of causing in vivo red cell clearance. However, the provision of antigen-negative blood for all patients immunized against one of these antigens is known

sometimes to represent overkill. We (331) have produced direct evidence that some Rh antibodies that are detectable in tests using enzyme-treated red cells, PEG, or Polybrene, but that fail to react in a LISS-IAT method, do not destroy antigen-positive red cells when such cells are transfused. Further, in most of the patients we studied, who were given antigen-positive blood in the presence of the "enzyme-active" Rh antibody, no secondary immune response was seen. Contreras et al. (332) used in vivo red cell survival studies to demonstrate the benign nature of some non-red cell stimulated Rh antibodies. Others (333) have shown that the elimination of antibody-screening tests using enzyme-treated red cells does not result in an increase in the rate of transfusion reactions and (334) that some antibodies detectable only in the manual polybrene test behave, in the monocyte monolayer assay, as if they too would be benign in vivo. However, at present there is no rapid in vitro test that distinguishes between potentially destructive and potentially benign alloantibodies so that, as mentioned above, antigen-negative blood is normally provided for these immunized patients once presence of the antibody has been established. Clearly, workers who do not wish to supply unnecessary antigen-negative units can avoid use of in vitro methods that detect too many benign antibodies.

In terms of HDN, it seems that those Rh antibodies (including anti-D) that are detectable only by ultra sensitive methods at the time of delivery of the infant, do not cause clinical HDN. Like van Dijk (335,336) our experience (337) has been that infants born to women with an Rh antibody present at that level at the time of delivery most often have a negative DAT in spite of the fact that their red cells carry the antigen to which the maternal antibody is directed. Garner et al. (338) have claimed that the use of enzyme-treated red cells to test the sera of pregnant women is advantageous since it identifies some who are immunized, early in the pregnancy. In the case they described an anti-E was detectable only in tests against enzyme-treated red cells at 11 and 20 weeks of gestation but had a titer of 256 by IAT at term and caused HDN. Judd et al. (339) disputed the value of early knowledge of immunization and pointed out that those Rh antibodies that cause clinical HDN are always detectable by methods less sensitive than the use of enzyme-treated red cells at term. We (337) agreed with the contentions of Judd et al. (339) and pointed out that we knew of no instance in which clinical intervention would have helped the fetus while just an "enzyme-only" antibody was present. This point is discussed again in Chapter 41.

Of the four antibodies being discussed here, anti-E is the most common and anti-c the next most frequently encountered. Anti-C as a single antibody in Rh- individuals and at all in Rh+ individuals is comparatively rare (anti-rh$_i$, see later, is more common) and only about 2 people in every 100 are able to make allo-anti-e. While anti-E may be the most common of the four antibodies it is frequently found in the sera of individuals who have not been transfused or pregnant. In other words, anti-E is often a non-red cell stimulated antibody (304,340-342). Many examples of this type of anti-E react only with enzyme-modified red cells, while others present as agglutinins active only at temperatures below 37°C. As advocated in many places in this book, we believe that antibody screening and compatibility tests at room temperature should not be performed. It follows, of course, that examples of room temperature-active anti-E agglutinins will not be detected if those tests are omitted. However, in those services where the tests have been excluded, this has not been a problem. In other words, delayed transfusion reactions due to anti-E have not been seen, nor has there been any increase in the number of examples of 37°C-active anti-E detected in patients previously transfused. As discussed elsewhere (331) one of us suspects that this type of antibody is not truly anti-red-cell in nature but cross-reacts with a red cell-borne structure (hence its apparent specificity) and is not subject to stimulation to an increase in titer or widening of thermal range, when antigen-positive red cells are introduced. The actions of anti-C in causing delayed transfusion reactions are described in the section below dealing with Rh antibodies in general.

A number of patients with anti-E in their serum will have c- red cells because the genotype R^IR^I is common, particularly among Whites. Some workers advocate the use of E- c- blood for transfusion to persons who have formed anti-E, to prevent immunization to c. Shirey et al. (343) addressed the validity of such a policy, directly. One hundred patients with R_1R_1 red cells and anti-E in the serum were seen in a six year period. Thirty two of them had both anti-E and anti-c present when first studied. Of the 68 who had anti-E alone, 27 were transfused with E- blood that had not been typed for c. Of the remaining 41 patients, 35 were not transfused and 6 were lost to follow-up. Among the 27 patients who were transfused, 5 (18.5%) formed anti-c. The authors (343) concluded that in spite of the reduction of acceptable donors from 70% (E-) to 14% (E- c-) and the extra expense involved, the routine use of E- c- blood for R_1R_1 patients with anti-E can be justified. However, in their paper they point out that since only 5 of 27 patients developed anti-c, their data can equally well be used to argue against the policy. Those of us (PDI) who believe that E- c- blood should be provided only after the patient has made both anti-E and anti-c, use the finding that none of the 5 patients in this study who made anti-c suffered a delayed transfusion reaction, to support their view.

Deliberate immunization studies have also shown that C, c, E and e are very much less immunogenic than is D. In a series in which injections were continued over a one and a half year period, Jones et al. (344,345) found that they could not stimulate production of anti-C or anti-E in any of 32 D+ subjects; produced anti-c in only two of nine c- volunteers during 10 months of injections; and had to inject an individual who had E+ e- red cells with e+ cells for six years before he made anti-e. Wiener (346) tried to produce anti-hr' in 19 rh'+ hr'- volunteers but not one made the antibody. van Loghem et al. (347) tried to produce anti-e in three R_2R_2 volunteers. Although one of these individuals eventually made anti-e, attempts to increase the level of that antibody by further injections, caused the person to make anti-K and anti-Fy^a as well. Similarly, as described in the next section, the transfusion of C+ D- and D- E+ blood to C- and E- recipients, regardless of their D status, very seldom results in the production of anti-C or anti-E.

The Transfusion of r'(Cde) and r" (cdE) Blood to D- Recipients

In most populations, the *Rh* haplotypes *r' (Cde)*, *r''(cdE)*, *r^y(CdE) and R^z(CDE)* are rare (17,22,28,29, 34,37,349-360). *R^o(cDe)* is considerably more common in Blacks than in Whites. As a result, most D+ persons have red cells that are also C+ and/or E+ while most D- red cells lack C and E. Because early studies clearly indicated the high immunogenicity of D, in D- recipients, it was feared that C and E might be similarly immunogenic in persons whose red cells lacked C, D and E. For this reason, most donor processing centers decided that for a unit of blood to be labeled as Rh-negative, it was necessary to show that the red cells of the donor were D- C- and E-. As more and more transfusions were given, it became apparent that C and E are not very immmunogenic in D+ persons. Routine transfusions of D+ blood to D+ patients (when no other Rh typings are performed) often involve the transfusion of R_1r or R_1R_1 blood to R_2R_2 or R_2r recipients and of R_2r or R_2R_2 blood to R_1R_1 or R_1r recipients. By these transfusions C, c, E and e are all introduced as foreign antigens. Since so few D+ transfused individuals formed anti-C or anti-E, it was reasoned that r' (C+ D-) and r" (D- E+) cells might not prove any more immunogenic in D- C- E- (rr) recipients. Accordingly, beginning in the early 1960s, many transfusion services in the USA elected to type donors only for D (including weak D) and label units negative in those tests as Rh-. The decision was obviously correct for there was no increase in the production of anti-C or anti-E, by D- recipients. To this day, there are some countries in which r' and r" donors are regarded as Rh+. Difficulties are encountered in trying to convince the workers involved that r′ and r″ units can be safely used as Rh- because the decision to do exactly that, in the USA, was largely an arbitrary one and not many studies were performed to prove the safety of the procedure.

The largest prospective study carried out was that of Schorr et al. (361,362) that was reported verbally, but never published in full. Schorr and his colleagues transfused 136 units of r′ blood to 66 D+ C- recipients. One made anti-K, none made anti-C. In the test series, 134 units of r′ blood were transfused to 64 D- C- E- recipients. None of them made anti-C. To control the r″ transfusion series, 71 units of r″ blood were transfused to 44 D+ E- recipients. One made anti-E and anti-K. Eighty-nine units of r″ blood were transfused to 47 D- C- E- recipients. None of them made anti-E. In the same series, 10 D- C- E- recipients were given, among them, 37 units of r′ and/or r″ blood. One made anti-C and a second (obviously a good responder, see Chapter 2) made anti-C, anti-E and anti-K.

Next, Schorr et al. (361,362) transfused r′ and r″ blood to D- C- E- patients who had already made anti-D. Five rr patients with anti-D received 94 units of r′ blood. One of the five made anti-C. Four rr patients who already had anti-D were given 49 units of r″, one of the four made anti-E. These 9 patients with anti-D are considered separately from those who had no anti-D before transfusion, since it is entirely possible that transfusion of the r′ and r″ units acted as a secondary immunization. Those patients with anti-D might well have mounted a primary immune response to C or E at the time that they were immunized to D, but failed to make serologically detectable anti-C or anti-E until after re-exposure to the antigens.

In 1971 Huestis (363) reported a study that involved 4 rr patients. The first was transfused with 281 rr, 7 r′ and 4 r″ units, the patient made anti-K. Another was transfused with 264 rr, 17 r′ and 4 r″ units. The two others, between them received 38 rr and 6 r′ units. These three patients did not make anti-C or anti-E.

One of us (310) compared the incidence of production of anti-C and anti-E in some older series (300-302,307) studied at the time that r′ and r″ donors were regarded as Rh+, with the incidence in his own service where r′ and r″ units were transfused as Rh-. When r′ and r″ units were considered Rh+, the incidence of anti-C was 1 in 9000, the incidence of anti-E was 1 in 850 (see earlier for a discussion of the production of non-red cell stimulated anti-E). When r′ and r″ units were considered Rh-, the incidence of anti-C was 1 in 11,000 and of anti-E, 1 in 1000. These findings occurred in spite of the fact that in the later studies, more sensitive tests for the detection of anti-C and anti-E were used than was the case when the earlier tests were done. Further, the examples of anti-C and anti-E in this author's series (310) were *all* made by D+ people.

The conclusion from these studies (310,361-363) is inescapable. There is no justification whatever for regarding C+ D- and D- E+ units as anything other than Rh- for transfusion purposes. First, typing tests for C and E on the D- units waste time, reagents and money. Second, the chronic shortage of Rh- blood should not be exacerbated by calling r′ and r″ units Rh+. Extremely rare findings (363) such as that in which a D- person made anti-G after being transfused with r′ blood (we have heard anecdotal reports of three other such instances in the last 30 years) do not alter this conclusion in any way. As discussed in a later section, G is even less immunogenic in D- persons than is C.

Rh Phenotypes and Genotypes

When red blood cells are typed for D, C, c, E and e, the results constitute an Rh phenotype. From that phenotype it is possible to determine the most likely *Rh* genotype of the individual involved. Since genes cannot be detected in serological typing tests and since red cells carry gene products and not genes anyway, red cells cannot be Rh genotyped. This fundamental point is overlooked by many blood bankers who should know much better, with alarming regularity.

Because there are several different *Rh* haplotypes that encode the production of similar sets of antigens, *Rh* genotypes can seldom be deduced with absolute certainty, from phenotyping studies. However, because some haplotypes are common while others are rare or very rare, the most probable genotype, as interpreted from a phenotype, is very often the correct one. As described later in this chapter, antibodies to the antigens rh$_i$(Ce), f(ce), cE and CE define additional gene products. In brief, red cells that react with anti-rh$_i$ must come from an individual with *RHCe* on at least one chromosome. Red cells that type as C+ e+ rh$_i$- must come from an individual who has *RHC* on one chromosome and *RHe* on the other. As can be seen antibodies to rh$_i$, f, cE and CE can sometimes be used to differentiate between different genotypes that are represented by the same phenotype.

Similarly and as also described later in this chapter, dosage studies can sometimes be of help in differentiating between possible genetic interpretations of a phenotype. Unfortunately the antibody that would be of most use in this respect, anti-D, does not yield reliable dosage results by conventional tests. Thus in D+ phenotypes, difficulties are often encountered in attempts to determine whether the individual involved has one or two *RHD* genes. This topic is discussed in more detail in the next section.

With the above limitations stated, table 12-5 lists the various Rh phenotypes that can be determined by use of antibodies to C, c, D, E and e and their interpretations in terms of most likely and alternative genotypes. Because of their extreme rarity, genes such as *Dc-, D--, $\overline{r}$ (---)*, et al., are not considered in table 12-5. However, it must be remembered that on very rare occasions the presence of such a gene will considerably complicate the interpretation of a phenotype as a probable genotype. In previous editions of this book, the equivalent table to 12-5 included Rh phenotypes described in the terminology originally proposed by Mourant (365). However, valid objections to that terminology have been raised. As examples, red cells typed as C+ c+ D+ E+ e+ were described as CcDEe, an exact reflection of the antigens shown to be present. Red cells typed as C+ c+ D+ E+ e- were described as CcDEE. Two objections can be made. First,

the designation EE implies that the individual's *Rh* haplotypes both make E. While this is likely given the frequency of *Rh* haplotypes, it is certainly not proved in a phenotyping study. Second, lack of any mention of e in the phenotype designation could be taken to indicate either that the red cells were e- or that no test with anti-e was performed. This latter consideration was particularly worrying when (not long ago) anti-e typing reagents were difficult to obtain. Even the compromise CcDE leaves the reader to guess about presence, absence, or not tested for e. Accordingly, phenotype designations such as C+ c- D+ E- e+ and C- c+ D- E- e+ are to be preferred over CCDee and ccee (or ccddee) respectively. Such listings are not given in table 12-5 since they can be inferred directly from the typing results that are shown.

TABLE 12-5 Interpretation of Rh Typing in Terms of Phenotypes and Possible Genotypes

Part 1: In which the most likely genotype is common and most of the alternatives are rare.

Reactions with Anti-						
D	C	E	c	e	Most Likely Genotype	Other Possible Genotypes
+	+	+	+	+	CDe/cDE	CDe/cdE, cDE/Cde, CDE/cde, CDE/cDe, cDe/CdE
+	+	0	+	+	CDe/cde	CDe/cDe, cDe/Cde
+	0	+	+	+	cDE/cde	cDE/cDe, cDe/cdE
+	+	0	0	+	CDe/CDe	CDe/Cde
+	0	+	+	0	cDE/cDE	cDE/cdE
+	0	0	+	+	cDe/cde*1	cDe/cDe*1
0	0	0	+	+	cde/cde	None

Part 2: In which all the genotypes are so rare that it is not possible to guess which is the most likely and where family studies may be essential to get the correct answer.

Reactions with Anti-					
D	C	E	c	e	Possible Genotypes
0	+	0	+	+	Cde/cde
0	0	+	+	+	cdE/cde
0	+	0	0	+	Cde/Cde
0	0	+	+	0	cdE/cdE
+	+	+	0	+	CDe/CDE, CDe/CdE, Cde/CDE
+	+	+	+	0	cDE/CDE, cDE/CdE, cdE/CDE
+	+	+	0	0	CDE/CDE, CDE/CdE
0	+	+	+	+	Cde/cdE, CdE/cde
0	+	+	0	0	CdE/CdE
0	+	+	0	+	CdE/Cde
0	+	+	+	0	CdE/cdE

*1   In Blacks, the frequency of *R⁰* is higher than that of *r*. Thus for the phenotype shown, *R⁰R⁰* will be about 1.5 times more common than *R⁰r* in Blacks.

Table 12-6 follows 12-5 for those workers who have antibodies to f, rh$_i$, cE and CE and use them to try to differentiate between genotypes represented by the same phenotype. These antibodies and the antigens they define are discussed again in a later section of this chapter. As mentioned earlier, the term *d* in tables 12-5 and 12-6 is used merely to indicate the absence of *D*.

Dosage Studies

Comparatively few, rather exceptional Rh antibodies, differentiate between red cells that carry single and double doses of an Rh antigen. For example, it might be expected that the red cells of an individual of *Rh* genotype R^2R^2 (*cDE/cDE*) would carry more c and E than would those of an individual of *Rh* genotype R^1R^2 (*CDe/cDE*). The difference in quantity of c and E might be expected because the R^2R^2 individual has two haplotypes encoding production of those antigens, while the R^1R^2 individual has only one. In titration studies (single tests with undiluted sera are almost never of value) certain anti-c and anti-E will make a differentiation between doses of antigen. The difference may be seen in one of two ways. First, the sera may react to a higher titer with the cells carrying a double dose of the antigen or second, they may give a higher titer score with those cells (see Chapter 3). While manual titration studies have been used to measure Rh antigen dose for years, more recent techniques (see below) have shown that the results obtained are not particularly reliable. There are three major reasons for this. First, as pointed out in the section on number of Rh antigen sites on red cells, there is considerable variation in the number of measurable antigen sites on the red cells of individuals of apparently the same genotype. Second, as stated, only exceptional Rh

antibodies demonstrate clear dosage effect. Third, manual titration studies suffer the disadvantages associated with all subjectively read tests.

Measurement of antigen levels, as associated with *Rh* haplotypes present, can be achieved with better results when the red cells of related individuals are tested. Rosenfield and his colleagues (59-65) have shown that the *Rh* haplotypes within one family will punctiliously transmit genetic information for not only which, but for exactly how much Rh antigen will be made. The measurements are highly reproducible, in different family members with the same *Rh* haplotype, in whom the *trans* position haplotype does not influence antigen production. However, dosage measurement in family members may not be necessary since phenotyping may reveal exactly which *Rh* haplotypes are present.

When dosage studies are considered, it is apparent that the most useful results would be generated if such studies could be used to differentiate between individuals homozygous and heterozygous for *RHD*. When a D- woman with potent anti-D in the serum is married to a D+ man, determination of *RHD* zygosity of the man would reveal whether the couple could produce a D- infant or whether all infants would be D+. Such information would be of particular value if the woman had previously delivered an infant suffering from severe HDN or a hydropic stillborn. As discussed below, the D type of a fetus can now be determined very early in pregnancy. Before such molecular techniques were available and even now when a couple such as the one described above are trying to decide whether to have another child, it would be extremely useful to be able to determine *RHD* zygosity of the male. Because such information would be so valuable, numerous attempts to measure dosage of D and correlate it with gene dose, have been reported. It has long been accepted that man-

TABLE 12-6 Some Antigens Encoded by the Eight Most Common *Rh* Haplotypes

Rh Haplotype	Phenotype Designation	Antigens Made								
		D	C	E	c	e	f	rh$_i$	cE	CE
R^1 or *CDe*	R$_1$ or CDe	+	+	0	0	+	0	+	0	0
R^2 or *cDE*	R$_2$ or cDE	+	0	+	+	0	0	0	+	0
R^0 or *cDe*	R$_0$ or cDe	+	0	0	+	+	+	0	0	0
R^z or *CDE*	R$_z$ or CDE	+	+	+	0	0	0	0	0	+
r or *cde*	r or cde	0	0	0	+	+	+	0	0	0
r′ or *Cde*	r′ or Cde	0	+	0	0	+	0	+	0	0
r″ or *cdE*	r″ or cdE	0	0	+	+	0	0	0	+	0
r^y or *CdE*	r^y or CdE	0	+	+	0	0	0	0	0	+

ual titration studies with anti-D are of no value in attempts to determine *RHD* zygosity. As a result other methods have been evaluated. Using ferritin labeled anti-IgG to measure the amount of anti-D bound to red cells, Masouredis et al. (366) were able to differentiate *RHD* homozygotes from heterozygotes within a family. As pointed out in the previous edition of this book, workers with great expertise in the use of capillary tube methods (359,379-382) using well characterized and much used anti-D, can sometimes differentiate between the red cells of *RHD* homozygotes and heterozygotes, based on the speed of the reaction of the red cells with anti-D. Again, this technique is more applicable to the study of red cells from family members than to the study of individual samples from unrelated persons. Other methods used have included rosetting assays (367,368) and enzyme-linked immunoadsorbant assays (369). It is the opinion of most workers that tests to determine *RHD* zygosity by in vitro serological methods are not sufficiently reliable for routine use. As described in the section of this chapter dealing with the molecular genetics of Rh, PCR amplification of genomic DNA from the cells of the fetus, if used carefully and by amplification of several regions of *RHD* DNA, will indicate the D status of an infant early in pregnancy. However, since D+ individuals have *RHD*, this technique cannot be used to differentiate between *RHD* homozygotes and heterozygotes if the father of the child is tested.

There is little doubt that the most reliable method yet devised for dosage measurements of antigens such as C, c, E, e and those of other blood group systems, involves use of the flow cytometer (370-374,387, 388,944). In some of these studies (370,373,387,944) it has been shown that manual titration studies can lead to erroneous interpretations, particularly if too few controls

(cells from known homozygotes and heterozygotes) are used. As examples, the variations in level of antigen expression are such that an unknown (actually C+ c+) sample may match C- c+ samples or that an unknown (actually C- c+) sample may match C+ c+ samples if only a few controls are run.

In view of the accuracy of dosage results obtained with the flow cytometer, several groups of workers (296,375,376,378) have used the instrument, often in conjunction with the use of monoclonal anti-D, to determine the level of D on the red cells of unrelated individuals. It has been found that D antigen expression is a continuum from very low to very high levels and that there is overlap in the amount of D between the red cells of *RHD* heterozygotes and homozygotes. This, of course, is not surprising. As discussed in the next section, it has been known for many years that, for example, some red cells of phenotype R_2r, express more D than some of phenotype R_1R_1.

As yet there is no report of any material replacing *RHD* in D- persons in whom *RHD* is deleted. If such material exists and if it can be identified and amplified by PCR, its presence could presumably be used, along with the presence of amplified genomic *RHD* DNA, to differentiate *RHD* heterozygotes from *RHD* homozygotes. Perhaps such speculation is science fiction or perhaps such a method will have been developed by the time this book is printed!

Numbers of Rh Antigen Sites on Red Cells

Much elegant work has been performed in attempts to determine the number of Rh antigen sites on the red cells of various Rh phenotypes. Sometimes the methods

TABLE 12-7 Estimated Number of Available Antigen Sites on Red Blood Cells

Phenotype	D	C	E	c	e	G
CDe/CDe	14,500-19,500	46,000-56,500	0	0	18,000-24,500	10,000-12,000
CDe/cde	10,000-15,000	21,500-40,000	0	37,000-53,000	18,000-24,500	6,000
cDE/cDE	16,000-33,500	0	25,500	70,000-85,000	0	3,500-6,000
cDE/cde	14,000-16,500	0	N.T.	70,000-85,000	13,500-14,500	4,000
CDe/cDE	23,000-31,000	25,500-40,000	N.T.	37,000-53,000	13,500-14,500	N.T.
cDe/cde	12,000-20,000	0	0	70,000-85,000	18,000-24,500	N.T.
cde/cde	0	0	0	70,000-85,000	18,000-24,500	0
-D-/-D-	110,000-200,000	0	0	0	0	N.T.

For comparison: A_1 cells, approx 2 x 10^6 A sites.
B cells, approx 2 x 10^6 B sites.
K+ k- cells approx 6,000 K sites.
K+ k+ cells approx 3,500 K sites.
Fy(a+) cells approx 12,000 Fy^a sites.

involved radio-labeled Rh antibodies and on other occasions used non-agglutinating IgG Rh antibodies and radio or ferritin-labeled anti-IgG. By counting the amount of label bound to the red cells, or the amount bound to the cell-bound IgG, it has been possible to estimate the number of Rh antigen sites on the cells. Table 12-7 presents a composite of results obtained from many different studies that used human polyclonal antibodies (265,266,369,383-386). When monoclonal antibodies are used in similar studies the results, particularly when the number of D sites is estimated, are likely to be directly affected by the epitope specificity of the antibody used. In spite of this, various studies (389-398) that often used monoclonal antibodies directed against high frequency markers on Rh polypeptides, have suggested that those polypeptides are present in numbers between 100,000 and 200,000 per red cell. Such estimates are in general agreement with the figures in table 12-7, if the haplotype products in a given genotype are totaled.

For the sake of comparison, table 12-7 shows some estimates (390,394,399-404) of the number of antigens of some other blood group systems, on red cells. As discussed in Chapter 6 (section on intravascular red cell destruction) and as mentioned in Chapter 8, there are reasons to believe (394,395) that the number of A and B antigens on red cells may be 2×10^6, that is twice the number originally estimated (399,400). Similarly, studies using more sophisticated methods and potent monoclonal antibodies may require that some other numbers in table 12-7 be changed. However, it seems likely that the ratios of numbers of AB:Rh:K:Fy^a antigen sites may remain as presently indicated.

Finally, it should be remembered that all methods that measure antigen site numbers using an antibody, will yield figures representing the number of available (to antibody) antigens. That is to say, more antigens than appears to be the case may be present, if the binding of antibody to some, blocks the access of antibody to others. Less likely, the figures may overestimate the number of antigens if more than one antibody can bind per antigen (i.e. via different epitopes) if a polyclonal antibody is used. Methods that do not use an antibody (i.e. calculations that estimate the number of antigen-bearing structures present) may produce different estimates to antibody-based calculations. This is of no moment at the practical level since the number of antigens available to antibody is of prime importance for both in vitro and in vivo antigen-antibody reactions.

Rh Antibodies: Non-red Cell Immune

The overwhelming majority of Rh antibodies are made by individuals exposed to foreign red cell antigens via transfusion or pregnancy. However, there is now a considerable body of data about non-red cell immune or "naturally-occurring" Rh antibodies. As described above, anti-E is often found in never-transfused, never-pregnant individuals (304,340-342). Although encountered less often than anti-E, both anti-C^w and anti-C^x are found in similar circumstances (405-408). Both antibodies also occur frequently as alloantibodies in the sera of patients with "warm" antibody-induced hemolytic anemia (49,50,409). Some of the non-red cell stimulated Rh antibodies that have been studied have been found to be, at least in part, IgM. However, weak Rh antibodies that are detected only in tests using enzyme-treated red cells, or by methods with similar sensitivity are more often IgG than IgM (74,331,410,411).

Although fairly rare, examples of non-red cell stimulated anti-D have been described (417-419). When tests were performed in the Autoanalyzer and in some in which the manual polybrene method was used, it was found (412-416) that some sera from D- individuals contain non-red cell stimulated, "cold-reactive", anti-D. When Lee et al. (416) gave multiple injections of D+ red cells to four males with "cold-reactive", non-red cell immune anti-D already present, they found that two of the subjects made anti-D with characteristics of the immune form of that antibody, one made no anti-D with such characteristics but cleared ^{51}Cr-labeled D+ red cells at an accelerated rate in an in vivo survival study while in the fourth no "immune" type anti-D was made and ^{51}Cr-labeled D+ red cells survived normally in vivo. Contreras et al. (33) described three individuals with non-red cell stimulated anti-D active at 37°C. In the two in whom the antibody could be detected by IAT, ^{51}Cr-labeled D+ red cells were cleared, in vivo, at an accelerated rate. In the third, in whom the anti-D was demonstrable in vitro only in tests against enzyme-treated red cells, the in vivo survival of ^{51}Cr-labeled D+ red cells was normal.

It seems that non-red cell immune Rh antibodies are rather accommodating for practical purposes. That is, those antibodies demonstrable by conventional methods seem often to be clinically relevant, while those detectable only by ultra-sensitive methods seem usually to be clinically benign.

Rh Antibodies: Immune

It would be expected that the production of Rh antibodies would follow the classical pathway described in Chapter 2, in which IgM antibody is made first and IgG later. One group of investigators (168) concluded that is what happens while another (158) found that early made Rh antibody was IgG or IgA. Certainly, if IgM antibody is made first, the switch to IgG production occurs early. Gunson et al. (377) found that by the time serologically detectable Rh antibody is present, at least part of it is IgG.

When IgG Rh antibodies are made it seems (420-430) that most of them are IgG1 or IgG3. In studies on antibodies made following immunization by pregnancy it was found (421) that IgG1 anti-D was more common than was the IgG3 type. From findings (421,425,430) that hyperimmunized individuals form mixtures of IgG1 and IgG3 anti-D it has been postulated that IgG1 anti-D is most often the first formed and that it is most frequently joined by IgG3 anti-D when repeated exposure to D occurs. There are also reports in the literature of IgG2 and IgG4 anti-D (431-434). For reasons discussed in detail in Chapter 6, IgG3 antibodies are more efficient than are those made of IgG1, in clearing antigen-positive red cells in vivo. In HDN the greater efficiency of IgG3 antibodies is somewhat offset by the fact that IgG1 crosses the placenta in greater quantity and earlier in gestation, than does IgG3 (435,436). Nevertheless, when a woman has a high titered IgG3 anti-D in her serum, severe HDN can result because of the rapid destruction of D+ red cells when that antibody reaches the fetal circulation (945).

Although Rh antibodies are most often IgG1 and/or IgG3 in composition and although those subclasses of IgG are usually efficient in initiating complement activation, Rh antibodies that bind complement in vitro, have only occasionally been reported (437-440). Possible reasons for the failure of Rh antibodies to activate complement have been discussed in Chapter 6. In addition to considerations of paucity of antigen sites, distance of antigens from the membrane and immunoglobulin molecule shape change after binding to antigen, it has now been suggested (74) that the size of the Rh epitope may be a limiting factor. That is to say, perhaps for K, more than one molecule of anti-K may be able to bind to a single antigen and thus two Fc pieces could become available to activate C1q. It is suggested (74) that for D, the epitope is small enough (209) that only a single molecule of anti-D can bind. In working with red cell ghosts, it was found (441) that Rh antibodies still did not activate complement, but it was claimed that treatment of the ghosts with papain caused the subsequently used antibodies to effect some complement activation. We are not aware of additional investigations concerning this observation. The puzzle created by the inability of IgG Rh antibodies to activate complement is compounded by observations (74) that IgM Rh antibodies similarly lack that ability.

Rh antibodies have been incriminated as causative of delayed transfusion reactions (442-455). Sometimes, particularly it seems when the antibody has anti-C specificity (447), the delayed reaction is associated with the presence of free hemoglobin in the plasma. This is unexpected because hemoglobinemia is most often associated with intravascular hemolysis and Rh antibodies do not activate complement. It is possible that the accumulation of hemoglobin in the plasma, when Rh antibodies destroy red cells, may represent no more than release of hemoglobin from the spleen (where red cell sequestration and destruction occur) at a greater rate than that at which it can be excreted (169). On the other hand, it is possible that some cell destruction by Rh antibodies occurs in the patient's circulation via the K-cell lysis mechanism (456-461) that is also described in Chapter 6.

Although the subject is discussed in more detail in Chapter 35, it should be mentioned here that in some of the cases of transfusion reactions cited earlier (450,451,453) no Rh antibody was demonstrable in serological tests either before or after the transfusion of incompatible blood. The specificity of the antibody presumed to be present was determined in each case by ^{51}Cr-labeled in vivo red cell survival studies. In other words, while most Rh antibodies are easy to detect (see below) and characterize (see above) there are rare examples that defy detection in vitro (462).

The In Vitro Detection of Rh Antibodies

Most Rh antibodies are relatively easy to detect and identify in vitro. The rare IgM examples mentioned earlier in this chapter will often agglutinate red cells suspended in saline, in tests at room temperature or 37°C. IgG Rh antibodies are hardly any more difficult to detect. The majority of them react well in IATs and are detected by the anti-IgG of antiglobulin reagents. Studies performed to evaluate different antiglobulin reagents (463-465) have nearly always found that the anti-IgG components of any reagent will detect Rh antibodies, even if those components have shortcomings in the detection of IgG antibodies of other blood group systems. The more potent examples of IgG Rh antibodies will agglutinate red cells in tests using high protein media (such as bovine albumin or human serum). The reactions of easily detected (via albumin or IAT methods) Rh antibodies can be further enhanced in tests using proteolytic enzymes. The advantages of using protease-modified red cells to detect Rh antibodies are seen most dramatically when weak antibodies are encountered. Some of these antibodies are detected in tests that use enzymes but cannot be demonstrated at all in IATs. There have been some claims that enzymes vary in their ability to enhance the reactions of weak Rh antibodies. However, it has been our experience (50,466,467) that if ficin, papain and bromelin are used under optimal conditions, each is as effective as the others in the detection of Rh antibodies.

Methods for the use of these enzymes are given by Judd (468). While the term "enzyme-only" is retained, below, it must be appreciated that the words are now relative. Originally enzyme-only Rh antibodies were those that reacted with enzyme-pretreated red cells but failed to give positive reactions in IATs (410,411,469). As IATs using LISS, PEG and Polybrene techniques were introduced, it became apparent that the previously called, enzyme-only Rh antibodies would react by some, many or all of these methods, dependent on their strength. Thus, as used here, the term "enzyme-only" describes an Rh antibody that gives visible reactions in tests against enzyme-pretreated red cells, but fails to give a visible reaction by LISS-IAT. Some, but by no means all of these antibodies react (visibly) in PEG or Polybrene IATs (331). One obvious advantage of using a method in which an antibody with a low binding constant is given the opportunity to agglutinate red cells, is that no washing (as in IATs) is required after the antigen-antibody reaction has taken place. The chance of antibody dissociation is thus considerably reduced. A more subtle advantage in the use of enzymes for the detection of Rh antibodies relates to the rate at which antibodies bind to red cells. Masouredis (470) demonstrated that enzyme-treated D+ red cells bind twice as much anti-D as do untreated cells. Hughes-Jones et al. (471) confirmed this observation and thought that it was due to an increase in the association constant between antibody and the red cells. This increase might occur because protease-treatment of red cells removes structures from the membrane that otherwise interfere with antigen-antibody complex formation (169,472).

While the use of enzyme-treated red cells for the detection of Rh antibodies is of great help in the identification of antibodies that give ambiguous reactions by less sensitive techniques and in the identification of antibodies in sera that contain multiple specificities, the method is too sensitive for routine use. In retrospective tests on samples from 10,000 patients, that had given negative antibody-screening tests by LISS-IAT, we (331) found 29 Rh antibodies. However, of the 19 patents who had already been transfused with antigen-positive blood before the Rh antibody was detected, none had an immediate and only one had a delayed transfusion reaction. Further, the presence of an "enzyme-only" antibody and transfusion with antigen-positive blood was not associated with a secondary immune response nor, among the 10,000 patients studied in whom there was a secondary immune response, were "enzyme-only" antibodies present, before transfusion. If we had used enzyme-treated red cells in routine pretransfusion tests on these 10,000 patients we would have: found 28 clinically-insignificant antibodies; had to investigate 77 sera in which positive reactions were seen but the antibody was too weak to

identify; perform typings on donor units to find 163 that lacked the antigen to which the patient had the antibody; and perform autoadsorption then repeat antibody-screening and/or identification studies on 216 samples that contained autoantibodies active against enzyme-treated red cells. All that work would have prevented one delayed transfusion reaction caused by anti-c. Clearly the use of enzymes in routine pretransfusion (or prenatal) serology is not cost effective.

The use of enzyme pretreated red cells provides a highly sensitive method for the detection of Rh antibodies. In our large study (331) on 29 Rh antibodies that reacted by IAT with ficin-treated red cells, but were nonreactive by LISS-IAT, we tested those sera available in sufficient quantity by Polybrene and PEG methods. Of 25 antibodies tested by Polybrene-IAT, nine (36%) were reactive; of 27 tested by PEG-IAT, 11 (41%) were reactive. In spite of this higher incidence of positive reactions of Rh antibodies by enzyme than by Polybrene or PEG methods, very rare Rh antibodies detectable by Polybrene but not by enzyme methods, have been reported (634-638). It should be added that some of these reports gave only scant details of the enzyme pretreatment methods used. As pointed out in Chapter 3, to obtain optimal results, fairly exact conditions must be used when red cells are treated with proteases. However, the fact that some of the "polybrene-only" antibodies caused in vivo red cell destruction, clearly indicates that the method should be included in the investigation of unexplained transfusion reactions.

The Rh System at a Complex Level

Thus far this chapter has dealt with aspects of the Rh system that apply in many instances in transfusion therapy. As blood bankers know, there is a huge amount of additional information available about the system at the serological level and in the last fifteen years much has been discovered about the biochemical structure of the Rh antigen-bearing red cell membrane components and the molecular genetic events that control their production. The remainder of this chapter deals with the complexities of Rh. Perforce some of the descriptions are abbreviated and in a few, interpretive descriptions are presented. Readers are strongly encouraged to read some of the references cited, in the original since our interpretations may not always be identical to those of the workers reporting new data.

A brief explanation of some terms used in this section is necessary. Now that it is known (40) that in D+ persons, two *Rh* genes, *RHD* and *RHCE* (alleles *RHCe*, *RHcE*, *RHce* and *RHCE*) are present while in most D-persons, *RHD* is deleted, use of the term gene can be more accurately applied. As examples, what used to be called the gene complex *CDe* or R^1 is now best described as a haplotype, i.e. *RHD* and *RHCe* genes on the same chromosome. What used to be called the gene complex *cde* or *r* is now best described as the gene *RHce*. Throughout the remainder of this chapter (and in portions of the preceding sections) the term haplotype indicates the (sometimes presumed) presence of at least two genes while the term gene indicates only one. The terms *RHD*, *RHCe*, *RHcE*, *RHce* and *RHCE* (with *RHCE* also used as a generic term for the locus or sublocus) are used whenever the descriptions relate to information obtained via biochemical or molecular biology studies. The terms *RHD* and *RHCE* were introduced (58) primarily for such use.

Epitopes of the D Antigen

In 1951, Shapiro (274,275) who used the Rh-Hr nomenclature, reported production of anti-Rh_0 by an individual with Rh_0+ red cells. Two years later, Argall et al. (276) found an allo-anti-D in the serum of a person with "D^u" red cells. It rapidly became apparent (117-120,478-484) that rare individuals with D+ red cells can make a form of anti-D that reacts with almost all D+ cells but not with their own. It is now appreciated that the D antigen comprises multiple epitopes, all of which are present on most D+ red cells. Those individuals with one or more of the epitopes missing from their red cells (partial D, see below) can mount an immune response to the missing epitope(s) when exposed to the common form of D+ red cells. Because most D+ red cells carry all the epitopes of D, the antibody produced will be seen to have anti-D specificity. Because anti-D typing reagents are prepared from pools of human anti-D or selected monoclonal anti-D and are designed to detect any epitope of D, the antibody-makers' red cells will type as D+. In some instances red cells that lack one or more epitopes of D will type as weakly positive for D. Much more frequently, the red cells will give unremarkable positive reactions when typed for D.

The Rh_0^{alphabet} Classification

Two groups of workers investigated the situation in which D+ people make alloimmune anti-D, by testing the red cells of the antibody-makers with the anti-D made by other D+ persons. Because of differences of opinion regarding the genetic control of Rh antigen production, different terminologies were introduced. Wiener and his colleagues (117-120,481,484-492) described the Rh_0 antigen as being made of four pieces, Rh^A, Rh^B, Rh^C

and Rh^D. When the portion of the antigen was present a capital letter was used, when it was absent a lower case letter was substituted. Thus red cells of the phenotype Rh^{ABcd} had Rh^A and Rh^B present but lacked Rh^C and Rh^D. The anti-Rh_0 made by a person with Rh^a red cells reacted with normal Rh_0+ red cells and with those described as Rh^A, but not with other Rh^a samples, and so on. That the system was inadequate to explain all the complexities was apparent from findings such as those that showed that some Rh^{abcd} red cells reacted with anti-Rh_0 made in Rh_0- individuals (26,484), Since it is no longer used, the $Rh^{alphabet}$ classification of Rh_0 will not be further described. As mentioned earlier in this chapter, the ISBT working party on terminology for red cell surface antigens has declared (58) the terms Rh^A, Rh^B, Rh^C and Rh^D obsolete, since antibodies to define the determinants are no longer available.

The Category Classification of Partial D

A different way of classifying the D+ red cells of persons who make anti-D was introduced by Tippett and Sanger (49,122,123) and later expanded by Tippett (124,493). These workers divided the antibody-makers into a series of categories in which, in each category, the red cells of the antibody-maker and the anti-D made were identical or very similar. This was accomplished, first by screening tests with selected and well characterized anti-D made in D- persons, that varied in their reactions and reaction strengths with the red cells of different categories. Next, the red cells of the antibody-maker and the anti-D made were cross-tested against other D+ red cells from persons who had made alloimmune anti-D. As mentioned earlier, many red cells that lack one or more epitopes of D, react unremarkably with anti-D made in D- persons. The category classifications made using human anti-D, included only such samples. Because the antibodies used did not always react well with weak D (formerly D^u) samples, such bloods were not classified even when the individual involved had made anti-D. As discussed below, the use of monoclonal anti-D to define presence or absence of D epitopes has largely overcome this problem and samples with weak D can ɔw often be characterized. Table 12-8 is included, partly for historical reasons. It shows the original division of red cells with partial D into six categories. The table also shows the percentage of anti-D made in D- persons, that reacted with the red cells of each category. Of particular note, the red cells of category VI reacted with the least number of such antibodies. This was an elegant serological demonstration that forecast a much later finding (see below) that category VI red cells carry fewer of the various epitopes of D, than do the red cells of any other category.

TABLE 12-8 Original Classification of D+ Red Cells of People who make Anti-D, into Categories (from Tippett and Sanger, 49, 67, 122)

Red blood cells of category	Reactions of anti-D made by people with red cells of category					Percent of anti-D made by D- people that react with the cells of each category
	II	III	IV	V	VI	
I	+	+	+	+	+	100
II	0	+	+	+	+	100
III	+	0	+	+	+	100
IV	+	(+)	0	+	+	96
V	+	0	+	0	(+)	74
VI	0	0	+	0	0	35

As more examples of D+ red cells from persons who had made anti-D were studied and as more examples of this type of anti-D became available, it became apparent that heterogeneity existed within some of the categories. In 1977, Tippett and Sanger (123) published an updated version of their classification of the subdivisions of D. It was shown that the majority of samples studied could still be assigned to one of the categories originally proposed and further, that common findings on different samples allowed subdivision of the categories to include similar but not identical reactivities, within three of the original categories. The updated findings of Tippett and Sanger (123) are reproduced in table 12-9. These addi-

tional studies showed very clearly that the category classification is much more flexible than the Rh^{alphabet} classification described above, in that it allows for the addition of new findings within the original framework. As can be seen from table 12-9, by 1977 the original category I had been excluded, it had been realized that some samples originally assigned to that category involved the transient presence of anti-D. Although the finding was reported much later (494) it can be added here that subcategory Vc has also now been abolished since monoclonal anti-D show that categories Vc and IVb are probably the same. The data shown in table 12-9 also constitute an elegant serological forecast as to what was later

TABLE 12-9 To Show Subdivisions within the Original Categories of D+ Red Cells of People who make Anti-D (from Tippett and Sanger (123))

Red blood cells of category	Reactions of anti-D made by people with red cells of category											
	II	IIIa	IIIb	IIIc	IVa some	IVa others	IVb	Va	Vb	Vc	VIi	VIii
II	0	+	+	+	+	+	(+)	+	+	(+)	+	+
IIIa	+	0	+	0	+	+	+	+	+	+	+	+
IIIb	+	0	0	0	+	+	+	(+)	+	+	+	+
IIIc	+	0	+	0	+	+	+	+	+	+	+	+
IVa	0	(+)	+	0	0	0	0	+	+	0	+	+
IVb	0	(+)	+	(+)	0	0	0	0	0	(+)	+	0
Va	+	0	+	0	+	(+)	+	0	(+)	0	+	0
Vb	+	0	+	0	+	0	0	0	0	0	0	0
Vc	+	0	+	0	(+)	0	(+)	0	0	0	+	0
VI	0	0	+	0	+	0	+	0	0	0	0	0

1. The red cells in category VI are similar, as shown, two different types of anti-D are made
2. Red cells of category IIIb are G-, others are G+
3. Red cells of category IVa are Go(a+), others are Go(a-)
4. Red cells of category Va are D^w+, others are D^w-
5. Subcategory Vc has now been abolished, see text

to be found using epitope specific monoclonal anti-D and by studying the genes involved in the production of partial D, at the molecular level.

Monoclonal Anti-D and Epitopes of the D Antigen

Monoclonal antibodies are, of course, epitope specific (see Chapters 2 and 5). Thus when a number of MAb to D became available, they were tested against the red cells of D+ persons who had made alloimmune anti-D. Different MAb to D gave different patterns when the red cells of various categories were tested. These studies thus identified the epitope specificities of the MAb to D and demonstrated the presence or absence of the various epitopes on the red cells of different categories. It was apparent that the term partial D, as introduced by Salmon et al. (495) in 1984, most accurately describes the situation. Fortunately the term partial D is now in widespread use and has replaced both the D mosaic term and the D variant term. Replacement of the term D variant is particularly appropriate since that term had been used (498) to describe both quantitative and qualitative variants of D, much to the rightful chagrin of some (263,496,497).

Gorick et al. (391) used seven MAb to D in competitive binding assays and identified the first three epitopes of D. Lomas et al. (209) then extended these studies by using 29 MAb to D in serological tests against partial D

red cells of categories III, IVa, IVb, Va, Vc, VI and VII (category Vc cells were later (494) reassigned to category IVb). The results showed the existence of at least seven epitopes of D (epD1 to epD7), the serological reactions of the antibodies to epD6 and epD7 were identical, differentiation between the two epitopes was based on the results of the earlier (391) competitive binding assays. The results from the study by Lomas et al. (209) provide the basis for table 12-10, as described below, additional findings have been added. Work with newly available MAb to D (210,241) resulted in the identification of epD8 and epD9 and additional phenotypes involving partial D were found when red cell samples gave unique patterns in tests with MAb that define epD1 to epD9. The new phenotypes DFR, DBT and the D made by R^{oHar} were not given category numbers. By the time that MAb to D were being used to characterize red cells for presence or absence of the various epitopes of D, some of the human polyclonal anti-D made by D+ persons were no longer available so that the partial D classifications are now based on D epitope profiles. Table 12-10 shows the presence or absence of epD1 to epD9 on the red cells of 12 different phenotypes of partial D, it by no means represents the end of the story. As can be seen from that table, many additional D epitopes must exist. First, category IIIa, IIIb and IIIc red cells carry all 9 epitopes of D listed in the table. However, individuals with D+ red cells of category III are able to make alloimmune anti-D (49,122-124,493) showing that their red cells

TABLE 12-10 Epitopes of D on Partial D Red Cells of Different Categories

Partial D Category	Reaction of red cells with monoclonal antibody to							
	epD1	epD2	epD3	epD4	epD5	epD6/7	epD8	epD9
II	+	+	+	0	+	+	+	0
IIIa	+	+	+	+	+	+	+	+
IIIb	+	+	+	+	+	+	+	+
IIIc	+	+	+	+	+	+	+	+
IVa	0	0	0	+	+	+	+	0
IVb	0	0	0	0	+	+	+	+
Va	0	+	+	+	0	+	+	+
VI	0	0	+	+	0	0	0	+
VII	+	+	+	+	+	+	0	+
DFR	+/0	+/0	+	+	+/0	+/0	0	+
DBT	0	0	0	0	0	+/0	+	0
D of R^{oHar}	0	0	0	0	+/0	+/0	0	0

+ = epitope present; 0 = epitope absent; +/0 positive with some, negative with other MAb with apparently the same epitope specificity.

must lack epitopes of D not listed in table 12-10. Second, some partial D cells listed in table 12-10 react with some but not with other MAb to D that, in tests with the other partial D red cells in the table, appear to have the same epitope specificity. These findings show that the MAb to D involved, have similar but not identical specificities. Daniels et al. (216) and Jones et al. (218) have published data that show differences among the MAb that initially appeared to define epD6/7. Daniels et al. (216) list eight different epitopes (epD6/7.1 to epD6/7.8) defined by these antibodies, differences in the specificities of the antibodies are all based on their patterns of reactions with partial D phenotypes DFR, DBT and the D made by R^{oHar}. Jones et al. (218) show two further specificities (their terminology is epD6/7a to epD6/7j) determined from tests that included two additional partial D phenotypes HMi and HMii. The basis for these subdivisions is shown in table 12-11, it should be noted that Jones et al. (218) describe their numbering system as temporary and comment that it will be revised at a future international workshop on monoclonal antibodies. Those workers who refer to the publication of Jones et al. (218) should be aware that a letter to the Editor (reference given with 218) was later published to correct some of the results printed in the original paper. While the data in tables 12-10 and 12-11 represent the current (December 1995) state of the art and are useful to illustrate the extreme complexity of the D antigen, there is little doubt but that

they will have been expanded, revised and/or corrected before this book is published.

As mentioned briefly above, the original subcategory Vc has been reassigned to the heterogeneous IVb category. This was done (494) when it was found that epitope specific monoclonal anti-D failed to demonstrate any difference between Vc and IVb red cells.

In concluding this section on detection of epitopes of D with monoclonal antibodies, it must be stressed that the serological reactions are very much technique dependent. Thus while an epitope may appear to be absent when the MAb is used by one method, it may be seen to be present when a different test system is used. It is hoped that the data given in table 12-11 represent the total positive reactions of the MAb used.

Which Epitopes of D are Most Immunogenic in D- Persons?

The answer to the question that heads this section is not known. However, some pertinent observations can be made. First, partial D category VI red cells react with fewer (i.e. 35%, see table 12-8) anti-D made by D- persons than do the red cells of other categories. Second, category VI red cells carry fewer epitopes of D than do those of other categories (see table 12-10). Third, category VI red cells fail to react with any of the 10 different

TABLE 12-11 Subdivision of Monoclonal Antibodies to epD6/7

Name used for the epitope		Present (+), absent (0) on partial D red cells of phenotype				
Daniels et al. (216)	Jones et al. (218)	DFR	DBT	D of R^{oHar}	HMi	HMii
epD6/7.1	epD6/7a	+	+	+	+	+
epD6/7.2	epD6/7b	+	+	0	+	+
epD6/7.3	epD6/7c	+	0	+	+	+
epD6/7.4		+	0	0		
	epD6/7d	+	0	0	+	+
	epD6/7e	+	0	0	+	0
epD6/7.5	epD6/7f	0	+	+	+	+
epD6/7.6	epD6/7g	0	+	0	+	+
epD6/7.7	epD6/7h	0	0	+	+	+
epD6/7.8		0	0	0		
	epD6/7i	0	0	0	+	+
	epD6/7j	0	0	0	+	0

1. Results of tests against partial D red cells HMi and HMii given by Jones et al. (218) but not by Daniels et al. (216). Concordance of epD6/7.1, .2, .3, .5, .6 and .7 with epD6/7a, b, c, f, g and h may not be as complete as shown.
2. epD6/7.4 of Daniels et al. (216) could correspond to epD6/7d or epD6/7e of Jones et al. (218)
3. epD6/7.8 of Daniels et al. (216) could correspond to epD6/7i or epD6/7j of Jones et al. (218).

specificity MAb to epD6/7 (216,218). Thus it is tempting to speculate that when the immune system of a D- individual is confronted with the constellation of D epitopes on D+ red cells, it recognizes epD6/7 somewhat more readily than other epitopes present.

It should be added that adsorption studies using red cells of different partial D categories do not split polyclonal anti-D made in D- persons into specificities that recognize different partial D phenotypes.

Low Incidence Rh Antigens on Partial D Red Cells

1. D^{Cor} or Go^a

In 1956, Rosenfield et al. (96) described an antigen, D^{Cor}, that is found in Blacks. In 1967, anti-Go^a was described (500). Eventually it became appreciated that D^{Cor} and Go^a are the same antigen but in spite of the priority of D^{Cor}, the name Go^a has persisted. Further, in spite of the report (500) to the contrary, it is now clearly established (103,501) that Go^a is an Rh system antigen and is found on red cells that carry partial D. The antigen has a frequency between 1.9 and 2.8% in American Blacks (500,502,503) and anti-Go^a sometimes (but not always (504)) causes severe HDN ((500,505); reference 505 lists four otherwise unreported cases).

The Go^a antigen is found on the red cells of category IVa people (see table 12-12). Indeed, it is the presence of Go^a that helps identify red cells of that category. Partial D, category IVa, Go(a+) red cells have been seen in persons with the Rh haplotypes R^o, R^1, R^2 and D(C)-. When Go^a is made by the haplotype R^2, the E antigen made by that haplotype may give weaker than usual reactions in serological tests (506). The $D^{IV}(C)$- haplotype encodes the low incidence antigens Go^a, Rh33, Riv (Rh45) and FPTT (Rh50) (107,114).

Although partial D, category IVa red cells lack (at least) epD1, epD2, epD3 and epD9 (see table 12-10) they react more strongly than do other D+ red cells, with most examples of human anti-D made by D- persons. Presumably the epitopes of D on category IVa red cells are either more readily accessible to anti-D or are present in higher numbers, than those on other D+ red cells.

2. Rh37 or Evans

Although this antigen is described in more detail in the later section on the D•• haplotype, it needs to be mentioned here. While partial D, category IVb red cells

TABLE 12-12 Low Incidence Rh Antigens Associated with Red Cells that Carry Partial D (for references, see text)

Partial D Category	Low Incidence Antigen
IVa	Go^a and see footnote 1
IVb	Perhaps Rh37, but see footnote 2
Va	D^w
VI	BARC, but see footnote 3
VII	Tar
DFR	FPTT
DBT	Rh32, but see footnote 4
D of R^{oHar}	Rh33

1. The rare haplotype $D^{IV}(C)$- encodes production of the low incidence antigens Go^a, Rh33, Riv (Rh45) and FPTT (Rh50).
2. At one time it was thought that some category IVb red cells would adsorb, and yield on elution, some examples of anti-Go^a. It is now believed that the cells react with sera that contain anti-Go^a and anti-Rh37 (anti-Evans) but not with those that contain only anti-Go^a. No serum containing anti-Rh37 alone, is available.
3. Anti-BARC reacted with 76 of 78 category VI red cells of individuals with the R^1 haplotype but not with those of 21 persons in whom D^{VI} was made by R^2.
4. Rh32 was first recognized as a product of the $\bar{\bar{R}}^N$ haplotype. However, partial D cells of the DBT phenotype carry Rh32 and some are from individuals who do not have $\bar{\bar{R}}^N$.

type as Go(a-) in direct typing tests, it had been noticed (507) that some of them would adsorb, and yield on elution, some examples of anti-Go^a. Daniels (508) reports that this finding may represent the presence of Rh37 on category IVb red cells and the presence of anti-Rh37 in some sera that contain anti-Go^a. The cells react with those sera that contain anti-Go^a and anti-Rh37 but not with those that contain just anti-Go^a. No example of anti-Rh37 without anti-Go^a is available, further to study the situation.

3. D^w (formerly D^{Wiel})

In 1962, Chown et al. (93) described the antigen Wiel that eventually became known as D^w. The antigen was found on the red cells of 9 of 235 Blacks, but none of 13,000 Whites (509). The original suspicion (93) that Wiel was an Rh antigen was soon confirmed (509,510). The antigen is present on partial D red cells of category Va, as far as we are aware, it has not been found on other red cells.

4. BARC or Rh52

This antigen was admitted to the Rh system, as Rh52, at the 1996 meeting of the ISBT working party on terminology for red cell surface antigens (943). Anti-BARC was initially seen (511) to define a low incidence antigen present on the partial D, category VI red cells of individuals with the haplotype $CD^{VI}e$. It is not present on the category VI red cells of individuals with $cD^{VI}E$. The most recent count (216) indicates that of 78 $CD^{VI}e$/cde samples, 76 were Rh:52 (BARC+). All of 21 $cD^{VI}E$/cde samples were Rh:-52 (BARC-). As described later in this chapter, the $cD^{VI}E$ haplotype, that is said to encode partial D, category VI, type 1, represents a different genetic change than $CD^{VI}e$, that is said to encode partial D, category VI, type II (211). Since category VI red cells are now identified via D epitope pattern, using monoclonal (epitope-specific) anti-D, it is possible that the two $CD^{VI}e$/cde Rh:-52 samples represent a new category with a similar epitope composition to $CD^{VI}e$/cde Rh:52. The gene conversion events that result in the formation of $CD^{VI}e$ and $cD^{VI}E$, are described later in this chapter.

5. Tar or Rh40

In 1975, Humphreys et al. (512) described the low incidence antigen Tar. Shortly thereafter Lewis et al. (52) showed that the antigen is part of the Rh system and it was assigned the number Rh40. Several examples of anti-Rh40 and Tar+ red cells had been reported (513-515) before it was shown (516) that the Tar antigen is present on red cells with partial D, the new category was called VII. One family in which Tar is encoded by D-- has been described (513). The D antigen on Tar+ red cells (other than those that are D--) gives slightly weaker than normal reactions with polyclonal anti-D but it is necessary to equal the expertise of Lewis et al. (52) in capillary tube typing, to demonstrate the weakening.

6. FPTT or Rh50

In 1988, Bizot et al. (114) described the low incidence antigen FPTT that was present on Rh:33 red cells and on some with previously undescribed phenotypes with depressed expressions of Rh antigens. In 1994, Lomas et al. (115) showed that FPTT, that was given the number Rh50, is present on red cells of a partial D phenotype that was named DFR. As can be seen from table 12-10, DFR red cells react with some but not other MAb to D, that otherwise appear to have the same epitope specificity. Clearly, DFR red cells will be useful in the further division of epitope specificity of MAb to D.

7. Rh32

The low incidence antigen Rh32 has long been recognized (98,99) as a product of the $\overline{\overline{R}}^N$ haplotype, that is described in detail later in this chapter. However, Rh32 has also now been found (245) on red cells with partial D, that were not from individuals who had $\overline{\overline{R}}^N$. The partial D phenotype, that differs in D epitope composition from any other (see table 12-10) has been named DBT.

8. Rh33

Among a number of highly unusual characteristics (see later in this chapter) the R^{oHar} haplotype, first described by Giles et al. (100) in 1971, encodes production of a difficult to detect form of D. Red cells from R^{oHar}/r individuals were often initially thought to be D- (244) although an occasional polyclonal anti-D reacted well with such cells (100,243). More recently, some monoclonal anti-D have been seen (245) to react with the red cells of individuals genetically R^{oHar}/r, as if those cells carry normal, unremarkable D antigen. Another product of R^{oHar} is the low incidence antigen Rh33. For many years it was not known if the D made by R^{oHar} differed from normal D in a qualitative, or merely a quantitative manner. Beckers et al. (246) have now shown that the D encoded by R^{oHar} is indeed partial D. The epitope composition of the D made, is shown in table 12-10. One of the three individuals with R^{oHar} studied, made anti-D (246), another example that caused mild HDN has since been seen (247). Further, as described in detail in a later section of this chapter, the molecular genetic basis of R^{oHar} is now known (248). Thus the low incidence antigen Rh33 is shown to be the product of another haplotype that makes partial D, as described above it had previously been seen to be made also by $D^{IV}(C)$- (114). Daniels (508) points out that the D made by R^{oHar} differs from other partial D in another respect. Generally, weak D is best detected by IgG anti-D using the IAT. The D of R^{oHar} was detected by four of four IgM but only 5 of 24 IgG, monoclonal anti-D (241).

9. Riv or Rh45

As mentioned several times above, one of the products of $D^{IV}(C)$- haplotype is the low incidence antigen Riv. Since no example of Riv+ red cells in an individual who does not have $D^{IV}(C)$- has been found, it is not yet possible to decide whether Riv is associated with partial D in the same manner as other antigens described in this section.

The low incidence Rh antigens whose presence is

associated with partial D phenotypes, are listed in table 12-12. Some other features of partial D red cells are shown in table 12-13.

TABLE 12-13 Some Other Features of Red Cells that Carry Partial D
Unless otherwise shown, data are from Tippett (493) and Daniels (508)

Category	Features
II	Three propositi studied were all White. Partial D encoded by $CD^{II}e$ in two families studied.
IIIa and IIIb	Most propositi are Black and are phenotypically C- E-. Some have red cells that react with all examples of anti-VS but only some examples of anti-V. IIIa red cells are G+.
IIIb	Cells are G-, some are hr^s-.
IIIc	All propositi are White, red cells are C+ G+ V- VS-.
IVa	Most propositi are Black, partial D most often encoded by $cD^{IV}e$.
IVb	Most propositi are White, the subcategory (that now includes that previously called Vc) is heterogeneous. Four IVb individuals found in tests on more than 5 million Japanese (521).
Va	More common in Blacks ($cD^{V}e$) than in Whites ($CD^{V}e$), one family with $cD^{V}E$ found (67).
Vb	One family only, family was White.
VI	Majority of propositi are White, $CD^{VI}e$ most common but $cD^{VI}E$ and $cD^{VI}e$ also found. Some category VI red cells may have an unusual form of G (122, 123). Fairly large scale tests in England, the Netherlands, Australia and the USA (242, 522-524) have established a frequency of category VI between 0.02 and 0.04% in (predominantly) White populations. One category VI sample was found (521) in tests on over 5 million Japanese blood donors.
VII	Propositi are predominently White and most have $CD^{VII}e$.

A Note on Formation of the Low Incidence Antigens Just Described

Although the topic is discussed in detail in a later section of this chapter, it can be mentioned here that production of Rh polypeptides that carry partial D has already been shown to result from three different genetic mechanisms. First, at the time of meiosis, misalignment of *RHD* and *RHCE* can result in gene conversion in which one or more exons of one gene replace the equivalent exons of the other. Second, missplicing of one or more exons within the gene may occur. Third, point mutation involving nucleotide substitution may produce

a codon that encodes an amino acid different from that in the wild type protein. Following any one of these three events, the polypeptide made will have an amino acid sequence different from that encoded by the common forms of *RHD* and *RHCE*. If a portion of the new sequence of amino acids is immunogenic, it may stimulate production of an antibody that recognizes the rare protein structure, i.e. an antibody to a low incidence antigen. Not only does such a hypothesis provide a highly plausible explanation of the antigens Go^a, D^w, Rh32, Rh33, Rh37, Tar, Riv, FPTT and BARC, it may also explain some other observations. First, gene conversion, missplicing or mutation involving exons common to more than one gene, might explain production of the same low incidence antigen by two originally dissimilar genes. Second, homology but not exact identity of the region containing the new amino acid sequence, might explain antibody cross-reactivity or the presence of inseparable antibodies of apparently different specificities in the same serum. As an example, the original Tillett serum appeared to contain anti-Go^a, anti-Rh32 and anti-Evans. However, red cells carrying Go^a or Rh32 or Evans, but lacking the other two, would adsorb the serum to exhaustion (104). Perhaps the serum actually contained an antibody to an amino acid sequence common to the three antigens, hence its apparent content of three antibodies. It is possible that the finding mentioned above, that category IVb red cells react with sera that contain anti-Go^a and anti-Evans, but not with those sera that contain anti-Go^a, represents a similar situation.

Recognition of Partial D Phenotypes via Presence of a Low Incidence Antigen

As the previous section shows, presence of certain low incidence antigens may be an indication that the red cells involved belong to a category of partial D. However, the finding of such an antigen by no means establishes that fact. Over the years, one of us (PDI) has been sent a number of Go(a+) samples that, it was assumed belonged to category IVa. In fact some them had normal D. The explanation, of course, was that the other *Rh* haplotype in the individual made D. In other words, while an individual genetically *CD$^{IV}e/cde$* who has Go(a+) red cells will have the category IVa phenotype, one who is genetically *CD$^{IV}e/cDe$* and has Go(a+) red cells, will have a normal D+ phenotype.

Clinical Significance of the Anti-D made by Individuals with Partial D on their Red Cells

There is no doubt that the anti-D made by persons

with partial D on their red cells are clinically important. Most of the recognized specificities have caused transfusion reactions (118,119,485,487,491,525,526) and HDN (117,119,120,184,497,527,529-533,566). Some of the cases of HDN have been fatal or particularly severe. These findings, of course, prompt the question (discussed below) as to whether Rh immune globulin should be used in women of partial D phenotypes, who deliver D+ infants.

Clinical Significance of Partial D on the Red Cells of Blood Donors

There seems little doubt that the red cells of some categories of partial D would be capable of stimulating production of anti-D, if transfused to D- individuals. However, this aspect of transfusion is not as much of a problem as it may at first appear. The major reason, of course, is that most red cells that carry partial D, react as D+ in currently used typing tests. In other words, most units from such donors are typed as D+ and are transfused to D+ recipients, usually without any knowledge that the red cells involved carry partial D. Recent experience (277) suggests that those red cells that carry qualitatively altered or quantitatively reduced amounts of D, such that they type as D- in current routine test systems, are either non-immunogenic or only poorly so, in D- recipients.

There is one report (535) of a D- woman making anti-D after delivery of an infant with partial D, category Va red cells. In another case (536) RhIG failed to remove the infant's partial D red cells from the maternal circulation but the woman did not make anti-D. As discussed below, it is not clear that RhIG works by clearing D+ red cells from the maternal circulation, anyway.

Quantitatively Reduced Expression of D

The clinical importance, or to be more precise the lack thereof, of the weak D phenotype (formerly D^u) when the difference between normal D and the weak D is purely quantitative, has been discussed at length, above. Accordingly this section will deal with the expression of D on weak D red cells and the mechanisms that bring about the down regulation of expression of D. As indicated earlier, these forms of weak D involve a reduced number of copies of D on red cells but presence of all the D epitopes. Thus individuals with red cells of these phenotypes are unable to make alloimmune anti-D.

Studies with both polyclonal and monoclonal anti-D have been used to determine the number of D antigen sites on red cells. When human polyclonal anti-D were used (265,266) normal D+ red cells of the R_1r and R_2R_2

phenotypes were found to carry about 10,000 and 30,000 sites per red cell, respectively. In contrast, on red cells of weak phenotypes, the D sites per red cell were found to vary over a range of about 300 to about 9000 (267-269).

Although the phenotypic situations that result in these forms of weak D are partially understood (see below), the exact mechanisms that cause down regulation of expression of D, when all epitopes of D are present, are not. Beckers et al. (537) studied six samples with weak D, in which it had been shown that the D antigen site number was between 500 and 1000 per red cell. Four of the samples were D+ C+ c+ E- e+, two were D+ C- c+ E+ e+. All six individuals had an *RHD* gene that was grossly normal when studied by Southern blot analysis and by PCR amplification of selected regions of the gene. Thus no obvious mechanism was apparent to explain the low number of copies of D on the weak D red cells of these individuals. Clearly additional studies will be necessary to determine whether an inefficient transcriptional process, an abnormality in post-transcriptional regulation, an inefficient translation process, or some other mechanism is involved. Eventually, the explanation of the weak D phenotype in individuals with apparently normal *RHD* genes may also explain the well established finding that expression of D is affected by the other gene in the *Rh* haplotype. As mentioned earlier (see table 12-7) R_1R_1 red cells carry between 15,000 and 20,000 D sites per cell, while those of individuals genetically R^2R^2 carry between 16,000 and 32,000 per cell.

The *trans* Position Type of Weak D

In 1952, Ceppellini et al. (270) reported that in some individuals, *C* on one chromosome affects the actions of *D* on the other to such a degree that the individuals concerned present with the weak D phenotype. That the phenotype involved gene interaction was clear for it was demonstrated that the *D* gene, in the parents or children of the weak D individual, encoded production of normal D when *C* was not in *trans*. Other examples of this weak D phenotype have been reported (271,296,382,538,539). In cases studied in detail, it has been noticed that this type of weak D is most often found in persons of genotypes *R_1r' (CDe/Cde)* or *$R^o r'$ (cDe/Cde)*. However, *r^y (CdE)* has also been shown to exert a depressing effect on *D* in *trans* (540). It is somewhat perplexing that on other occasions *C* in *trans* to *D* has had no effect on the function of *D* (382,541).

The Directly Inherited Form of Weak D

A different form of weak D, in which all epitopes of

D seem to be present so that the individuals involved cannot form alloimmune anti-D, involves the inheritance of a form of *D* gene that makes less than the usual amount of D. This is sometimes called the inherited form of weak D, a poor choice of terms since all forms of weak and partial D result from the genes inherited. In this type of weak D, the *D* gene present does not appear to be influenced by any other *Rh* genes in *trans* (or in *cis*) and seems to be passed as a normal character in families (256,257). As yet, nothing is known about the mechanism that results in this form of *D* encoding fewer than normal copies of the D antigen.

Rh Immune Globulin and the Weak D Phenotype

Because the weak D phenotype sometimes represents lack of some epitopes of the D antigen, a few people of that phenotype can form alloimmune anti-D. As a result, the question arises as to whether women with weak D red cells, who give birth to D+ infants, should be protected with Rh Immune Globulin. Some authorities (498,542) feel that the incidence of formation of anti-D by persons with weak D red cells is so low that Rh immune globulin need not be given. Further, it is sometimes argued that the anti-D, if injected, will bind to the woman's own weak D red cells so will not be protective. In fact, there are two established counters to such an argument. First, experimental studies (543) have shown that because of their partial D status, the womens' own cells bind relatively little of the injected anti-D. Second, it is far from clear how RhIG prevents immunization to D. It is entirely possible that the injected anti-D, even if bound in part to the womens' own weak D+ red cells, could still prevent immunization to D. Other workers (283,543,544) believe that women with partial D on the red cells should receive RhIG after delivery of a D+ infant. It is sometimes argued that the use of RhIG for women with weak D on the red cells is unnecessary and wastes money. However, it has also been pointed out (284,285) that the cost of performing tests for weak D on the blood of 15 to 17% of recently delivered women is probably far more than the cost of giving Rh immune globulin to the few who have weak D red cells. In other words, if all recently-delivered women whose red cells typed as D- were injected with the product and no tests for weak D were done, the total cost might be lower than that involved if tests for weak D were done and a few injections (to women with weak D) were not given.

One of us has pointed out elsewhere (311) that there is a middle road. If the woman's red cells that carry weak D are typed for C, those that fail to react must come from women whose weak D phenotype cannot by caused by *C*

in *trans* to *D*. Those women can then be injected with Rh immune globulin on the basis that many of them may have the partial D type of weak D. Those whose cells are C+ can be denied Rh immune globulin since it can be assumed that many of them have the *trans* position type of weak D so cannot form alloimmune anti-D. Obviously this method is not 100% accurate. Some of the C- weak D+ women will not be able to form anti-D while some whose cells are C+ will lack some epitopes of D. However, C-typing does provide some sort of division between people with weak D red cells, who can and cannot make anti-D.

It is probable that this subject is not as important as the controversy makes it appear. First, the formation of anti-D by an individual with weak D on the red cells is a rare event. Second, as already described, most women whose red cells lack epitopes of D will not be recognized in routine typing tests since their red cells will type as D+. However, a case can be made (543) for the use of RhIG in women with weak D on the red cells and it is difficult to understand the vehemence of those not wishing to use Rh immune globulin in this setting, in insisting that no others should use it either. It seems that the decision to use the prophylactic should be an individual one and that its use or non-use in women with weak D on the red cells, can both be justified.

It would be extremely useful if the weak D phenotype that represents lack of some epitopes of D could be distinguished serologically from the phenotype that represents a *trans* position effect of *C*. Obviously, the reason is that individuals of the partial D phenotype can form anti-D if transfused with D+ blood while those of the *trans* position type cannot. However, there is as yet no simple test for distinguishing between the two types of weak D.

Transient Auto-Anti-D Production by Persons with Partial D on their Red Cells

Throughout the earlier sections of this chapter, it has been stressed that the D+ people who make anti-D make alloantibodies. In contrast, it is well established that some individuals with autoimmune hemolytic anemia make auto-anti-D. Clinically significant autoantibodies and benign auto-anti-D in persons with normal D+, not partial D red cells, are described in Chapters 37 and 39 so will not be discussed further, here. However, some individuals with partial D red cells, when first immunized, do make anti-D that reacts with their own red cells. This situation was first recognized in 1963 (483) and has been reported sporadically since (548-552). In the experience of one of us (PDI), although the production of anti-D by a D+ subject is in itself a rare event (due to the rarity of the partial D phenotypes) the production of a benign auto-anti-D often precedes or accompanies early production of the allo-anti-D. From the cases studied, a number of observations have been made. First, the anti-D had true specificity and were not of the mimicking type described in Chapter 37. Second, in each instance, the auto-anti-D appeared benign in vivo. Third, the positive DAT was almost always seen (and anti-D eluted) in the first sample in which serum anti-D was detected. In spite of this, the cases did not involve the binding of allo-anti-D to remaining transfused D+ cells. The positive DAT reactions were not of the mixed-field type and in some cases the interval between transfusion and development of the positive DAT was too long for transfused cells still to be present. Fourth, the cases did not involve production of anti-LW (that in its weakest form can look like anti-D, see Chapter 13). Fifth, nearly all the cases followed the transfusion of D+ blood to individuals who had originally been typed as D+ and not as weak D. In some cases that were followed, the anti-D being made eventually became just an alloantibody. That is, it no longer reacted with the red cells of the antibody-maker or with those of others of a similar partial D phenotype. On other occasions, the anti-D continued to react with the antibody-maker's red cells but remained benign in nature. There are several reports in the literature of simultaneous production of allo and autoantibodies (51,327,549,550,552-561) some of which (327,553, 559,561) involved an autoantibody that did destroy the patient's own red cells. One of us (PDI) suspects, but cannot prove, that sometimes when alloimmunization occurs, the antibody first released is of poor fit (sloppy specificity). This antibody is often regarded as "non-specific" autoantibody. Later, as the immunocytes release slightly better refined molecules, the antibody may appear to have a definable specificity, but may still react with the antibody-maker's red cells if they carry an antigen similar to the one that elicited the immune response. It is to this place that this author (PDI) would assign auto-anti-D of the type being discussed, if later it can be shown that the individual is no longer producing autoantibody. Eventually, when the activated immunocytes make molecules of good fit, the antibody no longer binds to the antibody-maker's red cells. A similar argument is used in Chapter 13 to explain the anti-LW sometimes made by Rh- persons as a prelude to the production of anti-D. It should be added that not all cases of apparent autoantibody production can be explained in this manner. Before invoking this explanation it is necessary to exclude: true autoantibody production causing in vivo red cell destruction; alloantibodies bound to transfused red cells; mimicking specificity antibodies; injection of Rh immune globulin (it has been given to Rh+ infants and fathers instead of the Rh- mother (562-565)); and the

non-specific uptake of IgG by red cells.

Red Cells that React as if They Carry Increased Amounts of D

The red cells of individuals of certain blood group phenotypes react with anti-D as if they carry increased amounts of D antigen. Such is the reaction of some of these red cells that they are agglutinated in saline tests with selected anti-D, that otherwise behave as incomplete (antiglobulin test-active) antibodies. At one time it was believed that D+ red cells of the phenotype En(a-) and those from individuals with the M^k or Mi^V genes had greatly exalted amounts of D (567,568). Although such cells are strongly agglutinated by anti-D and will react in saline with some of them, it is now appreciated that this occurs because in certain MN system phenotypes (including those mentioned above) there is a reduction of sialic acid on the red cell membrane (569-576). Thus these cells behave somewhat like red cells treated with proteolytic enzymes, that do in fact remove sialic acid and other structures from the membrane. It has already been pointed out that the reactions of Rh antibodies are enhanced in serological tests against enzyme-premodified red cells. Thus in spite of the enhanced reactions of these cells with anti-D and other Rh antibodies, they will not be further considered here.

When enhancement of D is considered in terms of Rh phenotypes, it is seen that red cells of the phenotypes D--/D-- and D••/D•• react more strongly with anti-D than do any others. It was originally supposed (90,577) that the enhanced D on these cells represented the fact that the *D* genes present in the individuals involved, did not have to compete with *CcEe* genes for available precursor substance. However, now that it is known that *Rh* genes encode production of their antigen-bearing structures directly, and do not use a precursor substance, a different explanation is required. It seems probable that on D--/D-- and D••/D•• red cells, access of the D antigen to anti-D is easier than usual, because no CcEe-bearing structures are present to impede such access. As shown in table 12-7, D--/D-- red cells appear to have some 110,000 to 200,000 D sites. For R_2R_2 cells the number is in the order of 16,000 to 33,500. While this appears to indicate that D--/D-- red cells carry more D sites than do R_2R_2 red cells, it must be remembered that the site numbers were calculated from tests that measured the red cells' ability to bind molecules of anti-D. In other words, R_2R_2 cells may have more D sites than the figures suggest but the cE-bearing proteins present on those cells may block the access of anti-D to some of those sites. Alternatively, perhaps red cells need a certain number of Rh antigen-bearing proteins on the surface, to ensure membrane integrity. Perhaps in the absence of CcEe-bearing proteins, the *D* genes compensate by producing additional numbers of D-bearing structures.

Other red cell samples that give enhanced reactions with anti-D are those that are Go(a+) and those from individuals with $\bar{\bar{R}}^N$ and one form of a gene best written as *(C)D(e)* (i.e. similar to $\bar{\bar{R}}^N$, see later). As described above, Go(a+) red cells react more strongly with anti-D than do most other D+ red cells, although they lack some epitopes of D. For red cells from persons with $\bar{\bar{R}}^N$ and *(C)D(e)*, the same concept as that described above may apply, since in both instances less C and e than that made by $R^1(CDe)$ appear to be present. As shown in table 12-7, among red cells with common Rh phenotypes, R^2R^2 red cells react more strongly with anti-D than do those of other phenotypes. Occasionally the serum of a rr individual may appear to contain anti-E since it reacts with R_2R_2 red cells, but may actually be seen to contain anti-D when more sensitive tests are used (578). In such cases the positive reactions with R_2R_2 cells represent the presence of anti-D, of a strength such that it will react only with cells with stronger than usual D, by certain methods. Again, it is possible that the cE-bearing protein causes less impediment to access to D, than do the Ce and ce-bearing proteins.

At the beginning of this section it was mentioned that D--/D-- and D••/D•• red cells are agglutinated in saline test systems by some incomplete anti-D. It should not be assumed that all incomplete anti-D possess this ability. While human polyclonal anti-D that agglutinate D--/D-- red cells are relatively easy to find, only uncommon exceptional examples will similarly agglutinate the red cells of *D--* heterozygotes (i.e. R^1/D--). Indeed, in family studies involving searches for the presence of *D--* in the heterozygous form, methods such as those using the flow cytometer (371) are far more reliable. Fewer incomplete anti-D agglutinate D••/D•• than agglutinate D--/D-- red cells in saline systems. In one study (579), 98 incomplete anti-D were tested against red cells of both phenotypes. Of those sera 42 agglutinated D--/D-- and D••/D•• red cells, 38 agglutinated only D--/D-- red cells and 18 agglutinated neither. This finding correlates with the fact that D••/D•• red cells appear (579) to have about 56,000 available D sites per red cell, that is over twice as many as R_2R_2 cells but only a quarter to a half as many as D--/D-- cells.

G and Anti-G

Before 1958, many workers had been puzzled about the production and serological reactions of some antibodies with apparent anti-C plus anti-D (anti-CD) specificity. Sometimes rr individuals exposed to R_o (cDe) or r'

(Cde) cells, via pregnancy or transfusion, made anti-CD. When R_o cells carried the immunogen, production of anti-C was unexpected, when r' cells carried the immunogen production of anti-D was unexplained (580,581). When some examples of anti-CD were tested, in adsorption studies with R_o or r' cells, it was found that either cell type would adsorb the anti-CD to exhaustion. Further, eluates made from the R_o or the r' cells contained apparent anti-CD specificity. These unexpected findings were generally attributed to an assumed similarity between the C and D antigens and cross-reactivity of some examples of anti-CD. This was an unsatisfactory explanation for two reasons. First, many other examples of anti-C and anti-D, that showed no inclination to cross-react, had been found. Second, other examples of anti-CD behaved as expected in adsorption studies in that separable anti-C and anti-D could be shown to be present. Most of the answers were provided in 1958, when Allen and Tippett (86) described the Rh antigen, G. It was shown that genes that that make C and almost all those that make D, make G as well. Those genes that do not make C or D do not usually make G. Since R_o cells were now known to be cDeG and r' cells to be CdeG, it became clear that anti-G would look like anti-CD in antibody identification studies. Those rr individuals who had apparently made anti-CD following exposure to R_o or r' cells had actually made anti-G sometimes with and sometimes without anti-D and anti-C, respectively. Those examples of apparent anti-CD that could be adsorbed to exhaustion with R_o or r' cells were actually anti-G. Allen and Tippett (86) recognized existence of the G antigen when they found red cells of the very rare phenotype C- D- G+. Since that time the almost equally rare phenotype D+ G- has been found (67,92,582,583). As discussed in the section on partial D, category IIIb red cells are D+ G-, Cape Colored and Bantu people in South Africa have been reported (92,499,517) to have partial D cells of the $Rh_o{}^d$ phenotype, that are also G-. As far as we are aware there has been only one claim (589) that a C+ G- sample has been found. That report is discussed further in the last paragraph of this section. Vos (584) showed that red cells that carry weak D and are C-, often have reduced expression of G.

Red cells that are: r' or C+ D- G+; R_1 or C+ D+ G+; R_o or C- D+ G+; and r or C- D- G-; are normally used in antibody identification studies so that the identification of anti-G in the presence of anti-C and/or anti-D is not straightforward. Further, C- D- G+ and D+ G- cells are extremely rare and are not generally available for routine antibody identification work. However, it is possible to use R_o and r' cells in sequential adsorption-elution studies to determine which anti-CD sera contain anti-G and which lack that antibody (584). The serum is first adsorbed with R_o or r' cells. An eluate from the adsorbing cells is made.

The eluate is then adsorbed with the other cells (r′ or R_o dependent on which were used first) and a second eluate is made. Table 12-14 illustrates the principle of the double elution method and is sufficiently self-explanatory that the technique need not be described further here.

When Allen and Tippett (86) first described the G antigen, they reported that most of the anti-CD sera that they studied contained anti-G. One of us (PDI) became concerned that many workers subsequently assumed that all (or most) sera that behaved as anti-CD, had anti-G specificity. Accordingly, a study was undertaken (585) to

TABLE 12-14 Adsorption-Elution Procedure for the Recognition of Anti-G

Antibodies present in the raw serum.	Anti-D Anti-C Anti-G	Anti-D Anti-C
Phenotype of red cells used for the first adsorption.	cDeG	cDeG
Antibodies present in the first eluate.	Anti-D Anti-G	Anti-D
Phenotype of red cells used for the second adsorption.	CdeG	CdeG
Antibody present in the second eluate.	Anti-G	None

determine the incidence of anti-G in sera that behaved as anti-CD. We found that all of 11 commercially-available anti-CD or anti-CDE typing reagents contained a potent anti-G component. However, in tests on 50 single donor anti-CD sera we showed, by the double elution procedure, that only 15 (30%) contained anti-G. This, in spite of the fact that 37 of the raw sera reacted with C- D- G+ red cells. We concluded that the 22 sera that reacted in the raw state with C- D- G+ red cells, but from which no separable anti-G could be isolated, contained anti-C^G together with anti-C and/or anti-D (see later in this chapter for a description of the C^G antigen). We also concluded that while hyperimmune anti-CD and anti-CDE sera (those used in the pools from which the commercial reagents were made) almost always contain anti-G, the antibody is much less frequent in individuals (those from whom the single donor anti-CD were obtained) who have had less exposure to C, D and G. Our methods were subsequently criticized (586) but we pointed out (587) that first, there was no evidence to support the contention that there was anything inappropriate about our methods and that second, our findings that about 30% of single donor anti-CD contain anti-G were in complete agreement with earlier, smaller studies (177,584,588). Indeed, our study

(585) is the largest one performed to determine the true incidence of anti-G and probably established the frequency of that antibody more reliably than those that preceded it. Our study also showed that the sometimes expressed fear that r′ blood may be immunogenic in rr recipients because the cells carry G as well as C, does not constitute cause to regard r′ blood as Rh+. Indeed, G appears to be no more immunogenic than C, that is poorly immunogenic in rr individuals anyway. It is clear that in order for anti-G to be made, rr individuals who have already made anti-C and anti-D, must be exposed to additional G+ red cells before the antibody is made in appreciable amounts.

Although anti-G is most often seen as a component of a hyperimmune response in individuals with D- C- G- red cells, it can be made by others who have G- red cells. The antibody has been found (123,493) as a separable component in the sera of partial D, category IIIb individuals, in others (92,499,517) with partial D (i.e. $Rh_o{}^d$) and in some (582,583) described as phenotypically D+ G-. Several examples of monoclonal anti-G have been produced (224,518-520).

From what has been written above it will be abundantly clear that G has a close relationship to C and D. Additional early evidence of this fact was provided by Allen and Tippett (528) and by Nijenhuis (591) who showed that presence of anti-G on red cells would at least partially block the uptake of anti-C and anti-D, and more surprisingly sometimes anti-e, by those cells. As discussed in more detail later in this chapter, genetic control of G antigen production is now understood at the molecular level. Briefly, the Rh polypeptides that carry C and D share the same amino acid sequence from residue 50 to residue 103, the region encoded by exon 2 of *RHD* and *RHC*. When that sequence is encoded by *RHD* and *RHC* the exofacial amino acid at position 103 is serine. When the analogous sequence is encoded by *RHc*, proline occupies position 103 (41,204-207,545,546). In individuals with partial D, category IIIb red cells, exon 2 of the *RHD* gene is replaced by exon 2 of an *RHc* gene (560). The D-c-D hybrid protein encoded thus lacks some epitopes of D (not yet characterized, see table 12-10) and has proline at exofacial position 103, the red cells are D+ G-. Clearly the exofacial serine at position 103 of both the C-bearing and the normal (wild type) D-bearing polypeptides is involved in expression of both C and G. Daniels (508) makes the eminently logical suggestion that it appears that anti-C recognizes a serine 103-based structure on the C-bearing but not on the D-bearing polypeptide, while anti-G recognizes a serine 103-based structure on both the C and D-bearing proteins. The finding that G is apparently encoded by exon 2 of both *RHD* and *RHC* makes the single report (589) mentioned above, of an individual with D+ C+ c+ E+ e+

G- red cells, difficult to understand.

an anti-C^G component.

The r^G Gene

Allen and Tippett (86) assigned the term r^G to describe the gene that makes G but no D. Because the proposita in their study was $r^G r$, samples from other family members were studied in an attempt to define exactly the products of r^G. In one, in whom r^G was paired with a gene making E not e, it was shown that r^G makes e. However, no family member had r^G paired with a gene that did not make c, so it could not be determined whether r^G makes that antigen. In 1961, Levine et al. (87) reported an individual said to be genetically $r^G r^G$. The blood of the propositus was studied again in 1975 by Rosenfield et al. (63) who used quantitative methods (62,65) to determine the r^G gene products. It was shown that r^G is not simply a r gene that also encodes production of G. To summarize a very detailed study (63), it was shown that r^G makes: less G than do genes that make C or D; Hr and Hr_o (see later); and e. Earlier (87) it had been thought that r^G makes less e than other e-producing genes but in this study (63) it was shown that e production is near normal while production of two e-like antigens is abnormal. The r^G gene makes a reduced amount of hr^S and either no, or only a trace amount of hr^B (for hr^S and hr^B see later). The r^G gene does not make c, f (ce), E, C^W, C^X or rh_i (Ce). The question as to whether r^G makes some C, or another antigen called C^G, is discussed below in the section dealing with C^G. It has been reported (547) that the presence of r^G can result in serological findings that can be mistaken for exclusion of parentage. At least one woman of the r^G phenotype made anti-D following D+ pregnancies (590).

The r''^G Gene

Red cells of the phenotype D- C- E+ G+ in which production of G is sometimes reduced, had been found (67,592,593) but not reported in full when Case (594) described r''^G. Normally, r'' (cdE) does not make G so that these samples are highly unusual. Case (594) found that r''^G made normal c and that the red cells of an $r''^G r$ individual reacted with some anti-C sera. Rather than supposing that the r''^G gene was making a small amount of C, Case (594) preferred the explanation "that 'pure' anti-C is able, under appropriately sensitive conditions and in the absence of D, to recognize the G antigen in the products of atypical gene complexes, and thus to mistake it for C". As described in a later section, an alternative explanation is that G is often accompanied by a similar antigen, C^G, and that some but not all anti-C sera contain

Heterogeneity of r^G

After the description of r^G was published (86), other bloods from individuals with that gene were studied and it became apparent that considerable heterogeneity exists. In Blacks (123,590,595), r^G tends to make less G than does the equivalent gene in Whites (63,86,87). Rosenfield et al. (46) believed that some r^G genes make G without D or C while others make G without D but with a form of C that was named C^G. This distinction is far from clear and it is not certain whether the presence or absence of C^G or some form of C, is dependent on gene action or on the anti-C used to type the red cells. This subject is discussed in more detail in the next section.

In 1971, Beattie et al. (588) described a phenotype that they called r^{Gu}. The G antigen present was weak and best detected by IAT. It is entirely possible that the phenotype described is the r^G phenotype of Blacks. The r^G of Blacks may differ from the r^G of Whites in that the former but not the latter includes hr^H among its products (48). Beattie et al. (588) described r^{Gu} red cells as being V+ VS+, as discussed in a later section, it is probable that some "anti-VS" are, or contain, anti-hr^H. In describing the r^G phenotype that involves VS+ red cells, Daniels (508) uses the term r^{Gs} and points out that the phenotype is heterogeneous and may include the one described as r^{Gu}.

While the phenotypes expected when r^G, r^{Gu} and r'^S are present, can be described on paper, recognizing them at the practical level and differentiating between them can be exceedingly difficult. In addition to the similarities already described, the r'^S gene, whose actions are described below, encodes a remarkably similar phenotype. All the genes mentioned above make a form of C that may be difficult to detect, G that may vary considerably in amount made and e, some of them make VS. While the r^G series are said not to make c, while that antigen is made by r'^S, this will not help in the serological investigation if the paired haplotype makes c. If the paired haplotype makes C but not c, recognition of the atypical C made by the r^G or r'^S gene is impossible. One needs the luck of encountering a family in which the gene of interest (one of the r^G or r'^S genes) is paired with a C gene in some members and a c gene in others, to make the distinction with some degree of confidence.

The Antigen C^G

After several bloods from individuals with one or

two r^G genes had been studied, it became apparent that some of the red cells involved do react, albeit weakly, with some examples of anti-C. While the serological results have been similar in various laboratories, the names applied to the reactive antibodies are not the same. First, it must be pointed out that the anti-C sera that react with r^G cells are not simply the strongest examples of that antibody. In other words, the differences do not appear to be simply quantitative. Race and Sanger (49) regarded the positive reactions as indicating the presence of some form of C on the red cells. They described the reactive sera as anti-CC^G and the nonreactive ones as anti-C. However, the C^G designation in anti-CC^G was used simply to identify the reactive sera. It was not believed that anti-CC^G represented the presence of two antibodies. In the USA (44,48,63,87,311) the term anti-C^G is generally used to describe an antibody that defines an antigen similar to but not identical with C. In other words, all genes that make C also make C^G. Rare genes (such as r^G, r^{Gu} and perhaps r'^S) make C^G but not C. Again, the differences are largely semantic and will probably not be clarified until the structures of C and C^G (if indeed they differ) are understood at the biochemical level. Levine et al. (87) and Rosenfield et al. (46) felt that anti-C^G could be isolated from anti-CC^G, by adsorption on to and elution from, Rh:-1, -2,12,21 (D- C- G+ C^G+) red cells. However, they cautioned that few anti-Rh2 that lack anti-Rh1 and anti-Rh12 (anti-C without anti-D or anti-G), contain enough anti-C^G for the antibody to be isolated. These workers (46) also said that the anti-C agglutinin, active in anti-C plus anti-D agglutinin mixtures, that contain, or to which have been added, potent anti-D blocking antibodies, has anti-C^G reactivity. As mentioned above, it has been reported that some r^G cells are C- D- G+ C^G+ while others are C- D- G+ C^G-. However, an alternative way to describe those phenotypes, respectively, could be C+^{w} D- G+ and C- D- G+, with the proviso that the C+^{w} status can be recognized only with certain anti-C. An almost exactly parallel situation exists when the r'^S gene (previously r'^N and r'^n (46,596)) is considered. That gene produces either an unusual form of C, or C^G without C, dependent on one's interpretation. The gene is discussed in more detail below. Readers who have just read the sections beginning with G and anti-G, through to this point, may well wish they had taken Dramamine® before undertaking the trip. The lady who typed the manuscript (LAI) certainly does!

The Antigens f (ce), rh$_i$ (Ce), cE (Rh27) and CE (Rh22)

For the most part, understanding these antigens is a

straightforward matter. It was originally believed that they are *cis* gene products. That is to say, when c and e were on the same chromosome, c, e and f (ce) were all made. In an individual genetically *CDe/cDE*, c and e were present but were in the *trans* position (i.e. on opposite chromosomes). Thus c was made (by *cDE*), e was made (by *CDe*) but f was not made, i.e. red cells C+ c+ D+ E+ e+ f-. Now that it is known (41) that the D polypeptide is encoded by *RHD* and the CcEe polypeptides by alleles at the *RHCE* locus, understanding production of these antigens, in the overwhelming majority of individuals, is even more straightforward. The alleles at the *RHCE* locus are *RHce*, *RHCe*, *RHcE* and *RHCE*. As the names imply, these alleles encode production of: c, e and f (ce); C, e and rh$_i$ (Ce); c, E and cE (Rh27); and C, E and CE (Rh22) respectively. Table 12-6 illustrates production of these antigens by the eight common *Rh* haplotypes. One of us (PDI) has always disliked the term "compound antigens" to describe these determinants. A compound is made "by combining parts or elements" (597). The antigens under discussion are distinct entities, f or ce is not made whenever c and e are present (i.e. CDe/cDE, etc. red cells are f-). While the description of c and e in *cis* making f (ce) may no longer be totally accurate, it is clear that f is (usually) made when c and e are made by the same gene.

Just as the four antigens being described are not simple mixtures of parts of two other antigens, made whenever those two antigens are present, the antibodies that define them are not simple mixtures of two separable antibodies. As a single example (the other antibodies behave in an analogous manner) an R$_1$R$_1$ (CDe/CDe) individual, transfused with R$_2$R$_2$ (cDE/cDE) blood, is exposed to at least three foreign Rh antigens, c, E and cE (Rh27). If that individual makes anti-c, anti-E and anti-cE, the serum will behave as if it contains anti-c and anti-E. However, if the serum is adsorbed with R$_z$r (CDE/cde) or r^{y}r (CdE/cde) cells, until it no longer reacts with those cells, the anti-c and-E will have been removed while the anti-cE will be left unadsorbed (both R$_z$r and r^{y}r cells are c+, E+, cE-). Such adsorption studies (using appropriate red cells) have shown that the antibodies to f, rh$_i$, cE and CE define distinct antigens and are separable antibodies. The use of these four antibodies in differentiating between possible genotypes, to explain an observed phenotype, is described earlier in the section that includes table 12-6.

As mentioned, for the most part these four antigens are made and the antibodies that define them behave, according to the simple scheme outlined (79-82,598-602,618). However, there are a few complexities that have come to light. First, anti-f as made by an R$_1$R$_2$ (CDe/cDE) individual, who cannot make alloimmune anti-c or anti-e, might not have exactly the same specificity as anti-f made by an R_2R_2 (cDE/cDE) individual who can also make anti-e (49,598,603). Second, some (604-606) but not all (606,607) Dc-/Dc- bloods (in which D is enhanced and c is depressed) can be shown to be weakly f+. From studying one such blood that was f+ and one that was f-, Tessel et al. (606) suggested that genes that have been called *Dc-* are in fact a heterogeneous group. They thought that perhaps *Dc(e)f, Dc(e)(f)* and *Dc-* (the gene not making f) might all exist and that the antigens made by the genes shown in parentheses might be detectable only by adsorption-elution studies. This suggestion is perhaps supported by one other observation. Generally, the *Dc-* gene produces a depressed c (604-607). Indeed, the cells of one individual who had *Dc-* paired with R^1 were at first thought to be c-negative (607). In a different Dc-/Dc- individual (608) in whom the c antigen was present in normal or near normal amounts, the cells were clearly f+. As described later, the different *Dc-* genes also vary in terms of production of Hr and Hr_0 (606). A third complexity of the antigens under discussion is the finding (609) that an individual genetically R^1/Dc- made anti-f that caused fairly severe HDN in her infant. Fourth, a very rare gene called r^L (610,611) makes markedly reduced amounts of c and e, but normal f.

In terms of their clinical significance, antibodies directed against the antigens being described here are similar to other Rh antibodies. Anti-f has caused HDN (609,612,613) and has perhaps contributed to delayed transfusion reactions (614,615), other antibodies were present so that the exact role of anti-f could not be determined. Anti-rh_i has caused mild HDN (616) and perhaps a delayed transfusion reaction (617), again another antibody was present. One example (440) of anti-cE was highly unusual in that it appeared to be non-red cell stimulated and it caused complement activation. A form of anti-C initially called (596) anti-C^N, that was later (619) seen to have anti-rh_i specificity, is described in the next section.

The Gene r'^S

This gene that is rare in Whites but is not infrequent in Blacks (600,619-621) and in South African Bantu people (623,624), was originally named r'^S because it was thought to be a form of *r'(Cde)* that differed from the more usual *Cde* haplotype in that it made e^S instead of e (see later, in the section on V, VS and hr^H). Sturgeon et al. (596) found an anti-C, that they called anti-C^N, that divided C+ bloods from Blacks into two groups. Those that reacted with the antibody were called C^N, those that failed to react were called C^n. It was noted that red cells from individuals with r'^S (where the paired haplotype did

not make C) were always C^n. Eventually it became appreciated (619) that anti-C^N was actually an example of anti-rh_i (anti-Ce) as described earlier by Rosenfield et al. (81). Thus, it was seen that r'^S makes some form of C, but does not make rh_i (Ce). Further, r'^S has also been shown (600,619-621) to make some c and some f. As a result, there were different interpretations of r'^S. Those (49) who believed that the gene made some form of C interpreted it as $Ccde^S$. Those (311,622) who believed that the haplotype made C^G and that C^G differed from C, interpreted it as cde^SC^G. Since both haplotype designations list c and e as being part of the same gene, the production of f by r'^S is explained. However, the designation $Ccde^S$ is less explanatory of the lack of production of rh_i, than is the term cde^SC^G. While the difference between the gene symbols used is largely semantic, one of us (PDI) long preferred cde^SC^G since he regarded r'^S as a form of r and not as a form of r'. Again this interpretation was made because of the production of f and the lack of production of rh_i by r'^S.

In fact, it turns out that r'^S is probably not an altered form of r or r' but is probably derived from *RHD*. Blunt et al. (625) showed that r'^S contains at least exons 1, 2, 8, 9 and 10 of *RHD*; due to the fact that all the samples they studied came from individuals with a normal *RHce* on the paired chromosome, these investigators could not determine whether exons 3 to 7 of *RHD* had been deleted or had been replaced with exons 3 to 7 of *RHce*. Since no genetic material likely to encode C was found, the authors (625) suggested that the atypical C (or C^G in the terminology of others) made by r'^S might be a product of a remaining exon of *RHD*. It remains to be seen whether genes such as r^G, r^{Gu} and r^{Gs} represent similar gene rearrangements and whether the unusual C seen on the red cells of persons with such genes, is encoded by *RHC* or *RHD*-derived material.

Rh42

In 1980, Moulds et al. (54) described an antibody that reacted with red cells from individuals with r'^S but not with V+ or VS+ cells that lacked all representation of C. The antibody was called anti-Ce^S and later anti-Rh42 and differed from anti-Ce (anti-rh_i) in that it reacted with cells from individuals who had a gene making both C and e^S, but not with those who had a gene making both C and e. While the existence of Ce^S or Rh42 appears at first to suggest that r'^S is $Ccde^S$ rather than cde^SC^G, again the question is one of semantics. If C^G truly differs from C (perhaps it is encoded by an exon derived from *RHD* and not from *RHC*), anti-Rh42 can be thought of as anti-C^Ge^S. If Ce^S is likened to f, rh_i, cE and CE, as described above, r'^S becomes the first gene to make two such products, namely f and Ce^S (Rh42).

Rh41

In 1981, Svoboda et al. (53) described an antibody with a specificity similar to anti-rh$_i$ and anti-Rh42, the reactions of which are rather difficult to accommodate in the currently accepted patterns of Rh antigen production. Anti-Rh41 behaves like anti-rh$_i$ in reacting with red cells from persons with an *RHCe* allele. However, it was reported also to react with the C or C^G+ f+ rh$_i$- cells of persons with *r'^{S}* but not with the C+ f- rh$_i$+ cells of persons with *C^{W}De*. The antibody was made by a woman who apparently had a *CC^{W}De/cDE* genotype. No further work on Rh42 or Rh41 appears to have been published. As far as we are aware, no additional examples of either antibody have been found.

The Haplotype *R^{1s}*

As would be expected from what has been written about *r'^{S}*, C, C^G, rh$_i$ and f, there is a D+ equivalent to *r'^{S}* in Blacks. The haplotype can be thought of as *CcDe^S* or as *cDe^{S}C^G*. Like *r'^{S}*, *R^{1S}* makes f but not rh$_i$. While it was previously possible to use the same reasoning as applied to *r'^{S}* and argue as to whether *R^{1S}* was derived from *R^1* (*CcDe^S*) or *R^o* (*cDe^{S}C^G*), both those interpretations now seem in doubt, based on the findings of Blunt et al. (625) about the derivation of *r'^{S}* from *RHD* (see above). *R^{1S}* is quite different from a haplotype found (very rarely) in Whites that is best written *CDe^S* and makes rh$_i$ but no f or c (see later, section on V, VS and hr^H).

On the Fine Specificity of Anti-C

From what has been written in the several previous sections it is clear that when an antibody is identified as anti-C, using antibody identification red cells of common Rh phenotypes, a number of distinct possibilities exist. Many apparent anti-C are, in large part, anti-rh$_i$ (anti-Ce). This occurs because most people with C- red cells who receive C+ blood, are D+. In other words, exposure to C as a foreign antigen, via transfusion, most often represents the transfusion of R$_1$r (CDe/cde) blood to an R$_2$r (cDE/cde) recipient. In this setting, rh$_i$ (Ce) appears to be more immunogenic than C and much of the antibody produced has anti-rh$_i$ specificity. Differentiation of anti-rh$_i$ from anti-C can be made using adsorption studies. The serum under test is adsorbed with C+ rh$_i$- (CDE/cde or CdE/cde) red cells until it no longer reacts with those cells. If it still reacts strongly with C+ rh$_i$+ (CDe/cde or

CdE/cde) red cells, it is probable that anti-rh$_i$ has been isolated. However, an additional one or two adsorptions with the, now non-reactive, C+ rh$_i$- red cells are in order since it is probable that C is less well expressed on those cells, than on C+ rh$_i$+ cells. Once adsorption with the C+ rh$_i$- red cells no longer reduces the titer of the antibody, it can be assumed that only anti-rh$_i$ remains. Much less frequently, anti-C may contain an anti-CE (anti-Rh22) component, similar adsorptions with appropriately selected cells can be used. A number of examples of anti-C are anti-CC^G or anti-C plus anti-C^G, depending on one's interpretation; such sera often contain anti-rh$_i$ that is stronger than the anti-CC^G or anti-C plus anti-C^G components. Tests to determine the presence of absence of anti-C^G require use of red cells of the phenotypes described in earlier sections.

Commercially-obtained anti-C typing reagents are sometimes pools of different raw sera and often contain mostly anti-Ce (anti-rh$_i$). In spite of reports to the contrary, we (585) were able to detect C in the absence of rh$_i$ in tests with six different commercially-prepared anti-C reagents. Certainly, the anti-rh$_i$ components of the sera were stronger than the anti-C components in several instances, indicating that in critical cases (such as paternity studies) the use of C+ rh$_i$+ and C+ rh$_i$- control cells would be advisable.

The recognition of rh$_i$ (Ce), C^G, and CE, occurred after results of the original studies with anti-C had been incorporated into the pool of knowledge about Rh. It is now impossible to determine what specificity antibodies were used in the early studies. As an example, it is generally accepted that the C antigen produced by the *R^Z* (*CDE*) and *r^Y* (*CdE*) haplotypes, is less in quantity than that produced by *R^1* (*CDe*) (35,38,351-355,540,626-628). However, if, as is extremely probable, the antibodies originally used were predominantly anti-rh$_i$ in specificity, the actual difference in amount of C made by *R^Z*, *r^Y* and *R^1* may not be as much as has been assumed. In spite of this, as mentioned earlier, we believe that *R^Z* and *r^Y* make quantitatively reduced amounts of C, when compared to *R^1*.

In their last edition, Race and Sanger (49) included a table showing the heterogeneity of anti-C specificity (as opposed to the effects of quantitative differences in antigen production). They said that the reactions of anti-C (lacking anti-D and anti-G) cannot be fully explained in terms of just anti-C, anti-Ce and anti-CE. As will be apparent, the understanding of one of us (PDI) is considerably aided by the belief that anti-C and anti-C^G define different antigens.

In addition to the many complexities of C described above, there are reports (629,630) of the production of alloimmune anti-C by individuals with C+ (sometimes the C made by *r'^{S}*) red cells. This may (not proved) indicate the existence of red cells that carry partial C (see later sections, many Rh antigens other than D seem to exist in partial forms). The above references do not include cases in which anti-C was made by an individual with C^w+ or C^x+ red cells. Although, for many years, it was believed that all C^w+ or C^x+ red cells are also C+, it is now well documented (for references see later sections) that the phenotypes C^w+ C- and C^x+ C- both exist. Thus, when persons of such phenotypes make anti-C, there is no reason to regard them as being different from examples of anti-C made by persons with C- C^w- C^x- red cells.

One additional consideration regarding the apparent production of anti-C by persons with C+ red cells, is that adsorption studies are essential before anti-C specificity is assigned. As discussed in detail below, antibodies to partial e antigens (particularly those called anti-hr^B) not infrequently present in such a manner that they react visibly (IAT) only with C+ (or rh_i+) red cells. Such antibodies can be adsorbed to exhaustion with C- e+ red cells thus showing that they do not have anti-C specificity.

Some of the serological difficulties with C, that are described above, may be explainable at the molecular level. In studies of r'^S, Blunt et al. (625), and on genes that encode VS and weak C, Faas et al. (751), have shown that the genes (that differ from each other) are comprised of some exons from *RHD* and some from *RHCE*. Although the gene conversion events leading to formation of these genes are discussed more fully in later sections of this chapter, it can be said here that neither gene carries the information that normally encodes C. In other words, an exon derived from *RHD* may be responsible for production of the C-like (and perhaps the G) determinant. Recognition of the serological complexities involved, of course, led to introduction of the name C^G by Levine et al. (87) to explain the atypical reactions seen with anti-C.

The Genes r^M, r^L, r^t and the Haplotype R^{oL}

In addition to the genes and haplotypes described above, there are a number of other unusual and rare *Rh* genes and haplotypes whose actions can be conveniently mentioned here.

The gene r^M (601) is somewhat like r^G, except that it makes less G and C^G than does r^G and it makes a depressed form of E. Since r^M makes neither c nor e, the r in its title indicates its relationship to r^G, not to r.

The gene r^L (610) makes less c and e than does r, but makes normal f. From a study of the family in which r^L was first found, it was impossible to say whether the gene was r^L or R^{oL} (that can be written as *(c)d(e)f* and *(c)D(e)f*, respectively). No doubt both exist. Additional persons with r^L have been found (611).

The gene r^t makes an unusual form of c antigen (67) called c^t and some e and f. It was shown, in direct tests and by adsorption studies, that the c antigen made by the r^t gene is apparently qualitatively different from the usual c antigen. Some anti-c sera would react with and could be adsorbed by c^t cells, others would do neither. Another example of r^t *(c^tde)* was later found (631) and it was shown that c^t and Rh26 (next section) are not the same.

The Antigen Rh26 and Partial c

In 1964, Huestis et al. (94) described an antibody similar to anti-c. That the antibody was not anti-c was shown when rare bloods, with a weakened expression of c, were found neither to react with nor to adsorb the new antibody. The antibody was named anti-Rh26 and the c+, non-reactive samples, that also had weakened expressions of f, were described as Rh:w4,w6,-26. The authors found that such bloods were rare and that the majority of random samples were either c+ Rh:26, or c- Rh:-26. In addition to finding samples having c, but lacking Rh26, the authors found one example of the phenotype c- Rh:26 and reported that many examples of apparent anti-c were really mixtures of anti-c and anti-Rh26. The individual who made what is still the only reported example of pure anti-Rh26, was phenotypically C+ c- Rh:-26. The question posed as to whether a c+ Rh:-26 individual could make anti-Rh26, has not yet been answered.

Over the years, one of us (PDI) has been sent a number of samples that closely resembled anti-Rh26 as made by persons of the Rh:-26 phenotype. An alloimmune anti-c made by an individual with c+ Rh:-26 red cells, who probably had a *Dc-* haplotype, was described in an abstract (632). In addition, Reviron et al. (633) described a family in which the propositus and his sister had red cells that reacted, albeit weakly with, and would adsorb all polyclonal anti-c used in the tests, but would neither react with, nor adsorb, a monoclonal anti-c. Unfortunately, the original anti-Rh26 and red cells typed as c+ Rh:-26 and c- Rh:26, are no longer readily available for cross-testing. Nevertheless, the findings described seem to indicate the existence of partial c and the ability of persons of such partial phenotypes to make antibodies against the epitopes of c that their red cells presumably lack.

The Haplotypes $\overline{\overline{R}}^N$, Two Called *(C)D(e)* and The Antigens Rh32 and Rh35

In 1960, Rosenfield et al. (600) described a new *Rh* haplotype in a Black family. They called the haplotype $\overline{\overline{R}}^N$ and noted that it encodes production of much smaller quantities of C and e, than does R^I. Indeed, when $\bar{\bar{R}}^N$ was paired with a haplotype that did not make C, the amount of C was reduced to the point where it could easily have been overlooked. The paper is a classic description of the difficulties that can arise when attempts are made to follow the inheritance of *Rh* haplotypes in Blacks. Workers who use the Rh system, in paternity studies in Blacks would be well advised to read this paper. $\bar{\bar{R}}^N$ also encodes slightly more D than do other *Rh* haplotypes. However, the increased level of D is not marked and sensitive tests with selected anti-D may be necessary to demonstrate the increase.

In 1963, Broman et al. (639) found a haplotype, in the Swedish population, that had actions similar to $\bar{\bar{R}}^N$. The new haplotype was called *(C)D(e)*, the parentheses indicating that the haplotype makes less C and e than does R^I. In 1965, Heiken and Giles (611) expanded the findings of Broman et al. (639) by showing that there are two different *(C)D(e)* haplotypes in the Swedish and Danish populations. Although both encode reduced amounts of C and e, the presence of one results in slightly exalted D, while the presence of the other results in production of a more normal amount of D. Although $\bar{\bar{R}}^N$ and the two types of *(C)D(e)* had certain features in common, it was shown that they could not be identical for the C and e antigens encoded behaved differently when tests with the same anti-C and anti-e were performed (640). As would have been expected, some of these haplotypes were shown to code for production of reduced amounts of rh_i (Ce) (600,639). Indeed, in some instances rh_i appears not to be made at all (108,600,641) while in others (639) it can be shown to be present only by the use of adsorption-elution studies. In one unusual family (642) an $\bar{\bar{R}}^N$ haplotype appeared to produce no rh_i at all, even when adsorption-elution studies were used, in the father, but made a small amount of the antigen, that could be detected in IATs, in both of his children. The situation was considered possibly to represent the presence of an unusual *ce(f)* gene in *trans* to $\bar{\bar{R}}^N$, or presence of an unlinked suppresser of *Rh*, acting to prevent his $\bar{\bar{R}}^N$ haplotype from making rh_i, and to reduce the amount of f made by his *r* gene.

One major problem when attempts were made to study the antigens made by $\bar{\bar{R}}^N$ and the *(C)D(e)* haplotypes was that the products of the haplotypes could not be readily identified when the paired haplotype made C and/or e. Between 1965 and 1971, two important discoveries were made. First, Chown et al. (98,99) showed that several sera (Troll, Bill, Reynolds, Harper, Comacho and Garcia), that contain several antibodies (often Rh), also contain an antibody that defines a low incidence antigen, that is a product of $\bar{\bar{R}}^N$. The new antigen was called Rh32. It was shown (98,99) that Rh32 is present on the red cell of persons who inherit $\bar{\bar{R}}^N$, but not on those of individu-

als who inherit either of the *(C)D(e)* haplotypes found in the Scandinavian populations. It should be added that the haplotype is $\bar{\bar{R}}^N$, the antigen is Rh32 and the antibody anti-Rh32. Terms such as anti-$\bar{\bar{R}}^N$ and the $\bar{\bar{R}}^N$ antigen are incorrect.

In 1971, Giles and Skov (101) found another antibody directed against a rare Rh antigen, in a serum known as 1114. This antibody, that was subsequently named anti-Rh35, defines a low incidence antigen (Rh35) that is a product of the *(C)D(e)* haplotype that does not produce increased levels of D. The red cells of people who had inherited $\bar{\bar{R}}^N$ or a *(C)D(e)* haplotype making slightly enhanced D, were shown to be Rh:-35. The discovery of anti-Rh32 and anti-Rh35 meant that the presence of one of the three haplotypes under discussion could be recognized and that the presence of the other two could be excluded. Persons whose red cells typed as Rh:32,-35 had $\bar{\bar{R}}^N$; those whose red cells typed as Rh:-32,35 had *(C)D(e)* that makes normal D; while those whose red cells had slightly enhanced D and reduced C and e, but were Rh:-32,-35, might well have the other type of *(C)D(e)*. Even in the absence of absolute proof of presence of the last mentioned haplotype, it could be concluded that the Rh:-32,-35 phenotype meant that $\bar{\bar{R}}^N$ and *(C)D(e)* (normal D), were not present. In addition to providing a serological means for differentiation between persons with any one of the three haplotypes, the discovery of anti-Rh32 and anti-Rh35 resulted in another advance. By use of these antibodies it became possible to recognize the presence of $\bar{\bar{R}}^N$ and *(C)D(e)* (normal D) in the heterozygous state, even when the paired haplotype was a normal R^I.

One published abstract (715) has described the production of alloimmune anti-C in an individual with a form of *(C)D(e)* that encoded normal D. However, the individual's red cells were said to be Rh:-35, as described above the *(C)D(e)* haplotype making normal D, described by Giles and Skov (101), made Rh35. Thus it is possible that the *(C)D(e)* haplotype in this individual differed from that previously described. The abstract does not mention adsorption studies. As described elsewhere, antibodies to partial e antigens often resemble anti-C or anti-rh_i (Ce) in initial antibody identification studies but can be adsorbed by C- e+ Ce- red cells that carry normal e.

LePennec et al. (108) described 18 persons who were homozygous for $\bar{\bar{R}}^N$. Some of these individuals were first studied because their sera contained an antibody to a high incidence antigen. The study of LePennec et al. (108) confirmed the supposition (641,643) that Rh32 behaves as if it is an antithetical antigen to that defined by the antibody made by $\bar{\bar{R}}^N$ homozygotes. That antibody was called anti-Rh46, it is described in more detail in a later section. A case in which $\bar{\bar{R}}^N$ appeared to have arisen by de novo mutation of R^1 (99) is also discussed in more detail below.

The story with $\overline{\overline{R}}^N$ is now a little more complicated. Although at first apparently a marker only for $\overline{\overline{R}}^N$, Rh32 has now been found on the red cells of persons who do not have that gene. In describing the partial D phenotype, DBT, Tippett et al. (71) reported that red cells of that phenotype are Rh:32. Among nine DBT propositi, six had normal C, two had weak C (one also had weak e) and one was C-. As discussed in the section on low incidence antigens present on red cells of partial D phenotypes, it is relatively easy to guess how the same low incidence antigen can be encoded by different *Rh* genes. Because no second example of anti-Rh35 has ever been reported, less is known about Rh35 than about Rh32; anti-Rh32 is not a particularly uncommon antibody, especially when sera containing multiple antibodies to low incidence antigens are studied.

$\overline{\overline{R}}^N$ by Mutation

There exists in the literature, an eloquent report of a sophisticated investigation that revealed the de novo production of an $\overline{\overline{R}}^N$ haplotype. While studying the red cells of members of a family belonging to a strict religious order, to show the inheritance pattern of Bu^a, Chown et al. (99) found one of the few well authenticated cases of observed mutation at the *Rh* locus. The parents involved were almost certainly of the genotypes R^1R^2 and R^1R^1. Of their seven children, four were R^1R^1, two R^1R^2 and one $R^2\overline{\overline{R}}^N$. Non-parentage was satisfactorily excluded on several counts. The child with the $\overline{\overline{R}}^N$ haplotype had red cells that reacted with an eluate made using the Bill serum. That serum was already known to contain anti-C, anti-rh$_i$, anti-C^w, anti-V and anti-D^w (93). The investigation of the family showed that the Bill serum (like the famous Troll serum (98,406)) also contains anti-Rh32. The red cells of the $R^2\overline{\overline{R}}^N$ son were Rh:32, those of his parents and six sibs were Rh:-32. The mutation apparently involved an R^1 to $\overline{\overline{R}}^N$ change and the actions of the new $\overline{\overline{R}}^N$ haplotype were found to be identical to those of previously studied examples. In the study, Chown et al. (99) at first thought that they were using anti-D^w made by elution of the Bill serum from D^w+ C- C^w- rh$_i$- V- red cells. However, it was found that the eluate, in fact, contained anti-D^w and anti-Rh32 although the red cells from which it was made were Rh:-32. This failure to separate anti-D^w from anti-Rh32, by selective adsorption and elution has been mirrored using other sera that contain antibodies to more than one low incidence Rh antigen. The phenomenon is discussed further in the section on low incidence Rh antigens.

The *R¹-like* Haplotype that Encodes JAL (Rh48)

In 1990, Lomas et al. (111) and Poole et al. (112) described the low incidence antigen JAL that was given the number Rh48. Anti-JAL had caused HDN severe enough to necessitate exchange transfusion in one family and had perhaps caused the disease in a second (111). In Whites, JAL was encoded by an *R¹-like* haplotype that makes reduced amounts of C and e, and D and G antigens that are normal in some and slightly enhanced in other individuals with JAL+ red cells. In Switzerland, 90,000 donors were typed and four were found to be JAL+ for an incidence of 0.004% (112). However, all four JAL+ donors were French-speaking although such individuals comprised only 7.5% of the 90,000 donors tested. Thus the incidence of JAL+ in French-speaking Swiss was 0.06%.

The antigen JAL provides another example of a low incidence antigen encoded by different *Rh* haplotypes. As described later in this chapter, in Blacks, JAL is encoded by an *R⁰-like* haplotype.

The Antigen C^w

For many years after its discovery (83) in 1946, C^w was regarded as the product of an allele (C^w) at the *Cc* locus or sublocus (84,405,644,645). It was found that all genes that made C^w also made C and that C^w could occur in the alignments C^wDe, C^wde, C^wDE and C^wdE (405,644-651). Further, it was thought that many anti-C sera contained an anti-C^w component although this conclusion may have been reached because C^w+ cells were always C+. Indeed, the idea that all genes that make C^w also make C was so ingrained that when a gene making C^w without C was encountered, it was not immediately recognized. As described more fully below, the concept that C^w is an allele of C and c was first questioned by Giles and Skov (101) who wondered if C^w might be a low incidence marker antigen of an *R¹-like* gene, just as Rh32 and Rh35 seemed to be.

In 1976, Habibi et al. (652) described a blood sample that reacted with all of 17 examples of anti-C^w but that failed to react with any of 21 anti-C sera that reacted with other C^w+ samples. Rather than accept a suggestion made to them by Ruth Sanger (653) that the blood was from an individual with C^w in an unusual alignment (i.e. a haplotype making C^w without C) the authors (652) elected to propose a complex mosaicism involving C and what they called C^{w1} and C^{w2}. Shortly after the publication of Habibi et al. (652), a somewhat similar case was described by Leonard et al. (654). This time the patient's cells were clearly C^w+ but their C status could not be determined for sure since the cells reacted with 16 of 22 anti-C sera. The ability of the sera to react with the patient's cells was not correlated with the amount of anti-C they contained. However, the C- C^w+ status of the patient's cells seemed apparent since the patient made alloimmune anti-C.

In both cases cited (652,654) there was additional (indirect) evidence for the presence of a haplotype making C^w but not C. The red cells of the Habibi et al. (652) propositus carried more than a single dose of c and were f+ rh_i-. In other words, it appeared that both *Rh* haplotypes were making c and that one of them was also making C^w. The red cells of the Leonard et al. (654) proposita had reduced levels of e and hr^S. In other words, evidence of the presence of an unusual *Rh* haplotype. As can be seen from the sections earlier (on $\bar{\bar{R}}^N$, Rh32 and Rh35) *Rh* haplotypes that encode production of low incidence marker antigens often make less than the usual amount of standard antigens. That applied in these two cases, i.e. one and one half doses of c in one case (652) when both genes were making c and reduced levels of e and hr^S in the other (654) when both genes were making those antigens.

Like Ruth Sanger (653), one of us (622) concluded that in both cases a r or R^o haplotype making C^w was present. The haplotype in the Habibi et al. case (652) could be thought of as *(c)D* or *deC^w* while that in the case of Leonard et al. (654) could be forecast to be *cD* or *d(e)(hr^S)C^w*. In both cases the D or d designation is indicative of the fact that it was not possible to tell if the haplotype making c and C^w did or did not make D.

That the forecasts outlined above (622,653) were correct was seen when Sachs et al. (655) described a German family in which several members had a haplotype that made c and C^w but no C. There was no doubt, from a family study that involved extensive typing for many genetic markers, that the haplotype involved produces both c and C^w, but no C. Indeed, through three generations of the family studied, it was seen that when a haplotype producing C was passed, no C^w was made, while C^w was made each time a non-C-producing haplotype was transmitted. Since the *cC^w* gene was not partnered by a gene not making D, in the family involved, it was possible to decide whether a *rC^w* or an *R^oC^w* haplotype had been found. A second German family described (656) five years later left no doubt that the haplotype present in that family made D. The haplotype was *cC^wDe*, or a form of *R^o* making C^w. Since the reports cited above were published, other examples of c+ C^w+ C- red cells have been found (657).

As described in the section on the *Rh-deletion* genes, there is some evidence (67,658,659) that the C^w of DC^w-/DC^w- red cells may be qualitatively different from the C^w encoded by non-deleted genes. The possible role

of C^w as a low incidence marker antigen of certain *Rh* haplotypes is discussed below as is the antigen Rh51 or MAR, that behaves, at the serological level, as if it is antithetical to both C^w and C^x.

Anti-C^w is not uncommon; it is sometimes seen in individuals who have never been pregnant or transfused (405,407,408); at other times as an alloantibody in the sera of patients with "warm" antibody-induced hemolytic anemia (409); and sometimes following transfusion or pregnancy (408). Stimulation of production of anti-C^w by transfusion is perhaps most common in patients who have already made anti-c and require repeated transfusions. The selection of c- red cells for these patients will result in an increased probability that they will receive C^w+ red cells since, as stated above, C^w is most often produced by a gene that makes C and not c. Thus the combination of anti-c plus anti-C^w in a multiply transfused R_1R_1 patients is not particularly uncommon. When the antibody causes HDN, the disease is usually mild or subclinical (408,661-670).

The Antigen C^x

Like C^w, C^x, that was first described (84) in 1954, was long regarded as the product of an allele at the *Cc* sublocus. Indeed, the early examples of C^x were found in the alignments *C^xDe* and *C^xde* (84,406,409,671,672). However, lack of *C^xdE* and *C^xDE* may simply reflect the facts that the incidence of C^x is much lower than that of C^w and the haplotypes *r^Y* and *R^Z* are both rare.

In 1987, Sistonen et al. (673) described a gene, in four of 513 unrelated Somalis, that encodes production of c and C^x, but no C. The gene was further unusual in that it made V and VS (see later) but no f. These unusual features of the gene that makes c and C^x but no C, were reminiscent of those previously seen with other genes that make C^x. The haplotype *C^xDe* appears to encode weak e and no hr^S (674) while both *C^xDe* and *C^xde* encode weak C.

Anti-C^x occurs in circumstances similar to those described above for anti-C^w (406); alloimmune anti-C^x is often seen in the sera of patients with "warm" antibody-induced hemolytic anemia (409). Anti-C^x has also caused mild HDN (84,671).

A Change in Terminology for Haplotypes that make C^w or C^x

Once it is accepted that haplotypes that make c and C^w or c and C^x, but no C, exist, it becomes apparent that slightly different terminology should be used. By analogy to *cC^wDe* (i.e. the haplotype making c and C^w without C), R^{1w} is more correctly written as CC^wDe than as C^wDe, to indicate that it encodes C and C^w (without c). Similarly: r'^w should be CC^wde, not C^wde; R^{1x} should be CC^xDe and r'^x should be CC^xde. The previously used (in this chapter) $cdeC^w$ and $cDeC^w$, should be cC^wde and cC^wDe, respectively. We hope that we will remember these new rules in writing the rest of this chapter!

The Antigen MAR, Rh51

In 1994, Sistonen et al. (116) described an antibody to a very high frequency antigen. The antibody reacted with all red cells of common Rh phenotypes but not with those of C^w and C^x homozygotes, nor with those of individuals heterozygous for C^w and C^x. The antibody did not react with D-- or Rh_{null} red cells. The definitive study could, perhaps, only been performed in Finland because the incidence of C^w in that population is between 7 and 9% (49) and the incidence of C^x is almost 2% (116). As shown in table 12-2 the incidence of C^w does not exceed 1% in most other populations, the incidence of C^x varies from 0.1 to 0.3% (84,671,675). It is difficult to imagine that a C^wC^x heterozygote could be found anywhere other than in Finland.

The findings of Sistonen et al. (116) showed that the new antibody, that was called anti-MAR and, later anti-Rh51, defines a very common antigen with an antithetical relationship to both C^w and C^x. In other words, genes that make C^w or C^x, do not make MAR. Family studies confirmed this point, 20 children of a parent with Rh:-51 red cells, in eight different families, had red cells that were either C^w+ or C^x+. Anti-Rh51 showed some dosage effect by often reacting weakly with C^w+ C^x- Rh:51 and C^w- C^x+ Rh:51 red cells (i.e. those from persons heterozygous for C^w or C^x).

Eleven years before the publication (116) describing the antithetical relationship of Rh51 to C^w and C^x appeared, Mougey et al., in a published abstract (675) described a woman who was apparently homozygous for C^x and who had produced an antibody to a very common antigen, that caused HDN. A complete study was never possible, in part because the antibody was not produced in appreciable levels for very long and in part because of the rarity of C^w and C^x in the USA. A similar antibody was found by Larimore (676), similar reasons prevented a full investigation. Even if the two earlier found antibodies (675,676) had the same specificity as anti-Rh51, credit for establishing the Rh51, C^w, C^x relationship clearly belongs to Sistonen et al. (116).

As described in detail in the section on the molecular genetics of Rh, Mouro et al. (208) have shown that the amino acid changes encoded by exon 1 of *RHCE*, that result in expression of C^w and C^x, are at different posi-

tions on the polypeptide. In C^w, arginine replaces glutamine at position 41. In C^x, threonine replaces alanine at position 36. These findings could, perhaps, be taken to indicate that the antigens MAR(Rh51), C^w and C^x are not the products of alleles. Nevertheless, as described above, the antithetical relationships of MAR and C^w and of MAR and C^x, were clearly demonstrated at the serological level (116). If, in fact, the MAR determinant includes Ala36 and Gln41; the C^w determinant includes Ala36 and Arg41; and the C^x determinant includes Thr36 and Gln41, it could be equally well argued that the three antigens are indeed the products of alleles. Since the primary difference (41) between C and c involves position 103 on the same polypeptide (serine in C, proline in c) it becomes clear how C^w and C^x can be made by some genes that make C and some that make c. It is also tempting to speculate that the presence of Arg41 in C^w or Thr36 in C^x, results in a configurational change at Ser103 that is seen at the serological level as reduced production of C.

Rh Haplotypes in Series

As discussed in previous editions of this book, it is possible to arrange *Rh* haplotypes in series, based on similarities of their encoded products. This idea was first suggested by Heiken and Giles (611), was expanded by Giles and Skov (101) and was then further developed by one of us (311,622,686). Tables 12-15, 16, 17 and 18, that follow, illustrating this point, are not intended to be all inclusive, instead selected haplotypes are shown. For example $cD^{IVa}e$, $cD^{IVa}E$ and $(C)D^{IVa}$- are all included since most blood group serologists will have anti-Go^a so will be able to recognize presence of those haplotypes. In contrast, the haplotypes $cD^{Va}e$, $CD^{Va}e$ and $cD^{Va}E$ are not shown, although each is known to exist (493), since anti-D^w is not generally available. $CD^{VI}e$ is listed since it apparently encodes production of BARC (511), $cD^{VI}E$ is not listed since it is not (yet) known to encode production of a low incidence marker antigen. Most of the *Rh* haplotypes recognized but not included in the tables, are described in the text. Table 12-15 lists some haplotypes that can be considered to be similar to R^1 (CDe). Much of what is known about the haplotypes listed in that table has been described above. As can be seen, reading from the top to the bottom of the table, many of the haplotypes encode production of gradually decreasing amounts of C and e, sometimes but not always in conjunction with some increase in D. For haplotypes not previously described it can be added that: one making normal C but reduced e is known (101); that R^{1x} may have additional unusual characteristics (see section on C^x); and that the Rh-deletion gene $D\bullet\bullet$ makes the low incidence antigen

Evans (Rh37) (see later).

Because R^1 (*CDe*) is common and R^Z (*CDE*) is rare, $D^{IV}(C)$- and DC^w- have been included in table 12-15 although their ancestor may have been R^Z (*CDE*) and not R^1. For the same reason, *D--* and *D••* are included although they could have descended from R^2, R^Z or R^o instead of from R^1.

The Haplotype R^{oHar} and the Antigen Rh33

Some features of R^{oHar} have already been described in the section dealing with partial D. Indeed, as stated in that section, it is now known that the D made by R^{oHar} is partial and that persons with that form of D on their red cells can make alloimmune anti-D (246,247). In their original description, Giles et al. (100) reported that R^{oHar} makes a form of D that is difficult to detect; greatly diminished amounts of e, f and Hr_o; and no hr^S, G or Hr. As discussed earlier, haplotypes that make D but not G are rare. Similarly, those that make e but not hr^S and those that make Hr_o but not Hr, are also rare, R^{oHar} qualifies on

all three counts! The c antigen made appears to be normal, details about the form of D made were given earlier.

While reporting the first example of R^{oHar}, Giles et al. (100) described a "new" low incidence antigen, Rh33, that was apparently encoded only by R^{oHar}. Use of anti-Rh33 has permitted the identification of additional individuals with R^{oHar} (243,244) but workers involved in Rh serology should be warned that not all red cell samples labeled as being from an individual with R^{oHar} have been shown to be Rh:33. Because of the difficulties encountered in detecting the D made by R^{oHar}, many anti-D have been tested to see which ones have that ability. Unfortunately, some workers have then assumed that an anti-D with such an ability will automatically identify bloods from individuals with R^{oHar}. In testing such antibodies, we (243) demonstrated that some of the anti-D are able also to detect very weak forms of D on Rh:-33 red cells. In other words, such sera detect very weak expression of D, but not all such antigens are made by individuals who have inherited R^{oHar}. Both examples of separable anti-Rh33 that have been found (100,677) were present in sera that

TABLE 12-15 Some Haplotypes Apparently Related to R^1

Shorthand Name	*CDE* Term	Low Incidence "Marker" Antigen	Antigen Levels (Compared to R^1 (*CDe*) Products)
R^1	*CDe*		
R^{1IVb}	$CD^{IVb}e$	? Evans	
R^{1Va}	$CD^{Va}e$	D^w	
R^{1VI}	$CD^{VI}e$	BARC	D usually ↓
	CD(e)		e↓
R^{1w}	$(C)C^wD(e)$	C^w	C↓ e↓
R^{1x}	$(C)C^xD(e)$	C^x	C↓ e↓
	(C)D(e)	Rh35	C↓ e↓
	(C)D(e)	FPTT	C↓ e↓
R^{1Jal}	*(C)D(e)*	JAL	C↓ e↓ G↑ (in some)
R^{1Lisa}	*(C)D(e)*	? Rh33	C↓ e↓
	(C)D(e)		C↓ e↓ D normal
$\bar{\bar{R}}^N$	*(C)D(e)*	Rh32	C↓ e↓ D↑ Enhanced D difficult to demonstrate
	(C)D(e)		C↓ e↓ D↑
	$(C)D^{IVa}-$	Go^a, Rh33, Riv, FPTT	C↓ D↑ no e
$\bar{R}^{ow}$	$(C)(C^w)D-$	C^w	C↓ C^w↓ (compared to R^{1w}) D↑ no e
	•D•	Evans	D↑ no C, no e
	-D-	Tar	D↑ no C, no e
$\bar{\bar{R}}^o$	*-D-*		D↑ no C, no e

also contained anti-D. Thus red cells should not be said to be Rh:33 until they have been shown to react with anti-Rh33 from which all anti-D has been removed by adsorption with D+ Rh:-33 red cells. Similarly, anti-D that react with the red cells of individuals known to have R^{oHar} should not be assumed to contain anti-Rh33. That antibody can be identified when left unadsorbed in a serum, that originally contained anti-D and anti-Rh33, that has been adsorbed with D+ Rh:-33 cells until it no longer reacts with cells that carry D but not Rh33. Obviously, if anti-Rh33 is present it will react with the red cells of individuals with R^{oHar}. Since the D made by R^{oHar} is so hard to detect it seems certain that some individuals with that haplotype have been classified as D- blood donors. However, this probably does not represent any real danger. As far as we are aware, no D- individual transfused with red cells carrying the weak D made by R^{oHar} (or for that matter any other cells carrying that small an amount of D) has undergone a primary response to D. No doubt very rare exceptions may eventually be reported.

The second haplotype seen to encode production of Rh33, was $D^{IV}(C)$- (107). That haplotype and the series of low incidence antigens that it encodes are described in a later section. A third haplotype being a potential producer of Rh33 came to light during our studies (678) on the blood of a Black woman whose red cells were Rh:33. That the antigen was not encoded by R^{oHar} was suggested by a number of findings. First, the proposita's red cells reacted, in titration studies with anti-Rh33, as if they carried a double dose of Rh33. Second, the red cells were G+ f- and carried normal D. We tentatively assigned the name R^{oJoh} to describe a haplotype that appeared to produce normal D, G and c, Rh33, a reduced amount of e, but no f. If R^{oJoh} acts as we (678) supposed, it may also have been present in a White family that we (679) studied. Two sisters with Rh:33 red cells were found. In one, the red cells behaved as if they carried the products of R^{oHar}. In the other, Rh33 appeared to be encoded by a gene that made near normal D, G but no f or Hr_o. In this sister, who made an anti-Hr_o-like antibody, it seemed that Rh33 could have been the product of R^{oJoh}. As discussed in detail later in this chapter, the antigen Hr_o seems to comprise a series of epitopes and individuals with partial Hr_o on their red cells and alloimmune anti-Hr_o in their sera are not infrequent. A fourth haplotype potentially encoding Rh33 was invoked by Moores et al. (716). It was supposed that the German proposita had two haplotypes encoding Rh33, one was thought to be R^{oHar}, the other appeared to make D, weak C, very weak or no e and no Hr_o. The haplotype was tentatively called R^{1Lisa}, it was apparently different from $D^{IV}(C)$- (that also makes Rh33, see above) in that the proposita's red cells did not react with anti-Go^a.

However, in the paper it is mentioned that positive control cells were not available for antibodies to all low incidence Rh antigens. Thus further studies seem necessary to distinguish R^{1Lisa} from $D^{IV}(C)$-.

The production of separable anti-Rh33 has twice (the only two published examples) been seen to occur in unusual circumstances. The first example (100) was found in a serum that contained anti-D, the antibody-maker had C+ red cells. The second example (677) was found in a serum that contained alloantibodies to D, c, V and K and an autoantibody that mimicked anti-D. The antibody-maker in this case had partial D on the red cells, that were also C+. Since the incidence of persons with C+ D- or C+ partial D+ red cells is about one fortieth the incidence of persons with C- D- red cells, it follows that the chance of finding separable anti-Rh33, in a serum containing anti-D, made by a person with C+ red cells, is about 1 in 40 of the chance of finding the antibody in a serum containing anti-D, made by a person with C- D- red cells, if production of anti-Rh33 has nothing to do with the C status of the antibody-maker's red cells. The chance of finding two consecutive examples of separable anti-Rh33 (and the only two thus far reported) in sera containing anti-D, made by persons with C+ red cells, is about 1 in 1600 if the presence of C does not influence the production of anti-Rh33. The above calculations are based on the premise that persons with C+ D- and C- D- red cells are at equal risk of making anti-D. In fact, persons with C+ D- red cells also have G and C^G on their cells so may be at lower risk of making anti-D than those who have C- D- G- C^G- red cells. If that is the case, the chance of finding both examples of anti-Rh33 in the circumstances described, may be less than 1 in 1600. One possibility to be considered is that Rh33 may be structurally similar to C, G or C^G so that the immune system of an individual with C+ D- G+ C^G+ red cells can recognize Rh33 while that of an individual with D- C- G- C^G- red cells recognizes C, G or C^G instead.

As described in the section on partial D, the epitope composition of the partial D made by R^{oHar} is known (246) (table 12-10), as described in a later section, the molecular genetic event that resulted in the production of R^{oHar} has also been determined (248).

The *Santi* Haplotype

Another R^o variant of considerable interest is that known as *Santi*. In *CDE* terms this haplotype can, perhaps, best be described as $cD^{Variant}e(G)(V)$. In such a description, variant indicates partial D. Reports on the famous bloods from Mrs. Shabalala (26) and Mrs. Santiago (680,681) described the first studies on the products of this haplotype and because of the nature of the antibodies made by those two individuals, a separate section below describes the complexities. In considering *Santi* as a variant of *R⁰* it can be said that the haplotype encodes (among other things) the production of weak G and weak V. From his observation that G and V typings, on the red cells of individuals with the haplotype, are initially read as positive but rapidly become weakly positive or negative, Rosenfield (680,681) has suggested that the G and V antigens produced may be misshapen so that their ability to retain anti-G and anti-V is poor. Lewis et al. (682) in describing a family showing normal inheritance of the *Santi* haplotype (that was not apparent in the first cases studied), reported similar difficulties in G and V typings. The term $R^{ou(GV)}$ has also been used (682) to describe the *Santi* haplotype that, in addition to the above, is unusual in that it encodes production of some Rh$_o$ (the cells usually type as weak D+) but no Rh^A, Rh^C or Rh^D. In manual tests (682) no Rh^B can be found either, but tests in the AutoAnalyzer (683) suggested that a small amount of that antigen was present. The *Santi* haplotype makes e and hr^B but no Hr or hr^S. As mentioned above, these complexities are discussed in a later section.

The R^{oi} Haplotype

A haplotype called R^{oi} was found by Layrisse et al. (684,685) in a South American Indian tribe. This haplotype, that can be written as *cD(e)*, or *cDe^i*, encodes production of less e than that made by *R⁰*. Whether e^i is qualitatively different from e, or simply represents a quantitative reduction of e, is not known.

The R^o-*like* Haplotype that Encodes JAL (Rh48)

As described above, Rh48 in Whites, is encoded by a haplotype that can be described as *(C)D(e)*. In Blacks, the antigen is encoded by a form of *R⁰* (111) that can be written as *(c)D(e)*. The expression of D is slightly increased.

Other Variants of R^o

As mentioned elsewhere, it is not always possible to differentiate between unusual *r* genes and unusual *R⁰* haplotypes, in individuals who have a paired haplotype that makes D. Accordingly, D-producing haplotypes, equivalent to *r^L* and *r^t* (67,610,611,631) may well exist. R^{oL} could be written as *(c)D(e)f* (c and e production reduced, f production normal) and R^{ot} as *(c)D(e)(f)* (c, e and f production all reduced).

The haplotype called R^{1n} by some and R^{on} by one of us (311,622,686) encodes production of D, some C or C^G, c, e and f, but no rh$_i$. For the same reasons that *r'^{S}* was considered a variant of *r* and not a variant of *r'*, R^{on} was considered a variant of *R⁰* not of *R¹* (686). That interpretation is, of course, now called into question by the already described observation of Blunt et al. (625) that *r'^{S}* is probably derived from *RHD* and not from *r* or *r'*.

Champney et al. (687) reported a haplotype described as *cD(e)* in a Black individual and we (688) studied a Black family in which the proposita was apparently a *cD(e)* homozygote. It was noticeable that the e antigen made by the *cD(e)* homozygote was so depressed in expression that she was at first thought to be homozygous for *Dc-*. While attempting to perform dosage studies in the investigation we found that the red cells of Black e homozygotes, often carry similar levels of e to the red cells of White *Ee* heterozygotes. Table 12-16 shows the products of some haplotypes that appear similar to *R⁰*.

Variants of R^2, the Antigens E^T and E^W and the Phenotype E^u

There are fewer variants of this haplotype than of *R¹* and *R⁰*. Vos and Kirk (121) reported a non-red cell stimulated antibody in the serum of an Australian Aborigine that had a specificity close to that of anti-E, for it reacted with all of 130 E+ samples from Whites. However, the antibody was non-reactive with approximately half of a similar number of E+ red cells from Australian Aborigines. The antibody was called anti-E^T and it was concluded that all reactive samples from Whites were phenotypically E+ E^T+, while among Australian Aborigines the phenotypes E+ E^T+ and E+ E^T-, both exist. The haplotype making E and E^T was called *cDE^T* (presumably the same as the White *R²* (*cDE*) haplotype) while the one that made E without E^T was called *cDE '*. As mentioned in the introduction of this chapter, E^T has now been declared obsolete (could one say that ET went home?). The reason for declaring E^T obsolete is that no anti-E^T remains so that the E+ E^T- phenotype can no longer be recognized for comparison with other forms of partial E (see next section).

The haplotype R^{2w} (*cDE^w*) makes less E than does R^2 (85,689-692). Additionally, there is a qualitative difference between E and E^w since antibodies with anti-E^w specificity have been found (85,691). The E^w variant of E is rare and can perhaps be thought of as a low incidence marker antigen, made by certain rare R^2 haplotypes. As far as we are aware, a *cDE^w* haplotype has not yet been found, although it probably exists. Anti-E^w has caused HDN (85,691).

A variant form of R^2 was originally called R^{2u} to

TABLE 12-16 Some Haplotypes Apparently Related to R^o

Shorthand Name	CDE Term	Low incidence "Marker" Antigen	Some Antigen Levels (Compared to R^o)
R^o	cDe		
R^{oJal}	(c)D(e)	JAL	c↓ e↓ D slt↑
R^{oIVa}	$cD^{IVa}e$	Go^a	D↑
R^{oJoh}	cDe	?Rh33	
R^{oVa}	cDe	D^w	
R^{oi}	cDe^i		e↓
R^{on}	cDe^{s}C^G		e↓
R^{ow}	cDeC^w	C^w	c↓ e↓
	cD(e)		e↓↓
R^{oL}	(c)D(e)		c↓ e↓ f→
R^{ot}	(c)D(e)		c↓ e↓ f↓
Santi	$cD^{acd}e$		D↓ e↓ G↓ V↓
R^{oHar}	c(D)(e)	Rh33, FPTT	D↓↓ e↓

indicate that the amount of E made was reduced, the analogy was that E^u was to E as D^u was to D (693-696). In other words, what we would now prefer to call weak E, involved a quantitative not a qualitative difference from E. Another variant of R^2 is best described (697,698) as (c)D(E) since it makes less c and E than does R^2. Race and Sanger (49) pointed out that at least once the same individual was described in one publication (697) as having (c)D(E) and in another (695) as having cDE^u. As mentioned earlier, the R^2 haplotype that makes Go^a is thought to make less E than does R^2 (506).

Partial E

It is entirely probable that some of the phenotypes described above represent the presence of partial E on red cells. That the E antigen comprises a number of epitopes is apparent from reports (699,700) of the production of alloimmune anti-E by individuals with E+ E^T+ E^w- red cells and the finding (701) of E+ red cells that failed to react with two of eight monoclonal and four of 22 polyclonal anti-E. No doubt when a sufficient number of samples that carry partial E has been found, monoclonal antibodies will be used to determine their E epitope composition. Because such data are not yet available, table 12-17 lists the variants of R^2 recognized from tests with human Rh antibodies.

The Antigen Be^a (Rh36)

In 1953, Davidsohn et al. (102) described the low incidence antigen, Be^a, the antibody against which caused severe HDN (702). It was not until 24 years later when another example of the antibody caused HDN (703) that it was shown (49) that Be^a is part of the Rh system. In three generations of the family studied (49,703) Be^a was seen to be encoded by a r gene that also makes reduced levels of c, e and f. Before Be^a was shown

TABLE 12-17 Some Haplotypes Apparently Related to R^2

Shorthand Name	CDE Term	Low Incidence "Marker" Antigen	Some Antigen Levels (Compared to R^2)
R^2	cDE		
R^{2t}	cDE^t		no E^T
R^{2IVb}	$cD^{IVb}E$	?Evans	
R^{2Va}	$cD^{Va}E$	D^w	
R^{2VI}	$cD^{VI}E$		
	cDE	FPTT	
	cDE		partial E
R^{2w}	cDE^w	E^w	E↓
	cDE^u		E↓
R^{2IVa}	$cD^{IVa}(E)$	Go^a	D↑ E↓
	(c)D(E)		c↓ E↓

to be encoded from the Rh locus, another case of HDN caused by anti-Be^a was reported (704), an additional severe case has been reported since (705).

Other Variants of r

Once it was shown that a (c)d(e) gene, that also encodes production of a reduced amount of f, includes Be^a as one of its products, it became clear that not all (c)d(e) genes are the same for others are known that do not make Be^a. In other words, the presence or absence of Be^a divides individuals with two different forms of (c)d(e), just as the presence or absence of Rh35 divides individuals with two different forms of (C)D(e).

Other genes in the r series include r^L that, as mentioned earlier, encodes reduced expression of c and e, but a normal expression of f and r^t that encodes reduced production of c, e and f. Table 12-18 lists a number of vari-

TABLE 12-18 Some Genes Apparently Related to *r*

Shorthand Name	*CDE* Term	Low Incidence "Marker" Antigen	Some Antigen Levels (Compared to *r*)
r	*cde*		
	cde		partial c
	(c)de		c↓ Rh:-26
r^s	*cde^s*		e↓
r^L	*(c)d(e)*		c↓ e↓ f→
r^t	*(c)d(e)*		c↓ e↓ f↓
Be^a	*(c)d(e)*	Be^a	c↓ e↓
	(c)d(e)C^w	C^w	c↓ e↓
	(c)d(e)C^x	C^x	c↓ e↓
	(c)d(e)		c↓ e↓

ant genes thought to be related to *r* and includes *cC^wde* and *cC^xde* that have been described earlier.

Variants of *R^Z*, *r^Y*, *r′* and *r″*

Since the *R^Z* haplotype and the *r^Y*, *r′* and *r″* genes are all rare, it is not surprising that relatively few variant forms have been reported.

An unusual expression of an antigen, at first named c^V (35,38) was later shown (627) to be the C made by *R^Z* (*CDE*). As already discussed, while *R^Z* is generally said to make less C than does *R¹*, such observations may reflect, in part, the fact that many anti-C sera are largely anti-rh_i (anti-Ce) and that *R¹* makes rh_i while *R^Z* does not. The haplotype *CC^wDE* has been reported (648-650).

In the *r′* series *CC^Wde* (83,647) and *CC^xde* (672) have been described; in the *r^Y* series *CC^wdE* has been reported (646). A form of *r″* making a reduced amount of E was described (706) as *cdE^u*. In 1967, Morton and Rosenfield (707) described a gene that appeared to encode production of C, c and E, but no D. The gene was called *r^{Yn}* in analogy to *r′ n* and *R¹ⁿ*. In view of what has been written earlier, it seems that the gene could be interpreted as either *CcdE* or as *cdEC^G*.

Low Incidence Rh System Antigens

It is a tribute to blood group serologists, biochemists and geneticists, that most of the low incidence antigens of the Rh system have been, or will be, described in other sections of this chapter. That is to say, knowledge about

the Rh system is now such that most of the antigens are known to be encoded by certain *Rh* genes or are firmly established as being characteristic of certain phenotypes. Table 12-19 lists 16 low incidence Rh antigens and indicates the places of 15 of them within the Rh system. That table will also serve as an index so that readers will be able to see in which section each antigen is described. The table includes one other low incidence antigen that already has an Rh number (Craw or Rh43) and two (HOFM and LOCR) that are potential candidates for admission to the Rh system. HOFM and LOCR, together with Craw are described in this section. The antigens V, VS and hr^H are not included in table 12-19, while rare in Whites, the antigens are more common in Blacks and are described in their own section. The antigens CE (Rh22) and Ce^S (Rh42) are also excluded from the table since they have been considered in the section dealing with f, rh_i, et al.

1. Craw (Rh43)

In studies with the only examples of anti-Rh43 described in print, Cobb (105) found the antigen defined to be present on the red cells of about 1 in 950 random Blacks in the Southeastern part of the USA. Assignment of the number Rh43 may have been premature since the evidence that Craw is part of the Rh system is entirely circumstantial and not strong, at that. First, anti-Craw was found as a separable component in two lots of anti-D typing reagents. Second, reexamination of the pedigrees of families that included persons with Craw+ red cells showed that the encoding gene did not segregate from *Rh*, although it was originally reported (105) to do so. Third, it was found (708) that most Craw+ samples were from persons with *r′^S* but exceptions were seen. Clearly, more work is necessary to determine whether Craw is truly an Rh antigen, additional examples of anti-Craw do not seem to have been found.

2. HOFM (ISBT 700.50)

This antigen was described in 1990 (709) when the defining antibody caused mild HDN. In the family studied, those persons with HOFM+ red cells had depressed expression of C but not of E or e. No unrelated persons with HOFM+ red cells have been found (58).

3. LOCR (ISBT 700.53)

This antigen was described in 1994 (710) when, in two cases, the defining antibody caused mild HDN. In

TABLE 12-19 Low Incidence Antigens of the Rh System

Antigen	Some Characteristics
C^w and C^x	Most often present with C, rarely present on C- c+ red cells
E^w	E^w+ red cells react with most, but not all anti-E
D^w	Marker of partial D, category Va red cells
Go^a	Marker of partial D, category IVa red cells
Rh32	Encoded most often by $\bar{\bar{R}}^N$, also present on partial D, DBT red cells
Rh33	Encoded by R^{oHar} and $D^{IV}(C)$- and perhaps by R^{oJoh} and R^{ILisa}
Rh35	Made by a *(C)D(e)* haplotype that makes normal D
Be^a	Made by a gene that makes weak c and e
Evans	Made by *D••* and possibly present on partial D, category IVb red cells
Tar	Marker of partial D, category VII red cells, found on one D - -/D - - sample
Craw	Possibly made by some *r* genes, may not be an Rh system antigen
Riv	Thus far seen only as a product of $D^{IVa}(C)$-
JAL	Associated with *(C)D(e)* in Whites and *(c)D(e)* in Blacks
STEM	Present on some but not all red cells that are hr^S- or hr^B-
FPTT	Made by $D^{IV}(C)$-, R^{oHar} and some other rare haplotypes that make weak C and/or weak e
BARC	Made by $CD^{IV}e$ but not by $cD^{VI}E$
Low Incidence Antigens That May be Part of the Rh System	
HOFM	May be associated with haplotypes that make weak C
LOCR	May be associated with haplotypes that make weak c or e

two unrelated families with LOCR+ members and in a third unrelated proband, presence of the LOCR antigen was associated with reduced expression of c. In a fourth unrelated individual with LOCR+ red cells, e antigen expression was reduced. Although the gene encoding LOCR was seen to travel with *r* in all three families studied, statistical evidence fell just short of proving that LOCR is an *Rh* antigen.

4. Commentary

In considering both HOFM and LOCR, it should be remembered that a phenotypic relationship with Rh does not always extend to the genetic level. The low incidence antigen Ol^a (ISBT 700.43) was seen (711) to be associated with weakened expression of C and/or E and less marked weakening of D in 11 members of a family who had Ol(a+) red cells. In 9 members of the same family, who had Ol(a-) red cells, no reduction in expression of Rh antigens was seen. However, Kornstad (711) showed that *Ol^a* is not at the *Rh* locus (independently inherited suppressors of Rh are discussed in a later section). It

should be stressed that the investigators reporting HOFM and LOCR (709,710) pointed out that the antigens show a phenotypic association with Rh but that the data available at that time, did not allow assignment of *HOFM* or *LOCR* to the Rh locus.

Other Observations on Antibodies to Low Incidence Rh Antigens

In working with antibodies to low incidence antigens it should always be remembered that Rh antibodies cause (often severe) HDN. Accordingly, any time that an unidentified antibody to a low frequency antigen causes the disease, efforts are in order to see if an Rh antibody is involved. It should be remembered that anti-Go^a and anti-Be^a were initially thought to define non-Rh antigens. Both anti-Go^a (500) and anti-Be^a (102) caused HDN when first found; both (anti-Go^a,504,505) (anti-Be^a,703-705) have done so since. Later (49,103) it was shown that Go^a and Be^a are encoded from the *Rh* locus. Thus it comes as no surprise to find that: anti-C^w (83,408,644,661-663,666,668,669); anti-C^x (84,406,

671); anti-E^w (85,691); anti-Rh32 (99,642,712); anti-Rh33 (247); anti-Evans (104,713); anti-Tar (513-515); anti-Riv (107); anti-JAL (111); anti-STEM (113); and perhaps anti-D^w (923,924) have all caused varying degrees of HDN. Whenever we are called on to investigate a case of HDN caused by an antibody that is initially seen to react only with red cells of the infant and those of its father, our next step (642) is always to test red cells that carry low incidence Rh antigens, often we need look no further.

An antibody, anti-Zd, described in 1970 by Svanda et al. (714) fit many of the criteria above, *Zd* may have traveled with *r* in the family studied. However, we understand that Zd+ red cells and anti-Zd are no longer available so that the relationship of Zd to Rh, if any, will never be known.

As mentioned earlier, when Chown et al. (9) investigated the case in which $\bar{\bar{R}}^N$ arose by de novo mutation, they adsorbed a serum known to contain antibodies to C, rh$_i$, C^w, V and D^w on to red cells that were D^w+ but which lacked the other antigens to which antibodies were directed. The eluate from those cells contained anti-D^w and anti-Rh32 although the adsorbing red cells were then shown to be Rh:-32. Somewhat similarly, a serum Tillett, originally appeared to contain antibodies to Go^a, Rh32 and Evans (Rh37) although the antibody-maker had not been exposed to any of those antigens. When the serum was adsorbed with Rh:32 Go(a-) Rh:-37 red cells, all activity for Go^a and Rh37, as well as that for Rh32 was removed (493). A later batch of the Tillett serum contained activity for Go^a and Rh:37 but not for Rh:32 red cells. When that batch of serum was adsorbed with Rh:32 Go(a-) Rh:-37 red cells, no activity was removed. However, adsorption with either Go(a+) Rh:-37 or Go(a-) Rh:37 red cells removed all activity for both antigens (717). The Tillett serum also contains several antibodies to antigens that are not part of the Rh system (718), one of those antibodies is anti-Wr^a. When Wr(a+) Go(a-) Rh:-32,-37 red cells were used in adsorption studies, anti-Wr^a was removed, the Rh antibodies were not. When the Rh:32 cells adsorbed activity for all three Rh antigens, anti-Wr^a was not removed (493,717).

In the section dealing with low incidence antigens on partial D red cells, it is suggested that the low incidence antigens represent new sequences of amino acids on Rh polypeptides encoded by rearranged genes. Presumably, the adsorption studies just described represent the presence of amino acid sequences common to more than one antigen. The regular appearance of anti-Rh32 in sera that contain inseparable Rh antibodies, is noticeable. It is possible that, similarly to what has been suggested (508) for anti-C and anti-G, some of these antibodies recognize a structure of an *RHD*-encoded polypeptide, others recognize the same (or similar) structure on an *RHCE*-encoded protein, while still others recognize the structure on either type of protein.

Rh Haplotypes in Families and *Trans* and *Cis* Position Effects

The haplotypes described in tables 12-15 to 12-18 probably represent oversimplification, haplotypes intermediate to those shown probably exist. In quantitative studies, Rosenfield and his colleagues (59-65) have shown that, in the absence of *trans* position effects, an *Rh* haplotype in a family will produce the same amount of antigens in all members who inherit the haplotype.

In contrast to the above, there are known situations in which the haplotype on one chromosome affects the expression of that on the paired chromosome. The most dramatic *trans* position effect (see earlier) involves genotypes such as *r'R^o* or *r'R^1* in which *C* in *trans* to *D* can result in the weak D phenotype although the *D* gene involved makes normal *D* when *c* is in *trans* (270,271). Somewhat similarly, more C seems to be made by persons genetically *Cde/cde* than by those genetically *CDe/cDE* (719). In general, the presence of *D* in *trans* seems often to have a depressing effect on C, E and e (49).

There is no longer a need to speculate about *cis* position effects (formerly the effect of a gene on another on the same chromosome). Since combinations of C, c, E and e are encoded by the alleles of *RHCE*, it can now be presumed that different alleles, i.e. *RHCe*, *RHcE*, *RHce* and *RHCE* encode different amounts of antigen or, more likely, polypeptides on which the antigens are more, or less, accessible to their antibodies.

Independently Inherited Suppressor Genes

There are a number of reports that describe the actions of genes, apparently not at or linked to the *Rh* locus, that affect Rh antigen production. Dunsford and Tippett (720) showed that two sisters, who had inherited the same *R^1* haplotype, had noticeably different amounts of D, C, rh$_i$, c, f and e on their red cells (each sister had *r* paired with the *R^1*). Giles and Bevan (721) studied a family in which the actions of both *R^1* and *R^2* haplotypes were affected. Both haplotypes made the expected quantities of antigens in the parents. Their two daughters appeared to *(C)D(e)/(c)D(E)*, yet the son of one of the daughters inherited his mother's *R^2* haplotype that, in him, functioned normally. In a family, studied by Heiken and Giles (722) an *R^2* haplotype behaved normally in a mother and two of her children, but acted like *(c)D(E)* in a third child. The *R^1* haplotype of the affected child produced the expected amounts of C, D and e. In the families mentioned above, the evidence suggested that the suppressor genes were not at or linked to the *Rh* locus. That these conclusions were almost certainly correct is illustrated by findings regarding the most dramatic suppressors of Rh. As described in later sections, the $X^o r$ gene that, in double dose effects the modifier type of Rh_{null} and the X^Q gene that, in double dose causes the Rh_{mod} phenotype, have been shown, many times (references given in the later sections) to segregate independently of *Rh*. It is entirely possible that some of the cases referenced above involved the presence of X^Q or a similar gene.

The Antigen e and its Variants

The e antigen is of high incidence being found on the red cells of 98% of random Whites and on the cells of perhaps even more random Blacks. In the majority of, but not quite all cases, e and anti-e in Whites, are straightforward. The antibody can be formed by E+ e- (usually $R^2 R^2$) people and when made, reacts with all e+ samples. In Blacks the story is rather different for some of them, who have red cells that type as e+, make antibodies that closely resemble anti-e (or anti-f or anti-rh_i, see below) yet which do not react with the antibody-makers' own red cells. In this respect, it seems that the e antigen must involve many epitopes and that the state of lacking some of them, that is having red cells that carry partial e, is more common in Blacks than in Whites. Unfortunately, the situation involving the production of anti-e by persons with partial e on their red cells is not as well characterized as the situation in which persons with partial D make alloimmune anti-D. Instead, in many instances it seems that the antibodies made are individualistic in specificity. The complexity was recognized early. In the fifth edition of their textbook, Race and Sanger (723) included a table, prepared from the studies of Dr. Tippett, of the reactions of antibodies with specificities similar to anti-e made by Black women who had e+ red cells. Although only nine samples are listed, at least six different patterns of antibody reactivity can be seen. In the text, a tenth sample giving yet another reaction pattern is mentioned. In 1981 we (724,725) tried to classify the e+ red cells of the antibody-makers and the anti-e-like specificities made, in 16 persons. We needed 12 categories. If anything, since 1981 the situation has become more, instead of less complex. However, as explained below, the complexity is not entirely due to heterogeneity of the antibodies. An added complication is that not all red cell samples called hr^S- or hr^B-, or all antibodies called anti-hr^S or anti-hr^B, are as alike as the names imply.

The sections that follow, on e and its variants (660) are disproportionally long, compared to the way in which other Rh antigens are described in this chapter. These lengthy explanations have been included by design. First, the provision of blood for patients with e+ red cells and alloimmune anti-e-like specificities in the serum, is a fairly frequent problem for blood bankers. It is hoped that these sections will provide practical help. Second, one of us receives more telephone calls about this situation than about any other aspect of Rh. Third, there are no short answers!

The Antigen hr^S

In 1960, Shapiro (26) published the results of his studies on the blood of a Bantu lady, Mrs. Shabalala. In initial tests, the Shabalala serum reacted with all red cells that carried E or e; however, its reactions were noticeably weaker with E+ e- than with e+ red cells. After adsorption with $R_2 R_2$ red cells, the Shabalala antibody still reacted with most e+ but not with E+ e- red cells. Shapiro called the unadsorbed antibody anti-hr^S and reported that most bloods (including almost all samples from Whites) that are e+ are also hr^S+. E+ e- and E- e- samples are all hr^S-. In the Black South African population, e+ hr^S- samples were found. Shapiro used a carat sign to indicate haplotypes that make e but not hr^S; $\hat{R}^o$, $\hat{R}^{ou}$ and $\hat{r}$ were all described. Because it was not known (and is still quite hard to determine) which anti-e were mixtures of anti-e and anti-hr^S and which were anti-e without anti-hr^S, it was difficult to be certain that e+ hr^S- red cells carry less e than those that are e+ hr^S+. While subsequent studies have certainly suggested that this is the case, the difference appears most dramatic when an anti-e containing anti-hr^S is used to type e+ hr^S- samples.

The other antibody in the Shabalala serum, that was adsorbed by $R_2 R_2$ red cells, initially appeared to be identical to the anti-Hr$_o$ made by immunized Rh-deletion (*D--*, *Dc-*, etc., i.e. E- e-) homozygotes. However, Shapiro (26) was able to separate the antibodies in such sera by adsorption with the Shabalala red cells. He concluded that the Shabalala red cells were Hr$_o$+ Hr- and that the sera of many immunized Rh-deletion homozygotes contain both anti-Hr$_o$ and anti-Hr. He named the second antibody in the Shabalala serum anti-Hr. In a later publication (51) it was suggested that the portion of the Shabalala serum that was not anti-hr^S (i.e. that portion that could be adsorbed by $R_2 R_2$ red cells) could be thought of as anti-Hr^S.

The findings described above started an argument that has still not been resolved. While some workers (26,46,51,109,311,680,681) regard anti-Hr (anti-Hr^S) and anti-hr^S as defining distinct Rh antigens, others

(517,726,727) regard anti-hr^S as being contained within anti-Hr. Case (726) and Moores (739) believe that the Shabalala antibody defines a single character that has a graded strength on different red cells, i.e. greater on e+ than on e- samples. Unfortunately, adsorption studies have not resolved this point. While some workers (109,311,686) found that once anti-Hr had been removed from the Shabalala serum by adsorption with R_2R_2 red cells, further adsorption with red cells of that phenotype did not remove anti-hr^S, there are anecdotal reports that others, working with sera ostensibly containing the same antibodies, were able to achieve adsorption to exhaustion with R_2R_2 red cells.

Regardless of the explanation of the Shabalala serum, other individuals (presumably with Hr+ hr^S- red cells) appear to have made anti-hr^S without anti-Hr (728,729). The patient described by Grobbelaar and Moores (728) was genetically $R^2\hat{R^o}$ or $R^2\hat{r}$ and so presumably had Hr on her red cells (i.e. made by her R^2 gene). As described below, we (729) have described a number of immunized individuals who appeared to have partial e, partial Hr$_o$, and sometimes partial D on their red cells. In many instances these individuals at first presented with anti-e-like specificities. Following transfusion (often with R_2R_2 blood) some of them made an antibody very much like anti-Hr$_o$, presumably directed against the portion(s) of Hr$_o$ that their red cells lacked. However, other patients with anti-e-like (some of which failed to react with some hr^S- samples) continued to make just those antibodies, even after many transfusions. Thus, it seems that persons with partial e on their red cells, including those with e+ hr^S- and with e+ hr^B- phenotypes (see below), can be divided into two groups. Some have red cells that carry partial e and partial Hr$_o$ or partial Hr^B (see below). Such persons can make antibodies to the epitopes of e and Hr$_o$ or Hr^B that their red cells lack. The second group have red cells that carry partial e, again including some with e+ hr^S- and some e+ hr^B- red cells, but apparently all epitopes of Hr$_o$ and Hr^B. In these persons the immune response (in terms of partial e) appears to be limited to the production of anti-e-like specificities (including anti-hr^S and anti-hr^B).

The Antigen hr^B

In 1972 Shapiro et al. (97) published a report of their studies on the blood of a South African Cape Colored lady, Mrs. Anne Bastiaan. In many respects, the findings in this case were similar to the findings in the Shabalala case. The whole Bastiaan serum reacted with all red cell samples; again, the reactions with R_2R_2 red cells were notably weaker than those with e+ samples. After adsorption with R_2R_2 red cells to the point at which E+

e- cells were no longer reactive, the Bastiaan serum contained activity for a large majority of e+ samples. This isolated antibody was named anti-hr^B. This time it was found that in the South African Black population, the phenotype e+ hr^B- exists. Shapiro et al. (97) designated those *Rh* haplotypes that made e but not hr^B with a large period over the gene symbol. Presence of haplotypes $\dot{R^o}$, $\dot{R^{ou}}$ and $\dot{r}$ in the population was reported. Later, it was suggested (51) that the portion of the Bastiaan serum that is not anti-hr^B can be thought of as anti-Hr^B. However, Allen and Rosenfield (47) had applied the term anti-Rh34 to describe the total immune response of Bastiaan. Thus, it is important to realize that anti-Rh34 and anti-Hr^B are not the same thing. Unlike the situation described above for Shabalala, where anti-Hr and anti-Hr^S are alternative names for the same antibody and where the total immune response can be described as anti-Hr (or anti-Hr^S) plus anti-hr^S, anti-Rh34 represents anti-Hr^B plus anti-hr^B.

Essentially the same situation exists regarding the Bastiaan serum as that regarding the Shabalala serum. While some workers (47,51,31) regard anti-Hr^B plus anti-hr^B as defining separate entities, others (730) regard the entities as quantitatively different amounts of Rh34. So as not to belabor the point it will simply be stated that, as discussed above for Shabalala, one of us (729) has tested samples from patients who made anti-e-like specificities that failed to react with some hr^B- samples and that did not contain anti-Hr^B. This time it appears that some persons have e+ hr^B- red cells that do not lack any portions of Rh34 or Hr^B, so they can make just anti-hr^B (or an antibody closely related to it, see below).

Ostensible Similarities Between Anti-hr^S and Anti-f and Between Anti-hr^B and Anti-rh$_i$

For reasons discussed in the next section, it is somewhat hazardous (at least in the United States) to identify an antibody as anti-hr^S or anti-hr^B; far safer terms are anti-hr^S-like and anti-hr^B-like. However, based on the original reports (26,97) and on subsequent studies (46,47,311,686,724,725,731) there are a number of clues that suggest that an antibody of one of these types has been found. The antigen hr^S is better developed on red cells that are f+ than on those that are e+ f-. Thus, an antibody that reacts with rr, R_o and R_1R_1 cells, but gives stronger reactions with cells of the first two phenotypes, may well be anti-hr^S-like in nature. The antigen hr^B is better developed on red cells that are rh$_i$+ than on those that are e+ rh$_i$-. Thus, when an antibody reacts with R_1R_1, rr and R_o red cells, but gives its best reactions with cells of the first phenotype listed, anti-hr^B-like should be considered a very real possibility. In both cases an obvious additional initial clue is that the antibody in question does not react with R_2R_2 (e- f- rh$_i$-) red cells. The suggestive evidence can be taken further. One of us (686) has seen several examples of antibodies that appeared to be anti-f but were apparently alloimmune in nature and were certainly made by persons with f+ red cells. The facts that the antibodies could be adsorbed to exhaustion with R_1R_1 (e+ hr^S- f-) red cells and that the antibody makers had red cells that did not react (or react well) with some anti-e helped in pursuing evidence for the anti-hr^S-like specificities. Somewhat similarly, we (732) were sent a serum that appeared to contain only alloimmune anti-C or anti-rh$_i$ although the antibody maker had C+ rh$_i$+ red cells. The finding that the antibody could be adsorbed to exhaustion with rr red cells pointed to its actual anti-hr^B-like specificity. This second finding explains the admonition, made twice earlier in this chapter, that an apparent alloimmune anti-C, made by an individual with C+ red cells, should never be ascribed that specificity until it has been shown to resist adsorption by C- e+ hr^S+ h^B+ red cells.

Differentiation between hr^S, hr^B and Other Partial e Antigens

As would have been expected from the findings on partial D, red cells that lack one epitope of e, if that is how hr^S and hr^B can truly be described (see below), are more likely than not to lack more than one epitope. Thus, when e+ hr^S- and e+ hr^B- red cells first became available for use in serological studies, some anti-e-like specificities, made in persons with e+ red cells were called anti-hr^S or anti-hr^B because of their failure to react with (sometimes only one example of) hr^S- or hr^B- red cells. Those sera were then used to characterize other partial e samples and the designations e+ hr^S- or e+ hr^B- (or even e+ hr^S- hr^B-) were applied. In fact, in many instances the "new" examples of anti-hr^S and anti-hr^B were not exactly the same as the originals, meaning that the "new" e+ hr^S- and e+ hr^B- samples were not the same as the originals, either. When these antibodies and red cells samples were used to resolve new cases, and the materials from the new cases were used to resolve still others, the problem was magnified by a geometric progression. The net result is that now many cells and sera in the collections of immunohematologists are labeled in terms of hr^S and hr^B when they would be more correctly described as being red cells or sera from persons with partial e on their red cells. It is, of course, for these reasons that the admonition to use the terms anti-hr^S-like and anti-hr^B-like is given in the preceding section.

Further Complexities of Partial e

As indicated earlier, subdivision of the e antigen into the phenotypes e+ hr^S- hr^B+, e+ hr^S+ hr^B- and e+ hr^S- hr^B- represents a gross oversimplification of the actual state of affairs. As an example, when the blood samples of Shabalala (26) and Santiago (680,681) were studied, it appeared that both proposita were phenotypically e+ hr^S- and that both had made anti-hr^S. Later we (682) studied a family in which one gene made the hr^S defined by the Shabalala antibody but not that defined by the Santiago serum, while another gene did exactly the opposite. As mentioned earlier, Race and Sanger (723) documented six anti-e-like specificities made in nine individuals. In that table, the Shab and Santi antibodies gave the same reactions; the later studied red cells of our family members (682) subdivided one of the six anti-e-like specificities listed. Many other antibodies apparently recognizing additional epitopes of e have been found, names have not been applied because of the individualistic nature of many of the antibodies. As discussed in the next section, the complexity is further compounded since persons with partial e on the red cells seem often to have partial Hr and/or Hr$_0$ antigens as well. Thus the antibodies they make appear often to detect epitopes of more than one antigen. Resolution of this complexity will apparently need considerable input at the biochemical level. That is, how do the Rh polypeptides of these individuals differ and against which structures are their antibodies directed?

Partial e Associated with Partial Expression of Other Rh Antigens

We (660,729) have reported some of our observations on more than 50 cases of anti-e-like specificities that we have studied over the last 15 years. Several points are pertinent to this discussion. First, some 90 percent of the antibody-makers were Black. Clearly, lack of portions of the e antigen is more common in Blacks than in Whites. Second, from the finding that the situation was not totally confined to Blacks, it is clear that partial e is also encountered in Whites. Workers should not be overly surprised to find anti-e-like specificities in the sera of White patients who have e+ red cells (660,686,724, 725,733). Third, most of the patients making antibodies of this type had cDe, cD(e) or cD^{weak}e red cells. However, the phenotypes cde and cd(e) were also represented. Fourth, all the patients we studied had been transfused, and the majority had also been pregnant. Fifth, patients with sickle cell disease were overrepresented; this finding may simply have reflected the facts that 90 percent of the patients were Black and that multiple transfusions in patients with sickle cell disease are common. Sixth, as discussed more fully below, many of the antibodies failed to react with some red cell samples alleged to be hr^S- and/or hr^B-. Seventh, the red cells of the antibody makers often failed to react with sera alleged to have anti-hr^S or anti-hr^B specificity. Eighth, a minority of the antibody makers made alloimmune anti-D in spite of the D+ status of their red cells.

In studying this group of patients, we tried to identify persons with hr^S- or hr^B- red cells who had made anti-hr^S or anti-hr^B, respectively. Our efforts were seldom rewarded. Instead, we found many examples of persons whose red cells were nonreactive with some examples of purported anti-hr^S or anti-hr^B but whose antibodies did not correspond to the apparent phenotype of their red cells. In other words, as discussed earlier, failure of red cells to react with anti-hr^S or anti-hr^B and failure of the antibodies to react with hr^S- and/or hr^B- test cells often indicates no more than that the individual involved has partial e on the red cells and has made an antibody or antibodies to those epitopes of e that are missing from the red cells.

Of more interest was our finding that the immune responses of these persons can be (generally) divided into two categories. First are persons whose red cell antigen abnormality seems to be restricted to partial e. Such persons make allo-anti-e-like specificities that do not change (save for the fairly regular production of separable anti-E) when they are transfused with R_2R_2 blood. Second are persons whose red cells seem to have both partial e and partial Hr$_0$ (for a full description of Hr$_0$ see a later section). When these individuals are transfused, the specificities of their alloantibodies seem to broaden, or additional antibodies are made such that their sera then react with all except Rh-deletion and Rh$_{null}$ red cells. In tests on the red cells of these patients with a battery of anti-Hr$_0$ made by immunized Rh-deletion homozygotes, it was seen that like e, Hr$_0$ is apparently composed of a series of epitopes. About two thirds of the patients we studied apparently had both partial e and partial Hr$_0$, after transfusion with R_2R_2 blood, their antibodies that previously recognized only the portions of e that their red cells lacked, broadened in specificity to recognize the missing portions of Hr$_0$, as well. Tests with the anti-Hr$_0$ described above confirmed this conclusion by giving variable reactions with the red cells of the antibody makers. In retrospect, it seems highly likely that this situation also describes the immune response of Mrs. Shabalala. In other words, the antibody that was originally called anti-Hr was probably similar to what we (729) called anti-Hr$_0$-like; that is, an antibody made by a person with partial Hr$_0$ on the red cells. Lack of the original reagents will likely prevent this point from ever being proved; however, the close similarities of the sero-

logical observations make the explanation likely.

The situation described is relatively easy to recognize, but extremely difficult to categorize. In a typical case, a patient with e+ red cells presents with an alloimmune anti-e-like specificity. Often the antibody is nonreactive with R_2R_2 red cells. Following transfusion with such red cells, the patient's antibody is seen to have changed so that now only Rh-deletion and Rh$_{null}$ red cells are compatible. As indicated above, the patient has now made anti-e-like and anti-Hr$_0$-like specificities (arguably the same immune response) to epitopes lacking from the red cells. It should be remembered that heterogeneity of anti-Hr$_0$-like specificities has already been documented. Rosenfield (680,681) and Rosenfield et al. (46) reported that some of these antibodies prefer (i.e., give strongest reactions with) E+ e- red cells, while others prefer cells that are E- e+. Still others show no preference for E+ or e+ red cells. Similarly, some of the sera react preferentially with C+ red cells and initially appear to contain anti-C. Later we (734) showed that auto-anti-nl (which ostensibly at least have an anti-Hr$_0$-like specificity) behave similarly. In other words, just as anti-hr^S can resemble anti-f and anti-hr^B can resemble anti-rh$_i$ or anti-C in initial antibody identification studies, antibodies to epitopes of Hr$_0$ can resemble anti-E or anti-e. As already mentioned, in these settings adsorption studies are essential to establish actual antibody specificities.

Yet another complication to this story is that some of these patients have partial D as well as partial e and partial Hr$_0$ on their red cells. In such cases, following the transfusion of R_2R_2 red cells (or other compatible D+ blood, see below), the patient's serum reacts with all except Rh$_{null}$ red cells. The finding that Rh-deletion red cells (D--/D--, Dc-/Dc-, etc.) are now incompatible can be extremely confusing. We (720) resolved this particular conundrum by adsorbing the sera in question with rr red cells. Eluates made from the adsorbing red cells contained the anti-e-like and anti-Hr$_0$-like specificities, and the adsorbed sera contained anti-D. In all cases of this type that we have seen, the anti-D was easily separable from the other antibodies present. The same was not always true of the anti-e-like and anti-Hr$_0$-like antibodies made.

Heterogeneity of hr^S and hr^B

From what is written above, it is clear that some of the apparent heterogeneity of anti-hr^S and anti-hr^B relates directly to the labels that have been applied to various similar but not identical specificity antibodies. However, from our tests (739) with individual sera (often well categorized by Dr. Phyllis Moores in Durban, South Africa), it was apparent that hr^S and hr^B are unlikely to be single entities. One interpretation of such findings is that like e, D, and Hr_0; hr^S and hr^B may each be comprised of several epitopes. However, perhaps a more likely explanation is that hr^S- and hr^B- red cells lack a number of epitopes, one of which is common to each phenotype and perhaps more immunogenic than others in the group. Thus the forms of anti-hr^S and anti-hr^B most commonly seen may be directed against that epitope and the complexity may relate to the multiple epitope specificity of the antibodies and permutations of different epitopes missing from different examples of so-called hr^S- and hr^B- red cells.

Transfusions in Patients with Antibodies to Epitopes of e and Hr_0

In some patients with antibodies to the portions of e that their red cells lack, R_2R_2 red cells appear both serologically compatible and to survive normally in vivo. If the antibody specificity does not broaden after transfusion and if the patient does not make allo-anti-E, finding suitable blood for transfusion is no more difficult than finding blood for an R_2R_2 patient who has made anti-e. If the antibody-maker is of the type who has partial Hr_0 (and/or partial D) on the red cells and makes antibodies to the missing portions of those antigens, finding compatible blood becomes very difficult. Although the findings are not documented in the literature, we have heard several anecdotal reports of in vivo red cell survival studies performed in patients with antibodies to portions of e and Hr_0. It seems that such antibodies can be significant in vivo and sometimes effect clearance, at least of small labeled aliquots of incompatible red cells. However, screening tests on samples from selected donors are sometimes rewarded. It follows that if a number of persons with Rh phenotypes that lack portions of e and Hr_0 become immunized following transfusion (and less often following pregnancy), other individuals within the same ethnic group will have red cells of similar phenotypes. In working with patients of these phenotypes, we have sometimes been able to obtain large volumes of plasma. When we conducted mass screening studies (686,724,725), we found that in some instances, compatible units could be found (in selected donor groups) with an incidence of 1 or 2 in 100. With other antibodies the incidence was lower but compatible units could occasionally be found. Clearly, since most antibody-makers of this type are Black (739), the chances of finding compatible blood are increased if samples from Black donors are screened. Further, since the majority of persons who form antibodies of this type are R_0 or rr, initial Rh phenotyping studies can be used if sufficient low-cost reagents

(patients' sera) and time are available. Identification of R_0 and rr donors before the screening studies are performed is of particular value when a limited supply of the patient's serum is available or when the patient has partial or no D and has made anti-D in addition to anti-e-like and anti-Hr_0-like specificities. The use of diluted sera, rapid methods (LISS, Polybrene, PEG, etc.), and microtiter plates also facilitates mass screening with limited supplies of serum and time.

Monoclonal Antibodies to e and Closely Related Antigens

Now that monoclonal anti-e are available, the red cells of a number of blood donors, previously typed as E+ e-, have been seen to react with some, but not all, of the monoclonal-based anti-e and anti-e-like reagents. It is not yet clear whether the reactive monoclonal anti-e detect epitopes of e not recognized by human polyclonal reagents (that continue to give negative reactions with the red cells involved) or whether the reactions are more related to antibody strength. One speculative idea about these reactions relates to the molecular structure of e. As described in more detail in a later section of this chapter, the polypeptide that carries e has alanine at amino acid position 226. The polypeptide that carries E has proline at that position (41). Most D-bearing polypeptides also have alanine at position 226, yet that structure is not recognized by human polyclonal anti-e, e.g. D--/D-- red cells neither react with nor adsorb such anti-e. Thus it seemed at least theoretically possible that human polyclonal anti-e and the non-reactive monoclonal anti-e might recognize a structure based on Ala226 on *RHCe* and *RHce* encoded proteins while the reactive monoclonal anti-e might recognize that structure and one based on Ala226 on the *RHD* encoded protein. Attractive as this theoretical idea might be, there are no data to indicate that it represents the actual state of affairs. Neither we (753) nor others (41,754-756) have been able to demonstrate a positive reaction between the MAb to e involved, and D--/D-- red cells.

Sufficient studies have been performed with the monoclonal-based anti-e and anti-e-like reagents that it can be said that it does not seem that the reactive red cells, that type as e- with the polyclonal reagents, are all weakly e+ and hr^B- or hr^S-. Comfortingly, there are already several anecdotal reports that blood from some of these apparently R_2R_2 donors has been transfused to patients, with anti-e in the serum, without immediate or delayed transfusion reactions being seen and without post-transfusion increases of anti-e levels in the recipients.

Autoantibodies to e and Closely Related Antigens

As discussed in detail in Chapter 37, many Rh specificities that have been seen as alloantibodies have also been encountered in an autoimmune form. Antibodies to e and the related antigens discussed above, are no exception. Complicating the serological investigation of presumed alloantibodies of this type is the fact that on rare occasions an individual may make an anti-hr^B-like and/or an anti-Hr$_o$-like antibody at a time that antigen expression on the red cells is markedly depressed (735-737). These antibodies will thus appear to be alloimmune in nature and it may be necessary to wait, years in some cases, (736) until Rh antigen production on the patients' red cells returns to normal levels, to recognize the autoimmune nature of the antibodies. Since, at the time these antibodies are found, the patients' red cells may lack detectable representation of the antigens to which the antibodies are directed, it may still be necessary to use antigen-negative blood for transfusion (660,738).

The Antigen STEM (Rh49)

This low incidence antigen was described in 1993, by Marais et al. (113). The first example of anti-STEM caused mild HDN. The antibody apparently subdivides the hr^S- and hr^B- phenotypes. Among the STEM+ red cells found, 28 were hr^S- and 5 were hr^B-. However, 55 STEM+ hr^S+ and 78 STEM+ hr^B+ samples were also found. It is possible that those cells were from individuals heterozygous for haplotypes that do not encode hr^S or do not encode hr^B. The authors suggested that these findings might represent linkage disequilibrium. STEM was described as being a graded character as seen from tests with several of the anti-STEM studied, strength of expression of the antigen could not be related to zygosity of the apparently encoding gene. In reading the report about the discovery of STEM, it must be remembered that the authors (113) regard hr^S and hr^B differently from the way in which those antigens have been described above. They believe (730,739) that all hr^S- samples are Rh:-18,-19 (i.e. hr^S (Rh19) is part of Hr (Rh18)) and that all hr^B- samples are Rh:-31,-34 (i.e. hr^B (Rh31) is part of Rh34). As discussed in the previous sections we believe that the phenotypes hr^S- Hr- (Rh:-18,-19) and hr^S- Hr+ (Rh:18,-19) both exist and that some hr^B- red cells are Hr^B+ while others are Hr^B-. Regardless of the interpretation, it is possible that STEM is a marker antigen for some form(s) of partial e.

The Antigens V and VS

In 1955, DeNatale et al. (88) described an Rh antibody that they named anti-V. From use of the first anti-V and two examples found soon after (740) it was shown that V is present on the red cells of almost 30% of random American Blacks and up to 40% of those of other Black populations (44,88,92,154). In contrast, very few bloods from Whites were found that carried V (88). In addition, it was noted that V was the product of R^o (including examples of that haplotype that made weak D) and of *r*.

In 1960, Sanger et al. (89) described another new Rh antibody that they named anti-VS, after the name of the antibody-maker, Mrs. V.S. Anti-VS reacted with all V+ red cells and with most of those from Blacks with the r'^S gene. It was noticed (88,89) that VS+ red cells had an unusual form of e. The variant was called e^S and VS+ (e^S+) red cells were found to react with most, but not all examples of anti-e made by E+ e- persons. When the VS+ (e^S+) red cells were tested with e-like antibodies made in e+ persons, a higher proportion (but still a minority) of the sera were non-reactive. From these observations it was suggested that VS (e^S) might be encoded by a variant allele of *E* and *e*. Since V appeared to be made whenever c was encoded by the gene making e^S it was felt that V might be to e^S as f is to c. For a time observed serological findings fit with this assumption. However, as described in more detail below, additional findings were made that throw doubt on these interpretations.

Based on the original interpretations that VS equals e^S and V equals ce^S, it follows that all red cells that are V+ must also be VS+. Similarly red cells that are VS+ but are from individuals in whom the VS-producing gene makes C but not c, should be V-. Exceptions were first found to the latter of these concepts. A gene in Blacks that was at first thought to be *r'* was seen to make V and VS. Other Blacks who also appeared to have *r'* had red cells that were, as expected, V- VS+. These findings were usually explained by invoking the existence of two *r'*-like genes. The gene r'^S that can be written as $Ccde^S$ or as cde^SC^G (see an earlier section) was thought to encode VS (e^S) and V (ce^S). When anti-Rh42 was found (54) it was concluded that r'^S encodes both V (ce^S) and Rh42 (Ce^S or C^Ge^S). The *r'* gene that made VS without V was interpreted as *r'* or Cde^S.

A more difficult to explain finding came to light in about 1970 when a highly unusual sample was studied. Mr. L.I. is White and no paper has ever been written about him and his family. Accordingly, what is written below concerning his blood, has been extracted from textbooks (49,50,311,508) or represents results passed on from interested workers. Mr. L.I.'s *Rh* genotype was almost certainly $R^{1w}R^1$ and from a somewhat restricted family study it was apparent that his R^1 haplotype was unusual in terms of production of V and/or VS. Mr. L.I.'s red cells reacted strongly with all examples of anti-V with which they were tested. In studies using 9 different (and potent) examples of anti-VS, the L.I. cells were as strongly positive as control VS+ red cells with six, only weakly positive with two others and were non-reactive with one. Thus, Mr. L.I.'s R^1 (*CDe*) haplotype seemed certainly to have made V and may or may not have made VS. In tests with numerous different examples of the antibody, it was shown that Mr. L.I.'s red cells totally lacked c. Of course, if V equals ce^S and VS equals e^S, Mr. L.I.'s CDe^S haplotype cannot be explained, for it makes V(ce^S) (but no c) while it may or may not make VS(e^S). That it was L.I.'s R^1 not his R^{1w} that made V and perhaps VS, was seen from the study in which his sister was seen to have R^1 that made V while her son, who did not inherit her R^1 haplotype, had V- red cells. Two brothers with apparently the same CDe^S haplotype have been found (741).

The Antigens hr^v and hr^H

A different interpretation of findings similar to those described above, was made by Shapiro (92). From a study on the blood of South African Bantus, it was concluded that two quite distinct blood factors exist. One of these, hr^v, is probably identical to the V of DeNatale et al. (88). The second, hr^H, is most certainly not the same as the VS of Sanger et al. (89). Shapiro (92) found that hr^v and hr^H are common in Bantus. Further, he felt that either or both the blood factors could be produced by a variety of different haplotypes (most often *rh*, *rh'* or *Rh^o*). Thus, Shapiro felt that phenotypes hr^v+, hr^H-; hr^v+ hr^H+; hr^v- hr^H+; (and, of course, hr^v- hr^H-) all existed. As mentioned above, it had been noticed that VS+ red cells failed to react with rare examples of anti-e made by e-people and with a few of the anti-e-like antibodies made by e+ persons. The non-reactive sera often contained relatively weak anti-e or anti-e-like antibodies. Further, some potent examples of these antibodies reacted less strongly with VS+, than with e+ V- VS-, red cells. Thus if production of VS did not involve a variant allele of *E* or *e* (with participation of *c* for production of V) these findings might simply mean that genes that make hr^v or hr^H, encode production of less hr''(e), than do genes that make hr''(e) without hr^v or hr^H.

Shapiro (92) believed that much of the confusion about V and VS had arisen because the anti-VS used were not all of the same specificity. Some, that he studied, he felt were examples of just anti-hr^H. Others were examples of anti-hr^H plus anti-hr^v. Thus red cells of the phenotype hr^v- hr^H+, could be misclassified as hr^v+ hr^H+, if the presence of anti-hr^v in the anti-hr^H serum was not recognized. It is clear that the apparent V, VS, phenotype of a blood will be entirely dependent on the type of anti-VS used if

Shapiro's observations (92) are correct. For example, an hr^v+ hr^H-, sample will type as V+ VS+, if the anti-VS serum used contains anti-hr^v as well as anti-hr^H. The *same* sample will type as V+ VS-, if the anti-VS serum used contains anti-hr^H but no anti-hr^v. Thus it would seem that Shapiro's (92) concepts resolve the V, VS, difficulties. If V equals ce^s and VS equals e^s, then a CDe^s gene must make VS but not V. As will be seen from the above description of Mr. L.I.'s red cells, exactly the opposite seemed to occur. However, if the *CDe* haplotype involved encoded production of hr^v, but not hr^H, the serological findings could be explained. The blood would type as V+ with all anti-V (anti-hr^v) sera; as strong VS+ with those anti-VS that contained a potent anti-hr^v component; as weakly VS+ with those anti-VS sera that contained a weak anti-hr^v component; and as VS- with those anti-VS sera that were really anti-hr^H.

In the studies in which he separated anti-hr^v and anti-hr^H in certain anti-VS sera, Shapiro (92) found an occasional inseparable component, that could have been called anti-hr^{vH} and that could have been thought of as defining either a portion of the agglutinogen present on hr^v+, or hr^H+ red cells, or another blood factor normally present when either hr^v or hr^H is made.

Further Studies on V, VS, hr^H and hr^{vH}

In 1978, Tregallas and Issitt (742,743) described a series of studies designed to isolate and characterize the inseparable anti-hr^{vH}, mentioned by Shapiro (92). We took over 60 different blood samples that were V and/or VS+ and a series of anti-V and anti-VS sera. At least two of the anti-VS sera were ones that Shapiro (92) had said contained anti-hr^v and anti-hr^H. We ran adsorption studies in an attempt to remove ant-hr^v and leave anti-hr^H unadsorbed. We found that after three adsorptions with V- VS+ cells, no activity remained in any of the anti-VS sera. In contrast, after three adsorptions with V+ VS+ cells, anti-VS activity remained for V- VS+ but not for V+ VS+ red cells. Thus, the partially adsorbed anti-VS were behaving similarly to the anti-hr^H specificities found by Shapiro (92). However, when we (742,743) adsorbed the sera three more times with V+ VS+ red cells, all anti-VS activity, for both V- VS+ and V+ VS+ cells was removed. Thus it was apparent that in the majority of instances, the VS antigen of V- VS+ cells was stronger than the VS antigen of V+ VS+, red cells. Naturally, we had to answer the question as to whether hr^H was simply the enhanced VS of V- VS+ red cells that can be detected by partially adsorbed anti-VS sera. We were able to secure a small sample of the Hernandez serum, that contained the original and pure anti-hr^H described by Shapiro (92). This antibody behaved quite differently to the anti-VS sera we had studied. It could be totally adsorbed by hr^H+ red cells, but was not adsorbed at all by hr^H- red cells of the phenotypes V- VS+ or V+ VS+.

In trying to superimpose our findings (742,743) on those of Shapiro (92), DeNatale et al. (88) and Sanger et al. (89) we are well aware of potential pitfalls. First, from our studies (742,743) we know that the V and VS antigens of South African Bantus are stronger than those of American Blacks. Second, we may be comparing reactions of antibodies given the same names, that do not have exactly the same specificities. Third, we are dealing with data reported in two different terminologies. Exact translation from one to the other is not always possible. In spite of these difficulties, it seemed (to us (742,743) at least) that three distinct antigens must exist. One is V or hr^v. The second is hr^H and the third is VS. It seemed that whenever a haplotype encodes production of V(hr^v) or hr^H, VS is also made. While a simile may be dangerous, it does appear that VS may be to V(hr^v) and hr^H, as G is to D and C. Most haplotypes that make D and/or C, make G. At the moment, it seems that all haplotypes that make V(hr^v) and/or hr^H make VS. Whether a haplotype can make V(hr^v) or hr^H but not VS, we do not know. To continue the dangerous simile, it has been pointed out that rare haplotypes make G without C or D. We have encountered bloods that have VS but do not seem to have V(hr^v) or hr^H. Indeed, haplotypes that make VS without V (hr^v) or hr^H, may be more common than those that make G without D or C.

It has been pointed out elsewhere (311) that the V, hr^H, VS story might yet involve partial D. Of the various possible combinations of the antigens, the phenotype hr^H- VS+, seems to be the least common. Bloods of that phenotype that have been described (92,682,742,743) have all had weak D. There are three possible explanations for these findings. First, perhaps many anti-VS sera contain another antibody that defines an epitope of D or a replacement antigen similar to Go^a or D^w. Second, perhaps all haplotypes that encode VS without hr^H encode also for only partial D. Third, perhaps VS itself, when it is not part of hr^v or hr^H is a form of partial D or a replacement antigen.

A Better Suggestion About the Names VS and e^s

As mentioned several times in the previous sections, equating VS with e^s causes considerable difficulty in the interpretation of some serological findings. A more logical interpretation has now been suggested by Steers et al. (1004). These workers extended their previous studies (750) and showed that the *RHCE* gene of persons with VS+ red cells carries a single base change that predicts

that at position 245 of the *RHCE* encoded protein, valine will replace leucine. Since the amino acid at position 245 is predicted to lie within the red cell membrane bilayer it must be presumed that its presence causes a configurational change in an exofacial portion of the polypeptide. Position 245 is close to position 226 where an amino acid change is responsible for the difference between E (proline) and e (alanine). Steers et al. (1004) suggest that the VS antigen is based on Val245 and that in the presence of that residue a configurational change in Ala226 results in the alteration from e to e^s. In other words, although VS and e^s will, most often, occur together (on VS+ red cells) they are not the same antigen. Along somewhat similar lines, Faas et al. (751) who also describe the Leu245Val change associated with the presence of VS, suggest that the change may also affect the expression of C (at serine 103) such that the weak C often associated with the VS+ e^s+ phenotype, is seen. These suggestions are compatible with our own findings (described more fully below) that the hr^B- phenotype is overrepresented in individuals with r'^S (746) and that hr^B- red cells are often VS+ (747). In other words, perhaps the change associated with VS alters expression of e so that it is recognized as e^s, and perhaps the e^s version of e often lacks (or has a reduced level) of the epitope(s) that comprise(s) hr^B. Once again, serological findings about Rh have indicated an area ripe for study at the molecular level.

Antibodies to V, VS and hr^H

Anti-V and anti-VS, particularly the latter, are relatively common antibodies; unless one has well characterized red cells available, it is difficult to differentiate between them. Anti-hr^H is rare, indeed other than the original (92) we do not know of a pure example. Again, the determination as to which anti-VS contain anti-hr^H is difficult (or impossible) unless red cells of the appropriate phenotype are available.

While most of the antibodies mentioned in the publications cited above were red cell immune and reactive by IAT, a saline active anti-V has been reported (744). There is at least one report of mild HDN caused by anti-VS (752). Byrne and Howard (745) pointed out that when Black patients with sickle cell disease become immunized to many antigens as a result of multiple transfusions, subsequent transfusions often involve the use of blood from Black donors because of the higher incidence of compatible units. As a result, these patients are exposed to V (and Js^a) more frequently than would be the case if random units, largely from White donors, were used. The net result is that anti-V (and anti-Js^a) production is seen more frequently in this population of patients than in others. When they undertook a program to identify suitable donors, these investigators (745) found that of 438 Black donors, selected because they had C- E- (and K-, Fy(a-b-), Jk(b-)) red cells, 168 (39%) were V+. This incidence is higher than that seen (88) when random American Blacks are typed, reflecting the fact that V is encoded more often by R^o and r than by other haplotypes, in this population group.

A Relationship Between r'^s, VS and hr^B

Beal et al. (746) undertook a screening program to identify hr^B- donors for transfusion to patients immunized to that antigen. Among selected samples, 4 of 75 that were C+ D- were hr^B-, another 14 had aberrant expression of hr^B, i.e. either weakly positive for that antigen or positive with some and negative with other examples of anti-hr^B and anti-hr^B-like (see above) antibodies. Of these 18 individuals, 15 were V- VS+, 3 were V+ VS+. Among 90 donors with C- red cells, 26 of whom were V+ VS+ and one of whom was V- VS+, no hr^B- sample was found. A retrospective review of records at several large reference laboratories confirmed the overrepresentation of r'^s (i.e. persons with C+ c+ D- E- e+ V and/or VS+ red cells) among patients and donors with hr^B- or hr^B variant red cells. Prompted by these findings, Reid et al. (747) further investigated the relationship between hr^B and VS using a monoclonal antibody with anti-hr^B-like specificity (748), to identify additional hr^B- samples. Of 48 apparent hr^B- samples, 45 were VS+. Based on the results of typing for C, 32 of those samples could have been from individuals with r'^S. While these findings suggested a possible antithetical relationship between hr^B and VS, Reid (749) has subsequently found more hr^B- VS- samples. Thus it seems that if hr^B and VS are encoded by alleles, a third allele that makes neither, must exist. Alternatively, it is possible that the genetic rearrangement that results in production of VS, often but not always results in lack of production of hr^B. On reflection, the second suggestion may be identical to the first! Perhaps a different alternative is that the apparent hr^B- VS- samples actually represent lack of different epitopes of e than that associated with the hr^B- phenotype. Two studies (750,751) have indicated the genetic alteration that may be responsible for the VS+ (e^s+) phenotype (see above and in more detail in a later section of this chapter).

A Possible Relationship Between V and D or Between V and C and D

We and others have noticed a peculiar relationship between V and D or between V and C and D. When sera containing anti-D or anti-CD, production of which has been stimulated by pregnancy or transfusion, are studied, it is not particularly unusual to find that some of them contain an anti-V component (or at least react with C- D- V+ red cells). On investigation, it is nearly always found that the children of the women immunized by pregnancy, or the donors of those immunized by transfusion, have V- red cells. This phenomenon is particularly noticeable when high levels of anti-D or anti-CD are being made. Why the immune (perhaps hyperimmune) response to D (or CD) should involve production of anti-V (or a component of the anti-D or anti-CD reactive with C- D- V+ red cells) is not known. Again, this observation calls in to question a possible relationship between V (and VS, see above) and partial D.

The *Rh-deletion* Genes and Haplotypes

There are a number of rare *Rh* genes and haplotypes that behave as if part of the genetic material has been deleted. Indeed as described in a later section of this chapter, in some instances exactly that has happened. In other instances studies at the molecular level have shown that the genetic material is present but, for reasons that are not always clear, fails to encode production of detectable protein or antigens. At the serological level, the resulting phenotypes can be considered together since the red cells involved behave similarly, even when different genetic backgrounds are involved. In the previous edition of this book, these genes were called *D-deletion*. That was a terrible choice of terms, in many instances E and e or C, c, E and e are not produced, but D and G are made, often in exalted levels. As indicated above, the term *Rh-deletion* is used in this edition. Although in some cases *RHCE* is deleted and *RHD* is left, the term haplotype will be used so that those cases in which *RHCE* is present but appears not to encode a product, are included.

The first of these haplotypes recognized (90,577) was D-- and since the first example was described, numerous others have been reported (409,757-777,780). D-- encodes production of D and G but does not make any antigens in the Cc or Ee series. As discussed below, the red cells of D-- homozygotes also lack several high incidence Rh system antigens. A haplotype called D•• is similar, in many respects to D-- (104,579,713,778). Production of the low incidence antigen Evans (Rh37) and the high incidence antigen DAV (Rh47) by D•• is described below. In 1957, the haplotype DC^w- was described (779). DC^w- encodes production of D and G and a weak form of C^w that may differ qualitatively from the C^w made by R^{1w} (CC^wDe) (67,658,659). In 1960, Dc- was first reported (604), other examples have been found

(109,605-608,780). *Dc-* encodes production of D and G but different examples vary greatly in the amount of c that is made. As discussed above, in the section on f (ce), it is likely that some haplotypes that have been called *Dc-* might better have been described as *Dc(e)* or *Dc((e))*. The amount, if any, of f made, is sometimes seen to be proportional to the small amount of e made by some of these haplotypes. A summary of the actions of haplotypes that have been called *Dc-* is provided in table 12-20. Spielmann et al. (609) described a case of HDN caused by the anti-f made by a woman who apparently was of genotype $R^1/Dc-$. In 1969, Salmon et al. (781) described the haplotype $D^{IV}(C)-$ that makes the D typical of partial D category IVa, G and a markedly reduced amount of C. Production of the low incidence antigens Go^a, Rh33, Riv (Rh45) and FPTT (Rh50) by $D^{IV}(C)-$, and its possible production of rh$_i$ and some e, is discussed below. The ultimate *Rh-deletion* gene $\overline{\overline{r}}$ or --- that fails to encode production of any Rh antigens is discussed below in the section on Rh$_{null}$. Existence of a silent allele at the *Rh* locus had been invoked (782,828-833) to explain unusual inheritance of Rh antigens, before the first $\overline{\overline{r}}$ homozygote was found (783,784).

Race and Sanger (49) pointed out that the incidence of consanguinity among the parents of *Rh-deletion* homozygotes is higher than would be expected. Daniels (508) notes that if cases reported since 1975 are added, it can now be seen that consanguineous matings were involved in 24 of 33 families in which *D--, D••, DC^w-* and *Dc-* homozygotes were identified. Some degree of consanguinity is, of course, expected among the parents of persons who inherit two rare recessive haplotypes (the same rare haplotype is passed through different branches of the family). Why the consanguinity rate of parents of *Rh-deletion* homozygotes should be so much higher than that of parents of *hh*, *pp*, or *K^{o}K^o* individuals (49) is not understood. A second unusual finding in families with *Rh-deletion* homozygotes was also pointed out by Race and Sanger (49) and relates to the sibs of the homozygotes. If the *Rh-deletion* haplotypes are inherited in a normal manner and if the propositi are excluded from the counts, it would be expected that less than one quarter of the sibs of *Rh-deletion* homozygotes would be *Rh-deletion* homozygotes themselves. Again, Daniels (508) notes that if cases reported since 1975 are added to the original figures of Race and Sanger (49) it is seen that 31 of 77 (40%) of the sibs are homozygous for the *Rh-deletion* gene involved. Boettcher (785) suggested that the statistically significant excess of *Rh-deletion* homozygotes among the sibs might be related to early loss of fetuses with normal Rh phenotypes. However, the incidence of miscarriages reported in the families involved does not seem sufficient fully to explain the

TABLE 12-20 To Show the Heterogeneity of *Dc-* and Closely Related Haplotypes

Haplotype and Reference	D	c	e	f	Hr$_o$	Other
Dc- of Yamaguchi et al. (607)	↑	↓↓↓	0	0	0	
Dc- of Tessel et al. (606)	↑	(↓)	0	0	0	hr^B 0 hr^S 0
Dc- of Tate et al. (604)	↑	↓↓	0	↓↓	0	
Dc- of Leyshon (608)	+	+	0	*		
Dc((e)) of Tessel et al. (606)	↑	↓↓	↓↓↓	+	+	
Dc(e) of Issitt et al. (688)	+	+	↓↓	↓	+	hr^B↓ hr^S 0

↑   = antigen level elevated
+   = antigen level normal
(↓)   = antigen level slightly depressed
↓   = antigen level depressed
↓↓   = antigen level markedly depressed
↓↓↓   = antigen level even more markedly depressed
0   = antigen not present
*   = haplotype said to make f, antigen level not specified.

findings. As mentioned in the previous edition of this book, we would not like to believe that a sperm carrying only *RHD* would be able to outpace its competitors weighted down with both *RHD* and *RHCE*, in the race to the ovum.

The amount of D on the red cells of many persons homozygous for *Rh-deletion* haplotypes is such that those cells are agglutinated in saline systems by some anti-D that act only as incomplete, or sensitizing antibodies in tests with normal D+ red cells. Such anti-D will sometimes (49,577,786) but not always (759,787) agglutinate the red cells of persons heterozygous for an *Rh-deletion* gene. As pointed out earlier in this chapter, anti-D with this property have to be selected from tests with many examples of the antibody. While it was originally thought that Rh-deletion red cells might carry more D than other D+ red cells because the *D* gene present had no competition from *CcEe* genes for a precursor substance, it is now appreciated that *Rh* gene action does not involve conversion of a precursor. Perhaps the very high levels of D on these red cells (see table 12-7) reflects the ease with which anti-D can approach its antigen in the absence of hindrance from *RHCE* encoded polypeptides or perhaps, in the absence of a functional *RHCE* allele, *RHD* makes more than usual product.

The Antigens Hr_o and Hr

The *Rh-deletion* haplotypes fail to encode production of some antigens that are made by the overwhelming majority of other *Rh* haplotypes. Two of these high incidence antigens have been named Hr_o and Hr although, as discussed below, it now seems probable that Hr is an epitope of Hr_o and is expressed on some red cells that carry partial Hr_o. Since *Rh-deletion* homozygotes lack the antigens it follows that they can make alloantibodies against them when exposed to foreign red cells via transfusion or pregnancy.

From their study on the serum of the first found *D--* homozygote, Race et al. (577) concluded that some separable anti-e, anti-C and anti-c were probably present. However, since the serum was found to react with all red cells with normal (i.e. not-deleted) Rh phenotypes, it was concluded that "much of the antibody (was) directed against C and c indifferently". Hackel (788) reached a somewhat similar conclusion from a study of the sera of two other immunized *D--* homozygotes. While he felt that some anti-e, anti-C, anti-c, anti-E and anti-f could be isolated, the reactions of the sera with all cells of normal Rh phenotype again suggested the presence of an antibody reacting with an antigen common to those cells. That this antibody was the major (and sometimes the only) component of this type of serum became apparent when it was found (49, 759, 760, 763, 765, 779, 781, 789, 790) that the sera of immunized *D--*, *D••*, *DC^w-*, *Dc-* and *D^{IV}(C)-* homozygotes usually react strongly with red cells of normal Rh phenotypes but are non-reactive with all (or most) of the five types of deletion cells listed. For a while, mutual compatibility between the sera and red cells of these homozygotes was the rule. As described below in the sections on the antigens Nou and Dav, exceptions have now been seen.

In 1958, Allen and Corcoran (91) reported a detailed study on the sera of immunized *D--/D--* individuals. The sera were first adsorbed onto CDe/CDe red cells and an eluate was made. That eluate was adsorbed onto cDE/cDE cells and a second eluate was made. The second eluate was adsorbed onto cde/cde cells and a third eluate was made. From their findings that the third eluates reacted to approximately the same degree, with red cells of all common Rh phenotypes, Allen and Corcoran (91) concluded that the major portion of the original antibody was directed against a high incidence antigen made by all common *Rh* haplotypes. The antibody was called anti-Hr_o (91) and was said to define an antigen that Wiener (525) had suggested was produced in just such circumstances. Further advances were made from studies (26,680,681) on the antibodies made by Shabalala and Santiago and by other persons (Ellington, Fentry and Davis) with similarly unusual phenotypes. These antibodies have been

described in large measure in the previous section on partial e. Essentially, what was found was that rare haplotypes in addition to those of the *Rh-deletion* series, fail to encode production of the high incidence antigens. For example, the Shabalala cells adsorbed anti-Hr_o from the sera of immunized D--/D-- persons, but left a second antibody (that was called anti-Hr) of almost identical specificity, unadsorbed. As discussed in detail earlier, it is now apparent that like (at least) D and e, Hr_o is composed of a series of epitopes (561,660,729). Persons with partial e on their red cells often also have partial Hr_o and make antibodies to both the epitopes of e and the epitopes of Hr_o, that their red cells lack. Mrs. Shabalala had e+ Hr_o+ Hr-hr^S- red cells so that the antibody that she made that was named anti-Hr (26) can be seen, in retrospect, probably to have been directed against an epitope of Hr_o that her red cells lacked.

In 1961, Rosenfield (46,48,681) showed that the names anti-Hr and anti-Hr_o really describe groups of antibodies of similar but not identical specificities. Some of the sera studied appeared to contain anti-E and some appeared to contain anti-e. However, adsorption with E-e+, and E+ e- red cells, respectively, removed all antibody activity. Rosenfield concluded (681) that some anti-Hr and anti-Hr_o have a "preference" for E+ cells, some a "preference" for e+ cells, while still others react equally with E+ e- and E- e+ red cells. Clearly, these early studies portended the later observations on the concomitant lack of epitopes of e and of Hr_o from the red cells of rare individuals with unusual *Rh* haplotypes.

In studies on sera containing anti-Hr/Hr_o Moore et al. (789) compared the efficiency of red cells of different Rh phenotypes to adsorb the raw sera to exhaustion. They found that cde/cde red cells were more efficient in this respect than were CDe/CDe cells, but that the CDe/CDe cells were in turn, more efficient than CDE/CDE cells. In other adsorption studies Moore et al. (789) found that chimpanzee, baboon and vervet monkey red cells did not adsorb anti-Hr/Hr_o. Daniels et al. (791) felt that the strongest antibodies made by *Rh-deletion* homozygotes were somewhat alike in specificity. However, these workers also felt that some differences could be seen, a conclusion shown to be entirely correct when the antigens Nou and Dav (see below) were described.

The Antigen Rh34

As already described, the raw serum of Mrs. Bastiaan reacts with all red cells; the activity left after the serum is adsorbed with R_2R_2 cells is called anti-hr^B (97). The total antibody activity of the Bastiaan serum has been called (48) anti-Rh34 and we (51) have shown that *Rh-deletion* haplotypes do not make Rh34. It is not clear whether the sera of immunized D--/D-- etc., individuals contain separable anti-Rh34 and/or anti-Hr^B (see section on hr^B). However, since both antibodies show a marked preference for rh$_i$+ (Ce+) red cells and since several of the sera studied have been reported to contain "a difficult to isolate anti-C" (577,788) it would come as no surprise to find anti-Rh34 and/or anti-Hr^B as a component of those sera.

$D^{IV}(C)$- Revisited and the Antigen Nou (Rh44)

During the investigation of the only known $D^{IV}(C)$-homozygote, Salmon et al. (781) found that the haplotype encodes production of D, G and a markedly reduced amount of C. Whether $D^{IV}(C)$- makes some e and/or rh$_i$ is not entirely clear, the red cells involved reacted with 3 of 10 anti-e but the presence of anti-rh$_i$ in those sera was not excluded. As its name indicates, the authors (781) felt that $D^{IV}(C)$- does not make e. As described earlier, $D^{IV}(C)$-, when its products were studied on the red cells of individuals heterozygous for the haplotype, was seen to make Go^a (781), Rh33, Riv (Rh45) and FPTT (Rh50) (107,114).

Pertinent to this portion of the chapter is the fact that $D^{IV}(C)$- makes two high incidence antigens that are not encoded by other *Rh-deletion* haplotypes. (A third high incidence antigen, Rh29, that is made by all *Rh-deletion* haplotypes is considered separately, in a later section). Initially, it appeared that $D^{IV}(C)$- was like other *Rh-deletion* haplotypes since the red cells of Madam Nou, the homozygote, were non-reactive with the sera of some immunized *Rh-deletion* homozygotes. This and the fact that Madame Nou made anti-Hr$_o$, that caused fatal HDN in her third child, showed that her red cells were Hr$_o$- Hr- and probably Rh:-34. However, when Perrier et al. (792) and Habibi et al. (106) later tested four sera from immunized D-- homozygotes and two from immunized Dc- homozygotes against the red cells of Madam Nou, they found that one of each reacted with those cells. Presence of antibodies to Go^a, Rh33, Riv and FPTT was excluded by the finding that red cells lacking those antigens would adsorb the reactive sera to exhaustion. The red cells of the $D^{IV}(C)$- homozygote adsorbed all activity against them from the two reactive sera, but left anti-Hr$_o$ unadsorbed, again showing that $D^{IV}(C)$- does not encode Hr$_o$. The high incidence antigen defined on the red cells of the $D^{IV}(C)$- homozygote, that is also present on all red cells of normal Rh phenotype, but that is lacking from other Rh deletion cells, was called Nou and was later assigned the number, Rh44. It is important to appreciate that the very common antigen Rh44 is not antithetical to any of

the low incidence antigens, Go^a, Rh33, Riv or FPTT since all five antigens are encoded by $D^{IV}(C)$-. When a similar study was performed on the red cells of a D•• homozygote (see below) and the antigen Dav (Rh47) was recognized, it was shown that Nou and Dav are different and that $D^{IV}(C)$- encodes production of both of them.

D•• Revisited and the Antigen Dav (Rh47)

A story similar to that just recounted for $D^{IV}(C)$-emerged when the red cells of a D•• homozygote were studied. D•• was already known (49,104,579) to encode production of D, G and the low incidence antigen Evans (Rh37). When Daniels (109,110) tested the red cells of Helen Dav, a D•• homozygote, with sera from 25 immunized *Rh-deletion* homozygotes he found four, one each from persons D--/D--, Dc-/Dc-, DC^w-/DC^w- and D---/---, that reacted with those cells. Adsorption studies showed that the red cells of the D•• homozygote removed all activity for those cells, but left anti-Hr$_o$ unadsorbed. Again, the findings that the D••/D•• red cells did not react with the other 21 sera (one of which was from the D•• homozygote herself) and that they did not adsorb anti-Hr$_o$ from the four reactive sera, showed them to be Hr$_o$- Hr- and probably Rh:-34. That the reactive sera did not contain anti-Rh37 was demonstrated when they were adsorbed to exhaustion by Rh:-37 cells of normal phenotypes. The additional high incidence antigen made by D•• was called Dav and given the number Rh47. Daniels (110) then showed that Rh47 differs from Rh44. The reactive sera were adsorbed with D••/D•• red cells to remove anti-Rh47, the adsorbed sera still contained anti-Hr$_o$ and still reacted with the red cells of the $D^{IV}(C)$-homozygote, showing that D••/D•• red cells are Rh:-44,47. As mentioned above, the red cells of the $D^{IV}(C)$-homozygote adsorb such sera to exhaustion suggesting that they are Rh:44,47 or as Daniels (110) suggested, that anti-Rh44 may contain anti-Rh47. As with $D^{IV}(C)$-, the low incidence antigens it encodes and Rh44; Rh47 cannot be antithetical to Rh37. Rh37 and Rh47 are encoded by D••; Rh47 is encoded by all common *Rh* haplotypes but not by other *Rh-deletion* genes.

D - - and Another Candidate High Incidence Antigen

While studying the red cells of a newly found D--/D--individual, we (876) found that they reacted weakly with four of ten sera from immunized *Rh-deletion* homozygotes. The red cells in question were shown to be Hr$_o$-Hr- Rh:-34 and the reactive sera did not contain anti-Nou or anti-Dav. Those sera were adsorbed to exhaustion with red cells of normal Rh phenotypes. Thus it seems that there is at least one other high incidence antigen made in similar circumstances to production of Nou by $D^{IV}(C)$- and Dav by $D\bullet\bullet$. We used the term Hr_L as a working designation for the antigen involved but were never able to get repeat samples from the donor to complete the investigation.

$\bar{\bar{R}}^N$ Revisited and the Antigen Rh46 (Sec)

Although the relationship of Rh46 to $\bar{\bar{R}}^N$ is totally different to the relationship of Rh44 and Rh47 to $D^{IV}(C)$- and of Rh47 to $D\bullet\bullet$, it is, like Rh44 and Rh47, of very high incidence, so can conveniently be described here. As described earlier, $\bar{\bar{R}}^N$ encodes weak C and e, Rh32 and a form of D that can be shown (with difficulty) to be slightly enhanced when selected anti-D are used.

When $\bar{\bar{R}}^N$ homozygotes are immunized they can make an antibody that reacts with: all red cells of common Rh phenotypes; rare cells such as those that are Hr_o+ Hr- (Shabalala); Rh:-34 (Bastiaan); from R^{oHar} homozygotes; or from C^w homozygotes (Rh:-51) (108,641,643). The antibody does not react with Rh-deletion or Rh_{null} red cells. Since the red cells of $\bar{\bar{R}}^N$ homozygotes react with the sera of immunized *Rh-deletion* homozygotes, it follows that $\bar{\bar{R}}^N$ makes Hr_o and probably Hr and Rh34. The antibody made by $\bar{\bar{R}}^N$ homozygotes has been called anti-Rh46 and since such red cells are all Rh:32,-46 it appears that Rh32 and Rh46 have the same type of antithetical relationship as do C and c, E and e, C^w, C^x and Rh51. As with some of those pairs of antigens, an exception to the rule has been seen. Just as some genes encode neither C nor c, or neither E nor e, we (793) have encountered one individual, who did not appear to have *Rh-deletion* genes, whose red cells appeared to be Rh:-32,-46. However, we (794) also pointed out that since it is extraordinarily difficult to differentiate between antibodies that define Hr_o, Hr, Rh34, Rh44, Rh46 and Rh47, our interpretation (793) of the phenotype as Rh:-32,-46 was the most likely explanation but was not absolutely proved. Regrettably, a family study that might have been informative, could not be performed.

The important difference between the antigens of very high incidence described in the last three sections is that $D^{IV}(C)$- encodes production of Rh44 and Rh47; $D\bullet\bullet$ encodes production of Rh47; $\bar{\bar{R}}^N$ does not encode production of Rh46. Indeed, it is possible that the same structural change that effects the production of Rh32 results in no production of Rh46 and marked depression of expression (perhaps spatial rearrangement) of C and e (641,643).

The Antigen Rh29

Although the Rh_{null} phenotype is described in later sections of this chapter, Rh29 is also a high incidence antigen so can conveniently be mentioned here. The antigen is present on all other Rh-deletion cells but is missing from those that are Rh_{null}. Anti-Rh29 can be formed as an alloantibody by persons of the Rh_{null} phenotype (795, for additional references see a later section) and has been responsible for both mild (796-798) and severe (799) HDN. While the identification of anti-Rh29 is relatively straightforward, the antibody reacts with all except Rh_{null} red cells and the antibody-maker's cells are Rh_{null}, it should be remembered that some Rh_{null} individuals have made antibodies to other Rh antigens and not to Rh29.

The Antigen Rh39

In 1979, we (51) reported the existence of autoantibodies that defined a hitherto undescribed antigen associated with the Rh system. In testing a number of autoantibodies that seemed to be directed against C, c, D, E or e we (557,558,734) found many that could be adsorbed to exhaustion with red cells with which they did not react directly (see also Chapter 37). Since red cells of normal phenotypes but not Rh-deletion cells would adsorb these autoantibodies, we concluded that their specificities were the same as the allo-anti-Hr/Hr_o studied by Rosenfield (46,48,681) that reacted visibly only with E+ or e+ red cells, but could be adsorbed to exhaustion by any cells with normal Rh phenotypes. Two autoantibodies that gave visible reactions only with C+ red cells could be adsorbed to exhaustion with normal and with Rh-deletion cells. Since Rh-deletion cells are Hr- Hr_o- Rh:-34 it was clear that the two autoantibodies had a different specificity. We (51) called the specificity anti-Rh39 and pointed out that distribution of Rh39 is similar to that of Rh29. One of us (PDI) has since seen several further examples of auto-anti-Rh39 but an alloantibody with that specificity has not yet shown up. Allo-anti-Rh39 could, of course, only be made by an Rh_{null} individual and might well look like anti-C unless adsorption studies were performed. Rosenfield (800) has forecast that auto-anti-Rh39 with no preference for C+ red cells, may be found.

Rh-deletion Haplotypes, a Summary

Table 12-21 is an attempt to summarize many of the data described in the several previous sections. It attempts to describe the production of low incidence antigens by *Rh-deletion* (and closely related) haplotypes, and to list which high incidence antigens are made or not made. It should be remembered that the tabulation of such information unavoidably results in some oversimplification. For full details about the Rh haplotypes listed in table 12-21, the text above should be consulted.

Possible Production of Anti-LWᵃ as a Prelude to the Production of Anti-D and Rh Autoantibodies

These topics, both of which were included in this chapter in the third edition of this book, have moved to new homes. All aspects of the LW system, including the early production of anti-LWᵃ in persons who later make anti-D, are discussed in Chapter 13. The role of Rh autoantibodies in causing antibody-induced hemolytic anemia is described in Chapter 37, clinically benign Rh auoantibodies are discussed in Chapter 39.

Rh Mosaics in Healthy Individuals

There are a number of reports in the literature (49 (includes reports of unpublished cases), 801-805) of healthy individuals with two populations of red cells, as determined by Rh phenotyping, in whom no other differences in the red or other cell populations were found. In some of the cases chimerism was apparently excluded, as was later development of disease, and it was assumed that somatic mutation or proliferation of clones monosomic for an *Rh* gene were involved. In other cases (806-809) the mosaic situation involved Rh and other chromosome 1 markers.

Rh Mosaics and Disease

In a number of other cases (375,735,736,803,810-819) cessation of production of Rh antigens has clearly been associated with the patient's disease. In leukemia, polycythemia, myeloproliferative disorders and even in antibody-induced hemolytic anemia, it appeared that a clone of monosomic cells was producing red cells on which the products of only one of the patient's *Rh* haplotypes were expressed. In some, but by no means all these cases, chromosomal translocation was demonstrated. One of these cases is discussed further, below, in the section describing the assignment of the *Rh* locus to chromosome 1. In yet other cases (see the next section) simple depression of Rh antigen expression (particularly in leukemia) was seen.

Other Aspects of Rh and Disease

The red cell deficiency type of hemolytic anemia associated with the Rh_{null} and Rh_{mod} phenotypes is discussed below under the heading, Rh_{null} syndrome. The major role played by Rh antibodies in hemolytic disease of the newborn is described in Chapter 41; their role as autoantibodies causative of hemolytic anemia is discussed in Chapter 37.

Already mentioned are clonal disorders in which two populations of red cells differing in Rh phenotype have been seen. In addition, some cases of what is perhaps the same event have been reported to involve weakening of Rh antigen expression (810,815,822,823).

Mourant et al. (834) reported that Hodgkin's disease is more common in D- than in D+ persons. In studying a kindred of more than 1200 members in Newfoundland, Newton et al. (835) found more than a two fold excess of D- individuals over the expected number. In spite of this, the increased incidence of Hodgkin's disease in D- persons could still be seen. It has also been reported (820,821) that oral squamous cell carcinoma is twice as likely to result in mortality in persons who are D- than in those who are D+.

One report (935) has described an increased incidence of schizophrenia in adult D+ males born to D- women. Although data were not available (save in two cases) to show that the mothers of the affected males were immunized to D, the increased incidence was seen only in second or later born individuals. That is in first borns, delivered at a time when presence of maternal anti-D would be unlikely, the incidence of the disorder was the same as in the general population. Thus the report at least raises the possibility that either fetal hypoxia associated with anemia or the effects of increased bilirubin levels may sometimes result in permanent neurological damage. However, since there is now emerging evidence (936-939) that schizophrenia may be associated with second-trimester perturbations, the authors (935) felt that if anti-D HDN is a risk factor for the disorder at all, it is likely that the fetal phase of HDN is involved.

The Phenotype Rh_{null} and the Genes $X^o r$, $X^1 r$ and $\bar{r}$

In 1961, Vos et al. (824) reported the first example of a blood in which the red cells lacked all representation of Rh antigens. The phenotype was called ---/--- and the investigators pointed out that the phenotype could represent either the inheritance of rare suppressor or regulator genes at a locus other than *Rh*, or the inheritance of silent alleles at the *Rh* locus itself. The accuracy of that forecast

TABLE 12-21 An Oversimplified Summary of Rh-deletion Haplotypes (for exceptions, see text)[*1]

Haplotype or Phenotype	Polymorphic and Low Incidence Antigens														
	D	C	c	E	e	f	G	C^w	Go^a	Rh32	Rh33	Evans	Tar	Riv	FPTT
$D - -$	+	0	0	0	0	0	+	0	0	0	0	0	0[*2]	0	0
$D \bullet \bullet$	+	0	0	0	0	0	+	0	0	0	0	+	0	0	0
$Dc-$	+	0	(+)	0	0	(+)[*3]	+	0	0	0	0	0	0	0	0
DC^w-	+	0	0	0	0	0	+	(+)	0	0	0	0	0	0	0
$D^{IV}(C)-$	+	(+)	0	0	0	0	+	0	+	0	+	0	0	+	+
$\overline{\overline{R}}^{N\ *4}$	+	(+)	0	0	(+)	0	+	0	0	+	0	0	0	0	0
Rh_{null}(both types)	0	0	0	0	0	0	0	0	0	0	0	0	0	0	0

Haplotype or Phenotype	High Incidence Antigens							
	Hr_0	Rh29	Rh34	Rh39	Nou	Dav	Rh46	MAR
$D - -$	0	+	0	+	0	0	0	0
$D \bullet \bullet$	0	+	0	+	0	+	0	0
$Dc-$	0	+	0	+	0	0	0	0
DC^w-	0	+	0	+	0	0	0	0
$D^{IV}(C)-$	0	+	0	+	+	+	0	0
$\overline{\overline{R}}^{N\ *4}$	+	+	+	+	+	+	0	+
Rh_{null}(both types)[*5]	0	0	0	0	0	0	0	0

+ = antigen present (for elevated levels other than D, see text)
(+) = antigen present but at depressed level
0 = antigen not present (some assumptions made)
*1 Some assumptions made from published statements such as "antibody reacted with all except Rh-deletion and Rh_{null} red cells"
*2 One D - - sample was shown to be Rh:40, D was not elevated, G status not reported (513)
*3 f antigen variable, see table 12-20
*4 Included to illustrate specificties of anti-Rh32 and anti-Rh46
*5 Included to illustrate specificities of anti-Rh29 and anti-Rh39

is shown by the fact that both genetic situations are now known to exist. Because the original proposita was an Australian Aborigine with no immediate relatives, the genetic background of the phenotype was not immediately determined. Later studies (825,826) on members of the proposita's more distal relatives, strongly suggested that her Rh_{null} phenotype is of the modifier or regulator, X^orX^or, (see below) type. When it became apparent that the phenotype can be caused by genes not at the *CDE* locus, it was pointed out (827) that the term ---/--- is not suitable since it implies the presence of silent alleles at the *Rh (CDE)* locus, accordingly the term Rh_{null} was substituted. As will be apparent from what is written below, the term --- is suitable to describe the later discovered $\overline{\overline{r}}$ gene since that gene certainly behaves like a silent allele at the *Rh* locus.

In 1964, Levine et al. (836-838) reported the second

example of the Rh_{null} phenotype. This time a family study was possible and one of the genetic backgrounds that can cause the phenotype was recognized. Figure 12-1 shows some of the findings on informative family members, details about others are given in the original papers. A number of important observations were made. First, the father of the proposita had red cells that were C+ c+. While not proving the point absolutely, this strongly suggested that he had two normal *Rh* haplotypes, one making C and the other c. If that was the case, it meant that he must have passed one normal *Rh* haplotype to his Rh_{null} daughter in whom it failed to function. Second and equally important, the husband of the Rh_{null} proposita was *rr* and their daughter was R^1r. The R^1 haplotype that the child had inherited must have been transmitted by the Rh_{null} woman. Third, several sibs of the proposita's parents appeared to have normal *Rh* haplotypes but had reduced levels of Rh antigens on their red cells. Levine et al. (836-838) put all these facts together and proposed the modifier or regulator background for this type of Rh$_{null}$. Studies on families found since, that include Rh$_{null}$ members, have proved the accuracy of this proposal many times. It was supposed that at a locus other than *Rh*, a very common gene, X^lr exists. Most individuals are genetically X^lrX^lr. In that genotype the *Rh* haplotypes inherited function normally and Rh antigens are made. The rare allele of X^lr was called X^or and it was supposed that in individuals genetically X^orX^or, the normal *Rh(CDE)* haplotypes inherited were somehow prevented from functioning. Such a theory explained how the parents and child of the Rh$_{null}$ proposita could have two normal *Rh* haplotypes and how the proposita could be phenotypically Rh$_{null}$ although she carried two normal haplotypes at the *CDE* locus. Figure 12-2 expands figure 12-1, by showing the presumed X^lr and X^or genes inherited by the various individuals described in the figures. As can be seen, the X^lrX^or genotype (parents and child of the Rh$_{null}$ proposita and several of the parents' sibs) does not prevent either *CDE* haplotype inherited from functioning but can result in reduced amounts of Rh antigens being made.

The family studied by Levine et al. (836-838) also provided evidence that the X^lrX^or and *Rh(CDE)* loci are genetically independent. The R^lr genotype was found in four of the father's sibs, three of whom appeared to be genetically X^lrX^or while the other was apparently X^lrX^lr (i.e. normal expression of red cell Rh antigens). On the maternal side, the proposita's mother was apparently R^lR^l and must have been X^lrX^or since she produced an Rh$_{null}$ (X^orX^or) daughter. Two of her four R^lR^l sibs were apparently X^lrX^or and two apparently X^lrX^lr. Although

only one of the proposita's grandparents was available for testing, evidence that X^or did not always travel with the same *Rh* gene in the family was obtained. Studies on later found families in which the X^or regulator gene was present have also, many times, confirmed the genetic independence of the X^lrX^or and *Rh(CDE)* loci.

In 1966, Ishimori and Hasekura (783,784) described the Rh$_{null}$ phenotype in a Japanese boy. A complete family study was performed and some (but by no means all) of the pertinent findings are illustrated in figure 12-3. This time it was apparent that X^lrX^or genes did not provide an explanation for the genetic background of the Rh$_{null}$ phenotype. As figure 12-3 shows, the parents of the Rh$_{null}$ propositus appeared to be R^lR^l and R^2R^2. While each could have passed an *Rh* haplotype (R^l and R^2 respectively) and X^or to the Rh$_{null}$ child, the phenotype of the propositus' brother shows that this cannot have been so. The brother is apparently R^2R^2 and appears, at first, to have inherited no *Rh* haplotype from his mother but two R^2 haplotypes from his father. In fact, the serological findings on many of their immediate relatives (783,784) can be explained if a silent allele at the *Rh* locus is invoked. The silent gene has been named $\overline{\overline{r}}$ (it can also be described as ---) and the genotypes of the parents in figure 12-3 can be written as $R^l\overline{\overline{r}}$ and $R^2\overline{\overline{r}}$. The brother with D+ C- E+ c+ e- red cells can be seen to be genetically $R^2\overline{\overline{r}}$ (meaning that he got $\overline{\overline{r}}$ from his mother and one R^2 haplotype from his father) and the propositus can be seen to be genetically $\overline{\overline{rr}}$. In the original reports (783,784) the red cells of $R^l\overline{\overline{r}}$ and $R^2\overline{\overline{r}}$ people could not be shown to have reduced levels of Rh antigens. In the family studied by Seidl et al. (839) it did seem that the putative *Rh*$\overline{\overline{r}}$ heterozygotes (where *Rh* represents a normal haplotype at the *CDE* locus) had single doses of Rh

FIGURE 12-1 Part of the Family of the Rh$_{null}$ Proposita of Levine et al. (836-838)

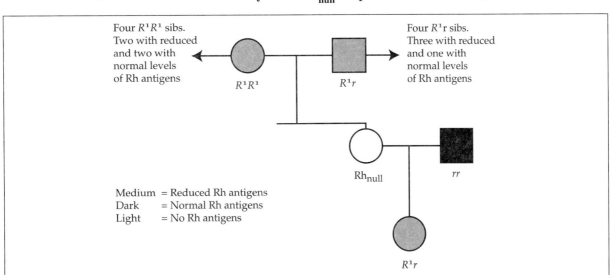

Four R^1R^1 sibs. Two with reduced and two with normal levels of Rh antigens

R^1R^1

R^1r

Four R^1r sibs. Three with reduced and one with normal levels of Rh antigens

Rh$_{null}$

rr

Medium = Reduced Rh antigens
Dark = Normal Rh antigens
Light = No Rh antigens

R^1r

FIGURE 12-2 To Show the Inheritance of *Rh* and *X¹rX⁰r* Genes in the Family Studied by Levine et al. (836-838)

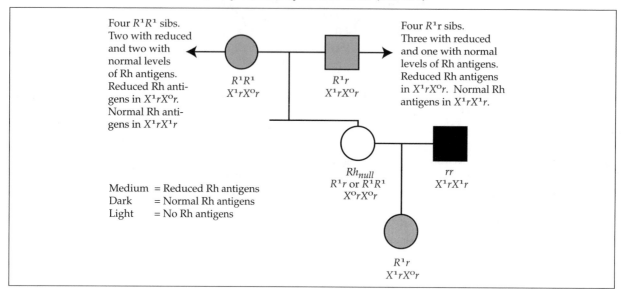

Four *R¹R¹* sibs. Two with reduced and two with normal levels of Rh antigens. Reduced Rh antigens in *X¹rX⁰r*. Normal Rh antigens in *X¹rX¹r*

R¹R¹
X¹rX⁰r

R¹r
X¹rX⁰r

Four *R¹r* sibs. Three with reduced and one with normal levels of Rh antigens. Reduced Rh antigens in *X¹rX⁰r*. Normal Rh antigens in *X¹rX¹r*.

Medium = Reduced Rh antigens
Dark   = Normal Rh antigens
Light   = No Rh antigens

Rh$_{null}$
R¹r or *R¹R¹*
X⁰rX⁰r

rr
X¹rX¹r

R¹r
X¹rX⁰r

antigens on their red cells. However, proof that such individuals were *Rh$\bar{\bar{r}}$* and not *X¹rX⁰r* heterozygotes could not be obtained. As mentioned above, the genotype *X¹rX⁰r* can result in decreased expression of Rh antigens.

The findings described above that prove that *$\bar{}r$* can act as a silent allele at the *Rh* locus substantiated interpretations of several observations made earlier. Family studies showing apparent maternal exclusions, when there was no chance that the supposed mother was not the real mother, and some serological findings, had been interpreted as indicating the heterozygous state of a silent allele at the *Rh* locus (782,828-833). It may be noticed that some care has been taken in describing *$\bar{\bar{r}}$*. It has been said that the gene can act as a silent allele, meaning that it encodes no production of Rh antigens. In fact, as described in more detail below, the gene may be grossly

normal in structure but is somehow prevented from acting, in terms of Rh antigen production. As discussed in a later section, some, but by no means all, *D--/D--* persons have been found to have a grossly normal, but apparently non-functional allele in the *RHCE* series. This has led to the tongue-in-cheek suggestion that the *$\bar{\bar{rr}}$* type of Rh$_{null}$ can be thought of as a D- form of D--/D--! More seriously, it is possible that a similar genetic aberration could result in the D--/D-- situation if a D producing genome was originally involved, and the *$\bar{\bar{rr}}$* type of Rh$_{null}$, if a genome lacking *RHD* was originally involved (i.e. a mutation in a D- person).

Since the original reports of Vos et al. (824), Levine et al. (836-838) and Ishimori and Hasekura (783,784) appeared, a substantial number of persons with Rh$_{null}$ red cells have been found. While both types, regulator and

FIGURE 12-3 To Show the Rh$_{null}$ Propositus of Ishimori and Hasekura (783,784)

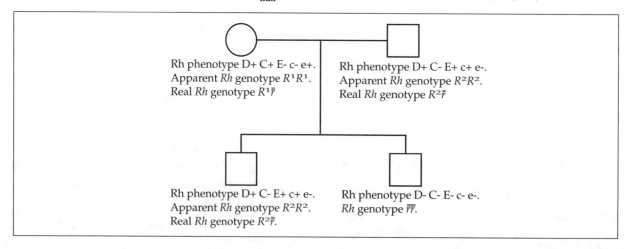

Rh phenotype D+ C+ E- c- e+.
Apparent *Rh* genotype *R¹R¹*.
Real *Rh* genotype *R¹$\bar{\bar{r}}$*

Rh phenotype D+ C- E+ c+ e-.
Apparent *Rh* genotype *R²R²*.
Real *Rh* genotype *R²$\bar{\bar{r}}$*

Rh phenotype D+ C- E+ c+ e-.
Apparent *Rh* genotype *R²R²*.
Real *Rh* genotype *R²$\bar{\bar{r}}$*.

Rh phenotype D- C- E- c- e-.
Rh genotype *$\bar{\bar{rr}}$*.

silent allele, are rare, the former have been found (95,796-799,841-849) considerably more often than the latter (850). In some instances, of course, family studies do not reveal the genetic background of the Rh_{null} phenotype (851-853), serological studies cannot be used reliably to differentiate between the two types. In addition to the examples referenced above, Daniels (508) lists 11 others known to him but otherwise unpublished. To the 32 propositi listed by Daniels (508) we can add one more. In 1992 at Duke University Medical Center, we (854) identified the Rh_{null} phenotype in a 76-year-old White man. His *rr* wife and two R^1r children showed that his phenotype had the regulator background. In tests on the propositus' three sibs and seven half-brothers, we found no other Rh_{null}. Normally, one would not expect to find the same rare genotype among half-sibs, in this case we looked because we had been told that the mother of the propositus and his three sibs and the mother of his seven half-brothers were cousins. Our patient was 76 years-old when first found to be Rh_{null} and died of unrelated causes soon after his phenotype was recognized. However, the fact that he lived to be 76 without being recognized as Rh_{null} indicates, as discussed below, that the hemolytic anemia associated with the Rh-deficiency syndrome can often be virtually symptomless. Among the 33 Rh_{null} propositi mentioned above, 20 were certainly and one probably of the regulator ($X^o r$) type, three certainly and one possibly of the amorph ($\overline{r}$) type, while in the remaining eight the genetic background could not be established.

As mentioned earlier, the genotype $X^1 r X^o r$ sometimes results in reduced expression of Rh antigens. In a number of studies (797,825,826,838,841,843,847,849) this has been demonstrated, in others (95,842,854, and see Daniels (508) for other unpublished cases) it has not. These findings, of course, explain the statement made above that serological studies cannot be used reliably to differentiate between the two types of Rh_{null}.

Anti-Rh29 and Other Antibodies Made by Rh_{null} Individuals

Anti-Rh29 was the term assigned by Haber et al. (95) and Bar-Shany et al. (796) to the antibody made by an immunized Rh_{null} proposita. The term anti-"Total Rh" was also used. As described above, Rh29 is present on all red cells of normal Rh phenotype and on those of *Rh-deletion* homozygotes. Rh_{null} red cells of the regulator ($X^o r X^o r$) and silent allele ($\overline{r}\overline{r}$) backgrounds are all Rh:-29. Thus, when Rh_{null} individuals become immunized, one of the alloantibodies they can make is anti-Rh29, the antibody has been found in Rh_{null} persons of both genetic backgrounds. That is to say, the presence of

normal *Rh* haplotypes in $X^o r X^o r$ individuals and of grossly normal but non-functional *Rh* genes in $\overline{r}\overline{r}$ persons, does not prevent immunization.

Production of anti-Rh29 differs somewhat from the production of antibodies by some other persons of null phenotypes. For example, anti-H is always present in the sera of O_h individuals (see Chapter 8), anti-$P+P_1+P^k$ is made by all persons of phenotype p (see Chapter 11). In contrast, anti-Rh29 is not always made by Rh_{null} individuals. Some such persons had been blood donors or patients for many years before their Rh_{null} phenotype was recognized and retrospective examination of records showed that antibody screening tests on their sera had been negative (783,784,824,841,854). The antibody can be made following pregnancy or transfusion (95,797-799,839,845,848,849,854). Anti-Rh29 has caused both mild (797,798) and severe (799) HDN. In the severe case, multiple exchange transfusions within the first 24 hours of life, followed by a simple transfusion at 8 weeks, with rr blood, were used successfully to treat the infant. In two Rh_{null} individuals not known to have been exposed to red cells, apparent anti-Hr_o was made (846,852); in another, anti-Hr_o caused HDN (850). Anti-e and anti-c plus anti-e have also been identified as the sole antibodies made by Rh_{null} individuals (838,839).

In tests on the Rh_{mod} (see below) red cells of two different individuals, with four different examples of anti-Rh29, we (855) thought that we had detected heterogeneity of anti-Rh29. While the reactions appeared to represent a qualitative difference of the determinants involved, we could not totally exclude the possibility that the difference was merely quantitative. The study foundered on the weakness of some of the anti-Rh29 available to us.

The Phenotype Rh_{mod} and the Gene X^Q

In 1971, Chown et al. (856,857) reported a case in which the proposita had a red cell deficiency type of hemolytic anemia (see later section on the Rh-deficiency syndrome) and marked depression of red cell Rh antigen levels. From a family study it was clear that the proposita was genetically R^1R^2 but phenotypically her red cells resembled those of the r^G homozygote described earlier in this chapter. The family data suggested but did not prove that the genes responsible for suppression of Rh antigen expression were located at a locus genetically independent of *Rh*. Chown et al. (856,857) named the phenotype Rh_{mod} (for modified) and suggested two possible genetic backgrounds to explain their findings. First, Rh_{mod} might arise when two genes called X^Q inhabit the $X^1 r X^o r$ locus. X^Q could thus be thought of as being intermediate between $X^1 r$ that permits normal Rh antigen expression and $X^o r$ that (in double dose) blocks such expression. Second, it was considered possible that the Rh_{mod} phenotype might represent the presence of two $X^o r$ genes in an environment different from that in which the genes cause the Rh_{null} phenotype. Both suggestions, of course, require that the modifying genes that cause the Rh_{null} and Rh_{mod} phenotypes are at the same locus. A third possibility would be that $X^o r$ and X^Q are at loci independent of each other.

A second family that included members with red cells of the Rh_{mod} phenotype was reported by Mallory et al. (64). In this family it was shown that the genes responsible for the Rh_{mod} condition (those genes are almost always called X^Q) do indeed segregate independently of those at the Rh locus. Further, it was shown that the same X^Q genes allow different amounts of Rh antigen to be made in related persons who inherit different Rh haplotypes. Mallory et al. (64) undertook careful studies to measure the amounts of 20 different Rh antigens and LW^a on Rh_{mod} cells and on the cells of family members heterozygous for X^Q. They found that on the Rh_{mod} cells, the only Rh antigens present in normal amounts were Hr_o and Rh29. Although the cells were D+ they carried only 1.2% of the expected quantity of D. The Rh_{mod} cells had an LW^a antigen level of about 50% of that seen on D-LW(a+) red cells. The amount of Rh antigen depression effected by X^Q in single dose was found to vary dependent on which Rh haplotypes had been inherited. As discussed below, it is now appreciated that there is great variation of Rh antigen expression on the Rh_{mod} red cells of different individuals. For example, in spite of the normal level of Rh29 on the red cells of the proposita of Mallory et al. (64), we (854) have tested an example of anti-Rh29 that failed to react at all with the Rh_{mod} cells of a different individual (858).

A third family with Rh_{mod} members was found in Japan (859). Although there was some evidence that the Rh_{mod} cells did not survive normally in vivo, it was clear that the individuals of that phenotype in this family were not as severely affected with the Rh-deficiency syndrome (see below) as those of the phenotype in the first two families studied (64,856,857).

Now that more individuals of the Rh_{mod} phenotype have been found (70,859-862) and see Daniels (508) for four additional, unpublished cases, it is clear that Rh antigen expression in this phenotype involves a continuum from the point at which adsorption-elution tests may be necessary to detect the antigen (858,860), to that at which weak but definite positive reactions are seen in direct tests (64,857). In retrospect it can be seen that the brother and sister reported by Stevenson et al. (860), who were described in the last edition of this book as being of the "not quite Rh_{null}" phenotype, were in fact of the Rh_{mod} phenotype at the lower end of the scale of antigen

production. Daniels (508) noted that including the unpublished cases of which he was aware, six of 11 Rh_{mod} propositi were Japanese and that eight of the 11 were products of consanguineous matings.

Probable Identification of $X^o r$ and X^Q

As described above, it has long been known that $X^o r$ and X^Q segregate independently of the Rh locus. It was not known if the genes are alleles of each other, nor indeed if they are different, or the same gene causing different phenotypes in different environments. As mentioned briefly below and as discussed in more detail later in this chapter, it is believed that in situ, the RHD and $RHCE$ encoded polypeptides form a complex with several other membrane components. Among the several components believed to be involved are the Rh-associated glycoproteins. These structures were first detected in 1982 (909) and were described in more detail later (893,901-903,920). Although there is some homology between the non-glycosylated Rh polypeptides and the Rh-associated glycoproteins, the glycoproteins are not simply glycosylated versions of the acylproteins. Somatic cell hybridization studies showed (903) that the genes encoding production of the Rh-associated glycoproteins are located on chromosome 6 at 6p21-qtr. The genes involved are most often called $Rh50$ to indicate the molecular size of the glycoproteins encoded; the $Rh50$ term should not be confused with Rh50, the numerical term for the FPTT antigen. The finding that the $Rh50$ genes are located on chromosome 6, while RHD and $RHCE$ are located on chromosome 1 (for details and references see below) indicated that the non-glycosylated polypeptides encoded by RHD and $RHCE$ must make the major contribution to Rh antigen structure.

Findings on the genetic independence of both $X^o r$ and X^Q, and of $Rh50$ from the $RHDRHCE$ locus have now been triumphantly combined by Chérif-Zahar et al. (1032) to provide a highly probable explanation of the modifier ($X^o r X^o r$) type of Rh_{null} and the Rh_{mod} phenotypes. These workers studied five unrelated Rh_{null} individuals, four of the $X^o r X^o r$ and one of the $\overline{rr}$ type, and one individual of the Rh_{mod} phenotype. In the four $X^o r X^o r$ and the one $X^Q X^Q$ individual mutant forms of $Rh50$ were identified. These varied among the individuals studied and involved a frameshift, nucleotide substitutions or failure of amplification. In the $\overline{rr}$ Rh_{null} individual the $Rh50$ transcript was normal. In other words, $X^o r$ and X^Q are almost certainly mutant forms of the chromosome 6-borne $Rh50$. Apparently in the absence of the Rh-associated glycoproteins the Rh antigens cannot be expressed (the $X^o r X^o r$ type of Rh_{null}); in the presence of greatly reduced amounts of Rh-associated glycoproteins, the Rh antigens are only poorly expressed (the $X^Q X^Q$ Rh$_{mod}$). The *Rh50* cDNA was used for in situ hybridization studies and showed that the *Rh50* gene is located at 6p11-p21.1 (1032). Clearly these findings are entirely compatible with those described in earlier sections that show that $X^o r X^o r$ Rh$_{null}$ and $X^Q X^Q$ Rh$_{mod}$ persons have normal *RHD* and/or *RHCE* genes that function in their parents and children who are heterozygous for the mutant *Rh50* genes.

Classical geneticists will no doubt be pleased if the discovery of mutant forms of *Rh50* eventually leads to abandonment of the terms $X^1 r$, $X^o r$ and X^Q. Those terms have long been viewed with disfavor since they imply a relationship to the X chromosome that has equally long been known not to exist.

The Rh-deficiency Syndrome

In 1967, Schmidt et al. (863) reported that the Rh$_{null}$ red cells of the second individual of the phenotype found, were serologically, morphologically and functionally abnormal. Instead of being biconcave, Rh$_{null}$ red cells are cup-shaped stomatocytes (851,864). From the original study (863) and from many performed since, it became clear that Rh$_{null}$ red cells do not survive normally in vivo. The red cell abnormality type of hemolytic anemia that can result (no autoantibody is involved in the red cell destruction) was at first called (865) Rh$_{null}$ disease but that name was later modified (866) to Rh$_{null}$ syndrome when it was seen that the condition is often clinically mild. Later still, after it became appreciated that Rh$_{mod}$ individuals also have the red cell deficiency hemolytic anemia, the term Rh-deficiency syndrome was introduced (867). Persons with this syndrome may present with anemia (796,843,845,850-852,868), with no anemia but with signs (such as an elevated reticulocyte count) of an accelerated rate of in vivo red cell destruction (784,795,838,869,870) or with only suggestive evidence (such as an increased level of red cell i antigen (869) that may indicate chronic marrow stress (871)) associated with accelerated in vivo red cell clearance and decreased maturation time of red cells in the bone marrow. The syndrome is sometimes mild enough that the Rh$_{null}$ individuals pass blood donor screening tests and a unit of blood is collected before the phenotype is recognized (841,842). The degree of anemia is quite variable in different Rh$_{null}$ individuals, even in sibs who have inherited the same genes causative of the phenotype (795,870). Further, the degree of anemia in one Rh$_{null}$ person is variable over time. The in vivo half life of Rh$_{null}$ cells (in Rh$_{null}$ individuals) has been found to range from as short as seven (842,870) to as long as 17 or 18 days (842,868,870) (normal 24 to 28 days) in dif-

ferent people of the phenotype. On rare occasions the hemolytic anemia may be severe enough that splenectomy is necessary (839). In addition to the reduced hemoglobin and hematocrit and increased reticulocyte count, features of the Rh deficiency syndrome may include increased levels of serum bilirubin and fetal hemoglobin and a decreased level of serum haptoglobin. The red cell osmotic fragility may be normal or only mildly abnormal when performed by a standard method (872). However, the incubation osmotic fragility and autohemolysis tests (873) often reveal the abnormality of Rh$_{null}$ red cells since increased rates of hemolysis may be seen in such tests. The increase of hemolysis seen is sometimes but not always corrected by the addition of glucose to the test system. The genetic background of the phenotype seems not to influence the clinical state for the red cell membrane abnormalities and the syndrome have been seen in both the $X^o r$ and $\overline{\overline{r}}$ types of Rh$_{null}$ (796,838,839,841-843,845,850,851,868,870,874,875). As mentioned above, the Rh-deficiency syndrome is also seen in persons with the Rh$_{mod}$ phenotype. Indeed in some such individuals the clinical disorder has been relatively severe and splenectomy has been necessary (64,857,858).

A very large number of investigations have been carried out to try to characterize the membrane defect of Rh$_{null}$ and Rh$_{mod}$ red cells. Clearly such information would help to answer the long asked question as to the function of Rh antigen-bearing, membrane proteins. A number of different defects of membrane structure and function in this setting, have been documented. They are discussed in detail below in the sections dealing with the biochemistry and function of Rh. One of us (877) has pointed out that in spite of the multiple functional defects associated with the membranes of Rh$_{null}$ and Rh$_{mod}$ red cells, explanation of the shortened in vivo life span of those cells might be much more straightforward. Perhaps the membrane abnormalities contribute simply by altering the shape of the red cells from biconcave discs, to stomatocytes. Perhaps the accelerated rate of red cell clearance then occurs as a result of the spleen's ability to filter abnormally shaped red cells. There are some observations that appear to support such a concept. First, the anemia of the Rh-deficiency syndrome is completely cured by splenectomy. Clearly, while such a surgical procedure removes a major site of red cell clearance, it does nothing to correct the membrane abnormalities of the red cells. In an Rh$_{null}$ individual described by Seidl et al. (839) the half life of the red cells was normal, following a splenectomy. Second, when Rh$_{null}$ red cells were labeled with ^{51}Cr and injected into an individual who had earlier had a splenectomy following an accidental injury, their survival was normal. In other words, the membrane abnormalities of Rh$_{null}$ red cells do not compromise survival of those red cells in an environment in which the red cells are not subject to splenic filtration.

Other Blood Group Antigens and Rh$_{null}$ Red Cells

In 1967, Schmidt et al. (863) reported that Rh$_{null}$ red cells give aberrant results in typing tests for some other red cell blood group antigens. The cells typed as weakly positive for s and as U-. As more Rh$_{null}$ bloods have been studied, it has become clear that many of them give aberrant results when typed for S, s and U and that as Schmidt et al. (863) suspected, the aberrations occur at the phenotypic and not the genetic level. Race and Sanger (49) noticed that although Rh$_{null}$ red cells may type as U- when antiglobulin-active anti-U are used, the cells will adsorb that antibody and yield it when eluates are made. Further, in typing tests with anti-U that act as agglutinins, the antigen can more easily be shown to be present on Rh$_{null}$ red cells. Somewhat similar findings have been made with anti-S and anti-s although the S and s antigens on Rh$_{null}$ cells are often not as difficult to detect as is U. The expression of U on different examples of Rh$_{null}$ red cells is quite variable, the variation is not correlated with the X^orX^or or $\overline{rr}$ background involved. Dahr et al. (878) showed that Rh$_{null}$ red cells of both genetic types carry only 30 to 40% of the amount of glycophorin B (the structure that carries S, s and U, see Chapter 15) found on U+ red cells of normal Rh phenotypes. We (879) showed that there is a similar reduction of glycophorin B on Rh$_{mod}$ red cells and that the cells of X^Q heterozygotes carry about 70% of the normal amount of glycophorin B. Another association between Rh and glycophorin B came to light when Le Pennec et al. (880) described a multiply transfused man with C+ c+ D+ E+ e+, S- s+ red cells who made an antibody that reacted only with D+, S+ red cells. The relationship between Rh and U disclosed by the Duclos antibody (68) is discussed in more detail in Chapter 31.

In 1971, Albrey et al. (881) described an antibody, anti-Fy3, that reacts with Fy(a+) and Fy(b+) cells, but not with those that are Fy(a-b-). The antibody was made by the second White found to have Fy(a-b-) red cells. In 1973, Colledge et al. (882) found another antibody that behaved similarly with Fy(a+), Fy(b+) and Fy(a-b-) red cells. However, the new antibody, that was called anti-Fy5, differed from anti-Fy3 in that it failed to react with Rh$_{null}$ red cells of the X^orX^or type and gave weaker than expected reactions with D--/D-- cells, although those samples carried Fy^a or Fy^b or both. Other examples of anti-Fy5 have been found (883-887) (see Chapter 14) and among other findings, it has been shown (883) that Rh$_{null}$ red cells of the $\overline{rr}$ genetic background are Fy:3,-5. It has also been claimed (885) but not confirmed, that red cells with variant e antigens fail to react with anti-Fy5.

The LW blood group system and its close phenotypic relationship to Rh are described in the next chapter of this book. Suffice it here to say that Rh$_{null}$ red cells, of both genetic types, are LW(a-b-ab-) (836). Again as described more fully below, the lack of any LW system antigens on Rh$_{null}$ red cells appears to represent total lack of the LW glycoprotein from those red cells (888-891).

In 1987, Miller et al. (892) described a monoclonal antibody, ID8, that reacted with the red cells of adults, when the Rh phenotype of those red cells was normal, but that failed to react with Rh$_{null}$ red cells and gave weaker than expected reactions with D--/D-- and cord red blood cells. It was clear from the start that ID8 was not defining an Rh antigen since studies using Chinese hamster ovary-human lymphocyte or fibroblast-hybrid cells, showed that the determinant recognized was encoded from a locus on human chromosome 3 (*Rh* is on chromosome 1, see below). Subsequent studies (893-896) using ID8 and similar specificity monoclonal antibodies have shown that the determinant involved (that does not have a blood group name) is carried on CD47, the integrin-associated protein (IAP) and that the amount of CD47 is reduced on Rh$_{null}$ red cells.

While the association between the Rh$_{null}$ phenotype and depression or absence of the antigens S, s, U; Fy5; LW^a, LW^b, LW^{ab}; and the determinant on CD47 have all been confirmed in independent studies, a possible relationship between Rh and the Ge antigens, has not. In 1988, we (897) described an antibody to a high incidence antigen that failed to react only with 9 of 10 Ge- samples that had normal Rh phenotypes and with Rh$_{null}$, Rh$_{mod}$, D--/D--, Dc-Dc-, DC(e)/DC(e), and e variant (supposedly hr^S- or hr^B-) red cells, all of which were Ge+. Although the antibody was weak, it resisted adsorption by the non-reactive red cells of Ge- or unusual Rh phenotypes. As far as we are aware, no other antibody suggesting a relationship between the Rh and Ge antigens (the latter of which are carried on glycophorin C, (see Chapter 16)) has been found.

This section has been written predominantly about serological observations made in tests on Rh$_{null}$ red cells. However, the association between the Rh antigen-bearing membrane components and glycophorin B, the Fy5-bearing component, the LW glycoproteins, CD47 and the Rh-associated glycoproteins (not mentioned above) is much more far-reaching than that described. In later sections of this chapter the possible arrangement of the Rh polypeptides in situ, on red cells, is discussed. As mentioned in those sections, there is evidence to suggest that all these components (and perhaps others, glycophorin C may make it yet) form a complex (898) or a cluster (840,899) that is not correctly assembled in the absence of the Rh polypeptides (i.e. on Rh$_{null}$ red cells). It is noticeable that while Rh$_{null}$ red cells usually have reduced levels of U, are Fy:-5, LW(a-b-ab-) and have a reduced level of CD47, red cells that are S- s- U-; or Fy(a-b-)Fy:-3,-5; or LW(a-b-ab-) all have normal Rh phenotypes. As one of us (guess which one, this time) has on a lecture slide: Rh, SsU, Fy5 and LW^{ab} are associated but the greatest of these is Rh.

Anti-A,D

In 1953, Ikin et al. (900) described a form of anti-D that gave reactions that have never been seen with any other anti-D. Although the antibody has nothing to do with the Rh$_{null}$ phenotype, it is described here because the Rh glycoproteins have just been mentioned. In tests in a saline system, the antibody agglutinated group A, D+ red cells but not those that were group A, D-, nor those that were group O, D+. When albumin was added to the test system, the antibody agglutinated group A and group O, D+, but not group A, D- red cells. The antibody was adsorbed to exhaustion with group O, D+ red cells but not at all with group A, D- cells. For the 34 years from 1953 to 1987 it hurt one's brain (942) even to think about the specificity of this antibody. In 1987, Moore and Green (901) in extending their earlier studies (909,915) reported that when the non-glycosylated Rh polypeptides are isolated by immunoprecipitation with Rh antibodies, associated glycoproteins that carry ABH antigens are co-precipitated. That specific immunoprecipitation and not formation of artefactual dimers was involved, was elegantly demonstrated (901). When immunoprecipitation with anti-D was performed using group A, D+ red cells, the glycoproteins precipitated carried A. When similar experiments were started with group O, D+ red cells, the isolated glycoproteins lacked A. When a mixture of equal parts of group A, D- and group O, D+ red cells was used in immunprecipitation with anti-D, the isolated glycoproteins lacked A. In other words, the glycoproteins involved show ABO specificity for the D+ red cells from which they are obtained. These observations have been confirmed and extended by others (902,903,920,921); the genes that encode production of the Rh-associated glycoproteins reside on chromosome 6. Now that an association between Rh and ABO-bearing Rh-associated glycoproteins has been established, it is less painful to think about the possible specificity of the antibody described by Ikin et al. (900). While the antibody was anti-D, its reactions were apparently influenced by the presence or absence of A, on Rh-associated glycoproteins. Now that it is finally possible, at least to speculate reasonably about the specificity of this antibody, perhaps other examples will be found.

A perhaps somewhat similar antibody was described

in 1990 by Le Pennec et al. (1067). This antibody apparently required the presence of D and S for formation of the epitope detected. As mentioned above, there are data that suggest that glycophorin B (that in one form carries S) is part of the Rh complex on red cells. Because this antibody may have detected an epitope formed by interaction between the Rh glycoproteins and glycophorin B, it is described in more detail in the section describing the Duclos antibody (68,69,396,893,1068) in Chapter 31.

Assignment of the *Rh* Locus to Chromosome One and Other Observations on Genes Linked to *Rh*

In 1953, Chalmers and Lawler (904) showed that a rare and benign condition called elliptocytosis, in which the individual has oval red cells, is controlled by a gene that in some families is linked to *Rh*. When linkage to *Rh* could be demonstrated, the gene causative of elliptocytosis was called *El$_1$*. In 1971, Weitkamp et al. (905) found that genes at the *6-PGD* locus, that control production of 6-phosphogluconate dehydrogenase, are also linked to *Rh*. In the same year, van Cong et al. (906) demonstrated linkage between the *Rh* and *PGM$_1$* loci, at the latter of which reside genes that control synthesis of a phosphoglutamatase enzyme. In 1972, Westerveld and Kahn (907) added the *PepC* genes, that control production of the enzyme peptidase C, to the *Rh* linkage group. All these linkages were demonstrated by conventional family studies. Thus by 1972 it was known that the *Rh*, *6-PGD*, *PGM$_1$* and *PepC* genes formed a linkage group. That is to say, although the genes were at different loci, the loci were situated close enough to each other on a chromosome that they traveled together most of the time. It was easy to show that the linkage group was not on the X or Y chromosome (the genes segregate independently of sex) but it was not known on which autosome the linkage group was located. A major advance was then made by Ruddle et al. (908) using cell hybridization studies. In this method, mouse and human (nucleated) cells are fused by treatment with the Sendai virus. The cells are then propagated in tissue culture. As the fused cells, that have two complete sets of chromosomes (one human and one mouse) grow, the human chromosomes are gradually expelled (perhaps, after all, mouse is mightier than man). By studying metabolic activities (such as enzyme production) of the cultured cells, it is possible to correlate loss of a particular function with loss of a recognizable human chromosome, thus showing that the genes that control that function must be carried on that chromosome. Triumphantly, Ruddle et al. (908) showed that loss of ability of the cultured cells to make the enzyme peptidase C was always associated with the loss of chromosome one. Since it was already known that the *Rh, 6-PGD* and *PGM₁* genes are linked to *PepC*, the whole linkage group had been shown to be carried on chromosome one.

Additional evidence to support and extend this conclusion was provided by Marsh et al. (814) in 1974. These workers studied a patient with myelofibrosis in whom about 7% of the red cells typed as D+ C+ E- c+ e+ and the other 93% as D- C- E- c+ e+. Marsh et al. (814) astutely realized that the patient did not have a mixture of R_1r and rr red cells. First, one of his parents was of the phenotype D+ C+ E- c- e+, so did not have a *r* gene to pass. Second, the patient had passed a normal R^1 haplotype to his son. This meant that in the patient's circulation the D+ C+ E- c+ e+ red cells must have descended from precursor cells in which both R^1 and *r* were functional. The D- C- E- c+ e+ red cells must have come from precursor cells in which *r* but not R^1 was functional. In chromosomal analysis of the nucleated cells of the patient it was shown that in 95% of them (a figure in very close agreement with the 93% of cde/- red cells) a deletion of the short arm of chromosome one had occurred. In other words loss (actually translocation in this case) of a small piece of the short arm of chromosome one had resulted in loss of a functional *Rh* (R^1) haplotype. Since the patient was heterozygous at the *PGM₁* locus and since all his cells contained both types of that enzyme, Marsh et al. (814) were able to conclude that the *Rh* locus must be further from the centromere on chromosome one, than is the *PGM₁* locus.

In 1975, Turner et al. (910) studied an American Indian family in which some members were homozygous for *D--*, some heterozygous for that haplotype and some had not inherited *D--* at all. In the homozygotes it was found that the short arms of both copies of chromosome one had been deleted. Heterozygotes showed a deletion of the short arm of one chromosome while relatives without *D--* had no deletions. However, this very convincing family is the exception rather than the rule. Chromosomal analyses of an Rh$_{null}$ individual and other individuals with *D--* (911,912) have not shown any abnormalities. There are several reasons that explain these negative findings. First, the chromosomal aberration may simply be too small to be seen with existing techniques. Second, reciprocal translocations of similarly staining chromosomal material might not be recognizable. Third, replacement of some genetic material by other material that is non-functional (silent) may not result in a change in physical appearance of the chromosomes. There are, in the literature, a number of reports of individuals who had two populations of red cells that differed only in their Rh antigens or who lost an Rh antigen during a disease process (for complete references see earlier). Only rarely can the double cell population or antigen loss be seen to be associated with an alteration of chromosome one (913). More often (823,914) no such change can be seen. Many of the cases (801,811,812,916,917) were studied before the location of the *Rh* locus was known so that chromosomal studies, when performed, had less chance of being informative. Once the molecular biology methods described in Chapter 5 became available, cDNA in situ hybridization was used (918,919) to confirm the assignment of the *Rh* locus to the short arm of chromosome one, namely to the region 1p34.3-1p36.13. As discussed (and referenced) in later chapters of this book, the *Fy* (*Duffy*); *Sc* (*Scianna*); *Cr* (*DAF, Cromer*); *Kn* (*CR1, Knops*) and *Rd* (*Radin*) blood group loci are also located on chromosome one. Genes that are on the same chromosome but that are far enough apart that the rate of crossing-over makes it seem that the genes segregate independently, are said to be syntenic. Such a description applies to *Rh* and *Fy*. Thus a case that at first (806) seemed possibly to represent somatic mutation involving *Rh* and *Fy* was later reinvestigated (807,922). While inactivation of part of chromosome one in erythrocytic precursors was postulated, it could not be proved.

Rh Antigens are Carried on Polypeptides of Mr 30,000

Early studies of the biochemical nature of Rh antigens were relatively unsuccessful because suitable techniques for isolating hydrophobic membrane proteins were lacking. Nevertheless some useful clues were obtained. Green (947,948) reported evidence that free thiol groups were necessary for the expression of the Rh antigens C and D, an observation which suggested that the antigens were protein in nature. These studies were based on the loss of antigenic activity after treatment of lyophilized red cell membranes with N-ethyl maleimide and parachloromercuribenzoate.

Green (949) also showed that when red cell membrane preparations were extracted with *n*-butanol, D antigen activity was not demonstrable in the butanol-soluble (lipid) fraction or the insoluble (protein) residue but that when these two fractions were recombined D activity was restored. He further showed that the critical component of the lipid fraction was phospholipid and concluded that Rh antigen activity is dependent on the presence of bound phospholipid containing at least one unsaturated fatty acid. The phospholipid dependence of Rh antigens was further demonstrated by Hughes-Jones et al. (950) and Kropp and Weicker (951) who showed that treatment of red cell membranes with phospholipases A2 and C destroyed D, Cc and Ee activity. Of particular interest is evidence that anti-D protects the D antigen from inactivation by treatment with phospholipase A2 (950,952) and that the number of Rh antigen sites can be modulated by cholesterol (953). These studies should be viewed in the light of subsequent studies on the presence of covalently linked fatty acids in Rh polypeptides (954,955 and see a later section).

Green's experiments (947,948) which demonstrated the thiol dependence of Rh antigens could not determine if the critical thiol groups were accessible on the outer surface of the red cell or the inner surface, or both. Abbot and Schachter (956) used glutathione-maleimides (membrane impermeable probes) to provide evidence that one or more exofacial thiol groups are necessary for the binding of anti-D since agglutination of D+ red cells by anti-D was inhibited by these membrane impermeable probes. The role of free thiol groups in Rh antigenicity has subsequently been questioned by Suyama et al. (957) who treated red cells with various sulfhydryl reagents and found no evidence of loss of the antigens D, c or E. Furthermore, these authors found that immune precipitation of D polypeptide with anti-D was not affected by previous treatment of the red cells with N-ethyl-maleimide. Suyama et al. (957) suggest that the difference between their findings and those of Green (947,948) may result from the use of red cell membranes rather than intact red cells in Green's studies. It seems clear from a detailed study carried out by Schmitz et al. (958) that inactivation of Rh antigens does occur when red cell membranes are treated with thiol reagents. As Suyama et al. (957) point out, the only evidence in the literature that the D antigen on intact red cells requires a free SH group is that reported by Abbott and Schachter (956, described above) and they suggest that this could be due to steric hindrance resulting from the bulky nature of the membrane impermeant maleimide used. Expression in K562 cells of D polypeptide in which the extracellular Cys 285 has been mutated to Ala did not result in the loss of D antigen (Smythe J and Anstee DJ, unpublished observations, 1997), a finding in support of the observations of Suyama et al. (957).

The breakthrough which led to the identification of the Rh proteins came in the early 1980s from the use of SDS-PAGE to separate the components of immune complexes obtained after detergent solubilization of red cells or red cell membranes coated with Rh antibodies. Soluble immune complexes containing anti-D had been obtained earlier by Lorusso et al. (959) using sodium deoxycholate as the detergent. Moore et al. (909) used Triton X-100 and described the immunoprecipitation of radioiodinated components of Mr 30kD from red cells of appropriate Rh phenotype using anti-D, anti-c and anti-E. Gahmberg (960) independently identified the same D-active component by immunoprecipitating from radioiodinated red cell membranes. At this time the first murine monoclonal anti-body with Rh specificity (R6A) was described and characterized by its failure to react with Rh_{null} cells (389). Ridgwell et al. (961) used R6A and human polyclonal anti-D in immunoprecipitation experiments with radioiodinated red cells and showed that R6A precipitated a radioiodinated component of Mr 34,000 while anti-D immunoprecipitated a component of Mr 32,000. These results suggested that Rh antigens were carried on two proteins, the R6A-polypeptide and the D-polypeptide. This conclusion was further supported by experiments using an ^{35}S-labeled membrane impermeable maleimide (*N*-maleoylmethionine sulfone) which showed that Rh_{null} membranes lacked two polypeptides of Mr 34,000 and 32,000 respectively and that each polypeptide had a least one exofacial thiol group (961). That the c and E antigens were located on a different polypeptide or polypeptides from that which carries D could also be inferred from the work of Moore et al. (909) since the D polypeptide was much more strongly radioiodinated than the c, E polypeptide(s). Further work (901) indicated that the c, E polypeptide(s) had a slightly higher Mr than the D polypeptide on SDS-PAGE suggesting that the c, E polypeptide(s) corresponded to the R6A polypeptide(s) described by Ridgwell et al. (961). This hypothesis has recently been confirmed in expression studies of *Rh* genes (described below).

Peptide mapping studies (962-964) established that polypeptides immunoprecipitated with anti-D, anti-c and anti-E are similar. However, while two-dimensional peptide maps of c and E polypeptides were almost identical, those of the D polypeptide revealed differences (964). These observations together with failure to demonstrate inhibition of binding of anti-c by anti-E or anti-D, inhibition of binding of anti-E by anti-c or anti-D and inhibition of binding of anti-D by anti-c or anti-E (965) led some workers to conclude that that D, c and E are each carried on different polypeptides. The peptide mapping results clearly demonstrated that the D polypeptide is different from the c, E polypeptide(s) a finding entirely consistent with the immunoprecipitation data described earlier in this section. The evidence that c and E are carried on different polypeptides is less convincing and this has remained a controversial point which will be discussed again in later sections.

Studies concerned with the identification and isolation of Rh proteins carried out before 1982 had given diverse results. Some authors reported that the D protein had an Mr in the range 7-10,000 (966,967) while others found evidence that Rh antigens were located on the anion transport protein, band 3 (389,968; band 3 is now known to carry Diego system antigens, see Chapter 17). These studies are most likely explained by proteolysis of D polypeptides during purification on the one hand (966,967) and problems with aggregation of band 3 on the other (389,968). The occurrence of Rh polypeptides in band 3 aggregates may simply reflect the fact that both proteins are very hydrophobic and co-migrate under the purification conditions used or a genuine association in the red cell membrane. Some tentative evidence for the latter comes from the observation that South East Asian ovalocytes which have a mutation in band 3 also have reduced expression of Rh antigens (969 and see Chapter 17 for further discussion).

Gahmberg (960,970) noticed that the D polypeptide appeared to lack carbohydrate, an unusual feature for a membrane protein which is accessible at the extracellular face of the plasma membrane (but see also Kx protein, Chapter 18). This conclusion was based on failure to label the D-polypeptide with either the galactose oxidase/NaB^{3}H$_4$ or periodate/NaB^{3}H$_4$ surface labeling techniques (960), by the failure of the purified polypeptide to bind to lectin columns comprising *Ricinus communis* or *Lens culinaris* and by the failure of treatment with endo-N-acetyl glucosaminidase H, endo-beta-galactosidase, or mild alkali to alter the apparent molecular weight of the polypeptide on SDS-PAGE (970). Glycosylation is a normal part of the processing of a membrane protein (see discussion in Chapter 4). It may be that the absence of glycosylation of Rh polypeptides reflects the fact that it is assembled as a complex containing the Rh glycoprotein (see below). Similarly, Kx appears to be covalently linked to the heavily glycosylated Kell glycoprotein (see Chapter 18).

Once the Rh polypeptides had been identified several research groups set about trying to purify them so that amino acid sequence information could be obtained, degenerate oligonucleotide probes synthesized and Rh cDNAs isolated. Some used preparative immunoprecipitation (902,963), an approach made possible by the availability of appropriate murine and human monoclonal antibodies, while others used non-immune methods (971). Saboori et al. (972), used hydroxylapatite chromatography to purify proteins structurally related to the Rh polypeptides from the red cells of rhesus monkeys, cows, cats, and rats. The purified poypeptides were labeled with ^{125}I, digested with chymotrypsin, and found to be 30-60% identical to human Rh polypeptides when compared by two-dimensional peptide mapping.

Protein sequence studies showed that the Rh polypeptide immunoprecipitated with anti-D had the same N-terminal sequence (up to residue 13) as the Rh polypeptide immune precipitated by mouse monoclonal antibody R6A (902). Since R6A reacts with D- red cells (389) these results suggested that the D antigen is on a different polypeptide from that which reacts with R6A and that anti-D and monoclonal antibody R6A defined two different but closely related polypeptides. Protein sequence studies of Rh polypeptides purified by hydrox-

yapatite chromatography from either D+ or D- red cells also gave the same N-terminal sequence (963,971).

The Rh Polypeptides are Associated with a Glycoprotein(s) (Rh Glycoprotein(s)) of Mr 45-70,000

The possibility that Rh polypeptides may be associated with a glycosylated component (Rh glycoprotein) in the red cell membrane was first suggested by the work of Gahmberg (970). He noticed that whereas purified D-polypeptide failed to bind to a lectin column containing *Ricinus communis*, D-polypeptide in solubilized whole membrane preparations did bind. The Rh glycoprotein was studied by Moore and Green (901) who used red cells labeled by the galactose oxidase-borohydride method to show that a glycoprotein of Mr 45-70,000 was immunoprecipitated in addition to a polypeptide of Mr 30,000 by anti-D, anti-c and anti-E. Moore and Green (901) also showed that the carbohydrate moiety on the Rh glycoprotein carried ABH activity. The fact that the glycosylated component had ABH activity allowed Moore and Green (901) to prove that the Rh polypeptides associated with the Rh glycoprotein in the native red cell membrane. Anti-D immunoprecipitates were prepared from two artificial red cell mixtures one comprising A, D+ and O, D- red cells and the other A, D- and O, D+ cells. Blood group A activity was found only (by immunoblotting with anti-A) in immunoprecipitates obtained from the mixture containing A, D+ cells proving that the association between Rh glycoprotein and Rh polypeptide occurred in the native cells and did not arise as an artifact of the experimental system. Avent et al. (893) used murine monoclonal anti-Rh (BRIC 69, an antibody similar to R6A) and human monoclonal anti-D to obtain essentially the same results. Treatment of BRIC 69 immunoprecipitates with endo F reduced the Mr of the Rh glycoprotein to 31,000, the same Mr as Rh polypeptides. The realization that Rh polypeptides are associated with Rh glycoprotein(s) in the native red cell raised the possibility that some antigens of the Rh blood group system might be expressed on the polypeptides while others might be expressed on the glycoprotein and that a third set of antigens might require the association of polypeptide and glycoprotein. However, subsequent studies discussed below have established that the critical protein sequences giving rise to Rh antigens are located on the polypeptides not the glycoprotein(s). Protein sequence studies on Rh glycoprotein purified by electroelution from SDS-PAGE from immunoprecipitates obtained with anti-D and with murine monoclonal antibodies having a similar serological specificity to R6A (BRIC 69 and BRIC 207) yielded the same N-terminal sequence, up to residue 30 (902). This Rh glycoprotein N-terminal protein sequence was different from the sequences obtained for Rh polypeptides (discussed in the previous section).

Rh Polypeptides are Major Fatty Acylated Red Cell Membrane Proteins

Early studies by Green (949) and Hughes-Jones et al. (950) described above, suggested that the proteins responsible for Rh antigens are complexed with lipid. These observations together with evidence that the asymmetry of the phospholipid bilayer is abnormal in Rh_{null} red cells (973) led de Vetten and Agre (954) to search for possible fatty acylation of the Rh polypeptides. They incubated intact red cells with tritiated palmitic acid and then prepared membranes, and looked for labeled bands after SDS-PAGE and fluorography. A major labeled band(s) of Mr 32,000 (accounting for 20-30% of the total label linked to membrane proteins) corresponding to the Rh polypeptides was found in D+ and D- red cells but not in Rh_{mod} cells indicating that both D and R6A polypeptides were labeled. Furthermore, a major labeled band could be immune precipitated from D+ red cells with anti-D. Similar observations were reported by Staufenbiel (974). Chemical deacylation studies suggested that the fatty acylation was through thioester linkages involving cysteine residues (954). The deduced protein sequence of the first Rh polypeptide to be cloned revealed six cysteine residues (see below) and five of these were predicted to be on cytoplasmic loops of the protein. Avent et al. (205) suggested that these were candidates for palmitoylation and noted that three of these cysteines formed part of the same sequence motif (Cys-Leu-Pro). Subsequent studies (955) using inside-out red cell membrane vesicles showed that fatty acylation is ATP and CoA dependent and that fatty acylation is a property of Rh polypeptides in all of five other mammalian species (monkey, dog, cow, goat, rat) examined. Direct evidence for the involvement of cytoplasmic cysteine residues in fatty acylation was obtained from experiments utilizing sulfhydryl reactive reagents (*N*-ethyl maleimide (NEM) and DTNB (5,5'-dithiobis (2-nitrobenzoic acid)). Both NEM and DTNB impaired fatty acylation when added to inside-out red cell membrane vesicles (955). Hartel-Schenk and Agre (955) also provide evidence that more than one of the 5 potential cysteines are fatty acylated under the conditions of their experiments. Inside-out red cell membrane vesicles from an individual with the D- phenotype were incubated with tritiated palmitic acid in the presence of ATP and CoA before digestion with trypsin, SDS-PAGE and fluorography. The band of Mr 32,000 corresponding to the R6A

(CE) polypeptide disappeared and two new palmitoylated bands of Mr 21,000 and 19,000 respectively were observed. These authors speculate that the trypsin cleavage occurs at a site in the cytoplasmic loop in the middle of the predicted protein and that the two fatty acylated bands correspond to fragments containing the N and C terminal portions of the protein respectively (see figure 12-4). Evidence that trypsin cleaves Rh polypeptides in this manner has been provided by others (975,976). Inspection of the predicted structure of the R6A/CE polypeptide (figure 12-4) shows that such trypsin cleavage would leave two of the five cysteines in the N-terminal fragment and three in the C-terminal fragment. Avent et al. (205) point to indirect evidence that the first cysteine (Cys-12) is palmitoylated because protein sequencing studies of Rh polypeptides failed to identify a residue at this position (902) and so it is likely to be modified. The function of fatty acylation is not fully understood. de Vetten and Agre (954) suggest that the Rh polypeptides probably require specific flanking phospholipid in order to attain the proper conformation on the membrane surface for immunogenicity, a proposal that implies that imunogenicity is a good thing. Nevertheless it seems likely that fatty acylation is relevant to the conformation of Rh polypeptides whatever their function(s).

Molecular Cloning of Rh Polypeptides

Once the polypeptides carrying Rh antigens were identified several groups purified the proteins and obtained partial protein sequence information which enabled the synthesis of degenerate oligonucleotide probes and the use of those probes to search for Rh cDNA. In 1990 two laboratories independently obtained exactly the same Rh polypeptide cDNA (204,205). Subsequent work has shown that this cDNA encodes the c and E antigens. Chérif-Zahar et al. (204) used oligonucleotide primers spanning amino acids 8-26 of the cE polypeptide in a PCR to isolate a cDNA fragment corresponding to amino acid residues 8-26. Avent et al. (205) used oligonucleotides primers spanning amino acids 28-54 of the D polypeptide and isolated two cDNA fragments, one corresponding to amino acids 37-47 of the cE polypeptide and the other to a fragment which encoded the same amino acid sequence as had been obtained for the D polypeptide. Both laboratories used the partial cDNAs corresponding to the cE polypeptide to obtain full length cDNAs from a human bone marrow cDNA library. However, extensive searches for a full length cDNA corresponding to the cDNA fragment obtained with D polypeptide sequence were unsuccessful. When full length clones corresponding to the D polypeptide were obtained (206,207,545) they did not encode the amino

FIGURE 12-4 The Structure of Rh Polypeptides

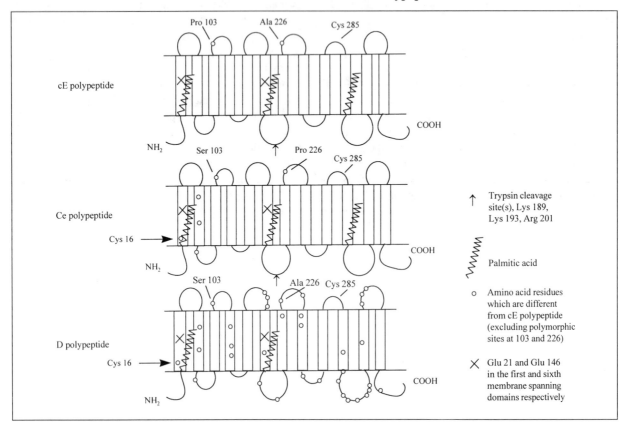

acid sequence reported by Avent et al. (205) nor did they encode a sequence corresponding to a tryptic peptide isolated from the C terminus of the D polypeptide which differed from the corresponding region of the CE polypeptide at two positions (Trp408-Asp, Lys409-Ile) (977). These discrepancies have not been explained but subsequent studies described below have confirmed unambiguously that the cDNAs do encode the D polypeptide.

When the sequence of cDNA corresponding to the CE polypeptide was first reported two different structures were proposed for the encoded polypeptide (204,205). The CE polypeptide comprises 417 amino acids. It lacks a signal peptide and the initiator methionine is postranslationally cleaved so that the mature protein has 416 residues, with serine at its N-terminus. Inspection of the amino acid sequence on the N-terminal side of the first membrane spanning domain reveals the presence of several basic amino acids, a feature consistent with an intracellular N-terminus (978, see also Chapter 4) and this interpretation is further supported by the observation that the tyrosine residue at position 4 of the mature protein is not radioiodinated when the polypeptide is labeled on intact red cells (902). When hydropathy plots were carried out to predict the membrane orientation of the rest of the polypeptide chain two

different interpretations were published. One predicted 12 transmembrane domains (205) and the other predicted 13 transmembrane domains (204). This difference is significant because a protein with 12 transmembrane domains would have its C-terminus in the cytoplasm while one with 13 domains would have an extracellular C terminus. The difference though significant, was not particularly surprising since hydropathy plots are not always easy to interpret (see Chapter 14 for discussion of the controversy over hydropathy plots and the structure of the Duffy glycoprotein). The two models could easily be tested by determining the position of the C-terminus. However, very surprisingly, experimental evidence in support of both orientations was forthcoming. Two groups argued that the C-terminus was extracellular (891,976) and one that it was intracellular (979). Bloy et al. (891) argued for an extracellular C-terminus because they failed to find radioactivity in anti-D immune precipitates obtained from radioiodinated intact red cells treated with carboxypeptidase Y, the assumption being that since the protein is radioiodinated in the absence of carboxypeptidase Y treatment and the enzyme specifically cleaves proteins at their C-terminii the C-terminus must have been altered on intact red cells and is therefore extracellular. Suyama and Goldstein (976) argued for an extracellular C-terminus because they could not detect a membrane-bound C-terminal fragment of the CE polypeptide after treatment of intact red cells with papain. Avent et al. (979) presented evidence that the C-terminus is intracellular by raising a rabbit antibody to a synthetic peptide corresponding to the predicted C-terminal sequence and showing that it would react with the polypeptide in red cell "ghosts" but would not react with intact red cells. Similar experiments by Hermand et al. (980) supported this conclusion and there is now general agreement that the Rh polypeptides (CE and D) have 12 membrane spanning domains and that both N and C-terminii are intracellular (754). It seems likely that the carboxypeptidase preparation used by Bloy et al. (891) may have been contaminated with endopeptidases since Suyama and Goldstein (976) showed that an N terminal chymotryptic fragment of the Rh polypeptide could be radioiodinated on the surface of intact red cells. The failure of Suyama and Goldstein (976) to detect a C-terminal membrane bound fragment after treatment of intact red cells with papain is likely to be because this small fragment (Mr 6,000) was not resolved on the SDS-gels that they used (979).

Inspection of the deduced structure of the CE polypeptide reveals a number of features of interest. Four acidic residues (Glu-21, Asp-95, Glu-156, Glu-340) are predicted to be located within membrane-spanning domains. Charged residues are often associated with the membrane spanning domains of proteins involved in ion transport. The multiple membrane spanning structure predicted for this protein suggests a transporter function (see Chapter 4 for further discussion). The CE polypeptide has six cysteine residues, five of these are predicted to be located on cytoplasmic loops and may be target sites for fatty acylation (see previous section), the sixth cysteine (Cys-285) is predicted to occur on the fifth extracellular loop (see figure 12-4), a feature consistent with evidence that the cE (R6A) polypeptide can be labeled with a membrane impermeant maleimide (961).

The isolation of a full length cDNA corresponding to the D polypeptide was reported independently by three groups (206,207,545). The protein sequences deduced from the three cDNAs were not identical but differed from the protein sequence of the cE polypeptide by 35 residues (clone Rh13) (207); 36 residues (clones RhII/RhXIII) (206); and 31 residues (clone RhPII) (545) respectively. These D polypeptides have the same number of amino acids as the cE polypeptides (417 residues) and the same structure (figure 12-4). The D and cE polypeptides are highly homologous, the D clone isolated by Arce et al. (207) was 96% identical to the cE clone at the nucleotide level and 92% identical at the protein level. The fact that D and cE clones are so

homologous suggested that they result from a common ancestral gene as a result of gene duplication, a hypothesis discussed in more detail below. Le Van Kim et al. (206) concluded that their clones were products of the *D* gene because they could detect the gene which corresponded to their cDNA clones in genomic DNA from individuals of D+ but not those of D- phenotype (evidence that the *D* gene is absent from individuals of the D- phenotype had previously been obtained from Southern blotting experiments (40)). Arce et al. (207) concluded that their clone corresponded to the product of the *D* gene because they could find the corresponding mRNA transcript in reticulocytes from D+ individuals but not from reticulocytes of D- individuals. Kajii et al. (545) concluded that their clone was *not* the product of the *D* gene because they could detect the cDNA in an individual of phenotype D- C+ c+ E+ e+ (545,981,982). These experimental differences were debated in letters published in the *Biochemical Journal* (983,984). The confusion that these discrepant results created may be apparent rather than real and result from the fact that while the D- phenotype found in Whites usually results from a deletion of the *D* gene (40) the D-phenotype in Japanese commonly occurs in the presence of a normal *D* gene. There is a phenotype found in Japanese known as D_{el}. Red cells with the D_{el} phenotype would type as D- by all the usual serological typing methods (they are not agglutinated by IgM anti-D typing reagents or by IgG anti-D used in an antiglobulin test) but a very weak D antigen can be detected by absorption /elution (293). Japanese individuals with the D_{el} phenotype have a normal *D* gene (985) but its polypeptide product must be expressed at very low levels in the red cell membrane for reasons as yet unknown. If the D- individuals studied by Kajii et al. (545) had the D_{el} phenotype then the differences would be explained.

The 30 or more sequence differences between the cE and D polypeptides are distributed throughout the protein (see figure 12-4). A cluster of sequence differences is found in the last predicted cytoplasmic loop one of which results in the loss of a cysteine residue in a Cys-Leu-Pro motif and hence a potential fatty acylation site. A single extracellular Cys-285 is found in the D polypeptide as well as the in cE polypeptide and this is consistent with evidence that membrane impermeable maleimides label the D polypeptide (956,961). Four acidic residues found in membrane spanning domains of the cE polypeptide (see above) are also found in the D polypeptide and a fifth (Asp-128) is found only in the D polypeptide. The D polypeptide contains a signal motif for N-glycosylation (Asn331-Phe-Ser) but this is predicted to be in the last cytoplasmic loop and therefore unlikely to be utilized.

Molecular Cloning of Rh Glycoprotein(s)

As discussed in an earlier section, immune precipitation experiments with anti-D and with monoclonal antibodies (901,893) demonstrated that the D polypeptide and cE polypeptide (syn R6A polypeptide) coprecipitate with N-glycosylated proteins (Rh glycoprotein(s)). The Rh glycoprotein components which precipitate with the D and cE polypeptides respectively have slightly different apparent molecular weights on SDS-PAGE which could be because they are different related proteins or because complexes involving D and CE polypeptides undergo differences in the processing of attached carbohydrate. Protein sequence studies showed that the two glycoprotein components have the same N-terminal amino acid sequence (at least to residue 30) (902). PCR primers based on the N-terminal amino acid sequence were used to isolate two cDNA fragments corresponding to the Rh glycoprotein and these were used to isolate full length cDNA clones from human erythroid cDNA libraries (903). The cDNA clones encoded a protein sequence of 409 amino acids with a predicted topology similar to that of the Rh polypeptides with 12 membrane spanning domains and intracellular N and C terminii (see figure 12-5). The predicted protein has three signal motifs for N-glycosylation (Asn-37, Asn-274, Asn-355) and two of these (Asn-37, Asn-355) on the first and last extracellular loops respectively, are predicted to be extracellular. The Rh glycoprotein does not contain any Cys-Leu-Pro motifs or the CCNR motif found in Rh polypeptides and so it is unlikely to be fatty acylated. Similarities in the overall structure of the Rh polypeptides and Rh glycoprotein extend to two acidic residues found in the same locations in the first and fifth membrane spanning domains (Glu-13 and Glu-146 in Rh glycoprotein; Glu-21 and Glu-146 in the Rh polypeptides) (903) and suggesting that the Rh glycoprotein may also be involved in ion transport. Eyers et al. (921) used rabbit antibodies to a synthetic peptide corresponding to the C-terminus of the Rh glycoprotein to provide experimental evidence that the Rh glycoprotein, like the Rh polypeptides, has its C-terminus in the cytoplasm. Eyers et al. (921) also showed that of the two possible extracellular N-glycan sites only the first is utilized. The *Staphylococcus aureus* V8 protease cleaves the deglycosylated Rh glycoprotein (deglycosylated by treatment with peptidyl N-glycanase) in the first extracellular loop at Glu-34 to create a large cleavage fragment containing the C terminus of the glycoprotein (see figure 12-5) of Mr 28,500. N-terminal amino acid sequence analysis of this fragment revealed an aspartic acid residue at the third residue which corresponds to Asn-37 in the intact protein. When peptidyl N-glycanase cleaves N-glycans from Asn residues the Asn is hydrolyzed to Asp (986)

and so this experiment shows that Asn-37 is glycosylated in the Rh glycoprotein (921). When red cell membranes are treated with trypsin the Rh glycoprotein is cleaved and at least 9 tryptic peptides result. The molecular size of the largest tryptic fragment containing the C-terminus of the Rh glycoprotein does not change after treatment with peptidyl N-glycanase indicating that Asn-355 on the last extracellular loop of the Rh glycoprotein is not glycosylated (921).

The Organization of the Genes Giving Rise to Rh Polypeptides

Once cDNAs corresponding to the Rh polypeptides had been obtained it was possible to use them as probes in Southern blotting studies of genomic DNA (gDNA) in order to investigate the structure of the *RH* locus. These studies showed that the *RH* locus comprises two very similar genes (now known as *CE* gene and *D* gene) and further showed that one of these genes was completely lacking from gDNA derived from several unrelated D-individuals (40). These studies established the basis of the common White D- phenotype, a phenotype resulting from the deletion of an entire gene (*D* gene). The organization of the *CE* gene was described by Chérif-Zahar et al. (987). These authors screened a human genomic placental library with cDNA corresponding to the CE polypeptide and with a PCR product specific for the N-terminal region common to both CE and D polypeptides. Ten positive clones were obtained two of which contained the *D* gene and eight the *CE* gene. Five of the eight *CE* gene clones and a sixth clone corresponding to the 3' end of the *CE* gene obtained from a different genomic library were used to determine the exon structure of the *CE* gene and to define the exon/intron junction sequences. The exon 4/intron 4 and intron 4/exon 5 junction sequences reported by Chérif-Zahar et al. (987) have been questioned by others (989,990) and probably reflect difficulties in manual DNA sequencing of GC-rich sequences in the former study. The *CE* gene comprises 10 exons ranging in size from 72-247bp and distributed over 75kb (see figure 12-6). The nine introns range in size from 1.5 to >10kb. The nucleotide sequence of the 5' end of the *CE* gene was determined for 600bp upstream of the transcription initiator site. This putative promoter region was shown to have transcriptional activity by CAT assay (see Chapter 5). The Rh(-600)-CAT construct was active in K562 cells (43.5% of control) but not in HeLa cells (6.9% of control) indicating that this region contains sequence motifs necessary for erythroid-specific transcription of the *CE* gene (987). Inspection of the nucleotide sequence of this promoter region revealed several putative transcription factor binding sites and in

FIGURE 12-5 Structure of the Rh Glycoprotein (from reference 921)

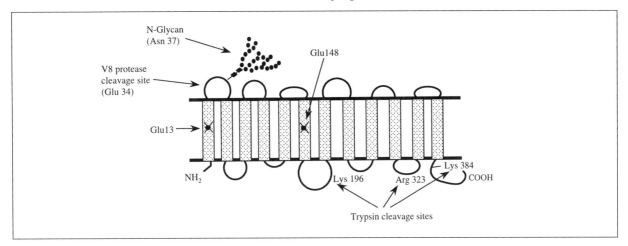

particular, three consensus GATA-1 binding motifs (at positions -2, -28 and -454).

The exon/intron structure of the *D* gene has not been formally published at the time of writing but it is clear from work in several laboratories that it is composed of 10 exons and has an organization which is extremely similar, though not identical, to that of the *CE* gene. The promoter sequence of the *D* gene (to 600bp upstream of the transcription initiator site) differs from that of the *CE* gene by only five nucleotides and contains the necessary sequence motifs for erythroid specific transcription (Rouillac and Chérif-Zahar, cited in 991). Arce et al. (207) noted that the *D* and *CE* genes differ with respect to intron 4. The *D* gene has a much smaller intron than the *CE* gene because of a 650bp deletion starting from nucleotide position 181 of the *CE* gene intron (intron 4 of the *CE* gene has 1076bp) (990,992). Nucleotide positions 1-181 and 831-1076 are nearly identical in the *CE* and *D* genes with only three nucleotide differences (992). The nucleotide sequence of intron 5 in the *D* and *CE* genes comprises 1,636bp and there are only 29 nucleotide differences between the two genes (98.2% homology) (992). It is clear from these studies that the extensive homology that exists between the coding sequences of the *D* and *CE* genes also extends to non-coding regions.

Given the level of homology between the two genes it would be expected that the *CE* and *D* genes arose by duplication of an ancestral *RH* gene. Interestingly, sequence analysis of Rh transcripts from non-human primates led Salvignol et al. (203) to suggest that an ancestral *RH* gene duplicated very early in evolution, in a common ancestor of man and African apes, giving rise to ancestral *CE* and *D* genes. This hypothesis is based on the observation that Rh transcripts in chimpanzees and gorillas are more like products of the *D* gene than of the *CE* gene.

The Molecular Basis of Cc and Ee Antigens

Southern blot analysis of human genomic DNA indicated that the *RH* locus is composed of two closely linked genes and that one of these genes is absent in most White individuals with the D- phenotype (40). The section above describing the cloning of the *Rh* genes explains that two related cDNAs (encoding CE and D polypeptides respectively) were described in 1990 (204,205) and 1992/93 (206,207,545) respectively. When it became clear that D antigen was associated with a separate gene which was absent in most White D-persons a simple strategy suggested itself for the determination of the molecular bases of Cc and Ee antigens. Mouro et al. (41) extracted mRNA from D- individuals of known CcEe phenotype and used synthetic oligonucleotide primers in the presence of reverse transcriptase to obtain full length cDNAs corresponding to the *CE* gene product. Nucleotide sequencing of these cDNAs revealed that the presence of E or e antigen correlated with a single nucleotide substitution which resulted in proline at position 226 when E was expressed and alanine at 226 when e was expressed. When cDNA sequences were compared with respect to C and c antigen expression the situation was more complex. Six nucleotide differences were observed of which four changed the nature of the amino acid in the polypeptide chain (Cys-16, Ile-60, Ser-68, Ser-103 when C is found, Trp-16, Leu-60, Asn-68, Pro-103 when c is found) (41). These findings were corroborated by amplification of exons 1 and 2 which encoded the Cc specific residues and exon 5 which encodes the Ee specific residues from genomic DNA derived from individuals of known phenotype. These results showed that the nucleotide sequence of the first Rh cDNA to be cloned would be expected to give rise to c and E antigens. Simsek et al. (546) came to the same conclusions independently. At

FIGURE 12-6 Structure of Genes Giving Rise to Rh Polypeptides

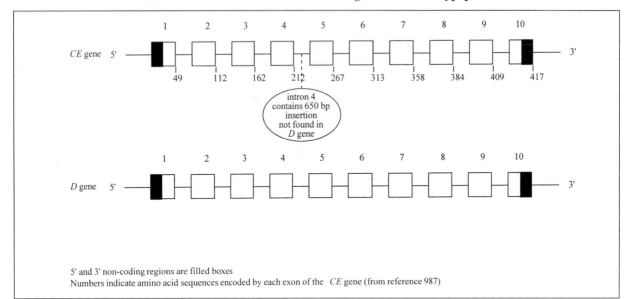

5' and 3' non-coding regions are filled boxes
Numbers indicate amino acid sequences encoded by each exon of the *CE* gene (from reference 987)

the time of these studies the cDNAs could not be expressed in a model system to prove that they did indeed encode the predicted antigens. Mouro et al. (204) put forward the hypothesis that although the Cc and Ee antigens were the products of the same gene and encoded by a single mRNA species, alternative splicing of the mRNA gave rise to several different protein products. It was suggested (204) that a full length polypeptide expressed Ee and not Cc, while a spliceoform lacking exon 5 encoded a polypeptide which expressed Cc and not Ee. Such a hypothesis could account for protein mapping evidence that Cc and Ee antigens were carried on different proteins (964) and was further supported by evidence that different splicing products of the CE gene could be isolated from preparations of mRNA (993). This hypothesis was criticized because such spliceoforms were detected only by PCR and had not been noted in Northern blotting studies of erythroid mRNAs suggesting that they were minor mis-spliced transcripts. Further, there were theoretical reasons why the protein products of such spliceoforms would not be expected to be assembled properly in the red cell membrane (898). Subsequent studies showed that spliceoforms were not restricted to products of the *CE* gene as had been suggested (993) but could also be found derived from the *D* gene (984). More significantly, spliceoforms could be isolated from immature erythroblasts but not from reticulocytes (981). The validity of the spliceoform hypothesis could most easily be addressed by expression studies but unfortunately early attempts to express the genes met with very limited success (980,994,995). These problems were overcome by the use of a retroviral expression system and direct evidence that the first Rh polypeptide cDNA to be cloned encoded production of c and E antigens, was obtained by transduction

of the erythroid cell line K562 (996). The c and E antigens were detected de novo on the surface of the transduced cells by flow cytometry. Since the cDNA used was full length and no smaller products could be detected in the transduced cells this result provides strong evidence that c and E antigens can be carried on a single polypeptide and that the expression of c antigen is not restricted to certain spliceoforms. Further evidence that Cc and Ee antigens can be carried on the same polypeptide chain was obtained from studies with antisera raised against different regions of the Rh polypeptides (997).

The critical residue responsible for E/e antigens (Pro226-Ala) is predicted to be in the fourth extracellular loop of the CE polypeptide (see figure 12-4) a location entirely consistent with its expected role in the structure of an antigen. It should be noted however that the antigens are not simply defined by a single amino acid. The D polypeptide has an alanine residue at position 226 but it does express e antigen because the antigen is defined by the environment in which the critical amino acids are contained (see also discussion of E/e variant antigens below). The structure of C and c antigens is more complicated because there are four different amino acids between polypeptides that express C and those that express c. Only one of these amino acids is predicted to be extracellular (Ser(C)103-Pro(c)).

The Molecular Basis of the G Antigen and its Relevance to an Understanding of the C Antigen

Almost all cells that carry D and/or C antigen also

express G antigen (86). Once it was shown that D and C are carried on different proteins it was clear that the G antigen must result from a common feature of the surface of D and C polypeptides. Inspection of the predicted amino acid sequences of D and C polypeptides reveals that three of the four amino acids that distinguish a C-active CE polypeptide from a c-active CE polypeptide (Ile-60, Ser-68, Ser-103) are also found in the D polypeptide. These three amino acids are encoded by exon 2 of the *CE* gene and exon 2 of the *D* gene. Assuming that the overall topology of the CE and D polypeptides is the same and that the many other sequence differences between the C and D polypeptides do not adversely affect the environment surrounding these three common residues it can be argued that the polypeptide sequence encoded by exon 2 of the *C* and *D* genes is critical for G antigen expression. Experimental support for this hypothesis has come from several sources. Faas et al. (998) studied genomic DNA and cDNA from two donors with the rare Rh phenotype C- c+ D+ E+ e+ G- and one with the phenotype C- c+ D- E+ e+ G+. In both ccDEe G- donors a single nucleotide substitution was found in exon 2 of the *D* gene which would result in a replacement of Ser-103 by Pro. The ccEe, G+ donor had a more complex genetic background and exhibited a hybrid *D-CE-D* gene in which exons 1,2,3,9 and 10 were derived from the *D* gene and exons 4,5,6,7 from the *CE* gene. The origin of exon 8 could not be ascertained because the sequence of this exon is the same in both *CE* and *D* genes. The occurrence of exon 2 derived from *D* gene in this donor would mean that Ile-60, Ser-68 and Ser-103 are present, a feature not inconsistent with their possible importance for the G antigen structure. Rouillac et al. (560) studied the rare phenotype D^{IIIb} in two unrelated individuals and found that the *D* gene of these individuals contained exon 2 derived from a *CE* gene in which exon 2 encodes a sequence associated with the expression of c antigen (Leu-60, Asn-68, Pro-103). Red cells of phenotype D^{IIIb} are G-. These results taken together provide evidence that G antigen is associated with Ile-60, Ser-68 and Ser-103 and that Ser-103 is critical for G antigen expression.

These results are relevant to an understanding of C antigen structure since the only residue found in C antigen which is not found in the unusual *D* gene of individuals with the rare phenotype D^{IIIb} or in the G+ donor of phenotype ccEe is Cys-16. Cys-16 is predicted to be located on the cytoplasmic face of the red cell membrane and so the interesting question is raised as to the mechanism by which Cys-16 could alter the surface structure of an Rh polypeptide to create C antigen. Inspection of the sequence in this region reveals that Cys-16 changes the sequence from C(12)LPLW to C(12)LPLC. As discussed in an earlier section, Cys-12 is known to be a site for fatty acylation in Rh polypeptides (205). The presence of Cys-16 creates another potential palmitoylation site. In fact it creates a palindromic sequence containing two possible Cys-Leu-Pro motifs. If the presence of Cys-16 alters the pattern of fatty acylation in this region of the molecule this might alter the conformation of the protein and create the novel surface structure called C antigen. Further support for a critical role of Cys-16 in C antigen expression comes from studies of red cells of persons with the rare genotype r^Gr. Nucleotide sequence analysis revealed that the r^G allele results either from a segmental DNA exchange between part of exon 2 of the *ce* gene and exon 2 of a *CE* or *D* gene or from a cross-over event between nt150 and nt178 of a *ce* and *Ce* gene (999). The predicted protein encoded by the r^G gene has Ile-60, Ser-68 and Ser-103 but not Cys-16 and of course, lacks C antigen. Studies of Rh polypeptide genes in primates have indicated that chimpanzee and gorilla have Cys-16, Ile-60, Ser-68, Pro-103 and yet type as c positive, C negative a result which implies that only Pro-103 is required for c structure (203). These primate studies led Salvignol et al. (203) to speculate that a proline residue at 102 is required for the presentation of c because the Rh polypeptides of crab-eating macaque and rhesus monkey have sequences that would predict c antigen and yet are c negative and these have Ser-102 not Pro-102. Other evidence indicates that c antigen expression is not dependent upon Trp-16 because Cys-16 can be found in Rh polypeptides which express c antigen (1000). To summarize, Ser-103 is required for G and Pro-103 for c whereas C requires Ser-103 and Cys-16. The availability of an expression system for Rh polypeptides (996) should allow the further definition of these antigens through the use of site-directed mutagenesis.

The Antigens C^W and C^X and MAR

Rh transcripts isolated from the blood of donors with the C^W antigen revealed a point mutation which changes a single amino acid (Gln41-Arg) in the product of the *CE* gene. This change results in the replacement of an uncharged amino acid with a basic amino acid on the predicted first extracellular loop of the CE polypeptide (208). Studies of the DC^W- phenotype revealed Rh transcripts which comprised exon 1 of the *CE* gene which contained the C^W mutation and exons 2-10 of the *D* gene (989). In another study the DC^W- phenotype was found to result from a hybrid gene comprising exons 1 and 10 of the *CE* gene and exons 2 (or 3) to 9 of the *D* gene (1001).

Rh transcripts isolated from the blood of donors with the C^X antigen revealed a point mutation which changes a single amino acid (Ala36-Thr) in the product of the *CE* gene (208). The sequence change would occur on the predicted first extracellular loop.

Red cells which lack the MAR antigen are either from persons who are homozygous for C^W, homozygous for C^X or heterozygous C^W/C^X (116). Since the critical residues for C^W and C^X are close together on the first extracellular loop of the CE polypeptide (sequence of first loop is H33YDA*SLEDQ**KGLVASYQLFQD where asterisks indicate critical residues for C^X * and C^W ** respectively) it seems likely that the MAR antigen is defined by some or all of this sequence.

Variants of E Antigen

A variant E antigen found in Japanese has been studied at the DNA level and found to result from a hybrid *cE-D-cE* gene in which part of exon 5 of the *cE* gene is replaced with part of exon 5 of a *D* gene (1002). This variant which presumably results from a gene conversion event causes nucleotides 697 and 712 to be replaced by their D-specific counterparts (Gln233Glu; Met238Val) with the result that some monoclonal anti-E react weakly with cells expressing the variant polypeptide.

A reciprocal event giving rise to a hybrid *D-cE-D* gene which encodes a polypeptide predicted to express partial D and partial E antigens was reported by Avent et al. (1003). This hybrid gene is identical to that reported as giving rise to D^{Va} (215) except that the encoded protein would contain proline and not alanine at residue 226.

The Molecular Basis of VS Antigen

The VS antigen is reported to correlate with a single nucleotide substitution at nt733 in exon 5 of the *CE* gene which changes Leu245 to Val (1004,1005).

Molecular Basis of the $\overline{\overline{R}}^N$ Phenotype

Roulliac et al. (991) examined genomic DNA and cDNA derived from three individuals with the $\overline{\overline{R}}^N$ gene (two homozygous and one heterozygous for the allele). Cells of this phenotype are characterized by weak C and e antigens and the presence of the low incidence antigen Rh32 (see earlier). Evidence was obtained that two different genetic mechanisms give rise to the $\overline{\overline{R}}^N$ phenotype. The two homozygous donors (Cou and Ba) had hybrid *Ce-D-Ce* genes in which exon 4 was derived from the *D* gene. The heterozygous donor (Maf) had a hybrid *Ce-D-Ce* gene in which the 3′ end of exon 3 and the entire exon 4 were derived from the *D* gene. This means that the *Ce-D-Ce* gene product in donors Cou and Ba differs from the normal White *Ce* gene product by seven amino

acids (at positions 169, 170, 172, 182, 193, 198 and 201) while that in donor Maf differs by eight amino acids (position 152 in addition to those listed for donors Cou and Ba). Clearly, these sequence differences are likely to explain the absence of Rh46 and the presence of Rh32 in this phenotype. If these hybrid *Ce-D-Ce* gene products are expressed at the same level as the *Ce* gene product then these results indicate that structure of C and e antigens are influenced by the protein sequence encoded by exon 4 of the *Ce* gene even though the critical amino acids required for antigen structure are not encoded by this exon. Which of the sequence differences are relevant to C and e expression is not known but this question could be addressed using site-directed mutagenesis and expression of the mutated genes.

Molecular Basis of D and Partial D Antigens

Once cDNA encoding the D polypeptide had been isolated (206,207,545) and it was realized that in most Whites the D- phenotype results from a deletion of the *D* gene (40) it was clear that much of the complexity associated with the D antigen was likely to reflect the fact that absence of D antigen, unlike most other polymorphic blood group antigens, results from the absence of a whole polypeptide. It follows from this that the immune response of a D- recipient to D+ red cells would be complex and could result in production of antibodies to several antigens on the polypeptide. This mixture of antibodies to several antigens is called anti-D. If anti-D is a mixture of antibodies to several antigens then someone with an unusual *D* gene might produce a D polypeptide with one antigen present and another missing. Such an individual when exposed to red cells containing a common D polypeptide could make an antibody to the antigen that was lacking and so a D+ person would make anti-D, not at all surprising, any confusion is created by man through his choice of nomenclature!

Nucleotide sequencing of D transcripts from individuals who are D+ but have made alloimmune anti-D would therefore be expected to reveal D polypeptides with different sequences from the normal D polypeptide and by comparing these sequence differences with the corresponding sequence in the normal D polypeptide, some information about the structure of the D antigen that is lacking can be inferred. Several studies of this type on partial D antigens have been published. One involving the lack of G antigen in D^{IIIb} red cells (560) has already been discussed above.

Rouillac et al. (215) analyzed Rh transcripts isolated from reticulocytes of individuals expressing several different partial D antigens (D^{IVa}, D^{IVb}, D^{Va}, DFR). In all cases evidence was obtained for replacement of *D* gene sequences by *CE* gene sequences. These replacements were postulated to occur via gene conversion between the two highly homologous genes at meiosis, a mechanism already well established for MNS antigens (see Chapter 15). All these hybrid genes predicted a polypeptide of 417 amino acids which would be expected to be incorporated into the red cell membrane normally. These results are summarized in table 12-10 and figure 12-7. Mouro et al. (211) studied red cells with the D^{VI} phenotype and found heterogeneity at the DNA level dependent upon whether the haplotype $CD^{VI}e$ or $cD^{VI}E$ was present. In the case of $CD^{VI}e$ a hybrid *D-CE-D* gene was found which contained exons 4, 5 and 6 of the *CE* gene. The predicted protein product of this gene would have 417 amino acids and would be expected to be incorporated into the red cell membrane normally. In the case of $cD^{VI}E$ these authors concluded that the *D* gene contained a deletion of exons 4, 5 and 6. This is a very surprising result since it is unlikely that a deletion of this type would allow the correct folding of the novel polypeptide for incorporation in the membrane (the same argument applies as in the case of spliceoforms giving rise to Cc antigens on different molecules from Ee antigens discussed in a previous section, and see ref 898). Subsequent studies from these authors (1006) and others (1003,1007-1009) have shown that in the $cD^{VI}E$ haplotype the abnormal *D* gene is a hybrid *D-CE-D* gene containing exons 4 and 5 of the *CE* gene and not a *D* gene with an internal deletion as previously reported.

Several other unusual D antigens have been shown to result from hybrid *D-CE-D* genes (table 12-10, figure 12-7). D^{IIIc} results from a hybrid *D-CE-D* gene containing exon 3 of the *CE* gene (1010). D^{DBT} results from a hybrid *D-CE-D* gene containing exons 5, 6, 7 and possibly 8 of the *CE* gene (1011).

Several partial D phenotypes result from point mutations in the *D* gene. D^{VII} results from a mutation in exon 2 of the *D* gene which changes Leu110 to Pro (214) whereas DNU and D^{HMi} result from point mutations in exon 7 of the *D* gene which change Gly353 to Arg and Ala354 to Asp respectively (1065, table 12-10, figure 12-7).

One of the more interesting partial D phenotypes is that encoded by the gene known as R^{oHar}. In this case the phenotype results from a *CE-D-CE* hybrid gene that contains exon 5 of the *D* gene (248). This phenotype is interesting because it results from a variant *CE* gene rather than a variant *D* gene serving as a reminder that antibodies detect antigens not genes and it does not necessarily follow that all D antigens will derive directly from a *D* gene.

Since cells with partial D phenotypes are frequently characterized by the expression of low incidence Rh antigens, molecular studies of the type described above also provide information about the location and structure of these infrequent antigens. The low incidence antigens Rh23 (in D^{Va}), Rh30 (in D^{IVa}), Rh32 (in D^{DBT}), Rh37 (in D^{IVb}) and Rh50 (in D^{DFR}) are likely to result from the presence of *CE* gene sequences in the context of a *D* gene whereas Rh33 (in R_o^{Har}) results from a *D* gene sequence in the *CE* gene. The structure of Rh40 is much easier to define since this results from the point mutation Leu110 to Pro found in the D^{VII} phenotype (214).

The results described above provide a great deal of information about the genetic mechanisms that give rise to the group of antigens collectively described as D. Unfortunately, these results are not very informative about the structure of the antigens themselves because there are many protein sequence differences between polypeptides deriving from a common *D* gene and from the hybrid genes of D+ individuals who have made alloimmune anti-D. If anti-D made by D+ individuals were widely available, which they are not, this problem could be approached using expression of normal and variant D genes together with site-directed mutagenesis.

The problem of defining the nature of the antigens that comprise D is further compounded by the widespread use of monoclonal anti-D for blood grouping. Monoclonal antibodies, by definition, react with epitopes not antigens (see Chapter 2). Occasionally, blood samples are found which fail to react with a particular monoclonal anti-D which means that the red cells of the individual concerned lack the epitope detected by the antibody. The epitope in question is part of an antigen since the monoclonal anti-D itself was derived from a polyclonal response to human D+ red cells but which antigen? Brave attempts have been made to bring order into chaos by carrying out cluster analysis, that is, by trying to determine how many different patterns of reactivity can be discerned among monoclonal anti-D and matching the patterns with molecular analyses of different partial D phenotypes. Some progress has been made (see figure 12-8, 1012,1013). There are, at the time of writing, more proposed D epitopes than sequence differences between the D and CE polypeptides! The availability of an expression system for the *D* gene (996) suggests an alternative approach. Mutant genes could be prepared by recombinant techniques in which sequences corresponding to each extracellular and adjacent transmembrane domains of the *D* gene are replaced by the corresponding sequences from the *CE* gene and expressed in K562 cells. Monoclonal anti-D could be grouped according to their reaction patterns. Key residues within a given segment could be identified by site-directed mutagenesis. A comprehensive study of this type would entail a great deal of work and it is arguable that it would be of limited value in the absence of a 3-dimensional structure of the Rh polypeptides. Nevertheless, evidence that the G

FIGURE 12-7 Genes Giving Rise to Partial D Antigens of Different Categories (references 992,1006)

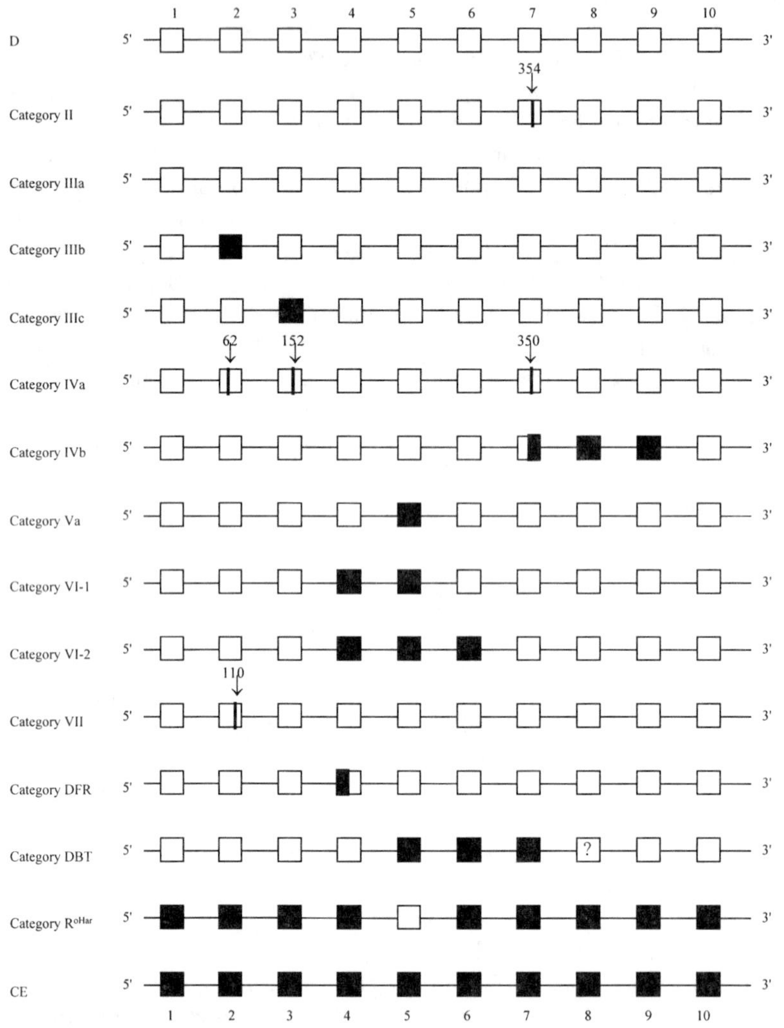

Open boxes exons derived from *D* gene, closed box exons derived from *CE* gene. Arrows indicate site of point mutations, numbers above arrows refer to the amino acid which is changed. ?= Exon 8 of *D* and *CE* gene are identical so origin of this exon unknown.

antigen can be expressed on both D and C polypeptides implies that the structure of the product of exon 2 of *D* and *CE* is retained in the context of either a CE or D polypeptide. Liu et al. (1014) introduced three amino acids found in the last extracellular loop of the D polypeptide (Asp350, Gly353, Ala354) into a cE or ce polypeptide (by site-directed mutagenesis) and showed, after expression of the resulting polypeptide in K562 cells, that some monoclonal anti-D react with the altered protein, a result which implies that the structure of the last extracellular loops of the D polypeptide and the CE polypeptide are largely independent of the structure of adjacent loops. These results suggest a model of an Rh polypeptide that can be assembled from pieces, each of which retain their own structure in the assembled whole

rather than the structure of one part in the final protein being dependent on the structure of another part. If this is so then the kind of mutation analysis proposed above may contribute greatly to the elucidation of the structure of the protein.

Molecular Basis of Weak D Antigens

The term weak D antigen refers to quantitative reduction in D antigen strength rather than the qualitative changes that occur in partial D antigens discussed above (264). Cells of the weak D phenotype (formerly D^u) have a selective depression of D but not Cc/Ee antigens. This depression of D does not result from any

FIGURE 12-8 Proposed Position of D Epitopes Relative to the Extracellular Loops of the D Polypeptide (from reference 1065)

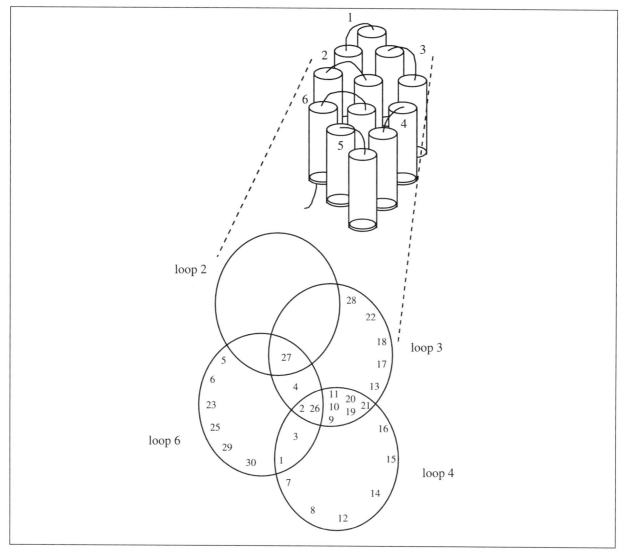

alteration in the structure of the *D* gene or the promoter sequence of the *D* gene (in the -600 to +41 region) and the *D* gene transcripts have a normal sequence (991,992). Roulliac et al. (991) compared the level of expression of D and CE transcripts in two donors with weak D phenotypes using a semi-quantitative PCR assay and concluded that the level of D transcripts in weak D is four to five-fold lower than in samples with a common D phenotype. Beckers et al. (992) also used a semi-quantitative PCR analysis to estimate the amount of full length D transcripts in weak D samples. In this study the level of D transcript in weak D, samples from *D* heterozygotes and homozygotes and from D-- phenotypes was compared with the level of glycophorin A transcripts and no difference was found between "weak D" and "normal D" although there were

more D transcripts in D-- cells. In one study (991) it was assumed that the level of CE transcripts would be the same as that in cells of common D phenotype and in the other study (992) it was assumed that the level of GPA would be constant. Further work will be required to resolve this discrepancy but it seems clear from these studies and from other work which demonstrates the presence of apparently normal *D* and *CE* genes in some examples of D-- and Rh$_{null}$ phenotypes (40,1015,1016) that there are as yet undefined regulatory elements in addition to the *RH* genes themselves which can influence the expression of the genes. It seems likely that one study which reported deletion of *D* gene sequences in a donor with the D^u phenotype (1017) describes the molecular basis of a partial D phenotype rather than a weak D phenotype.

The molecular basis of a very weak D antigen (D_{el}) found in Japanese has been investigated by Fukumori et al. (985). This phenotype is characterized by the presence of a D antigen that is so weak that it can only be detected by absorption-elution. PCR analysis of *D* gene exons in this phenotype have indicated that a normal *D* gene is present.

DNA-based Methods for Typing Rh Antigens and Their Value in the Management of Pregnancies at Risk of Hemolytic Disease of the Newborn

Knowledge of the molecular bases of Rh antigens described in previous sections allows for the determination of the Rh type of an individual by analysis of DNA and without the need for red cells. However, Rh typing from DNA is much more complicated than that for most other blood group antigens. Most blood group antigens are defined by single nucleotide substitutions in the relevant genes rather than the complex gene rearrangements which give rise to the appearance or disappearance of Rh antigens. Because of this complexity and the cost of PCR testing it seems unlikely that DNA-based methods will replace routine D typing of donors and patients by the use of antibodies, at least in the short term. Nevertheless, the application of DNA-based methods for Rh typing is well established as a useful aid to the management of pregnancies at risk from HDN. Despite the widespread use of prophylactic anti-D in the prevention of this disease (see Chapter 41) there remain some pregnancies where the mother has not been protected from making anti-D and thereby fetuses who are potentially at risk for the disease.

Early studies assumed that if the molecular basis of the D- phenotype is a complete deletion of the *D* gene it should be possible to type for D antigen simply by designing PCR tests which detect coding sequences which are found in the *D* gene but not in the *CE* gene. As has been discussed above the *D* and *CE* genes are highly homologous and so it is not particularly easy to find suitable regions of the *D* gene for amplification. One of the suitable regions is found at the 3' end of the *D* gene which differs from the 3' end of the *CE* gene. By careful selection of suitable oligonucleotide primers Bennett et al. (1018) developed a PCR test which yielded a 186bp product derived from the 3' end of exon 10 of the *D* gene but gave no product at all from the 3' end of exon 10 of the *CE* gene. In this particular test a second set of primers was included to amplify exon 7 from both *D* and *CE* genes yielding a product of 136bp from D+ and D-individuals to act as a control. Another method exploits sequence difference between the *D* and *CE* gene in exon

7 to produce products of 155bp from *D* gene and 146bp from *CE* gene (1019). Using this method under carefully controlled conditions it is possible to determine whether or not an individual is homozygous or heterozygous for the *D* gene (1019). A third method involves amplifying intron 4 of the *D* and *CE* genes (207,1020). The PCR product obtained from the *CE* gene is 1200bp while that from the *D* gene is 600bp because intron 4 of the *D* gene has a 650bp deletion. Yet another method involves exploitation of nucleotide sequence differences between exon 4 of the *D* and *CE* genes (1021).

When these various assays were evaluated on a large number of DNA samples derived from individuals of known D type it soon became clear that not all D-individuals have a deletion of the *D* gene. Simsek et al. (1020) reported finding three individuals with the haplotype *Cde* who typed as D+ and two subjects of phenotype CcDe who typed as D- using the exon 10 method. Hyland et al. (1022) reported two apparently White donors of phenotype Cde, one had *D* gene fragments present within the 5' upstream and exon 1 region and within the 3' non-coding region but lacked *D* gene exons between exons 7 and 10, the other appeared to have a normal *D* gene in the regions examined. Eight unrelated donors of African origin with the haplotype *Cde^s* had an internal deletion of the *D* gene but exons 8-10 at the 3' end were present so that these donors would type as D+ in an exon 10 specific PCR assay (625,1023). Carritt et al. (1023) also drew attention to the occurrence of Oriental donors with a normal *D* gene but whose D antigen was so weak that it could only be detected by absorption/elution. Rather surprisingly, the discrepant results reported by Simsek et al. (1020) were challenged on technical grounds (1024) but it is now generally accepted that such discrepancies do occur and that D typing from DNA should be carried out with at least two different tests which target different regions of the *D* gene or a multiplex PCR assay (988,990,1021,1025). Legler et al. (1026) have described a typing method which seeks to evaluate all D-specific nucleotide substitutions. Fortunately, the commonest White D- phenotype (cde) has been found to result from a complete deletion of the *D* gene in all studies reported at the time of writing and this explains why fetal D typing is a very useful diagnostic aid in the management of HDN in Europe and the USA.

DNA-based tests for c and E antigen typing have been reported (1027). These tests use allele-specific primers (ASP) in a PCR reaction. The c antigen test relies on the correlation of a single nucleotide substitution at nucleotide 307 giving Pro at residue 103 and a single nucleotide substitution at nucleotide 676 giving Pro at residue 226 for E.

Fetal DNA typing in potential HDN cases is usually

done on DNA extracted from amniocytes present in amniotic fluid samples but it can be done on DNA from chorionic villi if required. Attempts to obtain fetal DNA using non-invasive methods have been reported and these include assays of fetal cells in maternal peripheral blood (1028,1029) and in the cervical canal (1030) but neither of these approaches has given the reliability necessary for diagnostic use at the time of writing. Isolation of fetal erythroblasts from maternal blood and their successful use as a source of fetal DNA for antenatal typing of hemoglobinopathies has been reported (1031) and this provides a promising approach for fetal blood grouping in the future.

Nature of the Complex Formed Between Rh Polypeptides and Rh Glycoproteins and the Possible Role of Glycophorin B

Evidence that the Rh polypeptides and Rh glycoproteins coprecipitate indicates that they associate in the membrane (901). The fact that some individuals with the Rh_{null} phenotype have mutations in the Rh glycoprotein gene but normal *CE* and/or *D* genes (1032) and yet lack both glycoprotein and polypeptides from their red cells clearly shows that the Rh glycoprotein is necessary for the membrane assembly of the Rh polypeptides. The question then arises as to the stoichiometry of this association. Quantitative binding studies using radioiodinated monoclonal antibodies specific for Rh glycoprotein and Rh polypeptides respectively led Gardner et al. (398) to conclude that the Rh glycoprotein is found at about 150,000 copies/red cell while the Rh polypeptides were present at between 100,000 and 200,000 copies/red cell depending on which murine monoclonal antibody was used for the measurement. The measurements for Rh glycoprotein were made using three different monoclonal antibodies (MB-2D10, LA18.18, LA23.40) raised by von dem Borne et al. (69) and shown to react with purified Rh glycoprotein by immunoblotting (396). Two murine monoclonal antibodies (R6A, BRIC 209) reactive with Rh polypeptides gave values of ca 100,000 copies/red cell while a third (BRIC 69) gave values of 200,000 copies/red cell (398). Similar values were obtained by Chérif-Zahar et al. (1032). When BRIC 69, R6A and BRIC 209 are tested for reactivity with K562 cells expressing either a cE polypeptide or a D polypeptide, BRIC 69 reacts equally well with both cells but R6A and BRIC 209 react preferentially with the cells expressing the cE polypeptide (Smythe and Anstee, unpublished observations August, 1996).

These results suggest that Rh glycoproteins and Rh polypeptides are present in approximately equal amounts and the question then arises as to whether they exist in the membrane as heterodimers or higher oligomers. Hartel-Schenk and Agre (955) isolated the Rh-associated proteins by extraction of red cell membranes with non-ionic detergents and estimated the molecular weight of these extracts at 170,000 after correction for bound detergent. This value echoes an earlier study by Folkerd et al. (1033) who obtained a value of 174,000 by a completely different method. These values could be consistent with a tetrameric complex comprising two Rh polypeptides and two Rh glycoprotein molecules and such a model has been proposed (921). Obviously all such tetramers in the red cell membranes of a rr individual (with a deletion of the *D* gene) would comprise ce polypeptides and Rh glycoprotein. In a D+ individual, complexes of D polypeptide and Rh glycoprotein would also be present. The Rh glycoprotein associated with D polypeptide has a slightly higher apparent molecular weight than Rh glycoprotein associated with ce polypeptide (893). This may reflect differences in the glycosylation states of the Rh glycoprotein in the two associations.

In considering the possible arrangement of Rh polypeptides and Rh glycoprotein molecules in a tetrameric complex, Eyers et al. (921) note that the Rh glycoprotein can be cleaved by trypsin at Lys-196 (in the third predicted intracellular loop, figure 12-5) and that this cleavage effectively splits the glycoprotein into two polypeptides of similar organization, that is, each contains six transmembrane domains. The cE polypeptide can also be split into two halves by trypsin-treatment (976) probably in the cytosolic loop at Lys-189, Lys-193 or Arg-201) (921). Lys-189 (but not Lys-193 or Arg-201) is conserved in the D polypeptide and an additional Lys (198) is also found in this region of the D polypeptide. Eyers et al. (921) propose that the two halves of Rh glycoprotein and Rh polypeptides comprise sub-domains of the proteins and cite similar subdomain structures deduced for other multi-spanning membrane proteins from structural studies of two-dimensional crystals (for example, band 3) (1034). These authors also suggest that the N-terminal subdomain of the Rh glycoprotein interacts with the N-terminal subdomain of Rh polypeptides so that these portions of the proteins form the center of the Rh complex (921). Direct evidence for interaction between the N-terminal subdomain of the Rh glycoprotein and the Rh polypeptides was obtained from immune precipitation experiments. Tryptic cleavage of the Rh glycoprotein at Lys-196 separates the N-terminal and C-terminal subdomains of the Rh glycoprotein and when immune precipitations with monoclonal antibodies specific for Rh polypeptides (BRIC 69, BRIC 207) were carried out following tryptic cleavage, Rh glycoprotein tryptic fragments were not found in the immune precipitates (921). In contrast, immune precipitations from red cells previously treated with the V8 protease from *Staphylococcus aureus*, which cleaves the Rh glycoprotein at Glu-34 in the first extracellular loop, contained the 28.5kD Rh glycoprotein V8 peptide. These experiments did not yield direct evidence that the N-terminal subdomain of Rh polypeptides interacts with Rh glycoprotein because both N-terminal and C-terminal tryptic fragments of Rh polypeptides were found in the immune precipitates (921).

Dahr et al. (878) observed that red cells of phenotype Rh_{null} have a reduced content of glycophorin B (GPB) and suggested that GPB may associate with the proteins which carry Rh antigens. It seems likely that this association does occur and that it is mediated through interaction between GPB and the Rh glycoprotein. When the Rh glycoprotein in red cell membranes of phenotype S- s- was examined by immunoblotting with rabbit polyclonal antibodies to a synthetic peptide derived from the C-terminal sequence of the Rh glycoprotein, it was noted that the Rh glycoprotein migrated with a higher apparent molecular weight than that found in red cell membranes of normal Ss type (920). These results are reminiscent of the increased apparent molecular weight of band 3 observed in membranes from En(a-) cells which are deficient in glycophorin A (see Chapter 15 for further discussion). In this case the increased apparent molecular weight of band 3 is due to an increase in the average number of *N*-acetyllactosamine repeating units present in the N-glycan chain found on band 3 and results from the fact that band 3 and GPA associate during biosynthesis. The presence of GPA accelerates the movement of newly synthesized band 3 through intracellular membranes to the cell surface (1066). If band 3 moves more slowly through internal membranes in the absence of GPA there is more time for glycosylation to occur and a larger N-glycan results. Since some cells of phenotype S- s- lack GPB (see Chapter 15 for details) it seems likely that an analogous relationship to that between band 3 and GPA exists between GPB and the Rh glycoprotein, that is, GPB accelerates the movement of newly synthesized Rh glycoprotein through intracellular membranes to the cell surface.

In contrast to the effect of GPB, Rh polypeptides may retard the movement of newly synthesized Rh glycoprotein to the cell surface. Some examples of red cells with the Rh_{null} phenotype lack Rh polypeptides but contain some Rh glycoprotein and so it is clear that Rh polypeptides are not essential for surface expression of Rh glycoprotein (396,1032). However, the apparent molecular weight of the Rh glycoprotein in these Rh_{null} membranes is lower than that in normal membranes and the band is less diffuse indicating that it has a smaller N-glycan and therefore a shorter transit time through internal membranes (920). The very strong expression

of Rh glycoprotein in the virtual absence of Rh polypeptide expression in K562 cells (69,996) is further evidence that Rh polypeptides are not essential for Rh glycoprotein expression.

Estimates of the number of molecules of GPB in normal red cell membranes indicate approximately 250,000 copies/cell (1035) suggesting that Rh polypeptides, Rh glycoprotein and GPB occur in normal red cell membranes in the approximate ratio 1:1:1. Curiously, the number of molecules of Rh glycoprotein in D-- cells is reduced (398,1032). Murine monoclonal anti-Rh also show reduced binding (398) while the number of D antigen sites is reported at 100,000-200,000 (266). The reduced binding of murine monoclonal antibodies can be explained by their preferential reactivity with CE polypeptides but the apparently reduced levels of Rh glycoprotein is more difficult to explain. It may be that these antibodies preferentially bind to the glycosylated form of Rh glycoprotein associated with CE polypeptides over that associated with D polypeptides and so quantitative binding studies on D-- cells do not accurately reflect the number of Rh glycoprotein molecules on these cells. Evidence that the epitopes recognized by monoclonal antibodies to Rh glycoprotein are dependent on the presence of the N-glycan on Rh glycoprotein (treatment of red cells with preparations of peptidyl N-glycanase and/or endo F destroy the epitopes (396,1036)) would be consistent with this.

Other Molecules Associated with the Rh Complex: CD47, LW Glycoprotein and Duffy Glycoprotein

As discussed in the preceding section there is clear evidence for an association between the Rh polypeptides and the Rh glycoprotein in the red cell membrane and indirect evidence that this complex also includes glycophorin B. There is also evidence suggesting that three minor red cell membrane proteins, CD47, LW glycoprotein and Duffy glycoprotein, are associated with the Rh complex.

CD47 was first identified using murine monoclonal antibodies raised against intact red cells (893). Several monoclonal antibodies were obtained which gave weak reactions with Rh_{null} cells. These antibodies (originally termed BRIC 125-type) were different from antibodies of the R6A-type (described above) since the latter failed to react with Rh_{null} cells (389,893). Antibodies of the BRIC 125-type immune precipitated a glycoprotein of Mr 47,000-52,000 from radioiodinated normal red cells. The glycoprotein had a substantial content of N-glycans since treatment with a peptidyl N-glycanase/endo F preparation reduced the Mr of the protein to 28,000 (893). Antibodies of the BRIC 125-type gave normal reaction patterns with red cells of phenotype LW(a-b-) and Fy(a-b-) demonstrating that the BRIC 125 protein was a previously undescribed protein which appeared to be associated with the Rh complex. Immunofluorescence and immunocytochemical studies revealed that the BRIC 125 protein had a very wide tissue distribution, a feature which clearly distinguishes it from both the Rh polypeptides and the Rh glycoprotein (893,1037). This broad tissue reactivity led to the inclusion of two BRIC 125-type antibodies (BRIC 125 and BRIC 126) in the Fourth International Leukocyte Typing Workshop where they were clustered with a third antibody (CIKM1) to form a new cluster of antibodies known as CD47 (1038). At the fourth workshop it was confirmed that CD47 has a very broad tissue reactivity which includes virtually all hemopoietic cells, epithelial cells, endothelial cells, fibroblasts, and tumor cells lines (1039).

By the time of the Fifth Leukocyte Typing Workshop, held in Boston, USA in November 1993, it had become clear that CD47 was being studied under different names by several different research groups. At the fifth workshop, Mawby et al. (1040) reported that they had purified CD47 from red cells using immunoaffinity chromatography with monoclonal antibody BRIC 125. The amino terminus of the purified protein was blocked but a clear protein sequence was obtained for several peptides obtained after digestion of the purified glycosylated and deglycosylated protein with Lys-C. The sequences of these Lys-C peptides and the protein sequence of a tryptic peptide obtained when CD47 was purified from trypsin treated red cells, when used in database searches, revealed that CD47 from red cells had the same protein sequence, at least with respect to these peptides, as a previously described human ovarian tumor marker OA3 (1041). Mawby et al. (1040) noticed that the peptide sequences obtained for red cell CD47 were also found in a protein isolated from placenta called integrin-associated protein (IAP) (1042). Also at the fifth workshop Lindberg and Brown (1043) reported transfection studies which showed that CD47 was the same as IAP. Both groups subsequently published their studies in full in 1994 (896,1044).

Once it was realized that CD47 equaled OA3 it was not necessary to isolate a cDNA for CD47 since this had already been done by Campbell et al. (1041) for OA3. The cDNA sequence of OA3 predicts a signal sequence of 18 residues and a mature protein of 305 amino acids with a large N-terminal extracellular domain followed by five membrane spanning domains (see figure 12-9). The predicted protein contains six sequence motifs for N-glycosylation, five on the N-terminal extracellular domain and one on the extracellular loop between

membrane-spanning domains 2 and 3 (see figure 12-9). Protein sequence studies provide useful information concerning which of the 6 potential N-glycosylation sites are utilized in red cell CD47. Mawby et al. (1044) were able to obtain direct evidence that the potential N-glycosylation sites at Asn-16, Asn-55 and Asn-93 are utilized but that Asn-188 is not. Whether or not Asn-5 or Asn-32 are glycosylated was not determined although evidence that N-glycosylation occurs preferentially at sites near the N-terminus of proteins (1045) suggests that they are. The large N-terminal extracellular domain has significant homology with immunoglobulin V domains (1041). Inspection of the position of cysteine residues in CD47 led Mawby et al. (1044) to suggest that either Cys-15 or Cys-23 forms a disulphide bond with Cys-96 to make the immunoglobulin superfamily domain and that Cys-15 or Cys-23 might form a disulphide bond with Cys-241 or Cys-245 which are predicted to be on the extracellular loop between membrane-spanning domains four and five (see figure 12-9). A disulphide bond between a cysteine residue in the N-terminal extracellular domain and one on an extracellular loop between two membrane spanning domains is also found in the family of proteins which includes the Duffy glycoprotein (see Chapter 14). Lindberg et al. (894) constructed chimeric cDNAs (with a human Ig domain and a mouse membrane domain and vice versa) and showed that all of 7 anti-human CD47 monoclonal antibodies recognized epitopes on the human Ig domain confirming that this domain is extracellular. Linberg et al. (894) also used mouse monoclonal antibodies against the C terminus of CD47 to confirm its cytoplasmic location. CD47 occurs in four different alternatively spliced forms (894,1041,1046). Each isoform differs from the others only with regard to the sequence of the cytoplasmic C-terminal segment and each is generated by the inclusion or exclusion of three short exons (1046). The expression of isoforms is regulated in tissues. The bone marrow form is predominantly in bone marrow and endothelia and the neural form is predominantly expressed in the brain and peripheral nervous system.

The *CD47* gene is located on chromosome 3 (Williams cited in 1041,1047) at q13.1-q13.2 (896). The antigen recognized by monoclonal antibody 1D8 which has reduced expression on Rh$_{null}$ cells, was also mapped to chromosome 3 (892) and since cells transfected with CD47 react with 1D8 it can be concluded that the 1D8 antigen is on CD47 (896). The function of CD47 on red cells is far from clear. On some cell types CD47 is associated with integrins (hence integrin-associated protein, IAP) and would be expected to participate in adhesive interactions, a feature consistent with the presence of an Ig domain in the molecule, but since

FIGURE 12-9 Structure of CD47 (reference 1040)

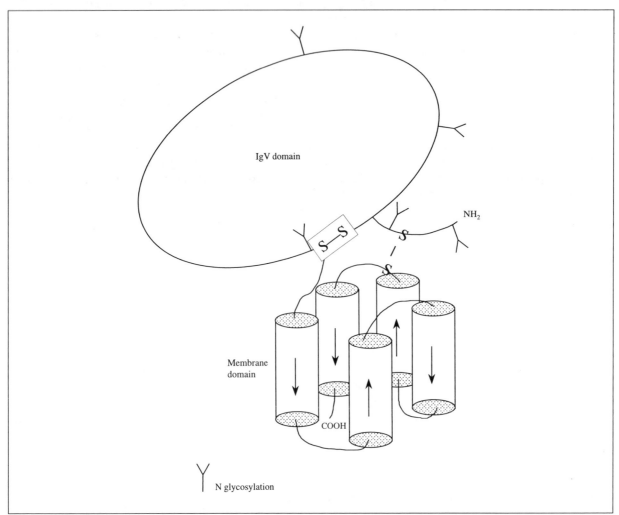

red cells lack integrins this function cannot occur in red cells (1042). Several functions for CD47 have been reported including a role in the migration of neutrophils through epithelia and endothelia (1048,1049), a role as a costimulatory molecule in T cell activation (1050,1051) and a role as a receptor for thrombospondin (1052). CD47 "knockout" mice show a defect in host defense mechanisms attributable to defects in neutrophil function (1053) but no specific defects in red cell function were noted. There are between 10,000 and 50,000 molecules of CD47 on a normal red cell (398), about one molecule per tetramer of Rh polypeptide/Rh glycoprotein.

The LW glycoprotein which also exhibits a phenotypic relationship with the Rh complex is present at lower levels (3,000 molecules/D- red cell, 4,400 molecules/D+ red cell (888)). Evidence that the presence of the D polypeptide is associated with a higher level of expression of the LW glycoprotein suggests that its involvement with the Rh complex may be mediated through interactions with the Rh polypeptides. However, the LW glycoprotein is not essential for assembly of the Rh complex since individuals with the rare LW(a-b-) phenotype have normal Rh antigen expression (see Chapter 13 for a detailed discussion of the LW glycoprotein). The association of the Duffy glycoprotein with the Rh complex relies on very tentative evidence, that is, the absence of an antigen Fy5 from Rh_{null} cells (discussed in more detail in an earlier section of this chapter). Fy(a-b-) cells have normal Rh antigens and since the Rh antigens can be expressed on the surface of the erythroid cell line K562 in the absence of the Duffy glycoprotein (996) one must conclude that the Duffy glycoprotein is not required for Rh antigen expression. It is possible that the antigen Fy5 results from some interaction between the Rh complex and the Duffy glycoprotein in the membrane.

The functional role of the minor glycoproteins

CD47, LW glycoprotein and Duffy glycoprotein is not understood although it seems certain that the LW and Duffy glycoproteins are not essential for the reasons given above. The role of CD47 is more uncertain because human red cells completely lacking CD47 have never been described. It would be of considerable interest to examine the red cells of CD47 "knockout" mice (1053) to see if the murine Rh polypeptides and Rh glycoproteins are expressed normally.

Deficiencies of Rh Antigens

The commonest deficiency involving Rh proteins is the D- phenotype which, as discussed above, commonly, though not exclusively, results from a complete deletion of the *D* gene (40). Deficiency of CcEe polypeptides but not of D polypeptide is much rarer but nevertheless several examples of this phenotype have been studied at the DNA level. The first example of the phenotype D-- (donor Gou of French origin) to be studied revealed the presence of a normal *D* gene and a normal *CE* gene with a normal *CE* gene promotor sequence (600bp sequenced upstream of the transcription initiation site) (1015). These authors concluded that the lack of Cc and Ee antigens in the red cells of this individual, confirmed by serological methods and immunochemical studies using antibodies to synthetic peptides (980) "might result from instability of mRNA or a mutation within transcription *cis*-acting elements located outside the proximal promoter region". A second individual with red cells of phenotype D-- was found to have a deletion of all but the extreme 5′ end of the *CE* gene (625). This individual was of Icelandic origin (775). In a note added in proof Blunt et al. (625) report that three other D-- genomes and one D•• genome that they had studied also had deleted *CE* genes. Huang et al. (1054) reported Southern blotting experiments on a D-- genome from an Italian donor (LM) which were interpreted as identifying a large deletion encompassing exon 2 through exon 9 of the *CE* gene. Subsequent studies on donor LM by Chérif-Zahar et al. (1055) led those authors to conclude that two unusual RNA transcripts were present in this donor. One of these was a hybrid derived from a *CE-D-CE-D* gene with exon 1 and exon 9 from the *CE* gene and exons 2-8 and exon 10 from the *D* gene. The other transcript derived from a hybrid *D-CE* gene with exons 1-9 derived from the *D* gene and exon 10 from the *CE* gene. Chérif-Zahar et al. (1055) suggest that the presence of two gene transcripts expressing D but not CcEe antigens explains why the D-- cells of donor LM have greater than the normal amount of D antigen. If this is so then the question is raised as to the mechanism by which increased numbers of D antigen sites are generated in other D-- donors.

Do the D-- donors studied by Blunt et al. (625) have similar RNA transcripts to those found in donor LM rather than a deletion of the *CE* gene? The results described by Chérif-Zahar et al. (1055) highlight the importance of analyzing RNA transcripts as well as genomic DNA. When RNA transcripts from a donor (Dav) of the D•• phenotype were analyzed, the product of a hybrid *D-CE* gene was found which comprised exons 1-6 of the *D* gene and exons 7-10 of the *CE* gene.

A donor of phenotype Dc- (donor Bol) was shown to have a normal *D* gene and a hybrid *CE-D-CE* gene in which exons 4 to 9 are derived from the *D* gene. This result explains the elevated D antigen in these cells and the absence of Ee antigens (1001,1055).

Rare cells of phenotype DC^W- (donor Glo) are reported to involve a normal *D* gene and a hybrid *CE-D-CE* gene in which exons 2 (or 3) to exon 9 are derived from the *D* gene (1001). A donor of phenotype DC^W- studied by Huang (989) was reported to have a *D-CE* hybrid gene on one chromosome (exon 10 derived from the *CE* gene) and a *CE-D* hybrid gene on the other (exon 1 derived from the *CE* gene). In this case the sequence of exon 1 from the *CE* gene corresponded to that predicted for C^W antigen (see above). These studies of rare phenotypes with deficiencies of common antigens suggest that several different genetic mechanisms can give rise to the same phenotype. Given the rarity of these phenotypes, the diversity of races in which they occur and the extensive homology that exists between the *CE* and *D* genes it is not surprising that they frequently result from different types of genetic event.

The molecular defect giving rise to the Rh_{null} phenotype has been investigated in several laboratories. At the time of writing none of the individuals with the Rh_{null} phenotype who have been studied have defects in the genes giving rise to Rh polypeptides (1015,1016,1032). This result, which is not unexpected in the case of Rh_{null} arising from a defect in a "regulator" gene unlinked to the *Rh* locus, has also been found in investigations of an Rh_{null} of the "amorphic" genetic background (1015,1016). The molecular background of Rh_{null} "amorph-type" is unknown at the time of writing. However, the molecular defect in four individuals with Rh_{null} resulting from a defect in a "regulator gene" and one individual with the Rh_{mod} phenotype has been shown to correlate with mutations affecting the gene giving rise to the Rh glycoprotein (1032). Three different types of mutation were found. Two apparently unrelated individuals from South Africa (SF and JL) had two nucleotide changes and a two base pair deletion which resulted in a frameshift after the codon for Tyr-51 and a premature stop codon at nt323-325. Rh glycoprotein could not be detected in the red cell membranes of these individuals using flow cytometry or immunoblotting indicating that the defective protein is not inserted into the membrane. One individual (TB) had a single base deletion at nt1086 resulting in a frameshift after Ala-362. This mutation was present in the heterozygous state and no transcript corresponding to the Rh glycoprotein could be amplified from the other allele. The mutation is predicted to give rise to an Rh glycoprotein of 376 amino acids including 14 novel residues at the C-terminus but the protein was not detected in the red cells of this individual either by flow cytometry or immunoblotting leading to speculation that the protein is unstable and is not transported to the membrane. The third mutation (Rh_{mod} donor VL) had a single base change which converted Ser79 to Arg. In this case the mutant protein was expressed at 20% of normal levels. No product of the Rh glycoprotein gene could be derived for an Rh_{null} individual (AL) suggesting that there is a defect in transcription in this case. In all of these individuals transcripts corresponding to CD47 could be obtained although the content of CD47 in the red cells was reduced.

Functions of Rh Proteins

It is clear from the foregoing discussion that a substantial amount is known about the proteins that give rise to antigens of the Rh blood group system and the genes that encode them. In marked contrast very little is known about the function of these proteins. Most attempts to elucidate the function of Rh proteins have focused on Rh_{null} cells in the hope of identifying functional deficiencies which could be attributed to the lack of Rh proteins in these cells. As discussed in an earlier section, some of the red cells of individuals with the Rh_{null} phenotype have abnormal shape, notably stomatocytes are present (851). Rh_{null} red cells are also reported to be dehydrated and have an abnormal permeability toward cations (874,845). The structure of Rh polypeptides and Rh glycoprotein suggests that they may be involved in membrane transport and the presence of conserved acidic amino acids in transmembrane domains (Glu-21 and Glu-146 in Rh polypeptides and Glu-13 and Glu-148 in Rh glycoprotein) suggests that the proteins are involved in the movement of a cationic component across the membrane (898,903). The number of molecules of Rh polypeptides and Rh glycoprotein/red cell (100,000-200,000) makes them major red cell membrane proteins on a par with the water transporter (aquaporin-1, Colton blood group-active protein, see Chapter 22) and stomatin which is also thought to play a role in cation transport in red cells (band 7.2) (1056). Since the Rh polypeptides and Rh glycoprotein appear to be restricted to red cells, any function that they perform would be expected to fulfil a specific need of the red

cell. The fact that individuals with Rh_{null} syndrome have only a mild and compensated hemolytic anemia suggests that the function(s) of the Rh complex in normal red cells can be carried out, at least in part, by other membrane proteins in Rh_{null} cells.

It has been suggested that Rh proteins may be involved in maintaining the phospholipid asymmetry of the normal red cell (973). This suggestion was based on the observation that Rh_{null} cells have an altered lipid organization with more phosphatidyl ethanolamine in the outer leaflet of the lipid bilayer and a faster transbilayer movement of phosphatidyl choline (973). Some studies (1057,1058) suggested that the Rh proteins may correspond to an ATP-dependent phosphatidyl serine (PS) translocase ("flippase") but Rh_{null} cells have normal PS flippase activity (1059) and this hypothesis is now considered most unlikely (754). Nevertheless, some association between the aminophospholipid transporter and Rh polypeptides has been suggested (1060).

Since the Rh polypeptides and Rh glycoprotein are major red cell membrane proteins it is possible that they play a structural role and there is evidence that these proteins remain associated with the red cell skeleton when red cell membranes are extracted with high concentrations of non-ionic detergents (893,1061-1063). However, the Rh polypeptides and the Rh glycoprotein lack a significant cytoplasmic domain (see figures 12-4 and 12-5) and so they are unlikely to interact directly with the skeletal network and any such role is likely to be mediated through other associated molecules (840,898).

The discussion above has focused on the functional role of the Rh proteins themselves rather than the functions of the blood group antigens that they express. The Rh system is the most polymorphic of all the blood group systems found on red cells (and thus puts Lewis, see Chapter 9, to shame) and this reflects the fact that the antigens derive from two adjacent and highly homologous genes (*CE* and *D*). The second most polymorphic system (MNS) also derives from two adjacent and highly homologous genes (*GYPA* and *GYPB*, see Chapter 15). The Rh system antigens, like the MNS system antigens, are only found on red cells and so whereas it can be argued that the function of carbohydrate antigens like A, B, H and Le^b are likely to be mediated through their distribution on cells and mucins in the gut and respiratory tract (see Chapters 8 and 9) the function of Rh antigens must be mediated through a property of the red cell. The idea that polymorphism is driven by infectious diseases was first propounded by Haldane (cited in 1064) and this theory is discussed further in Chapter 2. If cell surface variations in the structure Rh polypeptides are driven by selection against infectious disease then it follows that the relevant infectious disease or diseases must specifically involve red cells since these are the only cells which express the proteins. The obvious candidate disease is malaria. In the case of MNS antigens there is some direct evidence that some strains of the malarial parasite *Plasmodium falciparum* use glycophorin A as a receptor for attachment to red cells (see Chapter 15 for discussion). In the case of Rh antigens no direct evidence exists to the authors' knowledge. Investigation of the possible relationship between polymorphism in Rh polypeptides and susceptibility to malaria represents one of the most exciting and important challenges for future research in the field of human blood groups.

References

1. Bourgeois L. Cited by Bowman JM. In: Transf Med Rev 1988;2:129
2. von Gierke E. Verh Dtsch Pathol Ges 1921;18:232
3. Diamond LK, Blackfan KD, Baty JM. J Pediat 1932;1:269
4. Darrow RR. Arch Pathol 1938;25:378
5. Levine P, Stetson R. J Amer Med Assoc 1939;113:126
6. Rosenfield RE. Transfusion 1989;29:355
7. Landsteiner K, Wiener AS. Proc Soc Exp Biol NY 1940;43:223
8. Landsteiner K, Wiener AS. J Exp Med 1941;74:309
9. Levine P, Burnham L, Katzin EM, et al. Am J Obstet Gynecol 1941;42:925
10. Wiener AS, Peters HR. Ann Int Med 1940;13:2306
11. Rosenfield RE. Mt Sinai J Med 1974;41:626
12. Rosenfield RE. Am J Clin Pathol 1975;64:569
13. Domen RE. Arch Pathol Lab Med 1986;110:162
14. Buchbinder L. J Immunol 1933;25:33
15. Fisk RT, Foord AG. Am J Clin Pathol 1942;12:545
16. Murray J, Clark EC. Nature 1952;169:886
17. Wiener AS, Sonn EB, Belkin BB. Proc Soc Exp Biol NY 1943;54:238
18. Wiener AS. Proc Soc Exp Biol NY 1943;54:316
19. Wiener AS, Sonn EB. Genetics 1943;28:157
20. Wiener AS, Sonn EB. J Immunol 1943;47:461
21. Wiener AS, Sonn EB, Polivka HR. Proc Soc Exp Biol NY 1946;61:382
22. Wiener AS, Sonn EB. Ann NY Acad Sci 1946;46:969
23. Wiener AS, Sonn-Gordon EB, Handman L. J Immunol 1947;57:203
24. Wiener AS, Gordon EB, Handman L. Am J Hum Genet 1949;1:127
25. Wiener AS, Owen RD, Stormont C, et al. J Am Med Assoc 1956;161:233
26. Shapiro M. J Foren Med 1960;7:96
27. Race RR, Taylor GL. Nature 1943;152:300
28. Race RR, Taylor GL, Boorman KE, et al. Nature 1943;152:563
29. Race RR, Taylor GL, Ikin EW, et al. Ann Eugen 1944;12:206
30. Race RR. Nature 1944;153:771
31. Fisher RA. Ann Eugen 1946;12:150
32. Fisher RA, Race RR. Nature 1946;157:48
33. Fisher RA. Ann Eugen 1947;13:223
34. Race RR. Blood 1948;2(Suppl 3):27
35. Race RR, Sanger R, Lawler SD. Nature 1948;161:316
36. Race RR, Sanger R, Lawler SD. Nature 1948;162:292
37. Race RR, Mourant AE, Lawler SD, et al. Blood 1948;3:689
38. Race RR, Sanger R, Lawler SD. Heredity 1948;2:237
39. Race RR, Sanger R. Vox Sang 1982;43:354
40. Colin Y, Chérif-Zahar B, Le Van Kim C, et al. Blood 1991;78:2747
41. Mouro I, Colin Y, Chérif-Zahar B, et al. Nature Genet 1993;5:62
42. Smythe JS, Avent ND, Judson PA, et al. (abstract). Blood 1995;86 (Suppl 1):473a
43. Tippett P. Ann Hum Genet 1986;50:241
44. Mourant AE, Kopec AC, Domaniewska-Sobazak K. The Distribution of Human Blood Groups and Other Biochemical Polymorphisms, 2nd Ed. London:Oxford University Press, 1976
45. Walker RH, Ed. Technical Manual, 10th Ed. Arlington, VA:Am Assoc Blood Banks, 1990:201
46. Rosenfield RE, Allen FH Jr, Swisher SN, et al. Transfusion 1962;2:287
47. Allen FH Jr, Rosenfield RE. Haematologia 1972;6:113
48. Rosenfield RE, Allen FH Jr, Rubinstein P. Proc Nat Acad Sci USA 1973;70:1303
49. Race RR, Sanger R. Blood Groups in Man, 6th Ed. Oxford:Blackwell, 1975
50. Issitt PD, Issitt CH. Applied Blood Group Serology, 2nd Ed. Oxnard:Spectra Biologicals, 1975
51. Issitt PD, Pavone BG, Shapiro M. Transfusion 1979;19:389
52. Lewis M, Kaita H, Allerdice PW, et al. Am J Hum Genet 1979;31:630
53. Svoboda RK, West van B, Grumet FC. Transfusion 1981;21:150
54. Moulds JJ, Case J, Thorton S, et al. (abstract). Transfusion 1980;20:631
55. Lewis M, Allen FH Jr, Anstee DJ, et al. Vox Sang 1985;49:171
56. Lewis M, Anstee DJ, Bird GWG, et al. Vox Sang 1990;58:152
57. Daniels GL, Moulds JJ, Anstee DJ, et al. Vox Sang 1993;65:77
58. Daniels GL, Anstee DJ, Cartron J-P, et al. Vox Sang 1995;69:265
59. Kochwa S, Rosenfield RE. J Immunol 1964;92:682
60. Rosenfield RE, Kochwa S. J Immunol 1964;92:693
61. Gibbs MB, Rosenfield RE. Transfusion 1966;6:462
62. Berkman EM, Nusbacher J, Kochwa S, et al. Transfusion 1971;11:317
63. Rosenfield RE, Levine P, Heller C. Vox Sang 1975;28:293
64. Mallory DM, Rosenfield RE, Wong KY, et al. Vox Sang 1976;30:430
65. Rosenfield RE. In: A Seminar on Performance Evaluation 1976. Washington, D.C.:Am Assoc Blood Banks, 1976:93
66. Allen FH Jr, Anstee DJ, Bird GWG, et al. Vox Sang 1982;42:164
67. Tippett P. PhD Thesis, Univ London, 1963
68. Habibi B, Fouillade MT, Duedari N, et al. Vox Sang 1978;34:302
69. von dem Borne AEGKr, Bos MJE, Lomas C, et al. Br J Haematol 1990;75:254
70. Issitt PD, Crookston MC. Transfusion 1984;24:2
71. Tippett P, Lomas-Francis C, Wallace M. Vox Sang 1996;70:123
72. Pollack W, Ascari WQ, Crispen JF, et al. Transfusion 1971;11:340
73. Urbaniak SJ, Robertson AE. Transfusion 1981;21:64
74. Mollison PL, Engelfriet CP, Contreras M. Blood Transfusion in Clinical Medicine, 9th Ed. Oxford:Blackwell, 1993
75. Giblett ER. Clin Obstet Gynecol 1964;7:1044
76. Walker W, Murray S, Russell JK. J Obstet Gynaecol Brit Emp 1957;44:573

77. Wiener AS. Arch Pathol 1941;32:227
78. Mourant AE. Nature 1945;155:542
79. Rosenfield RE, Vogel P, Gibbel N, et al. Br Med J 1953;1:975
80. Dunsford I. Proc 8th Cong Europ Soc Haematol 1961
81. Rosenfield RE, Haber GV. Am J Hum Genet 1958;10:474
82. Gold ER, Gillespie EM, Tovey GH. Vox Sang 1961;6:157
83. Callender ST, Race RR. Ann Eugen 1946;13:102
84. Stratton F, Renton PH. Br Med J 1954;1:962
85. Greenwalt TJ, Sanger R. Br J Haematol 1955;1:52
86. Allen FH Jr, Tippett P. Vox Sang 1958;3:321
87. Levine P, Rosenfield RE, White J. Am J Hum Genet 1961:13:299
88. De Natale A, Cahan A, Jack JA, et al. J Am Med Assoc 1955;159:247
89. Sanger R, Noades J, Tippett P, et al. Nature 1960;186:171
90. Race RR, Sanger R, Selwyn JG. Nature 1950;166:520
91. Allen FH Jr, Corcoran PA. (abstract). Prog 11th Ann Mtg AABB, 1958
92. Shapiro M. J Foren Med 1964;11:52
93. Chown B, Lewis M, Kaita H. Transfusion 1962;2:150
94. Huestis DW, Catino ML, Busch S. Transfusion 1964;4:414
95. Haber GV, Bastani A, Arpin PD, et al. (abstract). Transfusion 1967;7:389
96. Rosenfield RE, Haber G, Gibbel N. Bibl Haematol 1958;7:90
97. Shapiro M, LeRoux M, Brink S. Haematologia 1972;6:121
98. Chown B, Allen FH Jr, Cleghorn TE, Giles CM, Tippett P. Unpublished observations 1965 to 1968 cited in Race RR, Sanger R. Blood Groups in Man, 5th Ed. Oxford:Blackwell, 1968:209
99. Chown B, Lewis M, Kaita H. Vox Sang 1971;21:385
100. Giles CM, Crossland JD, Haggas WK, et al. Vox Sang 1971;21:289
101. Giles CM, Skov F. Vox Sang 1971;20:328
102. Davidsohn I, Stern K, Strauser ER, et al. Blood 1953;8:747
103. Chown B, Lewis M, Kaita H, et al. Vox Sang 1968;15:264
104. Contreras M, Stebbing B, Blessing M, et al. Vox Sang 1978;34:208
105. Cobb ML. (abstract). Transfusion 1980;20:631
106. Habibi B, Perrier P, Salmon C. Blood Transf Immunohematol 1981;24:117
107. Delehanty C, Wilkinson SL, Issitt PD, et al. (abstract). Transfusion 1983;23:410
108. Le Pennec PY, Rouger PH, Klein MT, et al. Transfusion 1989;29:798
109. Daniels GL. PhD Thesis, Univ London, 1980
110. Daniels GL. Blood Transf Immunohematol 1982;25:185
111. Lomas C, Poole J, Salaru N, et al. Vox Sang 1990;59:39
112. Poole J, Hustinx H, Gerber H, et al. Vox Sang 1990;59:44
113. Marais I, Moores P, Smart E, et al. Transf Med 1993;3:35
114. Bizot M, Lomas C, Rubio F, et al. Transfusion 1988;28:342
115. Lomas C, Grässmann W, Ford D, et al. Transfusion 1994;34:612
116. Sistonen P, Sareneva H, Pirkola A, et al. Vox Sang 1994;66:287
117. Wiener AS, Geiger J, Gordon EB. Exp Med Surg 1957;15:75
118. Unger LJ, Wiener AS, Wiener L. J Am Med Assoc 1959;170:1380
119. Unger LJ, Wiener AS. J Lab Clin Med 1959;54:835
120. Sacks MS, Wiener AS, Jahn EF, et al. Ann Intern Med 1959;51:740
121. Vos GH, Kirk RL. Vox Sang 1962;7:22
122. Tippett P, Sanger R. Vox Sang 1962;7:9
123. Tippett P, Sanger R. Artzl Lab 1977;23:476
124. Tippett P. Med Lab Sci 1988;45:88
125. Goldfinger D, McGinniss MH. New Eng J Med 1971;284:942

126. Dausset J, Colombani J, Evelin J. Vox Sang 1958;3:266
127. Moulinier J, Servantie X. Vox Sang 1958;3:277
128. Ashurst DE, Bedford D, Coombs RRA. Vox Sang 1956;1:235
129. Gurevitch J, Neklen D. Vox Sang 1957;2:342
130. Lawler SD, Shatwell HS. Vox Sang 1962;7:488
131. Pfisterer H, Thierfelder S, Kottusch H, et al. Klin Wschr 1967;45:519
132. Lichtiger B, Hester JP. Haematologia 1986;19:81
133. Blanchette VS, Hume HA, Levy GJ, et al. Am J Dis Childh 1991;145:787
134. Bowman JM, Friesen AD, Pollock JM, et al. Canad Med Assoc J 1980;123:1121
135. Burnie KM, Barr RM. Unpublished observations cited by Mollison PL, Engelfriet CP, Contreras M. In: Blood Transfusion in Clinical Medicine, 9th Ed. Oxford:Blackwell, 1993:235
136. McBride JA, O'Hoski P, Blajchman M, et al. (abstract). Transfusion 1978;18:626
137. Barclay GR, Greiss MA, Urbaniak SJ. Br Med J 1980;2:1569
138. Dormandy K. Unpublished observations cited by Mollison PL. Blood Transfusion in Clinical Medicine, 6th Ed. Oxford:Blackwell, 1979:108
139. Clarke CA, Bradley J, Elson CJ, et al. Lancet 1970;1:793
140. Graham-Pole J, Barr W, Willoughby MLN. Br Med J 1977;1:1185
141. Isbister JP, Ting A, Seeto KM. Vox Sang 1977;33:353
142. Robinson AE, Tovey LAD. Br J Haematol 1980;45:621
143. van't Veer-Korthof ET, Niterink JSG, van Nieuwkoop JA, et al. Vox Sang 1981;41:207
144. Robinson AE. (Letter). New Eng J Med 1981;305:1346
145. Rubinstein P. In: Rh Hemolytic Disease: New Strategy for Eradication. Boston:Hall, 1982
146. Nicolaides KH, Rodek CH. Br J Hosp Med 1985;34:141
147. Bystryn JC, Graf MW, Uhr JW. J Exp Med 1970;132:1279
148. Bowman JM. Transf Med Rev 1990;4:191
149. Bowman JM. In: Immunobiology of Transfusion Medicine. New York:Marcel Dekker, 1994:553
150. Mollison PL, Reddy DJ. Nature 1946;158:629
151. Woo JK. Am J Phys Anthropol 1947;5:429
152. Simmons RT, Graydon JJ, Semple NM, et al. Med J Austral 1950;2:917
153. MacGregor A, Kelley A, Hornabrook MW. Hum Biol Oceania 1973;2:23
154. Tills D, Kopec AC, Tills RE. The Distribution of the Human Blood Groups and Other Polymorphisms. Suppl 1. Oxford:Oxford Unviersity Press, 1983
155. Diamond LK. Proc Roy Soc Med 1947;40:546
156. Cook K, Rush B. Med J Austral 1974;1:166
157. Pollack W. Unpublished observations 1972. Cited by Mollison PL. In: Blood Transfusion in Clinical Medicine, 6th Ed. Oxford:Blackwell, 1979
158. Davey MG, Campbell AL, James J. (abstract). Proc Austral Soc Immunol, 1969
159. Mollison PL, Frame M, Ross ME. Br J Haematol 1970;19:257
160. Nevanlinna HR. Ann Med Exp Fenn 1953;31:Suppl 2
161. Nevanlinna HR, Vainio T. Bibl Haematol 1962;13:281
162. Woodrow JC, Donohoe WTA. Br Med J 1968;4:139
163. Ascari WQ, Levine P, Pollack W. Br Med J 1969;1:399
164. Woodrow JC. Ser Haematol 1970;3:3
165. Archer GT, Cooke BR, Mitchell K, et al. Rev Fr Transf 1969;12:341
166. Archer GT, Cooke BR, Mitchell K, et al. Bibl Haematol 1971;38:877
167. Fletcher G, Cooke BR, McDowall J. Proc 2nd Mtg Asian

Pacific Div ISBT 1971:69

168. Jakobowicz R, Williams L, Silberman F. Vox Sang 1972;23;376

169. Mollison PL. Blood Transfusion in Clinical Medicine, 6th Ed. Oxford:Blackwell, 1979

170. Lehane D. Br J Haematol 1967;13:800

171. Tovey LAD, Taverner JM, Longster GH. Vox Sang 1982;42:131

172. Levine P. J Hered 1943;34:71

173. Race RR, Sanger R. Blood Groups in Man, 1st Ed. Oxford:Blackwell, 1950

174. Nevanlinna HR, Vainio T. Vox Sang 1956;1:26

175. Levine P. Hum Biol 1958;30:14

176. Clarke CA, Finn R, McConnell RB, et al. Int Arch Allgy 1958;13:380

177. Stern K, Berger M. Am J Clin Pathol 1961;35:520

178. Vos GH. Am J Hum Genet 1965;17:202

179. Bierme SJ, Blanc M, Arbal M, et al. Lancet 1979;1:604

180. Gold WR Jr, Queenan JT, Woody J, et al. Am J Obstet Gynecol 1983;146:980

181. Klarkowski DB. (abstract). Proc Austral Inst Med Lab Sci Mtg, 1983

182. Barnes RMR, Duguid JKM, Roberts FM, et al. Clin Exp Immunol 1987;67:220

183. Kenwright MG, Sangster JM, Sachs JA. Br Med J 1976;2:151

184. Hill Z, Vacl J, Kalasova E, et al. Vox Sang 1974;27:92

185. Johnson CA, Brown BA, Lasky LC. (Letter). New Eng J Med 1985;312:121

186. Ramsey G, Israel L, Lindsay GD, et al. Transplantation 1986;41:67

187. Solheim BG, Albrechtsen DA, Berg KJ, et al. Transplant Proc 1987;19:4236

188. Solheim BG, Albrechtsen D, Egeland T, et al. Transplant Proc 1987;19:4520

189. Swanson J, Sebring E, Sastamoinen R, et al. Vox Sang 1987;52:228

190. Albrechtsen D, Solheim BG, Flatmark A, et al. Transplant Proc 1988;20(Suppl 3):959

191. Oyonarte S, Cabello M, Clavero C, et al. Med Clin (Barc) 1988;90:545

192. Ramsey G. Transfusion 1991;31:76

193. Chown B. Canad Med Assoc J 1949;61:419

194. David MP, Milbauer B. Clin Pediat 1978;17:924

195. Aronsson S, Engleson G, Svenningsen NW. (Letter). Lancet 1965;2:847

196. Vontver LA. J Am Med Assoc 1973;226:469

197. Bichler A, Hetzel H. Gebrut Frauenh 1975;35:640

198. McVerry BA, O'Connor MC, Price A, et al. Br Med J 1977;1:1324

199. Wong LK, Smith LH, Jensen HM. Transfusion 1983;23:348

200. Köhler G, Milstein C. Nature 1975;256:495

201. Issitt PD. Murex Scientific Publication Series 1991;6:1

202. Wolter LC, Hyland CA, Saul A. (Letter). Blood 1994;84:985

203. Salvignol I, Calvas P, Socha WW, et al. Immunogenetics 1995;41:271

204. Chérif-Zahar B, Bloy C, Le Van Kim C, et al. Proc Nat Acad Sci USA 1990;87:6243

205. Avent ND, Ridgwell K, Tanner MJA, et al. Biochem J 1990;271:821

206. Le Van Kim C, Mouro I, Chérif-Zahar B, et al. Proc Nat Acad Sci USA 1992;89:10925

207. Arce MA, Thompson ES, Wagner S, et al. Blood 1993;82:651

208. Mouro I, Colin Y, Sistonen P, et al. Blood 1995;86:1196

209. Lomas C, Tippett P, Thompson KM, et al. Vox Sang 1989;57:261

210. Lomas C, McColl K, Tippett P. Transf Med 1993;3:67

211. Mouro I, Le Van Kim C, Rouillac C, et al. Blood 1994;83:1129

212. Rouillac C, Mouro I, Beolet M, et al. (abstract). Vox Sang 1994;67(Suppl 2):1

213. Colin Y, Bailly P, Cartron JP. Vox Sang 1994;67(Suppl 3):67

214. Rouillac C, Le Van Kim C, Beolet M, et al. Am J Hematol 1995;49:87

215. Rouillac C, Colin Y, Hughes-Jones NC, et al. Blood 1995;85;2937

216. Daniels G, Lomas-Francis M, Wallace M, et al. In: Molecular and Functional Aspects of Blood Group Antigens, Bethesda, MD:Am Assoc Blood Banks, 1995:193

217. Beckers EAM, Faas BHW, von dem Borne AEGKr, et al. (abstract). Transfusion 1995;35(Suppl 10S):51S

218. Jones J, Scott ML, Voak D. Transf Med 1995;5:171 and see 5:304 for corrections

219. Koskimies S. Scand J Immunol 1980;11:73

220. Boylston AW, Gardner B, Anderson RL, et al. Scand J Immunol 1980;12:355

221. Crawford DH, Barlow MJ, Harrison JF, et al. Lancet 1983;1:386

222. Bron D, Feinberg MB, Teng NNH, et al. Proc Nat Acad Sci USA 1984;81:3214

223. Melamed MD, Gordon J, Ley SJ, et al. Eur J Immunol 1985;15:742

224. Goosens D, Champomier F, Rouger P, et al. J Immunol Meth 1987;101:193

225. Kumpel BM, Leader KA, Merry AH, et al. Eur J Immunol 1989;19:2283

226. Crawford DH, Azim T, Daniels G, et al. In: Progress in Transfusion Medicine, Vol 3. Edinburgh:Churchill Livingstone, 1988:175

227. Thompson KM, Hough DW, Maddison PJ, et al. J Immunol Meth 1986;94:7

228. Rouger P, Goosens D, Champomier F, et al. Rev Fr Transf Immunohematol 1985;28:671

229. Doyle A, Jones TJ, Bidwell JL, et al. Hum Immunol 1985;13:199

230. Paire R, Monestier M, Rigal D, et al. Immunol Lett 1986;13:137

231. Thompson KM, Melamed MD, Eagle K, et al. Immunology 1986;58:157

232. Lowe AD, Green SM, Voak D, et al. Vox Sang 1986;51:212

233. Foung SKH, Blunt JA, Wu PS, et al. Vox Sang 1987;53:44

234. Melamed MD, Thompson KM, Gibson T, et al. J Immunol Meth 1987;104:245

235. McCann MC, James K, Kumpel BM. J Immunol Meth 1988;115:3

236. Rouger P, Anstee DJ. Vox Sang 1988;55:57

237. Bloy C, Blanchard D, Huet M, et al. Rev Fr Transf Immunohematol 1988;31:209 237

238. Kumpel BM, Poole GD, Bradley BA. Br J Haematol 1989;71:125

239. Kumpel BM, Wiener E, Urbaniak SJ, et al. Br J Haematol 1989;71:415

240. Thompson KM, Hughes-Jones NC. Ballière Clin Haematol 1990;3:243

241. Tippett P, Moore S. J Immunogenet 1990;17:309

242. Leader KA, Kumpel BM, Poole GD, et al. Vox Sang 1990;58:106

243. Issitt PD, Wilkinson-Kroovand S, Pavone BG. Afr J Clin Exp Immunol 1980;1:95

244. Schneider W, Tippett P. (abstract). Transfusion 1978;18:392

245. Issitt PD. (Letter). AABB News Briefs 1993;15:14

246. Beckers EAM, Porcelijn L, Ligthart P, et al. Transfusion 1996;36:104

247. Hazenberg CAM, Beckers EAM, Overbeeke MAM. (Letter). Transfusion 1996;36:478

248. Beckers EAM, Faas BHW, von dem Borne AEGKr, et al. Br J Haematol 1996;92:751

249. Armstrong SS, Wiener E, Garner SF, et al. Br J Haematol 1987;66:257

250. Walker MR, Kumpel BM, Thompson K, et al. Vox Sang 1988;55:222

251. Wiener E, Jollifee VM, Scott HCF, et al. Immunology 1988;65:159

252. Merry AH, Brojer E, Zupanska B, et al. Vox Sang 1989;56:48

253. Kumpel BM. J Immunogenet 1990;17:321

254. Thomson A, Contreras M, Gorick B, et al. Lancet 1990;336:1147

255. Callaghan TA, Fleetwood P, Contreras M, et al. (Letter). Transfusion 1993;33:784

256. Stratton F. Nature 1946;158:25

257. Stratton F, Renton PH. Nature 1948;162:293

258. Race RR, Sanger R, Lawler SD. Ann Eugen 1948;14:171

259. Renton PH, Stratton F. Ann Eugen 1950;15:189

260. Rosenfield RE, Vogel P, Miller EB, et al. Blood 1951;6:1123

261. Moore BPL. Vox Sang 1984;46(suppl 1):95

262. Agre P, Davies D, Issitt PD, et al. (Letter). Transfusion 1991;32:86

263. Moore BPL. (Letter). Transfusion 1992;32:593

264. Agre PC, Issitt PD, Lamy BM, et al. (Letter). Transfusion 1992;32:593

265. Rochna E, Hughes-Jones NC. Vox Sang 1965;10:675

266. Hughes-Jones NC, Gardner B, Lincoln P. Vox Sang 1971;21:210

267. Bush M, Sabo B, Stroup M, et al. Transfusion 1976;14:433

268. Merry AH, Hodson C, Moore S. (Letter). Transfusion 1988;28:397

269. Szymanski IO, Araszkiewicz P. Transfusion 1989;29:103

270. Ceppellini R. In: La Malattia Emolitica del Neonato. Milano, 1952

271. Ceppellini R, Dunn LC, Turri M. Proc Nat Acad Sci Wash DC 1955;41:283

272. van Loghem JJ. Br Med J 1947;2:958

273. Mollison PL, Cutbush M. Rev Hematol 1949;4:608

274. Shapiro M. S African Med J 1951;25:165

275. Shapiro M. S African Med J 1951;25:187

276. Argall CI, Ball JM, Trentleman E. J Lab Clin Med 1953;41:895

277. Issitt PD. In: Impact of New Technologies on Rh Typing. Raritan, N.J.:Ortho Diagnostic Systems, 1991:10

278. Schmidt PJ, Morrison EG. Shohl J. Blood 1962;20:196

279. Pavone BG, Issitt PD. Br J Haematol 1974;27:607

280. Wilkinson SL, Vaithianathan T, Issitt PD. Transfusion 1974;14:27

281. Eska PL, Grindon AJ. Br J Haematol 1974;27:613

282. Contreras M, Barbolla L, Lubenko A, et al. Br J Haematol 1979;41:413

283. Soloway HB. Med Lab Obs 1982;July p 21

284. Soloway HB. Med Lab Obs 1982;Sept-Oct p 13

285. Soloway HB. (abstract). Transfusion 1982;22:425

286. Schmidt PJ. Immunohematology 1987;3:49

287. van Rhenen DJ. Vox Sang 1990;58:254

288. Contreras M, Knight RC. Transfusion 1991;31:270

289. Stroup M. Transfusion 1991;31:273

290. Stroup M. Personal communication, 1991

291. Issitt PD. (Letter). AABB News Briefs 1995;17:9

292. Contreras M, Knight RC. Clin Lab Haematol 1989;11:317

293. Okubo Y, Yamaguchi H, Tomita T, et al. (Letter). Transfusion 1984;24:542

294. Ogasawara K, Yabe R, Mazda T, et al. (Letter). Transfusion 1988;28:603

295. Mak KH, Yan KF, Chen SS, et al. Transfusion 1993;33:348

296. Hasekura H, Ota M, Ito S, et al. Transfusion 1990;30:236

297. Steers F, Carritt B, Johnson P. Unpublished observations 1994. Cited by Daniels G. In: Human Blood Groups. Oxford:Blackwell, 1995:279

298. Yvart J, Gerbal A, Cartron J, et al. Rev Fr Transf 1974;17:201

299. Cronin CA, Harmon J, Miller WV. (abstract). Transfusion 1976;16:522

300. Vogel P. Bull NY Acad Med 1954;30:657

301. Kellner A. Obstet Gynecol 1955;5:499

302. Levine P, Robinson E, Stroup M, et al. Blood 1956;11:1097

303. Giblett ER. Transfusion 1961;1:233

304. Kissmeyer-Nielsen F. Scand J Haematol 1965;2:331

305. Myhre BA, Greenwalt TJ, Gajewski M. Transfusion 1965;5:350

306. Lostumbo MM, Holland PV, Schmidt PJ. New Eng J Med 1966;225:141

307. Sinclair M, Anderson C, Simpson S. Unpublished data cited in Moore BPL, Humphreys P, Lovett-Moseley CA. Serological and Immunological Methods 7th Ed. Toronto:Canadian Red Cross Society, 1972

308. Spielmann W, Seidl S. Vox Sang 1974;26:551

309. Giblett ER. Transfusion 1977;17:299

310. Issitt PD. In: A Symposium on the Rh Blood Group System. Groningen:Groningen Red Cross Blood Center, 1979:46

311. Issitt PD. Serology and Genetics of the Rhesus Blood Group System. Cincinnati:Montgomery, 1979

312. Blumberg N, Peck K, Ross K, et al. Vox Sang 1983;44:212

313. Blumberg N, Ross K, Avila E, et al. Vox Sang 1984;47:205

314. Walker RH, Lin DT, Hartrick MB. Arch Pathol Lab Med 1989;113:254

315. Hoeltge GA, Domen RE, Rybicki LA, et al. Arch Pathol Lab Med 1995;119:42

316. Abou-Elella AA, Camarillo TA, Allen MB, et al. Transfusion 1995;35:931

317. Economidou J, Constantoulakis M, Augoustaki O, et al. Vox Sang 1971;20:252

318. Orlina AR, Unger PJ, Koshy M. Am J Hematol 1978;5:101

319. Coles SM, Klein HG, Holland PV. Transfusion 1981;21:462

320. Lasky LC, Rose RR, Polesky HF. Transfusion 1984;24:198

321. Sirchia G, Zanella A, Paravicini A, et al. Transfusion 1985;25:110

322. Sarnaik S, Schornack J, Lusher JM. Transfusion 1986;26:249

323. Ting A, Pun A, Dodds AJ, et al. Transfusion 1987;27:145

324. Michail-Merianou V, Pamphili-Panousopoulou L, Piperi-Lowes L, et al. Vox Sang 1987;52:95

325. Spanos TH, Karageorga M, Ladis V, et al. Vox Sang 1990;58:50

326. Vichinsky EP, Earles A, Johnson RA, et al. New Eng J Med 1990;322:1617

327. Rosse WJ, Gallagher D, Kinney TR, et al. Blood 1990;76:1431

328. Wiener AS, Brancato GJ, Wexler IB. Exp Med Surg 1964;22:1

329. Pepperell RJ, Barrie JU, Fleigner JR. Med J Austral 1977;2:453

330. Chapman J, Waters AH. Vox Sang 1981;41:45

331. Issitt PD, Combs MR, Bredehoeft SJ, et al. Transfusion 1993;33:284

332. Contreras M, de Silva M, Teesdale P, et al. Br J Haematol 1987;65:475

333. Pereira A, Mazzara R, Gelabert A, et al. Haematologica 1991;76:475

334. Lown J, Willis J. Tranf Med 1995;5:281

335. Van Dijk BA. Doctoral Dissertation, Univ Leiden, Netherlands, 1991

336. Van Dijk BA. (Letter). Transfusion 1993;33:960

337. Issitt PD. (Letter). Transfusion 1993;33:960

338. Garner SF, Devenish A, Barber H, et al. (Letter). Vox Sang 1991;61:219

339. Judd WJ, Steiner EA, Nugent CE. (Letter). Vox Sang 1992;63:293

340. Malone RH, Dunsford I. Blood 1951;6:1135

341. Dybkjaer E. Vox Sang 1967;12:446

342. Harrison J. Vox Sang 1970;19:123

343. Shirey RS, Edwards RE, Ness PM. Transfusion 1994;34:756

344. Jones AR, Diamond LK, Allen FH Jr. New Eng J Med 1954;250:283

345. Jones AR, Diamond LK, Allen FH Jr. New Eng J Med 1954;250:324

346. Wiener AS. Proc Soc Exp Biol NY 1949;70:576

347. van Loghem JJ, Harkink H, van der Hart M. Vox Sang (Old Series) 1953;3:22

348. Moore BPL. Immunohematology 1988;4:42

349. Wiener AS, Landsteiner K. Proc Soc Exp Biol NY 1943;53:167

350. Race RR, Taylor GL, Cappell DF, et al. Nature 1944;153:52

351. Murray J, Race RR, Taylor GL. Nature 1945;155:112

352. Race RR, Taylor GL, Ikin EW, et al. Ann Eugen 1945;12:261

353. Wiener AS. Nature 1948;162:735

354. van den Bosch C. Nature 1948;162:781

355. Sussman LN, Wald N. Am J Hum Genet 1950;2:85

356. Miller EB, Rosenfield RE, Vogel P. Am J Phys Anthropol 1951;9:115

357. Hassig A, Rosin S, Rothlin A. Schweiz Med Wschr 1955;85:909

358. Shreffler DC, Sing CF, Neel JV, et al. Am J Hum Genet 1971;23:150

359. Lewis M, Kaita H, Chown B. Vox Sang 1971;20:500

360. Walker RH. In: Paternity Testing. Washington, D.C.:Am Assoc Blood Banks, 1978:69

361. Schorr JB, Schorr PT, Francis G, et al. (abstract). Prog 24th Ann Mtg, Am Assoc Blood Banks, 1971:100

362. Schorr JB. Personal communication 1976, cited by Issitt PD. In: Serology and Genetics of the Rhesus Blood Group System. Cincinnati:Montgomery, 1979

363. Huestis DW. Vox Sang 1971;21:186

364. Smith TR, Sherman SP, Nelson CA, et al. (abstract). Transfusion 1978;18:388

365. Mourant AE. Nature 1949;163:913

366. Masouredis SP, Dupuy ME, Elliot M. J Clin Invest 1967;46:681

367. Loren AB, Matsuo Y, Charman D, et al. Transfusion 1982;22:194

368. Horita M, Ricker AB, Jabs AD, et al. Afr J Clin Exp Immunol 1981;2:259

369. Caren LD, Bellevance R, Grumet FC. Transfusion 1982;22:475

370. Oien L, Nance S, Garratty G. (abstract). Transfusion 1985;25:474

371. Nelson J, Choy C, Vengelen-Tyler V, et al. Immunohematology 1985;2:38

372. Arndt P, Garratty G. (abstract). Transfusion 1987;27:514

373. Nance ST. In: Progress in Immunohematology. Arlington, VA:Am Assoc Blood Banks, 1988:1

374. Freedman J, Lazarus AH. Transf Med Rev 1995;9:87

375. van Bockstaele DR, Berneman ZN, Muylle L, et al. Vox Sang 1986;51:40

376. Kornprobst M, Rouger PH, Goosens D, et al. J Clin Pathol 1986;39:1039

377. Gunson HH, Stratton F, Cooper DG. Br Med J 1970;1:593

378. Nicholson G, Lawrence A, Ala FA, et al. Transf Med 1991;1:87

379. Chown B, Lewis M. Canad Med Assoc J 1946;55:66

380. Chown B, Lewis M, Peterson RF. Rev Hematol 1949;4:605

381. Chown B, Lewis M. J Clin Pathol 1951;4:404

382. Chown B, Lewis M. Ann Hum Genet 1957;22:58

383. Edgington TS. J Immunol 1971;106:673

384. Masouredis SP, Sudora EJ, Mahan L, et al. Transfusion 1976;16:94

385. Skov F. Vox Sang 1976;31:124

386. Skov F, Hughes-Jones NC. Vox Sang 1977;33:170

387. Oien L, Nance S, Arndt P, et al. Transfusion 1988;28:541

388. Wagner FF. Transfusion 1994;34:671

389. Anstee D, Edwards PA. Eur J Immunol 1982;12:228

390. Merry AH, Thompson EE, Anstee DJ, et al. Immunology 1984;51:793

391. Gorick BD, Thompson KM, Melamed MD, et al. Vox Sang 1988;55:165

392. Sonneborn HH, Ernst M, Tills D, et al. Vox Sang 1990;58:219

393. Gorick B, McDougall DCL, Ouwehand WH, et al. Vox Sang 1993;65:136

394. Anstee DJ. Vox Sang 1990;58:1

395. Anstee DJ. J Immunogenet 1990;17:219

396. Mallinson G, Anstee DJ, Avent ND, et al. Transfusion 1990;30:222

397. Hughes-Jones NC. Transf Med 1991;1:69

398. Gardner B, Anstee DJ, Mawby WJ, et al. Transf Med 1991;1;77

399. Greenbury CL, Moore DH, Nunn LAC. Immunology 1963;6:421

400. Economidou J, Hughes Jones NC, Gardner B. Vox Sang 1967;12:321

401. Hughes-Jones NC, Gardner B. Vox Sang 1971;21:154

402. Masouredis SP. In: Membrane Structure and Function of Human Blood Cells. Washington, D.C.:Am Assoc Blood Banks, 1976:37

403. Nichols ME, Rubinstein P, Barnwell J, et al. J Exp Med 1987;166:776

404. Jaber A, Blanchard D, Goosens D, et al. Blood 1989;73:1597

405. Chown B, Lewis M. Vox Sang (Old Series) 1954;4:41

406. Plaut G, Booth PB, Giles CM, et al. Br Med J 1958;1:1215

407. Korstad L, Ryttinger L, Hogman C. Vox Sang 1960;5:330

408. Bowman JM, Pollock J. Vox Sang 1993;64:226

409. Cleghorn TE. MD Thesis, Univ Sheffield 1961

410. Dodd BE, Eeles DA. Immunology 1961;4:337

411. Casey FM, Dodd BE, Lincoln PJ. Vox Sang 1972;23:493

412. Perrault R, Hogman C. Vox Sang 1971;20:340

413. Perrault R, Hogman C. Vox Sang 1971;20:356

414. Perrault RA, Hogman CF. Acta Univ Uppsal 1972:120

415. Nordhagen R, Kornstad L. (abstract). Book of Abstracts, 18th Cong ISBT 1984:218

416. Lee D, Remant M, Stratton F. Clin Lab Haematol 1984;6:33

417. Wiener AS. In: Abraham Levison Anniv Vol. Studies in Pediatrics and Medical History. New York:Froben, 1949

418. Grove-Rasmussen M, Levine P. Am J Clin Pathol 1954;24:145

419. Allen FH Jr, Newell JL. New Eng J Med 1958;259:236

420. Natvig JB, Kunkel HG. Ser Haematol 1968;1:66

421. Devey ME, Voak D. Immunology 1974;27:1073

422. Frankowska K, Gorska B. Arch Immunol Therap Exp

1978;26:1095

423. Zupanska B, Maslanka K, van Loghem E. Vox Sang 1982;43:243

424. Zupanska B, Thompson E, Brojer E, et al. Vox Sang 1987;53:96

425. Shaw DR, Conley ME, Knox FJ, et al. Transfusion 1988;28;127

426. Mattila PS, Seppala IJT, Eklund J, et al. Vox Sang 1985;48:350

427. Parinaud J, Blanc M, Grandjean H, et al. Am J Obstet Gynecol 1985;151:1111

428. Michaelsen TE, Korstad L. Clin Exp Immunol 1987;67:637

429. Francois-Gerard C, Opret-Meunier C. Vox Sang 1987;52:322

430. Gorick BD, Hughes Jones NC. Vox Sang 1991;62:251

431. Frame M, Mollison PL,Terry WD. Nature 1970;225:641

432. Abramson N, Schur PH. Blood 1972;40:500

433. Morell A, Skvaril F, Rufener JL. Vox Sang 1973;24:323

434. Dugoujon JM, de Lange GG, Blancher A, et al. Vox Sang 1989;57:133

435. Morell A, Skvaril F, van Loghem JJ, et al. Vox Sang 1971;21:481

436. Schur PH, Alpert E, Alper C. Clin Immunol Immunopathol 1973;2:62

437. Waller M, Lawler D. Vox Sang 1962;7:591

438. Ayland J, Horton MA, Tippett PA, et al. Vox Sang 1978;34:40

439. Graham HA, Davies DM Jr, Brower CE. In: An International Symposium on the Nature and Significance of Complement Activation. Raritan, N.J.:Ortho, 1976:107

440. Kline WE, Sullivan CM, Pope M, et al. Vox Sang 1982;43:335

441. Hidalgo C, Romano EL, Linares J, et al. Transfusion 1979;19:250

442. Roy RB, Lotto WN. Transfusion 1962;2:342

443. Joseph JI, Awer E, Laulicht M, et al. Transfusion 1964;4:367

444. Croucher BE, Crookston MC, Crookston JH. Vox Sang 1967;12:32

445. Moncrieff RE, Thompson WP. Am J Clin Pathol 1975;64:251

446. Snyder EL, Spivak M, Novodoff D, et al. Transfusion 1978;18:79

447. Pickles MM, Jones MN, Egan J, et al. Vox Sang 1978;35:32

448. Pineda AA, Taswell HF, Brzica SM Jr. Transfusion 1978;18:1

449. Moore SB, Taswell HF, Pineda AA, et al. Am J Clin Pathol 1980;74:94

450. Davey RJ, Gustafson M, Holland PV. Transfusion 1980;20:348

451. Baldwin ML, Barrasso C, Ness PM, et al. Transfusion 1983;23:40

452. Salama A, Mueller-Eckhardt C. Transfusion 1984;24:188

453. Harrison CR, Hayes TC, Trow LL, et al. Vox Sang 1986;51:96

454. Ness PM, Shirey RS, Thoman SK, et al. Transfusion 1990;30:688

455. Shirey RS, Ness PM. In: Clinical and Basic Science Aspects of Immunohematology. Arlington, VA:Am Assoc Blood Banks, 1991:179

456. Urbaniak SJ. Br J Haematol 1976;33:409

457. Handwerger BS, Kay NW, Douglas SD. Vox Sang 1978;34:276

458. Urbaniak SJ. Br J Haematol 1979;42:303

459. Urbaniak SJ. Br J Haematol 1979;42:315

460. Urbaniak SJ, Greiss MA. Br J Haematol 1980;46:447

461. Schreiber AD, Gomes F, Levinson AI, et al. Transf Med Rev 1989;3:282

462. Issitt PD, Gutgsell NS. In: Immune Destruction of Red Blood Cells. Arlington, VA:Am Assoc Blood Banks, 1989;77

463. Garratty G, Petz LD. Transfusion 1971;11:79

464. Issitt PD, Issitt CH, Wilkinson SL. Transfusion 1974;14:103

465. Issitt PD, Smith TR. In: A Seminar on Performance Evaluation. Washington, D.C.:Am Assoc Blood Banks, 1976:25

466. Issitt PD. Applied Blood Group Serology, lst Ed. Oxnard:Spectra Biologicals 1970

467. Judson PA, Anstee DJ. Med Lab Sci 1977;34:1

468. Judd WJ. Methods in Immunohematology, 2nd Ed. Durham:Montgomery, 1994

469. Adinolfi A, Mollison PL, Polley MJ, et al. J Exp Med 1966;123:951

470. Masouredis SP. Transfusion 1962;2:363

471. Hughes-Jones NC, Gardner B, Telford R. Vox Sang 1964;9:175

472. Steane EA. In: Blood Bank Immunology. Washington, D.C.:Am Assoc Blood Banks, 1977:61

473. Friesen AD, Bowman JM, Price HW. J Appl Biochem 1981;3:164

474. Bowman J. Clin Obstet Gynecol 1982;25:341

475. Kumpel BM, Goodrick MJ, Pamphilon DH, et al. Blood 1995;86:1701

476. Bierme SJ, Blanc M, Fournie A, et al. In: Rh Hemolytic Disease: New Strategy for Eradication. Boston:Hall, 1982:249

477. Beer AE, Quebbeman JF, Johnson MZ. Am J Reprod Immunol 1982;2:173

478. Argall CI. PhD Thesis, Univ Utah, 1955

479. Anderson LD, Race GJ, Owen M. Am J Clin Pathol 1958;30:228

480. Francis BJ, Hatcher DE, Marcuse PM. Vox Sang 1960;5:324

481. Wiener AS, Unger LJ, Jack JA. Rev Hematol 1960;15:286

482. Simmons RT, Krieger VI. Med J Austral 1960;2:1021

483. Chown B, Lewis M, Kaita H, et al. Vox Sang 1963;8:420

484. Sussman LN, Wiener AS. Transfusion 1964;4:50

485. Wiener AS, Unger LJ. J Am Med Assoc 1959;169:696

486. Unger LJ, Wiener AS. Am J Clin Pathol 1959;31:95

487. Unger LJ, Wiener AS, Katz L. J Exp Med 1959;110:495

488. Unger LJ, Wiener AS. Blood 1959;14:522

489. Unger LJ, Wiener AS. Acta Genet Med Gemell 1959;13 (Suppl 2):13

490. Sacks MS, Unger LJ, Wiener AS. J Am Med Assoc 1960;172:1158

491. Wiener AS, Unger LJ. Transfusion 1962;2:230

492. Wiener AS, Gordon EB. J Forens Med 1967;14:131

493. Tippett P. In: Blood Group Systems: Rh. Arlington, VA:Am Assoc Blood Banks, 1987:25

494. Lomas C, Tippett P, Mannessier L. (Letter). Transfusion 1993;33:535

495. Salmon C, Cartron J-P, Rouger P. The Human Blood Groups. New York:Masson, 1984:220

496. Zuck TF. (Editorial). Transfusion 1983;23:90

497. Lacey PA, Caskey CR, Werner DJ, et al. Transfusion 1983;23:91

498. Konugres AA, Polesky HF, Walker RH. Transfusion 1982;22:76

499. Shapiro M. Bibl Haematol 1965;23:299

500. Alter AA, Gelb AG, Chown B, et al. Transfusion 1967;7:88

501. Lewis M, Chown B, Kaita H, et al. Transfusion 1967;7:440

502. Lovett DA, Crawford MN. Transfusion 1967;7:442

503. Lassiter GR, Issitt PD, Garris ML, et al. (abstract). Transfusion 1969;9:282

504. Hossaini AA, Mirehandani I. (abstract). Book of Abstracts, 15th Cong ISBT 1978:192

505. Sabo BH. In: A Seminar on Perinatal Blood Banking. Washington, D.C.:Am Assoc Blood Banks, 1978:31

506. Tippett PA. Unpublished observations, cited in previous edi-

tions of this book.

507. Giles CM, Tippett P, Lomas C. Unpublished observations cited by Tippett P. In: Blood Group Systems: Rh. Arlington, VA:Am Assoc Blood Banks, 1987:33

508. Daniels G. Human Blood Groups. Oxford:Blackwell, 1995

509. Chown B, Lewis M, Kaita H, et al. Transfusion 1964;4:169

510. Lewis M, Macpherson CR, Gayton J. Canad J Genet Cytol 1965;7:259

511. Lomas C, Mougey R. (abstract). Transfusion 1989;29(Suppl 7S):14S

512. Humphreys J, Stout TD, Kaita H, et al. (abstract). Book of Abstracts, 14th Cong ISBT 1975:46

513. Humphreys J, Stout TD, Kaita H, et al. Vox Sang 1980;39:277

514. Levene C, Sela R, Grunberg L, et al. Clin Lab Haematol 1983;5:303

515. Lylloff K, Lundsgaard A, Lomas C, et al. Hum Hered 1984;34:194

516. Lomas C, Bruce M, Watt A, et al. (abstract). Transfusion 1986;26:560

517. Moores PP. MSc Thesis, Univ Natal, 1976

518. Rosenfield RE, Rubinstein P. In: Monoclonal Antibodies Against Human Red Blood Cell and Related Antigens. Paris:Arnette, 1987:205

519. Foung SKH, Blunt J, Perkins S, et al. Vox Sang 1986;50:160

520. Thompson K, Barden G, Sutherland J, et al. Immunology 1990;71:323

521. Okubo Y, Seno T, Yamano H, et al. (Letter). Transfusion 1991;31:782

522. van Rhenen DJ, Thijssen PMHJ, Overbeeke MAM. Vox Sang 1994;66:133

523. Watt J. (abstract). Transf Med 1993;3:72

524. Beck ML, Hardman JT. (abstract). Transfusion 1991;31(Suppl 8S):25S

525. Wiener AS. Science 1958;128:849

526. Morgan P, Bossom EL. Transfusion 1967;7:477

527. Lowes BCR. Vox Sang 1969;16:231

528. Allen FH Jr, Tippett P. Vox Sang 1961;6:429

529. Zaino EC, Applewhaite F. Transfusion 1975;15:256

530. Brandstadter W, Brandstadter M. Z Gynakol 1970;6:176

531. White CA, Stedman CM, Frank S. Am J Obstet Gynecol 1983;145:1069

532. Ostgård P, Fevang F, Kornstad L. Acta Paediat Scand 1986;75:185

533. Mayne KM, Allen DL, Bowell PJ. Clin Lab Haematol 1991;13:239

534. Hadley AG, Kumpel BM. Baillière's Clin Haematol 1993;6:423

535. Mayne K, Bowell P, Woodward T, et al. Br J Haematol 1990;76:537

536. Revill JA, Emblin KF, Hutchinson RM. Vox Sang 1979;36:93

537. Beckers EAM, Faas BHW, Overbeeke MAM, et al. (abstract). Transfusion 1995;35(Suppl 10S):50S

538. Levine P, Celano M, McGee R, et al. In P.H. Andresen Festskif. Copenhagen:Munksgaard, 1957

539. Gunson HH, Smith DS. Vox Sang 1967;13:423

540. McGee R, Levine P, Celano M. Science 1957;125:1043

541. Simmons RT. Vox Sang 1962;7:79

542. Jennings ER, Clear J. J Am Med Assoc 1982;247:367

543. Lubenko A, Contreras M, Habash J. Br J Haematol 1989;72:429

544. Anonymous. Technical Bulletin 61, Am Coll Obstet Gynecol, 1982

545. Kajii E, Umenishi F, Iwamoto S, et al. Hum Genet 1993;91:157

546. Simsek S, de Jong CAM, Cuijpers HTM, et al. Vox Sang 1994;67:203

547. Schornack JL, Beattie KM. (abstract). Transfusion 1978;18:379

548. Macpherson CR, Stevenson TD, Gayton J. Am J Clin Pathol 1966;45:748

549. Beard MEJ, Pemberton J, Blagdon J, et al. Med Genet 1971;8:317

550. Cook IA. Br J Haematol 1971;20:369

551. Holland PV, Gralnick MA. (abstract). Transfusion 1973;13:363

552. Issitt PD, Tessel JA. Unpublished observations 1980, cited by Mollison PL. In: Blood Transfusion in Clinical Medicine 7th Ed. Oxford:Blackwell 1983

553. Polesky HF, Bove JR. Transfusion 1964;4:285

554. Chown B, Kaita H, Lowen B, et al. Transfusion 1971;11:220

555. Lalezari P, Talleyrand NP, Wenz B, et al. Vox Sang 1975;28:19

556. Issitt PD. In: Blood Bank Immunology. Washington, D.C.:Am Assoc Blood Banks, 1977:17

557. Issitt PD, Zellner DC, Rolih SD, et al. Transfusion 1977;17:531

558. Henry RA, Weber J, Pavone BG, et al. Transfusion 1977;17:539

559. Sosler SD, Perkins JT, Saporito C, et al. (abstract). Transfusion 1989;29 (Suppl 7S):49S

560. Rouillac C, Le Van Kim C, Blancher A, et al. Br J Haematol 1995;89:424

561. Issitt PD. Br J Biomed Sci 1994;51:158

562. Marsh GW, Stirling Y, Mollison P. Vox Sang 1970;19:468

563. Chown B, Bowman JM, Pollock J, et al. Canad Med Assoc J 1970;102:1161

564. Sansone G, Veneziano G. Lancet 1970;1:952

565. Mollison PL. Blood Transfusion in Clinical Medicine, 7th Ed. Oxford:Blackwell, 1983

566. Davey MG. In: Proceedings of a Symposium on Rh Antibody Mediated Immunospression. Raritan N.J.:Ortho Research Institute, 1976

567. Darnborough J, Dunsford I, Wallace JA. Vox Sang 1969;17:241

568. Furuhjelm U, Myllylä G, Nevanlinna HR, et al. Vox Sang 1969;17:256

569. Sanger R. In: Blood and Tissue Antigens. New York:Academic Press, 1970:17

570. Metaxas MN, Metaxas-Bühler M. Vox Sang 1972;22:474

571. Dahr W, Uhlenbruck G, Leikola J, et al. J Immunogenet 1976;3:329

572. Issitt PD, Pavone BG, Wagstaff W, et al. Transfusion 1976;16:396

573. Dahr W, Issitt PD, Uhlenbruck G. In: Human Blood Groups. Basel:Karger, 1977:197

574. Metaxas MN, Metaxas-Bühler M. In: Human Blood Groups. Basel:Karger, 1977:344

575. Anstee DJ, Barker DM, Judson PA, et al. Br J Haematol 1977;35:309

576. Anstee DJ, Tanner MJA. Biochem J 1978;175:149

577. Race RR, Sanger R, Selwyn JG. Br J Exp Pathol 1951;32:124

578. Combs MR. Personal communication 1990

579. Contreras M, Armitage S, Daniels GL, et al. Vox Sang 1979;36:81

580. Jakobowicz R, Simmons RT. Med J Austral 1959;2:357

581. Jakobowicz R, Whittingham S, Barrie JU, et al. Med J Austral 1962;1:895

582. Stout TD, Moore BPL, Allen FH Jr, et al. Vox Sang 1963;8:262

583. Zaino EC. Transfusion 1965;5:320

584. Vos GH. Vox Sang 1960;5:472

585. Issitt PD, Tessel JA. Transfusion 1981;21:412

586. Case J, Moulds JJ. (letter). Transfusion 1982;22:258

587. Issitt PD, Tessel JA. (Letter). Transfusion 1982;22:259

588. Beattie KM, Neitzer GM, Zanardi V, et al. Transfusion 1971;11:152

589. Kusnierz-Alejska G. (abstract). Vox Sang 1994;67(Suppl 2):53

590. Huestis DW, Stern K. Transfusion 1962;2:419

591. Nijenhuis LE. Vox Sang 1961;6:229

592. Rosenfield RE. Unpublished observations cited by Race RR, Sanger R. Blood Groups in Man, 5th Ed. Oxford:Blackwell, 1968

593. Giles CM. Unpublished observations cited by Race RR, Sanger R. In: Blood Groups in Man, 5th Ed. Oxford:Blackwell, 1968

594. Case J. Vox Sang 1973;25:529

595. Kevy SV, Schmidt PG, Leyshon WC. Vox Sang 1959;4:257

596. Sturgeon P, Fisk R, Wintler C, et al. Bibl Haematol 1959;10:293

597. Fowler HW, Fowler FG. The Oxford Dictionary of Current English, 5th Ed. Oxford:Oxford Univ Press, 1964

598. Sanger R, Race RR, Rosenfield RE, et al. Proc Nat Acad Sci Washington D.C. 1953;39:824

599. Jones AR, Steinberg AG, Allen FH Jr, et al. Blood 1954;9:117

600. Rosenfield RE, Haber GV, Schroeder R, et al. Am J Hum Genet 1960;12:147

601. Tippett PA, Sanger R, Dunsford I, et al. Vox Sang 1961;6:21

602. Keith P, Corcoran PA, Caspersen K, et al. Vox Sang 1965;10:528

603. Grundorfer J, Kopchik W, Tippett P, et al. Vox Sang 1961;6:618

604. Tate H, Cunningham C, McDade MG, et al. Vox Sang 1960;5:398

605. Delmas-Marsalet Y, Goudemand M, Tippett P. Rev Fr Transf 1969;12:233

606. Tessel JA, Wilkinson SL, Hines SR, et al. (abstract). Transfusion 1980;20:632

607. Yamaguchi H, Okubo Y, Tomita T, et al. Proc Jpn Acad 1969;45:618

608. Leyshon WC. Vox Sang 1967;13:354

609. Spielmann W, Seidl S, von Pawel S. Vox Sang 1974;27:473

610. Metaxas MN, Metaxas-Bühler M. Vox Sang 1961;6:136

611. Heiken A, Giles CM. Hereditas 1965;53:171

612. Levine P, White J, Stroup M, et al. Nature 1960;185:188

613. Freda V, D'Esopo DA, Rosenfield RE, et al. Transfusion 1963;3:281

614. O'Reilly RA, Lombard CM, Azzi RL. Vox Sang 1985;49:336

615. Devenish A, Kay LA. Immunohematology 1994;10:120

616. Dahl JR, Giblett ER. Vox Sang 1963;8:452

617. Molthan L, Matulewicz TJ, Bansal-Carver B, et al. Vox Sang 1984;47:348

618. Race RR, Sanger R, Levine P, et al. Nature 1954;174:460

619. Sturgeon P. J Foren Sci 1960;5:287

620. Race RR, Sanger R. Vox Sang 1961;6;227

621. Rosenfield RE, Haber GV, Degnan TJ. Vox Sang 1964;9:168

622. Issitt PD. Canad J Med Tech 1978;40:52

623. Zoutendyk A, Teodorczuk H. Nature 1960;187:790

624. Zoutendyk A, Teodorczuk H. Bibl Haematol 1962;13:183

625. Blunt T, Daniels GL, Carritt B. Vox Sang 1994;67:397 625

626. Race RR, Sanger R. Heredity 1951;5:285

627. Race RR, Sanger R, Lawler SD. Vox Sang 1960;5:334

628. Metaxas MN, Metaxas-Bühler M, Butler R, et al. Vox Sang 1964;9:698

629. Vengelen-Tyler V, McGrath C, Nelson J. (abstract). Transfusion 1986;26:560

630. Lomas C, Storry JR, Spruell P, et al. (abstract). Transfusion 1994;34(Suppl 10S):25S

631. Albrey JA, Pollard M, Giles CM, et al. Unpublished observations. Cited in Race RR, Sanger R. Blood Groups in Man, 6th Ed. Oxford:Blackwell, 1975

632. Moulds JJ, Case J, Anderson TD, et al. (abstract). Book of Abstracts, 17th Cong ISBT 1982;289

633. Reviron M, Janvier D, Comte S, et al. (Letter). Transfusion 1989;29:464

634. Garratty G, Vengelen-Tyler V, Postoway N, et al. (abstract). Transfusion 1982;22:429

635. Steane SM, Montgomery S, Wiedermann J, et al. (abstract). Transfusion 1982;22:429

636. Fisher G. Transfusion 1983;23:152

637. Maynard BA, Smith DS, Farrar RP, et al. Transfusion 1988;28:302

638. Lin CK, Wong KT, Mak KH, et al. Am J Clin Pathol 1995;104:660

639. Broman B, Heiken A, Tippett PA, et al. Vox Sang 1963;8:588

640. Tippett PA. Unpublished observations, cited by Giles CM, Skov F. Vox Sang 1971;20:328

641. Issitt PD, Gutgsell NS, McDowell MA, et al. (abstract). Blood 1987;70(Suppl 1):110a

642. Issitt PD, Gutgsell NS, Martin PA, et al. Transfusion 1991;31:63

643. Issitt PD, Gutgsell NS. Immunohematology 1987;3:1

644. Lawler SD, van Loghem JJ. Lancet 1947;2:545

645. Collins JO, Sanger R, Allen FH Jr, et al. Br Med J 1950;1:1297

646. Dunsford I, Aspinall P. Nature 1951;168:954

647. van den Heide HM, Magnee W, van Loghem JJ. Am J Hum Genet 1951;3:344

648. Prokop O. Klin Wschr 1959;37:882

649. Prokop O, Rackwitz A. Blut 1959;5:279

650. Cleghorn TE. Vox Sang 1960;5:171

651. Jackobowicz R, Goldberg B, Simmons RT. Med J Austral 1967;2:738

652. Habibi B, Andre J, Fouillade MY, et al. Vox Sang 1976;31:103

653. Sanger R. Personal communication, cited by Habibi B, Andre J, Fouillade MT, et al. Vox Sang 1976;31:103

654. Leonard GL, Ellisor SS, Reid ME, et al. Vox Sang 1976;31:275

655. Sachs HW, Reuter W, Tippett P, et al. Vox Sang 1978;35:272

656. Giannetti M, Stadler E, Rittner C, et al. Vox Sang 1983;44:319

657. Wittman G, Zimmermann R, Wallace M, et al. Unpublished observations, 1994. Cited by Daniels, G. In: Human Blood Groups. Oxford:Blackwell, 1995:299

658. Rosenfield RE. Bibl Haematol 1959;10:557

659. Tippett P, Gavin J, Sanger R. Vox Sang 1962;7:249

660. Issitt PD. Immunohematology 1991;7:29

661. Sacks MO, Schulz C, Dagovitz H, et al. Pediatrics 1958;21:443

662. Geiger J. J Pediat 1959;54:484

663. Anderson GH, Fenton E. Canad Med Assoc J 1963;89:28

664. Polesky HF. Minn Med 1967;50:601

665. Beal RW. Clin Obstet Gynaecol 1979;6:493

666. Musialowicz J, Szmigiel M. Pol Tyg Lek 1980;35:1533

667. Hardy J, Napier JAF. Br J Obstet Gynaecol 1981;88:91

668. Hughes W, Pussell P, Klarkowski D. Austral NZ J Obstet Gynaecol 1982;22:161

669. Mogliner BM, Berrebi A, Levy A, et al. Acta Paediat Scand 1982;71:703

670. Zuliani G, Moroni GA, Buscaglia M, et al. Ric Clin Lab 1983;13:449
671. Finney RD, Blue AM, Willoughby MLN. Vox Sang 1973;25:39
672. Bevan B, Giles CM. Unpusblished observations, cited by Race RR, Sanger R. In: Blood Groups in Man, 6th Ed. Oxford:Blackwell, 1975
673. Sisteonen P, Aden Abdulle O, Sahid M. Transfusion 1987;27:66
674. Orjassaeter H, Gedde-Dahl T, Heisto ALG. Unpublished observations 1976. Cited by Daniels G. In: Human Blood Groups, Oxford:Blackwell, 1985:299
675. Mougey R, Martin J, Hackbart C. (abstract). Transfusion 1983;23:410
676. Larimore K. Unpublished observations 1987, cited by Issitt PD. Transf Med Rev 1989;3:1
677. Issitt PD, Wren MR, McDowell MA, et al. Transfusion 1986;26:506
678. Issitt PD, Gutgsell NS. (abstract). Blood 1987;70(Suppl 1):110a
679. Brown D, Hare V, Issitt PD, et al. (abstract). Transfusion 1987;27:548
680. Rosenfield RE. Proc 2nd Int Mtg Foren Path Med, New York, 1960
681. Rosenfield RE. Unpublished manuscript 1961, kindly provided by Dr. Rosenfield
682. Lewis M, Kaita H, Chown B, et al. Vox Sang 1976;30:282
683. Rosenfield RE. Unpublished observations 1976. Cited by Lewis M, Kaita H, Chown B, et al. Vox Sang 1976;30:282
684. Layrisse M, Layrisse Z, Garcia E, et al. Nature 1961;191:503
685. Layrisse M, Layrisse Z, Garcia E, et al. Vox Sang 1961;6:710
686. Issitt PD. Applied Blood Group Serology, 3rd Ed. Miami:Montgomery 1985
687. Champney A, Wilson B, Tippett P. Lab Med 1980;11:277
688. Issitt PD, Smith DL, McCollister LS, et al. Transfusion 1988;28:439
689. Kaita H, Lewis M, Chown B. Transfusion 1964;4:118
690. Winter N, Milkovich L, Konugres A. Transfusion 1966;6:271
691. Grobel RK, Cardy JD. Transfusion 1971;11:77
692. Henke J, Kasaluke D. Vox Sang 1976;30:305
693. Ceppellini R. Rev Hematol 1950;5:285
694. Ceppellini R, Ikin EW, Mourant AE. Bull Inst Siero Milanese 1950;29:123
695. Mourant AE, Ikin EW, Hassig A, et al. Schwiez Med Wschr 1952;82:1100
696. Sussman LN. Blood 1955;10:1241
697. Heiken A. Vox Sang 1967;13:158
698. Kornstad L, Øyen R. Vox Sang 1967;13:417
699. Skradski KJ, Rose RR, Balk MC, et al. (abstract). Transfusion 1989;29(Suppl 7S):35S
700. Lubenko A, Burslem SJ, Fairclough LM, et al. Vox Sang 1991;60:235
701. Okubo Y, Yamano H, Nagao N, et al. (Letter). Transfusion 1994;34:183
702. Stern K, Davidsohn I, Jensen FG, et al. Vox Sang 1958;3:425
703. Ducos J, Marty Y, Ruffie J, et al. Unpublished observations cited by Race RR, Sanger R. Blood Groups in Man, 6th Ed. Oxford:Blackwell, 1975
704. McCreary J, MacIlroy M, Courtenay DG, et al. Transfusion 1973;13:428
705. Clark J, Yorek H, Schuler S, et al. (abstract). Book of Abstracts, Joint Cong ISBT/AABB, 1990:81
706. O'Riordan JP, Wilkinson JL, Huth MC, et al. Vox Sang 1972;7:14
707. Morton NE, Rosenfield RE. Transfusion 1967;7:117

708. Moulds JJ, Wilkinson SL, Issitt PD. Unpublished observations, 1980. Cited by Issitt PD. Transf Med Rev 1989;3:1
709. Hoffman JJML, Overbeeke MAM, Kaita H, et al. Vox Sang 1990;59:240
710. Coghlan G, McCreary J, Underwood V, et al. Transfusion 1994;34:492
711. Kornstad L. Vox Sang 1986;50:235
712. Orlina AR, Unger PJ, Lacey PA. Rev Fr Transf Immunohematol 1984;27:613
713. Weiner W, Wrobel DM, Gavin J. Unpublished observations, cited in Race RR, Sanger R. Blood Groups in Man, 6th Ed. Oxford:Blackwell, 1975
714. Svanda M, Prochazka R, Kout M, et al. Vox Sang 1970;18:366
715. Brewer LG, Spruell P, Burton WC, et al. (abstract). Transfusion 1995;35(Suppl 10S):51S
716. Moores P, Smart E, Sternberger J, et al. Transfusion 1991;31:759
717. Contreras M, Tippett P. Unpublished observations 1980. Cited by Tippett P. In: Blood Group Systems: Rh. Arlington, VA:Am Assoc Blood Banks, 1987:25
718. Contreras M, Stebbing B, McGuire Mallory D, et al. Vox Sang 1978;35:397
719. Lawler SD, Race RR. Proc Int Soc Hematol 1950;168
720. Dunsford I, Tippett P. Unpublished observations, cited by Race RR, Sanger R. Blood Groups in Man, 6th Ed. Oxford:Blackwell, 1975
721. Giles CM, Bevan B. Vox Sang 1964;9:204
722. Heiken A, Giles CM. Nature 1967;213:699
723. Race RR, Sanger R. Blood Groups in Man, 5th Ed. Oxford:Blackwell, 1968;212
724. Tessel JA, Utz GL, Wilkinson SL, et al. (abstract). Book of Abstracts, 8th Ann Mtg, Ohio Assoc Blood Banks, 1981:6
725. Issitt PD. Proc 40th Anniv Symposium, Irwin Mem Blood Bank, 1981:14
726. Case J. Personal Communication 1978. In: Issitt PD. Serology and Genetics of the Rhesus Blood Group System. Cincinnati:Montgomery, 1979:127
727. Case J. In : Blood Group Systems: Rh. Arlington, VA:Am Assoc Blood Banks, 1987:55
728. Grobbelaar BG, Moores PP. Transfusion 1963;3:103
729. Issitt PD, Gutgsell NS. (abstract). Book of Abstracts, ISBT/AABB Joint Cong, 1990:29
730. Moores P, Smart E. Vox Sang 1991;61:122
731. Issitt PD. Transf Med Rev 1989;3:3
732. Issitt PD, Combs MR, Godwin J. Unpublished observations, 1991
733. Bell J, Mozeleski J. (abstract). Book of Abstracts, ISBT/AABB Joint Cong, 1990:81
734. Issitt PD, Pavone BG. Br J Haematol 1978;38:63
735. Issitt PD, Gruppo RA, Wilkinson SL, et al. Br J Haematol 1982;52:537
736. Issitt PD, Wilkinson SL, Gruppo RA. (Letter). Br J Haematol 1983;53:688
737. Vengelen-Tyler V, Mogck N. Transfusion 1991;31:254
738. Issitt PD. Immunohematology (Letter). 1991;7:83
739. Moores P. Vox Sang 1994;66:225
740. Giblett ER, Chase J, Motulsky AG. J Lab Clin Med 1957;49:433
741. Reid M, Tippett P. Personal communication to Daniels G. Cited in Daniels G. Human Blood Groups. Oxford:Blackwell, 1994:298
742. Tregellas WM. MS Thesis, Univ Cincinnati, 1974
743. Tregallas WM, Issitt PD. Transfusion 1978;18:15
744. Cheng MS. (Letter). Transfusion 1982;22:401

745. Byrne P, Howard JH. Immunohematology 1994;10:136

746. Beal CL, Oliver CK, Mallory DM, et al. Immunohematology 1995;11;74

747. Reid ME, Beal C, Mallory D, et al. (abstract). Transfusion 1995;35(Suppl 10S):51S

748. Blancher A, Reid ME, Tossas E, et al. (abstract). Transfusion 1995;35(Suppl 10S):23S

749. Reid ME. Personal communication, 1996

750. Steers F, Daniels GL, Johnson PH, et al. (abstract). Transfusion 1995;35(Suppl 10S):50S

751. Faas BHW, Beckers EAM, Wildoer P, et al. Transfusion 1997;37:38

752. Behzad O, Lee CL, Smith D. (letter). Transfusion 1982;22:83

753. Combs MR, Issitt PD. Unpublished observations, 1996

754. Cartron J-P. Blood Rev 1994;8:199

755. Bourel D, Lecointre M, Genetet N, et al. Vox Sang 1987;52:85

756. Fraser RH, Inglis G, Allen JC, et al. Transfusion 1990;30:226

757. Waller RK, Sanger R, Bobbitt OB. Br Med J 1953;1:198

758. Levine P, Koch EA, McGee RT, et al. Am J Clin Pathol 1954;24:292

759. Buchanan DI, McIntyre J. Br J Haematol 1955;1:304

760. Buchanan DI. Am J Clin Pathol 1956;26:21

761. Kuniyuki M, Takahara N. J Jpn Soc Blood Transf 1958;4:206

762. Allen FH Jr. J Pediat 1960;57:281

763. Moore BPL, McIntyre J, Brown F, et al. Canad Med Assoc J 1960;82:187

764. de Torregrosa M, Rullan MM, Cecile C, et al. Am J Obstet Gynecol 1961;82:1375

765. Read HC, Brown F, Linins I, et al. Vox Sang 1961;6:362

766. Yokoyama M, Solomon JM, Kuniyuki M, et al. Transfusion 1961;1:273

767. Charlton M, Humphreys P, Linins I, et al. Transfusion 1963;3:100

768. Unger LJ. Transfusion 1964;4:173

769. Nakajima H, Misawa S, Ota K. Proc Jpn Acad 1965;41:488

770. Yamaguchi Y, Tanaka S, Tsuji Y, et al. Proc Jpn Acad 1965;41:493

771. Badakere SS, Bhatia HM. Vox Sang 1973;24:280

772. Reali G, Avanzi G, Ghinatti C. Transf Sangue 1975;20:81

773. Sagisaka K, Tanaka H, Ohno T, et al. Acta Schol Med Univ Gifu 1978;26:403

774. Kendrick L, Dunstan-Adams C, Humphreys J, et al. J Immunogenet 1981;8:243

775. Olafsdottir S, Jensson O, Thordarson G, et al. Foren Sci Int 1983;22:183

776. Hesse R, Gathof B, Hoffman B. (abstract). Book of Abstracts, 20th Cong ISBT, 1988:160

777. Yuying D. (abstract). Book of Abstracts, 20th Cong ISBT 1988:295

778. Skradski K, Sabo B, Daniels G. (Letter). Transfusion 1981;21:472

779. Gunson HH, Donohue WL. Vox Sang 1957;2:320

780. Moores P, Vaaja U, Smart E. Hum Hered 1991;41:295

781. Salmon C, Gerbal A, Liberge G, et al. Rev Fr Transf 1969;12:239

782. Henningsen K. Nature 1958;181:502

783. Ishimori T, Hasekura H. Proc Jpn Acad 1966;42:658

784. Ishimori T, Hasekura H. Transfusion 1967;7:84

785. Boettcher B. Vox Sang 1964;9:641

786. Sturgeon P. J Immunol 1952;68:277

787. Lawler SD, Marshall R. Vox Sang 1962;7:305

788. Hackel E. Vox Sang 1957;2:331

789. Moore BPL, Cornwall S, Crockford J. (abstract). Book of Abstracts, 14th Cong ISBT 1975:58

790. Tippett P. Rev Fr Transf Immunohematol 1978;21:135

791. Daniels GL, Gavin J, Tippett P. (abstract). Book of Abstracts, 15th Cong ISBT, 1978:439

792. Perrier P, Habibi B, Salmon C. Blood Transf Immunohematol 1981;23:327

793. Storry JR, Gorman M, Maddox NI, et al. Immunohematology 1994;10:130

794. Issitt PD. Immunohematology 1994;10:117

795. Moulds J. In: A Seminar on Recent Advances in Immunohematology. Washington, D.C.:Am Assoc Blood Banks, 1973:63

796. Bar-Shany S, Bastani A, Cuttner J, et al. (abstract). Transfusion 1967;7:389

797. Gibbs BJ, Moores P. Vox Sang 1983;45:83

798. Gabra GS, Bruce M, Watt A, et al. Vox Sang 1987;53:143

799. Lubenko A, Contreras M, Portugal CL, et al. Vox Sang 1992;63:43

800. Rosenfield RE. Personal communication 1978. Cited in previous editions of this book

801. Vogt E. Nordisk Med 1964;71:510

802. Race RR, Sanger R. Haematologia 1972;6:63

803. Habibi B, Lopez M, Salmon C. Vox Sang 1974;27:232

804. Muller A, Serger J, Garretta A, et al. Rev Fr Transf Immunohematol 1978;21:151

805. Salaru NNR, Lay WH. Vox Sang 1985;48:362

806. Jenkins WJ, Marsh WL. Transfusion 1965;5:6

807. Marsh WL, Chaganti RSK. Transfusion 1973;13:314

808. Dodd BE, Lincoln PJ, Insley J. Proc 10th Cong Int Soc Foren Haemogenet 1983:131

809. Northoff H, Goldman SF, Lattke H, et al. Vox Sang 1984;47:164

810. Tovey GH, Lockyer JW, Tierney RBH. Vox Sang 1961;6:628

811. Levan A, Nichols WW, Hall B, et al. Hereditas 1964;52:89

812. Mannoni P, Bracq C, Yvart J, et al. Nouv Rev Fr Hematol 1970;10:381

813. Callender ST, Key HEM, Lawler SD, et al. Br Med J 1971;1:131

814. Marsh WL, Chaganti RSK, Gardner FH, et al. Science 1974;183:966

815. Cooper B, Tishler PV, Atkins L, et al. Blood 1979;54:642

816. Grabowska et al. (no other details of authors given) cited by Koscielak J. Vox Sang 1980;39:289

817. van't Veer MB, van Wieringen PMV, van Leeuwen I, et al. Br J Haematol 1981;49:383

818. Bracey AW, McGinniss MH, Levine RM, et al. Am J Clin Pathol 1983;79:397

819. Mohandas K, Najfield V, Gilbert H, et al. Immunohematology 1994;10:134

820. Bryne M, Eide GE, Lilleng R, et al. Cancer 1991;68:1994

821. Bryne M, Thrane PS, Lilleng R, et al. Cancer 1991;68:2213

822. Májsky A. Neoplasma 1967;14:335

823. Garner RJ, Rembe AM, Landells M. (abstract). Transfusion 1980;20:619

824. Vos GH, Vos D, Kirk RL, et al. Lancet 1961;1:14

825. Boettcher B, Hasekura H. Vox Sang 1971;21:200

826. Boettcher B, Watts S. Vox Sang 1978;34:339

827. Ceppellini R. Unpublished observations. Cited by Levine P, Chambers JW, Celano MJ, et al. Bibl Haematol 1965;23:350

828. Henningsen K. Bibl Haematol 1959;10:567

829. Prokop O, Schneider W. Dtsch Z Gerlicht Med 1960;50:423

830. Broman B, Heiken A. Unpublished observations, 1962. Cited by Race RR, Sanger R. Blood Groups in Man, 6th Ed. Oxford:Blackwell, 1975

831. Wiener AS, Wexler IB. An Rh-Hr Syllabus, 2nd Ed. New York:Grune and Stratton, 1963

832. Heiken A, Rasmuson M. Hereditas 1966;55:192

833. Rasmuson M, Heiken A. Nature 1966;212:1377

834. Mourant AE, Kopec AC, Domanienska-Sobczak K. Blood Groups and Disease. Oxford:Oxford Univ Press, 1978

835. Newton RM, Buehler SK, Crumley J, et al. Vox Sang 1979;37:158

836. Levine P, Celano MJ, Falkowski F, et al. Nature 1964;204:892

837. Levine P, Chambers JW, Celano MJ, et al. Bibl Haematol 1965;23:350

838. Levine P, Celano MJ, Falkowski F, et al. Transfusion 1965;5:492

839. Seidl S, Spielmann W, Martin H. Vox Sang 1972;23:182

840. Agre P, Cartron J-P. Blood 1991;78:551

841. Senhauser DA, Mitchell MW, Gault DB, et al. Transfusion 1970;10:89

842. Polesky HF, Moulds J, Hanson M. (abstract). Prog 24th Ann Mtg AABB 1971:83

843. Hrubisko M, Fabryova L, Lipsic T, et al. (abstract). Book of Abstracts, 13th Cong ISBT 1972:15

844. Gomez Casal G, Poderos Baeta C, Romero Colas MS, et al. Rev Clin Espan 1983;171:19

845. Ballas SK, Clark MR, Mohandas M, et al. Blood 1984;63:1046

846. Naoki K, Uda M, Uchiyama E, et al. Transfusion 1984;24:182

847. Sistonen P, Palosuo T, Snellman A. Vox Sang 1985;48:174

848. Kishi K, Yasuda T, Uchida M. J Immunogenet 1987;14:261

849. Bates AJ, Poole J, Day V, et al. (abstract). Transf Med 1994;4(Suppl 1):45

850. Pérez-Pérez C, Taliano V, Mouro I, et al. Am J Hematol 1992;40:306

851. Sturgeon P. Blood 1970;36:310

852. Nagel V, Kneiphoff H, Pekkers S, et al. Vox Sang 1972;22:519

853. Weise W, Ballowitz L, Martin W. Blut 1981;43:243

854. Eveland DJ, Combs MR, Issitt PD. Unpublished observations, 1992

855. Issitt PD, Gutgsell NS, Bruce M. (abstract). Blood 1987;70(Suppl 1):110a

856. Chown B, Lewis M, Kaita H. Lancet 1971;1:396

857. Chown B, Lewis M, Kaita H, et al. Am J Hum Genet 1972;24:623

858. Harrison CR, Issitt PD, Brendel WL, et al. (abstract). Book of Abstracts, 18th Cong ISBT 1984:167

859. Saji H, Hosoi T. Vox Sang 1979;37:296

860. Stevenson MM, Anido V, Tanner AM, et al. Br Med J 1973;1:417

861. Yamaguchi H, Okubo Y, Tanaka M, et al. Proc Jpn Acad 1975;51:763

862. Wallace M, Steers F, Mora L, et al. (abstract). Transf Med 1994;4(Suppl 1):46

863. Schmidt PJ, Lostumbo MM, English CT, et al. Transfusion 1967;7:33

864. Bessis M. Corpuscles. Atlas of Red Cell Shapes. Berlin:Springer-Verlag, 1974

865. Schmidt PJ, Holland PV. Bibl Haematol 1971;38:230

866. Rosenfield RE. Personal communication 1972. Cited by Moulds JJ. In: A Seminar on Recent Advances in Immunohematology. Washington, D.C.:Am Assoc Blood Banks, 1973:63

867. Marsh WL. In: Blood Group Antigens and Disease. Arlington, VA:Am Assoc Blood Banks, 1983:165

868. Hasekura H, Ishimori T, Furusawa S, et al. Proc Jpn Acad 1971;47:579

869. Schmidt PJ, Vos GH. Vox Sang 1967;13:18

870. Polesky HF, Moulds J. (abstract). Book of Abstracts, 13th Cong ISBT 1972:16

871. Hillman RS, Giblett ER. J Clin Invest 1965;44:1730

872. Dacie JV, Lewis SM. Practical Haematology, 5th Ed. New York:Longman, 1975

873. Selwyn JG, Dacie JV. Blood 1954;9:414

874. Lauf P, Joiner CH. Blood 1976;48:457

875. Nash R, Shojania AM. Am J Hematol 1987;24:267

876. Issitt PD, Gutgsell NS, Knight JM, et al. (abstract). Transfusion 1987;27:547

877. Issitt PD. Transf Med Rev 1993;7:139

878. Dahr W, Kordowicz M, Moulds J, et al. Blut 1987;54:13

879. Dahr W, Issitt PD, Wren MR. (abstract). Transfusion 1986;26:560

880. Le Pennec PY, Rouger P, Klein MT, et al. (abstract). Book of Abstracts, Joint Cong ISBT/AABB 1990:29

881. Albrey JA, Vincent EER, Hutchinson J, et al. Vox Sang 1971;20:29

882. Colledge KI, Pezzulich M, Marsh WL. Vox Sang 1973;24:193

883. DiNapoli J, Garcia A, Marsh WL, et al. Vox Sang 1976;30:308

884. Chan-Shu SA. Transfusion 1980;20:358

885. Meredith LC. (abstract). Transfusion 1985;25:482

886. Vengelen-Tyler V. (abstract). Transfusion 1985;25:482

887. Bowen DT, Devenish A, Dalton J, et al. Vox Sang 1988;55:35

888. Mallinson G, Martin PG, Anstee DJ, et al. Biochem J 1986;234:649

889. Bloy C, Blanchard D, Hermand P, et al. Mol Immunol 1989;26:1013

890. Bloy C, Hermand P, Chérif-Zahar B, et al. Blood 1990;75:2245

891. Bloy C, Hermand P, Blanchard D, et al. J Biol Chem 1990;265:21482

892. Miller YE, Daniels GL, Jones C, et al. Am J Hum Genet 1987;41:1061

893. Avent ND, Judson PA, Parsons SF, et al. Biochem J 1988;251:499

894. Lindberg FP, Gresham HD, Schwarz E, et al. J Cell Biol 1993;123:485

895. Poss MT, Swanson JL, Telen MJ, et al. Vox Sang 1993;64:231

896. Lindberg FP, Lublin DM, Telen MJ, et al. J Biol Chem 1994;269:1567

897. Issitt PD, Gutgsell NS, Bonds SB, et al. (abstract). Transfusion 1988;28(Suppl 6S):20S

898. Anstee DJ, Tanner MJA. Baillières Clin Haematol 1993;6:401

899. Cartron J-P, Agre P. Sem Hematol 1993;30:193

900. Ikin EW, Mourant AE, Pugh VW. Vox Sang (Old Series) 1953;3:74

901. Moore S, Green C. Biochem J 1987;244:735

902. Avent ND, Ridgwell K, Mawby WJ, et al. Biochem J 1988;256:1043

903. Ridgwell K, Spurr NK, Laguda B, et al. Biochem J 1992;287:223

904. Chalmers JNM, Lawler SD. Ann Eugen 1953;17:267

905. Weitkamp LR, Guttormsen SA, Greendyke RM. Am J Hum Genet 1971;23:462

906. van Cong N, Billardon C, Picard JY, et al. Acad Sci Series D, Paris 1971;272:485

907. Westerveld A, Khan MP. Nature 1972;236:30

908. Ruddle FH, Riccuti F, McMorris FA, et al. Science 1972;176:1429

909. Moore S, Woodrow CF, McClelland DBL. Nature 1982;295:529

910. Turner JH, Crawford MH, Leyshon WC. J Hered 1975;66:97

911. Marsh WL, Chaganti RSK, German J, et al. Vox Sang 1974;27:190

912. Moroni G, Margstakler E, de Virgiliis G, et al. (abstract). Book of Abstracts, 15th Cong ISBT 1978:190

913. Cooper B. Blood 1979;54:642

914. Marsh WL, Johnson CL, DiNapoli J, et al. (abstract). Transfusion 1980;20:619

915. Moore S. In: Red Cell Membrane Glycoconjugates and Related Genetic Markers. Paris:Arnette, 1983:97

916. Muller A. (abstract). Book of Abstracts,. 15th Cong ISBT, 1978:418

917. Muller A. (abstract). Book of Abstracts,. 15th Cong ISBT, 1978:442

918. Chérif-Zahar B, Mattéi MG, Le Van Kim C, et al. Hum Genet 1991;86:398

919. MacGeoch C, Mitchell CJ, Carritt B, et al. Cytogenet Cell Genet 1992;59:261

920. Ridgwell K, Eyers SAC, Mawby WJ, et al. J Biol Chem 1994;269:6410

921. Eyers SAC, Ridgwell K, Mawby WJ, et al. J Biol Chem 1994;269:6417

922. Marsh WL. Med Lab Sci 1976;33:125

923. George S, Gidden M, LeNoir D. (abstract). Proc 23rd Ann Mtg, South Central Assoc Blood Banks, 1981

924. Spruell P. Personal communication, 1991

925. Murray S, Dewar PJ, Lee E, et al. Vox Sang 1976;30:91

926. Darke C. Tissue Antigens 1977;9:171

927. Brain P, Hammond MG. Eur J Immunol 1974;4:223

928. Darke C, Street J, Sargeant C, et al. Tissue Antigens 1983;21:333

929. Wojtulewicz-Kurkus J, Zupanska B, Podobinska I, et al. Arch Immunol Ther Exp 1981;29:447

930. Hors J, Dausset J, Gerbal A, et al. Haematologia 1974;8:217

931. Petranyi GG, Ivanyi P, Hollan SR. Vox Sang 1974;26:470

932. van Rood JJ, van Hooff JP, Keuning JJ. Transplt Rev 1975;22:75

933. Kruskall MS, Yunis EJ, Watson A, et al. Transfusion 1990;30:15

934. Hildén J-O, Gottvall T, Lindblom B. Tissue Antigens 1995;46:313

935. Hollister JM, Laing P, Mednick SA. Arch Gen Psychiat 1996;53:19

936. Bogerts B. In: Fetal Neural Development and Adult Schizophrenia. Cambridge:Cambrdige Univ Press, 1991:153

937. Welham JL, McGrath JJ, Pemberton MR. Schizophr Res 1993;9:142

938. Adams W, Kendell RE, Hare EH, et al. Br J Psychiatry 1993;163:522

939. Mendick SA, Huttunen MO, Machon RA. Schizophr Bull 1994;20:263

940. Raum DD, Awdeh ZL, Page PL, et al. J Immunol 1984;132:157

941. Young NT, Street J, Darke C. Exp Clin Immunogenet 1995;12:88

942. Combs MR. Unpublished observations, 1996

943. Daniels GL, Anstee DJ, Cartron JP, et al. Vox Sang 1996;71:246

944. Garratty G. Baillières Clin Haematol 1990;3:267

945. Garratty G. In: Immune Destruction of Red Blood Cells. Arlington, VA:Am Assoc Blood Banks, 1989:109

946. Rosse WF. (Editorial). New Eng J Med 1987;317:704

947. Green FA. Vox Sang 1965;10:32

948. Green FA. Immunochemistry 1967;4:247

949. Green FA. J Biol Chem 1972;247:881

950. Hughes-Jones NC, Green EJ, Hunt VAM. Vox Sang 1975;29:184

951. Kropp J, Weicker H. Z Immun Forsch 1975;150:267

952. Green FA, Hui HL, Green LAD, et al. Mol Immunol 1984;21:433

953. Basu MK, Flam M, Schachter D, et al. Biochem Biophys Res Comm 1980;95:887

954. de Vetten MP, Agre P. J Biol Chem 1988;263:18193

955. Hartel-Schenk S, Agre P. J Biol Chem 1992;267:5569

956. Abbott RE, Schachter D. J Biol Chem 1976;251:7176

957. Suyama K, Lunn R, Goldstein J. Transfusion 1995;35:653

958. Schmitz G, Sonneborn HH, Ernst M, et al. Vox Sang 1996;70:34

959. Lorusso DJ, Binette JP, Green FA. Immunochemistry 1977;14:503

960. Gahmberg CG. FEBS Lett 1982;140:93

961. Ridgwell K, Roberts SJ, Tanner MJA, et al. Biochem J 1983;213:267

962. Krahmer M, Prohaska R. FEBS Lett 1987;226:105

963. Bloy C, Blanchard D, Dahr W, et al. Blood 1988;72:661

964. Blanchard D, Bloy C, Hermand P, et al, Blood 1988;72:1424

965. Hughes-Jones NC, Bloy C, Gorick B, et al., Mol Immunol 1988;25:931

966. Abraham CV, Bakerman S. Clin Chim Acta 1975;60:33

967. Plapp FV, Kowalski MK, Tilzer L, et al. Proc Nat Acad Sci USA 1979;76: 2964

968. Victoria EJ, Mahan LC, Masouredis SP. Proc Nat Acad Sci USA 1981;78:2898

969. Booth PB, Serjeantson S, Woodfield DG, et al. Vox Sang 1977;32:99

970. Gahmberg CG. EMBO J 1983;2:223

971. Saboori AM, Smith BL, Agre P. Proc Nat Acad Sci USA 1988;85:4042

972. Saboori AM, Denker BM, Agre P. J Clin Invest 1989;83:187

973. Kuypers F, van Linde-Sibenius-Trip M, Roelofson B, et al. Biochem J 1984;221:931

974. Staufenbiel M. J Biol Chem 1988;263:13615

975. Suyama K, Goldstein J. Blood 1990;75:255

976. Suyama K, Goldstein J. Blood 1992;79:808

977. Suyama K, Goldstein J, Aebersold R, et al. Blood 1991;72:411

978. Hartmann E, Rapoport TA, Lodish HF. Proc Nat Acad Sci USA 1989;86:5786

979. Avent ND, Butcher SK, Liu W, et al. J Biol Chem 1992;267:15134

980. Hermand P, Mouro I, Huet M, et al. Blood 1993;82:669

981. Umenishi F, Kajii E, Ikemoto S. Biochem Biophys Res Comm 1994;198:1135

982. Umenishi F, Kajii E, Ikemoto S. Biochem J 1994;299:203

983. Cartron J-P, Le Van Kim C, Chérif-Zahar B, et al. Biochem J 1995;306:877

984. Ikemoto S, Umenishi F, Iwamoto S, et al. Biochem J 1995;309:695

985. Fukumori Y, Hori Y, Ohnoki S, et al. Transf Med in press 1997

986. Alexander S, Elder JH. Meth Enzymol 1982;79:505

987. Chérif-Zahar B, Le Van Kim C, Rouillac C, et al. Genomics 1994;19:68

988. Lighten AD, Overton TG, Sepulveda W, et al. Am J Obstet Gynecol 1995;173:1182

989. Huang C-H. Blood 1996;88:2326

990. Avent ND, Martin PG, Armstrong-Fisher SS, et al. Blood 1997;89:2568

991. Rouillac C, Gane P, Cartron J, et al. Blood 1996;87:4853

992. Beckers EAM. Doctoral Thesis,Univ of Amsterdam, 1997:131

993. Le Van Kim C, Chérif-Zahar B, Raynal V, et al. Blood 1992;80:1074

994. Suyama K, Roy S, Lunn R, et al. Blood 1993;82:1006

995. Suyama K, Lunn R, Haller S, et al. Blood 1994;84:1975
996. Smythe JS, Avent ND, Judson PA, et al. Blood 1996;87:2968
997. Avent ND, Liu W, Warner KM, et al. J Biol Chem 1996;271:14233
998. Faas BHW, Beckers EAM, Simsek S, et al. Transfusion 1996;36:506
999. Mouro I, Colin Y, Gane P, et al. Br J Haematol 1996;93:472
1000. Hyland CA, Wolter LC, Liew YW, et al. Blood 1994;83:566
1001. Chérif-Zahar B, Raynal V, D'Ambrosio A-M, et al. Blood 1994;84:4354
1002. Noizat-Pirenne F, Mouro I, Gane P, et al. Transf Clin Biol 1996;3:517
1003. Avent ND, Finning KM, Liu W, et al. Transf Clin Biol 1996;3:511
1004. Steers F, Wallace M, Johnson P, et al. Br J Haematol 1996;94:417
1005. Faas BHW, Beckers EAM, Wildoer P, et al. (abstract). Vox Sang 1996;70 (Suppl 2):73
1006. Cartron J-P. Transf Clin Biol 1996;3:491
1007. Avent ND, Liu W, Jones JW, et al. Blood 1997;89:1779
1008. Armstrong-Fisher SS, Todd DH, Moss M, et al. Transf Clin Biol 1996;3:505
1009. Huang C-H. (Letter). Blood 1997;89:1834
1010. Beckers EAM, Faas BHW, Ligthart P, et al. Transfusion 1996;36:567
1011. Beckers EAM, Faas BHW, Simsek S, et al. Br J Haematol 1996;93:720
1012. Avent ND, Jones JW, Liu W, et al. Br J Haematol 1997;97:366
1013. Cartron J-P, Rouillac C, Le Van Kim C, et al. Transf Clin Biol 1996;3:497
1014. Liu W, Smythe JS, Jones JW, et al. (abstract). Transf Clin Biol 1996;3:35s
1015. Chérif-Zahar B, Le Van Kim C, Raynal V, et al. Blood 1993;82:656
1016. Carritt B, Blunt T, Avent ND, et al. Ann Hum Genet 1993;57:273
1017. Spence WC, Maddalena A, Demers DB, et al. Transfusion 1994;34:741
1018. Bennett PH, Le Van Kim C, Colin Y, et al. New Eng J Med 1993;329:607
1019. Wolter LC, Hyland CA, Saul A. (Letter). Blood 1993;82:1682
1020. Simsek S, Bleeker PMM, von dem Borne AEGKr. (Letter). New Eng J Med 1994;330:795
1021. Simsek S, Faas BHW, Bleeker PMM, et al. Blood 1995;85:2975
1022. Hyland CA, Wolter LC, Saul A. Blood 1994;84:321
1023. Carritt B, Steers FJ, Avent ND.(Letter). Lancet 1994;344:204
1024. Bennett PH, Warwick R, Cartron J-P.(Letter). New Eng J Med 1994;330:795
1025. Pope J, Navarrete C, Warwick R, et al. (Letter). Lancet 1995;346:376
1026. Legler TJ, Maas JH, Lynen R, et al. (abstract). Vox Sang 1996;70 (Suppl 2):73
1027. Le Van Kim C, Mouro I, Brossard Y, et al. Br J Haematol 1994;88:193
1028. Lo Y-MD, Bowell PJ, Selinger M, et al. (Letter). Lancet 1993;341:1148
1029. Lo Y-MD, Noakes L, Bowell PJ, et al. Br J Haematol 1994;87:658
1030. Adinolfi M, Sherlock J, Kemp T, et al. Lancet 1995;345:318
1031. Cheung M-C, Goldberg JD, Kan YW. Nature Genet 1996;14:264
1032. Chérif-Zahar B, Raynal V, Gane P, et al. Nature Genet 1996;12:168
1033. Folkerd EJ, Ellory JC, Hughes-Jones NC. Immunochemistry 1977;14:529
1034. Wang DN, Kuhlbrandt W, Sarabia VE, et al. EMBO J 1993;12:2233
1035. Dahr W. In: Recent Advances in Blood Group Biochemistry. Arlington, VA:Am Assoc Blood Banks, 1986:23
1036. Mallinson G. PhD Thesis. Univ West England, 1995
1037. Anstee DJ, Holmes CH, Judson PA, et al. In: Protein Blood Group Antigens of the Human Red Cell. Baltimore:Johns Hopkins Univ Press, 1992:170
1038. Knapp W, Rieber P, Dorken B, et al. Immunol Today 1989;10:253
1039. Hadam MR. In: Leucocyte Typing, 4th Ed. Oxford:Oxford Univ Press, 1989:658
1040. Mawby WJ, Anstee DJ, Spring FA, et al. In: Leucocyte Typing 5, Vol 2. New York:Oxford Univ Press, 1991:1691
1041. Campbell IG, Freemont PS, Foulkes W, et al. Cancer Res 1992;52:5416
1042. Brown E, Hooper L, Ho T, et al. J Cell Biol 1990;111:2785
1043. Lindberg FP, Brown EJ. In: Leucocyte Typing 5, Vol 2. New York:Oxford Univ Press, 1991:1693
1044. Mawby WJ, Holmes CH, Anstee DJ, et al. Biochem J 1994;304:525
1045. Gavel Y, von Hejne G. Protein Eng 1990;3:433
1046. Reinhold MI, Lindberg FP, Plas D, et al. J Cell Sci 1995;108:3419
1047. Anstee DJ, Spring FA. Transf Med Rev 1989;3:13
1048. Cooper D, Lindberg FP, Gamble JR, et al. Proc Nat Acad Sci USA 1995;92:3978
1049. Parkos CA, Colgan SP, Liang TW, et al. J Cell Biol 1996;132:437
1050. Ticchioni M, Deckart M, Mary F, et al. J Immunol 1997;158:677
1051. Reinhold MI, Lindberg FP, Kersh GJ, et al. J Exp Med 1997;185:1
1052. Gao A, Lindberg FP, Plas D, et al. J Biol Chem 1996;271:21
1053. Lindberg FP, Bullard DC, Caver TE, et al. Science 1996;274:795
1054. Huang C-H, Reid ME, Chen Y. Blood 1995;86:784
1055. Chérif-Zahar B, Raynal V, Cartron J-P. (Letter) Blood 1996;88:1518
1056. Stewart GW. Baillières Clin Haematol 1993;6:371
1057. Connor J, Schroit AJ. Biochemistry 1988;27:848
1058. Schroit AJ, Bloy C, Connor J, et al. Biochemistry 1990;29:10303
1059. Smith RE, Daleke DL. Blood 1990;76:1021
1060. Bruckheimer EM, Gillum KD, Schroit AJ. Biochim Biophys Acta 1995;1235:147
1061. Gahmberg CG, Karhi KK . J Immunol 1984;133:334
1062. Ridgwell K, Tanner MJA, Anstee DJ. FEBS Lett 1984;174:7
1063. Paradis G, Bazin R, Lemieux R. J Immunol 1986;137:240
1064. Howard JC. Nature 1991;352:565
1065. Scott ML, Voak D, Jones JW, et al. Transf Clin Biol 1996;3:391
1066. Groves J, Tanner MJA. J Biol Chem 1992;267:22163
1067. Le Pennec PY, Klein MT, Le Besnerais M, et al. (abstract). Book of Abstracts, Joint Cong ISBT/AABB 1990:29
1068. Le Pennec PY, Klein MT, Le Besnerais M, et al. Rev Fr Transf Immunohematol 1988;31:123
1069. Leader KA, Kumpel BM, Hadley AG, et al. Immunology 1991;72:481

13 | The LW Blood Group System

When Landsteiner and Wiener (1,2) immunized guinea pigs and rabbits with rhesus monkey red cells, it appeared that the antibody that they raised had the same specificity as human anti-D. In spite of some discrepant findings, many years passed before the difference between the animal anti-rhesus and human anti-D was clearly demonstrated. Among the early contradictory findings, Fisk and Ford (3) reported that the red cells of all newborn infants were agglutinated by guinea pig anti-rhesus although they could be divided into D+ and D- using human anti-D. Murray and Clark (4) showed that human D- red cells would stimulate production of the same antibody in guinea pigs, as that made when rhesus monkey red cells were injected. The same workers (4) showed that human D- red cells would adsorb the guinea pig anti-rhesus to exhaustion, although they would not adsorb anti-D. In 1961, Levine et al. (5,6) published additional data illustrating a difference between the antigens recognized by the guinea pig anti-rhesus and by human anti-D. First, they confirmed that human D- red cells stimulate production of the animal anti-rhesus when injected into guinea pigs. Second, D+ red cells were coated with incomplete anti-D until they were no longer agglutinable by complete anti-D, that is, all available D sites blocked. The anti-D coated red cells were still agglutinated by the guinea pig anti-rhesus, ergo, the guinea pig anti-rhesus was not complexing with D. The antigen defined by the guinea pig anti-rhesus became known (5-9) as D-like.

In 1955, Race and Sanger (10) had studied antibodies made in two D+ ladies, that had anti-D-like specificity, but could be adsorbed by D- red cells. Later, it was shown that the red cells of one of the antibody-makers were non-reactive with the guinea pig anti-rhesus of Levine et al. (5). The cells of the other antibody-maker were not available for testing. Thus, it became appreciated that these were the first known examples of human antibodies with the same specificity as the guinea pig anti-rhesus. In spite of the name change from anti-rhesus to anti-D-like for the guinea pig antibody, confusion continued. The antigen defined was present on D+ and D- red cells, albeit in greater quantity on the former (5,6,11). As a way to resolve the difficulties, Levine (12) introduced the term anti-LW to replace anti-D-like. The LW was said to be in honor of Landsteiner and Wiener who, Levine (12) claimed, had discovered the antigen in their studies with rabbit and guinea pig anti-rhesus. The honor was never accepted by Wiener (13) for it followed that if Landsteiner and Wiener (1,2) had discovered LW, Levine

and Stetson (14) must have discovered Rh. Wiener (13) and Wiener et al. (15) continued to believe that the antibody raised in guinea pigs and rabbits contained anti-Rh$_0$. Although the many additional serological findings made after the term LW was introduced are described below, and although several different terminologies have been used, table 13-1 lists the currently used terms and ISBT numbers for antigens of the LW system. An explanation as to why the ISBT terms begin at LW5 and not LW1, is also given below.

The (now obsolete) LW$_1$ LW$_2$ LW$_3$ LW$_4$ and LW$_0$ Phenotypes

When anti-D-like was first renamed anti-LW, only one antibody in the system was known. Because anti-LW reacted more strongly with D+ than with D- red cells, when samples from adults were tested, D+ LW+ red cells were said (11) to be of the LW$_1$ phenotype, D- LW+ red cells were said to be LW$_2$. Those individuals who made anti-LW (whether D+ or D-) were said to have LW- red cells. The state of being LW- was seen almost always to be the result of the inheritance of two rare recessive genes. The gene that encoded production of LW was called *LW*, the gene present in double dose in persons with LW- red cells was called *lw*. Tippett (16,17) was the first investigator to demonstrate that the *LW* and *Rh* genes are at different loci, a key observation in the distinction between the LW and Rh systems. The genetic independence between *LW* and *Rh* has subsequently been demonstrated in other families (18-21).

TABLE 13-1 Conventional and ISBT Terminology for the LW Blood Group System

Conventional Name: LW			
ISBT System Symbol: LW			
ISBT System Number: 016			
Historical (now obsolete) Terms	**Antigen Conventional Name**	**ISBT Antigen Number**	**ISBT Full Code Number**
D-like, LW	LW^a	LW5	016005
	LW^{ab}	LW6	016006
Ne^a	LW^b	LW7	016007

That not all persons who made anti-LW had red cells of identical phenotype soon became apparent. While the red cells of some of the early found antibody-makers were mutually compatible (16,17,22,23), in 1971, deVeber et al. (18) and deVeber (19) described a woman who made an anti-LW that reacted, albeit less strongly than with LW+ red cells, with the red cells of other individuals who had made anti-LW. The red cells of Mrs. Big, the lady described by deVeber (18,19) were non-reactive with all other examples of anti-LW. It was suggested (20,24) that those individuals who had made anti-LW yet whose red cells reacted with the serum of Mrs. Big, be said to be phenotypically LW_3 while Mrs. Big herself, be described as LW_4. As discussed in detail in the next section, persons originally described as being of the LW_3 phenotype are now recognized as being phenotypically LW(a-b+) and are able to make alloimmune anti-LW^a. Those originally called LW_4 are LW(a-b-) and are able to make alloimmune anti-LW^{ab}. In the older studies, Mrs. Big's anti-LW was used to differentiate between the LW_3 and LW_4 phenotypes. In more recent studies anti-LW^b has been used when available. While it would appear that LW_3 people can make anti-LW^a while LW_4 people can make anti-LW^{ab}, that difference cannot be used to distinguish the LW_3 and LW_4 phenotypes. As described below, some individuals who are genetically LW+ (i.e. LW_1 or LW_2) have been seen to have depressed expression of red cell antigen expression with concomitant production of either anti-LW^a or anti-LW^{ab}. When the (sometimes presumed) transient LW depression cases are excluded, it is seen that both types of genetic "LW-" are rare but that the one previously called LW_3 is more common (20-23,25,28,29) than the one previously called LW_4 (18,59).

As described in Chapter 12, all Rh_{null} red cells are LW- (in fact LW(a-b-), see next section) although all Rh_{null} persons must surely have *LW* genes. When the designations LW_1 LW_2 LW_3 and LW_4 were in use, Rh_{null} red cells were said (27) to be LW_o.

The Antigens LW^a and LW^b

In 1981, Sistonen et al. (35) described a low incidence antigen, that was initially named Ne^a. As described below, the discovery of Ne^a eventually brought order to the somewhat chaotic nomenclature for the LW system. The Ne(a+) phenotype was seen in a little under 6% of random Finns, in nearly 8% of 800 Estonians, in about 4% of Polish people living in Poland and in the USA (slightly higher in the former than in the latter) and in 3% of the Komi population (35,42). In tests on samples from Hungarian, Swiss and Belgian people, Ne^a was seen to have an incidence of less than 1%. The *Ne^a* gene

was shown to segregate independently of the *Rh* locus. Later in 1981, Sistonen (36) described a number of analogies between Ne^a and LW. First, the Ne^a antigen was found to be stronger on D+ than on D- red cells, when samples from adults were tested. Second, when cord blood Ne(a+) samples were tested, no difference in strength of Ne^a on D+ and D- red cells was seen. Third, like LW, expression of Ne^a was not influenced by presence or absence of C or E. Because of these similarities further studies were conducted and in 1982, Sistonen and Tippett (37,38) presented findings that definitively established the antithetical nature of Ne^a to LW, and the allelic nature of the genes that encode the antigens. Tests on families of four LW_3 propositi from the USA, Canada and Great Britain showed that all eight LW_3 individuals had Ne(a+) red cells. Further, the Ne^a antigen was found on the red cells of all the parents and children of the eight LW_3 people who were available for testing. Among 10,025 selected Finnish Rh+ blood donors, 11 (0.1%) were found to be LW_3, all were Ne(a+). A further 1000 Finnish blood donors were typed for Ne^a and LW: one was found to be Ne(a+) LW-; 60 were Ne(a+) LW+; 939 were Ne(a-),LW+.

Based on the findings of Sistonen and Tippett (37,38) and Sistonen et al. (50) LW was renamed LW^a and Ne^a became LW^b. The new terminology is shown in table 13-2. As can be seen the old LW_1 and LW_2 phenotypes can represent either LW(a+b-) or LW(a+b+). While the former will be much more common than the latter, distinction between them cannot be made unless anti-LW^b is available. The old LW_3 phenotype was seen to represent LW(a-b+) and the LW system alloantibody made by such persons was seen to be anti-LW^a. The former LW_4 phenotype was seen to be LW(a-b-) when the red cells of Mrs. Big, that were already known to be LW(a-) (i.e. LW-), were shown (38) to be non-reactive with anti-LW^b (i.e. Ne(a-)). The antibody made by persons of the LW(a-b-) phenotype reacts as if it is anti-LW^a plus anti-LW^b in an inseparable form, it is usually called anti-LW^{ab}.

As will be seen from table 13-2, it is suggested that the LW(a-b-) phenotype results from the inheritance of silent alleles (now called *LW* instead of *lw*) at the *LW* locus. Because of that suggestion the genotypes *LW^aLW* and *LW^bLW* are shown as possible rare alternatives to the much more likely *LW^aLW^a* and *LW^bLW^b* genotypes, to explain the LW(a+b-) and LW(a-b+) phenotypes, respectively. Sistonen and Tippett (38) pointed out that, based on family data, the LW(a-b-) phenotype could be equally well explained by postulating existence of a silent allele *LW* or by postulating that recessive suppressor genes were responsible for the phenotype. As discussed in more detail in the sections dealing with the molecular biology of LW, Hermand et al. (65) have now shown that two apparently normal *LW^a* genes are present in persons

TABLE 13-2 The LW System Updated to Include LW^b(Ne^a) (From Sistonen and Tippett (38))

Old Terms				New Terms	
Phenotype	Genotype			Phenotype	Genotype
LW+ or LW$_1$ (i.e. D+, LW+)	*LWLW or LWlw*	} Each can be either, see footnote 1 {		LW(a+b-)	*LW^{a}LW^a or LW^{a}LW*
LW+ or LW$_2$ (i.e. D-, LW+)	*LWLW or LWlw*			LW(a+b+)	*LW^{a}LW^b*
LW$_3$	*lwlw*			LW(a-b+)	*LW^{b}LW^b or LW^{b}LW*
LW$_4$	*lwlw*			LW(a-b-)	*LWLW*
Rh$_{null}$(LW$_0$)	See footnote 2			LW(a-b-)	See footnote 2

1. The old terms for LW+ (LW$_1$ and LW$_2$) can each represent either of the new terms LW(a+b-) or LW(a+b+). Differentiation cannot be made until the LW^b (Ne^a) status of the LW+ (LW(a+)) cells is known.
2. Most persons of the Rh$_{null}$ phenotype will be genetically *LW^{a}LW^a* (because of the high frequency of *LW^a* and the low frequencies of *LW^b* and *LW*). Their LW(a-b-) status is caused by suppressor (*X^{o}rX^{o}r*) genes not at the *CDE* locus, or silent alleles ($\overline{\overline{r}}\,\overline{\overline{r}}$) at the *CDE* locus.

of the LW(a-b-) phenotype although, clearly, LW^a is not expressed at the phenotypic level.

As discussed in Chapter 12, Rh$_{null}$ red cells of both the modifier (*X^{o}rX^{o}r*) and silent allele ($\overline{rr}$) type are LW(a-b-) (8,39). Clearly, the LW(a-b-) status of Rh$_{null}$ individuals could not represent the inheritance of two silent *LW* alleles. Family studies had strongly suggested that all Rh$_{null}$ individuals have *LW* (usually two *LW^a*) genes, that suggestion has now been confirmed at the molecular level (65). The Rh antigens on the red cells of Mrs. Big and on those of her LW(a-b-) brother, are normally expressed (18,38). As discussed in a later section of this chapter, it seems that the LW antigen-bearing glycoprotein cannot be incorporated into the red cell membrane in the absence of Rh antigen-bearing structures.

Findings that do not fit quite so well with the conclusions listed in table 13-2 involve (perhaps fittingly given the history of the discovery of the LW system) animal immunization experiments. When Polesky et al. (40) injected LW$_3$ (presumably LW(a-b+)) red cells into guinea pigs, the antibody raised appeared to have the same specificity as the animal anti-rhesus described in the introduction to this chapter. Obviously, production of anti-LW^a would not have been expected. Second, when Vos et al. (41) injected LW$_4$ (presumably LW(a-b-)) red cells into guinea pigs, the same antibody was made. Perhaps these findings simply mean that apparently negative red cells carry an antigen defective glycoprotein that is still immunogenic in animals and stimulates production of an antibody that can then react with antigen-bearing LW glycoprotein. Perhaps such a concept is supported by the finding (41) that when Rh$_{null}$ red cells were injected into animals, no anti-rhesus (anti-LW) was made.

In concluding this section of the chapter it can be said that when LW^a, LW^{ab} and LW^b were assigned ISBT numbers (see table 13-1) the terms LW1 LW2 LW3 and LW4 were avoided to prevent confusion with the phenotype designations with those numbers, that had been used in the past. Thus the LW and Gerbich (see Chapter 16) systems are the only ones whose first antigen is not number 1.

Development of the LW Antigens

As described above, when red cells from adults are tested with animal anti-LW and with some examples of human anti-LW^a and anti-LW^b, those that are D+ LW(a+) or LW(b+) react more strongly than do those that are D- LW(a+) or LW(b+). This distinction is not seen when blood samples from newborn infants are tested, that is to say the cells react equally with anti-LW^a or anti-LW^b, regardless of their D type. As would be expected from such observations, the LW^a, LW^b and LW^{ab} antigens are well developed at birth. Cord red blood cells carry more LW^{ab} antigen sites than do the red cells of adults of the same D type (48). When the level of LW^a on red cells is measured by titration with animal anti-LW^a, the amount on cord blood red cells is highest and the level on subsequently produced red cells gradually declines until the level seen on the red cells of adults is reached at about five years of life (23). In spite of the high levels of LW system antigens on the red cells of newborn infants, there are no documented cases of severe HDN caused by LW system antibodies.

Influence of Rh Phenotype on Expression of the LW Antigens

As already described, expression of LW^a, LW^{ab} and LW^b on red cells is profoundly affected by the presence or absence of D. In contrast, expression of those antigens does not seem to be influenced by the presence or absence of C, c, E or e, nor by zygosity of *D* (23). Expression of

LW^a is related not only to presence or absence of D, but to the amount of D expressed. Gibbs (43) showed that R$_2$R$_2$ red cells react more strongly with anti-LW^a than do cells that are R$_2$r. In turn, the R$_2$r red cells reacted more strongly than those that were R$_1$r. In these experiments, expression of LW^a clearly paralleled expression of D. Somewhat similarly, Swanson et al. (23) showed that the expression of LW^a on weak D (formerly D^u) red cells was similar to that on D- red cells. All these variations in expression of LW^a are more easily demonstrable with animal anti-LW^a than with human antibodies.

Identification of LW System Antibodies and Dosage Effects

Because LW^a is more strongly expressed on D+ than on D- red cells from adults, a weak example of anti-LW^a might be mistaken for anti-D (see table 13-3). Clearly, adsorption studies will allow differentiation. Although both weak anti-LW^a and anti-D may give visible reactions only with D+ red cells, anti-LW^a but not anti-D will be adsorbed by D- red cells. An additional method of differentiation is to test the antibody in question against D+ and D- cord blood red cells. While anti-D will react only with the D+ samples, anti-LW^a may react also with the D- red cells. However, it should be borne in mind that not all human anti-LW^a react with D- cord blood red cells.

TABLE 13-3 To Show Ostensible Similarities Between Weak Anti-LW^a and Anti-D

Test Red Cells from Adults	Visible Reactions of		
	Anti-D	Weak Anti-LW^a	Stronger Anti-LW^a
D+, LW(a+)	4+	1- 2+	2- 3+
D-, LW(a+)	0^{*1}	0^{*2}	1- 2+

*1   Red cells fail to react with or adsorb the antibody
*2   Red cells fail to react visibly but will adsorb the antibody to exhaustion

While the LW system antigens are not destroyed when red cells are treated with papain, ficin, trypsin or chymotrypsin, they are said to be denatured when red cells are treated with pronase (44). However, one of us (PDI) has not always been able to accomplish this and has heard anecdotal reports of others experiencing similar failures. Further, Green (45) has reported that all normal plasma and serum samples agglutinate pronase-treated red cells thus limiting the use of such cells in antibody identification studies. Treatment of red cells with dithiothreitol (DTT) or 2-aminoethylisothiouroni-

um bromide (AET) reduces or destroys LW^a and LW^{ab} antigen activity (46,47), treatment with neuraminidase has no effect on those antigens (47). While one group of investigators (48) reported that treatment of red cells with endoglycosidase-F destroyed their ability to react with a monoclonal anti-LW^{ab}, another group (49) did not find that to be the case. Clearly, some care is needed in the use of chemically-modified red cells for the identification of LW system antibodies.

In one family, we (25) were able to demonstrate a dosage effect when using anti-LW^a. The red cells of a D- parent of an LW$_3$ individual (the parent was presumably of the genotype LW^aLW^b) typed as LW(a-) in direct typing tests and could only be shown to be LW(a+) by the use of adsorption-elution studies. However, this finding seems to be the exception rather than the rule. In studying other families or obligate LW^a or LW^b heterozygotes, gene dosage effects have not been clearly (or at all) demonstrable (23,27,38,50). Certainly, presence or absence of D has a far more profound effect on LW^a, LW^{ab} and LW^b antigen expression than does zygosity of LW^a or LW^b.

Transient Production of Anti-LW^a

There are, in the literature, a considerable number of reports (26,27,31,51-56) that describe a transient reduction of expression of red cell LW system antigens, often to the point where the antibody-maker's red cells typed as LW(a-b-ab+) or LW(a-b-ab-) and the concomitant production of anti-LW^a or anti-LW^{ab}. In one case (50) transient depression of LW^b appeared to have occurred. Differentiation between the transient LW(a-b-ab+) and LW(a-b-ab-) states is somewhat dependent on the potency of the LW system antibodies available to test the patient's red cells.

In some instances, depression of antigen expression has been associated with an acute phase of a disease such as leukemia, lymphoma, sarcoma or Hodgkin's disease and remission, at least from the acute phase, has been associated with a return to normal (or near normal) expression of LW antigens. While this phenomenon has been seen in some seriously ill patients, there is no one disease or group of diseases with which it is most commonly associated. In a few cases, no disease state existed. As described below, the transient production of anti-LW^a has sometimes preceded the production of anti-D, by pregnant women. Daniels (57) points out that there is at least a partial reciprocal relationship between antigen loss and specificity of the antibody made. Individuals whose red cells type as LW(a-b-ab+) tend to make anti-LW^a while those whose red cells are depressed to the LW(a-b-ab-) phenotype tend to make anti-LW^{ab}.

However, intermediate examples are seen, perhaps related to the comment above, about measurement of antigen depression being influenced in part by the potency of the LW system antibodies available to test the red cells of the patients involved.

As discussed in the section on the clinical significance of LW system antibodies, none of those made by persons with transiently depressed red cell LW antigens has ever been seen to cause accelerated red cell destruction in vivo. In some instances, partial antigen suppression or concomitant production of antibody while the red cell antigen level was returning to normal, has resulted in the DAT being positive. In some such situations, anti-LW^a or anti-LW^{ab} has been recovered by elution from the patient's red cells. Again, in spite of these findings, appreciable red cell destruction by the antibodies has not been seen.

Does the Production of Anti-LW Sometimes Precede the Production of Anti-D?

A phenomenon perhaps associated with the transient production of anti-LW^a and anti-LW^{ab} involves the production of one of those antibodies as a prelude to the production of anti-D. When prenatal antibody screening studies were done, before RhIG was introduced and when immunization to D via pregnancy was fairly common, it was not particularly unusual to find a serum that reacted weakly with all red cells tested, especially if tests against enzyme-treated red cells were used. If women producing such antibodies were followed, it was seen that some of them later made anti-D. The early produced antibodies sometimes failed to react with Rh$_{null}$ red cells. In considering this generalization a number of points need to be made. First, not all women in whom the early antibodies were seen, went on to make anti-D. Second, while anti-LW specificity was suspected, it was not proved. Third, those individuals described in the previous section, who transiently made anti-LW^a or anti-LW^{ab} did not all go on to make anti-D. Nevertheless, some better documented findings described below, leave the impression that, at least in some cases, the initial response to D involves production of a wide specificity that may be related to LW. In the cases studied, the early produced antibody often reacted with the antibody-maker's own red cells but was always benign in vivo.

In the second publication reporting transient depression of LW antigen expression and concomitant production of anti-LW, Chown et al. (52) described three individuals in whom this occurred. Two of the three were D- and made anti-D, production of which was not transient. In 1971, Cook (58) reported results from a program in which male, D- volunteers, were injected with D+ red cells so that they would make anti-D that could then be used in the preparation of RhIG. Among 18 who produced antibody, 15 made anti-D, three made anti-D and a second antibody that reacted with all except Rh$_{null}$ red cells; LW$_3$ and LW$_4$ red cells were not tested. An antibody made in a different male who also made anti-D and was also part of a deliberate immunization program, was tested with appropriate red cells and was shown, by Napier and Rowe (30), indeed to have anti-LW^a specificity. Among those individuals described in the previous section, whose red cells had transient depression of LW antigen expression, at least one in addition to those already mentioned, made anti-D (51).

While the phenomenon that seems sometimes to involve the production of anti-LW as a prelude to the production of anti-D is not fully understood, it is possible to speculate. As discussed in Chapter 2, early released antibody molecules from clones of recently activated B cells, may be of poor fit. As subsequent generations of B cells are formed, antibody molecules of better fit (higher affinity) are synthesized. Perhaps the initial antibody made, when D is the foreign immunogen, can complex with LW, including the LW on the patient's own red cells. Perhaps as better (higher affinity) anti-D is made, it can no longer complex with D- LW+ cells. It can be speculated that in those individuals in whom anti-LW is transiently made and anti-D permanently synthesized, the early activated B cell clones are no longer functional. It can also be speculated that in those patients in whom alloimmune anti-D and autoreactive anti-LW are seen, the early stimulated clones of B cells continue to make antibody even after later developed clones are making higher affinity anti-D. Perhaps (and this simply stretches the speculation an additional step) the benign auto-anti-D sometimes seen in individuals with D+ red cells who eventually make allo-anti-D (see Chapter 12), is intermediate between auto-anti-LW and allo-anti-D. A somewhat parallel suggestion has been made (60,61) that production of auto-anti-Rh39 sometimes precedes the production of allo-anti-C.

Chown et al. (52) suggested that the phenomenon of transient production of a benign autoantibody as a prelude to the production of an alloantibody, may be more common than is generally supposed. In considering such a suggestion and the speculative mechanism suggested above, it should be remembered that production of an autoantibody of poor fit may take place only for a short period of time during the primary response. Thus, unless a blood sample happens to be drawn at an opportune time, the phenomenon may not be noticed at all. Perhaps, as suggested, it is most often seen when production of the early made autoantibody of poor fit is not shut down.

Monoclonal LW System Antibodies

At least four monoclonal anti-LW^{ab} have been produced (62-64). Three of the four reacted more strongly with D+ LW(a+) than with D- LW(a+) red cells (63,64), one of the four reacted with LW(a-b+) red cells only after those cells had been treated with papain (64). Shaw (65) used monoclonal anti-LW^{ab} and anti-D and the red cells of non-human primates to show that a series of different epitopes are recognized; somewhat similarly blocking experiments using human red cells were used to confirm that the LW and D determinants are different (63). As described later in this chapter, monoclonal anti-LW^{ab} was instrumental in the isolation of the red cell glycoprotein that carries LW^a, LW^b and LW^{ab}. That glycoprotein has been well characterized and the basis of the LW^a, LW^b polymorphism has been established (65), for details see below.

Immunoglobulin Types and Lack of Clinical Significance of LW System Antibodies

In the section describing LW system antibodies produced in individuals in whom red cell LW antigen expression is depressed, it is mentioned that none of those antibodies has ever caused accelerated red cell clearance in vivo. Some of the cases have been dramatic in their lack of clinical relevance of the antibodies. Tregellas et al. (26) transfused over 50 units of D- LW(a+) blood to a patient of this type, who had made anti-LW^a, without seeing any evidence of red cell destruction or any appreciable change in the level of anti-LW^a made. Devenish (31) transfused a 10 month-old child with D- LW(a+) blood, the anti-LW^a in the child's serum appeared not to cause any red cell destruction.

Alloantibodies made by persons genetically LW(a-b+) or LW(a-b-) seem usually also to be benign in vivo. Cummings et al. (28) transfused 7 units of D- LW(a+) blood to a patient who appeared to be genetically LW(a-) and who had made anti-LW^a. Although two different transfusion episodes were involved, the first did not appear to stimulate increased production of anti-LW^a since neither episode resulted in a transfusion reaction or any signs that in vivo red cell survival of the transfused cells was other than normal. A similar case was reported by Chaplin et al. (29) in which two units of D- LW(a+) blood were successfully transfused.

In some cases described in the literature, in which transfusions were given, it was not clear whether the anti-LW^a had been made during transient antigen depression or by a patient genetically antigen negative. The outcomes of those transfusions were similar to those described above. For example, Johnson et al. (33) described a patient who

had made antibodies to c, E, K and LW^{ab}. Because of the patient's immunization to c, D- LW(a+) blood could not be transfused. The patient, who had transfusion-dependent myelodysplasia, was transfused several times with D+ LW(a+) blood and on each occasion attained the expected increase in hematocrit that was maintained, showing that neither immediate nor delayed in vivo red cell destruction occurred.

In a few cases (30,32,34) in vivo red cell survival studies using ^{51}Cr labeled LW(a+) red cells and/or in vitro phagocytic cell assays (e.g. MMA) have suggested that the LW system antibody present might have limited ability to clear antigen positive red cells. However, in these cases, transfusions with LW(a+) blood were not given so that firm conclusions cannot be drawn. This is particularly true since in some of the cases in which LW(a+) blood was successfully transfused, ^{51}Cr survival studies and/or an MMA, had given similar suggestive findings (28,29). In one case involving anti-LW^{ab} (34), autologous transfusion was used because the MMA gave a result that suggested that some in vivo red cell destruction might occur. There are, of course, many good reasons to use autologous transfusion, that have nothing to do with the presence of anti-LW^{ab}. The first described example of anti-LW^b was described (38) as clearing LW(b+) red cells in an in vivo red cell survival study. Finding LW(b-) blood for a patient with anti-LW^b is, of course, very easy.

In spite of the apparently benign nature of most examples of LW system antibodies, many of them appear to be IgG in composition. IgG1 was the predominant constituent in three examples (28,30,54), another was a mixture of IgG and IgM (22) while still another was apparently just IgM (16). The two anti-LW^{ab} that were most efficient in clearing a small dose of ^{51}Cr-labeled LW(a+) red cells and that gave the strongest positive reactions in MMAs, were IgG3 in composition (32,34). Perhaps those two examples were more likely to have some clinical significance than the others described. The anti-LW^{ab} of Mrs. Big, when present in its highest level, caused only a 1+ DAT and a peak bilirubin level of 8.6 mg/100 ml, at two days of life, in her third child, who had D- red cells (18). Following a later pregnancy, Mrs. Big delivered twins. Both daughters had D+ red cells, in both the DAT was 3+ at birth and moderate anemia developed. However, neither twin needed any treatment other than phototherapy (19).

In tests using a low ionic polybrene method in the AutoAnalyzer, Perrault (66) found 10 examples of cold-reactive auto-anti-LW in tests on some 45,000 samples. Two of the antibodies were IgG, one IgM and the other seven were thought to be IgG. As expected from the fact that these autoantibodies were reactive only at 18° C, their presence was not associated with any pathological condition. These autoantibodies clearly differed from those that are active at 37°C and are found in patients with "warm" antibody-induced hemolytic anemia (12,41,67). Pathological auto-anti-LW are described in detail in Chapter 37.

The moral to be drawn from the story presented in this section seems to be to regard LW system alloantibodies (including those produced while red cell LW antigen expression is depressed) as innocent until proved guilty. Certainly there seems to be no justification for withholding necessary transfusions because a patient's serum contains anti-LW[a] or anti-LW[ab] and no antigen negative blood is available. The use of D- LW(a+) blood has always resulted in a satisfactory outcome to transfusion; based on the patient described by Johnson et al. (33) even the use of D- blood may represent overkill. While there are suggestive findings that a few examples of anti-LW[ab] may be clinically-significant (32,34) it should be remembered that the data are only suggestive, no antibody in the LW system has yet caused a transfusion reaction or HDN requiring transfusion. The usual characteristics of LW system antibodies are summarized in table 13-4.

The *LW* Locus and Chromosome 19

Sistonen (68) showed that the *LW* blood group locus is part of a linkage group on chromosome 19, an observation later confirmed, independently, by others (65,69). Other loci that reside on chromosome 19 and are also of interest to blood bankers are *Lu* (*Lutheran*, see Chapter 20), *Le* (*Lewis* or *FUT3*, see Chapter 9), *H* (*FUT1*, see Chapter 8), *Se* (*FUT2*, also see Chapter 8), *C3* (third component of complement, see Chapter 6) and *Ok* (see Ok[a] antigen, Chapter 31).

LW Antigens Are Located on a Novel Protein Which Is Homologous to Intercellular Adhesion Molecules (ICAMs)

The red cell membrane component carrying the LW antigens was first identified by Moore (70) who immunoprecipitated a component of apparent molecular weight 40,000 from radioiodinated LW(a+b-) red cells using human anti-LW[ab] serum (Big.). This experiment demonstrated that the LW antigens are located on a completely different molecule from those that are associated with D. Mallinson et al. (48) confirmed these findings in immunoblotting experiments with murine monoclonal anti-LW[ab] BS46 and BS56 that had been described earlier by Sonneborn et al. (63). In the immunoblotting experiments the LW component appeared as a diffuse band of 40,000-47,000kD which was sharper on blots of membranes from sialidase-treated red cells suggesting that the molecule was glycosylated. When immunoblots were carried out under reducing conditions the LW reactive bands were much weaker than in comparable experiments carried out under non-reducing conditions suggesting that the molecule is a protein containing intrachain disulphide bonds. The presence of intrachain disulphide bonds was also suggested by the previous studies of Konighaus and Holland (46) who reported that treatment of intact red cells with 100mM dithiothreitol (30 minutes at 37°C) destroyed LW antigen activity. Immunoblotting experiments with BS46 and BS56 on red cell membranes of phenotype Rh$_{null}$ and LW(a-b-) or on membranes from pronase-treated red cells of common LW type did not reveal any bands. Evidence was also presented that Endo F treatment of red cells resulted in the loss of the LW[ab] epitope(s) recognized by the monoclonal antibodies suggesting that the molecule contained one or more N-glycans. Subsequent studies (71,91) carried out with highly purified enzyme preparations showed that the molecule

TABLE 13-4 Usual Characteristics of LW System Antibodies

Antibody Specificity	Positive Reactions in In Vitro Tests				Usual Immunoglobulin		Ability to Bind Complement		Ability to Cause In Vitro Lysis		Implicated in		Usual Form of Stimulation		% of White Population Positive
	Sal	LISS	AHG	Enz	IgG	IgM	Yes	No	Yes	No	Transfusion Reaction	HDN	Red Cells	Other	
Anti-LW[a]	X	X	V	X		X		X		X	No	No*	X	Rare	>99
Anti-LW[b]	X	X	V	X		X		X		X	No	No*			<1
Anti-LW[ab]	X	X	V	X		X		X		X	No	No*	X		Almost 100

V = variable, see text.

* = no clinical disease.

contains N-glycans since the apparent molecular weight
was reduced after enzyme treatment but did not confirm
that the LW antigens were susceptible to N-glycanase. It
seems likely that the relatively crude Endo F preparation
initially used (48) may have had some residual protease
activity. Bloy et al. (91) reported that N-glycanase treatment reduced the Mr of the LW glycoprotein by 17kD
and that O-glycanase treatment reduced the Mr by 2kD.
Mallinson (71) found that the LW glycoprotein is rather
resistant to digestion with purified N-glycanase or purified Endo F and reported that when membranes from
enzyme-treated cells were examined on tricine gels, two
bands of Mr 42,000 and 39,000 in addition to a band corresponding to undigested glycoprotein of Mr 45-48,000
were observed. These results suggest the presence of at
least two N-glycans, each of Mr approximately 3,000 on
LW glycoprotein. In summary, these early results demonstrated that the LW antigens are carried on a glycoprotein
with at least two N-glycans and one or two O-glycans,
that contains intrachain bonds and is distinct from the
molecules expressing Rh antigens.

Quantitative binding assays using radioiodinated
BS46 indicated that the LW glycoprotein is a molecule of
low abundance in the red cell membrane. Mallinson et al.
(48) reported 4400 BS46 epitopes on R_2R_2 red cells and
2835 on rr red cells. When trypsin-treated cord red blood
cells were examined (LW antigens are trypsin-resistant)
D+ cord cells bound 5150 molecules of BS46 in comparison with 3620 molecules on D- cord cells. Trypsin treated Rh_{null} cells bound only 380 molecules and this probably represents "background" rather than specific binding.
Similar binding assays using Fab fragments of monoclonal anti-LW have not been reported. In other systems
(e.g. MN (93), Kell (94) and Indian (95)) it has often been
observed that Fab fragments give higher values (commonly 2-fold higher) than IgG presumably because of
problems with steric hindrance (one bound IgG molecule
obscuring access of another to an epitope situated nearby
on the membrane). The numbers noted above for LW
should therefore be treated as minimum values.

Bloy et al. (49) made the observation that if red cells
are incubated in the presence of EDTA, LW antigen
expression appears reduced and that reactivity can be
restored by reincubating the cells in the presence of Mg^{++}
but not Ca^{++} or Mn^{++} suggesting that bound Mg^{++} are
necessary for antigen activity. These observations were
confirmed by Mallinson (71) who noted some variability
in the effect with the reduction of activity being much
more marked with a human anti-LW[a] in comparison with
human anti-LW[b], anti-LW[ab] and monoclonal anti-LW[ab].

Bloy et al. (49) reported that the C-terminus of LW
glycoprotein was extracellular on the basis of experiments in which radiolabeled red cells and right-side-out
red cell membrane vesicles, treated with 50 units/ml car-

boxypeptidase Y for 18 hours at 22°C were shown to lose
label from the LW glycoprotein. Subsequent studies
described in detail below, have indicated that the C-terminus is cytoplasmic and it seems likely that the carboxypeptidase preparation used in these experiments
was contaminated with protease which degraded the LW
glycoprotein under the prolonged incubation conditions
used (96). Protease contamination is a known problem
with carboxypeptidase preparations.

In 1994 two groups (72,73) reported that the LW glycoprotein had structural features which suggested that it
was a novel member of the family of intercellular adhesion molecules (ICAMs). The groups used almost identical strategies. LW glycoprotein was purified from detergent solubilized red cell membranes by affinity chromatography on a monoclonal anti-LW[ab] column. The
purified protein and tryptic/Lys-C peptides were subjected to protein sequencing. Suitable peptide sequences
were used to generate synthetic oligonucleotide probes
that were then used to generate a partial cDNA from
mRNA by reverse transcription PCR. Anstee and
Mallinson (72) reported the isolation of a partial cDNA
clone of 248bp which corresponded to almost an entire
immunoglobulin-like C2 set domain. The predicted
domain showed remarkable homology with the N-terminal domains of ICAMs 1, 2 and 3. In particular, four cysteine residues that are conserved in the first C2 set
domain of ICAMs 1, 2 and 3 were also found in the LW
domain. Bailly et al. (73) used an almost identical partial
cDNA (245bp) to isolate a full length cDNA clone from
a human bone marrow cDNA library. The isolate predicted a protein of 241 residues consisting of an extracellular domain of 208 amino acids comprising two
immunoglobulin-like C2 set domains, a single membrane-spanning domain of 21 residues and a short cytoplasmic domain of 12 residues (see figure 13-1). The
nucleotide sequence of the 248bp cDNA reported by
Anstee and Mallinson (72) corresponded exactly with
the sequence of the first Ig domain in the protein predicted from the cDNA clone of Bailly et al. (73). The
nucleotide sequence reported by Bailly et al. (73) also
contained a signal peptide sequence of 29 amino acids.
Mallinson (71) isolated full length LW cDNA clones
from an EB virus-transformed lymphoblastoid cell line
and from a reticulocyte mRNA preparation derived from
Rh_{null} cells. The predicted protein sequence of these
clones differed from those reported by Bailly et al. (73)
with respect to 16 amino acid residues in the sequence
encoding the signal peptide. This discrepancy was due to
a sequencing error in the clones reported by Bailly et al.
(73) in which three bases were missed. This error was
subsequently corrected (65).

The predicted protein has a cleaved signal sequence
and has four potential sites of N-glycosylation, two in

FIGURE 13-1 Comparison of LW Glycoprotein with ICAM-1, 2 and 3

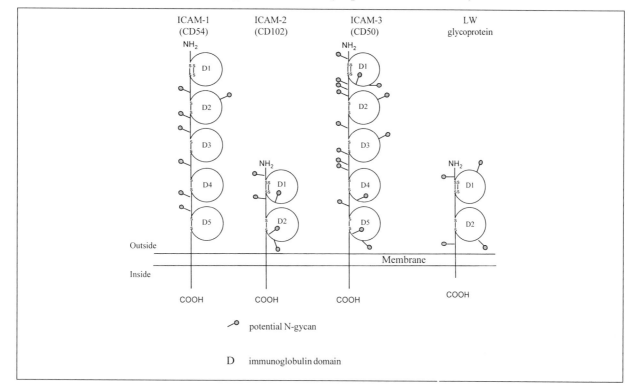

the first Ig-like domain (Asn38 and Asn 48) and two in the second Ig-like domain (Asn160 and Asn193, see figure 13-1). Studies on the electrophoretic mobility of LW glycoprotein after N-glycanase-treatment (described above) suggest that at least two of these potential N-glycosylation sites are utilized. Mallinson (71) was able to show that the first site (Asn38) is definitely utilized in the red cell. One of the peptides obtained after Lys-C digestion of Endo F-treated purified LW glycoprotein had the sequence SVQLDXSNSXP. The two residues not determined (X) are cysteines (cysteines are degraded by the sequencing chemistry) the sequence is therefore SVQLDCSNSCP that corresponds to residues 34 to 44 of LW glycoprotein but residue 38 is D(Asp) not N(Asn) as predicted by the nucleotide sequence. Endo F cleavage of N-glycans changes Asn to Asp on the polypeptide chain (81) and so Asn38 must be glycosylated in the LW glycoprotein.

Molecular Basis of LW Antigens

Hermand et al. (65) reported that the LW^a/LW^b polymorphism can be explained as a result of a single base change in the *LW* gene (A308 to G) which changes Gln70 to Arg in the E strand of the A-B-E face of the N-terminal C2 set domain (see figure 13-2). Arg70 was also found by Mallinson (71) in cDNA derived from the retic-

ulocyte mRNA of two Finns whose red cells had the phenotype LW(a-b+). Support for the conclusion that Gln70/Arg is the basis of the LW polymorphism was obtained (65) by expression of LW cDNAs in COS-7 cells and flow cytometric analysis with human anti-LW^a and human anti-LW^b. The predicted pattern of reactions was obtained although the levels of expression observed were rather low.

LW Typing From DNA

The A308G nucleotide substitution that correlates with the LW^a/LW^b polymorphism encompasses a restriction enzyme site for *Pvu* I. Hermand et al. (65) describe an RFLP test based on this enzyme that allows DNA based LW typing. When the genotype is *LW^{a}LW^a* the restriction enzyme site is cut. When the genotype is *LW^{b}LW^b* the restriction enzyme site is lost.

Organization of the *LW* Gene

The *LW* blood group locus was mapped to chromosome 19p13-p11 by Sistonen (68). A fragment of the LW cDNA was used (65) for in situ hybridization experiments with human chromosome preparations of phytohaemagglutinin (PHA)-stimulated lymphocytes in

FIGURE 13-2 Alignment of LW Glycoprotein (amino acid sequence domain 1) with Human ICAM 1, 2 and 3

```
                                                                                          52
LW                                M V P E F V A V Q P G K S V Q L N C S N S C P Q P Q N S S L R T P L R Q G K
Human ICAM 3          Q E F L L R V E P Q N P V L S A G G S L F V N C S T D C P S S E K I A L E T S L S K   E
Human ICAM 2    S D E K V F E V H V R P K K L A V E P K G S L E V N C S T T C N Q P E V G G L E T S L N K I L
Human ICAM 1                Q T S V S P S K V I L P R G G S V L V T C S T S C D Q P K L L G I E T P L P K K E

                               70                                     91
LW              T L R G P G   W V S Y Q L L D V R A W S S L A H C L V T C A G K T R W A T S R I T A Y A Y K
Human ICAM 3    L V A S G M G W A A F N L S N V   T G N S R I L C S V Y C N G S Q I T G S S N I T V Y G L P
Human ICAM 2    L D E Q A Q   W K H Y L V S N I   S H D T V L Q C H F T C S G K Q E S M N S N V S V Y Q P P
Human ICAM 2    L L L P G N N W K V Y E L S N V   Q E D S Q P M C Y S N C P D G Q S T A K T F L T V Y W T P
```

Conserved cysteines are boxed

metaphase to confirm the location of the gene on the short arm of chromosome 19 at p13.3. The partial LW cDNA clone described by Anstee and Mallinson (72) was also used to define the chromosomal location of the *LW* gene. In this case two LW-specific oligonucleotide primers corresponding to nucleotides 50-68 and 154-135 (antisense primer) of the 248bp clone were used to screen a panel of human monochromosomal somatic cell hybrids. A PCR amplified product was only obtained from the hybrid containing chromosome 19. A second panel of hybrids containing fragments of chromosome 19 was used (74) to localize the *LW* gene to the short arm at 19pter-p13.2.

LW is a small gene (approximately 2.65kb) comprising three exons (71,75). The first exon encodes production of the signal peptide and the first Ig domain. Exon 2 encodes production of the second Ig domain and exon 3 the transmembrane and cytoplasmic domain. The nucleotide sequence immediately upstream of the transcription initiation site has an inverted CAAT box (at -292), an inverted consensus sequence for GATA-1 binding (at -51). Binding sites for other transcription factors (SP-1,CACC and Ets) were also found (75) in the region of the GATA-1 binding site.

Molecular Basis of the LW(a-b-) Phenotype

Hermand et al. (75) examined the *LW* gene in two unrelated individuals (Big and Nic) who have the LW(a-b-) phenotype. No abnormality was detected in the *LW* gene from Nic but Big was homozygous for a deletion of 10bp in exon 1. This 10bp deletion altered the reading frame to generate a stop codon at the beginning of exon 2 which when translated would result in a truncated protein lacking a transmembrane domain. This explains why the phenotype of the donor's red cells is LW(a-b-). Since the absence of LW glycoprotein from the red cells of this donor results from a structural gene mutation, these results indicate that donor Big lacks the LW glycoprotein from all tissues in which it is normally expressed. There appears to be no evidence to indicate that donor Big is clinically affected as a result of this mutation so that the LW glycoprotein along with many other blood group active molecules, is apparently not, of itself, essential.

Comparison of LW Glycoprotein with ICAMs 1, 2 and 3

The structure of the LW glycoprotein is compared with those of ICAMs 1, 2 and 3 in figure 13-1. ICAM-1 (CD54) has 5 C2 set domains as does ICAM-3 (CD50), ICAM-2 (CD102) has two C2 set domains and therefore is the most similar to LW glycoprotein in terms of overall structure. The *ICAM-1* and *ICAM 3* genes are located at the same region of chromosome 19 as the *LW* glycoprotein gene suggesting a common ancestry (76). The gene for ICAM-2 is on chromosome 17 (77). All three ICAMs bind to the beta-2 integrin LFA-1 (CD11a/CD18) but this in itself is unremarkable since each of the ICAMs was discovered in a search for molecules capable of binding LFA-1. ICAM-1 is normally expressed at low levels on many tissues including leukocytes and endothelial cells and can be upregulated rapidly by cytokines. In contrast, ICAMs 2 and 3 are constitutive not inducible. ICAM-2 is found at low levels on leukocytes and endothelial cells while ICAM-3 is expressed at high levels on leukocytes but is absent from endothelial cells (reviewed in 78 and 79). The tissue distribution of LW glycoprotein is not well studied but the data that are available (80) suggest that it may be restricted to erythroid cells and placenta. There is some evidence of weak reactivity of monoclonal anti-LW with subsets of lymphocytes (62) and with monocytes and the monocyte cell line (80) but these reactivities may reflect interactions through Fc receptors rather than the presence of LW glycoprotein. Immunocytochemical studies suggested (80) that LW glycoprotein is expressed on hemopoeitic cells in fetal liver by the second trimester.

The functions of ICAMs have been studied in detail particularly those involving ICAM-1. The ICAM-1/LFA-1 interaction is central to current models of leukocyte endothelium interaction (78,79). The adhesive interaction between LFA-1 on leukocytes and ICAM-1 on endothelium appears to have a central role in the process of leukocyte migration into extravascular tissue at sites of inflammation/infection. The LFA-1 binding sites on each of the ICAMs have been studied and it appears that in each case LFA-1 binds the first domain (82-84). Since 30% of the amino acids in the first Ig-like domain of LW glycoprotein are identical to those found in the first domains of ICAMs 1, 2 and 3 it is pertinent to compare the critical residues for LFA-1 binding on ICAMs 1, 2 and 3 with the corresponding residues on LW glycoprotein (see figure 13-2). Holness et al. (84) identified Glu34 and Gln75 within ICAM-3 domain 1 as critical for LFA-1 binding and since homologous residues in ICAMs 1 and 2 are also critical for LFA-1 binding and these key residues are conserved across species (in chimpanzee, rat and mouse) they suggest that they represent a common essential ligand binding motif on all ICAMs. As can be seen in figure 13-2, the corresponding residues in LW glycoprotein are Arg52 and Thr91. The most striking aspect of this is the replacement of an acidic residue (Glu) in the ICAMs with a basic residue (Arg) in LW glycoprotein, they could hardly be more different! Nevertheless, Bailly et al. (85) have reported that purified LW glycoprotein will bind LFA-1. They also report that LW glycoprotein will bind another leukocyte integrin (Mac-1, CD11b/CD18) that binds to ICAM-1 but not ICAMs 2 and 3 and that monoclonal anti-LW[ab] will block the binding of both LFA-1 and Mac-1. This is also curious because the Mac-1 binding site on ICAM-1 has been mapped to the third Ig-like domain where the binding is affected by the degree of glycosylation of ICAM-1 (86). Clearly, these results if substantiated, bring into question previous studies on the specificity of LFA-1/ICAM interactions. If LW glycoprotein is an ICAM then the question arises as to the function of such a molecule on red cells. Studies on one individual (Big), with the LW(a-b-) phenotype, discussed above, show that the molecule is not essential on red cells or any other tissues, at least as far as that individual is concerned. Bailly et al. (85) speculate that LW glycoprotein may be involved in red cell senescence and suggest that splenic

macrophages containing CD11/CD18 integrins could bind and remove senescent red cells through interaction with LW glycoprotein. Other possibilities discussed (85) are a role in cytoadherence to *Plasmodium falciparum* infected red cells (ICAM-1 is known to bind such cells (87,88)) and a role in adhesive interactions relevant to erythroid development in bone marrow.

ICAMs 1, 2 and 3 have cytoplasmic domains of 27, 24 and 37 amino acids respectively whereas that for LW is only 12 residues. The cytoplasmic domain of ICAM-1 binds to the cytoskelton through an octapeptide sequence rich in basic amino acids. Carlos and Harlan (78) suggest that linkage with the cytoskeleton may localize ICAM-1 within regions of the endothelial cell membrane to facilitate leukocyte adherence and transmigration. It seems unlikely that the short cytoplasmic domain of LW interacts with the red cell skeleton. Evidence that 80% of LW is solubilized by extraction of red cell membranes with 0.5% Triton X-100 (91) is consistent with this conclusion.

Biochemical Relationship Between LW and Rh

There is a well documented serological relationship between the LW and Rh antigens which is discussed in detail earlier in this chapter. Recent molecular evidence concerning the nature of these antigens and the molecules that carry them has shown that the LW antigens are carried on a molecule with a completely different structure from those which carry Rh antigens. In addition, the *Rh* genes of individuals with the LW(a-b-) phenotype appear normal and the *LW* gene of individuals with the Rh[null] phenotype is also normal (65). Furthermore, Rh[null] individuals have normal *LW* gene transcripts (71). The Rh antigens D, c and E can be expressed in K562 cells, a cell line that has little or no LW antigen detectable by flow cytometry with monoclonal antibodies (89). LW antigens can be expressed, albeit at low levels, in COS-7 cells that lack Rh antigens (65). All these observations suggest that the LW are Rh are entirely independent entities. Why then, do D+ red cells give stronger reactions than D- cells when tested with anti-LW[a] and anti-LW[b]? One possibility is that the Rh proteins in general, and the D polypeptide in particular, though not essential for LW expression nevertheless facilitate the transport of LW glycoprotein to the plasma membrane (or vice versa).

Studies in which the LW glycoprotein and Rh proteins are co-expressed in a cell line that lacks both molecules are now feasible and should address this possibility. A precedent for such a hypothesis is already established. Glycophorin A is known (90) to facilitate transport of the anion transport protein, band 3, to the plasma membrane of *Xenopus* oocytes. Evidence for a direct association between the LW glycoprotein and Rh polypeptides was obtained from immunoprecipitation experiments in which monoclonal anti-LW^ab (BS46) co-precipitated the two proteins from radioiodinated red cells (49).

The predicted cytoplasmic domain of LW (sequence: YLCKCLAMKSQA) contains two cysteine residues, an observation that prompts one of us (DJA) to wonder if the LW glycoprotein is palmitoylated. The functions of protein palmitoylation are far from clear but may facilitate protein-protein interactions and/or protein-lipid interactions and may have a role in signal transduction (92 and see Chapter 29). Perhaps palmitoylation is relevant to the association of the LW glycoprotein with Rh polypeptides. The Rh polypeptides themselves are known to be extensively palmitoylated (see Chapter 12). Perhaps the transient loss of LW antigens so commonly reported and discussed earlier is a reflection of changes in palmitoylation.

References

1. Landsteiner K, Wiener AS. Proc Soc Exp Biol NY 1940;43:223
2. Landsteiner K, Wiener AS. J Exp Med 1941;74:309
3. Fisk RT, Foord AG. Am J Clin Pathol 1942;12:545
4. Murray J, Clark EC. Nature 1952;169:886
5. Levine P, Celano M, Fenichel R, et al. Science 1961;133:332
6. Levine P, Celano M, Fenichel R, et al. J Immunol 1961;87:747
7. Levine P, Celano M. Nature 1962;193:184
8. Levine P, Celano M, Vos GH, et al. Nature 1962;194:304
9. Levine P, Celano MJ, Wallace J, et al. Nature 1963;198:596
10. Race RR, Sanger R. Blood Groups in Man, 6th Ed. Oxford:Blackwell, 1975
11. Levine P, Celano MJ. Science 1967;156:1744
12. Levine P. In: Proceedings of an International Convocation on Immunology. Basel:Karger, 1969:140
13. Wiener AS. In: Blood and Tissue Antigens. New York:Academic Press, 1970:353
14. Levine P, Stetson R. J Am Med Assoc 1939;113:126
15. Wiener AS, Moor-Jankowski J, Brancato GJ. Haematologia 1969;3:385
16. Tippett P. PhD Thesis, Univ London, 1963
17. Tippett P. Unpublished observations cited by Race RR, Sanger R. Blood Groups in Man, 5th Ed. Oxford:Blackwell, 1968
18. deVeber LL, Clark GW, Hunking M, et al. Transfusion 1971;11:33
19. deVeber LL. (Letter). Transfusion 1971;11:389
20. Swanson JL, Azar M, Miller J, et al. Transfusion 1974;14:470
21. White JC, Rolih S, Wilkinson SL, et al. Transfusion 1975;15:368
22. Swanson J, Matson GA. Transfusion 1964;4:257
23. Swanson J, Polesky HF, Matson GA. Vox Sang 1965;10:560
24. Beck ML. In: A Seminar on Recent Advances in Immunohematology. Washington, D.C.:Am Assoc Blood Banks, 1973:83
25. Behzad O, Pothiawala M, Rolih SD, et al. Transfusion 1978;18:488
26. Tregellas WM, Moulds JJ, South SF. (abstract). Transfusion 1978;18:384
27. Giles CM. Immunol Comm 1980;9:225
28. Cummings E, Pisciotto P, Roth G. Vox Sang 1984;46:286
29. Chaplin H, Hunter VL, Rosche ME, et al. Transfusion 1985;25:39
30. Napier JAF, Rowe GP. Vox Sang 1987;53:228
31. Devenish A. Immunohematology 1994;10:127
32. Herron R, Bell A, Poole J, et al. Vox Sang 1986;51:314
33. Johnson ST, Davis HL, Gottschall JL. (abstract). Transfusion 1992;32(Suppl 8S):53S
34. Villalba R, Ceballos P, Fornés G, et al. (Letter). Vox Sang 1995;68:66
35. Sistonen P, Nevanlinna HR, Virtaranta-Knowles K, et al. Vox Sang 1981;40:352
36. Sistonen P. Med Biol 1981;59:230
37. Sistonen P, Tippett P. (abstract). Transfusion 1982;22:425
38. Sistonen P, Tippett P. Vox Sang 1982;42:252
39. Ishimori T, Hasekura H. Transfusion 1967;7:84
40. Polesky HF, Swanson J, Olson C. Bibl Haematol 1968;29:384
41. Vos GH, Petz LD, Garratty G, et al. Blood 1973;42:445
42. Sistonen P. PhD Thesis Univ Helsinki, 1984
43. Gibbs MB. Nature 1966;210:642
44. Lomas CG, Tippett P. Med Lab Sci 1985;42:88
45. Green C. Report to Special Interest Group of British Blood Transfusion Society, described by Daniels G. BBTS Newsletter No 38, Dec 1995:5
46. Konigshaus GJ, Holland TI. Transfusion 1984;24:536
47. Daniels G. Immunohematology 1992;8:53
48. Mallinson G, Martin PG, Anstee DJ, et al. Biochem J 1986;234:649
49. Bloy C, Hermand P, Blanchard D, et al. J Biol Chem 1990;265:21482
50. Sistonen P, Green CA, Lomas CG, et al. Ann Hum Genet 1983;47:277
51. Giles CM, Lundsgaard A. Vox Sang 1967;13:406
52. Chown B, Kaita H, Lowen B, et al. Transfusion 1971;11:220
53. Perkins HA, McIlroy M, Swanson J, et al. Vox Sang 1977;33:299
54. Reid ME, O'Day TM, Toy PTCY, et al. J Med Tech 1986;3:117
55. Poole J, Williamson LM, Clark N, et al. (abstract). Transfusion 1991;31(Suppl 8S):38S
56. Storry JR. Immunohematology 1992;8:87
57. Daniels G. Human Blood Groups. Oxford:Blackwell, 1995:519
58. Cook IA. Br J Haematol 1971;20:369
59. Kavitsky D, Gillotte T, Nance S. (abstract). Transfusion 1991;31(Suppl 8S):38S
60. Weber J, Caceres VW, Pavone BG, et al. Transfusion 1979;19:216
61. Issitt PD, Pavone BG, Shapiro M. Transfusion 1979;19:389
62. Oliveira OLP, Thomas DB, Lomas CG, et al. J Immunogenet 1984;11:297
63. Sonneborn H-H, Uthemann H, Tills D, et al. Biotest Bull 1984;2:145
64. Sonneborn H-H, Ernst M, Voak D. (abstract). Vox Sang 1994;67(Suppl 2):114
65. Hermand P, Gane P, Mattei MG, et al. Blood 1995;86:1590
66. Perrault R. Vox Sang 1973;24:150
67. Celano MJ, Levine P. Transfusion 1967;7:265
68. Sistonen P. Ann Hum Genet 1984;48:239
69. Lewis M, Kaita H, Philipps S, et al. Ann Hum Genet 1987;51:201

70. Moore S. Red Cell Membrane Glycoconjugates and Related Markers. Paris:Arnette 1983:97

71. Mallinson G. PhD Thesis, Univ West England 1995

72. Anstee DJ, Mallinson G. Vox Sang 1994;67 (suppl 3):1

73. Bailly P, Hermand P, Callebaut I, et al. Proc Nat Acad Sci USA 1994;91:5306

74. Spurr N, Warne D. Unpublished observations 1965 cited in Mallinson G. PhD Thesis Univ West England 1995

75. Hermand P, Le Pennec PY, Rouger P, et al. Blood 1996;87:2962

76. Bossy D, Mattei MG, Simmonds DL. Genomics 1994,23,712

77. Ropers HH, Pericak-Vance MA. Cytogenet Cell Genet 1991;58:751

78. Carlos TM, Harlan JM. Blood 1994;84:2068

79. Springer TA. Cell 1994;76:301

80. Anstee DJ, Holmes CH, Judson PA, et al. In: Protein Blood Group Antigens of the Human Red Cell. Baltimore:Johns Hopkins Univ Press 1992;170

81. Plummer TH, Elder JH, Alexander S, et al. J Biol Chem 1984;259:10700

82. Staunton DE, Dustin ML, Erickson HP, et al. Cell;1990:61:243

83. Li R, Nortamo P, Valmu L, et al. J Biol Chem 1993;268:17513

84. Holness CL, Bates PA, Littler AJ, et al. J Biol Chem 1995;270:877

85 Bailly P, Tontti E, Hermand P, et al. Eur J Immunol 1995;25:3316

86. Diamond MS, Staunton DE, Marlin SD, et al. Cell 1991;65:961

87. Berendt AR, McDowell A, Craig AG, et al. Cell 1992;68:71

88. Ockenhouse CF, Betageri R, Springer TA, et al. Cell 1992;68:63

89. Smythe JS, Avent ND, Judson PA, et al. Blood 1996;87:2968

90. Groves JD, Tanner MJA. J Biol Chem 1992;267:22163

91. Bloy C, Blanchard D, Hermand, P et al. Mol Immunol 1989;26:1013

92. Guo YJ, Lin S, Wang M, et al. Int Immunol 1994;6:213

93. Gardner B, Parsons SF, Merry AH, et al. Immunology 1989;68:283

94. Parsons SF, Gardner B, Anstee DJ. Transf Med 1993;3:137

95. Anstee DJ, Gardner B, Spring FA, et al. Immunology 1991;74:197

96. Hayashi R. Meth Enzymol 1977;247:84

14 | The Duffy Blood Group System

In 1950, Cutbush et al. (1) found an agglutinin, in the serum of a hemophiliac who had been transfused several times, that defined a hitherto unrecognized blood group antigen. The antibody was named anti-Fy^a (after the antibody-maker, Mr. Duffy) and was described in more detail in a later report (2). The following year, Ikin et al. (3) described anti-Fy^b, the antibody that defines the antithetical partner of Fy^a. In Whites, these antibodies define the phenotypes Fy(a+b-), Fy(a+b+) and Fy(a-b+) that most of the time, represent the genotypes Fy^aFy^a, Fy^aFy^b and Fy^bFy^b, respectively. In 1955, Sanger et al. (4) reported that the phenotype Fy(a-b-) is more common in American Blacks than is any phenotype in which Fy^a or Fy^b is present. It was thought that the Fy(a-b-) phenotype probably represented the $FyFy$ genotype, with Fy being a silent allele at the Fy^aFy^b (*Duffy*) locus. As described in detail below, it is now known (5-11) that the Fy gene in the vast majority of Blacks who have Fy(a-b-) red cells is an allele that is the same in its structural region as Fy^b but has a mutation in the GATA-1 site to which the erythroid transcription factor binds (see figure 14-2). The net result is that while this gene encodes production of Duffy glycoprotein in tissue cells, it never makes a red cell-borne Duffy glycoprotein. Thus, for reasons discussed in more detail below, the gene will continue to be called Fy in this section of this chapter. The Fy(a-b-) phenotype has also been found in Whites (12-15), in at least one such individual the genetic background leading to the phenotype was shown to differ from that seen in the majority of Fy(a-b-) Blacks (11). In some other Whites (16-18) it is assumed that the Fy(a-b-) phenotype represents admixture with genes from Blacks (for additional details see a later section). It has been estimated that the frequency of the Fy(a-b-) phenotype is between 100,000 (19) and 700,000 (20,21) times more common in Blacks than in Whites.

In 1965, Chown et al. (20) described a new allele, Fy^x at the *Duffy* locus. The actions of Fy^x were described more fully in a later paper (21) and it was shown that the gene does not encode production of an antigen that is distinct from others in the Duffy system. Instead, individuals who have inherited an Fy^x but not an Fy^b gene, have red cells that react poorly with some and not at all with other examples of anti-Fy^b. The red cells will adsorb and yield on elution, most or all examples of anti-Fy^b. In 1971, the antigen Fy3 (12) and in 1973, the antigens Fy4 and Fy5 (22,23) were described. In 1987, Fy6 was added to the system, existence of the antigen was recognized by use of a murine monoclonal antibody (24). The Duffy

system is number 008 in the ISBT terminology, table 14-1 lists the conventional and ISBT terms for antigens of the system. Additional information about each of the antigens is presented in later sections of this chapter.

TABLE 14-1 Conventional and ISBT Terminology for the Duffy Blood Group System

Conventional Name: Duffy		
Conventional Symbol: Fy		
ISBT Symbol: FY		
ISBT System Number: 008		
Antigen Conventional Name	ISBT Antigen Number	ISBT Full Code Number
Fy^a	FY1	008001
Fy^b	FY2	008002
Fy3	FY3	008003
Fy4	FY4	008004
Fy5	FY5	008005
Fy6	FY6	008006

In 1968, Donahue et al. (25) showed that the *Duffy* locus is on chromosome one. This was a momentous discovery for it represented the first instance in which a human red cell blood group locus was assigned to an autosome.

The Antigens Fy^a and Fy^b and the Antibodies that Define Them

At the level of practical blood transfusion, Fy^a and Fy^b are the most important antigens in the Duffy system. Anti-Fy^a is not a particularly uncommon antibody and is found both as a single entity in the sera of persons phenotypically Fy(a-b+) and as one of a mixture of antibodies made by good responders (see Chapter 2) when such individuals have Fy(a-b+) red cells. Although the first example of anti-Fy^a (1,2) was an agglutinin active in saline, most often the antibody is immune (red cell stimulated) and reacts optimally or only by IAT. In two different studies (26,27) it was found that anti-Fy^a is most often IgG1 in nature. It is also known (19) that about half of all examples of anti-Fy^a bind complement. The lower than expected incidence of production of

439

anti-Fy^a by Blacks of the Fy(a-b-) phenotype, is discussed in a later section, after Fy3 and anti-Fy3 have been described. Anti-Fy^b is found less frequently than anti-Fy^a and most examples seem to occur in individuals who make multiple antibodies after exposure to red cells. However, we (28) found a potent anti-Fy^b in the serum of a non-transfused male donor with no known exposure to foreign red cells. Thus, the antibody seemed, like an anti-Fy^a described by Rosenfield et al. (29), to be non-red cell stimulated (naturally-occurring). Although this seemed to apply to the anti-Fy^b we studied, it still reacted by IAT. Contreras et al. (30) have described the production of anti-Fy^b by a woman exposed to the antigen when the fetus she was carrying was given an intrauterine transfusion. The woman's husband was phenotypically Fy(a+b-) and the donor red cells used for the intrauterine transfusion were Fy(a+b+). It was concluded that the woman's only exposure to Fy^b was via the entry of donor red cells into her circulation at the time of the intrauterine transfusion.

Both anti-Fy^a and anti-Fy^b have caused immediate and delayed hemolytic transfusion reactions (29,31-41) rarely, immediate reactions have proved fatal (31,35). One case (42) has been reported in which the transfusion of donor blood containing anti-Fy^a was thought to have caused destruction of some of a patient's Fy(a+b+) red cells. Anti-Fy^a has caused HDN (43-49); in describing 23 pregnant women with anti-Fy^a in the serum, encountered during a 26 year period, Bowman (49) reports five cases of HDN, in four of which no treatment was required (50). In contrast, among 11 cases reviewed earlier by Greenwalt et al. (44), two were fatal. The literature seems to contain only one report (51) of HDN caused by anti-Fy^b, the affected infant was transfused to correct anemia.

Clearly anti-Fy^a and anti-Fy^b must be regarded as having the potential to be clinically significant when detected by serological methods whose positive results are associated with such significance. No doubt, like antibodies in other blood group systems, some examples of anti-Fy^a and anti-Fy^b detected only by ultra sensitive methods, will lack clinical relevance. Some characteristics of Duffy system antibodies, including some specificities described later in this chapter, are summarized in table 14-2. The selection of antigen-negative blood for patients with anti-Fy^a or anti-Fy^b in the serum presents no practical problem. Table 14-3 shows the incidence of Duffy system antigens and phenotypes in different populations. Occasional examples of Duffy system antibodies are particularly good at distinguishing the properties of various lots of anti-IgG in evaluation studies (52,53).

Development of Fy^a and Fy^b and Number of Antigen Sites per Red Cell

In spite of the facts that most cases of HDN caused by anti-Fy^a are mild and that anti-Fy^b has only once been incriminated (see previous section) both Fy^a and Fy^b are well developed at birth. The antigens have been detected on the red cells of fetuses as early as 6 or 7 weeks of life (57,58). The antigen levels do not appear to change

TABLE 14-2 Some Characteristics of Duffy System Antibodies

Antibody Specificity	Positive Reactions in In Vitro Tests				Usual Immunoglobulin		Ability to Bind Complement		Ability to Cause In Vitro Lysis		Implicated in		Usual Form of Stimulation		% of White Population Positive
	Sal	LISS	AHG	Enz	IgG	IgM	Yes	No	Yes	No	Transfusion Reaction	HDN	Red Cells	Other	
Anti-Fy^a	Very Rare	X	X	No	Most	Very Rare	Some	Some		X	Yes	Yes	Most	Very Rare	66
Anti-Fy^b		X	X	No	Most		Some	Some		X	Yes	Yes	Most	Very Rare	83
Anti-Fy3			X	X	Pres*1					X	Yes	Mild	X		100
Anti-Fy4			X	X		X				X			X		Approx 5%
Anti-Fy5			X	X	X					X			X		100
Anti-Fy6*2			X	No	X					X	No	No			100

*1. Presumed to be IgG since it has crossed the placenta and caused HDN
*2. Described thus far only as a murine monoclonal antibody.

TABLE 14-3 Fyᵃ and Fyᵇ Antigen and Phenotype Frequencies

Phenotype	% Frequency in		% Bloods from Whites Reactive with		% Bloods from Blacks Reactive with		% Bloods Non-reactive with anti-Fyᵃ and anti-Fyᵇ	
	Whites	Blacks	Anti-Fyᵃ	Anti-Fyᵇ	Anti-Fyᵃ	Anti-Fyᵇ	Whites	Blacks
Fy(a+b-)	17	9	66		10			
Fy(a+b+)	49	1		83		23		
Fy(a-b+)	34	22						
Fy(a-b-)	<0.1	68					<0.1	68

appreciably throughout life.

Using human source anti-Fyᵃ and anti-Fyᵇ and ferritin-labeled anti-IgG, Masouredis et al. (59) estimated that Fy(a+b-) and Fy(a-b+) red cells carry between 13,000 and 14,000 Fyᵃ or Fyᵇ sites, respectively. As expected, Fy(a+b+) red cells were found to have about half that number of Fyᵃ sites. Using a monoclonal antibody to Fy6 (see below), Nichols et al. (24) estimated that red cells carry some 12,000 copies of the Duffy glycoprotein per red cell, a figure in close agreement with those of Masouredis et al. (59). Using a different monoclonal anti-Fy6, Riwom et al. (60) estimated the number of copies per red cell to be about 6000. Somewhat confusingly, in their discussion, the latter authors conclude that each red cell carries in the order of 10,000 copies of Fy6.

Distribution of Fyᵃ and Fyᵇ

In Asian, unlike White and Black populations, the antigen Fyᵃ is of very high incidence; Won et al. (54) found 144 of 145 Japanese; Speiser (55) 393 of 394 Koreans; and Simmons (56) 1340 of 1341 Melanesians; to be Fy(a+). It is strange for blood bankers to have to realize that a rare Asian lacking Fyᵃ, who has produced anti-Fyᵃ, creates as great a transfusion problem in his home country, as say a patient with anti-Kpᵇ in a population of White European extraction.

Enzyme Sensitivity of Fyᵃ and Fyᵇ

It has been known for a long time that certain proteases either denature or remove the Fyᵃ and Fyᵇ antigens when those enzymes are used to treat red cells. There is no dispute that ficin, papain, bromelin, chymotrypsin, pronase and a neutral protease obtained from *Bacillus subtilis*, all render red cells non-reactive with anti-Fyᵃ and anti-Fyᵇ (61-72). One report (73) that claimed to show Fyᵃ and Fyᵇ present on ficin and papain-treated red cells, described tests in which the enzyme solutions used were too weak to effect antigen removal or denaturation.

The picture was not nearly as clear when trypsin was used to treat red cells. While some of the papers cited above reported that trypsin was as effective in this regard as ficin or papain, other investigators (66,70) found that Fyᵃ and Fyᵇ were still present on trypsin-treated cells. The explanation was provided in 1977 when Judson and Anstee (71) showed that trypsin does not remove or denature Fyᵃ or Fyᵇ, but that many trypsin preparations also contain small amounts of chymotrypsin that is active in this respect. If pure trypsin is used to treat red cells, Fyᵃ and Fyᵇ survive. If trypsin contaminated with chymotrypsin is used, the antigens are denatured or removed. As pointed out in Chapter 3, although chymotrypsin has a name that is similar to trypsin, its actions are more like those of ficin, papain and pronase, than like those of trypsin. Springer (74) reported that enzyme solutions that include neuraminidase but lack the proteases listed above, have no effect on red cell-borne Fyᵃ or Fyᵇ. In spite of the sensitivity of Fyᵃ to protease-treatment, Rosenfield et al. (15) found that anti-Fyᵃ could be detected without difficulty in an AutoAnalyzer system using bromelin. It seems likely that if anti-Fyᵃ binds to the Fyᵃ antigen before bromelin acts to cleave or denature the antigen, Fyᵃ may be protected, at least in part, from the actions of the enzyme. The trypsin resistance of Fyᵃ and Fyᵇ is now understood at the biochemical level and is described in detail later in this chapter.

Storage Properties of Fyᵃ and Fyᵇ

Williams et al. (76) reported that red cells stored in saline for two weeks lose some of their Fyᵃ, Fyᵇ and Fy3 antigens. Davies et al. (77) showed that storage of red cells in low pH, low ionic strength solutions results in a progressive loss of Fyᵃ and Fyᵇ activity. We have heard anecdotal reports that red cell samples stored frozen in liquid nitrogen may lose Fyᵃ and Fyᵇ antigen activity but our own experience has been to the contrary. We have seen no weakening of Fyᵃ or Fyᵇ on red cells stored in such a way for many years. The Fyᵃ, Fyᵇ and Fy3 antigens seem to be well preserved when red cells are stored in

ACD, CPD and CPD-A1 anticoagulated samples or in the preservative solutions used by commercial companies for the preparation of antibody identification panels (76,78).

Dosage of Anti-Fy^a and Anti-Fy^b

Some examples of these antibodies give reasonably reliable dosage results in tests using conventional serological procedures (3,79,80). Race and Sanger (81) note that agglutinating antibodies active in saline systems may give better dosage pictures than antiglobulin-active sera. More sophisticated techniques (immunoferritin labeling, HD 50 tests in the AutoAnalyzer and the enzyme-linked antiglobulin method) provide even more reliable dosage results in the system (59,82,83). As with other blood group systems, the most reliable dosage results in the Duffy system may be obtained when a flow cytometer is used (84,85).

Renal Transplant in a Patient with Anti-Fy^a

Ginsburg and Singer (86) described a patient with anti-Fy^a in the serum who received a kidney from her sister, who had Fy(a+) red cells. The recipient and donor were identical in terms of HLA type and compatible by mixed lymphocyte culture. Although the patient experienced an acute rejection episode (that was completely reversed by intravenous methylprednisolone) 17 days after the kidney was transplanted, the authors could find no evidence that the anti-Fy^a was associated with the rejection. They concluded that Fy^a is probably not an antigen that must be considered in renal transplantation. The investigation is a model example of how a possible true, true and unrelated situation should be investigated. It was true that the patient had anti-Fy^a. It was true that the kidney donor was Fy(a+). It would have been easy to conclude that the anti-Fy^a was responsible for the acute rejection. In fact, careful investigation showed that the two true events were unrelated. Blood bankers who find an antibody reactive with all cells except those of a null phenotype of one system, would do well to remember this lesson.

The Gene *Fy^x* and the Antigen Fy^b

Family studies in Whites provided evidence that the silent gene, *Fy*, might exist in such populations (81). In 1965, Chown et al. (20) and in 1972, Lewis et al. (21) showed that some of those data could be explained by inheritance of a different gene at the *Duffy* locus. It was shown that *Fy^x*, as the new gene was called, encodes

production of an antigen that can be detected in tests with some examples of anti-Fy^b. Red cells from individuals genetically *Fy^{a}Fy^x*, type as Fy(a+b+^{weak}) with the reactive anti-Fy^b. With the non-reactive sera, the cells type as Fy(a+b-) but can be shown to be capable of adsorbing the anti-Fy^b with which they do not react visibly. Obviously, it is usually possible to recognize the genotype *Fy^{b}Fy^x* only from a family study. Adsorption studies using cells from a person with an *Fy^x* gene and anti-Fy^b have not succeeded in separating an antibody from the anti-Fy^b sera that has the specificity of anti-Fy^x. Thus the evidence indicates that *Fy^x* is a variant form of *Fy^b*. Individuals genetically *Fy^{x}Fy^x* have been found (21,82,87,88) and as expected, their red cells carried more Fy^b than was present on the cells of persons genetically *Fy^{a}Fy^x*. Habibi et al. (82) used the AutoAnalyzer to show that red cells of persons genetically *Fy^{b}Fy^x* carry less Fy^b than do those of persons genetically *Fy^{b}Fy^b*. Less easy to understand are the findings (82,83,89) that red cells of individuals genetically *Fy^{b}Fy^x* seem to have less Fy^b antigen than those from persons genetically *Fy^{a}Fy^b*.

Based on their large series of typings, Chown et al. (20) and Lewis et al. (21) concluded that it is probable that both *Fy^x* and *Fy* are present in Caucasian populations. It seems that in such populations, *Fy^x* is more common than *Fy*. It has also been shown (13,82,89,90) that in the presence of *Fy^x*, less Fy3 and Fy5 (each of those antigens is described in a later section) is made than in the presence of *Fy^a* or *Fy^b*. Most recently it has been shown (9) that at the molecular level (also see a later section), *Fy^b* and *Fy^x* are identical in terms of their structural (coding) regions. This observation, of course, supports the already described serological findings that *Fy^b* and *Fy^x* encode production of a quantitatively different amount of the same antigen (Fy^b) and not different antigens. To conclude this section it can be said that the genes *Fy^b*, *Fy^x* and *Fy* are structurally the same in their coding regions: *Fy^b* encodes production of a standard amount of red cell-borne Fy^b antigen; *Fy^x* encodes production of a reduced amount of that antigen on red cells; *Fy* fails to encode production of any red cell-borne Fy^b. It seems probable that at the tissue cell level, all three genes encode production of the same Duffy glycoprotein.

Another Possibly Defective *Fy^b* Gene in Whites

Somewhat differently to the *Fy* gene in Blacks, that is a gene with the coding sequence of *Fy^b* that is permanently switched off at the red cell level (see below), Murphy et al. (201) showed that in Whites, a number of individuals have red cells that initially type as Fy(a+b-) but can be seen to have an Fy^b gene when PCR amplification of their DNA is performed. In tests on samples from 109 Whites with red cells of apparent Fy(a+b-) phenotype, 13 were found to have an Fy^b gene. That the gene was not the Fy gene seen in Blacks was clear since the red cells of some of these individuals would adsorb and yield on elution, selected examples of anti-Fy^b. While the gene involved behaved similarly to Fy^x (see above) the authors (201) felt that too many Fy(a+b+^{weak}) samples had been found for Fy^x to be the sole explanation, i.e. Fy^x is thought to be of very low frequency.

The *Fy* Gene in Blacks

As mentioned above, for many years it was believed (4) that the Fy(a-b-) phenotype, seen so often in Blacks, represented the inheritance of two *Fy* genes at the Fy^aFy^b locus. *Fy* was regarded as a silent allele that encoded no production of Fy^a or Fy^b. In spite of what has been learned about the structure of this gene, the above statement is still true. In Blacks, the Fy(a-b-) phenotype almost always represents the genotype *FyFy* in which *Fy* is defined as a gene failing to encode production of red cell-borne Duffy glycoprotein.

When it was shown (5-11) that Blacks with Fy(a-b-) red cells have genes that are identical to Fy^b in the region that normally encodes production of a glycoprotein carrying Fy^b and that such individuals express Duffy glycoprotein normally on their tissue cells, but have no red cell-borne Duffy glycoprotein, it became apparent that the gene, that was structurally the same as Fy^b in its coding region, must differ from Fy^b in some other way. Tournamille et al. (97) showed that a mutation disrupts the GATA-1 binding site for erythroid transcription so that the coding region of the gene (that is identical to that in Fy^b) is never transcribed at the red cell level. For this reason, as mentioned earlier, we continue to call the gene that is like Fy^b in its coding region but is permanently switched off by the GATA-1 mutation, *Fy* and not Fy^b. To us, at the red cell level, an Fy^b gene must, by definition, encode production of Fy^b antigen, *Fy* does not.

Because the mutation in *Fy* is in the binding site for an erythroid transcription factor, the gene is not silent with regard to production of Duffy glycoprotein in tissue cells. Perhaps for this reason, some workers (195-197) have called what used to be called *Fy*, Fy^b. As explained above, we prefer the term *Fy* because we are discussing red cells and because the gene never makes Fy^b on those cells.

It can perhaps be argued that the gene can be called Fy^b, although it never encodes production of red cell-borne Fy^b antigen, because Rh$_{null}$ individuals of the X^orX^or type have *CDE* genes and Bombay individuals

can have *A* and/or *B* genes, but in neither instance do the genes encode production of appropriate red cell-borne antigens. However, there is a fundamental difference. In the X^orX^or type of Rh$_{null}$, the *CDE* genes do not encode production of red cell-borne antigens because of the presence of mutant genes at an unlinked locus (198 and see Chapter 12). Further, it is clear that the *CDE* genes themselves are functionally normal since their products are expressed in the X^lrX^or parents and offspring of the Rh$_{null}$ individuals. Even more directly, it has long been known (199,200) that the *A* and/or *B* genes inherited by Bombay (*hh*) individuals function normally. That is, the transferase products of such genes can be detected in the individuals involved. Thus again the expected antigen is not seen because of the presence of abnormal genes at an unlinked locus, i.e. in the genotype *hh* no H is made so that no A or B immunodominant terminal carbohydrate can be added (see Chapter 8). With *Fy* (and Fy^b) the situation is quite different. Although the gene has the same coding region as Fy^b, the mutation that renders it unable to encode production of red cell-borne Fy^b (or Duffy glycoprotein) is part of the gene itself, i.e. in the erythroid transcription region. This means that non-action of the gene at the red cell level is not the result of genes at independent loci (i.e. no equivalents to X^or or *h*) and that the gene, when passed from parent to child will never encode production of red cell-borne Fy^b. For these reasons, in the section on the serology of the Duffy system in this book, *Fy* refers to the gene that has the same coding region as Fy^b but is permanently switched off and unlike Fy^b, the coding region of *Fy* is never transcribed in erythroid lines. In the section of this chapter on the biochemistry and molecular genetics of the Duffy system, the term *Fy* is sometimes used to describe the *Duffy* locus that can be occupied by Fy^a, Fy^b or *Fy*. However, the context in which *Fy* is used makes it abundantly clear when *Fy* the silent allele, and when *Fy* the locus is intended.

Fy3 and Anti-Fy3

Given the high incidence of the Fy(a-b-) phenotype in Blacks and the propensity of persons of null phenotypes in other blood group systems to form antibodies, it was surprising that anti-Fy^{ab} (i.e. anti-Fy^a and anti-Fy^b in an inseparable form) was not made by such individuals. In 1971, Albrey et al. (12) described just such an antibody but it was made by a White Australian woman who had been both transfused and pregnant. The antibody-maker was only the second White person with Fy(a-b-) red cells ever found. The antibody reacted with all Fy(a+b-), Fy(a+b+) and Fy(a-b+) red cells but not with those that were Fy(a-b-), it could not be split by adsorption into anti-Fy^a and anti-Fy^b components. Albrey et al. (12) named the antibody anti-Fy3 and not anti-Fy^{ab} for a number of reasons. First, anti-Fy3, unlike anti-Fy^a and anti-Fy^b reacted with enzyme-treated red cells suggesting that Fy^a and Fy^b were not part of Fy3. Second, it was suggested that Fy3 might be a precursor substance of Fy^a and Fy^b. Third, use of the term Fy3 allowed for further expansion of the Duffy system, that has occurred and is described below. The reactions of anti-Fy3 are shown in table 14-2.

A study (12) of the family of the White lady who made anti-Fy3 showed that the most simple explanation of her Fy(a-b-) phenotype was that she was genetically *FyFy*. However, subsequent studies (11, and see a later section of this chapter) have shown that the genetic background of her Fy(a-b-) phenotype differs from that of the vast majority of Black individuals who have Fy(a-b-) red cells.

In 1974, Oberdorfer et al. (91) reported the second example of anti-Fy3. This time the antibody was made by a Black lady who had Fy(a-b-) red cells and who had been transfused with one unit of Fy(a+b-) blood during her first pregnancy. The antibody differed from the original anti-Fy3 in that it failed to react with Fy(a+) or Fy(b+) cord blood samples. Other examples of anti-Fy3 have now been reported. Buchanan et al. (13) found the antibody in an Alberta Cree Indian lady who had Fy(a-b-) red cells; who had been transfused with two units of blood and who had been pregnant nine times. The antibody caused only mild HDN and her infant did not require treatment. This example of anti-Fy3, like the first, reacted strongly with Fy(a+) and Fy(b+) cord blood samples. The incidence of the Fy(a-b-) phenotype in Cree Indians is not known. While there were other individuals with Fy(a-b-) red cells in the proposita's family, her antibody reacted with all of 25 samples from Cree Indians believed to be unrelated. Reports of the fourth and fifth examples of anti-Fy3 appeared out of sequence in the literature. The fourth was described by Molthan and Crawford in 1977 (92) but, through no fault of the authors, their abstract (93) was not published until after the description of the fifth example by Oakes et al. (94) had appeared. These two examples of the antibody were both made in Blacks who had Fy(a-b-) red cells. Like the example described by Oberdorfer et al. (91) made by a Black, the one studied by Molthan and Crawford (93) was accompanied by separable anti-Fy^a in the serum. The example described by Oakes et al. (94) was present in the serum of a patient who had made anti-E and anti-C^w but no separable anti-Fy^a or anti-Fy^b. The fourth and fifth examples of the antibody were similar to the second in that the one studied by Molthan and Crawford (93) failed to react with Fy(a+) or Fy(b+) cord blood samples while that studied by Oakes et al. (94) reacted more strongly with red cells from adults than with

those from newborn infants. In other words, the anti-Fy3 made by a White and by a Cree Indian (12,13) reacted equally well with the red cells of adults and newborn infants while the three made by Blacks either failed to react (91,93) or reacted only weakly (94) with cord blood red cells.

Still more examples of anti-Fy3 have been described, one in an Algerian (18) and several in Blacks (96-99). One of these (98) was blamed for a severe transfusion reaction in a patient with sickle cell disease who had received an exchange transfusion. Vengelen-Tyler (97) described five Black patients who initially made anti-Fy^a. One of them subsequently made anti-Fy3, two made anti-Fy5 (see below) and two made an antibody that was not fully characterized but that could have been anti-Fy3 or anti-Fy5. When the anti-Fy3, anti-Fy5 and incompletely characterized antibodies were made, separable anti-Fy^a was no longer demonstrable in the patients' sera. Production of Duffy system antibodies by Black individuals is considered in more detail in the next section.

Paucity of Duffy System Antibodies in Blacks

There are many data in the literature that show that Black individuals, 68% of whom in the USA have Fy(a-b-) red cells, do not make Duffy system antibodies as frequently as would be expected. Molthan and Crawford (93) used the incidence of the Fy(a-b-) phenotype and the ratio of White to Black patients and donors, to calculate that each year, in the USA, some 231,000 Blacks but only 2 or 3 Whites with the Fy(a-b-) phenotype, are transfused with red cells that, in the vast majority of instances, carry Fy^a or Fy^b or both. In addition to the 68% of Blacks with Fy(a-b-) red cells, another 20% are phenotypically Fy(a-b+). In other words, when transfused with Fy(a+) blood, some 88% of Blacks should have the potential to make anti-Fy^a. In contrast, only 35% of Whites have Fy(a-) red cells, the overwhelming majority of those individuals are phenotypically Fy(a-b+). In spite of this there are a number of reports (95,100-106) that indicate that a higher proportion of transfused Whites, than transfused Blacks, make anti-Fy^a. The calculation (for additional details see 102) is as follows. If 100 Whites are each transfused with two random units of red cells, a total of 29 will be Fy(a-) and will have received at least one unit of Fy(a+) blood (i.e. based on the frequency of Fy^a in patients and donors). If 100 Blacks are each transfused with two random units of red cells, a total of 77 will be Fy(a-) and will have received at least one unit of Fy(a+) blood. Thus if Fy^a was equally immunogenic in Whites and Blacks, it would be expected that the incidence of anti-Fy^a would be more than two and a half times higher in transfused Blacks than in transfused Whites. In the study of Kosanke (100) four of 25 examples of anti-Fy^a were made by Blacks. In the study of Vengelen-Tyler (101) 14 of 130 anti-Fy^a were made by Blacks. Thus in the combined studies 18 (11.6%) of 155 anti-Fy^a were made in Blacks. Even allowing for the fact that more Whites than Blacks may have been transfused, the 11.6% incidence clearly falls very short of the calculated figure that suggests that 73% of anti-Fy^a should be seen in Blacks. Supportive data on the paucity of production of anti-Fy^a in Blacks compared to Whites, when exactly the opposite would be expected from the phenotype incidences, were found in other studies (103-105). As examples, in studying 110 Duffy system antibodies, Beattie (104) reported that although the ratio of White to Black patients from whom the samples were obtained was 1.7 to 1, 92 of the antibodies were made by Whites and only 18 by Blacks. Even more dramatically, Baldwin et al. (105) reported studies on approximately 10,000 patients, 53% of whom were Black and 47% White. Of 71 examples of anti-Fy^a identified, 56 (79%) were made by Whites and only 15 (21%) by Blacks. Of 6 examples of anti-Fy^b, five were made by Whites and only one by a Black. In tests on samples from 566 Black patients, 69 of whom had sickle cell disease and all of whom had Fy(a-b-) red cells and had been transfused, Le Pennec et al. (95) found no Duffy system antibodies. The only study to dispute these overwhelming findings is that of Sosler et al. (99). Tests were described on samples from 9876 patients, 47% of whom were Black, 29% White and 24% Hispanic. Forty-five examples of anti-Fy^a and two anti-Fy3 were found. Of the antibodies identified, 29 were made by Blacks, 12 by Whites and six by Hispanics. Thus the incidence of a Duffy system antibody was 1 in 160 in Blacks, 1 in 239 in Whites and 1 in 395 in Hispanics. While the study purports to show that Fy^a is as immunogenic in Blacks as in Whites, the numbers fall far short of the expected 2.7 times higher incidence expected in Blacks, that is described above.

In studying the specificity of alloantibodies made by multiply transfused patients with sickle cell disease, almost all of whom were Black, Rosse et al. (107) noted that the fourth most frequently made antibody was anti-Fy^a. This, of course, is not in conflict with the data described above that show that Fy^a is less immunogenic in Blacks than in Whites. None of the reports cited has ever claimed that Black individuals are unable to make Duffy system antibodies as has sometimes (100,101) been inferred. Instead, the data show that a considerably lower percentage of Blacks than Whites, with Fy(a-) red cells, make anti-Fy^a following exposure to the Fy^a antigen.

The incidence of immunization to Fy3 must also be considered in any review of the ability of Black individuals, who have Fy(a-b-) red cells, to make Duffy system antibodies. As stated above, the incidence of the Fy:-3 (i.e. Fy(a-b-)) phenotype in Blacks is between 100,000 and 700,000 times greater in Blacks than in Whites. In spite of this, two of the first three examples of anti-Fy3 were made by Whites (12,13). Clearly, no further calculation is necessary. The possibility that the two different genetic backgrounds that result in the Fy(a-b-) phenotype are both present in Blacks and that those who make anti-Fy3 are genetically similar to the White lady who made the first example (11,12) is considered below.

The lack of production of anti-Fy^b by Blacks who have Fy(a-b-) red cells is now better understood. As explained above, a number of investigators (5-11) have shown that the phenotype in Blacks is most commonly associated with a gentoype in which two *Fy* genes, that are the same as *Fy^b* in their structural regions but which do not encode production of red cell-borne Fy^b antigen, are present. The Duffy glycoprotein is present on many of the tissue cells of those individuals and although neither Fy^b nor Fy^a have been detected on such cells (108,158) it seems that the presence of tissue bound Duffy glycoprotein, encoded by the *Fy* genes of these individuals, prevents them from making anti-Fy^b. Those few examples of anti-Fy^b that are seen in Blacks may be made by *Fy^a* homozygotes (rare in this population) or by individuals whose Fy(a-b-) status has a different genetic background. Mallinson et al. (11) studied the genetic situation in the White Australian lady who has Fy(a-b-) red cells and who made the first example of anti-Fy3 (12). Unlike Blacks it was found that this lady has a partial deletion in her *Duffy* genes (for details regarding the deletion, frame shift and stop codon, see a later section) and probably makes no red cell or tissue bound Duffy glycoprotein.

It is entirely probable that the two genetic backgrounds that result in the Fy(a-b-) phenotype, that is the *Fy* gene that fails to encode red cell-borne Duffy glycoprotein and the partially deleted *Duffy* gene that encodes no red cell and probably no tissue-borne Duffy glycoprotein, both exist in Blacks. As described in the section on the Duffy system and malaria, there was considerable selective advantage in favor of the Fy(a-b-) phenotype in areas of the world where one form of malaria was endemic. Thus if both genetic events leading to the phenotype arose in those populations, both would have been selectively propagated. This raises the possibility (not yet proved) that those Blacks who make anti-Fy3 have the deleted form of the gene rather than the *Fy* that fails to encode production of red cell-borne Duffy glycoprotein. In other words, those individuals who have Fy(a-b-) red cells but are genetically similar to persons with two functional *Fy^b* genes but in whom the *Fy* genes are switched off at the red cell level, may be unable to recognize Fy3 (or Fy^b or Fy5, see below) as foreign because of the presence of Duffy glycoprotein on their tissue cells. It may take the Fy(a-b-) phenotype as dictated by genes that encode no production of Duffy glycoprotein on red or tissue cells, to equip an individual with the ability to mount an alloimmune response to Fy3. Such an argument does not alter the concept that persons who are genetically *Fy^{a}Fy^a* and therefore phenotypically Fy(a+b-) or *Fy^{b}Fy^b* with phenotypically Fy(a-b+) red cells, can recognize Fy^b and Fy^a, respectively, as foreign and mount an alloimmune response. It does say that those who are genetically *FyFy* and phenotypically Fy(a-b-) at the red cell level, are not similarly equipped. It seems probable that by the time this book is published the appropriate experiments to test this hypothesis will have been performed. In earlier editions of this book, a suggested, rather convoluted genetic pathway, was introduced as a possible explanation for the observed reduced production of Duffy system antibodies by Blacks. Fortunately, such a proposal is now redundant. However, it does appear that what was called (106) unconverted FYPS in that model was actually what is now recognized as tissue-bound Duffy glycoprotein in most Blacks with Fy(a-b-) red cells.

Fy4 and Anti-Fy4

In 1970, in the first edition of this book, it was reported that Harris et al. (109) had tested at least eight examples of antibodies that reacted preferentially with Fy(a-b-) red cells from Blacks. Due to the atrocious storage properties of those antibodies and difficulties encountered in trying to reproduce results with weakly reactive red cell samples, no definitive study could be performed. There is no doubt that the antibodies studied were examples of the specificity described in this section. In 1973, Behzad et al. (22) described anti-Fy4, an antibody that reacted with all Fy(a-b-) samples from Blacks and with most of those, from the same ethnic group of donors, that were Fy(a+b-) or Fy(a-b+). Anti-Fy4 did not usually react with Fy(a+b+) cells from Black donors nor with many cells from Whites, regardless of their Duffy phenotype (but see below). It was concluded that anti-Fy4 probably detects a product of the *Fy* gene that had hitherto been regarded as silent. In other words, the phenotype Fy(a-b-) in Blacks was now thought to represent the genotype *Fy^{4}Fy^4*. Because of the high frequency of *Fy* (now *Fy^4*) in Blacks, it was assumed that the phenotype Fy(a+b-) represented the genotype *Fy^{a}Fy^4* most of the time and *Fy^{a}Fy^a* only rarely. Similarly, most Fy(a-b+) cells of Blacks would be from individuals genetically *Fy^{b}Fy^4*, less frequently the phenotype would

represent the genotype *Fy^{b}Fy^b*. In Whites, in whom *Fy* (*Fy^4*) was already known to be rare, the phenotypes Fy(a+b-) and Fy(a-b+) would represent the genotypes *Fy^{a}Fy^a* and *Fy^{b}Fy^b* respectively, in the vast majority of individuals. If *Fy^4* was indeed an allele at the *Fy^{a}Fy^b* locus, the phenotype Fy(a+b+) must represent the genotype *Fy^{a}Fy^b* in both Blacks and Whites.

There are a number of observations that suggest that the situation is not as straightforward as *Fy^4* being an allele of *Fy^a* and *Fy^b*. First, not all examples of Fy(a-b-) red cells reacted as if they carried a double dose of Fy4. Second, some examples of Fy(a+b+) red cells reacted weakly with anti-Fy4. Third, like Fy3 but unlike Fy^a and Fy^b, Fy4 appeared to survive protease treatment of red cells. Fourth and of greatest significance, if the Fy(a-b-) phenotype in the majority of Blacks represents the *FyFy* genotype in which the *Fy* gene fails to encode production of red cell-borne Duffy glycoprotein, it becomes difficult to imagine what anti-Fy4 might define. Similarly, it was reported (22) that the Fy(a-b-) red cells of the Australian lady who made the first example of anti-Fy3 (12), reacted weakly with anti-Fy4. In the report of the Cree Indian who made anti-Fy3 it is mentioned (13) that the Fy(a-b-) cells behaved "as expected" in tests with anti-Fy4 but that the authors did not have red cells properly to control the tests. In the cases in which three Black individuals made anti-Fy3 (91,93,94) no data are given about tests on the Fy(a-b-) red cells of the antibody-makers with anti-Fy4. Taken together, these observations cast considerable doubt about the place (if any) of Fy4 in the Duffy blood group system.

Anti-Fs

Palatnik et al. (202) described an antibody made by a Brazilian mulatto woman whose red cells were Fy(a+b+), that reacted preferentially with Fy(a-b-) red cells. The antibody was called anti-Fs, the antibody-maker also had anti-D and anti-V in her serum. The reactions of anti-Fs, like those of anti-Fy4, were difficult to interpret because of extreme variability in the strengths of reactions. The report describes the presence of Fs on the red cells of children born to two parents whose red cells were Fs-negative. As far as we are aware, no other example of anti-Fs has been described.

The Fy(a-b-) Phenotype in Other Ethnic Groups

As already described, in American Blacks the Fy(a-b-) phenotype is the most common of those in the Duffy system (4). In some parts of tropical Africa the phenotype has a 100% incidence (110). However, the phenotype has also been found in other ethnic groups. Such populations can be roughly divided into those in which *Fy* was introduced by known admixture from Black populations and those in which the introduction of genes from Blacks cannot be proved. In the former group, Race and Sanger (111) found Fy(a-b-) members in four Yemenite Jewish and two Iraqi families studied. Sandler et al. (17) extended these findings when they studied blood samples from 1207 Jews and 509 Arabs living in Israel. The Fy(a-b-) phenotype was found in Moslem, Christian and Druze Arabs and in Jewish immigrants from Yemen and Iraq. The authors (17) pointed out that the incidence of *Fy* was consistent with the known admixture (16,112-118) of those groups with native African and admixed regional populations. The *Fy* gene was not found in Sephardi or Ashkenazi Jews in whom no admixture seems to have occurred.

In contrast, in addition to the two cases already described (12,13) in which the Fy(a-b-) phenotype was found in an Australian and a Cree Indian, Race and Sanger (111) described a White male in Texas with the phenotype. Although Black admixture could not be totally excluded, it was pointed out that at least the man's mother, who had emigrated from England, must have been a White capable of transmitting *Fy*. Libich et al. (15) found five members (spanning two generations) of a Czechoslovakian gypsy family to have Fy(a-b-) red cells. Mannessier et al. (18) found the phenotype in an Algerian who, as mentioned earlier, had made anti-Fy3.

Fy5 and Anti-Fy5

Another new antibody in the Duffy system, anti-Fy5, was reported in 1973 by Colledge et al. (23). Unlike anti-Fy3 and anti-Fy4 which could, because of what was already known about the Duffy system, be expected eventually to come to light, anti-Fy5 arrived as an almost complete surprise. There had been some clues that the Duffy and Rh systems might, in some way, be interrelated (119-123) but the reactions of anti-Fy5 were still largely unexpected.

Anti-Fy5 was formed by an Fy(a-b-) Black male child. At first, anti-Fy5 looked like a second example of anti-Fy3 for it reacted with all cells that were Fy(a+) or Fy(b+) but with none that were Fy(a-b-). However, the difference between anti-Fy3 and anti-Fy5 became apparent when Rh_{null} red cells were tested. Such cells have normal expressions of Fy^a and Fy^b and had all reacted with anti-Fy3. These same cells were shown to be Fy:-5. Further studies showed that the amount of Fy5 on D-- cells was less than that on cells with normal Rh phenotypes although the D-- cells carried normal quantities of

Fy^a and/or Fy^b and were Fy:3. Like Fy3 and Fy4 but unlike Fy^a and Fy^b, Fy5 was shown still to be detectable on protease-treated Fy:5 red cells.

When the second example of anti-Fy5 was found (124) it was shown that the Rh_{null} red cells of persons genetically X^orX^or and those genetically $\overline{rr}$ are Fy:-5. This finding, of course, removed any speculation that the *CDE* genes might be involved in encoding production of Fy5. In 1980, the third example of anti-Fy5 (that was mistakenly called the second example in the published report) was described (125). Like the first two examples of the antibody, this one was made by a Black with Fy(a-b-) red cells. Although the report (125) attributes a delayed transfusion reaction in the patient to the anti-Fy5, many workers will consider this far from proved. The Fy:5 unit transfused was also C+ E+ and anti-C and anti-E were found in the posttransfusion sample. Other examples of anti-Fy5 have subsequently been described (97,126), sometimes the antibody has been present in sera that also contained anti-Fy^a (124,126), twice it has been seen (97) in patients who had previously made anti-Fy^a but in whom no separable anti-Fy^a was detectable when the anti-Fy5 was made. As might have been anticipated, red cells from persons genetically Fy^xFy^x have a weaker than usual expression of Fy5 (90). Meredith (127) reported that all of 13 examples of red cells with variant e antigens gave negative reactions with two anti-Fy5 by albumin-IAT and manual polybrene tests although the red cells reacted normally with anti-Fy^a and/or anti-Fy^b and with anti-Fy3. We do not know if this observation has been confirmed by others.

In the report (23) describing the first example of anti-Fy5 it is stated that the Fy(a-b-) Fy:-3 red cells of the Australian lady who made the first example of anti-Fy3 (12) are Fy:5. In contrast, the Fy(a-b-) Fy:-3 red cells of the Algerian who made anti-Fy3, were Fy:-5 (18). While this at first provides a tentative clue that production or non-production of Fy5 may be associated with the partially deleted *Duffy* gene and the non-functional (in terms of red cell antigens) *Fy* allele, a problem exists. Since in both genetic situations it is believed that the red cells lack Duffy glycoprotein, no site on the membrane would seem to exist for Fy5. Two possible explanations exist. First, the Fy:5 status of the Australian lady's red cells was determined with an eluted form of anti-Fy5, this being necessitated because of ABO incompatibility. While the controls all gave the expected results and the authors concluded that there were no reasons to question the validity of the test, the anti-Fy5 was available in too small an amount for a second confirmatory test. If those red cells, like those of the Algerian, were actually Fy:5, the association of Fy5 and the Duffy glycoprotein might seem more secure. The second possible explanation is that Fy5 (as suggested in an earlier section for Fy4) is not encoded from the *Duffy* locus. Fy5 (and perhaps Fy4) might, perhaps, be directly associated with presence or absence of the Duffy glycoprotein and the Rh polypeptides in a manner somewhat like the association of Wr^b, that represents a protein band 3 polymorphism (see Chapter 17) but that also requires the presence of glycophorin A (see Chapter 15) for expression.

Fy6 and Anti-Fy6

The most recent addition to the Duffy blood group system, the antigen Fy6, was recognized by a murine monoclonal antibody (24). The antigen is present on red cells that carry Fy^a and/or Fy^b but is absent from red cells that are phenotypically Fy(a-b-) Fy:-3,-5. The antigens Fy3 and Fy6 differ in that Fy3 survives treatment of red cells by proteases, while Fy6 is removed or denatured. As described in the section on malaria and the Duffy system, the red cells of some non-human primates are Fy:-6, although they carry Fy3, some with and some without Fy^b. A second example of anti-Fy6, that was also a murine monoclonal antibody, was described by Riwom et al. (60). As far as we are aware no human example of anti-Fy6 has been found. The expanded reactions of Duffy system antibodies are listed in table 14-4.

Enzyme Sensitivity of Duffy System Antigens Revisited

As described in the earlier sections of this chapter, Duffy system antigens vary in their susceptibility to

removal or denaturation when red cells are treated with proteases. Fy^a, Fy^b and Fy6 are no longer detectable on ficin, papain or chymotrypsin red cells; Fy3, Fy4 and Fy5 survive such treatment. The most simple explanation for these findings would seem to be that Fy3, Fy4 and Fy5 are carried on the Duffy glycoprotein at a point closer to the red cell membrane than is the enzyme cleavage site. If Fy^a, Fy^b and Fy6 are all distal to that site, their removal when red cells are treated with a protease would be explained. While such an explanation may sound too simple to be true, epitope mapping of Fy^a, Fy^b, Fy3 and Fy6, as described in detail in later sections, supports such a straightforward concept.

The Duffy System and Malaria

It has been known (128-132) for a very long time that a high proportion of African and American Blacks are resistant to certain forms of malaria. In 1975, Miller et al. (133) made the first connection between malaria and the Duffy blood group system when they showed that Fy(a-b-) red cells are not invaded, in vitro, by *Plasmodium knowlesi* parasites. Although *P. knowlesi* does not cause malaria in humans it is similar to *Plasmodium vivax*, a parasite known (134,135) to cause the disease in man. Since, at the time of the discovery (133), *P. vivax* could not be cultured *P. knowlesi* merozoites were used for the initial in vitro experiments. Later, when methods had been developed (136) for the in vitro culture of *P. vivax*, the observations made using *P. knowlesi* were confirmed. It was shown (133,137,138) that *P. knowlesi* and *P. vivax* (136) invade red cells that are Fy(a+) or Fy(b+) but that Fy(a-b-) red cells are resistant to such invasion. The

TABLE 14-4 To Show the Reactions of Six Different Antibodies of the Duffy Blood Group System

Red Cells Phenotype and Source	Antibody					
	Anti-Fy^a	Anti-Fy^b	Anti-Fy3	Anti-Fy4	Anti-Fy5	Anti-Fy6
Fy(a+b-) White donor	+	0	+	Most 0, Very few +	+	+
Fy(a+b-) Black donor	+	0	+	Most +, Few 0	+	+
Fy(a+b+) White or Black donor	+	+	+	See text	+	+
Fy(a-b+) White donor	0	+	+	Most 0, Very few +	+	+
Fy(a-b+) Black donor	0	+	+	Most +, Few 0	+	+
Fy(a-b-) White donor who made anti-Fy3	0	0	0	See text	+	0
Fy(a-b-) Cree Indian donor who made anti-Fy3	0	0	0	See text		0
Fy(a-b-) Black donor	0	0	0	Almost all +	0	0
Fy(a+b+) Rh$_{null}$ donor	+	+	+		0	+
Fy(a+b+) D - -/D - - donor	+	+	+		Weak +	+

resistance to invasion was seen (138) with Fy(a-b-) red cells from Blacks and with those of the White Australian lady (12) and two Cree Indians (13). That the situation is not completely straightforward became apparent early when it was shown (133,138,139) that *P. knowlesi* parasites attach to Fy(a-b-) red cells but that no invasion occurs. This, of course suggested that two sites on the red cell membrane are involved, one for merozoite attachment and another for actual red cell invasion. The association between the Duffy system antigens and *P. vivax* malaria was confirmed at the clinical level, simultaneously with the in vitro studies. In a series of studies (140-143) it was shown that among 65 individuals who had *P. vivax* infection or malaria, all except one had red cells that carried Fy^a or Fy^b or both. In studying antibodies to *P. vivax* it was found (141) that they were present almost exclusively in persons with Fy(a+) or Fy(b+) red cells whereas antibodies to *Plasmodium falciparum*, that causes a severe form of malaria and in which infection is not associated with the Duffy phenotypes, were present in equal distribution in persons with Fy(a+), Fy(b+) and Fy(a-b-) red cells.

Once anti-Fy6 became available it was seen (24,136) that it is the presence of the Fy6 antigen that results in invasion of human red cells by *P. vivax* merozoites. In man, the presence or absence of Fy6 is completely correlated with presence or absence of Fy^a or Fy^b. That is, Fy(a+) or Fy(b+) red cells are always Fy:6, those that are Fy(a-b-) are Fy:-6. The invasion of Fy(a+) red cells by *P. vivax* can be partially blocked by coating the red cells with anti-Fy^a (133,136), it is totally blocked by anti-Fy6 (24,136,144). The exact role of Fy6 in malarial parasite invasion of red cells was revealed in studies using the red cells of some non-human primates. The red cells of the Rhesus monkey *Macaca mulatta* are Fy(b+) Fy:3,-6. Those cells are invaded by merozoites of *P. knowlesi*, they are resistant to invasion by merozoites of *P. vivax* (24,136,144). The red cells of the New World monkeys *Saimiri sciureus* (squirrel monkey) and *Aotus triviratus* (dourocouli monkey) are Fy:3,6 (the former are Fy(b-), the latter are Fy(b+)) and are susceptible to invasion by *P. knowlesi* and *P. vivax* merozoites. The red cells of *Cebus apella* (capuchin monkey) are Fy(a-b-), Fy:3,-6, they are not invaded by either *P. knowlesi* or *P. vivax* merozoites (24,136,138). Taken together, these findings seem to indicate (in an oversimplified form) that Fy^a, Fy^b and sometimes Fy3 are involved in invasion by *P. knowlesi* merozoites, while Fy6 in involved in invasion by *P. vivax*.

The proteins of the malarial parasites that enable the merozoites to bind to the human red cell Duffy antigens have been isolated and partially characterized (145,146). The protein of *P. knowlesi* is called PkDAP-1, that of *P. vivax* PvDAP-1. Pk and Pv indicate *P. knowlesi* and *P.*

vivax, respectively, DAP indicates Duffy-associating protein. Genes encoding production of the two proteins have been cloned and show some homology (147,148).

That the full story of the Duffy-malaria interaction is not yet to hand is apparent from a number of other observations. First, treatment of human Fy(a+) or Fy(b+) red cells with chymotrypsin results in their becoming resistant to invasion by *P. knowlesi* and *P. vivax* merozoites (133,136). While chymotrypsin is known to remove or denature Fy^a, Fy^b and Fy6, it has no effect on Fy3. Second, treatment of human Fy(a-b-) red cells with trypsin or neuraminidase results in their becoming susceptible to invasion by *P. knowlesi* merozoites (138). Third, while a considerable amount is known about the Duffy system antigens whose presence or absence results in merozoite invasion or non-invasion, far less is known about the sites to which the merozoites first attach. Perhaps some of the apparently contradictory effects of enzymes mentioned in this paragraph result from the actions of the enzymes on the attachment site and not the invasion receptor. Similarly, perhaps some of the resistance seen among the red cells of non-human primates relates to lack of an attachment site rather than lack of an invasion receptor.

Assignment of the *Duffy* Locus to Chromosome One

In 1963, Renwick and Lawler (149) reported studies on a family in which some members had a total nuclear cataract. The gene whose presence results in this condition is called *Cae* and it was shown that the *Cae* and *Duffy* genes are linked. In 1968, Donahue et al. (25) reported the existence of a gene whose presence results in a benign structural change of chromosome one. Presence of *Un-1* (*Un* for uncoiler) results in a localized thinning in the structure of chromosome one, near the centromere. Although the presence of *Un-1* does not result in any detectable phenotypic marker, in individuals with the gene, its presence can readily be determined by studies of the person's chromosomes. It was found that in Donahue's own family, *Un-1* and the *Duffy* genes were traveling together. Thus, the *Duffy* locus was assigned to chromosome one by virtue of linkage to a structural maker. This finding (25) represented the first assignment of a blood group gene to a specific autosome. Since that time, other genes have been added to the *Cae*, *Duffy*, *Un-1*, linkage group, by virtue of their linkage with one or more of those genes. Rivas et al. (150) added the *Amy$_1$* and *Amy$_2$* genes, whose presence controls the production of salivary and pancreatic amylase enzymes. Bird et al. (151) and Guiloff et al. (152) added *CMT 1* (Charcot-Marie-Tooth neuropathy, type 1), Winter et al. (153) *AT3* (antithrombin III) and Raeymaekers et al. (154) *SPTA* (alpha-spectrin). A suspected (155) linkage between the gene responsible for Darier's disease and the *Duffy* locus, was later excluded (156). The site of the *Duffy* locus on chromosome 1 was established as 1q22-23 by virtue of studies involving chromosomal rearrangements (88,157), chromosomal deletions (159,160), and lod score analysis (161) and was confirmed by in situ hybridization using *Duffy* cDNA (162).

The Syntenic Relationship Between the *Rh* and *Duffy* Loci

Although the *Rh* and *Duffy* loci are known to be on chromosome one, family studies show that there is no demonstrable linkage between them (163). Accordingly, the loci are said to be syntenic, that is on the same chromosome but far enough apart that the rate of crossing-over between them is such that no linkage can be demonstrated. The distance between the *Rh* and *Duffy* loci is such that when serological studies are interpreted, the genes can often be shown to have segregated independently. It is from use of methods listed in the previous section, that it is known that the *Rh* and *Duffy* loci are on the same chromosome.

The demonstration that the *Rh* and *Duffy* loci are syntenic, strengthened a claim made in 1965 by Jenkins and Marsh (120), that the observations that they had made on the blood of a healthy donor, could best be explained by postulating that a single genetic event had affected both the *Rh* and *Duffy* genes. The donor studied had a mixed population of red cells: 25% of his cells typed as C+ D+ E- c+ e+; Fy(a+b+); the other 75% typed as C- D- E- c+ e+; Fy(a-b+). The parents of the donor appeared to be genetically R^1R^1, Fy^aFy^a and R^1r, Fy^bFy^b. Thus the 25% of the donor's red cells that typed as C+ D+ Fy(a+) appeared to be those representing his highly probable R^1r, Fy^aFy^b genotype. Since at the time no known genetic relationship between the *Rh* and *Duffy* loci existed, Jenkins and Marsh (120) were obliged to conclude that the somatic mutation, that they believed had occurred, had affected a gene in some way involved with the production of a precursor substrate, on which both the *CDE* and *Duffy* genes act. It was supposed that the mutation had resulted in the production of a substrate from which C, D and Fy^a could no longer be made. In 1965, the alternative would have been to postulate two mutations, one affecting the *CDE* and the second affecting the *Duffy* locus. Certainly, such an explanation would have been far less plausible. Once the syntenic relationship between *Rh* and *Duffy* had been recognized, Marsh and Chaganti (122) retested the blood of this donor and proposed a revised explanation. It was found in 1973 (122) that the

donor's blood contained the same mixed population of red cells that had been observed in 1965 (120). The family study had established, with a high degree of probability, that the donor was genetically R^1r, Fy^aFy^b. The revised explanation was that the 25% of the donor's red cells that typed as C+ D+ Fy(a+), were the products of hematopoietic stem cells in which all the donor's *Rh* and *Duffy* genes were functioning. The 75% of red cells that typed as C- D- Fy(a-), were considered to be products of hematopoietic stem cells in which the R^1 haplotype and the Fy^a gene were no longer active. In other words, those cells were regarded as the products of monosomic cell lines, of genotypes $- /r$, $- /Fy^b$. Marsh and Chaganti (122) performed chromosomal analysis of the donor's leukocytes but found no abnormality of chromosome one. As the authors pointed out, this finding did not exclude the possibility that a chromosomal rearrangement, too small to be visualized, had occurred. However, they considered it more likely that the chromosomal change had occurred in an erythropoietic precursor cell (studies on that cell line were not possible) but not in other cell lines. As Marsh (123) has pointed out, the studies described (120,122) do not prove the *Rh* and *Duffy* genes to be syntenic. That other proof that they are, is available, allows a simple explanation of the above described case, an alternative explanation of which would be difficult to imagine.

Identification and Characterization of The Glycoprotein Carrying the Duffy System Antigens

The glycoprotein expressing the Duffy antigens was first identified by Moore et al. (164) in immunoprecipitation experiments with human anti-Fy^a and anti-Fy^b and radioiodinated red cells of appropriate Duffy phenotype. A major radioiodinated band of Mr 40kD was observed. In 1984, Hadley et al. (165) described immunoblotting experiments in which human anti-Fy^a identified a diffuse band of 35-43kD that was chymotrypsin sensitive and trypsin resistant. Sialidase-treatment of Fy(a+) red cell membranes altered the pattern of anti-Fy^a staining on subsequent immunoblots and gave a prominent band of 31kD indicating that the Duffy antigen-bearing molecule is a glycoprotein. Hadley et al. (165) further noted that if the red cell membranes used for immunoblotting were prepared in the presence of 2-mercaptoethanol the Duffy glycoprotein aggregated suggesting that disruption of disulphide bonds in the molecule caused aggregation. Dahr and Kruger (166) showed that the Duffy glycoprotein could be solubilized from red cell membranes with very low concentrations of Triton X-100 (0.05%) and bound to thiopropyl-Sepharose, an observation consistent with a cysteine-containing molecule. Lisowska et al.

(167) also demonstrated binding of Duffy protein to thiol-Sepharose although they report that higher concentrations of Triton X-100 (1%) were required to solubilize the glycoprotein. Lisowska et al. (167) also showed that one of three anti-Fy^a gave decreased reactivity with Fy(a+b-) red cells or membranes that had been treated with N-ethylmaleimide (6.6mM) suggesting that a free thiol group influenced the binding of this anti-Fy^a.

In 1988, Tanner et al. (68) showed that the Duffy glycoprotein is extensively glycosylated with polylactosaminyl N-glycans. The glycoprotein was extremely sensitive to digestion with Endo F which reduced and sharpened the Fy^a-active component from 40-50kD to 26-28kD. Treatment with endo-beta galactosidase reduced the size of the leading edge of the Fy^a-active component to 33kD showing that some or all of the N-glycans contained poly-N-acetyllactosaminyl chains. Sialidase-treatment of Endo F-treated cells did not cause a further reduction in Mr indicating that O-glycans were not present. These results suggested that some 40 to 50% of the Fy^a glycoprotein is carbohydrate.

Purification of the Duffy glycoprotein from Triton X-100 solubilized red cell membranes by preparative immunoprecipitation with a murine monoclonal antibody denoted anti-Fy6 (169) was the critical step that opened the way to clone the *Fy* gene. Amino acid sequence information from tryptic peptides obtained from this purified protein, was used to design oligonucleotide probes that eventually yielded cDNA clones for the Duffy protein from a human bone marrow cDNA library (5). A concatenation of two cDNA clones allowed deduction of an open reading frame of 1267bp giving a predicted amino acid sequence of 338 amino acids. The protein was predicted to have an amino-terminal extracellular domain of 65 amino acids with two potential N-glycosylation sites, 64 residues according to Chaudhuri et al. (5) because the authors assume that the N-terminal methionine is cleaved and the next residue (Ala) is the true amino terminus. Since the amino terminus of the isolated protein is blocked this has not been proved but would be expected. In the discussion presented here numbering is from the N-terminal methionine. The extracellular amino terminal domain is rich in acidic amino acids and contains three potential sites for N-glycosylation (Asn18-Ser-Ser, Asn29-Ser-Ser, Asn35-Asp-Ser). Chaudhuri et al. (5) believe that only two of these sites are utilized because the third sequence contains Asp that is not a favored residue in signal sequences for N-glycosylation. The remainder of the protein comprises a large multispanning membrane domain (60% of the protein) and a small cytoplasmic domain of 24 amino acids. A search of protein sequence databases (170) revealed that 27% of the amino acids in the predicted protein are identical with the human IL-8 low affinity receptor (IL-

8RB) and that the protein has greater than 23% sequence identity with other human chemokine receptors. Chaudhuri et al. (5) interpreted a hydropathy plot of the Duffy protein sequence as being consistent with 9 membrane spanning domains. Most other workers have taken a different view and consider that seven membrane spanning domains are more likely. Strong additional evidence for the seven membrane spanning model comes from analogy (170) with other members of the family of chemokine receptors which share homology with the Duffy glycoprotein. In particular, the Duffy glycoprotein has four cysteine residues that are conserved in all leukocyte and viral chemokine receptors. If a model of the Duffy protein is drawn with seven membrane spanning domains, there are three predicted extracellular loops each with one of the conserved cysteine residues (see figure 14-1). The fourth conserved cysteine is located in the N-terminal extracellular domain. By analogy with other chemokine receptors one would predict two disulphide bonds; one between cysteines on extracellular loops 1 and 2 and the other between the cysteine on extracellular loop 3 and the conserved cysteine in the N-terminal domain. In the nine membrane spanning model there are four extracellular loops of which only the first would have a cysteine residue. There is a fifth conserved cysteine residue located in the last membrane spanning domain that may be a site for palmitoylation.

Both models predict an intracellular cytoplasmic domain. Direct evidence for this was obtained by Mallinson (171) who used a rabbit antiserum raised to a synthetic peptide corresponding to the sequence of the last 16 amino acids of the protein and showed that pre-adsorption of the serum with intact red cells did not remove its ability to react with Duffy glycoprotein on immunoblots whereas pre-adsorption with red cell membranes removed all reactivity for the Duffy glycoprotein.

Baldwin (172) proposed a general structural model for G protein-coupled receptors based on the crystallographic structure of bacteriorhodopsin and rhodopsin. In this model the seven transmembrane helices are arranged clockwise and perpendicular to the membrane around an inter-helical pocket that might form a pocket for ligand binding and/or internalization.

The Duffy Glycoprotein is a Chemokine Receptor

It was known (173) that red cells are able to bind the chemokine interleukin 8 (IL-8) before isolation of cDNA clones corresponding to the Duffy protein. By 1993 it was clear that the red cell membrane contained a receptor capable of binding a wide variety of chemokines ("a promiscuous inflammatory peptide receptor", Neote

Chapter 14

FIGURE 14-1 Model of the Duffy Glycoprotein and Location of Antigens

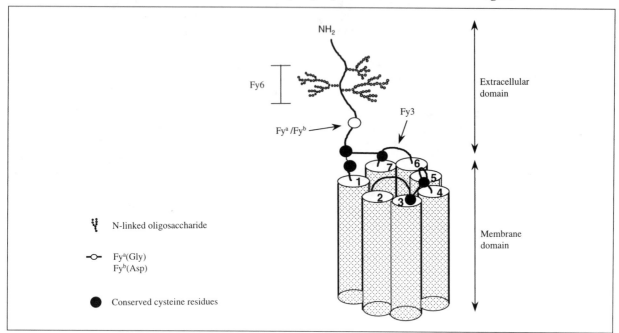

et al. (174)). In the August 1993 issue of *Science*, Horuk et al. (175) reported results indicating that the erythrocyte chemokine receptor and the Duffy glycoprotein were one and the same. Two of the authors of this paper (175) had noticed that red cells from the majority of African Americans did not bind IL-8. Since a high percentage of African Americans have the Fy(a-b-) phenotype (see earlier) the possibility that the failure to bind IL-8 correlated with the Fy(a-b-) phenotype was investigated and proved. Horuk et al. (175) also showed that the MAb denoted anti-Fy6 could block the binding of IL-8, MGSA, MCP-1 and RANTES (see below). Furthermore, MGSA and IL-8 inhibited the invasion of Fy(a+b-), Fy(a+b+) and Fy(a-b+) red cells by the simian malarial parasite *Plasmodium knowlesi*. These findings led Horuk et al. (175) to suggest that drugs modeled on the structure of IL-8 and MGSA might be therapeutically useful in areas of the world where chloroquine-resistant strains of *P. vivax* are found. In September 1993 one of us (DJA) was approached by Dr. Ken Soo from the Imperial Cancer Fund Laboratories in London. Dr. Soo had cloned the RANTES receptor and wished to obtain a monoclonal anti-Fy in order to test if RANTES corresponded to the Duffy glycoprotein. Using monoclonal anti-Fy3 provided by Dr Makoto Uchikawa, Red Cross Transfusion Service, Tokyo (the antibody was not described in print until 1996 (176)) Dr. Soo was able to show that the RANTES receptor he had cloned was the same as the Duffy glycoprotein but this work was overtaken by events when in November 1993, Chaudhuri et al. (5) published the cDNA sequence of the Duffy gly-

coprotein that was exactly the same as that of the RANTES chemokine receptor clone. Further proof that the Duffy glycoprotein and the red cell chemokine receptor are the same molecule was obtained by transfection studies in K562 cells (177) and in human embryonic kidney cells (178). Chaudhuri et al. (177) detected expression of Duffy glycoprotein using monoclonal anti-Fy6. Neote et al. (178) used anti-Fy6 and the anti-Fy3 described above. The Duffy glycoprotein is referred to as DARC (Duffy Antigen/Receptor for Chemokines) in some publications and ECKR (erythrocyte chemokine receptor) in others.

Duffy Glycoprotein (syn DARC, ECKR) Compared With Other Chemokine Receptors

The term chemokine is an abbreviation of chemoattractant cytokine. Chemokines are a large family of leukoattractants and activators. Nearly 30 distinct chemokines were known at the time of a 1994 review (179). All chemokines are small (8-10kD) polypeptides of about 350 amino acids sharing about 25% amino acid homology and most have four conserved cysteine residues that form the structure of the polypeptides through two disulphide bonds. The position of conserved cysteine residues forms the basis of a classification of the chemokines into two broad groups, the so-called C-C and C-X-C classes. This classification is based on whether or not the first two cysteines in the polypeptide are adjacent (C-C) or separated by an intervening residue

(C-X-C) where X is any amino acid. This structural distinction is related to the functions of the respective chemokines. Most C-X-C chemokines are chemoattractants for neutrophils not monocytes whereas most C-C chemokines appear to attract monocytes not neutrophils (179). Members of the C-X-C type include interleukin-8 (IL-8) and melanocyte growth-stimulating activity (MGSA). Members of the C-C group include RANTES, monocyte chemoattractant protein-1 (MCP-1) and macrophage inflammatory proteins (MIP) 1-alpha and 1-beta. Chemokines may also act as chemoattractants for subpopulations of lymphocytes. RANTES is a chemoattractant for memory T cells in vitro and MCP-1 is thought to induce T cell migration. The various selective effects of chemokines on different leukocyte populations are thought to be relevant to the process by which selected subpopulations of these cells migrate out of the blood stream into the tissues. The process by which leukocytes bind to endothelium before passage through junctions between the endothelial cells and entry into tissue is thought to involve three steps (180). Step 1 involves interaction between selectin molecules (discussed in Chapter 9) on the endothelium and mucin-like molecules on the circulating lymphocyte. This interaction triggers the release of chemoattractants from endothelial cells that bind to chemokine receptors on the lymphocytes. The binding of chemokine to chemokine receptor triggers a transmembrane signal that activates G proteins and a whole series of reactions that result in activation and upregulation of adhesive molecules (integrins) on the lymphocyte surface. This causes tight binding of the lymphocytes to endothelium through integrin on the lymphocytes and intercellular adhesion molecules (ICAMs, discussed in Chapter 13) on the endothelial cells.

Crucial to this process are the chemokine receptors. Chemokine receptors are a family of membrane glycoproteins characterized by the presence of seven membrane spanning domains (also known as the seven transmembrane domain receptors, STR (see 170, 179 and 181 for reviews)). Evidence that the Duffy glycoprotein is a member of this family of molecules was discussed above. In most chemokine receptors, binding of chemokine effects a conformational change in the receptor protein that causes a series of intracellular signaling events. These begin with the dissociation of trimeric GTP (guanosine triphosphate) binding proteins (G-proteins) and include the release of intracellular calcium and the phosphorylation of cellular proteins which eventually leads to activation of integrin molecules and binding of the leukocyte to ICAMs on the endothelium.

The Duffy glycoprotein does not effect release of intracellular calcium when it binds chemokines (178) and, as discussed elsewhere in this chapter, its role seems more likely to be as a scavenger for chemokines, the

chemokines garbage man! Perhaps the most persuasive argument for such a role is that the Duffy glycoprotein is the only chemokine receptor found to date, that will bind chemokines of either the C-C or C-X-C class.

Molecular Basis of Fy^a and Fy^b Antigens and The Location of The Binding Sites For Chemokines, Monoclonal Anti-Fy3 and Anti-Fy6

Once the sequence of Duffy cDNA was known, it was a comparatively simple matter to look for nucleotide sequence differences that might correspond to the Fy^a and Fy^b antigens respectively. Four different laboratories ran tests and all reached the same conclusions (6-9,182). When the *Duffy* genes of individuals of phenotype Fy(a+b-) and Fy(a-b+) are examined, a single nucleotide difference is found (G131A) that changes a single amino acid, Gly44 to Asp in the protein sequence. Direct evidence that this sequence change is responsible for the Fy^a/Fy^b polymorphism was obtained by transfection studies in COS-7 cells when the expected results were observed (6,7). These results locate the Fy^a/Fy^b antigens to the N-terminal extracellular domain of the protein (see figure 14-1). Inspection of the amino acid sequence of this domain reveals the absence of lysine and arginine residues and since trypsin specifically cleaves polypeptide chains at one or other of these residues, the well known trypsin-resistance of Duffy antigens is explained. The potential N-glycan sites are located in this domain and since the protein is known to be heavily N-glycosylated (see above) at least one of the sites and probably more must be utilized in the mature protein. Nevertheless Endo F treatment that removes the N-glycans, does not destroy Fy^a antigen activity (168) meaning that carbohydrate is not required for the formation of the antigen, a conclusion that suggests that the peptide region around residue 44 is exposed in the mature protein. There are two cysteine residues in the N-terminal domain (Cys53 and Cys56). Lisowska et al. (167) obtained evidence that the binding of one of three anti-Fy^a was reduced when red cells were treated with N-ethyl maleimide suggesting that a free thiol group was required for the reactivity of that antibody. Cys53 is conserved throughout the cytokine family and is likely to be disulphide bonded to the conserved cysteine on extracellular loop 3 (see above). However, it is possible that Cys56 is relevant to the antigen recognized by this antibody.

A murine monoclonal antibody denoted anti-Fy6 was described by Nichols et al. (24) in 1987. The antibody is of particular interest because it blocks invasion of red cells by the malarial parasite *Plasmodium knowlesi* (see above). The antibody fails to react with red cells of the

Fy(a-b-) phenotype and is distinguished from antibodies to Fy3, Fy4 and Fy5 because it does not react with red cells pre-treated with ficin, papain or chymotrypsin. A second monoclonal antibody with the same characteristics was described by Riwom et al. (60) and a third example was reported by Iwamoto et al. (183). Monoclonal anti-Fy6 blocks the binding of chemokines to the Duffy glycoprotein (175) suggesting that the binding site for chemokines is in the same region of the protein as the Fy6 epitope.

Zhao-hai et al. (184) demonstrated that chemokines and anti-Fy6 bind to the N terminal extracellular domain of the Duffy glycoprotein. These workers (184) prepared chimeric proteins comprising the entire N-terminal domain of the Duffy glycoprotein and the membrane domain and C-terminal domain of the IL-8 receptor B (IL-8RB). They exploited the amino acid sequence homology between residues 62-69 of the Duffy glycoprotein (S62ALPFFIL) and residues 27-34 of IL-8RB (S27TLPPFLL) to design a pair of complementary oligonucleotides (Duffy glycoprotein anti-sense, and IL-8RB sense) able to bind to either the Duffy glycoprotein or IL-8RB. This pair of oligonucleotides was used to generate two DNA fragments corresponding to the N-terminus of Duffy glycoprotein and the membrane domain and C-terminus of IL-8RB. The chimeric protein was then generated from the two fragments in a separate PCR. Stable transfectants of the chimeric protein were produced in K562 cells and used for chemokine and antibody binding experiments. Monoclonal anti-Fy6 bound to the chimeric protein but not to IL-8RB similarly expressed, demonstrating clearly that the epitope for the antibody is located in the N-terminal extracellular domain of the Duffy glycoprotein. The chimeric receptor bound IL-8 and MGSA with high affinity comparable to the native Duffy glycoprotein as well as RANTES, MCP-1 and a mutant MGSA(MGSA-E6A) which binds to the Duffy glycoprotein but not to IL-8RB. Monoclonal anti-Fy3 (176) did not bind to the chimeric protein nor did it inhibit chemokine binding. This result was not unexpected given the well documented observation that Fy3 is resistant to proteases. Zhao-hai et al. (184) went on to locate the Fy3 epitope recognized by the monoclonal antibody by preparing additional chimeric proteins containing the N terminal domain, the first extracellular loop and the N terminal domain of the Duffy protein and the first two extracellular loops. These chimeric proteins were expressed in insect cells using the baculovirus expression system. The results demonstrated that the Fy3 epitope was dependent on the third extracellular loop of the Duffy glycoprotein (see figure 14-1). The reactivity of human anti-Fy3 was not examined.

By comparing the sequences of *Fy* genes from chimpanzee and from rhesus, squirrel and aotus monkeys, the reactivity of their respective red cells with monoclonal anti-Fy6 and the susceptibility of their red cells to invasion by *Plasmodium vivax*, Chaudhuri et al. (8) concluded that the N-terminal region critical for anti-Fy6 reactivity involves residues 23 to 41 (22-40 in the paper because this group use a different numbering system as explained above) and that the binding site for *P. vivax* also involves residues 23-41 (figure 14-1). In the same paper it is suggested that residues 48, 57 and 60 may be relevant to Fy^b antigen structure because in squirrel monkey Duffy protein these residues are changed to Ala, Ser and Asn respectively and squirrel monkey cells fail to react with anti-Fy^b.

The N-terminal extracellular domain of chemokine receptors is rich in acidic amino acids (Glu/Asp) and this feature is thought (170) to be relevant to chemokine binding. Since the Fy^a antigen results from an Asp44 to Gly change, that is the loss of an acidic residue, Mallinson et al. (185) examined the binding of chemokines, RANTES, MGSA/gro, IL-8 and MCP-1 to Fy(a+) and Fy(b+) transfectants. No differences in chemokine binding were observed.

Duffy Typing From DNA

The single nucleotide difference (G131A) that defines the difference between the Fy^a and the Fy^b antigen, discussed in the previous section can be exploited for DNA based determination of the Duffy type of an individual. The nucleotide sequence corresponding to Fy^a but not that corresponding to Fy^b is a substrate for the restriction endonuclease *Ban I* (7-9,11). It is therefore possible to design an RFLP assay using *Ban I* that will determine the Duffy genotype of a individual. Mallinson et al. (11) described such an assay. Oligonucleotide primers were used to amplify a product of 583bp containing the polymorphic site from individuals of known Duffy phenotype. The products were digested with *Ban I* and subjected to electrophoresis on 2% agarose gels. DNA from individuals of phenotype Fy(a-b+) gave three bands of 364, 111 and 107bp while DNA from individuals of phenotype Fy(a+b-) gave four bands of 210, 154, 111 and 107bp. All bands were observed in digests of DNA from individuals of phenotype Fy(a+b+). As discussed earlier, anti-Fy^a is occasionally the causative antibody in cases of severe hemolytic disease of the newborn. The DNA based assay described above has been of value in the management of pregnancies at risk from HDN due to anti-Fy^a in the laboratory of one of the authors (DJA). DNA obtained by chorionic villus sampling or from amniocytes obtained at amniocentesis from pregnancies at risk (previously affected pregnancy and/or very high titer anti-Fy^a) can be typed for Duffy antigens and this information enables the obstetrician to plan an appropriate program of prenatal care. If the fetus is Fy(a-) there is no risk, if Fy(a+) a program of fetal monitoring can be instigated.

There is a very important caveat pertaining to the use of DNA based blood typing methods. The results obtained describe the genotype not the phenotype of the red cells of the fetus or patient. This aspect is particularly relevant to Duffy typing since the Fy(a-b-) phenotype is very common in Africans who type as Fy(a-b+) when DNA is used. This is because the Fy(a-b-) phenotype results not from an absence of the *Fy^a* and *Fy^b* genes but from a mutation outside the structural gene that prevents the transcription of the gene in erythroid cells (6, and see later in this chapter).

Organization of the *Fy* Genes

When Duffy glycoprotein DNA is amplified from genomic DNA using oligonucleotide primers based on the cDNA sequence published by Chaudhuri et al. (5) a product of the same size as that obtained from reticulocyte cDNA is obtained. When the genomic DNA is sequenced it gives the same sequence as cDNA. This means that the genomic sequence amplified is contained within a single exon (7-9,11). However, Iwamoto et al. (183,203) have shown that the situation is not quite as simple as these early results suggested. These workers set out to characterize the 5' end of Duffy mRNA and

using a technique known as 5' RACE (5' rapid amplification of cDNA ends) isolated seven clones from erythroblast RNA and nine clones from lung RNA. The clones revealed novel nucleotide sequences containing a small exon (denoted exon 0.1 in the paper). Exon 0.1 encodes seven amino acid residues initiated by a methionine and in the clones isolated by Iwamoto et al. (183) it is spliced into the sequence of the cDNA clone described by Chaudhuri et al. (5) at nucleotide 203. The result of this splicing event is the creation of a Duffy glycoprotein that is exactly the same as the protein predicted from the cDNA clone of Chaudhuri et al. (5) except that the first nine amino acids (MASSGYVLQ) are replaced by seven residues with the sequence MGN-CLHR (see figure 14-2). When this novel sequence was transfected into K562 cells the expressed protein reacted with monoclonal anti-Fy6 indicating that the N-terminal sequence is not relevant to the expression of the Fy6 epitope, a conclusion consistent with other studies described in a preceding section.

So there are two kinds of Duffy protein, differing only at their extreme N-terminus. This observation raises several questions. Are both proteins expressed in red cells? If so, which form predominates? Are the two forms differentially expressed in different tissues? Iwamato et al. (183,203) carried out Northern blotting studies to see which isoform predominates in erythroid cells and other tissues. In every case, the Duffy transcript containing the product of exon 0.1 was the predominant

FIGURE 14-2 Point Mutation in GATA-1 Binding Site of *FY* Gene Prevents Expression of FY Glycoprotein in Red Cells of Fy(a-b-) Individuals

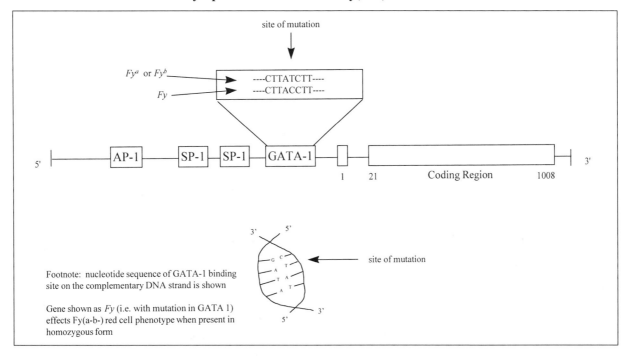

form. The authors concluded that the spliced-form Duffy mRNA encodes the predominant protein in red cells.

Tissue Distribution of Duffy Glycoprotein

Chaudhuri et al. (5) could detect the 1.3kb Duffy mRNA by Northern blotting in adult human bone marrow, spleen and kidney and in fetal liver. A 1.3kb mRNA is also found in adult human pancreas, skeletal muscle, lung, heart and colon. A larger 6.8kb species is found in placenta and brain (171,177,178). Duffy mRNA is not found in adult liver (5,171,178). Duffy mRNA is of low abundance in reticulocytes compared to bone marrow suggesting that little Duffy glycoprotein is produced in the later stages of erythroid maturation (185). The presence of Duffy glycoprotein in kidney membranes was demonstrated by immunoblotting with monoclonal anti-Fy6 (158). The kidney form of Duffy glycoprotein has a slightly larger Mr than that on red cells which is probably attributable to differences in glycosylation between the two molecules (the nucleotide sequence kidney Duffy mRNA is identical to the bone marrow sequence). Immunohistochemistry demonstrated that the Duffy glycoprotein in kidney is in small, thin-walled blood vessels (post-capillary venules) (158). Duffy glycoprotein is also expressed on endothelial cells of small venules in a wide variety if tissues except for liver (158). Duffy glycoprotein was also found in endothelial cells of small venules in breast tissue from one individual and in spleen from another individual, with the African Fy(a-b-) phenotype (10). These results are consistent with studies described above that show that the Duffy glycoprotein is absent only from the red cells of Fy(a-b-) individuals of this type because of a nucleotide substitution in a GATA-1 binding site (7,204). These results have also led to speculation that the absence of any clinical problems in individuals with the Fy(a-b-) phenotype can be explained because it is a selective deficiency from red cells only and the critical functions are carried out in other cells and tissues. This argument has to be reconciled with the occurrence of rare individuals with the Fy(a-b-) phenotype who have structural gene defects and may lack the protein from all their tissues, without apparent deleterious results (see later section).

Function of The Duffy Glycoprotein

Neote et al. (178) noted that although chemokines bound with high affinity to the Duffy glycoprotein they could not find evidence for signal transduction by looking for increases in intracellular calcium levels consequent upon chemokine binding. Other chemokine receptors (IL-8 receptor was used as the control in this study) mobilize intracellular calcium when chemokines are bound by a mechanism involving G-proteins. The general mechanism of signal transduction effected by chemokines was discussed in more detail in an earlier section. Several lines of evidence (170,181) suggest that the intracellular loops and cytoplasmic domain of chemokine receptors are involved in G-protein binding. It is therefore of interest to compare the sequence of the predicted cytoplasmic loops and C-terminal domain of Duffy glycoprotein with those of chemokine receptors known to effect signal transduction. Alignment of the sequence of the second intracellular loop of Duffy glycoprotein with those of other chemokines reveals the absence of a motif DRY-LAIVHA that is conserved in many other chemokine receptors. However, since many of the chemokine receptors were cloned by PCR amplification of mRNA using degenerate oligonucleotide primers to this region, it is difficult to know if this difference is relevant to function (170). The third intracellular loop of chemokine receptors is typically rich in positively charged amino acids. The Duffy glycoprotein has positively charged residues in this loop although there are fewer than in other chemokine receptors which may be significant. The C-terminal domain of Duffy glycoprotein, in common with other chemokine receptors, contains several serine residues that provide sites for phosphorylation. The last transmembrane domain of the Duffy glycoprotein contains a cysteine residue near the cytoplasmic face. This cysteine, that is conserved in the chemokine receptor family, may be a site for palmitoylation. Replacement of a conserved cysteine in the cytoplasmic domain of the beta 2 adrenergic receptor, and in rhodopsin, by site-directed mutagenesis, resulted (181) in a partial loss of G-protein coupling activity suggesting a possible functional role for palmitoylation. The regions of structure implicated in binding G-proteins are a highly conserved Asp/Glu-Arg-Tyr sequence in intracellular loop 2, intracellular loop 3, and the portion of the C-terminus near to the last transmembrane domain (186). Inspection of the Duffy protein sequence in each of these regions reveals differences from other members of the chemokine receptor family that might explain the lack of intracellular calcium mobilization in the experiments described by Neote et al. (178). In this context it is pertinent that Peiper et al. (10) found that K562 cells transfected with Duffy glycoprotein are able to internalize radioiodinated chemokines. Almost 40% of bound radioiodinated MGSA was internalized after 3 hours of incubation. These results raise the possibility that the Duffy glycoprotein functions as a clearance receptor for chemokines rather than as a signaling receptor. Red cells do not internalize chemokines (10). In this context it is interesting to note a report (187) that IL-2 immunotherapy induces circulating and red cell bound IL-8.

If the Duffy glycoprotein is a chemokine clearance receptor then one has to ask why Fy(a-b-) individuals are apparently not disadvantaged by the lack of such a huge chemokine sink as that provided by the large number of circulating red cells in an individual who does not have the Fy(a-b-) phenotype. There are reports (188,189) that chemokines, including IL-8 and MCP are released in in vitro models of hemolytic transfusion reactions and that chemokines, including IL-8 and MIP-1, are released by leukocytes present in blood components during storage and may have a role in febrile non-hemolytic transfusion reactions. These observations raise the question of whether or not individuals with the Fy(a-b-) phenotype suffer more severe transfusion reactions because of the absence of a chemokine clearance receptor on their red cells. If they do not then either the release of chemokines is not relevant to the transfusion reaction or individuals with the Fy(a-b-) phenotype can compensate for the absence of this chemokine clearance receptor in some as yet undiscovered way. Horuk et al. (175) cite evidence that Blacks have a lower peripheral neutrophil count than Whites as a possible lead in the search for such an explanation. Tanaka et al. (191) provide evidence that CD44 on endothelial cells can bind MIP-1 beta and that this bound chemokine can selectively trigger adhesion to lymphocyte subsets and other cell types. CD44 is expressed on red cells and is the molecule that expresses the Indian blood group antigens (see Chapter 29). It remains to be seen whether or not there are circumstances in which red cell CD44 can bind MIP-1 beta and/or other chemokines and to what extent such a mechanism can compensate for the deficiency of the Duffy glycoprotein in Fy(a-b-) red cells.

Molecular Basis of the Fy(a-b-) Phenotype

Elucidation of the molecular bases of null phenotypes is of interest in all the blood group systems because the information that results may throw light on the functional significance of the blood group active molecule in normal red cells and tissues. In the Duffy blood group system such studies are of special significance because of the selective advantage that the Fy(a-b-) phenotype confers on those who live in areas where *Plasmodium vivax* is found. In the paper (5) that described the Duffy cDNA clone, it was noted that the gene appeared normal in DNA from Blacks with the Fy(a-b-) phenotype but that Duffy mRNA was not detectable in the erythroid cells of these individuals. These results clearly indicated that there was a defect in the regulation of the *Fy* gene in the erythroid cells of these individuals. The molecular basis of this defect was elucidated (7) when it was shown that there was a nucleotide substitution in the 5′ noncoding region of the *Fy* gene which disrupts a binding site for the erythroid transcription factor GATA-1 and in so doing prevents normal transcription of the *Fy* gene in the erythroid cells of these individuals. Tournamille et al. (7) used the 5′ RACE method to identify a novel cap site in the *Fy* gene 484 nucleotides upstream from the first ATG identified by Chaudhuri et al. (5) and concluded that the *Fy* gene is a single exon. However, it appears from the work of Iwamoto et al. (183) that the cDNA isolated by Tournamille et al. (7) in fact corresponds to prespliced mRNA and contains the exon 0.1 sequence. Iwamoto et al. (183) confirmed the nucleotide substitution in the GATA-1 binding site described by Tournamille et al. (7) in DNA from three Blacks with the Fy(a-b-) phenotype and so the position of the critical mutation in figure 14-2 is based on the work of Iwamoto et al. (183).

The Fy(a-b-) phenotype so common in West Africans is extremely rare in other populations. It is therefore of interest to know if the genetic mechanism is the same as in Blacks when the Fy(a-b-) phenotype occurs in other populations. Two of the Fy(a-b-) members of a Czech family described by Libich et al. (15) have the same mutation in the same GATA-1 binding site as is found in Blacks (193). However, there are three other individuals of the Fy(a-b-) phenotype with different mutations in the *Fy* gene. Amplification of the *Fy* gene from the Fy(a-b-) individual AZ (12) revealed that a 14 bp deletion in the coding region (nucleotides 292-305) resulting in a frameshift that introduces a stop codon and produces a truncated protein of 118 amino acids. The predicted protein would contain the N-terminal extracellular domain and the first membrane spanning domain of the normal Duffy glycoprotein. Since this portion of the molecule contains the Fy^a/Fy^b polymorphism in the normal protein, it can be concluded that either the truncated protein cannot be incorporated into the plasma membrane or that the rest of the molecule is required for Duffy antigen activity in normal red cells. Another individual (NE) of phenotype Fy(a-b-) was shown (185) to have a single base change (G414A) which introduces a stop codon instead of Trp138. The Duffy glycoprotein produced by this individual would consist of the N-terminal domain and the first two membrane spanning domains. Analysis of the *Fy* gene in DNA from the Cree Indian Fy(a-b-) individual ML (13) also demonstrated a single nucleotide substitution that introduces a stop codon in place of a tryptophan, this time in codon 98 (194). The Duffy glycoprotein produced by this individual would be similar to that produced by donor AZ in that the N-terminal domain and the first transmembrane domain would be transcribed.

Unlike the situation in Fy(a-b-) individuals of African origin that results in an absence of Duffy glycoprotein from red cells but not from other cells and tissues, the mutations found in donors AZ, NE and ML are in the structural gene and would result in total absence or expression of a grossly abnormal Duffy glycoprotein in all the tissues of the affected individual. There are no reports of any clinical abnormalities associated with the Fy(a-b-) phenotype, a fact that raises questions about the functional significance of the Duffy glycoprotein.

References

1. Cutbush M, Mollison PL, Parkin DM. Nature 1950;165:188
2. Cutbush M, Mollison PL. Heredity 1950;4:383
3. Ikin EW, Mourant AE, Pettenkoffer HJ, et al. Nature 1951;168:1077
4. Sanger R, Race RR, Jack JA. Br J Haematol 1955;1:370
5. Chaudhuri A, Polyakova J, Zbrzezna V, et al. Proc Nat Acad Sci USA 1993;90:10793
6. Tournamille C, Colin Y, Cartron J-P. Nature Genetics 1995;10:224
7. Tournamille C, Le Van Kim C, Gane P, et al. Hum Genet 1995;95:407
8. Chaudhuri A, Polyakova J, Zbrzezna V, et al. Blood 1995;85:615
9. Iwamoto S, Omi T, Kajii E, et al. Blood 1995;85:622
10. Peiper SC, Wang Z, Neote K, et al. J Exp Med 1995;181:1311
11. Mallinson G, Soo KS, Schall TJ, et al. Br J Haematol 1995;90:823
12. Albrey JA, Vincent EER, Hutchinson J, et al. Vox Sang 1971;20:29
13. Buchanan DI, Sinclair M, Sanger R, et al. Vox Sang 1976;30:114
14. Hrubisko M, Mergancova O, Kusiková M. Vintrni Lekarstvi 1976;22:52
15. Libich M, Kout M, Giles CM. Vox Sang 1978;35:423
16. Sandler SG, Schilirò G, Russo A, et al. Acta Haematol 1978;60:350
17. Sandler SG, Kravitz C, Sharon R, et al. Vox Sang 1979;37:41
18. Mannessier L, Habibi B, Salmon C. Rev Fr Transf Immunohematol 1979;22:195
19. Mollison PL. Blood Transfusion in Clinical Medicine, 7th Ed. Oxford:Blackwell, 1983
20. Chown B, Lewis M, Kaita H. Am J Hum Genet 1965;17:384
21. Lewis M, Kaita H, Chown B. Vox Sang 1972;23:523
22. Behzad O, Lee CL, Gavin J, et al. Vox Sang 1973;24:337
23. Colledge KI, Pezzulich M, Marsh WL. Vox Sang 1973;24:193
24. Nichols ME, Rubinstein P, Barnwell J, et al. J Exp Med 1987;166:776
25. Donahue RP, Bias WB, Renwick JH. Proc Nat Acad Sci USA 1968;61:949
26. Hardman JT, Beck ML. Transfusion 1981;21:343
27. Szymanski IO, Huff SR, Delsignore R. Transfusion 1982;22:90
28. Issitt CH, Tessel JA, Issitt PD. Unpublished observations 1976, cited in previous editions of this book
29. Rosenfield RE, Vogel P, Race RR. Rev Hematol 1950;5:315
30. Contreras M, Gordon H, Tidmarsh E. (Letter). Br J Haematol 1983;53:355
31. Freiesleben E. Acta Path Microbiol Scand 1951;29:283
32. Hutcheson JB, Haber JM, Kellner A. J Am Med Assoc 1952;149:274
33. Giblett ER, Hillman RS, Brooks LE. Vox Sang 1965;10:448
34. Croucher BEE, Crookston MC, Crookston JH. Vox Sang 1967;12:32
35. Badakere SS, Bhatia HM. Ind J Med Sci 1970;24:562.
36. Badakere SS, Bhatia SM, Sharma RS, et al. Ind J Med Sci 1970;24:565
37. Magni E, Rossetti V. Minerva Medica 1972;63:2525
38. Moncrieff RE, Thompson WP. Am J Clin Pathol 1975;64:251
39. Pineda AA, Taswell HF, Brzica SM Jr. Transfusion 1978;18:1
40. Solanki D, McCurdy PR. J Am Med Assoc 1978;239:729
41. Boyland IP, Mufti GL, Hamblin TJ. (Letter). Transfusion 1982;22:402
42. Gover PA, Morton JR. Clin Lab Haematol 1990;12:233
43. Baker JB, Grewar D, Lewis M, et al. Arch Dis Childh 1956;31:298
44. Greenwalt TJ, Sasaki T, Gajewski M. Vox Sang 1959;4:138
45. Bevan B. Lancet 1959;1:914
46. Geczy A. Vox Sang 1960;5:551
47. Giblett ER. Clin Obstet Gynecol 1964;7:1044
48. Weinstein L, Taylor ES. Am J Obstet Gynecol 1975;121:643
49. Bowman JM. In: Immunobiology of Transfusion Medicine. New York:Marcel Dekker, 1994:553
50. Bowman J. Transf Med Rev 1990;4:191
51. Carreras Vescio LA, Farinas D, Rogido M, et al. (Letter). Transfusion 1987;27:366
52. Issitt PD, Issitt CH, Wilkinson SL. Transfusion 1974;14:103
53. Issitt PD, Smith TR. In: A Seminar on Performance Evaluation. Washington, D.C.:Am Assoc Blood Banks, 1976:25
54. Won CD, Shin HS, Kim SW, et al. J Phys Anthropol 1960;18:115
55. Speiser P. Wein Klin Wschr 1959;71:549
56. Simmons RT, Gajdusek DG, Gorman JG, et al. Nature 1967;213:1148
57. Toivanen P, Hirvonen T. Scand J Haematol 1969;6:49
58. Toivanen P, Hirvonen T. Vox Sang 1973;24:372
59. Masouredis SP, Sudora E, Mahan L, et al. Blood 1980;56:969
60. Riwom S, Janvier D, Navenot JM, et al. Vox Sang 1994;66:61
61. Rosenfield RE, Vogel P. Transact NY Acad Sci 1951;13:213
62. Unger LJ, Katz L. J Lab Clin Med 1951;38:188
63. Unger LJ, Katz L. J Lab Clin Med 1952;39:135
64. Morton JA. PhD Thesis, Univ London 1957
65. Haber G, Rosenfield RE. In: P.H. Andresen, Papers in Dedication of his 60th Birthday. Copenhagen:Munksgaard, 1957
66. Morton JA. Br J Haematol 1962;8:134
67. Issitt PD, Jerez GC. Transfusion 1966;6:155
68. Vyas GN, Fudenberg HH. Vox Sang 1968;15:300
69. Prager MD, Soules ML, Fletcher MA. Transfusion 1968;8:220
70. Chattoraj A, Kamat M, Summaria L. Proc Soc Exp Biol Med 1969;130:1315
71. Judson PA, Anstee DJ. Med Lab Sci 1977;34:1
72. Daniels GL. Immunohematology 1992;8:53
73. Strohm PL, Busch S. Transfusion 1969;9:93
74. Springer GF. Bact Rev 1963;27:191
75. Rosenfield RE, Szymanski IO, Kochwa S. Cold Spr Harb Symp Quant Biol 1964;29:427
76. Williams D, Johnson CL, Marsh WL. Transfusion 1981;21:357
77. Davies DM, Hall SJ, Graham HA, et al. (abstract). Transfusion 1979;19:638
78. Linnins I, McIntyre J, Moore BPL. Canad J Med Technol 1959;21:47
79. Race RR, Sanger R, Lehane D. Ann Eugen 1953;17:255
80. Chown B, Lewis M, Kaita H. Am J Hum Genet 1962;14:301
81. Race RR, Sanger R. Blood Groups in Man, 5th Ed.

Oxford:Blackwell, 1968

82. Habibi B, Fouillade MT, Levanra J, et al. Rev Fr Transf Immunohematol 1977;20:427

83. Caren LD, Bellavance R, Grumet FC. Transfusion 1982;22:475

84. Oien L, Nance S, Garratty G. (abstract). Transfusion 1985;25:474

85. Nance ST. In: Progress in Immunohematology. Arlington, VA:Am Assoc Blood Banks, 1988:1

86. Ginsburg JC, Singer MA. New Eng J Med 1978;299:775

87. Cedergren B, Giles CM. Vox Sang 1973;24:264

88. Cook PJL, Page BM, Johnston AW, et al. Cytogenet Cell Genet 1978;22:378

89. Habibi B, Perrier P, Salmon C. J Immunogenet 1980;7:191

90. Marsh WL. CRC Rev Clin Lab Sci 1975;5:387

91. Oberdorfer CE, Kahn B, Moore V, et al. Transfusion 1974;14:608

92. Molthan L, Crawford MN. (abstract). Prog 30th Ann Mtg, Am Assoc Bloods Banks, 1977

93. Molthan L, Crawford MN. (abstract). Transfusion 1978;18:386

94. Oakes J, Taylor D, Johnson C, et al. (Letter). Transfusion 1978;18:127

95. Le Pennec PY, Rouger P, Klein MT, et al. Vox Sang 1987;52:246

96. Kosinski KS, Molthan L, White L. Rev Fr Transf Immunohematol 1984;27:619

97. Vengelen-Tyler V. (abstract). Transfusion 1985;25:482

98. Jensen N, Crosson J, Grotte D, et al. (abstract). Transfusion 1988;28 (Suppl 6S):8S

99. Sosler SD, Perkins JT, Fong K, et al. Transfusion 1989;29:505

100. Kosanke J. Red Cell Free Press 1983;8:4

101. Vengelen-Tyler V. (Letter). Red Cell Free Press 1983;8:14

102. Issitt PD. (Letter). Immunohematology 1984;1:11

103. Beattie KM. (Letter). Red Cell Free Press 1983;8:13

104. Beattie KM. (Letter). Immunohematology 1984;1:14

105. Baldwin M, Shirey RS, Coyle K, et al. (abstract). Transfusion 1986;26:546

106. Issitt PD, Issitt CH. Applied Blood Group Serology, 2nd Ed. Oxnard:Spectra Biologicals, 1975

107. Rosse WF, Gallagher D, Kinney TR, et al. Blood 1990;76:1431

108. Rouger P, Salmon C. Rev Fr Transf Immunohematol 1982;25:643

109. Harris JP, Tegoli J, Jacobson G, et al. Unpublished observations 1966 to 1968, cited by Issitt PD. Applied Blood Group Serology, lst Ed. Oxnard:Spectra Biologicals 1970

110. Mourant AE, Kopec AC, Domaniewska-Sobczak K. The Distribution of the Human Blood Groups and Other Biochemical Polymorphisms, 2nd Ed. Oxford:Oxford Univ Press, 1976

111. Race RR, Sanger R. Blood Groups in Man, 4th Ed. Oxford:Blackwell, 1962:248 and 443

112. Bonne B, Ashbel S, Modai M, et al. Hum Hered 1970;20:609

113. Pollitzer WS. CRC Crit Rev Clin Lab Sci 1970;1:193

114. Bonne B, Godber M, Ashbel S, et al. Am J Phys Anthropol 1971;34:397

115. Pollitzer WS. Haematologia 1972;6:193

116. Gelpi AP. Ann Intern Med 1973;79:258

117. Gelpi AP, King MC. Science 1976;191:1284

118. Levene C, Rachmilewitz EA, Ezekiel E, et al. Acta Haematol 1976;55:300

119. Race RR, Sanger R. Blood Groups in Man, 2nd Ed. Oxford:Blackwell, 1954

120. Jenkins WJ, Marsh WL. Transfusion 1965;5:6

121. Sturgeon P. Blood 1970;36:310

122. Marsh WL, Chaganti RSK. Transfusion 1973;13:314

123. Marsh WL. Med Lab Sci 1976;33:125

124. DiNapoli J, Garcia A, Marsh WL, et al. Vox Sang 1976;30:308

125. Chan-Shu SA. Transfusion 1980;20:358

126. Bowen DT, Devenish A, Dalton J, et al. Vox Sang 1988;55:35

127. Meredith LC. (abstract). Transfusion 1985;25:482

128. Mayne B. Public Health Rep 1932;47:1771

129. Boyd MF, Stratman-Thomas WK. Am J Hyg 1933;18:485

130. Young MD, Eyles DE, Burgess RW. J Parasitol 1955;41:315

131. Bray RS. J Parasitol 1958;44:371

132. Young MD, Baerg DC, Rossan RN. Exp Parasitol 1975;38:136

133. Miller LH, Mason SJ, Dvorak JA, et al. Science 1975;189:561

134. Milan DF, Coggeshall LT. Am J Trop Med 1938;18:331

135. Miller LH, Dvorak JA, Shiroishi T, et al. J Exp Med 1973;138:1597

136. Barnwell JW, Nichols ME, Rubinstein P. J Exp Med 1989;169:1795

137. Miller LH, Haynes JD, McAuliffe FM, et al. J Exp Med 1977;146:277

138. Mason SJ, Miller LH, Shiroishi T, et al. Br J Haematol 1977;36:327

139. Miller LH, Aikawa M, Johnson JG, et al. J Exp Med 1979;149:172

140. Miller LH, Mason SJ, Clyde DF, et al. New Eng J Med 1976;295:302

141. Spencer HC, Miller LH, Collins WE, et al. Am J Trop Med Hyg 1978;27:664

142. Miller LH, McGinniss MH, Holland PV, et al. Am J Trop Med Hyg 1978;27:1069

143. Van Ros G. Ann Soc Belge Med Trop 1985;65(Suppl 2):45

144. Hadley TJ, Miller LH, Haynes JD. Transf Med Rev 1991;5:108

145. Haynes JD, Dalton JP, Klotz FW, et al. J Exp Med 1988;167:1873

146. Wertheimer SP, Barnwell JW. Exp Parasitol 1989;69:340

147. Adams JH, Hudson DE, Toril M, et al. Cell 1990;63:141

148. Fang X, Kaslow DC, Adams JH, et al. Mol Biochem Parasitol 1991;44:125

149. Renwick JH, Lawler SD. Ann Hum Genet 1963;27:67

150. Rivas ML, Merritt AD, Lovrein EW, et al. Am J Hum Genet 1972;24:40

151. Bird TD, Ott J, Giblett ER. Am J Hum Genet 1982;34:388

152. Guiloff RJ, Thomas PK, Contreras M, et al. Ann Hum Genet 1982;46:25

153. Winter JH, Bennet B, Watt JL, et al. Ann Hum Genet 1982;46:29

154. Raeymaeckers P, van Broeckhoven C, Backhovens H, et al. Hum Genet 1988;78:76

155. Munro CS, Mastana SS, Papiha SS. Ann Genet 1992;35:157

156. Craddock N, Burge S, Parfitt L, et al. Ann Genet 1993;36:211

157. Cook PJL, Robson EB, Buckton KE, et al. Ann Hum Genet 1974;37:261

158. Hadley TJ, Lu Z, Wasniowska K, et al. J Clin Invest 1994;94:985

159. Estevez de Pablo C, Garcia Sagredo JM, Ferro MT, et al. J Med Genet 1980;17:483

160. Schinzel A, Schmid W. Clin Genet 1980;18:305

161. Collins A, Keats BJ, Dracopoli N, et al. Proc Nat Acad Sci USA 1992;89:4598

162. Mathew S, Chaudhuri A, Murty VS, et al. Cytogenet Cell Genet 1994;67:68

163. Sanger R, Tippett P, Gavin J, et al. Ann Hum Genet

1973;36:353

164. Moore S, Woodrow CF, McClelland DBL. Nature 1982;295:259

165. Hadley TJ, David PH, McGinniss MH. Science 1984;223:597

166. Dahr W, Kruger J. Proc 10th Int Cong Soc Foren Haematogenet. Munich:Schmitt and Meyer, 1983:141

167. Lisowska E, Duk M, Wasniowska K. In: Red Cell Membrane Glycoconjugates and Related Genetic Markers. Paris:Arnette, 1983:87

168. Tanner MJA, Anstee DJ, Mallinson G, et al. Carbohyd Res 1988;178:203

169. Chaudhuri A, Zbrzezna V, Johnson C, et al. J Biol Chem 1989;264:13770

170. Murphy PM. Ann Rev Immunol 1994;12:593

171. Mallinson G. PhD Thesis, Univ West England, 1995

172. Baldwin JM. EMBO J 1993;12:1693

173. Darbonne WC, Rice GC, Mohler MA J. Clin Invest 1991;88:1362

174. Neote K, Darbonne WC, Ogez J, et al. J Biol Chem 1993;268:12247

175. Horuk R, Chitnis CE, Darbonne WC, et al. Science 1993;261:1182

176. Aisaka N, Uchikawa M, Tsuneyama H, et al. (abstract). Vox Sang 1996;70 (Suppl 2):128

177. Chaudhuri A, Zbrzezna V, Polyakova J, et al. J Biol Chem 1994;269:7835

178. Neote K, Mak JY, Kolakowski LF, et al. Blood 1994;84:44

179. Schall TJ, Bacon KB. Curr Opin Immunol 1994;6:865

180. Springer TA. Cell 1994;76:301

181. Dohlman HG, Thorner J, Caron MG, Et al. Ann Rev Biochem 1991;60:653

182. Mallinson G, Soo K, Anstee DJ. (abstract). Transf Med 1994;4 (Suppl 1):45

183. Iwamoto S, Li J, Omi T, et al. Blood 1996;87:378

184. Zhao-hai L, Zi-xuan W, Horuk R, et al. J Biol Chem 1995;270: 26239

185. Mallinson G, Burgess G, Hook S, et al. (abstract). Transf Med 1995;5 (Suppl 1):19

186. Hargreave PA. Curr Opin Struct Biol 1991;1:575

187. Tilg H, Shapiro L, Atkins MB, et al. J Immunol 1993;151:3299

188. Davenport RD, Strieter RM, Standiford TJ, et al. Blood 1990;76:2439

189. Davenport RD. In: Transfusion Immunology and Medicine. New York:Marcel Dekker, 1995:319

190. Snyder EL. In: Transfusion Immunology and Medicine. New York:Marcel Dekker, 1995:333

191. Tanaka Y, Adams DH, Hubscher S, et al. Nature 1993;361:79

192. Reid ME. In: Molecular and Functional Aspects of Blood Group Antigens. Bethesda:Am Assoc Blood Banks, 1995:111

193. Mallinson G, Anstee DJ. Unpublished observations 1996

194. Pogo O, Chaudhuri A. Unpublished observations cited by Reid ME. In: Molecular and Functional Aspects of Blood Group Antigens. Bethesda:Am Assoc Blood Banks, 1995:111

195. Sosler SD. In: Blood Groups: Refresher and Update. Bethesda:Am Assoc Blood Banks, 1995:112

196. Moulds JM, Hayes S, Wells TD. (abstract). Transfusion 1996;36 (Suppl 9S):48S

197. Reid ME, Lomas-Francis C. The Blood Group Antigen Facts Book. San Diego:Academic, 1997:220

198. Chérif-Zahar B, Raynal V, Gane P, et al. Nature Genet 1996;12:168

199. Race C, Watkins WM. FEBS Lett 1972;27:125

200. Schenkel-Brunner H, Chester MA, Watkins WM. Eur J Biochem 1972;30:269

201. Murphy MT, Templeton LJ, Fleming J, et al. Transf Med 1997;7:135

202. Palatnik M, Junqueira PC, Alves ZMS. Rev Fr Transf Immunohematol 1982;25:629

203. Iwamoto S, Li J, Sugimoto N, et al. Biochem Biophys Res Comm 1995;222:852

204. Orkin SH. Blood 1992;80:575

15 | The MN Blood Group System

MN was the second of the human blood systems to be discovered. Following tests with sera from rabbits that had been immunized with human red cells, Landsteiner and Levine in 1927, reported discovery of the antigens M and N (1,2). Since that time many excellent anti-M and anti-N typing reagents have been prepared from the sera of immunized rabbits. Indeed, such reagents were still in fairly wide use when the first monoclonal anti-M and anti-N (see later in this chapter) were made. In 1947, Walsh and Montgomery (3) described the first example of anti-S that was soon shown to define an antigen closely related to M and N (4,5) and in 1951, Levine et al. (6) described anti-s, the antibody that defines the antigen antithetical to S. It is now known that M and N represent one pair of antithetical antigens encoded from one locus, while S and s are encoded from a closely linked, but separate locus. As described and referenced below, crossing-over between the loci is rare but has been seen to occur. Thus a case can be made for calling MN one blood group system and Ss, another. Since hybrid genes that encode single membrane components that carry both M or N *and* S or s have been found and since crossing-over between the *MN* and *Ss* loci is rare, M, N, S and s are most often regarded as being part of the same blood group system. However, the above findings have led to a variety of names being used. Race and Sanger (7) used the term "The MNSs Blood Groups"; the ISBT Working Party on Terminology for Red Cell Surface Antigens (8) and Daniels (9) use "The MNS Blood Group System" while one of us (10,11) continues to use "The MN Blood Group System". It has always seemed illogical to one of us (10,11) to add S but not s to the name used for the system. However, if the term MNSs system was used, a case would surely be advanced for adding U, i.e., the MNSsU system and so on, through many other antigens. Thus, as in previous editions of this book, the MN Blood Group System will be described with full appreciation that two loci are involved. Actually the same can be said for Rh although there the two loci, *RHD* and *RHCE*, seem more tightly linked than do *MN* and *Ss*.

Since S and s were added, a large number of other antigens that belong to the MN system have been reported. Some of these are important in routine blood banking but many others are of very low incidence and most blood bankers will never have the opportunity to work with the antibodies that define them. However, the antibodies against these rare antigens occasionally present as a cause of compatibility testing difficulty and on rare

occasions as causative of HDN. Studies on these rare antigens also contribute to the overall picture of human genetics so that some of them have become important out of proportion to their frequency.

Beginning in 1976 (12-17) a great deal of data began to emerge about the red cell membrane structures, glycophorin A and glycophorin B, that carry the antigens of the MN system. Accordingly, it is possible to describe the system from two different perspectives, the serological and the biochemical. This chapter attempts to do exactly that. The first part of the chapter describes the MN system at the serological level, particularly the importance of the antibodies involved in routine and clinical transfusion practice. The second part of the chapter deals with the biochemical, molecular biological and molecular genetic aspects of the system. However, it will be added, in this early introductory section, that complete separation between the two sections is impossible. In order to make some of the serology understandable, some biochemical data must be considered. An attempt will be made to limit the number of biochemical findings described in the first portion of the chapter to a minimum. The findings mentioned early will be expanded, in greater detail, later.

In 1928, Landsteiner and Levine (18) discussed the relationship between the antigens M and N. Although they mentioned different genetic mechanisms that could explain the observed relationships, they concluded that the most likely was that M and N are the products of co-dominant alleles (*M* and *N*) that reside at a single genetic locus. As described later in this chapter, current serological, genetic and biochemical findings show that M and N are indeed antithetical and are the products of alleles at a single locus. That is not to say that the theory advanced by Landsteiner and Levine (18) was never challenged. Over the years, several findings were made (19-22) that seemed to indicate that N might be a precursor substrate from which M is made. Some investigators (21-24) suggested that *N* is located at one locus and encodes production of the N antigen. They further supposed that N is converted to M by the action of the *M* gene, that could be at a locus unrelated to that at which *N* is situated. In the absence of the *M* gene, it was supposed that no conversion of N occurred so that the allele of *M* was considered to be a silent gene that could be called *m*. Although some support continued (25-33) for the concept that M represented an N structure to which a second N-acetyl-neuraminic acid (NeuAc) residue was added by the actions of the *M* gene-specified sialyl transferase, such a view was abandoned by most investigators. Instead, it is now accepted as proved that *M* and *N* encode production of glycophorin A molecules that differ in amino acid composition at residues 1 and 5 (34-36 and see below). It is known that NeuAc (and other carbohydrate) residues that are present in side chains attached to the protein backbone of glycophorin A contribute to M and N structure. However, that contribution is usually secondary and may represent, at least in part, steric arrangement of the protein backbones. The trace of N antigen detectable on red cells that initially type as M+ N- S or s+, that was for many years regarded as unconverted N substance, has now been recognized (37) as being an antigen produced whenever a functional *S* or *s* gene is present. This antigen, now called (34,38) 'N' to distinguish it from N, is described in detail in a later section of this chapter.

As mentioned, S and s were found to be products of alleles that occupy a locus very close to that at which *M* and *N* reside. Linkage between the *MN* and *Ss* loci is not absolute; a number of well documented cases of crossing-over between the loci have been reported (see below). In addition, it has been found that the distribution of *S* and *s*, in pairings with *M* and *N*, is not equal. Of the four possible haplotypes *Ns* is the most common, *Ms* the next most frequent, *MS* third in incidence, and *NS* the least frequent. That does not mean that the complex producing N and S is rare, indeed all four haplotypes have been found in good incidence in most populations studied.

Another important antibody, later shown to define an MN system antigen, was described in 1953. Wiener et al. (39) reported that anti-U caused a fatal hemolytic transfusion reaction. In testing over 2000 random blood samples, they (40) found that all of 1100 samples from Whites were U+. However, in testing 989 samples from New York Blacks, they found 12 that were non-reactive with the antibody. They concluded that the phenotypes U+ and U- probably represented the existence of co-dominant alleles, *U* and *u*, (*u* has also been called *S^u*) at a single locus. At the time that anti-U was discovered, all blood samples previously tested with anti-S and anti-s had been shown to carry one, the other, or both of those antigens. From their observation that all twelve U- samples were also S-, Wiener et al. (40) supposed them to be of the phenotype S- s+. That this was not the case became apparent when Greenwalt et al. (41) discovered the second example of anti-U and showed that two U- samples were S- s-. This finding provided another indication (subsequently proved) that U might be an MN system antigen. Although many later found examples of S- s- red cells typed as U-, the situation is not straightforward. First, some S- s- samples are non-reactive with some anti-U but reactive, albeit weakly in terms of visible reactions, with others. Second, some S- s- samples

that fail to react visibly with anti-U can be shown to adsorb that antibody and yield it on elution. To distinguish these situations the terms S- s- U- and S- s- U+^{weak} and S- s- U+^{var} (for variant) have been used to describe the phenotypes. As described below, the S- s- U+^{var} phenotype is some four times more common in American Blacks, than is the phenotype S- s- U-. However, it is now clear that the S- s- U+^{var} phenotype is heterogeneous at the serological level and represents more than one genetic background. The S, s and U antigens are normally carried on glycophorin B. In one form of the U- phenotype that glycophorin is missing from the red cells (342,366-370). In other forms, that may explain all the S- s- U+^{var} phenotypes, variant forms of glycophorin B or hybrid sialoglycoproteins are present (341-344,370). Further, since some different hybrid glycophorins are comprised in part of material encoded by genes that normally encode production of glycophorin A and in part of material encoded by genes that normally encode production of glycophorin B, the phenotypes S+ and/or s+ U- have now been found (45-52).

The finding that glycophorin B normally carries S or s and U has allowed a different interpretation of the previously named *U* and *u* (*S^u*) genes. Instead of regarding *S* and *s* as one pair of alleles and *U* and *u* as another pair, it is clear that *u* (*S^u*) is a third allele at the *Ss* locus. That is to say, the usual form of *S* encodes production of glycophorin B that carries, at least, S and U. The usual form of *s* encodes production of glycophorin B that carries, at least, s and U. The *u* gene can thus be thought of as a silent allele at the *Ss* locus, that encodes no production of glycophorin B. Thus in *u* homozygotes, the S- s- U- phenotype is seen. It is more difficult briefly to describe the genetic situations that result in the S- s- U- or S- s- U+^{var} phenotypes in which an abnormal form of glycophorin B or a hybrid glycophorin is present. For the ease of communication in this early section on the serology of S, s and U, the term *u* will be used to describe the gene involved in both S- s- U- and S- s- U+^{var} phenotypes although it is appreciated that this is an oversimplification and that the same gene is not responsible for both phenotypes.

While the M, N, S, s and U antigens are the ones most often of relevance in transfusion practice, they by no means represent the entire system. Over the years a large number of other antigens in the system have been recognized. Not all these antigens have received ISBT numbers. For example antigens such as M$_1$, Tm, M' and N^A that probably represent different to usual glycosylation of the protein backbone of glycophorin A, have not been given ISBT terms. The genes that control production of the transferase enzymes that cause alternative glycosylation are perhaps independent of the *MN* and *Ss* loci. Antigens such as Hu and Sul do not have ISBT numbers because of lack of proof that they are encoded from the *MN* or *Ss* locus and/or because of a shortage of available reagents. The antigens En^{a}TS, En^{a}FS and En^{a}FR are all called MNS28 although they can readily be differentiated in serological studies. The ISBT Working Party adopted a rule that specified that antigens recognized only after treatment of red cells with an enzyme (or another chemical) would not be numbered. The specificities of anti-En^{a}TS, anti-En^{a}FS and anti-En^{a}FR are clearly apparent when tests against untreated, trypsin-treated and ficin-treated red cells are used. Nevertheless, there is no way to differentiate between them using ISBT terms. Because the purpose of this book is to provide information about any red cell antigen or antibody that may be encountered in blood bank studies, table 15-1 lists all the MN system antigens reported, blank spaces in the columns for ISBT terms indicate that no such terms exist. Table 15-1 also includes references to the original reports describing each antigen and/or the paper documenting that the antigen involved is part of the MN system, the year the antigen was reported and, when known, the approximate incidence of the antigen in the White and US Black Populations. Because table 15-1 lists all serologically defined MN system antigens, in the sequence in which they were reported and regardless as to whether an ISBT number has been assigned, the ISBT terms that are included in that table, do not appear in numerical sequence.

For many years it was thought that genetic control of MN system antigen synthesis involved a number of genes at closely-linked loci. At the first locus the genes were thought to be *M, N* or one of their alleles. At the second, the major genes seemed to be *S, s* or *u* (*S^u*), again additional alleles seemed to exist. The multitude of low incidence antigens (see table 15-1) seemed to be produced by a series of genes that could be seen to be closely-linked to the *MN* and *Ss* loci. However, since the presence of one gene encoding production of a rare antigen did not seem to exclude the presence of any other, it was never clear how many different linked loci might exist. It was clear that an uneconomical genetic arrangement was being postulated since most of the time none of the additional loci seemed to carry structural genes (most persons have M and/or N, S and/or s and U, but *none* of the low incidence antigens on their red cells). Now that the role of glycophorins A and B in carrying the MN system antigens is known, it can be seen that the genetic situation is much more simple. The common forms of *M, N, S* and *s* encode glycophorins that do not carry any of the low incidence antigens. Variant alleles of those genes encode glycophorins that carry M, N, S or s and one or more of the low incidence antigens in the system. Sometimes the M, N, S or s produced by the variant gene is normal, sometimes it differs either quantitatively or

qualitatively from normal. At the same time, a glycosylation change or an amino acid substitution on the glycophorin results in the presence of a different antigen. Such a change may affect expression of M, N, S or s. However, since some of these changes are at some distance from M, N, S or s on the glycophorins, no change in those antigens will be seen. On still other occasions hybrid glycophorins are formed following gene conversion at the *MNSs* loci. Genes comprised in part of exons from *M* or *N* and in part of exons from *S* or *s*, encode production of hybrid glycophorins on which antigen expression will vary dependent on the exon structure of the converted gene and the ability of the exons to encode a product, in their new environment. In other words, genetic control of MN system antigen synthesis devolves to two loci, *MN* and *Ss* with multiple alleles producing only standard (M, N, S, s and U) or standard and additional (M, N, S, s, U, He, M^g, Ny^a, etc., etc.) antigens, and a series of unusual genes that arose by mutation, gene conversion and/or unequal crossing-over of genes at the two loci. In even simpler terms, each gene (allele) encodes one glycoprotein that can carry a variable number of MN system antigens.

Anti-M and Anti-N

Many examples of anti-M and anti-N are cold-reactive, non-red cell stimulated antibodies. That is, they are found in the sera of never transfused, never pregnant individuals and act as agglutinins in tests performed at temperatures below 37°C. One report (176) has claimed that anti-M is often made by children with bacterial infections. Although they are usually non-red cell stimulated (177), both IgM (109-111) and IgG (112-113) anti-M and anti-N are seen. Indeed, when Smith and Beck (113) tested 50 examples of anti-M they found that 39 (78%) of them were IgG, or contained an IgG component. In our series (114) the percentage of anti-M with an IgG component was a little less (circa 50%) but we agreed that cold-reactive anti-M active as agglutinins in a saline system, are often IgG. Most examples of anti-M fail to activate complement (109,110) or cause only a small amount of such activation (110,115). The example described by Branch et al. (115) was unusual in that while it was IgM it was shown to "bind small amounts of complement (C3) under strict prewarmed (37°C) conditions". After the patient was transfused with M+ blood an IgG anti-M that did not bind complement was made. In 1991, we (116) described a highly unusual form of anti-M. The antibody activated so much complement that it hemolyzed M+ N-but not M+ N+ red cells in LISS tests at 37°C. The antibody was made by a patient with M+ N+ red cells and in spite of its activity at 37°C (it strongly agglutinated the

TABLE 15-1 Antigens of the MN System

			Percent Frequency				
Historical Derivation	Antigen Conventional Name	Year Reported	Whites	U.S. Blacks	References	ISBT Antigen Number	ISBT Full Code Number
				Conventional Names: MN System or MN and Ss Systems			
				ISBT System Symbol: MNS, ISBT System Number: 002			
	M	1927	78	74	1, 2, 18, 53	MNS1	002001
	N	1927	72	75	1, 2, 18, 53	MNS2	002002
Hunter	Hu	1934	1	7	54		
	S	1947	57	30	3, 4	MNS3	002003
	s	1951	88	93	6	MNS4	002004
Henshaw	He	1951	<1	3	55	MNS6	002006
Miltenberger	Mi^a *1	1951	<1	<1	56	MNS7	002007
	U *2	1953	>99.9	99.7	39, 40	MNS5	002005
	M^c *3	1953	<0.1	<0.1	57	MNS8	002008
Gr, Verweyst	Vw	1954	<0.1	<0.1	58	MNS9	002009
Gilfeather	M^g	1958	<0.01	<0.01	59	MNS11	002011
Verdegaal	Vr	1958	<0.1	<0.1	60	MNS12	002012
	M$_1$	1960	0.5	16.5	61		
Murrell	Mur	1961	<0.1	<0.1	62	MNS10	002010
	M^e	1961	0.5	1	63	MNS13	002013
Martin	Mt^a	1962	0.25	<0.1	64	MNS14	002014
Stones	St^a	1962	0.1	<0.1	65	MNS15	002015
Ridley	Ri^a	1962	<0.1	<0.1	65	MNS16	002016
Caldwell	Cl^a	1963	<0.1	<0.1	66	MNS17	002017
Nyberg	Ny^a	1964	<0.1	<0.1	67	MNS18	002018
Orris	Or	1964*5	<0.1	<0.1	68, 69	MNS31	002031
Sheerin	Tm	1965	25*6	31*6	70		
Hutchinson	Hut	1966	<0.1	<0.1	72	MNS19	002019
Hill	Hil	1966	<0.1	<0.1	72	MNS20	002020
Armstrong	M^v	1966	0.6*7		73, 74	MNS21	002021
	M^A	1966	78	74	75		
Sullivan	Sul	1967	<0.1	<0.1	76		
	Sj	1968	2	4	77		
	M′	1968	9*8		78		
Kamhuber*9	Far	1968	<0.1	<0.1	79-82	MNS22	002022
En^a *10	En^{a}TS	1969	>99.9	>99.9	62-64		
	En^{a}FS	1969	>99.9	>99.9	62-64	MNS28	002028
	En^{a}FR	1969	>99.9	>99.9	62-64		
	Shier	1969	25	30	86		
	N^A	1971	72	75	87		
Z	U^z	1972	>99.9	99.7	88		

TABLE 15-1 Antigens of the MN System Continued

Historical Derivation	Antigen Conventional Name	Year Reported	Percent Frequency		References	ISBT Antigen Number	ISBT Full Code Number
			Whites	U.S. Blacks			
	'N'	1977	>99.9	99.9	34, 37	MNS30	002030
Anek	Hop	1977	<0.1	<0.1	89, 90	MNS26	002026
Raddon/Lane	Nob	1977	<0.1	<0.1	90, 91	MNS27	002027
X	U^x	1978	>99.9	99.7	92		
Dryer	s^D	1978	<0.1	<0.1	93, 94	MNS23	002023
Canner	Can	1979	27[*11]	60[*11]	95		
Mitchell	Mit	1980	0.12	<0.1	96	MNS24	002024
	Dantu	1982	<0.1	0.5	45, 46	MNS25	002025
	Os^a	1983[*12]			97, 98	MNS38	002038
	UPR	1989	>99.9	99.7	340		
	UPS	1989	>99.9	99.7	340		
	Sext	1983	0	23.5	178		
	En^aKT	1986	>99.9	>99.9	99	MNS29	002029
	DANE	1991	0.4[*13]		100	MNS32	002032
	SAT	1991	0.01[*14]		101	MNS36	002036
	TSEN[*15]	1992			102	MNS33	002033
	MINY[*15]	1992			103	MNS34	002034
	MUT	1992	<0.1	<0.1	104	MNS35	002035
	AVIS	1992	>99.9	>99.9	757		
	MARS	1992	<0.1	<0.1	757		
	ERIK[*15]	1993			105	MNS37	002037
	ENEH	1993	>99.9	>99.9	106	MNS40	002040
	ENEP	1995	>99.9	>99.9	107	MNS39	002039
	HAG[*17]	1995			107		

*1. Mi^a may not be an antigen. The reactivities of those sera said to contain anti-Mi^a may represent cross-reactivities with other antigens of the Miltenberger series.

*2. The antigens previously called U^A and U^B are described later in this chapter.

*3. Not defined by a specific antibody. M^c+ red cells react with most anti-M and some anti-N.

*4. Anti-M^e reacts with all M+ red cells and with M- cells that are He+. Antigen incidence shown represents M- He+ only.

*5. The antigen Or was first studied (68) in 1964 but was not shown to be part of the MN System until 1987 (69).

*6. Antigen incidence shown from tests against untreated red cells. When anti-Tm is tested against neuraminidase-treated red cells it reacts with all that are N+ (71).

*7. The first example (73) of anti-M^v behaved as inseparable anti-NM^v and reacted with all N+ red cells. The second example (74) lacked anti-N and react with the red cells of 0.6% of English donors. The incidence in Blacks of M^v without N is not known.

*8. The incidence of M' in Blacks is not known.

*9. The Kamhuber antigen was reported in 1966 (79) no association with an established blood group system was noticed. The Far antigen was first reported in 1968 (81) and was shown probably to belong to the MN System. In 1977 (82) the Kamhuber and Far antigens were shown to be the same thing.

*10. Anti-En^a was first reported in 1969 (83, 84). By 1981 it was clear that anti-En^a are heterogeneous and the terms En^aTS, En^aFS and En^aFR were introduced (85) to describe three of the antigens defined.

*11. Antigen incidence shown from tests against untreated red cells. When anti-Can is tested against neuraminidase-treated red cells it reacts with all that are M+ (95).

*12. The antigen Os^a was first reported (97) in 1983 but was not shown to be part of the MN system until 1993 (98). The antigen has a frequency of less than 0.01% in the Japanese, frequency in other populations not known.

*TABLE 15-1 Footnotes Continued**

*13. Incidence of 0.4% in Danes, frequency in other populations not known.

*14. Incidence of 0.01% in Japanese, frequency in other populations not known.

*15. The antigens TSEN, MINY and ERIK are all of low incidence. Exact frequencies not known.

*16. Anti-MUT defines an antigen previously supposed to represent cross-reactivity of anti-Mur and anti-Hut, but that has now been recognized as a distinct antigen (104, 108).

*17. HAG is a low incidence antigen that was found (107) on red cells on which an amino acid change in glycophorin A results in non-production of the very common antigen ENEP, i.e. red cells that are MNS:-39. HAG is not yet (as of May 1996) an official member of the MN System.

*18. For further descriptions of En^{a}KT (MNS29), ENEH (MNS40) and ENEP (MNS39), each of which represents lack of a common antigen when an amino acid change on glycophorin A (or glycophorin A derived material) occurs, see the section on heterogeneity of En^a.

*19. Because they appear more likely to be quantitative variants than qualitatively different antigens, M_2, N_2, S_2 and S^B are not listed in table 15-1.

*20. Some of the low incidence antigens listed in table 15-1 may be associated with genes that have been called M^z, M^r and N^2.

*21. The silent alleles *En* (*MN* locus), *u* (*S^u*)(*Ss* locus) and M^k (*MNSs* loci) are described later in this chapter.

M+ N+ red cells that it did not hemolyze) there was no evidence that it caused in vivo destruction of the patient's own red cells. Although there are other claims (117) that anti-M acting as a hemolysin has been found, we (118) gave reasons for believing that those antibodies (119-122) actually had anti-Pr^M and not anti-M specificity. This view was, of course, advanced by the investigators describing (122) anti-Pr^M. While allo-anti-M and benign auto-anti-M are not expected to bind complement, autoantibodies causative of CHD (119-122) most certainly are. For additional details about anti-Pr^M see Chapter 34, for more information about CHD see Chapter 38. A second example of a clinically benign autoantibody that had anti-M and not anti-Pr^M specificity, that caused hemolysis in vitro, has been described (217).

Those examples of anti-M and anti-N that are not active at 37°C are clinically-insignificant and should be ignored in red cell transfusion therapy or, better yet, go undetected in pretransfusion tests because such tests were not performed at temperatures below 37°C. Mollison and his colleagues (123-128) conducted in vivo studies with a series of antibodies, including several in the MN system and showed that antibodies that are not active at 37°C, do not cause destruction of red cells carrying the antigens that they define. Fortunately, there is now a marked move (129-139) among blood bankers, away from the inclusion of a room temperature incubation period in antibody screening and compatibility tests. Thus, many cold-reactive antibodies in the MN system, that would have been detected and identified some years ago, go undetected today. The patient, the donor and the blood banker are no worse off for not knowing that these antibodies are present. Indeed, the patient is frequently better off in terms of costs of laboratory tests and both patient and blood banker are better off in terms of time saved in the selection of suitable blood for transfusion. That is not to say that anti-M and anti-N are never clinically significant. As described below, both antibodies have caused transfusion reactions and HDN. However, it should always be remembered that

in order for an antibody to destroy red cells in vivo, it must be able to complex with antigen-positive red cells at 37°C. In vitro, tests to demonstrate that ability have to be performed with a considerable amount of care (see below).

Although there are occasional reports of anti-M or anti-N being formed after the transfusion of blood (115,140-144), there are a number of points that must be considered in relation to that fact. First, the event is rare. Second, development of IgG warm-reactive (i.e. antibodies of potential clinical significance) does not regularly occur in patients in whom IgM cold-reactive antibodies were present before transfusion. Indeed, our experience (145) has been that on those very rare occasions that anti-M or anti-N causes a delayed transfusion reaction, the patients involved are ones who have undergone a de novo (apparently secondary) immune response and not ones in whom cold-reactive anti-M or anti-N was demonstrable before transfusion. Third, the immune response to N, in individuals phenotypically M+ N- S- s- U- (or U+^{wk}) who lack 'N' from their red cells (146-152) is quite different from the immune response in persons phenotypically M+ N- S or s+, who have 'N' on their red cells. Taken together, these findings indicate that there is no justification whatever for using units of blood, typed and selected to lack M or N, for patients with cold-reactive anti-M or anti-N in the serum. Instead, if only cold-reactive anti-M or anti-N is present, units (not typed for M or N) that are nonreactive in immediate spin compatibility tests, can be used with impunity. The selection of blood for patients with 37°C-reactive anti-M and anti-N in the serum is discussed in the next section. In addition to the cases cited above, Teesdale et al. (179) described the production of anti-M (and anti-D) in three of 20 males with M- N+ cells, who were injected with D+, M+ red cells, to raise anti-D for use in the preparation of Rh immune globulin.

Anti-M and Anti-N in Transfusion Therapy

While examples of anti-M can all be considered

together, in terms of the transfusion of blood, distinction must be made between two different types of anti-N. The first is the more common variety made by individuals with red cells that type as M+ N- and carry S or s. Although such cells type as N-, they carry 'N' on glycophorin B (34,37,38). Thus the anti-N made is actually an autoantibody. However, that fact can usually only be demonstrated by adsorption studies (i.e. with the patient's red cells or others that type as M+ N- and are S or s+). The anti-N made in this setting seldom reacts visibly with the patient's red cells, or others typed as N- in direct typing tests (149). The second type of anti-N is the one made by individuals with M+ N- S- s- red cells (i.e. cells that lack 'N'). This antibody is alloimmune, will often react with cells previously typed as M+ N- S or s+, albeit less strongly than those that are M- N+ or M+ N+. The type of anti-N made by persons with 'N'- red cells is usually of greater clinical importance than the type made by persons with 'N'+ cells. For the remainder of this section and in several that follow, the more benign form of anti-N, made by persons with 'N'+ red cells will be considered. That antibody is somewhat analogous to anti-M made by persons with M- N+ red cells in terms of clinical significance. A separate section later in the chapter describes the anti-N made by persons with 'N'- red cells.

Since IgG anti-M and anti-N are made, it would be expected that those examples able to bind to red cells at 37°C might cause in vivo red cell destruction. Indeed the literature contains some reports (142-144,153,154,156-161,175) of, mostly delayed, transfusion reactions that were attributed to anti-M or anti-N. However, such reports should be regarded with some degree of caution. First, some of them (153,154,158) document findings made many years ago, before the methods used today were introduced. In other words, while the patients clearly had anti-M, they might also have had other antibodies, not demonstrable by the techniques then available, that were actually the cause of the transfusion reactions. Second, in some of the more recent reports, the evidence that anti-M caused red cell destruction is not unequivocal. For example, one paper (142) purports to describe three cases of delayed transfusion reactions caused by anti-M. However, the findings were purely serological, there was no clinical evidence of hemolysis in any of the patients. In all three patients the post-transfusion DAT became weakly positive, in two of the three anti-M was recovered by elution. However, in the absence of any evidence of immune red cell destruction (no cell survival studies were done) the weakly positive DATs and findings with the eluates, might simply have meant that a small amount of (harmless) anti-M had become bound to the transfused red cells. As further evidence that anti-M and anti-N are seldom responsible for

delayed transfusion reactions, the findings of Pineda et al. (155) can be cited. These workers conducted careful evaluations in 23 patients in whom delayed transfusion reactions had occurred. Among the patients, 28 antibodies were identified, none was in the MN system. A more convincing case of a delayed transfusion reaction caused by anti-M was described by Alperin et al. (143) in a patient who had an IgG antibody reactive at 37°C. In addition to the clinical sequelae, this case was more convincing because a ^{51}Cr in vivo cell survival study was used to demonstrate the activity of the anti-M in the patient's circulation. Clearly, anti-M can sometimes cause accelerated in vivo clearance of M+ red cells (143,144,156,157). Equally clear, the event is rare and care in the investigation of suspected cases is necessary to avoid the true, true and unrelated phenomenon. Cases in which anti-N was said to have caused a transfusion reaction are considered later, in the section of the chapter dealing with 'N' and anti-N.

Considerable care is also necessary in performing serological tests to determine whether an anti-M or anti-N is truly reactive at 37°C. If the tests are set up at room temperature and then transferred to 37°C, agglutination seen after the 37°C incubation step may represent carry-over of agglutination that began at a lower temperature before the contents of the tubes reached 37°C. Carefully performed prewarmed tests are a much more suitable way of making the determination. It must also be remembered that the use of sensitive methods, i.e. those using LISS, PEG or Polybrene, etc., may result in an antibody reacting at 37°C when the same antibody may not have that capability in saline or albumin tests. No doubt this contributes to the finding that compatibility tests at 37°C are entirely suitable for the selection of blood for patients with anti-M and anti-N, including those with antibodies reactive at 37°C. That is to say, there is no need to type donor units for M and N and select those that lack the appropriate antigen. Instead, the patient's serum can be used in IATs, prewarmed to 37°C if necessary, and those units found to be compatible can be transfused with impunity. As discussed later, many examples of anti-M and anti-N display dosage effects. However, an anti-M or anti-N that failed to react with M+ N+ (i.e. single dose red cells) in an IAT at 37°C, would not be expected to destroy such red cells, in vivo. As already discussed, since secondary immune responses to M and N are rare, their consideration need not enter into the decision as to how blood will be selected for these patients. Table 15-2 lists phenotype frequencies when M and N are considered and 'N' is ignored (i.e. red cells non-reactive in direct tests with anti-N are called N-). As can be seen, compatibility tests against random donor units will identify the many that are suitable for transfusion.

TABLE 15-2 Approximate Frequencies of the MN Phenotypes

Phenotype	Whites	U.S.Blacks
M+N-	28%	25%
M+N+	50%	49%
M-N+	22%	26%

Anti-M and Anti-N in Patients in Whom Hypothermia Will Be Used

Because anti-M and anti-N often react only at temperatures below 37°C, the question sometimes arises as to whether they should be honored (in terms of transfusion of antigen-negative blood) in patients whose body temperature will be reduced during surgery. Although there are not abundant data available to answer the question, at least two patients with cold-reactive anti-M failed to effect any clearance of M+ red cells when the body temperature was reduced to 16°C (162). Equally comforting is the fact that most transfusion services providing blood for patients in whom hypothermia will be used do not perform any antibody screening tests below 37°C. In other words, many cold-reactive alloantibodies, including anti-M and anti-N, must go undetected and many units of antigen-positive blood must be transfused. Lack of any documented ill effects would appear to indicate that cold-reactive alloantibodies are as unimportant in patients to be cooled as in patients who will be treated at normal temperatures.

HDN Caused by Anti-M and Anti-N

As would be expected, since many examples of anti-M and anti-N are non-reactive at 37°C so are unable to complex with red cells in vivo and since some are IgM in nature, HDN caused by these antibodies is comparatively rare. Nevertheless cases caused by anti-M have been documented (164-169). Surprisingly, some of these cases have been exceptionally severe (perhaps less dramatic cases have simply not been described in print). In the case reported by Stone and Marsh (164) a woman with anti-M reactive to a titer of 1000 at 37°C in albumin tests, carried twins. One died in utero and the other required an exchange transfusion at birth. Other cases (167,168) of intrauterine deaths have been blamed on anti-M, in the second of these reports (details of the antibody given in (169)) it was claimed that the anti-M had caused the antibody-maker to deliver four consecutive stillborn infants. In her fifth pregnancy the patient was treated by plasma exchange from the 18th to the 21st week of gestation. Thereafter, 5 to 7 liters of plasma per week were removed, adsorbed with M+ red cells (170) and returned to the

patient. The plasma removal/adsorption procedure reduced the titer of the anti-M from 512 to 128 or 256 each week. At 33 weeks gestation a liveborn infant was delivered by Caesarean section. The DAT on the infant's M+ N+ red cells was only weakly positive, anti-M with a titer of 128 was present in the cord serum. The infant was given two exchange transfusions and made a complete recovery. The plasma removal/adsorption procedure was credited with having removed enough anti-M to allow the infant to survive until the Caesarean section was performed at 33 weeks. However, it should be noted that the woman's first pregnancies lasted 36, 36, 29 and 30 weeks respectively, in the absence of treatment. While the authors (170) advocated use of their adsorption method in cases in which anti-D is present in the maternal serum, Robinson (171) pointed out a very real danger. The procedure had been tried (172) in a woman in whom plasma exchange could not be used since the infusion of allogeneic plasma caused transfusion reactions. After an initial drop in level of anti-D, that antibody was suddenly produced at a much higher level. It seems entirely probable that when the adsorbed plasma was reinfused, it contained some D+ red cells or stroma from such cells, that acted as a secondary immunogen. It might not be possible always to remove stroma from such plasma, in spite of hard centrifugation (171,172) and while use of a filter during reinfusion of the plasma, as suggested by Yoshida et al. (173), might prevent intact D+ red cells from entering the maternal circulation, it might not serve to prevent the passage of fragments of stroma. Given the differing natures of secondary immune responses to D and to M, the procedure would seem much more dangerous in a woman already making potent anti-D than in one making anti-M.

In two other cases in which anti-M caused HDN severe enough to warrant exchange transfusion, the DAT on the infant's red cells was only weakly positive in one (164) and was negative in the other (166). In both cases, the red cells of the infants agglutinated spontaneously when suspended in high protein media.

HDN caused by anti-N seems even less frequent than that caused by anti-M. One mild case seen by Giblett (174) involved a woman with anti-N in her serum who gave birth to a child whose red cells typed as M+ N-. Presumably the anti-N found enoug. 'N' on the glycophorin B on the child's cells to cause a small amount of red cell destruction. Another mild case of HDN caused by anti-N involved an antibody made by a person with M+ N- S- s- 'N'- red cells and is described below.

Anti-N in Patients Undergoing Renal Dialysis

In 1972, Howell and Perkins (180) reported an increased incidence of formation of anti-N in patients undergoing renal dialysis. The observation was soon confirmed and the phenomenon has been studied by many others (181-195). The antibody made is found in some patients with red cells that type as N- and in some with red cells that type as N+. The antibody sometimes reacts with the 'N' antigen on glycophorin B so that red cells previously typed as M+ N- may react, albeit less strongly than those that type as N+. In one study (190) the antibody was found in 21% of renal dialysis patients, in another (191) in 27% of such patients. In 1975, it was reported (181,184-186) that formation of the anti-N was almost completely confined to those patients treated on dialysis machines that had been sterilized with formaldehyde. It was supposed (184) that residual red cells in the machines at the time of sterilization were modified by the formaldehyde and that the altered N on those red cells then acted as an immunogen. The antibody became known as anti-Nf and as anti-Nform. Dahr et al. (43,44,192) performed antibody binding studies and showed that anti-Nform has an affinity for formaldehyde-treated N+ red cells that is some one to two hundred times greater than its affinity for N on untreated cells. From the results of a later study, Dahr and Moulds (192) concluded that anti-Nform recognizes the terminal leucine on glycophorin A of N+ red cells and the terminal leucine on glycophorin B of S+ or s+ red cells after the free amino group of the leucine has been modified by formaldehyde. Although it seems probable that the immunogen that causes anti-Nform to be made is carried on red cells exposed to formaldehyde in the dialysis machines, it is possible that some in vivo alteration of red cells occurs. It has been suggested (198) that when the formaldehyde sterilized dialysis machines are re-used some of the formaldehyde enters the patients' circulation and modifies N (and 'N') on the patients' own red cells. Sandler et al. (191) pointed out that exposure of humans to formaldehyde is not particularly unusual. It has been used for local treatment in urology (199) and cardiovascular surgery (200) and occurs as a metabolite following the use of methenamine as a bacteriostatic agent in urinary tract infections (201). The evidence (192) that formaldehyde alters N and 'N' excludes an earlier suggestion (183) that anti-Nform might be directed against a precursor of N. Indeed, it is now clear that no such precursor exists (34,37,38).

In 1977, Bird and Wingham (187) reported that red cells of any MN phenotype would react with anti-Nform after those red cells had been treated with formaldehyde. Although this at first seems to exclude any role for modified N in the reaction, the full explanation emerged later. In 1978 and 1979, Sandler et al. (189,191) studied the sera of 22 patients treated on dialysis machines sterilized with formaldehyde. In six of the patients, anti-Nform was clearly present. In 20 of the 22 sera, including the six that contained anti-Nform, a second antibody, reacting with formaldehyde-treated red cells of any phenotype

was present. Since this antibody, that can be thought of as "anti-formaldehyde" reacted with M+ N- S- s-, i.e. N-'N'- red cells, its specificity clearly had no association with N. The "anti-formaldehyde" reactivity was completely removed by adsorption with formaldehyde-treated M+ N- S- s- 'N'- red cells. Lynen et al. (194) studied antibody formation in this group of patients and concluded that the usual immune response involves the formation of "anti-formaldehyde" first, followed in a smaller number of patients by the formation of separable anti-Nform. In their study on "anti-formaldehyde" and anti-Nform, Sandler et al. (191) also tested samples from 71 patients treated on machines that used a presterilized disposable dialysis membrane instead of formaldehyde; none of the patients had either of the antibodies.

It has been suggested (180,196) that anti-Nform may be of some importance in renal transplantation. In one patient with anti-Nform, a chilled kidney was rejected at transplantation, perhaps because red cells within the kidney were agglutinated by the anti-Nform. A second kidney, from the same donor, was warmed to 37°C before being transplanted in the same patient, that kidney graft was successful. As far as we have been able to determine, only one group of workers (190) felt that anti-Nform or "anti-formaldehyde" were of any significance in transfusion. Lynen et al. (194) reported that anti-Nform is usually made of IgM while "anti-formaldehyde" is often IgG. A cold-reactive IgM antibody (anti-Nform) would not be expected to be of any clinical significance, an IgG "anti-formaldehyde" would be equally harmless since red cells used for transfusion are not formaldehyde-treated! Dzik et al. (195) found that some of these antibodies are responsible for positive DATs in the patient involved.

One example of an auto-anti-M, in a patient who had been treated by hemodialysis and who had then received a renal transplant, has been reported (197). However, the immunological and serological findings on the auto-anti-M were quite different from those made on examples of anti-Nform. First, the auto-anti-M did not give enhanced reactions when tested against formaldehyde-treated red cells. Second, its production did not decrease following receipt of the allograft (cessation of dialysis) by the patient, as nearly always occurs with anti-Nform (180).

Anti-M and Anti-N in Persons with M+ and N+ Red Cells, Respectively

In addition to anti-M and anti-N made by persons with red cells that type as M- and N- respectively, a number of examples of anti-M made by persons with M+ and anti-N made by persons with N+ red cells have been found. Such antibodies can be divided into two major types. First, those antibodies that seemed to be alloimmune in nature, that is they reacted with all (or almost all) other M+ or N+ red cells, but not with those of the antibody-maker. The second type were clearly autoantibodies in that they reacted with the antibody-makers' red cells and with other M+ or N+ red cells.

Some of the antibodies that appeared to be alloimmune have been given their own names because it appeared that their specificity was different from ordinary anti-M or anti-N. For example, the M+ red cells of a child with allo-anti-M in the serum, were called M^a by Konugres et al. (75) and the antibody made was called anti-M^A. It was said that all normal M+ red cells, that reacted with the new antibody, carried the antigens M and M^A, while those of the child carried M but not M^A, hence their being designated M^a. Similarly, Booth (87) called an anti-N made by a person with N+ red cells, anti-N^A and said that the antibody-maker had N^a red cells because those cells did not react with the antibody. Use of such names implies that M and N may each be comprised of a number of different epitopes. There is now evidence from work with monoclonal anti-M and anti-N (see below) that those antibodies do indeed recognize different epitopes of M and N. It seems probable that human polyclonal anti-M and anti-N (like other polyclonal antibodies) contain antibody populations of different specificities, recognizing different epitopes of the antigen against which the antibody is directed. There are other reports of examples of allo-anti-M in persons with M+ red cells (202-204) and allo-anti-N in persons with N+ red cells (205-209).

In most instances where anti-M and anti-N appeared to be autoimmune in nature, they seemed (116,177,210-217,745) to be benign in vivo even when they acted as hemolysins in vitro (116,217). However, rare examples have been reported (120,216,218-222) where the presence of the antibody was associated with an accelerated rate of in vivo red cell destruction and/or anemia. Those autoantibodies are discussed in more detail in Chapters 37 and 38.

pH Dependent Anti-M and Anti-N

In 1965, Beattie and Zuelzer (223) described an anti-M that agglutinated red cells only when the pH of the test system was acid. The antibody was noticed when the plasma of a donor, obtained from an ACD sample and hence having an acid pH, agglutinated M+ red cells, but serum from the donor did not. In the subsequent investigation, the sera of 1000 donors with M- N+ red cells were screened and 21 examples of pH dependent anti-M were found. It was shown that the optimum test system for detection of these antibodies was one adjusted to pH 6.5

and that enhancement of different examples of the antibodies, at acid pH, varied. Other examples of anti-M were studied that were not affected by variation in pH. A few other reports about the effects of pH on the reactivity of anti-M and anti-N have appeared (10,222,224,225).

As discussed below, monoclonal anti-M and anti-N are affected by the pH of the test system to a greater degree than are their human polyclonal counterparts. In studies using monoclonal antibodies it has been found (226-228) that variations in pH affect charged groups on some amino acids of glycophorin A and some in the carbohydrate side chains attached to the protein backbone at positions very close to M and N.

Anti-M and Anti-N Agglutinins for Red Cells Exposed to Glucose

In 1975, Morel et al. (229) described three examples of anti-N that would agglutinate N+ red cells only after those cells had been exposed to glucose. In a full report published in 1981, these workers (230) added an example of anti-M with similar characteristics. M+ and N+ cells could be converted to become reactive with the antibodies by incubation in a 1 to 2% glucose solution, buffered to neutral or alkaline pH. Conversion of cells to the reactive form was time and temperature dependent occurring in hours at 37°C and in days at 4°C. The authors concluded that the antibodies were detecting structures in which interaction between glucose and the amino group of the NH_2 terminal amino acid of the M or N SGP had taken place. The actions of these antibodies were not the same as the pH dependent ones described above since changes in pH of the test system did not enhance the reactions of these antibodies. M+ N+ cells could be made to react with the anti-M by incubation in galactose but such incubation did not cause the cells to react with the anti-N active against red cells exposed to glucose. The anti-M studied was inhibited by the addition of 2% solutions of glucose, mannose and maltose but not by similar strength solutions of fructose, ribose, fucose, galactose, lactose or sucrose. One of the anti-N was inhibited by glucose, ribose, fucose and mannose but not by fructose, galactose, lactose, maltose or sucrose. The authors (230) suggested that the names M^D and N^D for the determinants defined, to indicate that they are sialic-acid-independent forms of M and N with alterations effected by dextrose (glucose) solutions. These terms have not been widely used.

Two other examples of anti-M reacting with red cells exposed to glucose have been documented (231,232). The patient with M- N+ red cells described by Reid et al. (231) had diabetes mellitus. The anti-M that she made agglutinated M+ red cells exposed to glucose in vitro and the untreated M+ red cells of six of seven other diabetic patients. In other words, the change of M effected by glucose can occur in vivo as well as in vitro. This study (231) also showed that the change is not permanent. Red cells exposed to glucose, then washed and suspended in saline, gradually lost the ability to react visibly with the anti-M.

Pallagut and Edwards (233) reported that the anti-M lectin made from *Iberis amara* is glucose-dependent and reacts optimally if prepared in a solution containing 7% polyvinylpyrrolidone (PVP). M+ red cells collected in a manner such that they were not exposed to glucose, were non-reactive with the lectin but could be made to react by incubation in a 20% glucose solution for 30 minutes at 37°C. M+ cells collected in modified Alsever's solution or CPDA-1 were reactive without further treatment.

Dosage Effects of Anti-M and Anti-N

Many examples of anti-M and anti-N react to higher titers and titer scores with the red cells of individuals homozygous for the genes producing those antigens (*MM* and *NN* respectively) than with the cells of individuals heterozygous for *M* and *N* (i.e. genetically *MN*). In our experience, anti-M and anti-N made in rabbits often give reliable dosage scores that can be extremely helpful in the investigation of unusual blood samples (i.e. M+ N-, cells that are in fact from an individual heterozygous for *M*, e.g. *MM^k*, *MEn*) and in further investigation of apparent indirect exclusions of parentage.

The dosage effects displayed by anti-M and anti-N relate, of course, directly to the number of copies of the antigens on red cells. One of us (234-236) has reviewed the data that show that glycophorin A is present in about 1×10^6 copies per red cell. If M and N antigens are accessible to their antibodies on all copies of the sialoglycoprotein it follows that: in almost all *M* homozygotes, M will be present in one million copies; in almost all *N* homozygotes, N ('N' is ignored in the calculation) will be present in a similar number; while in almost all *MN* heterozygotes 500,000 copies each of M and N will be present per red cell.

Effects of Enzymes on the M and N Antigens

As described in the section on the biochemistry of the MN system, glycophorin A, that normally carries M or N, has a number of sites that are susceptible to cleavage by proteolytic enzymes. Thus red cells treated with trypsin, papain, ficin, bromelin, chymotrypsin or pronase no longer carry glycophorin A-borne M or N. The fact that protease modified red cells do not react with anti-M or anti-N was, of course, known for many years (237-

240,242,243) before it became apparent why this is the case. Indeed, blood group serologists have long taken advantage of the fact in antibody identification studies.

Glycophorin B does not carry similar protease sensitive sites to glycophorin A. When red cells are trypsin-treated, the 'N' antigen survives. Thus potent examples of anti-N, particularly those made by persons with M+ N- S- s- 'N'- red cells (see below), may continue to react with trypsin or other protease modified red cells. Trypsin-treated red cells will adsorb anti-N unless they are of the N- 'N'- phenotype.

The early and now largely abandoned concept that M and N antigen structure is dependent wholly on N-acetyl-neuraminic acid (NeuAc residues) (244-246) was based, in large part, on the finding that anti-M and anti-N failed to react with neuraminidase-treated red cells (241,248-250). Unlike the proteases described above, neuraminidase does not cleave the protein backbone of glycophorin A. Instead, it specifically removes NeuAc residues, including those in the tetrasaccharide side chains attached to glycophorin A. The early experiments in which it was found that anti-M and anti-N did not react with neuramindase-treated red cells often used rabbit anti-M and anti-N or relatively weak examples of those antibodies made by humans. As more potent examples of anti-M and anti-N were tested it became apparent that some such antibodies do react with neuraminidase-treated red cells. Demonstration of that fact is not easy. Virtually all human sera contain anti-T and the T receptor is exposed when red cells are treated with neuraminidase (see Chapter 42). Thus in order to determine whether anti-M and anti-N are reactive with the treated cells it is necessary first to remove anti-T by adsorption. While this can be accomplished for sera containing anti-M by adsorption with M- N+ neuraminidase-treated red cells, it is not nearly as easy for sera that contain anti-N. Neuraminidase-treated red cells that type as M+ N- S or s+ will carry 'N' and will adsorb both anti-T and anti-N. Accordingly, such sera must be adsorbed with neuraminidase-treated M+ N- S- s- 'N'-red cells. Red cells of that phenotype are, of course, much more difficult to obtain than are M+ N- S or s+ cells. In 1979, Judd et al. (251) described a series of experiments using anti-M and anti-N, from which anti-T had been removed, in tests against neuraminidase-treated red cells. The results of those experiments are summarized in table 15-3. As can be seen, of 30 examples of anti-M tested, 21 (70%) reacted with neuraminidase-treated M+ red cells. Further, three of those antibodies reacted more strongly with treated than with untreated red cells. Of seven examples of anti-N, four (57%) still reacted with neuraminidase-treated N+ red cells although the reactions of two of them were weaker with the treated than the untreated red cells. In a later

TABLE 15-3 Reactions of Human Anti-M and Anti-N with Untreated and with Neuraminidase-treated Red Cells (from Judd et al. 251)

	Anti-M	Anti-N
Number tested	30	7
Number non-reactive with neuraminidase-treated red cells	9	3
Number giving weaker reactions with neuraminidase-treated than with untreated red cells	0	2
Number reacting equally with neuraminidase-treated and untreated red cells	18	2
Number giving stronger reaction with neuraminidase-treated than with untreated red cells	3	0

study we (252) showed that those anti-M and anti-N that fail to agglutinate neuraminidase-treated red cells are not adsorbed by those cells either. That is to say, the epitopes defined are no longer available once the cells have been neuraminidase-treated.

Taken together, these observations (251,252) show that the antigens defined by anti-M and anti-N can be divided into two rather broad types. First are those antigens (defined by the sera that fail to react with neuraminidase-treated red cells) for which the presence of NeuAc is essential. Such antigens may represent steric orientation of the NH$_2$ terminal end of glycophorin A that is dependent on the presence of NeuAc or may represent antigens in which NeuAc is an essential component. Second, are those antigens (defined by the antibodies that react with the neuraminidase-treated red cells) in which presence of the appropriate amino acids on glycophorin A imparts specificity regardless of presence or absence of NeuAc. It is possible that N-acetyl galactosamine and galactose residues, that are also present in the tetrasaccharides attached to glycophorin A in close proximity to the MN polymorphism (see below) and which are not removed when red cells are treated with neuramindase, participate in presentation or structure of this second form of M and N.

There are ample other data to support the concept outlined above regarding NeuAc-dependent and NeuAc-independent forms of M and N. Lisowska and Kordowicz (253) raised antibodies in rabbits using desialized M+ and N+ red cells. The anti-M and anti-N produced were used to phenotype desialized (neuraminidase-treated) red cells with results that were identical to those obtained using conventional anti-M and anti-N to type untreated red cells. Sandler et al. (254) showed that if NeuAc was removed from red cells then replaced, using animal source sialyl transferases, the

original MN phenotype of the cells was restored, this being demonstrated in tests using anti-M and anti-N defining NeuAc-dependent antigens. As discussed in later sections of this chapter, the above concepts are totally compatible with what is known about the structure of glycophorin A and the polymorphism of that glycoprotein that imparts M or N specificity.

Monoclonal Anti-M and Anti-N

A large number of monoclonal antibodies that at first appear to define M or N have been produced using spleen cells from immunized mice in the establishment of antibody-secreting hybridomas (226,227,254-267). As described below, while many monoclonal anti-N seem to have the same specificity as human and rabbit anti-N, a number of monoclonal antibodies that initially appeared to be anti-M, have been seen to have a specificity slightly different from human and rabbit anti-M. This has proved to be of no serious disadvantage and some of those MAb have been used to produce excellent anti-M typing reagents.

In describing two monoclonal antibodies that they claimed had anti-M specificity, Nichols et al. (260) reported that when used undiluted, the antibodies would agglutinate M- N+ red cells. At modest dilutions, i.e. 1 in 16 or greater, the antibodies were specific for M and indeed reacted with M+ red cells to titers between 64 and 256. Whether these antibodies should be called anti-M is debatable. As described later in this chapter, glycophorin A that carries M differs from glycophorin A that carries N in the amino acids at the first and fifth positions of the NH$_2$ terminal end. M and N-bearing glycophorin A have identical carbohydrate side chains attached at positions 2, 3 and 4. Thus it seemed to one of us (268,269) that these MAb were likely complexing with an epitope in one (or more) of the side chains common to the two types of glycophorin A. The preferential reactivity of the MAb with M+ over M- N+ red cells might have reflected orientation of the epitope in the side chains, as influenced by the differing amino acids in the polypeptide backbone of the glycophorins. When they described four somewhat similar monoclonal antibodies, Fraser et al. (227) approached the specificity question similarly to this author. The three that reacted, albeit weakly, with M- N+ red cells were described as defining an M related antigen. Both Fraser et al. (227) and one of us (268,269) pointed out that when used at appropriate dilutions and under controlled conditions, those MAb that in concentrated forms react with M- N+ red cells but at higher dilutions, only with M+ red cells, can be used as totally reliable anti-M typing reagents.

A MAb described by Jaskiewicz et al. (267) was different in that it would react only with red cells that had the *M* gene-specified amino acid at position 1 of glycophorin A. This MAb could, with more justification be called anti-M. While some MAb that have a preference for N may show some cross-reactivity with M it seems that a higher percentage of MAb with ostensible (at first) anti-N specificity can then be shown to have true anti-N specificity (255-258). Two MAb against N differed in their affinity for N and 'N' (261). Since those two antigens appear to be biochemically identical, presumably the MAb "saw" differences in steric presentation based on the glycophorin A and glycophorin B carrier proteins.

As mentioned earlier, MAb used to type red cells for M and N are more stringent than human or rabbit antibodies in their requirements in terms of pH and temperature of the test system. While full details need not be given, it is clear that following the reagent manufacturer's directions for use with these typing reagents is even more important than when using human-source reagents. As with human anti-M and anti-N, some MAb define NeuAc-dependent and others NeuAc-independent structures. Inhibition studies using preparations from Chinese hamster ovary cells transfected with *M* or *N* or variant cDNA have been used (270,271) to determine the requirements of various MN MAb in terms of amino acid sequence in the epitope defined. Monoclonal antibodies to M and N have also been used (272-281) in attempts to determine the incidence of somatic mutation in erythroid precursor cells.

The 'N' Determinant and Anti-N in Individuals with N- 'N'- Red Cells

In 1963, Allen et al. (282) reported that individuals homozygous for an *MN* haplotype (*Mu*) that produced M but no U (see below) had red cells that lacked the small amount of N found on red cells that initially typed as M+ N- U+. In 1966, Francis and Hatcher (283) described an antibody, made by an individual who had red cells that typed as M+ N- S- s-, that at certain dilutions reacted as anti-U (again see below) and at others as anti-N. Although these observations (282,283) could not be fully explained at the time, they were the first reports of the situation to be described in this section.

As mentioned briefly above, normal glycophorin B, that carries S or s, is identical at its NH_2 terminal end to the form of glycophorin A that carries N. This means that almost all red cells that type as S+ and/or s+ are actually N+. Those that initially type as M+ N- have a low level of N on glycophorin B, the antigen is usually called 'N' to distinguish it from the glycophorin A-borne form of N (34,37,38). Individuals who have red cells that initially type as M+ N- and who lack, or have a highly unusual

form of glycophorin B, have cells that are M+ N- 'N'-. Such cells were the ones originally described by Allen et al. (282), the antibody described by Francis and Hatcher (283) was the first reported example of anti-N made by an individual with N- 'N'- red cells.

Since the true nature of 'N' on red cells that initially type as M+ N- was recognized, a number of examples of the M+ N- 'N'- phenotype have been found. While the full biochemical explanations for the lack of 'N' are given later in this chapter, it can be stated here that absence of glycophorin B in the U- phenotype or the alteration of that sialoglycoprotein that occurs in the S- s- U+^{wk} phenotype, coupled with the presence of *M* and not *N* at the *MN* locus, are the most frequently encountered situations resulting in the 'N'- phenotype (20,146,148,282,283). Less frequently 'N' is missing from red cells because of a change in the structure of glycophorin B, for example, as seen on He+ red cells (147,284-286) or when certain hybrid sialoglycoproteins are made by genes comprised of some material from the *MN* and some from the *Ss* locus (287-295). In addition, the gene M^k encodes no production of glycophorin A or glycophorin B so that the red cells of M^k homozygotes lack 'N' (296-298). All the genes that fail to encode production of 'N' are rare. In a number of instances that antigen has been seen to be absent from the red cells of an individual heterozygous for haplotypes that do not encode production of 'N'. As examples, Judd et al. (147) studied one family in which the proposita with the 'N'- phenotype was genetically *MsHe/Mu*. In an unrelated family, Judd et al. (290) identified the 'N'- phenotype in an individual who was genetically Mi^V/M^k. These findings illustrate the fact that when attempts to determine the presence or absence of 'N' are undertaken at the serological level, the products of both haplotypes must be considered. While an individual genetically *Mu/Mu* (where *u* is the gene also called S^u that encodes no production of glycophorin B) will have 'N'- red cells, those genetically *Mu/MS* and *Mu/Ms* will have 'N' present since the former has S and the latter *s*. In the examples given above M^k makes no S, s, U or 'N'. Other haplotypes, e.g. *MsHe*, Mi^V, etc., can make s and U, without 'N'.

Complex as the genetic alterations that lead to nonproduction of 'N' may be, recognition as to whether an example of anti-N is causing agglutination because of the presence of glycophorin A-borne N, or because of the presence of that determinant and the presence of glycophorin B-borne 'N', is relatively straightforward at the serological level so long as red cells of common MNSs phenotypes are used. Glycophorin A has a trypsin-sensitive site so that when red cells are treated with trypsin, N is cleaved. Glycophorin B, when present on intact red cells, does not carry a similar site so that trypsin-treatment of red cells does not remove 'N'. Thus by testing untreated and trypsin-treated red cells it is possible to determine whether the anti-N is agglutinating N+ 'N'+ and N- 'N'+ red cells, or only the former, no antibody agglutinating only the latter exists. A number of provisos must be made regarding such tests. First, as stated, the tests determine the visible reactions of the anti-N (agglutination is described, IATs can also be used). If adsorption studies are used, trypsin-treated red cells of any common MNSs phenotype will adsorb anti-N because they are 'N'+. Second, red cells of common MNSs phenotypes must be used since rare cells carrying hybrid glycophorins may carry glycophorin A-derived N but may have lost the trypsin-sensitive site. In other words, on such red cells, ordinary N survives trypsin-treatment. In routine work, the danger that an unrecognized sample carrying a hybrid glycophorin will be inadvertently used can be obviated by testing three or more random samples of common MNSs phenotypes. The chance that an unrecognized variant will obfuscate the interpretation is then nil. Table 15-4 summarizes the N and 'N' phenotypes of untreated and trypsin-treated red cells of various MNSs phenotypes. For the sake of convenience, that table lists red cells that initially type as M+ N- as M+ N-. Those examples that (untreated) are 'N'+ are, of course, not truly N-.

As might be expected, anti-N made by persons with M+ N- 'N'- red cells is often a more potent antibody than the anti-N made by persons with red cells that initially type as M+ N- but are actually 'N'+. The net result is that few persons with this type of anti-N have been given N+ blood. Ballas et al. (148) described one example, in a patient with sickle cell disease, that caused reduced in vivo survival of ^{51}Cr-labeled N+ red cells, gave a positive reaction in a monocyte monolayer assay and was thought to have caused a delayed transfusion reaction. Earlier reports (299,300) of transfusion reactions attributed to anti-N do not give details about the S or s status of the patients' red cells so that it is not possible retrospective-

ly to assess the 'N' status of those red cells. Of course, at the time these cases were studied, the utility of typing for S and s to determine the probable 'N' status was not known. One case of HDN caused by anti-N made a woman with M+ N- 'N'- red cells has been reported (146). The infant was mildly affected and required only phototherapy. This was somewhat surprising since the anti-N had an IAT titer of 1024 against M+ N+ red cells (the baby's phenotype).

In concluding this section we will again stress, as have others (149), that no human anti-'N' has ever been made. The antibody made is always anti-N. Some examples react, visibly, only with N+ red cells, others react with cells that initially type as N- but carry 'N'. Terms such as anti-'N', anti-N'N', et al. are incorrect because the antigen defined is N. As mentioned in the previous section, two monoclonal antibodies to N were shown to differ in that one had a higher affinity for N than for 'N', while the other behaved in the reverse manner (261). Presumably these affinities were influenced by the steric presentation of N on glycophorin A and 'N' on glycophorin B. Human polyclonal anti-N showing such variation have not been found.

Anti-S and Anti-s

Anti-S and anti-s are encountered less frequently than anti-M and anti-N. When seen they are most often red cell stimulated via transfusion or pregnancy (3,4,6,301-305). However, at least some non-red cell stimulated anti-S have been found (302,306). Most examples of the antibodies are IgG (11,136,307), rarely IgM forms are seen (109). While most blood group serologists think of anti-S and anti-s as usually being 37°C active antibodies reactive best by IAT, there is evidence that some of the antibodies have somewhat different characteristics. For example, Lalezari et al. (309) studied seven examples of anti-s in tests in the AutoAnalyzer and

TABLE 15-4 N and 'N' Content of Red Cells of Various MN Phenotypes Before and After Treatment with Trypsin

Phenotype	N and 'N' content of untreated cells	Ability of untreated cells to adsorb anti-N	N and 'N' content after trypsin-treatment	Ability of trypsin-treated cells to adsorb anti-N
M+ N- S or s+	N- 'N'+	Yes	N- 'N'+	Yes
M+ N+ S or s+	N+ 'N'+	Yes	N- 'N'+	Yes
M- N+ S or s+	N+ 'N'+	Yes	N- 'N'+	Yes
M+ N- S- s- U-	N- 'N'-	No	N- 'N'-	No
M+ N+ S- s- U-	N+ 'N'-	Yes	N- 'N'-	No
M- N+ S- s- U-	N+ 'N'-	Yes	N- 'N'-	No

by manual techniques. They found that like anti-M, anti-N and some examples of anti-S, these antibodies were optimally reactive at temperatures below 37°C. In manual IATs (all the antibodies studied were IgG and none of them activated complement) each antibody was found to react to a higher titer when the tests were incubated at 4°C than when they were incubated at 37°C. While these findings may at first appear to be at odds with the experience of most workers, it must be remembered that different methods were used. Lalezari et al. (309) did not find any cold-reactive agglutinins. Instead, they performed IATs following incubation of the cell-serum mixtures at different temperatures. In other words, because most blood bankers use single tube tests that are incubated at 37°C, the tests that demonstrated optimal reactivity of anti-S and anti-s at reduced temperatures are not routinely performed. When Arndt and Garratty (310) ran tests on 140 IgG antibodies to determine optimal reaction temperatures of those antibodies, their results were a little different. Among eight examples of anti-S and one anti-s studied, two anti-S reacted significantly better at temperatures below 37°C than at 37°C when tests at normal ionic strength were used. When low ionic strength methods were used the reactions at 10°C, 22°C and 30°C were not significantly stronger, and with one anti-S were weaker, than those at 37°C. The moral of this story seems to be that if an antibody that looks like anti-S or anti-s is being studied, but cannot be identified for sure, tests below 37°C may be of help in determining antibody specificity. As discussed later in this chapter, the s antigen on M^V+ red cells may be difficult to detect (7,74). This finding relates to the fact that M^V+ cells have normal MN but abnormal Ss SGP (311-314). Beck and Hardman (315) showed that those anti-s that would not react with M^V+ s+ red cells in IATs incubated at 37°C, would invariably do so if the tests were incubated at 4°C or room temperature. The reactivity of the anti-s sera with the M^V+ cells was optimal at pH 6.0 (315).

While any phenotyping test using a human serum to type red cells can be subject to incorrect interpretation because of the unsuspected presence of an antibody to a low incidence antigen, tests with anti-S are particularly prone to this problem. Most experienced blood group serologists will have used different examples of anti-S to type the same red cell sample, only to see discrepant results because of the presence of another antibody in one, or more, of the anti-S. Lubenko (324) studied nine single donor anti-S. Four contained at least one antibody to a low incidence antigen, one other contained at least two such antibodies, and two contained multiple such antibodies, that is at least 15 in each serum. It is, of course, entirely possible that the two sera that appeared to contain only anti-S, were simply not tested against red cells carrying the low incidence antigen to which they

also contained the antibody because no S- red cells positive for the antigen(s) were available. While working with Dantu+ samples, we (347) found that seven of nine anti-S also contained anti-Dantu.

In addition to the anti-s mentioned above, an anti-S giving its strongest reactions in a test system at pH 6.5 has been reported (316). An anti-S reactive only in tests at low ionic strength has also been seen (317). Anti-s has been produced by immunizing rabbits (323), as far as we are aware, anti-S has not.

Anti-S and Anti-s in Transfusion Therapy and in Hemolytic Disease of the Newborn

There is no doubt that anti-S and anti-s active at 37°C must be taken seriously in the provision of blood for immunized patients. Anti-S has caused both immediate (301) and delayed (155,157,158) transfusion reactions, anti-s has been involved in delayed reactions (157) and perhaps in unreported immediate ones. There are no data regarding the clinical significance of anti-S and anti-s that are demonstrable only in tests below 37°C (see above). Presumably these antibodies do not cause immediate transfusion reactions (they are unable to bind to the transfused red cells at normal body temperature). We are not aware of any systematic study designed to determine if patients with cold-reactive anti-S or anti-s undergo an anamnestic response following transfusion with S+ or s+ red cells. In terms of selecting suitable units of blood for patients with 37°C reactive anti-S or anti-s in the serum, screening of random units with the patient's serum is an effective way of finding compatible blood. Although as described below, anti-S and anti-s often show dosage effect, we have not heard of a patient's serum failing to react with S+ s+ red cells, when anti-S or anti-s was present. For ideal transfusion practice, of course, units found to be non-reactive with the patient's serum in the initial screening tests, can be confirmed as antigen-negative by the use of reagent grade anti-S or anti-s.

Both anti-S and anti-s have caused hemolytic disease of the newborn (6,11,303-305,325). In some cases the disease has been particularly severe, at least one fatal case due to anti-S (303) and one due to anti-s (304) have been recorded.

The provision of antigen-negative blood for patients with anti-S is relatively easy, 45% of White and almost 70% of Black donors have S- red cells. Finding s- units is only a little more difficult, some 11% of Whites and 7.5% of Blacks have s- red cells. Table 15-5 lists the approximate phenotype frequencies of S and s. Because genes at the *MN* and *Ss* loci are in linkage disequilibrium, the distribution of S and s is not equal among persons of different MN phenotypes. As mentioned earlier, when the four

TABLE 15-5 Approximate Frequencies of the Ss Phenotypes

Phenotype	Whites	U.S. Blacks
S+ s-	11%	6%
S+ s+	44%	24.5%
S- s+	45%	68%
S- s-	<0.01%	1.5%

TABLE 15-6 Approximate Frequencies of the MNSs Phenotypes

Phenotype	Whites	U.S. Blacks
M+ N- S+ s-	6%	2.1%
M+ N- S+ s+	14%	7%
M+ N- S- s+	8%	15.5%
M+ N- S- s-	<0.01%	0.4%
M+ N+ S+ s-	4%	2.2%
M+ N+ S+ s+	24%	13%
M+ N+ S- s+	22%	33.4%
M+ N+ S- s-	<0.01%	0.4%
M- N+ S+ s-	1%	1.6%
M- N+ S+ s+	6%	4.5%
M- N+ S- s+	15%	19.2%
M- N+ S- s-	<0.01%	0.7%

common haplotypes are considered the incidences are such that *Ns>Ms>MS>NS*. Since patients are sometimes encountered with either anti-M or anti-N and anti-S or anti-s in the serum, table 15-6 lists the approximate frequencies of the *MNSs* phenotypes. While this table can be used to determine what percentage of random units will be compatible with the serum of a patient with anti-M or anti-N and anti-S or anti-s, it must be added that the given frequencies in Blacks are more approximate than those in Whites, having been calculated from just three reasonably sized surveys (77,283,326).

Anti-S in the Sera of Individuals with S+ Red Cells

There are reports (319,320) of benign autoantibodies with apparent anti-S specificity in which it was shown that the antibody mimicked anti-S but did not truly have that specificity. Those antibodies are described in the next section of this chapter. Auto-anti-S has been seen in patients with "warm" antibody-induced hemolytic anemia (327-329), those antibodies are discussed further in Chapter 37. We do not know of any reported example of benign or pathological auto-anti-s, presumably such antibodies will eventually come to light.

Antibodies That Resemble Anti-S

In 1978, Case (318) reported that some antibodies that behave as anti-S in tests against untreated red cells, react with S- s+ but not with S- s- U- or S- s- U+ red cells after those cells have been treated with ficin. In 1982, we (319) described an antibody made by an individual with M+ N+ S+ s+ U+ red cells that reacted only with ficin or papain-treated red cells. While the antibody had a marked preference for S+ red cells it could be adsorbed to exhaustion by S- s+ U+ and by the patient's own S+ s+ U+ red cells. It was not adsorbed at all by S- s- U- or S- s- U+ red cells. In 1987, Puig et al. (320) described an antibody that caused a delayed transfusion reaction and appeared to be anti-S, made by a patient with S- s+ red

cells. However, the antibody, which could be eluted from the patient's DAT- red cells three years after the transfusion, could be adsorbed to exhaustion with S- s+ red cells. It is possible that some or all the antibodies described in this paragraph had a specificity similar to anti-U^Z that is described later in this chapter.

All these observations (318-320) were mirrored by some findings made later using monoclonal antibodies directed against glycophorin B. While those findings are discussed below, it seems apparent that some antibodies are directed against glycophorin B but, under certain conditions behave as anti-S. One possible explanation relates to the finding (321,322) that *S* encodes production of about 1.5 times the number of copies of glycophorin B as are encoded by *s*. A second possibility is that the antibodies recognize a determinant on glycophorin B that is common to S-bearing and s-bearing forms of that structure. Perhaps in the presence of S, the determinant is simply more accessible to its antibody, than in the presence of s.

Dosage Effects with Anti-S and Anti-s

Many examples of anti-S and anti-s show dosage effects (6,303,330). Sometimes the effect is not as dramatic as that seen with anti-M and anti-N. At first this seems to be a paradox. It is known that *M* and *N* each encode production of about half a million copies of glycophorin A per red cell (234-236). That is to say, there is no difference in the amount of glycophorin A encoded by *M* and *N*. In contrast, the available data (321,322) show that *S* encodes production of about 125,000 copies of glycophorin B per red cell, while *s* encodes production of about 85,000 copies. Thus red cells from *S* homozygotes should carry some 250,000 copies of glycophorin B per red cell, while those of *s* homozygotes should carry some 170,000 copies. At first this seems to suggest that anti-S and anti-s should be more likely to show dosage effects than anti-M and anti-N. The reason that this is not necessarily the case relates, of course, to the total number of copies of antigen per cell. Red cells from *M* homozygotes should carry some 1 million copies of M, that is 500,000 encoded by each of their *M* genes. Red cells from *MN* heterozygotes should carry some 500,000 copies of M, encoded by the single *M* gene present. Thus the difference, for anti-M to see in dosage studies, is 500,00 copies of antigen. In contrast the red cells of *S* homozygotes should carry some 250,000 copies of S, that is 125,000 copies encoded by each of their *S* genes. The red cells of *Ss* heterozygotes should carry some 125,000 copies of S encoded by the single *S* gene, and some 85,000 copies of s encoded by the single *s* gene. Thus the difference in the number of S antigens on S+ s- and S+ s+ red cells, for anti-S to see in dosage studies is 125,000, far short of the 500,000 difference between M+ N- and M+ N+ red cells.

Amount of 'N' on Red Cells of Different Ss Phenotypes

As described in an earlier section, the 'N' determinant is located at the NH$_2$ terminus of glycophorin B. Since red cells of *S* homozygotes carry some 250,000 copies of that sialoglycoprotein, while those of *s* homozygotes carry some 170,000 copies, it is not surprising that S+ s- red cells react more strongly with those anti-N that agglutinate red cells originally typed as M+ N-, than do S- s+ red cells. Perhaps the most dramatic demonstration of this difference is that seen when potent examples of *Vicia graminea* lectin are used. At an appropriate dilution that lectin (see below) can be used to type red cells for glycophorin A-borne N, without interference by 'N'. If undiluted *Vicia graminea* lectin is used, it can be seen to agglutinate S+ red cells previously typed as M+ N- but not similarly typed M+ N- red cells that are S- s+ (7).

Effects of Enzymes on the S and s Antigens

As mentioned above, on intact red cells glycophorin B, that carries the 'N', S and s antigens, lacks the trypsin-sensitive site found on glycophorin A. Thus red cells treated with trypsin retain their 'N', S and s antigens (38,243). Once glycophorin B is extracted from red cells,

it has a number of trypsin-sensitive sites (321). Presumably while the sialoglycoprotein is in situ, those cleavage sites are not accessible to the actions of trypsin.

The enzymes chymotrypsin, papain, ficin, bromelin and pronase all cleave glycophorin B and, theoretically at least, should result in the treated red cells losing 'N', S and s (38,243,331). In practice, such antigen denaturation is not easy to achieve. In the experience of one of us (PDI), papain, ficin and bromelin-treated red cells often continue to react with anti-S and anti-s. The literature states that S is denatured by a lower concentration of chymotrypsin than that required to denature s (243,331) but that S is less easily denatured than s, when papain or ficin are used (38). Again, from personal experience, one of us (PDI) has found that while these enzymes may denature S, they must be used at relatively high concentrations, for extended periods of time, to have any effect on s. As far as we are aware, no one has ever seen any reduction in level of S or s on red cells from which NeuAc has been removed, i.e. neuramindase-treated red cells.

Monoclonal Anti-S

A murine monoclonal antibody was seen to have apparent anti-S specificity in agglutination and indirect antiglobulin tests (332,333). However, when immunoblotting studies or serological tests at pH 6.5 were used (334) the antibody was seen to react with S- s+ red cells and to have anti-glycophorin B specificity. As discussed above, in the section on human polyclonal antibodies that resemble (or mimic) anti-S, the reactions of the antibody may have been influenced by the number of copies of glycophorin B on red cells (see section on dosage of anti-S) or different steric orientation of the determinant recognized on S-bearing and s-bearing glycophorin B. The antibody (MAb 148, clone F84.3E8.E2, Immucor, Norcross, GA) was further unusual in that it reacted strongly with S- St(a+) and S- Dantu+ red cells but failed to react with S+ red cells of the Mi.IV (GP.Hop) phenotypes (332-334). An intelligible explanation of these reactions can only be provided by consideration of the biochemical structure of the glycophorins on these unusual red cells. Such an explanation is given in the section of this chapter dealing with the biochemistry of the MN system and the derivation and structure of hybrid sialoglycoproteins.

The U Antigen and Its Complexities in Blacks

In 1953, Wiener et al. (39) described an alloantibody made by a Black patient, that defined an antigen of very high incidence. The antigen detected was named U, to indicate that it was of near universal occurrence. In tests on samples from 989 Black donors, 12 were found to be non-reactive, for an incidence of 1.2% (40). In 1954, Greenwalt et al. (41), in describing the second example of anti-U, reported that all U- red cells were also S- s-; the place of U in the MN system had been established. Large scale typing studies on the red cells of random Blacks initially showed two distinct frequencies for the U- phenotype. Table 15-7 lists the results from six studies. As can be seen, the findings of Wiener et al. (40), Francis and Hatcher (283) and Issitt et al. (77) are in close agreement and show a total of 23 U- persons among 1811 tested, for an incidence of 1.27%. The findings of Sanger et al. (308), Greenwalt et al. (41,335) and Greenwalt (336) are in close agreement with each other, but not with those of the three earlier series. In the latter three series a total of 4683 samples were tested, among them 11 U- samples were found for an incidence of 0.23%. The explanation of these findings was provided by Allen et al. (282) and Francis and Hatcher (283) who showed that among the samples found in the series described above, two different phenotypes exist. One is S- s- U-; the other is S- s- U+^{var} (var indicates variant) in which the U antigen is weakly expressed and may be qualitatively different from the U antigen present on S+ or s+ red cells. If the type of anti-U that reacts visibly with S- s- U+^{var} red cells is used, the incidence of the U- phenotype is around 0.23% (i.e. 1 in about 425 samples). If the type of anti-U that fails to react visibly with S- s- U+^{var} cells is used, the incidence of the apparent U- phenotype is 1.27% (i.e. 1 in about 79 samples). S- s- U+^{var} cells that do not react visibly with some examples of anti-U will usually (but perhaps not with all examples of anti-U) adsorb and yield those antibodies on elution. It is possible, but does not seem to have been proved, that the anti-U that react visibly with S- s- U+^{var} red cells are made by persons phenotypically S- s- U-, while those that fail to react visibly with S- s- U+^{var} red cells may have been made by persons whose own red cells are of the U+^{var} phenotype. However, as described below, the situation is not as simple as presence of the same variant U antigen on all S- s- U+^{var} samples.

Goldstein (337,338) claimed that the U antigen could be divided into two portions that she called U^A and U^B. The U- samples defined by the most discriminating examples of anti-U (those that type only 0.23% of bloods as U-) were said to be U^{ab}. That is, they lacked U^A and U^B. Those selected as U- by the less discriminating sera (that identify 1.27% of bloods as U-) were said to be U^{Ab}, U^{aB} or U^{ab}. That is to say, if anti-U^A is used to type red cells, those that are U^{aB} or U^{ab} will type as U-. If anti-U^B is used, those that are U^{Ab} or U^{ab} will be classified as U-. If anti-U^{AB} (as made by an individual with red cells of the U^{ab} phenotype) is used, only U^{ab} samples will

TABLE 15-7 Variation in the Incidence of the U- Phenotype

Series and References	Number Tested	Number U-	Incidence U-
Wiener et al. (40)	989	12	1.21%
Francis and Hatcher (283)	322	4	1.24%
Issitt et al. (77)	500	7	1.4%
Total of 3 series above (40, 77, 283)	1811	23	1.27%
Sanger et al. (308)	605	1	0.17%
Greenwalt et al. (41, 335)	997	3	0.3%
Greenwalt (336)	3081	7	0.23%
Total of second series of 3 (41, 308, 335, 336)	4683	11	0.23%

type as U-, those that are U^{Ab} or U^{aB} will be classed as U+ (sometimes only by means of adsorption-elution studies). While the concept of U+ red cells being U^{AB} and the phenotypes U^{Ab}, U^{aB} and U^{ab} all existing, would explain the variance in the reported incidence of the U- phenotype (0.23% and 1.27%) the situation is not that simple. We (339) had the opportunity to repeat many of the studies of Goldstein (337) with the original sera, but were not able to duplicate the U^A or U^B findings. We and many others have performed multiple tests with samples carrying small amounts of atypical U antigen and have found that the situation is at least as complex as the situation with D, in which some individuals with partial D on their red cells make allo-anti-D. Indeed, in trying to look at U antigen epitopes with anti-U made by persons with some expression of U on their red cells, the situation sometimes looks as if each antibody is individualistic in specificity. As described later in this section, it is now appreciated (341,755) that some of the reactions of some anti-U with some red cells of the S- s- U+^{var} phenotype are due to the presence of antibodies directed against other epitopes of glycophorin B, in the "anti-U" sera.

We (340) described another complexity involving the U antigen. All the early studies had shown that the U antigen survives treatment of red cells with proteases. That is to say, protease-treated red cells had all reacted with anti-U, indeed sometimes the reactions of the antibody had been enhanced in such tests. We found one anti-U that was reactive with untreated red cells but was non-reactive with U+ red cells that had been treated with papain. In the subsequent investigation we tested another 41 examples of anti-U. One was similar to the index serum and failed to react with papain-treated U+ red cells; the other 40 all reacted with papain-treated red cells. In adsorption studies, we showed that 19 of those 40 anti-U could be adsorbed to exhaustion with papain-treated red cells. However, when the other 21 were adsorbed with papain-treated red cells to the point at which they no longer reacted with such cells, antibody activity for untreated U+ red cells remained unadsorbed. We (340) called those anti-U that reacted with papain-treated red cells, anti-UPR (for U papain-resistant). Those anti-U that failed to react with papain-treated red cells were called anti-UPS (for U papain-sensitive). Among the 42 anti-U studied (including the index case): two contained only anti-UPS; 19 contained only anti-UPR; while 21 contained separable anti-UPR and anti-UPS. In all 21 of those sera, the anti-UPR was stronger, often by a considerable margin, than the anti-UPS. In an extended adsorption experiment, an anti-UPR with a titer of 512 was adsorbed to exhaustion in three adsorptions with papain-treated red cells. An anti-UPS, that also had a titer of 512, was very slowly adsorbed by papain-treated red cells. Unlike the anti-UPR, a total of 12 consecutive adsorptions were necessary to adsorb that antibody to exhaustion. In other words, the determinant recognized by anti-UPS is markedly damaged but not totally denatured when U+ red cells are treated with papain. That the very slow and gradual adsorption of anti-UPS by papain-treated U+ red cells was specific and did not represent simple antibody dilution by the saline present with the adsorbing red cells, was shown in a control in the experiment. An anti-U containing anti-UPR and anti-UPS, that also had a titer of 512 before adsorption, was adsorbed 12 consecutive times with papain-treated U- red cells. The dilution effect of those adsorptions reduced the titer of the antibody from 512 to 64.

Our conclusion from these studies (340) was that glycophorin B carries at least two determinants recognized by anti-U. The UPR determinant is apparently located closer to the red cell membrane than is a papain-sensitive site on glycophorin B. The UPS determinant is either located further from the membrane than is the papain-sensitive site, or includes that site within its structure. From the different levels of anti-UPR and anti-UPS in anti-U, it seemed that UPR must be more immunogenic than is UPS. To our considerable disappointment we found no correlation between the S- s- U+^{var} phenotype and the presence or absence of UPR and/or UPS.

To the complexities revealed by anti-UPR and anti-UPS, Storry et al. (341) have now added another layer. These workers investigated a number of examples of anti-U in light of two other facts. First, as described above, individuals genetically *MuMu* (where *u* encodes no production of U) have red cells that lack U, N and 'N'. N is missing because both *glycophorin A* genes make M (34-36). 'N' and U are missing because *u* does not encode production of glycophorin B (or at very least

does not encode production of normal glycophorin B) (34,37,38). Second, again as described above, when the antigen He is present, it replaces 'N' at the NH$_2$ terminal end of glycophorin B. In individuals with hybrid glycophorins, He may replace 'N' and a portion of glycophorin A derived material may replace the portion of glycophorin B that normally carries U. Again, the N-'N'- U- phenotype may result, but this time will be He+. Storry et al. (341) studied 17 examples of antibodies previously thought to have anti-U specificity. Five of them contained only anti-U, the other twelve contained anti-U and anti-He, or anti-U, anti-N and anti-He in inseparable forms. These authors concluded that many sera that contain what initially appears to be anti-U, are in fact anti-glycophorin B and as such may define a variety of determinants, i.e. at least U, 'N' and He. The situation was described as being analogous to that involving anti-En^a. As described later in this chapter, antibodies made by persons whose red cells lack or have altered forms of glycophorin A, are actually anti-glycophorin A. Because En(a-) red cells lack that glycophorin, the antibodies have been called anti-En^a. In fact, different examples of anti-En^a complex with different portions of glycophorin A.

Storry et al. (341) found a fairly good correlation between their observations on the multispecific anti-glycophorin B forms of anti-U, and UPR and UPS. Those antibodies previously classified (340) as anti-UPR contained anti-U or inseparable anti-U and anti-He. Those sera previously classified as anti-UPR plus anti-UPS contained inseparable anti-U, anti-N and anti-He.

Although the full picture is not yet to hand, it seems reasonable to suppose that the reactions of some S- s- U+^{var} red cells, with some examples of anti-U, sometimes represent the presence of other determinants on altered glycophorin B on those red cells and the anti-glycophorin B specificity of the supposed anti-U. There are now a number of reports (16,17,42,342-345) of glycophorin B-derived material on red cells that initially type as S- s-, many (perhaps all) of which are U+^{var}. At the practical level the presence of some form of, presumably altered, glycophorin B on some S- s- red cells can be recognized if anti-He or one of the other anti-glycophorin B specificities (i.e. directed against N, U, UPR, UPS or other as yet unnamed epitopes) is available. It has been shown that between 23% (755) and 40% (341,343,370) of red cells that initially type as S- s- U- are He+. It is also known (342-344,370 and see later in this chapter for additional details) that there are at least two different genetic backgrounds that lead to the S- s- phenotype. Again it seems reasonable to suppose that the S- s- U- phenotype most often represents deletion or non-function (at the phenotypic level) of the *glycophorin B* gene, while the S- s- U+^{var} phenotype most often represents the actions of an altered form of that gene. However, it must be added that at the serological level, it is easy to mistake S- s- U+^{var} red cells as being of the S-s- U- phenotype. A solution to that particular problem is discussed in the section on anti-U in transfusion therapy.

Anti-U may contain MN system antibodies other than those described above. For example, part of the difficulties in determining whether the hybrid genes (there are several different ones, see later) that encode production of Dantu, do or do not make U (45-47,346) occurred because some anti-U also contain anti-Dantu. The situation may not be analogous to that described by Storry et al. (341). We (347) found that two of six anti-U contained anti-Dantu. Eluates made from Dantu+ red cells that had been exposed to those sera, contained anti-Dantu but no anti-U.

Most of the work described in this section has been done using the S- s- U- and S- s- U+^{var} red cells of Blacks in the USA. Indeed the given frequencies of those phenotypes relate to the US Black population. The S- s-U- phenotype has been found, with a widely divergent incidence, in other Black populations. For example, Fraser et al. (406) tested samples from 126 Pygmies in Zaire and found that 44 (35%) of them were S- s- U-. In contrast, Lowe and Moores (407) found no U- sample in tests on the blood of 1000 Bantu-speaking individuals in Natal. Between these two extremes Hoekstra et al. (408) found that three of 1000 Black prenatal patients in the Eastern Cape of South Africa, had S- s- U- red cells. From tests on the red cells of 840 Black blood donors in Martinique in the French West Indies, Mornex et al. (409) concluded that the incidence of U- in that population is the same as in US Blacks. However, a review of their results suggests that the 9 U- they found, for an incidence of 1.07%, were all S- s- U-, meaning that none was S- s- U+^{var}. Thus the incidence of S- s- U- would appear to be higher than the 0.23% incidence in US Blacks (see above). Such an interpretation would fit with the believed derivation of the Black Martinique population (410,411) from the Ivory Coast, Upper Volta and Gabon, where the incidence of U- is higher than in the USA.

The U- and U+^{var} Phenotypes in Whites

As described in the previous section, the phenotypes S- s- U- and S- s- U+^{var} are both uncommon occurring in about 1 in 425 and 1 in 79 Blacks, respectively. The phenotypes are even less common in Whites, indeed they are rare enough that no reliable estimates of their frequency can be made. Sondag-Thull et al. (356) reported that four members of a French family had S- s- U- red cells. Eriksson (357) found that among 324 Finnish Lapplanders, six had S- s- U- red cells, Constans et al.

(358) reported the S- s- phenotype in two of 63 Central American Indians in Honduras. Moores (359) found four examples of the S- s- U- phenotype in an Indian family living in Natal. Although no Black admixture was known and although no physical or serological characteristics to suggest such admixture were found, the Indian population may have been present in South Africa for many generations so that admixture cannot be totally excluded. The presence of u in Whites has several times (360-364) been invoked to explain otherwise unexplainable inheritance of S or s. In one such case, Dahr et al. (365) used biochemical methods to show that only half the expected amount of glycophorin B was being made, thus confirming the presence of u. As described later in this chapter, the S- s- U- and S- s- U+^{var} phenotypes can result from any one of several different genetic backgrounds (342,366-370). It is not yet known whether the different backgrounds that account for the S- s- phenotype in Blacks are all present in Whites.

Anti-U in Transfusion Therapy

There is no doubt that patients who form allo-anti-U must be transfused with compatible blood. The antibody is invariably red cell immune, no example in a never transfused, never pregnant individual has been reported. Anti-U is almost always IgG in composition, most examples contain an IgG1 component (307). The first reported example of anti-U caused a fatal transfusion reaction (39), other examples that caused delayed hemolytic reactions, have been described (175,348-352). Although two reports (309,310) describe anti-U that reacted better at temperatures below 37°C than at that temperature, in vitro, neither report was intended to imply that anti-U might be benign in vivo.

Exactly how the transfusion needs of patients with anti-U in the serum should be met, is still not entirely clear. Since screening programs designed to identify U-donors are conducted with whatever anti-U is available, it follows that some donors (and units) thought to be U-, will actually be S- s- U+^{var} (see earlier for a description of the reactions of various anti-U). When a patient with anti-U in the serum is encountered, it is customary to test donor units previously classified as U-, with the patient's serum. However, the studies are usually confined to IATs to determine compatibility. Thus, it seems probable that individuals who have produced anti-U, have been transfused with red cells that appear compatible in IATs, but that would have adsorbed the patient's anti-U had appropriate tests been performed. (Those examples of S- s-U+^{var} units that give positive IAT reactions with the patient's serum are not usually transfused.) Whether U+^{var} red cells that appear compatible by IAT, but that would adsorb the patient's anti-U, survive normally in vivo, or whether they have a reduced but acceptable in vivo survival time, is not known as far as we are aware. However, it can be guessed that even if survival of the cells is not normal, it is not grossly reduced for surely transfusion-related complications would have been recognized by now, if rapid in vivo red cell destruction was common. There are two case reports in the literature about anti-U that broadened in specificity after the transfusion of U- (presumably U+^{var}) blood. Beattie et al. (350) described one such patient. Their case was complicated by the fact that the patient also had sickle cell disease and it is notoriously difficult to differentiate between a delayed transfusion reaction and a sickle cell crisis in such patients. While it seemed that the patient's anti-U broadened in specificity after the transfusion and was able to react with S- s- U+^{var} cells with which it gave no visible reaction before transfusion, the fact that some U+^{var} red cells could be detected in the post-transfusion sample suggests that some of those cells had survived. In a case described by Miceli et al. (353) a patient with anti-U was transfused with 15 units of supposed U- blood, all of which were compatible with the patient's serum. Although following transfusion of the last five units a weakly positive, mixed-field reaction, DAT was seen, and anti-U could be eluted from the post transfusion samples, the only clinical evidence suggestive of a delayed transfusion reaction was that the leukemic patient's transfusion requirements increased. Again, it was supposed that the transfusion of some S- s- U+^{var} blood had resulted in a broadening in specificity of the patient's anti-U. In a serologically similar case described by Mentor and Richards (354) it was claimed that the anti-U involved was recognizing a "rare variant associated with the U- blood group". The fact that the anti-U reacted with 80% of samples classified as U-, some of which had been found to be non-reactive with earlier samples of serum from the patient showed, in fact, that the patient's anti-U had changed to the point that it now gave visible reactions with S- s- U+^{var} red cells (355). The numbers were exactly right. That is, if S- s- U- and S- s- U+^{var} units are included in the U- donor pool, an anti-U capable of reacting visibly with S- s- U+^{var} red cells will react with four of every five samples in the pool.

Based on our observations (340) on anti-UPR and anti-UPS and on those of Storry and Reid (341) that show that some anti-U contain antibodies to N, He and other epitopes on glycophorin B, it is now clear what happens when a patient's anti-U "broadens" in specificity. If the patient initially makes a form of anti-U that defines a glycophorin B-borne epitope missing from red cells of the S- s- U- and S- s- U+^{var} phenotypes, the patient may be transfused with S- s- U+^{var} red cells. Two factors will contribute to this event. First, the S- s- U+^{var} red cells may

well have been classified as S- s- U- based on the specificity of the anti-U originally used to type them. Second, since the red cells lack the epitope of U (glycophorin B) to which the patient has made an antibody, red cells from the units will be non-reactive in IATs used in compatibility testing. Following transfusion, the patient's anti-U may appear to "broaden" in specificity and may react visibly with S- s- U+^{var} red cells that were previously non-reactive. In fact, the patient has now made an additional anti-glycophorin B specificity antibody or antibodies, capable of detecting epitopes on the altered glycophorin on the S- s- U+^{var} red cells.

The findings just described have led to suggestions (350,353) that when screening tests to identify U- donors are undertaken, additional tests should be performed on those samples that type as U- in the initial studies. That is to say, it was suggested (350,353) that those cells be shown to be non-reactive in adsorption-elution studies with potent anti-U, before being called U-. Storry and Reid (341) suggested that an antibody with broad anti-U/GPB specificity be used in the screening studies and that adsorption-elution tests may be desirable. However, in a later study Reid et al. (836) showed that if a suitable anti-U/glycophorin B was used, almost all, i.e. 46 of 47, S- s- U+^{var} samples, gave visibly position reactions by PEG-IAT or in an anti-IgG GEL card. The 47 samples tested were known to be capable of adsorbing anti-U.

While it is now possible to differentiate between S- s- U- and S- s- U+^{var} units with reasonable ease (341,836) it would not seem to be wise to insist that all units to be classified as U- be shown not to be of the S- s- U+^{var} phenotype. Such a policy would reduce the incidence of U- donors from about 1 in 79 (i.e. S- s- U- plus S- s- U+^{var}) to about 1 in 425 (i.e. S- s- U-). While no one would disagree with such a policy if there was evidence that S- s- U+^{var} red cells are rapidly destroyed in the circulation of a patient with anti-U, evidence on that point is equivocal. As referenced above many (perhaps most) patients with anti-U, who must be transfused, derive the required benefits from the transfusion of S- s- U+^{var} red cells that are compatible by IAT with the pretransfusion serum. Further, it can be anticipated that if persons of the S- s- U+^{var} phenotype can make anti-U, the red cells of some S- s- U+^{var} donors will be identical to those of the antibody-maker.

In short, it would not seem wise to jeopardize the already limited supply of U- blood by insisting that all U- donors be shown to lack all representation of glycophorin B-borne epitopes. To argue that such a practice would prevent further immunization of patients who have already made anti-U flies in the face of current transfusion practice. Other than avoidance of transfusion of D+ red cells to D- patients and avoidance of certain antigen exposures in certain patients (e.g. C, E and

K in patients with sickle cell disease) blood for transfusion is not selected with the objective of prevention of alloimmunization. On the other hand, keeping S- s- U- and S- s- U+^{var} (many of which will appear to be S- s- U-) units in the U- donor pool and using, for transfusion, those units that are non-reactive by IAT, with the patient's pretransfusion serum, is exactly in line with current transfusion practice. To belabor the point, any blood banker who has had to supply blood for a patient with anti-D and anti-U in the serum (not too uncommon a finding in some prenatal clinics) will know that D- , S- s- U+^{var}, IAT-compatible blood, is a lot easier to find than D- units, shown by adsorption-elution methods truly to lack all glycophorin B epitopes.

A compromise policy for those workers with a suitable anti-U/glycophorin B available would be to transfuse S- s- U- patients with S- s- U- blood and S- s- U+^{var} patients with S- s- U+^{var} blood. While a practical solution, such measures would not entirely prevent the development of additional reactivity in patients who had already made anti-U since it has been shown (286,340,341,343,345,755,836) that not all S- s- U+^{var} bloods are identical. However, as pointed out by Reid et al. (836) there are good reasons for regarding S- s- U- and S- s- U+^{var} units as rare blood, albeit in different categories if necessary.

Anti-U and Hemolytic Disease of the Newborn

This antibody has several times (371-378) caused HDN and in at least one case (372) was responsible for in utero death of the fetus. Like those caused by anti-S and anti-s, but unlike those caused by anti-M and anti-N, cases of HDN caused by anti-U are characterized by a strongly positive DAT on the cord blood red cells. While discussing the severity of HDN caused by anti-U, it should be mentioned that if a severely affected infant is encountered and if no U- blood is available for exchange transfusion, the use of U+ blood should be seriously considered. It should be remembered that in vivo red cell destruction in the infant is caused by maternal antibody. After birth, no additional antibody will enter the infant's circulation. Although U+ red cells will appear incompatible if excess anti-U is present in the infant's serum, most of that antibody as well as the infant's antibody-coated red cells will be removed by the exchange transfusion. Thus, if the affected infant is severely anemic so that its survival is in doubt, an exchange transfusion with incompatible U+ blood can be undertaken. Similarly, if after birth the infant's bilirubin level starts to rise (because of continued in vivo destruction of the antibody-coated red cells) and is likely to reach a level at which kernicterus

may result, an exchange transfusion with U+ blood is indicated if U- blood is still not available. In performing an exchange transfusion with incompatible red cells, it may be necessary to use a larger volume of blood than when compatible red cells are available. This is because the first incompatible red cells infused will become coated with the excess maternal antibody in the infant's plasma and will be subject to sequestration and destruction if not removed. Generally, a two unit exchange transfusion with incompatible blood is as efficient as a single unit exchange with compatible red cells. At the time that the second unit of incompatible red cells is infused, it is probable that most (or all) of the maternal antibody will have been removed from the infant's circulation. Certainly, it is much better to perform an exchange transfusion with incompatible red cells than risk the infant's death or risk kernicterus, while searches for compatible red cells are undertaken. These considerations apply, of course, any time a maternal antibody to a high incidence antigen causes severe HDN. They are in no way peculiar to HDN caused by anti-U. The use of U+ blood for an infant with severe HDN caused by anti-U (376) was discussed in print by a number of experts (379-384). In addition to the points made above, several discussants noted that if she is able to donate, the mother's washed red cells can be used, if only a single exchange transfusion is necessary. In answer to the question as to whether blood ABO incompatible with the infant, that lacks the antigen to which the causative antibody is directed, should be used if no other antigen-negative blood was available, opinions differed. While Rosenfield (384) advocated the use of such blood, both Huestis (381) and Giblett (382) advised against it. While it was agreed that the ABO incompatibility would be of no importance at the time of the exchange transfusion, both respondents were concerned that major side ABO incompatible red cells would still be present in the child's circulation when the child became immunologically competent, and would be destroyed as the infant made ABO system antibodies. In discussing the use of serologically incompatible blood for exchange transfusion, Rosenfield (384) commented that he would use three or four units of such blood. He reported that infants thus treated have a stormy course but that almost all of them survive and none have kernicterus if handled adequately.

Autoimmune Anti-U

Auto-anti-U has been reported in a number of patients with "warm" antibody-induced hemolytic anemia (385-389) where it is often accompanied by other, non-MN system autoantibodies. Auto-anti-U has also been seen in at least one patient with aldomet-induced hemolytic anemia (390) and in one patient with myasthenia gravis, in whom the autoantibody appeared to be benign (391). The example of auto-anti-U described by Bell and Zwicker (388) was demonstrable only when the test system was adjusted to pH 6.5 and when an antiglobulin serum containing anti-complement was used to read the IATs. Wojcicki et al. (392) described an 8 year-old girl with hemolytic anemia who had produced autoantibodies of more than one specificity. The auto-anti-U component gave greatly enhanced reactions in tests using a low ionic strength system adjusted to pH 5 or 6, in which the tests were incubated at low temperatures. Roush et al. (827) described a most unusual auto-anti-U that caused life-threatening hemolytic anemia. The autoantibody was described as being IgG2 in composition yet it was said to have caused intravascular hemolysis in the patient, who also presented with reticulocytopenia. The patient's anemia was not corrected by transfusions with U+ blood, his hemoglobin went up when he was treated with steroids and transfused with seven units of U- blood. Although no serological evidence of drug-induced hemolytic anemia was found, the report mentions that the patient was being treated with a nonsteroidal anti-inflammatory drug. Such drugs are known (828-833) to have caused hemolytic anemia and while not totally specific on the point, the report (827) implies that the non-steroidal anti-inflammatory drug was withdrawn and not reinstituted when the patient responded to steroid therapy. McGinniss et al. (393) reported finding auto-anti-U in nine of 28 (32%) hospitalized patients with AIDS. The auto-anti-U were detected only in tests using papain-treated red cells. We do not know if this observation has been confirmed by others, we do know that the first reported example of anti-UPS (see earlier) was made by a patient with AIDS. That antibody was alloimmune in nature and ironically initiated a study because it failed to react with papain-treated U+ red cells. Daniels (9) points out that while persons who make alloimmune anti-U are invariably Black, most persons described as having made autoimmune anti-U are White. Auto-anti-U are discussed again in Chapters 37, 39 and 40.

Dosage Effects and Anti-U

Although there are occasional reports (363,394) that some examples of anti-U show dosage effects, we (395) were unable to find such antibodies. We tested 11 different examples of anti-U against random donor red cells and those of nine obligate *u* heterozygotes (i.e. the parents or children of U- individuals) from four unrelated families. In blind studies we were unable to differentiate between red cells from individuals genetically *UU*

and those genetically *Uu*. Metaxas and Metaxas-Bühler (396) used several of the same anti-U and were unable to demonstrate a single dose of U on the red cells of M^k heterozygotes (for a description of the M^k gene see later in this chapter). We do not know if the flow cytometer has been used to try to demonstrate dosage of U. As mentioned in an earlier section, densiometric scans of stained SDS-PAGE preparations can be used to measure the comparative amount of glycophorin B on red cells and thus help to differentiate red cells from persons genetically *UU* and *Uu* (16,17,42,365).

The Effect of Enzymes on the U Antigen

As mentioned earlier in the description of UPR and UPS, most examples of anti-U react strongly with protease treated red cells (340). Indeed, in the study on UPR and UPS, 40 of 42 (95%) anti-U reacted with papain-treated red cells, in those sera containing anti-UPR and anti-UPS, the anti-UPR, that reacted with papain-treated red cells, was always the stronger of the two antibodies (340). The enzymes trypsin, chymotrypsin, pronase and neuraminidase (sialidase) and the agent aminoethylisothiouronium bromide (AET) also fail to effect any denaturation of U (397), as that antigen is defined by the 95% of anti-U mentioned above.

The U Antigen, Glycophorin B and Soybean Lectin

In many places in the previous sections it has been stated that the U antigen is carried on glycophorin B. Indeed the evidence for such a conclusion is incontrovertible (17,42,44,291,332,356,366,367,398,399). When Ballas et al. (400) studied membranes from S- s- U+^{var} red cells, they were unable to detect glycophorin B and suggested that the U antigen is not carried on that structure. In fact, the conclusion was reached because the amount of glycophorin B on S- s- U+^{var} cells is too little for detection by the methods used (400). Earlier, Dahr et al. (17,44) had shown that if the SDS-PAGE method is used with overloading of the gels, membranes from S- s- U+^{var} red cells can be shown to carry between 2 and 4% of the normal quantity of glycophorin B, although, as described above, the glycophorin B present is probably qualitatively different from normal glycophorin B.

It seems probable that the U antigen requires a red cell membrane component in addition to glycophorin B for normal expression. Dahr and Moulds (401) showed that the U antigen is labile and that it may require the presence of lipids for full integrity. This, coupled with the finding that Rh$_{null}$ red cells carry only about one third of the normal amount of glycophorin B (437) led to the suggestion that in the absence of the Rh polypeptides, glycophorin B could not be properly incorporated into the red cell membrane. Hence the U antigen was regarded as requiring both glycophorin B and the Rh polypeptides for normal expression. More recently, studies (412,414) on a monoclonal antibody somewhat similar in specificity to the Duclos antibody (see below) have suggested (433) that the components missing (or altered) on Rh$_{null}$ red cells that are needed in addition to glycophorin B for expression of U, are the Rh glycoproteins (see Chapter 12). Blanchard and Dahr (433) suggest that the protease-resistant portion of glycophorin B is the portion of that structure that, with the Rh glycoproteins, constitutes the U antigen.

There is a close analogy with glycophorin A in this respect. Although the Wr^a/Wr^b polymorphism represents an amino acid difference on protein band 3 (402,404) the Wr^b antigen requires both band 3 and a portion of glycophorin A for expression (403). Further, the portion of glycophorin A required for expression of Wr^b and the portion of glycophorin B required for expression of U, are both resistant to protease treatment of red cells and both are situated close to the point at which the respective glycophorins enter the red cell membrane.

Since glycophorin B carries about 15% of the red cell's total sialic acid (17); many S- s- U- red cells lack glycophorin B; and S- s- U+^{var} red cells carry only 2 to 4% of the normal level of glycophorin B; it follows that in both phenotypes there is a reduction in red cell sialic acid level. McKeever et al. (405) took advantage of the known fact that the lectin of *Glycine soja* (soybean) agglutinates red cells with a lower than normal sialic acid level to screen random donors to try to identify those who were U- or U+^{var}. Although the soybean lectin does not have anti-U specificity (it also reacts, at least, with En(a-), T and Tn-activated, Cad+ and St(a+) red cells and with those of M^k and *En* heterozygotes and homozygotes, see below) it was hoped that it would prove useful in large scale screening tests. McKeever et al. (405) showed that all of 30 S- s- U- and 4 S- s- U+^{var} samples were consistently agglutinated by the soybean lectin. Thus large numbers of bloods could be tested with the lectin and among those agglutinated, some should be of the S- s- U- and S- s- U+^{var} phenotypes. Obviously, the soybean lectin is easier to obtain in quantity than is human serum containing anti-U. In spite of the promising results reported in the preliminary study, we are not aware of a large scale screening program that has used *Glycine soja* lectin to find U- and U+^{var} samples.

Glycophorin B and Monoclonal Antibodies

A monoclonal antibody with a specificity similar to anti-S has been described above. As far as we are aware, no example of a monoclonal antibody directed against the U antigen has been found. Three MAb with a specificity similar to but not identical with the Duclos antibody have been studied (412). The Duclos antibody was unusual in that it reacted with all except some examples of Rh$_{null}$ red cells (413). Those Rh$_{null}$ red cells on which the U antigen was reasonably well expressed reacted with the Duclos antibody, those that typed as U- (although they would adsorb and yield anti-U on elution) failed to react. One of the three MAb that were similar to the Duclos antibody, MB-2D10, has been further studied and has been shown to define a carbohydrate dependent epitope present on both the D-associated and the CE-associated Rh glycoproteins (414). The MB-2D10 and Duclos antibodies differ in that the Duclos red cells react with MB-2D10; and in that the MB-2D10-defined determinant, but not that defined by the Duclos antibody, is destroyed by chymotrypsin-treatment of red cells. Additional information about the Duclos antibody is given in Chapter 31.

In addition to the MAb described above, a number have been found (258,415-419) that react with determinants common to glycophorin A and glycophorin B. These antibodies define non-polymorphic regions of the glycophorins, that is to say they do not have anti-N specificity. Readers about to consult the above cited references should be warned that one of them (416), while discussing glycophorins A and B, makes the extraordinary statement that "These two sialoglycoproteins are closely linked on chromosome 4..." One hopes that the authors (and the reviewers and editor) meant that the encoding genes are closely linked. It would be hard to fit glycophorin A (MW circa 36kD) and glycophorin B (MW circa 20 - 24kD) on a chromosome!

Crossing-over Between the MN and Ss Loci

In the overwhelming majority of families in which inheritance of the *M N S* and *s* genes has been studied, it has been found that the gene at the *MN* locus and the gene at the *Ss* locus, on one chromosome, travel together. Thus, the haplotypes *MS Ms NS* and *Ns* have all been seen to exist and sufficient data are available on the transmission of each haplotype that there is no doubt that the *MN* and *Ss* loci are closely linked. In spite of this, well documented cases of crossing-over between the loci have been reported. Such events are usually recognized when, for example, an M+ N+ S+ s+ parent who has previously passed *MS* and *Ns* to his or her offspring, is seen to transmit *Ms* or *NS*. If other explanations, such as mistyping, non-parentage, etc., can be excluded, it follows that in separation of the chromosomes a portion of one that carries *M* has recombined with a portion of the other, that carries *s* and that another new alignment, *NS*, has been formed as the other half of the event. The first recorded cross-over between the *MN* and *Ss* loci was that of Chown et al. (420). Gedde-Dahl et al. (421) reported another and reviewed five additional cases of which they were aware (422-428). Race and Sanger (7) made the observation that crossing-over is the most likely explanation in the families involved. If the transmission of *M* and *S* and *M* and *s* from one parent with M+ N+ S+ s+ red cells represent mutation and not crossing-over, then children with M, N, S or s, born to two parents who lacked the encoding gene in question, would have been seen. The event has not been seen. Figure 15-1 is a diagrammatic representation of a cross-over between genes at the *MN* and *Ss* loci.

Unequal Crossing-Over or Gene Conversion Within the *MN* and *Ss* Loci

Although this topic is described in much more detail in the later sections of this chapter that deal with the biochemistry and molecular genetics of the MN system, a brief description is necessary here in order to make the sections on serology that follow, more intelligible. Once glycophorin A had been recognized as the red cell membrane glycoprotein that carries M, N, En[a] and related antigens, and glycophorin B as the carrier of ′N′, S, s, U and related antigens (12,14-16,42,44,429) it became possible to examine the membranes of red cells carrying other MN system antigens and variants for their glycophorin content and composition. In 1981, two glycophorins that seemed to be hybrids of glycophorin A and glycophorin B were recognized (287,288). Since that time a large number of other hybrid glycophorins have been found. In many instances composition of these hybrid proteins has been shown to explain the presence or absence of certain MN

FIGURE 15-1 Diagrammatic Representation of a Cross-over Between the *MN* and *Ss* Loci

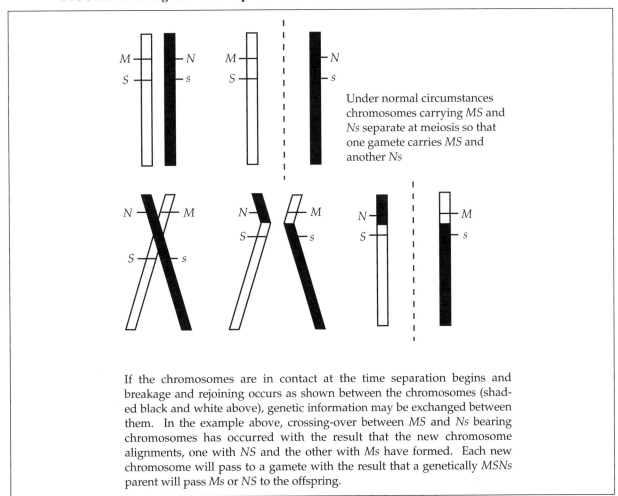

Under normal circumstances chromosomes carrying *MS* and *Ns* separate at meiosis so that one gamete carries *MS* and another *Ns*

If the chromosomes are in contact at the time separation begins and breakage and rejoining occurs as shown between the chromosomes (shaded black and white above), genetic information may be exchanged between them. In the example above, crossing-over between *MS* and *Ns* bearing chromosomes has occurred with the result that the new chromosome alignments, one with *NS* and the other with *Ms* have formed. Each new chromosome will pass to a gamete with the result that a genetically *MSNs* parent will pass *Ms* or *NS* to the offspring.

system antigens and/or abnormal characteristics of those antigens. As a single example, a hybrid glycophorin may carry trypsin-resistant M. This can occur on a hybrid protein that carries an M-bearing NH$_2$ terminal end encoded by a gene derived from part of a *glycophorin A* gene but on which the trypsin-sensitive site has been lost by replacement of another part of the *glycophorin A* gene by part of a *glycophorin B* gene.

When first encountered it seemed that these hybrid glycophorins represented the products of unequal crossing-over and of gene-fusion events (398). That is to say, at the time of meiosis, genes at the *MN* and *Ss* loci were misaligned. Following breakage of the chromosomes the repair mechanism caused gene fusion. However, instead of fusing say two broken parts of the same *M* gene, the misalignment resulted in fusion of part of an *M* gene with, say, part of an *s* gene. The resultant fused gene then comprised genetic material derived in part from *M* and in part from *s*. If functional, the fused gene would then encode a hybrid glycophorin carrying some material normally found on glycophorin A (*M* contribution) and some normally found on glycophorin B (*s* contribution). On some occasions this gene fusion event would result in a gamete carrying only the fused gene. On other occasions, because of the misalignment, a gamete would be produced carrying the reciprocal fused gene to that described above and one normal *glycophorin A* and one normal *glycophorin B* gene (i.e. the paired genes not involved in the original unequal cross-over and gene-fusion event). These events, that resemble the formation of Lepore and anti-Lepore hemoglobin genes (430), are described in more detail below.

More recently it has become appreciated (285,431-434) that some hybrid sialoglycoproteins are made following gene conversion. That is to say, during meiosis an exon from a *glycophorin A* gene replaces the equivalent exon of a *glycophorin B* gene, or vice versa. The complications provided by pseudo-exons and the *glycophorin E* gene are discussed later. An accepted terminology to describe hybrid glycophorins (and their encoding genes) has developed. A glycophorin A-B hybrid carries glycophorin A-derived material in its NH$_2$ terminal portion and glycophorin B-derived material in its C terminal portion. A glycophorin B-A hybrid, of course, carries glycophorin B and A-derived material in the opposite sequence. Not all glycophorin A-B hybrids are identical to each other, clearly they will differ dependent on the joining point of glycophorin A and B-derived material and the nature of the original genes contributing to the fusion. Obviously, the same applies to glycophorin B-A hybrids. Complex as the above situations may appear, they pale in comparison to some other findings. As described later, hybrid glycophorins with the sequences: A-B-A; B-A-B; and B-A-B-A, have all been found.

As mentioned above, presence of these hybrid glycophorins leads to some very interesting serological findings. Again, as examples: M and s (etc.) may be carried on the same glycophorin; the junction points of the glycophorin A and B (or B and A)-derived material represent new amino acid sequences and often antigens; on glycophorin A-B-A, B-A-B, and B-A-B-A hybrids there are multiple new arrangements that may represent antigens; changes in amino acid sequences from normal glycophorin A and B result in changes in glycosylation that may also affect antigen expression; loss or gain of an enzyme-sensitive site may reverse antigen characteristics from those normally seen.

MN System Antigens Beyond M, N, S, s and U

The next sections of this chapter comprise a series of descriptions of MN system antigens, antibodies and sometimes genes. As already explained, it is often impossible to write coherently about the antigens and genes without mentioning biochemical and/or molecular genetic aspects. It is hoped that the basic description of unequal crossing-over followed by gene fusion, and gene conversion, given in the previous section, will help to make some of the serological findings comprehensible. In many instances the antigens and genes described below are revisited in later sections of this chapter. Throughout the following sections the terms M SGP, N SGP, S SGP and s SGP will be used in addition to glycophorin A and glycophorin B. SGP is an abbreviation for sialoglycoprotein, glycophorins are sialoglycoproteins. Thus M SGP and N SGP are glycophorin A bearing M and N, respectively. Likewise S SGP and s SGP are glycophorin B bearing S and s respectively and, unless otherwise stated, both bearing 'N'.

In as far as possible, descriptions of these other MN system antigens will follow the sequence set out in table 15-1. Clearly some antigens will have to be advanced in the sequence when they have a close association with an antigen being described. Equally clear, any author would wish to delay writing about the Miltenberger-related antigens for as long as possible! Table 15-8 presents the most usual characteristics of MN system antibodies.

The M and N and The S and s Polymorphisms

Throughout the long (some will say long and tedious) introductory descriptions of M, N, S and s, and the antibodies that define them, care was taken to avoid mention of how those antigens differ from each other at the biochemical level. It was hoped that presentation of such information could be delayed until the full descrip-

TABLE 15-8 Characteristics of Some MN System Antibodies

Antibody Specificity	Positive Reactions in In Vitro Tests				Usual Immunoglobulin		Ability to Bind Complement		Ability to Cause In Vitro Lysis		Implicated in		Usual Form of Stimulation		% of White Population Positive
	Sal	LISS	AHG	Enz	IgG	IgM	Yes	No	Yes	No	Transfusion Reaction	HDN	Red Cells	Other	
Anti-M	X	X	Few	No	Some	Some	Very Rare	Most	Very Rare	Most	Rare	Rare	Few	Most	78
Anti-N	X	X	Few	No	Some	Some		Most		X	Poss.	Rare	Rare	Most	72
Anti-S	Some		Some	No	Some	Some	Few	Most		X	Yes	Yes	Some	Some	55
Anti-s	Rare		X		Most	Few	Few	Most		X	Yes	Yes	Most	Rare	89
Anti-U			X	Most	Most					X	Yes	Yes	Most		100
Anti-En^a			X	Some	Most					X	Prob		Most		100
Anti-M$_1$	Some	Some	Some	No	Scme	Some				X	No	No	Few	Most	5
Antibodies related to Anti-Mi^a	Some		Some		Some	Some				X	Some	Yes	Some	Some	
Most abs to rare antigens	Some	Some	Some	Some	Some	Most		Most		X		Some		Most	
Anti-N made by N- 'N'- persons	X	X	X		X					X		Yes			100

tion of the biochemistry of the system. However, since some of the other antigens about to be discussed differ from M and N, or from S and s, in terms of amino acid sequence and/or glycosylation of glycophorins A and B, the revelations can be withheld no longer! Figure 15-2 depicts the NH$_2$ terminal ends of glycophorin A when M or N is present. Figure 15-3 depicts the tetrasaccharide that is the most common carbohydrate-containing side chain attached to glycophorin A (circa 15 copies per glycophorin) and glycophorin B (circa 11 copies per glycophorin). Figure 15-4 depicts a portion of glycophorin B to illustrate the identity of 'N' with glycophorin A-borne N and lack of identity with M (both shown). Figure 15-5 depicts the amino acid difference that represents the polymorphism of S and s on glycophorin B. In addition to the methionine at position 29 in S-bearing glycophorin B and the threonine at that position in s-bearing glycophorin B, the carbohydrate side chain attached to threonine at position 25 and the glutamic acid at position 28, histidine at position 34 and arginine at position 35, all contribute to the structural integrity of S and s (321,436). As stated, these basic biochemical descriptions are provided here so that some variant antigens can be coherently described. The real biochemical explanations, particularly those involving complex hybrid glycophorins will be found later in this chapter.

The Antigen Hu

This was the third MN system antigen to be discovered (54) and was found with an antibody made in a rabbit immunized with human red cells. In tests using the first example of anti-Hu, the antigen was found on the red cells of approximately 7% of US Blacks and 23% of West Africans (438). In our study (77) on Tm and Sj, we used a different example of anti-Hu, made by immunizing rabbits with the red cells of Mr. Hunter, the same donor (54) whose cells had been used raise the first example of the antibody. We found 36 Hu+ samples in testing the red cells of 500 random New York Black donors, again an incidence of around 7%. In the same study (77), we found that five of 500 random White donors had Hu+ red cells. It is strange that the only examples of anti-Hu ever made have been produced following injections of the red cells of one donor, the original Mr. Hunter.

In the initial studies (54) all Hu+ red cells were

FIGURE 15-2 To Illustrate the Amino Acid Sequence at the NH₂ Terminal End of Glycophorin A when Produced under Control of an *M* (left) and *N* (right) Gene

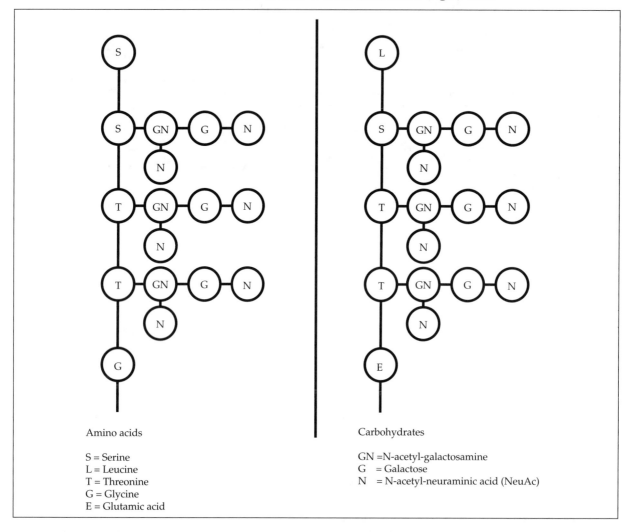

Amino acids

S = Serine
L = Leucine
T = Threonine
G = Glycine
E = Glutamic acid

Carbohydrates

GN = N-acetyl-galactosamine
G = Galactose
N = N-acetyl-neuraminic acid (NeuAc)

found among bloods of the phenotypes M- N+ and M+ N+. Although we (77) found one example of N- Hu+ red cells, all the others that were Hu+ (35 samples) were also N+. We pointed out that although the incidence of Tm was 31.4% in random Black donors, 19 of the 36 Hu+ samples were also Tm+, an incidence of 52.7%. Now that Tm is known (71) to be carried on the polypeptide portion of the N SGP and it is believed that those N+ samples that react with anti-Tm before they have been treated with neuraminidase, carry N in a different to usual steric arrangement, it is perhaps less surprising that the phenotype N+ Hu+ Tm+ is fairly common. Indeed, as discussed in later sections, it is possible that the antigens Hu, Tm, Shier and Sext (see below for the relationships of Shier and Sext to Hu) all represent different to usual glycosylation of N-bearing glycophorin A.

The Antigen He

Like Hu, He was initially identified (55) with a rabbit serum. The first example of the antibody was present in a serum containing anti-M, a second example was made (438) by deliberate immunization of rabbits with the red cells of Mr. Henshaw. Since that time, at least two human (7,439) and a number of monoclonal (286) anti-He have been described.

Several large scale screening studies have included tests with anti-He. In US Blacks, the incidence of the He+ phenotype has been reported (440) as 3.2% in 1000 samples tested (*He* traveling predominantly with *NS*), as 3.08% in 4510 samples tested (336) and as 2.0% in 500 samples tested (77) (*He* found in random distribution with regards to *M*, *N*, *S* and *s*). In Papua, He was seen (441) to travel predominantly with *Ns*; in Congo Blacks

FIGURE 15-3 To Show the Structures of O-linked Glycans found on Glycophorins A and B

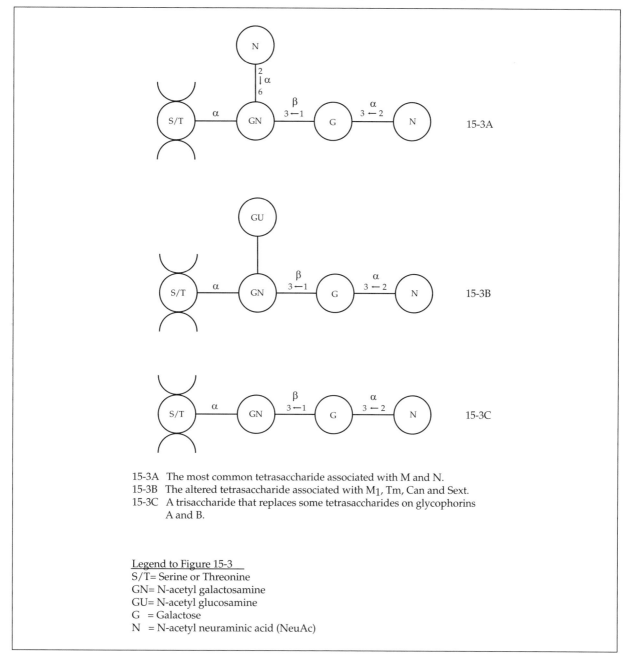

15-3A   The most common tetrasaccharide associated with M and N.
15-3B   The altered tetrasaccharide associated with M₁, Tm, Can and Sext.
15-3C   A trisaccharide that replaces some tetrasaccharides on glycophorins
           A and B.

Legend to Figure 15-3
S/T= Serine or Threonine
GN= N-acetyl galactosamine
GU= N-acetyl glucosamine
G = Galactose
N = N-acetyl neuraminic acid (NeuAc)

(441) and Hottentots (442) with *MS*; and in Cape Coloreds (443) with *Ms*. In studying seven large families, Shapiro (443) found *He* to travel with *MS*, *Ms* or *Ns*, but within any one family linkage between the *MNSs* haplotype and *He* was absolute. Although we (77) found only ten examples of He+ red cells in our study on Tm and Sj, the association seen between Hu and Tm was not seen between He and Tm. Three of the ten He+ bloods also carried Tm for an incidence of 30%, that is the same as the 31.4% incidence of Tm among random Black donors. Rosenfield et al. (444) found one example of a blood that carried He and Hu and had some evidence that the same *MNSs* haplotype might be making both antigens. We (77) found two further samples that typed as He+ Hu+ but did not perform the tests necessary to determine whether the *He* and *Hu* genes were on the same or different chromosomes.

In tests on the red cells of Pygmy Bush Negroes of Surinam, Nijenhuis and Wertel (445) found that 32 of 428 (7.5%) were He+. Of these samples, one had a markedly weak expression of He (as had some other samples found earlier in this population) but no qualita-

FIGURE 15-4 To Demonstrate the Identity Between N on Glycophorin A and 'N' on Glycophorin B

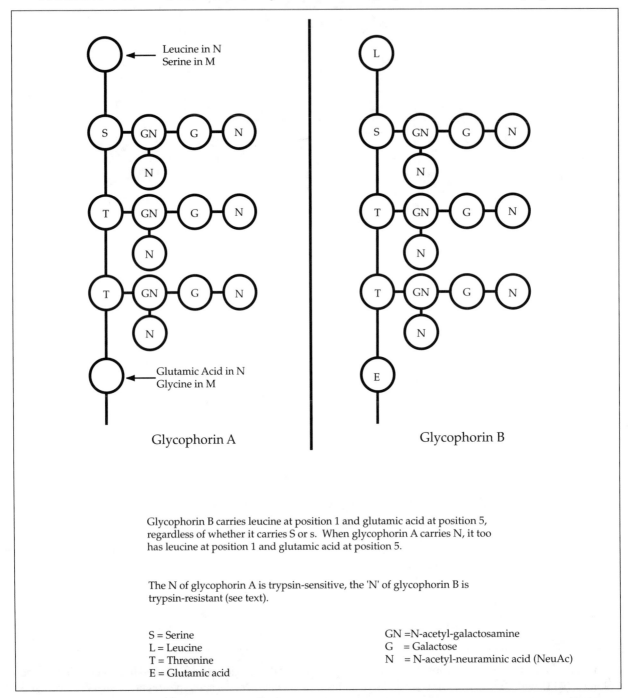

Glycophorin B carries leucine at position 1 and glutamic acid at position 5, regardless of whether it carries S or s. When glycophorin A carries N, it too has leucine at position 1 and glutamic acid at position 5.

The N of glycophorin A is trypsin-sensitive, the 'N' of glycophorin B is trypsin-resistant (see text).

S = Serine
L = Leucine
T = Threonine
E = Glutamic acid

GN = N-acetyl-galactosamine
G = Galactose
N = N-acetyl-neuraminic acid (NeuAc)

tive difference between the weakened expression of the antigen and normal He antigen, was found. In studies using human, rabbit and monoclonal anti-He, Reid et al. (286) confirmed this observation. Just as seen in the earlier studies mentioned in the paper of Nijenhuis and Wertel (445), Reid et al. (286) found that He is expressed at two levels, called weak and strong, for convenience. Among 39 He+ S+ samples (11 S+ s-, 28 S+ s+), 37 had a strong expression and two a weak expression of He. Among 10 He+ S- s+ samples, 3 had strong and 7 weak expression of He. Variation in strength of the reaction was seen a little more easily with the human and rabbit anti-He than with the MAbs. The original report should be consulted for results on exceptional samples such as those that were: S+^{w}; from *Su* and *su* heterozygotes; or were St(a+). Although less frequent than in Blacks, the

FIGURE 15-5 To Show the Positions of 'N', S and s on Glycophorin B

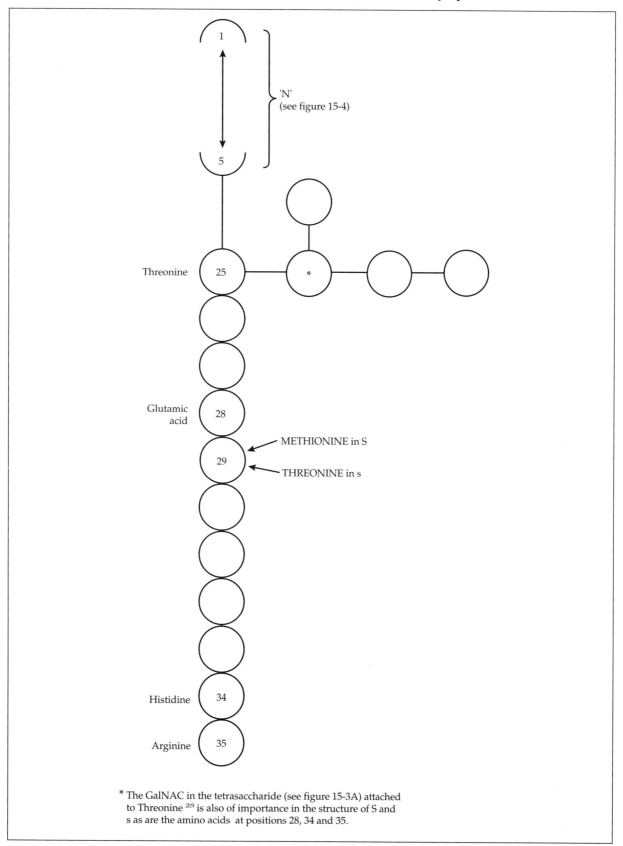

* The GalNAC in the tetrasaccharide (see figure 15-3A) attached
  to Threonine ²⁵ is also of importance in the structure of S and
  s as are the amino acids at positions 28, 34 and 35.

He antigen was found on the red cells of four of 500 (0.8%) random White donors in New York (77).

In 1976, in considering the haplotypes that encode production of He, Mourant et al. (446) wrote that "these considerations...suggest that the *Henshaw* locus is much nearer to that for *Ss* than to that for *MN*". As described below, this prophesy was correct for it has now been shown that *He* can be an allele at the *Ss* locus. In 1983, Judd et al. (147) studied a patient who was genetically *MsHe/Mu*. The fact that the patient's red cells lacked 'N' led the investigators to suppose that He had replaced 'N' on the glycophorin B encoded by her *MsHe* haplotype (her other haplotype made no glycophorin B). In the subsequent investigation, Dahr et al. (284) showed that the glycophorin encoded by the *MsHe* haplotype is in fact more like a hybrid SGP than like glycophorin B. The haplotype encoding s and He makes a glycophorin with tryptophan at position one, serine at position four and glycine at positive five. As shown in figure 15-4 the amino acids at those positions in normal glycophorin B are leucine, threonine and glutamic acid respectively. Huang et al. (285) have suggested that the encoding gene was originally a *glycophorin B* gene that was converted by the insertion of part of an exon from a *glycophorin A* gene. Additional events that apparently give rise to the formation of other haplotypes that encode production of a glycophorin that carries He (345,447) are discussed in the section on the biochemistry of the MN system.

The above observations were mostly made before it became appreciated that He is often present on S- s- red cells (286,343,370). In studying such red cells, Reid et al. (755) expanded the classification to include an intermediate expression of He (He+^{mod} for moderately strong) between He+^{s} and He+^{w}. It was found that the He+^{s} phenotype was seen only when S or s was expressed. All S- s- U- and S- s- U+^{var} red cells studied, that had He present, were of the He+^{mod} or He+^{w} phenotype. The presence of He on S- s- (U- or U+^{var}) red cells as it relates to the presence of some form of glycophorin B, or a related glycophorin on such red cells, was discussed above (section on U) in terms of serology and is revisited below in terms of biochemistry and molecular genetics of the MN system. It can be added that Reid et al. (755) and Reid (756) have found that some 90% of bloods that type as S- s- but carry some expression of U, are He+.

The Phenotype M^c

In this phenotype, the antigen that is present reacts with most anti-M and a few anti-N (57). There is no specific anti-M^c and the presence of M^c has to be deduced from tests with anti-M and anti-N known to react, or not

to react, with M^c bloods. Metaxas et al. (78) found that the presence of M^c was often associated with the presence of M$_1$ (see below). However, M^c and M$_1$ did not seem to be same thing for M$_1$N cells were found that reacted well with anti-M known not to react with M^c cells. Further, when Giles and Howell (448) found an anti-M$_1$ that lacked anti-M, they noted that it did not react with M^c cells. They suggested that the findings that showed that all (or almost all) M^c cells are M$_1$+, occurred because the anti-M$_1$ sera used contained anti-M (a known fact) and that the anti-M were of the type that react with M^c cells. The gene encoding the M^c phenotype has been found in alignment with *S* and *s* (57,78).

In 1981, Dahr et al. (449) and Furthmayr et al. (450) independently and apparently simultaneously, defined the biochemical structure involved in the M^c phenotype. The M^c SGP is intermediate between the M and N SGPs. Like M SGP it has serine at position one, like N SGP is has glutamic acid at position five. These findings correlate exactly with the serological characteristics of M^c as described above. M^c+ cells react with most but not all examples of anti-M and with a few but not many examples of anti-N. It is now clear that the reactive anti-M require serine at position one, the non-reactive examples require glycine at position five but in M^c that residue is glutamic acid. The minority of anti-N that react require glutamic acid at position five, the majority that do not react, need leucine at position one but in M^c that residue is serine. As Dahr et al. (449) pointed out, M^c can thus be thought of as an evolutionary step between M and N, or if one works out from the red cell membrane to the NH$_2$ terminus of the M^c SGP, between N and M. The requirements of human and rabbit anti-M for serine at position one or glycine at position five and those of human and rabbit anti-N for leucine at position one or glutamic acid at position five have been seen in monoclonal anti-M and anti-N (227,263,265,272,451). Some details about M^c are repeated in table 15-9.

The Antigen M^g

In 1958, Allen et al. (59) described M^g+ red cells and anti-M^g. M^g is perhaps the rarest blood antigen known, no M^g+ sample was found among some 144,000 donors tested (452-457). However, Metaxas et al. (458) found ten M^g+ samples in tests on 6,530 donors in Switzerland and Brocteur (459), while testing samples from approximately 6,300 Italian immigrants in Belgium, some 1,889 of whom were of Sicilian extraction, found that one non-Sicilian and three of Sicilian extraction, had M^g+ red cells. In tests on more than 9000 persons in Bombay (46) two more M^g+ samples were found.

In the original US family (59), in another US family

TABLE 15-9 Structures of Some Antigens on Glycophorin A

Amino Acid Present at Position (from NH$_2$ Terminus)	Antigens						
	M	N	M^g	M^c	M$_1$	Tm	Can
One	Serine	Leucine	Leucine	Serine	Serine	Leucine	Serine
Two	Serine*	Serine*	Serine°	Serine*	Serine**	Serine**	Serine**
Three	Threonine*	Threonine*	Threonine°	Threonine*	Threonine**	Threonine**	Threonine**
Four	Threonine*	Threonine*	Asparagine°°	Threonine*	Threonine**	Threonine**	Threonine**
Five	Glycine	Glutamic Acid	Glutamic Acid	Glutamic Acid	Glycine	Glutamic Acid	Glycine

*   Glycosylated residue
**   Probable glycosylation change, see text
°   Residue usually not glycosylated
°°   Residue never glycosylated

described later (462), in the Swiss families (458) and in the family from Italy (459) the alignment was *M^{g}s*. In the families of Sicilian extraction (459), it was *M^{g}S*. No abnormality of expression of S or s was noticed when *M^g* was present. In spite of the extreme rarity of *M^g*, one *M^{g}M^g* homozygote has been found (461).

The M^g antigen does not react with human or rabbit anti-M or anti-N. Thus the unrecognized presence of *M^g* and M^g can suggest an apparent, but actually false indirect exclusion of parentage, e.g. *MM^g* (appearing as M+ N-) x *NN* can produce an *M^{g}N* child, (appearing as M- N+). If the presence of the M^g antigen is recognized the apparent M+ N- parent can be seen to be M+ N- M^g+ and the apparent M- N+ child to be M- N+ M^g+. Because of the extreme rarity of *M^g* the case goes from an apparent indirect exclusion, to one in which parentage is virtually proved (but check to see if the brother is also M^g+)! Unlike human and rabbit anti-M, some monoclonal anti-M react with M- N+ M^g+ and M- N- M^g+ red cells (227,260,263,265,475). The critical residues involved in the positive reactions seem to be valine at position six and methionine at position eight, from the NH$_2$ terminus, when glycosylation is markedly reduced, as in M^g+ red cells. The same antibodies also require glycine at position five, to behave as anti-M when the M SGP is normally glycosylated, i.e. M+ N- M^g - and M+ N+ M^g - (476).

M^g encodes production of an antigen, M^g , that is recognized by a specific antibody, anti-M^g. Although the M^g antigen is exceedingly rare, anti-M^g is a common antibody. In studies performed in the USA, England and India (7,59,460,463) the published incidence was 45 examples of anti-M^g among 3157 sera tested, i.e. an incidence of 1 in 70 sera. The experience of one of us (PDI) is that if sensitive methods are used, anti-M^g can be seen to be twice as common as that. In Liberia 80 of 454 sera (i.e. more than

1 in 6) were found to contain anti-M^g, it was suggested (463) that the high incidence of the antibody might be associated with the high incidence of parasitic infections. Anti-M^g can also be made in rabbits (464). Dahr et al. (465,466) have suggested that the common occurrence of anti-M^g in human sera might be related to the clearance of normal red cells at the end of their in vivo lifespan. It is supposed that deglycosylation of normal glycophorin A might result in exposure of an M^g-like structure that is recognized as foreign by the immune system. As described below, the M^g SGP differs from M and N SGP by lacking or having reduced numbers of carbohydrate side chains.

In 1969, Nordling et al. (467) reported that M^g+ red cells have a reduced level of sialic acid when compared to M+ or N+ M^g- cells. Based on other studies of sialic acid levels and eletrophoretic mobility of M^g+ cells (468-470) and on the finding (470) that the terminal amino acid of the M^g SGP is leucine, Anstee et al. (471) forecast that the cells should lack three copies of the MN SGP-borne tetrasaccharides. When Dahr et al. (465) showed that the fourth residue of the M^g SGP is asparagine and not threonine, as in the N SGP of which the M^g SGP is a variant, they also showed that the second, third and fourth residues of the M^g SGP are either not glycosylated (see table 15-9) or that only a few copies (circa 25%) of those residues carry tetrasaccharide side chains. Further, these workers (474) found that 30% of the M^g SGP molecules lack the NH$_2$ terminal leucine residue and that some 10% also lack the serine residue that normally occupies the second position from the NH$_2$ terminus. Lack of the residues was thought (474) to represent a posttranslation change effected by amino peptidase. The findings of Dahr et al. (465) about lack of glycosylation of the M^g SGP have been duplicated by others (450,472). It seems (465,473) that *M^g* arose as a point mutation of *N* and in the encoded product, asparagine replaces threonine at position four from the NH_2 terminus. Asparagine at that position seems to prevent, or only allow 10% of the normal amount of glycosylation of the residues at positions two and three. Perhaps steric rearrangement due to the presence of asparagine at position four renders the other amino acids less accessible to the transferases that effect glycosylation. As would be expected from lack or reduced number of tetrasaccharides (see figure 15-3) attached to M^g SGP, anti-M^g does not usually require the presence of red cell-borne neuraminic acid to react with its antigen. Judd et al. (251) tested six examples of anti-M^g and found that five of them reacted to the same degree with untreated and with neuraminidase-treated red cells. The sixth example was non-reactive with the neuramindase-treated red cells and Dahr (322) later suggested that the antibody might be defining an epitope dependent on the glycosylation of some 25% of the copies of M^g SGP (see above).

A Variant Form of Mg

Dahr et al. (477) described a red cell sample that reacted with two of six examples of anti-M^g (no results regarding adsorption studies were given). The amino acid sequence at the NH_2 terminus was the same as in other M^g+ samples but in the variant some 75% of the copies M^g SGP were glycosylated. The authors suggested that the increase in glycosylation over other M^g+ samples might represent the presence of an altered glycosyl transferase, production of which was not encoded from the *MN* locus.

The Antigen Vr

In 1958, Hart et al. (60) described a new antibody, anti-Vr, that defines a rare MN system antigen. Two additional examples of the antibody were found in sera containing anti-S (one of which also contained anti-Vw and anti-M^g). No example of anti-Vr was found in tests on 202 sera from normal donors. Of 1200 random donors in the Netherlands, three had Vr+ red cells. In 1993, Poole et al. (478) described a family, believed to have some Dutch ancestry, in which *Vr* was traveling, as in the three original families (60), with *Ms*. Anti-Vr was again found (478) in a serum containing anti-S, this time the serum also contained anti-Mit (see below). Preliminary studies suggested (478) that Vr is carried on glycophorin A.

The Phenotype M₁+

Jack et al. (61) described the first example of anti-

M_1 that appears to detect a form of super M. However, the difference between M_1 and M is apparently not all quantitative for M+ N- M_1- and M+ N+ M_1+ cells were found. Had anti-M_1 simply detected a high level of M, non-reactive cells with a double dose of M and reactive cells with a single dose of that antigen would not have been expected. It was calculated (61,77,283,319,479, 480) that about 4% of Whites and 24% of American Blacks have M_1+ red cells. The Bantus of South Africa had an M_1 antigen incidence of 47% (481) and we (482,483) pointed out that unless care is taken in the serological tests, all M+ U- red cells appear to be M_1+. Early studies on anti-M_1 were performed with antibodies made by persons with M- N+ red cells, that were invariably mixtures of anti- M_1 and anti-M. Giles and Howell (448) found an anti-M_1 made a person with M+ red cells. The antibody lacked an anti-M component and from their study these workers (448) estimated that about 0.5% of Whites and 16.4% of Blacks have M_1+ red cells. When Molthan (484) described another example of anti-M_1 that lacked anti-M, she reported almost identical frequency figures to those of Giles and Howell (448). It is still possible that the later examples of anti- M_1 failed to detect all M_1+ samples for M_1 is very much a graded character (61) and some of the earlier discovered anti-M_1 seemed more potent than the later found examples.

There now seems little doubt that M_1 represents M SGP with different than usual glycosylation (see table 15-9). Dahr et al. (485) have shown that in some blood samples, the usual tetrasaccharide shown in figure 15-3, is replaced in variable numbers and at variable sites by one in which N-acetyl-glucosamine replaces the N-acetyl neuraminic acid residue normally attached to N-acetyl-galactosamine. Further, some of the copies of the usual tetrasaccharide are incompletely formed as trisaccharides or even disaccharides (485-487). When this occurs, antigens such as M_1 (or Tm, Can, Sext, etc., see below) are formed. Such antigens might represent different steric presentation of the polypeptide backbone of glycophorin A or epitopes of which the different carbohydrates are a part. The great variation in strength of M_1 on different M_1+ samples (61,77,448,484) might well be associated with the attachment site of the N-acetyl-glucosamine-containing tetrasaccharide, i.e. bound to glycophorin A at position two and/or three and/or four.

It is because antigens such as M_1, Tm, Can, Sext, etc., represent unusual glycosylation of SGPs bearing recognized MN system antigens, and because the transferase enzymes responsible for the atypical, and for that matter the typical glycosylation of the glycophorins are presumably not located at the *MN* locus, that these antigens do not have ISBT terms. However, in the admittedly limited number of family studies that have been performed, M_1, Tm, Can, Sext, etc., seem to have been inherited in a normal manner. This suggests, of course, that the genes that encode production of the transferases may be closely linked to the *MN* locus.

The Antigen Mᵉ

In 1961, Wiener and Rosenfield (63) tested an antibody made in a rabbit and found that it agglutinated all samples that were M+ and those M- N+ cells that carried the low incidence antigen He. The apparent anti-M and anti-He in the rabbit serum could not be separated by differential adsorption. The authors concluded that Mᵉ is made by all *M* genes and by the *N* gene that makes He (the *NHe* haplotype). In 1981, McDougall and Jenkins (488) described the first example of human anti-Mᵉ that, like the rabbit antibody, did not contain separable anti-M or anti-He. Since then, Levene et al. (489) have shown that the presence of anti-Mᵉ in anti-M is not that uncommon and have found that some human sera contain separable anti-M and anti-Mᵉ. Zelinkski et al. (492) reported that five of nine monoclonal anti-M reacted with M- He+ red cells.

When biochemical studies were performed (147,284,490,491) it was shown why Mᵉ is present whenever *M* or *He*, the latter of which is an allele of *S* and *s*, encodes a product. The amino acid at position five in glycophorin A encoded by *M* is glycine. The He-bearing form of Ss SGP has tryptophan at position one (see earlier section on the antigen He) and glycine at position five. Thus anti-Mᵉ reacts with red cells that carry an SGP with glycine at position five (see table 15-10). Those monoclonal anti-M that react with M- He+ red cells, recognize glycine at position five. These findings also explain the serological observation (489) that the reaction of anti-Mᵉ with M+ He- red cells is abolished when red cells are treated with trypsin (determinant carried within the trypsin-sensitive portion of glycophorin A) but that the reaction with He+ red cells survives such treatment (determinant carried on trypsin-resistant glycophorin B).

The serological study of Mᵉ and its original description (63) provide another outstanding example of the value of careful serological work and accurate reporting of the results. When Wiener and Rosenfield (63) described a single specificity antibody (i.e. not separable anti-M and anti-He) that reacted with all M+ red cells and those M- samples that were He+, there was no explanation of the serological conundrum. The presence of glycine at position five of M SGP and position five of the He (Ss) SGP, explains exactly the accurate results originally reported.

The Antigen Mtᵃ

In 1962, Swanson and Matson (64) described anti-Mtᵃ, an antibody defining a rare MN system antigen. No further example of anti-Mtᵃ was found in tests on 3500 sera from normal donors although the Guppy serum, that contains (at least) antibodies to V, Mᵍ, Swᵃ, Wrᵃ, By, Trᵃ, Bpᵃ and Ptᵃ and the Murrell serum, that contains (at least) antibodies to Mur, Miᵃ, Swᵃ, Cˣ and Wrᵃ both reacted with Mt(a+) red cells (493). The *Mtᵃ* gene was shown to travel with *Ns* in the original family. In 1963, Konugres et al. (494) succeeded in making anti-Mtᵃ in rabbits and in 1965 the results of population studies with the reagents were reported (495). Red cells from 12,914 Bostonians were tested and 29 of them were Mt(a+). Twenty-eight of the Mt(a+) bloods were among 11,625 samples from Whites, for an incidence of the Mt(a+) phenotype of 0.24%. Of 1007 samples from random Blacks only one was Mt(a+). None of the samples from 282 Orientals was Mt(a+), nor was the antigen found in any of 132 people belonging to 31 Samaritan families,

TABLE 15-10 Structures of Some Antigens on Glycophorin B

Amino Acid Present at Position (from NH₂ Terminus)	'N' and S	'N' and s	He and Mᵉ
One	Leucine	Leucine	Tryptophan
Two	Serine*	Serine*	Serine*
Three	Threonine*	Threonine*	Threonine*
Four	Threonine*	Threonine*	Serine*
Five	Glutamic Acid	Glutamic Acid	Glycine†
Twenty-nine	Methionine	Threonine	

* Glycosylated residue
† The amino acid at position five of M SGP is also glycine (see text re the Mᵉ antigen)

whose bloods were tested in Israel. Konugres et al. (495) found that in two informative families, Mt^a traveled with Ns and further, that all 29 Mt(a+) samples were N+ s+. Similarly, when Chandanayingyong et al. (456) found three of 318 samples from Thai blood donors to be Mt(a+), they studied one of the donor's families and found Mt^a to travel with Ns. Thus although some other rare genes in the MN system that encode production of antigens of low incidence have been seen to be part of different *MNSs* haplotypes in different families, it is possible that all Mt(a+) bloods found thus far, represent presence of the haplotype $NsMt^a$ (or NMt^as).

In 1972, Field et al. (496) described a case of HDN caused by anti-Mt^a that was severe enough that the infant required exchange transfusion with two units of blood. It has been reported (496,497) that Mt^a survives the treatment of red cells with trypsin but is denatured or removed when red cells are treated with papain or ficin. While this was taken (497) to indicate that Mt^a might be on glycophorin B rather than glycophorin A, considerable caution in such an interpretation is necessary. First, a trypsin-resistant, papain/ficin-sensitive antigen might be carried on normal glycophorin A at a point closer to the membrane than the trypsin-sensitive site but distal to the papain/ficin-sensitive site. Second an antigen with the enzyme sensitivity described might be carried on glycophorin A-derived material on a hybrid SGP that had lost its trypsin but retained its papain/ficin-sensitive site. In view of the serological findings with Mt^a, the first suggestion seems more likely than the latter. Because anti-Hu had been made only in rabbits immunized with red cells from the original Mr. Hunter, Konugres et al. (494,495) injected Mt(a+) red cells from two donors unrelated to the original Martin family, into rabbits. Both cell samples stimulated the production of anti-Mt^a.

The Antigens St^a and ERIK and the Genes M^z and M^r

In 1968, Metaxas et al. (78) described red cell samples that showed disturbances in the amounts of M and/or N that they carried. It was postulated that variant genes at the *MN* locus were involved. One gene was named M^z (498) and was said to produce an antigen that reacted with most anti-M and a few anti-N. Further, the red cells of persons with M^z were said to react with anti-M´ (see below) but not with anti-M$_1$. The second gene was named M^r (498) and was said to be similar in action to M^z except that the red cells of persons with M^r did not react with anti-M´ or anti-M$_1$. It is now known that persons who inherit either of the genes that were called M^z and M^r have red cells that are St(a+). Further, there are a number of different glycophorins, arising by a variety of

different mechanisms, that carry St^a.

In 1962, Cleghorn (65) described the rare MN system antigen, St^a. A total of 20 St(a+) samples (two of which were from related individuals) were found in tests on the blood of 17,013 English donors. The St^a antigen has a higher incidence in Oriental persons that in other populations. Madden et al. (499) found the antigen on the red cells of 14 of 220 Japanese and six of 420 Chinese, other examples in the Chinese have been reported (500) (and see below). No St(a+) blood was found in tests on samples from 386 Mexicans (499). Metaxas and Metaxas-Bühler (498) screened samples from 6202 Swiss donors using Rh antibodies that normally react only by IAT. Those red cells that were agglutinated in a saline system (in this instance a feature associated with a reduced level of red cell sialic acid) were selected for further study. Among 248 samples thus selected, six proved to be St(a+), with two of them being from related individuals. Vengelen-Tyler and Mogck (501) showed that all of eight ficin-treated St(a+) and four ficin-treated Dantu+ samples reacted strongly with *Vicia graminea* lectin. It was already known that both St(a+) (502) and Dantu+ (47) red cells carry hybrid B-A glycophorins. Ficin-treated red cells from 300 Oriental and 100 Black donors were then tested with *Vicia graminea*. Eight of the 300 Orientals but none of the 100 Blacks, were found to have St(a+) red cells, no Dantu+ was found in either group of donors.

The first example of anti-St^a was found (65) in a serum that contained separable antibodies to Wr^a, Sw^a and Ri^a. Other examples have subsequently been found (499) but the antibody is not common.

Anti-ERIK was first found (105) in the serum of a Danish woman whose husband has St(a+) ERIK+ red cells. The antibody caused a positive DAT in an infant born to the couple. Anti-ERIK was also present in two sera known to contain multiple antibodies to low incidence antigens. Four propositi with ERIK+ red cells were identified. In addition to the Danish family, the ERIK+ phenotype was found in: an Australian of Norwegian and English descent; a blood donor of Italian origin; and a woman of mixed ethnic background living in South Africa. All ERIK+ propositi and their ERIK+ relatives had St(a+) red cells, other tests on known St(a+) samples revealed 13 that were St(a+) ERIK-. Over 200 St(a-) samples were ERIK-.

As mentioned at the beginning of this section, it is now known that the St^a antigen is present on a number of variant glycophorins whose production is encoded by a series of genes that arose by different mechanisms. These glycophorins include: GP.Sch (502,503) (associated with the gene previously called M^r); GP.Zan (504,505) (associated with the gene previously called M^z); GP.EBH (105,506) (associated with perhaps more than one St(a+)

ERIK+ phenotype); and a hybrid B-A-B-A glycophorin that expresses St[a] and He (285). In view of the complexities, these glycophorins and the genes that encode them, are discussed in more detail later in this chapter, when the more complex biochemistry of the MN system is discussed. That section explains exactly the actions of M^r and M^z, actions that cannot easily be understood from the results of serological studies.

The Antigen Ri[a]

The first example of anti-Ri[a] was found by Cleghorn (65) in a serum that also contained antibodies to St[a], Wr[a] and Sw[a]. The four antibodies could be separated by appropriate adsorption. The original Ri(a+) propositus is unique. Other than members of his immediate family, no other Ri(a+) sample has been found. Cleghorn (65) tested 17,013 random samples, including 830 cord bloods in South London; Contreras et al. (507) tested 53,488 random donor samples and 1650 from Black and Indian prenatal patients in North London; as stated, no Ri(a+) sample was found. In the original study (65,508) no additional example of anti-Ri[a] was found in tests on some 100 sera. In the later study (507) one example of anti-Ri[a] was found in tests on the sera of 42,886 routine blood donors. The antibody was made by a woman with no history of pregnancy or transfusion. No anti-Ri[a] was detected in the sera of three Ri(a-) women from the original family, who among them had borne a total of five children with Ri(a+) red cells. Separable anti-Ri[a] was found (507) in 12 sera known to contain antibodies to other low incidence antigens, including the famous sera Tillett and Wilcox that contain, at least, 24 and 16 separable antibodies, respectively. While studying the 13 examples of anti-Ri[a] available to them (i.e., the one they had found in a donor and the 12 in the sera with multiple antibodies to low incidence antigens) Contreras et al. (507) found that 12 of them were IgM in nature; in the Wilcox serum the antibody was a mixture of IgM and IgG. However, in seven of the 13 sera the anti-Ri[a] was reactive by IAT and was detectable via the C3-anti-C3 reaction.

In addition to its extreme rarity, Ri[a] has a number of other unusual features for an MN system antigen. First, it is denatured or removed when red cells are treated with trypsin but survives the treatment of red cells with papain, pronase or chymotrypsin. The apparent reaction between anti-Ri[a] and trypsin-treated Ri(a+) red cells, when three examples of anti-Ri[a] were used, was explained when it was shown (507) that those sera also contained anti-S reacting only with trypsin-treated red cells. Anti-Ri[a] is also sometimes present in sera containing anti-S that react with untreated red cells. Indeed any time that anti-Ri[a] or, more frequently anti-S is used, it must be remembered that both antibodies are often present in the same serum. Second, as described, anti-Ri[a] are often IgM, complement binding antibodies, a rare feature of MN system antibodies.

In spite of the unusual enzyme sensitivity pattern of Ri[a], no glycophorin abnormalities were seen when the membranes of Ri(a+) red cells were studied by SDS-PAGE (509). While some of the features described above might appear to suggest doubt that Ri[a] is an MN system antigen, the family of the original propositus (65) contains 27 children in whom Ri^a appears to be part of the MS haplotype with a recombinant:non-recombinant score of 0:27.

The Antigen Cl[a]

In 1963, Wallace and Izatt (66) found the first example of anti-Cl[a] when an anti-B typing serum that they were using agglutinated a red cell sample that did not have B. Twenty-four other examples of anti-Cl[a] were found in tests on the sera of 5326 random British donors. In the two families studied, see below, no anti-Cl[a] was detected in the sera of five Cl(a-) women who had borne children with Cl(a+) red cells. In the two Scottish families studied, one of which was of Irish extraction, Cl^a traveled with Ms for an apparent $MsCl^a$ or a MCl^as haplotype. The Cl[a] antigen was denatured or removed when red cells were treated with trypsin or papain. No further Cl(a+) sample was found in tests on the red cells of 11,000 Scottish (66) and 1541 Swiss donors (510).

The Antigen Ny[a]

In 1964, Ørjasaeter et al. (67) described the first example of anti-Ny[a]. In tests on the sera of 3693 Norwegian donors, four other examples of the antibody were found, anti-Ny[a] was seen (519) to occur with a similar incidence in Germans. Anti-Ny[a] seems to be a non-red cell stimulated antibody, no example was found in seven Ny(a-) women who had borne children with Ny(a+) red cells (511). Because anti-Ny[a] can be made in rabbits (511) a large number of screening tests have been possible. With the exception (510) of one Swiss donor, these studies have shown that Ny[a] is almost exclusively the property of Norwegians. In separate studies, Ny(a+) red cells were found (67,511) in ten of 5931 and eight of 3746 Norwegian donors (512) (combined incidence, 1 in 538). Apart from the one Swiss donor with Ny(a+) red cells, a total of more than 46,500 bloods have been tested (510,513-519) without another Ny(a+) sample being found in a random survey. These bloods comprised more than 39,050 from predominantly White populations

(20,000 Germans, 9534 Swiss, 7400 Minnesotans, more than 1000 Bostonians, 800 British and 305 Laplanders); 6590 from Orientals (3281 Japanese, 1236 Taiwan Aborigines, 1041 Ryukyuans and 1032 Chinese); 650 from Blacks (350 in Boston, 300 in Britain) and 210 from American Indians. However, an Ny(a+) sample was found in the USA, when an ABO typing discrepancy was investigated (A_1 reverse typing cells Ny(a+) the group A patient's serum contained anti-Ny^a) (518). No Scandinavian ancestry of the individual with Ny(a+) red cells was known.

In 19 families in Norway (67,511,512) and in one in Switzerland (510) Ny^a was seen to travel with Ns for an NNy^as or an $NsNy^a$ haplotype. No unusual reactions of N or s on Ny(a+) red cells were noted (511), nor were any abnormalities seen when membranes from Ny(a+) red cells were subjected to SDS-PAGE (509). The Ny^a antigen is denatured or removed when red cells are treated with trypsin, papain or pronase (497,511,519).

The Antigen Or

In 1975, in the second edition of this book, the Or antigen was included in the MN chapter more on hunch than on science. In 1985, in the third edition, although no evidence that Or is an MN system antigen had emerged, tradition demanded that the antigen be kept in the MN chapter. In 1987, Bacon et al. (69) saved ours by documenting the evidence that resulted in Or being officially designated as an MN system antigen (520).

The first example of anti-Or was found (68) in the serum of a patient with "warm" antibody-induced hemolytic anemia. It reacted with the red cells of one of 163 Blacks but with none of those of 887 English donors. No further example of anti-Or was found in tests on 1405 sera from normal donors. In 1987, Bacon et al. (69) reported presence of the Or antigen on the red cells of a White blood donor in Australia. A study of the donor's family showed that Or was apparently transmitted via an Ms haplotype (i.e. $MOrs$ or $MsOr$). While the family was not large enough to prove that Or is located at the MN or Ss locus, other evidence that Or is indeed an MN system antigen, was found. First, glycophorins isolated from Or+ red cells specifically neutralized anti-Or. Second, all seven members of the family who had Or+ red cells, also had an M antigen that was more resistant to trypsin treatment of red cells than is the M antigen of Or- cells. Third, while the Or antigen was denatured or removed when Or+ red cells were treated with pronase or ficin, it was, like the M antigen of Or+ red cells, partially resistant to the actions of trypsin. Fourth, neuraminidase-treated Or+ red cells no longer reacted with anti-Or. The report (69) indicates that the Or+ red cells of an individual unrelat-

ed to the family described, reacted similarly to the Or+ red cells of the family members, as documented above. It is not clear whether those red cells, listed as Orriss D in the report, were from the original Or+ propositus of Cleghorn et al. (68) or from an unpublished source. Typing tests for MN system antigens and SDS-PAGE analysis of membranes from Or+ red cells revealed no abnormalities save for the increased resistance of M and Or to trypsin treatment, described above.

Bacon et al. (69) used the Or+ red cells of their propositus to screen random donor sera. Fifteen weak, saline-active anti-Or were found among 1152 samples tested. Anti-Or was also found in five of 50 sera containing antibodies to low incidence antigens but in no members of the family who had Or- red cells. One Or- woman in the family had borne two children with Or+ red cells. The anti-Or that was found in a compatibility test and that initiated the study, was shown to be IgM in composition. It was not inhibited by hydatid cyst fluid, human or guinea pig urine, secretor or non-secretor saliva, soluble AB substance, AB serum or serum from an individual with Or+ red cells.

The Antigen Tm

In papers published in 1965 and 1968, we (70,77) described an MN system antigen that we called Tm. Anti-Tm reacted with the red cells of 225 of 900 (25%) random White and 157 of 500 (31.4%) random Black donors. There was a marked association between Tm and N. Of the 382 Tm+ samples identified, 373 (97.6%) were from individuals with N+ red cells. Anti-Tm was not simply an example of weak anti-N for many M- N+ Tm- (i.e. double dose of N, no Tm) and M+ N+ Tm+ (i.e. single dose of N, Tm+) samples were found. Many M+ N+ Tm+ samples were also M_1+ (see description of glycosylation, below). The strength of the Tm antigen varied greatly on the red cells of different individuals. Between 1968 and 1980 several other examples of anti-Tm were encountered but not reported, in classifying weakly Tm+ red cells, their reactions were heterogeneous. One of us (PDI) has always believed that those antibodies that were called anti-Tm, that could be neutralized with hydatid cyst fluid, were weak examples of anti-P_1 detecting the strong P_1 antigen that is characteristic of the red cells of some Blacks.

In 1980, after participating in the study on the Can serum, we (71) decided to retest the original anti-Tm, against neuramindase-treated red cells. The removal of anti-T from anti-Tm was more complex than removal of anti-T from the Can serum (see below) because of the potential reactivity of anti-Tm with the N antigen. As explained earlier, red cells that are M+ N- and carry S or s, also carry 'N'. Thus, adsorption of the anti-Tm with neuraminidase-treated red cells of the phenotype M+ N- S or s+ would have been expected to remove any anti-N-related activity as well as anti-T. Accordingly, we (71) adsorbed the anti-T using neuramindase-treated M+ N- S- s- U- red cells. In this phenotype the red cells lack N and because they lack Ss SGP, also lack 'N'.

When tested against neuraminidase-treated red cells, the anti-Tm from which the anti-T had been removed, had simple anti-N specificity. In addition to agglutinating all red cells that were N+, but none that were N-, further studies (71) confirmed the anti-N specificity. In adsorption studies, neuraminidase-treated red cells of phenotypes M- N+ and M+ N+ removed all antibody in a single adsorption. Those that were M+ N- S or s+ required two adsorptions to exhaust the antibody, presumably because they carry 'N' but not N. Neuraminidase-treated M+ N- S- s- U- red cells did not adsorb the antibody at all. In inhibition studies (71), SGP preparations made from untreated M- N+ red cells failed to inhibit the adsorbed serum, while tryptic digests made from previously neuraminidase-treated M- N+ red cells caused total inhibition.

These findings (71) seemed to indicate that anti-Tm is anti-N polypeptide. That is to say, anti-Tm can recognize its antigen on N SGP under some but not all circumstances, when that SGP carries its normal, or close to normal content of N-acetyl-neuraminic acid (NeuAc). When NeuAc is removed by treatment of red cells with neuraminidase, anti-Tm can always recognize N SGP. Support for this conclusion was provided by the studies of Dahr et al. (485). As described in the section on the M_1 antigen, these workers showed that in some of the tetrasaccharides attached to glycophorin A on M_1+ or Tm+ or Can+, etc., red cells, N-acetyl glucosamine replaces one of the NeuAc residues (see figure 15-3 and table 15-9). Presumably, the absence of some NeuAc residues from glycophorin A, allows anti-Tm to recognize N SGP on untreated red cells. Perhaps in the presence of a full complement of NeuAc, the polypeptide backbone of N SGP is sterically oriented in a manner that prevents anti-Tm from binding. When some NeuAc residues are replaced by N-acetyl glucosamine, perhaps the polypeptide backbone is oriented in such a way that the antibody can bind, i.e. untreated red cells Tm+. When all or most of the NeuAc residues are removed, apparently the N polypeptide is oriented in a manner that allows anti-Tm to bind to all N+ red cells. It is tempting to speculate that the great variability in the strength of expression of Tm (70,77) relates directly to the replacement of NeuAc by N-acetyl glucosamine in the tetrasaccharides attached to the second and/or third and/or fourth residues from the NH_2 terminal end of the N SGP. The presence of NeuAc versus N-acetyl glucosamine at any,

some or all of those sites would presumably affect steric presentation of the polypeptide backbone of N bearing glycophorin A. This is a similar piece of reasoning to that applied to anti-M_1 above. However, in that instance it seems that anti-M_1 agglutinates all M+ red cells and that its reactions are enhanced when N-acetyl glucosamine replaces NeuAc.

The adsorption studies that showed (71) that anti-Tm is anti-N polypeptide also explained the original findings (70,77) of nine M+ N- Tm+ samples. Apparently the original anti-Tm also contained an anti-I that agglutinated those cells with the highest level of I. After adsorption with neuraminidase-treated M+ N- S- s- U- red cells, the serum did not agglutinate any N- samples. The adsorptions would, of course, be expected to remove both anti-T and anti-I (the I antigen survives neuraminidase-treatment of red cells, see Chapters 10 and 34).

The Antigen M^v

Although named as if it is a variant form of M, more recent data (see below) show that M^v is a low incidence antigen that is almost certainly carried on glycophorin B. In 1966, Gershowitz and Fried (73) described an antibody, that they named anti-M^v, that reacted with all M+ N+ and M- N+ red cells. In addition, it reacted with about one in 400 M+ N- bloods from Whites. In the original serum the anti-N and anti-M^v activity were inseparable. It was thought that the antibody had been produced following immunization during a pregnancy in which the child had M^v+ red cells. The maker of the anti-M^v was of the phenotype M+ N-. However, when M^v+ red cells (M+ N- M^v+) were injected into rabbits, anti-M was produced. In 1970, Crossland et al. (74) found an example of anti-M^v that lacked anti-N. This led Race and Sanger (7) to suggest that the original serum could now be thought of as anti-M^{v}N. In tests using the anti-M^v that lacked anti-N, the M^v antigen was found (74) to be present in 14 of 2371 (1 in 169) English donors.

In several families in which *M^v* was in alignment with *s*, the s antigen produced was weaker than normal (7,74,315). Indeed, in one study an anti-s was found that failed to give a visibly positive reaction with M^v+ S+ s+ red cells. The apparent indirect exclusion of paternity was shown to be false when other anti-s were shown to react, albeit less strongly than with M^v- s+ red cells, with the M^v+ S+ s+ red cells. In direct contrast, the S antigen present on M^v+ red cells appeared to be expressed normally (73,74,315).

In 1978, Dahr et al. (311,312) published findings that included SDS-PAGE analysis of the membranes of M^v+ red cells. They found that while the MN SGP of those cells appeared normal, the production of s SGP was only about 25% of that of a normal *s* gene. Thus, it seems that M^v might be thought of as an allele at the *Ss* locus, a sort of defective *s* gene. Mawby et al. (313) then produced evidence that the Ss SGP made by the M^v gene is different from normal Ss SGP in addition to being made in reduced amounts. They showed that the red cells of an Mi^V/M^v heterozygote did not react with *Vicia graminea* lectin after they had been treated with trypsin and that neither lactoperoxidase labeling nor PAS-staining, demonstrated normal Ss SGP on the cells, once those cells had been treated with trypsin. When these findings are reviewed in conjunction with those made on the red cells of the Mi^V homozygote (see below) they appear to indicate that M^v encodes production of a reduced level of abnormal, trypsin-sensitive Ss SGP. As already discussed, the s antigen of M^v+ red cells is detected by some but not all examples of anti-s in conventional test procedures.

Unlike the abnormal trypsin-sensitive s antigen encoded by the M^vs haplotype, the M^v antigen itself is resistant to trypsin treatment of red cells. However, M^v is denatured or removed when red cells are treated with chymotrypsin, papain, ficin or neuraminidase (314,497,521). All these findings point to s and M^v being carried on an abnormal form of glycophorin B, with the s antigen being distal to a trypsin-sensitive site and M^v being located between the trypsin and chymotrypsin/ papain/ficin sensitive sites and being, at least in part, dependent on the glycosylation of the abnormal form of glycophorin B. Less conjecture is possible about the M^vS haplotype, indeed there do not seem to be any data to indicate whether this haplotype encodes production of a normal or reduced amount of glycophorin B. From the serological results, one would suspect that M^vs and M^vS represent different genetic changes.

Anti-M^v can apparently be either red cell stimulated (73,521) or non-red cell immune (74). The antibody was blamed for mild HDN in two children born to a woman with anti-M^v in her serum (521).

The Phenotypes M^A, M^a, N^A, and N^a

Findings (75,87) that some people with M+ red cells make allo-anti-M and some with N+ red cells make allo-anti-N, have given rise to the use of different names. Thus, M^A and N^A red cells are said to carry M and M^A and N and N^A, respectively. Those called M^a and N^a are said to carry M without M^A and N without N^A, respectively. While limited findings suggest that the M^a and N^a conditions are inherited, it is not known whether the differences between M^A and M^a and between N^A and N^a, are qualitative or merely quantitative. Production of anti-

M and anti-N by persons of the M^a and N^a phenotypes, respectively, does not answer the question, people with A_2 red cells can make anti-A_1.

The Antigen Sul

When they investigated a White family of Lithuanian extraction, in which the propositus had Sul+ red cells, Konugres and Winter (76) found that the *Sul* gene traveled with *Ns*. In tests on 4935 samples (from Whites, Blacks, Chinese, Japanese, Mexicans, Filipinos, New Hebrides Islanders and including 320 cord bloods) they found no other Sul+ sample. Similarly, Metaxas (510) found no Sul+ sample in tests on the red cells of 6456 Swiss donors. In tests on the Sul+ red cells (17 such samples were found in four generations of the original family) Konugres and Winter (76) found that the antigen is destroyed when red cells are treated with ficin. In contrast to the rarity of the antigen, anti-Sul seemed fairly common, it was found in four of 119 normal sera and reacted as a room temperature, saline-active agglutinin. As far as we are aware, Sul+ red cells and anti-Sul are no longer available so that further work on the antigen is unlikely, unless the original family can be contacted.

The Antigen Sj

While investigating the first example of anti-Tm, we (77) realized that the serum contained a second MN system antibody, defining an antigen of low incidence. Adsorption studies with Tm+ Sj- red cells left anti-Sj unadsorbed, but adsorption with any Sj+ red cells removed both anti-Tm and anti-Sj. Since it is now known (71) that anti-Tm is anti-N polypeptide and since all 30 Sj+ red cells were also N+, it is no longer surprising that the Sj+ red cells adsorbed anti-Tm to exhaustion. In tests on the red cells of 500 random Whites we found 11 (2.2%) and in tests on the red cells of 500 random Blacks 19 (3.8%), that were Sj+. In the later investigation that showed that anti-Tm is a form of anti-N, we found no evidence to suggest that anti-Sj has a similar specificity. Indeed, the finding that N+ Tm+ Sj- red cells would adsorb anti-Tm but not anti-Sj, suggests that anti-Sj defines a low incidence antigen that is not a form of N. However, other than this serological clue, nothing is known about the structure of Sj.

The Phenotype M'

In 1968, Metaxas et al. (78) described an antibody,

that they named anti-M′, that was somewhat like anti-M_1. M+ N- and M+ N+ red cells that reacted with anti-M′ generally carried more M antigen than did red cells of similar phenotype that failed to react with the new antibody. In tests on the blood of an individual whom they described as genetically *M^zN*, these workers found that the red cells reacted with anti-M′ but not with anti-M_1. Conversely, M^c cells, that were thought to be M_1+, did not react with anti-M′. However, the anti-M_1 (448) that lacked anti-M was later shown to be non-reactive with M^c cells so that the already slight difference that existed between anti-M′ and anti-M_1, now seems even slighter. As discussed in other places in this chapter, the genes originally called *M^z* and *M^r* are known both to encode production of St^a, but via different backgrounds. The St(a+) red cells associated with the presence of *M^z* reacted with anti-M′, those associated with the presence of *M^r*, did not. The M′+ St(a+) red cells associated with *M^z* have a trypsin-resistant M antigen (105,504).

The Antigen Far, Previously Known as Kam

In 1966, a low incidence antigen, Kam, was reported (79) when the antibody against it caused a severe transfusion reaction in a multiply-transfused hemophiliac. The investigation of the case revealed that the patient had probably become immunized following transfusion with blood from the same donor, eleven years previously. The donor with Kam+ red cells had a brother whose cells were also Kam+ and a sister whose cells were Kam-. No other Kam+ sample was found in tests on 1100 bloods in Vienna.

In 1968, an antibody to a low incidence antigen caused severe HDN (80,81). The antibody was called anti-Far but in tests on 341 sera, including many from patients with WAIHA, SLE and other disorders in which the sera frequently contain antibodies to low incidence antigens, Cregut et al. (81) did not find another example. In the family that included individuals with Far+ red cells, it appeared that *Far* was traveling with *Ns*. Blood samples from 14,273 individuals in Paris and Liege were tested but no other Far+ sample was found. The Far antigen was shown to survive ficin and papain-treatment of red cells.

In 1977, the long list of low incidence antigens was reduced by one when Giles (82) showed that Kam and Far are the same thing. This study confirmed that the antigen survives ficin-treatment of red cells. While this finding suggests that Far is more likely to be carried on glycophorin B than on glycophorin A, it by no means proves the point. While not shown to be a part of the MN system when studied, examination of the test results showed that *Kam* traveled with *MS* in the original family (79).

An Introduction to the Heterogeneity of En^a

As will become apparent in the next section, the En^a antigens reside on glycophorin A. Since that glycoprotein has some 70 amino acids and multiple carbohydrate-containing side chains that extend out from the red cell membrane, it is not surprising that a number of different antigens (i.e. different portions of glycophorin A) are defined by antibodies called anti-En^a. Thus En^a is a group name that actually describes a series of different antigens and anti-En^a is a term encompassing several specificities. At the most straightforward level, En(a-) red cells are those that lack glycophorin A, anti-En^a are antibodies directed against any portion of normal glycophorin A. When hybrid SGPs are formed, comprised in part of material normally found on glycophorin A and in part of material normally found on glycophorin B, they may lack some but not all the En^a determinants. Similarly, mutations that alter the composition of glycophorin A (even by a single amino acid) have the potential to result in loss of one of the En^a determinants. In an attempt to make the next section as comprehensible as possible, En^a is initially treated as if it is a single entity (i.e. glycophorin A) and anti-En^a are treated as if they have a single specificity. The complications that arise when hybrid or mutated SGPs are present are described briefly in the section on anti-En^a and in more detail in the sections describing the biochemistry and molecular genetics of the MN system.

The En^a Series of Antigens

In back to back papers published in 1969, Darnborough et al. (83) described an English proposita and Furuhjelm et al. (84) a Finnish propositus, each with an alloantibody to a very high incidence antigen. The antibody was named anti-En^a and the red cell phenotype of the antibody-makers' red cells, En(a-). The red cells of the two individuals were mutually compatible. It was not immediately appreciated that En(a-) red cells lack normal M and N antigens. The red cells of the English proposita carried a weak, trypsin-resistant form of M, they were N-. The red cells of the Finnish propositus carried a weak, trypsin-resistant form of N, they were M-. The explanations of these findings are discussed later in this section.

It was recognized early (83,84) that there was some sort of perturbation of the membrane of En(a-) red cells. Indeed, the name En was introduced to indicate an abnormality of the envelope (membrane) of the red cells. Among many findings it has been shown that En(a-) red cells: are not aggregated or are aggregated only weakly by polybrene; have a reduced electrophoretic mobility due to a reduction of membrane-associated sialic acid; are agglutinated in saline systems by certain Rh antibodies that are reactive only by more sensitive methods, e.g. IAT, with En(a+) red cells; have increased glycosylation of protein band 3 (13-15,429). These findings all relate to the fact that En(a-) red cells lack glycophorin A.

SDS-PAGE studies of En(a-) red cells (12-15,34) quickly revealed that the cells either lacked glycophorin A or carried a non-glycosylated version of that protein. Additional studies (34,37) designed to detect the presence of glycophorin A whether or not it is glycosylated, revealed that the first of the two explanations applies, that is En(a-) red cells lack glycophorin A. Since glycophorin A carries some 60% of the sialic acid present on normal (i.e. En(a+)) red cells most of the abnormalities described above can be explained. First, polybrene does not aggregate red cells with a reduced sialic acid level. Second, the electrophoretic mobility of red cells is directly related to their sialic acid content. Third, when red cells are treated with ficin, papain, etc., glycophorin A is cleaved. Such treated red cells give enhanced reactions with Rh antibodies, untreated En(a-) red cells behave similarly, in this respect, to protease-treated En(a+) cells. The increased glycosylation of band 3 of En(a-) red cells is explained differently, as described below.

Since M and N are normally carried on glycophorin A and that glycoprotein is missing from En(a-) red cells, the presence of some N on the red cells of the Finnish propositus (84) and of some M on the red cells of the English proposita (83) require explanation. The gene present in the Finnish propositus is called *En*, it fails to encode production of glycophorin A so that in *En* homozygotes, the En(a-) phenotype results. *En* acts as a silent allele at the *MN* locus (369,526,527,529), its presence does not affect expression of glycophorin B. In other words, the weak, trypsin-resistant N, found on the red cells of the Finnish propositus (84) is the ′N′ antigen at the NH_2 terminal end of glycophorin B. Because, as described below, the genetic background in the English En(a-) proposita is different, the *En* gene in the Finnish propositus is often called *En(Fin)* to distinguish it from the gene in the English proposita.

While *En(Fin)* encodes no glycophorin A but does not affect expression of glycophorin B, the red cells of the English proposita were found (12,311,530) to carry a hybrid form of glycophorin B in which the only change from normal glycophorin B involved the presence of serine instead of leucine at the NH_2 terminal residue. This, of course, explained why the red cells of the proposita carried weak, trypsin-resistant M and not ′N′ (see figure 15-2). In order to distinguish this situation, from that in *En(Fin)* homozygotes, the gene in the English proposita is often called *En(UK)*. The phenotypes resulting from presence of these genes are sometimes written as

En(a-)(Fin) and En(a-)(UK). Studies on the family of the English En(a-) proposita strongly suggested that rather than being genetically *En(UK)En(UK)*, she is *En(UK)M^k*. While not yet described in this chapter, M^k serves as a silent allele at both the *MN* and *Ss* loci. That is, while *En(Fin)* encodes no production of glycophorin A but allows normal production of glycophorin B; *En(UK)* encodes no production of glycophorin A and encodes a hybrid SGP closely related to glycophorin B; M^k encodes no production of glycophorin A or glycophorin B. The red cells of M^k homozygotes (see below) are devoid of glycophorins A and B and carry no alternative hybrid SGP. The presence of M^k in the English proposita's family was deduced from perturbation of inheritance of antigens encoded from the *Ss* locus, *En(Fin)* and *En(UK)* apparently disrupt inheritance of M and N but not of S and s.

Another feature of red cells with reduced levels of sialic acid is that they react more readily than do red cells with normal levels, with the species antibodies in animal sera (84). Thus En(a-) red cells sometimes react with rabbit anti-M and anti-N not because of the anti-M and anti-N in those sera, but because of small amounts of anti-human reactivity present. En(a-) red cells also give stronger than normal reactions with the lectins *Sophora japonica* (adsorbed free of anti-A,B) and *Glycine soja* (that agglutinates red cells that have a reduced level of sialic acid). Similarly, the lectins *Bauhinia purpurea* (anti-N), *Dolichos biflorus* (anti-A, anti-A_1 when appropriately diluted), *Phaseolus lunatus* (anti-A) and *Arachis hypogea* (anti-T) all react better with En(a-) than En(a+) red cells (531). These reactions may all be based on the reduced sialic acid level of En(a-) red cells. The lectin *Maclura aurantiaca* binds to red cell glycophorins (14) and reacts less strongly with En(a-) than with En(a+) red cells (531). The reduced expressions of Ch and Rg antigens on En(a-) red cells and on those of M^k homozygotes (596) are discussed in Chapter 27.

As mentioned above, a different explanation may exist for the increased glycosylation of band 3 of En(a-) red cells. Groves and Tanner (532) used transfection experiments to show that glycophorin A facilitates expression of protein band 3 when *Xenopus* oocytes are used. Glycophorin A may be actively involved in the transport of band 3 to the cell surface. If this applies in human red cells, it is possible that the delay involved in band 3 reaching the membrane may allow time for additional glycosylation of that protein in the Golgi.

Since the original individuals of the En(a-) phenotype were reported (83,84) others have been found. A second En(a-) individual in Finland (533) and one in the USA (534) were eventually shown to be related to the original Finnish family (84) although that fact was not established until after the newly discovered En(a-) status of the individuals concerned, was known. In the large Finnish family there is a total of five *En(Fin)* homozygotes, two of the propositi are the products of cousin marriages. Two other persons with En(a-) red cells (both believed to be *En(Fin)* homozygotes) were identified when their sera were shown to contain anti-En^a, one was a French-Canadian, his parents were cousins (535), the other was a Pakistani (536,595). Two Japanese blood donors of the En(a-) phenotype, who did not have anti-En^a in the serum, were found in deliberate screening studies (537,538 and see below).

As mentioned above, En(a-) red cells carry only about 40% of the amount of sialic acid of normal red cells. The red cells of *En* heterozygotes carry about 70% of the normal level. Thus some of the unusual serological characteristics of En(a-) red cells that are described above, are seen to a lesser but still recognizable degree when red cells from *En* heterozygotes are tested. For example, such red cells may be agglutinated in a saline system using selected Rh antibodies that otherwise react by IAT. In the section above, on St^a, the screening tests of Metaxas and Metaxas-Bühler (498) using such antibodies, are described. Among 6202 donors tested, three possible *En* heterozygotes were found. Inglis et al. (539) used protamine sulphate in aggregation tests on red cell samples from 1300 Scottish donors. Since red cells with reduced sialic acid levels do not aggregate like those with normal levels of sialic acid, the tests led to the recognition of one *En(Fin)* and one *En(UK)* heterozygote. Hodson and Lee (540) identified two individuals with *En(UK)* in whom the hybrid SGP carried trypsin-resistant M and the s antigen. This indicates a different situation from that seen (83,539) in the other individuals with *En(UK)* in whom the hybrid SGP carried trypsin-resistant M and the S antigen. Presumably *En(UK)* arose at least twice. In one instance the converted gene encodes production of an S-bearing hybrid SGP with serine at its NH$_2$ terminus, in the other the converted gene encodes an s-bearing hybrid with the same NH$_2$ terminal change.

The En(a-) phenotype is extremely rare. In the original studies (83,84) tests on 12,500 English, 8800 Finnish and 200 Estonian donors identified no En(a-) sample. No En(a-) sample was found on the island of Espiritu Santo in the Republic of Vanuatu in the southwest Pacific when 214 samples (representing almost 1% of the population) were tested with monoclonal anti-M and anti-N (740). Shinozuka et al. (537) and Okubo et al. (538) used monoclonal anti-En^a to screen 250,000 Japanese blood donors, one En(a-) sample was found. As mentioned above, a second En(a-) propositus, not related to the first, has been found (541) in Japan in a separate study from the one involving tests on 250,000 donors.

Heterogeneity of Anti-En^a (Includes Antibodies to En^{a}TS, En^{a}FS, En^{a}FR, En^{a}KT, ENEP, ENEH, HAG, AVIS and MARS)

As stated in the previous section, the red cells and antibodies made by persons with the En(a-) phenotypes that represent the absence of glycophorin A (i.e. representing the genotypes *En(Fin)En(Fin)* and *En(UK)M^k*) are mutually compatible. That does not mean that the anti-En^a are all the same. The anti-En^a of the original English proposita (83) and the Finnish propositus (84) reacted with untreated, trypsin-treated and ficin or papain-treated En(a+) red cells. When the second Finnish propositus was found (533) a study of his antibody showed that two forms of anti-En^a exist. Both react with trypsin-treated En(a+) red cells but differ in that one reacts with ficin-treated En(a+) cells while the other does not. Adsorption studies showed that the first two examples of anti-En^a (83,84) contained both antibodies. When the French-Canadian propositus was found (535) it was seen that his anti-En^a did not react with trypsin or with ficin-treated En(a+) red cells. When an auto-anti-En^a was studied (542) it was seen to detect the trypsin-resistant, ficin-sensitive form of En^a. In order that these various specificities could be differentiated in verbal and written communications, we (85) proposed a modified terminology. Anti-En^{a}TS (trypsin-sensitive) described the form of anti-En^a that was non-reactive with trypsin-treated red cells. Anti-En^{a}FS (ficin-sensitive) described the form of anti-En^a that reacts with trypsin-treated but not with ficin-treated red cells. Anti-En^{a}FR (ficin-resistant) described the form of anti-En^a that reacts with trypsin and with ficin-treated En(a+) red cells. The explanation of these three specificities is straightforward. Glycophorin A has a trypsin-sensitive site at residue 39 and a ficin/papain-sensitive site at position 56. Thus the determinant recognized by anti-En^{a}TS must be between the NH$_2$ terminus and residue 39. Since the amino acids from positions 1 to 26 of glycophorin A and glycophorin B are the same (except for residues 1 and 5 on M SGP) and since most En(a-) red cells carry normal glycophorin B, it follows that anti-En^{a}TS when made as an alloantibody by an En(a-) individual, must recognize a determinant between residues 26 and 39 of glycophorin A. Since the determinant recognized by anti-En^{a}FS is trypsin-resistant but ficin-sensitive, it must be positioned between residues 39 and 56 of glycophorin A. Since the determinant recognized by anti-En^{a}FR is ficin-resistant, it must be positioned between residue 56 and about residue 70 (at which point glycophorin A enters the red cell membrane). The reactions of anti-En^{a}TS, anti-En^{a}FS and anti-En^{a}FR are summarized in table 15-11. For reasons that will become apparent later in this chapter, the

TABLE 15-11 To Show the Reactions of Three Types of Anti-En^a and of Anti-Wr^b Against Untreated and Protease-Treated Red Cells

Red Cells	Anti-En^{a}TS	Anti-En^{a}FS	Anti-En^{a}FR	Anti-Wr^b
Untreated En(a+)	+	+	+	+
Trypsin-treated En(a+)	0	+	+	+
Ficin-treated En(a+)	0	0	+	+
Untreated En(a-)	0	0	0	0
Untreated Wr(a+b-)	+	+	+	0

reactions of anti-Wr^b are also shown in table 15-11. Figure 15-6 is a simplified diagram that illustrates the locations of the trypsin and ficin-sensitive sites and those of En^{a}TS, En^{a}FS and En^{a}FR on glycophorin A.

Antibody inhibition studies using peptide fragments derived from glycophorin A have also been used (287,288,543-549) to determine the locations of En^{a}TS, En^{a}FS and En^{a}FR on glycophorin A. Dahr et al. (547) studied three examples of anti-En^{a}TS and, while the location of the determinants was seen to be similar to that described in the previous section, it was shown that each anti-En^{a}TS recognized a slightly different structure. The alloimmune anti-En^{a}TS made by the French Canadian En(a-) propositus (535) was best inhibited by a peptide containing the amino acids from position 31 to 39 with the tyrosine residue at position 34 being of particular importance. This anti-En^{a}TS was inhibited only by peptides on which the threonine at position 33 was not glycosylated. A transiently produced auto-anti-En^{a}TS, made by a patient with temporary suppression of antigen expression that apparently suppressed expression of En^{a}TS, but not of En^{a}FS or En^{a}FR (550 and see section on auto-anti En^a) was best inhibited by a peptide comprising amino acids from position 25 or 28 to 33 with the lysine residue at position 30 seeming to be of importance. The third anti-En^{a}TS, that caused a severe transfusion reaction (528,551), was best inhibited by a peptide containing the amino acids from position 36 to 42, with the arginine residue at position 39 apparently being critical for antigen integrity. In other words, while all three En^{a}TS determinants appeared to be within the amino acid

25 or 28 to 42 region (the trypsin-sensitive site is at residue 39) no two of them were exactly alike. Except as stated above, glycosylation of the peptides did not seem to play a major role in their abilities to inhibit anti-En^{a}TS.

The story with anti-En^{a}FS is a little more straightforward. In tests on six examples of this specificity, Dahr et al. (547) found that each of them could be inhibited by a peptide fragment comprising the amino acids from position 46 to 56 of glycophorin A. Five of the six anti-En^{a}FS were inhibited only when the threonine residue at position 50 was glycosylated. The anti-En^{a}FS made by the second Finnish propositus (533) required a larger peptide, i.e. from residues 42 to 56 for total inhibition. It is possible that this serum contained two antibodies directed against determinants in the trypsin-resistant, ficin-sensitive portion of glycophorin A. The glycophorin A derived peptides that inhibited the various anti-En^a specificities are depicted in table 15-12.

In early studies on the various anti-En^a, it was much harder to obtain evidence that En^{a}FR was a glycophorin A-borne structure, than to prove that point about En^{a}TS and En^{a}FS. Examples of anti-En^{a}FR made in humans were not inhibited by whole glycophorin A isolates. Indeed, for a time it appeared possible that anti-En^{a}FR was directed against a structure missing from En(a-) red cells, that was not on the MN SGP. The concept of a concomitant change (to lack of glycophorin A) on En(a-) red cells was not attractive and in 1980, Anstee and Edwards (552) produced the first piece of evidence that this idea could be abandoned. These workers showed that a monoclonal antibody with apparent anti-En^{a}FR specificity would precipitate isolated intact MN SGP. Later, Dahr et al. (402,545,546) produced direct evidence on this point. It was shown that when a peptide from the valine residue at position 62 to the glutamic acid at position 72 was incorporated into liposomes, it would inhibit anti-En^{a}FR and anti-Wr^b (see below). Earlier attempts at such inhibition had probably failed because of the method used to isolate the MN SGP. In order to achieve antibody inhibition, Dahr et al. (402,545,546) showed that SGP had to be isolated under non-denaturing conditions in the presence of Triton X-100. Further, incorporation of the peptide into liposomes was necessary before antibody inhibition could be demonstrated. En^{a}FR thus appeared to be a labile, lipid-dependent structure located within the residue 62 to 72 portion of glycophorin A.

As mentioned in the brief introductory paragraph about the heterogeneity of En^a, it is not necessary for red cells totally to lack glycophorin A in order to lack one or more of the antigens En^{a}TS, En^{a}FS and En^{a}FR. For example, when unequal crossing over or gene conversion occurs, involving the genes that normally encode production of glycophorin A and glycophorin B, the newly formed gene may encode a sialoglycopro-

FIGURE 15-6 To Show the Protease-sensitive Sites on Normal Glycophorin A and the Locations of En^a Antigens

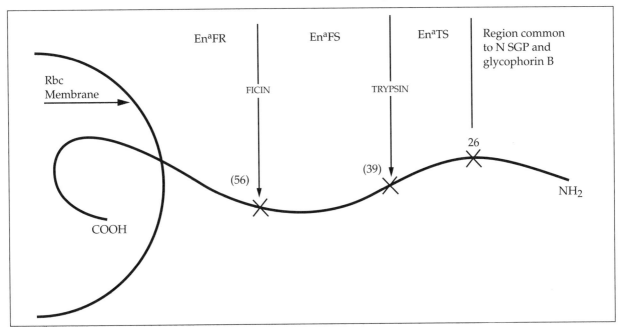

tein comprised in part of material usually found on glycophorin A and in part of material usually found on glycophorin B. If the material usually present on glycophorin A, now replaced by material usually present on glycophorin B, expresses one of the En^a antigens, that antigen will not be present on the hybrid glycophorin. In 1981, we described one woman homozygous for the Mi^V gene (287) (see below) and another (288) homozygous for a somewhat similar converted gene. Although both situations are described in more

detail in the section on the biochemistry of the MN system, it can be stated here that both women had hybrid glycophorins with their outer (NH$_2$) terminal portions derived from material normally present on glycophorin A and their inner (COOH) terminal portions derived from material normally present on glycophorin B (i.e. A-B hybrid glycophorins). In both instances the red cells typed as En^{a}TS+ En^{a}FS+ En^{a}FR-. The red cells of the Mi^V homozygote (287) would adsorb and yield on elution low levels of anti-En^{a}FR, those of the other individual (288)

TABLE 15-12 Peptides Shown to Inhibit Different Examples of Anti-En^a

Antibody Specificity	Paper Describing the Antibody	Paper Describing the Inhibition Study	Portion of Glycophorin A Shown to be Inhibitory	Other Observations
Anti-En^{a}TS	535	547	Residues 31 to 39	Inhibitory only when Thr^{33} not glycosylated. Tyr^{34} of major importance.
Anti-En^{a}TS	550	547	Residues 25 or 28 to 33	Inhibitory only when Thr^{33} not glycosylated. Lys^{30} of major importance.
Anti-En^{a}TS	551	547	Residues 36 to 42	Glycosylation or lack thereof of Thr^{33} not critical. Arg^{39} of major importance.
Anti-En^{a}FS	Multiple examples	547	Residues 46 to 56	Five of six examples inhibited only when Thr^{50} glycosylated.
Anti-En^{a}FS	533	547	Residues 42 to 56	Serum may have contained two different Anti-En^{a}FS.
Anti-En^{a}FR	Multiple examples	402	Residues 62 to 72	Peptide inhibitory only when isolated as part of liposomes.

would not. It is now known (for references see section on biochemistry) that the Mi^V hybrid SGP (now called GP.Hil) and the hybrid on the other patient's red cells (288) were probably comprised of the same portion of glycophorin A-derived material and a portion of glycophorin B that differed only in that the hybrid glycophorin of the Mi^V homozygote expressed s while that on the hybrid glycophorin of the other patient expressed S. Thus why one hybrid apparently carried a trace of En^{a}FR while the other did not, is not known. However, it should be added that the data inferred about the second patient (288) are largely based on studies on the genes and glycophorin of a different patient first described in 1989 (295,553) and believed to be the same as the one reported in 1981.

In 1986, Laird-Fryer et al. (99) described a woman homozygous for Mi^{VII}. The glycophorin A of her red cells has amino acid substitutions at residues 49 and 52 and possibly a glycosylation change (554). As a result her red cells do not carry the usual form of En^{a}FS and the alloantibody she made does not react with normal En^{a}FS. The name anti-En^{a}KT has been applied to those anti-En^{a}FS that do not react with the red cells of the Mi^{VII} homozygote. Somewhat similarly the name ENEPH (107), later modified to ENEP (555), has been introduced to describe the high incidence antigen missing from glycophorin A when proline replaces alanine at position 65. Again similarly, the name ENEH describes the high incidence antigen missing from glycophorin A when that structure is encoded by the Mi^I gene (106). A low incidence antigen apparently present on glycophorin A when ENEP is missing and perhaps antithetical to ENEP, has tentatively been named HAG. These changes in glycophorin A that lead to the absence of ENEP and ENEH are described in more detail in a later section.

A high incidence antigen tentatively called AVIS (757) apparently represents an interaction product of a different to usual glycophorin A and protein band 3 (834). That is to say, an amino acid substitution in glycophorin A near the point at which that glycoprotein enters the red cell membrane, seems to result in the AVIS-negative phenotype. A low incidence antigen present on AVIS- red cells that seems to result from the same amino acid change (834) was called MARS (757). In light of the possible glycophorin A-protein band 3 association, these antigens are discussed again in Chapter 17.

The Immune Response to En^a

It is probably more than coincidence that three persons (83,84,533) of the En(a-) phenotype who were immunized by the introduction of En(a+) red cells via transfusion or pregnancy, made at least anti-En^{a}FR and anti-Wr^b (see below) and perhaps anti-En^{a}FS and/or anti-

En^{a}TS as well, while one known example of allo-anti-En^a made by a non-transfused male (535) was just anti-En^{a}TS and that individual did not make anti-Wr^b. These observations are similar to the findings that anti-M and anti-N are often non-red cell immune, while anti-S, anti-s and anti-U are often red cell stimulated. The similarity, of course, relates to the similar locations of M, N and En^{a}TS on glycophorin A and the analogous locations of En^{a}FS and En^{a}FR on glycophorin A to those of S, s and U on glycophorin B.

The Wr(a-b-) Status of En(a-), Actually En^{a}FR- Red Cells

In 1975, after having worked on Wr^b for more than four years, we (556-558) made the totally unexpected finding that En(a-) red cells are Wr(a-b-). Since it is now known (404) that the Wr^a/Wr^b polymorphism represents an amino acid substitution at position 658 of protein band 3, meaning that Wr^a and Wr^b are antigens of the Diego blood group system, full details are given in Chapter 17. However, since persons who lack glycophorin A and some in whom a portion of that glycophorin is replaced with material normally carried on glycophorin B, often make anti-Wr^b in addition to anti-En^a, some mention of Wr^b is necessary here.

After many years of intense study, it was shown (322,402-404,559,560) that in order to be expressed at the serological level, Wr^b requires protein band 3 with glutamic acid at position 658 and the alpha helical portion of normal glycophorin A, from about residues 60 to 72. In other words, although glutamic acid at position 658 on band 3 may be present, Wr^b is not expressed in En(a-) red cells since no glycophorin A is present. Further, in those situations described in the previous section in which the portion of glycophorin A that carries En^{a}FR is replaced in a hybrid glycophorin with material normally present on glycophorin B, Wr^b is not expressed. In other words, red cells that are En^{a}TS+ En^{a}FS+ En^{a}FR- are often Wr(a-b-) (101,287,288). Some other haplotypes that would not be expected to encode the portion of glycophorin A necessary for expression of Wr^b have not yet been found in the homozygous state. Although it has not yet been described in this chapter, the M^k gene acts as a silent allele at both the MN and Ss loci. Thus the red cells of M^k homozygotes lack glycophorin A and B, as expected they are Wr(a-b-) (296-298,561). In contrast to the above situations, the Wr(a+b-) red cells of the Wr^a homozygote (557,562,565) carry normal glycophorin A and are En^{a}TS+ En^{a}FS+ En^{a}FR+; their Wr(b-) status represents the replacement of glutamic acid by lysine on all copies (i.e. encoded by both AE1 genes) of their protein band 3.

Since En(a-) and some En^aTS+ En^aFS+ En^aFR- red cells are Wr(a-b-) it is not surprising that some individuals of those phenotypes have made anti-Wr^b in addition to anti-En^a. When present, the antibodies are readily separable (287,288,548,549,556,564,565) but the rare En(a+) Wr(a+b-) red cells are needed to adsorb the anti-En^a and leave the anti-Wr^b unadsorbed.

Clinical Significance of anti-En^a

There is not very much information about the clinical significance of anti-En^a. One of the early found individuals with En(a-) red cells who had anti-En^a and anti-Wr^b in the serum had to be transfused and was given six units of En(a+) Wr(b+) blood, he suffered only a mild transfusion reaction (533). On the other hand, the patient mentioned above who had a transiently depressed expression of red cell En^a antigen and made anti-En^aTS, had a severe transfusion reaction (528,551) and died of the complications thereof. An anti-En^a comprised mostly of IgG1 but with an IgG3 component, made by an individual homozygous for M^k, caused severe HDN in her child (561). As discussed in the next section, auto-anti-En^a can also cause marked in vivo red cell destruction. Thus, when faced with anti-En^a in a patient who must be transfused, the blood banker would seem best advised to try to obtain En(a-) units, difficult as that task may be. However, as with virtually any other blood group antibody, if no compatible blood is available and the patient will die without transfusion, incompatible blood should be used. As mentioned above, at least once anti-En^a (accompanied by anti-Wr^b) was relatively benign in vivo (533).

Auto-Anti-En^a

In 1972, Worlledge (566) reported that some autoantibodies causative of WAIHA, that react with Rh_{null} red cells, have anti-En^a specificity. Shortly after the verbal report of Worlledge, we (556,557) showed that En(a-) red cells are Wr(a-b-). From these and subsequent studies (542,567-570) it became clear that both auto-anti-En^a and auto-anti-Wr^b can cause WAIHA. It is now well established (528,542,550,551,557,566-575) that autoantibodies directed against En^aTS, En^aFS, En^aFR, En^aKT and Wr^b cause often severe and sometimes fatal hemolytic anemia. In studying eight examples of auto-anti-En^aFS, Moulds et al. (572) found that while trying to prepare eluates from the patients' DAT positive red cells, they were unable to obtain a non-reactive last wash preparation, even after washing the patients' red cells 20 to 30 times. They suggested that this finding coupled with a non-reactive eluate, should alert the investigator to possible anti-

En^aFS specificity. When the anti-En^aFS were absorbed on to allogeneic red cells, the phenomenon did not occur.

It is, of course, difficult to differentiate auto-anti-En^a from auto-anti-Wr^b unless the rare En(a+) Wr(a+b-) red cells are available. Fortunately for the patients involved, determining the exact specificity is primarily an academic exercise. As discussed in Chapter 37 the amount, and to a lesser degree the subclass of an IgG autoantibody, are of some importance as regards severity of the disease, autoantibody specificity is not.

Monoclonal Anti-En^a

When monoclonal antibodies are made by injecting mice with human red cells then fusing spleen cells from the immunized mice with myeloma cells (576), the most common specificities produced are anti-Wr^b and anti-En^a. In 1982, one of us (577) described three monoclonal antibodies directed against glycophorin A. One had a specificity close to anti-En^aTS, a second behaved as anti-En^aFS and the third appeared to detect a determinant common to glycophorins A and B since it reacted with all red cells except those from M^k homozygotes. Many additional MAb to glycophorin A, that do not have anti-M or anti-N specificity, have been made (263,265,415,578-583). Much of the newer information included in this chapter thus far, and much of the information about the biochemistry and molecular biology of the MN system, has been generated by use of these antibodies.

The Serum Shier

In 1969, Beck (86) investigated a serum from a patient Shier and showed that it contained an antibody that reacted predominantly with N+ bloods. Many of the N+ Shier+ samples were also reactive with anti-Tm. In spite of the frequency of N+ Shier+ Tm+ cells, the Shier antibody and anti-Tm did not have the same specificity. Both N+ Shier+ Tm- and N+ Shier- Tm+ samples were found. Unfortunately, now that the behavior of anti-Tm as anti-N polypeptide is known, insufficient Shier serum remains for further investigation.

The Antigens U^z, Previously Known as Z, and U^x

In 1972, Booth (88) reported finding an antibody in the serum of a healthy, never transfused, young male Papuan blood donor, that defined a previously unrecognized MN system antigen. In tests on the blood of 1153 individuals, 890 of whom were Melanesian and 263 of whom were Europeans resident in Papua/New Guinea or New Zealand, Booth (88) found that the antigen, that he named Z, was present more often on S+ than on S- red cells. Three hundred and sixty-three of the samples carried S and Z, 27 carried S without Z, 120 carried Z without S and 643 lacked both S and Z. The Z antigen was more common in Whites than in Melanesians, 61% of the Whites and 36% of the Melanesians were shown to have Z+ red cells.

In a paper published in 1978, Booth (92) reported another new antibody, anti-U^x, also made by a never transfused Melanesian blood donor, and further studies on anti-Z, that resulted in that antibody being renamed anti-U^z. It was concluded that since there was evidence that anti-U blocks at least some of the sites with which anti-U^x and anti-U^z complex and since anti-s blocks some U^x sites, the antigens S, s, U, U^x and U^z might be in close proximity and that the steric configuration of each might affect the accessibility of (some of) the others. Through the kindness of Dr. Booth one of us (PDI) was able to test anti-U^x and anti-U^z. However, the positive reactions obtained were so weak that no definitive conclusions could be drawn. Both antibodies appeared to be non-red cell immune and both presented as agglutinins optimally reactive at reduced temperatures. It was difficult (in this author's hands) to distinguish between the reactivity of anti-U^x and anti-U^z and that of other cold-reactive agglutinins present in the sera.

From biochemical studies, Dahr (322,401,522) concluded that while anti-U^x and anti-U^z complex with determinants on glycophorin B, and in the case of anti-U^x on glycophorin A as well, they do not define polymorphisms of U as their names tend to imply. Indeed, the relationship of U^x and U^z to U seems primarily to reflect the fact that, since they do not have glycophorin B, S- s- U- red cells lack U^z and may have a reduced expression of U^x. Dahr (322,522) concluded that U^x is a NeuAc dependent residue carried on the portions of glycophorins A and B that are homologous, i.e. residues 1 to 26 of the NH_2 termini. Why anti-U^x reacts better with glycophorin B than with glycophorin A, is not known. Dahr (322) and Dahr and Moulds (522) produced evidence that U^z is probably located in the region of glycophorin B represented by residues 29 to 36. As mentioned elsewhere in this chapter, the S/s polymorphism occurs at residue 29 of glycophorin B but expression of S or s is also influenced by the amino acids at positions 25, 28, 34 and 35 (see figure 15-5). The U antigen appears to involve residues 33 to 40 of glycophorin B but its normal expression appears to be dependent also on the presence of membrane lipids (401).

The enhanced reactivity of anti-U^z with S+ s- red cells, compared to those that are S- s+ was considered (322,433) probably to represent the fact that S+ s- red cells carry about 1.5 times the number of copies of glycophorin B, as carried by S- s+ red cells (311,321,322,522,523). As mentioned earlier in this chapter, it is possible that those examples of anti-S that react with S- s+ red cells when different methods (e.g. tests against enzyme-treated red cells) are used, but that fail to react with or be adsorbed by S- s- U- and S- s- $U+^{var}$ red cells (318-320) are examples of the same antibody that is called anti-U^z in this section.

Read et al. (525) described a Hispanic woman with M+ N- S- s+ U+ He+(weak) red cells who made an antibody that was either anti-U^z or had a very similar specificity. The antibody-maker had never been transfused but had been pregnant four times. The antibody crossed the placenta and caused a 3+ DAT but no clinical HDN in the woman's fourth child. The facts that the antibody could be adsorbed onto and eluted from the woman's red cells, at the time it was being made in its strongest form and that three months before delivery, her serum had been found not to contain the antibody, caused the authors to wonder if the antibody had been made during a time when the mother's red cell antigen was transiently depressed. However, the second and third children born to the mother also had a positive DAT at birth with perhaps the same antibody being responsible.

The Antigen s^D

In 1978, Shapiro and LeRoux (93,94) studied an antibody that caused severe HDN, the antibody was named anti-s^D. In the large White South African family studied (the red cells of over 100 members were tested) 41 persons spanning four generations were found to have s^D+ red cells. The s^D antigen was seen always to be encoded by an *Ms* haplotype. Red cells of the S+ s+ s^D+ phenotype reacted weakly with some examples of anti-s and failed to react with others. In tests on samples from 1000 White South Africans, one s^D+ sample was found, the individual involved was then shown to be a member of the original family. In tests on samples from 1000 South Africans of mixed race, one other person with s^D+ red cells was found.

The Antigen Can

In 1979, Judd et al. (95) reported an antibody in a serum, Can. While the antibody had a specificity close to that of anti-M, it was not simply a weak example of that antibody. Some M+ N- (double dose of M) cells were Can- while some M+ N+ (single dose of M) cells were Can+. The antibody reacted with the red cells of 144 of 541 (27%) Whites and those of 268 of 447 (60%) Blacks.

Of the 412 Can+ samples, 359 (87%) were M+.

When anti-T was removed from the Can serum by adsorption with neuraminidase-treated M- N+ red cells and the adsorbed serum was tested against neuraminidase-treated red cells, it had simple anti-M specificity. Thus the antibody appeared to be defining a form of M that, when red cells carry their full complement of sialic acid (NeuAc), is sterically oriented in such a fashion that maximal antibody complexing cannot occur. Once NeuAc is removed, it appears that the M determinant recognized by the Can serum is oriented suitably on all M+ red cells for antibody binding to occur. When tested against untreated red cells, the Can serum agglutinated some that were M- N+. However, when the adsorbed Can serum was tested against neuramindase-treated samples, only M+ red cells were agglutinated. It is possible that the reactions of the unadsorbed serum with some M- N+ samples occurred because the serum contained another cold agglutinin not related to the MN system (such as anti-I reacting only with strongly I+ samples). That antibody may have been removed at the same time that the anti-T was adsorbed.

In 1991, Dahr et al. (485) showed that like M_1+ and Tm+ red cells, those that are Can+ carry some tetrasaccharide side chains in which N-acetyl-glucosamine replaces one of the N-acetyl-neuraminic acid residues (see figure 15-3). The way in which this change is presumed to affect orientation of the polypeptide backbone of glycophorin A has been discussed in detail in the section on Tm and need not be repeated. Suffice it here to say that when the normal amount of NeuAc is reduced (GNAc replacing some NeuAc) anti-Can can apparently sometimes recognize the M polypeptide (untreated red cells Can+). When most or all the NeuAc residues are removed, anti-Can can always recognize the M polypeptide (anti-Can is anti-M in tests against neuraminidase-treated red cells).

The Antigen Mit

In 1980, Battista et al. (96) described an antibody that caused a strongly positive DAT in the child born to the antibody-maker, but that apparently did not cause very much in vivo red cell destruction since the child required only phototherapy. The IgG antibody was called anti-Mit. In the subsequent investigation, Battista et al. (96) tested anti-Mit against more than 50 samples each of which carried a low incidence antigen and Mit+ red cells with more than 70 sera that contained antibodies to rare antigens. The Mit antigen was shown to differ from all antigens of low incidence carried on the red cell samples tested, or defined by the antibodies used. In tests on the red cells of random donors, three Mit+ samples were

found among 900 persons tested in Vancouver and one among 2411 tested in Winnipeg (i.e. 1 in 828 in the combined Canadian studies). Like the original family with Mit+ red cells, the four additional individuals of that phenotype were of western European extraction. No Mit+ sample was found in tests on red cells from 555 Manitoba Cree Indians, 662 African Blacks and 500 African East Indians. Lubenko et al. (584) tested the red cells of 17,951 North London blood donors with a rather weak anti-Mit and found four who were Mit+ (1 in 4488). The same authors (584) then tested red cells from an additional 8278 donors with a more potent anti-Mit and found seven with Mit+ red cells (1 in 1183). The ethnic backgrounds of the persons with Mit+ red cells were not mentioned.

In the Canadian study (96) no other example of anti-Mit was found by IAT screening of the sera of 500 pregnant women, nor by testing 660 samples from donors in an automated system.

In 15 informative families studied (96,584-586), *Mit* traveled with *MS* in 13, with *Ms* in one and with *NS* in one. The S antigen encoded by the *MSMit* haplotype may be difficult to detect. However, the degree of difficulty seems to vary greatly dependent on the particular anti-S used. In one study (587) two S+ Mit+ samples from unrelated persons failed to react with one anti-S but reacted with five other antibodies of that specificity. In a different study (586) the red cells of one S+ Mit+ individual reacted weakly with anti-S whereas those of an unrelated individual of the same phenotype reacted normally. In this study (586) it was pointed out that some anti-S contain anti-Mit. In spite of these clues that Mit may be carried on glycophorin B, SDS-PAGE studies (584,586) and immunoblotting (584) did not reveal any abnormality of glycophorin B of Mit+ red cells. Reduced staining intensity did suggest that Mit+ red cells may carry a reduced amount of, at least, S SGP (399). The Mit antigen survives trypsin and chymotrypsin treatment of red cells but is markedly reduced in reactivity on pronase-treated cells (584). The low incidence antigen Doughty, mentioned in the second and third editions of this book, is now known to be the same at Mit (597).

The Antigen Dantu

This is another MN system antigen that can only be described in a comprehensive manner at the biochemical level. Briefly, three different genetic events have been identified as resulting in haplotypes that produce Dantu. In the Dantu+ (Ph) type both a hybrid SGP and normal glycophorin A are present. It is believed that this anti-Lepore (see later) type situation represents the gene fusion or gene conversion of a normal *MN* gene with a *u* allele, i.e. no glycophorin B made by the anti-Lepore type haplotype (289,346,398). In the Dantu+ (NE) type, a hybrid SGP is again involved but is present in a much higher ratio to the normal glycophorin A that is also present, than in the Dantu+ (Ph) type (47,50,554,588-590). As in the Dantu+ (Ph) type, lack of normal glycophorin B suggests that the gene encoding production of the hybrid SGP arose by gene fusion or gene conversion of a normal *MN* gene with a *u* allele. The much higher ratio of hybrid SGP to glycophorin A in the Dantu+ (NE) type than in the Dantu+ (Ph) type suggests that in the NE type the gene encoding production of the hybrid SGP is duplicated. The third Dantu+ phenotype, known as Dantu+ (MD) has two major differences from the NE type. First, the ratio of hybrid SGP to normal glycophorin A is much lower. Second, the phenotype involves presence of the hybrid SGP and of normal glycophorin A and glycophorin B (48,52,590). This of course suggests that in the MD type the gene encoding production of the hybrid SGP arose by gene fusion or gene conversion of normal alleles at both the *MN* and *Ss* loci.

Support for the proposed derivations of the genes encoding production of the Dantu-bearing hybrid SGPs comes from the findings that the Ph and NE types have been found only in Blacks, where *u* is known to be present, while the MD type has been found only in a White, in Whites of course, *u* is very uncommon. It is probable that in all three Dantu+ phenotypes the hybrid SGP is the same and carries N and s, both of which survive protease, i.e. trypsin, chymotrypsin, papain, ficin or pronase treatment of red cells. In the Ph type the hybrid SGP is accompanied by glycophorin A but no glycophorin B. In the NE type, the hybrid SGP is apparently produced in large quantity following duplication of the encoding gene, it is accompanied by glycophorin A but not glycophorin B. In the MD type the hybrid SGP is accompanied by both glycophorin A and glycophorin B. Explanations as to how the genetic events that resulted in different haplotypes encoding production of the Dantu antigen occurred, together with an explanation of Lepore and anti-Lepore (that is not an antibody) for those who (like PDI) are not experts in hemoglobin genetics, are provided in a later section of this chapter.

Since the N antigen on Dantu+ red cells survives treatment of the red cells by ficin, screening for the Dantu+ phenotype can be accomplished by testing ficin-treated red cells with *Vicia graminea* lectin (51,501,591). Unger et al. (51) used this approach and found 16 Dantu+ samples in tests on 3200 (1 in 200) Black American donors, all 16 were of the NE type. Contreras et al. (47) tested 44,112 North London blood donors, most of whom were White and found only one Dantu+, that donor was from Mauritius and was of mixed Black, Indian, English and French extraction. In South Africa, Moores et al. (592) studied 57 Dantu+ persons. They found that the phenotype was rare in

Blacks, Whites and Asians but common, i.e. a 1.1% incidence in South Africans of mixed race. Since the mixed race individuals have Black, White, Asian and Khoi ancestry, it was concluded that *Dantu* was introduced into the population by the Khoi who were originally indigenous in Southern Africa but are now largely confined to the Kalahari desert. The Dantu+ (Ph) type was found (346) in a Zimbabwean family. Although all three Dantu+ phenotypes are rare, except in the mixed population in South Africa, the NE variety is much more common than the others (47,51). As far as we are aware, the Ph and MD varieties have each been found only in one family.

Anti-Dantu has thus far been found only in sera containing other antibodies. It is often present in sera containing multiple antibodies to low incidence antigens and is also seen (47) in sera that contain anti-S or anti-s. When we (347) tested some of the Dantu+ red cells described by Unger et al. (45) and by Skradski et al. (586) we found that seven of nine anti-S and two of six anti-U contained anti-Dantu. In tests on serum samples from 1348 normal donors, Contreras et al. (47) found no example of anti-Dantu. Other than causing a positive DAT but apparently no clinical HDN in a child born to a woman with anti-Dantu in the serum (47), nothing seems to have been published about the clinical significance of the antibody.

The Antigen Os^a

In 1983, Seno et al. (97) described a new low incidence antigen, Os^a. Although *Os^a* appeared to travel with *Ms* in the Japanese family studied, there were insufficient data to include Os^a in the MN system at that time. Tests on samples from some 50,000 Japanese donors failed to identify another Os(a+) blood. Anti-Os^a was found in several sera containing multiple antibodies to low incidence antigens but not in any of 100,000 sera from Japanese donors.

In 1993, Daniels et al. (98) used immunoblotting studies to show that Os^a is apparently carried on a form of glycophorin A of normal molecular weight. The monoclonal antibody-specific immobilization of erythrocyte antigens (MAIEA) method (524) was used to provide additional proof that Os^a is carried on glycophorin A. Two MAb to glycophorin A and anti-Os^a provided such evidence, a third MAb and anti-Os^a showed mutual blocking, the specificity of that MAb suggested that Os^a is carried in the region of glycophorin A close to residue 40 (98). Such a location would be consistent with the findings (97,98) that Os^a is resistant to trypsin treatment of Os(a+) red cells but is denatured or removed when red cells are treated with papain, ficin or pronase. As mentioned above, the trypsin-sensitive site of normal glycophorin A is at residue 39, the papain/ficin sensitive site is at residue 56 (see figure 15-6).

The Antigen Sext

In 1983, Wright et al. (178) described an IgG antibody made by a never transfused White male, that agglutinated the red cells of 79 of 335 (24%) Black donors. The antibody was provisionally called anti-Sext. All the Sext+ samples were also N+. Among 170 M+ N+ samples, 47 (28%) were Sext+, among 96 M- N+ samples, 32 (33%) were Sext+, all of 69 M+ N- samples were Sext-. Also among the Sext+ samples were 11 that were Tm+ but two Sext+ Tm- samples were also seen. Ant-Sext agglutinated 10 of 13 Hu+ samples, one non-reactive Hu+ was shown to adsorb anti-Sext. The Sext antigen was denatured or removed when red cells were treated with neuramindase, trypsin, papain or ficin. As can be seen, the Sext determinant had some of the features of Tm and some of Hu. However, it seemed that anti-Sext differed from anti-Tm in terms of specificity and in the fact that it failed to react with the red cells of any White donors (25% of White donors were found to be Tm+ in the original studies (70,77)). Anti-Sext seemed closer to anti-Hu than to anti-Tm in specificity but the incidence of Sext+ samples was much higher than that reported for Hu, in any study. As described above for M_1, Hu, Tm and Can, it seems likely (485) that expression of Sext is influenced, at least in part, by different to normal glycosylation of glycophorin A.

The Antigen SAT

In 1991, Daniels et al. (101) described the low incidence antigen, SAT, that was present in members of two Japanese families. Screening tests with a serum known to contain anti-NFLD (see Chapter 17) were performed on red cell samples from 10,480 Japanese donors. One reactive sample, Sat, was found but the reactive red cells were shown to be NFLD- in tests with other sera containing anti-NFLD. The newly defined antigen was called SAT and tests with SAT+ red cells revealed the presence of anti-SAT in three other sera. Two of these, Mess and Flo were known to contain multiple antibodies to low incidence antigens (at least 18 such antibodies in serum Mess and at least five in serum Flo), the third was found in screening tests on donor sera with SAT+ red cells.

The red cells of the proposita and those of her SAT+ sib were shown to carry a weakened form of M but otherwise appeared to have normal expressions of glycophorin A and B. When anti-SAT was used to test other samples, presence of the SAT antigen in a quite different circumstance was revealed. The red cells of a donor suspected of being En(a-) were found to be M- N+ S- s- U- En^{a}TS+ En^{a}FS+ En^{a}FR- Wr(a-b-) SAT+. Her serum was described as containing anti-En^{a}FR and/or anti-Wr^b. SDS-PAGE and immunoblotting studies suggested that the red cells of this individual and those of the members of her family who had SAT+ red cells, carried a GP.A-B hybrid glycophorin. Unlike all previously described A-B hybrids, this one appeared not to carry S, s or U. Analysis of cDNA showed that the SAT-carrying hybrid is the reverse of the Dantu-bearing B-A hybrid (593).

Uchikawa et al. (594) then found six more SAT+ propositi in Japan, three of them had the hybrid SGP described above, the other three had apparently normal glycophorin A and B. It is currently believed (593,594) that a three amino acid, glycophorin B derived insert, in the glycophorin A of the individuals who do not carry the hybrid SGP, creates a six amino acid sequence that is present in the hybrid SGP, at the junction of the glycophorin A and glycophorin B-derived material, and that this sequence creates the SAT antigen in two otherwise rather different phenotypes.

The Miltenberger Series of Antigens

In 1946, Graydon (598) described a low incidence antigen, that became known as Gr. The antigen was not recognized as being part of any known blood group system. In 1951, Levine et al. (56) described another low incidence antigen, to which they gave the name Mi^a. Again, no relationship between the antigen and any known blood group system was apparent. In 1954, Hart et al. (58) described a low incidence antigen that they called Vw. This time the investigation strongly suggested that the antigen was part of the MN blood group system. In 1959, Simmons et al. (599) showed that Gr and Vw are the same thing, in spite of the earlier discovery of Gr, the name Vw has persisted, perhaps because at the time of its discovery Vw was placed in the MN system. The association between Mi^a and Vw(Gr) that allowed Mi^a to be considered as an MN system antigen was that all known Vw+ samples were also Mi(a+). The reverse was not true, some Mi(a+) samples were Vw- (600). At this early stage in investigation of these antigens it was not clear whether the Mi(a-) Vw+ phenotype did not exist or whether all examples of anti-Mi^a contained anti-Vw. If the latter explanation obtained, it was clear that anti-Mi^a and anti-Vw were inseparable in the sera studied. By 1966, two more antibodies apparently defining antigens related to Mi^a had been described. Some Vw- Mi(a+) red cells reacted with the sera anti-Mur (62) and anti-Hil (601) while others reacted with anti-Mur but not with anti-Hil. In 1966, Cleghorn (72) published a summary of the findings made to that point and introduced the Miltenberger subsystem classification by which red cells were identified by class. In the 1966 publication, classes Mi.I to Mi.IV and antibodies to Vw, Mi^a, Mur and Hil were listed. Shortly thereafter, Cleghorn (508) added the red cell class Mi.V and the antibody anti-Hut. Primarily for historical interest the reactions of the first five Mi classes and those of the first five antibodies are shown in table 15-13. As described below (see footnote to table 15-14) the original interpretation of anti-Hut, as shown in table 15-13, has been changed. Since 1966 many new antigens and antibodies apparently related to the Miltenberger classes shown in table 15-13 have been described. By 1992, eleven Miltenberger classes (Mi.I to Mi.XI) had been defined using ten different antibodies to low incidence antigens (table 15-14) (for names of the antigens defined and references to publications describing the antibodies, see below). Throughout the history of the Miltenberger series, serological work has often been complicated by the fact that some sera contain monospecific antibodies while others contain mixtures of antibodies. In some sera containing more than one antibody, the specificities can be separated by appropriate adsorp-

tion. In others, with apparently identical mixtures of antibodies, the specificities are inseparable. The Miltenberger subsystem, as it used to be called, was held together by the facts that many of the antibodies involved reacted with the red cells of more than one Miltenberger class and that in nine of the eleven classes between two and five of the recognized antigens were shown to be present. In 1991, Daniels et al. (602) reported that M^g+ red cells

TABLE 15-13 The First Five Miltenberger Classes as Described by Cleghorn (72,508)

Red Cell Class	Antigens: +=Present, 0=Absent				
	Vw	Mi^a	Mur	Hil	Hut[*1]
Mi.I	+	+	0	0	0
Mi.II	0	+	0	0	+
Mi.III	0	+	+	+	+
Mi.IV	0	+	+	0	+
Mi.V	0	0	0	+	0

[*1] Anti-Hut is now interpreted differently. See footnote Number 1 in table 15-14.

TABLE 15-14 Proposed New Terminology for the Miltenberger Phenotypes (for derivation and references, see text)

Mi Class	First Proband	New Name for Glycophorin	Antigens: +=Present, 0=Absent, nt=not tested									
			Vw	Hut[*1]	Mur	MUT[*1]	Hil	TSEN	MINY	Hop	Nob	DANE
Mi.I	Vw	GP.Vw	+	0	0	0	0	0	0	0	0	0
Mi.II	Hut	GP.Hut	0	+	0	+	0	0	0	0	0	0
Mi.III	Mur	GP.Mur	0	0	+	+	+	0	+	0	0	0
Mi.IV	Hop	GP.Hop	0	0	+	+	0	+	+	+	0	0
Mi.V	Rog	GP.Hil[*2]	0	0	0	0	+	0	+	0	0	0
Mi.VI	Bun	GP.Bun	0	0	+	+	+	0	+	+	0	0
Mi.VII	Nob	GP.Nob	0	0	0	0	0	0	0	0	+	0
Mi.VIII	Joh	GP.Joh	0	0	0	0	0	nt	0	+	+	0
Mi.IX	Dane	GP.Dane	0	0	+	0	0	0	0	0	0	+
Mi.X	HF	GP.HF[*3]	0	0	0	+	+	0	+	0	0	0
Mi.XI	JR[*4]	GP.JL[*4]	0	0	0	nt	0	+	+	0	0	0

[*1] Anti-Hut as originally defined (72, 508) reacted with class II, III and IV red cells (see table 15-13). Giles (497) and Giles et al. (90) revised that definition and described anti-Hut as specific for class II (605). The reaction with classes III and IV was attributed to inseparable anti-Mur in the anti-Hut sera. The term anti-MUT is used to describe inseparable anti-Hut+Mur (606, 607) so that anti-MUT of Tippett et al. (104) is the same as the anti-Hut of Cleghorn (72, 508).

[*2] Although the original proband was Rog, Mi.V was long associated with the low incidence antigen Hil. Thus the glycophorin is called GP.Hil.

[*3] GP.HF was previously called GP.Mor (104).

[*4] Although JR was the first proband (288), the molecular basis of the phenotype was first determined on JL (295, 553). Hence the glycophorin is called GP.JL.

react with anti-DANE (see below) the eighth antibody added to the Miltenberger series. Further (475,602), M^g+ red cells reacted with the original anti-Mur (again see below) but not with 14 other examples of that antibody. Since M^g had long been established as an MN system antigen in its own right, its potential for admission into the Miltenberger subsystem proved to be the feather (59) that broke the subsystem's back. Tippett et al. (104) pointed out that still more phenotypes would be added to the subsystem and considered that regarding the antigens as members of a subsystem was a concept that had outlived its usefulness. Further, by 1992 the biochemical basis of many of the antigens was understood, they did not all have common features and in many instances it had been shown that various different genetic mechanisms were responsible for production of variant or hybrid glycophorins that carried the antigens. Tippett et al. (104) proposed that the glycophorins on which the various antigens were carried be used to describe each type. For example, GP.Vw would described the glycophorin carrying the Vw antigen. Such a terminology could then be used to describe other variants for which the glycophorin composition was known, whether or not the antigens associated with the variants had previously been considered to be part of the Miltenberger subsystem. An example of such additional use (603) would be GP.MEP to describe the hybrid glycophorin on the En(a-) red cells (En(a-)(UK)) of the English proposita (see section on En^a) although those red cells do not carry any known low incidence MN system antigen. Although the new terminology introduced by Tippett et al. (104) and used by Reid and Tippett (603) is clearly the most suitable for use in describing the old Miltenberger subsystem, it is equally clear that the original terminology will persist for some time. Further, most of the publications about the antigens and antibodies involved are written in the old terminology. Accordingly, in the following sections both terms for a given Miltenberger class will be used.

Ironically, by the time the new terminology was introduced, a time at which much had already been learned about the biochemistry involved, considerable doubt had arisen about the existence of a separate Mi^a antigen. It is now believed that the original serum from Mrs. Miltenberger (56) and others that appeared to have the same specificity, actually contained a variable number of antibodies defining (at least) the antigens Vw, Mur, Hut and MUT. Certainly no monospecific anti-Mi^a can be isolated from such sera. Thus the serum that gave its name to the subsystem is no longer considered to have contained a single antibody, anti-Mi^a, nor is an Mi^a antigen believed to exist (104,603).

Table 15-14 lists: the term originally used to describe the Miltenberger class; the name of the first proband of that class; the name proposed to describe the antigen-bearing glycophorin; then lists the antigens detected on the red cells. The table has been assembled from the publications of Tippett et al. (104), Reid and Tippett (603), Dahr (604) and Daniels (9). Clearly, given the complexity and even more importantly the variety of glycophorins on which the ten antigens listed in table 15-14 are carried, their description is best given at the biochemical level. Accordingly, the rest of this section will describe the incidence of the antigens (when known) and the reactions and clinical relevance of the antibodies directed against them. The glycophorins themselves and the molecular events leading to formation of the genes that encode their production, are described in later sections of this chapter.

Former Miltenberger Subsystem Members. 1. Anti-Mi^a

As described above, the antibody originally (56) called anti-Mi^a, and other examples of ostensibly the same specificity (600,608,609) are now regarded as having been mixtures of antibodies directed against Vw and/or Mur and/or Hut and/or MUT. From the results of serological studies, Sabo (610) and from the results of biochemical studies, Anstee (509), concluded that all reactivity previously attributed to anti-Mi^a could be explained by the actions of the other antibodies present. Thus the currently accepted view (104,603) is that Mi^a does not exist as a separate antigen. It is, of course, for this reason that Mi^a is not listed in table 15-14. Before anti-Mi^a was excluded as a distinct specificity a number of studies (56,58,72,598-600,611-613) had shown that in Whites the incidence of Mi.I (then Mi(a+) Vw+) was about 1 in 1800 and the incidence of Mi.II (then Mi(a+) Vw-) was about 1 in 1600. Again before thinking about anti-Mi^a changed, one example was reported (614) to have caused HDN.

Former Miltenberger Subsystem Members. 2. Vw and Anti-Vw

As can be seen from table 15-14, anti-Vw defines an antigen that is one of only three present on the red cells of a single former subclass. Anti-Vw was first described by Hart et al. (58) and as mentioned above defined the same antigen as anti-Gr (598). Race and Sanger (7) reviewed many published and unpublished data and found that 30 Vw+ bloods had been found in tests on 52,635 samples from Whites (i.e. an incidence of 1 in 1755). In South East Switzerland 22 Vw+ samples were found (510) among 1541 tested (1 in 70) while in Thailand one Vw+ sample was found in tests on red cells from 2500 individuals (615). This last finding contrasts sharply with the high incidence of Mur and Hop found in Oriental populations (see below). In 1993, Spruell et al. (106) described an individual apparently homozygous for the gene encoding GP.Vw (i.e. a V^w homozygote). The proposita's serum contained anti-En^{a}TS, a finding in complete agreement with the earlier findings of Dahr et al. (616) that the glycophorin A of Vw+ red cells contains an amino acid substitution (see below) within its trypsin-sensitive region, an observation subsequently confirmed by others (617-619).

In contrast to the rarity of the Vw antigen, anti-Vw is a common antibody (58,598,609); in deliberate searches anti-Vw has been found in one serum of about every hundred tested (62,599,620,621). Like other antibodies to low incidence antigens, anti-Vw is found frequently in sera that contain multiple antibodies to such antigens and as an alloantibody in the sera of patients with "warm" autoantibody-induced hemolytic anemia (72). Of eight samples tested by Smith et al. (622) seven were IgG and one a mixture of IgG and IgM. Anti-Vw has caused, sometimes severe, HDN (614,617,623-625). In one case, in which a double volume exchange transfusion was required, the DAT on the infant's red cells was negative (625), the findings were reminiscent of those described earlier in which anti-M has caused severe HDN with a negative DAT.

The literature contains one report (626) in which it is claimed that an anti-Mi^a plus anti-Vw caused a fatal transfusion reaction involving intravascular hemolysis. However, it is impossible to accept the conclusions drawn. First, the antibody was predominantly IgM but did not fix complement. By definition, intravascular hemolysis is complement mediated (136,627). Second, the antibody was optimally reactive at room temperature and no evidence was presented to show that the positive reactions seen at 37°C were not simply "carry-over" from tests at lower temperatures. Third, one of the major pieces of evidence to support the claim that intravascular hemolysis had occurred involved the post-transfusion plasma hemoglobin level. Avoy (628) pointed out that the level reported could have resulted from the destruction of as little as 27 ml of the packed red cells. Even when given a second opportunity to explain how a predominantly IgM, non-complement binding antibody (the IgG component did not bind complement either) could cause intravascular hemolysis, the author (629) failed to do so.

Former Miltenberger Subsystem Members. 3. Hut and Anti-Hut

When first described (72,508) anti-Hut was believed to detect an antigen on red cells at that time classified as being Mi.II, Mi.III and Mi.IV (see table 15-13).

However, in 1975, Chandanayingyong and Pejrachandra (605) described a serum containing anti-Mur (see below) and anti-Hut, from which the anti-Hut could be isolated. It was shown that once separated from the anti-Mur, the anti-Hut reacted with Mi.II but not with Mi.III or Mi.IV red cells. Giles (497) and Giles et al. (90) revised the definition of anti-Hut and described it as specific for an antigen on Mi.II cells (see table 15-14), that retained the name Hut, and is now described as being present on GP.Hut. The reactions of Mi.III and Mi.IV red cells with sera that contain anti-Hut and anti-Mur are now believed to represent the presence of Mur, not Hut, on the red cells. However, the explanation is not that simple. Some sera that at first appear to contain inseparable anti-Hut plus anti-Mur have a specificity that cannot be fully explained in those terms. That specificity is now (104) called anti-MUT, and is described below.

The Hut antigen, i.e. based on the new definition of GP.Hut, was found in: 1 in 1552 Whites from tests on over 29,000 samples (62,600,643); 1 of 3350 Japanese (644) and 1 of 2500 Thais (615). Anti-Hut has been incriminated as causative of HDN (600,645,646) but, in retrospect, it is difficult to determine whether anti-Hut or anti-MUT was involved.

Former Miltenberger Subsystem Members. 4. Mur and Anti-Mur

When anti-Mur was first found (62) it was seen to detect an antigen present on what were then called Mi.III and Mi.IV red cells (see table 15-13). The antibody was often present in sera described at that time as anti-Mi^a, sometimes anti-Mur was a separable component in such sera. Anti-Mur as an apparent single specificity was also found (72,609,613,630). As described above, it was later found that anti-Mur and anti-Hut frequently occur in the same sera, sometimes as separate entities and sometimes in an inseparable form. Again as described below, the sera containing inseparable anti-Mur and anti-Hut are now regarded as containing a different specificity, anti-MUT (104). As shown in table 15-14, anti-Mur was later shown to react with red cells given the Miltenberger class designations VI and IX.

The gene encoding GP.Mur (as present on the previously called Mi.III red cells) is common in Oriental peoples. Chandanayingyong and Pejrachandra (615) found 241 samples carrying GP.Mur in tests on 2500 donors in Thailand, i.e. 9.6%. Similarly, GP.Mur was found in 7.3% of Chinese people in Taiwan (631) and 6.3% of Chinese people in Hong Kong (632). In contrast, in four large studies (62,72,613,633) on the red cells of White donors, only six Mur+ were found in tests on 50,101 samples, i.e. 0.012%.

Anti-Mur has been incriminated as causative of hemolytic transfusion reactions (631,634,635) and HDN (631,635-638); in at least one case the antibody was probably responsible for hydrops fetalis. As would be expected, these cases occurred in Oriental populations. As would also be expected, anti-Mur is found frequently in these populations. It was found in: 99 of 49,750 (0.2%) patients in Thailand (609); 60 of about 21,500 (0.28%) patients in Taiwan; and 34 of 52,334 (0.06%) blood donors in Hong Kong (639). The higher incidence of the antibody in patients than in donors (as shown above the incidence of the antigen in Hong Kong approaches the incidences in Thailand and Taiwan) suggests that at least some examples of anti-Mur are red cell stimulated. The fact that Mur+ red cells and anti-Mur are common in the Hong Kong and Taiwan populations has engendered considerable debate (634,635,640-642) as to whether Mur+ (GP.Mur, Mi.III) red cells should be used in antibody screening tests in those countries. While the incidence figures for the antigen and antibody suggest that such a policy would be desirable, the situation is complicated by the fact that many of the antibodies are reactive only at temperatures below 37°C. Thus the cost effectiveness of adding an additional red cell sample to all antibody-screening tests, has been questioned.

Former Miltenberger Subsystem Members. 5. MUT and Anti-MUT

As mentioned in the previous two subsections, anti-Hut and anti-Mur often occur together. When they can be separated or when one of them occurs as a single specificity, their reactions are as shown in table 15-14. For some time it was thought that all the reactivity of sera containing anti-Hut and anti-Mur could be explained by the actions of those antibodies. However, it has now been shown (100) that GP.Dane (formerly Mi.IX) red cells react with separable anti-Mur but not with sera containing apparently inseparable anti-Hut plus anti-Mur. GP.HF (formerly Mi.X) red cells do not react with separated anti-Mur or anti-Hut but do react with sera containing those antibodies in an inseparable form (104,108). Thus it is now apparent that sera containing anti-Hut and anti-Mur in an inseparable form, contain an additional specificity that has been named (104,603) anti-MUT. GP.Dane (Mi.IX) red cells are Hut- Mur+ MUT-, while GP.HF (Mi.IX) red cells are Hut- Mur- MUT+. When sera ostensibly containing anti-Hut and anti-Mur are studied, various patterns are seen (104). Most such sera do not contain a separable anti-Hut (605) component. Many contain anti-MUT sometimes with separable anti-Mur. A few contain just separable anti-Hut and anti-Mur. One has been found (607) that appears to

contain just anti-MUT. As mentioned in an earlier section, it is no longer clear whether the cases of HDN attributed to anti-Hut (600,645,646) were due to that antibody or to anti-MUT. In retrospect, it seems very likely that the HDN that we (648) described in successive infants born to a Vietnamese woman living in Canada, were caused by anti-MUT. The antibody involved appeared to be inseparable anti-Vw plus anti-Hut plus anti-Mur, the red cells of the infants' father were Vw- but reactive with an anti-Hut/Mur serum and with anti-Hil (see below) i.e. probably GP.Mur.

Former Miltenberger Subsystem Members. 6. Hil and Anti-Hil

In 1963, Worlledge et al. (601) studied but did not describe in print, a new antibody that was later (72) named anti-Hil. The antibody reacted with red cells that at that time were called Mi.III. The antibody did not react with Mi.I, Mi.II or Mi.IV red cells so could be seen to lack antibody activity for Vw, Mi^a and Mur. In 1970, Crossland et al. (74) described a phenotype in which the red cells were Hil+ but Mi(a-) Mur- so clearly differed from Mi.III. The new phenotype (see table 15-13) was given the designation Mi.V (now GP.Hil). Mi.V red cells were the first ones associated with the Miltenberger subsystem that failed to react with then named anti-Mi^a reagents. That observation is now recognized as reflecting the fact that Mi.V (GP.Hil) red cells lack the antigens Vw, Hut, Mur and MUT (i.e. those recognized by the polyspecific sera originally called anti-Mi^a).

The original anti-Hil (74), that caused HDN, was the only one available for 12 years. In 1982, Ellisor et al. (650) described the second example, it was the only antibody detectable in the serum of a multiply transfused woman. Other anti-Hil have since been detected but not described in the literature. Although additional Hil+ red cell samples have been described (287,649), shortage of anti-Hil has prevented large scale studies.

Former Miltenberger Subsystem Members. 7. TSEN and Anti-TSEN

As far as we are aware, the example of anti-TSEN described by Reid et al. (102) is the only one to have been found. It was present in the serum of a woman who had been transfused many times. The antibody reacted strongly by IAT and following some initial clues that the antibody reacted with red cells carrying an A-B hybrid glycophorin, extension tests were performed. Anti-TSEN was found (102) to react with some other red cell samples that carried A-B hybrid glycophorins, if those cells were also S+. As shown in table 15-14 red cells with GP.Hop (Mi.IV) and those with GP.JL (Mi.XI) are TSEN+. As discussed in detail in the section on the biochemistry of the MN system, the initial investigation (102) of anti-TSEN resulted in recognition of the structure of the TSEN antigen.

Former Miltenberger Subsystem Members. 8. MINY and Anti-MINY

In a paper immediately following the one describing anti-TSEN, Reid et al. (103) described the only known example of anti-MINY. The antibody was made by a woman who had been pregnant three times and had also received transfusions. Her serum contained antibodies to S, Vw, Mit, Dantu, St^a and Wr^a and a saline agglutinin that reacted with a hitherto unrecognized low incidence antigen. The authors (103) named the new specificity anti-MINY and, as was the case with anti-TSEN, showed that it detected an antigen present on some glycophorin A-B hybrids. Unlike anti-TSEN, anti-MINY reacted with some cells carrying glycophorin A-B hybrids, regardless of the S or s status of those red cells. As shown in table 15-14, anti-MINY reacts with GP.Mur (Mi.III), GP.Hop (Mi.IV), GP.Hil (Mi.V), GP.Bun (Mi.VI), GP.HF (Mi.X) and GP.JL (Mi.XI) red cells. A number of Japanese individuals with GP.HF (Mi.X) red cells have been found but not yet described in full reports (594,657). As can also be seen from table 15-14, all red cells that are Hil+ are MINY+, not all MINY+ cells are Hil+. As discussed in the section on biochemistry, anti-MINY also reacts with some red cells that carry glycophorin A-B hybrids, that were never included in the Miltenberger subsystem. Again similarly to the situation with anti-TSEN, the initial investigation of anti-MINY resulted in characterization of the structure of the MINY determinant.

Former Miltenberger Subsystem Members. 9. Hop and Anti-Hop

In three papers published simultaneously in 1977 (89-91) the sera Anek, Raddon and Lane that among them contain various permutations of anti-Hop and anti-Nob (see below) were described. The Anek serum, from a Thai man who had never been transfused and whose red cells were of the Mi.III phenotype, was originally called anti-Hop. However, more recently the Anek serum has been described (104) as anti-Hop plus anti-Nob since it reacts with both GP.Hop (Mi.IV) and GP.Nob (Mi.VII) red cells. As shown in table 15-14 GP.Hop (Mi.IV) red cells are Hop+ Nob-, while GP.Nob

(Mi.VII) cells are Hop- Nob+. Other examples of anti-Hop found (497,652,653) since the Anek serum was described (89,90) have been seen to react with GP.Hop (Mi.IV, Hop+ Nob-) but not with GP.Nob (Mi.VII, Hop- Nob+) red cells. As shown in table 15-14, anti-Hop reacts with GP.Hop (Mi.IV), GP.Bun (Mi.VI) and GP.Joh (Mi.VIII) red cells. In tests on samples from 2500 Thai individuals, 17 (1 in 147) were found (89,615) to react with the Anek serum.

Former Miltenberger Subsystem Members. 10. Nob and Anti-Nob

In the three papers (89-91) mentioned in the introduction to the section on anti-Hop, two sera, Raddon and Lane were described as having anti-Nob specificity. More recently (104) the Raddon serum has been described as containing anti-Nob and a weak anti-Hop since it reacts weakly with GP.Hop (Mi.IV) and GP.Bun (Mi.VI) red cells. The Lane serum is still regarded as containing anti-Nob. A second example of the Raddon-type serum that may have caused a very mild transfusion reaction (654) appeared to have anti-Nob plus anti-Hop specificity, the red cells transfused were of the GP.Nob (Mi.VII) phenotype. As shown in table 15-14, anti-Nob reacts with GP.Nob (Mi.VII) and GP.Joh (Mi.VIII) red cells. In tests on samples from 4929 English donors, three (1 in 1643) were found (91) to have Nob+ red cells. In tests on 1766 donors in the USA, among whom the number of White and Black donors was not known, no Nob+ sample was found (654).

Former Miltenberger Subsystem Members. 11. DANE and Anti-DANE

Anti-DANE was found by Skov et al. (100) in the serum of a never transfused Danish man. Although relatively little of the antibody was obtained before the patient died, the fact that DANE+ red cells carry a trypsin-resistant M antigen allowed some screening to be done. Skov et al. (100) found two DANE+ samples by screening trypsin-treated red cells from 467 Danish blood donors with a monoclonal anti-M. In all, including the original DANE+ samples and the two found by deliberate screening, four families with members with DANE+ red cells, were studied. It was shown (100,655) that the presence of the DANE antigen was associated with yet another glycophorin A-B hybrid molecule, this time one from which the usual glycophorin A-borne trypsin-sensitive site had been lost and on which glycosylation changes had occurred. The GP.DANE (Mi.IX) hybrid (that probably arose by gene conversion (655)) molecule also carries Mur. It is possible that the presence of an asparagine residue in the M^g glycophorin A (see earlier) accounts for the reaction of M^g+ red cells with anti-DANE. As mentioned in an earlier section, M^g+ red cells reacted with anti-DANE and the original anti-Mur, but not with 12 others examples of anti-Mur (475). It is perhaps fitting that anti-DANE should be the last of the antibodies formerly considered to be part of the Miltenberger subsystem to be described. As mentioned in the introduction, it was the finding (475) that M^g+ red cells are DANE+ that called into question the usefulness of continuing to consider Miltenberger as a subsystem (104,603).

Close Relatives of the Now Extinct Miltenberger Subsystem

In spite of the length of these sections on the former Miltenberger subsystem, not all the available data have been included. Were the subsystem terms to continue to be used to describe antigens and antibodies, there are others that could be added (605). Indeed, in some instances a better case could be made for the inclusion of some new phenotypes than was made when some of the existing phenotypes were added. As a single example, red cells that carry GP.Kip were found (656) to be Mur+ Hil+ MINY+ MUT+ and to react with sera (Anek and Raddon) that contain anti-Hop and anti-Nob although they did not react with sera containing only anti-Hop or anti-Nob. Again, complexities such as this are best explained in biochemical terms and are discussed in more detail in later sections of this chapter.

The Former Miltenberger Subsystem, Additional Comments

Readers who have ploughed through the subsections on the former Miltenberger subsystem (who must thus be commended for perseverance and tenacity although their judgment may be questioned) will now understand the earlier comment that one of us (PDI) chose to delay writing those subsections for as long as possible. It may also be asked why an extinct subject should be discussed so exhaustively and exhaustingly. The answer, of course, is that the antigens and antibodies have not gone away, they are simply no longer regarded as being inexorably linked. In fact the biochemistry of the MN system is such that almost any combination of antigens may be able to occur on an unusual glycophorin. Complex and confusing as the serology may be, it represents reactions that can be logically and systematically explained at the biochemical and molecular genetic levels, as described below.

The M^k Gene and the $M^k M^k$ Genotype

In 1964, Metaxas and Metaxas-Bühler (659) presented evidence for the existence of a gene, M^k, that in the family studied appeared to be a silent allele at, at least the *MN* locus. Other individuals, who apparently had M^k were then found (78,457,467,633,660-663) and it became clear that the gene makes no M, N, S or s and probably no U. For many years no individual of the genotype $M^k M^k$ was known, which meant that the presence of M^k had to be recognized in the heterozygous state. This was usually first suspected in a family study in which an individual with say, M+ N- S+ s- red cells (and thus apparently of the genotype *MS/MS*), passed neither *M* nor *S* to his or her offspring. Supportive evidence for the assumption that M^k was present was then often obtained in serological tests although later (664) of course, biochemical data were used as well. An individual of the M+ N- S+ s- phenotype, who is genetically *MS/M^k* can usually be shown to have only single doses of M and S on his or her red cells. Further, it is now known that when the red cells of persons heterozygous for M^k and a normal *MNSs* haplotype are studied by PAS-staining of SDS-PAGE preparations of the membranes, the staining intensity is only about 50% of normal in the positions to which the MN and Ss SGPs and their complexes migrate (312,469,471). As expected since some 70% of red cell membrane sialic acid is carried on glycophorins A and B, the red cells of M^k heterozygotes have a sialic acid level that is some 35 to 40% below that of normal red cells and have reduced electrophoretic mobility (468). As mentioned several times in this chapter, red cells with a reduced level of sialic acid, such as those of M^k homozygotes and heterozygotes, are agglutinated in saline systems by some Rh antibodies that are otherwise reactive only by IAT or other sensitive methods (498).

As can be seen, M^k differs from both *En* and *u*. While *En* behaves as if it is a silent allele at the *MN* locus and *u* behaves as if it is a silent allele at the *Ss* locus, M^k acts as a silent allele that covers both the *MN* and *Ss* loci. The M^k gene was already known to exist in Whites and Orientals when Tokunaga et al. (292) found a Japanese blood donor and his brother to be of genotype $M^k M^k$. Virtually everything that had been concluded about the M^k gene, from its lack of action in M^k heterozygotes, was proved from the study of these men. No PAS staining bands corresponding to the carbohydrates (sialic acid) normally carried on glycophorin A and B were seen when SDS-PAGE preparations were examined. Further, when lactoperoxidase radioiodination was used, no polypeptide structures corresponding to the backbones of the MN or Ss SGP were seen, confirming the total absence of both glycophorins from the red cells. The sialic acid content of the red cells of the M^k homozygotes was about 30% of normal. There was no evidence to suggest that the MN or Ss SGPs had been replaced by hybrid forms. As a result of the absence of glycophorins A and B, the red cells of the M^k homozygotes typed as M- N- S- s- U- 'N'- and were non-reactive with all other MN system antibodies with which they were tested. As expected, the red cells were also Wr(a-b-) and since they totally lacked glycophorin A, were EnªTS- EnªFS- EnªFR-.

Probably because they had never been transfused, neither of the M^k homozygotes had anti-glycophorin A (anti-Enª) or anti-glycophorin B (anti-U, anti-N reacting with N and 'N') in the serum. One of them had a non-red cell immune antibody that was, in all probability anti-Pr. As explained in detail in Chapter 34, there are a series of antigens in the Pr series, that are sialic acid (N-acetyl neuraminic acid) dependent and are carried in the carbohydrate side chains (see figure 15-3) attached to red cell glycophorins. The red cells of M^k homozygotes are not Pr- since non-MN system related glycophorins (glycophorins C and D, see Chapter 16) carry similar carbohydrate side chains. However, the lack of glycophorins A and B from the red cells of M^k homozygotes results in those cells carrying a very markedly reduced level of the Pr antigens. Thus it is likely that M^k homozygotes with a reduced number of copies of the Pr antigens, can make anti-Pr, just as A_2 persons with a reduced number of copies of A, can make anti-A_1. Unfortunately, in the study on the red cells of the two M^k homozygotes (296) no tests were performed to prove the specificity of the supposed anti-Pr. That antibody would be expected to be adsorbed rapidly by red cells with normal levels of glycophorins A and B, slowly by En(a-) red cells because of their lack of glycophorin A and even more slowly by the red cells of the M^k homozygotes on which the Pr antigens would only be present on glycophorins C and D that are carried in far fewer copies than glycophorins A and B (see Chapter 16). Anti-Pr would also be expected to survive adsorption with neuramindase-treated red cells (NeuAc and hence Pr removed by the enzyme).

Since the report by Tokunaga et al. (296) appeared, the M^kM^k genotype has been found in two Japanese sisters (298) whose parents were, like those of the M^kM^k brothers of Tokunaga et al. (296) consanguineous. It has also been found in a Black American child (297) and a Turkish woman and her brother (561).

In some of the early reports on M^k in the heterozygous state, an antibody described as anti-M^k was mentioned (78,661). The antibody, found in a number of sera, reacted weakly with the red cells of M^k heterozygotes but not with normal red cells. Since it is now known that M^k encodes no production of glycophorin A or B, nor any replacement structure, it seems that anti-

M^k could not exist. In retrospect it seems probable that "anti-M^k" was actually a property of some normal sera that could cause agglutination of red cells with a reduced level of sialic acid. Less likely, the sera may have been recognizing the increased level of glycosylation of band 3 that is characteristic of the red cells of individuals with M^k and En (296,298,469).

The Allele N^2

In 1935, Crome (647) described an individual whose red cells carried a weakened form of N. In 1939, Friedenreich (651) found a second example of apparently the same phenotype, named it N_2 and showed that the condition was apparently controlled by an allele at the MN locus. A number of other bloods with weakened expression of N were also said (665-667) to be of the N_2 phenotype. In 1968, Metaxas et al. (78) presented results from a large study on bloods with unusual MN phenotypes. These workers (78) felt that the term N_2 had been used to describe a heterogeneous group of samples, so redefined the term. N^2 was now said to cause production of weak but "complete" N. In other words, the difference between N_2 and N was strictly quantitative. Metaxas et al. (78) believed that previous use of the term had implied the presence of "incomplete" N, that is there appeared to be a qualitative difference between some forms of N_2 and N. The new definition of N^2 also stated that it made weak N, but no M. The published descriptions of the N^2 gene and the N_2 phenotype are mostly rather old. The only one of which we are aware that has been published (737) since the biochemical nature of M and N was established did not include any biochemical findings. It is, of course, entirely possible that some alleles of M and N encode production of fewer copies of M and N SGP. Such differences would present at both the serological and biochemical level as simple quantitative variations.

Throughout their somewhat checkered history, the phenotype N_2 and the gene N^2 have been known to differ from the weak form of N, also called N_2 that, as described below, is associated with an inherited positive DAT.

The Allele S^2

In 1964, Hurd et al. (668) described a variant form of an antigen that they called S_2, that seemed to be a weakened form of S. S_2 did not seem to differ from S in any qualitative manner. Inheritance of the S_2 phenotype in the large family studied was such that production of the antigen could be explained by postulating an allele, S^2, at the Ss locus. The S^2 gene traveled with M in the

family studied and its presence did not seem to affect the actions of *M*. It is not known if the weakened form of S in the family was associated with presence of the Mit antigen (see above), that was discovered much later.

Inherited Positive DAT Associated with Weakened N and M

In 1962, Jensen and Freiesleben (669) described an individual whose red cells had a positive DAT and carried a weakened expression of N. As mentioned above, the phenotype was called N_2 although in the N_2 phenotype described earlier the DAT was negative. Two other families demonstrating the same phenomenon have been described (670,671). In the families studied the positive DAT was inherited in a dominant fashion but no evidence of an accelerated rate of in vivo red cell clearance was seen in any individual with the positive DAT. A similar phenomenon involving a weak expression of M, that was called M_2, had been described earlier (672,673) in a woman and her child. Again, neither the mother nor the child had hemolytic anemia. Although the positive DAT associated with weak M was described before that associated with N, more family members with weak N have been studied. As with the N_2 phenotype described earlier, no studies on this phenomenon seem to have been performed since the biochemical structure of M and N became known.

The Antigen Duclos

In 1979, Habibi et al. (413) described an antibody that reacted with almost all red cells tested. The antigen defined, that the investigators named Duclos, was poorly expressed on Rh_{null} red cells that typed as U+ and on U− cells that had normal Rh antigens. Rh_{null} red cells that typed as U− could be shown to carry the Duclos antigen only by use of adsorption-elution studies. Current thinking (412) is that expression of the antigen is dependent on the presence of normal glycophorin B and normal Rh glycoproteins (414). The antigen is described in more detail in Chapter 31.

Enzyme Sensitive Sites On and Number of Copies of Glycophorin A and B

Although these topics are both covered in more detail in the sections on biochemistry of the MN system, they are mentioned here in relation to the way in which they affect MN system serology. As shown in figure 15-6, the composition of normal glycophorin A (17,37,38, 235,322,398,471,509,674-649) is such that it has a trypsin sensitive site at residue 39 and a papain/ficin sensitive site at position 56. This means that any antigen carried just on glycophorin A, between residues 1 and about residue 39 will be removed when red cells are treated with trypsin, papain or ficin. Any antigen carried just on glycophorin A, between residues 39 and 56 will survive treatment of red cells with trypsin but will be removed when red cells are treated with papain or ficin. Any antigen carried on glycophorin A between residue 56 and residues 70 to 72, where glycophorin A enters the red cell membrane, will survive treatment of red cells with trypsin, papain and ficin. Because normal N-bearing glycophorin A and glycophorin B are identical from residues 1 to 26 and because glycophorin B lacks the trypsin-sensitive site at residue 39, any antigen common to glycophorin A and B between residues 1 and 26 will be weakened but not totally removed when red cells are treated with trypsin. That is to say, copies on glycophorin A removed, copies on glycophorin B, trypsin-resistant.

As stated, normal glycophorin B lacks the trypsin-sensitive site of normal glycophorin A while in situ on red cells. However, Dahr et al. (321,436) have shown that once isolated from red cells, glycophorin B can be cleaved into several pieces by trypsin. Apparently glycophorin B in situ is folded in such a way that its trypsin-sensitive sites are not accessible to the enzyme. Glycophorin B carries a papain/ficin sensitive site close to the point at which it enters the red cell membrane (321,436). Blood groupers will be well aware that the S and s antigens can be removed when red cells are treated with papain or ficin (17,680-683) but that if the enzymes are used under less than optimal conditions, removal of S and s may not be accomplished (684,685). Perhaps the papain/ficin sensitive site on glycophorin B is not readily accessible to the enzyme. Our finding (340) that one form of U (UPR) survives papain treatment of red cells while another form (UPS) is removed, suggests that the U antigen and the papain-sensitive site on glycophorin B are close to each other.

As mentioned several times in this chapter, the rules regarding trypsin, papain and ficin sensitivity of MN system antigens may become null and void when hybrid glycophorins are considered. As simple examples, on a glycophorin A-B hybrid, M antigen may be present on the glycophorin-A derived portion of the hybrid. The trypsin-sensitive site may have been lost since the portion of the hybrid on which it is normally present has been replaced by glycophorin B-derived material. The net result will be that the red cells carry trypsin-resistant M. Similarly in a glycophorin B-A hybrid, N ('N' on glycophorin B) may be present on the glycophorin B-derived material, the hybrid molecule may have a trypsin-sensitive site on its glycophorin A-derived material. The net result will be that the red cells lack the trypsin-resistant 'N'. It is easy to imagine the complexities that result when glycophorin A-B-A, B-A-B and B-A-B-A hybrids are formed or when the anti-Lepore type situations result in the presence of normal glycophorin A, normal glycophorin B and a hybrid glycophorin, all on the same cells!

Each normal *M* or *N* gene is believed (322,585,588) to encode production of about 500,000 copies of glycophorin A. Thus red cells of normal MN phenotype have about 1×10^6 copies of that glycoprotein per red cell. Since red cells from an individual genetically *MM* will carry about one million copies of M, while those from an individual genetically *MN* will carry about 500,000 copies of that antigen, it is easy to understand why some examples of anti-M (and anti-N, reverse the figures) show good dosage effects.

Glycophorin B is present in smaller numbers than glycophorin A, per red cell (322,582,588). Dahr et al. (321) have produced evidence that *S* encodes production of about 125,000 copies of glycophorin B, while *s* encodes production of about 85,000 copies. Thus red cells from an individual genetically *SS* will carry about 250,000 copies of glycophorin B while those from an individual genetically *ss* will carry about 170,000 copies of that glycoprotein. The red cells of *Ss* heterozygotes carry about 210,000 copies. This difference can be demonstrated at the serological level. The lectin *Vicia graminea* (686 and see below) can be diluted so that it reacts as an anti-N typing reagent. If used in a more concentrated form it will agglutinate M+ N- red cells that carry normal glycophorin B, because those cells carry 'N'. When used at such a strength the lectin agglutinates S+ s- red cells (250,000 copies of 'N' per cell) more strongly than it agglutinates S- s+ red cells (7) (170,000 copies of 'N' per cell).

Antigens of the Pr Series

While these antigens are not part of the MN system, they are carried primarily on glycophorins A and B so merit mention here. As stated in the section on *M^k*, the Pr antigens are sialic acid dependent structures expressed in the tetrasaccharide and trisaccharide side chains attached to glycophorins A and B (687). When red cells are treated with neuraminidase, that specifically cleaves N-acetyl neuraminic acid (NeuAc, a sialic acid), the Pr antigens are denatured. Red cells treated with papain or ficin will fail to react with most Pr system antibodies. This occurs not because papain and ficin specifically cleave NeuAc but because they cleave glycophorin A and B, the indirect carriers of the Pr antigens. In fact, some copies of the Pr determinants are probably left on papain and ficin

treated red cells, especially if the enzyme treatment does not completely remove glycophorin B (see previous section). Such is the profusion of glycophorin A compared to glycophorin B (again see previous section) that red cells that lack glycophorin A but carry glycophorin B (i.e. En(a-) red cells) or have had glycophorin A but not glycophorin B removed (i.e. protease treatment in less than optimal situations) may fail to react visibly with anti-Pr. Such cells will sometimes adsorb the anti-Pr with which they do not react visibly.

While most Pr antibodies detect their antigens equally well on M or N-bearing glycophorin A, there are two Pr specificities that show a preference for red cells based on MN phenotype. Anti-Pr^M (122,687) and anti-Pr^N (218,687) react equally well with M+ N- and M- N+ red cells at low temperatures. At higher temperatures the antibodies react better with M+ N- and M- N+ red cells respectively. Presumably the amino acids present in the NH₂ terminal region of glycophorin A that differ in M-bearing and N-bearing glycoproteins serve to orient the Pr^M and Pr^N determinants to allow access by the antibodies. While reporting the first antibody that was described as having anti-Pr^M specificity, Roelcke et al. (122) pointed out that previously reported examples of auto-anti-M could be divided into two groups. Some (10,197,203,210,211, 213,215,745) seemed truly to have anti-M specificity. Others (119-121) gave reactions similar to, or identical with the newly described (122) anti-Pr^M. For additional details about the Pr antigens and antibodies see Chapter 34.

MN System Antigens Affected by NeuAc

Just as the amino acids in the polypeptide backbone of glycophorin A influence presentation of some Pr antigens (see above), the presence or absence of NeuAc in the side chains attached to glycophorin A influences the presentation of some MN system antigens to their antibodies. In table 15-3 the reactions of 30 anti-M and 7 anti-N against untreated and neuraminidase treated red cells are shown. Table 15-15 presents data from the same study (251) showing the reactions of some other MN system antibodies in similar tests. As tables 15-3 and 15-15 illustrate, some MN system antibodies define NeuAc-dependent structures, others define epitopes that are not influenced to any measurable degree by the presence or absence of NeuAc.

The Cryptantigens T and Tn

Again these antigens are not part of the MN system but are present in the tetrasaccharide side chains attached to glycophorins A and B. Figure 15-7A shows the struc-

TABLE 15-15 Reactions of MN System Antibodies Other than Human Anti-M and Anti-N with Untreated (unttd.) and Neuraminidase-treated (ttd.) Red Cells. From Judd et al. (251)

Antibodies (human, polyclonal unless otherwise specified)	Number tested	Non-reactive with ttd. cells	Reaction weaker with ttd. than with unttd. cells	Reaction same with ttd. and unttd. cells	Reaction stronger with ttd. than with unttd. cells
Anti-M (Rabbit)	1	1	0	0	0
Anti-M (*Iberis amara* lectin)	1	0	0	0	1
Anti-M_1	3	0	0	2	1
"Dialysis" Anti-N (Anti-N_{form})	3	3	0	0	0
Anti-N (Rabbit)	5	1	2	2	0
"Anti-N" (*Vicia graminea* lectin)	1	0	0	0	1
Anti-M^g	6	1	0	5	0
Anti-M^v	1	0	0	1	0
"Anti-Mi^a"	2	0	0	2	0
Anti-Vw	5	0	0	1	4
Anti-Hut	2	0	0	1	1
Anti-He	4	0	1	3	0
Anti-Shier	1	0	0	0	1
Anti-Can[1]	1	0	0	0	1
Anti-Tm[2]	1	0	0	0	1

[1]   Had anti-M specificity in tests against neuraminidase-treated red cells
[2]   Had anti-N specificity in tests against neuraminidase-treated red cells

ture of the common tetrasaccharide. When NeuAc is removed (figure 15-7B) as occurs when red cells are treated with neuraminidase, the exposed galactose residue comprises the T antigen. Since all normal human sera from adults contain anti-T, such cells are polyagglutinable. This means that when neuraminidase treated red cells are tested, as described many times in this chapter, it is necessary to work with sera from which anti-T has been removed or with eluates. Failure to use one or the other of these maneuvers will result in all tests being positive due to T-anti-T reactions.

When the galactose residue is not added, a situation sometimes associated with certain disease states, the exposed N-acetyl-galactosamine residue (figure 15-7C) comprises the Tn antigen. Again, all normal human sera from adults contain anti-Tn and the red cells are polyagglutinable. Additional information about T and Tn and references to the statements made in this section will be found in Chapter 42.

Lectins

Over the years a number of lectins have proved useful in serological and biochemical studies on the MN system. With the advent of monoclonal antibodies, lectins will probably be used less than in the past. This section deals primarily with the use of lectins in serological tests. Their use in biochemical investigations is described in more detail in a later section.

Anti-M activity has been found in the seeds of *Iberis amara*, *Iberis umbellata*, *Iberis semperivens* and in the Japanese radish/turnip (688-690). Anti-N activity has been found (691) in the seeds of *Bauhinia candicans*, *Bauhinia variegata*, *Bauhinia bonatiana* and *Bauhinia purpurea*. Not all batches of lectins made from the above seeds are active (692) and one abstract (233) has suggested that the *Iberis amara* lectin is glucose-dependent and works best in a PVP augmented system. Fletcher (693) reported that the lectin *Bauhinia variegata* initial-

FIGURE 15-7 To Illustrate Derivation of the T and Tn Receptors

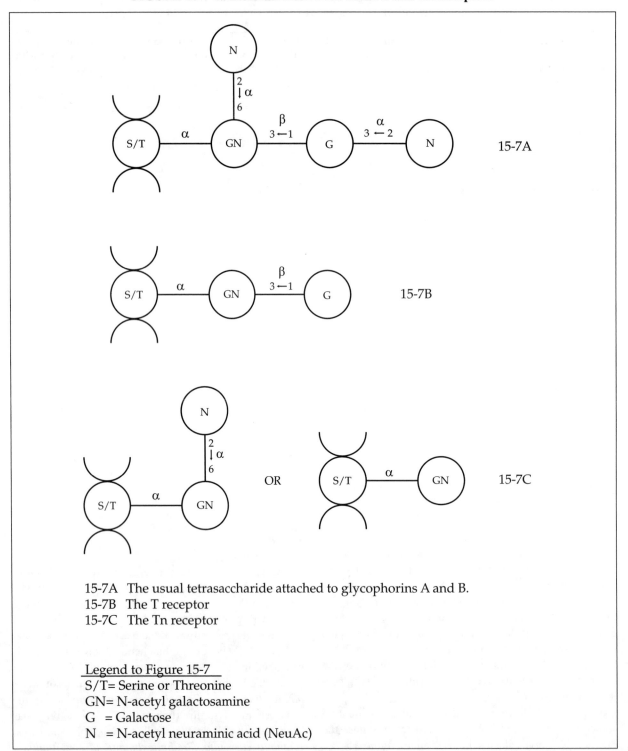

15-7A   The usual tetrasaccharide attached to glycophorins A and B.
15-7B   The T receptor
15-7C   The Tn receptor

Legend to Figure 15-7
S/T= Serine or Threonine
GN= N-acetyl galactosamine
G = Galactose
N = N-acetyl neuraminic acid (NeuAc)

ly agglutinated all red cells but that one specificity present could be inhibited by the addition of 0.1M glucose, leaving a second specificity that agglutinated only N+ red cells. Two lectins, *Molucella laevis* (694) and one component in *Bandeiraea* (now *Griffonia*) *simplicifolia*

extract (695) have the serological specificity of anti-A+N. The specificity of the lectin *Ricinus communis* is similar (37,509,696) to that of *Phaseolus vulgaris* as described below.

Although not useful in differential typing studies

because they complex with carbohydrates present on all red cells, other lectins have proved of value in screening tests and biochemical investigations. The lectin *Maclura aurantiaca* that is made from the Osage orange, appears to detect a structure carried in the tetrasaccharides attached to glycophorins A and B (14,697,698). Indeed, this lectin may bind to the same structure as does *Vicia graminea* and yet *Maclura aurantiaca* agglutinates all cells. If the two lectins do complex with the same determinant (possibly the galactose-galactosamine-serine or threonine structure) it seems that *Vicia* finds the determinant in a sterically favorable form on N compared to M SGP, while *Maclura* is able to bind equally well to the structure on N or M SGP. The major use of the *Maclura* lectin has been in the recognition of red cells that either lack the MN SGP, or have reduced numbers or variant forms of that molecule. For example, since En(a-) red cells lack the MN SGP (and hence many copies of the determinant recognized by *Maclura aurantiaca*) they react less strongly than do normal red cells with dilutions of the lectin. Individuals heterozygous for the genes that result in the En(a-) phenotype have only about 50% of the normal number of copies of MN SGP on their red cells. Those cells also yield weaker than usual (by titration) results than do normal red cells, when tests with the lectin are performed. It must be remembered that because this lectin defines a structure present as part of the carbohydrate-containing side chains attached to glycophorins A and B, a weaker than normal reaction will be seen in a variety of different genetic situations and unusual phenotypes (e.g. En(a-), *En* heterozygotes, M^k heterozygotes, Mi^V homozygotes, etc.). Thus the lectin does not specifically identify any one particular condition. Nevertheless it is a useful screening reagent. By virtue of yielding weaker than normal reactions with a variety of red cells of unusual phenotypes, it selects those deserving of further study without use of the much more difficult to obtain antibodies.

Because many variant phenotypes in the MN system are characterized by reduced levels of red cell membrane-associated NeuAc, the lectins *Glycine soja* (*Glycine max*) and *Sophora japonica*, both of which react optimally with sialic acid depleted red cells, have proved useful for screening for such cells (692,699). (See earlier for a description of the use (405) of *Glycine soja* in searches for S- s- U- red cells.) The reactions of this group of lectins are not blood group specific and identify sialic acid deficient red cells of all phenotypes (692) much as do tests in polybrene or tests with non-agglutinating Rh antibodies in saline systems. Some of the lectins that characterize different forms of polyagglutination also react preferentially with sialic acid depleted red cells (692,700).

Without doubt the most widely used lectin in MN serology is that made from the seeds of *Vicia graminea*. In 1953, Ottensooser and Silberschmidt (686) showed that this lectin preferentially agglutinates N+ red cells. Later, Mäkelä (691) demonstrated similar activity in the seeds *Vicia leganaya* and *Vicia picta* and Moon and Wiener (701) showed that an extract made from the leaves of *Vicia unijuga* is similarly active. Although hundreds of thousands of red cell N typings have been performed with the *Vicia graminea* lectin since that time, it is now known that the specificity of the extract is not anti-N. When a *Vicia graminea* lectin is prepared from suitable seeds (not all batches yield agglutinating activity) it can be shown, in titration studies, to react well with red cells of the phenotypes M- N+ and M+ N+. The lectin either fails to react, or reacts only weakly, with cells that are M+ N-. Accordingly, at a suitable dilution, *Vicia graminea* lectin is a reliable anti-N typing reagent. However, if other tests are performed it is seen that the lectin no longer behaves as anti-N.

First, if the lectin is used in titration studies against neuramindase-treated red cells, it is found that cells of the phenotypes M- N+, M+ N+, and M+ N-, react to about the same titer. Further, the titers are invariably higher than those in titrations against untreated N+ cells. Second, if untreated red cells are used to adsorb the lectin, it is found that M+ N- cells, as well as those that are N+, adsorb activity.

The explanation of these paradoxical findings seems to be that the lectin defines a receptor that is included in the carbohydrate-containing side chains attached to glycophorins A and B. Since the lectin reacts well with neuraminidase-treated red cells (and often with M+ N- red cells only after they have been treated with neuraminidase) it is apparent that NeuAc residues are not an integral part of the receptor defined. Instead, it seems (746) that the *Vicia* receptor is the galactose-N-acetyl-galactosamine-serine/threonine portion of the tetrasaccharide and backbone protein. There is suggestive evidence, discussed in detail later in this section, that the *Vicia* receptor may be restricted to those tetrasaccharides located at or near the NH_2 terminal portion of the M and N SGPs.

Neither galactose nor galactosamine alone neutralizes the activity of the lectin and even when the two are joined in the correct linkage only partial inhibition occurs. These findings suggest a role for the serine or threonine residue, to which the tetrasaccharide is attached, in the receptor defined by *Vicia graminea*. Since the exact nature of this receptor is suggested, but not yet fully characterized, it is not known which of its component parts are involved in complexing with the active molecules of the lectin and which contribute by orienting the structure into the required steric conformation for binding to occur.

Since the *Vicia* lectin complexes with a determinant that is common to M and N SGPs, it must be asked why, under suitable conditions, the lectin is such an efficient anti-N agglutinin. In other words, how does it find its determinant on untreated N+ but not on untreated N- red cells? Presumably, since removal of NeuAc abolishes the ability of the lectin to distinguish between N+ and N- cells, the determinant must be accessible on N+ cells when those cells carry their full complement of NeuAc and must be present but inaccessible on N- cells, when NeuAc is present in full amounts. It seems that this difference must relate directly to the serine/leucine and glycine/glutamic acid differences at positions one and five of the NH_2 terminal end of the M and N SGPs. It is not difficult to imagine that the leucine residue at position one and/or the glutamic acid residue at position five, orient one or more of the tetrasaccharide side chains bound to the serine, threonine and threonine residues at positions two, three and four respectively on the N SGP, in such a way that one or more of those tetrasaccharides is in a position in which the galactose-galactosamine-serine/threonine complex is accessible to the *Vicia* lectin. Conversely, in the M SGP, it would seem that the serine residue at position one and/or the glycine residue at position five, orient the three tetrasaccharides bound at positions two, three and four, so that the galactose-galactosamine-serine/threonine complex is not accessible. If this is the case, it is not difficult to imagine that removal of NeuAc would result in one or more of the necessary complexes bound to the M SGP, being reoriented in such a way that it (they) would now become accessible.

Because neuraminidase-treated red cells of any MN phenotype are agglutinated by *Vicia graminea* lectin, it has been suggested (702) that the lectin contains anti-T, in addition to its anti-N-like (sometimes called anti-N_{vg}) activity. We do not believe this to be the case and have performed experiments (703) that demonstrate the absence of anti-T from the lectin. First, we took a potent example of the lectin and tested it against untreated M+ N- S+ s+ red cell samples. We found that the lectin did not react visibly with those cells. Thus, the extract that we were studying was shown not to agglutinate red cells carrying the tetrasaccharide that includes the lectin's receptor, on their M or Ss SGPs. Next, we took the lectin and tested it against several M+ N- U- and M- N+ U- samples from different donors. As expected, the lectin agglutinated the latter but not the former of those samples. Since U- red cells lack the Ss SGP, our studies with U- red cells tested the ability of the lectin to define its receptor in tetrasaccharides attached to M or N SGPs. We then tested the *Vicia* lectin against the same M+ N- U- and M- N+ U- red cells, after those cells had been treated with trypsin. The lectin failed to react with any of the samples, indicating that the portion of the N SGP that carries the tetrasaccharide(s) containing the receptor with which *Vicia* complexes, had been removed from the M- N+ U- samples. Then we took the trypsin-treated M+ N- U- and M- N+ U- red cells and treated them with neuraminidase. All the samples now reacted strongly with *Arachis hypogea* (704) lectin (anti-T) and with human sera containing anti-T, showing that T-activation had occurred. None of the samples reacted with, nor would they adsorb the *Vicia graminea* lectin.

We (703) believe that these experiments allow two important conclusions to be drawn. First and most simply, they show that *Vicia graminea* lectin does not contain anti-T. Second and potentially of more significance, these experiments may mean that the *Vicia* receptor is confined to the tetrasaccharides near the NH_2 terminal end of the M or N SGP. It is known that other copies of the tetrasaccharide are present on the MN SGP, at a point closer to the red cell membrane than is any trypsin sensitive-site (12,17). Indeed, these tetrasaccharides were presumably among the ones involved in T-activation of the trypsin-treated red cells. However, it was apparent from the agglutination and adsorption experiments that those tetrasaccharides do not include a receptor with which *Vicia graminea* lectin can combine. Presumably, this last finding again relates to the amino acids present at positions one and five of the M and N SGPs and their ability to orient the receptor defined by the lectin into a suitable shape.

A slightly different interpretation would be that the *Vicia* receptor includes the galactose-galactosamine-serine/threonine complex already described and one or more of the amino acids leucine, glutamic acid, the serine at position one in the M SGP, and glycine. If this is the case, it would have to be supposed that the true *Vicia* receptor includes leucine and/or glutamic acid (N SGP) but that serine and/or glycine can act (M SGP) as alternatives, in the absence of NeuAc.

In spite of our conclusive serological studies, reports have continued to appear (741,742) stating that *Vicia graminea* lectin has a dual anti-N,T specificity. This conclusion is based primarily on the finding (741) that *Arachis hypogea* (anti-T) lectin (704) blocks the uptake of the *Vicia* lectin by neuraminidase treated red cells. We would interpret that finding as indicating that since the T (see figure 15-7) and the *Vicia* receptors (see above) are in such close proximity, the binding of one to its receptor sterically interferes with binding of the other (to a different but spatially close receptor). To repeat, we (703) showed that N- 'N'- red cells that were strongly T-activated, would not adsorb the *Vicia* lectin. The N- 'N'- T-activated red cells used in the adsorptions were, of course, not coated with anti-T.

The finding (7) that potent *Vicia* lectins that can agglutinate red cells that carry 'N' but not N, react more strongly (or only) with S+ s- than with S- s+ red cells has been explained in the earlier section describing the number of copies of glycophorin A and B on red cells. Since the number of copies of N SGP on M- N+ cells is four to five times greater than the number of copies of 'N' on S+ s- red cells, it is easy to see why *Vicia* agglutinates cells that carry N far more efficiently than it agglutinates those that carry 'N' without N.

Because *Vicia graminea* seeds are difficult to obtain, Moulds, Moulds and Moulds (705) have described details of home cultivation of *Vicia* plants and methods for obtaining maximum yields of seeds. In concluding this section on lectins a reminder should be added that the major contribution to MN system antigen structure seems to be protein (backbone of SGP), but that most (if not all) lectins complex with carbohydrates. Thus in considering these lectins, it should be borne in mind that most (or perhaps all) of them complex with carbohydrates attached to SGPs and not with the protein portions of the antigens. Extracts from *Limulus polyphemus* (horseshoe crab) have been shown (706-713) to complex with red cell membrane-borne N-acetyl neuraminic acid and are also useful in the recognition of NeuAc deficient red cells.

The MN System and Disease

Vaisanen et al. (714) reported that cultures of one strain of *Escherichia coli* (IH 11165) had the ability to agglutinate M+ but not M- red cells. The agglutination was not abolished by the addition of α-methyl-D-mannoside to the cultures although that substance does inhibit the reactions of some strains of *E. coli* with structures that carry P blood group system determinants (715-719). The authors (714) believed that the *E. coli* were complexing with the serine residue at the NH_2 terminal end of the M SGP and that persons with the M antigen were thus more susceptible to pyelonephritis caused by this organism than were persons without M. Ohyama et al. (722) reported that some strains of influenza A and B viruses complex best with glycophorin A while others complex best with glycophorins B and C. Kao et al. (176) described four children with bacterial infections, two of whom had meningitis, who produced anti-M that was no longer detectable following resolutions of the infections. In two cases the infections were with *Proteus mirabilis*, with a concurrent infection with *Staphylococcus aureus*, in one, in another the infecting organism was *Haemophilus influenzae* and in the fourth *Neisseria meningitidis*. In all four cases the anti-M, when present, were optimally reactive in agglutination tests at room temperature. Blajchmann et al. (720) reported that the proliferative response to mixed lymphocyte culture,

while dependent on genes at the *HLA-D* locus and affected by differences at the *HLA-A* and *HLA-B* loci, is also affected by the MN but not the Ss phenotypes of the donors from whom the lymphocytes are collected. Since it is not known for sure whether or not the MN sialoglycoprotein is present on lymphocytes (721) the authors suggested (720) that the effects seen might be due to *MN* or to closely linked genes. Planas et al. (743) believed that the amount of glycophorin A is decreased on the red cells of patients with sickle cell disease.

The claims (837-840) that glycophorin A is a complement regulatory protein have been discussed in Chapter 6. As mentioned there, it seems that if the protein does contribute to the regulation of complement activation its role must be relatively minor. We are not aware of any reports that suggest any perturbation of complement regulation in individuals who lack glycophorin A or have atypical red cell glycophorins.

There have been a number of reports that claim to show that the MN phenotypes serve as genetic markers for a propensity towards hypertension. However, the findings vary (747). In one study (748) hypertension caused by environmental factors was said to be most common in *N* homozygotes. In another (749) an excess of the MN phenotype was reported in young adults with essential arterial hypertension. In still other studies an association was reported in Whites but not Blacks (750) or the association was seen to be different in men and women (751). No doubt Dr. Alexander Wiener (752,753) would best have liked the study (754) that showed no association between *MN* and essential or secondary hypertension in Whites, Blacks, men or women.

Hill et al. (723) have described what they believe is suggestive evidence for linkage between the *MN* and *AS* (alcoholism susceptibility) genes. Golin et al. (724) had earlier looked for linkage between various human polymorphisms and genes associated with affective disorders and found that only *MN* gave any indication of linkage, however, the lod score was only 1.39 at q = 0.20. As described below, the *MN* locus is on chromosome 4. That chromosome also carries the genes that encode ADH (alcohol dehydrogenase) (725). However, it is not known if *MN* and *ADH* are linked. If alcohol consumption and *MN* are related it will be a surprise to one of us (PDI) who thought that writing textbooks was the cause!

Assignment of the *MN* Locus to Chromosome 4

In 1968, German et al. (726,727) studied a child with multiple congenital abnormalities. In cytogenetic studies it appeared that part of the long arm of chromosome 2 had been translocated to the long arm of chromosome 4. In phenotyping studies it was found that the child did not express products of the *Ns* haplotype that he should have inherited from his father who had M- N+ S- s+ red cells that carried a double dose of N. Thus the child appeared to be hemizygous for the maternal contribution of *MS* and his genotype was thought to be *MS/-*. In 1973 German and Chaganti (728) studied the child's chromosomes again using banding techniques that had not been available in 1968. The findings seemed to indicate that during the translocation a small piece of the long arm of chromosome 2 had been lost and it was deemed likely that the *MN* and *Ss* loci were on chromosome 2. However, other cases are known (729-733) in which there are abnormalities of chromosome 2. In some of these (729,730) it was shown that the aberrations of the chromosome were at positions 2q13 and 2q21. In reviewing all the cases, Weitkamp et al. (734) (in a paper in which German and Chaganti were co-authors) pointed out that there was no linkage between inheritance of the abnormality and genes at the *MN* and *Ss* loci. In 1979, while studying the chromosomes of the supposed *MS/-* child yet again, German et al. (735) showed that the deletion on chromosome 2 was at 2q14. Data from the studies of Weitkamp et al. (734) and Thompson et al. (733) showed that the 2q13 aberration must be at least 14 centimorgans from the *MN* locus, if that locus was on chromosome 2, so essentially excluded that chromosome as a carrier of *MN* and *Ss*. Thus it was concluded that the data of German et al. (726-728,735) probably represented the fact that the *MN* and *Ss* loci are on the long arm of chromosome 4, a tentative location at 4q28 to 4q31 was suggested (735).

Once it became apparent that glycophorin A carries the M and N et al. and glycophorin B the S and s et al. antigens and the *GYPA* and *GYPB* genes had been cloned and sequenced (see below), Rahuel et al. (526) used in situ hybridization to locate *GYPA* (the gene that encodes production of glycophorin A) on the q28 to q31 region of chromosome 4. A third gene, *GYPE* (again see below) that is closely linked to *GYPA* and *GYPB* was localized to the same region (736) again by in situ hybridization. What used to be so very difficult (726-728,735) is now not necessarily easy, but is so much more direct (526,736). It is clear that the genes that encode production of glycophorins A and B arose during in the evolutionary pathway that led to the current human state (see below). Rearden (739) and Rearden et al. (744) have studied glycophorin A in non-human primates and have described a sialoglycoprotein analogous to glycophorin B, in a chimpanzee.

Genetic Control of MN System Antigen Production

Although as described below, details regarding the

molecular genetics of the MN system are extraordinarily complex, recognition of the general principles involved has greatly simplified the overall concept. As a single example, an individual who has passed a haplotype encoding production of N, s, U, He, M^e, Tm and Mt^a to his/her offspring will be considered. Before the biochemical structures of glycophorin A and glycophorin B were understood, it would have been concluded that the individual had an *Ns* haplotype to which genes encoding He, M^e, Tm and Mt^a were closely linked. Since none of those antigens (nor the other low incidence antigens listed in table 15-1) appeared to be the products of alleles it would have been thought that six very closely linked loci (i.e. carrying *N, s, He, M^e, Tm* and *Mt^a*) were involved. Clearly such a situation is genetically uneconomical and since there is no evidence that presence of any of those antigens confers any selective advantage, is unlikely to exist. Now that the structures of glycophorins A and B are understood, production of all six antigens by the two genes in the *Ns* haplotype can be explained. The *N* gene encodes production of glycophorin A on which N, Tm and Mt^a are carried. N represents the NH$_2$ terminal amino acids of that structure, Tm represents unusual glycosylation in the NH$_2$ terminal region of the glycoprotein (see figure 15-3) and Mt^a probably represents an amino acid change (from glycophorin A that does not carry Mt^a) in the region of glycophorin A between residue 39 and residue 56 (i.e. Mt^a is trypsin resistant, papain/ficin sensitive). The *s* gene encodes production of a form of glycophorin B that carries s and U but in which the NH$_2$ terminal amino acids comprise the He instead of the usual 'N' antigen. Thus the haplotype involved could be rewritten, if one wished, as *NMt^a/sHe*. Production of Tm would not be included since that antigen apparently represents a glycosylation change and the location of the gene encoding production of the transferase involved is not known. Clearly the old concept of one gene-one antigen does not apply. In this case the description of one gene-one polypeptide-multiple antigens fits but, as described in the next Chapter, on the Gerbich blood group system, the old one gene-one polypeptide rule is no longer inviolate.

Early Studies on the Biochemical Nature of MN Antigens

Glycophorin A is a major component of the red cell membrane being expressed at approximately 1 million molecules/red cell. Only band 3, the major anion transport protein which carries antigens of the Diego blood group system is of equivalent abundance (see Chapter 4 for general review of the red cell membrane). In marked contrast to band 3 which is extremely hydrophobic and very difficult to extract from red cell membranes, glycophorin A can be extracted with relative ease since it is water-soluble. Glycophorin A was therefore one of the first membrane proteins to be isolated and characterized. Early extraction procedures involved the use of phenol-saline mixtures (23,758). When red cell membranes are extracted in this way the aqueous phase contains glycophorin A as the major component and such materials are able to inhibit MN system antibodies (23,759).

Winzler (760) isolated a sialic acid-rich glycopeptide by treatment of intact red cells with crystalline trypsin and demonstrated that the major component of this peptide preparation was derived from glycophorin A. The amino acid composition of this peptide showed that almost half the amino acid residues were either serine or threonine. Winzler further showed that the peptide contained two types of carbohydrate, O-glycan and N-glycan, and that the major O-glycan was a sialotetrasaccharide comprised of a core structure Galβ1,3-GalNAc-Ser/Thr to which two sialic acid residues are added, one in an α2,3 linkage to the Gal and the other in α2,6 linkage to the GalNAc (see figure 15-3A). Winzler (760) considered that these data were consistent with a structure of a glycoprotein which "was considered to be anchored in the membrane by the lipophilic portion of the molecule at its carboxyl end. The rest of the molecule is in the external environment of the cell, probably as a semi-rigid rod held extended by the many anionic sialyl groups". This structure has been modified in terms of detail in the intervening years but remains broadly correct. The term glycophorin was first proposed for this glycoprotein by Marchesi et al. (761).

Further progress in elucidating the structure of glycophorin A was facilitated to a large extent by the development of detergents for solubilizing and separating membrane proteins and in particular by the application of SDS-PAGE to the analysis of membrane proteins. SDS-PAGE allows the high resolution separation of membrane glycoproteins and when preparations of glycophorin A were subjected to SDS-PAGE and stained for sialic acid with the PAS stain, it became clear that these preparations of glycophorin A were not pure but contained other minor sialic acid-rich glycoproteins (now known as glycophorins B, C and D). Hamaguchi and Cleve (762) were the first to show that MN antigens are carried on a different glycoprotein from Ss antigens. This was achieved by gel filtration on columns of Sephadex G-100 in the presence of 1% sodium dodecyl sulfate. MN activity was found associated with the major glycoprotein peak (glycophorin A) while Ss activity was associated with a minor glycoprotein peak now known as glycophorin B. This simple distinction of MN on glycophorin A and Ss on glycophorin B was complicated by the demonstration of some N antigen activity on the Ss-active glycophorin B. This additional N activity is often referred to as 'N' (N

quotes) to distinguish it from N activity found on glycophorin A. Unlike N on glycophorin A, 'N' does not contribute to the MN polymorphism so cells from persons of genotype *MM* can still have 'N' activity. N and 'N' can also be distinguished because trypsin treatment of intact red cells removes M and N activity (releasing the glycopeptide studied by Winzler (760) that is described above) but does not remove 'N'. This is because glycophorin B does not have a trypsin sensitive site. Furthmayr et al. (763) used gel filtration in the presence of detergents to purify glycophorin A free of glycophorin B and other minor glycophorins.

The Nomenclature of Glycophorins and the Use of SDS-PAGE for Their Analysis

In this chapter the terms glycophorin A (GPA), glycophorin B (GPB) and glycophorin E (GPE) are used for the protein products of the three genes that give rise to antigens in the MN system. The reader may wonder why A, B, E and not A, B, C. This is an unfortunate legacy of the history of how these molecules were discovered. Glycophorin C and glycophorin D do exist but they have nothing to do with the MN system (see Chapter 16). Glycophorin was coined by Marchesi et al. (761) for the major sialic acid-rich glycoprotein of red cells. When it became clear that preparations of glycophorin contained other less abundant sialic acid-rich glycoproteins the major component was named glycophorin A and two minor components glycophorin B and glycophorin C (678). Other workers who examined red cell membranes using the high resolution SDS-PAGE system of Laemmli (764) were aware that there were four sialic acid-rich glycoproteins not three. Dahr et al. (676) referred to these four glycoproteins as the MN-sialoglycoprotein (= GPA), the Ss-sialoglycoprotein (= GPB), the D sialoglycoprotein (= GPC) and the E sialoglycoprotein. Anstee et al. (398) referred to the four sialoglycoproteins as α (GPA), δ (GPB), β (GPC) and γ. The use of α, β, γ, δ was convenient with regard to the naming of PAS-staining bands on SDS-PAGE because GPA and GPB formed homodimers ($α_2$, $δ_2$) and heterodimers (αδ) under the conditions of electrophoresis as well as running as monomers (α,δ). GPB was labeled δ rather than β because the bands were labeled according to the apparent molecular weights of their monomeric forms on the gel. These different nomenclatures were themselves modified by others so that, for example, sialoglycoprotein α became glycophorin α in some papers. Eventually, Dahr (322) proposed that the term glycophorin D be adopted for the E-sialoglycoprotein and sialoglycoprotein γ and the GPA, B, C, D nomenclature has been widely adopted since then. When DNA sequence analysis revealed the existence of a third gene at the *MN* locus its protein product had to be called glycophorin E because C and D had already been used (765).

It is still a matter of irritation to one of us (DJA) that the term glycophorin became applied to the products of the *Gerbich* locus. If the term is used for Gerbich glycoproteins it could equally well be used for the CD55 (Cromer) or CD44 (Indian) blood group active molecules since these are also sialic acid-rich glycoproteins and glycophorin is being used as a generic term for molecules of this type. Nevertheless, having just typed the αβγδ nomenclature on a laptop computer the author who introduced it has definitely gone off this nomenclature as well! Priority for naming what is now called GPC in fact lies with Mueller and Morrison (766) who proposed the name glyconnectin because of its association (connection) with the red cell skeleton (see Chapter 16).

The Structure of Glycophorin A (GPA)

The complete amino acid sequence of purified glycophorin A was reported in 1978 (677). This major achievement was accomplished by manual sequencing of a series of overlapping peptides derived from glycophorin A by treatment with cyanogen bromide, trypsin or chymotrypsin, a far cry from today's methods where a small amount of amino acid sequence information can be used to isolate cDNA and the protein sequence predicted from the cDNA sequence (see Chapter 5). Manual sequencing requires large amounts of purified protein and so could be applied successfully to a major red cell membrane protein like glycophorin A. These sequencing studies revealed that glycophorin A is a protein of 131 amino acids with a large N-terminal extracellular domain (residues 1-72), a single hydrophobic membrane-spanning domain (residues 73-95) and an intracellular cytoplasmic domain (residues 96-131). The N-terminal extracellular domain contained a single N-glycan at residue 26 and numerous O-glycans (15 were reported by Tomita et al. (677)). The sequence published by Tomita et al. (677) was revised at positions 11 and 17 in subsequent studies (322) and the revised sequence confirmed when cDNA was isolated and sequenced by Siebert and Fukuda in 1986 (767). Sequencing of cDNA also revealed the presence of a cleavable signal sequence (residues -19 to -1). GPA is therefore a typical type I membrane glycoprotein (see Chapter 4 for general discussion of the structure of membrane proteins).

The structure of the single N-glycan on GPA at residue 26 was determined independently by two groups (768, 769, see figure 4-4 in Chapter 4). The predominant O-glycan structure was the sialotetrasaccharide reported by Winzler and discussed above (435,770) (see figure

15-3A). This structure was also reported independently by Adamany and Kathan (771). Thomas and Winzler (435) also reported the presence of a trisaccharide containing one molecule of sialic acid (see figure 15-3C). Subsequent studies by others confirmed that the major O-glycan is the sialotetrasaccharide and that the linear trisaccharide of structure: sialic acid-α(2,3)Galβ(1,3) αGalNAc-Ser/Thr is also present in significant amounts (36,772,773). The exact number and composition of O-glycans on GPA is not constant for all GPA molecules, in fact there is considerable heterogeneity. Tomita et al. (677) noted differences in protease sensitivity of various sites on the GPA molecule which they attributed to carbohydrate heterogeneity and this has been noted by others. One of the clearest examples of heterogeneity is seen when GPA is digested with chymotrypsin. There is a chymotrypsin cleavage site at Tyr34 which is accessible in about 40% of GPA purified from red cells. The large chymotrypsin-resistant component probably results from the utilization of O-glycosylation sites at Thr33 and/or Thr37, thereby preventing access to Tyr34 in these resistant molecules (547,582). Extensive O-glycosylation of mucin-like molecules provides a well described mechanism of protecting the molecules from protease digestion (774) and GPA could be described as a membrane-bound mucin-like molecule. Recently the number of potential O-glycan sites on GPA has been revised to 16 (775). Whereas prediction of possible sites for N-glycosylation is clearly defined by the signal motif Asn-X-Ser/Thr it has proved extremely difficult to predict whether or not a given Ser or Thr residue in a polypeptide will be O-glycosylated (see Chapter 4 for further discussion). An explanation of this difficulty has recently emerged from studies of the glycosyltransferases that add GalNAc to Ser or Thr. It is now known that there is not one GalNAc transferase but many (up to 12 identified so far) and that these enzymes vary in their ability to utilize Thr and/or Ser according to the peptide sequence surrounding the Thr and/or Ser (776,777). As a general rule, sialotetrasaccharides are found towards the N-terminus of GPA and trisaccharides towards the lipid bilayer (36,547, 772,773). Extensive characterization of O-glycans in a mixture of glycophorins comprising 85% GPA using fast atom bombardment mass spectrometry (FAB-MS) has shown that small amounts of pentasaccharide are also found (778). Two pentasaccharides were identified each containing three sialic acids attached to the core Galβ(1,3)GalNAc-Ser/Thr structure (see figure 15-8). The pentasaccharides comprise about 5% of the total O-glycans, the sialotetrasaccharide 78% and the linear sialotrisaccharide 17%. These findings are of particular interest in relation to the structure of M and N blood group antigens and are discussed again in the section on M and N antigen structure.

The Structure of Glycophorin B (GPB)

As already discussed in an earlier section, the application of detergents and SDS-PAGE to the study of membrane proteins led to the realization first reported by Hamaguchi and Cleve (762) that the Ss antigens and the 'N' antigen are located on a minor glycoprotein (now called GPB) (678) which is distinct from the major sialic acid-rich glycoprotein (GPA). The amino acid sequence of an N-terminal tryptic peptide derived from GPB (residues 1-35) was first reported by Furthmayr in 1978 (37) and confirmed by Dahr et al. in 1980 (321). These results showed that the N-terminal 26 residues of GPB are identical to the N-terminal 26 residues of GPA showing that the two proteins are related. Amino acid sequence information up to residue 71 of GPB was subsequently reported by Blanchard et al. (779). When cDNA corresponding to GPB was isolated and sequenced it became clear that the protein comprises 72 amino acids and contains a cleavable leader sequence identical to that found in GPA (780,781). The cDNA sequence also revealed some minor corrections to the sequence obtained by amino acid sequencing. GPB differs from GPA in that it lacks an N-glycan at residue 26 (residue 28 is not Ser or Thr and so the signal sequence for N-glycosylation found in GPA is absent from GPB). GPB also lacks a cytoplasmic domain (see figure 15-9). GPB has about 11 O-glycans (322) with structures presumed to be the same as those found on GPA (see previous section).

The Structure of M and N Antigens

Early studies on the chemical nature of the MN anti-gens established that influenza viruses inactivated both M and N antigens (241,248). This inactivation is attributable to influenza-produced sialidase. However, not all anti-M and anti-N fail to react with sialidase-treated red cells (251). Studies on the structure of M and N antigens generated considerable controversy in the 1970s. Two apparently mutually exclusive hypotheses were extant. One predominantly espoused by Georg Springer in Evanston, Illinois and the other personified by Elwira Lisowska in Wroclaw, Poland.

The view according to Springer et al. (245-247) was that N is the precursor of M, not the product of its allele. It was believed that N is converted to M by addition of a sialic acid residue. The fact that red cells of persons of genotype *MM* also contain some N antigen whereas red cells of persons of genotype *NN* do not contain M antigen was taken as evidence that N is a precursor of M (247). When it became clear that red cells of persons of genotype *MM* have 'N' on GPB as well as M on GPA it could be seen that this argument was not valid. However, if M has a sialic acid residue not present in N it follows that it should be possible to isolate an oligosaccharide from M+ red cells which could not be found in N+ red cells and evidence was presented in support of this (782). In particular, it was argued that two terminal sialic acid residues located on different termini of a branched oligosaccharide and linked in different ways to the next sugar were required for M but not for N. One of us (DJA) has a very clear recollection of meeting Dr. Yang, one of Springer's collaborators, at the ISBT meeting held in Paris in 1978 and being impressed by the tremendous amount of work that had gone into isolating these large oligosaccharides and the obvious sincerity of Dr. Yang himself.

The opposing view was that M and N-active gly-

FIGURE 15-8 Sialopentasaccharides Found on Human Red Cell Glycophorins (reference 778)

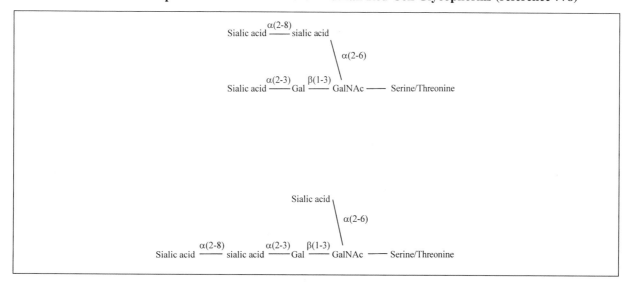

FIGURE 15-9 The Structures of Glycophorin A and Glycophorin B

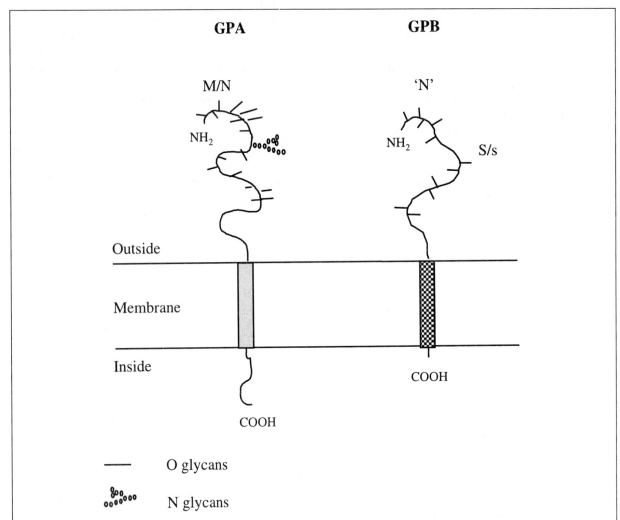

cophorins do not differ in their carbohydrate composition at all and differences in the amino acid sequence caused the oligosaccharide chains to adopt different conformations which were recognized as M or N (783,784). Interestingly, at least as far as this author (DJA) is aware, it is still not really known for certain if M-active glycophorin has any oligosaccharides that are different from those found in N-active glycophorin. The studies of Lisowska et al. (687,784) and several other workers including Winzler (760) did not reveal any oligosaccharides larger than the sialotetrasaccharide and no difference was found in the composition of oligosaccharides on GPA from M+ N-, M+N+, and M-N+ red cells but the methodology used would probably have precluded finding the pentasaccharides described much later by Fukuda et al. (778, see figure 15-8) because sialic acid linked to sialic acid as in these pentasaccharides is easily hydrolyzed (778). Unfortunately, the studies described by

Fukuda et al. (778) were carried out on glycophorins obtained from pooled red cells of unknown MN type and this question cannot be answered from their data. In any event, numerous studies (34-36,785) showed that the M and N antigens are antithetical and that antigen structure does depend on the amino acid sequence at two positions at the N terminus (Ser in M, Leu in N) and at position 5 (Gly in M, Glu in N) and most workers appear to be satisfied that the amino acid sequence differences are enough the explain the antigenic differences (see figure 15-2). There is no doubt that these amino acid sequence differences are critical for defining the antigens but one of us (DJA) would like to know if the structural changes effected by these amino acid sequence differences influence the glycosylation pattern at the N-terminus of GPA, before deciding that Dr. Yang was sincere but wrong. In this context it is interesting to note that Sadler et al. (786) were able to restore the MN antigens of sialidase-treated cells by incubation with either of the sialyltransferases required to synthesize the sialotetrasaccharide and the MN antigens restored always corresponded to the MN type of the starting material. They concluded that amino acid sequence must define the antigens but noted that there were wide variations in the reactivity of individual MN antisera with the resialylated cells "suggesting that the native M and N antigens may contain several determinants". Only about 60% of the sialic acid originally present on the red cells was restored by the transferases used in these experiments which were carried out before the occurrence of α(2,8) linked sialic acid on glycophorins was known. It seems that there is still more to learn about the structure of M and N. Inspection of the N-terminal amino acid sequence of GPB revealed that it is identical to that of GPA when GPA expresses N so that N is indistinguishable from 'N' at this level of comparison (see figure 15-4).

The Structure of Other Antigens Located at the N-terminus of GPA (M^c, M^g, M$_1$, Tm, Can and/or Hu) and the Epitope Recognized by Monoclonal Anti-M+M^g

Any comment to the effect that blood group serology is not a precise science can be refuted by consideration of studies of the M^c phenotype. Anti-M^c does not exist but the phenotype can be distinguished from M and N because it is recognized by most but not all anti-M and some but not all anti-N (57). Amino acid sequence studies revealed that the M^c phenotype has a very precise structural basis corresponding to Ser at position 1 of GPA and Glu at position 5 (450, and see table 15-9). The phenotype therefore derives from a hybrid sequence with the M-specific amino acid at position 1 and the N-specific amino acid at position 5. This information reveals something about the nature of the M and N antigens because anti-M that recognize M^c must ipso

facto recognize an antigen that is not dependent on the structure influenced by the Gly/Glu polymorphism at position 5. Likewise anti-N that recognize M^c are not dependent on the structure influenced by the Ser/Leu polymorphism at position 1. This is an interesting point because it underlines the fact that the extreme N-terminus of GPA is a large structure with three potential O-glycans (Mr 1,000 if sialotetrasaccharides) which can embrace many different antigens. In serological parlance it is convenient to distinguish M and N but the reality is much more complex with a range of possible antigenic stimuli of which the M^c phenotype is but one. The potential for heterogeneity in O-glycosylation patterns discussed in the previous section creates another set of possibilities in which certain anti-M or anti-N recognize only a subset of GPA molecules on a given red cell. A specific example of the influence of glycosylation pattern on antigenicity in this region of GPA is given by the group of antigens that includes M$_1$, Tm, Can and/or Hu. Blumenfeld and coworkers (472,787) isolated O-glycans from GPA derived from the red cells of two Black donors who were Tm+ and M$_1$+. These authors found that the O-glycans contained GlcNAc instead of sialic acid linked β(1,6) to GalNAc in the core structure of the O-glycans (see figure 15-10). Oligosaccharides in which the GlcNAc was further glycosylated by Gal and Gal-GlcNAc (lactosamine) units were also found. One of these GlcNAc containing oligosaccharides was found in the octapeptide released from GPA with cyanogen bromide (by cleavage at Met8) and so is located in the N-terminus of the molecule where the M, N-specific amino acids are located. Dahr (322) reports that such oligosaccharides can be found in Whites but at a much lower level (0.05-0.3 moles per mole of peptides) than in Blacks (4 moles per mole of peptides) exhibiting Tm, M$_1$, Can and/or Hu antigens and that these oligosaccharides are not found on GPB or GPC. These GlcNAc-containing O-glycans create a whole new potential for MN related antigenic variation which seems likely to reflect a selection process in the Black population.

FIGURE 15-10 N-acetylglucosamine-containing O Glycan Found on Glycophorin A (reference 787)

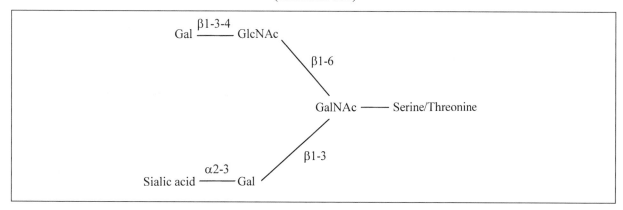

Since GPA is known to act as a receptor for some strains of the malarial parasite *Plasmodium falciparum* (788) and since these strains are known to bind through sialic acid, it is attractive to speculate that replacement of sialic acid-containing structures confers some selective advantage against malaria.

The antigen M^g is also defined by the N-terminal sequence of GPA. In this case the amino acid at position 4 in an N-specific sequence (Thr) is replaced by Asn (450,465,472). The replacement of Thr4 which is usually O-glycosylated by Asn obviously prevents glycosylation at position 4 but it appears that this substitution dramatically reduces O-glycosylation at the adjacent residues Ser2 and Thr3 (see table 15-9). Consistent with a lack of requirement for carbohydrate at least some anti-M^g can be inhibited by synthetic peptides and it appears that these antibodies bind primarily to the Leu at position 1 rather than Asn4 (789). At least one anti-M^g reacts with a sialic acid dependent antigen (251) and others will recognize a glycosylated structure (477).

Further complexity relating to the antigenicity of the N-terminal region of GPA is illustrated by some murine monoclonal antibodies which behave as if they are anti-M+M^g. This is at first sight a very surprising phenomenon because the antibodies require sialic acid to behave as anti-M and yet M^g is usually a peptide antigen lacking O-glycosylation at residues 2, 3 and 4. The specificity of these antibodies has been the subject of an elegant study by Jaskiewicz et al. (476). These authors showed that the sialic acid dependent anti-M activity requires Gly at position 5 but not Ser1. They further showed, using synthetic peptides, that the anti-M^g specificity requires Val6 and Met8. It appears that the Val6 and Met8 are accessible in the M structure but obscured in the N structure where Gly5 is replaced by the negatively charged Glu. This provides a very good example of how a single amino acid change (in this case Gly/Glu) can alter the conformation of a protein. Removal of sialic acid appears to change the conformation of this structure so that Val6 and Met8 are no longer accessible to the antibody in the M structure.

Structure of Ss Antigens

As described in an earlier section the S and s antigens are carried on GPB. Dahr et al. (436) demonstrated that the nature of the amino acid at position 29 in the GPB sequence is critical for defining the structure of S and s. If residue 29 is Met the molecule exhibits S activity, if residue 29 is Thr then s is expressed. The critical difference between S and s is therefore somewhat simpler than that between M and N since only a single amino acid is different. This pattern of antigen structure where a single amino acid change defines the products of two alleles of

a blood group, first demonstrated by these studies on S and s, has since been demonstrated for the majority of blood group antigens and numerous other examples will be found throughout this book.

In contrast to most anti-M and anti-N, the reactivity of anti-S and anti-s with red cells of appropriate phenotype is not affected by removal of sialic acid by sialidase treatment. Treatment of Ss-active glycopeptides with carbodiimide/glycine methyl ester destroyed both S and s suggesting that Glu28 is required for the formation of both antigens (436). Since Tn red cells have normal Ss antigen activity and since alkaline/borohydride-treatment of Ss-active peptides destroys Ss activity (alkaline/borohydride treatment releases O-glycans) Dahr et al. (321,436) suggest that the GalNAc core residue of the O-glycan on Thr25 may also influence the structure of the S and s antigens (see figure 15-5). The importance of residues other than Met/Thr29 in the structure of S and s has not received much attention in the intervening years. The techniques of molecular biology offer an obvious way of investigating the structure of these antigens in more detail. Expression of GPB cDNA of known Ss type in a eukaryotic expression system and the use of site-directed mutagenesis to test the importance of individual residues to the structure of both S and s should provide useful information in this regard.

Structure of Antigens at the Amino-terminus of GPB ('N', He, M^e)

The amino-terminal 26 residues of GPB are identical to those of GPA when GPA expresses N antigen and so the structure of 'N' is easily understood, it is the same as N, the use of ' ' does not describe a difference in structure but is a useful notation to distinguish N antigen when it occurs on GPB from N antigen when it occurs on GPA (17).

The He antigen is defined by the amino-terminal region of GPB. The probable location of He on GPB was flagged by studies on a woman with He+ red cells who made a potent anti-N and whose red cells lacked both N and 'N' (147). However, as mentioned in an earlier section, well before the structure of glycopι.rin B was known, Mourant (446) had suspected that He is more closely associated with S and s than with M and N. Subsequent amino acid sequence analysis of GPB peptides derived from the He+ red cells of the woman described by Judd et al. (147) revealed three amino acid sequence differences (at positions 1, 4 and 5) from those found in a normal N or 'N' antigen (284). Residue 1 of He was Trp not Leu, residue 4 was Ser not Thr and residue 5 was Gly not Glu (see table 15-10). This result was something of a surprise at the time because it was not obvious how three sequence changes could be effected in a single genetic event. Subsequent studies at the DNA level have provided an answer to this puzzle. It appears that the He antigen results from a gene conversion event in which a small segment of DNA from the *GYPA* gene is inserted into the *GYPB* gene at meiosis and that this DNA insertion changes the sequence of the translated protein to that observed when the He antigen is expressed (285). Gene conversion is a mechanism which gives rise to numerous antigens in the MN and Rh blood group systems and it is discussed in more detail later in this chapter.

The gene conversion event which gives rise to He results in a new N-terminal amino acid Trp, changes one O-glycosylation site Thr4 for another (Ser) and an N-specific residue (Glu5) for an M-specific residue (Gly). The change Glu5Gly explains why some anti-M react with M- N+ He+ red cells (63). The anti-M that are reactive, that have been said to be defining M^e, recognize an antigen defined by Gly5 rather than Ser1 of the M antigen sequence (see previous section on structure of M). The term M^e therefore defines an antigen which is part of the group of antigens described as M or put another way, M^e is part of M. Clearly most anti-He are likely to recognize the structure defined by Trp1 and the change Leu1Trp (one nonpolar amino acid for another) does not markedly affect the structure around Gly5. Sialic acid is not a necessary prerequisite for the binding of all anti-He, a property shared with some anti-M and anti-N (251)

Structure of the U Antigen

The structure of the U antigen is still not satisfactorily resolved. The absence of U antigen from the hybrid GPB-A glycophorin which gives rise to the Dantu antigen provides some of the most convincing evidence that the antigen is defined by the sequence of normal GPB (51). The hybrid glycophorin which creates the Dantu antigen is discussed in more detail in a later section. The relevant point here is that the hybrid contains residues 1-39 of GPB and 40-99 of GPA (434). This indicates that the U antigen may be defined at least in part, by that region of normal GPB which is closest to the lipid bilayer (residues 40-44). When GPB is isolated from the red cell membrane it does not inhibit anti-U (17,400) but this does not mean that the antigen is not defined by the sequence of GPB since the conformation of the protein may be dramatically changed when removed from the lipid bilayer. Dahr and Moulds (401) showed that inhibition of anti-U could be achieved with isolated GPB provided that lipid was added and concluded from a variety of experiments that the region corresponding to residues 33-40 of GPB is involved in U antigen activity.

A complication in the assignment of U antigen to GPB is provided by the occurrence of red cells, particularly in Blacks, of phenotype S- s- U+. Cells of this phenotype are variously reported as having no (400) or very little (2-3% of normal) (44) GPB. The U antigen on these cells although generally weaker than on cells of normal Ss phenotype is not difficult to detect in conventional serological tests. Some progress in understanding the molecular basis of the S- s- U+ phenotype has been made by Reid et al. (343) who noticed that cells of this phenotype are usually He+. Studies at the DNA level should provide an explanation for the small amount of GPB-like material observed by others in these cells. Some progress in this area has already been made with respect to cells of phenotype S- s- U- He+ (344 and see a later section).

Another area of difficulty in assigning the U antigen to GPB is provided by studies on red cells the of phenotype Rh$_{null}$. The GPB content of amorph-type and regulator-type Rh$_{null}$ cells is decreased by about 60-70% compared with that in cells of normal Rh phenotype (437) but whereas the amorph-type Rh$_{null}$ cells type as U+ with only slightly weakened U antigen, regulator-type Rh$_{null}$ cells often type as U- (437). Dahr et al. (44) proposed that GPB associates with a protein or proteins involved in the expression of Rh antigens and that this Rh-related protein might be required in addition to GPB to form the U antigen (and also Duclos, see Chapter 31). Support for this hypothesis came from immunoblotting studies which examined the expression of the Rh glycoprotein in Rh$_{null}$ U+ and Rh$_{null}$ U- red cells and showed that the Rh glycoprotein was present in the U+ but not the U- cells (414). Subsequent studies have shown that the Rh$_{null}$ phenotype most often results from mutations in the Rh glycoprotein gene which affect the level of its expression in the red cell membrane (790). These and other results (791) provide clear evidence that the Rh glycoprotein and GPB associate in the membrane but the correlation between Rh glycoprotein content and U antigen expression has not been further studied. There is also evidence for substantial heterogeneity in the specificity of antibodies described as anti-U (discussed in an earlier section). It seems possible that some anti-U will recognize GPB in the absence of the Rh glycoprotein while others will only recognize an antigen which is created by the association of the Rh glycoprotein and GPB (rather like the Wr^b antigen described in an earlier section). Clearly a detailed study of the nature of the U antigen is needed in order to clarify these issues.

The Structure and Organization of the Genes Giving Rise to Glycophorin A and B and the Putative GPE

Human GPA cDNA clones were first isolated by

Siebert and Fukuda (767) from a cDNA library derived from the erythroleukemic cell line K562. The largest cDNA was sequenced and the deduced amino acid sequence was that expected for a GPA with M antigen activity. The cDNA predicted a leader peptide sequence starting at Met -19. Human GPA cDNA clones were subsequently isolated from a human reticulocyte cDNA library (781) and a human fetal liver cDNA library (526). Human GPB cDNA clones were isolated by Siebert and Fukuda (780) and Tate and Tanner (781). Comparison of cDNA sequences for GPA and GPB showed that the two genes are remarkably similar except at their 3' ends and are likely to have resulted from gene duplication. Southern blotting demonstrated that GPA and GPB are encoded by separate and distinct single copy genes (792). Analysis of *GYPA* and *GYPB* in genomic clones isolated from a K562 genomic library revealed that *GYPA* and *GYPB* consist of 7 and 5 exons respectively and that the two genes have >95% identity in sequence from the 5' flanking region to the region approximately 1kb downstream from the exon encoding the transmembrane domains. The two genes are completely different in their 3' end sequences and the transition site from homologous to non-homologous regions is located within *Alu* repeat sequences (793). *Alu* repeat sequences are short stretches of DNA (about 300 nucleotides) distributed throughout the genome. There are about 500,000 copies in the haploid genome and together they comprise about 5% of human DNA (on average one copy every 5,000 nucleotide pairs (794)). Studies of genomic DNA revealed a third gene (*GYPE*) homologous to *GYPA* and *GYPB* (369,765). Although mRNA corresponding to

GPE is found in erythroid cells it is unclear at the time of writing as to whether or not this mRNA is translated into protein that is capable of insertion into the red cell membrane. The translated GPE protein would be predicted to be a polypeptide of 59 amino acids with blood group M specificity but lacking an N glycan or Ss antigen activity. There is doubt as to whether this protein could be inserted in the membrane because there is an eight amino acid insertion in the putative transmembrane domain which disrupts its overall hydrophobicity. One candidate GPE molecule of 20kDa has been proposed based on immunoblotting of red cell membranes with a monoclonal anti-M but protein sequence studies have not been carried out to confirm or deny this possibility (236) .

The genomic structures of *GYPA*, *GYPB* and *GYPE* are compared in figure 15-11, the order of the genes on chromosome 4 and the position of *Alu* repeat sequences is indicated in figure 15-12. The *GYPB* and *GYPE* genes are thought to have evolved from an ancestral *GYPA* gene by duplication of the ancestral *GYPA* gene and subsequent recombination (cross-over) events involving *Alu* repeat sequences. The first recombination event would create *GYPB* and the second *GYPE* (see figure 15-12). *Alu* repeat sequences provide a potent mechanism for generating novel proteins through recombinations of this type and are thought to have had a major impact on the pace of evolution in man (826). The series of recombination events outlined in figure 15-12 would explain why *GYPB* and *GYPE* are very similar at their 3' ends. The model for evolution of *GYPB* shown in figure 15-12 requires that *GYPB* acquires a new 3' sequence and this sequence was found adjacent to a second *Alu* repeat sequence 9.2kb

FIGURE 15-11 Structure of *GYPA*, *GYPB* and *GYPE*

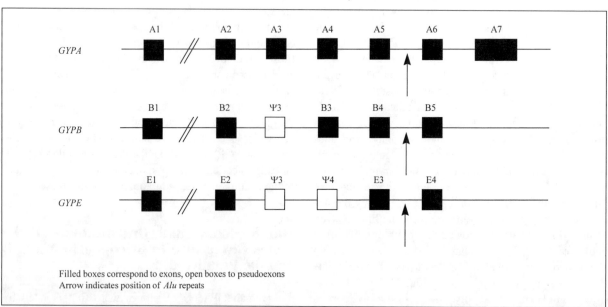

Filled boxes correspond to exons, open boxes to pseudoexons
Arrow indicates position of *Alu* repeats

FIGURE 15-12 Evolution of GYPA, GYPB and GYPE from an Ancestral GYPA gene (modified from reference 797)

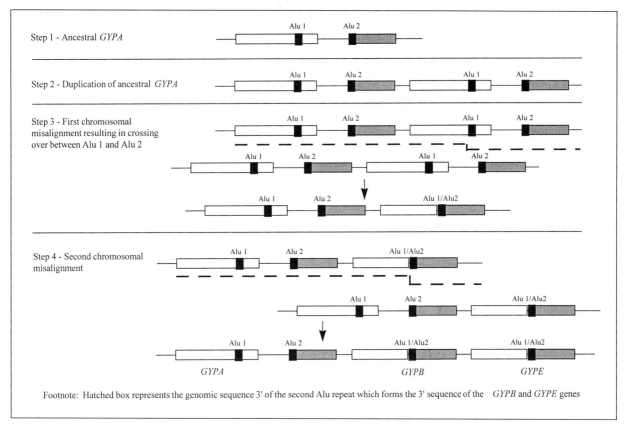

Footnote: Hatched box represents the genomic sequence 3' of the second Alu repeat which forms the 3' sequence of the *GYPB* and *GYPE* genes

downstream from the last exon of *GYPA* (826).

The series of recombination events outlined in the previous paragraph explains the origin of the genes for GPA, GPB and GPE but if these were the only changes to have occurred during evolution GPB and GPE would be identical to GPA with respect to their first 5 exons (i.e. all the exons 5' of the first *Alu* repeat, see figure 15-11). This is not the case. GPB lacks the product of the third exon of *GYPA* because of a subsequent point mutation which inactivates the 5' splice site of exon 3 and leads to ligation of the second exon to the fourth exon (for a general discussion of RNA splicing see Chapter 5). The third exon which is bypassed as a result is therefore a pseudoexon (ψ3). A nucleotide substitution in intron 3 of *GYPB* creates a new 5' splice site so that exon B4 encodes three amino acids (residues 40 - 42) not found in GPA. *GYPE* also has a pseudoexon 3 (presumably because the second recombination event which created *GYPE* occurred after the *GPB* splice site mutation) and a further mutation inactivates the 5' splice site for exon 4 which means that exon 4 in the *GYPE* gene is also a pseudoexon (ψ4). *GYPE* therefore comprises 4 exons (see figure 15-11).

The coding sequence of *GYPA* is contained within exon 2 (encoding amino acids 1-26), exon 3 (residues 27-58), exon 4 (residues 59-71), exon 5 (residues 72-100, transmembrane domain), exon 6 (residues 101-126, cytoplasmic domain), and exon 7 (residues 127-131, cytoplasmic domain). The coding sequence of *GYPB* is contained within exon 2 (residues 1-26), exon 3 (residues 27-39), exon 4 (residues 40-71, transmembrane domain), exon 5 (residue 72). The coding sequence of *GYPE* is contained within exon 2 (residues 1-26) and exon 3 (residues 27-58) and a single residue (residue 59) encoded by exon 4. The exon numbering system used here is shown in figure 15-11.

Since the protein sequence encoded by exon 2 of *GYPA* is common to all three proteins (for GPA it encodes either M or N, for GPB either N or He and for GPE only M) the amino acid sequence homology in this region of the proteins is explained. The absence of exon 3 of *GYPA* from *GYPB* explains GPB's much smaller extracellular domain. The absence of a cytoplasmic domain from GPB and GPE is explained because the *Alu* repeat sequence thought to be involved in the cross-over events which create *GYPB* and *GYPE* is situated between exon 5 and exon 6 of *GYPA* and since exons 6 and 7 encode the cytoplasmic domain these would be lost as a result of the recombination events.

The process of double recombination which gives rise to *GYPE* outlined in figure 15-12 is not entirely satisfactory because, as explained in the previous paragraph, GPE has an M-specific amino-terminus whereas GPB is N-specific. If the double recombination event occured as shown then it would be expected that GPE would be N-specific. GPE also differs from GPB in that it has an in-frame insert of 24 nucleotides in exon 3 (the equivalent of exon 5 in *GYPA*) which represents a duplication of an adjacent 3' coding sequence derived from an ancestral *GYPB* gene (744) and several sequences homologous to *GYPA* in other parts of the gene. Studies on glycophorin genes in other primates have shown that whereas *GYPA* can be detected in all primates tested, *GYPB* can only be detected in gorilla and higher primates and *GYPE* only in some gorillas and higher primates (744,795,796). These results clearly show that the *GYP* family evolved recently.

Studies on the genomic organization of the *GYP* genes have been hampered by the large size of the gene cluster. In fact exon 1 is so far away from the rest of the genes that conventional genomic libraries did not yield any clones which contained exon 1 and exon 2 in either the *GYPA*, *GYPB* or *GYPE* genes. Onda et al. (797) isolated large genomic sequences from yeast artificial chromosomes (YACs see also Chapter 5) and found that the whole gene family is contained in a gene segment of 330kb. Of approximately 1 million YAC clones that were screened with a probe that detects exon 1 of *GYPA, B* and *E* 10 positive clones were found. One of these clones contained all three genes while others contained various parts of the gene cluster. Five YAC clones were studied in detail. The results showed that the distance between exon 1 and the last exon of each member of this gene family is 40-45kb. The precursor 3' sequence is 9.2kb downstream of the *GYPA* gene which itself is about 70kb upstream of exon 1 of the *GYPB* gene. The *Alu* sequence in *GYPB* is about 70kb upstream of exon 1 of *GYPE* (797). These results led Onda et al. (797) to conclude that since only gorillas and higher primates possess *GYPB* but all primates tested have the precursor 3' segment, the unequal cross-over event through *Alu* repeats that created *GYPB* occurred approximately 8-10 million years ago. The genetic event giving rise to *GYPE* would have occurred before the divergence of chimpanzee from a human-gorilla ancestor about 6.3-7.7 million years. These authors seek to explain the presence of an M-specific sequence in GPE by suggesting that exon 2 of *GYPE* acquired a portion of exon 2 of *GYPA* through a gene conversion event. Experimental evidence in support of this hypothesis is provided by Kudo and Fukuda (798). These authors compared the nucleotide sequences of *GYPA, GYPB* and *GYPE* at the 3' end of intron 1, exon 2 and the entire intron 2 and found that this region of

GYPE is more like *GYPA* than like *GYPB*. An analogous gene conversion event involving the *GYPA* and *GYPB* genes has already been invoked to explain the origin of the He antigen (see an earlier section).

Regulation of Expression of *GYP* Genes

The *GYPA* and *GYPB* genes are expressed only in erythroid tissues (799,800) and appear at the same stage in erythropoiesis (801,802). The promoter regions of each of the glycophorin genes were studied by Vignal et al. (529) and Rahuel et al. (803). These authors found that the promoter regions of the three genes are highly homologous and differ only by a few point mutations in the sequence for 330bp upstream of the transcription start point. Each promotor sequence has functional regulatory sequences for transcription factors. These authors concluded that, in common with other erythroid-specific genes, the three glycophorin promoters are driven by GATA-1/Sp1 DNA binding proteins (transcription factors see Chapter 5 for further discussion).

Since GPA is much more abundant in red cells than GPB (4-fold higher) there must be other factors controlling the expression of these genes which are distinct from those that operate at the level of the promoter. Rahuel et al. (803) provide evidence that the difference in the relative amounts of GPA, GPB (and GPE ?) in the red cell membrane is a reflection of the relative stability of the individual mRNAs. These authors studied the stability of GPA, GPB and GPE mRNA in actinomycin-treated K562 cells (actinomycin binds to DNA and blocks the movement of RNA polymerase thereby inhibiting RNA synthesis). They found that GPA transcripts were very stable (at least 24hr), whereas the level of GPB transcripts was severely reduced after 17hr and GPE transcripts were barely detectable after 1hr. The differential stability of these mRNAs may be related to differences in the metabolism of the respective poly (A) tails (803,804). This would be consistent with GPB-A hybrid glycophorin found in Dantu cells of the NE type being expressed at the same levels as GPA (see later section).

Inherited Deficiencies of GPA and/or GPB (En(a-), S- s- Deletion and Non-Deletion Types, *M^k*)

En(a-) red cells have a total deficiency of GPA (12-14,37,429). S- s- red cells are deficient in GPB (16,42,398) and red cells from individuals homozygous for the *M^k* gene have a total absence of GPA and GPB (296,298). There are two different genetic backgrounds giving rise to the En(a-) phenotype, the so-called Finnish and English types. In the case of En(a-) red cells of the Finnish type the absence of GPA from the red cell membranes results from a large deletion which extends from intron 1 of *GYPA* to intron 1 of *GYPB* (527). The *GYPB* gene that is expressed is presumed to utilize exon 1 of *GYPA*. In the English type the genetic background appears more complex because the actual genotype of individuals with the En(a-) phenotype is *En(UK)/M^k*, that is one haplotype (*M^k*) results in the absence of GPA and GPB and the other (*En(UK)*) results in the absence of normal GPA and GPB but produces a GPA-B hybrid protein (Lepore-type, see next section for further discussion of this phenotype).

The genetic background of the S- s- phenotype is heterogeneous. Early studies carried out utilizing SDS-PAGE and subsequent PAS staining revealed that red cell membranes from individuals with the S- s- phenotype lacked staining bands corresponding to GPB suggesting that normal GPB is absent from the membranes of cells of this phenotype (16,42). In most cases, analyses carried out at the DNA level have demonstrated a large deletion extending from intron 1 of *GYPB* to intron 1 of *GYPE* (366,368,342). In other cases (referred to by Huang and Blumenfeld (434) as the "non-deletion" type) different genetic mechanisms are involved. In one report both the coding sequence and the promoter region of *GYPB* was said to be normal and an explanation for the S- s- phenotype (donor Del) was not found (342). Reid et al. (343) noted that red cells of phenotype S- s- are often He+. Since the He antigen is located at the amino-terminus of GPB this result presents something of a paradox. A detailed investigation of the glycophorin genes of one individual (P_2) of phenotype S- s-U- He+ was carried out by Huang et al. (344). These authors found two major structural changes in the S-active allele of a *GYPB* gene. The first change was caused by a gene conversion event which transferred a short sequence in the exon 2-intron 2 region from *GYPA* to *GYPB* and created the sequence associated with the He antigen. The second change involved two single nucleotide mutations 23bp apart affecting RNA splicing. One mutation occurred in a splice site at the 3' end of exon 5 and the other in the consensus sequence of a splice site in intron 5. These mutations in splice sites caused exon 5 to be spliced out so that the resulting translated glycophorin lacked the amino acid sequence encoded by exon 5 (the transmembrane domain) and the sequence encoded by exon 4 was directly ligated to that encoded by exon 6. This altered splicing event caused a shift in the open reading frame and resulted in translation of some of the 3' noncoding region. The resulting protein comprised residues 1-39 of an S-active *GYPB* gene encoding He antigen (residue 29 was Met), but the amino acid sequence downstream of exon 4 was completely changed from residue 40 to a new C-terminus at residue 81 (normal GPB has 72

residues). A hydropathy plot of the novel C-terminal sequence revealed that overall it had a hydrophobic character. Since the red cells of this individual typed as weakly positive with anti-He and since weak bands of the expected size were seen on immunoblots developed with a polyclonal antiserum raised to GPA, these authors concluded that some insertion of the abnormal glycophorin into the red cell membrane must occur. The absence of S activity on these cells was attributed to conformational affects caused by the novel C-terminal sequence. The apparent molecular weight on SDS-PAGE of the abnormal protein described by Huang et al. (344) is very similar to that of a band described by one of us (DJA) and colleagues (398) in 1979 in lactoperoxidase-labeled red cells of phenotype S- s- U-. The band was denoted ω (398). This is mentioned not so much because it adds to the reader's understanding of this phenotype but more because it provides a possible answer for the origin of band ω which the author has been waiting for almost 20 years! It will be of interest to examine the genetic basis of the S- s- U+ He+ phenotype to see if a related genetic mechanism gives rise to this phenotype. Information obtained from the examination of cells of these phenotypes should also contribute to our understanding of the structure of the U antigen.

Individuals homozygous for the *M^k* haplotype lack GPA and GPB and Southern blotting studies of DNA derived from one such donor (RS) demonstrated a gross deletion involving both *GYPA* and *GYPB* (368,369) which extends from intron 1 of *GYPA* to intron 1 of *GYPE*.

These three deficiency types (En(a-) (Finnish type), S- s- (deletion type) and homozygotes for *M^k*) result from different deletions involving the *GYP* family but, as Huang and Blumenfeld (434) have pointed out, the mechanism which creates these deletions has a common feature. The deletion which creates En(a-) (Finnish type) starts in intron 1 of *GYPA* and finishes in intron 1 of *GYPB*. The deletion which creates S- s- (deletion type) begins in intron 1 of *GYPB* and ends in intron 1 of GYPE. The deletion which creates *M^k* begins in intron 1 of *GYPA* and ends in intron 1 of *GYPE*. Intron 1 in each of these genes is very large indeed and genomic clones which contain the entire intron 1 of each of these genes have only recently been obtained and are not fully characterized (797). Nevertheless it is possible to envisage regions of sequence homology in the respective intron 1s that could effect unequal cross-over events at meiosis resulting in the deletions that are observed (434). A similar mechanism has already been discussed in relation to the role of *Alu* repeat sequences in the evolution of this gene family (see section on organization of the glycophorin genes).

An understanding of the nature of these deletions is relevant to the question as to whether GPE is ever expressed as a glycoprotein in the red cell membrane. The deletion giving rise to *M^k* would be predicted to result in a *GYPE* with exon 1 derived from *GYPA* and the product of the gene would be the only glycophorin expressed on the surface of red cells from an M^k homozygote. Immunoblotting studies carried out on red cell membranes from such red cells using a murine monoclonal anti-M (BS-38) identified a band or bands of 20kDa (236). The nature of these bands has not been further investigated.

Some MN System Antigens are Generated by Cross-over Events Between Misaligned *GYPA* and *GYPB* Genes at Meiosis (Hil, St^a, Dantu, SAT)

In an earlier section the structure and organization of the *GYP* gene cluster was described together with a mechanism whereby *GYPA*, *GYPB* and *GYPE* evolved. The evolution of these glycophorin genes appears to have occurred by duplication and non-homologous recombination involving *Alu* repeats when chromosomes have misaligned at meiosis. When chromosomes become misaligned at meiosis points of cross-over are not confined to regions containing *Alu* repeats. The regions of *GYPA*, *GYPB*, and *GYPE* which are immediately 5' to the *Alu* repeats (i.e. the regions corresponding to exons 2, 3, 4 and 5 of *GYPA*, see figure 15-11) are extremely homologous between the genes. Cross-over events and gene conversion events involving these regions of homology particularly between *GYPA* and *GYPB* have given rise to a large number of novel glycophorins and, ipso facto, novel antigens.

The existence of hybrid glycophorins comprising part of GPA and part of GPB was first noticed in the mid-1970s when SDS-PAGE was used in a fairly systematic way to look at the pattern of PAS-staining bands obtained when red cell membranes from individuals with unusual MN phenotypes were electrophoresed. The early studies concentrated on membranes from individuals whose phenotypes suggested the absence of normal MNSs antigens. In particular, cells of phenotype En(a-) were shown to lack PAS-staining bands corresponding to GPA (12-14,37,429) and cells of phenotype S- s- were shown to lack PAS-staining bands corresponding to GPB (16,42,398). These studies are described in more detail in the preceding section. When this type of analysis was extended to red cells with unusual MNSs antigens rather than red cells which lacked common MNSs antigens it was seen that in some cases novel PAS-staining bands were present. In the next few years SDS-PAGE proved to be a very useful tool for identifying unusual glycophorins. The reason that this approach was so successful is easy to see. GPA has a large cytoplasmic domain which is lacking from GPB and so GPA has a

larger molecular weight than GPB on SDS-PAGE. GPA also differs from GPB in that it has a larger extracellular domain because the amino acids encoded by exon 3 of *GYPA* (residues 27-58) are not present in GPB. These major differences in the size of GPA and GPB mean that hybrid molecules formed with an amino terminal segment derived from GPA and a carboxy terminal segment derived from GPB (or vice versa) would have a different apparent molecular weight from normal GPA and normal GPB and so would be detected as novel bands on SDS-PAGE. A similar approach, if applied to the study of Rh polypeptides which contain portions of the D polypeptide and portions of the CE polypeptide, would not work because the D and CE polypeptides are exactly the same size (417 residues) and run with almost the same apparent molecular weight on SDS-PAGE. Thus hybrid Rh polypeptides could not be distinguished from normal Rh polypeptides on the basis of size (see Chapter 12 for discussions of variant D and CE polypeptides created as a result of misalignment between the *D* and *CE* genes at meiosis).

In retrospect, the first evidence for hybrid GPA-GPB molecules came from the study of red cell membranes derived from individuals in an English family with the En(a-) phenotype (ME-P family) (83). The En(a-) phenotype in families with Finnish ancestry results in the absence of GPA from the red cell membranes but expression of an apparently normal GPB molecule (see previous section). The En(a-) phenotype in the English ME-P family (sometimes referred to as En(a-)UK to distinguish it from those of Finnish origin) clearly has a different genetic background because the absence of GPA is accompanied by a GPB molecule which carries an M blood group antigen (311,530). The suggestion that this M-active GPB was in fact a hybrid GPA-B molecule was made at the time (311) but it was difficult to prove because the molecular weight of this molecule was indistinguishable from that of normal GPB. Subsequent studies using murine monoclonal antibodies supported this prediction (451). Studies at the DNA level have shown that the molecule is indeed a hybrid GPA-B resulting from a cross-over event involving exon 2 of *GYPA* and exon 2 of *GYPB* (527).

The first unambiguous demonstration that hybrid GPA-B molecules exist came from studies of red cells with the phenotype known as Miltenberger Class V (289, 312,398,471). The early work was done on red cells from individuals heterozygous for the gene that encodes this phenotype but when rare cells from an individual homozygous for the gene were described (287) any doubts in interpretation were dispelled. Red cells from the *MiV* homozygote were totally deficient in normal GPA and GPB but contained a novel PAS-staining component of molecular weight intermediate between monomeric GPA and monomeric GPB. Immunoprecipitation studies with a monoclonal antibody (R18) specific for an epitope in the extracellular domain of GPA showed that the abnormal protein contained a region common to the extracellular domain of GPA. Parallel immuneprecipitation studies with a rabbit antiserum raised to the cytoplasmic domain of GPA failed to react with the abnormal protein in red cells of the *MiV* homozygote. These results suggested that the abnormal protein was composed of an N-terminus derived from GPA and a C-terminus from GPB (289). These results raised the obvious question as to the genetic mechanism that gave rise to this hybrid protein. If as seemed likely, the hybrid was created by a single genetic event then that event would have to explain not just the formation of the hybrid gene but also the concomitant loss of the normal *GYPA* and *GYPB* genes. Fortunately, a precedent for such a genetic event already existed. A hemoglobin variant known as HbLepore is a hybrid δβ globin which results from a cross-over event at meiosis between regions of homology in the δ globin and β globin genes. This cross over event creates one chromosome with a δβ globin gene and the other chromosome with normal δ and β globin genes and a hybrid βδ gene. This second chromosome represents the anti-Lepore haplotype (430). If the abnormal GPA-B molecule in the red cells of the *MiV* homozygote was created in an analogous fashion to HbLepore then individuals with an analogous "anti-Lepore" haplotype should exist and would be predicted to have normal *GYPA* and *GYPB* genes together with a hybrid *GYPB-A* gene which encoded a novel glycophorin containing the N-terminus of GPB and the C-terminus of GPA. At the time of this work a candidate "anti-Lepore" haplotype was found in the author's (DJA) laboratory. Red cells from an individual with the S- s- phenotype (MP Jnr) sent from Dr. Robert Lowe in Zimbabwe gave a unique and unexpected pattern of bands on SDS-PAGE. The pattern of staining and immunochemical investigation of the bands revealed an abnormal glycophorin of Mr 32,000 with properties that suggested it was a hybrid GPB-A molecule. The haplotype (denoted Ph variant) which contained the hybrid gene expressed normal GPA but lacked GPB (346). The absence of a normal GPB in this haplotype meant that the designation "anti-Lepore" was not certain since the abnormal band might have been some sort of GPB variant. The "anti-Lepore" haplotype exhibiting normal GPA and GPB as well as a hybrid GPB-A was subsequently found to correlate with expression of the St^a antigen (502). In 1981 Dominique Blanchard, then working in Jean-Pierre Cartron's laboratory in Paris, visited the author's laboratory to carry out experiments on a glycophorin variant denoted Pj. SDS-PAGE analysis of this variant was identical to that of St(a+) red cells and the cells were subsequently confirmed as St(a+) (503). The red cells of MP Jnr which expressed the Ph variant were subsequently shown

to have the Dantu antigen by Dr Patricia Tippett (47).

So it was that in the late 1970s and early 1980s it became clear that Lepore and anti-Lepore type haplotypes existed in the MN system. Lepore type haplotypes gave rise to MiV, a similar hybrid (JR) which lacked the Hil antigen (288), and probably also EnUK (311). Anti-Lepore type haplotypes correlated with the presence of the St^a antigen and probably the Dantu antigen as well. Since novel amino acid sequences would be created at the junction of GPA sequence and GPB sequence in the Lepore type, the Hil antigen was probably located in this unique sequence and similarly St^a and Dantu antigens were probably located in the junction sequences of GPB-A anti-Lepore type hybrids (see figure 15-13, 805). These results and conclusions were obtained before the cloning of the *GYP* genes and have since been largely confirmed at the DNA level.

Analysis of the predicted hybrid *GYPA-B* in the MiV phenotype gave the expected results. The gene comprises exons 1-3 of *GYPA* and exons 4-6 of *GYPB*. It was reported initially that the gene comprised exon 1 of *GYPB* rather than exon 1 of *GYPA* (292) but this rather surprising finding was in fact an error which was later corrected (529). The protein sequence of this GPA-B molecule comprises amino acids 1-58 of GPA and amino acids 27-72 of GPB. The cross-over point which creates the hybrid gene is located in intron 3 of *GYPA* (at the 5' end between nt 134-270) and intron 3 of *GYPB* (295)).

Another kind of GPA-B hybrid (JR) was described by Langley et al. (288). This hybrid was not associated with the expression of Hil antigen and so could not be classified as of the MiV phenotype. It was associated with S rather than s and the failure to express Hil antigen was related to this difference because the molecule behaved like the MiV hybrid in all other respects (288). A second similar example of this type of hybrid (AG) was soon reported but in this case weak reactivity with anti-Hil was observed (806). Protein sequence studies carried out on a third example (JL) which appeared to be identical to JR gave the expected results. It comprised residues 1-58 of GPA and residues 27-72 of GPB (only 27-68 were proved by sequence studies) (553). Kudo et al. (736) showed that, like the hybrid associated with MiV, the hybrid in JL red cells results from a cross-over event between regions of intron 3 of *GYPA* and *GYPB*. Kudo et al. (736) referred to this hybrid as MiV*. Similar results were reported by Huang et al. (295). When it was shown that GPA-B hybrids of this type express the antigen TSEN (102) the phenotype represented by GPA-B hybrids of the JR/JL type became Miltenberger Class XI. To summarize, the hybrid GPA-B molecule found originally in donor JR probably = JL = MiV* =

FIGURE 15-13 Chromosomal Misalignment at Meiosis Leading to Non-homologous Crossing-over between *GYPA* and *GYPB* and the Creation of Genes Encoding Hybrid Glycophorin Molecules

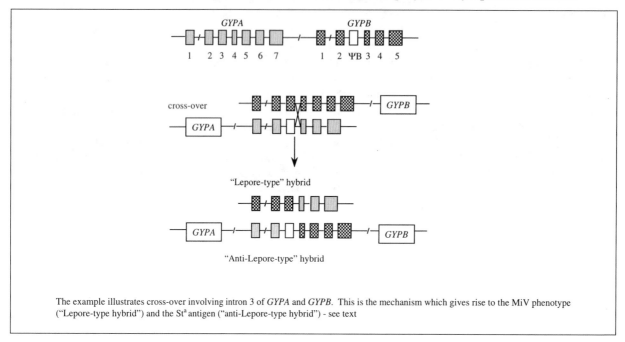

The example illustrates cross-over involving intron 3 of *GYPA* and *GYPB*. This is the mechanism which gives rise to the MiV phenotype ("Lepore-type hybrid") and the St^a antigen ("anti-Lepore-type hybrid") - see text

MiXI. This hybrid differs from that found in the MiV phenotype by a single amino acid. It has Met61 instead of Thr. This is because it results from a cross-over between *GYPA* and *GYPB* where *GYPB* encodes the S antigen. In MiV the analogous cross-over involved a *GYPB* which encodes s antigen.

Direct evidence that Hil and TSEN are defined by the novel amino acid sequences created at the cross-over sites has been obtained by hemagglutination inhibition experiments using synthetic peptides representing amino acids 54-67 of the hybrid molecules. If Thr61 is present the peptides inhibit anti-Hil but not anti-TSEN. If Met61 is present the peptide inhibits anti-TSEN but not anti-Hil (102,658).

Lepore-type hybrid GPA-B molecules are not confined to those resulting from cross-overs involving the respective intron 3s of *GYPA* and *GYPB*. Daniels et al. (101) described a Japanese family in which a novel MN system antigen SAT was inherited with a hybrid GPA-B molecule. Analysis of the gene giving rise to this hybrid molecule revealed that it resulted from a crossover between *GYPA* and *GYPB* within intron 4 and comprised exons 1-4 of *GYPA* and exons 5 and 6 of *GYPB* (593). The absence of exon 4 of *GYPB* explained why the hybrid glycophorin failed to express S or s antigens (and probably U). The hybrid gene encodes a polypeptide of 104 amino acids. A novel amino acid sequence (Ser-Glu-Pro-Ala-Pro-Val) is created at the GPA-B junction and this is likely to define the SAT antigen. The antigen SAT is not always found in association with a hybrid glycophorin (101,594). Nucleotide sequence analysis of *GYPA* cDNA from a SAT positive donor who lacked hybrid glycophorin revealed a 9 nucleotide insertion derived from the 5′ end of exon 5 of *GYPB* between the sequence encoded by exons 4 and 5 of *GYPA*. The 9 nucleotides effected an in-frame insertion of three amino acids (Ala-Pro-Val) thereby recreating the Ser-Glu-Pro-Ala-Pro-Val sequence found at the GPA-B junction in SAT positive hybrid glycophorins (594).

The cross-over events that give rise to these Lepore-type GPA-B hybrid molecules must ipso facto create another haplotype (anti-Lepore) containing normal *GYPA* and normal *GYPB* together with a hybrid *GYPB-A* gene (see figure 15-13). As discussed above, two MN system antigens (St^a and Dantu) were shown to mark such hybrid GPB-A molecules in the late 1970s and early 1980s (47,346,502,805). Subsequent protein and nucleotide sequencing studies have shown that the GPB-A hybrid found in St(a+) red cells is the anti-Lepore haplotype created when cross-overs occur between intron 3 of *GYPA* and *GYPB* (the event which creates the GPA-B hybrids with Hil or TSEN antigen activity). The GPB-A hybrid found in Dantu+ red cells corresponds to the anti-Lepore haplotype created when cross-overs occur between intron 4 of *GYPA* and *GYPB* (the event which creates the GPA-B hybrid with SAT antigen activity).

Genetic Mechanisms Giving Rise to the St[a] Antigen (or Different Ways of Eliminating Exon 3 From *GYPA*)

The structure of an St(a+) GPB-A hybrid was determined by protein sequence analysis and was found to contain residues 1-26 of GPB and 59-131 of GPA (807,808). Data consistent with these conclusions were obtained independently by Blumenfeld et al. (809) on an St(a+) GPB-A obtained from a Japanese donor homozygous for the gene encoding St[a]. The donor was first described by Macdonald et al. (810). Subsequent studies have revealed that the St[a] antigen can result from a variety of genetic backgrounds and so the GPB-A hybrid type referred to above is now known as GP.Sch (*M^r*) to distinguish it from other St(a+) glycophorins (see below). When examined at the DNA level the *GPB-A* gene giving rise to GP.Sch is seen to result from a cross-over event involving intron 3 of *GYPA* and intron 3 of *GYPB* encoding a hybrid GPB-A molecule with a novel protein sequence at the junction of GPB and GPA sequence (Gln-Thr-Asn-Gly-Glu-Arg-Val) which is presumed to form the basis of the St[a] antigen (295,811,812). Several different cross-over points within the respective intron 3s can create GP.Sch. Huang and Blumenfeld (813) found two different cross-over points in St(a+) Black Americans and a third in a Japanese. An St(a+) hybrid glycophorin formed by this mechanism but having the He antigen at its N-terminus rather 'N' was described by Huang et al. (285). This presumably arose by a cross-over involving an He+ *GYPB*.

The St(a+) glycophorin GP.Zan (*M^z*) has exactly the same protein sequence as GP.Sch but the genetic mechanism that creates this glycophorin is different from that which creates GP.Sch. The clue that led to the realization that this glycophorin was unusual was the presence of a trypsin-resistant M antigen (a conventional GPB-A hybrid glycophorin would have trypsin-resistant N ('N')). Dahr et al. (504) purified GP.Zan, determined its amino acid sequence, and showed that it is not a GPB-A hybrid but an abnormal GPA molecule which lacks amino acid residues 27-58. Since these residues are encoded by exon 3 of *GYPA* it was suggested that this exon is deleted in this abnormal *GYPA* gene. Subsequent DNA analysis revealed that exon 3 of *GYPA* and the 5′ end of intron 3 of *GYPA* were replaced by the corresponding region of the *GYPB* gene. Exon 3 of normal *GYPB* is a pseudoexon and is not spliced into the mRNA giving rise GP.Zan (505). When cDNA from these cells was examined, a minor transcript lacking the products of both exon 3 and exon 4 of *GYPA* was found which was membrane bound and would produce trypsin-resistant M antigen but not St[a].

A third genetic mechanism giving rise to the St[a] antigen is found in association with the low frequency antigen ERIK (105). Although SDS-PAGE revealed a band which would correspond to the expected GPB-A hybrid associated with St[a], immunoblotting studies revealed that the ERIK antigen was not found on this GPB-A band but on a band corresponding to normal GPA (105). Analysis at the DNA level provided the answer to this puzzle. A single point mutation in the last nucleotide of exon 3 of *GYPA* partially inactivates the 5′ splice site so that four different transcripts of this gene are produced (506). The full length transcript corresponds to a GPA molecule with a single amino acid sequence difference from normal GPA (Gly59Arg). This single amino acid change results from the point mutation in the last nucleotide of exon 3 of *GYPA* and it is this which creates the ERIK antigen. Since the point mutation which creates ERIK also partially inactivates a splice site a GPA transcript which lacks the sequence encoded by exon 3 is produced. The junction of exon 2 and exon 4 of GPA creates exactly the same sequence as the GPB-A hybrid which creates the St[a] antigen (GP.Sch) and the exon 3 deleted St(a+) abnormal GPA, GP.Zan described above. Thus this transcript explains the presence of the St[a] antigen on these cells. Two other transcripts were found, one lacked exons 2 and 3 of *GYPA* and the other exons 2, 3 and 4 of *GYPA*. The absence of the products of exon 2 from these transcripts would mean that they lack a complete leader sequence and so the polypeptides would not be inserted into the red cell membrane (506).

Yet another mechanism of generating St[a] and ERIK antigens has been found in an Australian family (434,814). This case is particularly interesting because it involves *GYPE*. The St[a]-active protein product is encoded by an altered *GYPA* lacking the product of exon 3 as it is in GP.Zan and the ERIK+, St(a+) case described in the previous paragraph. However, in this case the genetic event which causes the loss of exon 3 from *GYPA* results from insertion of the pseudoexon 3 and the inactive splice site in intron 3 from *GYPE*. The structure of the ERIK antigen in these cells has not been reported at the time of writing.

Genetic Mechanisms Giving Rise to the Dantu Antigen

As already mentioned, the Dantu antigen results from the anti-Lepore type haplotype which results from a cross-over between *GYPA* and *GYPB* involving their respective intron 4s (434,815). This anti-Lepore haplotype would be expected to comprise a normal *GYPA* gene, a normal *GYPB* gene and a hybrid *GYPB-A* gene. However, in most of the Dantu+ samples studied there is an absence of *GYPB* from the anti-Lepore haplotype because the cross-over occurred on a deletion-type S- s-background. This was true of the first candidate anti-Lepore haplotype (Ph variant) (346) which was subsequently shown to be Dantu+ (47) and the first haplotype studied because it produced the Dantu antigen (NE) (589). The occurrence of these GPB-A hybrids on this genetic background made interpretation of the molecular mechanism giving rise to the GPB-A hybrid more difficult (at this point one of us (DJA) should own up to the incorrect suggestion that the Dantu hybrid (NE-type) was a GPA-B-A molecule) (588). The expected anti-Lepore haplotype with normal *GYPA* and *GYPB* in addition to the hybrid *GYPB-A* was subsequently reported by Dahr et al. (52) in a White individual (MD) with Dantu+ red cells.

That the structure of the GPB-A glycophorin in Dantu+ red cells was different from that found in St(a+) red cells was clear from immunochemical studies. In particular, it was noted that the Dantu hybrid could not be immunoprecipitated with monoclonal anti-Wr^b whereas the St^a hybrid could (816). Since the Wr^b antigen had been located to a region involving residues 61-72 of GPA, it followed that this region would be predicted to be absent from the GPB-A Dantu hybrid but not from the GPB-A St^a hybrid (816). Subsequent protein sequence studies showed that the GPB-A hybrid in the Dantu+ donors comprises residues 1-39 of GPB and 71-131 of GPA (donor NE (554) donors MD and DA) (590). These protein sequence studies established the nature of the Dantu GPB-A hybrid but did not elucidate the reasons for other differences between different Dantu+ phenotypes. The Dantu+ haplotype found in the Ph variant produced a normal GPA and a Dantu GPB-A hybrid expressing 'N' and s but no GPB. The ratio of GPA to GPB-A was 1:1 (346). The Dantu+ haplotype found in donor NE also produces normal GPA and a Dantu GPB-A hybrid expressing 'N' and s and no GPB but in this case the amount of GPA produced was less than half of normal levels and the hybrid GPB-A molecule was produced at high levels (the ratio of GPA to GPB-A was 1:2.4) (589). In the White Dantu+ donor, MD, the molar ratio GPA to hybrid was similar to that in the Ph variant (1:0.6) (52). Quantitative binding studies using radioiodinated murine monoclonal antibodies showed that the amount of Dantu hybrid in cells of the NE type is significantly greater than that found in cells of the Ph variant type (315,000 copies/cell compared with 200,000 copies/cell) (588). These results clearly indicated that at least two molecular mechanisms can give rise to the Dantu+ phenotype.

An explanation for the higher level of Dantu hybrid GPB-A in cells of the NE type was provided by Huang and Blumenfeld (815) who found that the *GYPB-A* gene in individuals of this type is duplicated and arranged in tandem in the haplotype. If the hybrid genes are transcribed at the same level as normal *GYPA* and the translated hybrid mRNA is as stable as normal GPA mRNA (normal GPB mRNA is not as stable as normal GPA mRNA (803) and see section on regulation of *GYP* genes) and if the membrane assembly of the hybrid molecules is no less efficient than that of normal GPA (see later section on the association of glycophorins with band 3 and Rh glycoprotein) then the molar ratio of GPA relative to GPB-A in the red cell membrane would be 1:2 which is what is observed. The reduced level of GPA and hence weak M antigen in those Dantu+ cells which have M-active GPA presumably reflects the fact that the total amount of glycophorin that can be incorporated into the membrane is limited (perhaps by the amount of band 3) (589). It is assumed that duplication of the hybrid *GYPB-A* gene does not occur in the haplotype giving rise to the Ph variant and in the White donor MD, but this does not appear to have been formally proved at the time of writing.

Some MN System Antigens are Generated by Gene Conversion Events Occurring at Meiosis Which Create GPB-A-B and GPA-B-A Variants

I. GPB-A-B hybrid glycophorins (MiIII, MiIV, MiVI, MiX)

In the 1970s SDS-PAGE analysis of membranes from red cells of phenotypes Miltenberger III, IV and VI revealed the presence of an abnormal PAS-staining band of apparent molecular weight 38,000 which formed complexes with itself, GPA and GPB (312,398). Red cells from persons heterozygous for the Miltenberger gene in question had a reduced content of GPB suggesting that the abnormal band was an unusual form of GPB. SDS-PAGE analysis of red cells from individuals homozygous for the genes confirmed this impression since these cells lacked normal GPB (509). Amino acid sequence studies on the abnormal protein suggested that it comprised GPB with a small sequence insertion derived from GPA (99). Immunoblotting studies using murine monoclonal antibodies specific for different epitopes on GPA demonstrated that antibody R18 reacted with the abnormal glycoprotein providing further evidence that it contained a GPA insert (293). DNA sequence analysis demonstrated that the gene giving rise to the abnormal glycoproteins in MiIII and MiVI cells are indeed hybrid *GYPB-A-B* genes (818). The novel GPA sequence found in these proteins is in fact derived from a new exon created from the 5' portion of the pseudoexon 3 found in *GYPB* and the 3' portion of exon 3 from *GYPA*. The portion of *GYPA* found in the hybrid genes extends into intron 3 so the active splice site at the *GYPA* exon 3-intron 3 junction replaces the inactive splice site that prevents incorporation of pseudoexon 3 into the normal *GYPB* gene product (see figure 15-14). Subsequent studies revealed that the MiX phenotype is derived from a similar genetic event (108). In each of these phenotypes the *GYPB-A-B* gene is slightly different. In MiIII a 55bp segment from *GYPA* replaces the equivalent *GYPB* gene sequence. In MiVI the replacement sequence is 131bp and in MiX it is 98bp but in every case an active donor splice site derived from the *GYPA* exon 3-intron 3 junction is introduced into the *GYPB* gene so that a novel protein sequence results. In the case of MiIII (syn. GP.Mur) (104) the hybrid B-A-B glycophorin is comprised of residues 1-26 from GPB, residues 27-48 from ψexon 3 of GPB, residues 49-57 from GPA and residues

58-103 from a GPB gene which encodes the s antigenic sequence (434). In the case of MiVI (GP.Bun) (104) the hybrid GPB-A-B glycophorin comprises residues 1-26 of GPB, residues 27-50 from ψexon 3 of GPB, residues 51-57 from GPA and residues 58-103 from an s-active GPB. In the case of MiX (GP.HF) (9), formerly GP.Mor (104) the hybrid GPB-A-B glycophorin comprises residues 1-26 of GPB, residues 27-34 from ψexon 3 of GPB, residues 35-58 of GPA and residues 59-104 of an s-active GPB. The MiIII and MiVI hybrid glycophorins have different amino acid sequences at the junction formed by ψexon 3 of *GYPB* and exon 3 of *GYPA* but are otherwise identical. Since the two hybrids are distinguished by the fact that MiIII cells lack the Hop antigen whereas MiVI cells do not, it is logical to deduce that the Hop antigen is defined by the sequence at this junction in MiVI. Consistent with this assumption, a synthetic peptide corresponding to

FIGURE 15-14 Different Gene Conversion Events Give Rise to Hybrid Glycophorin Genes of Type *GYPA-B-A* and *GYPB-A-B*

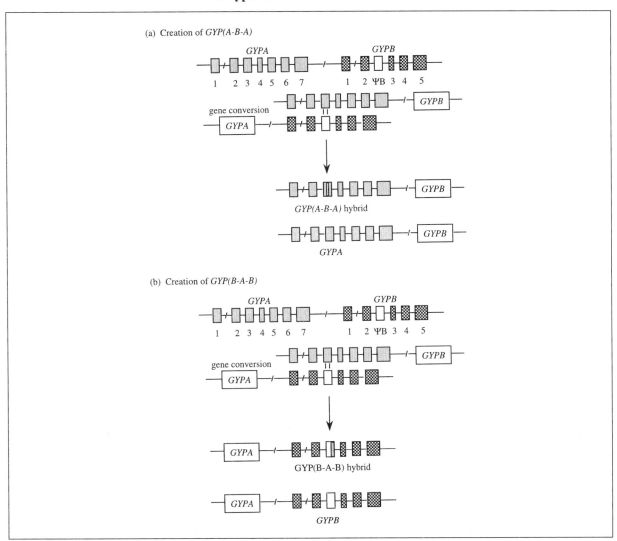

residues 45-54 of MiVI (GP.Bun) was shown to inhibit anti-Hop (658). MiX (GP.HF) differs from MiIII and MiVI in that it fails to react with anti-Mur. Inspection of the amino acid sequence of MiX at the ψexon 3 GPB-GPA junction in comparison with the corresponding junction sites in MiIII and MiVI would suggest that the Mur antigen is located in the region corresponding to residues 34-48 of MiIII and MiVI which is derived from the ψexon 3 sequence. Consistent with this, anti-Mur was shown to be inhibited by a synthetic peptide corresponding to residues 32-44 of the MiIII and MiVI hybrid glycophorin sequences (658). The inhibition of anti-Hop and anti-Mur by synthetic peptides indicates that O-glycans are not essential for the structure of these antigens despite the presence of Ser and Thr residues in the antigen. Indirect evidence suggests that the MiIV phenotype (GP.Hop) is derived from a mechanism identical to that which gives rise to MiVI except that the *GYPB* gene involved encoded S rather than s antigen. This also explains why GP.Hop lacks the Hil antigen.

II. GPA-B-A hybrid glycophorins (MiI, MiII, MiVII, MiVIII, MiIX)

Hybrid glycophorins also occur in which a short stretch of the *GYPB* pseudoexon is introduced into exon 3 of the *GYPA* gene. These insertions do not alter the reading frame or disrupt the 5′ and 3′ splice sites and so create GPA-B-A hybrid molecules (see figure 15-14). The insertions that produce hybrids of this type are, however, much smaller than those which give rise to GPB-A-B hybrids and range in size from 1 to 16 bp (434). Huang et al. (434,619) argue that small insertions of this type account for changes of a single amino acid in the GPA sequences that give rise to the antigens Vw (MiI, GP.Vw), Hut and Mut (MiII, GP.Hut) and Hop and Nob (MiVIII, GP.Joh). The Vw antigen is located on GPA and is known from protein sequencing studies to result from a single amino acid change Thr28 to Met. Similarly, the Hut antigen results from a single amino acid change at the same place Thr28 to Lys (616). The sequence changes that give rise to Vw and Hut destroy the signal sequence (Asn26-X-Thr) in normal GPA which gives rise to an N-glycan at Asn26 on GPA. The absence of this N-glycan means that GPA expressing either Vw or Hut antigens runs with an apparent molecular weight 3000 less than normal GPA on SDS-PAGE (616). The absence of this N-glycan is indicated by experimental evidence which shows that GPA expressing either the Vw or the Hut antigens fail to bind the *Phaseolus vulgaris* lectin (616) and is unaffected by treatment with N-glycanase (619). GPA in the MiVIII phenotype (GP.Joh) also differs from normal GPA at a single amino acid residue

(Arg49 to Thr) and this Thr49 is O-glycosylated (819). This single amino acid change creates two antigens Hop and Nob. The dependence of Hop on the nature of residue 49 is not unexpected since comparison of the sequences of hybrid B-A-B molecules MiIII, GP.Mur and MiVI, GP.Bun lead to similar conclusions. It is difficult to be certain that these single amino acid differences arose by gene conversion rather than by single nucleotide mutations but the fact that all of the nucleotide substitutions leading to these variants, except for GP.Vw, are present in the *GYPB* pseudoexon does suggest that gene conversion rather than point mutation is the most likely mechanism. The argument for gene conversion is stronger in the case of MiVII (GP.Nob). GP.Nob is an abnormal GPA molecule in which two amino acids differ from those found in normal GPA. The Arg49Thr change found in GP.Joh (MiVIII) is present in GP.Nob and an additional change Tyr52Ser is also present (554). GP.Nob expresses the antigen Nob but not Hop and so it must be concluded that the Tyr52Ser change results in the loss of Hop antigen. It is conceivable that GP.Nob could have resulted from a single point mutation in the gene giving rise to GP.Joh but it seems more likely that it results from a gene conversion event that produces an A-B-A hybrid gene which encodes a glycophorin comprising residues 1-48 derived from GPA, residues 49-52 derived from the GPB pseudoexon and residues 53-131 derived from GPA (434). Insertion of this small sequence from the *GYPB* pseudoexon would account for the two amino acid changes in a single event. Both Hop and Nob antigens are sialidase-sensitive (9,554) and since both are present on GP.Joh it seems likely that Thr49 is O-glycosylated and accounts for Hop and Nob. Since Hop is lost in GP.Nob when Tyr52 becomes Ser, Tyr52 is required for Hop but not for Nob. Curiously, anti-Hop is inhibited by synthetic peptides comprising residues 45-54 of GP.Joh (658) and Thr49 cannot be O-glycosylated on these synthetic peptides. This situation is rather reminiscent of the specificity of monoclonal antibodies with anti-M+M^g specificity (476) where the role of the sialic acid residue appears to be to maintain the conformation of a peptide epitope rather than participate directly in its structure. These considerations lead one to conclude that Tyr52 is the key residue defining Hop whereas Nob may depend directly on the glycosylated Thr49.

The GPA-B-A hybrid glycophorin with the largest GPB insert (16bp) is that which gives rise to the MiIX phenotype (GP.Dane). In this case 16bp from the *GYPB* pseudoexon are inserted into *GYPA* creating an alteration in six amino acids (residues 35-40) (655). The resulting GP.Dane expresses both the Mur antigen and a novel antigen DANE. GP.Dane was originally identified through studies of the DANE antigen which showed that it was associated with an abnormal GPA molecule with a

Mr of 1000 less than normal GPA and lacking the trypsin cleavage site at residue 39. Monoclonal antibodies which recognize epitopes in the region of residues 26-39 of normal GPA also failed to react with this abnormal glycophorin (100). A single sialotetrasaccharide has a molecular weight of approximately 1000 and so these results could be explained by a sequence change in the region 26-39 of normal GPA which resulted in the loss of a single O-glycosylation site. DNA sequence analysis identified an insertion from the *GYPB* pseudoexon into exon 3 of *GYPA*. The resulting hybrid glycophorin contains residues 1-34 derived from GPA, residues 35-40 derived from the *GYPB* pseudoexon and residues 41-130 from GPA so that Ala35-Ala-Thr-Pro-Arg-Ala-His in normal GPA is replaced with Pro35-Ala-His-Thr-Ala-Asn in the GPA-B-A glycophorin. This insertion which replaces seven amino acids with six, explains the loss of the trypsin-sensitive site at Arg39 in normal GPA since it is replaced by Ala in the hybrid glycophorin. Since the *GYPB* pseudoexon sequence contains one Thr and the GPA sequence that it replaces also contains one Thr, the loss of an O-glycan is not simply explained. It may be that the sequence of amino acids around Thr38 in the hybrid glycophorin is not a suitable acceptor for the available GalNAc transferases. Such a hypothesis can now be tested by experiment since several of the GalNAc transferases which are capable of initiating O-glycan synthesis have been cloned and it is possible to test their specificity using synthetic peptides (776,777). GP.Dane expresses the Mur antigen and it seems likely that the pseudoexon insert comprising residues 35-40 define Mur since this sequence is also contained in the GPB-A-B hybrids found in MiIII, IV and VI which are also Mur+ (see previous section). In addition to the pseudoexon insert comprising residues 35-40, GP.Dane also has an additional point mutation. Ile46 of GPA is replaced by Asn45 in GP.Dane (Asn 45 not 46 because of the loss of one amino acid as a result of the pseudoexon insertion). It has been suggested that the DANE antigen is defined by this Asn45 and that the mutation may have resulted from an error in DNA repair at the time of the gene conversion event which introduced the pseudoexon sequence (655). Anti-DANE also reacts with M^g cells prompting the suggestion that this relates to the requirement for Asn in both determinants (475).

MN System Antigens that Result from Cross-over or Gene Conversion Events: An Overview of How the Miltenberger Series Fits

Detailed discussion of the molecular mechanisms giving rise to a large number of different antigens, such as that in the preceding sections, is liable to the give the impression that the whole system is bewilderingly complex. It is not! For example, all the genetic events giving rise to antigens that have been collected together in the Miltenberger series result from either a cross-over or gene conversion event involving exon 3 of *GYPA* and pseudoexon 3 of *GYPB*. In the case of a cross-over event there are two possible products, GP.Hil (MiV) if the crossover involves a s-active *GYPB* or GP.JL (MiXI) if the cross-over involves a S-active *GYPB*. GP.Hil reacts with anti-Hil because of the s-active *GYPB* sequence. GP.JL reacts with anti-TSEN because of the S-active *GYPB* sequence. Both GP.Hil and GP.JL react with anti-MINY because this antibody recognizes the sequence at the GPA-B junction irrespective of whether it is derived from a S- or s-active *GYPB*.

In the case of gene conversion events there are two possibilities. In one case hybrid GPB-A-B glycophorins are produced and in the other GPA-B-A hybrid glycophorins are produced. When a segment of exon 3 from *GYPA* is inserted into *GYPB* so that it creates an acceptor splice site which allows the pseudoexon 3 of *GYPB* and the *GYPA* exon 3 insert to be translated into a GPB-A-B protein the resultant hybrid protein can be one of four types: GP.Mur (MiIII); GP.Hop (MiIV); GP.Bun (MiVI); or GP.HF (MiX). GP.Hop and GP.Bun differ only in their reactivity with anti-Hil (GP.Bun) and anti-TSEN (GP.Hop). This is because they are derived from a gene conversion event involving a s-active *GYPB* and S-active *GYPB* respectively and because the gene conversion event creates exactly the same GPA-GPB junction sequence as that found in the GPA-B hybrids GP.Hil and GP.JL which result from cross-over events and are also Hil+ and TSEN+ respectively. For the same reasons both GP.Hop and GP.Bun are MINY+. In GP.Mur the gene conversion event is slightly different so that the Hop antigen is not found but otherwise the hybrid glycophorin is the same as GP.Bun. In GP.HF the gene conversion creates an exon 3 with less material derived from the pseudoexon of *GYPB* and more from exon 3 of *GYPA* than is found in the other GPB-A-B hybrids. This has the effect of creating a hybrid glycophorin which lacks the sequence required for Mur antigen but because the GPA-GPB junction is the same as that found in the other GPB-A-Bs, and the GPB is derived from an s-active *GYPB*, the hybrid molecule expresses the Hil and MINY antigens. All GPB-A-B hybrid glycophorins are MUT+ because they all contain a Lys at residue 28 derived from the pseudoexon of *GYPB* (Lys28 is the critical residue which defines GP.Hut (MiII), see next paragraph).

When a segment of *GYPB* is inserted into *GYPA* a gene is created which encodes a GPA-B-A hybrid. Five examples of such insertions give rise to hybrid molecules with different Miltenberger phenotypes. They are GP.Vw (Mi.I), GP.Hut (MiII), GP.Nob (MiVII), GP.Joh (MiVIII) and GP.Dane (MiIX). Whether GP.Vw really fits into this scheme or results from an independent point mutation cannot be determined. It reacts with anti-Vw but no other antibodies in the Miltenberger series. GP.Hut presumably reacts with anti-Hut and anti-Mut because Lys28 is common to both antigens. GP.Joh and GP.Nob are distinguished by reactivity with anti-Nob and anti-Hop (GP.Joh) and anti-Nob alone (GP.Nob). GP.Dane reacts with anti-Mur because the inserted pseudoexon 3 from GPB encodes a sequence also found in Mur positive GPB-A-B hybrids (see previous paragraph).

All the Miltenberger antigens are therefore explained by three types of genetic events. Cross-overs creating GPA-B glycophorins or gene conversion events creating either GPB-A-B or GPA-B-A hybrids. In the case of cross-over events, as has been explained earlier, a GPB-A hybrid gene is created ipso facto on the other haplotype. The GPB-A hybrid resulting from the cross-over which creates GPA-B (GP.Hil or GP.JL) has St^a antigen activity.

The Functions of Glycophorins A and B

The discussion of the functions of GPA and GPB can be conveniently considered in two parts, the functions of GPA and GPB in the normal red cell and functions of the extensive polymorphism which derives from the fact that GPA and GPB are encoded by adjacent highly homologous genes.

The first evidence concerning the role of GPA and GPB in the normal red cell derived from studies of the GPA deficient cells (En(a-)), the GPB deficient cells (S-s- U-) and cells deficient in both proteins (red cells from persons homozygous for M^k). The most remarkable thing about studies of each of these cell samples was that deficiency of these proteins was not associated with any pathology. Each of the deficiency types has been found in individuals who appear perfectly healthy. Apparently healthy individuals with blood group null phenotypes are found in almost all the blood groups systems (835) but in the case of GPA and GPB-deficiency this is quite surprising because GPA and GPB are major red cell membrane molecules. Of course, it does not follow that because there are healthy individuals who lack these proteins that the proteins therefore do not have any function. It does follow that this function is not vital to the viability of the red cell.

Early studies on the membranes of En(a-) red cells and red cells from M^k homozygotes soon revealed that absence of GPA or GPA and GPB respectively was not the only abnormality. In particular, SDS-PAGE revealed that the anion transport protein band 3 had a higher apparent molecular weight in these cells than in normal cells. This increase in apparent molecular weight was soon shown to be due to the presence of a larger than normal N-glycan on band 3 and that the increase was probably due to a larger number of lactosaminyl repeating structures (13,15, and see figure 4-4 in Chapter 4). This shift in glycosylation of band 3 in the absence of GPA suggested that the two proteins were closely associated in the endoplasmic reticulum and competed for nucleotide sugars in that milieu (322). The converse situation was seen to occur in red cells exhibiting the anti-Lepore haplotypes producing Dantu or St^a antigen where the total amount of glycophorins A, B and B-A hybrids exceeds that of GPA and GPB alone in normal cells and consequently the size of the N-glycan on band 3 is reduced (589). The decrease in apparent molecular weight of band 3 is particularly striking in red cells from persons homozygous for St^a (Macdonald and Anstee, 1984 unpublished observations). Several other studies have provided evidence that band 3 and GPA associate in the red cell membrane and that this association is critical for the formation of the Wr^b antigen (see Chapter 17 for a detailed description of these associations and the structure of Wr^b). The fact that the two proteins associate does not of itself identify the function of GPA in such an association but direct evidence that GPA facilitates the membrane assembly of band 3 was provided by Groves and Tanner (532) who expressed band 3 with and without GPA in *Xenopus* oocytes (see Chapter 17 for a further discussion of band 3/GPA interaction). The absence of GPA from the red cells of persons homozygous for M^k also has a slight effect on the function of band 3. Bruce et al. (820) found that the sulfate transport activity of red cells from M^k homozygotes is approximately 60% of that of red cells with a normal MN phenotype. Evidence that GPB facilitates the membrane assembly of the Rh complex is less clear cut but available data suggest that this is likely (437,791 see also Chapter 12 for further discussion). The presence of GPA and GPB at the normal red cell surface provides the cell with a large mucin-like surface and it has been suggested that this provides a barrier to cell fusion and/or macromolecules (821,822). It seems possible that the enhanced glycosylation of band 3 that occurs in GPA and GPA/GPB deficiency states can effectively compensate for the absence of GPA and GPB.

One of the functions of GPA is often described, especially in the early literature, as an influenza virus receptor. The virus binds to red cells through sialic acid residues on GPA and presumably also GPB (760). The role of blood group antigens as receptors for microorganisms is discussed in Chapter 2 where it is argued that the binding of viruses and bacteria to cell surfaces is much more relevant in the context of the exposed surfaces of the respiratory, gut and urino-genital tracts where ABH, Lewis P and I antigens are found, than to the surface of a red cell. GPA and GPB appear to be restricted to erythroid cells (and possibly cells in kidney cortex (823)) so any functional role as receptors for microorganisms, or more to the point any functional role in the avoidance of acting as a receptor for microorganisms, is likely to be directed at microorganisms that infect red cells. The obvious candidate for avoidance is the malarial parasite. Surely the huge diversity of GPA/GPB structures that are found in man and which are described in this chapter are driven by the need to avoid the malarial parasites. The selection of the Fy(a-b-) phenotype because of the advantage it confers against *Plasmodium vivax* is well documented and discussed in Chapter 14. There is direct evidence that some strains of *Plasmodium falciparum* bind to GPA through a sialic acid-dependent interaction (824). The widespread occurrence of GPA/B polymorphisms in areas of the world where malaria is endemic (He antigen, S- s- phenotype and Dantu antigen in Africa and the St[a] antigen and Miltenberger III/VI phenotype in South-East Asia) and the absence of those same polymorphisms in areas where malaria is not endemic, must surely be a reflection of selective forces (825).

References

1. Landsteiner K, Levine P. Proc Soc Exp Biol NY 1927;24:600
2. Landsteiner K, Levine P. Proc Soc Exp Biol NY 1927;24:941
3. Walsh RJ, Montgomery C. Nature 1947;160:504
4. Sanger R, Race RR. Nature 1947;160:505
5. Sanger R, Race RR, Walsh RJ, et al. Heredity 1948;2:131
6. Levine P, Kumichel AB, Wigod M, et al. Proc Soc Exp Biol NY 1951;78:218
7. Race RR, Sanger R. Blood Groups in Man, 6th Ed. Oxford:Blackwell, 1975
8. Allen FH Jr, Anstee DJ, Bird GWG, et al. Vox Sang 1982;42:164
9. Daniels G. Human Blood Groups. Oxford:Blackwell, 1995
10. Issitt PD. The MN Blood Group System. Cincinnati:Montgomery, 1979
11. Issitt PD. Applied Blood Group Serology, 3rd Ed. Miami:Montgomery, 1985
12. Dahr W, Uhlenbruck G, Wagstaff W, et al. J Immunogenet 1976;3:383
13. Gahmberg CG, Myllylä G, Leikola J, et al. J Biol Chem 1976;251:6108
14. Tanner MJA, Anstee DJ. Biochem J 1976;153:271
15. Tanner MJA, Jenkins RE, Anstee DJ, et al. Biochem J 1976;155:701
16. Tanner MJA, Anstee DJ, Judson PA. Biochem J 1977;165:157
17. Dahr W, Issitt PD, Uhlenbruck G. In: Human Blood Groups. Basel:Karger, 1977:197
18. Landsteiner K, Levine P. J Exp Med 1928;48:731
19. Hirsch W, Moores P, Sanger R, et al. Br J Haematol 1957;3:134
20. Allen FH Jr, Corcoran PA, Ellis FR. Vox Sang 1960;5:224
21. Figur AM, Rosenfield RE. Vox Sang 1965;10:169
22. Springer GF, Desai PR. Biochem Biophys Res Comm 1974;61:420
23. Springer GF, Nagai Y, Tegtmeyer H. Biochemistry 1966;5:3254
24. Springer GF. Naturwissenschaften 1970;57:162
25. Desai PR, Springer GF. Glycocon Res 1972;2:659
26. Springer GF, Yang HJ, Desai PR. Naturwissenschaften 1978;65:547
27. Springer GF, Desai PR, Murthy MS, et al. Prog Allergy 1979;26:42
28. Springer GF, Desai PR, Murthy MS, et al. Transfusion 1979;19:233
29. Yang HJ, Springer GF. Glycocon Res 1979;1:573
30. Desai PR, Springer GF. Naturwissenschaften 1979;66:372
31. Desai PR, Springer GF. J Immunogenet 1979;6:403
32. Desai PR, Springer GF. J Immunogenet 1980;7;149
33. Springer GF, Yang HJ, Mbawa E, et al. Naturwissenschaften 1980;67:473
34. Dahr W, Uhlenbruck G, Janssen E, et al. Hum Genet 1977;35:335
35. Wásniowska K, Drzeniek Z, Lisowska E. Biochem Biophys Res Comm 1977;76:385
36. Blumenfeld OO, Adamany AM. Proc Nat Acad Sci USA 1978;75:2727
37. Furthmayr H. Nature 1978;271:519
38. Dahr W, Uhlenbruck G, Knott H. J Immunogenet 1975;2:87
39. Wiener AS, Unger LJ, Gordon EB. J Am Med Assoc 1953;153:1444
40. Wiener AS, Unger LJ, Cohen L. Science 1954;119:734
41. Greenwalt TJ, Sasaki T, Sanger R, et al. Proc Nat Acad Sci USA 1954;40:1126
42. Dahr W, Uhlenbruck G, Issitt PD, et al. J Immunogenet 1975;2:249
43. Dahr W, Issitt PD, Moulds J, et al. Forsch der Transf Immunohematol, Vol 4. Berlin:Medicus Verlag, 1978
44. Dahr W, Issitt PD, Moulds J, et al. Hoppe-Seyler's Z Physiol Chem 1978;359:1217
45. Unger PJ, Orlina AR, Dahr W, et al. (abstract). Transfusion 1981;21:614
46. Unger P, Orlina A, Dahr W, et al. (abstract). Foren Sci Int 1981;18:258
47. Contreras M, Green C, Humphreys J, et al. Vox Sang 1984;46:377
48. Pilkington P, Dahr W, Lacey P, et al. (abstract). Transfusion 1985;25:464
49. Moulds JJ, Dahr W, Unger PJ, et al. (abstract). Transfusion 1985;25:464
50. Dahr W, Moulds J, Unger P, et al. Adv Foren Haemogenet, Vol 1. Berlin:Springer-Verlag, 1986:3
51. Unger P, Proctor JL, Moulds JJ, et al. Blut 1987;55:33
52. Dahr W, Pilkington PM, Reinke H, et al. Blut 1989;58:247
53. Landsteiner K, Levine P. J Exp Med 1928;47:757
54. Landsteiner K, Strutton WR, Chase MW. J Immunol 1934;27:469
55. Ikin EW, Mourant AE. Br Med J 1951;1:456
56. Levine P, Stock AH, Kuhmichel AB, et al. Proc Soc Exp Biol NY 1951;77:402
57. Dunsford I, Ikin EW, Mourant AE. Nature 1953;172:688
58. Hart van der M, Bosman H, Loghem van JJ. Vox Sang (Old Series) 1954;4:108
59. Allen FH Jr, Corcoran PA, Kenton HB, et al. Vox Sang 1958;3:81
60. Hart van der M, Veer van der M, Loghem van JJ, et al. Vox Sang 1958;3:261
61. Jack JA, Tippett P, Noades J, et al. Nature 1960;186:642
62. Cleghorn TE. MD Thesis, Univ Sheffield, 1961
63. Wiener AS, Rosenfield RE. J Immunol 1961;87:376
64. Swanson J, Matson GA. Vox Sang 1962;7:585

65. Cleghorn TE. Nature 1962;195:297
66. Wallace J, Izatt M. Nature 1963;200:689
67. Ørjasaeter H, Kornstad L, Heier AM, et al. Nature 1964;201:832
68. Cleghorn TE, Jenkins WJ, Koster HG. Unpublished observations1964, cited in Race RR, Sanger R. Blood Groups in Man, 6th Ed. Oxford:Blackwell, 1975
69. Bacon JM, Macdonald EB, Young SG, et al. Vox Sang 1987;52:330
70. Issitt PD, Haber JM, Allen FH Jr. Vox Sang 1965;10:742
71. Issitt PD, Wilkinson SL. Transfusion 1981;21:493
72. Cleghorn TE. Vox Sang 1966;11:219
73. Gershowitz H, Fried K. Am J Hum Genet 1966;18:264
74. Crossland JD, Pepper MD, Giles CM, et al. Vox Sang 1970;18:407
75. Konugres A, Brown LS, Corcoran PA. Vox Sang 1966;11:189
76. Konugres AA,Winter NM. Vox Sang 1967;12:221
77. Issitt PD, Haber JM, Allen FH Jr. Vox Sang 1968;15:1
78. Metaxas MN, Metaxas-Bühler M, Ikin EW. Vox Sang 1968;15:102
79. Speiser P, Kühböck J, Mickerts D, et al. Vox Sang 1966;11:113
80. Cregut R, Lewin D, Lacomme M, et al. Rev Franc Transf 1968;11:139
81. Cregut R, Liberge G, Yvart J, et al. Vox Sang 1974;26:194
82. Giles CM. Vox Sang 1977;32:269
83. Darnborough J, Dunsford I, Wallace JA. Vox Sang 1969;17:241
84. Furuhjelm U, Myllylä G, Nevanlinna HR, et al. Vox Sang 1969;17:256
85. Issitt PD, Daniels G, Tippett P. (Letter). Transfusion 1981;21:473
86. Beck ML. Unpublished observations 1969 cited in Issitt PD, Issitt CH. Applied Blood Group Serology, 2nd Ed. Oxnard:Spectra Biologicals, 1975
87. Booth PB. Vox Sang 1971;21:522
88. Booth PB. Vox Sang 1972;22:524
89. Chandanayingyong D, Pejrachandra S, Poole J. Vox Sang 1977;32:272
90. Giles CM, Chandanayingyong D, Webb AJ. Vox Sang 1977;32:277
91. Webb AJ, Giles CM. Vox Sang 1977;32:274
92. Booth PB. Vox Sang 1978;34:212
93. Shapiro M, LeRoux ME. Unpublished observations 1978 cited in Issitt PD. The MN Blood Group System. Cincinnati:Montgomery, 1979
94. Shapiro M, LeRoux ME. (abstract). Transfusion 1981;21:614
95. Judd WJ, Issitt PD, Pavone BG. Transfusion 1979;19:7
96. Battista N, Stout TD, Lewis M, et al. Vox Sang 1980;39:331
97. Seno T, Yamaguchi H, Okubo Y, et al. Vox Sang 1983;45:60
98. Daniels GL, Green CA, Petty AC, et al. (abstract). Transf Med 1993;3 (Suppl 1):85
99. Laird-Fryer B, Moulds JJ, Dahr W, et al. Transfusion 1986;26:51
100. Skov F, Green C, Daniels G, et al. Vox Sang 1991;61:130
101. Daniels GL, Green CA, Okubo Y, et al. Transf Med 1991;1:39
102. Reid ME, Moore BPL, Poole J, et al. Vox Sang 1992;63:122
103. Reid ME, Poole J, Green C, et al. Vox Sang 1992;63:129
104. Tippett P, Reid ME, Poole J, et al. Transf Med Rev 1992;6:170
105. Daniels GL, Green CA, Poole J, et al. Transf Med 1993;3:129
106. Spruell P, Moulds JJ, Martin M, et al. Transfusion 1993;33:848
107. Poole J, Banks JA, Bruce LJ, et al. (abstract). Transfusion 1995;35 (Suppl 10S):40S
108. Huang C-H, Kikuchi M, McCreary J, et al. J Biol Chem 1992;267:3336
109. Adinolfi M, Polley MJ, Hunter DA, et al. Immunology 1962;5:566
110. Freedman J, Massey A, Chaplin H, et al. Br J Haematol 1980;45:309
111. Mollison PL. Blood Transfusion in Clinical Medicine, 7th Ed. Oxford:Blackwell, 1983
112. Mollison PL. Blood Transfusion in Clinical Medicine, 5th Ed. Oxford:Blackwell, 1972
113. Smith ML, Beck ML. Transfusion 1979;19:472
114. Duckett JB, Issitt PD. Unpublished observations 1979 cited in Issitt PD. The MN Blood Group System. Cincinnati:Montgomery, 1979
115. Branch DR, McBroom R, Jones GL. Rev Fr Transf Immunohematol 1983;26:565
116. Combs MR, O'Rourke MM, Issitt PD, et al. Transfusion 1991;31:756
117. Chapman J, Murphy MF, Waters AH. (Letter). Transfusion 1992;32:391
118. Combs MR, Issitt PD, Telen MJ. (Letter). Transfusion 1992;32:391
119. Bowes A. Proc 8th Cong NBTS, Session A, 1976
120. Sangster JM, Kenwright MG, Walker WP, et al. J Clin Pathol 1979;32:154
121. Chapman J, Murphy MF, Waters AH. Vox Sang 1982;42:272
122. Roelcke D, Dahr W, Kalden JR. Vox Sang 1986;51:207
123. Mollison PL, Cutbush M. Lancet 1955;1:1290
124. Cutbush M, Giblett ER, Mollison PL. Br J Haematol 1956;2:210
125. Cutbush M, Mollison PL. Br J Haematol 1958;4:115
126. Mollison PL. Br Med J 1959;2:1035
127. Mollison PL. Br Med J 1959;2:1123
128. Mollison PL. Acta Hematol 1959;10:495
129. Giblett ER. Transfusion 1977;17:299
130. Morel PA, Garratty G, Perkins HA. Am J Med Technol 1978;44:122
131. Issitt PD. In: Clinically Significant and Insignificant Antibodies. Washington, D.C.:Am Assoc Blood Banks, 1979:13
132. Garratty G. In: Clinically Significant and Insignificant Antibodies. Washington, D.C.:Am Assoc Blood Banks, 1979:29
133. Issitt PD. In: Pathology-Anatomical and Clinical. Oxford:Pergamon, 1982:395
134. Shulman IA. In: Immune Destruction of Red Blood Cells. Arlington, VA:Am Assoc Blood Banks, 1989:171
135. Petz LD, Swisher SN, Kleinman S, et al. Eds. Clinical Practice of Transfusion Medicine, 3rd Ed. New York:Churchill Livingstone, 1996
136. Mollison PL, Engelfriet CP, Contreras M. Blood Transfusion in Clinical Medicine, 9th Ed. Oxford:Blackwell, 1993
137. Walker RH, Ed. Technical Manual, 11th Ed. Bethesda, MD:Am Assoc Blood Banks, 1993
138. Judd WJ. Methods in Immunohematology, 2nd Ed. Durham:Montgomery 1994
139. Judd WJ. In: Pretransfusion Testing: Routine to Complex. Bethesda, MD:Am Assoc Blood Banks, 1995
140. Callender ST, Race RR. Ann Eugen 1946;13:102
141. Freiesleben E, Knudsen EE. In: PH Andresen. Papers in Dedication of his Sixtieth Birthday. Copenhagen:Munksgaard, 1957:26
142. Furlong MB, Monoghan WP. Transfusion 1981;21:45
143. Alperin JH, Riglin H, Branch DR, et al. Transfusion 1983;23:322

144. Chandanayingyong D, Pejrachandra S, Chongkolwatana V, et al. (abstract). Book of Abstracts, ISBT/AABB Joint Cong, 1990:109

145. Issitt PD, Combs MR, Telen MJ. Unpublished observations, 1989-1996

146. Telischi M, Behzad O, Issitt PD, et al. Vox Sang 1976;31:109

147. Judd WJ, Rolih SD, Dahr W, et al. Transfusion 1983;23:382

148. Ballas SK, Dignam C, Harris M, et al. Transfusion 1985;25:377

149. Judd WJ. Immunohematology 1986;2:49

150. Guizzo ML, Meadows S. Immunohematology 1986;2:116

151. Kosanke J, Behzad O. Immunohematology 1986;2:118

152. Judd WJ. Immunohematology 1987;3:25

153. Wiener AS. Rev Hematol 1950;5:3

154. Stahl M, Pettenkofer HJ, Hasse W. Vox Sang (Old Series) 1955;5:34

155. Pineda AA, Taswell HF, Brzica SM Jr. Transfusion 1978;18:1

156. Croucher BEE. In: A Seminar on Laboratory Management of Hemolysis. Washington, D.C.:Am Assoc Blood Banks, 1979:151

157. Moore SB, Taswell HF, Pineda AA, et al. Am J Clin Pathol 1980;74:94

158. Croucher BEE, Crookston MC, Crookston JH. Vox Sang 1967;12:32

159. Thomson S, Johnstone M. Canad J Med Technol 1972;34:159

160. Vogel RA, Worthington M. (Letter). J Am Med Assoc 1978;240:2432

161. Solanki D, McCurdy PR. J Am Med Assoc 1979;239:729

162. Kurtz SR, Ouellet R, McMican A, et al. Transfusion 1983;23:37

163. Jakobowicz R, Bryce LM. Med J Austral 1951;1:365

164. Stone B, Marsh WL. Br J Haematol 1959;5:344

165. Simmons RT, Krieger VL, Jakobowicz R. Med J Austral 1960;2:336

166. Freiesleben E, Jensen KG. Vox Sang 1961;6:328

167. Macpherson CR, Zartman ER. Am J Clin Pathol 1965;43:544

168. Yoshida Y, Yoshida H, Tatsumi K, et al. New Eng J Med 1981;305:460

169. Matsumoto H, Tamaki Y, Sato S, et al. Acta Obstet Gynaecol Jpn 1981;33:525

170. Yoshida Y, Yoshida H, Tatsumi K, et al. Vox Sang 1982;43:35

171. Robinson AE. (Letter). Vox Sang 1983;44:326

172. Robinson AE, Tovey LAD. Br J Haematol 1980;45:621

173. Yoshida Y, Yoshida H, Tatsumi K, et al. (Letter). Vox Sang 1983;44:327

174. Giblett ER. Unpublished observations cited in Mollison PL. Blood Transfusion in Clinical Medicine, 5th Ed. Oxford:Blackwell, 1972

175. Howard PL. Ann Clin Lab Sci 1973;3:13

176. Kao YS, Frank S, de Jongh DS. Transfusion 1978;18:320

177. Perrault R. Vox Sang 1973;24:134

178. Wright J, Lim FC, Freeman J, et al. Transfusion 1983;23:120

179. Teesdale P, de Silva M, Contreras M. Vox Sang 1991;61:37

180. Howell ED, Perkins HA. Vox Sang 1972;23:291

181. McLeish WA, Brathwaite AF, Peterson PM. Transfusion 1975;15:43

182. Harrison PB, Jansson K, Kronenberg H, et al. Austral NZ J Med 1975;5:195

183. Boettcher B, Nanra RS, Roberts TK, et al. Vox Sang 1976;31:408

184. Crosson JT, Moulds J, Comty CM, et al. Kidney Int 1976;10:463

185. Fassbinder W, Pilar J, Scheuermann E, et al. Proc Eur Dial Transplt Assoc 1976;13:333

186. Shalden S, Chevallet M, Maraoui M, et al. Proc Eur Dial Tranplt Assoc 1976;13:339

187. Bird GWG, Wingham J. Lancet 1977;1:1218

188. White WL, Miller GE, Kaehny WD. Transfusion 1977;17:443

189. Sandler SG, Sharon R, Stressman J, et al. Israel J Med Sci 1978;14:1177

190. Fassbinder W, Seidl S, Koch KM. Vox Sang 1978;35:41

191. Sandler SG, Sharon R, Bush M, et al. Transfusion 1979;19:682

192. Dahr W, Moulds J. Immunol Comm 1981;10:173

193. White WL, Meisenhelder J, Rivzi J. (Letter). Transfusion 1983;23:79

194. Lynen R, Rothe M, Gallasch E. Vox Sang 1983;44:81

195. Dzik WH, Darling CA. Am J Clin Pathol 1989;92:214

196. Belzer FO, Kountz SSL, Perkins HA. Transplantation 1971;11:422

197. Lown JAG, Barr AL, Kelly A. Vox Sang 1980;38:301

198. Ogden DA, Myers LE, Ekelson CKD, et al. Proc Clin Dial Transpl Forum 1973;3:141

199. Servadio C, Nissenkorn I. Cancer 1976;37:900

200. Rudolph AM, Heymann MA, Fishman N, et al. New Eng J Med 1975;292:1263

201. Musher DM, Griffith DP. Antimicrob Agents Chemotherapy 1974;6:708

202. Schmidt AP, Taswell HF. Transfusion 1969;9:203

203. Howard PL, Picoff RC. Transfusion 1972;12:59

204. Lawe JE, LaRoche LL. Vox Sang 1983;44:92

205. Metaxas-Bühler M, Ikin EW, Romanski J. Vox Sang 1961;6:574

206. Greenwalt TJ, Sasaki T, Steane EA. Vox Sang 1966;11:184

207. Lahmann N. Haematologia 1970;4:79

208. Moores P, Botha MC, Brink S. Am J Clin Pathol 1970;54:90

209. Booth PB, Moores P. Vox Sang 1973;25:374

210. Fletcher JL, Zmijewski C. Int Arch Allergy 1970;37:586

211. Tegoli J, Harris JP, Nichols ME, et al. Transfusion 1970;10:133

212. Nichols ME, Harris JP. (Letter). Transfusion 1971;11:66

213. Hysell JK, Beck ML, Gray JM. Transfusion 1973;13:146

214. Hysell JK, Gray JM, Beck ML. Transfusion 1974;14:72

215. Vale DR, Harris IM. Transfusion 1980;20:440

216. Sacher RA, Abbondanzo SL, Miller DK, et al. Am J Clin Pathol 1989;91:305

217. Judd WJ, Steiner EA, Knaff P, et al. (abstract). Transfusion 1992;32 (Suppl 8S):22S

218. Hinz CF, Boyer JT. New Eng J Med 1963;269:1329

219. Dube VE, House RF Jr, Moulds J, et al. Am J Clin Pathol 1975;63:828

220. Cohen DW, Garratty G, Morel P, et al. Transfusion 1979;19:329

221. Dickerman JD, Howard P, Dopp S, et al. Am J Dis Childh 1980;134:159

222. Bowman HS, Marsh WL, Schumacher HR, et al. Am J Clin Pathol 1974;61:465

223. Beattie KM, Zuelzer WW. Transfusion 1965;5:322

224. Reid ME, Ellisor SS, Barker JM. Transfusion 1984;24:222

225. Bowman HS. (Letter). Transfusion 1985;25:86

226. Fraser RH, Munro AC, Williamson AR, et al. J Immunogenet 1982;9:303

227. Fraser RH, Inglis G, Mackie A, et al. Transfusion 1985;25:261

228. Fraser RH, Inglis G, Mitchell R. (Letter). Transfusion 1986;26:118

229. Morel P, Hill V, Bergren M, et al. (abstract). Transfusion 1975;15:522

230. Morel PA, Bergren MO, Hill V, et al. Transfusion 1981;21:652

231. Reid ME, Ellisor SS, Barker JM, et al. Vox Sang 1981;41:85
232. Drzeniek Z, Kusnierz G, Lisowska E. Immunol Comm 1981;10;185
233. Pallagut SJ, Edwards JM. (abstract). Transfusion 1982;22:409
234. Anstee DJ, Spring FA. Transf Med Rev 1989;3:13
235. Anstee DJ. Vox Sang 1990;58:1
236. Anstee DJ. J Immunogenet 1990;17:219
237. Morton JA, Pickles MM. Nature 1947;159:779
238. Unger LJ, Katz J. J Lab Clin Med 1951;38:188
239. Löw B. Vox Sang 1955;5:94
240. Haber G, Rosenfield RE. In: PH Andresen. Papers in Dedication of his Sixtieth Birthday. Copenhagen:Munksgaard, 1957
241. Mäkelä O, Cantell K. Ann Med Exp Fenn 1958;36:366
242. Pirofsky B, Mangum MEJ. Proc Soc Exp Biol NY 1959;101:49
243. Judson PA, Anstee DJ. Med Lab Sci 1977;34:1
244. Springer GF, Huprikar SV. Haematologica 1972;6:81
245. Springer GF, Tegtmeyer H, Huprikar SV. Vox Sang 1972;22:325
246. Springer GF, Desai PR. Biochem Biophys Res Comm 1974;61:470
247. Springer GF, Desai PR. Carbohydr Res 1975;40:183
248. Springer GF, Ansell NJ. Proc Nat Acad Sci Washington, D.C. 1958;44:182
249. Romanowska E. Vox Sang 1964;9:578
250. Bird GWG, Wingham J. Vox Sang 1970;18:240
251. Judd WJ, Issitt PD, Pavone BG, et al. Transfusion 1979;19:12
252. Issitt PD, Wilkinson SL. Transfusion 1983;23:117
253. Lisowska E, Kordowicz M. Vox Sang 1977;33:164
254. Fraser RH, Munro AC, Williamson AR, et al. J Immunogenet 1982;9:295
255. Bigbee WL,Vanderlaan M, Fong SSN, et al. Mol Immunol 1983;20:1353
256. Allen RW, Nunley N, Kimmeth ME, et al. Transfusion 1984;24:136
257. Fletcher A, Harbor C. J Immunogenet 1984;11:121
258. Edelman L, Blanchard D, Rouger P, et al. Exp Clin Immunogenet 1984;1:129
259. Wásniowska K, Reichert CM, McGinniss MH, et al. Glycocon J 1985;2:163
260. Nichols ME, Rosenfield RE, Rubinstein P. Vox Sang 1985;49:138
261. Rubocki R, Milgrom F. Vox Sang 1986;51:217
262. Lisowska E, Messeter L, Duk M, et al. Mol Immunol 1987;24:605
263. Rouger P, Anstee D, Salmon C. Rev Fr Transf Immunohematol 1988;31:261
264. Wásniowska K, Duk M, Steuden I, et al. Arch Immunol Ther Exp 1988;36:623
265. Chester MA, Johnson U, Lundblad A, et al. Proc 2nd Int Workshop and Symposium on MAb, 1990
266. Jáskiewicz E, Lisowska E, Lundblad A. Glycocon J 1 990;7:255
267. Jáskiewicz E, Moulds JJ, Kraemer K, et al. Transfusion 1990;30:230
268. Issitt PD. Transfusion 1989;29:58
269. Issitt PD. Murex Sci Pub Ser 1991;6:1
270. Blackall DP, Ugorski M, Smith ME, et al. Transfusion 1992;32:629
271. Blackall DP, Ugorski M, Pählsson P, et al. J Immunol 1994;152:2241
272. Langlois RG, Bigbee WL, Jensen RH. J Immunol 1985;134:4009
273. Langlois RG, Bigbee WL, Jensen RH. Hum Genet 1986;74:353
274. Langlois RG, Bigbee WL, Kyoizumi S, et al. Science 1987;236:445
275. Kyoizumi S, Nakamura N, Hakoda M, et al. Cancer Res 1989;49:581
276. Langlois RG, Bigbee WL, Jensen RH. Prog Clin Biol Res 1990;340C:47
277. Bigbee WL,Wyrobeck AW, Langlois RG, et al. Mutat Res 1990;240:165
278. Langlois RG, Nisbet BA, Bigbee WL, et al. Cytometry 1990;11:513
279. Grant SG, Bigbee WL, Langlois RG, et al. Clin Biotech 1991;3:177
280. Bigbee WL, Jensen RH, Grant SG, et al. Am J Hum Genet 1991;49 (Suppl):446
281. Grant SG, Jensen RH: In: Immunobiology of Transfusion Medicine. New York:Marcel Dekker, 1994:299
282. Allen FH Jr, Madden HJ, King RW. Vox Sang 1963;8:549
283. Francis BJ, Hatcher DE. Vox Sang 1966;11:213
284. Dahr W, Kordowicz M, Judd WJ, et al. Eur J Biochem 1984;141:51
285. Huang C-H, Lomas C, Daniels G, et al. Blood 1994;83:3369
286. Reid ME, Lomas-Francis C, Daniels GL, et al. Vox Sang 1995;68:183
287. Vengelen-Tyler V, Anstee DJ, Issitt PD, et al. Transfusion 1981;21:1
288. Langley JW, Issitt PD, Anstee DJ, et al. Transfusion 1981;21:15
289. Mawby WJ, Anstee DJ, Tanner MJA. Nature 1981;291:161
290. Judd WJ, Geisland JR, Issitt PD, et al. Transfusion 1983;23:33
291. Lu Y-Q, Nichols ME, Bigbee WL, et al. Blood 1987;69:618
292. Vignal A, Rahuel C, El Maliki B, et al. Eur J Biochem 1989;184:337
293. King MJ, Poole J, Anstee DJ. Transfusion 1989;29:106
294. Habash J, Lubenko A, Pizzaro I, et al. (abstract). Book of Abstracts, ISBT/AABB Joint Cong 1990:155
295. Huang C-H, Blumenfeld OO. Blood 1991;77:1813
296. Tokunaga E, Sasakawa S, Tamaka K, et al. J Immunogenet 1979;6:383
297. Gutendorf R, Lacey P, Moulds J, et al. (abstract). Transfusion 1985;25:481
298. Okubo Y, Daniels GL, Parsons SF, et al. Vox Sang 1988;54:107
299. Singer E. Med J Austral 1943;2:29
300. Yoell JH. Transfusion 1966;6:592
301. Cutbush M, Mollison PL. Lancet 1949;2:102
302. Coombs HI, Ikin E, Mourant AE, et al. Br Med J 1951;1:109
303. Levine P, Ferraro LR, Koch E. Blood 1952;7:1030
304. Giblett E, Chase J, Crealock FW. Am J Clin Pathol 1958;29:254
305. Drachmann O, Hansen KB. Scand J Haematol 1969;6:93
306. Constantoulis NC, Paidoussis M, Dunsford I. Vox Sang (Old Series) 1955;5:143
307. Hardman JT, Beck ML. Transfusion 1981;21:343
308. Sanger R, Race RR, Greenwalt TJ, et al. Vox Sang 1955;5:73
309. Lalezari P, Malamut DC, Dreiseger ME, et al. Vox Sang 1973;25:390
310. Arndt P, Garratty G. Transfusion 1988;28:210
311. Dahr W, Uhlenbruck G, Leikola J, et al. J Immunogenet 1978;5:117
312. Dahr W, Longster G, Uhlenbruck G, et al. Blut 1978;37:129
313. Mawby WJ, Anstee DJ. Unpublished observations 1979 cited by Anstee DJ. In: Immunobiolgy of the Erythrocyte. New York:Liss, 1980:67

314. Dahr W, Longster G. Blut 1984;49:299
315. Beck ML, Hardman JT. (Letter). Transfusion 1980;20:479
316. Leigh K, de Ruiter K. (Letter). Transfusion 1988;28:86
317. Kernan S, Mullahy DE. Med Lab Sci 1981;38:269
318. Case J. (abstract). Transfusion 1978;18:392
319. Issitt PD, Tregellas WM, Wilkinson SL, et al. Transfusion 1982;22:174
320. Puig N, Carbonell F, Soler MA, et al. Vox Sang 1987;53:173
321. Dahr W, Beyreuther K, Steinbach H, et al. Hoppe-Seyler's Z Physiol Chem 1980;361:895
322. Dahr W. In: Recent Advances in Blood Group Biochemistry. Arlington, VA:Am Assoc Blood Banks 1986:23
323. Puno CS, Allen FH Jr. Vox Sang 1969;16:155
324. Lubenko A. (abstract). Proc 5th Ann Mtg Br Blood Transf Soc 1987: Section 01, No 17
325. Mayne KM, Boswell PJ, Green SJ, et al. Clin Lab Haematol 1990;12:105
326. Crawford MN. Unpublished observations 1967 cited by Race RR, Sanger R. Blood Groups in Man, 6th Ed. Oxford:Blackwell, 1975
327. Johnson MH, Plett MJ, Conant CN, et al. (abstract). Transfusion 1978;18:389
328. Alessandrino EP, Costamagna L, Pagani A, et al. (Letter). Transfusion 1984;24:369
329. Fabijanska-Mitek J, Kopec J, Seyfried H. (abstract). Vox Sang 1994;67 (Suppl 2):123
330. Sanger R, Race RR. Am J Hum Genet 1951;3:332
331. Voak D, Davies D, Sonneborn H, et al. In: Advances in Forensic Haemogenetics, Vol 2. Berlin:Springer-Verlag 1988:268
332. Green CA, Daniels GL, Khalid G, et al. Proc 2nd Int Workshop and Symposium on MAb Against Human Red Blood Cells and Related Antigens. Lund 1990:119
333. Poole J, Byrne P, Banks J, et al. Proc 2nd Int Workshop and Symposium on MAb Against Human Red Blood Cells and Related Antigens. Lund 1990:122
334. Hemming NJ, Reid ME. Transfusion 1994;34:333
335. Greenwalt TJ, Sasaki T, Sanger R, et al. Proc 6th Cong ISBT. Basel:Karger, 1958:104
336. Greenwalt TJ. Prog Hematol 1963;3:71
337. Goldstein EI. MS Thesis, Univ Cincinnati, 1966
338. Goldstein EI, Hoxworth PI. (abstract). Transfusion 1969;9:280
339. Issitt PD, Wilkinson SL, Weiland DL, et al. Unpublished observations 1972 to 1978 cited in Issitt PD. Applied Blood Group Serology, 3rd Ed. Miami:Montgomery, 1985:325
340. Issitt PD, Marsh WL, Wren MR, et al. Transfusion 1989;29:508
341. Storry JR, Reid ME. Transfusion 1996;36:512
342. Rahuel C, London J, Vignal A, et al. Am J Hematol 1991;37:57
343. Reid ME, Sausais L, Hoffer J, et al. (abstract). Transfusion 1993;33 (Suppl 9S):49S
344. Huang C-H, Reid ME, Blumenfeld OO. J Biol Chem 1994;269:10804
345. Reid ME, Huang C-H, Blumenfeld OO. (abstract). Transfusion 1994;34 (Suppl 10S):62S
346. Tanner MJA, Anstee DJ, Mawby WJ. Biochem J 1980;187:493
347. Moulds JJ, Wren MR, Issitt PD. Unpublished observations 1984 cited in Issitt PD. Applied Blood Group Serology, 3rd Ed. Miami:Montgomery, 1985:654
348. Meltz DJ, David DS, Bertles JF, et al. Lancet 1971;2:1348
349. Rothman IK, Alter HJ, Strewler GL. Transfusion 1976;16:357
350. Beattie KM, Sigmund KE, McGraw J, et al. (Letter). Transfusion 1982;22:257
351. Taliano V, Fleury M, Pichette R, et al. Rev Fr Transf Immunohemat 1989;32:17
352. Pillary GS, Womack B, Sandler SG. Immunohematology 1993;9:41
353. Miceli C, Diekamp U, Sosler SD. (Letter). Transfusion 1983;23:364
354. Mentor J, Richards HA. Vox Sang 1989;56:62
355. Issitt PD. (Letter). Vox Sang 1990;58:70
356. Sondag-Thull D, Girard M, Blanchard D, et al. Exp Clin Immunogenet 1986;3:181
357. Eriksson AW. Unpublished observations cited in Mourant AE, Kopec AC, Domaniewska-Sobczak K. The Distribution of the Human Blood Groups and Other Polymorphisms, 2nd Ed. London:Oxford Univ Press, 1976
358. Constans J, Quilici JC, Malaspina L, et al. Unpublished observations cited in Tills D, Kopec AC, Tills RE. The Distribution of the Human Blood Groups and Other Polymorphisms, Suppl 1. Oxford:Oxford Univ Press, 1983
359. Moores PP. Vox Sang 1972;23:452
360. Giblett ER, Gartler SM, Waxman SH. Am J Hum Genet 1963;15:62
361. Smerling M. Beitr Gericht Med 1971;28:237
362. Polesky HF, Moulds J. Am J Hum Genet 1975;27:543
363. Austin RJ, Riches G. Vox Sang 1978;34:343
364. Mauff G, Pulverer G, Hummel K, et al. Blut 1977;34:357
365. Dahr W, Weber W, Kordowicz M. In: Biomathematical Evidence of Paternity. Berlin:Springer-Verlag 1981:131
366. Huang C-H, Johe K, Moulds JJ. Blood 1987;70:1830
367. Huang C-H, Lu WM, Boots ME, et al. (abstract). Transfusion 1989;29 (suppl 7S):35S
368. Tate CG, Tanner MJA, Judson PA, et al. Biochem J 1989;263:993
369. Vignal A, Rahuel C, London J, et al. Eur J Biochem 1990;191:619
370. Huang C-H, Blumenfeld OO, Reid M. (abstract). Transfusion 1993;33 (Suppl 9S):46S
371. Alfonso JR, de Alvarez RR. Am J Obstet Gynecol 1961;81:45
372. Birki U, Degnan TJ, Rosenfield RE. Vox Sang 1964;9:209
373. Austin T, Finklestein J, Okada D, et al. J Pediat 1976;89:330
374. Dhandsa N, Williams M, Joss V, et al. Lancet 1981;2:1232
375. Magaud JP, Jouvenceaux A, Bertrix F, et al. Arch Fr Peidat 1981;38:769
376. Gottschall JL. (Letter). Transfusion 1981;21:230
377. Tuck S, Studd JWW. Br J Obstet Gynaecol 1982;89:91
378. Dopp SL, Isham BE. (Letter). Transfusion 1983;23:273
379. Schmidt PJ. (Letter). Transfusion 1981;21:231
380. Levine P. (Letter). Transfusion 1981;21:231
381. Huestis DW. (Letter). Transfusion 1981;21:231
382. Giblett ER. (Letter). Transfusion 1981;21:231
383. Allen FH Jr. (Letter). Transfusion 1981;21:231
384. Rosenfield RE. (Letter). Transfusion 1981;21:232
385. Nugent ME, Colledge KI, Marsh WL. Vox Sang 1971;20:519
386. Marsh WL, Reid ME, Scott EP. Br J Haematol 1972;22:625
387. Vos GH, Petz LD, Garratty G, et al. Blood 1973;42:445
388. Bell CA, Zwicker H. Transfusion 1980;20:86
389. Sacher RA, McGinniss MM, Shashat GG, et al. Am J Clin Pathol 1982;77:356
390. Kessey EC, Pierce S, Beck ML, et al. (abstract). Transfusion 1973;13:360
391. Beck ML, Butch SH, Armstrong WD, et al. Transfusion 1972;12:280
392. Wojcicki RE, Hardman JT, Beck ML, et al. (abstract). Transfusion 1980;20:628
393. McGinniss MH, Macher AM, Rook AH, et al. Transfusion

1986;26:405

394. McCreary J, Sabo B. Unpublished observations cited by Levine P, Tripodi D, Struck J Jr, et al. Vox Sang 1973;24:417

395. Issitt PD, Pavone BG, Rolih SD. Vox Sang 1976;31:25

396. Metaxas MN, Metaxas-Bühler M. Unpublished observations 1975 cited in Issitt PD, Pavone BG, Rolih SD. Vox Sang 1976;31:25

397. Daniels G. Immunohematology 1992;8:53

398. Anstee DJ, Mawby WJ, Tanner MJA. Biochem J 1979;183:193

399. Khalid G, Green CA. Vox Sang 1990;59:48

400. Ballas SK, Reilly PA, Murphy DL. Biochim Biophys Acta 1986;884:337

401. Dahr W, Moulds JJ. Biol Chem Hoppe-Seyler 1987:368:659

402. Dahr W, Wilkinson S, Issitt PD, et al. Biol Chem Hoppe-Seyer 1986;367:1033

403. Telen MJ, Chasis JA. Blood 1990;76:842

404. Bruce LJ, Ring SM, Anstee DJ, et al. Blood 1995;85:541

405. McKeever BG, Pochedley M, Meyer JD. (abstract). Transfusion 1980;20:634

406. Fraser GR, Giblett ER, Motulsky AG. Am J Hum Genet 1966;18:546

407. Lowe RF, Moores PP. Hum Hered 1972;22:344

408. Hoekstra A, Albert AP, Newell GAI, et al. Vox Sang 1975;29:214

409. Mornex JF, Lapierre Y, Biggio B, et al. (Letter). Transfusion 1983;23:272

410. Livingston FB, Gershowitz H, Neel JV, et al. Am J Phys Antrhopol 1960;18:161

411. Languillat G, Cartron J, Gerbal R, et al. Rev Fr Transf Immunohematol 1980;23:675

412. von dem Borne AEGKr, Bos MJE, Lomas C, et al. Br J Haematol 1990;75:254

413. Habibi B, Fouillade MT, Duedari N, et al. Vox Sang 1978;34:302

414. Mallinson G, Anstee DJ, Avent ND, et al. Transfusion 1990;30:222

415. Rearden A, Taetle R, Elmajian DA, et al. Mol Immunol 1985;22:369

416. Banyard MR, Shaw DC. Aust J Exp Biol Med Sci 1985;63:503

417. Anstee DJ. Rev Fr Transf Immunohematol 1988;31:359

418. Anstee DJ, Lisowska E. J Immunogenet 1990;17:301

419. Su S, Sanadi AR, Ifon E, et al. J Immunol 1993;151:2309

420. Chown B, Lewis M, Kaita H. Am J Hum Genet 1965;17:9

421. Gedde-Dahl T, Grimstad AL, Gundersen S, et al. Acta Genet 1967;17:193

422. Chown B, Lewis M, Kaita H. Unpublished observations 1967, cited by Gedde-Dahl T, Grimstad AL, Gundersen S, et al. Acta Genet 1967;17:193

423. Scholz W, Murken J-D. Z Menschl Vereb Konstit-Lehre 1963;37:178

424. Scholz W. Unpublished observations 1967 cited by Gedde-Dahl T, Grimstad AL, Gundersen S, et al. Acta Genet 1967;17:193

425. van der Weerdt CM. Thesis (Drukkerig Aemstelstad) Amsterdam, 1965

426. van der Weerdt CM. Unpublished observations 1965 cited by Gedde-Dahl T, Grimstad AL, Gundersen S, et al. Acta Genet 1967;17:193

427. Davison BCC. J Med Genet 1965;2:293

428. Davison BCC. Unpublished observations 1967 cited by Gedde-Dahl T, Grimstad AL, Gundersen S, et al. Acta Genet 1967;17:193

429. Dahr W, Uhlenbruck G, Leikola J, et al. J Immunogenet 1976;3:329

430. Bunn HF, Forget BG, Ranney HM. In: Human Haemoglobins. London:Saunders, 1977:151

431. Cartron J-P, Rahuel C. Transf Med Rev 1992;6:63

432. Chasis JA, Mohandas N. Blood 1992;80:1869

433. Blanchard D, Dahr W. In: Immunobiology of Transfusion Medicine. New York:Marcel Dekker 1994:37

434. Huang C-H, Blumenfeld OO. In: Blood Cell Biochemistry, vol 6. New York:Plenum 1995:153

435. Thomas DB, Winzler RJ. J Biol Chem 1969;244:5493

436. Dahr W, Gielen W, Beyreuther K, et al. Hoppe-Seyler's Z Physiol Chem 1980;361:145

437. Dahr W, Kordowicz M, Moulds J, et al. Blut 1987;54:13

438. Chalmers JNM, Ikin EW, Mourant AE. Br Med J 1953;2:175

439. MacDonald KA, Nichols ME, Marsh WL, et al. Vox Sang 1967;13:346

440. Pollitzer WS. Am J Phys Anthropol 1956;14:445

441. Nijenhuis LE. Vox Sang 1953;3:112

442. Zoutendyk A. Proc 5th Cong ISBT. Basel:Karger 1955:247

443. Shapiro M. J Foren Med 1956;3:152

444. Rosenfield RE, Haber GV, Schroeder R, et al. Am J Hum Genet 1960;12:143

445. Nijenhuis LE, Wortel L. Vox Sang 1968;14:462

446. Mourant AE, Kopec AC, Domaniewska-Sobczak K. The Distribution of Human Blood Groups and Other Biochemical Polymorphisms, 2nd Ed. Oxford:Oxford Univ Press, 1976

447. Daniels GL, Green CA, Mallinson G. (abstract). Transfusion 1994;34 (Suppl 10S):62S

448. Giles CM, Howell P. Vox Sang 1974;27:43

449. Dahr W, Kordowicz M, Beyreuther K, et al. Hoppe-Seyler's Z Physiol Chem 1981:362:363

450. Furthmayr H, Metaxas MN, Metaxas-Bühler M. Proc Nat Acad Sci USA 1981;78:631

451. Bigbee WL, Langlois RG, Vanderlaan M, et al. J Immunol 1984;133:3149

452. Chown B, Lewis M. Am J Phys Anthropol 1959;17:13

453. Kout M. Vox Sang 1962;7:242

454. Metaxas MN, Metaxas-Bühler M, Romanski J. Vox Sang 1966;11:157

455. Cleghorn TE. Unpublished observations 1966 cited by Metaxas MN, Metaxas-Bühler M, Romanski J. Vox Sang 1996;11:157

456. Chandanayingyong D, Sasaki TS, Greenwalt TJ. Transfusion 1967;7:269

457. Metaxas MN, Metaxas-Bühler M, Edwards JH. Vox Sang 1970;18:385

458. Metaxas MN, Matter M, Metaxas-Bühler M, et al. Proc 9th Cong ISBT. Basel:Karger 1964:206

459. Brocteur J. Hum Hered 1969;19:77

460. Joshi SR, Bharucha ZS, Sharma RS, et al. Vox Sang 1972;22:478

461. Metaxas-Bühler M, Cleghorn TE, Romanski J, et al. Vox Sang 1966;11:170

462. Winter NM, Antonelli G, Walsh EA, et al. Vox Sang 1966;11:209

463. Neppert J. Transfusion 1980;20:448

464. Ikin EW. Vox Sang 1966;11:217

465. Dahr W, Beyreuther K, Gallasch E, et al. Hoppe-Seyler's Z Physiol Chem 1981;362:81

466. Dahr W, Weinberg R, Roelcke D, et al. (abstract). Transfusion 1992;32 (Suppl 8S):54S

467. Nordling S, Sanger R, Gavin J, et al. Vox Sang 1969;17:300

468. Luner SJ, Sturgeon P, Szklarek D, et al. Vox Sang 1975;29:440

469. Dahr W, Uhlenbruck G, Knott H. J Immunogenet 1977;4:191

470. Dahr W, Metaxas MN. Unpublished obserations 1977 cited in Dahr W, Uhlenbruck G. Hoppe-Seyler's Z Physiol Chem 1978;359:835

471. Anstee DJ, Tanner MJA. Biochem J 1978;175:149

472. Blumenfeld OO, Adamany AM, Puglia KV. Proc Nat Acad Aci USA 1981;78:747

473. Dahr W, Metaxas-Bühler M, Metaxas MN, et al. J Immunogenet 1981;8:79

474. Dahr W, Beyreuther K, Bause E, et al. Prot Biol Fluids 1982;29:57

475. Green C, Daniels G, Skov F, et al. Vox Sang 1994;66:237

476. Jáskiewicz E, Czerwinski M, Syper D, et al. Blood 1994;84:2340

477. Dahr W, Collins P, Shin C, et al. (abstract). Transfusion 1983;23:422

478. Poole J, Banks J, Hemming N, et al. (abstract). Transf Med 1993;3 (Suppl 1):98

479. Yasuda NJ. Unpublished observations cited in Francis BJ, Hatcher DJ. Vox Sang 1966;11:213

480. Morton NE, Miki C. Vox Sang 1968;15:15

481. Le Roux ME, Shapiro M. J Foren Med 1969;16:135

482. Jackson VA, Issitt PD, Richmond RS, et al. (abstract). Prog 17th Ann Mtg Blood Bank Assoc NY State 1968

483. Issitt PD, Issitt CH. Applied Blood Group Serology, 2nd Ed. Oxnard:Spectra Biologicals, 1975

484. Molthan L. Vox Sang 1980;38:210

485. Dahr W, Knuppertz G, Beyreuther K, et al. Biol Chem Hoppe-Seyler 1991;372:573

486. Baumeister G, Dahr W, Beyreuther K, et al. (abstract). Prog German Soc Blood Transf Immunohematol, 1982

487. Dahr W, Baumeister G, Beyreuther K, et al. (abstract). Transfusion 1982;22:420

488. McDougall DCJ, Jenkins WJ. Vox Sang 1981;40:412

489. Levene C, Sela R, Laeser M, et al. Vox Sang 1984;46:207

490. Dahr W, Kordowicz M, Judd WJ, et al. (abstract). Transfusion 1982;22:412

491. Judd WJ, Rolih SD, Dahr W, et al. (abstract). Transfusion 1982;22:412

492. Zelinski T, Coghlan G, Becher E, et al. Rev Fr Transf Immunohematol 1988;31:273

493. Cleghorn TE. Unpublished observations 1962 cited by Swanson J, Matson GA. Vox Sang 1962;7:585

494. Konugres AA, Huberlie MM, Swanson J, et al. Vox Sang 1963;8:632

495. Konugres AA, Fitzgerald H, Dresser R. Vox Sang 1965;10:206

496. Field TE, Wilson TE, Dawes BJ, et al. Vox Sang 1972;22:432

497. Giles CM. Vox Sang 1982;42:256

498. Metaxas MN, Metaxas-Bühler M. Vox Sang 1972;22:474

499. Madden HJ, Cleghorn TE, Allen FH Jr, et al. Vox Sang 1964;9:502

500. Metaxas-Bühler M, Metaxas MN, Sturgeon P. Vox Sang 1975;29:394

501. Vengelen-Tyler V, Mogck N. Transfusion 1986;26:231

502. Anstee DJ, Mawby WJ, Parsons SF, et al. J Immunogenet 1982;9:51

503. Blanchard D, Cartron J-P, Rouger P, et al. Biochem J 1982;203:419

504. Dahr W, Blanchard D, Chevalier C, et al. Biol Chem Hoppe-Seyler 1990;371:403

505. Huang C-H, Reid ME, Blumenfeld OO. J Biol Chem 1993;268:4945

506. Huang C-H, Reid ME, Daniels G, et al. J Biol Chem 1993;268:25902

507. Contreras M, Armitage SE, Stebbing B. Vox Sang 1984;46:360

508. Cleghorn TE. Unpublished observations 1966 cited in Race RR, Sanger R. Blood Groups in Man, 6th Ed. Oxford:Blackwell, 1975

509. Anstee DJ. In: Immunobiology of the Erythrocyte. New York:Liss, 1980:67

510. Metaxas MN. Unpublished observations 1973 cited in Race RR, Sanger R. Blood Groups in Man, 6th Ed. Oxford:Blackwell, 1975

511. Ørjasaeter H, Kornstad L, Heier A. Vox Sang 1964;9:673

512. Kornstad L, Larsen-Heier AM, Weisert O. Am J Hum Genet 1971;23:612

513. Nakajima H, Ohkura K, Ørjasaeter H, et al. Jpn J Hum Genet 1967;11:263

514. Cleghorn TE. Unpublished observations 1964 cited by Nakajima H, Ohkura K, Ørjasaeter H, et al. Jpn J Hum Genet 1967;11:263

515. Matson GA. Unpublished observations 1964 cited by Nakajima H, Ohkura K, Ørjasaeter H, et al. Jpn J Hum Genet 1967;11:263

516. Brice CL. Unpublished observations 1966 cited by Nakajima H, Ohkura K, Ørjasaeter H, et al. Jpn J Hum Genet 1967;11:263

517. Ørjasaeter H. Unpublished observations 1967 cited by Nakajima H, Ohkura K, Ørjasaeter H, et al. Jpn J Hum Genet 1967;11:263

518. Pineda AA, Taswell HF. Vox Sang 1969;17:459

519. Schimmack L, Muller I, Kornstad L. Hum Hered 1971;21:346

520. Lewis M, Anstee DJ, Bird GWG, et al. Vox Sang 1990;58:152

521. Walsh TJ, Giles CM, Poole J. Clin Lab Haematol 1981;3:137

522. Dahr W. Rev Fr Transf Immunohematol 1981;24:53

523. Dahr W, Uhlenbruck G, Schmalisch R, et al. Hum Genet 1976;32:163

524. Petty AC. J Immunol Meth 1993;161:91

525. Read SM, Taylor MM, Reid ME, et al. Immunohematology 1993;9:47

526. Rahuel C, London J, d'Auriol L, et al. Eur J Biochem 1988;172:147

527. Rahuel C, London J, Vignal A, et al. Eur J Biochem 1988;177:605

528. Postoway N, Anstee DJ, Wortman M, et al. Transfusion 1988;28:77

529. Vignal A, London J, Rahuel C, et al. Gene 1990;95:289

530. Anstee DJ, Barker DM, Judson PA, et al. Br J Haematol 1977;35:309

531. Bird GWG, Wingham J. Vox Sang 1973;24:48

532. Groves JD, Tanner MJA. J Biol Chem 1992;267:22163

533. Furuhjelm U, Nevanlinna HR, Pirkola A. Vox Sang 1973;24:545

534. Walker PS, Bergren MO, Busch MP, et al. Vox Sang 1987;52:103

535. Taliano V, Guévin RM, Hébert D, et al. Vox Sang 1980;38:87

536. Rapini J, Howard C, Behzad O, et al. (abstract). Transfusion 1993;33 (Suppl 9S):23S

537. Shinozuka T, Miyata Y, Kuroda N, et al. Jpn J Legal Med 1992;46:301

538. Okubo Y, Seno T, Yamaguchi H, et al. Immunohematology 1993;9:105

539. Inglis G, Anstee DJ, Giles CM, et al. J Immunogenet 1979;6:145

540. Hodson C, Lee D. (abstract). Prog 2nd Mtg BBTS 1984:G50

541. Murata S. Unpublished observations cited in Okubo Y, Seno T, Yamaguchi H, et al. Immunohematology 1993;9:105

542. Pavone BG, Billman R, Bryant J, et al. Transfusion 1981;21:25

543. Dahr W, Moulds J, Müller T, et al. (abstract). Prog German Soc Blood Transf Immunohematol 1982

544. Dahr W, Müller T, Krüger J, et al. (abstract). Transfusion 1982;22:428

545. Dahr W, Wilkinson S, Issitt PD, et al. (abstract). Int Cong Soc Foren Haematogenet 1983

546. Dahr W, Wilkinson S, Issitt PD, et al. (abstract). Transfusion 1983;23:424

547. Dahr W, Müller T, Moulds J, et al. Biol Chem Hoppe-Seyler 1985;366:41

548. Daniels GL. PhD Thesis, Univ London 1980

549. Daniels GL. (abstract). Book of Abstracts 16th Cong ISBT, 1980:254

550. Garratty G, Brunt D, Greenfield B, et al. (abstract). Transfusion 1983;23:408

551. Postoway N, Anstee DJ, Wortman M, et al. (abstract). Transfusion 1982;22:412

552. Anstee DJ, Edwards PAW. (abstract). Book of Abstracts, 16th Cong ISBT, 1980:273

553. Johe KK, Smith AG, Vengelen-Tyler V, et al. J Biol Chem 1989;264:17486

554. Dahr W, Beyreuther K, Moulds JJ. Eur J Biochem 1987;166:27

555. Daniels G, Anstee DJ, Cartron J-P, et al. Vox Sang 1996;71:246

556. Issitt PD, Pavone BG, Wagstaff W, et al. Transfusion 1976;16:396

557. Issitt PD, Pavone BG, Goldfinger D, et al. Transfusion 1975;15:353

558. Issitt PD, Pavone BG, Goldfinger D. (abstract). Book of Abstracts 14th Cong ISBT, 1975:69

559. Rearden A. Vox Sang 1985;49:346

560. Rearden A. (Letter). Transfusion 1989;29:187

561. Leak M, Poole J, Kaye T, et al. (abstract). Book of Abstracts. Joint Cong ISBT/AABB 1990:57

562. Adams J, Broviac M, Brooks W, et al. Transfusion 1971;11:290

563. Wren MR, Issitt PD. Transfusion 1988;28:113

564. Pavone BG, Pirkola A, Nevanlinna H, et al. Transfusion 1978;18:155

565. Issitt PD, Wilkinson-Kroovand S, Langley JW, et al. Transfusion 1981;21:211

566. Worlledge SM. (abstract). Book of Abstracts 13th Cong ISBT, 1972:43. Note: The presentation included data about the first examples of auto-anti-En^a but those data do not appear in the abstract.

567. Goldfinger D, Zwicker H, Belkin GA, et al. Transfusion 1975;15:351

568. Dacie JV. Arch Int Med 1976;135:1293

569. Issitt PD, Pavone BG, Goldfinger D, et al. Br J Haematol 1976;34:5

570. Bell CA, Zwicker H. Transfusion 1978;18:572

571. Laird-Fryer B, Moulds JJ, Dahr W, et al. (abstract). Transfusion 1983;23:424

572. Moulds MK, Lacey P, Bradford MF, et al. (abstract). Book of Abstracts 19th Cong ISBT, 1986:653

573. Garratty G, Arndt P, Clark A, et al. (abstract). Book of Abstracts, Joint Cong ISBT/AABB, 1990:154

574. D'Orsogna DE, Heinz R, Wawryszczuk V, et al. (abstract). Transfusion 1991;31 (Suppl 8S):23S

575. Arndt P, Clarke A, Domen R, et al. (abstract). Transfusion 1991;31 (Suppl 8S):29S

576. Kohler G, Milstein C. Nature 1975;256:495

577. Anstee DJ, Edwards PAW. Eur J Immunol 1982;12:228

578. Ridgwell K, Tanner MJA, Anstee DJ. Biochem J 1983;209:273

579. Ochiai Y, Furthmayr H, Marcus DM. J Immunol 1983;131:864

580. Telen MJ, Scearce RM, Haynes BF. Vox Sang 1987;52:236

581. Wásniowska K, Schroer KR, McGinniss M, et al. Hybridoma 1988;7:49

582. Gardner B, Parsons SF, Merry AH, et al. Immunology 1989;68:283

583. Uchikawa M, Yabe T, Toyada C, et al. (abstract). Vox Sang 1996;70 (suppl 2):48

584. Lubenko A, Savage JL, Gee SW, et al. (abstract). Books of Abstracts. 20th Cong ISBT, 1988:116

585. Lewis M. Clinics in Lab Med 1982;2:137

586. Skradski K, McCreary J, Zweber M, et al. (abstract). Transfusion 1983;23:409

587. Eichhorn M, Cross DE, Moulds M. (abstract). Transfusion 1981;21:614

588. Merry AH, Hodson C, Thomson E, et al. Biochem J 1986;233:93

589. Dahr W, Moulds J, Unger P, et al. Blut 1987;55:19

590. Blumenfeld OO, Smith AJ, Moulds JJ. J Biol Chem 1987;262:11864

591. Yange E, Moore BPL. (abstract). Transfusion 1983;23:409

592. Moores P, Smart E, Marais I. (abstract). Transf Med 1992;2 (Suppl 1):68

593. Huang C-H, Reid ME, Okubo Y, et al. Blood 1995;85:2222

594. Uchikawa M, Tsuneyama H, Wang L, et al. (abstract). Vox Sang 1994;67 (Suppl 2):116

595. Rapini J, Batts R, Yacob M, et al. Immunohematology 1995;11:51

596. Tippett P, Storry JR, Walker PS, et al. Immunohematology 1996;12:4

597. Doughty RW. Personal communication to PDI from the propositus! 1984

598. Graydon JJ. Med J Austral 1946;2:9

599. Simmons RT, Albrey JA, McCulloch WJ. Vox Sang 1959;4:132

600. Mohn JF, Lambert RM, Rosamilia HG, et al. Am J Hum Genet 1958;10:276

601. Worlledge S, Giles CM, Cleghorn TE. Unpublished observations 1963 cited in Cleghorn TE. Vox Sang 1966;11:219

602. Daniels G, Green C, Skov F, et al. (abstract). Transf Med 1991;1 (Suppl 2):32

603. Reid ME, Tippett P. Immunohematology 1993;9:91

604. Dahr W. Vox Sang 1992;62:129

605. Chandanayingyong D, Pejrachandra S. Vox Sang 1975;28:149

606. Green C, Poole J. Unpublished observations cited in Tippett P, Reid ME, Poole J, et al. Transf Med Rev 1992;6:170

607. Poole J. Unpublished observations cited in Tippett P, Reid ME, Poole J, et al. Transf Med Rev 1992;6:170

608. Wallace J, Milne GR, Mohn J, et al. Nature 1957;179:478

609. Chandanayingyong D, Pejrachandra S. Vox Sang 1975;29:311

610. Sabo B. In: A Seminar on Perinatal Blood Banking. Washington, D.C.:Am Assoc Blood Banks, 1978:31

611. Walker ME, Tippett PA, Roper JM, et al. Vox Sang 1961;6:357

612. Mohn JF, Lambert RM, Rosamilia HG. Transfusion 1961;1:392

613. Cornwall S, Wright J, Moore BPL. Vox Sang 1968;14:295

614. Alcalay D, Tanzer J. Rev Fr Transf Immunohematol 1977;20:623

615. Chandanayingyong D, Pejrachandra S. Vox Sang 1975;28:152

616. Dahr W, Newman RA, Contreras M, et al. Eur J Biochem 1984;138:259

617. Rearden A, Frandson S, Carry JB. Vox Sang 1987;52:318

618. Herron R, Smith GA. Vox Sang 1991;60:118
619. Huang C-H, Spruell P, Moulds JJ, et al. Blood 1992;80:257
620. Darnborough J. Vox Sang 1957;2:362
621. Kornstad L, Ørjasaeter H, Heier-Larsen AM. Acta Genet 1966;16:355
622. Smith L, Hsi R, McQuiston D, et al. (abstract). Transfusion 1985;25:447
623. Bowley CC, Griffith RW. Vox Sang 1962;7:373
624. Taylor AM, Knighton GJ. Transfusion 1982;22:165
625. Judd WJ, Hoschner JA, Kahn SR, et al. (abstract). Transfusion 1992;32 (Suppl 8S):20S
626. Molthan L. Vox Sang 1981;40:105
627. Fairley NH. Br Med J 1940;2:213
628. Avoy DR. (Letter). Vox Sang 1982;42:54
629. Molthan L. (Letter). Vox Sang 1982;42:55
630. Bergren MO, Morel PA. (abstract). Book of Abstracts 15th Cong ISBT 1978:438
631. Broadberry RE, Lin M. Transfusion 1994;34:349
632. Poole J, King M-J, Mak KH, et al. Transf Med 1991;1:169
633. Sturgeon P, Metaxas-Bühler M, Metaxas MN, et al. Vox Sang 1970;18:395
634. Lin M, Broadberry RE. (Letter). Vox Sang 1994;67:320
635. Cheng G, Hui CH, Lam CK, et al. Clin Lab Haematol 1995;17:183
636. Spruell P, Yawn D, Leveque CM, et al. (abstract). Transfusion 1992;32 (Suppl 8S):21S
637. Lin CK, Mak KH, Szeto SC, et al. Clin Lab Haematol 1996;18:91
638. Lin CK, Mak KH, Yuen CMY, et al. Immunohematology 1996;12:115
639. Mak KH, Poole J, King MJ, et al. (abstract). Transfusion 1989;29 (Suppl 7S):14S
640. Feng CS. (Letter). Transfusion 1994;34:1013
641. Lin M, Broadberry RE. (Letter). Transfusion 1994;34:1013
642. Issitt PD. Transfusion 1994;34:1014
643. Lewis M, Kaita H, Uchida I. Vox Sang 1963;8:245
644. Mohn JF, Lambert RM, Iseki S, et al. Vox Sang 1963;8:430
645. Hart van der M. Unpublished observations 1971 cited in Race RR, Sanger R. Blood Groups in Man, 6th Ed. Oxford:Blackwell, 1975:113
646. Sausais L, Mann J. Unpublished observations 1971 cited in Race RR, Sanger R. Blood Groups in Man, 6th Ed. Oxford:Blackwell, 1975:112
647. Crome W. Dtsch Ztschr Gerichtl Med 1935;24:167
648. Telen MJ, Roy RB, Issitt PD, et al. (abstract). Transfusion 1991;31 (Suppl 8S):27S
649. Metaxas MN, Metaxas-Bühler M, Heiken A, et al. Vox Sang 1972;23;420
650. Ellisor SS, Zelski D, Sugasawara E, et al. (Letter). Transfusion 1982;22:402
651. Friedenreich V. Dtsch Ztschr Gerichtl Med 1939;25:358
652. Dybkjaer E, Poole J, Giles CM. Vox Sang 1981;41:302
653. Vengelen-Tyler V, Goya K, Green CA, et al. (abstract). Transfusion 1985;25:464
654. Baldwin ML, Barrasso C, Gavin J. Transfusion 1981;21:86
655. Huang C-H, Skov F, Daniels G, et al. J Biol Chem 1992;80:2379
656. Green C, Poole J, Ford D, et al. (abstract). Transf Med 1992;2 (Suppl 1):67
657. Uchikawa M. Unpublished observations 1992 cited in Daniels G. Human Blood Groups. Blackwell:Oxford 1995:170
658. Johe KK, Vengelen-Tyler V, Leger R, et al. Blood 1991;78:2456
659. Metaxas MN, Metaxas-Bühler M. Nature 1964;202:1123
660. Henningsen K. Acta Genet 1966;16:239
661. Heiken A, Ikin EW, Martensson L. Acta Genet 1967;17:328
662. Metaxas MN, Metaxas-Bühler M, Romanski Y. Vox Sang 1971;20:509
663. Metaxas MN, Metaxas-Bühler M. In: Human Blood Groups. Basel:Karger, 1977:344
664. Hodson C, Lee D, Cooper G, et al. J Immunogenet 1979;6:391
665. Wiener AS. Blood Groups and Transfusion, 3rd Ed. Springfield:Thomas 1943
666. Andresen PH. Acta Path Microbiol Scand 1947;24:545
667. Andresen PH. Menneskets Blodtyper Anvendelsini Retsmedicinen. Copenhagen:Munksgaard 1948
668. Hurd JK, Jacox RF, Swisher SN, et al. Vox Sang 1964;9:487
669. Jensen KG, Freiesleben E. Vox Sang 1962;7:696
670. Jeannet M, Metaxas-Bühler M, Tobler R. Schweiz Med Wschr 1963;93:1508
671. Jeannet M, Metaxas-Bühler M, Tobler R. Vox Sang 1964;9:52
672. Jakobowicz R, Bryce LM, Simmons RT. Med J Austral 1949;2:945
673. Jakobowicz R, Bryce LM, Simmons RT. Nature 1950;165:158
674. Tomita M, Marchesi VT. Proc Nat Acad Sci USA 1975;72:2964
675. Fujita S, Cleve H. Biochim Biophys Acta 1975;382:172
676. Dahr W, Uhlenbruck G, Janssen E, et al. Blut 1976;32:171
677. Tomita M, Furthmayr H, Marchesi VT. Biochemistry 1978;17:4756
678. Furthmayr H. J Supramol Struct 1978;9:79
679. Blanchard D. Transf Med Rev 1990;4:170
680. Morton JA, Pickles MM. J Clin Pathol 1951;4:189
681. Morton JA. PhD Thesis. Univ London 1957
682. Issitt PD, Jerez GC. Transfusion 1966;6:155
683. Dahr W, Uhlenbruck G, Schmalisch R, et al. Hum Genet 1976;32:727
684. Brigid Sister M. Transfusion 1961;1:321
685. Strohm PL, Busch S. Transfusion 1969;9:93
686. Ottensooser F, Silberschmidt K. Nature 1953;172:914
687. Roelcke D. Transf Med Rev 1989;3:140
688. Nakajima H, Nakayama T. Rep Jpn Nat Res Inst Police Sci 1968;21:111
689. Allen NK, Brilliantine L. J Immunol 1969;102:1295
690. Okada T, Nakajima H. Rep Jpn Nat Res Inst Police Sci 1970;23:207
691. Mäkelä O. Ann Med Exp Biol Fenn 1957;35 (Suppl II):1
692. Judd WJ. In: Critical Reviews in Clinical Laboratory Sciences, Vol 12, No 3. Boca Raton:CRC, 1980
693. Fletcher G. Austral J Sci 1959;22:167
694. Bird GWG, Wingham J. Vox Sang 1970;18:235
695. Judd WJ, Murphy LA, Goldstein IJ, et al. Transfusion 1978;18:274
696. Kornfeld R, Kornfeld S. J Biol Chem 1970;245:2536
697. Lisowska E. Eur J Biochem 1972;10:574
698. Dahr W, Uhlenbruck G, Bird GWG. Vox Sang 1975;28:133
699. Bird GWG, Wingham J, Beck ML, et al. Lancet 1978;1:1215
700. Judd WJ. Transfusion 1979;19:768
701. Moon GL, Wiener AS. Vox Sang 1964;26:167
702. Bird GWG. Plenary Session Lectures, 15th Cong ISBT. Paris:Arnette, 1978:87
703. Rolih SD, Issitt PD. (abstract). Transfusion 1978;18:637
704. Bird GWG. Vox Sang 1964;9:748
705. Moulds M, Moulds E, Moulds JJ. (abstract). Transfusion 1978;18:646
706. Cohen E. Ann NY Acad Sci 1968;30:427
707. Pardoe G, Uhlenbruck G, Bird GWG. Immunology 1970;18:73
708. Cohen E, Roberts SC, Nordling S, et al. Vox Sang

1972;23:300

709. Cohen E, Rozenberg, M, Massero EJ. Ann NY Acad Sci 1974;36:28
710. Cohen E, Minowda J, Pliss M, et al. Vox Sang 1976;31:117
711. Cohen E. Ann Clin Lab Sci 1980;10:248
712. Cohen E, Ilodi GHU, Vasta GR, et al. Prot Biol Fluids 1980;27:417
713. Cohen E, Vasta GR. In: Developmental Immunology: Clinical Problems and Aging. New York:Academic, 1982:99
714. Vaisanen V, Korhonen TK, Jokinen M, et al. Lancet 1982;1:1192
715. Kornhonen TK. FEMS Microbiol Lett 1979;6:421
716. Leffler H, Svanborg EC. FEMS Microbiol Lett 1980;8:127
717. Kornhonen TK, Leffler H, Svanborg EC. Infec Immunol 1981;32:796
718. Vaisanen V, Elo J, Tallgren LG, et al. Lancet 1981;2:1366
719. Kallenius G, Mollby R, Svenson SB, et al. Lancet 1981;2:1369
720. Blajchman MA, Heddle N, Naipul N, et al. Nature 1982;299:67
721. Anstee DJ. Sem Haematol 1981;28:13
722. Ohyama K, Yamauchi S, Endo T, et al. Biochem Biophys Res Comm 1991;178:79
723. Hill SY, Aston C, Rabin B. Alcohol: Clin Exp Res 1988;12:811
724. Goldin LR, Gershon ES, Targum SD, et al. Am J Hum Genet 1983;35:274
725. Kidd KK, Gusella J. Cytogenet Cell Genet 1985;40:107
726. German J, Walker ME, Stiefel FH, et al. Science 1968;162:1014
727. German J, Walker ME, Stiefel FH, et al. Vox Sang 1969;16:130
728. German J, Chaganti RSK. Science 1973;182:1861
729. Weitkamp LR, Janzen MK, Guttormsen SA, et al. Ann Hum Genet 1969;33:53
730. Ferguson-Smith MA. Ann Genet 1973;16:29
731. Mace MA, Noades J, Robson EB. Ann Hum Genet 1975;38:479
732. Higgins JV, Wisnieweski L, Hassold T, et al. Birth Defects Orig Article Ser 1976;12:314
733. Thompson MW, Falk CT,Worton RG, et al. Birth Defects Orig Article Ser 1976;12:355
734. Weitkamp LR, Ferguson-Smith MA, Guttormsen SA, et al. Ann Hum Genet 1978;42:183
735. German J, Metaxas MN, Metaxas-Bühler M, et al. Cytogenet Cell Genet 1979;25:160
736. Kudo S, Chagnovich D, Rearden A, et al. J Biol Chem 1990;265:13825
737. Henke J, Schweitzer H. Z Rechtsmed 1980;85:221
738. Henke J, Schweitzer H, Cleef S, et al. Forens Sci Int 1988;39:279
739. Rearden A. J Immunol 1986;136:2504
740. Brindle PM, Maitland K, Williams TN, et al. Hum Hered 1995;45:211
741. Prigent MJ, Blanchard D, Cartron J-P. Arch Biochem Biophys 1983;222:231
742. Bird GWG. Transf Med Rev 1989;3:55
743. Planas J, Denson D, Gomez R, et al. (abstract). Mol Biol Cell 1992;3 (Suppl):208A
744. Rearden A, Magnet A, Kudo S, et al. J Biol Chem 1993;268:2260
745. Boccardi V, Gaetano de G, Dolci G, et al. Haematol Lat 1962;5:191
746. Blanchard D, Asseraf A, Prigent M-J, et al. Hoppe-Seyler's Z Physiol Chem 1984;365:469

747. Gleiberman L, Gershowitz H, Harburg E, et al. J Hypertens 1984;2:337
748. Cruz-Coke R, Nagel R, Etecheverry R. Ann Hum Genet 1964;28:39
749. Delanghe J, Duprez D, de Buyzere M, et al. Eur Heart J 1995;16:1269
750. Heise E, Moore M, Reid Q, et al. Hypertension 1987;9:634
751. Wedner A, Schork N, Julius S. Hypertension 1991;17:977
752. Wiener AS. J Forens Med 1960;7:166
753. Wiener AS. Am J Hum Genet 1970;22:476
754. Miller J, Grim C, Corneally P, et al. Hypertension 1979;1:493
755. Reid ME, Storry JR, Ralph H, et al. Transfusion 1996;36:719
756. Reid ME. Personal communication 1996
757. Moulds JJ, Moulds MK, Lacey B, et al. (abstract). Transfusion 1992;32 (Suppl 8S):55S
758. Klenk E, Uhlenbruck G. Hoppe-Seyler's Z Physiol Chem 1960;319:151
759. Baranowski T, Lisowska E, Morawiecki A, et al. Arch Immunol I Terapii Dosw 1959;7:15
760. Winzler RJ. In: Red Cell Membrane Structure and Function. Philadelphia:Lippincott, 1969:157
761. Marchesi VT, Tillack TW, Jackson RL, et al. Proc Nat Acad Sci USA 1972;69:1445
762. Hamaguchi H, Cleve H. Biochim Biophys Acta 1972;278:271
763. Furthmayr H, Tomita M, Marchesi VT. Biochem Biophys Res Comm 1975;65:113
764. Laemmli UK. Nature 1970;227:680
765. Kudo S, Fukuda M. J Biol Chem 1990;265:1102
766. Mueller TJ, Morrison M. In: Erythrocyte Membranes. 2. Recent Clinical and Experimental Advances. New York:LISS, 1981:95
767. Siebert PD, Fukuda M. Proc Nat Acad Sci USA 1986;83:1665
768. Yoshima H, Furthmayr H, Kobata A. J Biol Chem 1980;255:9713
769. Irimura T, Tsuji T, Tagami S, et al. Biochemistry 1981;20:560
770. Thomas DB, Winzler RJ. Biochem Biophys Res Comm 1969;35:811
771. Adamany AM, Kathan RH. Biochem Biophys Res Comm 1969;37:171
772. Lisowska E, Duk M, Dahr W. Carbohydr Res 1980;79:103
773. Prohaska R, Koerner TAW Jr, Armitage IM, et al. J Biol Chem 1981;256:5781
774. Allen A. Br Med Bull 1978;34:28
775. Pisano A, Redmond J, Williams K, et al. Glycobiology 1993;3:429
776. Clausen H, Bennett EP. Glycobiology 1996;6:635
777. Bennett EP, Hassan H, Clausen H. J Biol Chem 1996;271:17006
778. Fukuda M, Lauffenburger M, Sasaki H, et al. J Biol Chem 1987;262:11952
779. Blanchard D, Dahr W, Hummel M, et al. J Biol Chem 1987;262:5808
780. Siebert PD, Fukuda M. Proc Nat Acad Sci USA 1987;84:6735
781. Tate CG, Tanner MJA. Biochem J 1988;254:743
782. Springer GF, Yang HJ. Immunochemistry 1977;14:497
783. Lisowska E, Duk M. Eur J Biochem 1975;54:469
784. Lisowska E, Kordowicz M. In: Human Blood Groups. Basel:Karger, 1977:188
785. Lisowska E, Wasniowska K. Eur J Biochem 1978;88:247
786. Sadler JE, Paulson JC, Hill RL. J Biol Chem 1979;254:2112
787. Adamany AM, Blumenfeld OO, Sabo B, et al. J Biol Chem 1983;258:11537
788. Sim BKL, Chitnis CE, Wasniowska K, et al. Science 1994;264:1941
789. Cartron J-P, Ferrari B, Huet M, et al. Expl Clin Immunogenet

1984;1:112

790. Cherif-Zahar B, Raynal V, Gane P, et al. Nature Genet 1996;12:168
791. Ridgwell K, Eyers SAC, Mawby WJ, et al. J Biol Chem 1994;269:6410
792. Siebert PD, Fukuda M. J Biol Chem. 1986;261:12433
793. Kudo S, Fukuda M. Proc Nat Acad Sci USA 1989;86:4619
794. Alberts B, Bray D, Lewis J, et al. Molecular Biology of the Cell, 3rd Ed. New York:Garland, 1994:395
795. Rearden A, Phan H, Kudo S, et al. Biochem Genet 1990;28:209
796. Lu WM, Huang CH, Socha WW, et al. Biochem Genet 1990;28:399
797. Onda M, Kudo S, Fukuda M. J Biol Chem 1994;269:13013
798. Kudo S, Fukuda M. J Biol Chem 1994;269:22969
799. Villeval JL, Le Van Kim C, Bettaieb A, et al. Cancer Res 1989;49:2626
800. Le Van Kim C, Colin Y, Mitjavila MT, et al. J Biol Chem 1989;264:20407
801. Gahmberg CG, Jokinen M, Andersson LC. Blood 1978;52:379
802. Loken MR, Civin CI, Bigbee WL, et al. Blood 1987;70:1959
803. Rahuel C, Elouet J-F, Cartron J-P. J Biol Chem 1994;269:32752
804. Manley JL, Proudfoot NJ. Genes Dev 1994;8:259
805. Anstee DJ, Mawby WJ, Tanner MJA. In: Membranes and Transport, A Critical Review. New York:Plenum, 1982;2:427
806. Morel PA, Vengelen-Tyler V, Williams EA, et al. Rev Franc Transfus Immunohematol 1982;25:597
807. Blanchard D, Dahr W, Cartron J-P. (abstract). 3rd Joint Meeting of the Biochem Soc of France, Germany and Switzerland 1985
808. Blanchard D, Dahr W, Beyreuther K, et al. Eur J Biochem 1987;167:361
809. Blumenfeld OO, Adamany AM, Kikuchi M, et al. J Biol Chem 1986;261:5544
810. Macdonald B, Anstee DJ, unpublished observations 1984 cited by Anstee DJ. Vox Sang 1990;58:1
811. Huang C-H, Guizzo ML, Kikuchi M, et al. Blood 1989;74:836
812. Rearden A, Phan H, Dubnicoff T, et al. J Biol Chem 1990;265:9259
813. Huang C-H, Blumenfeld OO. J Biol Chem 1991;266:23306
814. Huang CH, Reid M, Daniels GL, et al. (abstract). Blood

1994;84 (Suppl 1):238a

815. Huang C-H, Blumenfeld OO. Proc Nat Acad Sci USA 1988;85:9640
816. Ridgwell K, Tanner MJA, Anstee DJ. Immunogenet 1984;11:365
817. Dahr W, Beyreuther K, Moulds JJ. Eur J Biochem 1987;166:31
818. Huang C-H, Blumenfeld OO. J Biol Chem 1991;266:7248
819. Dahr W, Vengelen-Tyler V, Dybkjaer E, et al. Hoppe-Seyler's Biol Chem 1989;370:855
820. Bruce LJ, Groves JD, Okubo Y, et al. Blood 1994;84:916
821. Tanner MJA. Curr Topics Memb Transport 1978;11:279
822. Jentoft N. Trends Biochem Sci 1990;15:291
823. Anstee DJ, Holmes CH, Judson PA, et al. In: Protein Blood Group Antigens of the Human Red Cell. Baltimore:Johns Hopkins Univ Press, 1992:170
824. Sim BKL, Chitnis CE, Wasniowska K, et al. Science 1994;264:1941
825. Miller LH. Proc Nat Acad Sci USA 1994;91:2415
826. Onda M, Kudo S, Rearden A. et al. Proc Nat Acad Sci USA 1993;90:7220
827. Roush GR, Rosenthal NS, Gerson SL, et al. Transfusion 1996;36:575
828. Schulenburg BJ, Beck ML, Pierce SR, et al. (abstract). Transfusion 1989;29:638
829. Squires JE, Mintz PD, Clark S. Transfusion 1985;25:410
830. Johnson FP Jr, Hamilton HE, Liesch MR. Arch Int Med 1985;145:1515
831. van Dijk BA, Rico PB, Hoitsma A, et al. Transfusion 1989;29:638
832. DeCoteau J, Reis MD, Pinkerton PH, et al. Vox Sang 1993;64:179
833. Garratty G. In: Immunobiology of Transfusion Medicine. New York:Marcel Dekker, 1994:523
834. Jarolim P, Moulds JM, Moulds JJ, et al. (abstract). Blood 1996;88 (Suppl 1)182a
835. Issitt PD. Transf Med Rev 1993;7:139
836. Reid ME, Storry JR, Maurer J, et al. Immunohematology 1997;13:111
837. Okada N, Yasuda T, Tsumita H, et al. Biochem Biophys Res Comm 1982;108:770
838. Okada H, Tanaka H. Mol Immunol 1983;20:1233
839. Brauch H, Roelcke D, Rother U. Immunobiology 1983;165:115
840. Tomita A, Radike E, Parker CJ. J Immunol 1993;151:3308

16 | The Gerbich Blood Group System

In 1960, Rosenfield et al. (1) reported three examples of an antibody, that they named anti-Ge, that reacted with an antigen present on the red cells of most people. Rosenfield et al. (1) and Cleghorn (2) did not find any Ge- samples in tests on 33,831 random bloods. One year later, Barnes and Lewis (3) reported the fourth example of anti-Ge and it became apparent that more than one very high incidence antigen is involved and that antibodies in this system differ from each other. The fourth example (3) of anti-Ge was non-reactive with the red cells of the three previous antibody-makers, Mrs. Gerbich, Mrs. Esp. and Mrs. St., (1) but the red cells of the person making the fourth example (Mrs. Yus.) were reactive with the antibody made by Mrs. Gerbich. Thus, it was clear that the red cells of Mrs. Gerbich and those of the other two antibody-makers reported by Rosenfield et al. (1) are the same in that they lack both antigens detected by the antibody made by Mrs. Gerbich. Such cells became known as the Ge-type and the antibody made by Mrs. Gerbich was called the Ge-type antibody. The red cells of Mrs. Yus lacked one of the antigens (against which Mrs. Yus made the antibody) but carried the other. These cells were called Yus-type and the antibody made became known as the Yus-type antibody. Another unusual finding was that the other two propositae described by Rosenfield et al. (1) (Mrs. Esp and Mrs. St) had Ge-type red cells (the cells did not react with Mrs. Gerbich's antibody) but made the Yus-type antibody (their sera did not react with the red cells of Mrs. Yus). This difficult to remember terminology was later modified (4) and the antigens missing from Mrs. Gerbich's cells were called Ge2 and Ge3 (phenotype of the Ge-type cells Ge:-2,-3). The antigen present on the cells of Mrs. Yus was called Ge3 so that the Yus-type cells became Ge:-2,3. This meant that the antibody made by Mrs. Gerbich could be called anti-Ge2,3 while that made by Mrs. Yus, Mrs. Esp and Mrs. St could be called anti-Ge2. One further complication was that the red cells of Mrs. Yus, (Ge:-2,3) were capable of adsorbing the antibody made by Mrs. Gerbich (anti-Ge2,3) to exhaustion. It was assumed that Mrs. Gerbich had made anti-Ge2 and anti-Ge3 in an inseparable form.

Booth et al. (5) and Booth and McLoughlin (4) expanded the Gerbich system in studies on the blood of Melanesians in Papua/New Guinea. First, they showed that in some parts of the country over 50% of the population have Ge- red cells. Second, they found an antibody, that they called anti-Ge1, that defined an additional Gerbich system antigen that was missing from the Ge-

type and Yus-type red cells. In Melanesians the phenotype Ge:-1,2,3 is fairly common, it does not seem to exist in other populations. Ge+ red cells (that is Ge:2,3 cells that are incompatible with the Ge-type and Yus-type antibodies) are invariably Ge:1,2,3 in populations other than Melanesians. The discovery of anti-Ge1 (5) and the high incidence of some of the Gerbich-negative phenotypes in Papua/New Guinea (i.e. Ge:-1,2,3 and Ge:-1,-2,-3; the phenotype Ge:-1,-2,3 (previously the Yus-type) does not seem to exist there) paved the way for use of the Gerbich system phenotypes as anthropological markers (6-10). However, in recent years anti-Ge1 has not been available and the antigen defined was declared obsolete by the ISBT Working Party on Red Cell Surface Antigens (11) while Gerbich was still considered a collection and before it was officially recognized (12,13) as a blood group system.

Two papers published in 1984 (14,15) and one that appeared in 1985 (16) showed that antigens of the Gerbich system were almost certainly carried on two minor red cell glycoproteins, glycophorins C and D. A spate of supportive publications appeared, by 1987 at least ten papers (17-26) confirming and extending these findings had been published. Many others, most of which are referenced later in this chapter, have appeared since then. Although the names glycophorin C and glycophorin D might suggest that these glycoproteins are related to glycophorins A and B (see Chapter 15), genetic control of production of glycophorins C and D is independent of that controlling production of glycophorins A and B. Indeed, as described in Chapter 15, *GYPA* and *GYPB*, that encode production of glycophorin A and B, respectively, are located on chromosome 4 while *GYPC*, that encodes production of both glycophorin C and glycophorin D (see below) is located on chromosome 2 (18). In spite of their genetic independence, the glycophorins have some structural similarities. They comprise a family of heavily glycosylated proteins (27-29) that between them carry most of the red cell membrane's sialic acid. Primary glycosylation is via multiple O-linked carbohydrate side chains, glycophorins A and C each carry one N-linked carbohydrate side chain, glycophorins B and D do not. In terms of numbers, glycophorins C and D are minor red cell membrane constituents when compared to glycophorins A and B. Of all PAS (periodic acid Schiff) staining material of the red cell membrane, glycophorin A carries 85%; glycophorin B, 10%; glycophorin C, 4% and glycophorin D, 1%. Glycophorin C carries more carbohydrate-containing side chains per copy than does glycophorin B but less than the number on glycophorin A. Glycophorin D is the least heavily glycosylated of the four (29). In terms of copies per red cell, as indicated in Chapter 15 glycophorin A is present in about 1 million copies per red cell and glycophorin B from 170,000 to 250,000 copies per cell. In contrast, glycophorin C is present in the range of 50,000 to 100,000 copies per red cell and glycophorin D in about 20,000 copies per cell.

Although full details are given later in the sections on biochemistry and molecular genetics of the Gerbich system, it can be mentioned here that Ge-type (Ge:-2,-3) and Yus-type (Ge:-2,3) red cells lack normal glycophorin C and D but that each type carries a variant glycophorin. The variant form on Ge:-2,-3 red cells differs from that on Ge:-2,3 red cells.

In persons with Ge:-2,-3 red cells production of the variant glycophorin C-like structure is encoded by a *GYPC* gene from which the third exon has been deleted (21,30-32,34). The glycoprotein produced lacks Ge2 and Ge3. Lack of Ge2 is not fully understood since the *GYPC* gene with exon 3 deleted would be expected to encode production of glycophorin D (that would then be expected to carry Ge2) but it does not. It has been suggested (31) that if the *GYPC* gene responsible for the Ge:-2,-3 phenotype does encode production of glycophorin D, that protein may not reach the red cell membrane or may be degraded.

In persons with Ge:-2,3 red cells, production of the variant glycophorin C-like structure is encoded by a *GYPC* gene from which the second exon has been deleted (21,30,32,33). The glycophorin produced is smaller than normal glycophorin C but larger than normal glycophorin D and the variant glycophorin on Ge:-2,-3 red cells. The variant glycophorin encoded by the *GYPC* gene from which the second exon has been deleted carries Ge3. It fails to encode production of glycophorin D since the initiation site for production of that glycoprotein is in exon 2 of normal *GYPC*. Thus the lack of production of Ge2 by this gene is understood.

A number of monoclonal antibodies have been shown to have specificities within the Gerbich system (for references, see below). Anstee et al. (14,15) were using such antibodies (35) that agglutinated Ge:2,3 red cells but reacted with Ge:-2,3 and Ge:-2,-3 red cells only by indirect antiglobulin technique, when they found a third Ge-negative phenotype. The Ge:-2,-3 red cells of two unrelated women were found to be non-reactive with the monoclonal antibodies. The new specificity was called anti-Ge4, the new phenotype was Ge:-2,-3,-4 and was named the Leach phenotype. Red cells of the other two Ge-negative phenotypes were shown to be Ge:4. That is to say, red cells of the Yus phenotype were Ge:-2,3,4, those of the Gerbich phenotype were Ge:-2,-3,4. After the Leach phenotype had been reported a human allo-

anti-Ge4 (36) and an auto-anti-Ge4 (37) were found.

At least two different genetic backgrounds have been found in persons with red cells of the Leach phenotype (30,36,38,39). While it is somewhat of an over simplification, the Ge:-2,-3,-4 phenotype can be thought of, at the serological level, as a Ge$_{null}$ phenotype and the red cells involved can be thought of as lacking glycophorin C, glycophorin D and as having no replacement glycophorin.

Once glycophorin C and glycophorin D had been recognized as the red cell membrane components that carry the Gerbich system antigens, it became possible to identify other antigens on those structures, that must therefore also belong within the system.

The low incidence antigen Wb was first described by Simmons and Albrey (40) in 1963. In 1985, Reid et al. (41) and in 1986, Macdonald and Gerns (42) independently showed that Wb+ red cells carry a reduced level of an abnormal glycophorin C. Chang et al. (32) and Telen et al. (43) then showed that the presence of Wb represents an amino acid and glycosylation change on glycophorin C.

The Ls^a antigen is also of low incidence. Unfortunately in early work the confusing term Lewis II was sometimes used to describe this antigen. The antigen was first recognized between 1962 and 1967, was mentioned from a personal communication (44) by Race and Sanger (45) and was documented in an abstract published in 1975 (46). In 1990, Macdonald et al. (47) reported that Ls(a+) red cells carry normal glycophorin C, normal glycophorin D and abnormal forms of each of those glycophorins. The abnormal glycophorins C and D were larger than the normal forms. High et al. (30) and Reid et al. (48) then demonstrated that the abnormal glycophorins on Ls(a+) red cells are encoded by a *GYPC* gene in which exon 3 has been duplicated. Shortly before Ls^a joined the Gerbich system, the low incidence antigen Rl^a, first described in 1981 (49) was found (50) to be the same as Ls^a.

The low incidence antigen An^a, was described by Furuhjelm et al. (51) in 1972. In 1993, Daniels et al. (52) used immunoblotting methods to demonstrate that An^a is present on glycophorin D but not on glycophorin C. When the amino acid change that represents An^a was identified, it was seen (52) that the change occurs on both glycophorin C and glycophorin D. However, as described, the antigen was detected on glycophorin D but not on glycophorin C. Daniels et al. (52) suggested that anti-An^a recognizes a conformational change in the NH$_2$ terminal region of glycophorin D, that is not detected when the change occurs in glycophorin C further from the NH$_2$ terminus (see below for additional details).

The fourth low incidence antigen to join the Gerbich system was Dh^a. The first example of anti-Dh^a was found by Jørgensen et al. (53) in 1982. In 1991, Spring (54)

used immunoblotting to show that Dhᵃ is present on glycophorin C but not on glycophorin D. The mutation and
amino acid changes leading to expression of the Dhᵃ
antigen were identified (55) and it was shown that the
antigen is carried on the portion of glycophorin C encoded by the exon in *GYPC* that does not participate in
encoding production of glycophorin D (again, see later
for a complete explanation).

As one of us has pointed out elsewhere (56) the
chance that the antigens Wb, Lsᵃ, Anᵃ and Dhᵃ would
ever have been shown to be part of the Gerbich system
by classical family studies is virtually nil (with perhaps
the exception of Anᵃ, that may (52) be antithetical to
Ge2). The chance that any association would have been
suggested by classic serological studies is not much
higher. Clearly, biochemical and molecular genetic studies are the only way that these antigens could have been
taken out of limbo and into Gerbich!

Table 16-1 lists the conventional and ISBT terms for
antigens of the Gerbich blood group system. Although as
stated above, Ge1 is now considered to be obsolete, it is
included in that table for historical reasons. Table 16-2
equates the old (Ge type, Yus type) phenotypes with the
currently used terms.

The Antigen Ge1 and Gerbich Negative Phenotypes in Melanesians

As stated in the introduction of this chapter, anti-Ge1
and the Ge:-1 phenotype were found in Melanesians living
in Papua New Guinea (4,5). The Ge:-1 phenotype seemed
to be confined primarily to peoples living on the North
East Coast of the island. Some 15% of the inhabitants of
that area, whose red cells reacted with anti-Ge2 and/or
anti-Ge3, had Ge:-1 red cells. As far as we are aware, anti-
Ge1 has not been used in large scale studies on other populations but in the original studies no non-Melanesian

TABLE 16-1 Conventional and ISBT Terminology for the Gerbich Blood Group System

Conventional Name: Ge

ISBT System Symbol: GE

ISBT System Number: 020

Antigen Conventional Name	ISBT Antigen Number	ISBT Full Code Number
Ge1		
Ge2	GE2	020002
Ge3	GE3	020003
Ge4	GE4	020004
Wb	GE5	020005
Lsᵃ	GE6	020006
Anᵃ	GE7	020007
Dhᵃ	GE8	020008

individual with Ge:-1,2,3 red cells was found (4,5).
Samples from non-Melanesians that were already known
to be Ge:-2,3 or Ge:-2,-3 were all Ge:-1. In a later study
(110) it was stated that existence of the Ge:1,-2 phenotype
in Melanesians could not be ruled out.

In 1989, Gorman and Woody (109) described a 13
year-old Black female patient with sickle cell disease,
whose red cells typed as Ge:2,3 and whose serum contained an antibody that reacted with all red cells except
those that were Ge:-2,3 and Ge:-2,-3. No Ge:-1,2,3 red
cells or anti-Ge1 were available for the study but the antibody, as described, displayed most of the reactions expected of anti-Ge1. The case was complicated by the fact that
the patient, not atypically for one with sickle cell disease,
had also made antibodies to C, E, Fyᵃ, Jkᵇ and Leᵃ.

Other Gerbich-negative phenotypes were also found

TABLE 16-2 To Equate Previous and Current Terminologies for Gerbich System Phenotypes and Antibodies

Previous Name for Phenotype	Reactions of Red Cells with		New Name for Phenotype	Reactions of Red Cells with Antibody to		
	Yus-type Antibody	Gerbich-type Antibody		Ge2	Ge3*	Ge4
Ge+	+	+	Ge: 2, 3, 4	+	+	+
Ge- Gerbich type	0	0	Ge: -2, -3, 4	0	0	+
Ge- Yus type	0	+	Ge: -2, 3, 4	0	+	+
			Ge: -2, -3, -4 (Leach phenotype)	0	0	0

*   Some anti-Ge3 made by persons with Ge: -2, -3 red cells, contain anti-Ge2 (see text)

in the Melanesian population. In the Sepik, New Guinea, Madang and the Islands regions, 199 of 1182 (16.8%) people had Ge:-2 red cells. In the Morobe and northern Papua regions the incidence of the Ge:-2 phenotype was 531 in 1613 (33%). In sharp contrast, in the south Papua and Highlands regions, only one Ge:-2 person was found among 1542 tested. Booth and McLoughlin reported that 89 of 664 sera from Melanesians with Ge:-2 red cells contained anti-Ge. In most cases the antibodies were non-red cell immune being found as often in non-transfused males as in females who had been pregnant. In spite of this high incidence of Gerbich system antibodies in Melanesians, only two examples of anti-Ge1 have been described (4,110).

The Ge:-2,3 (Yus) and Ge:-2,-3 (Gerbich) Phenotypes

Other than as described above, these phenotypes are both extremely rare. In tests using anti-Ge2 no negative sample was found in tests on red cells from: 22,331 English (2); 22,000 Japanese (57); 5000 New Zealand (58); 500 Danish (1); 500 Californian (59); or 250 Polynesian (66) persons. Using anti-Ge3, one negative sample was found among 5912 French donors (45,60) but none among 11,000 New Yorkers (1) at least 1500 of whom were Black and about 100 Chinese. In tests in Thailand (69) using an anti-Ge that could have been either anti-Ge2 or anti-Ge3, one negative sample was found among 4253 donors. This means, of course, that most persons with Ge:-2,3 or Ge:-2,-3 red cells have been identified when they presented with anti-Ge in the serum, many such individuals have been found (1-3,15,57-68,125). Among those reports it can be seen that the Ge:-2,3 phenotype is more common than Ge:-2,3. The Ge:-2,-3 phenotype has been found in Whites and Blacks particularly in peoples of the Middle East, that is Arabs, a Turkish Cypriot and White and Black Jews. That the variant *GYPC* gene that in homozygotes results in the Ge:-2,-3 phenotype is more common than the variant *GYPC* gene that in homozygotes results in the Ge:-2,3 phenotype was also demonstrated by Moulds et al. (70). These workers used immunochemical studies and showed that among ten Ge:-2,3 propositi, five were heterozygous for the two variant *GYPC* genes described.

The Ge:-2,-3,-4 (Leach) Phenotype

As mentioned in the introduction of this chapter, red cells of the Ge:-2,-3,-4 phenotype, like those of the Ge:-2,3 and Ge:-2,-3 phenotypes, lack normal glycophorin C and glycophorin D. However, unlike Ge:-2,3

and Ge:-2,-3 red cells, those that are Ge:-2,-3,-4 carry no variant form of glycophorin encoded by an altered *GYPC* gene. Although there are at least two different genetic changes that can bring about the Ge:-2,-3,-4 phenotype, red cells of the phenotype behave similarly in serological tests, regardless of the genetic background. Also as mentioned earlier, the Ge:-2,-3,-4 phenotype was first recognized (14,15) by the use of monoclonal antibodies that: agglutinate Ge:2,3 red cells; react by IAT with those that are Ge:-2,3 and Ge:-2,-3; but fail to react at all with Ge:-4 red cells.

Six Ge:-2,-3,-4 propositi are known (15,36,71-73), all are White and all are European or of European extraction. An unusual feature of Ge:-2,-3,-4 red cells is that they are elliptocytic (14,15,20,38,71,72). It is known (74-80) that in Ge+ red cells glycophorins C and D are transmembrane proteins that are attached, via protein 4.1 to the cytoskeleton of the red cells. It is believed that this attachment is one of a number of features that stabilize red cell shape. In the absence of glycophorins C and D in the Ge:-2,-3,-4 phenotype, this attachment cannot occur and red cell elliptocytosis results. Since Ge:-2,3,4 and Ge:-2,-3,4 red cells are discoid not elliptocytic it is concluded that in those cells, the variant glycophorins present serve the function of normal glycophorins C and D in this respect. The elliptocytosis associated with the Ge:-2,-3,-4 phenotype is not the same condition as that known as South East Asian ovalocytosis (SAO). Since that condition involves a variant form of protein band 3, it is described in Chapter 17. It is not known if the high incidence of both the Ge- phenotypes and SAO in Papua New Guinea is a coincidence or if both are involved as resistance factors to malaria.

It is not yet clear whether the lack of glycophorins C and D from Ge:-2,-3,-4 red cells compromises survival of those red cells in vivo. Two brothers with Ge:-2,-3,-4 red cells, studied by Rountree et al. (73), had a history of mild anemia. In the family described by Telen et al. (38) a similar clinical picture was seen (81). If Ge:-2,-3,-4 red cells do have a shortened in vivo life span, the resultant anemia is not severe. Other reports on individuals of this phenotype have not contained any description of an associated clinical disorder.

Location and Enzyme Sensitivities of High Incidence Gerbich System Antigens

Early studies with Gerbich system antibodies and enzyme treated red cells gave confusing and at times conflicting results. Once the locations of Ge2, Ge3 and Ge4 on glycophorin C and/or glycophorin D were recognized, the earlier described reactions became understandable. While full details are given in the section on biochemistry of the Gerbich system later in this chapter, the major findings as they relate to serological studies can be described here.

As mentioned in the introduction to this chapter, production of glycophorin C and glycophorin D is encoded by the same *GYPC* gene (21,89). The initiation sites for production of the two glycophorins are different with the result that glycophorin C has 21 amino acids at its NH$_2$ terminus that are not present on glycophorin D (90). In simple terms, glycophorin D can be thought of as glycophorin C, missing the first 21 amino acids. This difference affects which antigens are present and the enzyme sensitivity of those antigens.

Ge2 is located near the NH$_2$ terminal end of glycophorin D (20,24). Although the same amino acids are present on glycophorin C, the Ge2 antigen is not detectable on that protein, presumably because of a steric alteration brought about by presence of the portion of glycophorin C that is missing from glycophorin D. That is to say, Ge2 is relatively exposed near the NH$_2$ terminus of glycophorin D. The same sequence of amino acids that comprise Ge2 on glycophorin D is at least 21 residues further away from the NH$_2$ terminus of glycophorin C. The Ge2 antigen is denatured when Ge:2,3 red cells are treated with trypsin or papain (82,91), it survives treatment of those red cells with chymotrypsin and pronase. About half of all examples of anti-Ge2 give weaker reactions with neuraminidase-treated than with untreated red cells (82) leading to the suggestion (92) that anti-Ge2 are probably heterogeneous. Apparently some examples define sialic acid dependent and others, sialic acid independent epitopes at the NH$_2$ terminus of glycophorin D.

Ge3 is present on both glycophorin C and glycophorin D (20,24,93-95). It is denatured when Ge:2,3 red cells are treated with trypsin but is resistant to treatment of such red cells with papain, chymotrypsin and pronase (82,91). Given these sensitivities, Ge:2,3 red cells, treated with papain will become Ge:-2,3 and can be used to identify anti-Ge3, when red cells of the Ge:-2,3 phenotype are not available. However, as described below, such red cells will also fail to react with anti-Ge4, they will, in fact, be Ge:2,3,-4 a phenotype not yet found in nature.

Ge4 is present on glycophorin C but not on glycophorin D, thus indicating that it is present within the first 21 residues of the NH$_2$ terminus of glycophorin C, i.e. the portion of glycophorin C that is not present on glycophorin D (14,15,37,94,96). Ge4 is denatured when Ge:2,3,4 cells are treated with trypsin or papain, a finding in agreement with the presumed position of the antigen within the NH$_2$ terminal region of glycophorin C.

The variant glycophorin seen on red cells of the Ge:-2,-3,4 phenotype differs from all those described above in that it lacks a trypsin-sensitive site. Thus when Ge:-2,-3,4 red cells are treated with trypsin, they continue to react with anti-Ge4 (15). Both Ge:2,3,4 and Ge:-2,3,4 red cells become non-reactive with anti-Ge4 once they have been treated with trypsin. As described below, this feature of Ge:-2,-3,4 red cells has been used to recognize presence of the variant *GYPC* gene that encodes a Ge:-2,-3,4 glycophorin, in the heterozygous state. The reactions of red cells of various Ge phenotypes with antibodies to Ge2, Ge3 and Ge4 before and after those cells have been treated with trypsin or papain are summarized in table 16-3. In using the data listed in that table it should be remembered that some Gerbich system antibodies contain anti-Ge2 and anti-Ge3 in an apparently inseparable form.

Antibodies to Ge2, Ge3 and Ge4

Although the Ge:-2,-3 phenotype is more common than Ge:-2,3 anti-Ge2 is more common than anti-Ge3. Daniels (82) reported that among 17 antibodies made by persons with Ge:-2,-3 red cells, 13 were anti-Ge2 while four were anti-Ge3. Among six immunized persons who had Ge:-2,-3,-4 red cells, four made anti-Ge2, one anti-Ge3 and one anti-Ge4 (15,36,71-73).

Gerbich system antibodies may be made following exposure to foreign red cells via transfusion or pregnancy or may be non-red cell immune. In the Melanesian Gerbich-negative individuals non-red cell stimulated antibodies were common, i.e. 89 of 664 individuals (4) and similar antibodies have been seen in others (57-59,83). Among those Gerbich system antibodies best reactive by IAT (84-88) many were IgG, IgG1 was the most common subclass seen (85). Nothing seems to have been published regarding the ability, or lack thereof, of Gerbich system antibodies to activate complement.

Gerbich system antibodies do not show dosage effects (67). As described above, individuals heterozygous for the gene that encodes production of Ge3 but not Ge2 and the gene that encodes production of neither, were recognized from the results of immunochemical studies (70). Reid et al. (68) used monoclonal anti-Ge4 and trypsin-treated red cells to identify individuals heterozygous for the *GYPC* variant gene that encodes production of a glycophorin that lacks Ge2 and Ge3 in a family with Ge:2,3 and Ge:-2,-3 members. As described above, when Ge:-2,-3 red cells are treated with trypsin, they continue to react with anti-Ge4; normal Ge:2,3 and Ge:-2,3 red cells do not. Reid et al. (68) found that the same was true of the red cells of persons heterozygous for the variant *GYPC* gene that fails to encode production of Ge2 and Ge3. That the method differentiates between individuals homozygous for the *GYPC* gene that makes Ge2 and Ge3 and heterozygous for

TABLE 16-3 To Show the Reactions of Untreated, Trypsin and Papain-treated Red Cells of Various Gerbich Phenotypes with Antibodies to High Incidence Gerbich System Antigens

Red Cells	Antibodies		
	Anti-Ge2	Anti-Ge3	Anti-Ge4
Untreated			
Ge: 2, 3, 4	+	+	+
Ge: -2, 3, 4	0	+	+
Ge: -2, -3, 4	0	0	+
Ge: -2, -3, -4	0	0	0
Trypsin-treated			
Ge: 2, 3, 4	0	0	0
Ge: -2, 3, 4	0	0	0
Ge: -2, -3, 4	0	0	+
Ge: -2, -3, -4	0	0	0
Papain-treated			
Ge: 2, 3, 4	0	+	0
Ge: -2, 3, 4	0	+	0
Ge: -2, -3, 4	0	0	0
Ge: -2, -3, -4	0	0	0

that gene and the variant gene that makes neither Ge2 nor Ge3, was confirmed in immunoblotting studies.

The most usual reactions of Gerbich system antibodies, including those directed against the low incidence antigens of the system (see later) are shown in table 16-4.

Clinical Significance of Antibodies to Ge2, Ge3 and Ge4

Although the data are not abundant, those that have been published suggest that antibodies to the high incidence Gerbich system antigens are benign in vivo, more often than they are clinically significant. There are no reports of antibodies to Ge2, Ge3 or Ge4 causing transfusion reactions but it is not known how many patients with the antibodies have been transfused with serologically reactive blood. In one patient (61) transfusion was associated with fever at the time of infusion. Ten days later the patient was found to have anti-Ge2 in the serum but there was no evidence of premature clearance of the transfused red cells. In another patient with anti-Ge2 (88), 16 units of Ge:2 blood were transfused during a three week period with no clinical evidence of a transfusion reaction. In one red cell survival study (84) an anti-Ge (specificity not further described) caused some destruction of the small test dose of red cells within the

first 24 hours after injection, thereafter the remaining 80% of the test dose survived normally. In contrast there are some reports (83,86,87) of red cell survival studies or monocyte monolayer assays that suggested that Ge+ red cells would be destroyed in patients with anti-Ge in the serum. In none of these cases were whole units transfused so that correlation (or lack thereof, see Chapter 35) of the test results with transfusion outcome was not possible.

In at least five cases (1,63-66) an antibody directed against a high incidence Gerbich system antigen has caused a positive DAT on the red cells of a newborn infant but in no instance did the antibody cause severe HDN. The Ge2 and Ge3 antigens are apparently fully developed at birth (1) and anti-Ge (exact type not known) was found to react with the red cells of fetuses at as early as 18 weeks (44).

Autoantibodies to High Incidence Gerbich System Antigens

Unlike some of the alloantibodies to high incidence Gerbich system antigens described above, some autoantibodies to those antigens have caused marked in vivo red cell destruction. Two auto-anti-Ge2 (97,98) one of which (98) was apparently IgA in composition, and one auto-anti-Ge3 (99) have been associated with severe

TABLE 16-4 Usual Characteristics of Gerbich System Antibodies

Antibody Specificity	Positive Reactions in In Vitro Tests				Usual Immuno-globulin		Ability to Bind Complement		Ability to Cause In Vitro Lysis		Implicated in		Usual Form of Stimulation		% of White Population Positive
	Sal	LISS	AHG	Enz[*1]	IgG	IgM	Yes	No	Yes	No	Trans fusion Reaction	HDN	Red Cells	Other	
Anti-Ge1			X		X					X	No	No	X		>99.9
Anti-Ge2	Some		Most		Most	Few				X	No	*2	Some	Some	>99.9
Anti-Ge3	Some		Most		Most	Few				X	No	*2	Some	Some	>99.9
Anti-Ge4			X		X					X	No				>99.9
Anti-Wb (Anti-Ge5)	X					X		X		X	No	No		X	<0.1
Anti-Ls[a] (Anti-Ge6)	X		X		Some	Some		X		X	No	Yes		X	<0.1
Anti-An[a] (Anti-Ge7)	X					X				X	No	No		X	<0.1
Anti-Dh[a] (Anti-Ge8)	X					X		X		X	No	No		X	<0.1

[*1] Different reactions when different enzymes used, see text
[*2] May cause positive DAT on cord red cells, no clinical HDN reported
[*3] Characteristics of antibodies to Ge1, Ge4, Wb, Ls[a], An[a], and Dh[a] based on few examples of each antibody

"warm" autoantibody-induced hemolytic anemia. In another case (100) anti-Ge2 was found in the serum of a patient with Ge:2 red cells that had a negative DAT. The auto-anti-Ge2 could be recovered by elution from the patient's red cells. Although the serological specificity of two of the autoantibodies described appeared to be anti-Ge2 (97,100) immunoblotting studies showed (100,101) that they bound to glycophorin C but not to glycophorin D. As described above, Ge2 as defined by alloantibodies, is carried on glycophorin D and is not expressed, serologically, on glycophorin C. In both cases, Ge2 antigen depression was noticed on the patients' red cells. The auto-anti-Ge3 described (99) immunoblotted to glycophorins C and D, like alloimmune anti-Ge3 (101).

In another case an autoantibody that either had anti-Ge4 specificity or closely resembled that antibody, was found in a patient with aplastic anemia who had elliptocytic red cells (37,102). The autoantibody did not cause hemolytic anemia and was produced transiently while the level of glycophorin C on the patient's red cells was temporarily reduced; the level of glycophorin D on the red cells was normal. Two years after the initial investigation (37) the patient's red cells carried normal levels of glycophorin C, were no longer elliptocytic and her serum no longer contained antibody. Her red cells were then reactive with the earlier sample of her serum.

Monoclonal Antibodies to High Incidence Gerbich System Antigens

As mentioned several times in this chapter, a number of monoclonal antibodies directed against glycophorin C have been developed. Indeed it was through the use of such reagents that the Ge:-2,-3,-4 phenotype was first recognized (14,15). Most of the monoclonal antibodies made have been directed against epitopes near to the NH_2 terminus of glycophorin C (14,15,35,94-96,103,104) in serological studies such antibodies behave as anti-Ge4. However, monoclonal anti-Ge3 have also been made (93-95) and one MAb directed against what appeared to be an epitope common to glycophorin C and protein band 3, has been described (105).

Association Between Red Cells That Lack High Incidence Gerbich System Antigens and the Kell Blood Group System

In 1973, Muller et al. (60) first reported that some Ge-negative red cells have weakened expressions of high incidence Kell system antigens. Many other investigators studied this phenomenon although few results were published. In some cases depression of Kell system antigen expression was confirmed, in others no weakening of those antigens was seen. Considerable order was brought to this rather chaotic situation in 1982, when Daniels (82) reported that among 11 Ge:-2,-3 samples weakening of Kell system antigens could be demonstrated in nine. In contrast, among six examples of Ge:-2,3 red cells, none showed any weakening of Kell system antigens. Since then, this observation has been confirmed by others (15,36,57,71). While all Kell system antigens including K and KL may be affected, K11 seems particularly prone to this effect. Depression of Kell system antigen expression has also been seen (15,36,71) in at least four individuals with the Ge:-2,-3,-4 phenotype. While nothing is known about the interaction that leads to weakening of Kell system antigens on some Ge-negative samples, it is noteworthy that the two Ge phenotypes involved, i.e. Ge:-2,-3,4 and Ge:-2,-3,-4 lack the portion of glycophorin C normally encoded by exon 3 of the GYPC gene. Red cells of the Ge:-2,3,4 phenotype, that carry the product of exon 3, do not show weakening of Kell system antigens. Thus it has been speculated (106) that the product of exon 3 of GYPC somehow alters the availability of antigens on the 93kD Kell glycoprotein (107,108) to their antibodies.

High Incidence Gerbich System Antigens, the Rh System and the Vel Antigen

In 1988, we (111) described a weak antibody that reacted with all red cell samples except those that were Ge-negative and some with unusual Rh phenotypes. In addition to Ge-negative samples, those that were Rh$_{null}$, Rh$_{mod}$, D--/D--, Dc-/Dc-, Dc(e)/Dc(e), hr^S- and hr^B- were non-reactive. Although the antibody was weak, it resisted adsorption by Ge-negative and Rh$_{null}$ red cells. While we hoped that the apparent association might parallel that described above involving Gerbich and Kell system antigens, that possibility seemed to be excluded since: Ge:-2,3,4; Ge:-2,-3,4; and Ge:-2,-3,-4 red cells were all non-reactive with the antibody. In using other Gerbich and Rh system antibodies we were unable to find any abnormality of Ge antigens on Rh$_{null}$, Rh$_{mod}$, D--/D--, Dc-/Dc-, Dc(e)/Dc(e), hr^S- and hr^B- red cells or any abnormality of Rh antigens on Ge:-2,3,4; Ge:-2,-3,4; and Ge:-2,-3,-4 red cells. Thus we do not know how to interpret the finding with this, thus far unique, antibody.

In 1994, we (126) described a patient with Ge:-2,-3 red cells who had made anti-Ge (exact specificity not determined). In the initial stages of the investigation, the red cells of the antibody-maker were seen to be non-reactive with some examples of anti-Vel (see Chapter 31). In the subsequent investigation we tested 14 examples of anti-Vel against: one Ge:-2,3,4; eight Ge:-2,-3,4; one Ge:-2,-3,-4; and three unclassified Ge-negative samples.

Three of the anti-Vel failed to react with at least four Ge:-2,-3,4 samples while two others were non-reactive with some of those samples. The other nine anti-Vel reacted with all eight Ge:-2,-3,4 samples. All 14 of the anti-Vel reacted with the single examples of Ge:-2,3,4 and Ge:-2,-3,-4 samples available.

Taken together, the weakening of some Kell system antigens on Ge:-2,-3,4 samples (60,82), the failure of some Ge:-2,-3,4 samples to react with some anti-Vel (126) and the antibody (111) that failed to react with Ge:-2,3,4; Ge:-2,-3,4; and Ge:-2,-3,-4 and red cells with unusual Rh phenotypes, suggest that perhaps when glycophorin C is altered (Ge:-2,3,4 and Ge:-2,-3,4 red cells) or absent (Ge:-2,-3,-4 red cells) a general membrane alteration results in a non-specific (perhaps steric) change of other membrane components and the antigens that they carry. Somewhat ironically, the Mexican donor described by Biro et al. (127) (for full details see Chapter 17) who had depressed antigens in so many systems (including Vel) was described as having a normal expression of Ge.

Low Incidence Antigens of the Gerbich System. 1. Wb

In 1963, Simmons and Albrey (40) found anti-Wb as an unexpected contaminant in an anti-A typing serum. In tests on 3550 unrelated White Australians, two Wb+ samples were found (i.e. 1 in 1775). No Wb+ sample was found in tests on the red cells of 92 Australian Aborigines and 105 Melanesians in New Guinea (40). Cleghorn (44) found 3 Wb+ samples in tests on red cells from 15,815 English adults (i.e. 1 in 5272) but none in tests on 395 cord blood samples. Bloomfield et al. (112) found 8 Wb+ samples among 10,117 Welsh donors (i.e. 1 in 1265) for an incidence similar to that seen in White Australians (were all the British convicts sent to Australia, Welsh?). In Japan, Ikemoto et al. (113) found no Wb+ sample in 513, and Nakajima et al. (114) none in 2957 donors. Ørjasaeter et al. (115) found no Wb+ sample among 42 Tibetans. While a commercially available anti-A used in the USA for many years was found to contain anti-Wb, no count of the number of Wb+ bloods nor the total number of samples tested, was ever made. The Wb antigen is destroyed when red cells are treated with trypsin or neuraminidase but remains intact on red cells treated with chymotrypsin.

Simmons and Albrey (40) did not find an example of anti-Wb in tests on 2000 sera from Australian donors, but Cleghorn (44) found three among 2400 normal sera in England. Nothing seems to be known about the clinical significance or lack thereof, of anti-Wb.

In 1985, Reid et al. (41) and in 1986, Macdonald and

Gerns (42) independently showed that Wb is carried on glycophorin C. The change (32,43) in that glycoprotein that results in the expression of Wb is described below in the section on biochemistry of the Gerbich system.

Low Incidence Antigens of the Gerbich System. 2. Ls^a

Cleghorn and Dunsford (116) found anti-Ls^a in an anti-B typing serum that was subsequently shown (46) also to contain anti-Cl^a (see Chapter 15). Initially it appeared that Ls^a is primarily an antigen of Blacks, it was found (44) in: nine of 878 Black West Indians (i.e. 1 in 98); two of 81 Black West Africans; and one of 110 American Blacks. In the same study (44) no Ls(a+) sample was found among 5887 English and 226 other European donors. One Ls(a+) was found among 160 donors in Finland (44). However, in subsequent tests (46) 17 Ls(a+) samples were found in tests on red cells from 1053 Finnish donors (i.e. 1 in 62) and 8 among 7151 samples (49) from Norwegian donors (i.e. 1 in 894). In the Norwegian study, the antibody used was called anti-Rl^a (49), it was later shown (50) that anti-Rl^a is the same as anti-Ls^a, the name Ls^a has priority. The Ls^a antigen is destroyed when red cells are treated with trypsin but is resistant to treatment of red cells with ficin and neuraminidase (47).

In screening tests on 4000 normal sera one additional example of anti-Ls^a was found (44,46). The antibody has also been found in sera containing multiple antibodies to low incidence antigens (49), as the cause of a positive antibody screening test (117) and once (118) as causative of HDN. The anti-Ls^a detected in pretransfusion antibody screening tests (117) was present in the serum of an 87 year-old, White male. It was IgG in nature and reactive by IAT. Although, as described above, Ls^a has been reported (47) to survive ficin treatment of red cells, the anti-Ls^a found in the 87 year-old male did not react with two Ls(a+) samples pretreated with ficin or papain (117). The anti-Ls^a that caused HDN was said to have caused severe enough disease to necessitate exchange transfusion in the second child born to a woman with anti-Ls^a in the serum. The third child had Ls(a+) red cells and a positive DAT at birth, no treatment was described.

Again, the genetic and biochemical changes that result in the production of an abnormal glycophorin that carries Ls^a (30,47,48) are described in detail below. It can be mentioned here that the mechanism is of particular interest since it involves duplication of an exon of the *GYPC* gene.

Low Incidence Antigens of the Gerbich System. 3. An^a

In 1972, Furuhjelm et al. (51) described anti-An^a that defined an antigen present on the red cells of six of 10,000 Finnish and two of 3266 Swedish donors (i.e. 1 in 1667 and 1 in 1633 respectively). The An^a antigen is denatured or removed when red cells are treated with trypsin, papain or neuraminidase (52).

Anti-An^a was found in the sera of six of 5350 Finnish donors, two of 1868 Finnish patients and five of 1693 Swedish donors. The authors (51) pointed out that the incidences of the antibody are not significantly different and that most persons who made anti-An^a had never been exposed to An(a+) red cells. Nothing seems to have been reported about the clinical significance, or lack thereof, of anti-An^a.

In 1993, Daniels et al. (52) showed that An^a is present on glycophorin D but not on glycophorin C. This somewhat difficult to explain finding is discussed more fully below. As will be seen from the biochemistry and molecular genetics of An^a, it is possible that the antigen is antithetical to Ge2.

Low Incidence Antigens of the Gerbich System. 4. Dh^a

The IgM non-red cell immune antibody to this antigen was first found in Denmark in 1968 but was not described in print until 1982 (53). Dh(a+) red cells and anti-Dh^a were sent to laboratories all around the world, soon after the antibody was found, but it was not until 1980 that additional Dh(a+) red cells and additional examples of anti-Dh^a were found (119). In the original study (53) no Dh(a+) sample was found in tests on samples from 2493 Danish donors. In an English family (120) eight persons, spanning three generations, had Dh(a+) red cells. The Dh^a antigen is denatured or removed when red cells are treated with trypsin, papain, ficin, pronase or neuramindase, it survives treatment of red cells with chymotrypsin (52,120).

In 1991, Spring (54) showed that Dh^a is present on glycophorin C but not on glycophorin D. Again the genetic and biochemical change that results in the expression of Dh^a on glycophorin C, is described below.

Table 16-5 shows some incidences of low incidence Gerbich system antigens and the antibodies that define them.

The *Gerbich* Locus is on Chromosome 2

Traditional family studies had been used to show that the *Gerbich* locus is independent of the loci for many blood group systems (1,44,60,61,121-123). After recognition of the fact that the glycophorin C gene (*GYPC*) encodes production of both glycophorin C and

TABLE 16-5 Some Studies on the Freqency of Low Incidence Gerbich System Antigens and the Antibodies that Define Them[*1]

Antigen	Number Red Cell Samples Tested	Population	Number Positive	Refs	Antibody	Number Sera Tested[*2]	Population	Number Abs Found	Refs
Wb	3550	Australians	2	40	Anti-Wb	2000	Australian	0	40
	15,815	English	3	44		2400	English	3	44
	10,117	Welsh	8	112					
	3470	Japanese	0	113,114					
Ls[a]	878	Black West Indians	9	44	Anti-Ls[a]	4000	Europeans	1	44, 46
	81	Black West Africans	2	44					
	110	Black Americans	1	44					
	6113	Europeans (non-Finnish)	0	44					
	1213	Finns	18	44, 46					
	7151	Norwegians	8	49					
An[a]	1000	Finns	6	51	Anti-An[a]	7218	Finns	8	51
	3266	Swedes	2	51		1693	Swedes	5	51
Dh[a]	2493	Danes	0	53					

[*1] For smaller studies not included in this table, see text.
[*2] Random sera, those known to contain antibodies to other low incidence antigens, not included.

glycophorin D and that the Gerbich system antigens are carried on those glycoproteins (or their variants encoded by mutated or altered *GYPC*) it followed that the *Ge* and *GYPC* loci are the same thing. In 1986, Mattei et al. (18) used in situ hybridization to localize *GYPC* to chromosome 2, between 2q14 and q21. Since no other blood group locus was known to be on chromosome 2, this almost established Gerbich as an independent blood group system. The final step for Gerbich to achieve such status was achieved in 1991, when Zelinski et al. (124) demonstrated recombination between *GYPC*, via a *Taq*I polymorphism, and loci for the Diego, Dombrock and Cartwright (Yt) blood group systems. At that time the now recognized loci for *DI* (*Diego*) (see Chapter 17), *YT* (*Cartwright*) (see Chapter 23), and *DO* (*Dombrock*) (see Chapter 22) were not known. Thus, demonstration that *GYPC* was genetically independent of *DI*, *YT* and *DO* allowed Gerbich to be recognized as an independent blood group system (12,13).

Identification of Glycophorins C and D

Originally, the red cell sialoglycoproteins were described as a single polypeptide (129,130). The methods available to early workers did not readily allow the recognition or purification of minor components in the "sialoglycoprotein fraction" and so the data obtained were related to the major component which was subsequently called glycophorin (sugar-bearing) by Marchesi and colleagues (131). When biochemical methods like gel filtration and SDS-PAGE were applied to study the "sialoglycoprotein fraction" in the 1970s it became clear that glycophorin is not one protein but several. However, it took some time for different workers in the field to agree on the number of unique proteins partly because of the suspicion that some minor proteins might be proteolytic degradation products of others rather than novel, partly because some workers were using more sensitive electrophoretic methods and so could detect bands that others could not and partly because the proteins had a tendency to form dimers and heterodimers which survived the process of SDS-PAGE! As a result several different nomenclatures (see table 4-3 in Chapter 4 and Chapter 15 for discussion of nomenclatures) were used to describe what eventually became four proteins now known as glycophorins A, B, C and D. These names are far from satisfactory. Glycophorin A (GPA) and glycophorin B (GPB) are the products of adjacent genes on chromosome 4 and give rise to MN system antigens whereas glycophorin C (GPC) and glycophorin D (GPD) are the products of a single gene on chromosome 2 and give rise to Gerbich system antigens. The two sets of proteins are completely different in terms of amino acid sequence but share some structural similarities in that they are type I membrane proteins which are rich in O-glycans and therefore sialic acid-rich. Unfortunately, these names still cause confusion and the reader may well come across contemporary publications which talk of glycophorin without specifying which one or, less frequently, incorrectly refer to GPA instead of GPC.

GPC and GPD form the subject of this chapter. Recognition of the existence of GPC and GPD came from the application of the discontinuous buffer system of Laemmli (132) for the electrophoretic analysis of red cell membrane proteins. This buffer system gave a much better resolution of proteins than other systems available at the time and when gels were stained with the periodic acid Schiff's Base stain (PAS stain) to detect sialic acid-rich components several bands were consistently obtained. Most of these bands could be accounted for as monomeric GPA, monomeric GPB and homo- or heterodimers of GPA and GPB (see Chapter 15) but two bands of Mr 35,000 (GPC) and 27,000 (GPD) respectively, could not be explained in this way. GPC was denoted PAS 2′ (133), D SGP (134), GPC (28) and sialoglycoprotein beta (135). GPD was denoted E SGP (134) and sialoglycoprotein gamma (135).

The Structure of Glycophorin C

Clear evidence that GPC is a novel protein unrelated to GPA and GPB was obtained from determination of the N-terminal amino acid sequence of a tryptic peptide (residues 1 to 48) derived from GPC (28,136,137). GPC and GPB could be separated from GPA by gel filtration in detergents but it was extremely difficult to separate the minor components GPC and GPB. Subsequently, purification of GPC was achieved using high-performance liquid chromatography (HPLC) and the amino acid sequence of GPC was obtained through residue 88 (25).

The N-terminal sequence of GPC was used to design oligonucleotide probes to screen bone marrow cDNA libraries and clones were obtained which allowed deduction of the complete amino acid sequence of GPC (17,19). The protein comprises 128 amino acids, has a single membrane spanning domain (24 residues) and is oriented with its N-terminus extracellular (57 residues) and its C-terminus in the cytosol (47 residues; see figure 16-1).

The protein contains a single N-glycan at Asn8 and there are numerous serine and threonine residues in the extracellular domain that accommodate approximately

12 0-glycans (26). The protein is not translated with an N-terminal signal sequence that is cleaved during insertion of the protein into the membrane and it is thought that the membrane domain acts as an internal signal sequence (89).

Glycophorin C and Glycophorin D are Related Proteins

Clear evidence that GPC and GPD are related proteins and that they are responsible for Gerbich blood group antigens came from the demonstration that the red cells of certain rare individuals (PL and KW) lacked Gerbich blood group antigens and have a complete deficiency of GPC and GPD (14). Red cells of this phenotype were named Leach phenotype after the first individual found (PL). Patient PL was known to be Gerbich-negative. Recognition of her unique phenotype was achieved by testing the patient's red cells with a panel of monoclonal antibodies of unknown specificity that had been raised against normal red cells. Two antibodies (BRIC 4 and BRIC 10) failed to react with the red cells of PL and subsequently a second Gerbich-negative patient (KW) was tested and found to have the same phenotype. SDS-PAGE and subsequent staining with PAS stain revealed that membranes from the red cells of PL and KW lacked bands corresponding to GPC and GPD. When the sialic acid-containing components of PL and KW red cells were labeled with the periodate/tritiated sodium borohydride method and the electrophoretically separated components subjected to prolonged fluorography, GPC and GPD were again undetectable and an additional minor band found in normal cells (denoted beta 1) was also absent from PL and KW cells. It is likely that beta 1 represents a proteolytic fragment of GPC. Immunoprecipitation experiments revealed that the monoclonal antibodies BRIC 4 and BRIC 10 recognized epitopes on GPC but not on GPD thereby explaining their lack of reactivity with red cells of Leach phenotype and also demonstrating that GPC and GPD had different extracellular domains.

The concomitant absence of GPC and GPD from the red cell membranes of PL and KW was extremely unlikely to be a coincidence and so the red cells of other individuals with the Gerbich-negative phenotype were examined with remarkable results (15,16). BRIC 4 and BRIC 10 were tested for their ability to agglutinate eleven additional Gerbich-negative red cell samples, eight of phenotype Ge type (Ge:-2,-3; phenotypically the same as PL and KW) and three of the Yus type (Ge:-2,3; see previous section for discussion of the serological definition of these types). All 11 were agglutinated by the monoclonal antibodies. However, whereas BRIC 10

FIGURE 16-1 Structure of Glycophorins C and D and the Location of Common Gerbich System Antigens

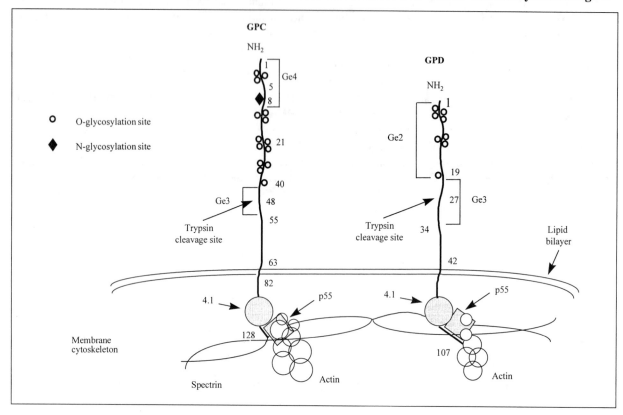

agglutinated normal cells directly it agglutinated these Gerbich-negative cells only in the indirect antiglobulin test. None of the 11 samples was of the Leach phenotype. When membranes from the red cells of Ge:-2,-3 and Ge:-2,3 cells were examined by SDS-PAGE both were found to lack GPC and GPD but both contained different novel proteins (Mr 30,500-34,500 and 32,500-36,500 respectively) of Mr intermediate between that of GPC and GPD. BRIC 4 and BRIC 10 reacted with the novel proteins present in both phenotypes demonstrating that both contained epitopes common to GPC (15,16).

The relationship between GPC and GPD was further clarified when it was shown that GPC and GPD have common sequences in their cytoplasmic domains (20,24). Rabbit antisera raised against purified GPC were absorbed with intact red cells to produce a reagent specific for the cytoplasmic/transmembrane domain of GPC. When this reagent was used for immune precipitation experiments with periodate/tritiated sodium borohydride labeled red cell "ghosts" from normal cells both GPC and GPD were precipitated. Similar experiments established that the cytoplasmic domains of the novel proteins found in Ge:-2,-3 and Ge:-2,3 cells were like those of GPC and GPD in normal red cells. Some human anti-Ge sera (anti-Ge3, see below) immunoblotted GPC and GPD in normal red cells demonstrating that part of

the extracellular domains of GPC and GPD had common sequences (20,24). In summary, these immunochemical studies indicated that GPC and GPD have similar cytoplasmic domains and that parts of their extracellular domains are also similar.

As discussed above it was known from protein sequencing studies that GPC has a single N-glycan at Asn8 (136). Treatment of intact normal red cells with preparations containing endo F and peptidyl N-glycanase reduced the Mr of GPC by 3,500 whereas the Mr of GPD was unchanged. Treatment with endo-beta galactosidase had no effect on either molecule indicating that the N-glycan on GPC lacks poly-N-acetyl lactosaminyl repeating units (41,138). The novel proteins found in red cell membranes from individuals of the Ge:-2,-3 or Ge:-2,3 phenotypes have broader bands on SDS-PAGE than GPC and GPD suggesting heterogeneity in carbohydrate content. When red cells from individuals with these phenotypes were treated with endo-beta galactosidase the novel proteins gave sharper bands when immunoblotted with BRIC 10. When these cells were treated with endo F preparations a new band of lower Mr was observed in both Ge:-2,-3 cells (Mr 24,500 -27,000) and Ge:-2,3 cells (Mr 26,000-27,000(20)). These results show that unlike normal GPC the novel proteins in these Gerbich-negative cells have one or more N-glycans with poly-N-acetyl lactosaminyl units.

The relationship between GPC and GPD and the structure of the abnormal proteins found in Ge:-2,-3 and Ge:-2,3 cells was further elucidated by analysis at the DNA level. Southern blot analysis of the *GYPC* gene in DNA from individuals with Ge:-2,-3 and Ge:-2,3 red cells led to the conclusion that the novel proteins found in these cells result from different internal deletions in the *GYPC* gene (89,21). Since these cells also lack GPD it must be concluded that GPD is a product of the *GYPC* gene since it would be difficult to explain the absence of GPD from these Ge-negative cells if it were the product of a separate gene. Inspection of the RNA sequence around the initiator codon for GPC revealed that it does not conform closely with the consensus sequence found in eukaryotic mRNAs and led to the suggestion that the methionine codon downstream of this initiator codon (at amino acid 22) could act as an alternative initiator since it is contained within a sequence that fits the consensus initiator sequence (139,140) better than the sequence around codon 1 (89).This would mean that the protein sequence of GPD would be identical to that of GPC from residue 22 of GPC onwards. Formal proof that this is the mechanism giving rise to GPD was obtained by Le Van Kim et al. (141) who expressed GPC cDNA in COS-7 cells and showed that both GPC and GPD were produced. If a mutation was introduced into codon 1 then GPD alone was expressed. If a mutation was introduced into codon 22 then only GPC was expressed in the transfected cells.

Organization of the *GYPC* Gene in Gerbich-positive and Gerbich-negative Phenotypes

The *GYPC* gene in Ge-positive individuals spans 13.5kb and comprises four exons (30,31 and see figure 16-2). Exons 1 and 2 and most of exon 3 encode the extracellular domain of GPC/D whereas exon 4 encodes the membrane domain and the cytoplasmic domain. Exon 2 and exon 3 have highly homologous DNA sequences and the homology extends to both the 5′ and 3′ flanking intronic sequences. These sequences are likely to have arisen by duplication of an ancestral gene. The homology between exons 2 and 3 and the surrounding sequences provides an explanation for the molecular mechanisms giving rise to the Ge-type (Ge:-2-3,4) and Yus type (Ge:-2,3,4) phenotypes. In the Ge-type exon 3 is deleted and in the Yus type exon 2 is deleted (21,30,31,89). It seems likely that different genetic events involving unequal crossing-over at meiosis occurring between the highly homologous regions 5′ and 3′ to exons 2 and 3 account for the Ge:-2,-3,4 and the Ge:-2,3,4 phenotypes. If the *GYPC* genes on adjacent chromosomes

align during meiosis so that exon 2 and its environs on one chromosome are next to exon 3 and its environs on the other chromosome then several different gene variants are possible (see figure 16-3). In one scenario a crossover occurring 5′ of exon 2 on one chromosome and 5′ of exon 3 on the other would generate one chromosome with a deletion of exon 2 and another with a duplication of exon 2. Similarly a cross-over occurring between regions of homology 3′ would generate one chromosome with a deletion of exon 3 and another with a duplication of exon 3. The deletions of exon 2 and exon 3 explain the Ge:-2,3,4 and Ge:-2,-3,4 phenotypes but if such cross-overs are indeed the genetic mechanisms giving rise to these phenotypes then there should be variant *GYPC* genes with duplicated exon 2 and duplicated exon 3. Duplicated exon 3 was shown to be the mechanism that gives rise to the Ls[a] antigen (30 and see above). Duplicated exon 2 has also been found but in this case without an associated antigen (128,142). The absence of an antigen that marks the duplication of exon 2 is not unexpected since the sequences around the exon junctions would not differ from those found in normal GPC (30).

When the structure of the *GYPC* gene in Leach phenotype donor PL was examined it was shown to have a large deletion encompassing exons 3 and 4 (30,89). Since exon 4 encodes the membrane-spanning domain and this also acts as the membrane insertion signal, any translated products of this gene would not be targeted to the red cell membrane and consequently the membrane would lack GPC and GPD. Subsequent studies demonstrated the same deletion in four other individuals with the Leach phenotype (Cud, MWB, TL, JC) (39,43). Surprisingly, Winardi et al. (39) could isolate a stable mRNA corresponding to the predicted translated product of the partially deleted *GYPC* gene from the reticulocytes of Leach phenotype individuals. They hypothesize that this mRNA arises because the Leach gene rearrangement has "serendipitously juxtaposed a polyadenylation signal close to exon 2 (or the downstream intron) allowing normal mRNA 3′ end processing to occur". These authors suggest that the protein product of this truncated mRNA could either be degraded in the cytoplasm or translocated across the membrane and secreted.

Telen et al. (43) described an individual with the Leach phenotype (LN) whose membrane deficiency of GPC and GPD resulted from a different defect in the *GYPC* gene. Northern blots using mRNA from the donor's lymphocytes revealed a GPC mRNA of normal size. Nucleotide sequencing of this RNA revealed four mutations. Two mutations were silent, the third was a single nucleotide substitution that changed Trp44 to Leu and the fourth a single nucleotide deletion in codon 45 that altered the reading frame and caused a premature stop signal at codon 56. The resultant protein would lack

FIGURE 16-2 Structure of *GYPC* and the Synthesis of GPC and GPD by the Use of Different Initiator Codons

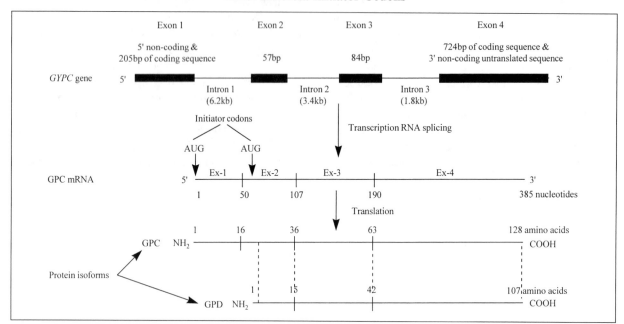

a transmembrane domain and would probably be secreted or degraded in the cytoplasm. Pinder et al. (143) immunoblotted LN membranes with a monoclonal antibody to the C terminus of GPC/D and demonstrated the presence of a component of Mr 12,000 that was not found in the membranes of Leach phenotype donor PL. This remarkable finding suggested that reinitiation of translation has occurred on the LN GPC/D mRNA after chain termination at the stop codon (codon 45). Pinder et al. (143) remark that, to their knowledge, this phenomenon has not been described before in eukaryotes and point out that inspection of the mRNA sequence shows the presence of two possible initiation codons downstream of the stop codon and a third initiation codon that

FIGURE 16-3 *GYPC* Variants Resulting from Unequal Cross-over Events at Meiosis (reference 30)

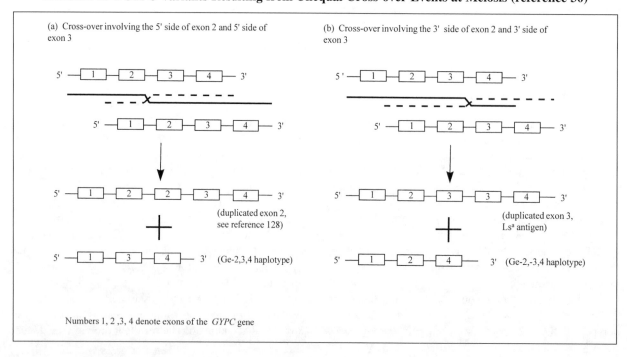

overlaps the stop codon.

Molecular Bases of Gerbich Blood Group Antigens

Reid et al. (20) found in immunoblotting experiments that 16 of 19 anti-Ge sera were specific for an antigen found on GPD while 3 reacted with an epitope common to GPC and GPD. Similar data were reported by Dahr et al. (24). Since antibodies specific for GPD failed to react with either Ge:-2,-3 or Ge:-2,3 type cells they have the specificity anti-Ge2. Antibodies reactive with both GPC and GPD reacted with Ge:-2,3 cells but not Ge:-2,-3 cells and are therefore anti-Ge3. Murine monoclonal antibodies BRIC 10 and BRIC 4 were specific for epitopes on GPC and the novel proteins found in Ge:-2,3 and Ge:-2,-3 cells but did not react with GPD (15). A human antibody present in the serum of a donor with the Leach phenotype that behaved like the murine monoclonal antibodies BRIC 10 and BRIC4 was subsequently reported by McShane and Chung (36) and denoted anti-Ge4. Rodent monoclonal anti-Ge3 has also been described (93, 95).

Inspection of the structure of GPC, GPD and the novel proteins found in Ge:-2,3 and Ge:-2,-3 cells provides an explanation for the different patterns of reactivity found with human and monoclonal antibodies (see figure 16-1). Anti-Ge4 must recognize an antigen found on a sequence of GPC not present in GPD and the antigen is therefore likely to be located in the N terminal region of GPC. Anti-Ge2 is specific for GPD and must therefore recognize a region of GPD not found in GPC. Since GPD is derived from the *GYPC* gene and has an identical sequence to residues 22-128 of GPC, the only point of difference is at the extreme N terminus of the protein where there is a free amino group. Thus the Ge2 antigen is likely to be defined by the extreme N-terminal region of GPD. The location of Ge2 to this region is consistent with the failure of anti-Ge2 to react with the novel protein in Ge:-2,3 cells. The *GYPC* gene of individuals with Ge:-2,3 cells has a deletion of exon 2 (see previous section) and the N terminus of GPD is encoded by exon 2 in persons with normal cells. Anti-Ge3 recognizes an antigen common to GPC and GPD that is absent from Ge:-2,-3 cells but not Ge:-2,3 cells. Since the *GYPC* gene of individuals with Ge:-2,-3 cells lacks exon 3 but the gene of persons with Ge:-2,3 cells does not, it can be inferred that anti-Ge3 recognizes an antigen that is defined by the protein sequence encoded by exon 3 (see figure 16-1).

Ge2 ,Ge3 and Ge4 are sialidase-sensitive (24,36,93) and so the antigens are not defined by protein sequence alone but by a structure that depends on a conformation resulting from carbohydrate:protein interaction in a manner analogous to MN antigens (see Chapter 15). Ge3 is trypsin sensitive, a property that locates it to the region of GPC around residue 48, the trypsin cleavage site. Dahr et al. (24) consider that the antigen requires an O-glycan on Ser42. Daniels et al. (52) found that 2 of 10 anti-Ge2 failed to agglutinate red cells treated with acetic anhydride a procedure that acetylates free amino groups. These results suggest that anti-Ge2 are a heterogeneous group and that a minority require the free amino group on residue Met1 for reactivity.

The structures of Ge2, Ge3 and Ge4 have not yet been defined in more detail. More information could probably be obtained by in vitro expression of artificial mutants in which individual amino acids are changed and changes in antigen expression examined. There is always a problem with in vitro expression of highly glycosylated proteins because the glycosylation pattern of the expressed proteins may not be identical to that of the native proteins. However, provided a eukaryotic expression system is used and appropriate controls included useful information should be obtained.

The molecular basis of several low frequency antigens in the Gerbich system have been elucidated and each has yielded interesting information from the biochemical point of view. The antigens fall into three categories: antigen common to GPC and GPD (Ls[a]), antigens unique to GPC (Wb and Dh[a]) and antigen unique to GPD (An[a]).

The Ls[a] antigen is of interest because it marks red cells from individuals who have a *GYPC* gene containing a duplicated exon 3. The occurrence of such a gene would be predicted if the Ge-type and Yus-type of Gerbich-negative phenotypes arose because of crossover between misaligned genes at meiosis (see previous section and figure 16-3). Macdonald et al. (47) examined the membranes of Ls(a+) red cells by SDS-PAGE and noted after staining the gel with the PAS stain that in addition to GPC and GPD there were two bands with Mr 5500 greater than normal GPC and normal GPD respectively. The band of greater Mr than GPC was an abnormal GPC molecule because it reacted with monoclonal anti-GPC and the other abnormal band was related to GPD because it reacted with anti-Ge2. These workers further observed that these abnormal bands reacted more strongly with anti-Ge3 than normal GPC and GPD when the antibody was used for immunoblotting experiments. When the *GYPC* gene from Ls(a+) individuals was examined it was found that exon 3 was duplicated (30,48). This explained why the abnormal GPC and GPD were larger than normal and why anti-Ge3 bound to the abnormal molecules with greater intensity. Inspection of the predicted amino acid sequence of the abnormal GPC and GPD molecules revealed that duplication of exon 3 would create a novel amino acid sequence encoded by the junction of the two exons and that the Ls[a] antigen was likely to result from this novel sequence (30). Direct evidence that this is indeed the case was obtained by Reid et al. (48) who showed that a synthetic peptide corresponding to the amino acid sequence predicted at the exon 3:exon 3 junction, inhibited anti-Ls[a]. Unlike Ge2, 3 and 4, Ls[a] is not sialidase sensitive and since the antibody is inhibited by a synthetic peptide the antigen appears to be defined by protein sequence alone (but see discussion of Dh[a] below).

When Wb+ red cell membranes were examined by SDS-PAGE a reduced level of GPC staining was observed together with a novel component of Mr 3000 less than GPC (41,42). The abnormal component reacted with monoclonal antibodies to GPC but unlike normal GPC it lacked an N-glycan since treatment of Wb+ red cells with endo F preparations did not reduce the Mr of the abnormal band. Reid et al. (41) noticed that the reduction in Mr of normal GPC after endo F treatment was greater than 3000 and speculated that the abnormal protein resulted from a mutation that resulted in the loss of the N-glycan and simultaneously created an additional O-glycosylation site. Subsequent studies identified a point mutation A to G that changes Asn8 to Ser (39,43) and thereby destroys the N-glycosylation site found on normal GPC and replaces it with a serine that could form an additional O-glycan site. The Wb antigen is sialidase sensitive.

The Dh[a] antigen was shown to be located on GPC by immunoblotting with human anti-Dh[a] (54). The antigen does not appear to require the presence of the N-glycan on Asn8 since endo F treatment does not affect it (54). Nucleotide sequencing of cDNA derived from two Dh(a+) individuals identified a single nucleotide change (C40 to T) in exon 1 that changes Leu14 to Phe (55). Somewhat surprisingly (Dh[a] is sialidase sensitive), it has been reported that a synthetic peptide corresponding to residues 8-21 of GPC (with Phe at residue 14) inhibits anti-Dh[a] (144). Inspection of the sequence of GPC in this region reveals two potential sites for O-glycosyslation (Thr10 and Ser15). It is possible that the presence of Phe14 prevents glycosylation of Ser15 and/or that the synthetic peptide can take up a conformation in solution that is the same as that induced by sialylation of the native protein. An analogous situation occurs in the MN system where Lisowska et al. (145) have shown that certain monoclonal antibodies of specificity anti-M+M[g] recognize a critical peptide motif (Met8/Val6) that is present in M, N and M[g] structures but only exposed in M and M[g]. The fact that Wb and Dh[a] are found on GPC but not GPD is entirely to be expected given their dependence on Ser8 and Phe14 respectively since, as discussed above, the N terminal residue of GPD corresponds to Met22 of GPC.

Immunoblotting with human anti-An[a] showed that the An[a] antigen is located on GPD but not on GPC (52). In this respect An[a] is like Ge2 (see above) and the same reasoning would lead one to suppose that the An[a] antigen is located at the extreme N-terminus of GPD. Sequence analysis of cDNA from two An(a+) individuals revealed a single nucleotide substitution (G67 to T) that would correspond to a change of a single amino acid Ala2 to Ser on GPD. Since GPD is derived from the same gene as GPC, the same amino acid sequence change is present in GPC but in this case it corresponds to Ala23 to Ser. Why then if the same amino acid change is present in GPC and GPD is the antigen only expressed on GPD? One obvious possibility is that the free amino group of Met1 in GPD (Met 22 in GPC does not have a free amino group) is required for An[a] activity. However, two anti-An[a] sera reacted normally with acetic anhydride-treated An(a+) red cells, a procedure that acetylates free amino groups and destroys the epitope recognized by monoclonal antibody BRIC 10 (52). The change Ala2 to Ser creates an additional O-glycosylation site but there is no evidence regarding whether or not it is utilized in either GPC or GPD. The An[a] antigen is sialidase-sensitive and such additional sialylation might be relevant to the antigenic structure. Notwithstanding these considerations it is clear that conformation of the GPD protein at its N-terminus must be completely different from the corresponding region of GPC and this conformational difference defines the antigen An[a].

Tissue Distribution of GPC/GPD and Regulation of the *GYPC* Gene

Even before it was appreciated that the Gerbich antigens are on GPC/GPD Sieff et al. (146) used a monoclonal antibody (GERO) that was known to give weaker reactions with Ge-negative cells to show that the epitope recognized by this antibody was expressed on erythroid precursors at an earlier stage than GPA. It was subsequently shown that GERO recognizes a similar sialic acid-dependent epitope at the N-terminus of GPC to that recognized by BRIC 10 (described above), as well as several other monoclonal antibodies (MR4-130, APO 2 and 7G11) (96,147). Another monoclonal anti-GPC (APO 3) that recognized a sialic acid-independent epitope mapped to the region involving Glu17 or Asp19 (96,147), was found to react with mature BFU-e prompting the suggestion that the degree of sialylation of GPC changes as erythroid cells mature (148).

GYPC mRNA is expressed in human erythroblasts, erythroid cell lines (K562, HEL, KU812) and fetal liver (17). Its presence in fetal liver may reflect expression in hematopoietic progenitor cells because immunocytochemical staining of fetal liver with BRIC 10 revealed reactivity in hematopoietic progenitor cells in first and second trimester but no reactivity with non-hematopoietic cells (149). However, the *GYPC* gene is expressed in several non-hematopoietic tissues including kidney (19), thymus, stomach, breast and adult liver (150). Sequencing of cDNAs indicated that the primary structure of GPC in erythroid and non-erythroid cells is the same (151) but the sialic acid-independent antibody APO 3 reacted with a much wider variety of cells and tissues than the sialic acid-dependent antibody MR4-130 prompting the suggestion that the GPC/D protein in different tissues is differently sialylated. BRIC 10 that also recognizes a sialic acid-dependent epitope was reported to stain brain cerebellum, ileum, blood vessels and kidney (medulla and cortex) but not tongue, stomach, pancreas or adult liver (149). It is well established that the same protein may be differently glycosylated in different tissues (152) and so failure to demonstrate tissue reactivity with a glycosylation-dependent antibody cannot be regarded as proof that any particular glycoprotein is not expressed. One way of overcoming the potential problem of tissue variations in glycosylation of a given protein is to use an antibody specific for the cytoplasmic domain. When a monoclonal antibody (BGRL 100) raised to a synthetic peptide corresponding to the C-terminal 15 amino acids of GPC/D was used in immunocytochemical studies, staining was observed in kidney glomeruli, brain cerebellum and brain stem and hepatic sinusoids as well as hematopoietic progenitor cells in fetal liver (153).

Although the *GYPC* gene is expressed in a wide variety of tissues it appears that the level of transcription is greater in cells of erythroid origin. Higher levels of GPC mRNA were found in erythroid cell lines (K562, HEL, KU812) than lymphoid (Jurkat), myeloid (U937) or megakaryocytic (MEG01) (150) lines. Furthermore, GPC mRNA was initiated at a different CAP site in erythroid cells than in non-erythroid cells (150). A search for motifs that bind transcription factors at the 5′ end of the *GYPC* gene revealed three GATA-1 binding sites and a binding site for a novel erythroid/megakaryocyte regulatory protein NF-E6 in a region comprising 200 nucleotides (see figure 16-4) (154). GATA-1 is a transcription factor essential for erythroid development (155, see also Chapters 5 and 14). Inspection of figure 16-4 suggests that the GATA-1 binding site immediately 5′ to the erythoid CAP site may be critical for the enhanced expression of GPC in erythroid cells. Colin and Le Van Kim (156) quote unpublished observations to the effect that this GATA-1 site is indeed necessary and that the NF-E6 site is also required for accurate transcriptional activity of the GYPC promoter in erythroid cells.

Function of GPC/GPD

Red cells require substantial strength and stability to withstand the shearing forces imposed on them during their 120 day circulation in the body. In addition, they have to be flexible and deformable in order to pass through narrow capillaries. These properties are largely the result of a network of structural proteins located beneath the membrane and known as the red cell skeleton. The skeleton is anchored to the membrane through at least two sets of protein:protein interactions. One set of interactions involves a proportion of band 3 molecules linked to spectrin through ankyrin and protein 4.2 (see Chapter 4 and figure 4-1 in that Chapter) and the other involves GPC/D linked to protein 4.1 and p55.

The first evidence indicating association of GPC/GPD with the red cell skeleton via protein 4.1 was

FIGURE 16-4 Binding Sites for Transcription Factors in the *GYPC* Gene Promoter (reference 156)

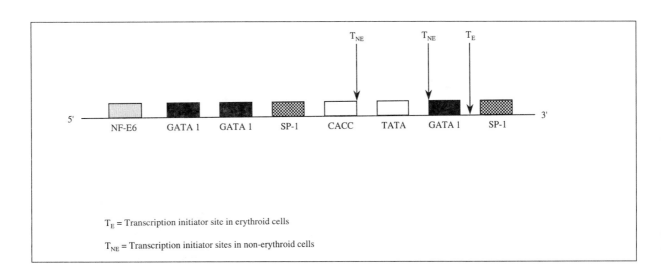

T_E = Transcription initiator site in erythroid cells

T_{NE} = Transcription initiator sites in non-erythroid cells

reported by Mueller and Morrison (75) who showed that GPC (that they termed PAS 2′) was present in the pellet that remains after extraction of normal red cell membranes with Triton X-100. This pellet contains all the structural proteins that comprise the red cell skeleton. When a similar extraction was carried out on red cell membranes from an individual with elliptocytosis who had a complete absence of protein 4.1, they observed that GPC was no longer found in the Triton insoluble pellet. Mueller and Morrison (75,133) concluded that GPC in the red cell membrane was likely to be connected to protein 4.1 in the skeleton and suggested the name glyco-connectin for GPC. In retrospect, it is a great pity that this name was not taken up and used by other workers in the field because it could have prevented a lot of the confusion that has resulted from using the name glycophorin for two sets of completely unrelated proteins. Unfortunately it took a long time (more than 15 years!) for these observations to be accepted by the established workers in the red cell skeleton field and by that time the name GPC was in common use.

As discussed above, individuals with the Leach phenotype have a total deficiency of GPC and GPD. A proportion of the red cells in the peripheral blood of these individuals are elliptocytic supporting the proposition that GPC/GPD is involved in the maintenance of cell shape in normal red cells (14,71). Studies of the deformability of Leach phenotype red cells in the ektacytometer have shown that the membranes of these cells are, on average, 40% less deformable than normal cells and are substantially more susceptible to fragmentation by shear stress (23). Red cells with the Ge-type or Yus-type Ge-negative phenotypes do not show abnormalities in the ektacytometer suggesting that the abnormal GPC molecules found in these cells are able to carry out the same function as GPC and GPD in normal cells (157). Beattie and Sigmund (102) described a patient with anemia and elliptocytosis who was receiving gold therapy for rheumatoid arthritis and had produced an anti-Ge4-like antibody. Subsequent studies showed that the red cells of this patient were markedly deficient in GPC although the level of GPD appeared normal (37). Two years after presentation, the patient's red cells were no longer elliptocytic, had a normal content of GPC as judged by agglutination tests with monoclonal anti-GPC and the patient was no longer anemic. These authors suggest that the transient loss of GPC was directly related to the occurrence of elliptocytes in the peripheral blood and if this is so then this case provides further evidence of a direct relationship between GPC and the maintenance of red cell shape.

Red cells that are deficient in protein 4.1 have a marked reduction (60-70%) in the amount of GPC/GPD in their membrane (158) and a careful analysis of the level of protein 4.1 in red cells of the Leach phenotype revealed that they have a 10-20% deficiency (76). Furthermore, protein 4.1 is much more easily extracted from the membranes of red cells with the Leach phenotype than from normal membranes. When Leach phenotype membranes (PL) were extracted at low ionic strength, approximately 70% of the 4.1 was extracted compared with 25% from normal membranes (143). All these results provide indirect evidence for an interaction involving the cytoplasmic domain of GPC/GPD and protein 4.1 that is necessary to maintain the normal shape, flexibility and deformability of the red cell. In 1993, evidence emerged that suggested that an additional protein might be involved in the interaction between GPC/GPD and protein 4.1. Alloisio et al. (76) showed that the membranes of individuals with hereditary elliptocytosis as a result of absence of 4.1 and Leach phenotype membranes lacked a protein denoted p55 and suggested that it was involved in the GPC/D:4.1 interaction. Independently, Pinder et al. (143) came to the conclusion that GPC/D contains two types of binding site for 4.1 because of differences observed between the extractability of 4.1 from the red cell membranes of two individuals with the Leach phenotype (PL, LN). As discussed above, the molecular mechanism giving rise to GPC/D deficiency in donor LN is different from that in other individuals with the Leach phenotype (43). Pinder et al. (143) noticed that whereas 70% of the 4.1 in PL membranes was extracted at low ionic strength only 50% was extracted from LN membranes. When membranes from LN were subjected to immunoblotting with a monoclonal antibody to the carboxy terminus of GPC/D, a component of Mr 12,000 was observed. These authors proposed that the component of Mr 12,000 corresponded to a membrane bound C-terminal fragment of GPC/D present in LN membranes and that the reduced extractability of 4.1 in these cells compared with those of PL was due to a proportion of 4.1 binding to this fragment. These experiments raise two major questions, first, how is the Mr 12,000 component bound to the membranes of LN cells and second, what is the molecular mechanism that allows the C terminal fragment of GPC/D to be expressed in LN cells? Given the findings of Alloisio et al. (76), the answer to the first question seemed likely to be p55. In order to answer the second question Pinder et al. (143) proposed that reinitiation of translation occurs after the stop codon (codon 45) in GPC mRNA of LN so that a C terminal peptide is generated (see section on molecular bases of Ge-negative phenotypes above for further discussion).

Subsequent studies showed that p55 can bind to 4.1 and to GPC/D with high affinity (79,80). Localization of the binding sites for protein 4.1 and p55 on GPC/D have shown that protein 4.1 binds to a region of GPC/D close to the bilayer (the interaction is inhibited by a synthetic peptide corresponding to residues 82-98 of GPC, 61-77 of GPD) while p55 binds to the extreme C-terminal region of GPC (residues 112-128) and GPD (residues 91-107) (77-80). The mild elliptocytosis found in cells of the Leach phenotype has been attributed to the small reduction (10-20%) in 4.1 found in these cells rather than to the absence of GPC/D. Addition of purified protein 4.1 or the isolated spectrin-actin binding domain of 4.1 restores the mechanical stability of Leach phenotype red cells (159).

The functional roles of the extracellular domains of GPC and GPD are poorly understood. GPC and GPD together comprise approximately 200,000 molecules in a normal red cell (95). This compares with about 250,000 molecules of GPB and 1,000,000 molecules of GPA (see Chapter 15). Sialic acid-rich glycoproteins are found at the surface of most circulating cells where they are thought to provide a barrier to microorganisms (160). As far as red cells are concerned the most serious microbial agent is the malarial parasite *Plasmodium falciparum* and so in vitro experiments have been carried out to assess the possible role of GPC/D as receptors for this parasite. Different strains of *P. falciparum* show reduced ability to invade red cells of Leach phenotype (161,162). It is not clear whether this reduction is related to the reduced content of protein 4.1 or the absence of GPC/D. Protein 4.1-deficient red cells that have a reduction of GPC/D content are also refractory to invasion by *P. falciparum* (and *P. knowlesi*, 163). GPC and GPD are certainly not essential for the viability of red cells as evidenced by the absence of disease associated with the Leach phenotype.

References

1. Rosenfield RE, Haber GV, Kissmeyer Nielsen F, et al. Br J Haematol 1960;6:344
2. Cleghorn TE. MD Thesis, Univ Sheffield, 1961
3. Barnes R, Lewis TLT. Lancet 1961;2:1285
4. Booth PB, McLoughlin K. Vox Sang 1972;22:73
5. Booth PB, Albrey JA, Whittaker J, et al. Nature 1970;228:462
6. Simmons RT, Booth PB. Commwlth Serum Labs, papers 546 to 549. Parkville, Austral:Commwlth Serum Labs, 1971
7. Booth PB, Wark L, McLoughlin K, et al. Hum Biol Oceania 1972;1:215
8. Booth PB, Hornabrook RW, Malcolm LA, et al. Hum Biol Oceania 1972;1:259
9. Booth PB, Hornabrook RW, MacGregor A, et al. Hum Biol Oceania 1972;1:267
10. Booth PB, Hornabrook RW. Hum Biol Oceania 1973;2:72
11. Lewis M, Anstee DJ, Bird GWG, et al. Vox Sang 1990;58:152
12. Lewis M, Anstee DJ, Bird GWG, et al. Vox Sang 1991;61:158
13. Daniels GL, Anstee DJ, Cartron J-P, et al. Vox Sang 1995;69:265
14. Anstee DJ, Parsons SF, Ridgwell K, et al. Biochem J 1984;218:615
15. Anstee DJ, Ridgwell K, Tanner MJA, et al. Biochem J 1984;221:97
16. Dahr W, Moulds J, Baumeister G, et al. Biol Chem Hoppe Seyler 1985;366:201
17. Colin Y, Rahuel C, London J, et al. J Biol Chem 1986;261:299
18. Mattei MG, Colin Y, Le Van Kim C, et al. Hum Genet 1986;74:420
19. High S, Tanner MJA. Biochem J 1987;243:277
20. Reid ME, Anstee DJ, Tanner MJA, et al. Biochem J 1987;244:123
21. Le Van Kim C, Colin Y, Blanchard D, et al. Eur J Biochem 1987;165:571
22. Sondag D, Alloisio N, Blanchard D, et al. Br J Haematol 1987;65:43
23. Reid ME, Chasis J, Mohandas N. Blood 1987;69:1068
24. Dahr W, Kiedrowski D, Blanchard D, et al. Biol Chem Hoppe Seyler 1987;368:1375
25. Blanchard D, Dahr W, Beyreuther J, et al. J Biol Chem 1987;262:5808
26. Dahr W. In: Recent Advances in Blood Group Biochemistry. Arlington, VA:Am Assoc Blood Banks, 1986:23
27. Furthmayr H. Nature 1978;271:519
28. Furthmayr H. J Supramol Struct 1978;9:79
29. Cartron J-P, London J. In: Protein Blood Group Antigens of the Human Red Cell. Baltimore:Johns Hopkins Univ Press, 1992:101
30. High S, Tanner MJA, Macdonald EB, et al. Biochem J 1989;262:47
31. Colin Y, Le Van Kim C, Tsapis A, et al. J Biol Chem 1989;264:3773
32. Chang S, Reid ME, Conboy J. Blood 1991;77:644
33. Daniels GL, Johnson P, Levene C. (abstract). Vox Sang 1994;67 (Suppl 2):53
34. Serjeantson SW, White BS, Bhatia K, et al. Immunol Cell Biol 1994;72:23
35. Daniels GL, Banting G, Goodfellow P. J Immunogenet 1983;10:103
36. McShane K, Chung A. Vox Sang 1989;57:205
37. Daniels GL, Reid ME, Anstee DJ, et al. Br J Haematol 1988;70:477
38. Telen MJ, Le Van Kim C, Chung A, et al. Blood 1991;78:1603
39. Winardi R, Reid ME, Conboy J, et al. Blood 1993;81:2799
40. Simmons RT, Albrey JA. Med J Austral 1963;1:8
41. Reid ME, Shaw M-A, Rowe G, et al. Biochem J 1985;232:289
42. Macdonald EB, Gerns LM. Vox Sang 1986;50:112
43. Telen MJ, Le Van Kim C, Guizzo ML, et al. Am J Hematol 1991;37:51
44. Cleghorn TE. Unpublished observations 1962-1967 cited in Race RR, Sanger R. Blood Groups in Man, 6th Ed. Oxford:Blackwell, 1975
45. Race RR, Sanger R. Blood Groups in Man, 6th Ed. Oxford:Blackwell, 1975
46. Cleghorn TE, Contreras M, Bull W. (abstract). Book of Abstracts, 14th Cong ISBT, 1975:47
47. Macdonald EB, Condon J, Ford D, et al. Vox Sang 1990;58:300
48. Reid ME, Mawby W, King M-J, et al. Transfusion 1994;34:966
49. Kornstad L. Immunol Comm 1981;10:199
50. Green CA, Sistonen P, Kornstad L, et al. Unpublished observations 1989 cited in Daniels G. Human Blood Groups. Oxford:Blackwell, 1995
51. Furuhjelm U, Nevanlinna HR, Gavin J, et al. Med Genet

1972;9:385

52. Daniels G, King M-J, Avent ND, et al. Blood 1993;10:3198
53. Jørgensen J, Drachmann O, Gavin J. Hum Hered 1982;32:73
54. Spring FA. Vox Sang 1991;61:65
55. King MJ, Avent MD, Mallinson G, et al. Vox Sang 1992;63:56
56. Issitt PD. Transfusion 1994;34:462
57. Okubo Y, Yamaguchi H, Seno T, et al. Transfusion 1984;24:274
58. McLoughlin K, Rogers J. Vox Sang 1970;19:94
59. Hindmarsh C, Jennings ER, Tippett P, et al. Unpublished observations 1962 cited in Race RR, Sanger R. Blood Groups in Man, 6th Ed. Oxford:Blackwell, 1975
60. Muller A, André-Liardet J, Garretta M, et al. Rev Fr Transf 1973;16:251
61. Nunn HD, Giles CM, Seidl S. Vox Sang 1967;13:23
62. Fermepin GH, Perez-Prado A, de Pippig TF, et al. Vox Sang 1968;14:228
63. Peddle LJ, Josephson JE, Lawton A. Vox Sang 1970;18:547
64. Reid M, Rector D, Danneskiold T. Immunohematology 1984;1:7
65. Sacks DA, Johnson CS, Platt LD. Am J Perinatol 1985;2:208
66. Pinder L, Coleman R, Woodfield DG. Vox Sang 1992;63:74
67. Reid ME, Sullivan C, Taylor M, et al. Am J Hum Genet 1987;41:1117
68. Reid ME, Poole J, Liew YW, et al. Immunohematology 1992;8:29
69. Chandanyingyong D, Pejrachandra S, Metaseta P, et al. SE Asia J Trop Med Pub Health 1979;10:209
70. Moulds M, Dahr W, Kiedrowski S, et al. (abstract). Transfusion 1987;27:533
71. Daniels GL, Shaw M-A, Judson PA, et al. Vox Sang 1986;50:117
72. Reid ME, Martynewycz MA, Wolford FE, et al. Transfusion 1987;27:213
73. Rountree J, Chen J, Moulds MK, et al. (abstract). Transfusion 1989;29 (Suppl 7S):15S
74. Owens JW, Mueller TJ, Morrison M. Arch Biochem Biophys 1980;204:207
75. Mueller TJ, Morrison M. In: Erythrocyte Membranes. 2. Recent Clinical and Experimental Advances. New York:Liss, 1981:95
76. Alloisio N, Venezia ND, Rana A, et al. Blood 1993;82:1323
77. Hemming NJ, Anstee DJ, Mawby WJ, et al. Biochem J 1994;299:191
78. Marfatia SM, Lue RA, Branton D, et al. J Biol Chem 1994;269:8631
79. Marfatia SM, Lue RA, Branton D, et al. J Biol Chem 1995;270:715
80. Hemming NJ, Anstee DJ, Staricoff MA, et al. J Biol Chem 1995;270:5360
81. Telen MJ. Personal communication 1995
82. Daniels GL. (abstract). Transfusion 1982;22:405
83. Pearson HA, Richards VL, Wylie BR, et al. Transfusion 1991;31:257
84. Tilley CA, Crookston MC, Haddad SA, et al. Transfusion 1977;17:169
85. Vengelen-Tyler V, Morel PA. Transfusion 1983;23:114
86. DiNapoli J, Gingras A, Diggs E, et al. (abstract). Transfusion 1986;26:545
87. Nance SJ, Arndt P, Garratty G. Transfusion 1987;27:449
88. Mochizuki T, Tauxe WN, Ramsey G. J Nucl Med 1990;31:2042
89. Tanner MJA, High S, Martin PG, et al. Biochem J 1988;250:407

90. Cartron J-P, Le Van Kim C, Colin Y. Semin Hematol 1993;30:152
91. Daniels G. Immunohematology 1992;8:53
92. Daniels G. Human Blood Groups. Oxford:Blackwell, 1995
93. Loirat MJ, Gourbil A, Frioux Y, et al. Vox Sang 1992;62:45
94. Loirat MJ, Dahr W, Muller JY, et al. Transf Med 1994;4:157
95. Smythe J, Gardner B, Anstee DJ. Blood 1994;83:1668
96. Dahr W, Blanchard D, Kiedrowski S, et al. Biol Chem Hoppe Seyler 1989;370:849
97. Reynolds MV, Vengelen-Tyler V, Morel PA. Vox Sang 1981;41:61
98. Göttsche B, Salama A, Mueller-Eckhardt C. Vox Sang 1990;58:211
99. Shulman IA, Vengelen-Tyler V, Thompson JC, et al. Vox Sang 1990;59:232
100. Poole J, Reid ME, Banks J, et al. Vox Sang 1990;58:287
101. Reid ME, Vengelen-Tyler V, Shulman I, et al. Br J Haematol 1988;69:61
102. Beattie KM, Sigmund KE. Transfusion 1987;27:54
103. Anderson SE, McKenzie JL, McLouglin K, et al. Pathology 1986;18:407
104. Telen MJ, Scearce RM, Haynes BF. Vox Sang 1987;52:236
105. Loirat MJ, Blanchard D. (abstract). Rev Paulista Med 1992;110:IH-07
106. Issitt PD. Transf Med Rev 1993;7:139
107. Redman CM, Avellino G, Pfeffer SR, et al. J Biol Chem 1987;261:9521
108. Lee S, Zambas ED, Marsh WL, et al. Proc Nat Acad Sci USA 1991;88:6353
109. Gorman M, Woody B. Immunohematology 1989;5:55
110. Macgregor A, Booth PB. Vox Sang 1973;25:474
111. Issitt PD, Gutgsell N, Bonds SB, et al. (abstract). Transfusion 1988;28 (Suppl 6S):20S
112. Bloomfield L, Rowe GP, Green C. Hum Hered 1986;36:352
113. Ikemoto S, Nakajima H, Furuhata T. Proc Jpn Acad 1964;30:432
114. Nakajima H, Ikemoto S, Tokunaga E, et al. Proc Jpn Acad 1965;41:86
115. Ørjasaeter H, Kornstad L, Larsen AMH. Vox Sang 1966;11:726
116. Cleghorn TE, Dunsford I. Unpublished observations 1963 cited in Race RR, Sanger R. Blood Groups in Man, 6th Ed. Oxford:Blackwell, 1975
117. Clark AL, Dorman SA. Transfusion 1986;26:368
118. Sistonen P. (abstract). Book of Abstracts, 19th Cong ISBT, 1986:652
119. Green C, Tippett P. Unpublished observations 1980 cited by Jørgensen J, Drachman O, Gavin J, et al. Hum Hered 1982;32:73
120. Spring F, Poole J, Liew YW, et al. (abstract). Transf Med 1990;1 (Suppl 1):66
121. Hindmarsh C, Jennings ER, Tippett P, et al. (abstract). Prog 15th Ann Mtg Am Assoc Blood Banks 1962
122. Brocteur J. Unpublished observations 1973 cited in Race RR, Sanger R. Blood Groups in Man, 6th Ed. Oxford:Blackwell, 1975:412
123. Colpitts P, Cornwall S, Moore BPL. Unpublished observations 1974 cited in Race RR, Sanger R. Blood Groups in Man, 6th Ed. Oxford:Blackwell, 1975:412
124. Zelinski T, Kaita H, Lewis M, et al. Vox Sang 1991;61:62
125. Moores P, de Beer R, Marais I, et al. Hum Hered 1990;40:242
126. Issitt PD, Combs M, Carawan H, et al. (abstract). Transfusion 1994;34 (Suppl 10S):60S
127. Biro V, Garratty G, Johnson CL, et al. Transfusion 1983;23:65
128. Uchikawa M, Tsuneyama H, Onodera T, et al. Transf Med, in

press 1997

129. Winzler RJ. In: Red Cell Membrane Structure and Function. Philadelphia:Lippincott, 1969:157
130. Marchesi VT, Andrews EP. Science 1971;174:1247
131. Marchesi VT, Tillack TW, Jackson RL, et al. Proc Nat Acad Sci USA 1972;69:1445
132. Laemmli UK. Nature 1970;227:680
133. Mueller TJ, Dow AW, Morrison M. Biochem Biophys Res Comm 1976;72:94
134. Dahr W, Uhlenbruck G, Janssen E, et al. Blut 1976;32:171
135. Anstee DJ, Mawby WJ, Tanner MJA. Biochem J 1979;183:193
136. Dahr W, Beyreuther K, Kordowicz M, et al. Eur J Biochem 1982;125:57
137. Dahr W, Beyreuther K. Biol Chem Hoppe-Seyler 1985;366:1067
138. Tanner MJA, Anstee DJ, Mallinson G, et al. Carbohydrate Res 1988;178:203
139. Kozak M. J Mol Biol 1987;196:947
140. Kozak M. J Cell Biol 1989;108:229
141. Le Van Kim C, Piller V, Cartron J-P, et al. Blood 1996;88:2364
142. Tsuneyama H, Uchikawa M, Suzuki Y, et al. (abstract). Vox Sang 1996;70 (Suppl 2):129
143. Pinder JC, Chung A, Reid M, et al. Blood 1993; 82:3482
144. Storry JR, Reid ME, Mawby WJ. (abstract). Transfusion 1994;43(Suppl 10S):24S
145. Jaskiewicz E, Czerwinski M, Syper D, et al. Blood 1995;84:2340
146. Sieff CA, Greaves MF. In: Red Cell Membrane Glycoconjugates and Related Markers. Paris:Arnette, 1983:243
147. Dahr W, Blanchard D, Kiedrowski S, et al. In: Monoclonal Antibodies Against Human Red Blood Cell and Related Antigens. Paris:Arnette, 1987:289
148. Villeval JL, Le Van Kim C, Bettaieb A, et al. Cancer Res 1989;49:2626
149. Anstee DJ, Holmes CH, Judson PA, et al. In: Protein Blood Group Antigens of the Human Red Cell. Baltimore:Johns Hopkins Univ Press, 1992:170
150. Le Van Kim C, Colin Y, Mitjavila MT, et al. J Biol Chem 1989;264:20407
151. Le Van Kim C, Mitjavila MT, Clerget M, et al. Nucleic Acids Res 1990;18:3076
152. Parekh RB, Tse AGD, Dwek RA, et al. EMBO J 1987;6:1233
153. King MJ, Holmes CH, Mushens RE, et al. Br J Haematol 1995;89:440
154. Colin Y, Joulin V, Le Van Kim C, et al. J Biol Chem 1990;265:16729
155. Orkin SH. Blood 1992;80:575
156. Colin Y, Le Van Kim C. In: Blood Cell Biochemistry. New York:Plenum 1995;6:331
157. Reid ME, Anstee DJ, Jensen RH, et al. Br J Haematol 1987;67:467
158. Alloisio N, Morle L, Bachir D, et al. Biochim Biophys Acta 1985;816:57
159. Discher D, Knowles D, McGee S, et al. (abstract). Blood 1993;82 (Suppl 1):309a
160. Jentoft J. Trends Biochem Sci 1990;15:291
161. Pasvol G, Anstee DJ, Tanner MJA. Lancet 1984;1:907
162. Chishti AH, Palek J, Fisher D, et al. Blood 1996;87:3462
163. Hadley TJ, Erkman Z, Kaufman BM, et al. Am J Trop Med Hyg 1986;35:898

17 | The Diego Blood Group System

In 1955, Layrisse et al. (1) described a case of HDN caused by an antibody to a low incidence antigen. The antibody had a specificity different from any other previously recognized and was called anti-Di^a, existence of the antibody had been noted briefly, one year earlier (2). A large number of population studies (2-28,48) have shown that Di^a is found primarily in persons of Mongolian extraction although, as described in later sections of this chapter, rare exceptions have been seen. In 1967, Thompson et al. (29) reported the first two examples of anti-Di^b, that defines an antigen antithetical to Di^a. Given the rarity of Di^a in other than Mongolian populations, Di^b is, of course, of almost universal occurrence in Whites and Blacks. In 1992, Spring et al. (30) reported that Di^a is carried on protein band 3. Two years later, Bruce et al. (31), in the same research team, described the Di^a/Di^b polymorphism. When protein band 3 expresses Di^a, leucine occupies position 854 on the protein. When protein band 3 expresses Di^b, proline is at position 854. However, as discussed later in this chapter, other mechanisms can also lead to the Di(a+b-) phenotype (198).

In 1953, Holman (32) had described a low incidence antigen that he named Wr^a. Although numerous studies had been performed on Wr(a+) red cells, that are found with an incidence of around 1 in 1000 in Whites and hundreds of examples of anti-Wr^a had been identified (for references see later in this chapter) there was no suspicion that Di^a and Wr^a had anything in common, save being rare in most populations. In 1971, Adams et al. (33) described an antibody to a very common antigen, made by a woman with Wr(a+) red cells. Dosage studies suggested that the antibody maker was genetically *Wr^{a}Wr^a* and the antibody in her serum was tentatively called anti-Wr^b. After many false leads and side trips that appeared to indicate that the so-called Wr^b antigen was part of the MN system (for the full story, see below), Wren and Issitt (34) produced objective serological evidence that Wr^a and Wr^b are antithetical. Since it was already known (for references see below) that *Wr^a* segregates independently of the *MN* locus, it followed that production of Wr^b could not be encoded solely by a gene at the *MN* locus. Following early evidence (35-39) that Wr^b required the presence of at least one other red cell membrane component in addition to glycophorin A, for serological expression, Telen and Chasis (40) showed that the other required component is protein band 3. Bruce et al. (41) then showed that the Wr^a/Wr^b polymorphism represents lysine and glutamic acid, respectively, at position 658 of protein band 3. As discussed below, under certain conditions a portion of glycophorin A, in addition to glutamic acid 658 of band 3, is necessary for Wr^b antigen expression. It is not yet known if glycophorin A is necessary, in addition to lysine 658 of band 3, for Wr^a to be expressed.

Recognition of the facts that protein band 3 carries the polymorphisms that represent Di^a and Di^b, and Wr^a and Wr^b, has led other investigators to look for still other blood group antigens on that protein. Two approaches have been used. One has been to try to show identity of genes encoding low incidence antigens with *AE1*, the gene that encodes production of protein band 3, the anion exchange protein, or AE1 protein. The second approach has been to look for amino acid differences in protein band 3 on low incidence antigen positive and negative red cells. A number of these investigations have already yielded fruit, similar successes can be expected in the future. As described in more detail later in this chapter, where references are given, the rare antigens Wd^a, Rb^a, WARR, ELO, Wu, Bp^a, Mo^a, Hg^a, Vg^a, Tr^a, Sw^a, NFLD and Jn^a are all now known to be carried on protein band 3, and hence to be part of the Diego blood group system. There is already preliminary evidence (again see later for references) that several other antigens of low incidence will find homes on protein band 3.

It is, of course, not surprising that band 3 should be the home to so many red cell blood group antigens. It is a large protein of some 911 amino acids, is glycosylated, is present on red cells in approximately one million copies per cell and functions in the rapid exchange of HCO_3 and Cl ions in CO_2 transport across the membrane. Any mutation in the encoding *AE1* gene that alters the composition or sequence of amino acids in the anion exchanger protein, but does not affect or seriously impair function of that protein, is likely to be propagated since it imparts no selective disadvantage. Thus with such a large protein, MW circa 100,000 (42-44) it is not surprising to find that a number of changes in the protein can be recognized by blood group antibodies. The conventional and current ISBT terminology for the Diego blood group system are shown in table 17-1.

The Di^a and Di^b Antigens

As mentioned in the introduction of this chapter, Di^a is found predominantly among individuals of Mongolian extraction. Table 17-2 lists the number of Di(a+) bloods found in a series of surveys, in descending order of fre-

TABLE 17-1 Conventional and ISBT Terminology for the Diego Blood Group System
Conventional Name: Diego; ISBT System Symbol: DI; ISBT System Number: 010

| Antigen Name | | | ISBT | |
Historical	Conventional	Antigen Number[*1]	Full Code Number	Previous Number(s)[*2]
Diego	Di^a	DI1	010001	
Luebano	Di^b	DI2	010002	
Wright	Wr^a	DI3	010003	700001, 211001
Fritz	Wr^b	DI4	010004	900024, 901010, 211002
Waldner	Wd^a	DI5	010005	700030
Redelberger	Rb^a	DI6	010006	700027
Warrior	WARR	DI7	010007	700055
	ELO	DI8	010008	700051
Wulfsberg	Wu	DI9	010009	700013
Bishop	Bp^a	DI10	010010	700010
Moen	Mo^a	DI11	010011	700022
Hughes	Hg^a	DI12	010012	700034
Van Vugt	Vg^a	DI13	010013	700029
Traversu	Tr^a	*3		700008
Swann	Sw^a	*3		700004
Newfoundland	NFLD	*3		700037
Nunhart	Jn^a	*3		700014
Bowyer	BOW	*3, *4		700046
Froese	Fr^a	*3, *4		700026
	SW1	*3, *4		700041

*1   For assignment of DI1 and DI2 see Lewis et al. (213); for DI3 and DI4 see Daniels et al. (254); for DI5 to DI7 see Daniels et al. (174); and for DI8 to DI13 see Daniels (271).

*2   The 700, 900 and 901 series numbers become obsolete when a system number (010, Diego) is assigned.

*3   No ISBT number assigned as of July 1997, the 700 series numbers continue in use until a system number is assigned.

*4   Not yet (July 1997) formally proved to be part of the Diego system.
    For additional Diego system antigens see Chapter 46, the Addendum.

quency. Although the table lists a descending order, some caveats should be borne in mind when the data are reviewed. First, the number of samples tested varied widely, i.e. from 24 to 5259 in the various studies. Thus tests on larger numbers of some of the populations would likely change the sequence of frequencies. Second, although one survey (25) found 32 Di(a+) samples in 1000 Chinese persons in Taiwan, a different survey (26) found none in 772. The reason for this difference is not known. Third, a number of other surveys that found a very low incidence of Di^a or no Di(a+) samples are not listed in table 17-2. These comprised surveys in which the incidence of Di^a was: 1 in 4462 Europeans (2,3,13,22,24); 1 in 827 American Blacks (18); and none

in 1741 Papuans in New Guinea (19), 1374 Australian Aborigines (19), 1000 American Whites (3), and 107 Ghanaians (7). However, the Di^a antigen has been found in some of these populations by means other than large scale testing. Often such findings have been made when anti-Di^a caused HDN, or when anti-Di^a or anti-Di^b was encountered in pretransfusion tests. Thus Di^a has been found in an English family (24), in persons of Irish, Austrian and Slavic extraction in whom there was no known history of Mongolian ancestry (15,45,46) and in an American White (22). One White German of Hungarian extraction, has been found to have Di(a+b-) red cells (47). Many of the cases referenced above are revisited in the section below on anti-Di^a and anti-Di^b.

When we (23) tested samples from 784 donors of Hispanic extraction, who were living in southern Florida, we found that they were all Di(b+). Eleven in whom the Di^b antigen appeared to be weaker than normal were typed for Di^a, one was Di(a+).

The finding (28) that among 9661 Poles tested, 45 (0.47%) had Di(a+) red cells, an incidence much higher than that seen in any other White population tested, was attributed to gene admixture resulting from the invasion of Poland by Tartars of Mongolian background in the thirteenth and fifteenth to seventeenth centuries. This supposition was supported by the findings (see table 17-2) that in Southeastern Poland, the area closest to the home of the invading Tartars, the incidence of Di^a was 0.66%, while in Western Poland it was 0.3%. The original publication (28) includes a map of Poland and the antigen frequency can be seen clearly to follow the route of the invading Tartars.

As expected from the low incidence of Di^a in non-Mongolian populations and the fact that the Di(a-b-) phenotype has not been found, the incidence of Di^b in those populations is very high. In fairly recent studies, Edwards-Moulds and Alperin (22) found six (0.14%) Di(a+b-) samples among 4225 Mexican Americans living in Texas. As mentioned, we (23) found no Di(b-) sample in tests on the blood of 784 Hispanic Americans.

Both Di^a (8,50) and Di^b (22,29) seem to be as fully developed on the red cells of newborn infants as on the red cells of adults. Both antigens also survive the treatment of red cells with trypsin, chymotrypsin, papain, bromelin, pronase, neuraminidase and 2-aminoethylisothiouronium bromide (AET) (8,51-54). Masouredis et al.

TABLE 17-2 Incidence of the Di^a Antigen in a Number of Different Population Groups[*1]

Population	Number Tested	Number Di(a+)	Percent Di(a+)	References
Kainganges Indians (Brazil)	48	26	54.0	3
Carajas Indians (Brazil)	36	13	36.1	18, 21, 49
Caribe Indians (Venezuela)	121	43	35.5	3
Mayan Indians (Guatemala)	255	57	22.4	16
Inuits (Siberia)	86	18	20.9	18, 21
Mexican Indians	152	31	20.4	48
Guanibo Indians (Venezuela)	76	11	14.5	18, 21, 49
Piaroa Indians (Venezuela)	24	3	12.5	18, 21, 49
Chippewa Indians (USA)	148	16	10.8	6
Mexicans (USA)	1685	172	10.2	22
Penobscots Indians (USA)	249	20	8.0	12
Ciudad Bolivar Indians	100	7	7.0	18, 21, 49
Koreans	277	17	6.1	13
Arawaco Indians (Venezuela)	152	8	5.3	3
Chinese (Mainland)	617	32	5.2	18
Japanese	1594	78	4.9	18
Indians (Northern India)	377	15	4.0	18
Chinese (Taiwan)[*2]	1000	32	3.2	25
Caracas Indians (Venezuela)	500	10	2.0	18, 21, 49
Pregonero Indians	148	1	0.68	18, 21, 49
Poles (South-eastern Poland)	4402	29	0.66	28
Poles (Western Poland)	5259	16	0.30	28
Inuits (Alaska and Canada)	1477	2	0.14	18

[*1]   For other population groups with a lower incidence of Di^a, see text
[*2]   For a study (26) that found no Di(a+) among 722 Chinese in Taiwan, see text
[*3]   For additional studies see references 18, 21 and 49

(55) used quantitative immunoferritin microscopy to study Di^b. They estimated that Di(a-b+) red cells carry in the order of 15,000 Di^b sites per red cell. As mentioned above and as discussed in more detail below, it is now known that Di^b is carried on protein band 3. There are data (42-44,56-59) that indicate that band 3 is present in circa one million copies per red cell. It is not yet clear how the estimated 15,000 copies of Di^b can be reconciled with the estimated one million copies of band 3.

Phenotypes with a Weak Expression of Di^b

In 1983, Biro et al. (60) described a healthy Mexican blood donor whose red cells initially appeared to be Di(a-b-). Further tests with a battery of sera showed that the donor's red cells were Di(a-) and carried only a weak expression of Di^b. In tests using eight different anti-Di^b the donor's red cells reacted visibly with six, but always less strongly than the Di(a+b+) and Di(a-b+) control samples. The donor's red cells failed to react visibly with two of the anti-Di^b but were able to adsorb those antibodies and yield them on elution. The donor's red cells also had reduced expressions of D, LW, H, I, i, Vel, JMH, Sd^a and Rx antigens. As the authors (60) pointed out, the pattern of antigen depression differed from that seen in Melanesians with ovalocytosis (see below) and from that effected by *In(Lu)* (see Chapter 20). The woman in question had passed all donor fitness and hemoglobin requirements to donate blood, attempts to trace her to see if the red cell phenotype was associated with any form of hematological abnormality, were unsuccessful. Other investigators (22,23) have noticed weakened expressions of Di^b on the Di(a-b+) red cells of some individuals, but not to the same degree as that reported by Biro et al. (60). It is not known whether the weak Di^b phenotype represents a genetically determined or an acquired condition.

Anti-Di^a, Anti-Di^b and their Clinical Significance

These antibodies are most often red cell stimulated, are IgG in composition and give their best reactions in antiglobulin tests. Several examples of the antibodies have been shown to contain IgG1 and IgG3 components (24,28,53,61,62). While some examples have been shown (29,52,63) not to activate complement, others with the ability to do so, have been seen (28,64,65). Indeed, anti-Di^a capable of hemolyzing untreated red cells in vitro, have been described (65). As mentioned

above, Di^a and Di^b survive protease treatment of red cells. Some examples of anti-Di^a and anti-Di^b give stronger reactions with protease-treated than with untreated red cells, sometimes to the point of causing direct agglutination of the enzyme-treated red cells (63,66). In spite of the most usual characteristics of Diego system antibodies, as described above, exceptions are seen. Both anti-Di^a (15) and anti-Di^b (67) have been seen as agglutinins, at least twice (15,68) anti-Di^a has been produced by individuals with no known exposure to foreign red cells. In one of these cases (68), the IgG anti-Di^a had a titer of 128. Anti-Di^a is sometimes found in sera that contain multiple antibodies to low incidence antigens but does not seem to be as common, in such sera, as say anti-Wr^a or anti-Mi^a. It has been reported (29,62,63,69-71) that anti-Di^b may show dosage effects more readily than anti-Di^a.

Anti-Di^a has once (52) been thought to have caused an immediate transfusion reaction but the case was complicated by the fact that the patient also had anti-c. The major evidence that anti-Di^a was involved in the in vivo red cell destruction was that the titer of the antibody increased after transfusion. A different example of anti-Di^a was tested in an in vitro macrophage binding assay (64) and yielded a result that suggested that it would be capable of destroying Di(a+) red cells in vivo. One of the first two examples of anti-Di^b was thought (29) perhaps to have caused a delayed transfusion reaction.

Anti-Di^a has caused many cases of HDN (1,3,15,24, 28,46,51,53,61,71-73,270) at least one of which (3) was fatal and others of which were particularly severe (1,3, 15,51,72,73). Because of the low incidence of Di^a, finding compatible blood for an affected infant is not difficult. More difficult is finding the maternal anti-Di^a in prenatal tests. Clearly, antibody screening cells will all be Di(a-) in locations in which the Di^a antigen, and hence immunization to it, is rare. In those regions in which immunization to Di^a is more likely, it may be necessary to add a local Di(a+) sample to the set of screening cells.

Anti-Di^b seems more benign than anti-Di^a in terms of HDN. Two cases (63,73) have been described in which exchange transfusions were necessary, in one of these (73) incompatible Di(b+) blood had to be used. More often, HDN caused by anti-Di^b is relatively mild (66,74), in a number of cases (29,62,70,74) positive serological findings, e.g. positive DAT on the newborn's red cells, have been seen in the absence of clinical HDN.

The most usual characteristics of anti-Di^a and anti-Di^b and those of other Diego system antibodies not yet described in this chapter, are shown in table 17-3. For reasons that will become apparent in the section itself, auto-anti-Di^b is described in a later section, together with the much more common auto-anti-Wr^b.

TABLE 17-3 Usual Characteristics of Diego System Antibodies

Antibody Specificity	Positive Reactions in In Vitro Tests				Usual Immuno-globulin		Ability to Bind Complement		Ability to Cause In Vitro Lysis		Implicated in		Usual Form of Stimulation		% of White Population Positive
	Sal	LISS	AHG	Enz[*1]	IgG	IgM	Yes	No	Yes	No	Trans-fusion Reaction	HDN	Red Cells	Other	
Anti-Di[a]	Few		Most		Most	Rare	Rare	Most	Rare	Most	?	Yes	Yes	Rare	<0.1
Anti-Di[b]	Rare		Most		Most	Rare	Rare	Most		X	?	Yes[*2]	X		>99.9
Anti-Wr[a]	Some		Some		Some	Some		Most		X	Yes	Yes	Few	Many[*3]	0.1
Anti-Wr[b]			X		X			Most		X			X		>99.9
Antibodies to Wd[a], Rb[a], WARR	Most		Few		Some	Some		Most		X				Most[*3]	<0.1
Antibodies to Sw[a], SW1, Fr[a], ELO	Some		Some		Most	Few		Most		X		Yes	Some	Many[*3]	<0.1
Antibodies to Wu, NFLD, BOW, Vg[a], Bp[a], Hg[a], Mo[a], Tr[a], Jn[a]	Most		Few		Some	Some		Most		X				Most[*3]	<0.1

[*1] Most antibodies react with red cells treated with trypsin, papain or ficin. Some fail to react with chymotrypsin-treated red cells, see text.

[*2] Usually only mild HDN, one exception, see text.

[*3] Often found in sera containing multiple antibodies to low incidence antigens. Some of those sera are from persons with no known exposure to foreign red cells.

Wr[a]

Since Holman (32) described the first example of anti-Wr[a] in 1953, many hundreds, perhaps thousands of examples of the antibody have been found. As a result, long before Wr[a] became part of the Diego system, it became perhaps the most studied, at the serological level, of all low incidence antigens.

Many thousands of typing tests have been performed with anti-Wr[a]. By adding the test series reported in the literature (10,11,32,75-93) it can be seen that documentation exists of typing tests on 94,124 blood samples, 63 of which (1 in 1494) were Wr(a+). If these series are subdivided into ethnic groups (and this cannot be done with complete accuracy since some series report tests on mixed populations) it is seen that the 63 Wr(a+) bloods were found in about 86,000 Whites (either European or of primarily European extraction) for an incidence of 1 in 1365. This figure agrees well with the incidence found in the largest series reported (78,79,88,93). Although far fewer people have been tested, the Wr[a] antigen has not been found in Blacks (79), Eskimos (10,11), Alaska Indians (11), Tibetans (87), Bhutanese (89), Caribs in Dominica (90), Australian Aborigines (86,92) or natives

of New Guinea (83,92). Relatively large numbers of these last two groups have been typed.

Many studies (32,79,80,85,94-97) had shown independent segregation of *Wr[a]* from other blood group loci, well before Wr[a] was recognized (41) as being a Diego system antigen. That finding, of course, meant that production of Wr[a] is controlled by a gene on chromosome 17 (98,99). Of particular importance to the discussion below about the dependence of Wr[b] (the antithetical partner to Wr[a]) on the presence of portions of both band 3 and glycophorin A for expression, were those findings (79,80,85,95,96) that demonstrated independent segregation of *Wr[a]* from the *MN* locus. One family (100) suggested that *Wr[a]* might be linked to the gene that encodes the Sd(a++) ("super Sid") phenotype (see Chapter 31). We are not aware of further investigations of this suggestive finding.

Wr[a] survives treatment of red cells with trypsin, chymotrypsin, papain, pronase, neuraminidase and 2-aminoethylisothiouronium bromide (54,101). The antigen appears to be fully developed at birth, see below for cases of HDN caused by anti-Wr[a]. Although Wr[b] is known (39-41) to require band 3 and a portion of glycophorin A for expression, it is not known if the same requirement applies to Wr[a]. No person with Wr(a+) red cells who also lacks glycophorin A, or carries that sialo-glycoprotein in a form that abrogates expression of Wr^b, has been found. Of course, if Wr^a has the same dependence as Wr^b on the presence of glycophorin A, it would be necessary to detect the *Wr^a* gene in an individual lacking, or with altered glycophorin A, since the antigen would not be expressed. Such biochemical evidence as exists (39) suggests that Wr^a might not require glycophorin A for its expression at the serological level (see a later section in this chapter).

Anti-Wr^a and its Clinical Significance

Anti-Wr^a is a relatively common antibody. Its incidence in the sera of healthy individuals is approximately 1 in 100 (78,79,88,93,102) although, as described below, the incidence varies if the antibody-makers are subdivided. The antibody occurs in many forms from an IgM agglutinin optimally reactive at temperatures below 37°C (79,88,102), to an IgG antibody reactive only by IAT at 37°C (88,102,103). All of nine IgG anti-Wr^a studied by Hardman and Beck (103) were IgG1 in composition.

Anti-Wr^a has caused severe HDN (32,75,104,105) and hemolytic transfusion reactions (85,106). However, other examples of anti-Wr^a must be benign. While anti-Wr^a is common, it is seldom detected in antibody-screening tests since Wr(a+) red cells are not used. Widespread use of the immediate spin compatibility test and computer matching of units for patients in whom antibody screening tests are negative, must, by now, have resulted in some patients with undetected anti-Wr^a in the serum, receiving Wr(a+) blood in spite of the low incidence of that phenotype. However, transfusion reactions caused by anti-Wr^a in this setting, have not been reported.

The occurrence of anti-Wr^a in different groups of individuals provides a fascinating study. Cleghorn (79,107) showed that if sera from normal donors are tested, the incidence of anti-Wr^a is between 1 in 100 and 1 in 200. In the sera of recently delivered women, the incidence is about 1 in 50 except if recently delivered women who have formed anti-D are separated from the series, then the incidence rises to about 1 in 14. If the sera of patients with "warm" autoimmune hemolytic anemia are studied, one in every two or three contains anti-Wr^a. These findings are listed in table 17-4. However, the source of immunization that results in production of anti-Wr^a remains obscure. The husbands and children of the recently delivered women who produce anti-Wr^a (with or without anti-D) show no higher an incidence of Wr^a than the normal population. If the red cells of donors of blood given to the patients with WAIHA are typed, there too a normal distribution of Wr^a is seen. Two conjectures can be made from these observations. First, as the immune

**TABLE 17-4 The Incidence of Anti-Wr^a
(from Cleghorn 79, 107)**

	Approximate frequency of antibody
Normal blood donors	1 in 100 to 1 in 200
Recently delivered women	1 in 50
Recently delivered women who have made Rh antibodies	1 in 14
Patients with antibody-induced hemolytic anemia	1 in 2 to 1 in 3

system in different groups of people becomes more active (normal—pregnant no Rh antibodies—pregnant with Rh antibodies—autoimmune hemolytic anemia) the incidence of anti-Wr^a increases. Second, as the amount of red cell destruction in different groups of people becomes greater (normal—remove old cells at end of 120 day life span; pregnant—no Rh antibodies—destroy ABO incompatible fetal cells entering the maternal circulation; pregnant with Rh antibodies—destroy ABO and Rh incompatible fetal cells; WAIHA—abnormal rates of destruction of all cells) the incidence of anti-Wr^a increases. Thus in patients with hyperactive immune systems who are exposed to the breakdown products of Wr(a-) cells the incidence of formation of anti-Wr^a increases. It seems that surely this information must be important at some basic level of the immune response and antibody production. These findings, together with the fact that sera that contain an antibody to one rare antigen are more likely than not to contain antibodies to other antigens of low incidence, are considered again in Chapter 32. As described in Chapter 6, there is one school of thought (108) that maintains that senescent red cell removal is mediated by a physiological IgG antibody directed against an antigen on protein band 3, that becomes exposed as red cells age in vivo. Whether this mechanism is in any way related to the facts that Wr^a is carried on band 3, and that anti-Wr^a is frequently seen in persons never exposed to foreign red cells, is not known. At least one murine monoclonal anti-Wr^a has been made (101).

Wr^b, The Short Story

Since one of us (PDI) has frequently been accused of having an obsession with Wr^b, this brief section listing only final conclusions is included for those who do not wish to read the long story, in the next section. Wr^b is antithetical to Wr^a (33,36,39,109-111,113) and as such, is obviously of very high incidence. Based on the incidence of *Wr^a* it was calculated (97) that the Wr(a+b-) phenotype, representing the *Wr^{a}Wr^a* genotype, would occur in approximately 1 in 8 million individuals. The blood of one such individual (33) has been extensively studied (36,39,109-111,113), that of a second such person was available only for limited testing (114). The Wr^a/Wr^b polymorphism has been shown (41) to represent an amino acid difference at position 658 on protein band 3; lysine occupies that position when band 3 carries Wr^a, glutamic acid is at position 658 when the protein expresses Wr^b.

In spite of the extreme rarity of the Wr(a+b-) phenotype, other Wr(b-) samples, and ones on which expression of Wr^b was markedly reduced, have been found. In 1975, we (109,115) showed that En(a-) red cells (see Chapter 15) are phenotypically Wr(a-b-). Since that time, other samples that lack glycophorin A (116-119) or have an altered form of that sialoglycoprotein (120-124) have also been shown to be phenotypically Wr(a-b-). Further, some samples on which glycophorin A is altered, express Wr^b only weakly (125,126).

The explanation of the above findings is that although the Wr^a/Wr^b polymorphism represents the amino acid difference at position 658 on the fourth external loop of protein band 3, that is described above, the Wr^b antigen is not expressed at the serological level unless the portion of normal glycophorin A, from about residue 60 to residue 72 is also present (37-41). It initially appeared (41) that presence of the arginine residue at position 61 of glycophorin A was key for the interaction between band 3 and glycophorin A, that results in the expression of Wr^b. More recently a blood sample has been described (126) in which the alanine normally present at residue 65 of glycophorin A, was replaced by proline. The red cells involved reacted with 8 of 15 anti-Wr^b. Thus it seems that more than one amino acid in the residue 60 to 72 portion glycophorin A, interacts with the glutamic acid at position 658 of band 3, to form Wr^b. Huang et al. (127) have suggested that any change in the alpha-helical region and transmembrane junction of glycophorin A (residues 59-71) has the potential to affect the protein-protein interaction between band 3 and glycophorin A and thus abrogate or alter expression of Wr^b.

Wr^b, The Long Story, Now Including ENEP, HAG, AVIS and MARS

Some of the details mentioned in this section are included, in part, for historical reasons. The story of the gradual evolution of the understanding of Wr^b antigen structure provides a good example of how serological studies, when correctly performed and accurately reported, can eventually be seen to be totally correct and explainable although, at the time they were made, they seemed contradictory in nature.

In 1971, we (33) described an antibody that we thought defined Wr^b, the antigen antithetical to Wr^a. Additional findings of our study were published in 1976 (109). We described a lady with Wr(a+) red cells who had made an antibody that reacted with all red cells tested except her own. The serological evidence that the antibody had anti-Wr^b specificity seemed excellent. First, the red cells of the antibody-maker were Wr(a+) and in titration studies with dozens of examples of anti-Wr^a, reacted as though they carried a double dose of that antigen, when compared to Wr(a+) red cells from unrelated individuals. Second, the antibody made by the lady with Wr(a+) red cells gave double dose reactions with Wr(a-) cells from random donors and a single dose score with Wr(a+) cells from unrelated persons. Third, the sibs of our patient whom we supposed had Wr(a+b-) red cells, almost all had Wr(a+) cells suggesting that her parents (who were not available for study) could each have been of the Wr(a+) phenotype. Fourth, the patient's only child had Wr(a+) cells. Fifth, although not known to have been related, the patient's parents had come to the USA from the same small region in Germany, close to the Polish border. In 1975, we (109,115,128) made the totally unexpected finding that En(a-) red cells are phenotypically Wr(a-b-). Since this finding was made at about the same time as it was shown (134-141) that En(a-) red cells lack glycophorin A, the carrier of M, N and many other MN system antigens (see Chapter 15) it was natural that intensive investigations of the En(a-) Wr(a-b-) phenotype and the relationship between the MN and Wright antigens would be performed (97,109,111,129-133).

It was already known (79,80,85,95,96) that *Wr^a* segregates independently of the *MN* locus. However, the lack of Wr^b from En(a-) red cells certainly suggested that Wr^b might be an MN system antigen and thus not antithetical to Wr^a at all. Additional studies on glycophorin A (142-144) led to the suggestion (145) that Wr^b must be located in the alpha helical region of MN SGP between residues 55 and 70. Direct evidence that this is the case was obtained by Dahr et al. (35,39,145) who showed that a peptide fragment of MN SGP, that contains residues 62 to 72, inhibits anti-En^{a}FR and anti-Wr^b once it has been incorporated in liposomes. These findings seemed to show that Wr^b must be an MN system antigen (a form of En^{a}FR) and that the maker of anti-Wr^b must have rare alleles at the *MN* locus. Accordingly, the amino acid sequence of glycophorin A, extracted from the red cells of the Wr(a+b-) proposita was determined. It was found (36,39) to be identical to that of Wr(a-b+) and Wr(a+b+) red cells! Since one of us (PDI) never doubted that Wr^b is antithetical to Wr^a (and therefore not encoded from the *MN* locus) we (34) repeated the dosage studies using anti-Wr^a and anti-Wr^b that we had performed earlier (109) by manual titrations, using a quantitative, objectively read method. We used the enzyme-linked antiglobulin test to measure the amounts of Wr^a and Wr^b on red cells of different phenotypes. Studies on 24 Wr(a+b+) and 23 Wr(a-b+) samples using the original anti-Wr^b (33) as an eluate (to free it of the weak anti-D also made by the proposita) showed that, on average, the Wr(a+b+) red cells bound a little over a half of the amount of anti-Wr^b as bound by the Wr(a-b+) samples (that were traveled controls and thus matched to the Wr(a+b+) samples sent by colleagues). In similar tests using six different anti-Wr^a, 10 Wr(a+b+) samples bound about half the amount of anti-Wr^a as bound by the Wr(a+b-) red cells. In spite of evidence that put our original interpretation (109) in doubt, it was again clear that Wr^a and Wr^b have an antithetical relationship. When the second person with phenotypically Wr(a+b-) red cells was found (114), it was at first thought that she was genetically *Wr^{a}Wr^a*. However, her red cells differed from those of the original proposita in that they reacted weakly with six examples of mouse monoclonal anti-Wr^b. Since the patient, who was 82 years-old, died soon after her phenotype was recognized, only limited studies were possible. In retrospect, it seems likely that this patient had an altered form of glycophorin A and that her Wr(b-) status could have had the same background as that (126) described below. If that was the case, the idea is conjectural, it might mean that Wr^a does not need normal glycophorin A, for its expression at the serological level (see section above on Wr^a).

The long held belief of one of us (PDI), that was challenged many times between 1971 and the 1990s, that Wr^a and Wr^b are antithetical, was vindicated in 1995 when Bruce et al. (41) showed that when protein band 3 expresses Wr^b it has glutamic acid at position 658 whereas, when it expresses Wr^a, lysine occupies that position. The explanation for the findings described above was to hand! For the benefit of readers who skipped "Wr^b, The Short Story" above, the final explanation will be repeated here.

Although the Wr^a/Wr^b polymorphism represents the amino acid difference at position 658, just mentioned, on the fourth external loop of protein band 3, the Wr^b antigen is not expressed at the serological level unless the portion of normal (wild type) glycophorin A, from about residue 60 to 72 is also present (37-41). It initially appeared (41) that presence of the arginine residue at position 61 of glycophorin A was the requirement for the interaction between band 3 and glycophorin A, that results in expression of Wr^b. More recently a blood sample has been described (125,126) in which the alanine normally present at residue 65 of glycophorin A, was replaced by proline. The red cells involved reacted with 8 of 15 anti-Wr^b and lacked the high incidence antigen ENEP (see Chapter 15). Thus it seems that more than one amino acid in the residue 60 to 72 portion of gly-

cophorin A, interacts with the glutamic acid at position 658 of band 3, to form Wr^b. The red cells on which expression of Wr^b was altered, presumably by the change from alanine to proline at position 65 of glycophorin A, carry a previously undescribed low incidence antigen, tentatively called HAG. Presumably this antigen could represent the same change in the amino acid sequence of glycophorin A (i.e. proline instead of alanine at position 65) that results in alteration of Wr^b. A case that is perhaps similar to that described by Poole et al. (125,126) was reported in 1992 by Moulds et al. (161). The patient, a 46 year-old Indian lady, made an antibody to a very high frequency antigen that was not present on red cells that lack or have an altered expression of glycophorin A (En(a-) and those from *M^k* and *Mi^V* homozygotes). The antigen defined was apparently expressed normally on Wr(a+b+) red cells. The red cells of the antibody-maker reacted only weakly with human anti-Wr^b but normally with monoclonal antibodies with apparently that specificity. Again it is apparent (246) that a change in the alpha-helical region of glycophorin A, that is proximal to the red cell membrane and presumed to interact with band 3, was responsible for lack of the high incidence antigen, provisionally called AVIS, to which the patient was immunized. A previously unidentified low incidence antigen, provisionally called MARS, was found on the antibody-maker's red cells, presumably it was produced as a result of the change in glycophorin A (246). Huang et al. (127) have suggested that any change in the alpha-helical region and transmembrane junction of glycophorin A (residues 59-71) has the potential to affect the protein-protein interaction between glycophorin A and band 3 and thus abrogate or alter expression of Wr^b. This means, of course, that antibodies that fail to react with En(a+) Wr(a+b+) and En(a-) Wr(a-b-) red cells and will thus be called anti-Wr^b, may have slightly different specificities. While the En(a+) Wr(a+b+) red cells of the original proposita represent the *Wr^{a}Wr^a* genotype and while En(a-) red cells represent the absence of glycophorin A, other samples will have alterations in the alpha-helical region of glycophorin A and will thus lack determinants different from Wr^b. Antibodies against such determinants may, ostensibly at least, appear to have anti-Wr^b specificity. Differences in specificity of some monoclonal antibodies that appear, at first, to be directed against Wr^b, have been reported (146-148).

Anti-Wr^b and its Clinical Significance

Although only two examples of allo-anti-Wr^b made by persons with Wr(a+b-) red cells have been described (33,109,115), a number of other examples have been found (67,109,132,133,149) as separable antibodies in the sera of immunized En(a-) individuals who have also formed anti-En^a or in the sera of persons with glycophorin A-B hybrids whose red cells were Wr(b-) (120,121). The antibodies are usually IgG in nature and react best in IATs. Our experience has been that the antibodies are readily detected with anti-IgG but we have not looked specifically to see whether they activate complement. As discussed below, some examples of auto-anti-Wr^b have caused intravascular hemolysis, clearly those antibodies did activate complement.

Not very much is known about the in vivo characteristics of allo-anti-Wr^b. One patient with anti-En^a and anti-Wr^b suffered a mild delayed transfusion reaction after receiving six units of En(a+) Wr(b+) blood (150). A woman with allo-anti-Wr^b in her serum gave birth to a child with Wr(b+) red cells. The DAT on the cord blood red cells was positive but the infant did not have to be transfused. In spite of the paucity of evidence, allo-anti-Wr^b should probably be regarded as having the potential to destroy Wr(b+) red cells in vivo. This assumption is based on the evidence described below about the pathological nature of some examples of auto-anti-Wr^b. Many murine monoclonal anti-Wr^b have been produced, some of them have been described in print (153-156).

Red Cell Ovalocytosis and Protein Band 3

As mentioned briefly in Chapter 16, in addition to the comparatively high incidence of some Ge-negative phenotypes in Papua New Guinea, there is a fairly high incidence of hereditary red cell ovalocytosis in that population. The condition is also seen in surrounding areas and is known as South East Asian Ovalocytosis or SAO. In this inherited state the red cells are oval rather than round (229-232). In 1977, Booth et al. (233) reported that the ovalocytes have depressed expression of many red cell blood group antigens. Among the antigens whose expression was less than normal were: Di^b; Wr^b; I^F, I^T; D, C, e; LW; S, s, U, En^a; Kp^b; Jk^a, Jk^b; Xg^a and Sc1. Antigens expressed normally on ovalocytes included: A$_1$; I^D, i; P$_1$; M, N; k; Lu^b; Fy^a; Co^a; Vel and Ge (presumably Ge2 and Ge3).

Presence of the ovalocytosis condition in the region seems to have resulted from selective advantage since the red cells involved are more resistant than normal red cells to invasion by *Plasmodium falciparum* parasites (234,235). It is likely that in addition to any alteration in parasite receptors, rigidity of the ovalocytes in comparison to normocytes, contributes to this resistance (236). Once the structure of normal protein band 3 had been established (42,43) an abnormality of that protein in SAO red cells was found. Jarolim et al. (237) showed that protein band 3 of SAO red cells lacks the amino acids present

from positions 400 to 408 on normal band 3. Although this deletion results in a defect in anion transport across the red cell membrane, the defect is apparently less disadvantageous than the resistance to malarial invasion is advantageous. In other words, the mutant form of *AE1* that encodes production of the altered form of band 3, seems to have been selectively propagated.

It will be noticed that among the antigens whose expression is depressed on SAO red cells are two, Di^b and Wr^b, now known to be carried on band 3. While the deletion on band 3 SAO involves the amino acids at positions 400 to 408 and the Di^a/Di^b and Wr^a/Wr^b polymorphisms are at positions 854 and 658, respectively, it is not known whether the regions involved are proximal or distal when band 3 is folded in situ. However, in view of the many other genetically independent red cell antigens involved, it seems most likely that the alteration in red cell shape, that can be attributed to abnormal attachment of the altered band 3 to the cytoskeleton, affects orientation of several different red cell antigen-bearing membrane components. In other words, depression of red cell antigen expression in SAO seems to be a rather non-specific orientation effect and thus differs from the defect in the Leach (Ge:-2,-3,-4) phenotype. As described in Chapter 16, lack of glycophorins C and D, that are normally attached via protein 4.1 to the red cell cytoskeleton, seems directly to cause elliptocytosis of Ge:-2,-3,-4 red cells. The depression of expression of antigens in the Mexican donor (60) described earlier in this chapter seems to resemble SAO more closely than Ge:-2,-3,-4 since antigens of several genetically independent blood group systems were involved.

Diego System Autoantibodies

At about the same time as the Wr(a-b-) status of En(a-) red cells was recognized, thus allowing anti-Wr^b specificity to be recognized from tests with more than one known Wr(b-) sample, we were sent an autoantibody from a patient with "warm" antibody-induced hemolytic anemia (WAIHA). Helen Zwicker in Los Angeles had astutely noticed that although the antibody reacted with all red cell samples, its reactions were noticeably weaker with a Wr(a+) sample than with Wr(a-) red cells. The antibody was indeed the first recognized example of auto-anti-Wr^b (130). Having seen this specificity causing WAIHA, we (131) undertook a large study. Among 150 consecutively studied persons with a strongly positive DAT and an IgG "warm" reactive autoantibody, we found 46 examples of auto-anti-Wr^b. Four of the autoantibodies were "pure" anti-Wr^b, the other 42 were present as components of anti-dl (see Chapter 37) and were identified when they remained unadsorbed after the other autoantibodies present had been adsorbed to exhaustion with Wr(a+b-) red cells. Of the 150 individuals studied, 87 had WAIHA. Among those 87 patients, two were seen in whom anti-Wr^b was the only autoantibody present, another 32 had auto-anti-Wr^b as a component of their anti-dl. Another 33 of the 150 persons had made autoantibodies as a result of alpha methyldopa therapy (see Chapter 40). Among those 33 patients, none of whom had hemolytic anemia, four examples of auto-anti-Wr^b as a component of anti-dl, were found. The remaining 30 individuals with a positive DAT and a "warm" reactive IgG autoantibody were hematologically normal. Among those 30 individuals, two had made only auto-anti-Wr^b while another six had a separable auto-anti-Wr^b as a component of their anti-dl. In other words, auto-anti-Wr^b is sometimes pathological and sometimes benign. Even if the auto-anti-Wr^b that occur as components of anti-dl are excluded from consideration it can be seen that in two patients with WAIHA, auto-anti-Wr^b was the only antibody present (pathological) while in two hematologically normal individuals, auto-anti-Wr^b was the only autoantibody present (benign).

Since our large study that described 46 examples of auto-anti-Wr^b was published (131), other examples of auto-anti-Wr^b have been encountered. In two cases (151,152) the antibody presented as an auto-hemolysin active at 37°C and in both cases intravascular hemolysis resulted in a fatal outcome.

In 1993, Leddy et al. (157) described the results of tests in which they had used 20 autoantibodies causative of WAIHA in immunoprecipitation studies. Among the autoantibodies, nine precipitated the Rh polypeptides, some with and some without coprecipitation of protein band 3. Another five precipitated just band 3 while the remaining six precipitated both band 3 and glycophorin A. One year later, the same group of investigators (158) reported serological studies on the six autoantibodies that had precipitated both band 3 and glycophorin A. Of the six autoantibodies one was anti-Wr^b, two were anti-Wr^b with one or more additional components while in three no specificity was apparent although one of them may have included an anti-Wr^b component. We theorized that since not all autoantibodies that precipitate band 3 have anti-Wr^b specificity, some may be anti-Di^b. We (159) tested eluates from 119 patients in whom the DAT was positive, IgG was present on the red cells and in whom the autoantibody reacted with all red cells of normal phenotype. In tests against Di(a+b+) red cells all 119 autoantibodies reacted, showing that no patient had made just anti-Di^b. We had sufficient materials to perform adsorption studies on 74 of the autoantibody-containing eluates. Seventy-two of them were adsorbed to exhaustion with Di(a+b+) red cells. In the other two, anti-Di^b remained unadsorbed after all activity for the

Di(a+b-) red cells had been removed. Thus, two of 74 patients had made auto-anti-Di^b as a component of their anti-dl (see Chapter 37). One of the patients with auto-anti-Di^b had hemolytic anemia secondary to his myelocytic leukemia. The DAT on his red cells was positive with both anti-IgG and anti-C3. However, since his auto-anti-Di^b was present with other autoantibodies, it was not clear whether the auto-anti-Di^b had activated complement. The second patient with auto-anti-Di^b had coronary artery disease, rheumatoid arthritis and hypothyroidism. There was no evidence of hemolytic anemia showing that like auto-anti-Wr^b, auto-anti-Di^b can be benign in vivo. In this patient the DAT was positive with anti-IgG and negative with anti-C3, suggesting that this auto-anti-Di^b did not activate complement. It is perhaps significant that both patients who made auto-anti-Di^b were also alloimmunized. The patient with leukemia had made antibodies to D, C and E following multiple transfusions of HLA-matched platelets from D+ donors, his serum also contained anti-Wr^a (i.e. he had one auto and one allo Diego system antibody). The second patient had made allo-anti-C following transfusions during earlier surgery. Her eluate contained auto-anti-e and anti-dl, in addition to the auto-anti-Di^b. While it is tempting to speculate that both these individuals made auto-anti-Di^b because they are good responders, it must be remembered that some 23% of persons who make autoantibodies, make alloantibodies as well (170).

It is not clear why auto-anti-Wr^b is so common and auto-anti-Di^b so infrequent. Our study (131) on auto-anti-Wr^b included 110 examples of anti-dl, 46 (42%) of them were, or contained, anti-Wr^b. Our study (159) on auto-anti-Di^b included 119 examples of anti-dl, none was just anti-Di^b and only two of 74 (2.7%) contained anti-Di^b. Wr^b is situated on the fourth external loop of band 3, Di^b is located on the seventh external loop of that protein. Wr^b is located close to a major glycosylation site of band 3. It is not known if this fact has any bearing on the relative immunogenicity of Wr^b and Di^b as targets for autoantibody production. It is known that Wr^b represents an interaction product of band 3 and glycophorin A (see above). On the other hand, Di^b seems to need only band 3 for expression. As described in detail in Chapter 12, expression of red cell Rh antigens requires the presence of several membrane components. Some 50% of all autoantibodies are directed against Rh associated antigens (131). Perhaps antigens that arise via complex red cell membrane component interactions are simply more likely to serve as targets for autoantibodies than those that represent more simple amino acid substitutions. The above suggestion is, of course, purely speculative.

Although we have been credited in one publication (93) with having described auto-anti-Wr^a, we (160) have not seen such an autoantibody, nor do we expect to do so.

Wd^a, a Diego System Antigen

The antibody defining this antigen was found by Lewis and Kaita (162) in a serum being used to type red cells for Fr^a (see below). The Wd^a antigen was not found in any of 4000 unrelated North American Whites but was present in many members of two large Hutterite families with the surname Waldner (from whence comes Wd^a). No Wd(a+) sample was found in tests on 7151 Norwegians (163) but two sisters in a Black Hei//om Khoisan family in Namibia had Wd(a+) red cells (164).

Later studies (165) on seven nuclear Hutterite families showed absolute linkage (i.e. no recombinants) between *Wd^a* and a *Pst1* RFLP of *AE1* (the gene that encodes production of the red cell anion exchanger (protein band 3)) and the Diego system antigens. Thus Wd^a was seen to be a low incidence antigen in the Diego system. In 1995, Bruce et al. (166) reported that when protein band 3 expresses Wd^a, methionine is present at position 557 of the protein. When protein band 3 does not express Wd^a, i.e. the wild type protein present on the common form of band 3 of Wd(a-) red cells, the amino acid at positive 557 is valine. Since the amino acid change at position 557 is close to the chymotrypsin cleavage sites on band 3, i.e. Tyr 553 and Tyr 555, it became clear why Wd^a is inactivated when red cells are treated with that enzyme. Localization of the Wd(a-) to Wd(a+) change in the third ectoplasmic loop of the red cell band 3 protein was later confirmed by others (167,247,248,250).

Anti-Wd^a is not an uncommon antibody in sera that contain other antibodies to low incidence antigens and was also found (162) in a commercially-supplied anti-S typing serum. In tests on the sera of pregnant women, one example of anti-Wd^a was found among 358 samples tested. Anti-Wd^a most often presents as a saline-active agglutinin but at least one IgG example optimally reactive in IATs has been found (162). In six Wd(a-) Hutterite women who among them bore 30 children with Wd(a+) red cells, none made anti-Wd^a (162).

Rb^a, a Diego System Antigen

In 1978, Contreras et al. (168) described the low incidence antigen Rb^a. Anti-Rb^a is often present in sera that contain antibodies to other antigens of low incidence. The antigen is named for Mr. Redelberger (from whence comes Rb^a) who at the time that the antigen was found was a donor recruiter for the Community Blood Center of Dayton (Ohio). It tests on 13,500 random donor samples, two that were Rb(a+) were found, both in the United Kingdom. In tests on 6200 random donor sera, six examples of saline-active anti-Rb^a were identified. However, anti-Rb^a was present more often in sera

known to contain antibodies to other low incidence antigens. No anti-Rb^a was found in the sera of five Rb(a-) women who had borne Rb(a+) children (168).

In 1995, Jarolim et al. (167) reported that sequencing studies on protein band 3 showed that when that protein carries Rb^a, leucine occupies position 548. When protein band 3 does not express Rb^a, i.e. the wild type protein present on the common form of band 3 of Rb(a-) red cells, the amino acid at position 548 is proline. Like the Wd(a-) to Wd(a+) change, the Rb(a-) to Rb(a+) change occurs in the third ectoplasmic loop of protein band 3 and close to the Tyr 553 and Tyr 555 chymotrypsin sensitive sites. Before recognition of the Rb(a-) to Rb(a+) change, it had been noticed that some, but not all examples of anti-Rb^a gave reduced strength reactions with protease-treated Rb(a+) red cells (168). It seems that to denature Rb^a, chymotrypsin and not papain, ficin or bromelin, should be used. It should be added that in the abstract (167) describing the amino acid difference between Rb(a+) and Rb(a-) red cells, the term Rb(a+b+) is used. However, anti-Rb^b has not been found (169) and the term Rb(a+b+) was incorrectly used to describe red cells from individuals heterozygous for *Rb^a* and the wild type *AE1* allele, that does not encode production of Rb^a. In other words, individuals described in the abstract as Rb(a+b+) have one set of copies of protein band 3 with leucine at position 548 and another (equal number) set with proline at that position. The amino acid change involved in formation of Rb^a has been described in other publications (247,250).

WARR, a Diego System Antigen

In 1991, Crow et al. (171) reported briefly on a low incidence antigen, WARR, the antibody to which caused mild HDN. Shortage of material prevented further studies until several years later when the father of the child presented as a routine blood donor. Use of his red cells allowed additional examples of anti-WARR to be identified. In the ensuing study, Coghlan et al. (172) tested a total of 8275 individuals, the only WARR+ sample found was from the sister of the original propositus. Among the WARR- samples, 1082 were from Native Americans, 319 from African Americans, 189 from Whites, 67 from Orientals and 8 from Hispanics. The remaining 6609 samples were from donors whose race was not known, it was presumed that almost all, or all, were White. The eldest WARR+ member of the kindred with WARR+ members is reported to be of pure Absentee Shawnee ancestry; it was considered likely (172) that the antigen may be unique to Native Americans. The WARR antigen was not denatured by ficin or dithiothreitol (DTT) treatment of red cells, indeed the WARR-anti-WARR reaction was enhanced when ficin-treated WARR+ red cells were used. Plasma from an individual with WARR+ red cells did not inhibit anti-WARR.

In contrast to the rarity of the WARR antigen, anti-WARR is a common antibody. The antibody was found in the plasma of 5 of 166 random units collected in Oklahoma. The antibody was also present, and readily separable, in 26 of 47 sera containing multiple antibodies to low incidence antigens, in the collections of such antibodies in reference laboratories in Houston and Winnipeg. A total of 15 individuals with WARR+ red cells was found in the two related kindreds (those of the original propositus and his sister). Tests with the sera containing multiple antibodies to low incidence antigens against many of the 15 WARR+ samples were used to show that the same low incidence antigen was being detected, i.e. the reactive sera all contained anti-WARR.

In 1996, Jarolim et al. (173,250) reported that a C→T mutation in codon 522 leads to a threonine to isoleucine substitution at residue 552, in the third ectoplasmic loop of protein band 3, in individuals with WARR+ red cells. Thus like Wd^a and Rb^a, as described above, WARR was admitted to the Diego blood group system (174).

ELO, a Diego System Antigen

In 1979, the ELO+ red cells of the original proposita were recognized (219) as carrying a previously undescribed low incidence antigen. Over the next eleven years seven additional and unrelated propositi with ELO+ red cells were found and in 1990 an abstract (220) describing the antigen, was published. In 1993, a more complete report appeared (221). Of the then known eight persons with ELO+ red cells, the ancestry was described as: Anglo-Saxon in three; Belgian in one; Greek in one; Iranian in one; and as unknown in the two others. One of the propositi had been found in tests on 16,223 donors (ethnic mix not known) in North London. No ELO+ sample was found in tests on the red cells of 958 pregnant women in Manitoba. One ELO+ propositus in Manitoba was the husband of a woman who had produced anti-Wr^a but not anti-ELO. The ELO antigen was found (221) to survive treatment of red cells with papain, trypsin and 2-aminoethylisothiouronium bromide (AET) but was denatured or removed when red cells were treated with alpha-chymotrypsin. Plasma from a person with ELO+ red cells did not inhibit anti-ELO.

No example of anti-ELO was found in screening tests on the sera of 9024 donors in London, two examples were found in Manitoba during tests on the sera of 858 pregnant women. In tests on sera containing antibodies to other low incidence antigens (sera containing single

and multiple specificities were included) four examples of anti-ELO were found among 96 sera tested in London and two others (in addition to one found in the pregnant woman and mentioned above) among 29 samples tested in Manitoba.

In 1992, Ford et al. (222) described a case of mild HDN that seemed to have been caused by anti-ELO but in which jaundice due to prematurity could not be excluded. In 1993, Better et al. (223) reported that the same lady, with IgG3 anti-ELO in the serum, had been delivered of another child by caesarean section. Such delivery was undertaken because analysis of amniotic fluid at 35 weeks had indicated that the infant would be seriously affected with HDN. The infant had a positive DAT, anti-ELO was eluted from the cord blood red cells and a two volume exchange transfusion was performed seven hours after delivery of the child. The IAT titer of the maternal anti-ELO at the time of delivery was 2048, an IgM anti-ELO with a titer of 16 was also present. Red cells from the father of the infant were included in the study (221) on ELO and anti-ELO, described above.

In 1996, Coghlan et al. (227) reported that expression of the ELO antigen is controlled by the *AE1* (anion exchanger 1 or band 3) gene. Jarolim et al. (228) showed that in the wild type protein band 3 arginine is present at residue 432, when band 3 carries the ELO antigen, tryptophan occupies that position in the first ectoplasmic loop of the protein. Thus as shown in tables 17-1 and 17-6, the ELO antigen is now part of the Diego system (271).

The Antigens Wu (previously known as Hov and Haakestad) and NFLD, both Diego System Antigens and the Antigen BOW

In 1973, Szaloky et al. (199) described anti-Hov, an antibody to a low incidence antigen, present with anti-Fy^a in the serum of a woman who gave birth to twins, one of whom had HDN caused by the anti-Fy^a. In tests on 1155 donors in the Netherlands, two with Hov+ red cells were found. In tests on three families, 28 persons with Hov+ red cells were identified. The Hov antigen was fully developed at birth and survived enzyme treatment of red cells.

The first mention of the low incidence antigen Haakestad seems to be in the 1972 abstract (222) describing Mo^a (see below). Although no full report of Haakestad was ever published, the antigen was mentioned in a number of other papers (201-203) describing rare antigens.

The antigen Wu was described in its own right by Kornstad (201) in 1976 although its existence and even some information about it, had been mentioned earlier (204-206). In the 1976 publication (201) tests on more than 12,800 random donor samples in Norway and

England that yielded one Wu+ sample, are described. However, since different examples of anti-Wu, that varied in strength were used, the figures most often cited are those from tests using the most potent anti-Wu. Those tests identified one Wu+ sample in 7000 Norwegian and none in 1323 English donors. Additional Wu+ samples were found when compatibility tests yielded unexpected positive reactions and the 1976 paper (201) describes three families that among them had 18 persons with Wu+ red cells. Tests on 8813 donor sera yielded five examples of anti-Wu, four of them in sera that contained multiple antibodies to low incidence antigens. In 1980, Young et al. (207) reported the results of tests performed in South Australia. Four Wu+ bloods were found in tests on 16,476 samples for an incidence of about 1 in 4000, that is higher than the incidence of the antigen in Europeans. Using figures from unpublished data (204,205) the incidence of anti-Wu was 1 in 2400 sera; in the published report from Europe (201) it was 1 in 1763; in the Australian study (207) six examples of anti-Wu were found in tests on 4200 donor sera for an incidence of 1 in 700. However, of those six antibodies, four reacted only in an automated test system. Thus if manual test-active anti-Wu are considered the Australian figure of two examples in 4200 sera is the same as the European figures, i.e. 1 in 2100 (207) compared to 1 in 2400 (204,205) and 1 in 1763 (201). In sharp contrast, Broman (208) found 10 examples of anti-Wu in tests on samples from 700 Swedish donors.

The Wu antigen is apparently well developed at birth and survives papain treatment of red cells (201). The antigen has been found in at least one Black (208). One family was studied (209) in which the parents, who were second cousins, both had Wu+ red cells. Dosage studies suggested that the propositus, his non-identical twin brother, and his sister, were homozygous for *Wu*. All seven children of the apparent *Wu* homozygotes had Wu+ red cells. As described above, the Hov antigen was first identified in the Netherlands. In the family just described (209), both sets of grandparents of the propositus had come to the USA from the Netherlands.

In 1987, Kornstad et al. (210) published data that showed that the Haakestad and Hov antigens are the same thing. During the study, 4 of 2021 Danish blood donors were shown to have Hov+ red cells. Anti-Hov was found in 10 sera that contained antibodies to other low incidence antigens (including the famous examples Kirk, Blombley, Mess and Wilcox). Among them, the 10 sera were reported to contain at least 111 antibodies. However, that number must be reduced by eight since anti-Wu was identified in eight of the sera and, as described below, anti-Hov and anti-Wu define the same antigen.

In 1992, Moulds et al. (211) published data that showed that the Hov and Wu antigens are the same thing.

A total of 153 sera with multiple antibodies to low incidence antigens were tested. Twenty-two of the sera reacted with red cells previously shown to be either Hov+ or Wu+, 131 sera reacted with neither. Adsorption studies with cells previously typed as Hov+ or Wu+, confirmed that the same antibody was involved. In spite of the priority of the name Hov (and Haakestad although no paper describing that antigen in its own right was ever published), the name Wu has persisted for the antigen (196,213). Because several studies had been performed in different population groups, on the incidence of Hov, Haakestad and Wu before the antigens were shown to be the same thing, table 17-5, showing the incidence of Wu, can be constructed.

In 1984, Lewis et al. (214) described a new low incidence antigen, NFLD, present in a White family. The first example of anti-NFLD was found in the serum Mess that also contains antibodies to, at least, Ri^a, Fr^a, Hg^a, Jn^a, Sw^a, Tr^a, Vg^a, Wd^a, Wu, BOW, SHIN and SAT (210,215). Anti-NFLD was then identified in six of twelve other sera that contain multiple antibodies to low incidence antigens. The propositus with NFLD+ red cells was of French extraction, no other NFLD+ sample was found in tests on the red cells of 1125 random Whites, 500 Hutterites, 111 Cree Indians and 30 unrelated Canadians of Japanese ancestry. The NFLD antigen was not denatured when red cells were treated with 2-aminoethyliosthiouronium bromide (AET).

In 1988, Okubo et al. (216) found the NFLD antigen in the Japanese population. In screening tests on 45,825 donor samples with anti-Os^a, two were found to react, but were shown to be Os(a-) when tested with other examples of anti-Os^a. In tests on those red cells, using 33 sera containing multiple antibodies to low incidence antigens, 22 known to contain anti-NFLD gave positive reactions, 11 known not to contain anti-NFLD were nonreactive. Adsorption-elution tests confirmed that the two samples were NFLD+ and that the initially used anti-Os^a also contained anti-NFLD. In tests on 153,387 serum samples from blood donors in Osaka, Fukuoka, Ohita and Miyagi, 67 examples of anti-NFLD were found, i.e. an incidence of 1 in 2289. Unlike most of the other sera that contain anti-NFLD, many of these examples did not have multispecific activity for rare antigens. An NFLD-Japanese lady who delivered three children with NFLD+ red cells, did not make anti-NFLD (216).

In 1988, Chaves et al. (217) described the first example of anti-BOW in a serum that also contained anti-Reiter (see Chapter 32). A total of 65 other sera containing antibodies to low incidence antigens (not all of which were multispecific) were tested against BOW+ red cells and 16, all of which contained multiple specificities, were found to contain anti-BOW. The first example of BOW+ red cells was found following an unexpected positive

TABLE 17-5 Incidence of the Wu Antigen in Different Population Groups

Name of antibody at time tests were performed	Country of individuals tested	Number tested	Number Wu+	Incidence Wu+	References	Year reported
Anti-Wu	Norway	1511	0		205	1967
Anti-Hov	Netherlands	1155	2	1 in 577	199	1973
Anti-Wu	Norway	7000	1*	1 in 7000	201	1976
Anti-Wu	England	1323	0*		201	1976
Anti-Wu	Norway	4477	0*		201	1976
Anti-Wu	Australia	16,476	4	1 in 4119	207	1980
Anti-Wu	Norway	7151	1	1 in 7151	163	1986
Anti-Hov/Wu	Denmark	2021	4	1 in 505	210	1987

*   See text for division of 12,800 donors tested

reaction in a compatibility test. A second example from an unrelated individual was found when an anti-Wr^a reagent that also contained anti-BOW was used. In tests on papain-treated red cells from more than 50,000 donors, no other example of BOW+ red cells was found. The BOW antigen was shown (217) to survive treatment of red cells with papain, ficin, trypsin, chloroquine diphosphate, dithiothreitol (DTT) and 2-aminoethylisothiouronium bromide (AET). However, the antigen was denatured when the BOW+ red cells were treated with alpha-chymotrypsin or pronase.

In 1991, Kaita et al. (218) described a serological relationship among Wu, NFLD and BOW; this relationship is, of course, the reason that the descriptions of NFLD and BOW are included in this section. Although specific antibodies exist that react with either Wu+ or NFLD+ or BOW+ red cells, adsorption studies show that red cells with any one of the three antigens will remove activity for all three antigens from sera that, before adsorption, react with red cells carrying any one of the antigens. In the experiments described (218) the cross-reactivity of antibodies to Wu, NFLD and BOW, did not extend to Wd^a and Sw^a, two other antigens described in this chapter. That is to say when a serum that, unadsorbed, reacted with Wu+ or NFLD+ or BOW+ or Wd(a+) or Sw(a+) red cells was adsorbed with Wd(a+) or Sw(a+) red cells, activity for Wd(a+) or Sw(a+) red cells, respectively was removed, activity for Wu+ or NFLD+ or BOW+ red cells was not. While not mentioned in the paper (218) it is noticeable that the red cells used to control the experiments of antibody crossreactivity, carried low incidence antigens (Wd^a and Sw^a) that have also now found their way into this chapter on the Diego system. One wonders if the authors already suspected that this state of affairs might eventually come to pass.

In 1996 Coghlan et al. (227) showed that production of Wu is controlled from the *AE1* (band 3) locus and Jarolim et al. (228) showed that the Wu antigen represents replacement of glycine at position 565 in the wild type band 3, with alanine at that position on Wu+ red cells. Thus like Wd^a, Rb^a, WARR and ELO, Wu was recognized as a Diego system antigen (271). At the time that Wu was recognized as a member of the Diego system, NFLD and BOW appeared to be associated only through their serological relationship to Wu, that is described above. Since that time, convincing evidence that NFLD is a Diego system antigen has been obtained. Zelinski et al. (275) have shown that the glutamic acid residue at position 429 in wild type protein band 3 is replaced by aspartic acid at that position when the protein carries the NFLD antigen. Presumably more news about BOW will be forthcoming. As shown in table 17-6, Wu is on the third and NFLD on the first external loop of band 3.

Bp^a, a Diego System Antigen

When Cleghorn (94) found that the famous serum Gu, that came from a patient with "warm" antibody-induced hemolytic anemia (WAIHA) and that was already known to contain at least antibodies to the low incidence antigens Wr^a, By, Mg, Mi^a, Tr^a and Sw^a, also contained an antibody defining a previously unreported rare antigen, he named the new specificity anti-Bp^a. Two other examples of anti-Bp^a were found in the sera of patients with WAIHA and two more in tests on 2796 normal sera. Anti-Bp^a occurs in sera that contain multiple antibodies to low incidence antigens and is present in the famous Tillett, D'Ar and Wilcox sera that have been mentioned above.

In tests on samples from 75,000 blood donors in England, only one Bp(a+) sample was found (94). No Bp(a+) blood was found in tests on samples from 42 Tibetans (87). In 1974, Kornstad (206) reported that no Bp(a+) sample was found in tests on 7000 Norwegian donors. In a 1996 publication, Kornstad (163) mentions that no Bp(a+) sample was found among 7151 Norwegians. We do not know, but presume that this makes the score, no Bp(a+) among 14,151 Norwegians.

In 1996, Jarolim et al. (228) showed that a nucleotide substitution (ACA to AAA) in band 3 cDNA forecasts an asparagine 569 change to lysine in the change from wild type to Bp(a+) band 3 in the third external loop of that protein.

Mo^a, a Diego System Antigen

Kornstad and Brocteur (200) found the first example of anti-Mo^a in a serum being used to screen random donors for presence of the low incidence antigen Jn^a. Five sera that contained other antibodies to low incidence antigens were shown also to contain anti-Mo^a. In screening tests on the sera of 5010 donors in Oslo, Norway, one further example of anti-Mo^a was found. The Mo^a antigen was found in two of 9793 Belgians but in none of 9000 Norwegians.

In 1996, Jarolim et al. (228) reported that a CGT to CAT nucleotide substitution in band 3 cDNA forecasts an arginine 656 change to histidine in the change from wild type to Mo(a+) band 3 in the fourth external loop of that protein.

Hg^a, a Diego System Antigen

In 1983, Rowe and Hammond (226) described a serum that contained benign auto-anti-e reactive only against enzyme-treated red cells (the DAT on the patient's red cells was negative) and alloantibodies to Pt^a, Wd^a and BOW. An additional antibody that was IgM in nature and was directed against a low incidence antigen was detected in the serum and was named anti-Hg^a. In tests on the red cells of 5434 group O, but otherwise unselected Welsh donors, two additional Hg(a+) samples were found. No example of anti-Hg^a was found in the sera of 6580 random donors but the antibody was present in 18 sera (including the famous examples Troll, Wilcox, Binge, Miles, Blomley and S2117 that among them and including anti-Hg^a, contain at least 57 antibodies) that contain antibodies to other low incidence antigens. It was reported (226) that Hg^a was removed or denatured when red cells were treated with enzymes (specific enzymes not named in the paper but papain

was used in other studies described) and that the antigen was fully developed on cord blood red cells. During the investigation it was shown that the low incidence antigen, Tarp or Tarplee that was mentioned by Young (224) and in the third edition of this book, is the same as Hg^a.

In 1996, Jarolim et al. (228) reported that a CGT to TGT nucleotide substitution in band 3 cDNA forecasts an arginine 656 change to cysteine in the change from wild type to Hg(a+) band 3. It will be noticed from the descriptions of Mo^a and Hg^a that the mutations giving rise to those antigens occur in the same place. In the wild type band 3 the amino acid at position 656 is arginine, when Mo^a is present it is histidine, when Hg^a is present it is cysteine. One of us (PDI) finally understands what Dr. Hal Allen told him in 1964 when he said that two very rare antigens could be the products of alleles. As shown in table 17-6, Mo^a and Hg^a differ from most of the other low incidence antigens described in this section in that they are carried on the fourth external loop of protein band 3.

Vg^a, a Diego System Antigen

The antibody defining Vg^a was reported in 1981 by Young (224). It was present in a serum known to contain anti-Wu. Anti-Vg^a is also present in other sera (including the famous examples Tillett, Wilcox and Kirk that among them and including anti-Vg^a, contain at least 66 antibodies) that contain antibodies to many low incidence antigens. In screening tests using an automated method, 11 examples of anti-Vg^a were found among 1669 donor sera. Eight of the 11 antibodies reacted by manual methods and five of them were found also to contain anti-Wr^a. In tests on the red cells of 17,209 random donors in South Australia, only one Vg(a+) sample was found. The Vg^a antigen was said to survive enzyme treatment of red cells, the enzyme(s) used was (were) not specified.

In 1996, Jarolim et al. (228) reported that a TAC to CAC nucleotide substitution in band 3 cDNA forecasts a tyrosine 555 change to histidine in the change from wild type to Vg(a+) band 3 in the third external loop of that protein.

Tr^a, a Diego System Antigen

Cleghorn (94) found anti-Tr^a to be present in 12 of 18 sera that contained anti-Wr^a. In each instance the antibodies could be separated by differential adsorption. In tests on sera from 700 normal donors, one example of anti-Tr^a was found (94). Tests on samples from 38,069 random English donors revealed two with Tr(a+) red cells. No Tr(a+) sample was found on the red cells of 9500 Norwegians (205). An antigen that has been called

Lanthois in some publications, is the same as Tr^a.

In 1997, Jarolim et al. (247) published data to the effect that the lysine residue at position 551 of wild type protein band 3 is replaced by asparagine when the protein carries Tr^a in the third external loop of that protein.

Sw^a, a Diego System Antigen and the Apparently Related Antigen SW1

In 1959, Cleghorn (180) described the first example of anti-Sw^a. The antigen it detects is rare. By combining the results of five surveys (78,79,94,112,180) it is seen that 10 Sw(a+) samples were found in tests on 73,071 English donors for an incidence of about 1 in 7300. In a study in Switzerland (181), three Sw(a+) samples were found among about 7000 donors. Anti-Sw^a is frequently present in sera that contain antibodies to other low incidence antigens. The original anti-Sw^a was found (180) in the serum Guppy that has been shown (94,182) to contain, at least, antibodies to Wr^a, By, M^g, Mi^a, Tr^a, Bp^a and Sw^a.

At one time, family data (182,183) apparently showing linkage between *Sw^a* and the *Sese* and/or *Lutheran* loci, raised the possibility that Sw^a might be a Lutheran system antigen. *Sese* and *Lutheran* had long been known (184-189) to be linked, recent data (190-193) have confirmed that linkage. Naturally it was hoped that Sw^a might prove to be a low incidence antithetical partner to one of the high incidence Lutheran antigens (see Chapter 20). However, this hope was not realized. First, Metaxas and Metaxas-Bühler (181) found a family in which *Sw^a* segregated independently of the *Lutheran* locus. Second, Judd et al. (194) showed that the apparent Sw^a-Lutheran system association had occurred because of the presence of both the low incidence antigens Sw^a and Lu14, on the red cells of one of the critical family's members. Third, Lewis et al. (197) studied a large family that reduced the mathematical probability that *Sw^a* and *Lutheran* are linked.

In 1987, Contreras et al. (195) published data that showed heterogeneity among anti-Sw^a and documented the existence of a second antigen, related to Sw^a. It was found that some Sw(a+) red cells reacted with all examples of anti-Sw^a, while others reacted with only some of those sera. The difference was shown to be qualitative not quantitative. The red cells that reacted with all examples of anti-Sw^a were said to carry two antigens, Sw^a and SW1. Those that reacted with only some anti-Sw^a were said to carry Sw^a but to lack SW1. Since Sw^a already had an ISBT number, 700004, the second antigen, SW1, was allocated (196) the number 700041. Thus in some publications, the term 700:4,41 indicates the phenotype Sw(a+) SW:1. The term 700:4,-41 indicates the pheno-

type Sw(a+) SW:-1. Sw(a-) red cells carrying the SW1 antigen have not been found, all anti-Sw^a react with Sw(a+) red cells. Family studies showed that Sw^a and SW1 are encoded from the same locus or from very closely linked loci. In different families the Sw(a+) SW:1 and Sw(a+) SW:-1 phenotypes were inherited in a normal fashion. That is to say in families in which the phenotype was Sw(a+) SW:1, all persons with Sw(a+) red cells were of that phenotype. In families in which the phenotype was Sw(a+) SW:-1, all persons with Sw(a+) red cells were of that phenotype. These findings, of course, confirmed that the difference between Sw^a and SW1 is qualitative not quantitative. However, those anti-Sw^a that react with both Sw(a+) SW:1 and Sw(a+) SW:-1 red cells cannot be split, by adsorption, into separable anti- Sw^a and anti-SW1 components. Instead, red cells of both Sw(a+) phenotypes (i.e. Sw(a+) SW:1 and Sw(a+) SW:-1) adsorb the antibodies to exhaustion.

At the serological level, a relationship between Sw^a, SW1 and the low incidence antigen Fr^a (see a later section) has been found (195). Both Sw(a+) SW:1 and Sw(a+) SW:-1 red cells will adsorb both anti-Sw^a and anti-Fr^a from sera that contain the two antibodies. In contrast, Sw(a-), Fr(a+) red cells adsorb anti-Fr^a but not anti-Sw^a, for either type of Sw(a+) red cells, from those sera. This shows, of course, that Sw^a and Fr^a are not the same antigen. Further, as described in the later section, anti-Fr^a that do not contain anti-Sw^a have been found (176-178).

In 1995 Coghlan et al. (179) and in 1996 Zelinski et al. (249) published data that showed that production of Sw^a (and Fr^a, see below) is controlled from a locus on chromosome 17q. Although the data were highly suggestive that Sw^a is a Diego system antigen, they were short of absolute proof. Such proof was provided in 1997 when Zelinski et al. (276) reported that a G to A mutation in *AE1* (the band 3 gene) forecasts a change from arginine 646 in wild type band 3 to glutamine in the fourth external loop of band 3 that expresses Sw^a.

Jn^a, a Diego System Antigen

When Kornstad et al. (269) found a new antibody that they named anti-Jn^a, in a serum containing anti-Wr^a and anti-Bp^a, they used Jn(a+), Wr(a-), Bp(a-) red cells to test other sera that contain antibodies to low incidence antigens. They found two more examples of anti-Jn^a, one in a serum that contained antibodies to Wr^a, Bp^a and C^w and the second in a serum that contained antibodies to Wr^a and St^a. No Jn(a+) sample was found in tests on the red cells of 13,824 random Norwegian donors (163,210,269). It was reported (269) that anti-Jn^a gives enhanced reactions with Jn(a+) red cells treated with some proteases but it is now known that Jn^a is no longer detectable on red cells treated with alpha-chymotrypsin (268).

In 1997 Poole et al. (268) described studies on samples from three unrelated individuals with Jn(a+) red cells. In two of them a nucleotide substitution forecast that Pro556 of wild type band 3 would be replaced by Ser in band 3 from Jn(a+) persons. In the third person with Jn(a+) red cells the forecast change was Pro556 to Ala. It was shown (268) that Jn^a could be subdivided serologically as well as by recognition of the amino acid change. Thus the Pro556Ser change was said to represent Jn^a while Pro556Ala was said to represent a subtype of Jn^a (268). As can be seen from table 17-6 a similar situation applies at position 656. An Arg656Cys change accounts for Hg^a while an Arg656His change explains Mo^a (228). That Hg^a and Mo^a have different names represents the fact that each was recognized by an antibody, and hence given a name, before the biochemical basis of the polymorphisms was established. No doubt had the Pro556Ser and Pro556Ala changes been differentiated at the serological level before being detected at the biochemical level, Jn^a and the other change, if it is immunogenic, would have separate names. It is, of course, entirely likely that antibodies to the two changed structures exist in the same sera. Thirteen sera containing antibodies to multiple low incidence antigens reacted with red cells in which the change was Pro556Ser or Pro556Ala, one reacted with red cells representing the Pro556Ser but not with those representing the Pro556Ala change (see also the addendum).

Fr^a, Probably a Diego System Antigen

In 1978, Lewis et al. (175) reported studies on a serum from a male Mexican patient that contained antibodies to the low incidence antigens Mit, Wr^a and Rb^a. The serum reacted strongly with a Mit-, Wr(a-), Rb(a-) sample, thus showing that it contained yet another antibody to a low incidence antigen. The new antibody was called anti-Fr^a, the Mit-, Wr(a-), Rb(a-), Fr(a+) red cells that allowed recognition of anti-Fr^a were from the matriarch of a large Mennonite kindred. In the initial study red cells from 415 unrelated individuals were tested, no other Fr(a+) sample was found. In extension studies (176,177) 650 unrelated individuals (parents in families being studied for other genetic markers) and 1400 Manitoba Red Cross blood donors were tested, one Fr(a+) sample was found in each group. Both persons with Fr(a+) red cells were Mennonite, but were not known to be related. In 1983, Harris et al. (178) described a White woman with anti-Fr^a in her serum. Her husband and their second, fourth and sixth children had Fr(a+) red cells. The fourth and the sixth children had a positive DAT at birth but neither suffered from clinical HDN.

As mentioned in the previous section, the antigen Fr^a is somehow related to the antigen Sw^a. Both Sw(a+) SW:1 and Sw(a+) SW:-1 red cells will adsorb anti-Sw^a and anti-Fr^a from sera that contain both antibodies. Fr(a+) red cells will adsorb anti-Fr^a but not anti-Sw^a, from such sera.

In 1996, Zelinski et al. (249) reported that the gene that encodes production of Fr^a is located on chromosome 17q. The odds in favor of *Fr^a* being at the *AE1* locus were calculated as being 10^6:1. In view of all the other low incidence antigens described in this chapter that have been shown to be part of the Diego system, it seems virtually certain, though not yet formally proved, that Fr^a is also a Diego system antigen.

A Summary About Low Incidence Antigens in the Diego System

When this chapter was first drafted, the low incidence antigens Di^a, Wr^a, Wd^a, Rb^a and WARR were known to be part of the Diego system. While it was suspected that some other rare antigens belonged within the system, formal proof of such suspicions was absent. By the time some of the rest of the book had been written such proof was available. A year after it had first been drafted this chapter had to be revised to list ELO, Wu, Bp^a, Mo^a, Hg^a, Vg^a, Tr^a, Sw^a, NFLD and Jn^a as proved members of the Diego system and Fr^a, SW1 and BOW as probable members.

As will be apparent, there are a number of ways in which the presence of an antigen on protein band 3 can be established or anticipated. First, as described, presence of a different to wild type amino acid at a particular position on the protein. Second, nucleotide substitutions in *AE1* from persons with the antigen involved can be used to forecast which amino acid will be encoded by the substituted codon and at which position in the protein. While this method is less certain than amino acid sequencing, when the same nucleotide substitution is seen in two or more unrelated individuals with the same rare antigen, the chance that the substitution correlates with antigen production is greatly increased. Third, linkage or identity between the gene encoding the rare antigen and *AE1* can be used to show that the antigen involved is encoded from the *Diego* locus. Having listed which antigens are and which probably are, members of the Diego system, it can be said that table 17-1 lists all the antigens discussed and shows which have ISBT numbers (174,271), table 17-3 lists the usual characteristics of the definitive antibodies, table 17-6 summarizes the evidence that the antigens belong to the Diego system or the indications that show that is probably the case, table 17-7 lists frequencies of some of the antigens while figure 17-1 indicates the supposed location of a few of the antigens on band 3. For the sake of clarity, figure 17-1 shows examples of positions on band 3 at which amino acid substitutions represent antigens. By using table 17-6 (amino acid residue and external loop involved) in conjunction with figure 17-1, location of each of the Diego system antigens can be recognized.

It is very highly probable that by the time this book is printed, this chapter and the tables listed above will be out of date. The reader is invited to the addendum to see if additional low incidence antigens joined the Diego system before this book went to the printer.

Antigens of the Diego Blood Group System are Carried on the Red Cell Anion Transporter Protein (Band 3, syn AE1)

There are about one million molecules of band 3 in the red cell membrane (44). Only glycophorin A (GPA) is expressed at similar levels. Both band 3 and GPA have been extensively studied for several decades but whereas GPA was known as the MN glycoprotein (238) long before the name glycophorin was coined by membrane biochemists (239) the association of blood group antigens with band 3 did not occur until 1992. A blood sample from an elderly male patient of Polish origin was referred from Manchester, U.K. to the International Blood Group Reference Laboratory in Bristol and found to have the phenotype Di(a+b-). This phenotype is extraordinarily rare in Whites (although not in South-East Poland) (28 and see earlier) and so the membranes from these cells were subjected to a routine analysis by SDS-PAGE to see if there was anything unusual about the pattern of protein staining bands. Remarkably, the protein staining band corresponding to band 3 had a slower electrophoretic mobility than the corresponding band in control cells. There are two well established reasons for such a pattern, increased glycosylation as occurs in red cells of the En(a-) phenotype and in red cells of persons homozygous for the M^k gene (see Chapter 15) and presence of the band 3 variant known as Memphis (240). Band 3 Memphis results from a single nucleotide mutation in the band 3 gene which causes a single amino acid change (Lys56 to Glu) in the N-terminal cytoplasmic domain of the protein (241,242). The Memphis variant is easily identified because if red cells treated with pronase or chymotrypsin are subjected to SDS-PAGE and stained for protein, the band 3 fragment containing the Memphis mutation has an apparent molecular weight of 63,000 whereas the corresponding fragment from band 3 lacking the Memphis change has an apparent molecular weight of 60,000. When red cells from the Di(a+b-) patient were pronase-treated and subjected to SDS-PAGE it was clear

that the patient was homozygous for the Memphis variant (a single band of 63,000 was observed). The Memphis variant is not uncommon in some populations (25% in American Indians, 15% in African Americans, 29% in Japanese) (243, 244) and the Di^a antigen is common in American Indians and Japanese though not in African Americans (see earlier sections). Thus the question was raised as to whether or not the occurrence of homozygosity for band 3 Memphis and the Di(a+b-) phenotype was purely coincidental or indicative of a relationship between band 3 Memphis and the Di^a antigen. A further six Di(a+b-) samples from unrelated donors were homozygous for band 3 Memphis and 11 samples of Di(a+b+) red cells were heterozygous for band 3 Memphis. However, 7 of 37 Di(a-b+) samples were also heterozygous for band 3 Memphis (30). Clearly, band 3 Memphis is not always associated with the Di^a antigen and in any case, it was difficult to see how a mutation in the N-terminal cytoplasmic domain (see figure 17-1) could influence the expression of an antigen on the outer surface of the red cell. However, Hsu and Morrison (245) showed that there are two types of band 3 Memphis and that these could be distinguished by covalently labeling red cells with 4,4'-di-isothiocyanato-1,2-diphenylethane-2,2'disulphonic acid (H$_2$DIDS) because variant 2 was much more readily labeled with H$_2$DIDS than variant 1. When red cells of known Diego phenotype were labeled with (^{3}H)-H$_2$DIDS the results clearly showed that the presence of Di^a antigen correlated with Memphis variant 2 and that it was therefore extremely likely that the Di^a antigen was carried on band 3 in these cells (30). When the entire coding sequence of band 3 from a Mexican-American with the Di(a+b-) phenotype was elucidated, a homozygous mutation at nucleotide 2561 (C to T) was found (in addition to the band 3 Memphis mutation) which would change amino acid Pro854 to Leu (31). Exactly the same change was found in Di(a+) donors from Japan and Brazil (31).

Subsequent studies by Jarolim et al. (167,198) confirmed the correlation between the presence of Di^a and Pro854 to Leu in 11 North American Choctaw Indians and four South American Indians. These authors also found examples (in two White families from the USA and Czech Republic respectively) of the Di(a+b-) phenotype resulting from heterozygosity for the Pro854 to Leu mutation and a mutation in the other band 3 allele that prevented expression of that allele in the plasma membrane, and evidence for heterozygous expression of the Pro854-Leu mutation in two Mexicans with the Di(a+b-) phenotype where the other band 3 allele was expressed. One of us (DJA) has also seen a Mexican Di(a+b-) of this type. The mechanism which abrogates expression of Di^b in these individuals is, as yet, unexplained.

TABLE 17-6 Findings that Show that Antigens are or may be Part of the Diego Blood Group System

Antigen	Observations	Located on Band 3 Ectoplasmic Loop Number	References
Di^a (DI1)	Leucine at position 854	7	31
Di^b (DI2)	Proline at position 854	7	31
Wr^a (DI3)	Lysine at position 658	4	41
Wr^b (DI4)	Glutamic acid at position 658[*1]	4	41
Wd^a (DI5)	Methionine in Wd(a+) replaces valine in Wd(a-) at position 557	3	166, 167
Rb^a (DI6)	Leucine in Rb(a+) replaces proline in Rb(a-) at position 548	3	167
WARR (DI7)	Isoleucine in WARR+ replaces threonine in WARR- at position 552	3	173
ELO (DI8)	CGG to TGG nucleotide substitution forecasts tryptophan in ELO+ replacing arginine in ELO- at position 432	1	227, 228
Wu (DI9)	GGC to GCC nucleotide substitution forecasts alanine in Wu+ replacing glycine in Wu- at position 565	3	227, 228
Bp^a (DI10)	ACA to AAA nucleotide substitution forecasts lysine in Bp(a+) replacing asparagine in Bp(a-) at position 569	3	228
Mo^a (DI11)	CGT to CAT nucleotide substitution forecasts histidine in Mo(a+) replacing arginine in Mo(a-) at position 656[*2]	4	228
Hg^a (DI12)	CGT to TGT nucleotide substitution forecasts cysteine in Hg(a+) replacing arginine in Hg(a-) at position 656[*2]	4	228
Vg^a (DI13)	TAC to CAC nucleotide substitution forecasts histidine in Vg(a+) replacing tyrosine in Vg(a-) at position 555	3	228
Tr^a	AAG to AAC nucleotide substitution forecasts asparagine in Tr(a+) replacing lysine in Tr(a-) at position 551	3	247
Sw^a	G to A nucleotide substitution forecasts glutamine in Sw(a+) replacing arginine in Sw(a-) at position 646	4	179, 249, 253
NFLD	Nucleotide substitution forecasts aspartic acid in NFLD+ replacing glutamic acid at position 429	1	252
Jn^a	C to T nucleotide substitution forecasts serine in Jn(a+) replacing proline in Jn(a-) at position 566 in two Jn(a+) donors. In a third a C to G substitution forecasts alanine replacing proline at postion 566. If serine at 566 represents Jn^a, presumably alanine at that position represents a different antigen (see addendem).	3	268
BOW	Serological association with Wu, see text		218
Fr^a	Encoding gene at or very tightly linked to *AE1*. Antigen has serological association with Sw^a, see text		179, 195, 249
SW1	Serological association with Sw^a and Fr^a, see text		195

[*1] Also requires a portion of wild type glycophorin A, see text.
[*2] The nucleotide substitutions that purportedly lead to genes encoding production of Hg^a or Mo^a, occur in the same codon. For additional Diego system antigens see Chapter 46, the Addendum.

TABLE 17-7 Some Studies of the Frequency of Low Incidence Diego System (and related) Antigens and the Antibodies that Define Them

Antigen	Number Red Cell Samples Tested	Population	Number Positive	Refs	Antibody	Number Sera Tested[*1]	Population	Number Abs Found	Refs
Di^a		See TABLE 17-2							
Wr^a	circa 86,000	Whites	63	See text	Anti-Wr^a	Incidence around 1 in 100 sera			see text
	circa 8,000	Blacks	0	See text					
Wd^a	4000	N. American Whites	0	162	Anti-Wd^a	358	N. American Whites	1	162
	7151	Norwegians	0	163					
Rb^a	13500	English	2	168	Anti-Rb^a	6200	English	6	168
WARR	8275	Mixed Canadians (circa 6500 White)	1[*2]	172		166	N. American Whites	5	172
Sw^a	73,071	English	10	See text					
	7000	Swiss	3	181					
Sw1	Less frequent than Sw^a, see text								
Fr^a	2465	Mixed Canadians	2	175-177					
Wu		See TABLE 17-5			Anti-Wu	8813	Norwegian and English	5	201
						4200	Australian	6[*3]	207
						700	Swedes	10	208
NFLD	1776	Canadians (mixed ancestry)	0	214	Anti-NFLD	153,387	Japanese	67	216
	45,825	Japanese	2	216					
BOW	50,000	Mixed English	0	217					
ELO	16,223	Mixed English	1	221	Anti-ELO	9024	Mixed English	0	221
	958	Canadian	0	221		858	Canadian[*4]	2	221
Vg^a	17,209	Australian	1	224	Anti-Vg^a	1669	Australian	11[*5]	224
Bp^a	75,000	English	1	94	Anti-Bp^a	2796	English	2	94
	14,151	Norwegians	0	163, 206					
Hg^a	5434	Welsh	2	226	Anti-Hg^a	6580	Welsh	0	226
Mo^a	9793	Belgians	2	200	Anti-Mo^a	5010	Norwegians	1	200
	9000	Norwegians	0	200					
Tr^a	38,069	English	2	94	Anti-Tr^a	700	English	1	94
	9500	Norwegians	0	205					
Jn^a	13,824	Norwegians	0	163, 210					

[*1] Random sera, those known to contain antibodies to other low incidence antigens, not included.
[*2] Later found to be sister of the propositus with WARR+ red cells.
[*3] Four of the six antibodies reacted only in an automated system.
[*4] Pregnant women.
[*5] All detected in an automated system, eight of the 11 also reacted in manual tests.

Other Blood Group Antigens on Band 3

As discussed above there are many antigens of low frequency that belong to the Diego blood group system. Classical methods of linkage analysis through family studies are not feasible when low frequency antigens occur in populations lacking the Di^a antigen. However, once the Diego system antigens were assigned to band 3 a relatively straightforward method became available. The structure of the band 3 gene is known (44). It comprises 20 exons and spans18kb on chromosome 17q12-q21 (98). In 1995 Bruce et al. (166) showed that Wd^a is

FIGURE 17-1 Location of Some Blood Group Antigens on the Anion Transport Protein Band 3

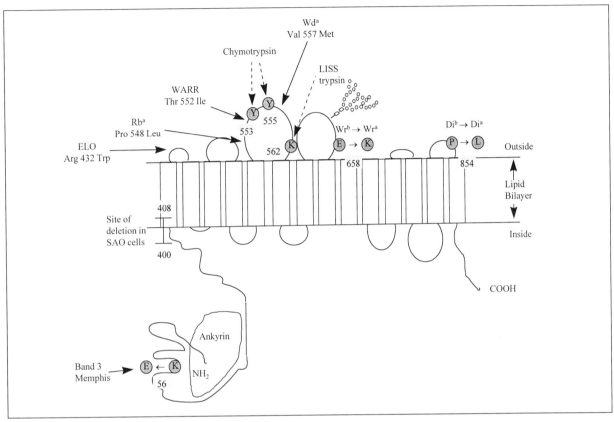

encoded by the band 3 gene (table 17-6). By using intronic primers spanning exons 11 to 20 of the band 3 gene (the entire membrane domain), screening the amplified product of each exon for single strand conformational polymorphisms (SSCPs) and determining the nucleotide sequence of any exons showing SSCPs, Petr Jarolim in Boston, has set up something of a production line for assigning low frequency antigens to the Diego system (167,173,228,247,250). At the time of writing, single nucleotide changes in the band 3 gene which change a single amino acid in the membrane domain appear to account for the Wd[a], Rb[a], WARR, ELO, Wu, Bp[a], Mo[a], Hg[a], Vg[a], Tr[a], Sw[a], NFLD and Jn[a] antigens (166,167,173,227,228,247-250,252,253,268). The relevant nucleotide substitutions and their corresponding amino acid changes are summarized in table 17-6. The position of some of these critical residues on the predicted topology of the band 3 protein are shown in figure 17-1. Two antigens, ELO and NFLD are defined by the sequence of extracellular loop 1, eight, Wd[a], Rb[a], WARR, Wu, Bp[a], Vg[a], Tr[a] and Jn[a] by the extracellular sequence of loop 3, four, Wr[a], Mo[a], Hg[a] and Sw[a] by that of loop 4, and one, Di[a], by that of loop 7. It is not certain if or how much of loops 5 and 6 extend above the red cell membrane. If a Diego system antigen was located to

such a position it would indicate that at least one residue is extracellular. However, as shown in figure 17-1, no such finding has yet been made.

A series of rodent monoclonal antibodies raised to the extracellular domain of band 3 by immunization with intact red cells appeared to recognize epitopes on the third extracellular loop (274). The epitopes recognized by these antibodies fell into two groups by virtue of their different susceptibilities to proteases. One group was very susceptible to chymotrypsin treatment while the other group failed to react with red cells treated sequentially with chymotrypsin and trypsin under low ionic strength conditions (274). Chymotrypsin treatment of intact red cells cleaves the membrane domain of band 3 after Tyr553 and Tyr555 (251,273). Pronase also cleaves in this region whereas trypsin under low ionic strength conditions cleaves after Lys562 (252). None of the monoclonal antibodies was reactive with pronase-treated cells. All these protease cleavage sites are on the third extracellular loop (see figure 17-1). Quantitative binding studies using these monoclonal antibodies showed that the number of molecules bound to Wd(a-) cells was twice that bound to Wd(a+) cells (Spring, Gardner, Anstee, unpublished) and since Wd[a] is located on the third loop of band 3 these results provide further evidence for location of the relevant epitopes on the third loop and a critical role for Val557 which in Wd(a+) cells is methionine. By analogy, it might be anticipated that the blood group antigens located on loop three would differ from antigens assigned to other loops by being susceptible to protease treatment and in particular, chymotrypsin. However, ELO (loop 1) is reported to be chymotrypsin-sensitive. Inspection of the amino acid substitution which gives rise to ELO shows that it results when Arg432 is converted to Trp. It may be that this Trp creates a novel chymotrypsin cleavage site on loop 1 (chymotrypsin cleaves at Phe, Trp or Tyr).

The Wr[b] Antigen is Formed by the Interaction of Band 3 and Glycophorin A (GPA)

The historical development of our understanding of the relationship between Wr[a], Wr[b], band 3 and GPA has been described in detail above. Early biochemical studies had shown that the Wr[b] antigen was dependent on the presence of GPA in the red cell membrane and yet family studies clearly demonstrated that the Wr[a] antigen segregates independently from the M and N blood group antigens which are located on GPA. These results suggested that the antigens were defined by a membrane component which required interaction with GPA in order to create the structure recognized by anti-Wr[b]. Band 3 is the only red cell membrane protein present at the same level of abundance as GPA and seemed a good candidate for such a role (38). There are several different experiments which suggest that the two molecules are associated in the membrane. Antibodies to GPA reduce the rotational mobility of band 3 in red cell membranes (253). Band 3 in red cells which lack GPA (En(a-) and those from M^k homozygotes) has a larger N-glycan than cells with a normal GPA content (136,138,272). Band 3 in red cells which effectively have more GPA than normal (Dantu, St(a+) (38,255)) has a smaller N-glycan than in cells with a normal GPA content. These results suggest that the two proteins interact during their biosynthesis (38). Monoclonal antibodies to GPA were shown to immunoprecipitate just GPA, those to band 3 just band 3, while monoclonal anti-Wr[b] were seen to precipitate both band 3 and GPA (41,146,148). Direct evidence that GPA accelerates the movement of newly synthesized band 3 to the plasma membrane was obtained by Groves and Tanner (256) who expressed band 3 with and without GPA in *Xenopus* oocytes. Bruce et al. (41) settled the matter by determining the nucleotide sequence encoding band 3 from donor MF Wr(a+b-) and several individuals of the Wr(a+b+) phenotype. In every case the presence of Wr[a] antigen corresponded with a single nucleotide sub-

stitution G1972 to A which results in a change of amino acid Glu658 to Lys. Residue 658 is close to Asn642, the site of the N-glycan, on the fourth extracellular loop of band 3 (see figure 17-1). That a lysine is the critical residue for Wr[a] antigenic activity is consistent with earlier experiments which showed that reagents which block free amino groups on proteins destroy Wr[a] activity but have no effect on the Wr[b] antigen (257). The change of Glu658 for Lys involves the replacement of a negatively charged amino acid with a positively charged residue. It is not clear whether such a major charge difference abolishes the association of Wr[a]-bearing band 3 with GPA. Anti-Wr[b] are extremely effective in rigidifying red cell membranes (258-260) but similar experiments with anti-Wr[a] have not been reported. Some indirect evidence suggesting that the interaction between band 3 and GPA in Wr(a+b-) red cells differs from that in Wr(a-b+) cells was obtained by Paulitschke et al. (261) who observed that the monoclonal anti-GPA, R18 was much less effective in rigidifying Wr(a+b-) cells than rigidifying Wr(a+b+) or Wr(a-b+) cells. This experiment could be interpreted as providing evidence that R18 rigidifies Wr(b+) cells through interaction with band 3 and thereby with the red cell skeleton and that the alteration Glu658 to Lys disrupts this interaction. However, when these authors carried out the same experiment using another monoclonal anti-GPA, R10, Wr(a+b-) red cells were rigidified at a comparable level to Wr(a-b+) cells suggesting that cells either can be rigidified through a GPA/band 3 interaction which is independent of the Wr[a]/Wr[b] antigens or that rigidification can occur directly through the cytoplasmic domain of GPA and the red cell skeleton.

Immunoprecipitation studies with monoclonal anti-Wr[b] have shown that whereas the variant glycophorin which carries the St[a] blood group antigen is found in the precipitate, the variant glycophorin associated with Dantu antigen is not (262). These results suggested that the Wr[b] antigen is associated with residues 61-70 of GPA and led Bruce et al. (41) to propose that Arg61 of GPA, which is present in St[a] glycophorin but not in Dantu glycophorin, might form a charge pairing with Glu658 of band 3, i.e. when band 3 expresses the Wr[b] antigen. Huang et al. (127) studied a glycophorin variant which expresses the SAT antigen and showed that despite the presence of residues 61-70 of GPA including Arg61 and Glu658 on band 3 in the same red cells, the Wr[b] antigen was not expressed. The most likely explanation was the insertion of three residues (Ala72-Pro-Val) derived from GPB, at the junction between the extracellular domain and the transmembrane domain. The insertion of such a sequence, particularly one containing a proline residue, would be likely to alter the interaction between GPA.SAT and band 3 and thereby result in the loss of the

Wr^b antigen. This experiment does not preclude a role for Arg61 in normal GPA per se. Huang et al. (127) went on to compare GPA and band 3 sequences in several other primates and, of those tested with human anti-Wr^b (serum of the Wr(a+b-) individual MF) only chimpanzee red cells were positive. This observation is in contrast to a previous report which used a monoclonal anti-Wr^b (R7) and found chimpanzees to be Wr(b-) (153). Nucleotide sequencing of chimpanzee band 3 and GPA revealed the presence of Glu658 in band 3 as would be expected for Wr^b expression but the region of GPA comprising residues 61-70 differed in 3 positions from its human counterpart, i.e. 61Gly, 65Val, 67Arg in chimpanzee compared with Arg, Ala, His respectively in human suggesting that an arginine at 61 is not critical for Wr^b expression in chimpanzees but raising the question of whether or not Arg67 is involved in a charge pair with Glu658 on band 3. As Huang et al. (127) point out, the most useful approach to determining the critical residues involved in Wr^b expression would appear to be coexpression of human band 3 and human GPA in a suitable cell line and then the use of site-directed mutagenesis to assess the role of individual amino acids on each protein.

Yet another complication arises from the differences between monoclonal and polyclonal anti-Wr^b. The human anti-Wr^b used by Huang et al. (127) in the study described above would be expected to recognize the several epitopes which comprise the Wr^b antigen and so if chimpanzee red cells express only one of those epitopes then they would be recorded as Wr(b+). Monoclonal anti-Wr^b see only a single epitope and the failure of antibody R7 to react with chimpanzee red cells (153) may reflect the absence of the relevant epitope rather than polymorphism between chimpanzees in New York and those in Bristol. Clear and unambiguous evidence that monoclonal anti-Wr^b are heterogeneous in terms of their epitope specificity has come from studies of a low frequency antigen found on GPA. Poole et al. (126) described a case study of a patient with a low frequency antigen (HAG) the presence of which correlated with a single nucleotide substitution in *GYPA* which changed Ala65 to Pro in the encoded GPA and showed that human anti-Wr^b (MF) and some but not all, monoclonal anti-Wr^b failed to react with the patient's cells while others (including R7 see above) gave positive reactions. Nucleotide sequence analysis of the band 3 gene in this patient revealed that he was homozygous for Glu658 and would therefore be expected to have the phenotype Wr(a-b+). The change Ala65 to Pro would be expected to disrupt the alpha helix predicted for residues 61 to 70 of normal GPA and clearly destroys the epitopes recognized by human anti-Wr^b and some but not all monoclonal anti-Wr^b.

These results showing that an amino acid sequence change on GPA can destroy the Wr^b epitope recognized by human anti-Wr^b and some but not all monoclonal anti-Wr^b raise the amusing question of whether or not the antibodies failing to react with HAG+ cells should be called anti-Wr^b, or something else. The question is based on the fact that the antibodies define antigens not determined by the amino acid sequence of band 3, but by that of GPA. In other words, do the antibodies recognize a determinant in the MN, not the Diego system? The validity of the question is illustrated by the fact that the low incidence antigen MARS and the high incidence antigen AVIS represent an amino acid polymorphism in the same region of GPA (161,246). Those antigens are described above and in Chapter 15 on the MN system as, indeed at the serological level, is the antigen HAG.

Band 3 Variants in Hereditary Spherocytosis

A large number of molecular defects result in hereditary spherocytosis (HS) and several of these are associated with band 3 variants (Prague I, II, III, Hradec Kralore, Jablonec, Tuscaloosa) which are either not expressed or are expressed at lower than normal levels in the red cell membranes of the affected individuals (263,264). It would therefore be expected that the red cells of these patients would have weakened expression of Wr^b and Di^b antigens. In a study of 70 unrelated Czech subjects with autosomal dominant HS, Jarolim et al. (264) reported 17 subjects who had a band 3 deficiency ranging from 50-70% of normal and so in this population up to 25% cases of HS would be predicted to have weakened Wr^b and Di^b antigens. However, in the only study of these antigens in HS known to us, samples from 19 US patients from eight different kindreds, were examined but none showed any weakening of Wr^b or Di^b antigens (265).

Why No Null Phenotype in the Diego System?

Band 3 has a very restricted tissue distribution being found only in red cells and kidney. In the red cell it has two main functions, first, interaction through ankyrin with the red cell skeleton to maintain the integrity of the membrane and second, increasing the capacity of the blood to carry CO_2 as HCO_3^- from the tissues to the lungs. In the kidney its anion exchange activity may play a role in regulating the pH of urine. The structure and function of the protein has been reviewed in detail by Tanner (44). The complete absence of band 3 has not been described (i.e., the Di(a-b-) phenotype) and it has been thought that such an absence would be incompatible with life. As discussed above there are a number of examples of reductions in the level of band 3 expression in human red cells (the hemizygous expression of a mutant band 3 incapable of anion transport in SAO cells, and the reduction of normal band 3 in several kinds of HS) but no null phenotype. The assumption that absence of band 3 would be incompatible with life has been brought into question by the discovery of band 3 deficient cattle (266) and the creation of band 3 "knockout" mice (267). Although not incompatible with life, the absence of band 3 from the red cells of these animals is not without severe consequences. Both animals have severe spherocytosis with unstable red cell membranes which shed membrane as vesicles. The red cells have little or no anion transport activity. The newborn animals have high levels of mortality and those that survive have growth retardation.

References

1. Layrisse M, Arends T, Dominguez SR. Acta Med Venezuela 1955;3:132
2. Levine P, Koch EA, McGee RT, et al. Am J Clin Pathol 1954;24:292
3. Levine P, Robinson EA, Layrisse M, et al. Nature 1956;177:40
4. Layrisse M, Arends T. Nature 1956;177:1083
5. Junqueira PC, Wishart PJ, Ottensooser F, et al. Nature 1956;177:41
6. Lewis M, Ayukawa H, Chown B, et al. Nature 1956;177:1084
7. Layrisse M, Arends T. Nature 1957;179:478
8. Layrisse M, Arends T. Proc 6th Cong ISBT. Basel:Karger, 1958:114
9. Iseki S, Masaki S, Furukawa K, et al. Gunma J Med Sci 1958;7:120
10. Chown B, Lewis M. Am J Phys Anthropol 1959;17:13
11. Corcoran PA, Allen FH Jr, Allison AC, et al. Am J Phys Anthropol 1959;17:187
12. Allen FH Jr, Corcoran PA. Am J Phys Anthropol 1960;18:109
13. Won CD, Shin HS, Kim SW, et al. Am J Phys Anthropol 1960;18:115
14. Lewis M, Chown B, Kaita H. Am J Hum Genet 1963;15:203
15. Simmons RT, Albrey JA, Morgan JAG, et al. Med J Austral 1968;1:406
16. Cann HM, Van West B, Barnett CR. Science 1968;162:1391
17. Iseki S, Masaki S, Furukawa K, et al. Vox Sang 1970;19:483
18. Mourant AE, Kopéc AC, Domaniewska-Sobczak K. The Distribution of Human Blood Groups and Other Polymorphisms, 2nd Ed. London:Oxford Univ Press, 1976
19. Simmons RT. Vox Sang 1970;19:533
20. Yokoyama M, Murakata M, Ueno N. Nature 1980;188:591
21. Tills D, Kopéc AC, Tills RE. The Distribution of the Human Blood Groups and Other Polymorphisms, Suppl 1. Oxford:Oxford Univ Press, 1983
22. Edwards-Moulds JM, Alperin JB. Transfusion 1986;26:234
23. Issitt PD, Wren MR, Rueda E, et al. (Letter). Transfusion 1987;27:117
24. Riches RA, Laycock CM, Poole J. (abstract). Book of Abstracts, 20th Cong ISBT 1988:299
25. Lin-Chu M, Broadberry RE, Chang FJ. Transfusion 1988;28:350
26. Yung CH, Chow MP, Hu HY, et al. Transfusion 1989;29:233
27. Lee TD, Zhao TM, Chow MP, et al. Transfusion 1990;30:728
28. Kusnierz-Alejska G, Bochenek S. Vox Sang 1992;62:124
29. Thompson PR, Childers DM, Hatcher DJ. Vox Sang 1967;13:314
30. Spring FA, Bruce LJ, Anstee DJ, et al. Biochem J 1992;288:713
31. Bruce LJ, Anstee DJ, Spring FA, et al. J Biol Chem 1994;269:16155
32. Holman CA. Lancet 1953;2:119
33. Adams J, Broviac M, Brooks W, et al. Transfusion 1971;11:290
34. Wren MR, Issitt PD. Transfusion 1988;28:113
35. Dahr W, Wilkinson SL, Issitt PD, et al. (abstract). Transfusion 1983;23:424
36. Wren MR, Issitt PD, Dahr W. (abstract). Transfusion 1984;24:425
37. Rearden A. Vox Sang 1985;49:346
38. Dahr W. In: Recent Advances in Blood Group Biochemistry. Arlington, VA:Am Assoc Blood Banks, 1986:23
39. Dahr W, Wilkinson S, Issitt P, et al. Biol Chem Hoppe-Seyler 1986;367:1033
40. Telen MJ, Chasis JA. Blood 1990;76:842
41. Bruce LJ, Ring SM, Anstee DJ, et al. Blood 1995;85:541
42. Tanner MJA, Martin PG, High S. Biochem J 1988;256:703
43. Lux SE, John KM, Kopito RR, et atl. Proc Nat Acad Sci USA 1989;86:9089
44. Tanner MJA. Semin Hematol 1993;30:34
45. Lewis M, Kaita H, Chown B, et al. Am J Hum Genet 1976;28:18
46. Graninger W. Vox Sang 1976;31:131
47. Luboldt W, Henneberg-Quester K-B. Proc 10th Int Cong Soc Forens Hematogenet 1983:123
48. Mallén MS, Arias T. Science 1959;130:164
49. Zafar M, Reid ME. Immunohematology 1993;9:35
50. Buchanan DI, Patterson M, Turc JM. (Letter). Transfusion 1983;23:80
51. Layrisse M, Arends T. Blood 1957;12:115
52. Hinckley ME, Huestis DW. Rev Fr Transf Immunohematol 1979;22:581
53. Alves de Lima LM, Bertheir ME, Sad WE, et al. Transfusion 1982;22:246
54. Daniels G. Immunohematology 1992;8:53
55. Masouredis SP, Sudora E, Mahan L, et al. Blood 1980;56:969
56. Steck TL. J Cell Biol 1974;62:1
57. Anstee DJ, Spring FA. Transf Med Rev 1989;3:13
58. Anstee DJ. Vox Sang 1990;58:1
59. Anstee DJ. J Immunogenet 1990;17:219
60. Biro V, Garraty G, Johnson CL, et al. Transfusion 1983;23:65
61. Zupanska B, Brojer E, McIntosh J, et al. Vox Sang 1990;58:276
62. Habash J, Devenish A, Macdonald S, et al. Vox Sang 1991;61:77
63. Nakajima H, Hayakawa Z, Ito H. Vox Sang 1971;20:271
64. Kusnierz-Alejska G, Bochenek S, Zukowsa B. Mater Med Pol 1990;22:15
65. Mollison PL, Engelfriet CP, Contreras M. Blood Transfusion in Clinical Medicine, 9th Ed. Oxford:Blackwell, 1993
66. Ishimori T, Fukumoto Y, Abe K, et al. Vox Sang 1976;31:61
67. Daniels GL. PhD Thesis, Univ London, 1980:310
68. Steffey NB. (abstract). Red Cell Free Press 1983;8:24
69. Layrisse M, Sanger R, Race RR. Am J Hum Genet 1959;11:17
70. Feller CW, Shenker L, Scott EP, et al. Transfusion 1970;10:279

71. Uchikawa M, Shibata Y, Tohyama H, et al. Vox Sang 1982;42:91

72. Levine P, Robinson EA. Blood 1957;12:448

73. Tatarsky J, Stroup M, Levine P, et al. Vox Sang 1959;4:152

74. Gottlieb AM. Vox Sang 1971;21:79

75. Wiener AS, Brancato GJ. Am J Hum Genet 1953;5:350

76. Dunsford I. Vox Sang (Old Series) 1954;4:160

77. Wallace J, Milne GR. Unpublished observations 1956 cited by Race RR, Sanger R. Blood Groups in Man, 6th Ed. Oxford:Blackwell, 1975

78. Cleghorn TE. Vox Sang 1960;5:556

79. Cleghorn TE. MD Thesis, Univ Sheffield 1961

80. Kornstad L. Vox Sang 1961;6:129

81. Juel E. . Unpublished observations 1961 cited in Korstad L. Vox Sang 1961;6:129

82. Walker ME, Tippett PA, Roper JM, et al. Vox Sang 1961;6:357

83. Simmons RT, Graydon JJ, Zigas V, et al. Am J Trop Med Hyg 1961;10:92

84. Kout M. Vox Sang 1962;7:242

85. Metaxas MN, Metaxas-Bühler M. Vox Sang 1963;8:707

86. Vos GH, Kirk RL. Occ papers in Aboriginal Studies No 4. Canberra:Austral Inst Aboriginal Studies, 1965

87. Ørjasaeter H, Kornstad L, Heier-Larsen AM. Vox Sang 1966;11:726

88. McGuire D, Funkhouser JW. (abstract). Transfusion 1967;7:385

89. Glasgow BG, Goodwin MJ, Jackson F, et al. Vox Sang 1968;14:31

90. Harvey RG, Godber MJ, Kopec AC, et al. Hum Biol 1969;41:342

91. Liotta I, Purpara M, Dawes BJ, et al. Vox Sang 1970;19:540

92. Simmons RT. Vox Sang 1970;19:533

93. Greendyke RM, Banzhaf JC. Transfusion 1977;17:621

94. Cleghorn TE. Unpublished observations 1962 to 1967 cited by Race RR, Sanger R. Blood Groups in Man, 6th Ed. Oxford:Blackwell, 1975

95. Allen FH Jr. Transfusion 1961;1:24

96. Stout TD, Moore BPL, Kaita H. Transfusion 1961;1:393

97. Pavone BG, Issitt PD, Wagstaff W. Transfusion 1977;17:47

98. Solomon E, Ledbetter DH. Cytogenet Cell Genet 1991;58:686

99. Zelinksi T, Coghlan G, White L, et al. Genomics 1993;17:665

100. Lewis M, Kaita H, Chown B, et al. Vox Sang 1973;25:336

101. Ring SM, Green CA, Swallow DM, et al. Vox Sang 1994;67:222

102. Lubenko A, Contreras M. (Letter). Transfusion 1992;32:87

103. Hardman JT, Beck ML. Transfusion 1981;21:343

104. Daw E. J Obstet Gynecol Br Commwth 1971;78:377

105. Jørgensen J, Jacobsen L. Vox Sang 1974;27:478

106. Loghem JJ van, Hart M van der, Bok J, et al. Vox Sang (Old Series) 1955;5:130

107. Cleghorn TE. Unpublished observations 1963 cited by Issitt PD. Applied Blood Group Serology, 3rd Ed. Miami:Montgomery 1985:409

108. Kay MMB. In: Immunobiology of Transfusion Medicine. New York:Marcel Dekker 1994:173

109. Issitt PD, Pavone BG, Wagstaff W, et al. Transfusion 1976;16:396

110. Issitt PD, Pavone BG, Dahr W, et al. (abstract). Transfusion 1978;18:393

111. Issitt PD. Med Lab Sci 1978;35:3

112. Contreras M, Lubenko A, Armitage S, et al. Vox Sang 1980;39:225

113. Issitt PD. In: Red Cell Antigens and Antibodies. Arlington, VA:Am Assoc Blood Banks, 1986:99

114. Dahr W, Schütt KH, Arndt-Hanser A, et al. (abstract). Transfusion 1992;32 (Suppl 8S):55S

115. Issitt PD, Pavone BG, Goldfinger D, et al. Transfusion 1975;15:353

116. Tokunaga E, Sasakawa S, Tamaka K, et al. J Immunogenet 1979;6:383

117. Gutendorf R, Lacey P, Moulds J, et al. (abstract). Transfusion 1985;25:481

118. Okubo Y, Daniels GL, Parsons SF, et al. Vox Sang 1988;54:107

119. Leak M, Poole J, Kay T, et al. (abstract). Book of Abstracts, Joint Cong ISBT/AABB 1990:57

120. Vengelen-Tyler V, Anstee DJ, Issitt PD, et al. Transfusion 1981;21:1

121. Langley JW, Issitt PD, Anstee DJ, et al. Transfusion 1981;21:15

122. Judd WJ, Geisland JR, Issitt PD, et al. Transfusion 1983;23:33

123. Habash J, Lubenko A, Pizzaro I, et al. (abstract). Book of Abstracts, Joint Cong ISBT/AABB 1990:155

124. Daniels GL, Green CA, Okubo Y, et al. Transf Med 1991;1:39

125. Poole J, Banks J, Levene C, et al. (abstract). Vox Sang 1994;67 (Suppl 2):115

126. Poole JA, Banks JA, Bruce LJ, et al. (abstract). Transfusion 1995;35 (Suppl 10S):40S

127. Huang C-H, Reid ME, Xie S-S, et al. Blood 1996;87:3942

128. Issitt PD, Pavone BG, Goldfinger D. (abstract). Book of Abstracts 14th Cong ISBT 1975:69

129. Goldfinger D, Zwicker H, Issitt PD, et al. (abstract). Book of Abstracts 14th Cong ISBT 1975:68

130. Goldfinger D, Zwicker H, Belkin GA, et al. Transfusion 1975;15:351

131. Issitt PD, Pavone BG, Goldfinger D, et al. Br J Haematol 1976;34:5

132. Pavone BG, Pirkola A, Nevanlinna HR, et al. Transfusion 1978;18:155

133. Issitt PD, Pavone BG. Transfusion 1978;18:761

134. Dahr W, UhlenbruckG, Leikola J, et al. J Immunogenet 1976;3:329

135. Dahr W, Uhlenbruck G, Wagstaff W, et al. J Immunogenet 1976;3:383

136. Gahmberg CG, Myllylä G, Leikola J, et al. J Biol Chem 1976;251:6108

137. Tanner MJA, Anstee DJ. Bichem J 1976;153:271

138. Tanner MJA, Jenkins RE, Anstee DJ, et al. Biochem J 1976;155:701

139. Anstee DJ, Barker DM, Judson PA, et al. Br J Haematol 1977;35:309

140. Dahr W, Uhlenbruck G, Leikola J, et al. J Immunogenet 1978;5:117

141. Furthmayr H. Nature 1978;271:519

142. Perkins M. J Cell Biol 1981;90:563

143. Pasvol G, Wainscoat JS, Weatherall DJ. Nature 1982;297:64

144. Pasvol G, Jungery M, Weatherall DJ, et al. Lancet 1982;2:947

145. Dahr W, Wilkinson S, Issitt PD, et al. (abstract). Proc Int Soc Forens Immunogenet 1983

146. Rearden A. (Letter). Transfusion 1989;29:187

147. Wainwright SD, Tanner MJA, Martin GEM, et al. Biochem J 1989;258:211

148. Ring SM, Tippett P, Swallow DM. Vox Sang 1994;67:226

149. Daniels GL. (abstract). Book of Abstracts 16th Cong ISBT 1980:254

150. Furuhjelm U, Nevanlinna HR, Pirkola A. Vox Sang 1973;24:545

151. Dankbar DT, Pierce SR, Issitt PD, et al. (abstract).

Transfusion 1987;27:534

152. Ainsworth BM, Fraser ID, Poole GD. (abstract). Book of Abstracts 20th Cong ISBT 1988:82
153. Anstee DJ, Edwards PAW. Eur J Immunol 1982;12:228
154. Ridgwell K, Tanner MJA, Anstee DJ. Biochem J 1983;209:273
155. Rouger P, Anstee D, Salmon C, et al. Rev Fr Transf Immunohematol 1988;31:261
156. Gardner B, Parsons SF, Merry AH, et al. Immunology 1989;68:283
157. Leddy JP, Falany JL, Kissel GE, et al. J Clin Invest 1993;91:1672
158. Leddy JP, Wilkinson SL, Kissel GE, et al. Blood 1994;84:650
159. Issitt PD, Combs MR, Allen J, et al. Transfusion 1996;36:802
160. Issitt PD, Goldfinger D. (Letter). Transfusion 1979;19:350
161. Moulds JJ, Moulds MK, Lacey B, et al. (abstract). Transfusion 1992;32 (Suppl 8S):55S
162. Lewis M, Kaita H. Am J Hum Genet 1981;33:418
163. Kornstad L. Vox Sang 1986;50:235
164. Moores P, Smart E, Marks M, et al. Hum Hered 1990;40:257
165. Zelinski T, Coghlan G, White L, et al. Genomics 1995;25:320
166. Bruce LJ, Tanner MJA, Zelinski T. (abstract). Transfusion 1995;35(Suppl 10S):52S
167. Jarolim P, Murray JL, Rubin HL, et al. (abstract). Blood 1995;86 (Suppl 1):445A
168. Contreras M, Stebbing B, Mallory DM, et al. Vox Sang 1978;35:397
169. Moulds JM. Personal communication 1995
170. Issitt PD, Combs MR, Bumgarner DJ, et al. Transfusion 1996;36:481 170.
171. Crow M, Spruell P, Moulds JJ, et al. (abstract). Transfusion 1991;31 (Suppl 8S):52S
172. Coghlan G, Crow M, Spruell P, et al. Vox Sang 1995;68:187
173. Jarolim P, Murray JL, Rubin HL, et al. (abstract). Transfusion 1996;36 (Suppl 9S):49S
174. Daniels G, Anstee DJ, Cartron J-P, et al. Vox Sang 1996;71:246
175. Lewis M, Kaita H, McAlpine PJ, et al. Vox Sang 1978;35:251
176. Kaita H, Lewis M, McAlpine PJ. Transfusion 1980;20:217
177. Zelinski T, Kaita H, Philipps S, et al. (abstract). Book of Abstracts 20th Cong ISBT 1988:301
178. Harris PA, de la Vega S, Clinton BS, et al. Transfusion 1983;23:394
179. Coghlan G, Philipps S, McAlpine PJ, et al. (abstract). Transfusion 1995;35 (Suppl 10S):59S
180. Cleghorn TE. Nature 1959;184:1324
181. Metaxas MN, Metaxas-Bühler M. Vox Sang 1976;31 (Suppl 1):39
182. Cleghorn TE. Br J Haematol 1960;6:433
183. Metaxas-Bühler M, Metaxas MN, Giles CM. Vox Sang 1972;23:429
184. Mohr J. Acta Path Microbiol Scand 1951;28:207
185. Mohr J. Acta Path Microbiol Scand 1951;29:339
186. Ceppellini R. Ric Sci Mem 1955;25:3
187. Ceppellini R. Proc 5th Cong ISBT. Basel:Karger 1955:207
188. Ceppellini R, Siniscalco M. Rev d'Inst Serio Ital 1955;30:431
189. Mohr J. A Study of Linkage in Man. Copenhagen:Munksgaard 1956
190. Lewis M, Kaita H, Philipps S, et al. Ann Hum Genet 1987;51:201
191. Zelinski T, Coghlan G, Greenberg CR, et al. Transfusion 1989;29:304
192. Ball SP, Tongue N, Gibaud A, et al. Ann Hum Genet 1991;55:225
193. Zelinski T. Transfusion 1991;31:762

194. Judd WJ, Marsh WL, Øyen R, et al. Vox Sang 1977;32:214
195. Contreras M, Teesdale P, Moulds M, et al. Vox Sang 1987;52:115
196. Lewis M, Allen FH, Anstee DJ, et al. Vox Sang 1985;49:171
197. Lewis M, Kaita H, Philipps S, et al. Vox Sang 1988;54:184
198. Jarolim P, Rubin HL, Moulds JM. (abstract). Transfusion 1996;36 (Suppl 9S):49S
199. Szaloky A, Sijpesteign NK, Hart van der M. Vox Sang 1973;24:535
200. Kornstad L, Brocteur J. (abstract). Book of Abstracts Joint Cong ISBT/AABB 1972:58
201. Kornstad L, Howell P, Jørgensen J, et al. Vox Sang 1976;31:337
202. Kornstad L. Immunol Commun 1981;10:199
203. Korstad L. (abstract). Book of Abstracts 17th Cong ISBT 1982:290
204. Heisto H. Unpublished observations 1967 cited by Race RR, Sanger R. Blood Groups in Man, 6th Ed. Oxford:Blackwell, 1975:436
205. Kornstad L, Wolthuis K. . Unpublished observations 1967 cited by Race RR, Sanger R. Blood Groups in Man, 6th Ed. Oxford:Blackwell, 1975:435
206. Kornstad L. Unpublished observations 1974 cited by Race RR, Sanger R. Blood Groups in Man, 6th Ed. Oxford:Blackwell, 1975:435
207. Young S, Mallan M, Case J, et al. Vox Sang 1980;38:213
208. Broman B. Unpublished observations 1973 cited in Race RR, Sanger R. Blood Groups in Man, 6th Ed. Oxford:Blackwell, 1975:436
209. Moulds M, Chovanec D, Kaita H, et al. (abstract). Transfusion 1989;29 (Suppl 7S):14S
210. Kornstad L, Jerne D, Tippett P. Vox Sang 1987;52:120
211. Moulds M, Kaita H, Kornstad L, et al. Vox Sang 1992;62:53
212. Jørgensen J, Kissmeyer-Nielsen F. . Unpublished observations 1975 cited in Race RR, Sanger R. Blood Groups in Man, 6th Ed. Oxford:Blackwell, 1975
213. Lewis M, Anstee DJ, Bird GWG, et al. Vox Sang 1990;58:152
214. Lewis M, Kaita H, Allderdice PW, et al. Hum Genet 1984;67:270
215. Daniels G. Human Blood Groups. Oxford:Blackwell, 1995:638
216. Okubo Y, Yamaguchi H, Seno T, et al. Hum Hered 1988;38:122
217. Chaves MA, Leak MR, Poole J, et al. Vox Sang 1988;55:241
218. Kaita H, Lubenko A, Moulds M, et al. Transfusion 1992;32:845
219. Green C, Tippett P. Unpublished observations 1979 cited in Coghlan G, Green C, Lubenko A, et al. Vox Sang 1993;64:240
220. Coghlan G, Kaita H, Zelinski T. (abstract). Book of Abstracts Joint Cong ISBT/AABB 1990:124
221. Coghlan G, Green C, Lubenko A, et al. Vox Sang 1993;64:240
222. Ford DS, Stern DA, Hawksworth DN, et al. Vox Sang 1992;62:169
223. Better PJ, Ford DS, Frascarelli A, et al. (Letter). Vox Sang 1993;65:70
224. Young S. Vox Sang 1981;41:48
225. Green CA, Glameyer T. Unpublished observations 1989 cited in Daniels G. Human Blood Groups. Oxford:Blackwell, 1995:636
226. Rowe GP, Hammond W. Vox Sang 1983;45:316
227. Coghlan G, Punter F, Zelinski T. (abstract). Transfusion 1996;36 (Suppl 9S):49S
228. Jarolim P, Rubin HL, Reid M. (abstract). Transfusion 1996;36

(Suppl 9S):49S

229. Pryor DS, Pitney WR. Br J Haematol 1967;13:126
230. Lei-Injo LE, Kosasih EN, Siregar A. SE Asian J Trop Med Pub Health 1973;4:560
231. Amato D, Andrews S. Proc Asian-Pacific Div Cong Int Soc Haematol 1975:124
232. Isbister J, Amato D, Woodfield DG. Papua New Guinea Med J 1975;18:47
233. Booth PB, Serjeantson S, Woodfield DG, et al. Vox Sang 1977;32:99
234. Kidson C, Lamont G, Saul A, et al. Proc Nat Acad Sci USA 1981;78:5829
235. Hadley T, Saul A, Lamont G, et al. J Clin Invest 1983;71:780
236. Mohandas N, Lie-Injo LE, Friedman M, et al. Blood 1984;63:1385
237. Jarolim P, Palek J, Amato D, et al. Proc Nat Acad Sci USA 1991;88:11022
238. Baranowski T, Lisowska E, Morawiecki A, et al. Arch Immunol I Terapi 1959;7:15
239. Marchesi VT, Tillack TW, Jackson RL, et al. Proc Nat Acad Sci USA 1972;69:1445
240. Mueller TJ, Morrison M. J Biol Chem 1977;252:6573
241. Yannoukakos D, Vasseur C, Driancourt C, et al. Blood 1991;78:1117
242. Jarolim P, Rubin HL, Zhai S, et al. Blood 1992;80:1592
243. Ranney HM, Rosenberg GH, Morrison M, et al. Br J Haematol 1990;76:262
244. Ideguchi H, Okubo K, Ishikawa A, et al. Br J Haematol 1992;82:122
245. Hsu L, Morrison M. Biochemistry 1985; 24:3086
246. Jarolim P, Moulds JM, Moulds JJ, et al. (abstract). Blood 1996;88 (Suppl 1):182a
247. Jarolim P, Murray JL, Rubin HL, et al. Transfusion 1997;37:607
248. Bruce LJ, Zelinksi T, Ridgwell K, et al. Vox Sang 1996;71:118
249. Zelinski T, McKeown I, McAlpine PJ, et al. Transfusion 1996;36:419
250. Jarolim P, Murray J, Rubin H, et al. (abstract). Vox Sang 1996;70 (Suppl 2):72
251. Jennings ML, Adams-Lackey M, Denney GH. J Biol Chem 1984;259:4652
252. Brock CJ, Tanner MJA, Kempf C . Biochem J 1983;213:577
253. Nigg EA, Bron EA, Girardet M, et al. Biochemistry 1980;19:1887
254. Daniels GL, Anstee DJ, Cartron J-P, et al. Vox Sang 1995;69:265
255. Macdonald B, Anstee DJ,1984, unpublished observations cited in Anstee DJ. Vox Sang 1990;58:1
256. Groves JD, Tanner MJA. J Biol Chem 1992;267:22163
257. Dahr W, Wilkinson S, Issitt PD, et al. Biol Chem Hoppe Seyler 1986;367:1033
258. Chasis JA, Reid ME, Jensen RH, et al. J Cell Biol 1988;107:1351
259. Pasvol G, Chasis JA, Mohandas N, et al. Blood 1989;74:1936
260. Clough B, Paulitschke M, Nash GB, et al. Mol Biochem Parasitol 1995;69:19
261. Paulitschke M, Nash GB, Anstee DJ, et al. Blood 1995;86:342
262. Ridgwell K, Tanner MJA, Anstee DJ. J Immunogenet 1984;11:365
263. Jarolim P, Rubin HL, Liu SC, et al. J Clin Invest 1994;93:121
264. Jarolim P, Rubin HL, Brabec V, et al. Blood 1995;85:634
265. Ward MJ, Issitt PD. Biotest Bull 1982;30:174
266. Inaba M, Yawata A, Koshino I, et al. J Clin Invest 1996;97:1804
267. Peters LL, Shivdasani RA, Liu SC, et al. Cell 1996;86:917
268. Poole J, Hallewell H, Bruce L, et al. (abstract). Transfusion 1997;37 (Suppl 9S):90S
269. Kornstad L, Kout M, Larsen AMH, et al. Vox Sang 1967;13:165
270. Orlina AR, Unger PJ. Am J Clin Pathol 1979;71:713
271. Daniels G. BBTS Newsletter No 44, Spring 1997:14
272. Bruce LJ, Groves JD, Okubo Y, et al. Blood 1994;84:916
273. Steck TL. J Supramolec Struct 1978:8:311
274. Smythe J, Spring FA, Gardner B, et al. Blood 1995; 85:2929
275. Zelinski T, Pongoski J, Coghlan G. (abstract). Transfusion 1997;37 (Suppl 9S):90S
276. Zelinski T, Rusnak A, McManus K, et al. (abstract). Transfusion 1997;37 (Suppl 9S):89S

18 | The Kell and Xk Blood Group Systems

Following discovery of the K antigen by Coombs et al. (1) in 1946 and its antithetical partner k by Levine et al. (2) in 1949, the Kell system remained a simple two antigen system for eight years. This period was brought to an abrupt end in 1957 when Allen et al. (3) described Kp^a a new antigen in the system and Chown et al. (4) found the first K$_o$ (i.e. Kell$_{null}$) blood. Shortly after this Allen et al. (5) added Kp^b the antithetical partner to Kp^a. In 1965 Stroup et al. (6) and Morton et al. (7) showed that Js^a, discovered in 1958 by Giblett (8,9) and Js^b, discovered in 1963 by Walker et al. (10), also belonged in the Kell system. After eight years of relative dormancy the Kell system suddenly blossomed into a complex polymorphism of red cell antigens. Since that time a large number of additional antigens in the Kell system have been discovered. The antigen detected by an antibody often produced by immunized K$_o$ persons and present on most cells, was named Ku by Corcoran et al. (11). An antigen that was named K^w was tentatively assigned to the Kell system by Bove et al. (12) but genetic evidence that the antigen belonged in the system was never obtained. The antigen is now regarded as obsolete (13) since no anti-K^w is available. KL, an antigen present on most cells was described in 1968 by Hart et al. (14). For reasons that are discussed in detail later in this chapter, Marsh (15) suggested that the term anti-KL be used to describe the total immune response of individuals of the McLeod phenotype (16,17) (again see later). In most instances, anti-KL can be shown to be a mixture of two separable antibodies, one of which has anti-Kx specificity and for the other of which the term anti-Km was suggested (15). Accordingly, the term KL is now also considered obsolete (13). As discussed below, anti-Km is also known as anti-K20 while anti-Kx is known to detect an antigen that is phenotypically related to the Kell system, but is encoded by an X chromosome-borne gene that is genetically independent of the Kell system (see the XK system, later in this chapter).

Since 1968 a considerable number of antigens have been added to the Kell system. The new antigens fall into one of two categories. Some are like Kp^a and Js^a in that they are of low incidence in almost all populations. Others are like Kp^b and Js^b in that they are of very high occurrence in all populations studied. In some, but regrettably rather few instances, an antithetical relationship has been shown to exist between one of the low and one of the high incidence antigens.

As described in more detail in the sections that follow, the earlier found antigens of low incidence were

shown to be part of the Kell system via traditional family studies, i.e. linkage of the encoding gene to a gene known to be at the *Kell* system locus. More recently, immunoprecipitation studies and the monoclonal antibody-specific immobilization of erythrocyte antigen (MAIEA) (18) technique have been used. Thus the rare antigen Ul^a, first described by Furuhjelm et al. (19) in 1968, was shown, one year later and by the same investigators (20), to be encoded from the *Kell* complex locus. The low incidence Wk^a was detected by an antibody first studied in 1967 (34). In 1974, Strange et al. (21) published data showing that in five families with Wk(a+) K+ members, transmission to all of 13 children was either *kWk^a* or *K* without *Wk^a*. The probability of this being a chance occurrence (if *Wk^a* was not at the *Kell* complex locus) was 1 in 8192. As described in a later section, Wk^a or K17 is now known (21,35,36) to be the low incidence antithetical partner to the high incidence antigen, K11. In 1979, Yamaguchi et al. (22) described a Japanese family in which the proposita and three of her sibs had red cells of the Kp(a-b-) phenotype. The individuals concerned were not *K^o* homozygotes since their red cells carried normal expressions of k and Js^b. In an accompanying paper, Gavin et al. (23) showed that the Kp(a-b-) red cells of all four individuals carried the low incidence antigen Levay. That antigen had initially been described in 1945 (24,25) and was the first apparently independent low incidence antigen ever reported. Thus in 1979, 34 years after its discovery, the antigen Levay became Kp^c, or the 21st antigen of the Kell blood group system. Since Levay was reported (24) one year before K (1,26) the name Levay had priority over Kell. Some (who shall remain nameless) suggested that the Kell system should be renamed. Levay would become Le^a, K would be Le^b, k Le^c and so forth. The idea never caught on! The next low incidence antigen to be included in the Kell system was K23. The antibody to this antigen caused a positive DAT on the red cells of the third infant born to the woman with anti-K23 in her serum, but did not cause clinical HDN (27). Association of K23 with the Kell system is based solely on the fact that the anti-K23 in the woman's serum immunoprecipitated the 93kD Kell glycoprotein from her husband's red cells. Thus, as is true for some of the high incidence Kell system-associated antigens described below, there is, as yet, no genetic evidence that K23 is part of the Kell system. Such antigens are called para-Kell by some (28,29) although, as shown in table 18-1, they have been given ISBT numerical terms (13,30). When Eicher et al. (31) studied a "new" antibody to a low incidence antigen, they found that it reacted with three known K:-14 samples. At that time (see below) K14 was known to be a high incidence antigen that was not present on K_o red cells and had certain other characteristics of a Kell system antigen (again see below). The new specificity, anti-Cls, was thus thought to be defining an antigen antithetical to K14 and was called anti-K24. Additional evidence that the antibody was defining a Kell system antigen was provided by the fact that, like other antigens of the Kell system (once again see below), Cls (K24) was no longer detectable on red cells treated with 2 aminoethylisothiouronium bromide (AET). The most recent low incidence antigen added to the Kell system is VLAN that was shown (32), by use of the MAIEA assay, to be located on the Kell glycoprotein. The antigen has been given the number KEL25 in the ISBT terminology (33).

Since 1971, ten different antigens of very high incidence have been described; each may be a part of the Kell system although absolute proof of that situation is available for only one of them. In several instances the initial association between the high incidence antigen and the Kell system occurred at the phenotypic level when the defining antibody reacted with all red cells tested except those of the antibody-maker (and in some instances those of sibs) and those of K^o homozygotes (i.e. Kell$_{null}$ red cells). Clearly such a finding does not prove that the antigen defined is part of the Kell system. For example, Rh$_{null}$ red cells do not react with anti-LW^a, anti-LW^b or anti-Fy5 but none of those antibodies defines an Rh system antibody (see Chapter 12). Thus in the absence of genetic proof, the structures defined by these antibodies have been described (28,29) as para-Kell antigens. Over the years some evidence that some of these antigens do belong in the Kell system has emerged. As mentioned above, one of them, K11, has been shown (21,35,36) to be antithetical to Wk^a (K17), an antigen firmly established in the Kell system. In other instances the supporting evidence is less direct. For example, as described later, absence of some of these high incidence antigens is associated with a weak expression of Kp^b on the red cells involved. The same is true of K13 but that determinant is, itself, a para-Kell antigen. Second, the findings that all Kell system antigens are inactivated when red cells are treated with AET (37) and are either inactivated or markedly weakened when red cells are treated with dithiothreitol (DTT) (56) or ZZAP, a reagent containing DTT and papain (57), has allowed additional studies to be performed. Clearly, if an antibody defining a so-called para-Kell antigen is truly defining a Kell system antigen, it will be non-reactive with AET-treated red cells and either non-reactive or only very weakly reactive with red cells treated with DTT or ZZAP. Third, two phenotypes, McLeod (16,58 and see later for references to

many other examples) and Kell$_{mod}$ (58-63) have been described in which expression of all Kell system antigens (k, Kp^b, Js^b, K11, etc.) is very markedly (McLeod) or markedly (Kell$_{mod}$) depressed. Again if an antibody defining a so-called para-Kell antigen is actually directed against a Kell system antigen, it should react weakly with red cells of these phenotypes. Fourth, the MAIEA assay (18) has been used to indicate location of some of these antigens on a red cell membrane component immobilized by use of a monoclonal Kell system antibody. Fifth and most recently, biochemical recognition and isolation of the red cell glycoprotein that carries antigens of the Kell system (38-41) has allowed use of some of the antibodies to para-Kell antigens in immunoprecipitation studies, to see if they do indeed precipitate the Kell glycoprotein. The supportive evidence for promotion of the so-called para-Kell antigens to full Kell system antigen status is given in each section describing such an antigen. For historical reasons, eight of the antigens described between 1971 and 1982 are listed below. The Kell system number is used as the primary name but the name used in the original publication, that is referenced for each antigen, is also shown. Some of these antigens became fairly well known using terms such as Côté and Bøc. After this reversion to use of original names, and a similar listing in table 18-1, these antigens are called by their conventional or numerical term in the rest of this chapter. The antigen K11 (Côté) was described in 1971 (42). K12 (Bøc) and K14 (San) were described in the same paper (43) in 1973, that paper included additional details about K11. The antigen K13, sometimes but not always also called Sgro, was reported in a 1973 abstract (44) and more fully in a 1974 paper (45). The antigen K16 may be a quantitative variant of k (46). The antigen K18 (sometimes but not often also called V.M.) was reported in 1975 (47) and K19 (Sub) in 1979. The last high incidence antigen to be given a Kell system ISBT number was K22 (N.I.), that was reported in 1982 (49). However, there are two additional high incidence antigens, discovered since 1982, that qualify as para-Kell antigens. The antigen TOU was described in 1994 (55). It is present on all except red cells from K^o homozygotes, is weakly expressed on K$_{mod}$ and McLeod phenotype red cells, is denatured when red cells are treated with DTT and can be located to the Kell glycoprotein by the MAIEA assay. The antigen RAZ was also described in 1994 (64). It is of high incidence, being present on all red cells tested except those of the antibody-maker and those of K^o homozygotes. The antigen was denatured when normal red cells were treated with AET, was only weakly expressed on McLeod phenotype red cells and was localized to the Kell glycoprotein by use of the MAIEA assay. Neither the TOU nor the RAZ antigen has yet been shown to be inherited although two unrelated probands with TOU- red cells have been found (55). Thus neither antigen has been given an ISBT number, but both are included in table 18-1 (now see Addendum). Readers with good memories will recall that K18 has not been shown to be inherited either but somehow got through the screening process and was given the ISBT number 006018 or KEL18.

While the references listed above are to papers or abstracts in which first mention of the antigens K11, K12, K13, K14, K18, K19 and K22 was made, there are many other reports, sometimes describing additional examples of antibodies to these antigens, that provide more information than that given in some of the references already cited. Each of these papers is referenced in the sections below, giving specific details about each of the antigens.

The original (historical) names (that should not be used (50) except in a historical review, such as that above), the conventional, numerical (17) and ISBT terms (13,30,33) for the Kell system antigens are given in table 18-1. That table also shows the incidence of each antigen in a White (European or primarily European extraction) population, the year that the antigen was reported and gives references to the original reports. In some instances, the footnotes to the table include references to reports that documented the fact that the antigen involved is part of the Kell blood group system.

Anti-Kell Does Not Exist

Of all the misuses of blood group terminology that one sees written (even in some peer-reviewed journals of which the editors should know much better) and hears spoken, perhaps use of anti-Kell when anti-K is intended, is the most common. Close behind are phenotypes described as Kell+ and Kell- when K+ and K- would be correct. Kell is the name of the blood group system that contains the antigens listed in table 18-1. Anti-Kell would be an antibody to an entire blood group system. Throughout this chapter the terms anti-K, K+ and K- are used exclusively in the section on serology. In the section on the molecular biology of the system the term Kell protein describes the 93kD glycoprotein that carries all antigens of the Kell system. Dependent on the haplotype that encodes production of the Kell protein, the protein may carry K or k, Kp^a or Kp^b, Js^a or Js^b, etc. In the section on biochemistry an antibody to the Kell protein is one that defines, e.g. by immunoprecipitation, the glycoprotein although some antibodies to individual Kell system antigens have this same property. The *Kell* gene is a gene that encodes production of the Kell glycoprotein. Different alleles (haplotypes) exist, e.g. *kKp^{b}Js^b*, *KKp^{b}Js^b*, etc., that among them will encode

production of polymorphic glycoproteins. The *Kell* gene encodes production of the Kell glycoprotein, the *K* (not *Kell*) gene encodes production of the K (not Kell) antigen. The *Kell* locus (sometimes called the *Kell* complex locus) is the site of different *Kell* genes (haplotypes).

At one time one of us (PDI) responded to comments such as "he has Kell in the serum" with the comment "how interesting that the serum contains an entire blood group system". When the original statement was revised to "he has anti-Kell in the serum" the response became "how interesting that he has an antibody to an entire blood group system in the serum". Eventually the author gave up using the responses since their intent was seldom appreciated. Even now in listening to experienced and technically excellent blood groupers talk about the use of Kell-negative blood, he wonders where all the *K^{o}K^o* donors will be found.

Kell System Haplotypes, Absence of Some Expected Combinations

Given that the *Kell* complex locus involves the presence of genes that either, from a single locus, or from a series of subloci, encode production of antigens, several of which have antithetical relationships to each other, it might be expected that haplotypes would exist that produce these antigens in all various combinations and permutations. The available evidence (38-41) suggests that each *Kell* system haplotype encodes production of a glycoprotein and that in many instances (for details see section on biochemistry) antigen differences (K versus k, Kp^a versus Kp^b versus Kp^c, etc.) represent amino acid differences in the protein backbone of the glycoprotein. However, haplotypes producing the antigens in all combinations have not been found. Table 18-2 lists the Kell system antigens in terms of their antithetical relationships or lack thereof. As can be seen there are five low incidence Kell system antigens with known antithetical partners, one with a tentative partner and three for which no antithetical partner has been identified. No Kell system haplotype has ever been found that encodes production of more than one of those low incidence antigens. In considering the four established sets of antithetical antigens, that comprise a total of nine antigens since Kp^a and Kp^c are both antithetical to Kp^b (it is not known if Kp^a and Kp^c can be antithetical to each other), it is seen that the common Kell system haplotype *kKp^{b}Js^{b}K11* does not encode production of any of the rare antigens. It is probable that this common haplotype can actually be written *kKp^{b}Js^{b}K11K12K13K14K18K19K22* since the red cells of most persons carry all the high incidence and none of the low incidence antigens of the system (i.e. most persons are homozygous for the common haplotype

TABLE 18-1 Antigens of the Kell Blood Group System[1]

Historical Term	Antigen Name	Numerical Term	ISBT Term	% Whites Positive	Year of Discovery	References[2]
Kelleher	K	K1	KEL1	9	1946	1, 26
Cellano	k	K2	KEL2	99.8	1949	2
Penney	Kp^a	K3	KEL3	2	1957	3
Rautenberg	Kp^b	K4	KEL4	99.9	1958	5
Peltz[3]	Ku	K5	KEL5	>99.9	1957	4, 11
Sutter	Js^a	K6	KEL6	<0.1	1958[4]	8, 9
Matthews	Js^b	K7	KEL7	>99.9	1963[4]	10
For K^w (formerly K8) and KL (formerly K9) see footnote number 5						
Kahula	Ul^a	K10	KEL10	2.6[6]	1968	19
Côté		K11	KEL11	>99.9	1971	42, 52
Bøc[7]		K12	KEL12	>99.9	1973	43, 53
Sgro[7]		K13	KEL13	>99.9	1973	44, 45
Santini[7]		K14	KEL14	>99.9	1973	43, 54
The Kx antigen (formerly K15) is now known not to be encoded from the *Kell* complex locus, see text						
k-like[7]		K16	KEL16	99.8	1976	46
Weeks	Wk^a	K17	KEL17	0.3[8]	1974	21, 34
V.M.[7]		K18	KEL18	>99.9	1975	47
Sub[7]		K19	KEL19	>99.9	1979	48
Km[5]		K20	KEL20	>99.9	1979	15
Levay	Kp^c	K21	KEL21	<0.1	1945[9]	24, 25
N.I.[7]		K22	KEL22	>99.9	1982	49
Centauro[7]		K23	KEL23	<0.1	1987	27
Callois[7]	Cls	K24	KEL24	<0.1	1985	31
RAZ[7],[10]				>99.9	1994	64
TOU[7],[10]				>99.9	1994	55
VLAN[7]		K25	KEL25	<0.1	1996	32

[1] ISBT System Symbol KEL; ISBT System Number 006; ISBT Antigen Numbers (full code) 006001 to 006025 (see ISBT Term, in table).

[2] References given are to papers reporting the antigen. References assigning an antigen to the Kell system (where different from the original report) are given in these footnotes.

[3] Mrs. Peltz was the first *K*^{o} homozygote to be described (4). Four years later, the antibody in her serum was named anti-Ku (11).

[4] Data showing that Js^a and Js^b are part of the Kell system were published in 1965 (6, 7).

[5] K^w (12) was originally K8; it is now considered obsolete. KL (Claas)(14) was originally K9. It is now recognized that those antibodies called anti-KL were actually separable mixtures of anti-Kx (51) and anti-Km (anti-K20)(15).

[6] Antigen frequency 2.6% in Finns but less than 1% in other Whites. Shown to be part of the Kell system in 1969 (20).

[7] Genetic evidence that antigen is part of the Kell system not yet reported.

[8] Incidence 0.3% in English donors, incidence not known in other Whites.

[9] Shown to be part of the Kell system in 1979 (22, 23).

[10] Not yet shown to be inherited so not yet eligible for an ISBT number (but see the addendum).

TABLE 18-2 Kell System Antigens and Antithetical Relationships

Part 1. Antigens with Antithetical Relationships

Low Incidence	High Incidence
K	k
Kp^a, Kp^c	Kp^b
Js^a	Js^b
Wk^a	K11
Cls(K24)*	K14*

Part 2. Kell and Para-Kell Antigens with No Known Antithetical Partner

Low Incidence	High Incidence
Ul^a	
K23	
VLAN(K25)	
	K12
	K13
	K18
	K19
	K22

* Antithetical relationship suspected but not proved.

described). Each Kell system haplotype that has been seen to encode production of one low incidence antigen has been seen also to encode production of the high incidence partners of the other low incidence antigens. Thus the haplotype that makes K, always makes Kp^b, Js^b and K11, never Kp^a, Kp^c, Js^a or Wk^a. The haplotype that makes Kp^a, always makes k, Js^b and K11, never K, Js^a or Wk^a, etc. This observation can probably be extended through the rest of the Kell system although far fewer families have been studied than has been the case in following transmission of *K*, *Kp^a*, *Js^a* and *Wk^a*. It is known that the haplotype that makes Ul^a always also makes k, Kp^b, Js^b and K11. Indeed, it is this absolute association (linkage if subloci are involved) that initially resulted in recognition of the facts that Wk^a and Ul^a are Kell system antigens (20,21). Table 18-3 lists those Kell system haplotypes that have been found and indicates in which populations they have been identified. The table also lists some theoretically possible haplotypes that have not been found. For the sake of simplicity and because most studies have considered production of K, k, Kp^a, Kp^b, Kp^c, Js^a, Js^b, Ul^a, Wk^a and K11, the data given in table 18-3 include only findings about production of those antigens. As mentioned above, the findings probably apply beyond the antigens shown.

The above findings do not mean, of course, that samples carrying more than one of the antigens K, Kp^a, Kp^c, Js^a, Wk^a, and Ul^a do not exist. Although the phenotype K+

TABLE 18-3 Recognized and Theoretically Possible Haplotypes in the Kell Blood Group System

Haplotype	Incidence
k, Kp^b, Js^b, K^{ll}	Very common in all populations studied.
K, Kp^b, Js^b, K^{ll}	Less common than the haplotype that makes k, more than twice as common in Whites as in Blacks, very rare in Orientals.
k, Kp^a, Js^b, K^{ll}	Rare in Whites, extremely rare in Blacks.
k, Kp^b, Js^a, K^{ll}	More common than *K, Kp^b, Js^b, K^{ll}* but considerably less common than *k, Kp^b, Js^b, K^{ll}* in Blacks. Extremely rare in Whites.
k, Kp^c, Js^b, K^{ll}	Extremely rare in Whites, perhaps more common in Japanese, not yet found in Blacks.
k, Kp^b, Js^b, Ul^a, K^{ll}	Rare in Whites and Orientals, not yet reported in Blacks.
k, Kp^b, Js^b, Wk^a	Very rare in Whites, not yet reported in Blacks.
K^o	Extremely rare in all groups. The silent allele at the *Kell* complex locus.

Some theoretically possible haplotypes that have never been found			
K, Kp^a, Js^b, K^{ll} *K, Kp^b, Js^a, K^{ll}*	*K, Kp^b, Js^b, Ul^a, K^{ll}*	*K, Kp^b, Js^b, Wk^a*
k, Kp^a, Js^a, K^{ll}	*k, Kp^a, Js^b, Ul^a, K^{ll}*	*k, Kp^a, Js^b, Wk^a*
	k, Kp^b, Js^a, Ul^a, K^{ll}	*k, Kp^b, Js^a, Wk^a*
		k, Kp^b, Js^b, Ul^a, Wk^a

Not shown (for the sake of simplicity) but this section would include any haplotype that encoded production of more than two of the antigens K, Kp^a, Js^a, Ul^a, Wk^a.

k+ Kp(a+b+) is rare, it is found in Whites. The phenotype K+ k+ Js(a+b+) is rare, but is found in Blacks. In all cases in which family studies have been performed (2,6,7,28,65-69) it has been shown that persons with K+ k+ Kp(a+b+) red cells are genetically *KKp^b/kKp^a*, while those who are phenotypically K+ k+ Js(a+b+) are genetically *KJs^b/kJs^a*.

At present there is no explanation as to why no Kell system haplotype that encodes more than one of the antigens K, Kp^a, Kp^c, Js^a, Wk^a and Ul^a has been found. Chown (70) suggested that *kKp^bJs^b* represents the original *Kell* gene (haplotype) so that *KKp^bJs^b*, *kKp^aJs^b*, and *kKp^bJs^a* would each represent a single mutation. Thus *KKp^a* or *KJs^a* or *Kp^aJs^a* would each represent a double mutation and might, accordingly, be extremely rare given the low incidence of *K, Kp^a* and *Js^a* anyway. However, it does seem that sufficient time has elapsed and sufficient studies have been performed, that if such double mutations (mutation of a previous mutant) existed, they should have been found by now. Details obtained to date, about the structure of the Kell glycoprotein (38-41) do not provide an explanation as to why any one amino acid change that results in the presence of a rare low incidence antigen instead of the common high incidence one, should be mutually exclusive of all other such changes.

The Antigens K and k and the Antibodies That Define Them

K is the least infrequent of the low incidence Kell system antigens in Whites. As shown in table 18-4, the antigen is found on the red cells of about 9% of European Whites (28,71) although the incidence in Finland appears to be only about half of that (19). In Blacks, K has an incidence between 1.5 and 2.5% (6,72), in Japanese the incidence is even lower, i.e. circa 1 in 4850 (73). Accordingly the incidence of k, the antithetical partner to K, is very high. The phenotype K+ k- has been seen to have an incidence of about one in 500 Whites in some studies (2,74) although in tests on 1340 Welsh donors, only one k- blood was found (75). Clearly, given the low incidence of K in Blacks and Orientals, the incidence of the K+ k- phenotype in those populations is extremely low.

Anti-K is a common antibody and is most often produced by K- individuals following exposure to K+ red cells via transfusion or pregnancy. Kornstad and Heisto (76) conducted a survey that led them to conclude that of all K- persons transfused with one unit of K+ blood, some 10% form anti-K. As described in Chapter 12, of all D- subjects transfused with one unit of D+ blood, some 80% make anti-D. Thus it might appear that D is about eight times more immunogenic than K. However, Mollison et al. (77) give reasons for supposing that the above calculation may over estimate the immunogenicity of K. Giblett (78) estimated that D is fourteen times more immunogenic than K but the calculation was based on the conclusion that 5% of K- persons form anti-K

TABLE 18-4 Some Antigen and Phenotype Frequencies in the Kell System

Antigen	% Incidence in		Phenotype	% Incidence in	
	Whites	**Blacks**		**Whites**	**Blacks**
K	9.0	3.5	K+k-	0.2	<0.1
k	99.8	>99.9	K+k+	8.8	3.5
			K-k+	91.0	96.5
Kp^a	2.0	<0.1	Kp(a+b-)	<0.1	<0.1
Kp^b	>99.9	>99.9	Kp(a+b+)	2.0	<0.1
			Kp(a-b+)	98.0	>99.9
Js^a	<0.1	19.5	Js(a+b-)	<0.1	1.1
Js^b	>99.9	98.9	Js(a+b+)	<0.1	18.4
			Js(a-b+)	>99.9	80.5

For frequencies in other populations, see text.
Frequencies of other phenotypes are mostly <0.1 or >99.9 and can be determined from the antigen frequencies given in table 18-1 and the text.

after being transfused with one unit of K+ blood. Regardless of whether the immunogenicity of K is one eighth or one fourteenth that of D, it is clear that K is highly immunogenic. In the calculations of Giblett (78) K was estimated to be some 2.5 times more immunogenic than c, most practical blood bankers will be aware that they encounter anti-K more frequently than they encounter anti-c in the sera of previously transfused or pregnant patients. In a number of other series (79-87), Rh antibodies, other than anti-D, anti-CD, anti-DE and anti-CDE, have outnumbered anti-K in the total numbers of antibodies found. However, such studies invariably include anti-E in the Rh antibodies found and as discussed in Chapter 12, as many as 60% or more of anti-E may be non-red cell stimulated (88). Thus although in a routine transfusion service anti-E may be more common than anti-K, that is in turn more common than anti-c, it is likely that after D and C in D- persons, K is the most immunogenic red cell blood group antigen. One point not considered above is that in transfusion therapy, there is a greater chance that a c- patient will be exposed to c, than that a K- patient will be exposed to K (94). On the other hand, fewer transfusion recipients will have c- red cells than will have K- cells.

Most examples of red cell immune anti-K are IgG in nature and react well by IAT (see a later section for tests at low ionic strength). In subclassing studies (89-93) all anti-K were either IgG1 or contained an IgG1 component, about half of them also had an IgG3 and/or an IgG4 component. About 20% of anti-K activate complement to the C3 stage (96), no example that was hemolytic in vitro has been described (77). There is no doubt that anti-K is often a clinically significant antibody. At least one fatal transfusion reaction has been blamed on anti-K (95) other severe but non-fatal reactions have been documented (77,96,97,100). In some other cases (84-87) anti-K caused delayed transfusion reactions and at least six times (101-103,157-159) the antibody has caused a transfusion reaction due to interdonor incompatibility. That is to say, the same patient was transfused with one unit of blood that contained anti-K in the plasma and another unit of which the red cells were K+. There is little doubt that other examples of anti-K are benign in vivo. Some anti-K are detected only in tests using enzyme-treated red cells (104) so must be missed, with some units of K+ blood inadvertently transfused, when other methods of antibody screening and compatibility testing are used. However, we are not aware of an anti-K that has caused a transfusion reaction in this setting. Because it is so easy to find K- blood, most workers elect to transfuse such blood to any patient with anti-K in the serum, without undertaking any tests to determine the likely in vivo activity of the anti-K. While this is easy for patients with anti-K, attempts to prevent immunization to K, in women of

child-bearing age, would involve more time, effort and cost. This topic is addressed again, below.

As would be expected from what has been written above about the role of anti-K in causing transfusion reactions, the antibody has also been incriminated as causative of HDN (1,26,77,98,99,105-111,138). However, although some severe cases have been reported (98,105,109,111) they are the exception rather than the rule. In most cases HDN caused by anti-K is much less severe than the disease as caused by anti-D. Three surveys (108,110,111) covering many years, describe among them 45 infants with K+ red cells born to women with anti-K in the serum. Thirty five of the 45 infants (78%) were so mildly affected that no treatment was necessary. In one study (110) none of 10 infants with K+ red cells born to women with a titer of anti-K of less than 32, was affected. It is because of these findings that most workers do not agree with the suggestion (109,126,127) that females before and during child-bearing ages, who have K- red cells, should be transfused only with K- blood. First, even if K- donor units were identified from previous typing of the donors, thus avoiding additional typing costs, a separate inventory of blood would have to be maintained. Second, an additional cost in terms of labor, reagents and supplies would be involved in typing all female potential transfusion recipients below a certain age. Third, performing an additional test might delay the issue of blood in emergency situations. Fourth, of those K- women currently transfused with K+ blood, no more than 10% make anti-K. Fifth, anti-K HDN when it does occur, requires no treatment in over 75% of cases. Sixth, and perhaps most important of all, the incidence of the K antigen among the men who will father their children is no more than 9%, and much lower in non-White populations. Since almost all the K+ men involved are genetically *Kk*, only 50% of their children will have K+ red cells. In other words, of all K- women, only four or five in every 100 will carry a child with K+ red cells.

While the majority of examples of anti-K are, as described above, IgG red cell stimulated antibodies, both IgM anti-K, and anti-K in the sera of individuals who have never been exposed to K+ red cells have been described (112-123). In some cases, production of anti-K has been thought to have been provoked by bacteria or viruses infecting the antibody-maker. Thus anti-K arising without exposure to K+ red cells has been seen in patients infected with: *Mycobacterium tuberculosis* (114,116); *Escherichia coli* (115); *Enterococcus faecalis* (122); *Morganella morgani* (123); unidentified organisms causing septicemia (120); and an unknown virus causing an upper respiratory tract infection (119). Savalonis et al. (124) studied examples of 23 gram-negative bacteria, representing the genera: *Citrobacter*; *Edwardsiella*; *Escherichia*; *Klebsiella*; *Proteus*; *Salmonella*; *Serratia* and *Shigella* but found evidence of a K-like substance only in *E. coli* 0125:B15, subtype 12808. It was *E. coli* 0125:B15, subtype unknown, that apparently stimulated production of anti-K in the 20-day-old child with enterocolitis, described by Marsh et al. (115). The infant was group B and while infected had both IgM anti-A and IgM anti-K in the serum. Once the infection was cured, neither antibody was detectable in the infant's serum. In the patient infected with *M. morganii*, the anti-K was said to be IgA in nature (123). The authors wondered if some of the other non-red cell stimulated examples of anti-K might also have been IgA. In spite of the associations between bacterial infections and production of anti-K described (some of which may have been true, true and unrelated) other individuals have been found (113,118, 121) to have non-red cell stimulated anti-K but no evidence of any infection. In a different case, a patient with terminal sepsis caused by *Streptococcus faecium* did not form anti-K but his red cells, that were known to be K-, became K+ (125). Transfused K- red cells underwent the same conversion that could be reproduced in vitro using a culture of the infecting organism.

Since no more than two in every 100 Whites, and fewer persons in other population groups can form alloimmune anti-k, the antibody is rare. Nevertheless, since the first example was reported (2) many others have been found (77,100,111,128-137,142-144). In most instances anti-k is produced following exposure of persons with K+ k- red cells to k+ red cells, via transfusion and much less frequently, via pregnancy. Most anti-k are IgG in nature, IgG1 predominates in their composition (91,92). However, exceptions to the situations described above exist and a number of IgM anti-k, capable of agglutinating red cells in a saline system, sometimes at temperatures below 37°C, have been encountered (130,133,136,143). The antibody has been incriminated as causative of both hemolytic transfusion reactions (77,96,97,100) and HDN. In some reported cases (2,128,132,134) the HDN was relatively mild, in others it was much more severe. Rigal et al. (142) described one woman who lost two infants to hydropic deaths due to anti-k; Bowman et al. (144) described a case in which three intrauterine intravascular fetal transfusions were necessary to prevent hydrops fetalis from developing. In the same paper Bowman et al. (144) report that in a 20 years and 8 months period only one anti-k was seen among 3246 alloimmunized pregnant women in Manitoba. The most usual characteristics of anti-K, anti-k and other Kell system antibodies are listed in table 18-5.

Variants of K

Given the hundreds of thousands of typings for K that must have been performed and the enormous num-

ber of examples of anti-K that have been identified, it is not surprising that a few unusual findings have come to light. While attempting to find compatible blood for a patient with multiple antibodies, including anti-K, Hawley et al. (281) found one donor whose red cells would adsorb and elute some anti-K and not others, but would not give a visibly positive reaction with any example of anti-K. McDowell et al. (282) described a woman with K+ k+ red cells who made what appeared to be anti-K. The antibody did not react with the woman's own cells nor the K+ k+ red cells of her daughter. It did react with the K+ k+ red cells of the woman's son. When the maternal antibody was adsorbed onto the son's red cells and an eluate was made, anti-K was recovered but it still failed to react with the red cells of the antibody-maker and those of her daughter. The red cells of the antibody-maker and those of her daughter would adsorb, and yield on elution, other examples of anti-K. Although the original abstract (282) includes no mention of the strength of the K antigen on the red cells of the antibody-maker and her daughter, a later communication from the senior author (283) notes that no noticeable difference was seen in the strength of their K antigens and those on the K+ red cells of random unrelated donors. The original abstract (282) mentions that no abnormality of other Kell system antigens was seen on the red cells of the antibody-maker or those of her two children.

Kline et al. (284) found a donor on whose red cells K was only weakly expressed. In comparative studies the red cells of the White woman were seen to carry normal levels of k, Kp^b, Js^b and Kx. The weak K antigen was present in the donor's mother, her daughter and her grandson. The red cells that carried the weak expression of K were capable of adsorbing, and yielding on elution, all examples of anti-K.

Most recently, Skradski et al. (285) described a White male whose red cells reacted with eight of 72 anti-K. In adsorption-elution studies it was shown that the propositus' red cells would adsorb those anti-K with which they reacted visibly and would yield anti-K on elution. After incubation of the red cells of the propositus with anti-K that did not react visibly, no anti-K was recovered by elution. The k, Kp^b, Ku, Js^b, K11, K12, K13, K14, K18, K19 and K22 antigens on the red cells of the propositus were normal, his red cells lacked Kp^a, Kp^c, Js^a, Ul^a, Wk^a and K23 thus ruling out a *cis* position effect like that seen between *Kp^a* and *k* and *Js^b* (see later in this chapter). Three sisters of the propositus also had K+ k+ red cells that carried the variant form of K. The variant K antigen found in this family was a little weaker, but not markedly so, than the K antigen on K+ red cells of unrelated donors, when tested with the anti-K that gave visible reactions. The red cells of the proposi-

TABLE 18-5 Most Usual Characteristics of Kell System Antibodies

Antibody Specificity	Positive Reactions in In Vitro Tests				Usual Immuno-globulin		Ability to Bind Complement		Ability to Cause In Vitro Lysis		Implicated in		Usual Form of Stimulation		% of White Population Positive
	Sal	LISS	AHG	Enz	IgG	IgM	Yes	No	Yes	No	Trans-fusion Reaction	HDN	Red Cells	Other	
Anti-K	Rare	*1	X	Some	Most	Some	Some	Some		X	X	X	X	Rare	9.0
Anti-k	Rare		X		X					X	X	X	X		99.8
Anti-Kpᵃ	Rare		X		X					X	X	X	X	Rare	2.0
Anti-Kpᵇ			X		X					X	X	X	X		>99.9
Anti-Kpᶜ	Rare		X	X	X					X			X	Rare	<0.1
Anti-Ku			X		X					X	X	X	X		>99.9
Anti-Jsᵃ	Rare		X		X					X	X	X	X	Rare	<0.1
Anti-Jsᵇ			X	Some	X					X	X	X	X		>99.9
Anti-Ulᵃ			X	X	X					X			X		2.6
Anti-Wkᵃ			X		X					X			X		0.3
Anti-K23, K24, K25*2			X		X					X			X	Rare	<0.1
Anti-K11, K12, K13, K14, K18, K19, Km, K22, RAZ, TOU*2			X		X					X			X		>99.9

*1 Some workers have reported that anti-K and some other Kell system antibodies do not react well in LISS. Others have reported that some anti-K are enhanced in LISS, see text.

*2 Reactions of these antibodies based on few examples of each specificity.

tus were non-reactive with three human IgG and four human IgM, monoclonal anti-K. Of the eight anti-K that reacted with the red cells of the propositus, six were from antibody-makers with a positive DAT and one was from a woman whose anti-K titer increased dramatically during pregnancy with a K- fetus. The authors (285) wondered what was the immunogenic stimulus for the reactive anti-K. In tests on over 55,000 individuals with one of the reactive anti-K, no other sample was found that reacted with that anti-K but not with others.

The findings described in this section strongly suggest that two quite different situations exist. The study of Kline et al. (284) is best explained by postulating that there is a *K* gene that encodes production of a reduced number of copies of normal K antigen. That is to say a K antigen that differs quantitatively but not qualitatively from normal K. The studies of McDowell et al. (282), those of Skradski et al. (285) and perhaps those of Hawley et al. (281) are best explained by postulating that variant *K* genes exist that encode production of some but

not all the epitopes of normal K. That is to say, the K antigens found differ both quantitatively and qualitatively from normal K. This conclusion is perhaps supported by the finding (285) that seven monoclonal anti-K failed to react with red cells carrying the variant K antigen. Again, in view of the huge number of K+ red cells and examples of anti-K that have been studied over the years, it is perhaps surprising that epitope variation among K+ bloods is not more commonly encountered. Perhaps almost all K+ red cells carry the most immunogenic K epitope so that perhaps human polyclonal anti-K almost always contain the antibody to that epitope. Perhaps epitope variation among K+ red cells will be seen more often as more monoclonal anti-K are used.

The depression of expression of K, k and other Kell system and para-Kell antigens associated with the McLeod phenotype, the *cis* effect of *Kpᵃ* on k and Jsᵃ in the same haplotype, and weakening of Kell system and para-Kell antigens in the Kell$_{mod}$ phenotype, are each described in later sections of this chapter.

Anti-K and Tests at Low Ionic Strength

As mentioned in the previous section, most examples of anti-K are IgG antibodies. They are usually detected without difficulty using indirect antiglobulin tests on red cells suspended in saline or albumin at normal ionic strength. As attempts have been made to increase the sensitivity of in vitro antibody detection tests, some problems in the continued detection of anti-K have been reported. The difficulties stem from the fact that most of the methods that are more sensitive in terms of detecting other antibodies, involve tests at low ionic strength. Apparently such tests do not provide optimal conditions for the detection of anti-K. Merry et al. (145) used a radio-labeled anti-IgG to show that K+ red cells bound fewer molecules of IgG anti-K at low ionic than at normal ionic strength. It must be remembered (see Chapter 3) that tests such as those using PEG or Polybrene and those involving solid phase or gel technology, use a low ionic strength system in the antigen-antibody binding stage.

A number of publications (102,139,146-152) have described examples of anti-K not detectable by LISS methods or by automated methods based on low ionic strength conditions. In two cases (102,149) the missed anti-K was said to have caused a transfusion reaction. In one of them (102) the patient had been transfused with a K+ unit and was alleged to have had a reaction when transfused with a unit of whole blood, with the undetected anti-K in the plasma, four weeks later. In the other case (149) the anti-K that went undetected in LISS tests was in the patient's plasma. Voak et al. (151) claimed that the problem of non-detection of anti-K in LISS tests could be overcome by performing indirect antiglobulin tests in tubes. First, it was claimed that the increased serum to cell ratio (weaker suspension of cells used in the one volume of serum to one volume of LISS-suspended cells for tube tests than when cells are incubated with serum preparatory for reading on tiles) enhances the chance of antibody detection. Second, it was claimed that the use of two drops of antiglobulin serum instead of one, to read the test, results in the anti-K being detected. It is unlikely that workers in the USA will be convinced by these data since the "improved" antiglobulin test described by these authors (151) seems identical to the one that has been in routine use in the USA since the early 1960s.

While it at first seems alarming that some anti-K are missed in LISS tests, the problem may not be as serious as the reports tend to suggest. Most large transfusion services in the USA have been using antibody screening methods that in one way or another, involve reduction of ionic strength in the test system, for a least the last 20 years. There has been no noticeable increase in the number of transfusion reactions caused by anti-K. Perhaps the answer is that only weak anti-K are missed in LISS or that the use of LISS methods results in compensation since some anti-K are detected in LISS but not by other methods. Dankbar et al. (153) performed tests on 195 known examples of anti-K. Among them: 189 were detected in tests at low and normal ionic strength; two were detected in tests at normal ionic strength but not in LISS; four were detected in LISS tests but not in tests at normal ionic strength. As blood group serologists well know, there is no single in vitro method that detects all antibodies.

The reactions of anti-K and other Kell system antibodies against protease-treated red cells and the use of AET and DTT in Kell system serology, are described in a later section.

The Antigens Kp^a, Kp^b and Kp^c and the Antibodies That Define Them

As discussed in the introduction to this chapter, Kp^a has been found in Whites but not in Blacks or Orientals, Kp^c has been found almost exclusively in Orientals. Both Kp^a and Kp^c are of low incidence in the populations in which they have been found meaning that an overwhelming majority of Whites, Blacks and Orientals are phenotypically Kp(a-b+c-).

In tests on 18,934 Whites in Europe, Canada and the USA the incidence of Kp^a was found (3,28,68,153) to be one in 43 or just over 2%. In tests on 10,416 Japanese, the incidence of Kp^c was found (154,155) to be one in 417. The Kp^c antigen has also been found in one English family (the original one in which the Levay antigen was found (24,25)) and in a Spanish-American man whose red cells were Kp(a+b-c+) and whose serum contained anti-Kp^b (156). Other Kp(a+) and Kp(c+) bloods have, of course, been found. Individuals who are genetically *Kp^a/Kp^a* or *Kp^a/K^o* and those who are genetically *Kp^c/Kp^c* or *Kp^c/K^o* (see later for details about *K^o* that behaves as a silent allele at the *Kell* complex locus) have Kp(b-) red cells and will draw attention to themselves if they have made anti-Kp^b.

As will be apparent from the frequencies of Kp^a and Kp^b shown in table 18-4, when searches for Kp(b-) blood are undertaken, there is no point in screening samples from other than White donors. As described in the next section, there is no point in looking for Js(b-) samples in other than Blacks. Unfortunately searches for bloods of these rare phenotypes are made more difficult, at least in the USA, where noting the race of random donors on a regular basis is proscribed. Attempts to convince those who object to racial information on donors being recorded is in the best interests of patients of all races, but particularly those of minorities, are not always successful.

The first example of anti-Kp^a was found (3) in the serum of a man who had never been transfused; in spite of this the antibody reacted best by IAT. Two other examples of anti-Kp^a were described in the original report (3) and many others have been found (28,77,100,160,165) since then. In many cases the antibody appears to be red cell stimulated, it is often IgG and best reactive by IAT. Although we are not aware of any reported transfusion reaction caused by anti-Kp^a, the antibody has caused HDN. In some cases (107,111,160) the disease has been mild, in at least one (160) it caused a positive DAT on the red cells of an infant who required no treatment. In contrast, Smoleniak et al. (165) described a case in which repeated intrauterine transfusions were necessary to prevent death from hydrops fetalis.

Although the Kp(b-) phenotype is rare in all populations studied, many examples of alloimmune anti-Kp^b have been found (3,5,22,28,67,164,166-179). Most are red cell stimulated, IgG antibodies, best reactive by IAT. In subclassing studies (91,92) IgG1 has been seen to be the predominant component although IgG4 has sometimes been involved as well. Two examples of the antibody, that were apparently non-red cell stimulated and that failed to react by IAT, have been found (178,179). While anti-Kp^b does not seem to have been incriminated as causative of a hemolytic transfusion reaction, in vivo red cell survival studies and the monocyte monolayer assay have suggested (173,175) that at least some examples have the potential to cause accelerated clearance of Kp(b+) red cells in vivo. When Steane et al. (171) encountered a patient with anti-Kp^b whose blood needs were so great that sufficient Kp(b-) units were not available from the combined resources of several rare donor files, they elected to reduce the patient's level of anti-Kp^b by plasma exchange. The patient was then transfused with Kp(b+) blood and the plan was to perform an exchange transfusion with the Kp(b-) units that were available, once the causes of the patient's bleeding had been corrected. The plan was not completed because the patient died of sepsis before the Kp(b-) blood was used. However, the Kp(b+) blood apparently enjoyed some in vivo survival when transfused following the plasma exchanges.

At least two other patients with anti-Kp^b in the serum were transfused with Kp(b+) blood and seemed to gain the expected benefits of transfusion. In both cases the transfusion needs of the patient were acute enough that transfusions had to be given before suitable Kp(b-) units could be delivered from international rare donor files. In the patient in Argentina (174), IVIG and corticosteroids were used before transfusion of the Kp(b+) units. In the patient in Australia (177), who had anti-E and anti-S as well as anti-Kp^b, E- S- Kp(b+) units were transfused without pretreatment of the patient with IVIG or corticosteroids. As stated, the transfused Kp(b+) blood appeared to survive normally or near normally in vivo, in both patients the titer of the anti-Kp^b increased considerably after transfusion of the Kp(b+) units. As mentioned in several other places in this book, regardless of the specificity of the antibody, it is better to transfuse serologically incompatible red cells and hope that some of them will survive for some period of time in vivo, than to let the patient die of anemia while searches for antigen-negative blood are undertaken or until such blood arrives from a rare donor file.

Anti-Kp^b has also been incriminated as a cause of HDN. Like other Kell system antibodies (indeed like those of many blood group systems) anti-Kp^b has sometimes caused such mild HDN that no treatment was required (67,166) but on other occasions (170,176) has caused severe disease.

As mentioned in the introduction of this chapter, the first example (24,25) of anti-Kp^c was known as anti-Levay for some 34 years. It was made by a patient with systemic lupus erythematosus who had been transfused many times. The patient also made the first examples of anti-Lu^a, anti-C^w, human anti-N and incomplete anti-c. Cleghorn (66) found no example of anti-Levay (anti-Kp^c) in tests on 5774 sera from English donors. Daniels (168) found additional examples of the antibody in Japanese donors, all were apparently stimulated by exposure to Kp(c+) red cells.

The Antigens Js^a and Js^b and the Antibodies That Define Them

While it is rare in all except Black populations, Js^a is more common in Blacks than is K in Whites, and much more common than Kp^a in Whites and Kp^c in Orientals. In tests on samples from 1298 Black Americans (6,9,180), 206 that were Js(a+) were found, i.e. 15.9% or 1 in 6.3. In tests on samples from 1379 Black Africans (181,182) 205 that were Js(a+) were found, i.e. 14.9% or 1 in 6.7. When Byrne and Howard (183) typed 438 Black American donors selected because they had C- E- S- K- Fy(a-b-) Jk(b-) red cells (that is donors selected for other systems but not for the Kell system, the incidence of K is too low to influence selection) they found that 71 (16.2%), 1 in 6.2 were Js(a+). Using the figures from American Blacks to calculate the gene frequencies of Js^a and Js^b in that population, it can be seen (table 18-4) that in 1000 random donors from that population, seven should be phenotypically Js(a+b-), 152 Js(a+b+) and 841 Js(a-b+) (the K^o gene is rare enough to be ignored in the calculation). In three studies on samples from American Blacks using anti-Js^b (10,184,185,192) 5844 bloods were typed and 52 Js(b-) samples were found, 42 would have been expected, i.e. the observed and expected numbers are not significantly different. In a later study (186) on samples from 10,848 American Blacks only 34 that were Js(b-) were found, 76 would have been expected. In a follow-up report (319) on the same study, in which a computer program had been used to exclude repeat donors, it was said that 21 of 7341 samples were Js(b-). Again the number is low, among 7341 donors, 51 individuals with the Js(b-) phenotype would have been expected. It is not known if this significantly low number of Js(b-) samples represents a different incidence of *Js^a* and *Js^b* in different areas of the USA or whether the microplate method used in the later study failed to identify all Js(b-) samples. As will be apparent, the figure of only 34 Js(b-) individuals among 10,848 Blacks tested (186) has not been used in the calculation of Kell system phenotype frequencies given in table 18-4. Js^a has been found in at least one White European (28) and in an Arab family living in Israel (190). No Oriental with Js(a+) red cells seems to have been found and, as described below, all examples of anti-Js^b reported have been made by Blacks.

Anti-Js^a is not infrequent, many examples have been described (8,9,180-183,187-191). Most examples of the antibody are red cell stimulated via transfusion or pregnancy but at least one non-red cell immune example has been found (189). Like other antibodies in the Kell system, anti-Js^a usually react well in IATs. Byrne and Howard (183) pointed out that when patients with sickle cell disease are transfused repeatedly, they often make antibodies (among others) to C, E and Fy3. As a result, they are then transfused repeatedly with R_0 (C- D+ E-), Fy(a-b-) blood, all of which is from Black donors. As a result, these patients are frequently and repeatedly exposed to Js^a (and V) and many of them make anti-Js^a (and anti-V).

Anti-Js^a has been incriminated as causative of a delayed hemolytic transfusion reaction (191) and of HDN. As will, by now, be a familiar story, some examples of the antibody have caused only mild HDN (77,190) while others (77,188) have caused more severe disease.

Although the Js(b-) phenotype is more common in Blacks than is the Kp(b-) phenotype in Whites, anti-Js^b is still a comparatively rare antibody. Since the original examples were described (10,140) others have been documented in the literature (184,192-197). Like many other antibodies in the Kell system, most anti-Js^b are IgG in nature and optimally reactive by IAT. Waheed and Kennedy (141) described an alloimmune anti-Js^b, made in a patient with Js(b+) red cells, that caused a delayed transfusion reaction following the transfusion of Js(b+) red cells. It is not known if this finding means that the Js^b antigen comprises more than one epitope and if rare persons with Js(b+) red cells can make an alloantibody to

epitopes of Js^b that their red cells lack. If such a situation exists, it was not revealed in a study of the family of this antibody-maker. Ratcliff et al. (197) described a woman with anti-Js^b in the serum who gave birth to an infant with hydrops fetalis caused by that antibody. Because no Js(b-) units were immediately available and because transfusion was considered essential to save life, the baby was transfused with 100 ml and the mother with 275 ml of Js(b+) red cells. The baby died five hours later. The mother had no obvious clinical reaction to the transfusion with Js(b+) red cells and was transfused with five units of Js(b-) blood, when it became available, over the next four days. Survival of the Js(b+) red cells in the mother was followed retrospectively using flow cytometry. Although the Js(b+) red cells did not survive normally in vivo, their destruction was not immediate. At 19 hours posttransfusion just over 50% of the expected number of Js(b+) red cells, had those cells survived normally, were still present. By the fourth post transfusion day, no Js(b+) red cells remained in circulation. Again, it is better to give incompatible blood, when nothing else is available, than to let a patient hemorrhage to death.

Anti Js^b has caused HDN. By now it will come as no surprise that in one case (194) no treatment was required, in two others (195,196) the disease was moderately severe, while in the case described above (197) the anti-Js^b caused hydrops fetalis.

The Gene *K^o*, the Phenotype Kell_null or K_o and the Antigen Ku

In 1957, Chown et al. (4) described their study on the blood of Mrs. Peltz. At that time only four Kell system antigens K, k, Kp^a and Kp^b were known. Mrs. Peltz had the previously undescribed phenotype K- k- Kp(a-b-). A family study showed that the Peltz phenotype, as it was first called, apparently represented the homozygous state of silent alleles at the *Kell* complex locus. The gene involved became known as *K^o* and individuals of the *K^o K^o* genotype are now said to have the Kell_null phenotype. The term K_o phenotype is often used instead of Kell_null. In 1965, the first clue that Js^a and Js^b are a third pair of antithetical antigens in the Kell system was provided by the finding (6) that the red cells of *K^o* homozygotes are Js(a-b-). Family studies were then undertaken (6,7) and it was demonstrated that all persons who are phenotypically K+ k+ Js(a+b+) are genetically *kJs^a/KJs^b*. As new Kell system and para-Kell antigens have been found, it has been shown that the red cells of *K^o* homozygotes lack them all, i.e. they are phenotypically K- k- Kp(a-b-c-) Js(a-b-) Ul(a-) K:-11,-12,-13,-14,-16, Wk(a-) K:-18,-19,-20,-22,-23,-24,-25. The red cells of *K^o* homozygotes carry the antigen Kx (that was originally called K15). Indeed, Kx is expressed much more strongly on $Kell_{null}$ red cells than on any others. However, as described in more detail later in this chapter (where full references are given), production of Kx is now known to be encoded by a gene at a locus on the X chromosome, not from *Kell* complex locus. The Kx antigen is also known to be carried on a different red cell membrane component than the glycoprotein on which Kell system antigens are carried.

A number of other persons of the K^oK^o genotype have been reported (73,153,198-201) in their own right, several more were listed by Race and Sanger (28) via personal communications from other workers. The family described by Nunn et al. (200) was highly unusual. The red cells of the father were K- k+, those of the mother K+ k- and those of their three children K+ k+, K+ k- and K- k-. The explanation, of course, is that the k/K^o and K/K^o parents had produced one child of each of the genotypes K/k, K/K^o and K^o/K^o. The K^o gene has also been seen to be present in the heterozygous state in a number of individuals (45,51,198,202,203). Its presence can be suspected when an individual apparently homozygous for a *Kell* system gene fails to pass that gene to his or her offspring. For example, most persons with Kp(a+b-) red cells are Kp^a homozygotes. If such a person produces offspring with Kp(a-) red cells, the Kp^a/K^o genotype provides an explanation. The reason that most persons phenotypically Kp(a+b-) are Kp^a/Kp^a and not Kp^a/K^o is, of course, because Kp^a is more common than K^o.

Chown et al. (153) used the original anti-Ku (see below) made by the first $Kell_{null}$ proposita (4) to look for other K^o homozygotes. In tests on samples from 16,518 random White individuals, one K^o homozygote was found. Race and Sanger (28) compiled data from tests with various Kell system antibodies that would have detected the $Kell_{null}$ phenotype and reported that in tests on samples from 24,953 White donors, only one such sample had been found. In Japan, one $Kell_{null}$ person was found (73) among 14,541 tested. Although most K^o homozygotes are White and are European or of European extraction, the genotype has been found in a Canadian Indian (212) and in a Black American and her brother (213).

The proposita in the case of Chown et al. (4) had several Kell system antibodies in her serum. By adsorbing and eluting a serum aliquot sequentially with K- k+; K+ k-; and Kp(a+b-); red cells, it was shown that an antibody was present that, when separated from the other Kell system antibodies present, reacted with all red cells except those of the $Kell_{null}$ phenotype. This antibody was named anti-Ku (11) and was said to define an antigen present on all cells that carried Kell system antigens, regardless of the phenotype of those cells. While it is apparent that anti-Ku (anti-K5) is different from anti-Js[b], it is not clear that

studies to show that anti-Ku is not a mixture of antibodies directed against K11, K12, K13, K14, K18, K19, K20 and/or K22 have been performed. Clearly the difference is not important. Anti-Ku (anti-K5) can be regarded as the antibody made by immunized K^o homozygotes, with the proviso that the sera of such persons may also contain separable antibodies to other high incidence Kell system antigens. Quite differently from the situation just described, at least two K^o homozygotes (164,172) have made anti-Kp[b] and one (204) anti-k, without anti-Ku. These antibodies are, of course, easy to differentiate from anti-Ku since they fail to react with Kp(a+b-) and K+ k- red cells, respectively; anti-Ku reacts strongly with cells of each of those phenotypes.

From the studies that have been completed there are no reasons to suppose that K^o is anything other than a gene that acts as a silent allele at the *Kell* complex locus. That is to say, there is no evidence for independent suppression in the $Kell_{null}$ phenotype. All persons of that phenotype thus far found appear to be K^o homozygotes. Race and Sanger (28) reported that in 14 families in which a K^o homozygote had been identified, at least four involved cousin marriages. The sib count of nine K^o homozygotes and 29 who were not, was as expected and was different from the excess of Rh-deletion sibs of Rh-deletion probands, described in Chapter 12. No morphological or functional abnormality of $Kell_{null}$ red cells has been reported. Most studies (39,41,205) have suggested that $Kell_{null}$ red cells are devoid of Kell glycoprotein, but one (206) has produced evidence to suggest that an altered non-antigen-bearing structure may be present. The major phenotypic differences between the red cells of K^o homozygotes and those of the McLeod phenotype (see below) are listed in table 18-6.

The Antigen Ul[a] and the Antibody That Defines It

In 1968, Furuhjelm et al. (19) described an antigen with an incidence of 2.6% in the Finnish population, they named the antigen Ul[a]. One year later the same investigators (20) reported that in three families with K+ Ul(a+) members, *K* without Ul^a or k/Ul^a had been passed to all of 13 children. Ul^a has been excluded as an allele of *K* and *k*, and of Kp^a, Kp^b and Kp^c. Suitable family data have not yet been found to exclude the possibility that Ul^a is an additional allele of the genes that encode the antithetical pairs of antigens: Js[a] and Js[b]; Wk[a] and K11; or K14 and K24, if indeed that last pair are antithetical to each other (see below). Unfortunately, anti-Ul[a] does not appear to define an antithetical antigen to the high incidence Kell and para-Kell antigens K12, K13, K18, K19, K20 or K22, none of which yet have recognized antithetical partners.

In the original (19) and subsequent (207) studies, Ul^a was found on the red cells of 68 of 2620 Finns, one of 501 Swedes, one of 12 Chinese but on none of those of 140 Lapps, 66 Blacks, 5000 English and 314 other non-Scandinavian Whites. In a different study (161) Ul^a was found on the red cells of 37 of 8000 Japanese donors.

The two examples of anti-Ul^a found in Finland (19,20) were present in the sera of patients who had received many transfusions. The first anti-Ul^a found in Japan (161) was present in the serum of a male blood donor who had been transfused 15 years earlier. In screening tests on more than 66,000 serum samples from Japanese blood donors, no other example of anti-Ul^a was found (161). However, a second example of the antibody was found in Japan (162) in the serum of a never transfused woman, during her third pregnancy. In Finland, Furuhjelm et al. (19) tested the sera of 19 women of the Ul(a-) phenotype who had borne children with Ul(a+) red cells; none of the sera contained anti-Ul^a. However, one case of moderately severe HDN caused by the antibody has been described (162). An earlier study (163) had shown that, like other antigens of the Kell blood group system, Ul^a is fully developed at birth.

The Antigens Wk^a and Kll and the Antibodies That Define Them

The low incidence antigen Wk^a had been known (34) for some seven years before it was shown (21) to be a part of the Kell system. As mentioned in the introduction, in 1974, Strange et al. (21) used family studies and showed that in five unrelated families in which there were persons with K+ Wk(a+) red cells, the alignment was always *K* without *Wk^a* and *k/Wk^a*. In the initial studies 11,076 samples from English donors were tested, 32 were Wk(a+) for an incidence of 1 in 346. It was noticed that none of the Wk(a+) samples was K+ so additional typings for Wk^a were performed. Among 6956 K+ samples, 7 were Wk(a+) for an incidence of 1 in 994. The significant difference in the incidence of Wk^a in K- and K+ people was then explained by the family studies described above. In further studies no Wk(a+) sample was found among approximately 1000 donors with Kp(a+) red cells.

In 1971, Gúevin et al. (42) described an antibody to a very common antigen, additional details were given in a 1976 publication (52). The antibody, that is now known as anti-K11, reacted with all red cells tested except those of the antibody-maker, two of her sibs and those of *K^o* homozygotes. Red cells of the McLeod phenotype that express all their Kell system antigens very weakly (see below) did not react directly with anti-K11, but were able to adsorb that antibody.

Gavin (35) then found that two K:-11 samples were Wk(a+). Sabo et al. (36) added three more K:-11 Wk(a+) samples from unrelated individuals and used family studies to confirm the allelic relationship between *Wk^a* and *K^11*.

The original anti-Wk^a seems to be the only one described in print, Daniels (29) mentions that others are known. A number of examples of anti-K11 have been published (36,52,208,209). The first example (52) was made by a woman who had never been transfused but who had been pregnant nine times. The second (208), third and fourth (36) examples were formed by women who had been pregnant and transfused, the fifth (36) was made by a woman who had been pregnant but who had not been transfused. That example caused a positive DAT on the red cells of her third child who required no treatment for HDN. No details are given about the history of the 38 year-old woman who made the sixth example (209). It does not seem that K:11 blood has even been transfused to a patient known to have anti-K11 in the serum so that nothing is known about the clinical significance of the antibody in that setting.

The Antigens K14 and K24 and the Antibodies That Define Them

An antibody to a very common antigen, that reacted with all red cells tested except those of the antibody-maker, those of two of her four sibs, and those of *K^o* homozygotes was mentioned briefly in 1973 (43), then described in full in 1976 (54). The antibody was called anti-K14 and was then shown (210) to be the same as anti-Dp, an antibody described in 1970 (211) but not then associated with any known blood group system. The K:-14 probands (54,211), one of whom (211) was originally described as Dp-, were both White.

An antibody to a low incidence antigen, to which the name Cls was given, was described by Eicher et al. (31) in 1985. The antibody reacted with the red cells of the White antibody-maker's two children, those of the childrens' father and several of his direct relatives. In tests on 34 samples known to carry different low incidence antigens and 26 examples known to lack high incidence antigens, the only sample that reacted with anti-Cls, was one known to be K:-14. Two other K:-14 samples were then tested and were shown to react with anti-Cls. Titration studies appeared to support the interpretation that Cls is antithetical to K14. Red cells of the K:-14 phenotype (i.e. assumed to be from *Cls* homozygotes) reacted to higher titer than those phenotypically K:14 Cls+ (i.e. assumed to be from *Cls* heterozygotes). Anti-Cls was named anti-K24 and it is believed that K14 and K24 are the products of alleles.

The first antibody to be named anti-K14 was made by a White woman of French-Cajun extraction who had been pregnant seven times but who had never been transfused (54). Her fourth and fifth pregnancies ended in abortions, her sixth and seventh pregnancies resulted in live births, in both instances the infants had a positive DAT due to the anti-K14. Transfusion was contemplated for the infant resulting from the seventh pregnancy because of anemia and hyperbilirubinemia but was avoided when the clinical condition of the infant improved spontaneously. The K:-14 woman's parents were not known to be related. The lady who made what was originally called anti-Dp (211) that was later shown (210) to be the same as anti-K14 was also White and was also from the Bayou country of Louisiana. She too had been pregnant but never transfused, her parents were known (211) to be first cousins. In neither patient with anti-K14 was transfusion necessary so that the clinical significance of the antibody in a transfusion setting is not known.

The ethnic background of the White woman who made the only known example of anti-Cls is not given in the abstract describing the antibody (31). However, the case was reported out of New Orleans so that a Cajun or Bayou connection for Cls would surely support the presumption that Cls and K14 are the products of alleles. The antibody was made by a woman who had been pregnant but never transfused. The anti-Cls (anti-K24) caused a positive DAT on the red cells of the antibody-maker's second child but no treatment other than phototherapy was required.

The McLeod Phenotype and the Antigens Kx and Km

Although it is now known that the Kx antigen is not carried on the Kell glycoprotein and that the gene that encodes its production is on the X chromosome so is not at the *Kell* complex locus, lack of the glycoprotein on which Kx is carried has a dramatic effect on red cell expression of Kell system antigens. Accordingly the McLeod phenotype, the name used to describe the phenotype that results when no Kx is made, is described here. Genetic control of Kx production (the Xk blood group system) and some of the clinical effects associated with lack of Kx are described later in this chapter.

In 1961, Allen et al. (16) described a new phenotype in the Kell system. At first it was thought that the McLeod cells were representative of the K^oK^o genotype but it soon became apparent that the cells in fact carried weak expressions of some Kell system antigens. The revised terminology for the McLeod phenotype was K-k+^{w} Kp(a-b+^{w}). The expression of k and Kp^b on McLeod cells was such that adsorption-elution studies were

sometimes necessary to demonstrate their presence. Nunn et al. (200) and Stroup et al. (6) respectively showed that red cells of the McLeod phenotype carry weak expressions of Ku and Js^b. When discovered (16), it was apparent that the McLeod phenotype was not controlled from the *Kell* complex locus. The parents of the propositus had red cells of the phenotype K- k+ Kp(a-b+) and no evidence emerged to suggest other than that both of them were homozygous for the common Kell system haplotype *kKp^{b}Js^b*. As additional antigens have been added to the Kell system it has been seen that those that are present on McLeod phenotype red cells are very weakly expressed. Adsorption-elution studies are often necessary to demonstrate the presence of antigens such as K11, K12, K13, etc., on red cells of the phenotype.

In 1968, Hart et al. (14) described a young boy (Claas) with red cells of the McLeod phenotype, who had been transfused before his rare Kell system phenotype was recognized. Although, in retrospect, it can be seen that Claas was the first described patient with X-linked chronic granulomatous disease (CGD) and the McLeod phenotype, this section will describe just the red cell alloantibodies that he made. The Claas serum reacted with all red cells with normal Kell system phenotypes and with those of K^o homozygotes. It failed to react with the cells of the antibody-maker and with those of the original McLeod propositus (16). The antibody was named anti-KL and was later also called anti-K9. It was, of course, difficult to explain why a Kell system antibody reacted with Kell$_{null}$ red cells. Seven years later, during extensive investigations of the association of the McLeod phenotype with CGD, Marsh et al. (51) found that McLeod red cells lack an antigen that they called Kx. Immunized individuals of the McLeod phenotype are able to make anti-Kx (that at one time was also called anti-K15). The Kx antigen is present in large amounts on the red cells of persons genetically K^oK^o, in smaller amounts on the red cells of persons heterozygous for K^o and in smallest amounts on the red cells of persons with two fully expressed haplotypes at the *Kell* complex locus. Thus it was clear (51) that anti-KL and anti-Kx were not identical in specificity for anti-KL had been shown (14) to react equally with all cells except those of the McLeod phenotype, regardless of the presence (rare) or absence (very common) of a K^o gene in the individuals involved. The situation with regard to the antibody specificities was clarified by Marsh (15). He pointed out that Hart et al. (14) had suspected that anti-KL might include more than one specificity. Marsh et al. (51) and Marsh (15) showed that if anti-KL is adsorbed on to the red cells of K^o homozygotes, one antibody, anti-Kx, is removed and can be recovered as a single specificity by elution from the cells used in the adsorption. A second antibody, for which the terms anti-Km and anti-K20 were suggested (15), is not removed from anti-KL by adsorption with Kell$_{null}$ red cells. Anti-Km defines an antigen (Km or K20) that is present on all cells with normal Kell system phenotypes but is missing from Kell$_{null}$ and McLeod phenotype red cells. In short, anti-KL could now be regarded as a mixture of anti-Kx and anti-Km with the two antibodies being separable by differential adsorption.

Again as discussed in more detail below, production of Kx is encoded by a gene on the X chromosome. It is believed that presence of the glycoprotein on which Kx is carried is essential for the Kell glycoprotein, that carries all the antigens of the Kell system, to attach to or to be expressed normally on red cells. In the common situation, the Kx-bearing glycoprotein is made, then the Kell glycoprotein is somehow attached to it, or expressed near it, thus sterically blocking the access of anti-Kx to its antigen. In other words, red cells with normal expressions of Kell system antigens, react only weakly with anti-Kx. In individuals homozygous for K^o no Kell glycoprotein is made. The Kx glycoprotein is made normally (by a gene genetically independent of the *Kell* locus). Thus no Kell glycoprotein blocks access of anti-Kx to its antigen on the Kx glycoprotein and Kell$_{null}$ red cells reacted strongly with anti-Kx. The red cells of K^o heterozygotes give intermediate reactions between those of K^o homozygotes and those of people with two common *Kell* system haplotypes, when tested with anti-Kx. In the McLeod phenotype, no Kx glycoprotein is made. Although such individuals have normal *Kell* system haplotypes on both chromosomes, their Kell glycoprotein is not expressed normally (perhaps because no Kx glycoprotein is present to allow attachment of the Kell glycoprotein). As a result, those Kell system antigens that are present are all poorly expressed in the McLeod phenotype.

Since the loci involving the production of the Kx-bearing and Kell glycoproteins are independent, it would be expected that most persons with the McLeod phenotype would be genetically kKp^bJs^b/kKp^bJs^b, i.e. homozygous for the common *Kell* system haplotype. This expectation has been borne out in fact. Most of the more than 60 known McLeod bloods (14,16,51,58,200, 202,216-238) that have been carefully studied at the serological level, have been found to carry weak expressions of k, Kp^b, Js^b and the other high incidence antigens of the system and to lack K, Kp^a, Js^a and the other low incidence Kell system antigens. Indeed it was becoming a little worrying, if the Kell glycoprotein and the Kx-bearing structure interact in the manner described above, that no K+ or Kp(a+) McLeod phenotype had been found. Fears were put to rest when Marsh et al. (239) found an individual of the McLeod phenotype who had K+ red cells. As had been anticipated, the phenotype in the man involved was K+^{w} k+^{w} Kp(a-b+^{w}) with the K, k and Kp^b antigens all being very weakly expressed. The

family also provided additional evidence of independence of the gene responsible for the McLeod phenotype from the *Kell* complex locus. The McLeod individual of the K+^{w} k+^{w} Kp(a-b+^{w}) phenotype had a brother, who was also of the McLeod phenotype but his red cells were K- k+^{w} Kp(a-b+^{w}). In other words, the *Kk* father of the brothers, who had normal expressions of K and k on his red cells, had passed *K* to one son and *k* to the other. Neither gene influenced expression of the McLeod phenotype present in the sons following their inheritance of a non-Kx producing gene on one of their mother's X chromosomes.

Eleven years after an individual with the McLeod phenotype and with *K* in one of his *Kell* system haplotypes was reported (239) a propositus was found (279,280,390) in whom the mutant X-borne gene leading to the McLeod phenotype appears to be present in an individual who has Kp^a in both of his *Kell* system haplotypes. The red cells of the propositus carry no detectable Kell system or para-Kell antigens but the man cannot be a K^o homozygote. First, he has passed Kp^a to each of his three children. Second, his red cells react only weakly with anti-Kx. His two daughters have red cells that are Kp(a+b+) but have reduced expressions of all the Kell system and para-Kell antigens. Presumably the daughters are carriers of the mutant allele of the McLeod phenotype having received a normal paternal X chromosome. The son of the propositus has Kp(a+b+) red cells and expresses his red cell Kell system and para-Kell antigens in normal or near normal amounts. Presumably the son makes normal Kx glycoprotein having inherited a maternal X and the paternal Y chromosome. As described in a later section, when Kp^a is present it exerts a depressing effect on the amount of antigens encoded by other Kell system genes in the haplotype (i.e. a *cis* position effect). Thus the most likely explanation in this case seems to be that the propositus has the X chromosome-borne gene whose presence results in the McLeod phenotype and two kKp^aJs^b haplotypes. If that is the case, it seems that this combination results in no production of detectable red cell-borne Kell system or para-Kell antigens.

Marsh et al. (51) have pointed out that anti-Kx can be used to recognize the presence of K^o in individuals heterozygous for that gene and a normal *Kell* haplotype. Such differentiation cannot usually be made by titrations with antibodies to high incidence Kell system antigens (51,240). As mentioned above, red cells from K^o heterozygotes react more strongly with anti-Kx than do cells from individuals with two common *Kell* haplotypes, but less strongly than do cells from K^o homozygotes. Daniels (29) has pointed out that use of this differentiation method is limited by two factors. First, anti-KL (actually anti-Km plus anti-Kx) from immunized McLeod individuals is always in short supply. Second, separation of the two antibodies by adsorption with red cells from K^o homozygotes is often difficult to achieve. Clearly, common Kell phenotype bloods cannot be used in the adsorptions. Although such cells carry a strong expression of Km, they also carry a weak expression of Kx, so would be capable of adsorbing both antibodies. The difficulty in separating anti-Kx from anti-Km may relate to the nature of the Km determinant. A speculative model regarding formation of that antigen is presented in the next section.

The McLeod phenotype is rare and is predominantly a characteristic of Whites. As mentioned above, more than 60 individuals with the phenotype are known (58). Almost all are White but the phenotype has been seen in at least one American Black (225) and one Japanese (237). Since the phenotype is determined by an X chromosome-borne gene it is seen almost exclusively in males, one full blown McLeod phenotype female has been reported (236) and, as described in a later section, the carrier state in females can be recognized. The clinical relevance of anti-Kx and anti-Km in transfusion therapy is discussed in a later section. Table 18-6 lists the antigens most commonly present in the McLeod phenotype and contrasts red cells of that phenotype with those of K^o homozygotes.

The Antigen Km, a Theoretical Model

As mentioned in the previous section, both McLeod phenotype red cells and those from K^o homozygotes lack the antigen Km, i.e. they are K:-20. Further, Km is the only Kell or Xk system antigen missing from both phenotypes (except, of course, when one antigen of an antithetical pair replaces the other, e.g. Kp(a+b-) red cells lack Kp^b). Because it is not present on the red cells of K^o homozygotes and because like other Kell system antigens, it is denatured when red cells are treated with AET (see below), Km is often regarded as a high incidence Kell system antigen whose production is encoded from the *Kell* complex locus. Such an assumption means that Km should be carried on the Kell glycoprotein. A flaw in such a concept is that McLeod phenotype red cells are Km- although such cells must carry a small amount of the Kell glycoprotein. Even if antibodies such as those directed against k, Kp^b, Js^b, Ku, K11, K12, etc., do not react visibly with McLeod phenotype red cells, they can be adsorbed onto and eluted from those cells. Thus if Km (K20) was analogous to K11, K12, K13, etc., it should be present in small amounts on red cells of the McLeod phenotype. This is clearly not the case. First, anti-Km is not adsorbed by McLeod phenotype red cells. Second, individuals of the McLeod phenotype, when immunized, make anti-Km. By definition (15), anti-KL as made by

TABLE 18-6 To Compare Kell System and Kx Antigens on the Red Cells of K^o Homozygotes and those of the McLeod Phenotype

K^o Homozygotes	McLeod[*1]
K- k-	K- k+[w*2]
Kp(a-b-c-)	Kp(a- b+[w] c-)
Js(a-b-)	Js(a-b+[w])
Ku-	Ku+[w]
K_x +[strong] K:-20	K_x- K:-20
Ul(a-) Wk(a-)	Ul(a-) Wk(a-)
K:-12, -13, -14, -18, -19, -22, -23, -24, -25	K: w12, w13, w14, w18, w19, w22, -23, -24, -25
RAZ-, TOU-	

[*1]　Most common McLeod phenotype shown. Rare examples will carry weak expression of K (239) or Kp^a (279) or one of the other low incidence Kell system antigens.

[*2]　Those antigens shown as +[w] can sometimes only be detected via adsorption-elution studies.

these individuals is anti-Kx plus anti-Km. In at least one case (234) anti-KL (containing anti-Km) was made by a McLeod phenotype male who had never been transfused. In at least two other cases (224,235) McLeod phenotype individuals who had been transfused, made anti-Km without anti-Kx. One of these patients was further transfused with blood from K^o homozygotes (i.e. strongly Kx+, Km-) after he had made anti-Km, but still did not make anti-Kx (235). Clearly, McLeod phenotype red cells carry some Kell glycoprotein but not the Km antigen.

Km cannot be present on the Kx glycoprotein. Red cells of K^o homozygotes carry that protein, are strongly Kx+, but are Km-. Indeed, in this respect, Km, again resembles the high incidence antigens encoded from the *Kell* complex locus.

Since Km is clearly associated with the Kell and Xk blood group systems, the data that suggest that it is not present on either the Kell or the Kx glycoprotein, create a dilemma. The findings could all be explained if Km actually represents an interaction product between the Kell and Kx glycoproteins. In other words, it would be supposed that in order for Km to be expressed at the serological level, both Kell and Kx glycoproteins must be present. Absence of Km from the red cells of K^o homozygotes (no Kell glycoprotein) and those of the McLeod phenotype (no Kx glycoprotein) would thus be explained as would the denaturation of the antigen by AET (Kell glycoprotein altered or removed). The suggestion that Km requires presence of both the Kell and Kx glycoproteins for expression is not harmed by the findings of supposed interactions between those components, as described above. There is, of course, precedence for the supposition that interaction between two red cell membrane components, whose production is encoded from genetically independent loci, can result in expression of a red cell antigen. As described in Chapter 17, the Wr^a/Wr^b polymorphism represents an amino acid difference on protein band 3. However, Wr^b is not expressed at the serological level unless a portion of normal glycophorin A is present. The gene that encodes production of band 3 is on chromosome 17, the gene that encodes production of glycophorin A is on chromosome 4. The gene that encodes production of the Kell glycoprotein is on chromosome 7, the gene that encodes production of Kx is on the X chromosome.

The Clinical Significance of Anti-Kx and Anti-Km

Anti-KL, that is anti-Kx plus anti-Km, the most common immune response of McLeod individuals, has twice been incriminated as causative of a hemolytic transfusion reaction (14,221). It is of course, impossible to know which of the antibodies was destructive of red cells. As mentioned above, one untransfused male of the McLeod phenotype (234) made anti-Km plus anti-Kx and two who had been transfused (224,235) made anti-Km without anti-Kx. In one of these patients (235) further transfusions were required. An in vivo red cell survival study using ^{51}Cr labeled red cells, showed that the test dose of normal Kell phenotype red cells (i.e. Km+ Kx+^{w}) was completely cleared within 24 hours of injection. Similar survival studies using red cells from a K^o homozygote (i.e. Km- Kx+^{s}) showed much slower clearance (i.e. 57% of the test dose present 48 hours after injection) and the patient was transfused with four Kell$_{null}$ and one Kell$_{mod}$ (see below) units. The transfusion outcome was satisfactory and, surprisingly, the patient did not make anti-Kx. The apparent ease with which some McLeod phenotype individuals make anti-Kx and anti-Km (14,214,215,234) and the fact that others seem to make only anti-Km, in spite of exposure to Kx+ red cells, could conceivably mean that there is an as yet unrecognized heterogeneity of the McLeod phenotype. Since alloimmune anti-Km and anti-Kx can be made only by individuals of the McLeod phenotype, all except one (236) of whom have been male, neither antibody has had the opportunity to cause HDN.

The Antigen K12 and the Antibody That Defines It

In 1973, Heisto et al. (43) described the serum Bøc that defined a high incidence antigen present on all except the red cells of the antibody-maker and those of K^o homozygotes. The antibody was called anti-K12. In the same year, Marsh et al. (53) described the serum Sp, that contained the second example of anti-K12. The Sp anti-K12 reacted with all of 1000 random samples, most of which were from Whites and with 33 selected samples from Blacks (53). In 1982, Beattie et al. (241) described two brothers with K:-12 red cells, both of whom had been transfused and both of whom had anti-K12 in the serum. In 1995, Reid et al. (242) described another male with K:-12 red cells and anti-K12 in his serum. They used immunoprecipitation studies and the MAIEA assay to demonstrate that K12 is on the Kell glycoprotein and thus concluded that K12 can be moved from para-Kell status, into the Kell system proper. These observations were, of course, in line with earlier findings that K12 is only weakly expressed on red cells of the McLeod phenotype and is denatured when red cells are treated with AET (see below). The K:-12 phenotype has been found thus far only in Whites. An original report (53) that a man with K:-12 red cells was Black, was later corrected (243), the patient was White.

Anti-K12 seems to be made following the transfusion of blood. However, once made the antibody does not seem to be clinically significant. On at least two occasions (241,242) K:12 red cells have been transfused to individuals with anti-K12 in the serum, with no untoward effects and no evidence of accelerated red cell clearance. Following transfusion the DAT may become positive and the anti-K12 may (but does not invariably) increase in titer. However, as stated, there are no reported clinical sequelae associated with these laboratory findings. Anti-K12 does not seem ever to have had an opportunity to cause HDN.

The Antigen K13 and the Antibody That Defines It

The antibody to the high incidence antigen K13 was described briefly in a 1973 abstract (44) and more fully in a 1974 report (45). It was made by a White American of Italian extraction, who had been transfused in the past. The antibody reacted with all red cells of common Kell system phenotype, weakly with those of the McLeod phenotype but was non-reactive with the red cells of K^o homozygotes, those of the antibody-maker and those of one of his five sibs. The compatible sib had not been transfused but had been pregnant seven times; her serum did not contain anti-K13. In screening tests the anti-K13 was found to react with the red cells of 1000 random donors, most of whom were White.

In studying the family of the K:-13 propositus, Marsh et al. (45) produced evidence that the two individuals with K:-13 red cells were heterozygous for K^o. The K:-13 red cells had weak expressions of k, Kp^b, Js^b, Ku and K12. This weakening was attributed to the presence of the K^{-13} haplotype, not to the presence of K^o, since other members of the family who were K^{13}/K^o had normal expressions of k, Kp^b, Js^b, Ku and K12 on their red cells. Similarly, others (28,198) had already reported that K^o/kKp^bJs^b heterozygotes have red cells with essentially normal expressions of k, Kp^b, and Js^b. The whole story of *cis* modifying effects in various *Kell* haplotypes is given in a later section of this chapter. Similarly, an example of auto-anti-K13 (244) is described below. Nothing is known about the clinical significance of alloimmune anti-K13.

The Antigen K16 and the Antibody That Defines It

In 1976, Marsh (46) listed K16 as being a k-like antigen found on the k+ red cells of 99.8% of Whites. The antigen was said (245) to be present when k was present and absent from k- cells. The difference between k and K16 was that McLeod phenotype red cells were k+^{w} K:-16. It was not clear whether the difference was qualitative or quantitative and, as far as we are aware, no further studies on K16 have been reported.

The Antigen K18 and the Antibody That Defines It

In 1975, Barrasso et al. (47) described yet another antibody directed against a high incidence antigen, that reacted with all red cells tested except those of the antibody-maker and those of K^o homozygotes. The antibody reacted with all previously described samples (K:-12, K:-13, etc.) lacking such antigens so was seen to have a new specificity, that the authors named anti-K18. The IgG antibody was made by a White woman who had been pregnant eight times and had been transfused 22 years earlier. Her serum contained anti-K and anti-K18, in tests on 2000 K- samples, no further K:-18 blood was found. It was noticed (47) that K18 was expressed less strongly on Kp(a+b-) and K:-13 red cells than on those that were Kp(b+) K:13 (again see below). The K18 antigen was very weakly expressed on McLeod phenotype red cells. In 1983, Barrasso et al. (246) described additional studies undertaken when they were asked to assess the clinical significance of the anti-K18 found in 1975 and to determine whether donors with K:-18 red cells could be found. The antibody was shown to be a mixture of mostly IgG4 and some IgG1. In an in vivo red cell survival study using ^{51}Cr-labeled K- K:18 red cells it was

found that only 31% of the test dose was present in the patient's circulation, 24 hours after injection. A monocyte assay forecast that K:18 red cells would be destroyed in vivo. Tests on 54,450 donors revealed none with K:-18 red cells. In view of these findings and because red cells from K^o homozygotes were not available to provide long term support, the patient's physicians elected to modify treatment so that transfusion could be avoided.

In 1990, Pehta et al. (247) described the second example of anti-K18. The antibody was made by a 78 year-old White male who had been transfused. Both anti-K and anti-K18 were present in his serum. In tests in a flow cytometer, the K:18 red cells of the patient's son reacted less strongly than random K:18 samples thus providing the only evidence to date that K18 is an inherited character. Immunoprecipitation studies with the anti-K18 showed that the antigen defined is apparently present on the Kell glycoprotein, thus strengthening the supposition that this para-Kell antigen is part of the Kell blood group system. The abstract (247) describing this second individual with K:-18 red cells mentioned that the patient's red cells were non-reactive with four examples of anti-Yt^a and two examples of anti-Yt^b. As discussed in Chapter 23, the only other known example of the Yt(a-b-) phenotype represented transient depression of expression of Yt^a. It is not known if this case (247) represented a similar phenomenon.

The Antigen K19 and the Antibody That Defines It

The first example of anti-K19 was found (48) in the serum of a 40-year-old woman (race not mentioned in the paper) who had delivered one live child, had six miscarriages (ranging from two to five months gestation) but had not previously been transfused. Her serum, that also contained a weak anti-K, reacted with all red cells of common Kell system phenotypes and with those lacking other high incidence Kell and para-Kell antigens. Her serum was non-reactive with the red cells of K^o homozygotes, her own cells and those of one of her three sibs. The antigen defined was shown to be weaker on Kp(a+b-) and K:-13 red cells than on Kp(b+) and K:13 red cells, it was very weakly expressed on red cells of the McLeod phenotype. The expression of k, Kp^b, Js^b and other high incidence Kell system and para-Kell antigens was normal on K:-19 red cells. In tests on the red cells of 7294 random donors, no K:-19 sample was found.

Later in 1979, Marsh et al. (248) described the second example of anti-K19. The antibody was made by a 47-year-old Black male who had been transfused many times. The anti-K19 caused a delayed transfusion reaction and was reported to have cleared four units of K:19 blood within 10 days of their transfusion. However, hemorrhage secondary to hepatic disease caused by alcohol abuse, may have contributed to loss of some of the transfused K:19 red cells. Since their patient's serum contained anti-C as well as anti-K19 (the K:19 cells transfused were C-) Marsh et al. (248) continued to screen random donors with the original anti-K19. To the 7294 donors already screened by them and reported by Sabo et al. (48), Marsh et al. (248) added another 3463 random samples but found no other K:-19 blood. While a total of 10,757 samples had thus been tested without finding a K:-19 donor, Marsh et al. (248) pointed out that most of those samples were from Whites and, at least their patient with K:-19 red cells, was Black.

The Antigen K22 and the Antibody That Defines It

The first example of anti-K22 was identified by Bar Shany et al. (49) in the serum of an Israeli woman of Persian Jewish extraction. The antibody was found when the proposita donated blood. The lady had four sons, none of whom had jaundice or HDN at birth, but had never been transfused. The antibody detected an antigen of high incidence that was present on all red cells of normal Kell system phenotypes and on those of individuals lacking other high incidence Kell system or para-Kell antigens. The antibody was non-reactive with the red cells of K^o homozygotes, those of one of two McLeod phenotype individuals, the donor's own cells and those of one of three sibs. It was then shown that the non-reactive McLeod phenotype sample adsorbed anti-K22. Red cells of the Kp(a+b-) and K:-13 phenotypes expressed K22 normally. In tests on samples from 500 donors of mixed races in Israel, no further example of K:-22 red cells was found.

In 1985, Manny et al. (249) described another K:-22 proposita, like the first, the lady was an Iranian Jew living in Israel. The anti-K22 was found in her serum during her fourth pregnancy, she had been transfused after her first pregnancy. In the family studied, a little more evidence that K22 is a Kell system antigen was obtained. The consanguineous parents of the proposita were both phenotypically K+ k+ and throughout the family K always traveled with K^{22}, the gene not encoding production of K22 always traveled with k. That is, the proposita and her two K:-22 sibs were K- k+, her two K:22 sibs were both K+ k+. However, while suggestive, the data were too few in number to achieve statistical significance. Tests on 217 unrelated people from the Iranian Jewish ethnic group did not reveal another K:-22 sample. In this second study it was shown that

like other Kell system antigens, the expression of K22 is reduced on the red cells of persons genetically Kp^a/K^o (see also a later section). Redman et al. (28) have shown that K22 is carried on the 93kD Kell glycoprotein. As also discussed in a later section, many sera that contain alloimmune or autoimmune antibodies to high incidence Kell and para-Kell antigens, also contain anti-K. Often this is the case although the antibody-maker has never been exposed to K+ red cells. Neither proposita who made anti-K22 made anti-K (49,249). This was of particular note in the second case. The lady involved was D-, K- and had borne four D+ children, one of whom was also K+. The only antibody she made was anti-K22.

At the time of the full report, the second proposita with anti-K22 had delivered four children. The fourth had a positive DAT at birth and became mildly jaundiced but no treatment for HDN was described (249). In a later publication (250) events surrounding the birth of her fourth, fifth and sixth children were more fully documented. During the fourth and fifth pregnancies the anti-K22 in her serum was IgG1 in nature. Both infants had a positive DAT at birth and both were treated with phototherapy. When the sixth child was born, the DAT on the cord blood red cells was positive with both anti-IgG1 and anti-IgG3. The infant was severely affected and an exchange transfusion was performed using washed red cells from the mother, the child was also treated with high doses of IVIG.

The Antigen K23 and the Antibody That Defines It

In 1987, Marsh et al. (27) studied a case in which a gravida 4, para 3 White woman of Italian ancestry had an antibody that caused a strongly positive DAT on the red cells of her third child. The maternal antibody and an eluate made from the infant's red cells reacted with the red cells of one of the two previous children, those of the father of the children and those of his mother. The antibody did not react with numerous red cell samples known, among them, to carry a large number of different published and non-published antigens of low incidence, others known among them to lack a large number of antigens of high incidence, nor with any of 2116 samples from normal donors. Thus the case appeared to involve an antibody directed against a previously unrecognized antigen of low incidence.

The antigen involved was inactivated when the paternal red cells were treated with AET or ZZAP (see below). When the maternal antibody was used in immunoprecitation studies with the paternal red cells, a 93kD glycoprotein was precipitated. That glycoprotein was then shown to react with a rabbit antibody, specific for the Kell glycoprotein. The low incidence antigen involved was named K23. Disappointingly, K23 did not prove to be antithetical to any of the high incidence Kell system antigens described in the previous few sections and in table 18-2, that lack such partners. Although the maternal anti-K23 caused a strongly positive DAT on the red cells of the woman's third child, it did not cause clinical HDN.

The Antigen VLAN and the Antibody That Defines It

In 1996, Jongerius et al. (32) described anti-VLAN, that detects an antigen of low incidence. The VLAN antigen was found to be present on the red cells of a Dutch blood donor (race not specified), those of two of his sisters and those of a daughter of one of those women. Although not all the family members could be tested, VLAN was seen to be an inherited characteristic. In screening tests on random samples (race of the donors not given) no VLAN+ sample was found among 1068 tested. Because treatment of red cells with AET was shown to denature the VLAN antigen, it was suspected that the antigen might be in the Kell blood group system. Accordingly, six monoclonal antibodies to epitopes on the Kell glycoprotein and anti-VLAN were used in the MAIEA assay. It was shown (32) that the antigen is indeed carried on the 93kD Kell glycoprotein, blocking effects suggested that VLAN might be located at or close to the site of Kp^a, Kp^b and Kp^c on the glycoprotein. Anti-VLAN did not react with any red cell sample lacking a high incidence antigen so that VLAN does not seem to be antithetical to any common Kell system antigen that currently lacks such a partner. Based on the blocking studies mentioned above, it was considered possible (32) that the gene that encodes production of VLAN might be a fourth allele at the *Kp^{a}Kp^{b}Kp^c* sublocus. Based on the findings described above, VLAN was assigned the term KEL25 (33) in the ISBT terminology, it would be called K25 in the ordinary numerical terminology.

The only known example of anti-VLAN was made by a 60 year-old White Dutch patient whose transfusion history was not known. The antibody was composed of IgG1 and IgG2 and reacted by multiple methods including virtually all forms of IAT.

The incidences of the low incidence Kell system antigens in different populations, are summarized in table 18-7.

The Antigens RAZ and TOU and the Antibodies That Define Them

In 1994, Daniels et al. (64) described an antibody found in the serum of a woman of Kenyan-Indian origin, that defined an antigen of very high incidence. The antibody-maker's parents were first cousins. The antibody was provisionally called anti-RAZ and was reactive with

TABLE 18-7 Some Studies on the Incidence of Low Frequency Kell System Antigens

Antigen	Number of Red Cell Samples Tested	Population	Number Positive	References
K		Whites (US, Canada, Europe)	Circa 9%	Multiple, see text
		Whites (Finland)	Circa 4.5%	19
		Blacks (mostly in US)	1.5 to 2.5%	6, 72
	4850	Japanese	1	73
Kp^a	18,934	Whites (US, Canada, Europe)	440	3, 28, 68, 153
Kp^c	10,416	Japanese	25	154, 155
		Much lower in other populations		See text
Js^a	1736	Blacks in US	277	6, 9, 180, 183
Ul^a	2620	Finns	68	19, 207
	501	Swedes	1	19, 207
	5000	English	0	19, 207
	8000	Japanese	37	161
Wk^a	11,076	English	32	21, 34
K23	2116	Random New York donors	0	27
K24	No random survey reported			
K25	1068	Europeans	0	32

all red cells of common Kell system phenotype, those lacking previously described high incidence Kell and para-Kell antigens and the red cells of all available members of the proposita's family. Several lines of evidence qualify RAZ as a para-Kell antigen. First, anti-RAZ is non-reactive with the red cells of K^o homozygotes. Second, the antibody reacts only weakly with red cells of the McLeod and Kell$_{mod}$ (see below) phenotypes. Third, anti-RAZ does not react with AET-treated red cells. Fourth, the MAIEA assay was used to localize the RAZ antigen to the Kell glycoprotein.

The patient who formed anti-RAZ had been pregnant twice. While an exact transfusion history was not available, she had heart surgery 30 years before the antibody was found, at a time when transfusion was commonly used to support the surgical procedure involved. An in vivo red cell survival study using ^{51}Cr-labeled RAZ+ red cells showed that the half-life of the injected dose was three hours and that virtually no cells survived beyond 24 hours. The patient donated her own blood and received five units of that blood at surgery.

Since no RAZ- blood except that of the proposita is known, the antigen has not yet been shown to be inherited. Accordingly RAZ has not yet been given an ISBT Kell system number.

The story with TOU is somewhat similar to that of RAZ. The antibody provisionally called anti-TOU was found (55) in the serum of a 47-year-old Native American admitted to hospital for hip surgery. His serum reacted with all red cells of common Kell system phenotypes but was non-reactive with the red cells of K^o homozygotes and normal red cells treated with DTT (see below). The antibody was weakly reactive with red cells known to have depressed expressions of Kell system antigens, that is: McLeod phenotype; Kell$_{mod}$ (see below); Kp(a+b-); and K:-13 (also see below). The TOU antigen was localized to the Kell glycoprotein by use of the MAIEA assay. The TOU red cells were non-reactive with another antibody, IAN, believed to define a high incidence Kell system antigen, the IAN red cells were non-reactive with anti-TOU. IAN is a Hispanic female hospitalized for a hysterectomy. The red cells of IAN's three sibs and her son were incompatible with her antibody. Thus, like RAZ, TOU (IAN) has not yet been shown to be inherited so has not been given an ISBT Kell system number (but see the addendum).

Kell System Antigens, Proteases and Reducing Agents

The reactions of some Kell system antibodies are enhanced in tests against protease treated red cells. When we (104) tested 10,000 samples from patients, that had given negative antibody screening tests by LISS-IAT, in an IAT system with ficin-treated red cells, we found that seven of them contained an otherwise undetected anti-K. Among those seven antibodies, six were IgM and one IgG as judged by DTT treatment of the sera. The study was retrospective, the tests against ficin-treated red cells were performed on pretransfusion sera, after the patients had been transfused with units compatible by LISS-IAT. By chance, none of the patients in whom anti-K was detected had received K+ blood so we were unable to draw any conclusions about the clinical significance, or lack thereof, of the anti-K. However, in the same study we identified 19 patients with Rh antibodies, detectable in identical circumstances, who among them had received a total of 32 antigen-positive units. Among those 19 patients, one had a delayed transfusion reaction, in the other 18 there were no findings indicative of any untoward reaction. If those findings can be extrapolated to include the anti-K, it would seem that antibodies found in such tests are clinically benign.

Similar enhancement of the reactivity of some Kell system antibodies is seen when papain is used instead of ficin. Trypsin-treatment of red cells does not denature Kell system antigens but use of trypsin-treated red cells does not seem to enhance the reactivity of Kell system antibodies to the same degree as seen when ficin or papain-treated red cells are used. Treatment of red cells with a mixture of trypsin and alpha-chymotrypsin or sequential treatment of red cells with one enzyme, then the other (the sequence does not seem to matter) renders the cells non-reactive with antibodies to Kell system and para-Kell antigens (251,252). Treatment of red cells with chymotrypsin alone or with pronase alone, produces variable results (252), it is not clear if the variation relates to the antibodies used or to the source and methods of use of the enzymes. Some monoclonal antibodies to Kell system antigens continue to react with enzyme-treated red cells that are no longer reactive with human polyclonal antibodies (253).

In 1982, Advani et al. (37) showed that normal red cells treated with 6% aminoethylisothiouronium bromide (AET) at pH8, behave like those of K^o homozygotes. That is to say, the red cells are no longer reactive with any antibody to Kell system or para-Kell antigens but are strongly reactive with anti-Kx (untreated red cells of common Kell system phenotype react weakly with anti-Kx). This ability to make artificial Kell$_{null}$ red cells has greatly facilitated serological studies on Kell system antibodies. Since K^o is so rare, natural Kell$_{null}$ red cells are difficult to obtain. It has been pointed out that some other antigens are denatured or removed when red cells are treated with AET. These include antigens of the: LW (254,255); Lutheran (255-258); Dombrock (255,259-262); Cartwright (255,263); and Knops (255,259) blood group systems and the JMH (255,259) series. While some workers (254,259) have used these observations to caution against the use of AET-treated red cells in antibody identification studies, Marsh et al. (264,265) have pointed out that the danger that confusion will arise is not very great. First, many of the antibodies in the other systems mentioned above give relatively weak reactions in IATs and are not likely to be confused with potent IgG Kell system antibodies. Second, while AET-treated red cells are non-reactive with all antibodies directed against Kell system and para-Kell antigens, their reactions with antibodies in the other systems listed are variable. That is to say, some examples of the antibodies involved will fail to react with AET-treated red cells while others of the same specificity will continue to react. Third, when doubts do arise, adsorption studies can be used. AET-treated red cells will often adsorb antibodies directed against JMH, Gy^a, Hy, Kn and McC antigens even when they fail to give visibly positive reactions with those antibodies (264), see table 18-8. Correctly prepared AET-treated red cells will not adsorb antibodies directed against Kell system and para-Kell antigens.

In 1982, Branch and Petz (57) published a full description of their reagent ZZAP, that had already been used by many blood group serologists following its description in a 1980 abstract (266). The ZZAP reagent is a mixture of papain and dithiothreitol (DTT) and among other actions, renders treated red cells non-reactive with antibodies to Kell system and para-Kell antigens. In 1983, Branch et al. (56) showed that treatment with DTT alone will render red cells non-reactive with those antibodies. Many of the publications cited above describing antigen denaturation by AET also describe similar activities by DTT, other reports (267-271) describe the actions of DTT but not those of ZZAP.

Clearly, both AET and DTT act by reducing inter and intrapolypeptide disulfide bonds that are necessary for antigen expression at the serological (phenotypic) level. The finding (56) that Js^a and Js^b are denatured by much lower concentrations of DTT than those that are necessary to disrupt some other Kell system antigens, relates to the location of the various antigens on the Kell glycoprotein and is discussed in detail in the section on biochemistry of the system.

A solution containing glycine, hydrochloric acid and EDTA can also be used (272,273) to treat red cells to denature Kell system and para-Kell antigens. It was claimed (273) that some of the antigens outside the Kell system, that were listed above, survive glycine-HCl-EDTA treatment of red cells, better than they survive treatment of the cells with AET.

Number of Antigens Sites per Red Cell

From studies using polyclonal anti-K labeled with ^{125}I, Hughes-Jones and Gardner (274) estimated that K+ k- red cells have about 6000 available K sites while the number on K+ k+ cells is about 3500. In tests in which polyclonal IgG antibodies were bound to the red cells, then ferritin-labeled anti-IgG was bound to the cell-bound antibody, Masouredis et al. (275) estimated that K+ k+ red cells carry between 2300 and 6000 K sites. The number of available k sites on K+ k+ and K- k+ red cells was thought to be in the order of 2000 to 5000. Similar figures for K were obtained when a monoclonal anti-K was used (276). When monoclonal antibodies to the Kell glycoprotein were used (253) estimates of around 4000 copies per cell were obtained using intact antibody molecules, but higher numbers were estimated when isolated Fab portions of those antibodies were used, i.e. 4000 to 8000 copies estimated by three of the MAb and 18,000 per cell estimated by a fourth.

Some Position Effects in the Kell System

From the time that Kp^a was first reported (3) it was apparent that the presence of *Kp^a* in a *Kell* complex haplotype results in altered expression of other antigens encoded by that haplotype, i.e. a *cis* position effect. Allen et al. (5) reported that on K- k+ Kp(a+b-) red cells the k antigen was sufficiently depressed that its presence could have been overlooked had not a potent anti-k been used. In the same study, the expression of k on K- k+ Kp(a+b+) red cells was seen to be weaker than that on K- k+ Kp(a-b+) samples. In later studies the effect of *Kp^a* in *cis* to other genes encoding antigens of high incidence has been seen. Reported examples include weakened

TABLE 18-8 Antigens Denatured or Reduced in Strength on Red Cells Treated with AET or ZZAP (DTT plus Papain)

1. Antigens totally denatured	K, k, Kp^a, Kp^b, Kp^c, Ku, Js^a, Js^b, Ul^a, K11, K12, K13, K14, K16, Wk^a, K18, K19, K20, K22, K23, K24, K25, RAZ, TOU
2. Antigen phenotypically related to the Kell System, not denatured[*1]	Kx
3. Genetically independent antigens denatured or weakened[*2]	LW^a, LW^b, LW^{ab}, Lutheran, Dombrock, Cartwright, Knops and JMH antigens

[*1] Reaction of normal Kell system phenotype red cells with anti-Kx enhanced when red cells treated with AET.

[*2] For references, see text.

expression of: Ku (203); Js^b (203,240,277); K18 (47); K19 (48); TOU (55); and all high incidence Kell para-Kell antigens (278). In the first report of anti-K22 (49) the antigen defined was said to be normally expressed on Kp(a+b-) red cells; using the second anti-K22 found, Kp(a+b-) red cells were seen (249) to have a reduced expression of K22.

The effect of Kp^a in cis is, obviously, seen only with high incidence antigens. As described in the second section of this chapter, a haplotype producing Kp^a and any other low incidence antigen in the system, or for that matter a haplotype producing any two low incidence antigens of the system, has never been found. The depressing effect of Kp^a on the other antigens encoded by genes in cis with the Kp^a is not always readily demonstrable in serological studies (203). Tippett (240) used titration studies with selected anti-k and anti-Js^b in tests on five Kp(a+b-) red cells. The Kp(a+b-) sample from an individual thought to be genetically kKp^aJs^b/K^o had marked weakening of k and Js^b. Those from individuals thought to be genetically kKp^aJs^b/kKp^aJs^b showed only slight weakening of k and Js^b. Other investigators (28,202,203,278) have also reported that presence of K^o on one chromosome allows the depressing effect of Kp^a on other genes in its haplotype, to be recognized more easily. Somewhat similarly, the depressing effect of Kp^a on the expression of k is easier to recognize in persons genetically KKp^b/kKp^a than in those kKp^b/kKp^a.

As described above, in the section on the Kell system and para-Kell antigens of the McLeod phenotype, one individual, apparently of the McLeod phenotype, who is homozygous for Kp^a has been found (29,279,280,390). The fact that his red cells differed from those of other individuals of the McLeod phenotype in that they carried no traces of Kell system or para-Kell antigens, suggests that lack of Kx-bearing glycoprotein and presence of Kp^a in the Kell complex haplotype are additive in their effects of depressing expression of Kell system and para-Kell antigens.

Quite unlike Kp^a, the allele Kp^c seems (155) to have no effect on genes with which it finds itself in cis, i.e. in the same haplotype. That is to say, no depression of expression of k, Js^b or any other high incidence Kell system or para-Kell antigen has been noticed on Kp(a-b-c+) red cells.

The phenotype K:-13 is also associated with depression of expression of other Kell system and para-Kell antigens (45). Although the first individual with K:-13 red cells was believed to be heterozygous for K^o, Marsh et al. (45) concluded that the presence of K^o was not the cause of weakening of the other antigens. First, individuals in the same family who were K^{13}/K^o had normal expressions of k, Kp^b, Js^b, etc. Second, Kaita et al. (198) had already shown that individuals genetically

kKp^bJs^b/K^o, express k, Kp^b and Js^b normally. In other words, it appears that the gene that encodes production of the as yet unrecognized antithetical low incidence partner to K13, behaves similarly to Kp^a in causing the other genes in its company (i.e. in cis) in the Kell complex haplotype, to encode weaker than normal expressions of their antigens. K:-13 red cells (i.e. from homozygotes for the gene encoding the unknown low incidence antigen just mentioned or from individuals heterozygous for that gene and K^o) have been shown to have weaker than normal expressions of k, Kp^b, Js^b, Ku, K12 (45), K18 (47), K19 (48) and TOU (55). It seems probable that when enough K:-13 samples have been found and studied the depression of expression of high incidence antigens on those cells will extend to all such Kell system and para-Kell antigens. Clearly such information would be obtained more quickly if the low incidence antithetical partner to K13 could be found. The effects of the gene that fails to encode K13 could then be studied in heterozygotes.

An Effect of Kp^a Not Due to Cis Position, the Allen Phenotype

One family in which Kp^a was present and depression of expression of Kell system and para-Kell antigens was seen, did not fit the situation described in the previous section. Norman and Daniels (286) studied a healthy blood donor and his sister, both of whom had Kp(a+b+) red cells. In both individuals, expression of k, Kp^b, Js^b and K11 was markedly reduced; in the propositus but not in his sister expression of K12, K14, K18 and K19 was reduced as well. In both individuals, expression of Kp^a was slightly enhanced as compared to the level of that antigen on Kp(a+b+) red cells from unrelated persons. When the propositus, who was presumably Kp^a/Kp^b, passed Kp^a to his daughter, no suppression of expression of Kell system or para-Kell antigens was seen. Those red cells with depression of antigen expression were said to be of the Allen phenotype. It seems that K^o could not have been involved since both persons of the Allen phenotype had Kp(a+b+) red cells. One possibility (29,286) is that the propositus and his sister were heterozygotes for kKp^aJs^b and K^{mod}, a gene described in the next section, that appears to encode production of reduced amounts of k, Kp^b, Js^b, et al.

The Kell$_{mod}$ Phenotypes, Including the Day and Mullins Phenotypes

Over the years a number of individuals, in whom Kp^a and the gene failing to encode K13 were not present, have been seen to have variable degrees of suppression of expression of Kell system and para-Kell antigens. Marsh and Redman (58) have suggested that Kell$_{mod}$ can be used as an umbrella term to describe these phenotypes, that are not all identical. In some of the phenotypes the expression of Kell system and para-Kell antigens is such that adsorption-elution tests are necessary to detect their presence. In the Kell$_{mod}$ phenotypes as designated by Marsh and Redman (58) red cell Kx expression is greater than that on red cells of normal phenotypes (59-63). This suggests that less or altered Kell glycoprotein is present on the red cells so that access of anti-Kx to its antigen is not as hindered as is the case on normal red cells. Although the genetic background (or backgrounds) of the Kell$_{mod}$ phenotypes has (or have) not yet been fully elucidated, the most likely explanation seems to be a gene (or a series of genes) at the *Kell* complex locus, that encode(s) production of reduced amounts of Kell glycoprotein. The phenotype seems to involve recessive inheritance so that in individuals homozygous for the gene (or genes) the Kell$_{mod}$ phenotype is seen. As is always the case, conventional family studies will not differentiate between aberrant genes at the blood group locus and very closely linked suppressor genes. Perhaps molecular genetic studies will show which type of mechanism is involved.

Some individuals among those with Kell$_{mod}$ phenotypes have produced an antibody with a specificity similar to that of anti-Ku (58-60,62,63). However, the anti-Ku-like made by Kell$_{mod}$ individuals does not usually react with other Kell$_{mod}$ red cells. Anti-Ku usually reacts, albeit weakly, and sometimes only as demonstrated by adsorption-elution tests, with such red cells.

The first of the Kell$_{mod}$ phenotypes to be described was called (59) the Day phenotype. The patient was an 84 year-old White woman who had no close relatives available for testing. Her red cells were shown to carry weak expressions of k, Kp^b, Js^b, Ku, K11, K12, K13, K14, K18, K19 and K22. These weakly expressed antigens excluded her from being genetically K^oK^o, the fact that her red cells carried only low levels of Kx, excluded the McLeod phenotype. That the condition represented an inherited one, unlike the acquired phenotypes described in a later section of this chapter, was made more likely by the fact that her parents were first cousins. The second individual of the Kell$_{mod}$ phenotype to be described (60) was a 62 year-old male patient. Two of the patient's four brothers but none of seven children in the next generation of the family, nor any of 13 in the generation after that, had red cells of the same phenotype. Since the antibody made by this patient reacted weakly with red cells of the Day phenotype it was thought that the phenotypes differed and this one was named the Mullins phenotype. Other patients with red cells similar

to those of the Day and Mullins phenotypes have been found but not described in full in the literature.

In 1989, Winkler et al. (61) described the first example of the Kell$_{mod}$ phenotype to be found in a healthy blood donor. The propositus was a 28 year-old White male of primarily Anglo-Saxon extraction although a minor component of his background was American Indian; his parents were known to be related but the exact degree of consanguinity was not known. The mother, brother, daughter and four paternal siblings of the propositus had red cells on which the Kell system antigens were expressed normally. Also in 1989, Pehta et al. (62) described the Kell$_{mod}$ phenotype in a woman and her brother thus adding to the earlier evidence (60) that the phenotype is inherited (almost certainly as a recessive condition). In 1993, Byrne et al. (63) described an 88 year-old White woman whose Kell$_{mod}$ phenotype differed from those described earlier in that her red cells carried a weak expression of K, in addition to their weak expression of k, Kp^b, Js^b, etc.

In concluding this section it should be stressed that not all examples described herein as Kell$_{mod}$ are identical. As examples, the patient in the last case cited (63) had K+^{w} red cells. Her cells carried weak expressions of K11, K12, K13, K14, K18, K19 and K22. In contrast, in the patient described by Pehta et al. (62) k, Kp^b, Ku, Js^b, K14 and K22 were weakly expressed, the levels of K11, K13 and K18 were normal or near normal. These differences do not decrease the probability that all cases represent the same phenomenon. If there are genes at the *Kell* complex locus that can be thought of as *Kell$_{mod}$*, it is likely that most of them will be variants of *kKp^{b}Js^b*, the common *Kell* haplotype. However, others obviously exist, including at least one (63) that is an apparent variant of *KKp^{b}Js^b*. Further, it is likely that different *kKp^{b}Js^b* variants will encode production of different amounts of Kell glycoprotein and/or glycoproteins on which different antigens vary in the amount of suppression.

A Phenotypic Association Between the Kell and Gerbich Systems

The association between the Kell and Gerbich systems is described in some detail in Chapter 16. Suffice it here to say that since Muller et al. (287) described a woman and her brother who had weakened expressions of K, k and Kp^b on their red cells, that were of the Ge:-2,-3 phenotype, others have reported similar findings (for references see Chapter 16). The situation was confusing since some workers found that the Ge-negative phenotype was often associated with weakened expressions of Kell system antigens, while others found no such association. Some order was brought to the situation in 1982 when Daniels (288) reported that nine of 11 samples of the Ge:-2,-3 phenotype showed some weakening of Kell system antigens while no weakening was seen on any of six Ge:-2,3 samples. The weakening of Kell system and para-Kell antigens was quite variable on the Ge:-2,-3 samples, sometimes all antigens were affected, sometimes only K11 was involved; in no case was weakening as marked as that seen in the McLeod phenotype. From findings (289-291) that Ge:-2,-3,-4 red cells also have depressed expression of Kell system antigens it seems that absence of the product of exon 3 of a normal *glycophorin C (GYPC)* gene is involved in the failure of Ge:-2,-3,4 and Ge:-2,-3,-4 red cells to express Kell system and para-Kell antigens normally. Formation of glycophorin C variants that lack the product of exon 3 of *GYPC* and total absence of glycophorins C and D, are described in Chapter 16. Jaber et al. (276) estimated that K+ k+ red cells of the Ge:-2,-3 phenotype carried about half the number of K antigen sites of K+ k+, Ge:2,3 red cells.

Kell System Autoantibodies

Over the years a large number of autoantibodies directed against Kell system and para-Kell antigens have been reported. The circumstances in which they have been found have been quite variable. In some instances the autoantibodies have been seen in patients with apparently normal levels of red cell antigens, in others autoantibody production has occurred concomitantly with marked depression of Kell system and para-Kell antigen expression. In some cases apparent autoantibodies have been seen in patients whose red cells lacked the antigen against which the autoantibodies appeared to be directed. Like virtually all other specificities for which autoantibodies have been seen, some of those directed against Kell system and para-Kell antigens have been pathological in vivo while others have been totally benign. The autoantibodies described in this section are grouped according to some of the characteristics just mentioned. However, it must be remembered that different tests were done in different cases so that some of the variation reported may be more apparent than real. As a single example, Marsh (292) has noted that depression of antigen expression concomitant with transient autoantibody production is the rule rather than the exception in the Kell system. In a case in which the patient's blood has a positive DAT and in which studies cannot be performed over a lengthy period, neither the antigen depression nor the transient nature of autoantibody production may be noticed.

Marsh et al. (293,294) studied more than 3000 samples referred to them, in which the DAT was positive and IgG was detectable on the patients' red cells. In about one in 170 patients an autoantibody eluted from the red cells or present in the patient's serum was non-reactive with the red cells of K^o homozygotes and/or normal red cells that had been treated with AET. In one case (293) the autoantibody seemed to define a previously unreported Kell system-related antigen of very high incidence. However, since no negative red cells (other than those if K^o homozygotes or those treated with AET) were found, the antigen defined was not given a new name. It was noted (58) that in about 15% of the patients with a Kell system-related autoantibody, there was clinical evidence of "warm" antibody-induced hemolytic anemia (WAIHA). This low incidence of hemolytic anemia in this subgroup of patients probably reflects the fact that the patients were selected because their eluates or sera contained only a Kell system-related antibody. It has been shown (295,296) that the most common finding in patients with WAIHA is that multiple autoantibodies (including anti-dl, see Chapter 37) are present and that specific reactivity for a recognizable blood group antigen is most often only seen following adsorption. Indeed, following adsorption with AET-treated red cells, a higher proportion of eluates or sera from these patients can be shown to contain a Kell system-related autoantibody component. A common finding among patients with Kell system-related autoantibodies is the presence of alloimmune anti-K. In the series reported by Marsh et al. (293,294) 75% of such patients had anti-K in the serum. The high incidence of anti-K of patients with Kell system-related autoantibodies and in the sera of many individuals who make alloantibodies to high incidence Kell system and para-Kell antigens, although most such persons have never been exposed to K+ red cells, is discussed in the next section of this chapter.

In addition to the cases cited above, Marsh et al. (244) described a patient with WAIHA caused by auto-anti-K13. At first it was thought that the Kell system and para-Kell antigens were expressed normally on the patient's red cells but in another report (293) that conclusion is reconsidered. While the strongly positive DAT made the determination difficult, it was considered possible that some depression of antigen expression had occurred. Krickler et al. (297) described an auto-anti-Ku and Sullivan et al. (298) an auto-anti-Kx, both of which were found in patients in whom there was no apparent depression of antigen expression and neither of which caused in vivo red cell destruction. Somewhat similarly Eveland (318) described auto-anti-Js^b in a patient in whom the DAT was weakly positive. Reactivity of the antibody was enhanced in tests using PEG. When the patient's Js(a-b+) red cells were separated from recently transfused cells by microhematocrit centrifugation and treated with chloroquine diphosphate to remove the auto-anti-Js^b, their expression of Js^b antigen was similar to that of normal Js(b+) red cells. The older literature contains at least two reports (299,300) of auto-anti-K in patients with WAIHA. However, both cases were studied long before the characteristics of autoantibodies that mimic a specificity (in antibody identification studies) that they do not actually possess, were recognized. Given the frequent occurrence of autoantibodies that appear to have anti-K specificity but that can be adsorbed on to and eluted from, K- red cells (see below), the early reports of auto-anti-K must now be interpreted with some caution.

In 1972, Seyfried et al. (301) described a young male patient who had WAIHA. In addition to forming auto-anti-Kp^b, the patient had red cells on which the k, Kp^b, Js^b and Ku antigens were depressed during the hemolytic episode. The weakening of Kp^b was such that the DAT was only weakly positive but a hemolytic transfusion reaction resulted when Kp(b+) blood was transfused. As the patient went into remission, production of the auto-anti-Kp^b stopped and expression of Kell system antigens on his red cells became normal. Since that time a number of similar cases of transient Kell system antigen depression and concomitant temporary production of Kell system antibodies have been reported (302-307). In the case described by Beck et al. (302) the patient, who had gastro-intestinal bleeding, made anti-Kp^b while her red cells had depressed expression of k, Kp^b and Js^b. There was no indication that the auto-anti-Kp^b caused in vivo clearance of the patient's own cells but the patient died before any return of her antigens to normal strength was seen. The patient described by Brendel et al. (304) formed auto-anti-Kp^b during a post-surgical period. Her red cells had a weakly positive DAT and carried weak expressions of k, Kp^b and Js^b while the antibody was being made, again there was no evidence that the autoantibody was pathological in vivo. Some two weeks after the initial finding, no autoantibody was detectable in the patient's serum and k, Kp^b and Js^b expression on her red cells was normal. This case was the first in which it was shown that red cells transfused during the period of temporary suppression of antigen expression also developed weakened expression of Kell system antigens. As discussed below, that finding and the fact that the patient had a bacterial infection offer important clues as to the mechanism of antigen weakening. In the case described by Rowe et al. (306) the patient had slight weakening of Kell system and para-Kell antigens, the autoantibody made, that again was benign in vivo, was close to, or was, anti-Ku. Vengelen-Tyler et al. (305) described a patient with idiopathic thrombocytopenic purpura (ITP), a negative DAT, an antibody to an antigen of very high incidence and very marked depression of Kell system antigens. As in the case described by Brendel et al. (304), red cells transfused to this patient lost their Kell system antigens. When samples from the patient were tested five months later, no antibody was detectable and the patient's red cells carried normal expressions of Kell system anti-

gens. This patient too had a bacterial infection at the time of depression of antigen expression. A somewhat similar case was reported by Williamson et al. (307). Again the patient had ITP, depressed expression of red cell Kell system antigens and an antibody with apparent anti-Ku specificity. When the patient was treated and his ITP was in remission, antibody was no longer detectable in his serum and his red cell Kell antigen expression was normal. However, when the patient suffered a relapse his red cells lost their Lutheran system and LW^a antigens and the patient made an antibody with apparent anti-Lu3 specificity (see also Chapter 20).

In two other cases involving depression of expression of Kell system and para-Kell antigens, the findings were a little different. Manny et al. (308) described a patient with Kp(a+b-) red cells in whom the expression of Kp^a was slightly increased and the expression of k and Js^b was depressed. The patient's DAT+ red cells yielded anti-Kp^b when eluates were made. There was no evidence of accelerated red cell destruction in vivo and a cell survival study showed that ^{51}Cr-labeled Kp(b+) red cells survived normally in vivo. Nine months after the initial investigation, no antibody was detectable in the patient's serum and the red cells typed as Kp(a+b-) and carried the expected levels of k and Js^b. In the case described by Puig et al. (309) the patient had depression of expression of red cell Kell system antigens and a positive DAT. His red cells were Kp(a+b-) and an eluate from those red cells appeared to contain anti-Kp^b. The patient's serum contained alloimmune anti-K. The eluted antibody could be adsorbed and eluted on to and from other Kp(b-) red cells. There was no evidence to suggest that the autoantibody was causing hemolysis in vivo. The authors concluded that the autoantibody mimicked anti-Kp^b but did not have that specificity. The finding that the autoantibody could be adsorbed on to and eluted from AET-treated red cells casts some doubt as to whether it was related to the Kell system at all. The weakening of Kell system antigens on the patient's red cells could have occurred because he was homozygous for the kKp^aJs^b haplotype, that is, Kp^a in *cis* to k and Js^b on both chromosomes (see earlier).

There are a number of possible explanations for the phenomenon that involves transient depression of expression of Kell system and para-Kell antigens and concomitant production of antibody. Two of them are unlikely and a third likely, but not proved. First it is possible that the individuals involved are heterozygotes for K^o. This explanation is unlikely on two counts. First, the phenomenon is seen more often than the frequency of K^o would allow. Second and more important, the phenomenon is usually transient and reversible which would appear to exclude a genetic background. A second possibility is that the patients' disease states somehow interfere with the synthesis of production of red cell-borne Kell system and para-

Kell antigens. This concept is also unlikely on two counts. First, no antigens other than the Kell system and para-Kell antigens are affected contrary to what might be expected if a non-specific modification of red cell membrane components was at play. Second and again of more importance, in at least two patients (304,305) in whom this phenomenon has been seen, transfused red cells also lost expression of Kell system antigens. Thus the third explanation, while unproved, seems the most likely. That is, an external agent, such as a microbial enzyme, somehow modifies the Kell glycoprotein on red cells and reduces the expression of antigens on that structure. There are three lines of evidence that support such a theory. First, it is well known that enzymes produced by infecting bacteria modify red cell membrane components (see Chapter 42 and various other Chapters about the blood groups in this book). Second, as already mentioned, in at least two patients in whom antigen depression was seen, transfused red cells suffered the same fate (304,305) strongly suggesting an extrinsic rather than an intrinsic cause. Third, several of the patients in whom reduced expression of Kell system and para-Kell antigens was seen were known (293,302,304,305,308, 311) to be infected at the time. Further, in some cases (293,304,305,311) when the bacterial infection was eradicated, antigen expression returned to normal.

In addition to the antibodies already described, there have been several instances in which an apparent anti-K has been recovered by elution from DAT+, K- red cells. The case described by Garratty et al. (310) was of particular interest. The patient had K- red cells and was a carrier of the X chromosome-borne gene that results in the McLeod phenotype in males. The anti-K that she made could be adsorbed on to and eluted from K- as well as K+ red cells. The patient described by Hare et al. (311) had apparently normal levels of k, Kp^b and Js^b on his DAT+, K- red cells. His serum contained what looked like anti-K and an eluate from his red cells appeared to contain anti-K and an antibody to a high incidence Kell system-related antigen. Adsorption studies showed that his serum contained an antibody mimicking anti-K, that could be adsorbed on to K- red cells and a true specificity anti-K that could not. The eluate from his red cells could be adsorbed to exhaustion with K- red cells showing that the apparent anti-K that it contained was all mimicking in nature. Some years earlier, while studying autoantibodies that mimic Rh alloantibodies, we (312) had shown that particular situation to be relatively common. That is, the eluate made from the patient's antigen-negative red cells contains only the mimicking antibody while the patient's serum contains a mixture of the mimicking antibody and an antibody of real specificity directed against the antigen that the mimicking antibody appears to define. The situation is recognized (312,313) when the eluate can be adsorbed to exhaustion with antigen-negative red cells while antibody activity in

the serum is partially adsorbed (mimicking antibody) then adsorption stops, i.e. the serum cannot be adsorbed to exhaustion with antigen-negative red cells when only real specificity alloantibody remains. Another antibody mimicking anti-K was described by Viggiano et al. (314). The patient involved had DAT+, K- red cells but no clinical evidence of hemolytic anemia. An eluate made from the red cells appeared to contain anti-K but the antibody was adsorbed by both K+ and K- red cells.

It seems that autoantibodies that mimic anti-K in antibody identification studies are not rare. In 1996, we (315) published the results of a large study designed to determine the true incidence of alloimmunization in patients who have made red cell autoantibodies. Full details of the study are given in Chapter 37. However, it is pertinent here to mention that among 138 samples studied, nine appeared to contain anti-K after initial adsorptions to remove the panagglutinating autoantibodies had been performed. Additional adsorptions, with K- red cells in those nine cases revealed that six of the patients had indeed formed alloimmune anti-K, i.e. antibody not adsorbed by K- red cells. However, in the other three, adsorption with K- red cells removed all antibody activity showing that in those patients a partially adsorbed autoantibody mimicked anti-K although that was not the real specificity of the antibody involved.

In discussing one of our cases (311) of an autoantibody that mimicked anti-K, with colleagues who had seen but not reported similar examples, we were struck by the fact that too many of them had been seen in patients who had suffered head injuries or had growths in the brain. One of us (PDI) is not yet convinced that the association is purely coincidental and cannot help but wonder if damaged brain tissue carries an immunogenic structure that, when encountered by macrophages and immunocytes, causes an autoantibody directed against a common Kell system antigen to be made and if the specificity of the antibody is such that it reacts optimally with K+ red cells. It has been shown (317) that certain brain cells, oligodendrocytes, share antigens with suppressor T cells so that there is a tenuous link between brain cells and the immune response. The idea that damage to or alteration of brain cells might lead to the production of anti-K or an antibody reacting best with K+ red cells is, of course, entirely speculative. Should this concept eventually prove to have merit, please remember where you read it first (316).

Anti-K in Sera That Contain Other Kell System Antibodies

As mentioned several times in earlier sections of this chapter, anti-K is found more often than might be expected in sera that contain antibodies to other Kell system and para-Kell antigens. The first two examples (5,167) of anti-Kp^b to be found contained anti-K, others have been seen (28). The first examples of anti-K18 (47) and anti-K19 (48) were found in the sera of individuals who had also made anti-K. Marsh et al. (293,294) found that apparently alloimmune anti-K was present in some 75% of individuals who had formed Kell system-related autoantibodies. Anti-K was present in the serum of the patient (244) who formed auto-anti-K13. In considering these findings, two observations are pertinent. First, as pointed out in an early section in this chapter and as illustrated in table 18-3, the *Kell* system haplotype that encodes production of K, always also encodes production of all the high incidence Kell system and para-Kell antigens. This means, of course, that no K+ cells lacking one of these high incidence antigens exist. Thus when a serum contains an antibody to a high incidence antigen, the simultaneous presence of anti-K may be suspected because of variation of strength of the serum with K+ and K- red cells but can only be proved by adsorption studies. For example all K+ red cells are Kp(b+) so will adsorb a serum containing anti-K and anti-Kp^b to exhaustion. K- Kp(b+) red cells will adsorb anti-Kp^b and leave anti-K unadsorbed. If a serum containing an antibody to the high incidence antigen reacts equally with K+ and K- red cells, the presence of anti-K may not be suspected and the adsorption studies may not be done. Indeed in some of the reports describing such antibodies, appropriate adsorption studies are not mentioned. In other words, presence of anti-K in sera containing antibodies to high incidence Kell system and para-Kell antigens may be more common than has been reported. Second and different to the observation just made, it is possible that some of the apparent anti-K that have been reported in this setting, were antibodies mimicking anti-K. As described in the previous section, several such antibodies have been described (310,311,314,315). When a serum containing an antibody to a high incidence Kell system or para-Kell antigen is adsorbed with antigen-positive, K- red cells, and apparent anti-K remains in the adsorbed serum, the investigation usually stops because it is concluded that separable anti-K is present. The literature does not contain reports of further adsorptions with K- red cells to determine whether the apparent anti-K had or merely mimicked that specificity. In other words, in contrast to the first suggestion that anti-K may be more common in this setting than has been reported, it is possible that the common occurrence of the antibody may be more apparent than real. Regardless of the eventual resolution of this situation, there is currently no explanation as to why anti-K or an antibody reacting preferentially with K+ red cells should be made in this circumstance when usually the antibody-maker has not been exposed to K+ red cells.

Monoclonal Antibodies and the Kell System

As would be expected in a complex system that is characterized by high immunogenicity of many of its antigens, numerous examples of Kell system and Kell system-related monoclonal antibodies have been made. While monoclonal anti-K has not been produced using spleen cells from mice, at least two antibodies of that specificity have been made by EBV-transformation of human B cells (320,321). Murine anti-k have been produced (322,323) as have a number of monoclonal antibodies that react with all except red cells from K^o homozygotes but react to higher titer against K- k+ and K+ k+ than against K+ k- red cells. At appropriate dilutions and when used by controlled techniques, these antibodies can be used as reliable anti-k typing reagents (253,324,325,328). Clearly some of these antibodies, particularly those that do not show a preference for k, can be used as anti-Ku (253,324-326). A murine monoclonal antibody described by Parsons et al. (253) reacted with Kp(a-b+c-) and Kp(a-b-c+) but not with Kp(a+b-c-) red cells so appeared to be defining an epitope shared by Kp^b and Kp^c that is not present in the Kp^a antigen. The workers who first described anti-Levay (24,25) could never have guessed that one day there would be a monoclonal antibody with anti-Kp^{bc} specificity! Two murine monoclonal anti-K14 have been described (322) and other MAb directed against the Kell glycoprotein are known. As is fairly typical for MAb, the use of different techniques in different laboratories has produced results that are not always in total agreement as to the specificity of the MAb under study. As a single example, some MAb show apparently different specificities when tested against untreated and protease-treated red cells. As mentioned earlier, a few MAb with apparent Kell system specificity continue to react with AET-treated red cells. Readers with a particular interest in this topic are referred to a number of additional reports from the international workshop in which these MAb were studied (252,329,330,332-335).

As described in the section on biochemistry of the Kell system, monoclonal antibodies to the Kell glycoprotein have been instrumental in recognition of the structure of that red cell membrane component (39,327). As mentioned in several earlier sections of this chapter, the antibodies have also been used in the monclonal antibody immobilization of erythrocyte antigen (MAIEA) assay to demonstrate the presence of several of the para-Kell antigens on the Kell glycoprotein. If it can ever be made as a monoclonal antibody, anti-Kx would be particularly useful. In addition to its potential application to biochemical studies (see below) the antibody would be valuable for tests at the serological level. As described earlier, tests with anti-Kx are the best way of recognizing presence of K^o in individuals heterozygous for that gene. At present such studies are limited because of the shortage of anti-Kx.

The Kell System and Disease

The acquisition of a K-like antigen on red cells and the production of anti-K in patients with bacterial infections are described above in the section on the K and k antigens. Immune hemolytic anemia caused by Kell system antibodies is mentioned above and described in more detail in Chapter 37. The clinical abnormalities seen in individuals of the McLeod phenotype are described below.

As mentioned in the section describing the K and k antigens, McGinniss et al. (125) reported that K- red cells incubated in vitro with disrupted *Streptococcus faecium* organisms, acquired a K-like antigen. The conversion did not occur when whole bacteria were used. It is not clear how or if this observation is related to that of Byrd et al. (336) who reported a significant correlation between urinary tract infections with *S. faecium* and renal graft failure.

The Kell Locus is on Chromosome 7

The *Kell* complex locus was one of the last blood group loci to be assigned to a specific autosome. In 1991, Zelinski et al. (337,338) described tight linkage between the *Kell* locus and that at which the genes that encode production of prolactin-inducible protein (PIP) reside. The *PIP* locus had already been localized to chromosome 7 at 7q32-7q36. The *Kell* locus was then shown (339) to be linked to the cystic fibrosis gene that was also known to be located on the long arm of chromosome 7. In situ hybridization studies with cDNA encoding production of the Kell glycoprotein were then used (340,341) to confirm the assignment of the *Kell* locus to 7q33-q35.

The Xk Blood Group System

The Xk blood group system contains one antigen, Kx. In the ISBT terminology (see table 18-9) the system number is 019, the antigen is 019001. The reason that the system is included in this chapter with the Kell system is, of course, that in the absence of Kx, the McLeod phenotype results. The aberrations of Kell system antigens that are seen in the McLeod phenotype have been described above. As the name of the system implies, the gene that encodes production of the Kx antigen-bearing glycoprotein is located on the X chromosome. For the sake of this

TABLE 18-9 The Xk Blood Group System

Conventional Name: Kx
Conventional Symbol: Kx
ISBT System Symbol: XK
ISBT System Number: 019

Historical (now obsolete) Terms	Antigen Conventional Name	ISBT Antigen Number	ISBT Full Code Number
KL, K15	Kx	XK1	019001

discussion, the gene that encodes production of the Kx glycoprotein will be called *Xk*, the gene that fails to encode production of the glycoprotein will be called *Xk^o*. Since *Xk* and *Xk^o* are X chromosome-borne it follows that the McLeod phenotype (i.e. lack of Kx) will be seen almost exclusively in males. The phenotype in males arises from the genotype *Xk^o/Y*, in females *Xk^o* will almost always be accompanied by *Xk* on the other X chromosome, i.e. female carriers of the McLeod phenotype will be genetically *Xk^o/Xk*. Over 60 males with the McLeod phenotype are known (58), only one female of the McLeod phenotype (i.e. genetically *Xk^o/Xk^o*) has been reported (236).

Recognition of an Association Between the McLeod Phenotype and X-Linked Chronic Granulomatous Disease

Allen et al. (16) first described the McLeod phenotype in a healthy dental student who had no atypical antibody in his serum. The McLeod red cells were typed as K- k+^{w} Kp(a-b+^{w}) Ku+^{w}. The parents of the propositus had red cells that typed as K- k+ Kp(a-b+) Ku+ and expressed all their Kell system antigens normally. There were no reasons to suppose that the parents were other than kKp^bJs^b homozygotes. It was believed, from the start, that the McLeod phenotype represented the presence of genes at a locus unlinked to the *Kell* locus, that prevented the normal *Kell* complex genes that were presumed to be present, from expressing themselves at the phenotypic level. While the McLeod phenotype was thought probably to be a recessive characteristic, the original family was too small for the X-borne nature of the gene affecting expression of the Kell system antigens to be seen.

Seven years after the McLeod phenotype was reported (16), Hart et al. (14) described a five year-old male with a history of recurrent severe bacterial infections. His red cells were of the McLeod phenotype, his serum contained a potent antibody, that caused a hemolytic transfusion reaction and that reacted with all cells tested except his own and the original McLeod red cells. Three years later Giblett et al. (214) described a similar patient. Although the phenotype was described as that of a K^o homozygote, it can be seen in retrospect that the boy almost certainly had the McLeod phenotype and the same antibody in his serum as that in the patient of Hart et al. (14). The first associations between the McLeod phenotype and X-linked chronic granulomatous disease (CGD) had been seen. Since these early observations, other individuals with red cells of the McLeod phenotype have been seen, some but not all of them had X-linked CGD.

Chronic Granulomatous Disease (CGD)

This inherited disorder is characterized by severe and often fatal bacterial infections early in life. The white cells of the patients are able to phagocytose bacteria but are not able to kill them. There are two different genetic backgrounds that lead to CGD. One involves a gene on an autosome, the other a gene on the X chromosome (342). Only the X-linked form of the disease is associated with the McLeod phenotype. However, not all males with McLeod phenotype red cells have CGD. The reasons for this and other clinical manifestations that accompany the red cell McLeod phenotype are discussed below.

The Kx Antigen

As mentioned earlier, the Kx antigen is located on a glycoprotein to which the Kell glycoprotein either becomes attached or is present in close proximity. On red cells that carry normal expressions of Kell system and para-Kell antigens, Kx is poorly expressed. It is believed that this finding may represent steric interference by the Kell glycoprotein in the approach of anti-Kx to its antigen. The red cells of K^o homozygotes react strongly with anti-Kx, it is believed that absence of Kell glycoprotein from those cells allows anti-Kx easy access to the Kx antigen-bearing glycoprotein. In keeping with this supposition it has been found that the red cells of K^o heterozygotes react with anti-Kx in a manner intermediate between the reactions of those of K^o homozygotes and those of individuals with normally expressed Kell system and para-Kell antigens (51). Again in keeping with the concept described, red cells on which temporary depression of Kell system and para-Kell antigens occurs (see section above on Kell system autoantibodies) show increased levels of Kx, that declines to the normal low level as Kell system antigen expression returns to normal (244).

The Kx antigen is not denatured or removed when red cells are treated with proteases. Anti-Kx reacts much more strongly with AET or DTT-treated than with untreated red cells (37,343). Again, it is believed that removal or denaturation of Kell glycoprotein renders Kx readily available to its antibody.

Kx Antigen and Granulocytes

During early studies on the relationship between the McLeod phenotype and CGD, it was believed (51,216-218,344-346) that the primary defect leading to CGD might be lack of Kx antigen on granulocytes. Adsorption studies appeared to show (51,217) that all granulocytes except those from males with X-linked CGD carried Kx. Thus the antigen bearing structure was considered perhaps to be of importance in bacterial killing. However, it now seems that adsorption of anti-Kx by the leukocyte preparations occurred because those preparations contained some red cells. First, the genes involved in the McLeod phenotype and CGD have been shown both to be on the X chromosome but not to be the same (see below). Second, later studies (347) have produced data that indicate that normal granulocytes do not carry Kx.

Anti-Kx and Anti-Km (Anti-KL)

These antibodies have been described in detail earlier in this chapter and will be mentioned only briefly here. Anti-KL (formerly anti-K9) was the name given by Hart et al. (14) to the antibody made by their McLeod/CGD patient. At the time of their report, the serum was thought to contain two specificities. Marsh (15) and Marsh et al. (51) split anti-KL by adsorption onto and elution from the red cells of K^o homozygotes. The antibody that bound to and was eluted from those red cells was called anti-Kx (formerly anti-K15). The antibody not adsorbed by those red cells was called anti-Km (still anti-K20). Kx is said to be present on normal red cells and those of K^o homozygotes but is not present on McLeod red cells. Km is said to present on normal red cells but not those of K^o homozygotes or those of the McLeod phenotype (for a conjecture on the nature of Km, see earlier). The clinical relevance of these antibodies is described in an earlier section.

The McLeod Phenotype and X-linked CGD

As mentioned above, at one time it was thought that males with Xk^o had CGD because they had the McLeod phenotype. That is to say the Kx antigen or, more likely, its carrier protein was thought to have a functional role on granulocytes. The findings that some males had X-linked CGD but normal Kell system phenotypes (214,226,345,349) while others had the red cell McLeod phenotype but did not have CGD (16,223,224, 226,348) led to the suggestion (217,345) that a series of alleles of Xk existed. The X^1k gene was thought to encode Kx production on red cells and granulocytes, i.e. the common normal condition. X^2k was said to cause type II CGD, that is CGD and the McLeod phenotype, i.e. Kx missing from red cells and granulocytes. X^3k was said to cause type I CGD, that is Kx on red cells but not on granulocytes, i.e. X-linked CGD but a normal red cell Kell system phenotype. X^4k was said to encode no red cell Kx but normal Kx on granulocytes, i.e. McLeod red cell phenotype but no CGD. The situation is now known to be different. A series of genes on the X chromosome are indeed involved but they are not alleles at a single locus. Instead, the genes seem each to have a function and in the absence of the gene and its function, a different clinical abnormality occurs. That is to say, in the absence of different genes, all of which are normally carried in the Xp21 region of chromosome X, retinitis pigmentosa, chronic granulomatous disease, the McLeod phenotype, Duchenne's muscular dystrophy and adrenal hypoplasia are seen (229-232). Various combinations of these disorders (based on the sequence of the genes on the chromosome) are seen when small partial deletions in the Xp21 region of the X chromosome occur. In other words, if only Xk is deleted (i.e. what has been called here replacement by Xk^o) the individual will have the McLeod phenotype (actually the McLeod syndrome, see below) but not the other entities. In one patient studied by Frey et al. (231) the Xp21 deletion was such that the patient had CGD and the McLeod phenotype. In another patient described in the same report (231) the Xp21 deletion was larger and the patient had retinitis pigmentosa, chronic granulomatous disease, the McLeod phenotype and Duchenne's muscular dystrophy. The common occurrence of several of these disorders in the same patient in a number of cases (229-232) indicates that the genes are in close proximity and that a relatively small chromosomal deletion can have several effects. Marsh et al. (217) have estimated that between 20 and 30% of patients with X-linked CGD have a deletion that also results in the McLeod phenotype.

Although distinct from Xk^o that effects the McLeod phenotype, it can be added that X-linked CGD results from an abnormality at the $CYBB$ locus that results in a deficiency of cytochrome B (342,351-353).

The McLeod Syndrome

Young boys with X-linked CGD tend to succumb to overwhelming bacterial infections, such as those that cause lung abscesses, at an early age. Males with the McLeod phenotype who do not have CGD live longer but it is now realized that they do not enjoy perfect health. Instead, as they grow older they are afflicted with a number of conditions that are collectively known as the McLeod syndrome. McLeod red cells are acanthocytic, that aspect of the syndrome is described in the next section. Men of the McLeod phenotype also suffer muscular and neurological abnormalities that include muscle wasting, reduction in deep tendon reflexes, choreiform movements and cardiomyopathy. There is also an increase in serum creatine kinase (227-229,331,354,355). The muscular abnormalities are similar to those seen in Duchenne's muscular dystrophy, the creatinine phosphokinase (isoenzyme MM) increase is also typical of diverse forms of muscular dystrophy. High serum levels of this enzyme often indicate a lesion in cardiac or skeletal muscles or in the brain. The serum level of carbonic anhydrase III is also increased in individuals of the McLeod phenotype (227,350) again this is a feature seen in patients with muscular dystrophy. At present there is no explanation as to why individuals of the McLeod red cell phenotype who do not have a chromosomal deletion that also affects the Duchenne muscular dystrophy (DMD) locus, develop these abnormalities. However, the close proximity of the Xk and DMD loci must call into question the possibility of gene duplication and perhaps a functional role for the Kx glycoprotein on other than red cells.

The McLeod Phenotype, Hereditary Acanthocytosis and The Lyon Effect

McLeod phenotype red cells are morphologically abnormal, a high percentage of them are acanthocytic (218,229,236) (i.e. shaped like acanthus leaves, so look in the dictionary like I had to!). Since the McLeod phenotype is inherited as a recessive condition the term hereditary acanthocytosis can be used but it must be remembered that other forms of hereditary acanthocytosis, that are also associated with neuropathy but in which the red cells are not of the McLeod phenotype, exist (236). Perhaps hereditary, and certainly acquired red cell acanthocytosis has been associated with beta lipoprotein deficiency, hypothyroidism, hepatic diseases, hemolytic anemia and neonatal hepatitis. While as described below, some membrane phospholipid abnormalities have been reported in McLeod phenotype red cells, beta lipoprotein deficiency has not been seen.

As would be expected, acanthocytic McLeod phenotype red cells have reduced deformability (356). However, SDS-PAGE studies show that the red cell membranes are normal (357-359) suggesting that the membrane cytoskeleton is not altered. Gross phospholipid levels of the membranes are normal (360,361) but there is evidence for increased transmembrane passage of phosphatidylcholine (361) leading to an abnormality in composition of the membrane bilayer (362). McLeod red cells also take up ^{32}P more rapidly than normal red cells, particularly in incorporation of that compound into spectrin and protein band 3 (357). Protein methylation in the membranes of McLeod red cells is altered (363); while electrolyte transport across the membrane is normal, osmotic water permeability is reduced (360).

While the in vivo survival of red cells of the McLeod phenotype is said to be reduced (221) there is a paucity of reports of red cell deficiency type hemolytic anemia in these patients. Presumably, as in the Rh$_{null}$ condition (see Chapter 12) the hemolytic state is well compensated in most individuals of the McLeod phenotype. As far as we are aware there is only one report (223) of marked hemolytic anemia in a young male with the McLeod phenotype.

As indicated above, many of the red cells of a male with the McLeod phenotype (i.e. genotype *Xk^o/Y*) are acanthocytic. If the *Xk* locus is subject to the Lyon effect (see below), it should be possible to recognize a female carrier of the McLeod condition (i.e. genetically *Xk^o/Xk*) by the presence of acanthocytes and/or the presence of both Kx+ and Kx- red cells in her blood. The Lyon effect is one of chromosomal inactivation. That is to say, in females (XX) one X chromosome in somatic cells is inactivated so that all products in that line of cells are encoded by genes on one, but not both, of the X chromosomes (364-367). Modifications to the theory as originally proposed have been necessary since it has now been shown (368-372) that some, but not all loci on the given X chromosome are inactivated. Since Lyonization is random, if the *Xk* locus is subject to the effect it would be expected that some red cell precursor lines would make normal Kx+ biconcave red cells (*Xk^o* inactivated) while others would make Kx- acanthocytes (*Xk* inactivated). Exactly such a situation is seen in practice and many carriers of *Xk^o* have been identified from their mixed population of Kx- acanthocytic and Kx+ normocytic red cells (168,218,221,223-225,229,237,239,310). If the exercise is undertaken serologically, better success results from the use of anti-Kx than from the use of a Kell system antibody to a high incidence antigen that seeks to identify the weakened antigen expression on the McLeod phenotype population of red cells. However, since anti-Kx is in short supply, the latter approach must sometimes be tried. Use of the flow cytometer invariably results in a more accurate determination of the percentage of McLeod phenotype red cells present (58). If microscopic examination of blood films for the presence of acanthocytes and normocytes is used, a hematologist

with considerable skills in differentiating red cell morphology is a requirement equal to that of a flow cytometer for serological differentiation. Using the various methods it has been found that the percentage of red cells of the McLeod phenotype in *Xk^o/Xk* carriers, varies from 5% to 85%, Lyonization is truly random!

Linkage Between *Xk*, *CGD* and *Xg*

Since CGD is such a devastating disease there would be considerable advantages if tests during the prenatal period could be used to determine whether the fetus in utero will have the disease. A couple, in whom it was known that the female was an *Xk^o/Xk* carrier of CGD, could at least consider termination of the pregnancy if a reliable test showed that the child would have the disease. Since the *Xk*, *CGD* and *Xg* loci (see Chapter 25) are all located on the X chromosome and since *Xk* and *CGD* are proximal, close linkage would allow appropriate genetic counseling. If, for example, the *Xk^o/Xk* woman with a deletion involving both the *Xk* and *CGD* loci was also an *Xg^a/Xg* heterozygote, data from a previous male child, with or without CGD and with or without *Xg^a* could be used to determine the probable outcome in the current pregnancy. While linkage between the *Xk* and *Xg* loci has been reported (373,374) it is not close enough to permit reliable counseling advice. Recombination between the *Xk* and *Xg* loci (224,229) and between the *CGD* and *Xg* loci (168,375) has been reported. Further, linkage between *Xk* and *CGD* is not absolute. Densen et al. (226) studied a family in which five brothers had red cells of the McLeod phenotype. Four of them had CGD, the fifth did not. Apparently recombination between *Xk^o* and *CGD* had occurred. It is to be hoped that a molecular biological method can be developed to differentiate between the cDNA of *Xk* and *Xk^o*, so that reliable counseling can be provided.

The Biochemical Nature of Kell Blood Group System Antigens

Our present understanding of the biochemical nature of the Kell blood group system antigens is almost entirely due to the work of Colvin Redman and his colleagues working at the New York Blood Center. Early studies demonstrated that the Kell antigens were lost if red cells were treated with trypsin and chymotrypsin either as a mixture or sequentially (251). These results suggested that Kell antigens are dependent on a protein structure. When it was shown that the antigens were also lost when red cells were treated with thiol reagents (2-

aminoethylisothiouronium bromide, AET (37); or dithio-threitol, DTT (56) and that a combination of DTT and papain was extremely effective in destroying the antigens (343) a picture emerged of the Kell protein as a membrane protein with an extracellular domain having a tightly folded structure maintained by extensive disulphide bonding. Since the antigens Js^a and Js^b were markedly more susceptible to DTT treatment than the other Kell system antigens (56) it appeared that at least two disulphide bonds were involved, one more exposed on the surface of the protein than the other. The Kell protein was identified in 1984 by immunoprecipitation from radiodinated intact red cells using human alloimmune Kell system antibodies (38) and from Triton X-100 solubilized red cell membranes (40). When SDS gels were run under reducing conditions a single radioiodinated band of 93kD was observed. When gels were run under non-reducing conditions a different result was obtained with iodinated bands of 85-90kD, 115-130kD and some of higher molecular weight which did not penetrate a 7.5% polyacrylamide gel. By cutting each of these bands from non-reducing gels and re-electrophoresis of the excised bands under reducing conditions it could be shown that each band contained the 93kD band (39). These results suggested that the Kell protein is linked by disulphide bonds to another protein or proteins in the 29-40kD range. These early immunochemical studies have since been confirmed in several different laboratories (253,276,377) with several murine monoclonal antibodies to Kell protein and with human monoclonal Kell system antibodies. When it was shown that the Kx protein has an apparent molecular weight of 37 kD (359) it seemed likely that Kx is covalent linked to Kell protein and this has recently been confirmed (see below).

Like most membrane proteins the Kell protein is glycosylated. Deglycosylation with N-glycanase reduces its apparent molecular weight on SDS-PAGE to 79-80kD (362). O-glycanase is without effect. These results suggest that one or more N-glycans account for the 12% carbohydrate (by weight) found in the protein.

Kell is a Type II Membrane Glycoprotein

Lee et al. (41) obtained a full length cDNA corresponding to the Kell protein from a human bone marrow cDNA library. Attempts to obtain amino acid sequence from the amino-terminus of the purified protein were unsuccessful and so tryptic peptides were prepared and sequenced. An oligonucleotide probe corresponding to the sequence of one of these peptides was used to screen the library and of four positive clones obtained one had a full length open reading frame coding for the Kell protein. As deduced from the cDNA,

the Kell protein consists of 732 amino acids (molecular weight calculated from the protein sequence is 82,802). The protein lacks a signal sequence. The initiator methionine is followed by glutamic acid. By comparison with other membrane proteins it would be expected that the methionine is post-translationally cleaved and that the glutamic acid is the N-terminal amino acid of the mature protein. A hydropathy plot revealed a region of hydrophobic amino acids (residues 48 to 67) which form a likely membrane spanning domain and inspection of the protein sequence suggested that the Kell protein is a type II membrane protein with a small cytosolic N-terminal domain (residues 1-47, the N-terminal domain is extremely hydrophilic and contains two arginine residues immediately preceding the transmembrane domain). The predicted protein contains a very large extracellular carboxy terminal domain of 666 residues. Inspection of the sequence of this large extracellular domain revealed several interesting features. There are 15 cysteine residues, a feature consistent with an extensively folded disulphide bonded domain and with the earlier observations discussed above, which demonstrated the sensitivity of all Kell antigens to thiol reagents. Incidentally, there is an additional cysteine residue in the transmembrane domain, a feature which is often found in membrane proteins and has been implicated as a site of palmitoylation and dimerization in other proteins (see Chapters 12 and 29). The extracellular domain also contains six potential sites for N-glycosylation (Asn-X-Ser/Thr) although one of these (that closest to the carboxy terminus at Asn724) is unlikely to be utilized because in this case X = proline (N-glycosylation does not normally occur when X = Proline). The presence of N-glycosylation sites is consistent with studies described above which showed sensitivity of the Kell protein to N-glycanase. By far the most interesting feature of the extracellular domain is the presence of a consensus sequence H581EXXH found in the catalytic sites of zinc dependent endopeptidases. The Kell protein is homologous along its whole sequence with the membrane metalloproteinases endothelin converting enzyme 1 and 2 (ECE-1, ECE-2) and neutral endopeptidase-24.11 (NEP, syn. CALLA, CD10) and together these proteins form a subfamily of metalloproteinases (M13) (378). A model of the Kell protein based on that for ECE-1 (379) is given in figure 18-1. That the Kell protein is indeed a type II protein oriented as described above was formally proved using rabbit antibodies raised to synthetic peptides corresponding to different regions of the protein. An antibody to the N-terminal peptide reacted with inside-out red cell membrane vesicles but not with right-side-out vesicles or intact red cells (380). Some possible functions of the Kell protein are discussed in a later section.

The Location, Organization and Expression of the *Kell* Complex Gene

Zelinksi et al. (253) showed that the *Kell* locus is linked to the prolactin-inducible protein locus and therefore maps to the long arm of chromosome 7(q32-36). This assignment was confirmed by Purohit et al. (339) by linkage analysis between *Kell* and 3 DNA markers linked to the cystic fibrosis locus. Lee et al. (340) used fluorescence in situ hybridization (FISH) with labeled Kell-specific genomic DNA clones to define the locus at 7q33. Murphy et al. (341) also used FISH and mapped the Kell locus to 7q33-35.

The *Kell* complex gene comprises 19 exons and spans approximately 21.5 kb. The first exon contains the 5' untranslated region and the codon for the initiator methionine. The single transmembrane region is encoded by exon 3. The HEXXH motif characteristic of zinc-dependent metalloproteinases is encoded by a 68bp exon (exon 16) which shares 54.5% base identity with the corresponding exon in *NEP* (381).

Northern blot analyses of RNA from several tissues (bone marrow, fetal liver, brain, kidney, lung and adult liver) revealed Kell transcripts in bone marrow and fetal liver (major transcript 2.5 kb) but not elsewhere, suggesting that the expression of Kell protein is restricted to erythroid tissues (340). Similar conclusions were reached by Anstee et al. (382) in a study of the reactivity of a murine monoclonal anti-Kell protein with hematopoietic cell lines, fetal liver and a variety of other tissues. These authors noted that Kell expression was detectable on isolated hematopoeitic cells in fetal liver during the second trimester but not during the first trimester. Immunohistochemical staining of brain, tongue, trachea, stomach, pancreas, ileum, skin, spleen, liver, kidney and placenta failed to demonstrate Kell protein expression although some reactivity was observed on blood vessels.

The restricted expression of Kell protein suggests that the gene is regulated by erythroid transcription factors. Lee et al. (381) demonstrated promoter activity by CAT assay for the 5' flanking region -176 to -1. This region contains three potential GATA-1 binding sites, two of which are close to a CACCC box. GATA-1 is a transcription factor which is essential for erythroid development (383) and as discussed elsewhere, (see Chapters 5 and 14) mutation in a GATA-1 binding site is responsible for the absence of Duffy glycoprotein from the red cells of most individuals with the Fy(a-b-) phenotype. It will be interesting to see if similar mutations are responsible for the absence of Kell protein from the red cells of any individuals with the K_o phenotype.

The Molecular Basis of Kell Blood Group System Antigens

All the Kell antigens antigens so far studied at the molecular level have been found to result from mutations

FIGURE 18-1 Structure and Association Between XK and KELL Proteins (references 379,391)

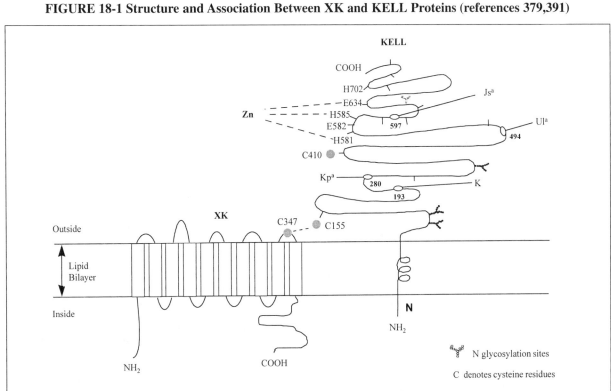

of a single nucleotide which change a single amino acid in the coding sequence of the Kell protein. The K antigen is extremely immunogenic, about 5% of K- adults transfused with one unit of K+ blood will make anti-K. Excluding ABO, K antigen is second only to D in its immunizing potential (78). Lee et al. (384) compared the sequences of the 19 exons which comprise the *Kell* complex gene in individuals homozygous for the *K* gene (*KK*) and homozygous for the *k* gene (*kk*). The sequences differed in only a single base in exon 6. *K* DNA encodes methionine at position 193 whereas *k* DNA encodes threonine at this position. The point mutation C to T in exon 6 which defines the K antigen creates a novel restriction enzyme site that can be cut by *BsmI* and this allowed the development of an RFLP analysis to confirm that the mutation does indeed identify the K antigen in an analysis of 42 individuals of known *Kk* status. If K is defined by a single amino change in the protein like numerous other antigens described in this book, why is it so much more immunogenic than other antigens? One possible explanation may be that this amino acid change affects a consensus sequence for N-glycosylation. Thr193 in k protein is part of the consensus sequence Asn191-Arg-Thr. If this site is glycosylated in the Kell protein expressing k then the Kell protein expressing K would have one less N-glycan than k-bearing protein. The absence of an N-glycan might result in a considerable change in the tertiary structure of the protein in this region and/or the exposure of parts of the protein not accessible at the surface of k-bearing protein. K protein might therefore appear to be very different from k protein and hence more immunogenic. Lee et al. (384) report that the Kell protein that carries K has a slightly faster electrophoretic mobility than the Kell protein that lacks K suggesting that k protein does indeed have a greater content of N-glycans.

A similar analysis of *Kell* gene exons from individuals of the Js(a+b-) phenotype revealed two nucleotide mutations in exon 17 only one of which changed the amino acid sequence of the protein (385). The base substitution T to C at nt1910 changes leucine 597 to proline. Protein sequence changes involving proline are not uncommon as the basis of novel antigens (see C/c; E/e; Di[a]/Di[b]; In[a]/In[b]). Proline residues induce bends in polypeptide chains and may as a consequence significantly alter the tertiary structure of a protein. In the case of Js[a] the proline residue is adjacent to one cysteine residue and close to another and so, as Lee et al. (385) point out, it is conceivable that the change could alter disulphide interactions and thereby markedly change the secondary and tertiary structure of the protein. As already mentioned, Js[a] and Js[b] are known to be far more sensitive to thiol reagents than other Kell system antigens, a feature consistent with the location of residues

critical for antigenic activity close to cysteines involved in disulphide bonding. Also noted by Lee et al. (385) is the interesting possibility that this change might alter the kinetics of the proteins' enzyme activity since the critical consensus sequence for zinc binding endopeptidases is close by in the linear sequence at H581-585.

Kp[a] and Kp[c] result from point mutations in exon 8. Kp[a] has a C961T substitution resulting in an Arg281Trp change. Kp[c] has a G962A substitution resulting in an Arg281Gln change. The antigen Ul[a] results from a point mutation in exon 13 (A1601T) resulting in a Glu493Val change (386). The Wk[a] antigen results from a single nucleotide substitution in exon 8 (T1025C) which changes a single amino acid Val302 to Ala (386). The positions of all the antigenic changes are indicated on the model of Kell protein given in figure 18-1.

Further information regarding the spatial arrangement of antigens on the Kell protein can be obtained from competitive binding studies. Parsons et al. (253) showed that murine monoclonal antibodies could be separated into two non-overlapping epitope groups, one containing antibodies with anti-k-like specificity and the other group associated with a monoclonal antibody denoted anti-Kp[bc]. These data indicate that regions of Kell protein containing the K/k polymorphism are spatially distinct from those defining the Kp[a]/Kp[b]/Kp[c] polymorphism. DNA sequencing studies described above showed that the critical residues for these two antigenic groups are 88 residues apart in the linear sequence of the protein. Clearly if these residues are themselves part of the epitopes (rather than indirectly causing a change to another region of the protein and thereby creating novel epitopes) the protein does not fold in such a way as to bring these two regions close enough together to be blocked by a molecule of the size of IgG. Petty et al. (18) expanded this approach by employing the MAIEA assay to carry out competitive binding assays involving human alloantibodies and murine monoclonal antibodies. These and other authors (242) distinguish four non-overlapping groups of antigens on the Kell protein. One group comprises K, k, Js[a], Js[b], Ul[a] and K22, another K14, a third K18 and the fourth the antigens Kp[a], Kp[b], Kp[c] and the antigen defined by the monoclonal anti-Kp[bc].

The molecular basis of the other Kell antigens had not been determined at the time of writing but it is clear from experiments involving immunoprecipitation (58) and those using MAIEA discussed above that all the high incidence antigens tested are carried on the same protein. K562 cells transfected with Kell cDNA express Kell system antigens whereas untransfected K562 cells do not (380). The cDNA expressed encoded both k and K14 thereby providing further proof that all the Kell system antigens are carried on a single protein.

Fetal DNA Typing

Elucidation of the molecular basis of the K/k polymorphism described above opened up the possibility of determining the K/k type of a fetus from DNA. Typing for K in this way has considerable practical value. Erythroblastosis fetalis caused by antibodies to Kell system antigens is rare but when it does occur it can be very severe. A particular problem is that severe disease may be associated with low titer antibody (8-16 by IAT) in the maternal serum (144). A further complication is that the disease due to Kell system antibodies, unlike that caused by Rh antibodies, is associated with minimal hemolysis. Indeed, there is evidence that fetal anemia caused by anti-K results not solely from destruction of red cells but also from inhibition of erythroid progenitor cell growth (387) (see also Chapter 42). These factors make it difficult for clinicians to assess the potential risk in a pregnancy where the mother has anti-K and it is often necessary to take a fetal blood sample to assess the level of anemia. Fetal blood sampling is not without risk and so the ability to determine the K type of a fetus from DNA (usually obtained from fetal cells in amniotic fluid) and thereby discern whether or not it is really at risk from maternal antibody is of considerable value. The K type of a fetus can be determined by RFLP analysis as originally described by Lee et al. (381) and modified by Murphy et al. (388) or by the use of allele specific primers (ASP) (389, 402). The International Blood Group Reference Laboratory, Bristol, UK received 23 requests for fetal K typing in 1996.

Molecular Basis of K_o Phenotype

K_o, the null phenotype phenotype of the Kell system has not yet yielded to analysis at the molecular level. Lee et al. (41) report studies on two individuals of K_o phenotype. They were able to isolate normal Kell mRNA (the sequence of the RNA from the initiator codon to the poly A tail was identical to RNA obtained from individuals of common Kell system phenotype) from the peripheral blood of both individuals. These workers did not report on the level of Kell mRNA expression in the K_o individuals. The situation in these K_o individuals is reminiscent of that observed in many examples of the weak D phenotype (see Chapter 12).

As discussed earlier, Daniels et al. (390) described an individual (MD) who typed as K_o by conventional serology but unlike other examples of K_o, the red cells of MD had a very weak expression of Kx. MD had three children whose red cells typed as Kp(a+b+) and since their mother's red cells typed as Kp(a-b+) the children must have inherited a Kp^a allele from the father. Weakened expression of Kell system antigens is known to be associated with the presence of the Kp^a allele (see earlier) and Daniels et al. (280,390) speculate that this weakening may be related to some general conformational change in the Kell protein effected by the replacement of arginine 281 with tryptophan in the Kell protein which creates the Kp^a antigen. In addition to being homozygous for the the Kp^a allele, MD was shown to be hemizygous for a mutation in the *Xk* gene. This mutation (a nucleotide substitution of G to A at nucleotide 5 of intron 2) is in a donor splice site sequence and would be expected to cause some degree of abnormal splicing of the *Xk* gene product and could thus account for the marked reduction in Kx antigen observed on the red cells of the patient. Two unrelated men (FD and ED described in the next section) with a mild form of McLeod syndrome, whose red cells had weak but detectable Kell antigens, had different single base mutations within consensus splice site sequences in intron 2 of the *Xk* gene (390,391). Daniels et al. (390) conclude that the K_o-like phenotype of MD is a consequence of the concomitant occurrence of two rare events, homozygosity for the Kp^a allele and a mutation in the *Xk* gene. These studies are of particular interest because they provide strong evidence that Kell protein and Kx protein associate together as a complex in the red cell membrane. In this context it is interesting to note that mutations in the *Xk* gene affect the expression of Kell antigens in an analogous manner to the way in which mutations in the gene giving rise to the Rh glycoprotein affect the expression of Rh polypeptides in Rh_{null} cells of the regulator type (see Chapter 12).

Kx Antigen and the McLeod Syndrome

The extreme paucity of anti-Kx made it very difficult to study the biochemical nature of the antigen and the molecule it identifies. Nevertheless Redman et al. (359) were able to report the location of the antigen on a molecule of 37kD, by immunoprecipitation from K_o and normal red cells with human allo-anti-Kx. Cloning of the gene giving rise to Kx protein was, however, achieved without the use of anti-Kx (391). Absence of the Kx protein from red cells is accompanied by several red cell abnormalities which contribute to the distinctive characteristics of the McLeod phenotype: reduced red cell survival in vivo; presence of acanthocytes; a 30% decrease in membrane permeability to water (358); increased phosphorylation of some membrane proteins and lipids (357); and enhanced exchangeability of membrane phosphatidylcholine with an exogenous source (361). The acanthocytes can be converted to discocytes by incubation with dimyristoyl phosphatidylserine which preferentially partitions into the inner half of the lipid bilayer suggesting that there is a lipid deficiency in the inner half of the bilayer (362). As discussed above, the McLeod phenotype occurs almost exclusively in males and may be accompanied by chronic granulomatous disease (CGD) and/or Duchenne's muscular dystrophy (DMD). Mapping of the genes for these associated X-linked diseases facilitated the mapping of McLeod (*Xk*) gene to the X chromosome at Xp21 between the CGD and DMD genes (233,376). Abnormalities associated with the McLeod phenotype are not confined to red cells. Patients have associated muscular (elevated serum creatinine kinase and carbonic anhydrase III, cardiomegaly sometimes followed by cardiomyopathy and skeletal muscle wasting) and neurological (choreiform and dystonic movements, caudate nucleus atrophy, cognitive deterioration, decreased binding of striatal dopamine D2 receptors) abnormalities (58,391,392). These associated abnormalities clearly suggest that the Kx protein, unlike the Kell protein, is not confined to erythroid cells but is also expressed in skeletal and cardiac muscle and neurological tissue.

The first step in cloning the *Xk* gene was the screening of a yeast artificial chromosome library (YAC) with cDNA probes (DXS709 and CYBB) which flanked the region of the X chromosome containing the gene. Three overlapping YAC clones were obtained which formed a contig of about 1200kb. The YAC clones were then used to screen a human X chromosome cosmid library to obtain a contig of about 360kb which extended from DXS709 to CYBB. Radiolabeled whole cosmids from this contig were hybridized to genomic DNA from patients with McLeod syndrome. One patient (MT) was found to have a large deletion (50kb) which identified the region containing the *Xk* gene. To search for transcription units within this region genomic fragments that spanned the deletion endpoints of patient MT were used to screen a human bone marrow cDNA library. Three cDNA clones hybridized to an mRNA transcript of 5.2kb when subjected to Northern Blot analysis. Eventually a consensus full-length transcript for the *Xk* gene was derived from 7 cDNA clones. DNA sequence analysis revealed a single open reading frame of 1335 nucleotides encoding a predicted protein of 444 amino acids. Sequence comparisons between cDNA clones and genomic DNA clones revealed that the gene contains three exons. Hydropathy analysis of the predicted protein suggested the presence of 10 membrane spanning regions (see figure 18-1). The predicted topology of the protein is indicative of a membrane transport function. The predicted protein lacks any motif for N-glycosylation. In this sense the protein is unusual for a membrane protein although the Rh polypeptides also lack N-glycans (see Chapter 12). It may be that the heavily glycosylated Kell protein facilitates membrane assembly of Kx protein in red cells thereby negating the need for N-glycans on the protein itself.

To prove that the isolated gene was responsible for the McLeod syndrome, Ho et al. (391) looked for point mutations in genomic DNA derived from patients in whom Southern blot analysis had not revealed the presence of gene deletions or rearrangements. Nucleotide sequence analysis of two patients (FD and ED) revealed point mutations in intron 2. The mutation in FD was in the 5' donor splice site while that in ED was at the 3' acceptor splice site. These mutations would be expected to result in reduced levels of Kx protein expression and provided strong evidence that the gene cloned was indeed the *Xk* gene. Further evidence was obtained by Khamlichi et al. (377) who purified Kx protein from red cells and showed that the N-terminal amino acid sequence (22 residues) of purified Kx protein is identical to that predicted from the cDNA sequence obtained by Ho et al. (391).

There is only one recorded exception to the rule that the McLeod syndrome is found exclusively in males. The index patient of family L was a lady with neuroacanthocytosis who presented with seizures at age 51 years and who was subsequently shown to have McLeod syndrome. Analysis of the *Xk* gene in family L revealed a novel mutation (393). A deletion of a single nucleotide at codon 90 (exon 2) caused a frameshift leading to premature termination of translation. The resultant protein would have only 128 amino acids of which the C-terminal 38 would be incorrect. The lady in question was heterozygous for this mutation. She died at age 60. Her two sons, both of whom inherited the mutation, died at age 31, after an illness of 6 to 8 years duration comprising seizures, areflexia and, in one, a personality change and involuntary movements. Female carriers of a variant *Xk* gene do not normally have McLeod syndrome. Ho et al. (393) provide experimental evidence that in this particular case the X chromosome carrying the normal *Xk* gene had been inactivated. Ho et al. (393) also point out that there is a vast excess of affected males among patients with neuroacanthocytosis and suggest that the peripheral blood of these patients should be examined for acanthocytes as a preliminary screening test for possible involvement of the mutations in the *Xk* gene.

Northern blot analysis with *Xk* cDNAs identified a common mRNA transcript of 5.2kb in several tissues. The highest levels of expression were observed in fetal liver and adult skeletal muscle, the RNA was also expressed in brain, heart and pancreas and at low levels in adult lung, liver, kidney and spleen.

The Kell Protein/Kx Protein Complex

It is clear from earlier sections in this chapter that there is considerable evidence to suggest that the Kell and

Kx proteins form a covalently linked complex in normal red cells. Khamlichi et al. (377) point out that only one of the 16 cysteine residues in the Kx protein is predicted to be extracellular (Cys347). Cysteine 347 is in the fifth extracellular loop (see figure 18-1). Inspection of the Kell protein sequence reveals 15 cysteine residues in the extracellular domain any one of which might form a disulphide bond with Cys347 of the Kx protein. In the model shown in figure 18-1, Cys155 of the Kell protein is shown as forming the disulphide bond but this is for the purposes of illustration only, there is no direct evidence for this!

Other functional complexes involving proteins encoded by unrelated genes are also found in the red cell membrane. The Diego blood group antigens are found on the anion transport protein, band 3, which associates with glycophorin A, a carrier of MN system antigens (see Chapters 15 and 17). The Rh polypeptides associate with the Rh glycoprotein and probably glycophorin B as well (see Chapter 12). Band 3, the Rh polypeptides, the Rh glycoprotein and the Kx protein are all multiple membrane spanning proteins. Glycophorin A and glycophorin B are sialoglycoproteins. It is clear that GPA facilitates the membrane assembly of band 3 (394). In this context it is interesting to note that there is some, albeit rather tentative, evidence that the sialoglycoproteins glycophorin C and D may be associated with Kell protein and ipso facto with Kx protein. This evidence derives from serological investigations which showed that Kell system antigen expression is depressed on the red cells of some individuals with Gerbich-negative phenotypes (see earlier section for a more detailed discussion). Jaber et al. (276) estimate that K+ k+ red cells of the Ge:-2,-3 phenotype have approximately half the number of K antigen sites as K+ k+, Ge:2,3 red cells. The antigen K11 seems to be particularly affected. K11 has recently been shown to depend on Val302 in the Kell protein (386). The critical region of GPC/D would appear to be that encoded by exon 3 of the *GYPC* gene (395). Whether or not these regions associate in such a complex remains to be proved. What is clear is that the Kell and Kx proteins are not required for GPC/D expression since Gerbich antigens are not depressed on red cells of either the K_o or McLeod phenotype. Earlier suggestions that Kx expression is increased on K_o cells have been questioned by Carbonnet et al. (396) who used a rabbit antibody to the Kx protein to show that K_o cells carry a lower amount of Kx protein. These results suggest that membrane insertion of Kx protein is facilitated by Kell protein. The stoichiometry of a complex between Kx protein, Kell protein and GPC/D is unbalanced. Kx protein is reported to be of very low abundance in red cells (500 copies/cell) (359), Kell protein is variously reported at between 3000 and 18,000 copies/cell (253,274) and GPC/D at 200,000 copies/cell (397) suggesting that a large proportion of GPC/D molecules are not associated with the putative complex and that a proportion of Kell protein molecules are similarly not associated. The Kell protein remains tightly associated with the red cell skeleton when immunoprecipitation is carried out using low concentrations of Triton X-100 (58,276). Whether or not this association is indirect through GPC/D and its interaction with proteins 4.1 and p55 (see Chapter 16), direct through interactions involving its N-terminal cytosolic domain, or via some other mechanism, is unknown.

Possible Functions of the Kell Protein/Kx Protein Complex

The functions of the Kell and Kx proteins are unknown but it is possible to infer likely functions by inspection of the protein sequences predicted from nucleotide sequencing of isolated cDNA clones.

The most striking feature of the Kell protein is the occurrence of a consensus motif HEXXH found in other proteins which are known to be zinc binding endopeptidases. The Kell protein has homology along its whole length with endothelin converting enzyme-1 (ECE-1), endothelin converting enzyme-2 (ECE-2) and neutral endopeptidase-24.11 (NEP, syn. CALLA, CD10). It is therefore instructive to consider the properties of ECE-1, ECE-2 and NEP since these are well characterized enzymes, in order to seek understanding of the likely function of the Kell protein. ECE-1 is a membrane-bound metalloproteinase which is expressed at high levels in vascular endothelial cells and functions by converting a 38 residue peptide produced by endothelial cells (big endothelin-1) into a 21 residue peptide (endothelin-1, ET-1). ET-1 is the most potent vasoconstrictor substance known (398). In contrast to ECE-1 which is highly specific, NEP has a very broad specificity. It cleaves and degrades many small biologically active peptides. Alignment of the amino acid sequences of ECE-1, NEP and Kell reveals other striking similarities in addition to the HEXXH motif. Each molecule has a cluster of cysteine residues proximal to the extracellular face of the membrane domain. A second cluster of three cysteine residues occurs at the extreme C terminus. Yet another cysteine (Cys155 in Kell) appears conserved in all three proteins. These similarities in the distribution of cysteine residues indicate that the three proteins have similar tertiary structures.

The residues critical for enzyme activity in NEP and ECE-1 have been studied in detail using site-directed mutagenesis. In this way the His, Glu and His residues of the HEXXH consensus motif in NEP and ECE-1 have been confirmed as part of the active site of the enzyme (379). The two histidines and a second glutamic acid some distance away in the linear sequence are necessary for binding the zinc atom. There is a second glutamic acid in a corresponding place in the Kell protein sequence (Glu634) and this is shown in the model of Kell protein in figure 18-1. A third histidine residue necessary for enzymic activity of NEP and ECE-1 also appears to be conserved in Kell protein (His702, figure 18-1). Both ECE-1 and NEP form dimers in the membrane. The dimer of NEP is formed by noncovalent interactions whereas that of ECE-1 is formed through a disulphide bond involving a cysteine which appears to be conserved between ECE-1 and Kell protein (Cys410 in Kell). There is, however, no direct evidence that the Kell protein forms homodimers in the red cell membrane. The foregoing structural considerations lead to the conclusion that the Kell protein must be a peptidase. What is its substrate? The answer to this question is not known but there are some clues which suggest a hypothesis which is amenable to experiment. It appears that Kell protein is expressed early in erythropoiesis. Manning et al. (387) report that anti-K inhibits the growth of erythroid progenitor cells (BFU-e) in in vitro culture and hypothesize that this may be the mechanism in vivo which gives rise to fetal anemia in pregnancies where a mother with anti-K carries a K+ fetus. Perhaps a peptidase function of the Kell protein is required for erythoid development. Preece et al. (399) in a paper brought to the attention of one of us (DJA) by Professor Jim Wiley, report evidence for the presence of a membrane-bound metalloproteinase on activated leukocytes which effects the endoproteolytic release of L-selectin from the leukocyte surface. These authors refer to the metalloproteinase as L-selectin sheddase. Since L-selectin is an important molecule which mediates the binding of leukocytes to endothelium (400) an attractive role for L-selectin sheddase would be to regulate the expression of L-selectin on the leukocyte surface and thereby regulate its adhesive interactions. Could it be that Kell protein has an analogous function in regulating adhesive interactions between erythroid progenitors and other cells in the marrow during erythroid development? L-selectin is known to be expressed on BFU-e (401).

These speculations must be tempered with the knowledge that individuals with K_o red cells, which lack Kell protein, are perfectly healthy. If Kell protein has an important function in mature red cells then one would have to argue that there is some other mechanism which can compensate for its deficiency in individuals with the K_o phenotype. Alternatively, Kell protein might be expressed during early erythropoeisis in individuals with the K_o phenotype and the defect in these individuals might be due to some abnormality in regulation at the later stages of erythropoiesis. Evidence that normal Kell mRNA was found in two individuals of K_o phenotype (384) would not be inconsistent with this hypothesis.

The predicted membrane topology of the Kx protein suggests that it functions as a membrane transport protein (see figure 18-1). An identical topology is predicted for the rabbit sodium-dependent glutamate transporter (391). Both proteins have a large putative second extracellular loop and multiple consensus phosphorylation sites in regions predicted to be cytoplasmic. Ho et al. (391) compared the transport properties of red cells of McLeod phenotype and normal red cells with respect to a variety of amino acids (arginine, alanine, glutamine, glutamate, glycine, tryptophan, valine) as well as potassium, choline, nucleoside adenosine, L-lactate, chloride and sulphate without discovering any differences between the two cell types. Ho et al. (391) also noted that the tissue distribution of Kx is almost identical to that of a brain sodium-dependent neutral amino acid transporter and conclude that the Kx protein may be involved in sodium-dependent transport of amino acids or oligopeptides. As has been discussed above, it seems likely that some, if not all, the Kx protein in red cells is covalently linked to Kell protein (see figure 18-1) and that the two proteins together may form a functional complex. However, the same complex could not occur in all cells and tissues which express Kx because Kell expression is much more restricted than that of the Kx protein. Perhaps the Kx protein is associated with a different protein or proteins in these other tissues and these other associations confer different functional properties on the complex. If such Kell protein analogues do occur their study may provide important clues to the underlying pathology of the neurological and skeletal muscle abnormalities in the McLeod syndrome. This subject is of considerable interest not least because the neurological and muscular abnormalities found in McLeod syndrome bear a striking resemblance to those seen in Huntington's Disease and Muscular Dystrophy respectively (391,393).

References

1. Coombs RRA, Mourant AE, Race RR. Lancet 1946;1:264
2. Levine P, Backer M, Wigod M, et al. Science 1949;109:464
3. Allen FH Jr, Lewis SJ. Vox Sang 1957;2:81
4. Chown B, Lewis M, Kaita H. Nature 1957;180:711
5. Allen FH Jr, Lewis SJ, Fudenberg HH. Vox Sang 1958;3:1
6. Stroup M, MacIlroy M, Walker RH, et al. Transfusion 1965;5:309
7. Morton NE, Krieger H, Steinberg AG, et al. Vox Sang 1965;10:608
8. Giblett ER. Nature 1958;181:1221
9. Giblett ER, Chase J. Br J Haematol 1959;5:319
10. Walker RH, Argall CI, Steane EA, et al. Transfusion 1963;3:94
11. Corcoran PA, Allen FH Jr, Lewis M, et al. Transfusion 1961;1:181
12. Bove JR, Johnson M, Francis BJ, et al. (abstract). Transfusion 1965;5:370.

13. Lewis M, Anstee DJ, Bird GWG, et al. Vox Sang 1990;58:152
14. Hart van der M, Szaloky A, Loghem van JJ. Vox Sang 1968;15:456
15. Marsh WL. (Letter). Vox Sang 1979;36:375
16. Allen FH Jr, Krabbe SMR, Corcoran PA. Vox Sang 1961;6:555
17. Allen FH Jr, Rosenfield RE. Transfusion 1961;1:305
18. Petty AC. J Immunol Meth 1993;161:91
19. Furuhjelm U, Nevanlinna HR, Nurkka R, et al. Vox Sang 1968;15:118
20. Furuhjelm U, Nevanlinna HR, Nurkka R, et al. Vox Sang 1969;16:496
21. Strange JJ, Kenworthy RJ, Webb AJ, et al. Vox Sang 1974;27:81
22. Yamaguchi H, Okubo Y, Seno T, et al. Vox Sang 1979;36:29
23. Gavin J, Daniels GL, Yamaguchi H, et al. Vox Sang 1979;36:31
24. Callender ST, Race RR, Paykoc CV. Br Med J 1945;2:83
25. Callender ST, Race RR. Ann Eugen 1946;13:102
26. Race RR. Br Med Bull 1946;4:188
27. Marsh WL, Redman CM, Kessler LA, et al. Transfusion 1987;27:36
28. Race RR, Sanger R. Blood Groups in Man, 6th Ed. Oxford:Blackwell, 1975
29. Daniels G. Human Blood Groups. Oxford:Blackwell, 1995
30. Daniels GL, Anstee DJ, Cartron J-P, et al. Vox Sang 1995;69:265
31. Eicher C, Kirkley K, Porter M, et al. (abstract). Transfusion 1985;25:448
32. Jongerius JM, Daniels GL, Overbeeke MAM, et al. Vox Sang 1996;71:43
33. Daniels GL, Anstee DJ, Cartron J-P, et al. Vox Sang 1996;71:246
34. Giles CM. Unpublished observations 1971 cited in Issitt PD. Applied Blood Group Serology, 3rd Ed. Miami:Montgomery 1985:289
35. Gavin J. Unpublished observations 1974 cited in Strange JJ, Kenworthy RJ, Webb AJ, et al. Vox Sang 1974;27:81
36. Sabo B, McCreary J, Gellerman M, et al. Vox Sang 1975;29:450
37. Advani H, Zamor J, Judd WJ, et al. Br J Haematol 1982;51:107
38. Redman CM, Marsh WL, Mueller KA, et al. Transfusion 1984;24:176
39. Redman CM, Avellino G, Pfeffer SR, et al. J Biol Chem 1986;261:9521
40. Wallas C, Simon R, Sharpe MA, et al. Transfusion 1986;26:173
41. Lee S, Zambas ED, Marsh WL, et al. Proc Nat Acad Sci USA 1991;88:6353
42. Gúevin RM, Taliano V, Waldmann O. (abstract). Prog 24th Ann Mtg Am Assoc Blood Banks, 1971
43. Heisto H, Gúevin RM, Taliano V, et al. Vox Sang 1973;24:179
44. Stroup M, Gellerman M, Marsh WL, et al. (abstract). Transfusion 1973;13:349
45. Marsh WL, Jensen L, Øyen R, et al. Vox Sang 1974;26:34
46. Marsh WL. Adv Immunohematol Vol 4, No 3, Oxnard:Spectra Biologicals, 1976
47. Barrasso C, Eska P, Grindon AJ, et al. Vox Sang 1975;29:124
48. Sabo B, McCreary J, Stroup M, et al. Vox Sang 1979;36:97
49. Bar Shany S, Porath DB, Levene C, et al. Vox Sang 1982;42:87
50. Issitt PD, Crookston MC. Transfusion 1984;24:2
51. Marsh WL, Øyen R, Nichols ME, et al. Br J Haematol 1975;29:247
52. Gúevin RM, Taliano V, Waldmann O. Vox Sang 1976;31 (Suppl 1):96
53. Marsh WL, Stroup M, MacIlroy M, et al. Vox Sang 1973;24:200
54. Wallace ME, Bouysou C, de Jongh DS, et al. Vox Sang 1976;30:300
55. Jones J, Reid ME, Øyen R, et al. (abstract). Transf Med 1994;4 (Suppl 1):45
56. Branch DR, Muensch HA, Sy Siok Hian AL, et al. Br J Haematol 1983;54:573
57. Branch DR, Petz LD. Am J Clin Pathol 1982;78:161
58. Marsh WL, Redman CM. Transf Med Rev 1987;1:4
59. Brown A, Berger R, Lasko D, et al. Rev Fr Transf Immunohematol 1982;25:619
60. Peloquin P, Yochum G, Hagy L, et al. (abstract). Transfusion 1988;28(Suppl 6S):19S
61. Winkler MM, Beattie KM, Cisco SL, et al. Transfusion 1989;29:642
62. Pehta JC, Johnson CL, Giller RL, et al. (abstract). Transfusion 1989;29(Suppl 7S):15S
63. Byrne PC, Deck M, Øyen R, et al. (abstract). Transfusion 1993;33 (Suppl 9S):55S
64. Daniels GL, Petty AC, Reid M, et al. Transfusion 1994;34:818
65. Lewis M, Kaita H, Duncan D, et al. Vox Sang 1960;5:565
66. Cleghorn TE. Unpublished observations 1961 to 1967 cited in Race RR, Sanger R. Blood Groups in Man, 6th Ed. Oxford:Blackwell, 1975
67. Wright J, Cornwall SM, Matsina E. Vox Sang 1965;10:218
68. Dichupa PZ, Anderson C, Chown B. Vox Sang 1969;17:1
69. Lewis M, Kaita H, Chown B. Vox Sang 1969;17:221
70. Chown B. 13th John G. Gibson II Lecture. New York:Columbia Presbyterian Medical Center, 1964
71. Garretta M, Gener J, Muller A. Rev Fr Transf Immunohematol 1978;21:379
72. Mourant AE, Kopéc AC, Domaniewska-Sobczak K. The Distribution of the Human Blood Groups and Other Biochemical Polymorphisms, 2nd Ed. London:Oxford Univ Press, 1976
73. Hamilton HB, Nakahara Y. Vox Sang 1971;20:24
74. Ball M, Cant B, Garwood P, et al. Biotest Bull 1989;4:15
75. Gale SA, Rowe GP, Northfield FE. Vox Sang 1988;54:172
76. Kornstad L, Heisto H. Proc 6th Cong Eur Soc Haematol, 1957:754
77. Mollison PL, Engelfriet CP, Contreras M. Blood Transfusion in Clinical Medicine, 9th Ed. Oxford:Blackwell 1993:112 and 250
78. Giblett ER. Transfusion 1961;1:233
79. Grove-Rasmussen M. Transfusion 1964;4:200
80. Grove-Rasmussen M, Huggins CE. Transfusion 1973;13:124
81. Tovey GH. Haematologia 1974;8:389
82. Pineda AA, Taswell HF, Brzica SM Jr. Transfusion 1978;18:1
83. Issitt PD. In: Rhesus Problems in Clinical Practice. Groningen-Drenthe: Red Cross Blood Bank, 1979:46
84. Croucher BEE. In: A Seminar on Laboratory Management of Hemolysis. Washington, D.C.:Am Assoc Blood Banks 1979:151
85. Moore SB, Taswell HF, Pineda AA, et al. Am J Clin Pathol 1980;74:94
86. Taswell HF, Pineda AA, Moore SB. In: A Seminar on Immune-Mediated Cell Destruction. Washington, D.C.:Am Assoc Blood Banks, 1981:71
87. Pineda AA, Chase CJ, Taswell HF. In: Thalassemia Today. The Mediterranean Experience. Milano:Centro Transfusionale Ospedale, 1987

88. Harrison J. Vox Sang 1970;19:123
89. Frame M, Mollison PL, Terry WD. Nature 1970;225:641
90. Abramson N, Schur PH. Blood 1972;40:500
91. Engelfriet CP. Unpublished observations 1978 cited in
     Mollison PL. Blood Transfusion in Clinical Medicine, 7th Ed.
     Oxford:Blackwell, 1983
92. Hardman JT, Beck ML. Transfusion 1981;21:343
93. Michaelsen TE, Kornstad L. Clin Exp Immunol 1987;67:637
94. Allen FH Jr, Warshaw AL. Vox Sang 1962;7:222
95. Ottensooser F, Mellone O, Biancalana A. Blood 1953;8:1029
96. Garratty G. In: Immune Destruction of Red Blood Cells.
     Arlington, VA:Am Assoc Blood Banks, 1989:109
97. Pineda AA, Brzica SM, Taswell HF. Mayo Clin Proc
     1978;53:378
98. Leventhal ML, Wolf AM. Am J Obstet Gynecol 1956;71:452
99. Wenk RE, Goldstein P, Felix JK. Obstet Gynaecol
     1985;66:473
100. Schultz MH. In: Blood Group Systems: Kell. Arlington,
     VA:Am Assoc Blood Banks, 1990:37
101. Zettner A, Bove JR. Transfusion 1963;3:48
102. West NC, Jenkins JA, Johnston BR, et al. Vox Sang
     1986;50:174
103. Reiner AP, Sayers MH. Arch Pathol Lab Med 1990;114:862
104. Issitt PD, Combs MR, Bredehoeft SJ, et al. Transfusion
     1993;33:284
105. Pepperell RJ, Barrie JU, Fliegner JR, et al. Med J Austral
     1977;2:453
106. Beal RW. Clin Obstet Gynaecol 1979;6:493
107. Hardy J, Napier JAF. Br J Obstet Gynaecol 1981;88:91
108. Walker RH. In: Hemolytic Disease of the Newborn.
     Arlington, VA:Am Assoc Blood Banks, 1984:173
109. Leggat HM, Gibson JM, Barron SL, et al. Br J Obstet
     Gynaecol 1991;98:162
110. Strohm P, O'Shaughnessy R, Moore J, et al.
     Immunohematology 1991;7:40
111. Bowman JM. In: Immunobiology of Transfusion Medicine.
     New York:Marcel Dekker 1994:553
112. Springer GF, Williamson P, Reader BL. Ann NY Acad Sci
     1962;97:104
113. Morgan P, Bossom EL. Transfusion 1963;3:397
114. Tegoli J, Sausais L, Issitt PD. Vox Sang 1967;12:305
115. Marsh WL, Nichols ME, Øyen R, et al. Transfusion
     1978;18:149
116. Kanel GC, Davis I, Bowman JE. Transfusion 1978;18:472
117. Schmelter S, Freed P. Lab Med 1978;9:53
118. Mukumoto Y, Konishi H, Ito K, et al. Vox Sang 1978;35:275
119. O'Brien M, King G, Dube VE, et al. Transfusion 1979;19:558
120. Judd WJ, Walter WJ, Steiner EA. Transfusion 1981;21:184
121. Clark A, Monaghan WP, Martin CA. Am J Med Technol
     1981;47:983
122. Doelman CJA, Westermann WF, Voorst tot Voorst E van, et al.
     Transfusion 1992;32:790
123. Pereira A, Monteagudo J, Rovira M, et al. Transfusion
     1989;29:549
124. Savalonis JM, Kalish RI, Cummings EA, et al. Transfusion
     1988;28:229
125. McGinniss MH, MacLowry JD, Holland PV. Transfusion
     1984;24:28
126. Contreras M, Knight RC. Clin Lab Haematol 1989;11:317
127. Contreras M, Knight RC. Transfusion 1991;31:270
128. Levine P, Kuhmichel AB, Wigod M. Blood 1952;7:251
129. Shapiro M. S Afr Med J 1952;26:951
130. Schmidt PJ, McGinniss MH, Leyshon WC, et al. Vox Sang
     1958;3:438
131. Newstead PH, Bruce N. Canad J Med Technol 1961;23:127

132. Bryant LB. Bull South Cent Assoc Blood Banks 1965;8:4
133. Thomas MJ, Konugres AA. Vox Sang 1966;11:227
134. Kulich V. Cesk Pediatr 1967;22:823
135. Kluge A, Jungfer H. Blut 1970;21:357
136. Hopkins DF. Br J Haematol 1970;19:749
137. Lee RS. J Am Osteopath Assoc 1975;75:313
138. Rodesch F, Lambermont M, Donner C, et al. Am J Obstet
     Gynecol 1987;156:124
139. Letendre PL, Williams MA, Ferguson DJ. Transfusion
     1987;27:138
140. Walker RH, Argall CI, Steane EA, et al. Nature 1963;197:295
141. Waheed A, Kennedy MS. Transfusion 1982;22:161
142. Rigal D, Juron-Dupraz F, Biggio B, et al. Rev Fr Transf
     Immunohematol 1982;25:101
143. Dinning G, Doughty RW, Collins AK. Vox Sang 1985;48:317
144. Bowman JM, Harman FA, Manning CR, et al. Vox Sang
     1989;56:187
145. Merry AH, Thomson EE, Lagar J, et al. Vox Sang
     1984;47:125
146. Lown JAG, Barr AL, Davis RE. J Clin Pathol 1979;32:1019
147. Confida S, Hurel C, Chesnel N, et al. Vox Sang 1981;40:34
148. Voak D. Biotest Bull 1981;1:24
149. Molthan L, Strohm P. Am J Clin Pathol 1981;75:629
150. Molthan L. Canad J Med Technol 1981;43:176
151. Voak D, Downie M, Haigh T, et al. Med Lab Sci 1982;39:363
152. Szymanski I, Gandhi JG. Am J Clin Pathol 1983;80:37
153. Chown B, Lewis M, Kaita H, et al. Vox Sang 1965;8:378
154. Okubo Y. Unpublished observations cited in Daniels G.
     Human Blood Groups. Oxford:Blackwell, 1995:387
155. Kikuchi M, Endo N, Seno T, et al. Transfusion 1983;23:254
156. Lawson J, Gavin J. Unpublished observations cited in Daniels
     G. Human Blood Groups. Oxford:Blackwell, 1995:390
157. Franciosi R, Awer E, Santana M. Transfusion 1967;7:297
158. Abbott D, Hussain S. Canad Med Assoc J 1970;103:752
159. Morse EE. Vox Sang 1978;35:215
160. Jensen KG. Vox Sang 1962;7:476
161. Okubo Y, Yamaguchi H, Seno T, et al. (Letter). Transfusion
     1986;26:215
162. Sakuma K, Suzucki H, Ohto T, et al. Vox Sang 1994;66:293
163. Miyata Y, Nakanura J, Kumazawa K, et al. J Jpn Soc Blood
     Transf 1987;33:430
164. Kuze M, Scott M. Unpublished observations 1967 cited in
     Race RR, Sanger R. Blood Groups in Man, 6th Ed.
     Oxford:Blackwell, 1975:303
165. Smoleniek J, Anderson N, Poole GD. (abstract). Transf Med
     1994;4:(Suppl1):48
166. Anderson L, White J, Liles B, et al. Am J Med Technol
     1959;25:184
167. Scudder J, Sargent M, Cahan A, et al. Unpublished observa-
     tions cited in Race RR, Sanger R. Blood Groups in Man, 6th
     Ed. Oxford:Blackwell, 1975:303
168. Daniels GL. PhD Thesis Univ London 1980
169. Sabo B, Keeling MM, Winkler MA, et al. (abstract). Book of
     Abstracts 17th Cong ISBT 1982:235
170. Dacus JV, Spinnato JA. Am J Obstet Gynecol 1984;150:888
171. Steane EA, Sheehan RG, Brooks BD, et al. In: Therapeutic
     Apheresis and Plasma Perfusion. New York:Liss, 1982:347
172. Bradley PM, Henry H, Speake L. (abstract). Book of
     Abstracts 20th Cong ISBT 1988:229
173. Wren MR, Issitt PD. (abstract). Transfusion 1986;26:548
174. Kohan A, Reybaud J, Salamone H, et al. Vox Sang
     1990;59:216
175. Eby CS, Cowan JL, Ramon RR, et al. (abstract). Book of
     Abstracts Joint Cong ISBT/AABB 1990:156
176. Gorlin JB, Kelly L. Vox Sang 1994;66:46

177. Watt J, Moffatt P, Chatfield S, et al. Immunohematology 1994;10:87

178. Darnborough J, Dunsford I. Unpublished observations 1959 cited in Race RR, Sanger R. Blood Groups in Man, 6th Ed. Oxford:Blackwell, 1975:303

179. McNeil C, Newman M. Unpublished observations 1966 cited in Race RR, Sanger R. Blood Groups in Man, 6th Ed. Oxford:Blackwell, 1975:303

180. Jarkowski TL, Hinshaw CP, Beattie KM, et al. Transfusion 1962;2:423

181. Fraser GR, Giblett ER, Motulsky AG. Am J Hum Genet 1966;18:546

182. Spielmann W, Teixidor D, Renninger W, et al. Humangenetik 1970;10:304

183. Byrne PC, Howard JH. Immunohematology 1994;10:136

184. Huestis DW, Busch S, Hanson ML, et al. Transfusion 1963;3:260

185. Crawford MN. Unpublished observations 1967 cited in Race RR, Sanger R. Blood Groups in Man, 6th Ed. Oxford:Blackwell, 1975:289

186. Beattie KM, Shafer AW, Sigmund K, et al. (abstract). Book of Abstracts 19th Cong ISBT 1986:312

187. Gerard Sister M. Transfusion 1965;5:359

188. Donovan LM, Tripp KL, Zuckerman JE, et al. Transfusion 1973;13:153

189. Ito K, Mukumoto Y, Konishi H. Vox Sang 1979;37:350

190. Levene C, Rudolphson Y, Shechter Y. Transfusion 1980;20:714

191. Taddie SJ, Barrasso C, Ness PM. Transfusion 1982;22:68

192. Lovett DA, Crawford MN. Transfusion 1967;7:442

193. Marshall G. Vox Sang 1968;14:304

194. Wake EJ, Issitt PD, Reihart JK, et al. Transfusion 1969;9:217

195. Purohit DM, Taylor HL, Spivey MA. Am J Obstet Gynecol 1978;131:755

196. Lowe RF, Musengezi AT, Moores P. Transfusion 1978;18:466

197. Ratcliff D, Fiorenza S, Culotta E, et al. (abstract). Transfusion 1987;27:534

198. Kaita H, Lewis M, Chown B, et al. Nature 1959;183:1586

199. Chown B, Lewis M, Kaita H, et al. Vox Sang 1961;6:620

200. Nunn HD, Giles CM, Dormandy KM. Vox Sang 1965;11:611

201. Simmons RT, Young NAF, Med J Austral 1968;2:1040.

202. Marsh WL. Med Lab Technol 1975;32:1

203. Ford DS, Knight AE, Smith F. Vox Sang 1977;32:220

204. Marsh WL, Redman CM. Transfusion 1990;30:158

205. Marsh WL. Transfusion 1992;32:98

206. Merry AH, Thomson EE, Anstee DJ, et al. Immunology 1984;51:793

207. Bowell PJ, Strange JJ. Unpublished observations 1974 cited in Race RR, Sanger R. Blood Groups in Man, 6th Ed. Oxford:Blackwell, 1975:290

208. McCreary J, Vogler AL, Gellerman M, et al. (abstract). Transfusion 1973;13:349

209. Gaudry LE, Watt JM, Bryant JA, et al. (abstract). Book of Abstracts 19th Cong ISBT 1986:651

210. Sabo B, McCreary J, Harris P. Vox Sang 1982;43:56

211. Frank S, Schmidt RP, Baugh M. Transfusion 1970;10:254

212. Humphreys PA, Moore BPL, Chown B. Unpublished observations 1963 cited in Race RR, Sanger R. Blood Groups in Man, 6th Ed. Oxford:Blackwell, 1975:293

213. Judd WJ. Personal communication 1994

214. Giblett ER, Klebanoff SJ, Pincus SH, et al. Lancet 1971;1:1235

215. Poole J. Med Lab Technol 1972;29:62

216. Marsh WL, Uretsky SC, Douglas SD. J Pediat 1975;87:1117

217. Marsh WL, Øyen R, Nichols ME. Vox Sang 1976;31:356

218. Wimer BM, Marsh WL, Taswell HF, et al. Br J Haematol 1977;36:219

219. Taswell HF, Lewis JC, Marsh WL, et al. Mayo Clin Proc 1977;52:157

220. Marsh WL. Mayo Clin Proc 1977;52:150

221. Brzica SM, Rhodes KH, Pineda AA. Mayo Clin Proc 1977;52:153

222. Bowell PJ, Hill FGH. Br J Haematol 1978;39:351

223. Symmans WA, Shepherd CS, Marsh WL, et al. Br J Haematol 1979;42:575

224. White W, Washington ED, Sabo BH, et al. Rev Fr Transf Immunohematol 1980;23:305

225. Fikrig SM, Phillipp JCD, Smithwick EM, et al. Pediatrics 1980;66:403

226. Densen P, Wilkinson-Kroovand S, Mandell GL, et al. Blood 1981;58:34

227. Marsh WL, Marsh NL, Moore A, et al. Vox Sang 1981;40:403

228. Faillace RT, Kingston WJ, Nanda NC, et al. Ann Int Med 1982;96:616

229. Swash M, Schwartz MS, Carter ND, et al. Brain 1983;106;717

230. Francke U, Oschs HD, de Martinville B, et al. Am J Hum Genet 1985;37:250

231. Frey D, Mächler M, Seger R, et al. Blood 1988;71;252

232. de Saint-Basile G, Bohler MC, Fischer A, et al. Hum Genet 1988;80:85

233. Bertelson CJ, Pogo A, Chaudhuri A, et al. Am J Hum Genet 1988;42:703

234. Carstairs K, Ruthledge Harding S, Lue K, et al. (abstract). Transfusion 1988;28 (Suppl 6S):20S

235. Sharp D, Rogers S, Dickstein B. (abstract). Transfusion 1988;28(Suppl 6S):37S

236. Hardie RJ, Pullon HWH, Harding AE, et al. Brain 1991;114:13

237. Uchida K, Nakajima K, Shima H, et al. (Letter). Transfusion 1992;32:691

238. Pehta J, Panesar N, Huima T, et al. (abstract). Transfusion 1992;32(Suppl 8S):19S

239. Marsh WL, Schnipper EF, Johnson CL, et al. Transfusion 1983;23:336

240. Tippett P. In: Human Blood Groups. Basel:Karger, 1977:401

241. Beattie KM, Heinz B, Korol S, et al. Rev Fr Transf Immunohematol 1982;25:611

242. Reid ME, Øyen R, Redman CM, et al. Vox Sang 1995;68:40

243. Taylor HL. (Letter). Transfusion 1979;19:787

244. Marsh WL, DiNapoli J, Øyen R. Vox Sang 1979;36:174

245. Marsh WL, Allen FH Jr. Unpublished observations 1973 cited in Issitt PD, Issitt CH. Applied Blood Group Serology, 2nd Ed. Oxnard:Spectra Biologicals, 1975

246. Barrasso C, Baldwin ML, Drew H, et al. Transfusion 1983;23:258

247. Pehta JC, Valinksy J, Redman C, et al. (abstract). Book of Abstracts Joint Cong ISBT/AABB 1990:57

248. Marsh WL, DiNapoli J, Øyen R, et al. Transfusion 1979;19:604

249. Manny N, Levene C, Harel N, et al. Vox Sang 1985;49:135

250. Levene C, Sela R, DaCosta Y, et al. (abstract). Book of Abstracts 20th Cong ISBT 1988:295

251. Judson PA, Anstee DJ. Med Lab Sci 1977;34:1

252. Daniels G. Rev Fr Transf Immunohematol 1988;31:395

253. Parsons SF, Gardner B, Anstee DJ. Transf Med 1993;3:137

254. Moulds JJ, Moulds MK, Patriquin P. (Letter). Transfusion 1986;26:305

255. Daniels G. Immunohematology 1992;8:53

256. Parsons SF, Mallinson G, Judson PA, et al. Transfusion

1987;27:61

257. Levene C, Karniel Y, Sela R. (Letter). Transfusion 1987;27:505

258. Daniels G. In: Blood Group Systems: Duffy, Kidd and Lutheran. Arlington, VA:Am Assoc Blood Banks, 1988:119

259. Moulds JJ, Moulds MK. (Letter). Transfusion 1983;23:274

260. Brown D. (abstract). Transfusion 1985;25:462

261. Spring FA, Reid ME. Vox Sang 1991;60:53

262. Spring FA, Reid ME, Nicholson G. Vox Sang 1994;66:72

263. Levene C, Harel N. (Letter). Transfusion 1984;24:541

264. Marsh WL, Johnson CL, Mueller KA. (Letter). Transfusion 1983;23:275

265. Marsh WL, DiNapoli J, Øyen R, et al. (Letter). Transfusion 1986;26:305

266. Branch DR, Petz LD. (abstract). Transfusion 1980;20:642

267. Konigshaus GH, Holland TI. Transfusion 1984;24:536

268. Shulman IA, Nelson JM, Lan HT. Transfusion1986;26:214

269. Toy EM. Immunohematology, 1986;2:57

270. Eckrich RJ. Immunohematology 1988;4:12

271. Greene M, Lloyd L, Popovsky MH, et al. (abstract). Transfusion 1989;29 (Suppl 7S):16S

272. Judd WJ. Methods in Immunohematology, 1st Ed. Miami:Montgomery 1988

273. Julleis J, Sapp C, Kakaiva R. (abstract). Transfusion 1992;32 (Suppl 8S):14S

274. Hughes-Jones NC, Gardner B. Vox Sang 1971;21:154

275. Masouredis SP, Sudora E, Mahan LC, et al. Haematologia 1980;13:59

276. Jaber A, Blanchard D, Goossens D, et al. Blood 1989;73:1597

277. Prewitt PL, Brendel WL, Moore RE, et al. Unpublished observations 1983 cited in Issitt PD. Applied Blood Group Serology, 3rd Ed. Miami:Montgomery, 1985:296

278. Walsh TJ, Daniels GL,Tippett P. Foren Sci Int 1981;18:161

279. Weinauer F, Jahn-Jochem H, Offner R, et al. (abstract). Transfusion 1994;34(Suppl 10S):25S

280. Daniels GL, Monaco AP, Weinauer F, et al. (abstract). Vox Sang 1996;70 (Suppl 2):42

281. Hawley WC, Blanda E, Kennedy MS. (abstract). Transfusion 1975;15:521

282. McDowell MA, Mann JM, Milakovic K. (abstract). Transfusion 1978;18:389

283. McDowell MA. Unpublished observations 1978 cited in Skradski K, Reid ME, Mount M, et al. Vox Sang 1994;66:68

284. Kline WE, Sullivan CM, Bowman RJ. Vox Sang 1984;47:170

285. Skradski K, Reid ME, Mount M, et al. Vox Sang 1994;66:68

286. Norman PC, Daniels GL. Transfusion 1988;28:460

287. Muller A, Andre-Liardet J, Garretta M, et al. Rev Fr Transf 1973;16:251

288. Daniels GL. (abstract). Transfusion 1982;22:405

289. Anstee DJ, Ridgwell K, Tanner MJA, et al. Biochem J 1984;221:97

290. Daniels GL, Shaw M-A, Judson PA, et al. Vox Sang 1986;50:117

291. McShane K, Chung A. Vox Sang 1989;57:205

292. Marsh WL. Unpublished observations 1984 cited in Issitt PD. Applied Blood Group Serology, 3rd Ed. Miami:Montgomery, 1985

293. Marsh WL, Øyen R, Alicea E, et al. Am J Hematol 1979;7:155

294. Marsh WL, Mueller KA, Johnson CL. (abstract). Transfusion 1982;22:419

295. Issitt PD, Pavone BG, Goldfinger D, et al. Br J Haematol 1976;34:5

296. Petz LD, Garratty G. Acquired Immune Hemolytic Anemias. New York:Churchill Livingstone, 1980

297. Krickler SH, Turner-Lienaux K, Godin T, et al. (Letter). Vox Sang 1987;52:157

298. Sullivan CM, Kline WE, Rubin BI, et al. Transfusion 1987;27:322

299. Dausset J, Colombani J. Blood 1954;14:1280

300. Fluckinger P, Ricci L, Usteri L. Acta Haematol 1955;13:53

301. Seyfried H, Gorska B, Maj S, et al. Vox Sang 1972;23:528

302. Beck ML, Marsh WL, Pierce SR, et al. Transfusion 1979;19:197

303. McCall L, Sobol RS, Ross D, et al. (abstract). Red Cell Free Press 1983;8:25

304. Brendel WL, Issitt PD, Moore RE, et al. Biotest Bull 1985;2:201

305. Vengelen-Tyler V, Gonzalez B, Garratty G, et al. Br J Haematol 1987;65:231

306. Rowe GP, Tozzo GG, Poole J, et al. Immunohematology 1989;5:79

307. Williamson LM, Poole J, Redman C, et al. Br J Haematol 1994;87:805

308. Manny N, Levene C, Sela R, et al. Vox Sang 1983;45:252

309. Puig N, Carbonell F, Marty ML. Vox Sang 1986;51:57

310. Garratty G, Sattler MS, Petz LD, et al. Rev Fr Transf Immunohematol 1979;22:529

311. Hare V, Wilson MJ, Wilkinson S, et al. (abstract). Transfusion 1981;21:613

312. Issitt PD, Pavone BG. Br J Haematol 1978;38:63

313. Issitt PD, Zellner DC, Rolih SD, et al. Transfusion 1977;17:539

314. Viggiano E, Clary NL, Ballas SK. Transfusion 1982;22:329

315. Issitt PD, Combs MR, Bumgarner DJ, et al. Transfusion 1996;36:481

316. Issitt PD. Applied Blood Group Serology, 3rd Ed. Miami:Montgomery, 1985:301

317. Oger J, Szuchet S, Antel J, et al. Nature 1982;295:66

318. Eveland D. (abstract). Book of Abstracts Joint Cong ISBT/AABB 1990:156

319. Winkler MM, Hamilton JR. (abstract). Book of Abstracts Joint Cong ISBT/AABB 1990:158

320. Goossens D, Champomier F, Rouger P, et al. J Immunol Meth 1987;101:193

321. Paire-Dante J, Martel F, Montcharmont P, et al. In: Monoclonal Antibodies Against Human Red Blood Cells and Related Antigens. Paris:Arnette, 1989:293

322. Nichols ME, Rosenfield RE, Rubinstein P. Vox Sang 1987;52:231

323. Chester MA, Johnson U, Lundblad A, et al. Proc 2nd Int Workshop on Monoclonal Antibodies Against Human Red Cell and Related Antigens 1990:126

324. Rouger P, Anstee D, Salmon C. Rev Fr Transf Immunohematol 1988;31:381

325. Inglis G, Fraser RH, McTaggart S, et al. Transf Med 1994;4:209

326. Parsons SF, Judson PA, Anstee DJ. J Immunogenet 1982;9:377

327. Jaber A, Loirat M-J, Willem C, et al. Br J Haematol 1991;79:311

328. Sonneborn HH, Uthemann H, Pfeffer S. Biotest Bull 1983;4:328

329. Marsh WL, Johnson CL, Rabin BI. Rev Fr Transf Immunohematol 1988;31:383

330. Zelinski T, Kaita H, Coghlan G, et al. Rev Fr Transf Immunohematol 1988;31:391

331. Marsh WL. In: Progress in Immunohematology. Arlington, VA:Am Assoc Blood Banks, 1988:93

332. Parsons SF, Judson PA, Spring F, et al. Rev Fr Transf Immunohematol 1988;31:401

333. Lubenko A, Gee S, Contreras M. Rev Fr Transf Immunohematol 1988;31:407

334. Sonneborn HH, Ernst M. Rev Fr Transf Immunohematol 1988;31:411

335. Marsh WL. Rev Fr Transf Immunohematol 1988;31:417

336. Byrd LH, Cheigh JS, Stenzel KH, et al. Lancet 1978;2:1167

337. Zelinski T, Coghlan G, Myal Y, et al. Ann Hum Genet 1991;55:137

338. Zelinski T, Coghlan G, Myal Y, et al. Cytogenet Cell Genet 1991;58:1927

339. Purohit KR, Weber JL, Ward LJ, et al. Hum Genet 1992;89:457

340. Lee S, Zambas ED, Marsh WL, et al. Blood 1993;81:2804

341. Murphy MT, Morrison N, Miles JS, et al. Hum Genet 1993;91:585

342. Babior BM, Woodman RC. Sem Hematol 1990;27:247

343. Branch DR, Sy Siok Hian AL, Petz LD. Br J Haematol 1985;59:505

344. Marsh WL. In: Cellular Antigens and Disease. Washington, D.C.:Am Assoc Blood Banks, 1977:52

345. Marsh WL. In: The Red Cell. New York:Liss, 1978:493

346. Marsh WL. Birth Defects Orig Article Series 1978;14:9

347. Branch DR. Gaidulis L, Lazar GS. Br J Haematol 1986;62:747

348. Marsh WL, Shepherd S, Øyen R. (abstract). Transfusion 1976;16:528

349. Ito K, Mukumoto Y, Konishi H, et al. Vox Sang 1979;37:39

350. Rouger P. In: Blood Group Systems: Kell. Arlington, VA:Am Assoc Blood Banks, 1990:77

351. Segal AW, Cross AR, Garcia RC, et al. New Eng J Med 1983;308:245

352. Ohno Y, Buescher ES, Roberts R, et al. Blood 1983;67:1132

353. Bohler MC, Seger R, Moug R, et al. J Clin Immunol 1986;6:136

354. Schwartz SA, Marsh WL, Symmans A, et al. (abstract). Transfusion 1982;22:404

355. Marsh WL. In: Blood Groups and Other Red Cell Surface Markers in Health and Disease. New York:Masson, 1982:17

356. Ballas SK, Bator SM, Aubuchon JP, et al. Transfusion 1990;30:722 356.

357. Tang LL, Redman CM, Williams D, et al. Vox Sang 1981;40:17

358. Glaubensklee CS, Evan AP, Galey WR. Vox Sang 1982;42:262

359. Redman CM, Marsh WL, Scarborough A, et al. Br J Haematol 1988;68:131

360. Galey WR, Evan AP, Van Nice PS, et al. Vox Sang 1978;34:152

361. Kuypers FA, Linde-Sebenius Trip M van, Roelofsen B, et al. FEBS Lett 1985;184:20

362. Redman CM, Huima T, Robbins E, et al. Blood 1989;74:1826

363. Wainfan E, Milkenny M, Johnson C, et al. Transfusion 1991;31:805

364. Lyon MF. Nature 1961;190:372

365. Lyon MF. Lancet 1961;2:434

366. Lyon MF. Am J Hum Genet 1962;14:135

367. Lyon MF. Biol Rev 1972;47:1

368. Gorman JG, di Re J, Treacy AM, et al.. J Lab Clin Med 1963;61:642

369. Fialkow PJ, Lisker R, Giblett ER, et al. Nature 1970;226:337

370. Lawler SD, Sanger R. Lancet 1970;1:584

371. Fialkow PJ. Am J Hum Genet 1970;22:460

372. Race RR. Proc 4th Int Cong Hum Genet, 1971:311

373. Marsh WL. Cytogenet Cell Genet 1978;22:531

374. Wolff G, Müller CR, Jokke A. Hum Genet 1980;54:269

375. Marsh WL. Unpublished observations cited in Wolff G, Muller CR, Jobke A. Hum Genet 1980;54:269

376. Ho M, Monaco AP, Blouden LAJ, et al. Am J Hum Genet 1992;50:317

377. Khamlichi S, Bailly P, Blanchard D, et al. Eur J Biochem 1995;228:931

378. Rawlins ND, Barrett AJ. Biochem J 1995;290:205

379. Shimada K, Takahashi M, Turner AJ, et al. Biochem J 1996;315:863

380. Russo DCW, Lee S, Reid M, et al. Blood 1994;84:3518

381. Lee S, Zambas E, Green ED, et al. Blood 1995;85:1364

382. Anstee DJ, Holmes CH, Judson PA, et al. In: Protein Blood Group Antigens of the Human Red Cell. Baltimore:John Hopkins Univ Press, 1992:170

383. Shivdasani RA, Orkin SH. Blood 1996;87:4025

384. Lee S, Wu X, Reid ME, et al. Blood 1995;85:912

385. Lee S, Wu X, Reid ME, et al. Transfusion 1995;35:822

386. Lee S, Wu X, Son D, et al. Transfusion 1996;36:490

387. Manning M, Warwick R, Vaughan J, et al. (abstract). Br J Haematol 1996;93 (Suppl 1):13

388. Murphy MT, Fraser RH, Goddard JP. Transf Med 1996;6:133

389. Avent ND, Martin PG. Br J Haematol 1996;93:728

390. Daniels GL, Weinauer F, Stone C, et al. Blood 1996;88:4045

391. Ho M, Chelly J, Carter N, et al. Cell 1994;77:869

392. Danek A, Uttner I, Vogl T, et al. Neurology 1994;44:117

393. Ho M, Chalmers RM, Davis MB, et al. Ann Neurol 1996;39:672

394. Groves J, Tanner MJA. J Biol Chem 1992;267:22163

395. Anstee DJ. Vox Sang 1990;58:1

396. Carbonnet F, Hattab C, Collec E, et al. (abstract). Transf Clin Biol 1996;3 (Suppl):54s

397. Smythe J, Gardner B, Anstee DJ. Blood 1994;83:1668

398. Xu D, Emoto N, Giaid A, et al. Cell 1994;78:473

399. Preece G, Murphy G, Ager A. J Biol Chem 1996;271:11634

400. Springer TA. Cell 1994;76:301

401. Simmons PJ, Zannettino A, Gronthos S, et al. Leukemia Lymphoma 1994;12:353

402. Hessner MJ, McFarland JG, Endean DJ. Transfusion 1996;36:495

19 | The Kidd Blood Group System

In 1951, Allen et al. (1) described the antibody that defines Jk^a. Two years later, Plaut et al. (2) reported the first example of anti-Jk^b that defines the antithetical partner to Jk^a. In 1959, Pinkerton et al. (3) described the phenotype Jk(a-b-). Their studies, plus others described below, suggested that the phenotype represents the inheritance of two silent *Jk* alleles at the *Jk^{a}Jk^b* locus. Individuals with this form of the Jk(a-b-) phenotype can make anti-Jk3, an antibody that behaves, at the serological level, as anti-Jk^{ab} in an inseparable form. In other words, *Jk^a* appears to encode production of Jk^a and Jk3 while *Jk^b* encodes production of Jk^b and Jk3. As described below, the amount of Jk3 made by *Jk^{a}Jk* and *Jk^{b}Jk* heterozygotes is not always as expected. In 1986, Okubo et al. (4) described their studies on a number of persons phenotypically Jk(a-b-), found in the Japanese population. While some of these individuals could be seen to be genetically *JkJk*, others had apparently inherited a dominant suppressor or modifier gene that effected the Jk(a-b-) phenotype. The gene was called (4) *In(Jk)* in analogy to *In(Lu)* (see Chapter 20). Persons genetically *JkJk* and those with *In(Jk)* could be differentiated by serological tests. In both situations the red cells type as Jk(a-b-). However, the red cells of *Jk* homozygotes do not adsorb, or yield on elution, anti-Jk^a or anti-Jk^b. The red cells of persons who have inherited *In(Jk)* may type as Jk(a-b-) but will adsorb and yield on elution, anti-Jk^a or anti-Jk^b, or both, dependent on which *Kidd* system genes have been inherited. No doubt when potent monoclonal anti-Jk^a and anti-Jk^b are developed, the Jk(a-b-) red cells of persons with *In(Jk)* will be seen to react weakly with some of them. As would be expected, since the red cells of *Jk* homozygotes are truly Jk(a-b-), such individuals can make anti-Jk3. Since the red cells of persons with *In(Jk)* carry small amounts of Jk^a and/or Jk^b, such individuals do not make anti-Jk3.

The Kidd system has remained relatively straightforward at both the serological and genetic levels. Table 19-1 lists the conventional and ISBT terms for the system. As described below, anti-Jk^a and anti-Jk^b can complicate transfusion therapy because antibody production at serologically demonstrable levels is often short-lived. Thus the antibodies are not infrequently associated with delayed transfusion reactions (see below). Until recently an additional problem was that anti-Jk^a and anti-Jk^b of sufficient potency reliably to type donor red cells, were difficult to obtain. That problem has been overcome by the production of monoclonal anti-Jk^a and anti-Jk^b (5,6).

TABLE 19-1 Conventional and ISBT Terminology for the Kidd Blood Group System

Conventional Name: Jk		
ISBT System Symbol: JK		
ISBT System Number: 009		

Antigen Conventional Name	ISBT Antigen Number	ISBT Full Code Number
Jk^a	JK1	009001
Jk^b	JK2	009002
Jk3	JK3	009003

The Antigens Jk^a and Jk^b

Table 19-2 shows antigen and phenotype frequencies in the Kidd system. The figures for Whites are derived from data published by Race and Sanger (7) and by Chown et al. (8,9). The listed frequency for Jk^a in American Blacks was derived from the figures of Rosenfield et al. (10) and of Sanger et al. (11), there do not seem to be any other published frequencies of Kidd antigens or phenotypes in Blacks.

Race and Sanger (7) noticed that in the series that they studied there was a slight shortage of the phenotype Jk(a+b-) and a slight excess of Jk(a+b+). It was considered possible that this might indicate heterogeneity of Jk^b. However, in the study of Chown et al. (9) the phenotype figures were exactly as expected from calculated gene frequencies. Along similar lines, Boyd (12) tested a large number of samples with several different examples of anti-Jk^b. Although a few samples (some of which were Jk(a+) and some Jk(a-)) gave weaker than standard reactions with one or more of the anti-Jk^b, no evidence of qualitative difference among Jk^b antigens was found. Each of the samples carrying a weaker than standard Jk^b antigen was shown capable of adsorbing each of the anti-Jk^b to exhaustion.

Toivanen and Hirvonen (13) showed that Jk^a and Jk^b develop early in fetal life. The Jk^a antigen was found on the red cells of a fetus of about 10 weeks gestation and Jk^b was found on the red cells of one of about six weeks. The antigens appeared to be as well developed as those on the red cells of adults, this condition persists until birth. As described the next section, both anti-Jk^a and anti-Jk^b have caused HDN.

TABLE 19-2 Antigen and Phenotype Frequencies in the Kidd System

Phenotype	% Frequency in Whites	% of Bloods Reactive with	
		Anti-Jk^a	Anti-Jk^b
Jk (a+b-)	27.5	76.9 in Whites	Circa 93% in American Blacks
Jk (a+b+)	49.4		
			72.5 in Whites
Jk (a-b+)	23.1		
Jk (a-b-)		<0.01 in most populations studied	

The Kidd system antigens survive treatment of red cells with proteases. Indeed, some examples of anti-Jk^a and anti-Jk^b are easier to detect and identify in tests using enzyme-treated, than in tests using untreated red cells. The antigens also survive treatment of red cells with neuraminidase and 2-aminoethylisothiouronium bromide (AET). Using IgG anti-Jk^a and ferritin-labeled anti-IgG, Masouredis et al. (46) estimated that Jk(a+b-) red cells carry in the order of 14,000 Jk^a sites per cell. As discussed in a later section of this chapter, it is now known that the Kidd antigens reside on the red cell urea transporter protein. Mannuzzu et al. (146) estimated that there are some 32,000 copies of that protein per red cell, clearly a number much higher than the estimate of Jk^a sites.

Anti-Jk^a and Anti-Jk^b

Of the two antibodies, anti-Jk^a is the more common and is seen both as a single specificity and in the sera of individuals who have formed other antibodies to red cell antigens. Anti-Jk^b is sometimes found as a single entity but is somewhat more frequently seen as one of a mixture of antibodies formed by one person, for references to many early examples of anti-Jk^a and anti-Jk^b, see the third edition of this book. Of 1469 antibodies studied by one of us (14), 403 were apparently red cell stimulated. Among those 403 antibodies, 41 were anti-Jk^a or anti-Jk^b. However, the figures may not be suitable for use in a calculation of the frequency of Kidd system antibodies since bias exists in the numbers. The totals include referred samples (i.e. 39% of the immune antibodies were Rh because of the author's known habit of collecting such oddities).

Anti-Jk^a and anti-Jk^b are almost always produced as a response to the introduction of foreign red cells via transfusion or pregnancy. A number of cases have been reported (15,16) in which it was believed that women made anti-Jk^a after having been exposed to Jk(a+) red cells, when the D+ fetuses that they were carrying were given intrauterine transfusions because of anticipated severe anti-D HDN.

However, it is also known (17) that the formation of anti-Jk^a by women with D- Jk(a-) red cells, who have already made anti-D, is not particularly uncommon. In at least one (16) of the cases mentioned, the infant was subsequently found to have Jk(a+) red cells.

Kidd system antibodies have caused immediate transfusion reactions (18-26,157), many delayed ones (for references see the next section in this chapter) and HDN (1,27-35). While occasional cases of severe HDN caused by Kidd system antibodies have been reported (29,35), many others have been so mild that no treatment was required, i.e. four of seven involving anti-Jk^a and one of two involving anti-Jk^b (35,36). Given the often severe immediate or delayed transfusion reactions caused by Kidd system antibodies, it is somewhat surprising that the degree of HDN caused by the antibodies is so often mild. As discussed below, it has previously been stated (41,50) that virtually all Kidd system antibodies activate complement. Although that statement has now been modified, again see below, it is accepted that many of the antibodies do activate complement. Perhaps the fact that at birth, infants have only about half the level of the complement components C1q, C4 and C3 and only one fifth the level of C9 of adults (37,38), serves to limit the degree of red cell destruction caused by Kidd system antibodies. Alternatively, it is possible that renal failure in adults attributed (60,64,69, see below) to transfusion reactions caused by Kidd system antibodies, involved localized damage of antibody-coated cells in the kidney (see later in this chapter for a description of the role of the Kidd antigen-bearing glycoprotein in urea transport). Lack of severity of Kidd system antibody-induced HDN might then represent the fact that while the fetus is in utero, urea excretion is handled by the mother. As already mentioned, most examples of antibodies in this system are of the red cell stimulated immune variety. However, IgM forms are occasionally encountered (39-41). In testing 15 examples of anti-Jk^a, Polley et al. (39) found that 12 were IgG, two IgM and one a mixture of IgG and IgM. Engelfriet (42) tested three examples of

IgG Kidd system antibodies and found that each of them was predominantly IgG3. Hardman et al. (43,44) tested 17 examples of such antibodies and found that 16 of them were mixtures of IgG3 and IgG1. This high incidence of IgG3 among Kidd system antibodies is presumably one of the reasons that the antibodies sometimes cause marked in vivo red cell destruction while yielding comparatively weak reactions in in vitro tests. This propensity for considerable in vivo activity also correlates with findings (41) that many Kidd system antibodies activate complement. Mollison et al. (41) have reported that although anti-Jk^a and anti-Jk^b only rarely present as in vitro hemolysins in standard tests against untreated red cells, in vitro hemolytic activity can sometimes be demonstrated in tests using enzyme-treated red cells or in ones in which animal serum is used as a source of complement. Haber and Rosenfield (45) reported that antigen dose may be of great influence in in vitro hemolysis by Kidd system antibodies. For example, an anti-Jk^a caused 100% lysis of ficin-treated Jk(a+b-) cells but only 25% lysis of similarly treated Jk(a+b+) cells. It would seem that the ability of anti-Jk^a and anti-Jk^b to activate complement may relate to the large number that contain an IgG3 fraction. Further, the fact that many anti-Jk^a and anti-Jk^b activate complement, while IgG3 Rh antibodies almost never do so, presumably relates to the position of Jk^a and Jk^b, compared to Rh antigens, at the red cell membrane surface (see Chapters 6 and 12). However, as mentioned earlier, the role of urea transport across red cell membranes has not been fully investigated in the in vivo hemolysis caused by Kidd system antibodies. As stated above, at one time it was believed (41,50) that virtually all Kidd system antibodies activated complement. More recently it has been accepted that this is not the case. Garratty (148) cites otherwise unpublished observations (149) that among 55 examples of anti-Jk^a tested, 25 (45%) were shown to cause C3 to become red cell bound. In an abstract Yates et al. (147) claimed that complement is activated by IgM but not by IgG Kidd system antibodies. Clearly, in view of previous reports (39-44,50) this latest claim will require careful investigation.

There is no doubt that anti-Jk^a and anti-Jk^b must be regarded as having potential clinical significance when found in the sera of patients requiring red cell transfusions. As discussed in detail below, compatibility tests with the patients' sera are not always adequate for the selection of units for transfusion. Also discussed below are some other difficulties encountered in working with these antibodies and their frequent role in causing delayed transfusion reactions.

Table 19-3 summarizes the characteristics of antibodies of the system. For the sake of completeness, anti-Jk3 is included in that table although it is not fully described until a later section of this chapter.

Difficulties in Working With Anti-Jk^a and Anti-Jk^b and the Role of Those Antibodies in Causing Delayed Hemolytic Transfusion Reactions

The in vitro detection and characterization of these two antibodies can be among the more difficult tasks that confront blood bankers. There are a number of reasons for the difficulties and many of them also contribute to the fairly regular role of the antibodies in causing delayed hemolytic transfusion reactions.

First, examples of anti-Jk^a and anti-Jk^b giving potent reactions in vitro are the exception rather than the rule. It is not uncommon to find a serum that reacts (often weakly) with some but not all Jk(a+b-) or Jk(a-b+) red cells, but with none that are Jk(a+b+). Sometimes, tests against protease-modified red cells or tests in LISS or polybrene enhance the positive reactions to the point that anti-Jk^a or anti-Jk^b can be identified. Fisher (47) described two examples of anti-Jk^b that could be identified by the polybrene but no other method. As described below, some examples of anti-Jk^a detected in similar situations have been seen to be clinically benign. Sometimes antibody identification has to be based on the reactivity of the serum with red cells carrying double doses of Jk^a or Jk^b (that is Jk(a+b-) and Jk(a-b+) respectively). On other

TABLE 19-3 Characteristics of Kidd System Antibodies

Antibody Specificity	Positive Reactions in In Vitro Tests				Usual Immuno-globulin		Ability to Bind Complement		Ability to Cause In Vitro Lysis		Implicated in		Usual Form of Stimulation		% of White Population Positive
	Sal	LISS	AHG	Enz	IgG	IgM	Yes	No	Yes	No	Trans-fusion Reaction	HDN	Red Cells	Other	
Anti-Jk^a			X	X	Most	Few	Many		Rare		Yes	Yes	All	No	77
Anti-Jk^b			X	X	Most	Few	Many		Rare		Yes	Yes	All	No	73
Anti-Jk3			X	X							Yes	Yes	Most	Rare	100

occasions no enhancement is seen and the question as to whether anti-Jk^a or anti-Jk^b is present cannot be satisfactorily resolved. Because both antibodies are capable of causing considerable in vivo destruction of antigen-positive red cells (18-26 and see below for references to delayed transfusion reactions) and because there is no quick, easy and reliable in vitro method to differentiate clinically-significant from clinically-insignificant forms, the safest decision would seem to be to transfuse only antigen-negative units when the presence of anti-Jk^a or anti-Jk^b is suspected. Until recently, this in itself created a catch 22 situation. Since potent anti-Jk^a and anti-Jk^b were difficult to obtain, it was not always easy to type donor units for patients thought possibly to have anti-Jk^a or anti-Jk^b in the serum. Unlike the situation with anti-Le^a and anti-Le^b where compatibility tests at 37°C reliably identify suitable units for transfusion, the anamnestic response so often associated with antibodies to Jk^a and Jk^b makes such a practice unsafe where those antibodies are concerned. As mentioned earlier, this problem has been largely overcome by the development of monoclonal anti-Jk^a and anti-Jk^b (5,6). However, such reagents are not inexpensive and cost containment considerations dictate that donor units not be typed for Jk^a and Jk^b unless there is good evidence that antigen-negative units are necessary for transfusion. One maneuver that is of help, when it is thought that anti-Jk^a or anti-Jk^b might be present, it to type the patient's red cells. Since some 77% of random individuals have red cells are Jk(a+) and some 73% cells that are Jk(b+), there is a three in four chance that misidentification of what is thought to be alloimmune anti-Jk^a or anti-Jk^b can be caught.

Second, even when the presence of anti-Jk^a or anti-Jk^b has been established beyond reasonable doubt and when the patient's cells have been shown to lack the antigen against which the alloantibody has been made, the patient's serum may not be reliable for use in the selection of units for transfusion. As mentioned above, some examples of anti-Jk^a and anti-Jk^b will react in vitro only with red cells carrying a double dose of the antigen involved. Thus Jk(a+b+) red cells may appear compatible in in vitro tests. However, transfusion of such units may well result in a, sometimes severe, transfusion reaction. Accordingly, when anti-Jk^a or anti-Jk^b is known to be present, compatibility tests should be performed using donor samples already typed for Jk^a or Jk^b, or units that have not already been typed but appear compatible with the patient's serum, should be typed with reagent grade antisera before being issued for transfusion. While the second of these methods may be more time consuming it is cheaper since the patient's serum, that is free, is used in an initial screening test thus reducing the number of units that need to be typed with purchased reagents.

Third, the difficulties in identifying these two antibodies are often compounded by the fact that either of them may be present in a serum that contains many other antibodies. If, for example, it is thought that anti-Jk^b may be present in a serum that also contains antibodies directed against c, E, K, s and Fy^b, it will not be easy to find sufficient c- E- K- s- Fy(b-) samples that have been typed for Jk^b, to confirm the presence of the antibody.

Fourth, anti-Jk^a and anti-Jk^b do not store particularly well. Careful hoarding of samples of antibodies, that reacted strongly when first identified, is sometimes a frustrating experience since antibody activity may have deteriorated before the precious sera are recovered from the freezer. Since both antibodies often activate complement, activity can sometimes be restored by adding fresh serum as a source of complement, to the stored samples of anti-Jk^a or anti-Jk^b. The addition of fresh serum is often more effective than use of the EDTA two-stage method (48) since the reactions of Kidd system antibodies are not particularly enhanced by that method.

Fifth and of great importance in the mechanism of delayed hemolytic transfusion reactions, continued in vivo production of potent anti-Jk^a or anti-Jk^b seems to be the exception rather than the rule. It is not uncommon to find that a patient who made one of the antibodies (following transfusion or pregnancy) has no serologically demonstrable antibody present in the serum a few weeks or months after the antibody was originally identified. Clearly, accurate blood bank records are essential to ensure that such patients receive appropriate antigen-negative units if the need for additional transfusion arises. This, in itself, creates another difficult situation. When a patient arrives at a hospital with a card that indicates that anti-Jk^a or anti-Jk^b was previously made, but has no antibody activity in the serum, the blood banker faces a dilemma. If the previous antibody identification was correct, the patient must now be transfused with Jk(a-) or Jk(b-) blood as appropriate. If the previous identification was incorrect (not a rare event, see points one and three above) the blood bank may use its precious (and/or expensive) supply of anti-Jk^a or anti-Jk^b unnecessarily. Again, typing the patient's red cells for Jk^a or Jk^a is worthwhile since the chance of catching a previous antibody misidentification is three in four. Exceptions to the situation in which Kidd system antibodies are synthesized for only a short period of time will, of course, be seen. One of us (49) has seen a case in which anti-Jk^a with a titer of 64 was still being made by a woman 16 years after her last exposure to Jk(a+) red cells.

Sixth, if saline systems (with or without the addition of albumin) are used, too little IgG anti Jk^a or anti-Jk^b may become red cell bound for subsequent detection by anti-IgG in IATs (33,34,50,51). One solution to this problem is to read the tests with a broad spectrum antiglobulin reagent that contains anti-C3. IgG Kidd system antibodies will sometimes cause enough C3 to become red cell bound that the positive reaction is seen with or amplified by the C3-anti-C3 reaction. While antibodies in the system detectable only by the C3-anti-C3 portion of the test were always rare, it was shown (51) that the IAT reaction was often stronger and thus more easily seen, if both cell-bound IgG and C3, rather than IgG alone, were detected. Current wisdom states that methods such as those that use LISS, PEG, Polybrene or similar, enable detection of clinically significant Kidd system antibodies via the detection of cell bound IgG in IATs performed in conjunction with use of those potentiators. While there is no doubt that such tests read with anti-IgG detect some of these difficult to detect Kidd system antibodies, there is little in the way of formal proof that all such examples are found. Continued use of these anti-IgG-based IATs for antibody screening and compatibility tests is predicated on the common experience that the incidence of immediate and delayed transfusion reactions caused by Kidd system antibodies has apparently not increased since the use of antiglobulin reagents containing anti-C3 was abandoned.

Based on what is written above it should come as no surprise that anti-Jk^a and anti-Jk^b are often incriminated as causative of delayed hemolytic transfusion reactions. What happens is that the patient forms anti-Jk^a or anti-Jk^b as a result of exposure to foreign red cells via transfusion or pregnancy. Antibody production then declines to a point at which serologically demonstrable antibody is no longer present in the patient's serum. Thus, antibody screening and compatibility tests yield negative results and apparently compatible red cells are transfused. Because the primary immune response has already occurred, the introduction of Jk(a+) or Jk(b+) red cells then causes a secondary response and additional antibody is rapidly made (usually within 24 to 48 hours of the transfusion). Once anti-Jk^a or anti-Jk^b production reaches a sufficient level (probably not very high if the antibody is IgG3, see section on macrophage recognition of IgG-coated red cells in Chapter 6) the transfused antigen-positive red cells are cleared and a delayed transfusion reaction is existant. Exactly this circumstance has been reported many times (41,52-69,158,159) in the literature. The high frequency with which anti-Jk^a and anti-Jk^b are involved in this situation is also clear from reviews of the subject. Mollison (70) found that 30% of the cases that he included in his review were caused by those antibodies. Croucher (67) reviewed cases in which a total of 109 antibodies were involved. Thirty-one (28%) of them had a specificity within the Kidd system. Pineda et al. (64) reported that over one-third of the delayed reactions they studied were caused by anti Jk^a. To these reports, one of us (PDI) would add his own

observations that if delayed transfusion reactions with clinical sequelae, as opposed to delayed serological reactions (69), are considered, the percentage caused by Kidd system antibodies is even higher, probably in the order of 50 to 60%.

There is relatively little that the blood banker can do to prevent genuine delayed hemolytic transfusion reactions; that is those in which the antibody is truly below serologically detectable levels in carefully performed sensitive tests, at the time of transfusion. As mentioned above, properly kept blood bank records and the issue of antibody cards to immunized patients help but the latter system is not without some disadvantages. The fact that some delayed transfusion reactions cannot be avoided must not be used as an excuse for not trying to prevent them. As already described, when there are indications that anti-Jk^a or anti-Jk^b might be present, additional tests using the most sensitive techniques available for demonstration of those antibodies must be undertaken. When there is real doubt and when the patient's red cells lack the antigen to which the antibody may be directed, the patient must be given the benefit of that doubt and must be transfused with antigen-negative blood. One of us (DJA) believes that Kidd system antigen-antibody incompatibility might better be demonstrated by incubating the patient's serum with red cells from the prospective donors and then testing those red cells for resistance to lysis by 2M urea. The other of us (PDI) is skeptical that the weak anti-Jk^a and anti-Jk^b, not detectable by current sensitive serological tests, would significantly alter the resistance of the red cells to 2M urea by blocking Jk^a and Jk^b antigen sites. Thus the authors do not agree as to the practicality of such a test in a routine situation. Readers are encouraged to perform the appropriate investigations and let us know which one of us is correct.

Kidd System Monoclonal Antibodies

As mentioned earlier, monoclonal antibodies to Jk^a and Jk^b have been produced. Lecointre-Coatmelec et al. (5) produced an anti-Jk^b, Thompson et al. (6) produced three anti-Jk^b and one anti-Jk^a. All the antibodies were made by EBV-transformation of lymphocytes from immunized individuals. All were IgM in nature and the most avid ones reacted by immediate spin methods against saline suspended red cells, including those of the Jk(a+b+) phenotype. Having spent so much of his professional career hoarding half-way decent anti-Jk^a and anti-Jk^b from immunized patients, one of us (PDI) may never get used to the idea that typing for Jk^a and Jk^b is now as easy (albeit more expensive) as typing for A and B; so much for the good old days!

The Phenotype Jk(a-b-) and the Recessive Allele, *Jk*

In 1959, Pinkerton et al. (3) reported that an individual of Filipino-Spanish-Chinese extraction, had red cells that typed as Jk(a-b-) and that failed to adsorb either anti-Jk[a] or anti-Jk[b]. Shortly thereafter, Pinkerton (71) found the phenotype in two other persons who, like the original propositus, lived in Hawaii. One was of Chinese-Hawaiian and the other of Spanish-Filipino extraction. Hawaii has since proved a rich source of Jk(a-b-) blood and Dr. Julia Frohlich and Ms. Ann Stegmaier of the Blood Bank of Hawaii have generously supplied samples of such blood to many reference laboratories around the world. In 1960, Silver et al. (72) found that five Indians of Mato Grosso, Brazil, among 88 tested, had Jk(a-b-) red cells. Since, at that time, all the evidence suggested that the Jk(a-b-) phenotype represented the *JkJk* genotype, with *Jk* being a silent allele of *Jk[a]* and *Jk[b]*, it seemed that *Jk* must have a high incidence in the Indians of Mato Grosso. However, as described in a later section, it is now known that a dominant suppressor gene, *In(Jk)*, also causes an (ostensible) Jk(a-b-) phenotype. Since both *Jk* and *In(Jk)* seem to have their highest incidence in Oriental peoples, it is no longer clear which of the early examples of the Jk(a-b-) phenotype, in non-immunized individuals, represented the *JkJk* genotype and which, the inheritance of *In(Jk)*. Figure 19-1 demonstrates the inheritance pattern of the Jk(a-b-) phenotype when the silent *Jk* gene is involved. In 1967, we (73) found the phenotype in a New Zealand Maori woman whose blood had been sent to us by Dr. Jock Staveley of Auckland. Subsequent to that observation, Woodfield et al. (74) ran large scale tests on the blood of New Zealand Polynesians and reported 66 examples of the Jk(a-b-) phenotype from tests on 7425 blood samples. The incidence of Jk(a-b-) blood was apparently 0.889%. More recently, Henry and Woodfield (75) have examined the records of some 17,300 random Polynesian blood donors and have found that the incidence of the Jk(a-b-) phenotype is 0.27%. It is now appreciated that the original series included samples from family members of the Jk(a-b-) propositi. Table 19-4 is taken from the report of Henry and Woodfield (75) and shows the frequency of Jk(a-b-) among Polynesians of different ethnic groups. It should be added that in the original report (75) the ethnic groups were listed as percentages of Polynesian donors. In table 19-4 the reported percentage is expressed as an approximate number of the 17,300 random donors included. It was felt (75) that increasing frequencies of the Jk(a-b-) phenotype in the various groups correlated directly with decreasing amounts of genetic admixture from European Whites and others.

In 1975, Sussman et al. (76) described what they

FIGURE 19-1 To Illustrate the Recessive Form of Jk(a-b-)

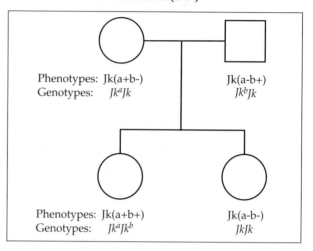

Phenotypes: Jk(a+b-)	Jk(a-b+)
Genotypes: *Jk[a]Jk*	*Jk[b]Jk*

Phenotypes: Jk(a+b+)	Jk(a-b-)
Genotypes: *Jk[a]Jk[b]*	*JkJk*

TABLE 19-4 To Show the Incidence of the Jk(a-b-) Phenotype in Some Polynesian Ethnic Groups (from reference 75)

Ethnic Group	Approximate Number Tested	Number Jk(a-b-)	Percent Jk(a-b-)
New Zealand Maoris	10,380	7	0.07
Samoans	4,325	14	0.32
Cook Islanders	865	4	0.46
Tongans	1,038	12	1.16
Niueans	692	10	1.45

See text for recalculation of some figures.

believed to be the first example of the Jk(a-b-) phenotype in a White person. However, later we (77) had the opportunity to test the red cells of the proposita described and found them to be Jk(a-b+) with a normal (double dose) level of Jk[b]. Further, although the proposita's serum was said (76) to contain anti-Jk3 (see below) we (77) found that it contained only anti-Jk[a]. At the time of the later tests the patient was transfused with Jk(a-b+) blood with no evidence of red cell destruction. We believe that in 1975 a mixture of anti-Jk[a] and anti-I in the patient's serum was mistaken for anti-Jk3. However, the Jk(a-b-) phenotype does exist in Whites; it has been found in such persons in France (78), Finland (79) and Australia (80). As mentioned above, discovery of the *In(Jk)* gene introduced the possibility that some persons thought to be genetically *JkJk* might actually have had *In(Jk)*. That possibility seems to have been excluded in the cases cited above. In one (79) a family study provided evidence for the presence of *Jk*, in all three (78-80) production of anti-Jk3 by a Jk(a-b-) person apparently excluded the *In(Jk)* genotype. Similarly, in cases reported from other parts of the world, production of anti-Jk3 often led to the recognition of the Jk(a-b-) phenotype. Bearing in mind that *In(Jk)* can sometimes be responsible, the Jk(a-b-) phenotype has been reported in: Polynesians (3,71,73,74,81-83); South East Asians (84-87); Japanese (4); Chinese (55); Asian Indians (85,88); South American Indians (72,85); an American Black (89); and the Whites described above (78-80). In the White family in which the *In(Lu)* gene (see Chapter 20) was first recognized, inheritance patterns showed that *Jk* was probably also present (90). Other cases in which presence of *Jk* may have explained unusual inheritance of Kidd system antigens have been seen (7,94,95). As an example, Behzad et al. (95) described a Black woman with Jk(a+b+) red cells whose child's cells were Jk(a-b+). The mother's red cells appeared to carry a single dose of Jk^a, dosage of Jk^b on the child's red cells was not reported. Tests for other genetic markers and subsequent calculations seemed to exclude non-maternity so that the most likely explanation was a *Jk^{a}Jk* mother with a *Jk^{b}Jk* child.

Anti-Jk3

In the first case in which the Jk(a-b-) phenotype was found (3), the propositus had made a Kidd system antibody that reacted equally with Jk(a+b-), Jk(a+b+) and Jk(a-b+) red cells but which failed to react with those that were Jk(a-b-). The antibody was not a mixture of separable anti-Jk^a and anti-Jk^b so was initially called anti-Jk^{ab} in an inseparable form. It is now more commonly known as anti-Jk3. As described earlier, it seems that *Jk^a* and *Jk^b* encode production of Jk^a and Jk3; and Jk^b and Jk3, respectively. The only red cells that are phenotypically Jk:-3 are those that are Jk(a-b-). Several other examples of anti-Jk3 have been reported. The antibody is most often produced as a result of immunization by transfusion or pregnancy. It is usually IgG in nature and, like anti-Jk^a and anti Jk^b, reacts well with protease-treated red cells. Some examples of anti-Jk3 have been present in sera that contained separable anti-Jk^a or anti-Jk^b. Anti-Jk3 has caused immediate (92) and delayed (55,74) transfusion reactions and HDN (74,82,86,88). The cases of HDN have all been mild; Woodfield et al. (74) reported that successive children born to immunized Jk(a-b-) mothers were affected to about the same degree.

The anti-Jk3 described by Arcara et al. (84,91) was unusual in that it was made by a Jk(a-b-) male who had never been transfused. Further, his Jk(a-b-) sister had made no antibody although she had borne seven children with Jk(a+), Jk:3 red cells. As discussed below, the

Jk(a-b-) phenotypes in the family involved may not have been as straightforward as in some others.

Humphrey and Morel (93) performed titration studies on the red cells of obligate *Jk* heterozygotes, using antibodies directed against Jk^a, Jk^b and Jk3. They were able to show that the red cells of *Jk^{a}Jk* and *Jk^{b}Jk* people carried single doses of Jk^a and Jk^b respectively, but that the cells behaved similarly to those expected to carry a double dose of antigen, when tested with anti-Jk3. One Oriental individual had Jk(a+b-) red cells that apparently carried a single dose of Jk^a and a reduced amount of Jk3. However, no family study was possible so that the significance of the finding is not known.

The Phenotype Jk(a-b-) and the Dominant Gene, *In(Jk)*

In 1986, Okubo et al. (4) found 14 Jk(a-b-) persons in tests on samples from 638,460 blood donors in Osaka, Japan. In two of the cases the serological and inheritance patterns were seen to be different from those expected when the Jk(a-b-) phenotype represents the *JkJk* genotype. First, although the red cells typed as Jk(a-b-) they would adsorb and yield on elution anti-Jk^a and/or anti-Jk^b, dependent on which *Kidd* system genes had been inherited (as revealed by family studies). Second, some of the samples that typed as Jk(a-b-) reacted, albeit weakly, with anti-Jk3. Third, family studies showed that the Jk(a-b-) phenotype represented inheritance of a single gene that was dominant in effect. The gene was named (4) *In(Jk)* in analogy to *In(Lu)* that acts as a dominant suppressor of (among other things) expression of Lutheran system antigens (see Chapter 20). A family study performed showed that *In(Jk)* does not reside at the *Kidd* (*Jk^{a}Jk^{b}Jk*) locus. Although other examples of *In(Jk)* were found in Japan (96), Okubo et al. (4) calculated that among the 35 Jk(a-b-) people known in Japan at that time, the *JkJk* genotype was six times more common than the *In(Jk)* gene. A fourth difference between the Jk(a-b-) status representing *JkJk* and that representing presence of *In(Jk)* is that persons of the former type can form anti-Jk3, while those of the *In(Jk)* type cannot. This, of course, is exactly as expected from the Jk:-3 status of the red cells of *Jk* homozygotes, and the presence of small amounts of that antigen on the red cells of persons with *In(Jk)*. Figure 19-2 demonstrates the inheritance pattern of the Jk(a-b-) phenotype when *In(Jk)* is responsible.

An Unusual Family with Jk(a-b-) Members

As mentioned above, family studies undertaken in

FIGURE 19-2 To Illustrate the Dominant Form of
Jk(a-b-)

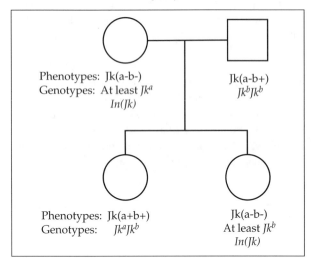

Phenotypes: Jk(a-b-)
Genotypes: At least *Jk^a*
In(Jk)

Jk(a-b+)
Jk^bJk^b

Phenotypes: Jk(a+b+)
Genotypes: *Jk^aJk^b*

Jk(a-b-)
At least *Jk^b*
In(Jk)

many of the cases described, provided evidence that the Jk(a-b-) phenotype represented the *JkJk* genotype. In 1969, we (84,91) studied a family of Filipino-Chinese-Spanish extraction in which three sibs were phenotypically Jk(a-b-) but in which the *JkJk* genotype did not provide a satisfactory explanation. At the time of the study, the existence of *In(Jk)* was not known. Although not documented in the abstract (84) a number of unusual findings were made (91) in the family. The propositus was a male with Jk(a-b-) red cells who had predominantly IgM, anti-Jk3 in his serum although he had never been transfused. Two of his sisters were also phenotypically Jk(a-b-). One of these women had borne seven children, all of whom were phenotypically Jk(a+b+). The father of the children was phenotypically Jk(a+b+). The Jk(a+b+) red cells of five of the children reacted as if they carried a double dose of Jk^a, the red cells of the other two reacted as if they carried a single dose of that antigen. Thus the mating did not appear to be *JkJk* X *Jk^aJk^b* producing *Jk^aJk* children. Now that the existence of *In(Jk)* has been recognized it becomes possible to provide a speculative explanation of inheritance in the family. If the mother of the seven children was genetically *Jk^aJk* and carried *In(Jk)*, she could have passed *Jk^a* to the five children whose red cells carried a double dose of Jk^a , and *Jk* to the two whose red cells carried a single dose of that antigen (see figure 19-3). If this is the correct explanation it must be accepted that the *Jk^aJk^b* father of the children passed *Jk^a* to all seven (a 1 in 128 chance); that the mother passed *Jk^a* five times and *Jk* twice (a 1 in 8 chance); and that she failed to pass *In(Jk)* to any of her children (another 1 in 128 chance). Unusual as such a postulate may be, there is some possibly supportive evidence. First, although the Jk(a-b-) mother had borne seven

Jk(a+b-) children, she had not made anti-Jk^a or anti-Jk3. A *Jk^aJk, In(Jk)* genotype would explain such a finding better than would a *JkJk* genotype. Second, the other Jk(a-b-) woman in the family had been pregnant (children not available for testing) but had not formed anti-Jk3 either. Against this evidence was the finding that the Jk(a-b-) propositus had made anti-Jk3 so that, using the same reasoning, he would have to be supposed to be genetically *JkJk*. This would mean that both of his (and his sisters') parents (who were deceased) must have carried *Jk* with one of them having *In(Jk)* as well (again, see figure 19-3). Another saving grace for this speculative explanation is that the family was of Filipino-Chinese-Spanish extraction, in the first two of those population groups, both *Jk* and *In(Jk)* have a higher incidence than in other populations. It should be added that this author (PDI) developed the courage to advance this explanation in part by reading the account of Daniels et al. (140) of a *Kp^a* homozygote who also had a mutant allele at the *Xk* locus that effected the McLeod phenotype. In other words, the inheritance of rare genes at genetically independent loci, that then exert an effect on each other at the phenotypic level, does sometimes occur in a single individual. Since the postulated explanation for the Kidd phenotypes in this family (89,91) involves the passage of *Jk^a* from a *Jk^aJk^b* heterozygote seven times out of seven, the non-passage of *In(Jk)* also seven times out of seven, the presence of *Jk* and *In(Jk)* in at least one and perhaps two women and in one of their parents and the presence of *Jk* in the other parent, skeptics will be excused!

A Transient Form of the Jk(a-b-) Phenotype

To return to reality, in 1990 we (92) described a patient with myelofibrosis and bleeding secondary to carcinoma of the colon, whose red cell Kidd system phenotype changed during a two year period, at least once, and probably twice, from Jk(a+b-) to Jk(a-b-). During the time that her red cells typed as Jk(a-b-) the patient made anti-Jk3 and later both anti-Jk3 and anti-Jk^b. The anti-Jk3 caused a transfusion reaction when the patient was given two units of Jk(a+b-) blood at a hospital where the anti-Jk3 had not been detected. During the time that the patient was making anti-Jk3, she was transfused uneventfully with a total of 39 units of Jk(a-b-) blood. When her red cell phenotype reverted to Jk(a+b-), production of both the anti-Jk3 and the anti-Jk^b stopped and the patient was uneventfully transfused with 11 units of Jk(a+b-) blood.

The first series of samples that typed as Jk(a-b-) were collected before the patient had received any Jk(a-b-) blood so that loss of her own Jk^a antigen, that was present in later samples, was conclusively shown.

FIGURE 19-3 Observed Phenotypes and Speculative Genotypes in a Family with Jk(a-b-) Members. From References 84 and 91 and the Fertile Mind of One of the Authors (PDI)

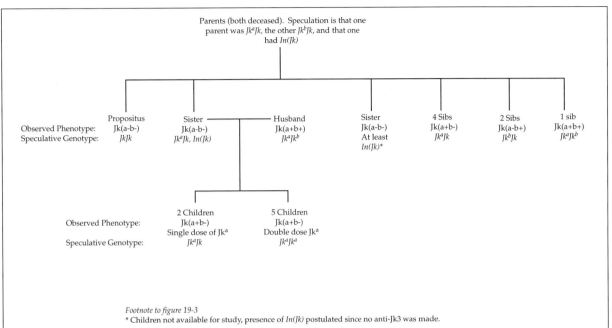

Footnote to figure 19-3
* Children not available for study, presence of *In(Jk)* postulated since no anti-Jk3 was made.

After one full four month reversion to the Jk(a+b-) phenotype, the patient's red cells again typed as Jk(a-b-). However, because of the patient's myelofibrosis and hemorrhages it was not entirely clear whether the second episode of the Jk(a-b-) phenotype, that lasted over a year, always represented loss of the patient's antigen, or presence of the Jk(a-b-) blood that was used for transfusion. Hemoglobin values during the year that her red cells typed as Jk(a-b-) in the second episode, strongly suggested that she was making blood, thus supporting the conclusion that a second loss of Jk^a antigen production had occurred.

The Jk(a-b-) Phenotype and Red Cell Resistance to Lysis by Solutions of Urea

In 1982, Heaton and McLoughlin (83) noticed that a few blood samples appeared to have extraordinarily high platelet counts when such counts were performed in automated machines, although blood films from the same patients did not show increases in platelets. The method being used involved the lysis of red cells by 2M urea, so that platelets could be counted in the cell counters. These workers then showed that unlike Jk(a+b-), Jk(a+b+) and Jk(a-b+) red cells, those that are Jk(a-b-) have a degree of resistance to urea-induced lysis. The resistant red cells were being counted as platelets in the machine! The Jk(a-b-) red cells in question were from *Jk* homozygotes. Later when the *In(Jk)* form of Jk(a-b-) red cells were found

they were shown (4) to have increased resistance to urea-induced lysis but not to the same degree as those from *Jk* homozygotes. Somewhat similarly, red cells from *Jk^{a}Jk* and *Jk^{b}Jk* heterozygotes have a lysis time intermediate between red cells from *Jk^a* or *Jk^b* homozygotes (or *Jk^{a}Jk^b* heterozygotes) and those of *Jk* homozygotes (97). It should be stressed that the resistance to urea-induced lysis is not complete. In the method used, Jk(a+) and Jk(b+) red cells are totally lysed within 1 or 2 minutes, i.e. minor variation between samples. When Jk(a-b-) red cells from *Jk* homozygotes are treated, lysis does not begin for some 15 to 30 minutes and is not complete for 45 minutes or longer, i.e. considerable variation between samples (83).

The resistance of Jk(a-b-) red cells to lysis by 2M urea has been studied by several groups of investigators (97-104). Clearly, the simplest explanation of the phenomenon was to assume that Jk(a-b-) red cells have a defect in urea transport across the membrane. However, the finding (97) that 2M urea prepared in phosphate-buffered saline and citrate buffer did not cause lysis of Jk(a+) or Jk(b+) red cells raised the possibility that water movement rather than urea transport might explain the resistance factor. In other words, in the presence of a small amount of urea it seemed possible that water movement across the membranes of Jk(a-b-) red cells might be restricted (97,99). However, other workers (100) found that if red cells were first exposed to urea and then to an excess of phosphate-buffered saline, Jk(a+) and Jk(b+) red cells were not lysed while Jk(a-b-) red cells were. This was taken to indicate that urea transport in Jk(a-b-)

red cells is slower than in other red cells and the reequilibration following exposure to excess saline was not sufficiently rapid to prevent lysis. In other words, the resistance factor in Jk(a-b-) red cells did indeed involve impairment of urea transport. The question now seems to have been resolved. Additional evidence has accumulated (101-103) that indicates that in Jk(a+) and Jk(b+) red cells, urea is actively transported across the membrane. In Jk(a-b-) red cells, urea traverses the membrane only by simple diffusion, the rate of such diffusion is some 1000 times slower than the rate of active transfer. Further, Olivès et al. (105) have shown that the Kidd blood group antigens and the urea transport function of red cells involve the same membrane protein and that the gene encoding that protein and the Kidd system antigens is the same thing.

Well before the resistance of Jk(a-b-) red cells to urea-induced lysis was understood at the biochemical or molecular level, blood group serologists took advantage of the observation and several large studies (4,74,88,100) conducted to find Jk(a-b-) individuals used urea lysis as a screening test, with serological confirmation on the red cells of resistant samples.

As would be expected, additional details about the structure of the Kidd glycoprotein, that is the urea transporter protein, and the difference between Jk^a and Jk^b on that protein, are given in the later sections of this chapter on the biochemistry, molecular biology and genetics of the system.

The *Kidd* Locus is on Chromosome 18

It proved somewhat more difficult to assign the *Kidd* blood group locus to a specific autosome than was the case with some other blood group loci. In 1973, tentative evidence (106) suggested that the *Kidd* locus might be on chromosome 7. In 1975, evidence was presented (107) that the *Co* (*Colton*, see Chapter 21) locus might be on chromosome 7. Since it was thought (108,109) that *Jk* and *Co* might be syntenic (i.e. on the same chromosome but not within measurable distance as determined by conventional family studies) this seemed to strengthen the tentative assignment of *Jk* to chromosome 7. However, evidence against such an assignment was found (110,111) and chromosome 7 was excluded as a home for *Jk*. Next, evidence emerged (112) that *Jk* might be on chromosome 2, but that site was also later (113) excluded. In 1987, it was shown (114,115) that *Jk* is linked to two RFLPs assigned to chromosome 18. After *Jk* had been assigned to chromosome 18 and Olivès et al. (116) had cloned *HUT11*, the gene that encodes production of the urea transporter protein, the same group of investigators showed (105) that *HUT11* and *Jk* are the

same thing and used in situ hybridization to localize the locus to 18q12-q21. Berg (141) has reported finding higher total serum cholesterol levels in persons homozygous for *Jk^a* than in persons homozygous for *Jk^b* or those heterozygous for *Jk^a* and *Jk^b*.

The Kidd System, Autoantibodies, Drugs and Bacteria

Although autoantibodies, including those with Kidd system specificities, that cause "warm" antibody-induced hemolytic anemia (WAIHA) are discussed in detail in Chapter 37 (and benign forms in Chapter 39), there are a number of observations that relate to serology of the Kidd system so require mention here.

Auto-anti-Jk^a has been incriminated as causative of WAIHA on a number of occasions (117-122) including one in which the patient had Evan's syndrome (see Chapter 37), and had in vivo red cell destruction but a negative DAT (122). We (125) were somewhat surprised to find that when we adsorbed 35 examples of anti-dl with Jk(a-b-) red cells, none of them could be shown to contain an anti-Jk3 component. Based on the findings that both pathological auto-anti-Jk^a (117-122) and auto-anti-Jk^b (126,127) can be made and given the general nature of autoantibodies causative of WAIHA (see Chapter 37), we fully expected that auto-anti-Jk3 would exist. In 1983, Ellisor et al. (128) described a previously untransfused, 25 year-old White primipara who was found to have a positive DAT when prenatal blood testing was performed. A heat eluate made from her red cells appeared to contain anti-Jk^b, an ether eluate appeared to contain anti-Jk3. The patient's red cells were Jk(a-b+), Jk:3. Although the antibodies were clearly autoimmune in nature, specificity was not as it at first appeared. The eluted antibody could be adsorbed to exhaustion with Jk(a-b-) red cells, it could not be split into separable antibodies resembling anti-Jk^b and anti-Jk3. Clearly in this case, the autoantibody mimicked both anti-Jk^b and anti-Jk3 but did not truly have either of those specificities. Such findings are not uncommon in patients with WAIHA (134). The patient in this case (128) clearly had hemolytic anemia that was exacerbated by her pregnancy. Some five months after delivery of the infant the patient was seen to have a reasonably well compensated form of WAIHA. In 1987, O'Day (129) (who was one of the co-author's of the Ellisor et al. (128) report) described what was said to be the second example of auto-anti-Jk3. The antibody was found in a 31 year-old White, para 1, gravida 2 woman. The patient's red cells were Jk(a+b-), Jk:3 and her serum contained anti-Jk^b. The DAT was positive and an eluate contained an antibody that reacted with all except Jk(a-b-) red cells. A single adsorption with Jk(a+b-) or Jk(a-b+) red cells removed all the apparent anti-Jk3 from the eluate, a single adsorption with Jk(a-b-) red cells did not remove antibody. Since multiple adsorptions with antigen-negative red cells may be necessary to adsorb autoantibodies with mimicking specificities (134), it is not clear whether this case represented a second example of an autoantibody mimicking anti-Jk3, the case described by Ellisor et al. (128) being the first, or the first example of auto-anti-Jk3. Although, as mentioned above, anti-Jk3 has caused mild HDN (74,82,86,88), in the two cases just described (128,129) the infants required no treatment. In the case described by O'Day (129) the maternal alloimmune anti-Jk^b was eluted from the cord blood red cells of her infant.

Auto-anti-Jk^a has also been incriminated as causative of in vivo red cell destruction in one patient being treated with alpha methyldopa (aldomet) (123) and in another being treated with chlorpropamide (124). In the patient receiving aldomet an acute hemolytic episode was curtailed by withdrawal of the drug, eventually production of auto-anti-Jk^a stopped. The patient receiving chlorpropamide also had acute hemolysis. When first studied her antibody reacted more strongly with Jk(a+) red cells in the presence of the drug but also reacted with such cells in its absence. After chlorpropamide treatment was withdrawn the antibody declined in strength and at one point would react with Jk(a+b+) red cells only in the presence of drug. Three other sulphonylureas acted similarly to chlorpropamide in enhancing the reactivity of the auto-anti-Jk^a. The antibody was not inhibited by chlorpropamide leading the authors (124) to suggest that drug plus antibody complexes were binding to Jk^a on the red cells. Chlorpropamide and the other drugs that enhanced autoantibody reactivity all contain urea. This case was studied long before it became known that the Kidd glycoprotein is the red cell urea transporter protein.

Autoantibodies in the Kidd system are not all pathological in their activities. Examples of auto-anti-Jk^a in individuals with no evidence of accelerated in vivo red cell destruction have been documented (125,130-132). Judd et al. (131) described three examples of auto-anti-Jk^a that reacted only in the presence of parabens (butyl, ethyl, methyl and propyl esters of parahydroxybenzoate) or certain other neutral aromatic compounds. Each of the antibodies was detected in tests using commercially prepared LISS solutions that included parabens as preservatives. As already mentioned, the findings obtained showed that the autoantibodies were not causing accelerated rates of in vivo red cell clearance thus leading the authors to suppose that it is unlikely that examples of paraben-dependent anti-Jk^a will be of any clinical significance. In the case described by Halima et al. (132) the auto-anti-Jk^a reacted only in the presence of methyl esters of hydroxy benzoic acid. Again, the antibody was first detected in tests with a LISS solution that included methyl paraben (a methyl ester of hydroxy benzoic acid) as a preservative. In this case, the positive IATs caused by the antibody were due to cell bound C3, no IgG was detected on the reactive Jk(a+) red cells. The authors concluded that immune complexes of the antibody and the chemical, formed in the serum and were then bound by Jk(a+) red cells because of some complementary aspect of the immune complexes and the Jk^a antigen. Once bound, the complexes were presumed to activate complement so that cell-bound C3 could be detected with anti-C3 in IATs. This autoantibody was also clinically benign.

McGinniss et al. (126) tested the blood of a patient who experienced a transient hemolytic episode apparently caused by auto-anti-Jk^b. Because the patient had a history of urinary tract infections caused by Proteus organisms and had blood cultures positive for those organisms in the past, the authors ran in vitro tests with *Proteus mirabilis*. They found that Jk(b-) red cells incubated with *P. Mirabilis* cultures became reactive with anti-Jk^b. None of 28 other red cell antigens studied was changed. The authors stated that they had found *Streptococcus faecium* to have the same transforming property. One of us (133) has seen one case in which a bacterially contaminated serum sample behaved as if it contained a very potent complement-binding anti-Jk^a. New, non-contaminated samples from the same patient contained no antibody activity. These findings, like those cited above concerning paraben-associated anti-Jk^a, are not yet fully understood at the biochemical level. It is to be hoped that recognition of identity between the Kidd glycoprotein and the urea transporter protein, will eventually lead to such understandings.

Kidd System Antigens and Other Cells

In 1974, Marsh et al. (135) reported that while granulocytes from persons with Jk(a+) or Jk(b+) red cells would not adsorb anti-Jk^a or anti-Jk^b, they would adsorb anti-Jk3. Other investigators (136-138) found that granulocytes, lymphocytes, monocytes and platelets lack Jk^a and Jk^b; Gaidulis et al. (137) could not detect Jk3 on granulocytes. While it seems that other tissue cells lack Kidd system antigens (139) the possibility now seems to exist that at least some cells will be found to be able to transport urea across the cell membrane via mechanisms that do not involve presence of the Kidd glycoprotein.

Kidd Antigens Are Carried On The Urea Transporter HUT11

The first clear lead as to the biochemical nature of

the Kidd antigens came from the observations of Heaton and McLoughlin (83) when they demonstrated that red cells of the phenotype Jk(a-b-) are markedly more resistant to lysis in the presence of urea than red cells of the phenotypes Jk(a+b-), Jk(a+b+) or Jk(a-b+). This observation suggested that the molecule expressing Kidd antigens is a urea transporter. Subsequent transport studies, discussed in detail in a previous section, have supported this hypothesis. Excretion of urea is the mechanism by which mammals dispose of waste products containing nitrogen. Urea is synthesized in the liver and excreted by the kidneys. Facilitated urea transport is important in the kidney as a mechanism for stabilizing osmotic gradients in the renal medulla created during the process of concentrating urine before excretion. It is thought that facilitated urea transport functions in the red cell to protect it from the osmotic gradients to which it is exposed during passage through the kidney.

The first indications as to the nature of this transporter were provided by Sinor et al. (142) who reported that Kidd antigens were located on a molecule of apparent molecular weight 45kD. Gunn et al. (103) reported the isolation a cDNA clone by screening a human reticulocyte cDNA expression library with a pool of human anti-Jk[a] and anti-Jk[b] sera. The sequence of the clone was not published but the authors reported that a protein with five putative transmembrane domains was predicted from the nucleotide sequence and that the protein lacked potential N-glycosylation sites. Some preliminary evidence that the clone corresponded to a urea transporter was obtained by transport studies carried out with LMTK-fibroblasts transfected with the clone.

The breakthrough that led to the unambiguous assignment of the Kidd antigens to a urea transporter came from the studies of You et al. (143) who cloned a rabbit urea transporter (UT2) by microinjecting cRNA from rabbit renal medulla into *Xenopus* oocytes and screening for transport activity. The nucleotide sequence of the UT2 clone predicted a protein of 397 amino acids. Hydropathy analysis suggested 10 membrane spanning domains with the amino and carboxy termini in the cytoplasm and one large extracellular domain of 47 residues between membrane spanning domains five and six. The sequence contained two potential N-glycosylation sites only one of which was predicted to be extracellular (Asn210 on the large extracellular loop). Apart from the one large loop the extracellular loops are very small and several lack charged residues (see figure 19-4). You et al. (143) point out that it is possible that most of the protein is totally embedded in the membrane rather than as represented in figure 19-4. As with all the multi-spanning membrane proteins described in this book, it is important to remember that a hydropathy plot is a useful way to build a picture of a protein's topology because it provides

a model that can be used to design experiments to elucidate structure. It does not mark the end of a process but provides a good starting place for further studies. One of the most useful aspects of determining the molecular basis of a blood group polymorphism is that it identifies a region of protein sequence that must, because it defines an antigen, be accessible on the outside of a cell. Information like this can be of great value in trying to understand the structure of multi-spanning membrane proteins (see for example, Chapter 17, the Diego Blood Group System).

The nucleotide sequence of this rabbit urea transporter was used by Olivès et al. (116) to isolate cDNA encoding the human equivalent. Two oligonucleotide primers corresponding to amino acids 67-74 and 242-247 of UT2 were used in a reverse transcribed PCR with mRNA derived from human spleen erythroblasts from a patient with beta-thalassemia, to isolate a 540bp fragment that encoded a peptide sharing 71.4% sequence homology with the UT2 protein. The 540bp fragment was then used to screen a human bone marrow cDNA library in order to obtain a full length cDNA clone. The largest clone obtained (HUT11) had a open reading frame of 1173 bases encoding a predicted protein of 391 amino acids. The predicted HUT11 protein had 62.4% sequence homology with the UT2 protein. Neither UT2 nor HUT11 had a peptide signal sequence. Hydropathy analysis of HUT11 predicted a very similar topology to that of UT2 (see figure 19-4) with an N-glycan (Asn211) in the large extracellular loop. Seven cysteine residues are conserved between the two proteins, six in membrane spanning domains and one in the large extracellular loop (see figure 19-4).

Formal proof that HUT11 is the human equivalent of the rabbit urea transporter was obtained by expression of HUT11 in *Xenopus* oocytes. HUT11 cRNA injected oocytes had a 20-fold greater plasma membrane urea (14C-urea) permeability than water injected control oocytes. Known inhibitors of urea transport (phloretin, para-chloromercuribenzene sulfonate (pCMBS), and analogues of urea), inhibited urea uptake by HUT11-cRNA injected oocytes. It was also shown that HUT11 cannot act as a water channel (compare CHIP which carries the Colton system antigens, see Chapter 21).

In a subsequent paper Olivès et al. (105) showed that HUT11 carries the Kidd blood group antigens. By in situ hybridization to human chromosomes in metaphase it was possible to map the *HUT11* gene to the q12-q21 region of chromosome 18, the same region as the *Kidd* blood group locus previously mapped by Leppert et al. (115). Direct evidence that the proteins are the same was obtained using coupled transcription-translation assays. HUT11 cDNA was subcloned into the pT7TS plasmid and HUT11 protein synthesis of the T7 promoter was

FIGURE 19-4 Model of the Urea Transporter Depicting the Location of the
Jk^a/Jk^b Blood Group Polymorphism (from references 105,116,150,151)

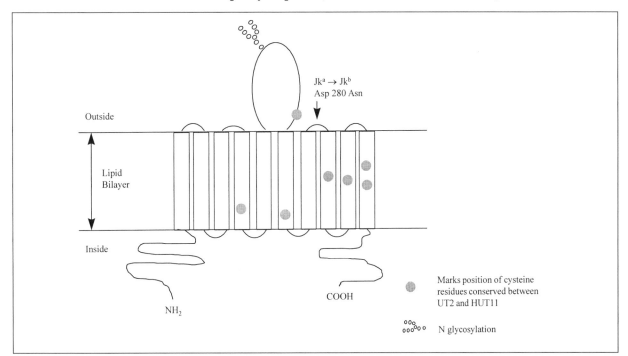

achieved in a reticulocyte lysate containing L-(35S)-methionine. On SDS-PAGE, a 35S labeled band of apparent molecular weight 36kD was observed, if the assay was performed in the presence of microsomal membranes an additional band of 40kD was observed. The 40kD band was assumed to be a glycosylated form of the 36kD band. Human anti-Jk3 precipitated the 36kD band. When the anti-Jk3 was used in immunoprecipitation experiments with red cells, a diffuse band of 46-60kD was obtained from cells of normal Kidd system phenotype but not from Jk(a-b-) cells. Extensive treatment of the immune precipitate with N-glycanase reduced the apparent molecular weight to 36kD. Olivès et al. (105) also used a rabbit antiserum made to a synthetic peptide corresponding to residues 16-31 (amino terminal cytoplasmic domain) of the HUT11 protein and showed, in immunoblotting studies, that the antibody identified a component of 46-60kD in membranes of normal Kidd system phenotype but not in membranes of Jk(a-b-) red cells. The authors conclude that their findings "provide compelling evidence that the urea transporter encoded by the HUT11 cDNA is the product of the *Kidd* locus" surely no one could disagree with that!

Northern blot analysis with the HUT11 probe revealed the presence of transcripts of 2.5kb and 4.7kb in human adult spleen erythroblasts and tumoral kidney but not in adult liver or monocyte and B-lymphoid cell lines. It is not known (116) if the two transcripts result from alternative splicing or different poly(A) usage.

Just as in the case of other blood group "null" phenotypes (see, for example, discussion of the absence of the water channel protein CHIP in Co(a-b-) cells in Chapter 21) these results raise the question of the functional importance of HUT11 since the Jk(a-b-) phenotype is apparently not associated with any pathology. There is evidence (144) that Jk(a-b-) individuals have moderately impaired urea recycling and thereby a reduced ability to concentrate urine but there is no evidence of any disease. One possibility is that other urea transporters can compensate and this may be particularly true in the kidney where there is evidence for other transporters. It is not yet known if HUT11 is absent from the kidneys of Jk(a-b-) individuals and at the time of this writing (June 1996) the mechanism giving rise to this phenotype has not been elucidated at the DNA level. Nevertheless, an explanation for the fact that the protein can be absent from red cells without deleterious consequences is required - answers on a postcard to the authors please! The relatively high frequency of the Jk(a-b-) phenotype in Polynesians suggests that some selective factor has been operating and one of us (DJA) cannot help wondering if this is another evidence of selective pressure from malaria. In this context it is of note that Roberts (145) reports an association between the Jk^b antigen and susceptibility to malaria in a small study carried out in West Africa

Given that the urea transporter is such a hydrophobic protein, it is not surprising that Kidd antigens are protease resistant but nevertheless there are potential cleavage sites on the large extracellular loop. It may be that they are covered by the N-glycan or that they are cleaved without affecting the organization of the protein outside the immediate locality as is the case for the third extracellular loop on band 3 (see Chapter 17). Inhibition of urea transport by pCMBS indicates a critical cysteine or cysteines in the process. There are seven cysteines conserved between UT2 and HUT11. Those that are important could be identified using site-directed mutagenesis (compare similar studies on CHIP described in Chapter 21).

Note Added at Proof Stage: The Jk^a/Jk^b Polymorphism

The molecular basis of the Jk^a/Jk^b polymorphism has now been described by Olivès et al. (150,151). It results from a single nucleotide change (G838A) in *HUT11* that results in an Asp280Asn (Jk^a to Jk^b) substitution in the fourth predicted extracellular loop of the urea transporter protein (the Kidd glycoprotein, see figure 19-4). This finding is of particular interest in that it confirms that the short peptide sequence, predicted by hydropathy analysis to form the fourth extracellular loop, is indeed accessible on the extracellular side of the red cell membrane. The location of the polymorphic site close to the surface of the lipid bilayer rather than on the third extracellular loop (see figure 19-4) is consistent with the serological properties of Kidd antibodies (see discussion of agglutination in Chapter 2). When Asn is present (i.e. Jk^b-bearing glycoprotein) it is not N-glycosylated because it is not part of an N-glycosylation signal motif.

In the full paper in which they described the basis of the Jk^a/Jk^b polymorphism, Olivès et al. (151) also showed that the polymorphism is not in linkage disequilibrium with a gene conferring susceptibility to type 1 diabetes mellitus. Previously, some data had suggested linkage (152-154) while other data had not (155,156).

References

1. Allen FH Jr, Diamond LK, Niedziela B. Nature 1951;167:482
2. Plaut G, Ikin EW, Mourant AE, et al. Nature 1953;171:431
3. Pinkerton FJ, Mermod LE, Liles BA, et al. Vox Sang 1959;4:155
4. Okubo Y, Yamaguchi H, Nagao N, et al. Transfusion 1986;26:237
5. Lecointre-Coatmelec M, Bourel D, Ferrette J, et al. Vox Sang 1991;61:255
6. Thompson K, Barden G, Sutherland J, et al. Transf Med 1991;1:91
7. Race RR, Sanger R. Blood Groups in Man, 6th Ed. Oxford:Blackwell, 1975
8. Chown B, Lewis M, Kaita H, et al. Vox Sang 1963;8:378
9. Chown B, Lewis M, Kaita H. Transfusion 1965;5:506
10. Rosenfield RE, Vogel P, Gibbel N, et al. Am J Clin Pathol 1953;23:1222
11. Sanger R, Race RR, Cahan A, et al. Unpublished data cited in Race RR, Sanger R. Blood Groups in Man, 6th Ed. Oxford:Blackwell, 1975
12. Boyd PA. MS Thesis, Univ Cincinnati, 1980
13. Toivanen P, Hirvonen T. Vox Sang 1973;24:372
14. Issitt PD. In: Rhesus Problems in Clinical Practice. Groningen:Groningen-Drenthe Red Cross, 1977:46
15. Simpson MB, Pryzbylik JA, Denham RA, et al. Obstet Gynecol 1978;52:616
16. Harrison KL, Popper EI. Transfusion 1981;21:90
17. Issitt PD. Transfusion 1965;5:355
18. Andre R, Salmon C, Malassenet R. Rev Hematol 1956;11:495
19. Lundevall J. Acta Path Microbiol Scand 1956;38:39
20. Kronenberg H, Kooptzoff O, Walsh RJ. Austral Ann Med 1958;7:34
21. Mazalton A, Philippon J. Bull Soc Med Hop Paris 1962;113:727
22. Derot M, Salmon J, Rosselin G. Bull Soc Med Hop Pris 1962;113:1113
23. Polesky HF, Bove JR. Transfusion 1964;4:285
24. Degan TJ, Rosenfield RE. Transfusion 1965;5:245
25. Pineda AA, Brzica SM, Taswell HF. Mayo Clin Proc 1978;53:378
26. Maynard BA, Smith DS, Farrar RP, et al. Transfusion 1988;28:302
27. Greenwalt TJ, Sasaki T, Sneath J. Vox Sang 1956;1:157
28. Kornstad L, Halvorsen K. Vox Sang 1958;3:94
29. Matson GA, Swanson J, Tobin JD. Vox Sang 1959;4:144
30. Geczy A, Leslie M. Transfusion 1961;1:125
31. Geczy A, Matheson WA. Am J Obstet Gynecol 1965;92:576
32. Zodin V, Anderson RE. Pediatrics 1965;36:420
33. Stratton F, Gunson HH, Rawlinson V. Transfusion 1965;5:216
34. Dorner I, Mare JA, Chaplin H. Transfusion 1974;14:212
35. Bowman J. In: Immunobiology of Transfusion Medicine. New York:Marcel Dekker, 1994:565
36. Bowman J. Transf Med Rev 1990;4:191
37. Ewald RA, Williams JH, Bowden DH. Vox Sang 1961;6:312
38. Adinolfi M, Zenthon J. Rev Perinatal Med 1984;5:61
39. Polley MJ, Mollison PL, Soothill JF. Br J Haematol 1962;8:149
40. Szymanski IO, Huff SR, Delsignore R. Transfusion 1982;22:90
41. Mollison PL, Engelfriet CP, Contreras M. Blood Transfusion in Clinical Medicine, 9th Ed. Oxford:Blackwell, 1993
42. Engelfriet CP. Unpublished observations 1978 cited in Mollison PL. Blood Transfusion in Clinical Medicine, 7th Ed. Oxford:Blackwell, 1983
43. Hardman JT, Beck ML, Pierce SR. (abstract). Book of Abstracts, 18th Cong ISBT. Basel:Karger, 1984:265
44. Hardman JT, Beck ML. Transfusion 1981;21:343
45. Haber G, Rosenfield RE. In: PH Andresen, papers in dedication of his 60th birthday. Copenhargen:Munksgaard, 1957:45
46. Masourdesis SP, Sudora E, Mahan L, et al. Blood 1980;56:969
47. Fisher GA. Transfusion 1983;23:152
48. Polley MJ, MollisonPL. Transfusion 1961;1:9
49. Issitt PD, Mollison PL, Chanarin I. Unpublished observations, 1962. Mentioned in the previous editions of this book
50. Issitt PD. Adv Immunohematol 1977;4:No 4
51. Wright MS, Issitt PD. Transfusion 1979;19:688
52. Cutbush M, Mollison PL. Br J Haematol 1958;4:115
53. Tenczar FJ, Bushch S, Loken B. Bull AABB 1960;13:445
54. Gohier M, Hayeur H. Canad J Med Technol 1964;26:102

55. Day D, Perkins HA, Sams B. Transfusion 1965;5:315
56. Giblett ER, Hillman RS, Brooks LE. Vox Sang 1965;10:448
57. Kurtides ES, Salkin MS, Widen AL. J Am Med Assoc 1966;197:816
58. Morgan P, Wheeler CB, Bossom EL. Transfusion 1967;7:307
59. Rauner TA, Tanaka KR. New Eng J Med 1967;276:1486
60. Holland PV, Wallerstein RO. J Am Med Assoc 1968;204:1007
61. Thomson S, Johnstone M. Canad J Med Technol 1972;34:159
62. Magni E, Rossetti V. Minerva Medica 1972;63:2525
63. Mollison PL, Newlands M. Vox Sang 1976;31:54
64. Pineda AA, Taswell HF,Brzica SM Jr. Transfusion 1978;18:1
65. Solanki D, McCurdy PR. J Am Med Assoc 1978;239:729
66. Vogel RA, Worthington M. (Letter). J Am Med Assoc 1978;240:2432
67. Croucher BEE. In: A Seminar on Laboratory Management of Hemolysis. Washington, D.C. Am Assoc Blood Banks, 1979:151
68. Moore SB, Taswell HF, Pineda AA, et al. Am J Clin Pathol 1980;74:94
69. Ness PM, Shirey RS, Thomas SK, et al. Transfusion 1990;30:688
70. Mollison PL. Blood Transfusion in Clinical Medicine, 7th Ed. Oxford:Blackwell, 1983
71. Pinkerton FJ. Unpublished observations 1960, cited by Race RR, Sanger R. Blood Groups in Man, 6th Ed. Oxford:Blackwell, 1975
72. Silver RT, Haber JM, Kellner A. Nature 1960;186:481
73. Sausais L, Issitt PD. Unpublished observations 1967, cited in previous editions of this book
74. Woodfield DG, Douglas R, Smith J, et al. Transfusion 1982;22:276
75. Henry S, Woodfield G. (Letter). Transfusion 1995;35:277
76. Sussman LN, Solomon R, Grogan S. Transfusion 1975;15:356
77. Issitt PD, Brendel WL, Sonkin D, et al. (Letter). Transfusion 1983;23:361
78. Habibi B, Avril J, Fouillade MT, et al. Haematologia 1976;10:403
79. Sistonen P. (abstract). Book of Abstracts, 18th Cong ISBT. Basel:Karger, 1984:164
80. Klarkowski DB. Austral J Med Lab Sci 1984;5:26
81. Yokoyama M, Mermod LE, Stegmaier A. Vox Sang 1967;12:154
82. Kuczmarski CA, Bergren MO, Perkins HA. Vox Sang 1982;43:340
83. Heaton DC, McLoughlin K. Transfusion 1982;22:70
84. Arcara PC, O'Connor MA, Dimmette RM. (abstract). Transfusion 1969;9:282
85. Tills D, Lopec AC, Tills RE. The Distribution of the Human Blood Groups and Other Biochemical Polymorphisms, 2nd Ed. London:Oxford Univ Press, 1976
86. Pierce SR, Hardman JT, Steele S, et al. Transfusion 1980;20:189
87. Ford DS, Stern DA, Duraisamy G. (abstract). Rev Paulista Med 1992;110:18
88. Smart EA, Moores PP, Reddy R, et al. (abstract). Transf Med 1993;3 (Suppl 1):84
89. Oliver CK, Sexton T, Joyner J. (abstract). Transfusion 1993;33 (Suppl 9S):23S
90. Crawford MN, Greenwalt TJ, Sasaki T, et al. Transfusion 1961;1:228
91. Garris ML, Issitt PD, Arcara PC. Unpublished observations 1968 cited in Issitt PD, Issitt CH. Applied Blood Group Serology, 2nd Ed. Oxnard:Spectra Biologicals, 1975:181
92. Issitt PD, Obarski G, Hartnett PL, et al. Transfusion 1990;30:46

93. Humphrey AJ, Morel PA. Transfusion 1976;16:242
94. Chandanayingyong D, Sasaki T, Greenwalt TJ. Transfusion 1967;7:269
95. Behzad O, Wong C, Gaucys G, et al. (Letter). Transfusion 1980;20:119
96. Kataoku, Taguchi (Initials not given). Unpublished observations cited by Okubo Y, Yamaguchi H, Nagao N, et al. Transfusion 1986;26:237
97. Edwards-Moulds J, Kasschau M. Transfusion 1988;28:545
98. Edwards-Moulds J, Kasschau MR. Vox Sang 1988;55:181
99. Edwards-Moulds J. In: Blood Group Systems: Duffy, Kidd and Lutheran. Arlington, VA:Am Assoc Blood Banks, 1988:73
100. McDougall DCJ, McGregor M. (Letter). Transfusion 1988;28:197
101. McGregor M, Gale SA. (abstract). Proc 7th Ann Mtg BBTS, 1989:95
102. Fröhlich O, Macey RI, Edwards-Moulds J, et al. Am J Physiol 1991;260:C778
103. Gunn RB, Gargus JJ, Frøhlich O. In: Protein Blood Groups Antigens of the Human Red Cell. Baltimore:Johns Hopkins Univ Press, 1992:88
104. Moulds JM. In: Blood Cell Biochemistry, Vol 6. New York:Plenum 1995:267
105. Olivès B, Mattei MG, Huet M, et al. J Biol Chem 1995;270:15607
106. Shokeir MHK, Ying LK, Pabello P. Clin Genet 1973;4:360
107. de la Chapelle A, Vuopio P, Sanger R, et al. Lancet 1975;2:871
108. Mohr J, Eiberg H. Clin Genet 1976;10:375
109. Mohr J, Eiberg H. Clin Genet 1977;11:372
110. Robson EB, Khan PM. Cytogenet Cell Genet 1982;32:144
111. Zelinski T, Kaita H, Lewis M, et al. Transfusion 1988;28:435
112. McAlpine PJ, Bootsma D. Cytogenet Cell Genet 1982;32:121
113. Lewis M, Kaita H, Phillips S, et al. Ann Hum Genet 1982;46:349
114. Geitvik GA, Høyheim B, Gedde-Dahl T, et al. Hum Genet 1987;77:205
115. Leppert M, Ferrell R, Kamboh MI, et al. Cytogenet Cell Genet 1987;46:647
116. Olivès B, Neau P, Bailly P, et al. J Biol Chem 1994;269:31649
117. Loghem JJ van, Hart M van der M. Vox Sang (Old Series) 1954;4:2
118. Dausset J, Colombani J. Blood 1959;14:1280
119. Guillausseau PJ, Wautier JL, Boizard B, et al. Sem Hop Paris 1982;53:803
120. Hoffman M, Berger MB, Menitove JE. Lab Med 1982;13:674
121. Sander RP, Hardy NM, Van Meter SA. Transfusion 1987;27:58
122. Ganley PS, Laffan MA, Owen I, et al. Br J Haematol 1988;69:537
123. Patten E, Beck CE, Scholl C, et al. Transfusion 1977;17:517
124. Sosler SD, Behzad O, Garratty G, et al. Transfusion 1984;24:206
125. Issitt PD, Pavone BG, Frohlich JA, et al. Transfusion 1980;20:733
126. McGinniss MH, Leiberman R, Holland PV. (abstract). Transfusion 1979;19:663
127. Roberston V, Hill M, Bryant J, et al. (abstract). Transfusion 1987;27:525
128. Ellisor SS, Reid ME, O'Day T, et al. Vox Sang 1983;45:53
129. O'Day T. (Letter). Transfusion 1987;27:442
130. Holmes LD, Pierce SR, Beck ML. (abstract). Transfusion 1976;16:521

131. Judd WJ, Steiner EA, Cochrane RK. Transfusion 1982;22:31
132. Halima D, Garratty G, Bueno R. Transfusion 1982;22:521
133. Issitt PD. Unpublished observations, 1961, cited in previous editions of this book
134. Issitt PD, Pavone BG. Br J Haematol 1978;38:63
135. Marsh WL, Øyen R, Nichols ME. Transfusion 1974;14:378
136. Dunstan RA, Simpson MB, Rosse WF. Transfusion 1984;24:243
137. Gaidulis L, Branch DR, Lazar GS, et al. Br J Haematol 1985;60:659
138. Dunstan RA. Br J Haematol 1986;62:301
139. Rouger P, Salmon C. Rev Fr Transf Immunohematol 1982;25:643
140. Daniels GL, Weinauer F, Stone C, et al. Blood 1996;88:4045
141. Berg K. Clin Genet 1988;33:102
142. Sinor LT, Eastwood KL, Plapp FV. Med Lab Sci 1987;44:294
143. You G, Smith CP, Kanai Y, et al. Nature 1993;365:844
144. Sands JM, Gargus JJ, Frohlich O, et al. J Am Soc Nephrol 1992;2:1689
145. Roberts DJ. (abstract). Transf Med 1996;5 (Suppl 2):53
146. Mannuzzu LM, Moronne MM, Macey RI. J Mem Biol 1993;133:85
147. Yates J, Howell P, Overfield J, et al. (abstract). Transf Med 1996;6 (Suppl 2):29
148. Garratty G. In: Immune Destruction of Red Cells. Arlington, VA:Am Assoc Blood Banks, 1989:109
149. Petz LD. Garratty G, Branch D. Unpublished observations, cited by Garratty G. In: Immune Destruction of Red Cells. Arlington, VA:Am Assoc Blood Banks, 1989:109
150. Olivès B, Cartron J-P, Bailly P. (abstract). Transf Clin Biol 1996;3 (suppl):57s
151. Olivès B, Merriman M, Bailly P, et al. Hum Mol Genet 1997;6:1017
152. Hodge SE, Anderson CE, Neiswanger K, et al. Lancet 1982;2:893
153. Barbosa J, Rich S, Dunsworth T, et al. J Clin Endocrinol Metab 1982;55:193
154. Davies JL, Kawaguchi Y, Bennett ST, et al. Nature 1994;371:130
155. Hodge SE, Anderson CE, Neiswanger K, et al. Am J Hum Genet 1983;35:1139
156. Dunsworth TS, Rich SS, Swanson J, et al. Diabetes 1982;31:991
157. Ouldamar AK, Cesaire R, Haustant G, et al. Transf Today 1997;July:p16
158. Takeuchi K, Suzuki S, Koyama K, et al. Thorac Cariovasc Surg 1993;41:104
159. Shahian DM, Werner MJ, Karts SR. Panminerva Med 1995;37:95

20 | The Lutheran Blood Group System

In 1945, Callender et al. (1) described an antibody, anti-Lu^a, that detects an antigen of fairly low incidence. Additional details were published a year later (2); as well as making the first example of anti-Lu^a, the patient made anti-c, anti-N, the first example of anti-C^w and what was for 35 years the only example of anti-Levay, an antibody now known (3,4) to detect Kp^c, the product of a third allele at the *Kp* sublocus of the Kell system (see Chapter 18). Before the antibody defining the antigen antithetical to Lu^a was found, the Lutheran system had been used to make significant contributions to human genetics. Mohr (5-7) showed that the *Lu (Lutheran) and Sese (Secretor)* loci are linked, this being the first recorded example of any (i.e. not just blood group) autosomal linkage in man. Once the *Lu:Se* linkage was established, it became possible to recognize the first known example of autosomal crossing-over in man. At the time of the early studies it appeared that linkage involved the *Lu* and *Le (Lewis)* loci, later it became appreciated (8-12) that the linkage was, in fact, between the *Lu* and *Se* loci. As described later in this chapter, it is now known (13-19,194,205) that the *Lu:Se* linkage group is carried on chromosome 19.

In 1956, Cutbush and Chanarin (20) described anti-Lu^b, the antibody that defines the high incidence antithetical partner to the low incidence antigen Lu^a. Since most blood bankers will encounter anti-Lu^a and anti-Lu^b more frequently than they will encounter antibodies to other Lutheran system antigens, table 20-1 shows Lutheran system antigen and phenotype frequencies as determined by just those two antibodies.

In 1961, Crawford et al. (21) described the first example of blood of the phenotype Lu(a-b-). It was shown that, in the family studied, the gene responsible for that phenotype differed from many others that cause minus-minus blood group phenotypes, by being dominant in action. It is now known (see a later section in this chapter) that *In(Lu)*, as the dominant gene has become known, is not situated at the *Lutheran* locus (22,23) and

that its presence causes marked suppression of production of Lutheran system antigens, but not their total absence (24). *In(Lu)* has also been shown to exert a suppressive effect on the expression of blood group antigens of several other systems (see below). In 1963, Darnborough et al. (25) studied a family that included the Lu(a-b-) phenotype and concluded that the phenotype might not always represent the inheritance of *In(Lu)*. Their (25) suggestion that a recessive silent allele, *Lu*, at the *Lutheran* locus might also exist was confirmed when Brown et al. (26) described a large inbred family in Nova Scotia in which the phenotype was present. Unlike the Lu(a-b-) red cells of persons who have inherited *In(Lu)*, those of individuals genetically *LuLu* are totally devoid of Lutheran antigens. Also different from *In(Lu)*, the *LuLu* genotype results only in the absence of Lutheran system antigens, those of other blood group systems are unaffected. Since these early studies many other families with individuals genetically *In(Lu)* or *LuLu* have been described. References to many of the papers describing them are given in later sections of this chapter. In 1986, Norman et al. (27) described an Australian family in which the Lu(a-b-) phenotype was seen to be caused by yet a different genetic event. In this family the phenotype represented inheritance of an X chromosome-borne suppressor gene. The normal gene that allows production of Lutheran system antigens was named *XS1*, the suppressor gene was called *XS2*. Thus sons of an *XS1/XS2* mother can be Lu(a-b-) (*XS2/Y*) or can have normal expression of Lutheran system antigens (*XS1/Y*). All daughters of an *XS1/XS2* mother will have normal expression of Lutheran antigens if their father expresses those antigens normally, that is *XS1/XS2* X *XS1/Y*, producing *XS1/XS1* (normal) or *XS1/XS2* (carrier) daughters. The Lu(a-b-) phenotype associated with the X chromosome-borne suppressor gene is more like the *In(Lu)* caused Lu(a-b-) phenotype than like the one caused by homozygosity of *Lu*. That is to say, the Lu(a-b-) red cells of males with *XS2* were shown capable of adsorbing and yielding on elution, anti-Lu^b. As described in more detail below, the trace amounts of Lutheran system antigens on the red cells of persons who have inherited *In(Lu)* or *XS2* seem to prevent them from making antibodies to high incidence Lutheran system antigens. An antibody at first called anti-Lu^{ab} but later renamed anti-Lu3, has been found in the sera of many persons genetically *LuLu* (see below).

In 1971, Bove et al. (28) described another Lutheran system related antibody, anti-Lu4. The antibody-maker

TABLE 20-1 Antigen and Phenotype Frequencies in Whites as Determined by Antibodies to Lu^a and Lu^b

Phenotype	% Frequency	% of Bloods Reactive with	
		Anti-Lu^a	Anti-Lu^b
Lu (a+b-)	0.15	7.65	
Lu (a+b+)	7.50		
Lu (a-b+)	92.35		99.85

671

had red cells of the common Lu(a-b+) phenotype and made an antibody that reacted with all except Lu(a-b-) red cells. In other words, the antibody-maker's cells were Lu(a-b+) Lu:3,-4, while Lu(a-b-) red cells are Lu:-3,-4. At a reference laboratory meeting in 1970 (held after the work on anti-Lu4 had been performed but before the paper was printed) it became appreciated (29) that a number of other previously unidentified antibodies to very common antigens, had a similar relationship to the Lutheran system to that displayed by anti-Lu4. Again, the red cells of the antibody-makers were Lu(a-b+) and again the antibodies reacted with all except Lu(a-b-) red cells. Because the red cells of the individual who made anti-Lu4 and those of the persons who had made the new antibodies were not mutually compatible, it was apparent that three new specificities had been found. These antibodies were called anti-Lu5, anti-Lu6 and anti-Lu7. Since 1970, several other antibodies that react with all except Lu(a-b-) red cells and that do not have the same specificity as the antibodies that define the antigens called Lu4, Lu5, Lu6 or Lu7 have been found. However, it must be remembered that failure of an antibody to react with the null red cells of a system shows only a phenotypic association between the antibody and the system. Genetic or biochemical evidence is required before the antigen defined can be assigned to the system with complete certainty. Thus like the Kell system, the Lutheran system has collected a considerable number of antigens regarded as being para-Lutheran in nature. In addition to Lu4, Lu5, Lu6 and Lu7, high incidence antigens named Lu8, Lu11, Lu12, Lu13, Lu16, Lu17 and Lu20 were considered, at one time or another, to fit this category. Genetic evidence has been found that Lu6 and Lu8 are indeed encoded from the *Lutheran* locus. Lu6 was found (30) to be antithetical to the low incidence antigen Lu9; Lu8 was found (31) to be antithetical to the rare antigen Lu14. As described below, family studies showed that *Lu^9* and *Lu^14* are at the *Lutheran* locus meaning that their alleles, *Lu^6* and *Lu^8* respectively, must be similarly situated. While the term para-Lutheran is still used to describe many of the other high incidence antigens there is evidence at the serological and/or biochemical level, in a number of instances, that the antigens are indeed part of the Lutheran system. Such evidence is described below in the sections describing the antigens.

In 1961, Salmon et al. (32) described the antigen Au^a that is present on the red cells of some 80 to 90% (see later for an explanation of this wide range in incidence) of White Europeans (32,33). Au^a was known to have some sort of relationship with the Lutheran system since by 1976 the red cells of 32 of 35 persons with the *In(Lu)* form of the Lu(a-b-) phenotype had been shown (34) to be Au(a-). In spite of this significantly low incidence of Au^a on *In(Lu)* Lu(a-b-) red cells, one family had been

found (35) in which it appeared that *Au^a* segregated independently of the *Lutheran* locus. In 1989, Frandson et al. (36) described anti-Au^b, the antibody defining the antithetical partner to Au^a. Evidence of an association between Au^a and Au^b and the Lutheran system continued to mount when red cells of the Lu(a-b-) phenotype with the *In(Lu)*, *LuLu* and *XS2* genetic backgrounds were all found to lack both Au^a (27,37,38) and Au^b (36,38). A major step in resolving the puzzle was made in 1990 when Daniels (39) reported that immunoblotting and immunoprecipitation studies showed that Au^a and Au^b are carried on the Lutheran glycoprotein (for details about that membrane structure, see a later section of this chapter). While these findings (39) did not prove that Au^a and Au^b are part of the Lutheran system, they made such a conclusion very much more likely than unlikely. The French family in which recombination between *Lu^a* and *Au^a* had been seen (35) was reinvestigated (40) and some red cell typing errors made in the original investigation were found. The new investigation supported the conclusion that production of Au^a and Au^b is encoded from the *Lutheran* complex locus. Zelinski et al. (41) then reviewed data from seven informative families and showed that there is no doubt that the *Au* and *Lutheran* loci are the same thing. The antigen Au^a thus became Lu18 and Au^b became Lu19 (42) and *Au^a* and *Au^b* became a fourth pair of alleles at the *Lutheran* complex locus.

To conclude this introductory section, table 20-2 lists: the conventional and ISBT terminology for the Lutheran system; lists the year in which the antigen was first described; gives a reference to the original description; and shows the incidence of the antigen in a White and, where known, a Black population. Because many of the para-Lutheran antigens were assigned numbers and were studied for many years before any publication about them appeared and because Au^a was added to the Lutheran system long after being discovered, table 20-2 breaks with tradition and lists the antigens in sequence of their numbers, rather than sequence of their discovery. Table 20-3 shows the relationships of the antigens of the system to each other and to the system as a whole. For historical interest, table 20-4 lists a number of "firsts" achieved by the Lutheran system over the years.

The Antigens Lu^a and Lu^b

As indicated in table 20-1, the Lu^a antigen is present on the red cells of between 7 and 8% of Whites (2,59-63). While fewer samples from Blacks have been tested (61) there are no indications that the Lu(a+) phenotype frequency is appreciably different in such people. The Lu^b antigen is very common and is found on the red cells of some 99.85% of random donors (61-66). This means

TABLE 20-2 Antigens of the Lutheran System

	Conventional Name: Lutheran				Conventional Symbol: Lu		
	ISBT System Symbol: LU				ISBT System Number: 005		
Historical Derivation	Antigen Conventional Name	Year Reported	Percent Frequency		References	ISBT Antigen Number	ISBT Full Code Number
			Whites	Blacks[*1]			
	Lu^a	1945	7.7		1	LU1	005001
	Lu^b	1956	99.9		20	LU2	005002
Lu^{ab}	Lu3	1963	>99.9	>99.9	25	LU3	005003
Ba	Lu4	1971	>99.9		28	LU4	005004
Be and Fo	Lu5	1972	>99.9		29	LU5	005005
Jan	Lu6	1972	>99.9	>99.9	29	LU6	005006
Ga	Lu7	1972	>99.9		29	LU7	005007
M.T.	Lu8	1972	>99.9		43	LU8	005008
Mull	Lu9	1973	1.7		30	LU9	005009
Re	Lu11	1974	>99.9		44	LU11	005011
Much	Lu12	1973	>99.9		45	LU12	005012
Hughes	Lu13	1983	>99.9		46, 47	LU13	005013
Hof	Lu14	1977	1.5 to 2.4[*2]		31	LU14	005014
	Lu16	1980	>99.9		48	LU16	005016
Pataracchia	Lu17	1979	>99.9		49	LU17	005017
Auberger	Au^a, Lu18	1961	80-90[*2]		32	LU18	005018
	Au^b, Lu19	1989	51	68	36	LU19	005019
	Lu20	1992	>99.9		50	LU20	005020

Lu10 was originally reserved (51-53) for a low incidence antigen defined by a serum, Singleton. The antibody was thought to define the antithetical partner to Lu5 but Crawford (54) found that five Lu:-5 samples (from four unrelated persons) were nonreactive with the Singleton serum.

Lu15 was originally reserved for the antigen now called AnWj (55-58) see Chapter 29.

[*1]   Frequency in Blacks often determined from tests on a limited number of samples and/or represents the unpublished observations of one of us (PDI).

[*2]   For comments on antigen frequency ranges, see text.

that the incidence of the Lu(a+b–) phenotype is about 1 in 667 random (primarily White) donors. In tests on 922 Chinese in Taiwan (67) all had Lu(a-b+) red cells. However, the phenotype Lu(a-b–) has been found in a Chinese individual (68).

The Lu^a and Lu^b antigens are not fully developed during fetal life (69,70) or at birth (71-73). As described in the next section, this fact no doubt contributes to the mildness of cases of HDN associated with anti-Lu^a and anti-Lu^b. As also more fully described in the next section, the Lu^a antigen is not evenly distributed on the red cells of persons of the Lu(a+) phenotype. Both Lu^a and Lu^b, in common with other Lutheran system and para-

Lutheran antigens, are denatured or removed when red cells are treated with trypsin, chymotrypsin or pronase. The antigens may be slightly weakened but are still detectable on papain-treated red cells (74-76). Both 2-aminoethylisothiouronium bromide (AET) and dithiothreitol (DTT) treatment of red cells renders them nonreactive with antibodies to Lutheran system and para-Lutheran antigens (75-78). However, it may be necessary to use AET or DTT under optimal conditions in order to effect total denaturation of the antigens (79),

Merry et al. (92) tested Lu(a+b+) and Lu(a-b+) red cells with a monoclonal anti-Lu^b to determine the number of Lu^b antigens sites per red cell. On Lu(a+b+) red

TABLE 20-3 Relationships of Lutheran and Para-Lutheran Antigens

Pairs of Alleles	Antigens Encoded	
	Low Incidence	High Incidence
Lu^a, Lu^b	Lu^a	Lu^b
Lu^6, Lu^9	Lu9	Lu6
Lu^8, Lu^14	Lu14	Lu8
Polymorphic		
Au^a, Au^b		Au^a, Au^b

Antigens that may be encoded from the *Lutheran* locus

Lu3, Lu4, Lu5, Lu7, Lu11, Lu12, Lu13, Lu16, Lu17, Lu20
(All are of very high incidence)

Other genes at the *Lutheran* locus: *Lu*

Genes not at the *Lutheran* locus: *In(Lu), XS2* and those that encode production of the low incidence antigen Singleton and the high incidence antigen AnWj.

TABLE 20-4 "Firsts" Associated with the Lutheran System

1. First example (with *Sese*) of autosomal linkage in man.

2. First example of autosomal crossing-over in man.

3. First example of unlinked dominant suppression of blood group antigen expression.

4. First example of X-linked suppression of blood group antigen expression.

5. First blood group system with three different genetic backgrounds for the minus-minus phenotype.

cells the range was 850 to 1820, on Lu(a-b+) cells the range was 1640 to 4070. These wide ranges are compatible with serological studies that often show wide variation in the reactions of different red cell samples when tested with anti-Lu^b.

Anti-Lu^a, Anti-Lu^b and Their Clinical Significance

Many examples of anti-Lu^a have been found, some of them have been described in print (1,2,59,72,81-91). The antibody most frequently presents as an agglutinin, active in tests using saline-suspended red cells at temperatures below 37°C. In such a form the antibody is clinically-benign since it is unable to attach to transfused Lu(a+) red cells at body temperature. When encountered as an agglutinin, anti-Lu^a often gives an unusual reaction pattern (2). The agglutinated red cells may be seen to be in small clumps superimposed on a background of unagglutinated cells. However, if the agglutinates are removed and the previously unagglutinated red cells are mixed with more anti-Lu^a, new agglutinates form showing that the cells all carry Lu^a antigen. Agglutination of Lu(a+) red cells by anti-Lu^a in capillary tube tests has been said (192) to produce a "pine tree-like" appearance. This atypical agglutination, that apparently results from unequal distribtuion or unequal access of Lu^a on Lu(a+) red cells, is often a useful clue to the blood group serologist that the antibody under investigation has anti-Lu^a specificity. Some anti-Lu^a appear to react by IAT in addition to behaving as agglutinins. However, it is not always clear that the IAT reactions represent detection of anti-Lu^a by the antiglobulin serum or whether they simply represent carry-through of agglutination that occurred during the initial incubation of the test and was not dispersed in the cell washing steps. One anti-Lu^a was described (87) as being reactive only by IAT. There is also a report (93) that anti-Lu^a reacts less strongly in PEG than in other low ionic strength test systems. One of us (PDI) has not seen this to be a constant feature of anti-Lu^a in PEG tests. Anti-Lu^a is often IgM in nature but IgG forms are also seen. The antibody only rarely (82,84) increases in strength following transfusion.

Those examples of anti-Lu^a that are active at 37°C do not often seem of any greater clinical significance than those detectable only at lower temperatures. There is one published report (88) of normal (or near normal) survival of Lu(a+) red cells in a patient whose serum contained anti-Lu^a and who was transfused with a unit of Lu(a+) blood. In a subsequent cell survival study, the 37°C-active anti-Lu^a failed to clear labeled Lu(a+) red cells. In another case (94) anti-Lu^a was blamed for a rather mild delayed transfusion reaction. However, it seems that some patients with anti-Lu^a must receive Lu(a+) blood without that fact being known. When deliberate screening tests with Lu(a+) red cells are undertaken (72,86) anti-Lu^a is seen to be more common than is generally supposed. However, many sets of commercially prepared antibody screening cells do not contain one that is Lu(a+). Thus a patient with only anti-Lu^a in the serum will often appear not to have any antibodies present on routine screening and will thus qualify to receive blood issued following an immediate spin compatibility test (see Chapter 35) or following computer matching. Since seven or eight random donors in every 100 will have Lu(a+) red cells, it follows that the unknowing transfusion of Lu(a+) blood to a patient with (sometimes 37°C-active) anti-Lu^a in the serum must occur not too infrequently. The fact that there are no documented immediate and only rare and mild delayed transfusion reactions attributed to anti-Lu^a must surely indicate that the vast majority of such antibodies are benign in vivo.

Similarly, those cases of HDN that have been reported as having been caused by anti-Lu^a have all been mild, (72,87,90) in none of them was transfusion necessary.

Although the Lu(a+b-) phenotype is rare, many examples of alloimmune anti-Lu^b have been documented in the literature (20,71,72,86,96-103). Production of the antibody can be stimulated by transfusion or pregnancy, the latter seems to be a particularly common route for immunization to Lu^b (72). The antibody is sometimes seen as a saline-active agglutinin (20,71,72,97) and is then often optimally reactive at temperatures below 37°C. It seems that a higher percentage of anti-Lu^b, than of anti-Lu^a, are IAT reactive. The literature contains mixed reports about the immunoglobulin type of anti-Lu^b. While some examples are undoubtedly IgG in composition (72,86,99,100,104) others have been described (72,102,103,105) as being predominantly IgA and/or partly IgM. At the practical level this seems to matter little, anti-Lu^b can usually be detected and identified in IATs read with anti-IgG. In one study (106) it was found that all of eleven anti-Lu^b contained an IgG4 component. However, more recently, Garratty et al. (107) have reported that among seven antibodies to high incidence Lutheran system and para-Lutheran antigens studied, three were IgG1 alone, while the other four contained an IgG1 component, three with IgG2, two with IgG3 and only one with IgG4 components.

As mentioned in an earlier section there is considerable variation in the number of Lu^b antigen sites detectable on different Lu(b+) samples. As a result anti-Lu^b may react to different strengths with different red cells, the pattern seen in an antibody identification study will sometimes resemble that seen when two or more antibodies are present in the serum under test. Some anti-Lu^b may fail to give visibly positive reactions with Lu(a+b+) red cells, others may react but may show a considerable dosage effect.

Anti-Lu^b seems only a little more likely than anti-Lu^a, to be of clinical importance. No serious transfusion reaction caused by the antibody has been reported and those delayed reactions in which it was believed that the antibody was involved, have been relatively mild (86,100). In a number of in vivo red cell survival studies (96,101,102) it has been shown that sometimes a few of the injected Lu(b+) red cells are rapidly cleared while the others enjoy a much closer to normal survival. It can be anticipated, based on what is written above, that the Lu(b+) red cells of different donors would show different rates of survival (i.e. proportional to antigen site numbers on the red cells of different persons). Clearly, in a life-saving emergncy, when no Lu(b-) blood was available, a patient with anti-Lu^b would be better served by being transfused with serologically incompatible red cells than by having transfusion withheld until antigen-negative

blood became available. For example, Tilley et al. (101) described an anti-Lu^b, with a titer of 256 at 37°C, that cleared Lu(a+b+) red cells but took eight days to eliminate 54% of a 1.0 ml labeled test dose.

As with anti-Lu^a, no example of anti-Lu^b has caused HDN severe enough to necessitate transfusion. In a number of infants with Lu(b+) red cells, born to women with anti-Lu^b in the serum, the DAT on the cord blood red cells was positive and mild jaundice developed (71,99,103). In no case was treatment other than phototherapy required. In other infants no signs of clinical HDN were seen (72,95,109). In one of these cases (109) the anti-Lu^b titer increased and an ADCC assay forecast that the infant would be affected but there was no clinical disease. Herron et al. (206) studied two pregnant women, one with anti-Lu^b comprised primarily of IgG1 but with an IgG2 component, and the other with an IgG1 anti-Lu6 (see below). The anti-Lu^b had a titer of 128 throughout the pregnancy, the anti-Lu6 increased from a titer of 32 at 28 weeks to 128 at term. Both women delivered infants in whom the DAT was negative and in whom no maternally-derived Lutheran system antibody was present in the cord serum. Neither infant had any symptoms of HDN. In both instances the cord blood red cells were shown to be antigen-positive (i.e. Lu(b+) and Lu:6, respectively) using the maternal antibodies. Since the anti-Lu^b was predominantly, and the anti-Lu6 apparently only IgG1, and since IgG1 is known (207-209) to cross the placenta and be present in higher levels in cord than in maternal serum, the authors (206) suggested that in these two cases (and perhaps in others involving Lutheran system antibodies) the placenta had acted as a barrier in preventing transfer of the Lutheran system antibodies. Similar suggestions have been made about antibodies in the Cromer system (210 and see Chapter 24) and the Indian system (211 and see Chapter 29). Certainly the suggestion is compatible with the fact that no Lutheran system antibody has ever caused clinically significant HDN. Table 20-5 lists the most usual characteristics of Lutheran system antibodies and those that define para-Lutheran antigens and includes many antibodies that are described later in this chapter.

The Antigens Lu6 and Lu9 and the Antibodies That Define Them

Anti-Lu6 is directed against an antigen of very high incidence. The first example was described by Marsh et al. (29) in 1972 and several others have been described since then (110-113). The antibodies were made by individuals with Lu(a-b+) Lu:-6 red cells and reacted with all except Lu(a-b-) cells. All three types of Lu(a-b-) cells (i.e. *In(Lu)*, *LuLu* and *XS2* backgrounds) typed as Lu:-6. As

TABLE 20-5 Characteristics of Antibodies that Define Lutheran System and Para-Lutheran Antigens

Antibody Specificity	Positive Reactions in In Vitro Tests				Usual Immuno-globulin			Ability to Bind Complement		Ability to Cause In Vitro Lysis		Implicated in		Usual Form of Stimulation		% of White Population Positive
	Sal	LISS	AHG	Enz	IgG	IgM	IgA	Yes	No	Yes	No	Trans-fusion Reaction	HDN	Rbc	Other	
Anti-Lu^a	Most	Most	Rare		Few	Some		Some	Some		X	No	Very mild		Most	7.65
Anti-Lu^b	Few		Most		Some	Some	Some	Some	Some		X	Mild	Very mild	Most		99.85
Anti-Lu3			X		Most			Some	Some		X	Mild	No	X		>99.9
Anti-Lu9			X		X						X	No	No	X		1.7
Anti-Lu6			X		X						X	Poss	No	X		>99.9
Anti-Lu14			X		X						X	No	No	Most	Rare	1.5 to 2.4
Anti-Lu8			X		X						X	No	No	X		>99.9
Anti-Au^a			X		X						X		No	X		82-90
Anti-Au^b			X		X						X	No	No	X		51
Abs to Lu4, Lu5, Lu7, Lu11, Lu12, Lu13, Lu16, Lu17, Lu20	Very rare		Most		Most	Very rare					X	Poss	No	Most	Very rare	>99.9

expected, the Lu(a-b-) red cells of persons with *In(Lu)* were shown to adsorb and yield on elution, the more potent examples of anti-Lu6. The Lu6 antigen was seen to be inherited when first recognized (29), two sibs of the Lu:-6 proposita also had Lu:-6 red cells. In 1973, Molthan et al. (30) studied the serum of a Mrs. Mull. The serum contained anti-Lu^a and another antibody that reacted with the red cells of nine of 521 random donors. Mrs. Mull's husband had Lu(a+b+) red cells that also carried the antigen defined by the second antibody in his wife's serum. An extensive family study showed that when *Lu^a* was transmitted by any individual who was Lu(a+) and positive for the new antigen, it traveled without the gene encoding production of the new antigen. Whenever the gene encoding production of the new antigen, in an individual with Lu(a+) red cells was transmitted, it traveled with *Lu^b*, never with *Lu^a*. In the three generation family there were 14 non-recombinants and no recombinants. Since this proved that the new antigen was encoded from the *Lutheran* complex locus and that it was not an allele of *Lu^a* and *Lu^b*, the new antigen was called Lu9 and the encoding gene was called *Lu^9*. In the same study (30) it was shown that the red cells of the original Lu:-6 proposita, those of her two Lu:-6 sibs, and those of the second

Lu:-6 proband were Lu:9. Thus not only was Lu9 (originally called Mull) seen to be encoded from the *Lutheran* complex locus, it was also seen that *Lu^6* and *Lu^9* represent a second pair of alleles at that locus. In other words, in the family described above, all individuals with Lu(a+) Lu:9 red cells were genetically *Lu^{a}Lu^6/Lu^{9}Lu^b*.

Lu(a-b-) red cells are Lu:-6,-9. With one exception, all Lu:-6 red cells that are not Lu(a-b-), have been found to react strongly with anti-Lu9. The one exception involves a family (111) in which the proposita's Lu:-6 red cells reacted only weakly with anti-Lu9. The red cells of the proposita's sib, that were also Lu:-6 reacted strongly with anti-Lu9 but the mother, who one would expect to be an *Lu^{6}Lu^9* heterozygote also had red cells that reacted only weakly with anti-Lu9. At present these findings are not fully understood, the Lu(weak) phenotype (see below) did not seem to be involved. If the findings represent existence of a third allele at the *Lu^{6}Lu^9* sublocus, it might have to be postulated that the product of that allele cross-reacts with anti-Lu9 or that the original and still the only anti-Lu9 (the Mull serum) contains another antibody. In terms of another antibody, the Mull serum is known (91) to contain anti-HLA-B7. While presence of that antibody would not explain the findings in the unusual family (111) described above, its presence does mean that the estimate that 1.7% of random donors (i.e. nine of 521 (30)) have Lu:9 red cells, might be too high.

Not very much is known about anti-Lu6 and anti-Lu9 in terms of their clinical significance. Gibson et al. (112) studied a Pakistani infant who had thalassemia and had IgG1 and IgG2 anti-Lu6 in the serum. Because an in vivo red cell survival study and a macrophage binding assay suggested that the antibody would not clear antigen-positive red cells, several transfusions with Lu(a-b+), presumably Lu:6, red cells were given. No untoward effects were noticed and production of the anti-Lu6 eventually stopped. In sharp contrast, we (113) studied a 76 year-old White lady who had metastatic carcinoma of the lung and anemia caused by chemotherapy. She had been pregnant once but had never been transfused, her serum contained an IgG1 anti-Lu6 with a titer of 64. The patient was transfused with one unit of Lu(a-b-) blood from a donor with *In(Lu)*, suffered no untoward reaction and had the expected increment in hemoglobin. Because further transfusions were anticipated we performed an in vivo red cell survival study with Lu(a-b+) Lu:6 red cells. The survival of the injected cells was followed by the ^{51}Cr method and by differential labeling in a flow cytometer. Some 20% of the injected red cells were cleared in the first hour after injection and some 80% in the first 24 hours. An in vitro monocyte monolayer assay was also positive. The study proved two points. First, this example of anti-Lu6 was clearly of clinical significance, Lu:6 blood could not be used to support this patient. Second, although Lu(a-b-) red cells of the *In(Lu)* type will adsorb and yield on elution some examples of antibodies to high incidence Lutheran system and para-Lutheran antigens, such cells apparently survived normally or near normally in this patient with a clinically-significant anti-Lu6. Whether that means that such cells will survive normally in all patients with antibodies of this type, is not clear. In this instance red cells from the *In(Lu)* donor whose blood was transfused would not adsorb the patient's anti-Lu6.

The only known example of anti-Lu9 caused a weakly positive DAT on the red cells of Mrs. Mull's three infants but did not cause clinical HDN in any of them (30). As mentioned in the previous section, an anti-Lu6 with a titer of 128 by IAT, apparently failed to cross the placenta (206).

The Antigens Lu8 and Lu14 and the Antibodies That Define Them

Anti-Lu8 is directed against an antigen of very high incidence. The first example was described by MacIlroy et al. (43) in 1972 and others have been found (80,108).

The antibodies were made by individuals with Lu(a-b+) Lu:-8 red cells and were initially recognized when they reacted with all red cells except those of the Lu(a-b-) phenotype that were from individuals with *In(Lu)*. The Lu:-8 phenotype was shown to be an inherited condition when it was found (43) that the sister of the original proposita also had Lu:-8 red cells.

In 1977, Judd et al. (31) described a serum from Mrs. Hoff a White patient who had received many transfusions. Her serum reacted with the red cells of some 2.4% of random White donors. During specificity tests on the Hof serum, two important observations were made. First, the serum reacted strongly with Lu:-8 red cells, the reactions were stronger than those of other reactive samples that were Lu:8. This suggested, of course, that the antibody detected an antigen antithetical to Lu8 that was present in double dose on Lu:-8 red cells and in single dose on the reactive Lu:8 cells. Second, the Hof serum reacted with the Sw(a+) red cells of the original propositus with that antigen (114). Thus for a while it seemed that Lu8 and Sw^a might be antithetical. Earlier family studies (115-117) had suggested that Sw^a might be a Lutheran system antigen but this possibility had been excluded when a family was found (118) in which recombination between *Lu^a* and *Sw^a* was convincingly demonstrated. Judd et al. (31) then showed that: other Sw(a+) red cells were non-reactive with the Hof serum; the original Sw(a+) propositus had passed *Sw^a* to both of his children, but the Hof-defined antigen to only one of them; and that the original Sw(a+) propositus had a second low incidence antigen, i.e. that defined by the Hof serum, on his red cells. The antigen defined by the Hof serum was called Lu14, adsorption-elution studies using Sw(a+), Lu:14 and Sw(a+), Lu:-14 red cells confirmed that anti-Sw^a and anti-Lu14 have different and distinct specficities.

Additional evidence that *Lu^8* and *Lu^{14}* represent a third pair of alleles at the *Lutheran* complex locus (table 20-3) is available. First, linkage disequilibrium was noted when it was found that 14 of 580 random donors (1 in 41) had Lu:14 red cells but that only one Lu:14 sample was found when 220 selected Lu(a+b+) samples were tested (31). Second, Skov et al. (119) studied a family in which the non-recombinant:recombinant score between *Lu^{14}* and *Lu^9* was 4:0. Skov et al. (119) also found that 9 of 615 Danish and 11 of 600 English donors had Lu:14 red cells. One finding (120) that currently awaits explanation is that Lu:14 red cells gave higher titration scores than Lu:-14 red cells when tested with the monoclonal anti-Lu^b, BRIC 108.

Little is known about the clinical significance of anti-Lu8 and anti-Lu14. One of the published examples (108) of anti-Lu8 caused both a delayed and an immediate transfusion reaction, as expected retrospective

MMAs on the three units of least incompatible Lu:8 blood transfused, were positive. Another example found (80) in a pregnant woman did not cause clinical HDN in her infant. In addition to the original anti-Lu14 (31) at least 10 others are known (91) but few details about them have been published. The example reported by Marsh et al. (121) was made by a pregnant woman but the infant delivered after the antibody was made had Lu:-14 red cells. Ballem et al. (122) studied three women who had made anti-Lu14, each had a child with Lu:14 red cells but none of the infants suffered HDN.

The Antigens Au^a (Lu18) and Au^b (Lu19) and The Antibodies That Define Them

In 1961, Salmon et al. (32) described the first example of an antibody that reacted with the red cells of about 82% of random Whites and probably (70) with a similar percentage of those of random Blacks. The antigen defined was named Au^a for the antibody-maker, Madame Auberger (see 123, pronounced O-ber-ghay not Owberger!). Determining the exact frequency of the Au(a+) and Au(a-) phenotypes was difficult since the Auberger serum also contained antibodies to E, K, Fy^b and at least one of the Bg antigens (see Chapter 30). When the second example of Au^a was found (124) it was present in a serum that, in addition, contained antibodies to Lu^a, K, Fy^b, Yt^b and HLA-A7 (anti-Bg^a). The third example (33) was found in a serum that contained anti-Fy^a and anti-HLA-A2. Using the third example of anti-Au^a, Drachman et al. (33) found that 362 of 400 (90.5%) of random donors in Denmark had Au(a+) red cells. They found that the strength of Au^a varies greatly on the Au(a+) red cells of different donors. Thus it is not known if the 82% incidence of Au^a in France and England (32) is truly different from the 90.5% incidence in Denmark (33) or if the lower incidence in the earlier study represents the fact that the anti-Au^a had to be separated from many other antibodies and then, in the separated form, was unable to detect Au^a on red cells with the lowest expression of that antigen. For this reason, table 20-2 shows an incidence of 80 to 90% for Au^a.

That Au^a was associated with the Lutheran system was long suspected. As mentioned earlier, by 1976 (34,37) it was known that the red cells of 32 of 35 persons with the *In(Lu)* form of the Lu(a-b-) phenotype had Au(a-) red cells. Whether the incidence of Au^a is 82% or 90.5%, an incidence of 91.5% Au(a-) in the *In(Lu)* Lu(a-b-) phenotype was clearly indicative of some type of association. After anti-Au^b was found (36) (see below), it was shown (27,36-38) that Lu(a-b-) red cells of the *In(Lu)*, *LuLu* and *XS2* types are all Au(a-b-). It is not know if the three *In(Lu)* type Lu(a-b-) samples men-

tioned above as being Au(a+), reacted with the anti-Au^a serum because of the presence of one of the other antibodies (e.g. anti-Bg) or whether like some of the Lutheran system antigens, Au^a was weakly expressed on those red cells. When the above studies were performed it was believed that Au^a (and later Au^b) were phenotypically related to the Lutheran system but that their production was not encoded from the *Lutheran* complex locus. This belief was based on the finding (35) that in one French family, *Au^a* and *Lu^a* segregated independently. As described below, that family has since been reinvestigated (40) and it has been shown that such independent segregation did not occur.

In 1989, Frandson et al. (36) described the first example of anti-Au^b, the antibody defining the antigen antithetical to Au^a. The original anti-Au^b and three examples found (125) since the first, were all present in sera that contained anti-Lu^a. In tests with anti-Au^b, 112 of 220 (51%) of White donors in London and 59 of 87 (68%) Black Americans were found (36) to have Au(b+) red cells.

In 1990, Daniels (39) used immunoblotting and immunoprecipitation methods (see Chapter 4) to demonstrate that Au^a and Au^b are carried on the Lutheran glycoproteins. While this strongly suggested that production of the antigens is encoded from the *Lutheran* complex locus, it did not prove that point. However, the findings of Daniels (39) were sufficient to prompt reinvestigation of the family (35) in which segregation between the *Au^a* and *Lu^a* genes had been reported. The new investigation (40) showed that the phenotypically Lu(a+b+) Au(a+b+) father transmitted either *Lu^{a}Au^b* or *Lu^{b}Au^a* to five of his six children (the sixth child was non-informative). In the original investigation (35) two persons with Au(a+) red cells had been mistyped as Au(a-) (see above for a description of the difficulties encountered in typing tests with the original anti-Au^a, i.e. exactly as in this family in that some Au(a+) phenotypes were not detected). Zelinski et al. (126) had already shown that the gene encoding production of Au^b is located on chromosome 19 (as is the *Lutheran* locus, see below). The same investigators (41) then reviewed data from seven informative families and provided final proof that *Au^a* and *Au^b* represent a fourth pair of alleles at the *Lutheran* complex locus (see table 20-3).

Nothing is known about the clinical significance of anti-Au^a or anti-Au^b. The first two examples of anti-Au^a were found (32,124) in multiply transfused patients, neither had to be transfused with Au(a+) blood after the antibodies were recognized. The third example (33) was present in the serum of a woman who had never been transfused. It seems that the anti-Fy^a and anti-Au^a in her serum had been stimulated by a single pregnancy, 37 years earlier. The patient had to be transfused after the anti-Au^a had been detected, but before it had been identified. She was given two units of Fy(a-), IAT-compatible blood. The efficacy of this approach was demonstrated later when it was shown that both units transfused were Au(a-). All four individuals who made anti-Au[b] had been transfused earlier in their lives. Two were female but the abstract (125) describing the cases does not mention whether either had been pregnant. In none of the published cases did anti-Au[a] or anti-Au[b] have the opportunity to cause HDN.

The Lu(a-b-) Phenotypes. 1. The *In(Lu)* Variety

In 1961, Crawford et al. (21), while studying samples from the senior author's family members, showed that the Lu(a-b-) phenotype can be caused by presence of a single gene that is dominant in effect. The gene became known as *In(Lu)* (23) and it has been shown (22,23) that it does not reside at the *Lutheran* complex locus. Indeed, from various studies (62,63) it has been shown that *In(Lu)* is not at the *ABO*, *Se*, *Rh*, *Kell*, *Jk*, *MN*, *P^1*, *Yt*, *Co* or *HLA* loci, nor does it seem to be closely linked to any other blood group locus. Although as discussed in more detail below, *In(Lu)* does not always totally prevent expression of Lutheran system antigens (those present can usually only be demonstrated by adsorption-elution studies) the description of the red cells of persons with *In(Lu)* as Lu(a-b-) remains convenient. As also described more fully below, it is now well established that *In(Lu)* depresses expression of some red cell antigens that are genetically unrelated to the Lutheran system.

Since the original report by Crawford et al. (21), many other examples of the *In(Lu)* form of Lu(a-b-) red cells have been described (22-25,62,63,127-134). There are, of course, three major clues that suggest the presence of a dominant inhibitor gene in a family. First, its effects are seen in successive generations, a situation not usually associated with the inheritance of rare recessive genes. Indeed for a rare recessive condition to be seen in successive generations it is necessary for the mating to involve a homozygote and a heterozygote for the gene involved. Such an event occurs regularly when the recessive gene is common, e.g. *OO* X *AO* producing *OO* offspring. Second, when enough families are studied, it is seen that about 50% of the offspring of parents with a dominant gene, inherit that gene themselves (one in two chance in each conception). Again, this is unlike recessive inheritance where roughly 25% of the offspring of two parents heterozygous for a silent allele are homozygous for that gene and therefore display its full effects. Third, an individual with a dominant suppressor gene that is not at a blood group locus, can pass a normal allele at that locus to his or her children and in the

absence of inheritance of the dominant suppressor, that gene will function (antigen made) in the child. Because *Lu^a* is rare and *Lu^b* is very common, most persons whose red cells type as Lu(a-b-) because they have inherited *In(Lu)*, are genetically *Lu^bLu^b*. Thus, when such an individual passes a functional *Lutheran* gene, it is *Lu^b*. However, the passage of a functional *Lu^a* gene from an individual with *In(Lu)* has been seen (22,23). Because, in those families, there were double heterozygotes, that is *Lu^aLu^b* and heterozygous for *In(Lu)*, it was possible to show that *In(Lu)* is not at the *Lutheran* locus.

Although it is still rare, the Lu(a-b-) phenotype has a higher incidence than that of minus-minus phenotypes in most other blood group systems. In two surveys in England the incidence was 79 in about 250,000 donors (1 in 3164) (62) and 1 in 3197 (130). However, in another large survey in Wales the incidence was lower, i.e. 15 in 75,614 or 1 in 5040 (63) and in another, lower still, i.e. 1 in 18,069 (25). In Houston, when anti-CD44 (see below) was used (132) to screen 42,000 bloods, eight Lu(a-b-) (1 in 5250) samples were found while in a study in Portland using anti-AnWj (again see below and Chapter 29) three Lu(a-b-) samples were found among 2400 tested, i.e. 1 in 800 (134). In the only reported study on samples from Black donors, two in 7341 (1 in 3670) tested in Detroit were Lu(a-b-) (133). In Taiwan, one of 1922 Chinese donors was found to have the Lu(a-b-) phenotype (67,68). As mentioned above and as described in more detail below, there are three genetic backgrounds that lead to the Lu(a-b-) phenotype. Thus the figures given above cannot be taken to represent only the incidence of *In(Lu)*. However, as described below, *In(Lu)* is considerably more common that *XS2* and the *LuLu* genotype (34,387) and it can be anticipated that most of the Lu(a-b-) samples found in surveys on random donors, represented individuals with *In(Lu)*.

In 1967, Stanbury and Francis (24) reported that Lu(a-b-) red cells of the *In(Lu)* variety would adsorb and yield on elution, anti-Lu[b]. In many of the subsequent studies on high incidence Lutheran system and para-Lutheran antigens (references given in later sections) it has been found that the same is true of antibodies directed against those antigens. On those rare occasions that the individual with *In(Lu)* also has a gene for one of the low incidence Lutheran system antigens, a similar finding may be made. For example, in the family described by Taliano et al. (23), the red cells of genetically *In(Lu)*, *Lu^aLu^b* individuals were found to adsorb and yield on elution, both anti-Lu[a] and anti-Lu[b]. As with other individuals with *In(Lu)*, the red cells typed as Lu(a-b-) in direct tests. In a later section of this chapter, the Lu(w) (for Lu(weak)) phenotype is described. In that phenotype expression of Lutheran system, para-Lutheran and some other antigens is markedly depressed but the antigens can be shown to be present when direct tests are performed. It is not yet known, but it is strongly suspected that the phenotype results from the inheritance of a gene similar in effect to *In(Lu)* but less efficient in its inhibitory abilities. It would not be surprising to find that *In(Lu)* represents a number of alleles (like *h*, see Chapter 8).

Again as mentioned below, the Lu(a-b-) red cells of persons genetically *LuLu* lack all representation of Lutheran and para-Lutheran antigens. Those of individuals with *XS2* are like those of persons with *In(Lu)* in that they will adsorb and yield on elution, antibodies to the depressed antigens that they carry. Some workers have taken these observations to mean that the genetic background of an individual with red cells that type as Lu(a-b-) can be determined at the serological level. This is not true. While red cells that type as Lu(a-b-) but adsorb and yield anti-Lu^b can be said, with confidence, not to represent the *LuLu* genotype, the converse does not apply. That is to say, the red cells of some persons proved by family study to be of the *In(Lu)* type of Lu(a-b-) have failed to adsorb any Lutheran system antibodies (21,128). Again it is tempting to speculate that the Lu(a-b-) phenotype in this setting may represent the presence of different alleles of *In(Lu)*.

Individuals with Lu(a-b-) red cells of the *In(Lu)* variety do not make Lutheran system antibodies. Many women with *In(Lu)* have delivered infants who had Lutheran system antigens on their red cells. Many people with *In(Lu)* must have been transfused with antigen positive (most often Lu(a-b+), Lu:3,4 etc.) blood before (or perhaps after) their Lu(a-b-) status was recognized. It is presumed that the trace amount of Lutheran system and para-Lutheran antigens (at least those of high incidence) on the red cells of persons with *In(Lu)* results in the immune system of those individuals not recognizing the antigens as foreign. The production of say anti-Lu^a by an individual genetically *In(Lu)*, *Lu^{b}Lu^b*, while never reported, would not violate the presumed rule.

The Lu(a-b-) Phenotypes. 2. The *LuLu* Variety and Anti-Lu3

In 1963, Darnborough et al. (25) described a woman with Lu(a-b-) red cells whose serum contained an antibody that reacted with all except her own and *In(Lu)* type Lu(a-b-) cells. Although the point was not proved for certain, the antibody made and the facts that the proposita's children had Lu(a-b+) red cells that appeared to carry a single dose of Lu^b and that no other family members had the Lu(a-b-) phenotype, suggested that the proposita's phenotype represented the presence of two silent alleles (*Lu*) at the *Lutheran* locus. Such a conclusion was supported by the finding of other families (26,135,136) in

which the *LuLu*, genotype could be seen to be present. In the Canadian family described by Brown et al. (26) one Lu(a-b-) X Lu(a+b+) mating had produced one child with Lu(a+b-) and one with Lu(a-b+) red cells. In other words, the mating was *LuLu* X *Lu^{a}Lu^b* producing *LuLu^a* and *LuLu^b* children. Brown et al. (26) also mention a family studied but not published by Crookston and Crookston (137) in which the mating Lu(a+b+) X Lu(a-b+) produced two Lu(a+b-) children, i.e. *Lu^{a}Lu^b* X *LuLu^b* producing *Lu^{a}Lu* children. Thus the first family in which the *LuLu* genotype was present was English (25), the second (26) was Canadian while *Lu* was clearly present in another Canadian family (137). The next three families found to have *LuLu* members were Japanese (135,136). All except the English family are predated by a 1965 abstract (138) in which a Black patient with Lu(a-b-) red cells and anti-Lu3 (see below) in the serum, is described. Although no family study could be performed, presence of anti-Lu3 (called anti-Lu^{ab} in 1965) in the serum was highly suggestive of the fact that the patient was genetically *LuLu*. As expected for a rare recessively inherited condition, consanguinity was known in several of the families in which the *LuLu* genotype was found (26,135,136).

There are a number of indications that suggest the presence of *Lu*. First, the Lu(a-b-) individuals never pass *Lu^a* or *Lu^b* to their children because they lack those genes (*Lu* is at the *Lutheran* locus). Second, obligate heterozygotes for *Lu* (the parents and children of *LuLu* individuals) have red cells on which single doses of Lutheran antigens (usually Lu^b) may be demonstrated by serological means. Third, the Lu(a-b-) phenotype is not expected to be seen in successive generations. This is because the mating *LuLu* X *Lu^{b}Lu* is rare, even in inbred families. The Lu(a-b-) phenotype, when it represents the genotype *LuLu*, differs from the Lu(a-b-) phenotype representing *In(Lu)* in some other ways as well. The red cells of persons genetically *LuLu* are Lu(a-b-) Lu:-3,-4,-5,-6,-7,-8, -9,-11,-12,-13,-14,-16,-17,-20 Au(a-b-). They lack the trace amounts of Lutheran system and para-Lutheran antigens found on the Lu(a-b-) red cells of persons with *In(Lu)* and *XS2*.

As a result of total lack of Lutheran system antigens from their red cells, persons genetically *LuLu* can make Lutheran system antibodies. The first example of anti-Lu3 was found in the serum of the proposita studied by Darnborough et al. (25). The antibody behaved like anti-Lu^{ab} in that it reacted equally well with Lu(a+b-) and Lu(a-b+) red cells. That it was not a mixture of separable anti-Lu^a and anti-Lu^b became clear when it was shown that the antibody could be adsorbed by either Lu(a+b-) or Lu(a-b+) red cells and that eluates made from the adsorbing cells reacted equally with cells of the two phenotypes. As will already be apparent, Lutheran system and related antigens beyond Lu^a and Lu^b are generally described in the numerical terminology. Accordingly, the antibody made by genetically *LuLu* persons is most often called anti-Lu3 and not anti-Lu[ab]. The antibody is often found in the sera of *LuLu* type Lu(a-b-) persons, indeed such persons are sometimes identified as being phenotypically Lu(a-b-) during investigation of an antibody, to a very common antigen, in their serum. Not very much is known about the clinical significance of anti-Lu3. The patient described by Myhre et al. (135) was transfused with several units of Lu(a-b-) blood on two different occasions. While no details about the genetic backgrounds of the donors are given, it is mentioned that the first four units were obtained from the National Reference Laboratory of the Canadian Red Cross and a later transfused four from the rare donor file of the US Red Cross and the New York Blood Center. Perhaps this means that the first four were from *LuLu* donors since persons of that genotype had been found in Canada, while the latter four were from *In(Lu)* donors since most Lu(a-b-) bloods in the USA are from such individuals. Regardless of the source of the units (the above is a guess), all units were transfused without incident and effected the expected increments in hemoglobin. As with the anti-Lu6 described in an earlier section, we hope that this means that the traces of Lutheran system and para-Lutheran antigens on the red cells of persons with *In(Lu)* are of no moment when such blood is transfused to persons with antibodies directed against those antigens. It is also worthy of comment that anti-Lu3 is usually seen in *LuLu* type Lu(a-b-) individuals who have previously been exposed to foreign red cells via transfusion or pregnancy (26,135,136,138). In a number of instances males and females who have not been transfused and females who have not been pregnant have been seen to be of the *LuLu* type of Lu(a-b-) with no anti-Lu3 in the serum. The antibody does not ever seem to have caused clinical HDN.

In addition to the serological data described above, the place of Lu3 in the Lutheran system has been strengthened by other findings. Both human (163) and monoclonal (39,164) antibodies have been used in immunoblotting experiments to show that Lu3 is carried on the Lutheran glycoproteins (see below). A similar finding was made using the monoclonal antibody-specific immobilization of erythrocyte antigen (MAIEA) method (165).

The Lu(a-b-) Phenotypes. 3. The *XS2* Variety

In 1986, Norman et al. (27) reported their study on five Lu(a-b-) samples found in a large Australian family. *In(Lu)* was excluded as the cause because three of the Lu(a-b-) individuals were the results of two Lu(a-b+) X Lu(a-b+) matings, i.e. neither of the parents had *In(Lu)*. *LuLu* was excluded as the cause since, for it to be responsible, five unrelated individuals would have had to have

been *Lu* heterozygotes, obviously an impossible coincidence since *Lu* is no more common in Australia than elsewhere. The inheritance of the Lu(a-b-) phenotype was explained by the presumption that an X-borne inhibitor gene prevents normal expression of Lutheran antigens by the independently inherited *Lutheran* genes. It was already well established (22-25,62,63,127-134) that *In(Lu)* is not carried on the X-chromosome. In the family studied (27) all Lu(a-b-) members were male, none of them passed the phenotype directly to a child. This, of course, reflects the fact that sons of males receive the paternal Y chromosome while daughters receive both a paternal and a maternal X. In other words, daughters of an Lu(a-b-) male of this type may be carriers of the condition (paternal X) but will be unaffected since they will receive a normal maternal X chromosome. The family showed that all five Lu(a-b-) males would have received a maternally donated X traceable to a common original ancestor. The locus at which the suppressor gene must be located was called *XS* (27), the common allele that allows the *Lutheran* genes present to express their products (antigens) was called *XS1*, and the rare inhibitor or suppressor gene was called *XS2*.

Lu(a-b-) red cells of the *XS2* variety are serologically similar to those of the *In(Lu)* variety in that while they initially type as Lu(a-b-), they are capable of adsorbing and yielding on elution anti-Lu[b]. No individual in the family had *Lu[a]*. None of the Lu(a-b-) individuals had a Lutheran antibody in the serum, again it would be presumed that the trace of Lu[b], and presumably other high incidence Lutheran system and para-Lutheran antigens, on their red cells, would serve to prevent their recognition of those antigens as foreign. Lu(a-b-) red cells of the *XS2* variety do not yet seem to have been tested with antibodies to Lu11, Lu13, Lu16 or Lu20. Red cells representing this genetic background do differ in other respects from Lu(a-b-) red cells representing the *In(Lu)* background. Those differences are described below in a section dealing with the effects of *In(Lu)* and *XS2* on expression of non-Lutheran system antigens. If other examples of the *XS2* type of the Lu(a-b-) phenotype have been found, they do not appear to have been described in print. In a genetic analysis study, it was found (139) that the *XS* locus is apparently close to that of *DXS14*, a DNA marker that is near to the centromere, but that *XS* is not close to *Xg* (see Chapter 25).

The Lu(a-b-) Phenotypes. 4. An Acquired Example and Depression of Expression of Lu[b]

Williamson et al. (161) described a patient with autoantibody-induced thrombocytopenia whose red cells had marked depression of expression of Kell system antigens and whose serum contained an antibody with an anti-

Ku-like specificity. At the time that the Kell system anti-gens were depressed the patient's red cells expressed their Lutheran system and LW^a antigens normally. When the patient was treated, the expression of Kell system antigens on his red cells returned to normal and production of the anti-Ku-like specificity stopped. However, during a subse-quent relapse, the patient's red cells typed as Lu(a-b-) and his serum contained an anti-Lu3-like specificity. At that time the expression of LW^a on his red cells was markedly depressed. A somewhat similar case was reported by Leger et al. (212). A 74 year-old dialysis patient was thought to have had a delayed transfusion reaction caused by anti-Lan (see Chapter 31) at a time that her red cells typed as Lan-. Some time later, the patient's red cells were found to type as Lan+ and anti-Lan was no longer detectable in her serum. Five months after that, the patient's red cells typed as Lan+, Lu(a+b-) and her serum contained weak anti-Lu^b. Four years later, the patient's blood was studied again, her red cells now typed as Lu(b+) and no antibodies were detectable in her serum.

The Lu(w) or Lu(weak) Phenotype

The term Lu(w) was introduced (29) when it was noticed that some Lu(a-b-) red cells of the *In(Lu)* type react, albeit weakly, with anti-Lu3. Other examples have been found (38,140) that react similarly with anti-Lu3, appear to be Lu(a-b-) when tested with some anti-Lu^a and anti-Lu^b, but give weak reactions when tested (140) with other examples of those specificities. As described in the next section, the presence of *In(Lu)* results in depression of expression of antigens in several systems genetically independent of Lutheran. Red cells of the Lu(w) phenotype often show depression of expression of those antigens as well. However, as others (34,38,70,91) have pointed out, many of those antigens, like Lu^a and Lu^b themselves, show considerable varia-tion in strength of expression on the red cells of normal individuals (i.e. those without *In(Lu)*) anyway. Nevertheless it is entirely possible that the Lu(w) phe-notypes represent the presence of *In(Lu)* in different environments or (perhaps more likely) the existence of alleles with slightly different effects, all of which have been grouped under the banner of *In(Lu)*. The Lu(w) phenotype, if it exists as a separate entity can, perhaps, be classified as one in which the antigen AnWj (see below and Chapter 29) can be detected in direct tests (29,38) whereas in the *In(Lu)* determined Lu(a-b-) phe-notype, the presence of AnWj can be detected only by very sensitive (e.g. adsorption-elution) methods. The relationship of Lu(w) to the *In(Lu)* type of Lu(a-b-) is further illustrated by the fact that both are dominantly inherited characteristics.

In(Lu), *XS2* and Non-Lutheran System Antigens

As mentioned already, the presence of *In(Lu)* or *XS2* results in depression of expression of all Lutheran system and para-Lutheran antigens. In addition, presence of one of these genes is often associated with decreased expression of other, genetically independent red cell anti-gens. Crawford et al. (37) noted an excess of the pheno-type P$_2$ and a reduction in the expected incidence of the antigen P$_1$, in persons with *In(Lu)*. Others (62,130) con-firmed that P$_1$, if detectable at all, is weakened on the red cells of persons with *In(Lu)*. In 1974, Contreras et al. (129) described a, by-then expected, event in which a phenotypically P$_2$, Lu(a-b-) X P$_2$, Lu(a-b+) mating pro-duced a phenotypically P$_1$, Lu(a-b+) child. Clearly, *P^1* was donated by the *In(Lu)* Lu(a-b-) parent in whom that gene made too little antigen for detection with anti-P$_1$. Other similar findings have since been reported (62,63). It has been shown (37,62,63,130) that in this situation, the same *P^1* gene produces the expected amount of P$_1$ antigen when inherited by a family member who does not inherit *In(Lu)*. Further, the distribution of *P^1* is exact-ly as expected among the relatives of persons with *In(Lu)* who do not inherit that inhibitor gene (70). In the only family with the *XS2* form of the Lu(a-b-) phenotype, P$_1$ expression was depressed (27) but it was not clear whether *XS2* depressed the expression of P$_1$ or whether the *P^1* gene in the family made only low levels of the antigen. No depression of expression of P$_1$ was seen on the Lu(a-b-) red cells of persons genetically *LuLu* (37).

The i antigen on the red cells of adults reacts only weakly with most anti-i (see Chapter 10). In individuals who inherit *In(Lu)*, i antigen expression is even weaker (37,62,129) as judged by many but not all anti-i. As described in Chapter 10, cord blood cells have a high expression of i; there was no marked suppression of expression of that antigen on the red cells of three of four newborns who had inherited *In(Lu)* and only modest depression on the red cells of the fourth (141). Lu(a-b-) red cells of persons genetically *LuLu* express i in a normal (for adults) level (37). The red cells of individuals with the *XS2* type of the Lu(a-b-) phenotype carried normal or enhanced levels (again for adults) of i (27). I antigen levels do not seem to be affected by the presence of *In(Lu)* (37).

As described in Chapter 29, the In^a and In^b antigens are carried on a glycoprotein called CD44 (142). Telen et al. (131,143) showed that the presence of *In(Lu)* marked-ly reduces expression of CD44 on red cells. As a result, Lu(a-b-) red cells of the *In(Lu)* type have reduced, but nev-ertheless detectable (131,142) levels of In^a and In^b. The CD44 glycoprotein and the In^b antigen were found to be present in normal levels on the Lu(a-b-) red cells of per-sons genetically *LuLu* (142,144) and those genetically *XS2*

(27). As also described in Chapter 29, the high incidence antigen AnWj (55,56,145-148) may well also be carried on CD44 (160). One of the pieces of evidence pointing to such a conclusion is that Lu(a-b-) red cells of the *In(Lu)* variety type as AnWj- (145,146,148 at that time the antigen was known as both Anton and Wj). Indeed, the term Lu15 was originally (151) reserved for Anton (later shown (55,56) to be the same as Wj) but the antigen was excluded from the Lutheran system and the term Lu15 was declared obsolete after Poole and Giles (147) showed that Lu(a-b-) red cells of the *LuLu* type express Anton (AnWj) normally. It is now appreciated (148) that Lu(a-b-) red cells of the *In(Lu)* type express AnWj similarly to the way in which they express Lu^b, Lu3, Lu4, et al. In the only family in which inheritance of AnWj has been documented, the gene that encodes its production was shown (152) to segregate independently of *Lu^a*.

Although less widely investigated, one study (153) has documented the fact that antigens of the Knops system, Kn^a, McC^a, Sl^a and Yk^a (see Chapter 28) and the antigen Cs^a (see Chapter 30) are depressed on Lu(a-b-) red cells of the *In(Lu)* type. The authors point out that the suppression of antigen expression is less marked than that seen with P$_1$ and i. Indeed family studies, comparing expression of these antigens on the red cells of persons in the same family, some of whom have *In(Lu)* and some of whom are of the Lu(a-b+) phenotype, may be necessary to recognize suppression.

In one family with nine individuals of the *In(Lu)* variety of the Lu(a-b-) phenotype, evidence was obtained (75) that *In(Lu)* may suppress expression of the MER2 (see Chapter 31) antigen.

The findings discussed in this section have called into question the suitability of the name *In(Lu)* for the inhibitor, modifying or suppressor gene involved. As mentioned earlier it has long been known (22,23) that *In(Lu)* does not reside at the *Lutheran* complex locus. The fact that antigens of so many different blood group systems are affected is not conveyed by the term *In(Lu)* that implies (70) a somewhat exclusive relationship to the Lutheran system. Marsh et al. (154) proposed that the locus involved be renamed *SYN-1* (for synthesis and the first gene at that locus). *SYN-1A* would be used to describe the gene at that locus that allows normal synthesis of the antigens, *SYN-1B* would be the allele (*In(Lu)*) that blocks such synthesis. However, Shaw and Tippett (155) pointed out that nothing is known about how *In(Lu)* exerts its effects and to claim that it interferes with antigen synthesis might result in the introduction of yet another term, later, if *In(Lu)* acts in some other manner. No general agreement has been reached and the name *In(Lu)* has continued to be used by most workers. We agree with sentiments expressed by Daniels (75) who points out that at the rate that biochemical understanding

of the nature of antigens affected by *In(Lu)* is increasing it is likely that soon the mechanism of action of *In(Lu)* will be understood. He (75) writes "Surely the renaming of the gene could wait until then, to avoid the danger of introducing another inappropriate notation".

In later sections of this chapter on the biochemistry of the Lutheran system, the effects of the presence of *In(Lu)* on some red cell membrane-borne structures are discussed in detail. To complete this section it will be mentioned that one such structure, CDw75 is increased on Lu(a-b-) red cells of the *In(Lu)* type. CDw75 is present on lymphocytes and red cells and is recognized by a number of monoclonal antibodies (156). An alpha-2→6-sialic acid residue is an essential portion of the CDw75 determinant (157). Red cell agglutination and binding assays with radiolabeled antibody were used (158) to show that the level of CDw75 is higher on Lu(a-b-) red cells of the *In(Lu)* type than on those from persons who do not have *In(Lu)*. The level of CDw75 was normal on Lu(a-b-) red cells of the *LuLu* type, the determinant was not detected on Lu(a-b-) red cells of the *XS2* variety (159). Cord red blood cells including those from infants with *In(Lu)* were non-reactive with monoclonal anti-CDw75 (159). In spite of the essential nature of the sialic acid residue to CDw75 structure mentioned above (157), one of three monoclonal anti-CDw75 continued to react with sialidase-treated red cells (159). A reason for including these brief details about CDw75 here relates to the name *In(Lu)*. As discussed in the previous paragraph, the *(Lu)* portion of that name is no longer very suitable since antigens of so many other systems are affected by the presence of the gene. In terms of CDw75 the *In* portion of the name is no more suitable since CDw75 is increased, not inhibited, on Lu(a-b-) red cells of the *In(Lu)* variety. This observation also suggests that *SYN-1B* would have been no more appropriate than *In(Lu)* unless the *SYN* designation could have been regarded as increasing synthesis of some antigens and decreasing that of others.

The Antigen Lu4 and the Antibody That Defines It

In 1971, Bove et al. (28) described a White woman who had been pregnant twice and who had been transfused in the past. Her red cells were phenotypically Lu(a-b+) and her serum contained anti-K and an antibody to a high frequency antigen. That antibody reacted with all except Lu(a-b-) red cells and was named anti-Lu4. Among 17 non-reactive Lu(a-b-) samples, three were from persons genetically *LuLu*, the remaining 14 were from persons with *In(Lu)* or persons in whom the genetic background of the Lu(a-b-) phenotype was not known.

Two of the proposita's five sibs had Lu(a-b+) Lu:-4 red cells, in the other three the phenotype was Lu(a-b+) Lu:4. Thus Lu4 has been shown to be an inherited characteristic. Evidence supporting but not proving the conclusion that Lu4 is a Lutheran system antigen has been obtained in other studies. Immunoblotting with human (163) and monoclonal (39,164) antibodies indicated that Lu4 is carried on the Lutheran glycoproteins (for details about those structures, see below). A similar conclusion was reached in studies using the monoclonal antibody-specific immobilization of erythrocyte antigens (MAIEA) method (165). In spite of this evidence, Lu4 is still regarded as a high incidence para-Lutheran antigen since its production has not yet been proved to be encoded from the *Lutheran* locus. As far as we are aware the Lu:-4 individuals and anti-Lu4 described by Bove et al. (28) are still the only known examples.

The Antigen Lu5 and the Antibody That Defines It

The first two examples of anti-Lu5 were identified at an ICII wet workshop in 1970 and described in print in 1972 (29). Both were made by women, one of whom was Black and the other White, who had been pregnant and transfused and both of whom had Lu(a-b+) Lu:3,4 red cells. The antibodies and red cells of the two women were mutually compatible. The anti-Lu5 reacted with all except Lu(a-b-) red cells, both *In(Lu)* and *LuLu* type samples were included in the original investigation. Another example of anti-Lu5 was described later in 1972 (162) this time in the serum of a Black woman who had been pregnant three times but who had not been transfused. The antibody-maker's red cells were Lu(a-b+) Lu:3,4,-5,6,7,8 (for Lu6 and Lu8 see earlier in this chapter, for Lu7, see below). A sister of the proposita had red cells of the same Lutheran phenotype; the sister had never been pregnant or transfused and her serum contained no atypical antibodies. The proposita's brother had red cells of the same Lutheran phenotype as his sisters save that they were Lu:5. While the family study did not prove linkage between *Lu5* and the *Sese* locus (*Lutheran* and *Secretor* are known to be linked, see earlier) the findings were compatible with such linkage. In addition to the cases cited above, at least five other examples of anti-Lu5 have been found (91). In the original study (29) 423 random samples, mostly from White donors, were tested, all were Lu:5. The Lu5 antigen has been shown to be inherited (162), the Lu:-5 phenotype has been found in both Whites and Blacks (29,91,162) but the encoding gene has not yet been shown to be part of the *Lutheran* complex locus. Thus Lu5 is still considered to be a high incidence para-Lutheran antigen.

The Antigen Lu7 and the Antibody That Defines It

The first example of anti-Lu7 was made by a White woman who had been pregnant five times but who had never been transfused (29). Her red cell phenotype was Lu(a-b+) Lu:3,4,5,6. Her antibody reacted with all cells except those that were Lu(a-b-), samples from donors with *In(Lu)* and the *LuLu* genotype were included in the original study. The antibody-maker had three sibs all of whom had Lu(a-b+) red cells. One brother had Lu:-7 red cells, another brother and a sister had Lu:7 cells. Thus Lu7 was seen to be inherited from the time it was first found (29). Another woman with Lu(a-b+) Lu:3,4,5,6,-7,8 (for Lu8 see earlier) red cells and an antibody reactive with all except *In(Lu)* and *LuLu* type Lu(a-b-) red cells was described later (166) but Lu:-7 red cells from the original family were not available to confirm the specificity of her antibody. In the original study (29) all of 285 random samples, most of which were from Whites, were found to be Lu:7. In view of the above data, Lu7 remains as a high incidence para-Lutheran antigen.

The Antigen Lu11 and the Antibody That Defines It

Gralnick et al. (44) described the first example of anti-Lu11 in the serum of a White woman who had been pregnant four times and who had received transfusions in the past. The patient's medical records suggested that the transfusions not the pregnancies provided the immunizing event. The antibody-maker's red cells were Lu(a-b+) Lu:3,4,5,6,7,8,-9. The anti-Lu11 in her serum was IgM in nature and caused agglutination similar to that seen with anti-Lu^a (see earlier). The anti-Lu11 reacted with all red cells from adults tested, except the patient's own and those of 11 persons with *In(Lu)* and those of two persons with the *LuLu* form of Lu(a-b-). Red cells of the *XS2* type of Lu(a-b-) have not yet been tested with anti-Lu11. The Lu11 antigen is apparently less well developed at birth than Lu^b for in tests on 20 cord blood samples, all of which were Lu(a-b+), anti-Lu11 reacted weakly with two and failed to agglutinate the other 18. At least two other examples of anti-Lu11 have been identified (91) but in none of the cases could Lu11 be shown to be an inherited characteristic. In the original study (44) 500 random samples that were mostly from Whites and 32 known to be from Blacks, were Lu:11. Thus Lu11 remains as a high incidence para-Lutheran antigen and like some others, described below, has not yet been shown to be inherited.

The Antigen Lu12 and the Antibody That Defines It

The story of Lu12 is a little different from those about other high incidence para-Lutheran antigens. The first example of anti-Lu12 was found by Sinclair et al. (45) in the serum of a woman of Polish and Ukrainian extraction during the antibody-maker's second pregnancy, the woman had never been transfused. The red cells of the antibody-maker were Lu(a-b+^{w}), that is their Lu^b antigen was only weakly expressed. The same Lu(a-b+^{w}) phenotype was seen in the proposita's sister whose red cells were also Lu:-12 and in her father, whose red cells were Lu:12. Two other sibs and the proposita's mother had Lu(a-b+) red cells on which Lu^b was expressed normally, all three had cells that were Lu:12. In tests with antibodies to Lu3, Lu4 and Lu6, the red cells of the three persons of the Lu(a-b+^{w}) phenotype reacted generally less strongly than those of the three family members with Lu(a-b+) cells that had a normal expression of Lu^b. The red cells of the proposita also gave only weakly positive reactions when tested with antibodies to Lu5, Lu7, Lu8, Lu11 and Lu13 (see below). As expected, her red cells lacked the low incidence antigen Lu9. One possibility seemed to be that in the presence of the gene that fails to encode production of Lu12 (i.e. proposita and her sister homozygotes, the father a heterozygote) other Lutheran system antigens are poorly expressed. The main argument against such a conclusion is that recombination between the gene failing to make Lu12 and the *Sese* genes was seen in the family. Since the *Lutheran* and *Secretor* loci are known to be linked (see earlier) this finding provided odds of 9 to 1 against the gene not making Lu12 being at the *Lutheran* complex locus. It was suggested (45) that in this family the Lu(w) phenotype (see above) and the Lu:-12 phenotype were genetically unrelated events.

The anti-Lu12 made by the proposita, like the second example described below, reacted with all cells except those of the Lu(a-b-) phenotype. Both *In(Lu)* and *LuLu* varieties of Lu(a-b-) red cells were tested. In screening tests on 1050 random Canadian donors, all except one sample reacted strongly with the proposita's anti-Lu12. The red cells of one donor reacted weakly and, like the red cells of the proposita's father (an obligate heterozygote for the gene not making Lu12) were of the Lu(a-b+^{w}) phenotype.

The second example of anti-Lu12 was found (167) in the serum of a White woman, two of whose sibs were also phenotypically Lu:-12. The abstract states that the antibody-maker's red cells were Lu(a-b+) no comment is made about the strength of the Lu^b antigen on her cells nor are details given regarding the Lutheran phenotypes of her two sibs with Lu:-12 red cells. Thus the findings in the original family (45) remain unexplained in terms of whether the presence of a gene failing to make Lu12 results in down regulation of expression of other Lutheran system and para-Lutheran antigens.

The anti-Lu12 in the serum of the original proposita (45) did not cause HDN, indeed her infant who was of the Lu(a-b+) Lu:12 phenotype, had a negative DAT at birth. The second anti-Lu12 reported (167) was non-reactive in a mononuclear phagocytic assay but caused accelerated clearance of Lu:12 red cells in an in vivo red cell survival study. One ml of ^{51}Cr labeled Lu:12 red cells were injected, survival rates were: 96.1% at 10 minutes; 85.4% at 1 hour; 50% at 24 hours and 38.3% at 96 hours.

Because of the findings in the original family (45) the authors forecast that *Lu^{12}* would eventually be shown not to be at the *Lutheran* complex locus. In the paper describing the case the term Much (after the antibody-maker) was preferred to the term Lu12. Others (70,123) similarly concluded that Lu12 was probably not encoded from the *Lutheran* locus. However, it now seems that those forecasts may have been incorrect since immunoblotting studies have shown (163) that Lu12 is present on the Lutheran glycoproteins.

Of particular note, in the original Much family (45) the red cells of the three members with the Lu(a-b+^{w}) or Lu(w) phenotype and those of the three members with the Lu(a-b+) phenotype in which Lu^b was expressed normally, reacted to the same degree with the Anton serum. At the time that the investigation was performed, the Anton serum had the provisional name of anti-Lu15 and was thought to define a high incidence para-Lutheran antigen. As discussed earlier in this chapter (section on *In(Lu)*, *XS2* and non-Lutheran system antigens) and in more detail in Chapter 29, the Anton (now AnWj) antigen (145-150) is now believed (160) to be carried on CD44. AnWj expression is down regulated in the presence of *In(Lu)* but AnWj is not a Lutheran system or a para-Lutheran antigen. Thus in retrospect, it is easy to understand why Anton (AnWj) was not depressed on the red cells of the individuals homozygous or heterozygous for the gene not producing Lu12, *In(Lu)* was not involved and AnWj is not encoded from the *Lutheran* locus.

The Antigen Lu13 and the Antibody That Defines It

The high incidence para-Lutheran antigen Lu13 has never been published in its own right. The Lu13 designation was reserved (168,169) for an antigen present on all except Lu(a-b-) red cells and defined by an antibody in a serum Hughes. The Lu:-13 phenotype is mentioned in other publications about the Lutheran system (148,170) and in one abstract (47) it is stated that a patient with Wj-, Lu:-13 red cells had two sibs with Wj+, Lu:-13 and three with Wj+, Lu:13 red cells. We do not know if the Hughes serum, the only one ever described as containing anti-Lu13, is still available. Red cells of the *XS2* variety of the Lu(a-b-) phenotype have not been tested with anti-Lu13.

The Antigen Lu16 and the Antibody That Defines It

Anti-Lu16 differs from other antibodies to high incidence Lutheran system and para-Lutheran antigens in that the three known examples (48) were all made by women with Lu(a+b-) red cells. All three antibody-makers were Black and all three made anti-Lu^b as well as anti-Lu16. The red cells and antibodies of the three antibody-makers were mutually compatible. Thus it is possible that just as *Lu^a* and *Lu^b* encode production of Lu^a and Lu3, and Lu^b and Lu3, respectively, *Lu^b* also encodes production of Lu16. Anti-Lu16 reacted with all red cells except those of the Lu(a-b-) phenotype, both *In(Lu)* and *LuLu* types were non-reactive, those of the *XS2* type were not tested. Anti-Lu16 specificity was assigned based on the finding that anti-Lu16 reacted with other Lu(a+b-) red cells but neither abstract published (48,172) about these antibodies mentioned whether adsorption with Lu(a+b-) red cells left anti-Lu^b unadsorbed or enabled isolated anti-Lu16 to be recovered by elution. Only one family study was possible and it yielded no information about the inheritance of Lu16.

The Antigen Lu17 and the Antibody That Defines It

A single example of anti-Lu17 has been reported (49). It was made by an Italian woman living in Canada, the family study included samples from family members in Canada and Italy. The antibody-maker had been pregnant four times but had never been transfused. None of her infants had HDN but it was not known when the anti-Lu17 was made. The antibody-maker had Lu(a-b+) red cells on which Lu^b was expressed normally. The family study failed to show inheritance of Lu17. The proposita's mother, an obligate heterozygote for the gene that fails to make Lu17 if that antigen is inherited, had Lu(a-b+) red cells that reacted to the same degree as red cells from presumed *Lu^{17}* homozygotes, in titration studies with anti-Lu17. The proposita's father was deceased but it was known that her parents were consanguineous. The anti-Lu17 was non-reactive with Lu(a-b-) red cells of the *In(Lu)* and *LuLu* varieties but reactive with cells lacking other high incidence Lutheran system and para-Lutheran antigens. Unexpectedly for an antibody directed against a para-Lutheran antigen, anti-Lu17 reacted with the same strength and to equal titers with Lu(a-b+) cord blood red cells and those from adults. In a follow-up study performed seven years after the anti-Lu17 was first found, it was shown (173) that the antibody was still reactive. It gave a 1+ reaction when tested undiluted but reacted weakly to a dilution of 1 in 256. Antibodies with characteristics such as this are often benign in vivo (149,150) so an in vivo red cell survival study using ^{51}Cr labeled Lu:17 red cells was performed (173). The study showed a survival time of the injected red cells of 12.5 days (normal by the method used described as 25 days) thus suggesting that the antibody might cause modest destruction of antigen-positive transfused red cells.

The Antigen Lu20 and the Antibody That Defines It

A thalassemic patient in Israel who had made antibodies to C, K and Fy^b was found (50) to have another antibody in the serum that reacted with all cells tested except those of the *In(Lu)* and *LuLu* forms of Lu(a-b-), those of the *XS2* type were not available. The antibody-maker's red cells were Lu(a-b+) and the antibody to the high incidence antigen had a specificity different to those that define other high incidence Lutheran system and para-Lutheran antigens. The new specificity was called anti-Lu20. The Lu20 antigen has not yet been shown to be inherited but was shown (50) to be located on the Lutheran glycoproteins.

Farewell to Lu10 and Lu15

The number Lu10 was originally reserved (but apparently not used) for a low incidence antigen defined by an antibody in a serum Singleton (51-53). Initial excitement was generated when the serum Singleton was found to react strongly with an Lu:-5 sample. Naturally it was hoped that Singleton (Lu10) and Lu5 would be shown to be encoded by another pair of alleles at the *Lutheran* complex locus and thus join the pairs of alleles listed in table 20-3. Alas these hopes were dashed when Crawford (54) showed that five Lu:-5 samples, four of which came from unrelated individuals, were non-reactive with the Singleton serum.

As already mentioned in several earlier sections (where references are given) the term Lu15 was originally reserved for the high incidence antigen Anton. That antigen, now known as AnWj, has found a better home in Chapter 29 and its number (Lu15) has been retired.

Monoclonal Antibodies and the Lutheran System

A number of murine monoclonal antibodies that behave as anti-Lu[b] in serological tests have been described (77,174,175). While at least one of these antibodies has been shown (176-178) to bind to some degree to Lu(a+b-) red cells and Lu(a-b-) red cells of the *LuLu* variety, there is no doubt that they can be adjusted to serve as reliable anti-Lu[b] typing reagents by appropriate techniques. Two murine monoclonal antibodies that behave in serological tests as anti-Lu3, that is they react with all except Lu(a-b-) red cells, have been made (179). As mentioned in an earlier section, the expression of CD44 is depressed on Lu(a-b-) red cells of the *In(Lu)* variety. Thus monoclonal antibodies to CD44 (131,132, 142,144) can be used to screen random samples for red cells of that phenotype (132). In addition to the monoclonal antibodies described above, others directed against the Lutheran glycoproteins and other membrane components whose expressions are altered in individuals who inherit *In(Lu)*, have proved of great value in studies on the biochemistry of the Lutheran glycoproteins and phenotypically related structures. Such monoclonal antibodies are described in later sections of this chapter.

Autoantibodies and the Lutheran System

There are apparently no reports of true autoantibodies to Lutheran system or para-Lutheran antigens being made because of the failure of the immune system of an individual. However, there are a few observations that can be conveniently considered under the above heading. Anderson et al. (180,222) described three patients who received kidney transplants from cadaveric donors and then produced autoantibodies that failed to react only with Lu(a-b-) red cells so perhaps had anti-Lu3 specificity. Production of the antibodies (that in the transplant recipients behaved as if they were autoimmune) was transient, at 35 days post transplant no patient had demonstrable antibody and the DATs were only microscopically positive. It was supposed that the antibodies were made by donor lymphocytes transplanted with the kidneys. The abstract describing two of these cases (180) mentions that at 8 weeks post transplant, both recipients rejected the kidneys. The authors do not mention whether they believe that graft rejection was in any way associated with the transient antibody production.

Anti-lymphocyte globulin (ALG) made in horses is used by some transplant surgeons and immunologists to try to prevent allograft rejection. The use of this product is known to cause positive DATs and IATs in some patients because the ALG binds to red cells and is then detected in tests using anti-IgG (181-183). This occurs because anti-human-IgG reagents made in rabbits also contain anti-IgG that reacts with horse IgG. The problem can be circumvented by using anti-IgG that has been adsorbed with red cells coated with equine ALG. The antibodies that react with the horse IgG can be removed by such adsorption that does not result in significant loss of anti-human IgG (182-184). The equine ALG apparently binds less well to red cells of the Lu(a-b-) phenotype than to other red cells and its presence in serum may result in a situation in which it appears that the patient has made an antibody such as anti-Lu3 (185). In fact, it seems that the phenomenon has nothing to do with the Lutheran system but merely mimics that situation because of the detection of equine IgG on red cells (183,184).

The *Lutheran* Locus is on Chromosome 19

As mentioned in the introduction of this chapter, early studies (5-7) showed that the *Lutheran* and *Secretor* loci are linked. The linkage was at first thought to involve the *Lutheran* and *Lewis* loci but, of course, Lewis system phenotypes are directly correlated with the presence or absence of *Se* (see Chapter 9). After the early studies of Mohr (5-7) the *Lutheran-Secretor* linkage was confirmed by others (12,97,185,186) but it was not known on which chromosome the linkage group was carried. An early observation by Mohr (7) that the *Lutheran* and *Lewis* loci are closely linked to *DM*, a gene whose presence results in a dominantly inherited neuromuscular disorder, was then confirmed by others (187,188). The *Lewis* locus was added to the linkage group when it was shown (189) that *DM* and *Lewis* are loosely linked. Linkage between the *Lewis* locus and the *C3* gene, that encodes production of the third component of complement, had been demonstrated earlier (190) so that when Whitehead et al. (191) assigned *C3* to chromosome 19, it followed that the entire *Lutheran-Secretor-DM-Lewis-C3* linkage group must reside on that chromosome. Confirmation of this assignment was provided when the *Secretor* and *DM* loci were shown to be linked (13) and when *DM* and *PEPD* (the gene that encodes production of peptidase D that was already known to reside on chromosome 19 (193)) were also shown to be linked (14). Later still, Southern blot analysis of somatic cell hybrids was used to show that the *Lewis* locus and hence the rest of the linkage group, is on chromosome 19 (195). As described in Chapter 8, the *Hh* locus is also known to be on chromosome 19 (196-199), as described in Chapter 13, the *LW* locus lives there too (200). Still to be described in this book is the high incidence antigen Ok[a] (see Chapter 31), it can be mentioned here that the gene that encodes its production is also on chromosome 19

(201). While there is not yet full agreement, Daniels (202) suggests that based on published data (16,19,203,204) the order of the blood group loci beginning from the tip of the short arm, may be *Lewis-C3-LW-centromere-Lutheran-Secretor-H.*

The Biochemical Nature of Lutheran Blood Group System Antigens

Early studies on the nature of the Lutheran system antigens demonstrated that they were susceptible to digestion with trypsin and chymotrypsin (74,178) and to treatment with thiol reagents (77,78,178). These data provided hints that the antigens were carried on a protein whose structure was maintained by disulphide bonds. Identification of the protein(s) which carry the antigens was achieved by immunoblotting red cell membranes subjected to SDS-PAGE under reducing conditions with a murine monoclonal antibody (BRIC 108) which had anti-Lu[b] specificity (77) (BRIC 108 identified two bands of 85kd and 78kd respectively). These bands were not observed when membranes from red cells of phenotype Lu(a+b-) or Lu(a-b-) were similarly treated. The apparent molecular weights of the 85kd and 78kd bands were reduced to 73kd and 66kd respectively when membranes from red cells treated with a preparation containing endoglycosidase F and peptidyl N-glycanase were used, indicating that the proteins were glycosylated with N-glycans.

Subsequent immunoblotting studies with human alloantibodies showed that the Lutheran antigens Lu[a], Lu[b], Lu3, Lu4, Lu6, Lu8, Lu12, Lu18 and Lu19 were also carried on glycoproteins of 85kd and 78kd (39,163). It could be shown that several of these antigens reside on the same glycoproteins by using another murine monoclonal Lutheran antibody (BRIC 221). Purified Lutheran glycoproteins prepared by immunoprecipitation from intact red cells with BRIC 221 were reactive with antibodies to Lu[a], Lu[b], Lu3, Lu4, Lu18 and Lu19 on immunoblots (39) and the same antibodies reacted with Lutheran glycoproteins bound to BRIC 221 in the MAIEA assay (165).

The Lutheran Glycoprotein is a Novel Member of the Immunoglobulin Superfamily

Full-length cDNA which allowed the prediction of the protein sequence of the Lutheran (Lu) glycoprotein was obtained by Parsons et al. (213). Monoclonal antibody BRIC 221 was used to purify Lu glycoproteins from Triton X-100 solubilized red cell membranes by immunoaffinity chromatography. The purified protein(s) were then subjected to N-terminal amino acid sequence analysis. In addition, peptides obtained after digestion of the purified protein(s) with lysyl endoproteinase C (Lys C) were purified and subjected to amino acid sequence analysis. Synthetic oligonucleotides corresponding to the expected DNA sequence of the N-terminal peptide and one of the Lys C peptides were then used to amplify a 459bp product from a human placental cDNA library. The 459bp product was labeled and used to screen a placental cDNA library. Two positive clones were obtained one (2.4kb) of which was almost full length. The extreme 5′ end sequence was determined from human placental poly(A) mRNA using the 5′ RACE procedure. The open reading frame predicted a protein with a putative leader sequence of 17 amino acids and a mature protein of 597 residues with a calculated molecular weight of 64,219. Inspection of the sequence and hydropathy plot analysis indicated a protein with a large extracellular N-terminal domain of 518 residues, a single membrane-spanning domain (residues 519-538) and a cytoplasmic domain of 59 residues.

A computer search of protein sequence databases revealed that the sequence was unique but shared similarity with several members of the immunoglobulin superfamily (IgSF) of receptor proteins. The predicted extracellular sequence was compared with that of 27 known IgSF variable region domains (V-set) and 37 known IgSF constant domains (C-set). It could be inferred that the extracellular region of the Lutheran glycoprotein comprised five IgSF domains, 2 V-set (at the N-terminus) and 3 C2-set domains. The predicted protein contained five signal sequences for N-glycosylation in its predicted extracellular domain, one in the third domain and four within the fourth domain (see figure 20-1).

Immunochemical studies suggested that the cloned sequence corresponded to the 85kd band observed on immunoblots with Lutheran antibodies rather than the 78kd band. This conclusion was based on the observation that a rabbit antiserum raised to purified Lu glycoproteins (85kd and 78kd) and extensively absorbed with intact red cells to render it specific for cytoplasmic/transmembrane domain(s) reacted with the 85kd band but not the 78kd band (213). It could not be inferred from these experiments whether the 78kd band represented an isoform of the 85kd band or simply a degradation product of the 85kd produced by proteolysis during membrane preparation.

Independently of the studies described above Campbell et al. (214) isolated a cDNA clone corresponding to a cell surface glycoprotein denoted B-CAM. The cDNA was obtained from a cDNA library derived from the colon carcinoma cell line HT29 by expression cloning using a monoclonal antibody (G253). G253 had been characterized previously as recognizing an epitope which is highly expressed on ovarian carcinomas. Inspection of the cDNA sequence corresponding to B-

CAM reveals it to be identical to the Lutheran cDNA except that it lacks the last 40 residues of the predicted cytoplasmic domain. These results raised the possibility that B-CAM corresponds to the isoform of the Lutheran glycoprotein corresponding to the 78kd band described above. That B-CAM is indeed an isoform of the Lutheran glycoprotein was demonstrated by Rahuel et al. (215) who concluded that the two proteins are generated through the use of alternative internal donor and acceptor splice sites within exon 13 of the *LU* gene.

The Location and Organization of the *LU* Gene

As discussed in a previous section, linkage analysis places the *LU* gene on chromosome 19q13.2 (13,16). Direct confirmation of this was obtained by Campbell et al. (214) who used a cosmid containing the B-CAM locus in fluorescence in situ hybridization (FISH) to localize the gene to 19q13.2-13.3.

The *LU* gene comprises 15 exons spanning 11kb (216). The first exon encodes the leader sequence, exons 2 and 3 encode the first IgSF domain, exons 4, 5 and 6 the second IgSF domain, exons 7 and 8, the third domain, exons 9 and 10 the fourth and exons 11 and 12 the fifth. Exon 13 encodes the transmembrane domain and the 5′ end of the cytoplasmic domain, the remainder of the cytoplasmic domain is encoded by exons 14 and 15 (see figure 20-2).

The Molecular Basis of Lutheran Blood Group Antigens

Several Lutheran system antigens have been mapped to particular IgSF domains by flow cytometric analysis of K562 cells transfected with a set of domain-deletion mutants (216). Four mutants comprising domains 1, 2, 3, 4; domains 1, 2, 3; domains 1 and 2 and domain 1 only were used to show that: Lu^b and Lu5, map to domain 1; Lu4 and Lu8 to domain 2; Lu20 to domain 3; Lu7 to domain 4; and Lu13 and Lu19 to domain 5 (see figure 20-1). Lu 6 was tentatively assigned to domain 3 and Lu12 to domain 1. The epitope recognized by monoclonal BRIC 221 mapped to domain 4. These results show that the Lutheran system antigens are distributed throughout the extracellular region of the protein and are not confined to a "hot spot".

Nucleotide sequencing of exons 2 and 3 (the exons which encode domain 1) amplified from genomic DNA from four individuals of phenotype Lu(a+b-), two of Lu(a-b+) and two of Lu(a+b+) revealed a nucleotide substitution (G230 to A) in all six Lu(a+) individuals (216).

This substitution converts arginine 77 (Lu^b) to histidine (Lu^a) and defines the molecular basis of the Lu^a/Lu^b polymorphism. A similar analysis of exons 11 and 12 (the exons which encode domain 5) revealed that the Au^a/Au^b (Lu18/Lu19) polymorphism is defined by a single base substitution G1615(Au^b) to A, which converts alanine 539 (Au^b) to threonine (Au^a). In the next issue of *Blood* to that in which the above findings of Parsons et al. (216) were reported, El Nemer et al. (223) documented the results of their studies on organization of the *LU* gene. They too found that an Arg77His change represents the Lu^b to Lu^a polymorphism.

Tissue Distribution of Lutheran Glycoproteins

Northern blot analysis using both Lu and B-CAM probes revealed the presence of Lu mRNA in human heart, brain, placenta, lung, liver, skeletal muscle, kidney and pancreas (213,214). These studies reported a single mRNA species (2.5kb (213); 3.0kb, (214)). Rahuel et al. (215) report that the 2.5kb transcript corresponds to the Lu cDNA cloned by Parsons et al. (213) and that a 4.0kb transcript could also be found in the same tissues. The 4.0kb transcript which corresponds to the B-CAM isoform, was very weakly expressed compared to the 2.5kb species except in the colon carcinoma cell line HT29 (B-CAM was cloned from a cDNA library derived from the HT29 line) (214) suggesting that there may be differential regulation of expression of the two isoforms in some tumor tissues.

Flow cytometric analysis lines using murine monoclonal antibodies indicated that expression of Lu glycoprotein is confined to red cells in peripheral blood and that it is not expressed on the hematopoietic cell lines K562, HEL, HL-60, IM-9 or Molt-4 (177). Attempts to isolate Lu cDNA from human bone marrow libraries were unsuccessful (213). The Lu protein is expressed in kidney glomeruli and its expression appears to be under developmental control in human liver. Immunocytochemical staining revealed that it is strongly expressed in first trimester fetal hepatocytes, less strongly expressed in second trimester fetal hepatocytes while hepatocytes from adults showed little or no activity (174,213). Immunoblotting experiments revealed that fetal liver reactivity is associated with a single band of 85kd (213). Extensive immunocytochemical staining was observed in placental tissue and this was why Parsons et al. (213) looked for Lu cDNA in a placental cDNA library. In full term placentae the antibodies stained arteries within the cores of chorionic villi. Intense staining of arterial walls was observed in a wide variety of tissues including tongue, trachea, esophagus, skin, cervix, ileum, colon, stomach and gall bladder. Staining was sometimes appar-

FIGURE 20-1 Structure of the Lutheran Glycoprotein and Location of the
Lutheran Blood Group Antigens

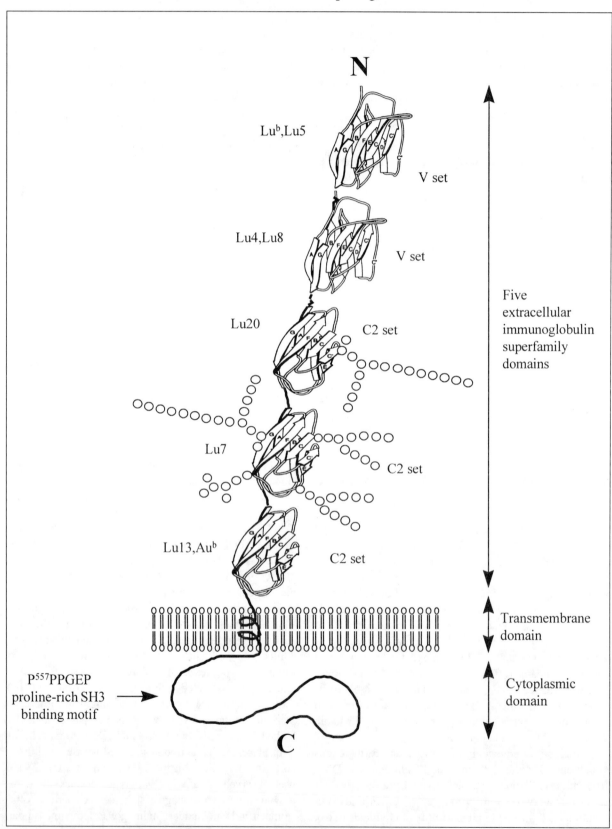

FIGURE 20-2 Structure of the LU Gene and Derivation of the Isoform B-CAM

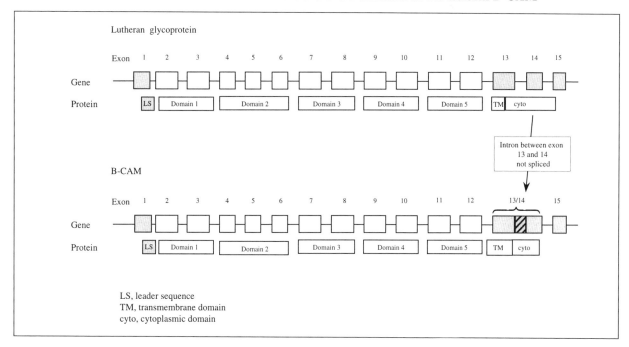

LS, leader sequence
TM, transmembrane domain
cyto, cytoplasmic domain

ent in the basement membrane region of epithelial cells.

An extensive immunocytochemical study of B-CAM expression (217) demonstrated a similar broad reactivity with normal tissues and in addition, strong reactivity with 27 of 31 samples of ovarian carcinoma and some examples of other tumors including breast, lung and melanoma. Renal, bladder, gastric and testicular tumors, neuroblastomas and lymphomas were unreactive.

The Function of the Lutheran Glycoproteins

The functions of the Lutheran glycoproteins are largely unknown. However, since the glycoproteins are members of the Ig superfamily it would be expected that like other members of the family, they are involved in adhesive and/or receptor functions. Evidence (221) that the Lutheran glycoprotein on red cells will bind to the extracellular protein laminin is consistent with such a role. Two other human IgSF family members have been described which have a similar organization of Ig domains (V-V-C2-C2-C2) to the Lutheran glycoprotein. These are MUC 18, a marker of tumor progression in melanoma (218), and ALCAM (activated leukocyte cell adhesion molecule) a molecule found on thymic epithelial cells, activated T cells, B cells and monocytes and in brain, which is known to bind to itself (homotypic adhesion) and to CD6 (219). Bowen et al. (219) speculate that since ALCAM and CD6 are

expressed by cells involved in immune recognition and in cells of the nervous system they may function as a ligand pair in cellular interactions between the immune and nervous systems.

Molecules that have a receptor function on cell surfaces frequently mediate signal transduction. In this context, it is of note that the cytoplasmic domain of the Lutheran glycoprotein contains a consensus motif (P557PPGEP) for the binding of Src homology 3 (SH3) domains. Interaction between such proline-rich motifs and SH3 domains of other proteins is a well established mechanism in intracellular signaling pathways (220). Although, at the time of writing, the function or functions of the Lutheran glycoproteins is not known, the foregoing discussion together with a consideration of the proteins' wide tissue distribution, developmental regulation in liver and elevated expression in some cancers (discussed in an earlier section) suggests that the proteins have important roles in cell:cell and cell:extracellular matrix interactions in a wide variety of tissues.

Lu$_{null}$ Phenotypes

The Lutheran null phenotypes described in an earlier section have yet to be studied at the DNA level. Now that the organization of the *LU* gene is known it is a comparatively straightforward exercise to see if there are any defects in the gene itself in individuals with the Lu(a-b-) phenotype resulting from the recessive form of inheritance and studies of this type are underway in our (DJA) laboratories. The genetic mechanisms giving rise to the Lu(a-b-) phenotype as a consequence of the *InLu* and *XS2* genes are far less amenable to study. The *InLu* type of Lu(a-b-) is also discussed in Chapter 29 because there is a deficiency of the Indian blood group glycoprotein (CD44) as well as Lutheran glycoproteins in cells of this phenotype.

References

1. Callender S, Race RR, Paykoc ZV. Br Med J 1945;2:83
2. Callender ST, Race RR. Ann Eugen 1946;13:102
3. Gavin J, Daniels GL, Yamaguchi H, et al. Vox Sang 1979;36:31
4. Yamaguchi H, Okubo Y, Seno T, et al. Vox Sang 1979;36:29
5. Mohr J. Acta Path Microbiol Scand 1951;28:207
6. Mohr J. Acta Path Microbiol Scand 1951;29:339
7. Mohr J. A Study of Linkage in Man. Copenhagen:Munksgaard 1954
8. Ceppellini R. Proc 5th Cong ISBT. Basel:Karger 1955:207
9. Ceppellini R. Ric Sci Mem 1955;25:3
10. Ceppellini R, Siniscalco M. Rev Inst Serioterapic Ital 1955;30:431
11. Race RR, Sanger R. Blood Groups in Man, 4th Ed. Oxford:Blackwell, 1962
12. Sanger R, Race RR. Heredity 1958;12:513
13. Eiberg H, Mohr J, Staub Nielsen S, et al. Clin Genet 1983;24:159
14. Westerveld A, Naylor S. Cytogenet Cell Genet 1984;37:155
15. Shaw D, Eiberg H. Cytogenet Cell Genet 1987;46:242
16. Zelinski T, Coghlan G, Greenberg CR, et al. Transfusion 1989;29:304
17. Le Beau MM, Ryan D, Pericak-Vance MA. Cytogenet Cell Genet 1989;51:338
18. Ropers HH, Pericak-Vance MA. Cytogenet Cell Genet 1991;58:751
19. Ball SP, Tongue N, Gibaud A, et al. Ann Hum Genet 1991;55:225
20. Cutbush M, Chanarin I. Nature 1956;178:855
21. Crawford MN, Greenwalt TJ, Sasaki T, et al. Transfusion 1961;1:228
22. Tippett P. Vox Sang 1971;20:378
23. Taliano V, Gúevin RM, Tippett P. Vox Sang 1973;24:42
24. Stanbury A, Francis BJ. Vox Sang 1967;13:441
25. Darnborough J, Firth R, Giles CM, et al. Nature 1963;198:796
26. Brown F, Simpson S, Cornwall S, et al. Vox Sang 1974;26:259
27. Norman PC, Tippett P, Beal RW. Vox Sang 1986;51:49
28. Bove JR, Allen FH Jr, Chiewsilp P, et al. Vox Sang 1971;21:302
29. Marsh WL. Transfusion 1972;12:27
30. Molthan L, Crawford MN, Marsh WL, et al. Vox Sang 1973;24:468
31. Judd WJ, Marsh WL, Øyen R, et al. Vox Sang 1977;32:214
32. Salmon C, Salmon D, Liberge G, et al. Nouv Rev Fr Haematol 1961;1:649
33. Drachmann O, Thyme S, Tippett P. Vox Sang 1982;43:259
34. Tippett P. In: Human Blood Groups. Basel:Karger, 1977:401
35. Salmon C, Rouger P, Liberge G, et al. Rev Fr Transf Immunohematol 1981;24:339
36. Frandson S, Atkins CJ, Moulds M, et al. Vox Sang 1989;56:54
37. Crawford MN, Tippett P, Sanger R. Vox Sang 1974;26:283
38. Tippett P. Transf Med Rev 1990;4:56
39. Daniels G. Vox Sang 1990;58:56
40. Daniels GL, Le Pennec PY, Rouger P, et al. Vox Sang 1991;60:191
41. Zelinski T, Kaita H, Coghlan G, et al. Vox Sang 1991;61:275
42. Lewis M, Anstee DJ, Bird GWG , et al. Vox Sang 1991;61:158
43. MacIlroy M, McCreary J, Stroup M. Vox Sang 1972;23:455
44. Gralnick MA, Goldfinger D, Hatfield PA, et al. Vox Sang 1974;27:52
45. Sinclair M, Buchanan DI, Tippett P, et al. Vox Sang 1973;25:156
46. Marsh WL. Unpublished observations 1983 cited in Issitt PD. Applied Blood Group Serology, 3rd Ed. Miami:Montgomery, 1985:381
47. Marsh WL, Johnson CL, Mueller KA, et al. (abstract). Transfusion 1983;23:423
48. Sabo B, Pancoska C, Myers M, et al. (abstract). Transfusion 1980;20:630
49. Turner C. Canad J Med Technol 1979;41:43
50. Levene C, Gekker K, Poole J, et al. (abstract). Rev Paulista Med 1992;110 (Suppl 1):13
51. Marsh WL. Unpublished observations 1972 cited in Reid ME. Adv Immunohematol Vol 2, No 2, 1973
52. Reid ME. Adv Immunohematol Vol 2, No 2, 1973
53. Crawford MN. Unpublished observations 1975 cited in Issitt PD. Applied Blood Group Serology, 3rd Ed. Miami:Montgomery, 1985:381
54. Crawford MN. Unpublished observations 1983 cited in Issitt PD. Applied Blood Group Serology, 3rd Ed. Miami:Montgomery, 1985:381
55. Poole J, Giles C. (Letter). Transfusion 1985;25:443
56. Marsh WL, Johnson CL. (Letter). Transfusion 1985;25:443
57. Mannessier L, Rouger P, Johnson CL, et al. Vox Sang 1986;50:240
58. Telen MJ, Rao N, Udani M, et al. (abstract). Transfusion 1993;33 (Suppl 9S):48S
59. Mainwaring UR, Pickles MM. J Clin Pathol 1948;1:292
60. Bertinshaw D, Lawler SD, Holt HA, et al. Ann Eugen 1950;15:234
61. Mourant AE, Kopéc AC, Domaniewska-Sobczak K. The Distribution of Human Blood Groups and Other Polymorphisms 2nd Ed. London:Oxford Univ Press 1976
62. Shaw MA, Leak MR, Daniels GL, et al. Ann Hum Genet 1984;48:229
63. Rowe GP, Gale SA, Daniels GL, et al. Ann Hum Genet 1992;56:267
64. Chown B, Lewis M, Kaita H, et al. Vox Sang 1963;8:378
65. Dublin TD, Bernanke AD, Pitt EL, et al. Br Med J 1964;2:775
66. Chown B, Lewis M, Kaita H. Vox Sang 1966;11:108
67. Yung CH, Chow MP, Hu HY, et al. Transfusion 1989;29:233
68. Broadberry RE, Lin-Chu M, Chang FC. (abstract). Book of Abstracts. 20th Cong ISBT 1988:301
69. Toivanen P, Hirvonen T. Vox Sang 1973;24:372
70. Race RR, Sanger R. Blood Groups in Man, 6th Ed. Oxford:Blackwell, 1975
71. Kissmeyer-Nielsen F. Vox Sang 1960;5:532
72. Greenwalt TJ, Sasaki TT, Steane EA. Transfusion 1967;7:189
73. Henke J, Basler M, Baur MP. Foren Sci Int 1982;20:233
74. Judson PA, Anstee DJ. Med Lab Sci 1977;34:1
75. Daniels G. In: Blood Group Systems: Duffy, Kidd and Lutheran. Arlington, VA:Am Assoc Blood Banks, 1988:119
76. Daniels G. Immunohematology 1992;8:53
77. Parsons SF, Mallinson G, Judson PA, et al. Transfusion

1987;27:61

78. Levene C, Karniel Y, Sela R. (Letter). Transfusion 1987;27:505
79. Marsh WL, Johnson CL, Mueller KA. (Letter). Transfusion 1983;23:275
80. Shirey RS, Buck S, Niebyl J, et al. (abstract). Book of Abstracts. 18th Cong ISBT 1984:168
81. Heide HM van der, Loghem JJ van. Proc 4th Cong ISBT. Basel:Karger 1951:383
82. Shaw S, Mourant AE, Ikin EW. Lancet 1954;2:170
83. Vogel P. Bull NY Acad Med 1954;30:657
84. Gozenbach R, Hassig A, Rosin S. Blut 1955;1:272
85. Hollander L. Schweiz Med Wschr 1955;85:10
86. Greenwalt TJ, Sasaki T. Blood 1957;12:998
87. Francis BJ, Hatcher DE. Transfusion 1961;1:248
88. Greendyke RM, Chorpenning FW. Transfusion 1962;2:52
89. Hartmann O, Heier AM, Kornstad L, et al. Vox Sang 1965;10:234
90. Inderbitzen PE, Windle B. (Letter). Transfusion 1982;22:542
91. Crawford MN. In: Blood Group Systems: Duffy, Kidd and Lutheran. Arlington, VA:Am Assoc Blood Banks, 1988:93
92. Merry AH, Gardner B, Parsons SF, et al. Vox Sang 1987;53:57
93. Fisher FS, Rolih SD. (abstract). Book of Abstracts. Joint Cong ISBT/AABB 1990:153
94. Castillo L, Leveque C. (abstract). Book of Abstracts. Joint Cong ISBT/AABB 1990:162
95. Boulton FE. Vox Sang 1990;59:61
96. Cutbush M, Mollison PL. Br J Haematol 1958;4:115
97. Metaxas MN, Metaxas-Bühler M, Dunsford I, et al. Vox Sang 1959;4:298
98. Croucher BEE, Scott JG, Crookston JH. Vox Sang 1962;7:492
99. Scheffer H, Tamaki HT. Transfusion 1966;6:497
100. Molthan L, Crawford MN. Transfusion 1966;6:584
101. Tilley CA, Crookston MC, Haddad SA, et al. Transfusion 1977;17:169
102. Peters B, Reid ME, Ellisor SS, et al. (abstract). Transfusion 1978;18:623
103. Dube VE, Zoes CS. Transfusion 1982;22:251
104. Chattoraj A, Gilbert R, Josephson AM. Transfusion 1967;7:355
105. Adkins D. (abstract). Transfusion 1989; 29 (Suppl 7S):16S
106. Hardman JT, Beck ML. Transfusion 1981;21:343
107. Garratty G, Arndt P, Nance S. (abstract). Transfusion 1996;36 (Suppl 9S):50S
108. Kobuszewski M, Wallace M, Moulds M, et al. (abstract). Transfusion 1988;28 (Suppl 6S):37S
109. Novotny VMJ, Kanhai HHH, Overbeeke MAM, et al. Vox Sang 1992;62:49
110. Wrobel DM, Moore BPL, Cornwall S, et al. Vox Sang 1972;23:205
111. Dybkjaer E, Lylloff K, Tippett P. Vox Sang 1974;26:94
112. Gibson M, Devenish A, Daniels GL, et al. (abstract). Prog Ann Mtg Br Blood Transf Soc 1983:27
113. Issitt PD, Valinsky J, Marsh WL, et al. Transfusion 1990;30:258
114. Cleghorn TE. Nature 1959;184:1324
115. Cleghorn TE. Br J Haematol 1960;6:433
116. Cleghorn TE. MD Thesis. Univ Sheffield 1961
117. Metaxas-Bühler M, Metaxas MN, Giles CM. Vox Sang 1972;23:429
118. Metaxas MN, Metaxas-Bühler M. Vox Sang 1976;31 (Suppl 1):39
119. Skov F, Jørgensen J, Torreggiani L, et al. Unpublished observations 1982 cited in Daniels G. Human Blood Groups.

120. Zelinski T, Kaita H, Lewis M. Rev Fr Transf Immunohematol 1988;31:429
121. Marsh WL, Øyen R, Rosso M, et al. Transfusion 1976;16:633
122. Ballem PJ, Stout TD, Battista N, et al. (abstract). Blood 1987;70 (Suppl 1):107a
123. Issitt PD. Applied Blood Group Serology, 3rd Ed. Miami:Montgomery, 1985
124. Salmon C, Gerbal A, Tippett P. Unpublished observations 1971 cited in Race RR, Sanger R. Blood Groups in Man, 6th Ed. Oxford:Blackwell, 1975:383
125. Moulds M, Moulds J, Frandson S, et al. (abstract). Transfusion 1988;28 (Suppl 6S):20S
126. Zelinski T, Kaita H, Johnson K, et al. Vox Sang 1990;58:126
127. Brice CL, Hoxworth PI. (abstract). Prog 18th Mtg AABB 1965
128. Wright J, Moore BPL. Vox Sang 1968;14:133
129. Contreras M, Tippett P. Vox Sang 1974;27:369
130. Gibson T. Hum Hered 1976;26:171
131. Telen MJ, Eisenbarth GS, Haynes BF. J Clin Invest 1983;71:1878
132. Udden MM, Umeda M, Hirano Y, et al. Blood 1987;69:52
133. Winkler MM, Hamilton JR. (abstract). Book of Abstracts. Joint Cong ISBT/AABB, 1990:158
134. Lukasavage T. Immunohematology 1993;9:112
135. Myhre B, Thompson M, Anson C, et al. Vox Sang 1975;29:66
136. Yamaguchi H, Okubo Y, Seno T. Unpublished observations 1980 cited in Daniels G. Human Blood Groups. Oxford:Blackwell, 1995
137. Crookston JL, Crookston M. Unpublished observations 1972 cited in Brown F, Simpson S, Cornwall S, et al. Vox Sang 1974;26:259
138. Melonas K, Noto TA. (abstract). Transfusion 1965;5:370
139. Mulley JC, Norman PC, Tippett P, et al. Hum Genet 1988;78:127
140. Tippett P. Unpublished observations cited in Race RR, Sanger R. Blood Groups in Man, 6th Ed. Oxford:Blackwell, 1975:272
141. Crawford MN, Wilfert K, Tippett P. (abstract). Transfusion 1992;32 (Suppl 8S):20S
142. Spring FA, Dalchau R, Daniels GL, et al. Immunology 1988;64:37
143. Telen MJ, Shehata H, Haynes BF. Hum Immunol 1986;17:311
144. Telen MJ, Green AM. Transfusion 1988;28:430
145. Boorman KE, Tippett P. Unpublished observations 1972 cited in Race RR, Sanger R. Blood Groups in Man, 6th Ed. Oxford:Blackwell, 1975:274
146. Daniels GL. PhD Thesis. Univ London 1980
147. Poole J, Giles CM. Vox Sang 1982;43:220
148. Marsh WL, Brown PJ, DiNapoli J, et al. Transfusion 1983;23:128
149. Mollison PL, Engelfriet CP, Contreras M. Blood Transfusion in Clinical Medicine, 9th Ed. Oxford:Blackwell 1993
150. Rolih SD. Transf Med Rev 1989;3:128
151. Marsh WL. Personal communication to Tippett PA, cited by Poole J, Giles CM. Vox Sang 1982;43:220
152. Poole J, Levene C, Bennett M, et al. Transf Med 1991;1:245
153. Daniels GL, Shaw MA, Lomas CG, et al. Transfusion 1986;26:171
154. Marsh WL, Johnson CL, Mueller KA. Transfusion 1984;24:371
155. Shaw MA, Tippett P. Transfusion 1985;25:170
156. Guy K, Andrew JM. Immunology 1991;74:206
157. Bast BJEG, Zhou L-J, Freeman GF, et al. J Cell Biol 1992;116:423

Oxford:Blackwell, 1995:373

158. Guy K, Green C. Immunology 1992;75:75
159. Tippett P, Guy K. (abstract). Transfusion 1993;33 (Suppl 9S):48S
160. Rao N, Udani M, Telen MJ. (abstract). Transfusion 1994;34 (Suppl 10S):25S
161. Williamson LM, Poole J, Redman C, et al. Br J Haematol 1994;87:805
162. Bowen AB, Haist AL, Talley LL, et al. Vox Sang 1972;23:201
163. Daniels GL, Khalid G. Vox Sang 1989;57:137
164. Daniels G. Unpublished observations cited in Daniels G. Human Blood Groups. Oxford:Blackwell, 1995:379
165. Petty AC. J Immunol Meth 1993;161:91
166. Hoffer J, Reid ME, Tossas E, et al. (abstract). Transfusion 1993;33 (Suppl 9S):23S
167. Shirey RS, Øyen R, Heeb KN, et al. (abstract). Transfusion 1988;28 (Suppl 6S):37S
168. Marsh WL. In: A Seminar on Recent Advances in Immunohematology. Washington, D.C.:Am Assoc Blood Banks, 1973:108
169. Allen FH Jr, Marsh WL. Personal communication cited by Issitt PD, Issitt CH. Applied Blood Group Serology, 2nd Ed. Oxnard:Spectra Biologicals, 1975
170. Marsh WL. In: Clinical Practice of Blood Transfusion, 1st Ed. New York:Churchill Livingstone, 1981:101
171. Reid ME. Adv Immunohematol Vol 2, No 1, 1973
172. Sabo B, Pancoska C, Myers M, et al. (abstract). Book of Abstracts. 16th Cong ISBT, 1980:206
173. Heddle N, Murphy W. (Letter). Transfusion 1986;26:306
174. Anstee DJ, Mallinson G, Yendle JE, et al. (abstract). Book of Abstracts. 20th Cong ISBT 1988:263
175. Inglis G, Fraser RH, Mitchell R. (abstract). Transf Med 1993;3 (Suppl 1):94
176. Telen M. Rev Fr Transf Immunohematol 1988;31:421
177. Judson PA, Spring FA, Parsons SF, et al. Rev Fr Transf Immunohematol 1988;31:433
178. Daniels G. Rev Fr Transf Immunohematol 1988;31:447
179. Parsons SF, Anstee DJ. Unpublished observations cited in Daniels G. Human Blood Groups. Oxford:Blackwell, 1995:363
180. Anderson HJ, Meisenhelder J, Stevens J. (abstract). Transfusion 1983;23:436
181. Draper EK, Dignam CM, Yang S, et al. (abstract). Transfusion 1982;22:415
182. Swanson JL, Mann EW, Condie RM, et al. (abstract). Transfusion 1982;22:415
183. Swanson JL, Issitt CH, Mann EW, et al. Transfusion 1984;24:141
184. Postoway N, Garratty G. (abstract). Transfusion 1984;24:427
185. Lawler SD, Renwick JH. Br Med Bull 1959;15:145
186. Greenwalt TJ. Am J Hum Genet 1961;13:69
187. Renwick JH, Bundey SE, Ferguson-Smith MA, et al. J Med Genet 1971;8:407
188. Harper PS, Rivas ML, Bias WB, et al. Am J Hum Genet 1972;24:310
189. Simola K, de la Chapelle A, Pirkola A, et al. Cytogenet Cell Genet 1982;32:317
190. Weitkamp LR, Johnston E, Guttormsen SA. Cytogenet Cell Genet 1974;13:183
191. Whitehead AS, Solomon E, Chambers S, et al. Proc Nat Acad Sci USA 1982;79:5021
192. Moore BPL, Humphreys P, Lovett-Moseley CA. Serological and Immunological Methods, 7th Ed. Toronto:Canadian Red Cross 1972
193. McAlpine PJ, Mohandas T, Ray M, et al. Cytogenet Cell Genet 1976;16:204
194. Gedde-Dahl T Jr, Olaisen B, Teisberg P, et al. Hum Genet 1984;67:172
195. Kukowska-Latallo JF, Larsen RD, Nair RP, et al. Gene Dev 1990;4:1288
196. Oriol R, Danilovs J, Hawkins BR. Am J Hum Genet 1981;33:421
197. Oriol R, Le Pendu J, Bernez L, et al. Cytogenet Cell Genet 1984;37:564
198. Larsen RD, Ernst LK, Nair RP, et al. Proc Nat Acad Sci USA 1990;87:6674
199. Rouquier S, Lowe JB, Kelly RJ, et al. J Biol Chem 1995;270:4632
200. Sistonen P. Ann Hum Genet 1984;48:239
201. Williams BP, Daniels GL, Pym B, et al. Immunogenetics 1988;27:322
202. Daniels G. Human Blood Groups. Oxford:Blackwell, 1995:708
203. Lewis M, Kaita H, Philipps S, et al. Hum Genet 1987;51:201
204. Zelinski T. Transfusion 1991;31:762
205. Tippett P. In: Human Genetics 1984: A Look at the Last Ten Years - and the Next Ten. Arlington, VA:Am Assoc Blood Banks, 1985:1
206. Herron B, Reynolds W, Northcott M, et al. (abstract). Transf Med 1996;6 (Suppl 2):24
207. Oxelius VA, Svenningsen NW. Acta Paediat Scand 1984;73:626
208. Einhorn MS, Granoff DM, Natim MH, et al. J Paediat 1987;111:783
209. Lubenko, Contreras M, Rodeck CH, et al. Vox Sang 1994;67:291
210. Reid ME, Chandrasekaran V, Sausais L, et al. Vox Sang 1996;71:48
211. Longster GH, Robinson EAE. Clin Lab Haematol 1981;3:351
212. Leger R, Garratty G, Vengelen-Tyler V. (abstract). Transfusion 1994;34 (Suppl 10S):69S
213. Parsons SF, Mallinson G, Holmes CH, et al. Proc Nat Acad Sci USA 1995;92:5496
214. Campbell IG, Foulkes WD, Senger G, et al. Cancer Res 1994;54,5761
215. Rahuel C, Le Van Kim C, Mattei MG, et al. Blood 1996;88:1865
216. Parsons SF, Mallinson G, Daniels G, et al. Blood 1997;89:4219
217. Garin-Chesa P, Sanz-Moncasi M-P, Campbell IG, et al. Int J Oncol 1994;5:1261
218. Lehmann JM, Riethmuller G, Johnson JP. Proc Nat Acad Sci USA 1989;86:9891
219. Bowen MA, Patel DD, Li X, et al. J Exp Med 1995;181:2213
220. Yu H, Chen JK, Feng S, et al. Cell 1994;76:933
221. Udani M, Jefferson S, Daymont C, et al. (abstract). Blood 1996;88 (Suppl 1):6a
222. Anderson HJ, AuBuchon JP, Draper EK, et al. Transfusion 1985;25:47
223. El Nemer W, Rahuel C, Colin Y, et al. Blood 1997;89:4608

In 1967, Heisto et al. (1) described three examples of an antibody directed against an antigen of high incidence. The antibody was named anti-Co^a and in tests on 4767 random donors in Norway, Holland, England and Minnesota, twelve with Co(a-) red cells were found. The antibody defining Co^b, the antithetical partner to Co^a, was described by Giles et al. (2) in 1970. Since that time many additional examples of anti-Co^a (3-10) and anti-Co^b (11-18) have been reported in the literature, no doubt many others have been found since the need to describe each new example in print passed. In 1974, Rogers et al. (19) described a woman whose red cells were Co(a-b-) and whose serum contained an antibody, that was named anti-Co3, that behaved as anti-Co^{ab} in an inseparable form. As listed below, several other examples of anti-Co3 have subsequently been described. As also described in a later section of this chapter, the Colton system antigens are now known (20) to reside on a water transport protein (Aquaporin-1 or AQP-CHIP) on red cells. Table 21-1 lists the conventional and ISBT terminology for the Colton blood group system.

The Antigens Co^a and Co^b

The incidence of Co^a, Co^b and the Colton phenotypes in Whites (1-4,13,21,22) are shown in table 21-2; one study (23) not included in the calculations used for table 21-2 found only 16 Co(a-) samples in tests on approximately 20,300 Welsh blood donors. The incidence of Co(a-) may have been a little higher than it seemed since some Co(a+) donors may have been included more than once during the year of the study. Although there are few supportive data, it seems that Co^a may be even more frequent in some other ethnic groups than in Whites. Crawford (24) tested samples from 1706 American Blacks, all were Co(a+). We (25) tested samples from 799 Hispanics living in Miami, with anti-Co^b, 37 (4.6%) were positive. Among those 37, one was Co(a-b+). Thus from this, admittedly small study, the incidence of Co^b in Hispanics seems to be a little over half that seen in Whites, this agreed with our finding of one Co(a-) in 799 (assuming that no Co(a-b-) was included in the group not tested with anti-Co^a) since the figure in Whites (see table 21-2) is about 1 in 498. All of 100 Cree Indians had Co(a+) red cells, two were Co(a+b+) (26).

Co^a and Co^b seem to be fully developed at birth (27,53), as described in the next section anti-Co^a has caused severe and anti-Co^b mild, HDN. The antigens are readily detected on red cells treated with proteases, sial-idase or AET (28) indeed, again as discussed in the next section, early examples of anti-Co^a were detected best, or only, in IATs using enzyme-treated red cells (1). Co^a was not detected on granulocytes, lymphocytes or monocytes (29). Somewhat like the Kidd glycoprotein as discussed in Chapter 19, it now seems possible (but certainly not proved) that the Colton glycoprotein, that is known to be the water transport protein (for references see below), is present on tissue cells in a form that does not express Co^a or Co^b. Also as discussed in more detail below, the red cell Co^a/Co^b polymorphism has been characterized at the molecular level (20). At position 45 on the water transporter protein, the amino acid is alanine when the protein expresses Co^a, and valine when it expresses Co^b.

Anti-Co^a and Anti-Co^b

These antibodies are most often IgG in nature and some of them bind complement. They usually react most strongly in IATs and their reactions are enhanced in tests against protease-treated red cells. At least one IgM anti-Co^a has been described (10). The antibodies are most often found in the sera of individuals who have been pregnant or transfused. While anti-Co^a is seen as the only antibody present, anti-Co^b is seen more frequently in sera that contain other blood group antibodies.

One example of anti-Co^a caused a delayed transfusion reaction (9), another caused severe HDN (6) and yet another brought about accelerated clearance of Co(a+b-) red cells in an in vivo survival study (10). One example of anti-Co^b caused an acute transfusion reaction (16), another caused a mild delayed transfusion reaction (17) and two others were shown to cause accelerated clearance of Co(b+) red cells in in vivo survival studies

TABLE 21-1 Conventional and ISBT Terminology for the Colton Blood Group System

Conventional Name: Co		
ISBT System Symbol: CO		
ISBT System Number: 015		
Antigen Conventional Name	ISBT Antigen Number	ISBT Full Code Number
Co^a	CO1	015001
Co^b	CO2	015002
Co3	CO3	015003

TABLE 21-2 Approximate Antigen and Phenotype
Frequencies for the
Colton System in Whites

Phenotype	% Frequency	% Bloods Reactive with	
		Anti-Co^a	Anti-Co^b
Co(a+b-)	91.2		
Co(a+b+)	8.6	} 99.8	
Co(a-b+)	0.2		} 8.8
Co(a-b-)	<0.01		

(18,54). Anti-Co^b has not yet been blamed for significant clinical HDN, no doubt such a case will eventually be seen. Taken together these findings suggest that anti-Co^a and anti-Co^b should be regarded as having potential clinical significance unless there is good evidence (e.g. a normal red cell survival study) to the contrary. Typical reactions of Colton system antibodies, including anti-Co3 that is described in more detail in the next section, are listed in table 21-3.

The Phenotype Co(a-b-), the Allele *Co* and Anti-Co3

Since 1974, when Rogers et al. (19) described the first examples (the proposita and two of her four sibs) of the Co(a-b-) phenotype, a number of others have been reported (30-34). In those cases in which family studies have been possible it has usually appeared that the Co(a-b-) phenotype represents homozygosity for the rare silent *Co* allele. However, as discussed in a later section of this chapter, *Co* alleles have been seen to have arisen via three different mutations of the *AQP1* gene (35). Other families in which there was suggestive evidence of the presence of *Co* have been described (36-38). In the family studied by Swanson and Eckman (37), the proposita's Co(a-b+^{w}) phenotype was thought to represent the presence of *Co* and a *Co^b* gene encoding less than the normal amount of

Co^b. However, a contribution to the unusual phenotype by the patient's clinical condition, paroxysmal nocturnal hemoglobinuria, could not be completely excluded.

In 1996, Mathai et al. (52) reported studies on aquaporin-1 deficient (Co(a-b-) Co:-3) red cells. The red cells appeared morphologically normal but laboratory studies revealed that the cells have a slightly reduced in vivo life span and a slight reduction in membrane surface area.

Many of the individuals with Co(a-b-) red cells were recognized (30-33) when it was found that their sera contained anti-Co3. As mentioned in the introduction of this chapter, anti-Co3 behaves as if it has anti-Co^{ab} specificity, but cannot be split into anti-Co^a and anti-Co^b by differential adsorption. Race and Sanger (39) found that the serum Swarts, that contained an antibody to a high incidence antigen, was non-reactive with the Co(a-b-) red cells found by Rogers et al. (19). The patient Swarts died in 1964, three years before the Colton system was discovered and ten years before Co(a-b-) cells were identified so that the Swarts red cells could not be typed for Co^a or Co^b. However, since the Swarts serum had been tested against so many red cell samples and had reacted with all except those that were Co(a-b-), it seems highly probable that the first example of then unrecognizable anti-Co3, predated the discovery of anti-Co^a and anti-Co^b. Like anti-Co^a and anti-Co^b, anti-Co3 has been found to be of clinical significance. An example described by Savona-Ventura et al. (32) caused severe HDN. An antibody closely resembling anti-Co3, that is described below, did the same thing (33).

Antibodies That Resembled Anti-Co3

In 1987, Lacey et al. (33) described a White woman of Scottish, Irish, and English extraction whose red cells typed as Co(a-b-) and whose serum contained an antibody that reacted strongly with Co(a+b-), Co(a+b+) and Co(a-b+) red cells, very weakly with Co(a-b-) red cells but not at all with her own cells. The antibody, that had an IAT titer of 32,000, caused severe HDN, the infant

TABLE 21-3 Characteristics of Colton System Antibodies

Antibody Specificity	Positive Reactions in In Vitro Tests				Usual Immuno-globulin		Ability to Bind Complement	Ability to Cause In Vitro Lysis		Implicated in		Usual Form of Stimulation		% of White Population Positive
	Sal	LISS	AHG	Enz	IgG	IgM	Yes / No	Yes	No	Transfusion Reaction	HDN	Red Cells	Other	
Anti-Co^a			X	X	X		Many		X	X	X	X		99.8
Anti-Cob			X	X	X	Rare	Many		X	X	Mild	X		8.8
Anti-Co3			X	X	X		Many	Rare		X	X	X		100

was given an exchange transfusion using the mother's red cells. From tests on the proposita's papain-treated red cells with a number of different anti-Co3, Lacey et al. (33) concluded that those cells may have had a weak expression of Co3. In a family study it was found that some relatives of the proposita had red cells on which Co[a] and Co3 were more weakly expressed than normal. It was suggested that the findings in the proposita and her family might represent presence of an inhibitor gene. The anti-Co3-like antibody reacted with many other rare samples, in addition to those that were Co(a-b-) and with the red cells of more than 40,000 random donors.

In 1988, Moulds et al. (40) described a White woman suffering from non-Hodgkins lymphoma in whom temporary depression of red cell Colton antigen expression was accompanied by transient production of anti-Co3. Since the patient's red cells typed as Co(a-b-) at some points during the investigation, although they would adsorb anti-Co[a] and yield that antibody on elution, the anti-Co3 that was, in fact, autoimmune in nature, mimicked an alloantibody.

The *Colton* Locus in on Chromosome 7

In 1977, Mohr and Eiberg (41) suggested that both *Co* and *Jk* might be located on chromosome 7. While, as described in Chapter 19, the *Jk* locus was eventually assigned to chromosome 18 (evidence against linkage between *Co* and *Jk* had already been presented (42)) *Co* has indeed been shown to be located on chromosome 7. The early evidence for this location of *Co* included lack of Colton antigens from the red cells of some patients with monosomy 7 (see below). In 1990, Zelinski et al. (43) reported that *Co* is closely linked to *ASSP11* (argininosuccinate synthetase pseudogene 11), a gene known to be located on the short arm of chromosome 7 (44). After the Colton antigens had been shown (20) to be carried on red cell aquaporin (the water transport protein, see also below) more precise location of the *Co* locus became possible. Moon et al. (45) used in situ hybridization studies to locate *AQP1*, the gene that encodes the water transport protein, to 7p14.

Monosomy 7 and the Colton Antigens

The loss of one chromosome 7 from hematopoietic stem cells is a rare abnormality associated with acute myeloid leukemia or a preleukemic syndrome. The phenotypes Co(a-b-) Co:-3 and Co(a+[w]) Co:w3 have been seen in a number of patients with monosomy 7 (46-48). It is not clear why the loss of one chromosome 7 can result in the loss of all Colton system antigens. Zelinski

et al. (43) suggested that the situation represents the loss of one *Colton* gene due to monosomy and alteration of the product of the other due to the patient's disease. Daniels (49) reports that of 35 monosomy 7 patients tested at the MRC Blood Group Unit, eight had loss or weakening of Colton antigens. None of the eight had been recently transfused. Among the remaining patients, 21 had transfused cells present at the time of the test. In none of those could weakening of Co[a] be seen. It was suggested (49) that either the depressed antigen expression cannot be seen in the presence of transfused cells or that transfusion confers some beneficial effect on the expression of Colton antigens.

The Colton System and Other Clinical Conditions

In 1994, Parsons et al. (34) described a child with a unique form of congenital dyserythropoietic anemia (CDA) whose red cells were deficient in CD44 protein. The phenotype of the patient's red cells was highly unusual, i.e. Co(a-b-) Co:3 (when tested with the anti-Co3-like antibody described above); In(a-b-); AnWj-; and only weakly reactive with anti-LW[ab]. Since it is known (for references see Chapter 29) that In[a], In[b] and AnWj are carried on CD44, the In(a-b-), AnWj- status of the red cells was at least partially understood. Their Co(a-b-) Co:3 phenotype and their weak expression of LW[ab] was not. Subsequent studies, discussed in more detail below, demonstrated that the patient's red cells had a marked reduction in CHIP (66). Since red cells from patients with other forms of CDA have normal expression of Colton system antigens, the meaning of the findings in this case are not clear but see also Chapter 29.

We (50,51) thought it no more than coincidence that when we tested the red cells of 19 patients with hereditary spherocytosis (HS), who represented among them eight unrelated kindreds, we found three samples that were Co(b+). Two were from members of one family, the other was from an unrelated individual. In a sample of this size, at the most one Co(b+) blood would be expected. Now with the known association between the Colton system and acute myeloid leukemia (see monosomy 7, above) and very tentative possible links with CDA (34) and PNH (37) our degree of suspicion against coincidence for an association between the Colton system and HS, is raised just a fraction.

The Biochemical Nature of the Colton Antigens

Clues concerning the biochemical nature of the

Colton antigens first emerged in 1992 when Frances Spring, working at the International Blood Group Reference Laboratory in Bristol, England, observed that antibodies to Co[a], Co[b], and Co3 immunoprecipitated a component of apparent molecular weight 28kD from radioiodinated human red cells of appropriate Colton phenotype. As already discussed, Zelinski et al. (43) had demonstrated, in 1990, that the *Colton* blood group locus is on the short arm of chromosome 7. When, in 1993, Moon et al. (45) described the structure, organization and chromosomal localization of the human Aquaporin-CHIP gene on chromosome 7p14, the possibility that CHIP carried the Colton antigens seemed likely since CHIP was known (55,56) to have an apparent molecular weight of 28kD. Subsequent studies by Smith et al. (20) established that the Colton antigens are on CHIP (see figure 21-1) and that the *Colton* blood group and the *Aquaporin-CHIP* loci are identical. Smith et al. (20) immunoblotted membranes from red cells of phenotype Co(a+b-), Co(a-b+) and Co(a-b-) with affinity-purified rabbit antibodies to CHIP. Rabbit anti-CHIP gave the expected band at 28kD (and a minor band of 40-60kD corresponding to the glycosylated form of CHIP, gly-CHIP) with Co(a+b-) and Co(a-b+) but not with Co(a-b-) membranes. When immunoprecipitates obtained with human anti-Co[a], anti-Co[b] and anti-Co3 were analyzed on immunoblots with anti-CHIP, the Colton antibodies were shown to precipitate CHIP in every case. Anti-Co[a] could immunoprecipitate Triton X-100 solubilized CHIP protein but attempts to immunoprecipitate SDS-denatured, nonglycosylated CHIP subunits were unsuccessful. Since Triton X-100 is known (57) to solubilize CHIP in its tetrameric form these results suggested that the native surface conformation of CHIP protein is required for antigen activity.

In order to investigate the molecular basis of Colton antigens, Smith et al. (20) amplified the four exons that comprise the CHIP gene, from genomic DNA derived from individuals of known Colton phenotype. Sequence analysis of the amplified products demonstrated a single difference at nucleotide 134 (C in DNA from Co(a+b-) samples and T in Co(a-b+) samples). DNA from Co(a+b+) individuals contained both nucleotides. The nucleotide substitution at 134 changes the coding sequence at amino acid residue 45 of the CHIP protein from alanine in Co(a+b-) individuals to valine in Co(a-b+) individuals (see figure 21-1).

Colton Typing from DNA

The nucleotide sequence substitution C134 to T described in the preceding section creates a second restriction site in exon 1 of the CHIP gene for the restric-

tion enzyme PflMI. This means that whereas digestion of amplified exon 1 from an individual of type Co(a+b-) yields two fragments of 300bp and 144bp, digestion of exon 1 from an individual of type Co(a-b+) with the same enzyme yields three fragments of 174bp, 144bp and 126bp (20). The ability to determine Colton phenotypes from DNA may be of practical value when the relatively rare Colton antisera are not available, when red cells are in poor condition or when large numbers of samples are to be typed for population or disease association studies.

Structure of CHIP

CHIP is an extremely well characterized protein. Detailed studies, most notably from Peter Agre's group at the Johns Hopkins University School of Medicine in Baltimore, have elucidated the structure of the encoding gene and the structure and function of the protein. Aquaporin-CHIP was the first known molecular water channel (reviewed by Agre et al. (58)). The protein was originally isolated as a byproduct during the purification of Rh polypeptides (59,60). On SDS-PAGE the protein has an apparent molecular weight of 28kD. A minor band of 40-60kD is also observed that corresponds to a glycosylated form of the 28kD protein. The protein exists as a tetramer in the membrane. Each tetramer contains one glycosylated monomer. There are approximately 200,000 copies of the protein in normal red cells (glycosylated and non-glycosylated monomers). The protein sequence was deduced from cDNA sequence (56). Amino terminal amino acid sequence was used to design degenerate oligonucleotide primers which ultimately led to the isolation of an almost full length cDNA (2.9kb) from a human bone marrow library. Northern blots of RNA from human bone marrow contained a single major transcript of 3kb. The cDNA contained an 807bp open reading frame encoding a protein of 28.5kD. Hydropathy analysis of the deduced amino acid sequence predicted six transmembrane domains with three extracellular and two intracellular loops (see figure 21-1). The N and C termini are intracellular. The critical residues defining the Colton antigens are located at residue 45 on the first and smallest predicted extracellular loop. There is an ABH active N-glycan at Asn42 on one monomer in each tetramer (20). Whether or not the N-glycan influences the expression of Colton antigens is presently unclear although failure to detect Co[a] antigen on CHIP expressed in *Xenopus* oocytes suggests that altered glycosylation may obscure access to the antigen (20). CHIP contains no known extracellular cleavage sites, a feature consistent with the use of protease-treated red cells for detection of Colton system antibodies. The use of the antiglobulin test in conjunction with protease treated cells for optimum sensitivity in anti-

FIGURE 21-1 The Structure of Aquaporin-1 and the Location of
Colton Blood Group Antigens (from reference 61)

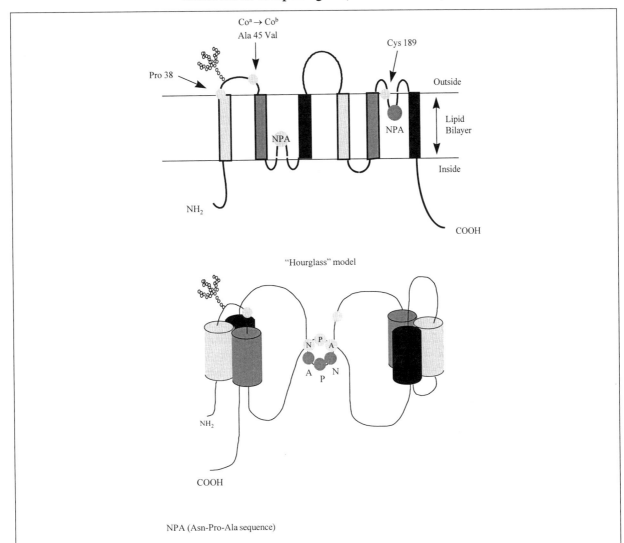

body detection is discussed above. The location of the critical residues for Colton antigens at a site very close to the lipid bilayer provides an explanation of the validity of this approach. Protease treatment would facilitate access of antibody by removing the extracellular domains of proteins of the glycocalyx, notably glycophorins (see Chapters 15 and 16).

Inspection of the amino acid sequence of CHIP revealed an internal homology between the amino terminal half of the molecule and the carboxyl terminal half. There is a three amino acid motif (Asn-Pro-Ala) in the first cytoplasmic loop which is repeated at a corresponding point in the third extracellular loop. This motif is characteristic of other members of the water channel family like MIP26, the major intrinsic protein of the lens. Agre et al. (58) and Jungi et al. (61) have suggested, on

the basis of site directed mutagenesis experiments, that the two loops containing the Asn-Pro-Ala motif may be physically associated when the polypeptide is folded within the membrane bilayer with the Asn-Pro-Ala motifs forming the aperture of the water channel (Hourglass model, see figure 21-1). CHIP is one of the few integral membrane proteins for which crystallographic data are available. Two groups (62,63) have reported electron crystallographic studies that are consistent with a tetrameric structure containing monomers each with 6 or 8 alpha-helices.

Function of CHIP

That CHIP could act as a water channel was first

demonstrated in the *Xenopus* oocyte system (64). The oocytes are suitable for the study of channel mediated water transport because they have only a low diffusional water permeability surviving in freshwater ponds (58). In vitro transcribed CHIP RNA in 50nl of water was microinjected into oocytes and control oocytes were injected with 50nl of water without RNA. Maximum expression of CHIP was observed after 72 hours of incubation. When the oocytes were transferred from 200 to 70 mosmol/kg H_2O buffer, the oocytes expressing CHIP increased in volume by 30-50% before rupturing after 3 to 5 minutes. The coefficient of osmotic water permeability (Pf) at 22°C was approximately eight-fold higher than that of control oocytes. CHIP permeability appeared selective for water, oocytes expressing CHIP failed to absorb urea or glucose when placed in an osmotic gradient (58). Site directed mutagenesis was used by Preston et al. (65) and Jungi et al. (61) to identify the amino acids critical for the water transport function. Initial studies focused on cysteine residues because water channels were known to be inhibited by mercurial sulfhydryl reagents such as mercuric chloride and p-chloromercuribenzene sulfonate (pCMBS). These studies identified cysteine 189 as the mercurial sensitive site (65). Cysteine 189 is close to one of the Asn-Pro-Ala motifs discussed above (Asn192, see figure 21-1). Jungi et al. (61) showed that if Cys189 was mutated to serine and Ala73 to Cys (Ala73 is near the second Asn-Pro-Ala motif at Asn76) this double mutant, when expressed in oocytes, resulted in the oocytes having a high Pf similar to the natural CHIP. These and other studies led Jungi et al. (61) to formulate the Hourglass model depicted in figure 21-1 and discussed above, whereby the first cytoplasmic loop and the third extracellular loop associate to form the water channel.

Organization of the CHIP Gene

The organization of the CHIP gene was elucidated by Moon et al. (45). The gene encompasses 17kb and was located at chromosome 7p14 by fluorescence in situ hybridization (FISH) using a genomic probe. The gene comprises four exons corresponding to amino acids 1-128,129-183,184-210 and 211-269.

CHIP in Erythroid and Renal Development

CHIP is a major component of proximal renal tubules where its function appears to be reabsorbtion of water from the glomerular filtrate. Red cells may use CHIP for rapid rehydration as the cells leave the markedly hypertonic renal medulla (66). CHIP is expressed at low levels in second trimester fetal red cells (17 weeks). Nearly adult levels of CHIP expression are reached by birth (66). This would be expected since Colton antigens are known to be fully developed at birth and anti-Co^a has been the cause of severe HDN. Renal tubules also contain nearly adult levels of CHIP at birth (66). It is not known if the Colton antigens are expressed on kidney cells. It is possible that an altered glycosylation pattern in kidney and other tissues precludes expression of the antigens. CHIP is already abundantly expressed by the CFU-e stage of erythroid differentiation (66).

Individuals with the Rare Co(a-b-) Phenotype Lack CHIP but are in Apparently Normal Health

The assignment of Colton blood group antigens to CHIP contributed little to the understanding of the structure of this protein other than to provide confirmation that the first predicted extracellular loop is indeed accessible on the outside of the red cell. In contrast, the assignment has had a marked affect on an understanding of the function of the protein because it drew attention to individuals with the rare Co(a-b-) phenotype as possible cases of CHIP deficiency. Preston et al. (35) studied three individuals with the Co(a-b-) phenotype none of whom had experienced hematological, renal, ocular, respiratory, gastrointestinal, reproductive or neurological dysfunction. Two of these individuals lacked detectable CHIP as judged by immunoblotting of their red cell membranes. The third had less than 1% of normal levels. In addition, one of the individuals who lacked CHIP from her red cell membranes was examined for the presence of CHIP in urine sediment. None was found although CHIP was evident in urine from normal controls. The osmotic water permeability of Co(a-b-) red cells was reduced by approximately 80% when compared with normal red cells.

Analysis of the CHIP gene using genomic DNA from each of the three Co(a-b-) individuals demonstrated that three different genetic mechanisms were responsible for the CHIP deficiency. Exon 1 could not be amplified from the first patient whereas exons 2, 3 and 4 were normal. Southern blot analysis indicated that most of exon 1 was absent. The second individual examined had a single base insertion in exon 1 at position 307 that produced a frameshift mutation starting after Gly104. The third individual had a C to T substitution at position 113 which resulted in a Pro38 to Leu substitution. In many ways the third individual has the most interesting mutation. It is clear that the first two cannot produce CHIP but why does a Pro to Leu change have such a dramatic effect on the level of CHIP in the red cells? Preston et al. (35) expressed mutant Pro38Leu cRNA in *Xenopus* oocytes and two days after injection could show that the osmotic water permeability of the mutant was three times higher than in control oocytes not given cRNA but eight times less than that obtained with normal CHIP cRNA. Three days after injection the total amount of the mutant protein in oocytes was substantially reduced when compared to those expressing normal CHIP. Pro38 is at the end of the first membrane spanning alpha helix (see figure 21-1). It seems likely that this residue is critical for stable insertion of the polypeptide in to the membrane. These studies raise difficult questions about the functional significance of CHIP. It clearly has a major role as a water channel in normal red cells and yet individuals who lack the protein entirely do not have any serious health problems. Mathai et al. (52) carried out a detailed functional analysis and confirmed the absence of any major functional lesions in CHIP deficient cells. They found evidence for a slight reduction in red cell lifespan and reduced membrane surface area and concluded that "the movement of water across the red cell membrane may reflect the complex behaviors of multiple membrane components in addition to AQP1".

A fourth individual with the Co(a-b-) phenotype was studied by Agre et al. (66). This patient was a child with a novel form of CDA characterized by membranous inclusion bodies in erythroid cells (Wickramasinghe et al. (67)), persistent expression of epsilon and zeta embryonic globins and large amounts of fetal hemoglobins (Tang et al. (68)). The patient's red cells were also In(a-b-) and AnWj-, a feature that correlated with CD44 deficiency, (34, and see Chapter 29). The patient's red cells had less than 10% of the normal level of CHIP and a markedly low osmotic water permeability. Sequencing of the four exons of the CHIP gene did not identify any abnormality. The existence of an erythroid-specific mutation in the CHIP promoter was not excluded. Agre et al. (66) suggest that the patient has a fundamental defect in erythroid ontogeny that might be related to a mutated form of an erythroid transcription factor that is required to suppress embryonic and fetal globin genes but induces expression of CD44 and CHIP. Agre et al. (66) also point out that juvenile chronic myelogenous leukemias may exhibit fetal and embryonic erythroid features (69,70). These observations taken together with the occurrence of the Co(a-b-) phenotype in association with monosomy 7 and myelogenous leukemia (see earlier) suggest that further study of the factors that regulate the CHIP gene and a detailed analysis of the Colton phenotypes of patients with erythroid/myeloid disorders may be a profitable avenue for future research.

References

1. Heisto H, Hart M van der, Madsen G, et al. Vox Sang 1967;12:18
2. Giles CM, Darnborough J, Aspinall P, et al. Br J Haematol 1970;19:267
3. Wray E, Simpson S. Vox Sang 1968;14:130
4. Smith DS, Stratton F, Howell P, et al. Vox Sang 1970;18:62
5. Thomas MJ, Deveney L, Wurzel HA. (abstract). Prog 24th Ann Mtg AABB, 1971:100
6. Simpson WKH. S Afr Med J 1973;47:1302
7. McIntyre C, Finigan L, Larsen AL. Transfusion 1976;16:76
8. Beattie KM, Adams G, Sigmund KE, et al. (abstract). Transfusion 1978;18:37
9. Kitzke HM, Julius H, Delaney M, et al. (abstract). Transfusion 1982;22:407
10. Kurtz SR, Kuszaj T, Ouellet R, et al. Vox Sang 1982;43:28
11. Ikin WE, Metaxas-Bühler M, Metaxas MN, et al. Vox Sang 1970;19:537
12. Lewis M, Kaita H, Anderson C, et al. Transfusion 1971;11:223
13. Case J. Vox Sang 1971;21:447
14. Wilson MJ, Miller WV, Issitt CH. Unpublished observations 1972, cited in Issitt PD, Issitt CH. Applied Blood Group Serology, 2nd Ed. Oxnard:Spectra Biologicals, 1975
15. Clausen J. (abstract). Book of Abstracts, 25th Ann Mtg AABB, 13th Cong ISBT, 1972:45
16. Lee EL, Bennett C. Transfusion 1982;22:159
17. Squires JE, Larson PJ, Charles WT, et al. Transfusion 1985;25:137
18. Dzik WH, Blank J. Transfusion 1986;26:246
19. Rogers MJ, Stiles PA, Wright J. (abstract). Transfusion 1974;14:508
20. Smith BL, Preston GM, Spring F, et al. J Clin Invest 1994;94:1043
21. Lewis M, Kaita H, Chown B, et al. Vox Sang 1977;32:208
22. Brackenridge CJ, Case J, Sheehy AJ. Hum Hered 1975;25:520
23. Gale SA, Rowe GP, Northfield FE. Vox Sang 1988;54:172
24. Crawford MN. Unpublished observations 1967, cited by Race RR, Sanger R. Blood Groups in Man, 6th Ed. Oxford:Blackwell, 1975
25. Issitt PD, Wren MR, Rueda E, et al. (Letter). Transfusion 1987;27:117
26. Lucciola L, Kaita H, Anderson J, et al. Canad J Genet Cytol 1974;16:691
27. Henke H, Basler M, Baur MP. Foren Sci Int 1982;20:233
28. Daniels G. Immunohematology 1992;8:53
29. Dunstan RA. Br J Haematol 1986;62:301
30. Fuhrmann U, Kloppenburg W, Kruger H-W. Geburtsch Frauenheilk 1979;39:66
31. Theuriere M, de la Camera C, DiNapoli J, et al. Immunohematology 1985;2:16
32. Savona-Ventura C, Grech ES, Zieba A. Obstet Gynecol 1989;73:870
33. Lacey PA, Robinson J, Collins ML, et al. Transfusion 1987;27:268
34. Parson SF, Jones J, Anstee DJ, et al. Blood 1994;83:860
35. Preston GM, Smith BL, Zeidel ML, et al. Science 1994;265:1585
36. Moulds JJ, Dykes D, Polesky HF. (abstract). Transfusion 1974;14:508
37. Swanson JL, Eckman JR. (abstract). Transfusion 1978;18:376
38. Moulds JJ. Personal communication 1976, cited by Issitt PD.

Applied Blood Group Serology, 3rd Ed. Miami:Montgomery 1985:391

39. Race RR, Sanger R. Blood Groups in Man, 6th Ed. Oxford:Blackwell, 1975

40. Moulds M, Strohm P, McDowell MA, et al. (abstract). Transfusion 1988; 28 (Suppl 6S):36S

41. Mohr J, Eiberg H. Clin Genet 1977;11:372

42. Zelinski T, Kaita H, Lewis M, et al. Transfusion 1988;28:435

43. Zelinski T, Kaita H, Gilson T, et al. Genomics 1990;6:623

44. Zelinski TA, White LJ, Coghlan GE, et al. Cytogenet Cell Genet 1991;58:1927

45. Moon C, Preston GM, Griffin C, et al. J Biol Chem 1993;268:15772

46. de la Chapelle A, Vuopio P, Sanger R, et al. Lancet 1975;2:817

47. Boetius G, Hustinx TWJ, Smits APT, et al. Br J Haematol 1977;37:101

48. Pasquali F, Bernasconi P, Casalone R, et al. Hum Genet 1982;62:40

49. Daniels G. Human Blood Groups. Oxford:Blackwell, 1995:509

50. Ward MJ. MS Thesis, Univ Cincinnati, 1980

51. Ward MJ, Issitt PD. Biotest Bull 1982;1:174

52. Mathai JC, Mori S, Smith BL, et al. J Biol Chem 1996;271:1309

53. Jerne D. Lylloff K. Acta Path Microbiol Scand 1980;88 (Section C): 57

54. Hoffmann JJML, Overbeeke MAM. Immunohematology 1996;12:11

55. Denker BM, Smith BL, Kuhajda FP, et al. J Biol Chem 1988;263:15634

56. Preston GM, Agre P. Proc Nat Acad Sci USA 1991;88:11110

57. Smith BL, Agre P. J Biol Chem 1991;266:6407

58. Agre P, Preston GM, Smith BL, et al. Am J Physiol. 1993;34:F463

59. Agre P, Saboori AM, Asimos A. J Biol Chem 1987;262:17497

60. Saboori AM, Smith BL, Agre P. Proc Nat Acad Sci USA 1988;85:4042

61. Jungi JS, Preston GM, Smith BL, et al. J Biol Chem 1994;269:14648

62. Mitra AK, van Hoek AN, Weiner MC, et al. Nat Struct Biol 1995;2:726

63. Walz T, Typke D, Smith BL, et al. Nat Struct Biol 1995;2:730

64. Preston GM, Carroll TP, Guggino WB, et al. Science 1992;256:385

65. Preston GM, Jung JS, Guggino WB, et al. J Biol Chem 1993;268:17

66. Agre P, Smith BL, Baumgarten R, et al. J Clin Invest 1994;94:1050

67. Wickramasinghe SN, Illum N, Wimberley PD. Br J Haematol 1991;79:322

68. Tang W, Cai SP, Eng B, et al. Blood 1993;81:1636

69. Weinberg RS, Leibowitz ME, Weinblatt ME, et al. Br J Haematol 1990;76:307

70. Papayannopoulou T, Nakamoto B, Anagnou NP, et al. Blood 1991;77:2569

22 | The Dombrock Blood Group System

In 1965, Swanson et al. (1) published a preliminary report describing anti-Do^a that defined a hitherto unreported antigen present on the red cells of some 67% of random White donors. Additional details about the antigen and antibody were published shortly thereafter (2-4). In 1973, Molthan et al. (5) described anti-Do^b, the antibody defining the antigen antithetical to Do^a. The incidence of Do^a and Do^b was found to be quite variable in different populations (see below). Other than that variation, the Dombrock system remained straightforward as a two allele, two antigen system for many years. In 1992, Banks et al. (6) announced their highly exciting finding that Gy(a-) red cells (see below) represent the null phenotype, i.e. Do(a-b-) and more (again see below) in the Dombrock system. A full report of this study appeared in 1995 (7). The high incidence antigen Gy^a had been described in 1967 (8) and some relatively complex serology (9,10) had shown that another high incidence antigen, Hy, described briefly in 1967 (11) and in more detail in 1970 (12) was closely related to Gy^a at the phenotypic level. In 1981, Laird-Fryer et al. (13) added Jc^a, another antigen of high incidence to the Gy^a, Hy phenotypic association. Weaver et al. (14,15) then showed that Jc^a is the same as Jo^a, an antigen that had first been described by Jensen et al. (16) in 1972. Since the name Jo^a clearly has priority over Jc^a, the term Jo^a is now used to the exclusion of Jc^a. The study by Banks et al. (7) showed that the null phenotype in the system is Do(a-b-) Gy(a-) Hy- Jo(a-).

Since the names Gy^a, Hy and Jo^a had been widely used before it was shown that the antigens involved are part of the Dombrock system, they have continued in use. The terms DO3, DO4 and DO5, respectively, were assigned by the ISBT Working Party on Terminology for Red Cell Surface Antigens (17) but have not been widely applied. Table 22-1 lists the conventional and ISBT terms for antigens of the system and shows the incidence of each in White and Black populations.

In 1990 Telen et al. (18) described some studies on the red cells of patients with paroxysmal nocturnal hemoglobinuria (PNH). Such patients have several populations of cells that can be separated by various means (see Chapter 4). PNH I red cells are essentially normal and phenotyping studies on those cells reveal which blood group genes the individual has inherited. PNH III red cells either lack or have grossly reduced amounts of all glycosylphosphatidyl-inositol-linked proteins. Such proteins (hereinafter PI-linked) are anchored to the red cell membrane via phosphatidylinositol and it is that structure that is defective in PNH III red cells. Thus lack of red cell

TABLE 22-1 Conventional and ISBT Terminology for the Dombrock Blood Group System

Conventional Name: Dombrock
Conventional Symbol: Do
ISBT System Symbol: DO
ISBT System Number: 014

Antigen Conventional Name	ISBT Antigen Number	ISBT Full Code Number	% Random Samples Positive for the Antigen	
			Whites	Blacks
Do^a	DO1	014001	67	55
Do^b	DO2	014002	82	89
Gy^a	DO3	014003	>99.9	>99.9
Hy	DO4	014004	>99.9	>99.9
Jo^a	DO5	014005	>99.9	>99.9

Thus far the phenotype Gy(a-) has been found only in Whites and Orientals, while the phenotypes Hy- and Jo(a-) seem to be almost exclusively confined to Blacks (see text).

blood group antigens from PNH III red cells is highly suggestive of the fact that such antigens are carried on one of several different PI-linked proteins. Additional support for such a conclusion is provided if the antigens are shown to be present on the PNH I red cells of the same patient. Such a finding shows that the individual concerned has the genes encoding production of the antigens and that lack of a PI-linked protein explains absence of the antigens from the PNH III population of red cells. Among a considerable number of findings (see also Chapter 23, The Cartwright System and Chapter 24, The Cromer System) Telen et al. (18) showed that PNH III red cells lacked Do^a, Do^b, Gy^a, Hy and Jo^a although the PNH I red cells of the individuals involved carried those antigens. This work was then extended by others (19,20) who showed that Do^a, Do^b, Gy^a, Hy and Jo^a are all carried on the same PI-linked protein.

The Antigens Do^a and Do^b and the Antibodies That Define Them

Although several examples of anti-Do^a (see below) and a few examples of anti-Do^b have been found, they have not been particularly strong and have often been present in

703

sera containing other antibodies. Thus although family studies (4,21,22) have clearly shown that *Do^a* and *Do^b* are codominant alleles that are inherited in a normal Mendelian fashion, less complete data are available regarding the frequency of Do^a and Do^b in different population groups. Such information as is available is listed in table 22-2, it must be remembered that far more tests have been performed with anti-Do^a than with anti-Do^b and that while the frequencies shown in the table have been supported by the somewhat limited serological studies performed, the incidence of Do^b sometimes represents a calculation from gene frequency figures. The probability that the calculated figures are close to correct is enhanced first by the fact that no evidence has emerged to suggest that there is a third functional allele at the *Do^aDo^b* locus and second, from the finding that the Do(a-b-) phenotype (i.e. the Gy(a-) phenotype) seems to be rare in all populations studied.

The Do^a and Do^b antigens appear to be fully developed at birth (1,5). Both antigens survive papain and ficin treatment of red cells (1-3,5) indeed examples of antibodies directed against them often react optimally, and sometimes only, in indirect antiglobulin tests using enzyme-treated red cells. In contrast, the antigens are either denatured or markedly reduced in expression when red cells are treated with trypsin, chymotrypsin or pronase (7,19,20). N-acetyl-neuraminic acid seems to play no role in the structure of Do^a or Do^b since both antigens survive treatment of red cell with neuramindase. Do^a and Do^b are both denatured when red cells are treated with 2-aminoethylisothiouronium bromide (AET) and dithiothreitol (DTT) (19,20,25).

In addition to the early discovered examples of anti-Do^a and anti-Do^b (1,3,5) many other examples of anti-Do^a (26-33) and fewer examples of anti-Do^b (34-36) have been described in the literature. The antibodies are usually IgG in nature, they are best detected in indirect antiglobulin tests and, as mentioned above, usually react more strongly with papain or ficin-treated, than with untreated red cells. Those examples studied for such ability, have been shown (3,29,34) not to bind complement. Some but by no means all examples of the antibodies show dosage effects (3,5,34,35), care is needed in the interpretation of such tests (as is the case with any studies designed to detect antigen dose) since Do^a shows considerable variation of expression on Do(a+b-) red cells from unrelated persons. As mentioned in the introduction of this chapter, anti-Do^a and anti-Do^b are most often seen in sera that contain other antibodies. Anti-Do^a has been encountered as the only antibody present on at least three occasions, each time production of the antibody was stimulated by pregnancy (28,29,33), in one of the cases (28) the antibody was made during a first pregnancy in which the infant had Do(a+) red cells. No non-red cell stimulated example of anti-Do^a or anti-Do^b has been described.

A few examples of anti-Do^a (3,30,32) and anti-Do^b (35,36) have been described as being clinically significant, among them the antibodies caused immediate and delayed transfusion reactions, shortening of in vivo survival of ^51Cr-labeled antigen-positive red cells and reactions in in vitro phagocytic cells assays that suggested that the antibodies were clinically significant. In contrast, in at least one case (31) an in vivo red cell survival study using Do(a+) red cells in a patient with anti-Do^a showed normal survival of those red cells at 24 hours and subsequent transfusions with Do(a+) blood produced no untoward effects at the time of or following transfusion. Although anti-Do^a has caused a positive DAT on the red cells of some Do(a+) infants born to women with anti-Do^a in the serum (28,29,33) neither anti-Do^a nor anti-Do^b has been reported as causing clinical HDN.

The Antigen Gy^a and the Antibody That Defines It

In 1967, Swanson et al. (8) described anti-Gy^a that

TABLE 22-2 Do^a and Do^b Phenotype Frequencies in Different Populations*

Population	Percent Do(a+b-)	Percent Do(a+b+)	Percent Do(a-b+)	Percent Do(a+)	Percent Do(b+)	References
Northern Europeans and White Americans	18	49	33	67	82	1-4,21
Black Americans	11	44	45	55	89	3,4
Japanese	1.5	22	76.5	23.5	98.5	22,23
Thais	0.5	13	86.5	13.5	99.5	24

*   These phenotype frequencies are based primarily on tests with anti-Do^a and calculated frequencies of the *Do^b* gene assuming that all (or almost all) persons with Do(a-) red cells are genetically *Do^bDo^b*.

defines an antigen of high incidence. In the original family of Americans of Czech extraction, the proposita who made the antibody had seven children four of whom had Gy(a-) red cells. The proposita and her husband were second cousins. The proposita's sister who had borne two children, was also Gy(a-) with anti-Gy^a in the serum. Swanson (37) then found another American family, also of Czech extraction, in which two sisters, both of whom had been pregnant, had Gy(a-) red cells and anti-Gy^a in the serum. An English family with possible similar Romany extraction was studied by Clark et al. (38) who found that six of twelve sibs a (a thirteenth was deceased) had Gy(a-) red cells. The four Gy(a-) female sibs had all been pregnant and each had anti-Gy^a in the serum. The two Gy(a-) male sibs had not been transfused and neither had made anti-Gy^a. Additional individuals with Gy(a-) red cells had previously been described by Moulds et al. (9) in Minnesota and by Massaquoi and Cornwall (39,42) in two probably related families in Newfoundland, Canada. Records of one of the Newfoundland families, both of which came from isolated populations, over a six generation period, revealed a total of 44 matings, 20 of which were consanguineous (42). More than 300 members of the kindred were tested and two, in addition to the proposita, were found to have Gy(a-) red cells. Clark et al. (38) discussed findings that suggested that the various families reported (8,9,37-39,42) might share a common Romany (Bohemian gypsy) ancestor. In their family (38) the recurrence of some surnames suggested the possibility of consanguinity.

That the Gy(a-) phenotype exists in populations other than those described above became apparent when Okubo et al. (40) described six apparently unrelated Japanese women with Gy(a-) red cells and anti-Gy^a in the serum. Each of the women had been pregnant, they were found at various blood centers in Japan (Osaka, Okayama, Sasebo, Kawasaki, Hokkaido and Okinawa) when five of them presented as blood donors and the sixth as a patient with an antibody to a very common antigen. One Chinese Gy(a-) male with what was presumed to be transfusion-induced anti-Gy^a, was identified in Hong Kong (41).

In deliberate screening studies 10,145 Americans (including 611 Native Americans and 75 Blacks) (8) and 9350 Japanese blood donors (40) were tested, no Gy(a-) sample was found. As mentioned briefly in the introduction of this chapter and as discussed in more detail below, the Gy(a-) phenotype has not been found in Blacks. The related Hy- phenotype (see below) that is associated with very weak expression of Gy^a is found exclusively in Blacks.

Unlike Do^a and Do^b that appear to be fully developed at birth, Gy^a has been said (10,38) to be poorly expressed on cord blood red cells (but see also the section on monoclonal anti-Gy^a). Other characteristics of Gy^a are similar to those of Do^a and Do^b. The antigen survives treatment of red cells with papain, ficin or neuraminidase but is partially sensitive to trypsin, chymotrypsin and pronase (19,20) and to the actions of AET and DTT (19,25,46,47) but again see the section on monoclonal anti-Gy^a .

It will be noticed from the above descriptions that anti-Gy^a seems almost always to be made when a woman with Gy(a-) red cells carries an infant whose red cells are Gy(a+). This, of course, suggests that Gy^a is highly immunogenic. Most examples of anti-Gy^a are IgG in nature, react optimally in indirect antiglobulin tests and do not fix complement (8,10,38,43). The example described by Clark et al. (38) was exceptional in that it contained both IgG and IgA components and was shown to bind complement when tested by an EDTA two-stage antiglobulin test (see Chapter 3). There are few data about the clinical significance of anti-Gy^a. The patient studied by Mak et al. (41) had an IgG anti-Gy^a with a titer of 512 by IAT. However, the antibody showed the characteristics of those said to be of high titer and low avidity (HTLA, see 44) and the patient was transfused uneventfully with ten units of Gy(a+) blood. A male patient who had never been transfused was found to have an IgG1 anti-Gy^a that was produced transiently (43). Three months after its initial identification, the antibody was no longer detectable in the patient's serum. While the anti-Gy^a was being made, an in vivo red cell survival study showed normal survival of Gy(a+) red cells (43). An additional finding (45) in this case was that the patient's red cells would adsorb, and yield on solution, anti-Hy. As discussed below, Gy(a-) red cells are truly Hy- and will not adsorb anti-Hy. Thus in this case (43) the transient production of non-red cell stimulated anti-Gy^a and the presence of some Hy on the antibody-maker's red cells strongly suggested (45) that the case represented temporary suppression of Gy^a red cell antigen production with concomitant transient production of anti-Gy^a. Like anti-Do^a and anti-Do^b, anti-Gy^a has never caused clinical HDN although as described above, anti-Gy^a has often been present in the sera of women who have delivered infants with Gy(a+) red cells.

The Antigen Hy and the Antibody That Defines It

Anti-Hy, that defines an antigen of high incidence, was first described in an abstract in 1967 (11). Workers interested in the history of discovery of the blood groups may recall that the abstract in question described four hitherto unreported high incidence antigens So, El, Hy and Dp. The antigen So is now known to be the same as Lan (see Chapter 31); El is known to be the same as At^a (also see Chapter 31); Dp is known to be the same as K14 (see Chapter 18); only Hy continues under the name used in the abstract. To add to the historical interest, the first description of At[a] (i.e. El, see above) appears as an abstract on the same page of the journal (48).

Several other examples of anti-Hy were subsequently described (49-51) all were made by Blacks. Moulds et al. (10) described a number of otherwise unpublished studies (52-56) that used anti-Gy[a] at a dilution at which it would not react with Gy(a-) Hy- or with Gy(a+[w]) Hy- (see below) red cells, to screen samples from random donors. No negative sample was found among: 13,989 American Whites; 683 Whites in Durban, South Africa; 735 Czechs; 1121 American Blacks; 1023 Blacks (Bantu) in Durban; 1679 Pima (American) Indians; 611 American Indians in Minneapolis; and 633 Asian Indians in Durban. Two of 597 Apache (American) Indians were found to have non-reactive red cells, both samples were subsequently shown to be Gy(a+[w]) Hy-. It was suspected (10) that in both cases, Black admixture explained the Hy- phenotype.

The Hy antigen appears to be less than fully developed at birth (10,38), like Do[a], Do[b] and Gy[a] the antigen survives treatment of red cells with papain, ficin or neuraminidase, it is partially sensitive to trypsin, chymotrypsin, pronase and treatment of red cells with AET or DTT (7,19,20,25,46,57).

Anti-Hy is usually an IgG antibody that is optimally reactive in IATs (10,49-51). One hemolytic transfusion reaction has been blamed on anti-Hy (49), another example of the antibody caused accelerated clearance of Hy+ red cells in an in vivo survival study (50). We have heard anecdotal reports of anti-Hy with HTLA characteristics, that were benign in vivo but such occurrences do not appear to have been described in print. While anti-Hy has caused a positive DAT on the Hy+ red cells of infants born to women with anti-Hy in the serum (11,51) it has not caused clinical HDN. The phenotypic relationships of Hy to Gy[a] and to Do[a] and Do[b] are described in a later section.

The Antigen Jo[a] (Jc[a]) and the Antibody That Defines It

In 1972, Jensen et al. (16) described the first two examples of anti-Jo[a], that defines an antigen of high incidence, when they studied mutually compatible samples from two unrelated Black individuals. A third example of the antibody was reported in 1976 (59) and a family study performed during the investigation showed that Jo[a] is an inherited characteristic. In 1981, Laird-Fryer et al. (13) described five unrelated Black women with an antibody to a high incidence antigen. The red cells and antibodies of the five women were mutually compatible, the antibody involved was named anti-Jc[a]. Weaver et al. (14,15) then showed that Jc[a] and Jo[a] are the same thing

(but see the addendum), the name Jo[a] had priority and the name Jc[a] has been abandoned. Jensen et al. (16) tested red cell samples from 3000 predominantly White New York blood donors and 7689 American Blacks and found no Jo(a-) sample.

Like Do[a] and Do[b] but unlike Gy[a] and Hy, Jo[a] seems to be fully developed at birth (16,17). Like other antigens of the system, Jo[a] survives papain, ficin or neuraminidase treatment of red cells, it is denatured or markedly weakened when red cells are treated with trypsin, chymotrypsin, pronase, AET or DTT (7,16,19,20,59).

Anti-Jo[a] is usually an IgG, non-complement binding, red cell stimulated antibody that reacts optimally in IATs. One example of anti-Jo[a] was shown (60) to be made in part of IgG1 and in part of IgG2. In in vivo red cell survival studies in a patient with sickle cell disease, who had anti-Jo[a] in the serum, it was found (61) that Jo(a+) red cells were cleared significantly faster than Jo(a-) cells. In contrast, we (62) recently studied a patient in whom anti-Jo[a] appeared to be clinically benign. The patient had hemoglobin SC disease and other disorders, one of which had resulted in several episodes of life-threatening thrombocytopenia. The patient had D- C- E- red cells and, because she had been transfused with platelets from Rh+ donors, had made antibodies to D, C and E. In addition, red cell transfusions necessitated by her HbSC disease had resulted in her forming anti-S and an IgG anti-M active at 37°C. The anti-S and anti-M had each caused delayed hemolytic transfusion reactions at different times. The patient was then found to have made anti-Jo[a] in addition to her antibodies to D, C, E, M and S. An in vitro monocyte monolayer assay using D- C- E-; M- S-; Jo(a+) red cells forecast that her anti-Jo[a] would bring about accelerated clearance of Jo(a+) red cells. Twice, in emergency situations, the patient required red cell transfusions and in the absence of units lacking all the antigens to which she had made antibodies, we were obliged to issue rr, M- S-, Jo(a+) blood. Four units of such blood were transfused with no obvious ill effects although the patient's clinical condition made it impossible to determine whether the transfused red cells survived normally. As the patient's clinical condition deteriorated, it was determined that a splenectomy was necessary to prevent further thrombocytopenic episodes. Because of her HbSC disease, a red cell exchange transfusion was deemed necessary before the splenectomy could be performed. A ten unit exchange using rr, M- S-, Jo(a+) blood (no rr, M- S-, Jo(a-) blood was available from any rare donor file) was performed and splenectomy was successfully undertaken one day later. Determinations of HbS, HbC and HbA (donor) levels before and after the exchange transfusion and after the splenectomy suggested that survival of the transfused blood was either normal or close to normal. As of this writing the patient is alive and in much better clinical condition than was the case before the "incompatible" transfusions. Like antibodies to Do^a, Do^b, Gy^a and Hy, anti-Jo^a has thus far failed to cause clinical HDN.

A Monoclonal Antibody Related to Gy^a

In 1993, Rao et al. (63) described a monoclonal antibody (5B10) that was produced using spleen cells of a mouse immunized with ficin-treated human red cells. The antibody bound to an epitope present on all human red cells except those that were Gy(a-) and PNH cells lacking PI-linked proteins (see above). Thus although the antibody ostensibly had anti-Gy^a specificity, it differed from human examples of that antibody in a number of ways. First, 5B10 was strongly reactive with Gy(a+) red cells treated with trypsin, chymotrypsin or AET. Second, neuramindase treatment of Gy(a+) red cells enhanced the binding of 5B10. Third, 5B10 reacted equally well with cord blood red cells and Gy(a+) red cells from adults. The 5B10 antibody reacted equally well with Do(a+b-) and Do(a-b+) red cells (as does human anti-Gy^a) and binding of 5B10 to Gy(a+) red cells was not blocked by human anti-Do^b or anti-Hy. In Western blots, 5B10 bound to a diffuse 54-57kD protein band, apparently the Do/Gy/Hy/Jo PI-linked protein. One possible explanation for the specificity of the MAb is that it is directed against an epitope on the Dombrock protein that is located closer to the red cell membrane than is (are) the trypsin, chymotrypsin, pronase sensitive sites and that the epitope defined is not dependent on the presence of disulfide bonds for its antigenic integrity (i.e. 5B10 recognized epitope not denatured by AET or DTT). Such a supposition is supported by the assumption that all red cells except those that are Gy(a-) (i.e. Do$_{null}$) and the PNH III population of PNH red cells, carry the PI-linked Do glycoprotein, regardless of their Do^a, Do^b, Gy^a, Hy and Jo^a status. For the sake of completeness it will be added that 5B10 did not bind to platelets, neutrophils, peripheral blood T lymphocytes or EBV-transformed B lymphocytes when tested by RIA. 5B10 failed to react with K562 but reacted weakly with HEL erythroleukemia cell lines. Thus the tissue distribution and molecular weight of the 5B10-defined epitope was seen to be similar to that of Gy^a.

Phenotypic Relationships Within the Dombrock System

Thus far, for practical reasons, the antigens Do^a, Do^b, Gy^a, Hy and Jo^a have been considered as separate entities. The information presented will enable workers to handle a situation in which an antibody to any one of the antigens is found in a patient's serum. In fact, there are some complex relationships between the antigens, at the phenotypic level, the first of which were recognized long before Gy^a, Hy and Jo^a were seen to be part of the Dombrock system.

When first discovered, Gy^a, Hy and Jo^a appeared to be independent antigens of high incidence. With regard to Gy^a and Hy, Moulds et al. (10) quickly realized that this is not the case. They showed that in Whites, Gy(a-) red cells are always Hy- was well. In Blacks, in whom the Gy(a-) phenotype is not known, Hy- red cells always have a markedly weakened expression of Gy^a, that is to say the phenotype is Gy(a+^{w}) Hy-. Neither the early nor later studies found red cells that are Gy(a-) Hy+, nor have any Hy- red cells expressing Gy^a at normal levels, come to light. Jo^a was added to the Gy^a/Hy story when it was found (13-15) that Hy- red cells (i.e. those of the phenotypes Gy(a-) Hy- and Gy(a+^{w}) Hy-) are always Jo(a-). Although all Hy- red cells are Jo(a-), the phenotype Gy(a+) Hy+^{w} Jo(a-) also exists (60). Just as the absence of Hy seems to result in weak expression of Gy^a, the absence of Jo^a seems to result in weakened expression of Hy. Thus the three rare phenotypes involving Gy^a, Hy and Jo^a are: Gy(a-) Hy- Jo(a-); Gy(a+^{w}) Hy- Jo(a-); and Gy(a+) Hy+^{w} Jo(a-). The lack of Jo^a in the last of these three phenotypes does not appear to prevent normal expression of Gy^a.

Obviously the phenotype of the antibody-maker affects the specificity of the antibody made. Moulds et al. (10) studied anti-Gy^a made by a person or persons with Gy(a-) Hy- red cells. Three adsorptions with Gy(a+^{w}) Hy- red cells removed all antibody activity (i.e. no separable anti-Hy left unadsorbed). Eluates made from the red cells used in the adsorption contained anti-Gy^a. The report does not specify how many examples of anti-Gy^a were studied so that it is not clear whether persons of the Gy(a-) Hy- phenotype always make just anti-Gy^a or whether this applied only the example(s) studied. Before Jo^a was shown to be associated with Gy^a and Hy it was assumed that persons with Gy(a+^{w}) Hy- red cells made just anti-Hy. However, Weaver et al. (14) studied a Black female who had Gy(a+^{w}) Hy- Jo(a-) red cells and had both anti-Hy and anti-Jo^a in the serum. Adsorption with Hy+^{w} Jo(a-) red cells left anti-Jo^a unadsorbed, an eluate made from the red cells used to adsorb the serum, contained anti-Hy. Before the Hy+^{w} Jo(a-) phenotype was recognized, a mixture of anti-Hy and anti-Jo^a could easily have been thought to be just anti-Hy since all Hy- red cells are Jo(a-). When Banks et al. (6,7) made the observation that the Gy(a-) phenotype represents the Do$_{null}$ situation (i.e. Do(a-b-) Gy(a-) Hy- Jo(a-)) they further extended some phenotypic associations that were later confirmed at the biochemical level (18-20,63). First, it was shown that the phenotype Gy(a+^{w}) Hy- also involves the absence of Do^a and a weakened expression of Do^b. Second, the phenotype Gy(a+) Hy+^{w} Jo(a-) also involves weak expression of Do^a and even weaker expression of Do^b. The phenotype Do(b+^{w}) Gy(a+^{w}) Hy- Jo(a-) (at first recognized (10) simply as Gy(a+^{w}) Hy-), has not yet been seen to involve any expression of Do^a. Whether this relates to the paucity of Gy(a+^{w}) Hy- Jo(a-) samples studied or whether the phenotype always totally prevents expression of Do^a is not yet known. No doubt the answer to the question will eventually be found at the biochemical level. Table 22-3 summarizes the currently known Dombrock system phenotypes and table 22-4 lists the most usual characteristics of antibodies of the system.

The Dombrock Locus is on Chromosome 12

Of the 23 blood group systems recognized by the ISBT Working Party (17), Dombrock was the last for which the chromosomal location of the encoding locus was recognized. Early suggestions (64) that *DO* might be linked to *GC* (65) on chromosome 4 were not supported by later studies (66). Hints (21,66) that suggested that *DO* might be linked to *PDG* and therefore located on chromosome 1 turned out to be false leads (58,67-71). In 1996, Eiberg and Mohr (79) showed tight linkage between *DO* and two flanking DNA polymorphisms (D12S358 and D12S364) and assigned *DO* to the region 12p13.2 to 12p12.1. Although the loci that encode CD9, CD27 and CD4 have all been assigned to chromosome 12 (80) none of them is apparently the same as *DO* (79).

The Biochemical Nature of the Dombrock Protein

Well before the assignment of the *DO* locus to chromosome 12 (79 and see above), it was known that the DO protein on red cells was likely to have a GPI tail because the Do^a, Do^b, Gy^a and Hy antigens are absent or reduced on the red cells of patients with PNH (18). PNH is an acquired hematopoietic stem cell disorder. Most, if not all, patients with PNH have a gross deficiency of all GPI-linked proteins because of deficiency in an enzyme (PIG-A) needed for the biosynthesis of the GPI tail itself (see Chapter 4 for a discussion of GPI-anchors). At least 17 GPI-anchored proteins are known to be deficient on various hematopoietic cells (72,73). Of the well characterized GPI-anchored proteins found on red cells, two others are known to carry blood group antigens (Cartwright antigens, Chapter 23; Cromer antigens, Chapter 24) and two are not (CD58, CD59, see Chapter 4). There is evidence that the JMH antigens and the Emm antigen are also carried on GPI-linked proteins (18).

Immunoblotting experiments with human anti-Gy^a and anti-Hy showed that under non-reducing conditions, the antibodies recognize a diffuse band of Mr 46,750-57,750 (19). The band was not observed on membranes from red cells treated with pronase or trypsin and was much weakened on membranes prepared from chymotrypsin-treated cells. When membranes treated with an Endo F preparation were examined the Mr of the Gy^a and Hy reactive band was reduced by 10,000 (19). These results suggest that the Gy^a and Hy antigens are carried on a glycoprotein which contains one or more N-glycans and requires one or more intrachain disulphide bonds to maintain its structure. When immunoblotting experiments were

TABLE 22-3 Currently Known Dombrock System Phenotypes

Antigens					Frequency (Percent)		
Do^a	Do^b	Gy^a	Hy	Jo^a	Whites	Blacks	Orientals[*1]
+	0	+	+	+	18	11	1
+	+	+	+	+	49	44	18
0	+	+	+	+	33	45	81
0	0	0	0	0	>0.1	NF	>0.1
0	w	w	0	0	NF	>0.1	NT
w	vw	+	w	0	NF	>0.1	NT
		0	vw		See footnote[*2]		

[*1]   Average for reported studies in Japan and Thailand (22-24)
     NF = Not yet found in this population
[*2]   Found only once and thought then to represent temporary depression of antigen expression
     NT = No reports of tests in this population

TABLE 22-4 Usual Characteristics of Dombrock System Antibodies

Antibody Specificity	Positive Reactions in In Vitro Tests				Usual Immuno-globulin			Ability to Bind Complement		Ability to Cause In Vitro Lysis		Implicated in		Usual Form of Stimulation			% of White Population Positive
	Sal	LISS	AHG	Enz[*1]	IgG	IgM	IgA	Yes	No	Yes	No	Trans-fusion Reaction	HDN	Red Cells	Other	
Anti-Do[a]		X	X	X					X		X	X	No	X	No	67
Anti-Do[b]		X	X	X					X		X	X	No	X	No	82
Anti-Gy[a]		X	X	X	Rare	Rare	Most				X		No	X	No	>99.9
Anti-Hy		X	X	X					X		X	X	No	X	No	>99.9
Anti-Jo[a]		X	X	X					X		X	X	No	X	No	>99.9

[*1] Reactions enhanced when papain- or ficin-treated red cells are used, depressed or abolished when trypsin-, chymotrypsin- or pronase-treated red cells are used

attempted with human anti-Jo[a] no reactive bands were observed indicating that the antigen is denatured under the conditions of SDS-PAGE (20). Immunoprecipitation experiments with radioiodinated red cells using anti-Jo[a], anti-Gy[a] and anti-Hy gave identical results with major bands of Mr 46,750-57,750 and Mr 85,000. When the electrophoretically separated components of these immune precipitates were immunoblotted with anti-Gy[a] and anti-Hy, the band of Mr 46,750-57,750 was stained in all cases (20). These results clearly established that the Jo[a] antigen is carried by the same molecule as the Gy[a] and Hy antigens. The nature of the band of Mr 85,000 observed in immunoprecipitates is not known. It is possible that it represents a dimer of the band of Mr 46,750-57,750. Alternatively it may be a different protein which associates with the Gy[a] glyco-protein in the red cell membrane.

Proof that the antigens Do[a] and Do[b] are carried on the same glycoprotein as Gy[a], Hy and Jo[a] was obtained by Banks et al. (7) who showed that anti-Do[b] gave the same pattern of staining on immunoblots as anti-Gy[a]. These authors further showed that immune precipitates prepared with anti-Do[a] and anti-Do[b] from radioiodinated red cells of appropriate phenotype gave the same broad band (Mr 48,750-59,750 in these experiments) as that observed with anti-Gy[a] and anti-Hy and that immunoblotting of the electrophoretically separated components of these immune precipitates with anti-Gy[a], and where appropriate anti-Do[b], also stained the same broad component. As discussed above, a monoclonal antibody that appears to recognize the same membrane glycoprotein as human anti-Gy[a] has been described (63). The availability of such a monoclonal antibody should facilitate the purification and ultimately the cloning of this protein.

Spring (74) raised the possibility that the Do protein may be identical to the complement regulatory protein HRF60 or MIP (75,76). HRF60 is reported to have a similar molecular weight and to be reduced in expression on PNH red cells (77,78). If this proves to be the case then the null phenotype of the Dombrock system (Do(a-b-), Gy(a-), Hy-, Jo(a-)) may be of value in studies of the function of HRF60.

References

1. Swanson JL, Polesky HF, Tippett P, et al. Nature 1965;206:313
2. Tippett P, Sanger R, Swanson J, et al. Proc 10th Cong Europ Soc Haematol 1965
3. Polesky HF, Swanson JL. Transfusion 1966;6:268
4. Tippett P. J Med Genet 1967;4:7
5. Molthan L, Crawford MN, Tippett P. Vox Sang 1973;24:382
6. Banks JA, Parker N, Poole J. (abstract). Transf Med 1992;2 (Suppl 1):68
7. Banks JA, Hemming N, Poole J. Vox Sang 1995;68: 177
8. Swanson JL, Zweber M, Polesky HF. Transfusion 1967;7:304
9. Moulds JJ, Ellisor SS, Reid ME, et al. (abstract). Transfusion 1973;13:363
10. Moulds JJ, Polesky HF, Reid M, et al. Transfusion 1975;15:270
11. Schmidt RP, Frank S, Baugh M. (abstract). Transfusion 1967;7:386
12. Frank S, Schmidt RP, Baugh M. Transfusion 1970;10:254
13. Laird-Fryer B, Moulds MK, Moulds JJ, et al. (abstract). Transfusion 1981;21:633
14. Weaver T, Kavitsky D, Carty L, et al. (abstract). Transfusion 1984;24:426
15. Weaver T, Lacey P, Carty L. (abstract). Transfusion 1986;26:561
16. Jensen L, Scott EP, Marsh WL, et al. Transfusion 1972;12:322
17. Daniels GL, Anstee DJ, Cartron J-P, et al. Vox Sang 1995;69:265
18. Telen MJ, Rosse WJ, Parker CJ, et al. Blood 1990;75:1404

19. Spring FA, Reid ME. Vox Sang 1991;60:53
20. Spring FA, Reid ME, Nicholson G. Vox Sang 1994;66:72
21. Lewis M, Kaita H, Giblett E, et al. Cytogenetic Cell Genet 1978;22:313
22. Nakajima H, Moulds JJ. Vox Sang 1980;38:294
23. Nakajima H, Skradski K, Moulds JJ. Vox Sang 1979;36:103
24. Chandanayingyong D, Sasaki TT, Greenwalt TJ. Transfusion 1967;7:269
25. Greene M, Lloyd L, Popovsky MA, et al. (abstract). Transfusion 1989 (Suppl 7S):16S
26. Webb AJ, Lockyer JW, Tovey GH. Vox Sang 1966;11:637
27. Williams CH, Crawford MN. Transfusion 1966;6:310
28. Polesky HF, Swanson J, Smith R. Vox Sang 1968;14:465
29. Moulds J, Futrell E, Fortez P, et al. (abstract). Transfusion 1978;18:375
30. Kruskall MS, Greene MJ, Strycharz DM, et al. (abstract). Transfusion 1986;26:545
31. Gudino M, Kranwinkel R, Lenart S, et al. (abstract). Transfusion 1986;26:546
32. Judd WJ, Steiner EA. (Letter). Transfusion 1991;31:477
33. Roxby DJ, Paris JM, Stern DA, et al. Vox Sang 1994;66:49
34. Yvart J, Cartron J, Fouillade MT, et al. Rev Fr Transf Immunohematol 1977;20:395
35. Moheng MC, McCarthy P, Pierce SR. Transfusion 1985;25:44
36. Halverson G, Shanahan E, Santiago I, et al. Vox Sang 1994;66:206
37. Swanson J. Unpublished observations 1967 cited in Race RR, Sanger R. Blood Groups in Man, 6th Ed. Oxford:Blackwell, 1975:423
38. Clark MJ, Poole J, Barnes RM. Vox Sang 1975;29:301
39. Massaquoi JM, Cornwall S. (abstract). Transfusion 1973;13:362
40. Okubo Y, Nagao N, Tomita T, et al. (Letter). Transfusion 1986;26:214
41. Mak KH, Lin CK, Ford DS, et al. Immunohematology 1995;11:20
42. Massaquoi JM. Transfusion 1975;15:150
43. Ellisor SS, Reid ME, Avoy DR, et al. Transfusion 1982;22:166
44. Rolih SD. Transf Med Rev 1989;3:128
45. Reid ME, Ellisor SS, Sabo B. Transfusion 1982;22:528
46. Eckrich RJ. Immunohematology 1988;4:12
47. Daniels G. Immunohematology 1992;8:53
48. Ginsberg V, Applewhaite F, Gerena J, et al. (abstract). Transfusion 1967;7:386
49. Beattie KM, Castillo S. Transfusion 1975;15:476
50. Hsu TCS, Jagathambal K, Sabo BH, et al. Transfusion 1975;15:604
51. Lacey P, Moulds M, Sobonya J. (abstract). Transfusion 1978;18:379
52. Swanson J. Unpublished observations 1966 cited in Moulds JJ, Polesky HF, Reid M, et al. Transfusion 1975;15:270
53. Moulds JJ. Unpublished data 1966 cited by Moulds JJ, Polesky HF, Reid M, et al. Transfusion 1975;15:270
54. Dept Army, Fort Knox. Unpublished data 1974 (investigators not specified) cited by Moulds JJ, Polesky HF, Reid M, et al. Transfusion 1975;15:270
55. Moulds JJ, Polesky HF, Reid M, et al. Transfusion 1975;15:270
56. Moores PP. Unpublished observations 1975 cited by Moulds JJ, Polesky HF, Reid M, et al. Transfusion 1975;15:270
57. Moulds JJ, Moulds MK. (Letter). Transfusion 1983;23:274
58. Rey-Campos J, Rubinstein P, Rodriguez de Cordoba S. J Exp Med 1987;166:246
59. Morel P, Myers M, Marsh WL, et al. (abstract). Transfusion 1976;16:531
60. Brown D. (abstract). Transfusion 1985;25:462
61. Viggiano E, Jacobson G, Zurbito F. (abstract). Transfusion 1985;25:446
62. Issitt PD, Combs MR, Telen MJ. Unpublished observations 1996
63. Rao N, Bumgarner J, Telen MJ. (abstract). Transfusion 1993;33 (Suppl 9S):48S
64. Olaisen B, Gedde-Dahl T Jr, Tippett P, et al. Cytogenet Cell Genet 1979;25:194
65. Falk CT, Martin MD, Walker ME, et al. Cytogenet Cell Genet 1978;22:313
66. Lewis M, Kaita H, Philipps S, et al. Ann Hum Genet 1983;47:49
67. Rodriguez de Cordoba S, Rey-Campos J, Dykes DA, et al. Immunogenetics 1988;28:452
68. Rao DC, Keat BJB, Laloulel JM, et al. Ann Hum Genet 1979;31:680
69. Keats BJB, Rao DC, Morton NE. Human Gene Mapping 1979;5:171
70. Mohr J, Eiberg H, Nielsen LS. Cytogenet Cell Genet 1985;40:701
71. Lewis M, Kaita H, Philipps S, et al. Vox Sang 1989;57:210
72. Kinoshita T, Inoue N, Takeda J. Adv Immunol 1995;20:367
73. Rosse WF, Ware RE. Blood 1995;86:3277
74. Spring FA. Transf Med 1993; 3:167
75. Schonermark S, Rauterberg EW, Shin ML, et al. J Immunol 1986;136:1772
76. Zalman LS, Wood LM, Müller-Eberhard HJ. Proc Nat Acad Sci USA 1986;83:6975
77. Hansch GM, Schonermark S, Roelcke D. J Clin Invest 1987;80:7
78. Zalman LS, Wood LM, Frank MM, et al. J Exp Med 1987;165:572
79. Eiberg H, Mohr J. Hum Genet 1996;98:518
80. Raeymaekers P, Zand KV, Jun L, et al. Genomics 1995;29:170

23 | The Cartwright Blood Group System

In 1956, Eaton et al. (1) described anti-Yt^a, an antibody detecting an antigen present on the red cells of most people. Many additional examples of anti-Yt^a had been found before Giles and Metaxas (2) described anti-Yt^b, the antibody detecting the low incidence antithetical partner to Yt^a. From the published work and from results obtained in a large unpublished series (3) the phenotype and antigen frequencies shown in table 23-1 can be calculated. It seems that in the USA at least, those figures apply in both Whites and Blacks and in Canada and Europe in Whites (1,3-8). Table 23-1 also includes the conventional and ISBT terms for antigens of the system. As discussed in detail later in this chapter, Yt^a and Yt^b were shown (9) to be carried on a red cell phosphatidylinositol-linked (PI-linked) glycoprotein that was then identified (10) as the enzyme, acetylcholinesterase (AChE). The difference between Yt^a and Yt^b involves a single amino acid change at position 322 of the acetylcholinesterase molecule: when the protein expresses Yt^a, histidine occupies that position, when it expresses Yt^b, asparagine is present (11). The Yt^a/Yt^b polymorphism does not affect activity of the enzyme (12).

The Antigens Yt^a and Yt^b

Because anti-Yt^a is more common than anti-Yt^b, more large scale screening studies have been done with anti-Yt^a than with anti-Yt^b. In tests (1,6,8) on samples from 39,880 European Whites, 99.8% were seen to be Yt(a+). In a large unpublished study in the USA (3) the incidence of Yt^a was 99.7%. In that study no difference in the incidence of the Yt(a-) phenotype among Whites and Blacks was seen. Based on the incidence of the Yt(a-) phenotype and using the fact that the first discovered example of anti-Yt^a appeared to show a dosage effect, it was calculated (1) that if an antigen antithetical to Yt^a existed and if a silent allele in the system did not exist or was very rare, the antithetical antigen should have an incidence of around 7 to 8% in European Whites. After anti-Yt^b was found (2), it was used in two surveys of such persons. Giles et al. (4) found 113 Yt(b+) samples among 1399 tested (8.1%); Salmon et al. (6) found 608 Yt(b+) samples among 7510 tested (8.1%). Lewis et al. (7) tested samples from 659 White Canadians with anti-Yt^a and anti-Yt^b, 589 were Yt(a+b-), 70 were Yt(a+b+), none was Yt(a-b+). Wurzel and Haesler (5) tested samples from 714 American Blacks with anti-Yt^b and found that 60 (8.4%) were Yt(b+). Again, this finding suggests that the incidence of Yt^a and Yt^b is the same among Whites and Blacks in the USA.

Two populations in which the incidence of Yt^a and Yt^b does differ from those described above, have been found. Nakajima et al. (13) tested samples from 5000 Japanese donors, all were Yt(a+). Seventy of the samples were tested with anti-Yt^b and were non-reactive. Thus it seems that in Japan the Yt(a+b-) phenotype is almost universal. In 1985, Levene et al. (14) noticed a higher than expected number of anti-Yt^a among problem samples submitted to the National Reference Laboratory in Jerusalem. When anti-Yt^b became available it was found that the incidence of that antigen was considerably higher in Israel than elsewhere. Clearly a higher incidence of Yt^b would mean a higher incidence of persons of the Yt(a-b+) phenotype able to form anti-Yt^a. As described in the next section, available data suggest that Yt^a is quite immunogenic and that anti-Yt^a is frequently made by Yt(a-) persons exposed to Yt(a+) red cells. In 1987, a full report of the study in Israel was published (15). Among 1683 Israeli Jews, Arabs and Druse tested, 26 had Yt(a-b+) red cells. That is, the phenotype had an incidence of 1 in 65; the incidence among European Whites and US Whites and Blacks is around 1 in 500. Among Israeli Jews 22 of 1521 (1 in 69) were phenotypically Yt(a-b+); the phenotype was seen in 2 of 85 Israeli Arabs and 2 of 77 Israeli Druse. The Yt^b antigen (i.e. persons phenotypically Yt(a-b+) and Yt(a+b+)) was found on the red cells of 26% of Israeli Jews, 24% of Israeli Arabs and 26% of Israeli Druse. These figures are some three times higher than those seen in European and US popula-

TABLE 23-1 Terminology and Antigen and Phenotype Frequencies in the Cartwright Blood Group System

Conventional Name of System: Cartwright

Conventional Symbol for System: Yt

ISBT System Symbol: YT

ISBT System Number: 011

Antigens Conventional	Yt^a Yt^b	ISBT	YT1, 011001 YT2, 011002

Phenotype	% Frequency	% Bloods Reactive with	
		Anti-Yt^a	Anti-Yt^b
Yt(a+b-)	91.9	} 99.7	
Yt(a+b+)	7.8		} 8.1
Yt(a-b+)	0.3		

tions. Few differences in the incidence of Yt[b] were seen when the country of birth of the donors was considered. Those readers interested in the finer points are referred to the original report (15), it will be mentioned here that among Jews born in may different countries the lowest incidence of Yt[b] was seen in those from Rumania and the highest among those born in India and Pakistan. We are not aware if workers in Europe and the USA have related the findings of Levene et al. (15) to the 1 in 500 donors in their populations who have Yt(a-) red cells. Among such donors it might be expected that Jews would predominate.

Data in the literature about the effects of enzyme treatment of red cells on the Yt[a] and Yt[b] antigens are often conflicting and sometimes outright contradictory. The first reported example of anti-Yt[a] failed to react with papain-treated red cells (1). In contrast, Giles et al. (4) found that papain or ficin-treated red cells reacted more strongly with the first two examples of anti-Yt[b] (2,16) than did untreated red cells. In the same study, Giles et al. (4) found that the reactions of some examples of anti-Yt[a] were enhanced in tests against papain or ficin-treated red cells. Vengelen-Tyler and Morel (17) studied 14 examples of anti-Yt[a]. Trypsin-treatment of red cells seemed to enhance the reactions of four of them and did not lessen the reactions of the others. Four of the anti-Yt[a] were non-reactive with ficin-treated red cells, three of the same antibodies failed to react with papain-treated cells. Of the remaining 10 anti-Yt[a], four reacted less strongly with ficin or papain-treated than with untreated red cells, the other six reacted about equally with ficin or papain-treated red cells. Among the six antibodies in this last group were all four examples that gave enhanced reactions with trypsin-treated red cells. Somewhat similar findings have been made in other studies. There seems no doubt (18,19) that Yt[a] and Yt[b] survive trypsin treatment of red cells but are removed or denatured when red cells are treated with chymotrypsin. As mentioned elsewhere in this book, less than pure preparations of trypsin often contain chymotrypsin. The reactions of anti-Yt[a] with ficin or papain-treated cells appear to vary based on the anti-Yt[a] used. It is not yet known whether this indicates the existence of enzyme-resistant and enzyme-sensitive Yt[a] epitopes and/or whether glycosylation of the antigen-bearing protein plays a role in epitope formation. As far as we are aware, no alloimmune anti-Yt[a] in an individual with Yt(a+) red cells, that might indicate partial Yt[a] antigen based on epitope variation, has been reported.

There is no doubt about the effects of some other chemicals on Yt[a] and Yt[b]. Both antigens survive sialidase treatment of red cells (18,19) showing that presence of NeuAc is not essential for their structure. Both antigens are denatured when red cells are treated with the reducing agents DTT and AET. Denaturation of Yt[a] and Yt[b] is concentration-dependent when DTT is used to treat red cells.

When 200 mM dithiothreitol is used both Yt[a] (20) and Yt[b] (21) are denatured. When 100 mM and 50 mM solutions of DTT are used, Yt[a] antigen strength is reduced proportional to the strength of the DTT solution, but is not completely abolished. It has also been found (22) that Yt[b] is denatured when red cells are treated with 500 mM 2-mercaptoethanol. As mentioned in Chapter 18, the use of 2-aminoethylisothiouronium bromide (AET) to create artificial Kell[null] cells has been criticized because that compound destroys some other (non-Kell system) antigens. However, when Levene et al. (21) treated Yt(a+) red cells with AET, it was found that denaturation of Yt[a] is not as complete as denaturation of all Kell system antigens (23). That is to say, while nine of 15 anti-Yt[a] did not react with AET-treated red cells, the other six still reacted, albeit less strongly than with untreated red cells.

The Yt[a] antigen appears not to be fully developed at birth (1,24,25) although cord blood red cells can be shown to be Yt(a+). In contrast, both Giles et al. (4) and Ferguson et al. (25) reported that Yt[b] antigen levels are similar on the red cells of newborns and those of adults. Gobel et al. (24) tested red cells from fetuses of less than 32 weeks gestation. Eight of 10 samples failed to react with anti-Yt[a], the other two reacted only weakly.

Spring et al. (10) used a monoclonal antibody to acetylcholinesterase (AChE) to determine the number of copies of the Yt glycoprotein per red cell. When whole antibody molecules were used the copy number ranged from 3000 to 5000 per cell. When Fab fragments of the antibody were used the copy numbers ranged from 7000 to 10,000 per cell leading the authors to suggest that the protein exists on the red cells in a dimeric form.

Two groups of workers (26,27) have reported decreased levels of AChE on the red cells of patients with diabetes, a third group (28) were unable to confirm this observation. In a considerably larger study, Whittaker (29) and Whittaker and Telen (30) found no significant decrease in AChE on the red cells of diabetics nor any decrease in expression of Yt[a]. Whittaker (29) suggests that the apparent reduction of AChE found in the earlier studies (26,27) may have resulted because fasting blood samples from diabetics were collected before insulin injections were given. Indeed the decrease of AChE was said to be inversely proportional to the increase in blood glucose levels. Insulin is known to increase red cell membrane fluidity independently of the blood glucose level (31,32). In one of the studies (27) it was shown that AChE levels returned to normal in diabetics injected with insulin.

Anti-Yt[a], Anti-Yt[b] and their Clinical Significance

In spite of the rarity of individuals of the phenotype Yt(a-b+), three in 1000, who can form alloimmune anti-

Yt^a, the antibody is not uncommon. A number of reports (37,39-41) have described multiple examples. In one reference service, 80 anti-Yt^a were identified and/or tested in a monocyte monolayer assay in a six year period (41). In 1968, Bettigole et al. (33) after finding 12 anti-Yt^a in four years, in one hospital, postulated that Yt^a is highly immunogenic and readily stimulates the production of anti-Yt^a in Yt(a-b+) persons who are transfused with Yt(a+) blood. In sharp contrast, anti-Yt^b is uncommon. In reviewing published reports describing anti-Yt^b we found no example described as the only antibody present in a patient's serum. Indeed in one serum containing anti-Yt^b, anti-Fy^b and anti-Bp were present (2,4); in another anti-C and anti-Hov (4,16); in a third anti-c (42); in a fourth anti-K (25) and in a fifth anti-E and anti-Le^a (43). Some examples of anti-Yt^b have been mentioned in reports of use of the monocyte monolayer assay to forecast in vivo clinical significance of an antibody (40,44-46) but not published in their own right. We do not know if any of those examples occurred as a single specificity in a serum. However, it is clear from the literature that Yt^b is a poor immunogen and that anti-Yt^b is made only by good responders to blood group antigens (see Chapter 2). All reported examples of anti-Yt^a and anti-Yt^b have been found in persons previously exposed to foreign red cells via transfusion or pregnancy.

Anti-Yt^a is almost always an IgG antibody best detected by IAT. While not many examples have been studied in this respect, at least one example was found (33) to activate complement, while two others were found (24,47) not to do so. As described below, many examples of anti-Yt^a have been shown to be benign in vivo. For many years it was thought that this feature represented the fact that anti-Yt^a was often predominantly IgG4 in nature. From some early studies (17,34-47) it appeared that while some anti-Yt^a contained an IgG1 component, most also contained or were exclusively (17) IgG4. However, more recently Garratty et al. (38) have reviewed their data from 15 years of subclassing studies. In tests on a total of 33 anti-Yt^a, 16 were shown by agglutination tests to be composed only of IgG1, a 17th was shown by flow cytometry to be the same, while the remaining 16 were too weak to be subclassed. No example of IgG4 anti-Yt^a was found. These latest findings correlate rather better with the clinical findings about anti-Yt^a than do the earlier ones. As discussed below, some anti-Yt^a clear Yt(a+) red cells in vivo while many others do not. If all (or most) anti-Yt^a were IgG4, few (if any) would be expected to be pathological in vivo. In contrast, as discussed in detail in Chapters 2 and 37, one of the most characteristic features of IgG1 antibodies is variability of different examples in their in vivo reactions. Although the correlation is not absolute, strongly reactive IgG1 antibodies are often pathological, weaker examples are more often benign. If

all (or most) anti-Yt^a are (or contain) IgG1, the extreme variability of their in vivo activities, as described below, would be more understandable.

The first example of anti-Yt^a to be found (1) was of the benign variety. The patient involved was transfused with Yt(a+) blood, did not suffer any untoward effects and apparently experienced the expected beneficial effects of the transfusions. That story has been repeated many times and many patients with anti-Yt^a in the serum have been successfully transfused with Yt(a+) red cells (37,39,41, numerous patients transfused in the studies cited). On the other hand, some examples of anti-Yt^a have reacted so strongly in vitro, that in vivo red cell survival studies have been undertaken. The results cover a very broad spectrum. They vary from markedly shortened in vivo survival of the Yt(a+) red cells (e.g. 24,33,47), to limited initial destruction of the injected red cells but definitely shortened half-life survival of the cells (e.g. 48-50), to limited initial destruction of the injected cells and only mildly reduced half-life survival (e.g. 37,51), to apparently normal survival (e.g. 37,40,49) (studies on multiple cases explain the appearance of the same reference in more than one category). One delayed hemolytic transfusion reaction has been blamed on anti-Yt^a (52).

In an attempt to bring some order to the situations outlined above, table 23-2 attempts to summarize the published data. The table lists: the report referenced; the number of examples of anti-Yt^a and the smaller number of examples of anti-Yt^b described in each of the reports, and the conclusions reached regarding the clinical significance of each antibody. In listing the conclusions drawn, the bases on which those conclusions were reached are shown. That is, transfusion of antigen positive blood, results of an in vivo cell survival study using ^{51}Cr labeled antigen-positive red cells, results of an in vitro assay using phagocytic cells (e.g. the monocyte monolayer assay) and effects on an infant in those cases in which an immunized woman delivered an infant with antigen positive red cells. In planning the table it was hoped that two categories, i.e. clinically significant and clinically benign, could be used for the antibodies. In preparing the table it became apparent that a third category, in which equivocal findings were made, was necessary. Having set out the data in table 23-2 it is now necessary to make a number of observations about those data. First, for those anti-Yt^a called clinically significant on the basis of in vivo red cell survival studies using ^{51}Cr labeled Yt(a+) red cells, it should be added that full transfusions with Yt(a+) red cells were not tried. Thus it is possible than when a 1 to 5 ml test dose was cleared relatively slowly, a whole unit may have had better survival. Davey and Simpkins (48) found that the survival of a test dose of Yt(a+) red cells was 80% at one hour and 63% at 24 hours but that the half

TABLE 23-2 To Illustrate the In Vivo Activities of Anti-Yt^a and Anti-Yt^b

Investigators, Reference and Year	Antibody(ies) Studied	Reasons for Concluding Antibody		Findings Equivocal (see text)
		Clinically Significant	Clinically Benign	
Eaton et al. (1) 1956	1 x Anti-Yt^a		Tx	
Bergvalds et al. (53) 1965	1 x Anti-Yt^a		Tx	
			No HDN	
Allen and Alter (55) 1966	1 x Anti-Yt^a		No HDN	
Bettigole et al. (33) 1968	1 x Anti-Yt^a	^{51}Cr		
Dobbs et al. (39) 1968	3 x Anti-Yt^a		Tx	
			No HDN	
Lavellée et al. (54) 1970	1 x Anti-Yt^a		No HDN	
Gobel et al. (24) 1974	1 x Anti-Yt^a	^{51}Cr		
Ballas and Sherwood (47) 1977	1 x Anti-Yt^a	^{51}Cr		
Silvergleid et al. (51) 1978	1 x Anti-Yt^a			^{51}Cr
Ferguson et al. (25) 1979	1 x Anti-Yt^b		No HDN	
Davey and Simpkins (48) 1981	1 x Anti-Yt^a	^{51}Cr		
Mohandas et al. (37) 1985	1 x Anti-Yt^a	^{51}Cr		
	3 x Anti-Yt^a		^{51}Cr	
	1 x Anti-Yt^a		Tx	
Nance et al. (40) 1987	2 x Anti-Yt^a	^{51}Cr, MMA		
	3 x Anti-Yt^a		^{51}Cr, MMA	
	1 x Anti-Yt^b			^{51}Cr, MMA
AuBuchon et al. (49) 1988	1 x Anti-Yt^a			see text
Levy et al. (43) 1988	1 x Anti-Yt^b			^{51}Cr
Kakaiya et al. (50) 1991	1 x Anti-Yt^a	^{51}Cr, MMA		
Hillyer et al. (52) 1991	1 x Anti-Yt^a	DxTxRx		
		^{51}Cr		
Eckrich and Mallory (41) 1993	15 x Anti-Yt^a		Tx, MMA	
	3 x Anti-Yt^a	Tx, MMA		

Legend to table 23-2

Reasons for conclusions regarding significance of the antibodies.

Tx = Transfusion with antigen positive red cells.

DxTxRx = Delayed transfusion reaction.

^{51}Cr = In vivo red cell survival study using radiolabeled antigen positive red cells.

MMA = Monocyte monolayer assay.

No HDN = Mother with antibody, infant with antigen positive red cells, some DAT+, some DAT-, no clinical disease.

life of the labeled red cells was only 96 hours. The authors recommended that the patient donate blood for autologous use in the future but that in an emergency, Yt(a+) blood could be transfused without risk of a catastrophic transfusion reaction. Second, for those antibod-ies called clinically significant on the basis of transfusion, no severe or immediate transfusion reactions were report-ed. In the case reported by Hillyer et al. (52) the picture of a delayed transfusion reaction was complicated by the presence of several other antibodies. In the three cases of

Eckrich and Mallory (41) the ill effects of transfusion involved lack of, or lack of maintenance of, expected hemoglobin increments, not frank transfusion reactions. Third, in those cases in which the antibodies were considered benign because of successful transfusions with Yt(a+) units, most of the observations related to the time at which the blood was transfused and short post transfusion periods. In other words, some of those patients may have cleared the Yt(a+) red cells several days after transfusion at a time at which the red cell clearance was clinically irrelevant. As discussed in Chapter 36, many workers feel that if transfused red cells survive long enough to fulfill the purpose for which they were used (i.e. to sustain life following trauma, to get the patient through a surgical procedure) but are then cleared say seven to ten days later, when the patient is making blood, the transfusions were successful. Thus under some circumstances (e.g. trauma, surgery) a case can be made for regarding such antibodies as clinically insignificant. Indeed, it is possible that some of the anti-Yt^a listed in table 23-2 behaved similarly in vivo but have been assigned to different categories in the table, simply because different tests were done. Fourth, the case described by AuBuchon et al. (49) merits special comment. In this patient the anti-Yt^a initially appeared to be clinically benign and the patient was successfully transfused with four units of Yt(a+) blood. However, 12 weeks after the transfusion the IgG1 anti-Yt^a had increased in strength and gave indications in both a ^{51}Cr survival study and an MMA that is should now be regarded as clinically significant. Such a secondary immune response in patients making anti-Yt^a seems to be the exception rather than the rule. Fifth, the antibodies described in table 23-2 as giving equivocal results would, no doubt, be regarded by some workers as being clinically significant and by others as being clinically benign. For example, the anti-Yt^b described by Levy et al. (43) was studied by an in vivo red cell survival study. At one hour post injection 100% and at 24 hours 93%, of the test dose of Yt(b+) red cells was still present in the patient's circulation. However, the half-life of the injected dose of red cells was 21 days (normal 28 to 32 days) indicating that slow and mildly abnormal clearance of the Yt(b+) red cells did occur. Similar findings (i.e. good initial survival but slightly reduced half-life) have been reported by others (40). Whether one regards such antibodies as clinically significant or insignificant relates to one's philosophy and expectations of the transfusions. Sixth, the anti-Yt^a studied by Silvergleid et al. (51) is in the equivocal column for a different reason. When a ^{51}Cr survival study was performed only 49% of the test dose was present at one hour. When the test was repeated with red cells from the same donor, in vivo survival was 65% at one hour. However, when Yt(a+) red cells from a different donor were used, in vivo survival was 95% at one hour. It is not

known if this difference represented variation of Yt^a antigen strength on the red cells of two donors or presence of another antibody in the patient's serum. Attempts to find such a second antibody were not successful.

In summarizing the transfusion data in table 23-2 a number of points can be made. First, if a patient with anti-Yt^a in the serum is in urgent need of transfusion and no Yt(a-) units are immediately available, Yt(a+) blood should be used. In the majority of cases, as exemplified by 27 of 39 anti-Yt^a in table 23-2 about which fairly firm conclusions can be reached, the transfused red cells would be expected to survive normally or near normally in vivo. In the minority of cases, i.e. exemplified by 12 anti-Yt^a in table 23-2, in which accelerated clearance of the Yt(a+) red cells would be expected, no severe transfusion reactions are likely. Second, if the patient with anti-Yt^a requires blood on a non-urgent basis, in vivo red cell survival studies and/or a phagocytic cell assay should be performed. There is no point in delaying elective surgery or using a rare resource (Yt(a-) units from a rare donor file) if the patient's anti-Yt^a is of the clinically benign variety. However, it should be remembered that in vivo red cell survival studies and MMAs are like antibody-screening and serological compatibility tests in that they need to be repeated after each series of transfusions in case the characteristics of the antibody have changed.

If the individual with anti-Yt^a or anti-Yt^b in the serum is pregnant, severe, or even clinical HDN can be regarded as a highly unlikely outcome. In addition to those cases shown in table 23-2 as causing no HDN, the anti-Yt^a described by Gobel et al. (24) that caused accelerated clearance of ^{51}Cr-labeled Yt(a+) red cells, did not cause HDN in the patient's Yt(a+) infant. The patient described by Davey and Simpkins (48) bore four infants, none of whom had clinical HDN, but it was not known if the later found, clinically significant anti-Yt^a was present when the patient delivered her children. In the case described by Allen and Alter (55) an anti-Yt^a with a titer of 500 caused no clinical disease in an infant with Yt(a+) red cells. Similarly, no case of HDN caused by anti-Yt^b has been reported. Table 23-3 summarizes the most usual serological characteristics of Cartwright system antibodies. For reasons that will be abundantly apparent, the columns listing the abilities of these antibodies to cause transfusion reactions refer the reader back to table 23-2.

A Transient Yt(a-b-) Phenotype

The only Yt(a-b-) phenotype described in detail in the literature (56,57) involved transient depression of expression of Yt^a in an individual with Yt(b-) red cells; no inherited form of the Yt(a-b-) phenotype has been reported. The patient described by Oxendine et al. (56)

TABLE 23-3 Usual Characteristics of Cartwright System Antibodies

Antibody Specificity	Positive Reactions in In Vitro Tests				Usual Immuno-globulin		Ability to Bind Complement		Ability to Cause In Vitro Lysis		Implicated in		Usual Form of Stimulation		% of White Population Positive
	Sal	LISS	AHG	Enz	IgG	IgM	Yes	No	Yes	No	Trans-fusion Reaction	HDN	Red Cells	Other	
Anti-Yt^a			X		X		Some	Some		X	*1	No	X		99.7
Anti-Yt^b			X		X					X	*1	No	X		8.1

*1   See table 23-2.

and by Rao et al. (57) had red cells that typed as Yt(a-b-) but that adsorbed and yielded on elution, two of four anti-Yt^a used in such studies. The patient's serum contained an antibody that reacted with both Yt(a+b-) and Yt(a-b+) red cells. Presumptive evidence that the antibody could be regarded as anti-Yt^{ab} came from the finding that it failed to react with PNH III red cells. As described above, Yt^a and Yt^b are carried on a phosphotidylinositol linked (PI-linked) protein on red cells. As described below, the PNH III population of red cells from patients with paroxysmal nocturnal hemoglobinuria (PNH) is deficient in PI-linked proteins (9,58,59) so that the red cells behave, among other things, as Yt(a-b-). The red cells of PNH patients are not all Yt(a-b-), PI-linked proteins and the antigens that they carry can be detected on the PNH I and PNH II populations of red cells from those patients. The patient described (56,57) did not have PNH. At the time that his red cells typed as Yt(a-b-) and anti-Yt^{ab} was detectable in his serum, ^{51}Cr survival studies indicated that neither Yt(a+b-) nor Yt(a-b+) red cells would survive normally in vivo. At that time the level of acetylcholinesterase on his red cells was about 10% of normal and the enzyme's activity was about 15% of normal (57). Autologous blood was collected to cover the patient's heart transplant surgery and four months after the initial findings, the patient's red cells were found to be weakly reactive when tested with anti-Yt^a. Those red cells, that had an acetylcholinesterase level of some 54 to 60% of normal were shown capable of adsorbing the anti-Yt^{ab} made earlier by the patient. However, the cells would not adsorb the antibody to exhaustion.

An abstract (67) describing the second example of anti-K18 (see Chapter 18) mentions that the antibody-maker, a 78 year-old previously transfused White male, (not the patient described above) had red cells that were non-reactive with four examples of anti-Yt^a and two examples of anti-Yt^b. No additional details are given about the patient's disease state or his apparent Yt(a-b-) phenotype.

Since acetylcholinesterase (AChE) is essential for the function of certain muscle and brain cells, it might be thought that a gene deletion that would lead to lack of the enzyme and the Yt(a-b-) phenotype would be lethal. However, it is known (60) that unlike on red cells, acetylcholinesterase is not PI-linked on muscle and brain cells. One exon of the encoding *AChE* gene (for additional details see below) specifies production of that portion of the protein that is required for attachment to the red cell membrane PI anchor. If a mutation occurred in that exon or if, in the transcription of mRNA to be translated into AChE that exon was skipped, the protein made would be able to attach to muscle and brain, but not to red cells. Thus the red cell Yt(a-b-) phenotype would be associated with no clinical sequelae because AChE function on muscle and brain cells would be normal (82). As one of us has pointed out elsewhere (61) this finding with *AChE*, Yt^a and Yt^b provides an important lesson for blood group serologists. Absence of a red cell membrane component, as suggested or proved by a null phenotype, does not mean that the antigen-bearing component is absent from all other cell lines. Alternative splicing and other genetic mechanisms dictate tissue-specific expression of functional molecules. Such findings may explain why many apparently major changes, at the red blood cell phenotypic level, are not associated with pathological sequelae.

The *Yt* Locus is on Chromosome 7

In 1989, Coghlan et al. (62) reported that among 31 informative families there was evidence for linkage between the *Yt* and *Kell* blood group loci, at that time the location of the *Kell* locus was unknown. In 1991, the *Kell* locus was provisionally assigned to chromosome 7 (63) and the same group of investigators in Winnipeg who produced evidence for that assignment, also showed (64) that *Yt* is closely linked to the chromosome 7 markers *COL1A2* and *D7S13*. As described earlier in this chapter, in 1992 it was shown (10) that Yt^a and Yt^b are carried on acetylcholinesterase. Also in 1992, the *AChE* gene, that encodes production of that protein, was shown by in situ hybridization (65,66) and by PCR-based somatic cell hybridization (66), to be located on chromosome 7 at 7q22.

The Molecular Basis of Cartwright System Antigens

Immune precipitation experiments with human anti-Yt[a] and anti-Yt[b] and radioiodinated intact human red cells revealed that the antigens are carried on a membrane component of 72kd if SDS-PAGE of the precipitates is carried out under reducing conditions or 160kd under non-reducing conditions (10). Spring et al. (10,68) noticed the similarity between the apparent molecular weight of the Cartwright (hereinafter YT) component under reducing and non-reducing conditions and the well characterized red cell membrane surface enzyme acetylcholinesterase (hereinafter AChE) and went on to prove that the YT component was indeed AChE. When monoclonal antibodies (AE1 and AE2 (69)) raised to AChE were used for immune precipitation experiments carried out under identical conditions to those used for anti-Yt[a] and anti-Yt[b] a component of the same apparent molecular weight under reducing and non-reducing conditions was obtained.

In order to show that the Yt[a] and Yt[b] antigens were carried on AChE itself and not on another component of the same size which also formed a disulphide-bonded dimer under non-reducing conditions, immune precipitates obtained with anti-Yt[a] and anti-Yt[b] were analyzed for AChE activity in comparison with similar immune precipitates prepared with AE1 and AE2. The results clearly demonstrated enzyme activity in Yt[a] and Yt[b] precipitates at about 50% of the level in AE1 precipitates. AE2 precipitates showed only 8% of the activity found with AE1. This was not unexpected because AE2 is known to inhibit enzyme activity (69). Whether or not the lower activity of Yt[a] and Yt[b] precipitates compared with AE1 precipitates was due to suboptimal conditions in the former experiments or because of partial inhibition of the enzyme, could not be discerned.

Rao et al. (57) described a patient with a transient Yt(a-b-) phenotype and showed that the patient's red cells had low levels of AChE by using a radioimmunoassay with monoclonal antibodies to AChE (AE1, 2, 3, 4) and by enzyme assay. Inheritance of the Yt(a-b-) phenotype has not been described but there are reports of patients with low levels of AChE activity where other family members also have lower than normal levels (70,71). The patient described by Shinoara and Tanaka (71) had AChE levels of 20% of normal in association with a mild hemolytic anemia. A similar patient described by Johns (70) did not have anemia and so studies of these cases did not throw any light on the functional significance of red cell AChE. Petty et al. (79) used a different method (MAIEA assay) to confirm that Yt[a] and Yt[b] are located on AChE.

Bartels et al. (11) amplified and sequenced the entire coding region of the *AChE* gene in DNA derived from an individual of type Yt(a+b-) and another of type Yt(a-b+). Three point mutations were found. The first mutation, in exon 1, changed His322 to Asn. The second mutation, in exon 2 changed the third base in codon 446 without changing the amino acid sequence and the third mutation, in an alternatively spliced fourth exon, changed Pro561 to Arg (number of the exons follows reference 72, see section on organization of the *AChE* gene below; Bartels et al. (11) use a different numbering system and described the mutations in exon 2, exon 3 and exon 5 respectively). Only the His322/Asn mutation would be present in the mature protein found on red cells. The Pro561/Arg mutation is in a region of the translated protein which is cleaved before attachment of the GPI anchor. Analysis of 17 DNA samples from individuals of known Yt[a]/Yt[b] phenotype gave complete concordance with the His322/Asn mutation. His is found when Yt[a] is expressed and Asn is found when Yt[b] is expressed.

As discussed below, AChE from *Torpedo californica* has been crystallized and the crystal structure determined (73). Bartels et al. (11) note that the amino acid residue corresponding to His322/Asn in *Torpedo* AChE is Lys 315 and that this residue is located on the outer surface of the protein. It would therefore be expected that His322/Asn are similarly located in human red cell AChE, a feature consistent with a role for these amino acids in defining Yt[a] and Yt[b].

The Structure of Acetylcholinesterase

Sussman et al. (73) determined the structure of AChE from the electric fish *Torpedo californica* by X-ray analysis of crystals of the protein. The form crystallized was the GPI-anchored homodimer which is highly homologous to the human red cell enzyme and its structure is therefore likely to be highly relevant to considerations regarding the structure of the human enzyme. The protein has an ellipsoidal shape and dimensions of 4.5nm by 6nm by 6.5nm. It consists of a central 12-stranded mixed beta sheet surrounded by 14 alpha helices. The AChE homodimer appears to be held together by a four helix bundle and one interchain disulphide bond involving the carboxy terminal Cys537. These authors (73) obtained evidence that at least one (Asn416) of the four possible N-glycosylation sites is utilized. The active site of the enzyme forms a deep and narrow gorge 2nm in length that penetrates halfway into the protein. The critical residues for enzyme activity His440, Ser200, Glu327 line this gorge. As discussed above, the amino acids critical for Yt[a]/Yt[b] expression are predicted to be at the surface of the structure and it seemed unlikely that the polymorphism would have a significant effect on enzyme activity. Masson et al. (12) examined red cells of the Yt(a+b-) and Yt(a-b+) phenotypes and showed that, as expected, there is no difference in AChE activity between the two phenotypes.

Organization of the Human Acetylcholinesterase Gene

The open reading frame of the human *AChE* gene encompasses 4.5-4.7kb. Three exons encode the signal peptide and the amino terminal 535 amino acids which are common to all forms of the enzyme found in different tissues. Different forms of the enzyme are found and each of these is generated by the use of different fourth exons (alternative exon usage). The major mRNA species found in mammalian brain and muscle contains a cysteine near the carboxy terminus which facilitates the formation of soluble disulphide-linked homodimers and tetramers and disulphide linkage to membrane-bound collagen-containing filamentous subunits.

The mouse *AChE* gene is organized in the same way as the human gene but in mouse bone marrow the most abundant mRNA species is produced when the third exon is not spliced before it reaches a termination codon 90bp from the 3' end of the exon. This results in a soluble AChE which lacks the cysteine near the carboxy terminus and is therefore likely to be monomeric. The human gene does not have a stop codon in the corresponding position and the predominant form in human red cells results from splicing in a novel fourth exon which encodes a stretch of hydrophobic amino acids upstream of a stop codon. This carboxyterminal hydrophobic sequence is then posttranslationally cleaved and a GPI anchor attached. Amino terminal to the cleaved peptide sequence is a cysteine residue necessary for dimer formation (60,72).

The Function of Acetylcholinesterase

In neuromuscular junctions and brain cholinergic synapses AChE functions by effecting the rapid hydrolysis of the neurotransmitter acetylcholine (74). When acetylcholine binds to the acetylcholine receptor in the membrane of a skeletal muscle cell it provokes an electrical change and then dissociates from the receptor whereupon it is hydrolysed by AChE and impulse transmission is terminated. The acute toxicity of organophosphorus compounds is a direct consequence of the fact that they are potent inhibitors of AChE.

The function of AChE in hematopoietic cells is, however, far from clear. It has been known for many years that AChE is deficient in the red blood cells of patients with PNH but this deficiency is unrelated to the extreme sensitivity of such cells to complement-mediated lysis which is primarily attributable to deficiency of another GPI-linked protein CD59 (75). There are hints in the literature that AChE may play a role in hematopoiesis. Abnormalities in chromosome 7 are frequently found in patients with acute non-lymphocytic leukemia and myelodysplastic syndromes and the commonest chromosomal breakpoint in these conditions is at 7q22, site of the *AChE* gene (76).

Alterations at the *AChE* locus induced by exposure to chemotherapy, radiation and organophosphorus compounds have been linked with abnormal megakaryocytopoeisis (77) and such a role for AChE in megakaryocytopoiesis is supported by in vitro experiments carried out in mice (78). In contrast to most of the blood group systems described in this book there is no true null phenotype (Yt(a-b-)) in the Cartwright system although, as discussed above, some partial deficiencies and transient deficiencies have been reported. Now that it is possible to culture erythroid cells in vitro (80) it may be feasible selectively to inhibit the expression of the *AChE* gene in such cultures (for example by the use of anti-sense oligonucleotides) (81) and thereby elucidate its function in blood cells more clearly.

References

1. Eaton BR, Morton JA, Pickles MM, et al. Br J Haematol 1956;7:333
2. Giles CM, Metaxas MN. Nature 1964;202:1122
3. Adebahr M, Allen FH Jr. Unpublished observations 1966 to 1968 cited in Issitt PD. Applied Blood Group Serology, 1st Ed. Oxnard:Spectra Biologicals, 1979:93
4. Giles CM, Metaxas-Bühler, Romanski Y, et al. Vox Sang 1967;13:171
5. Wurzel HA, Haesler W Jr. Vox Sang 1968;15:304
6. Salmon C, Cartron J-P, Rouger P. The Human Blood Groups. New York:Masson, 1984:289
7. Lewis M, Kaita H, Philipps S, et al. Vox Sang 1987;53:52
8. Gale SA, Rowe GP, Northfield FE. Vox Sang 1988;54:172
9. Telen MJ, Rosse WF, Parker CJ, et al. Blood 1990;75:1404
10. Spring FA, Gardner B, Anstee DJ. Blood 1992;80:2136
11. Bartels CF, Zelinski T, Lockridge O, et al. Am J Hum Genet 1993;52:928
12. Masson P, Froment M-T, Sorenson RC, et al. Blood 1994;83:3003
13. Nakajima H, Saito M, Murata S. J Anthropol Soc Nippon 1980;88:455
14. Levene C, Cohen T, Manny N, et al. (Letter). Transfusion 1985;25:180
15. Levene C, Bar-Shany S, Manny N, et al. Transfusion 1987;27:471
16. Ikin EW, Giles CM, Plaut G. Vox Sang 1965;10:212
17. Vengelen-Tyler V, Morel PA. Transfusion 1983;23:114
18. Rouger P, Dosda F, Girard M, et al. Rev Fr Transf Immunohematol 1982;25:45
19. Daniels G. Immunohematology 1992;8:53
20. Branch DR, Muensch HA, Sy Siok Hian AL, et al. Br J

Haematol 1983;54:573

21. Levene C, Harel N. (Letter). Transfusion 1984;24:541
22. Shulman IA, Nelson JM, Lam H-T. (Letter). Transfusion 1986;26:214
23. Advani H, Zamor J, Judd WJ, et al. Br J Haematol 1982;51:107
24. Gobel U, Drescher KH, Pottgen W, et al. Vox Sang 1974;27:171
25. Ferguson SJ, Boyce F, Blajchman MA. Transfusion 1979;19:581
26. Testa I, Rabini RA, Fumelli P, et al. J Clin Endocrinol Metab 1988;67:1129
27. Suhail M, Rizvi SI. Ind J Exp Biol 1990;28:234
28. Kamada T, McMillan DE, Yamashity T, et al. Diabetes Res Clin Pract 1992;16:1
29. Whittaker DS. MHS Thesis, Duke Univ 1994
30. Whittaker DS, Telen MJ. (abstract). Transfusion 1994;34 (Suppl 10S):63S
31. Bryszewska M, Leyko W. Diabetologia 1983;24:311
32. Dutta-Roy AD, Rany TK, Shinha AK. Biochem Biophys Acta 1985;816:187
33. Bettigole R, Harris JP, Tegoli J, et al. Vox Sang 1968;14:143
34. Hardman JT, Beck ML, Pierce SR. (abstract). Book of Abstracts, 16th Cong ISBT 1980:265
35. Pierce SR, Hardman JT, Hunt JS, et al. (abstract). Transfusion 1980;20:627
36. Hunt JS, Beck ML, Hardman JT, et al. Am J Clin Pathol 1980;74:259
37. Mohandas K, Spivak M, Delehanty CL. Transfusion 1985;25:381
38. Garratty G, Arndt P, Nance S. (abstract). Transfusion 1996;36 (Suppl 9S):50S
39. Dobbs JV, Prutting DL, Adebahr M, et al. Vox Sang 1968;15:216
40. Nance SJ, Arndt P, Garratty G. Transfusion 1987;27:449
41. Eckrich RJ, Mallory DM. (abstract). Transfusion 1993;33 (Suppl 9S):18S
42. Wurzel HA, Haesler W Jr. Vox Sang 1968;14:460
43. Levy GJ, Selset G, McQuiston D, et al. Transfusion 1988;28:265
44. Garratty G. In: Clinical and Serological Aspects of Transfusion Reactions. Arlington, VA:Am Assoc Blood Banks, 1982:81
45. Branch DR, Gallagher MT, Mison AP, et al. Br J Haematol 1984;56:19
46. Branch DR, Gallagher MT. (Letter). Br J Haematol 1986;62:783
47. Ballas SK, Sherwood WC. Transfusion 1977;17:65
48. Davey RJ, Simpkins SS. Transfusion 1981;21:702
49. AuBuchon JP, Brightman A, Anderson HJ et al. Vox Sang 1988;55:171
50. Kakaiya R, Sheahan E, Julleis J, et al. Immunohematology 1991;7:107
51. Silvergleid AJ, Wells RF, Hafleigh EB, et al. Transfusion 1978;18:8
52. Hillyer CD, Hall JM, Tiegerman KO, et al. Immunohematology 1991;7:102
53. Bergvalds H, Stock A, McClure PD. Vox Sang 1965;10:627
54. Lavellée R, Lacombe M, D'Angelo C. Rev Fr Transf 1970;13;71
55. Allen FH Jr, Alter A. Proc 11th Cong ISBT 1966, Bibl Haematol Basel:Karger 1968;29:973
56. Oxendine SM, Telen MJ, Rao N, et al. (abstract). Transfusion 1992;32 (Suppl 8S):18S
57. Rao N, Whitsett CF, Oxendine SM, et al. Blood 1993;81:815
58. Telen MJ, Rosse WF. Baillières Clin Haematol 1991;4:849
59. Rosse WF. Sem Hematol 1993;30:219
60. Li Y, Camp S, Rachinsky TL, et al. J Biol Chem 1991;266:23083
61. Issitt PD. Transf Med Rev 1993;7:139
62. Coghlan G, Kaita H, Belcher E, et al. Vox Sang 1989;57:88
63. Zelinski T, Coghlan G, Myal Y, et al. Ann Hum Genet 1991;55:137
64. Zelinski T, White L, Coghlan G, et al. Genomics 1991;11:165
65. Getman DK, Eubanks JH, Camp S, et al. Am J Hum Genet 1992;51:170
66. Ehrlich G, Viegas-Pequignot E, Ginzberg D, et al. Genomics 1992;13:1192
67. Pehta JC, Valinksy J, Redman C, et al. (abstract). Book of Abstracts ISBT/AABB Joint Cong, 1990:57
68. Spring FA, Anstee DJ. (abstract). Transf Med 1991;1 (Suppl 2):42
69. Soreson K, Brodbeck U, Rasmussen AG. Biochem Biophys Acta 1987;912:56
70. Johns RJ. New Eng J Med 1962;267:1344
71. Shinohara K, Tanaka KR. Am J Hematol 1979;7:313
72. Taylor P. J Biol Chem 1991;266:4025
73. Sussman J, Harel M, Frolow F, et al. Science 1991;253:872
74. Massoulie J, Bon S. Ann Rev Neurosci 1985;5:57
75. Yamashina M, Ueda E, Kinoshita T, et al. New Eng J Med 1990;323:1184
76. Kere J, Ruutu T, Davies KA, et al. Blood 1989;73:230
77. Lapidot-Lifson Y, Prody CA, Ginzberg D, et al. Proc Nat Acad Sci USA 1989;86:4715
78. Patinkin D, Seidman S, Eckstein F, et al. Mol Cell Biol 1990;10:6046
79. Petty AC. J Immunol Meth 1993;161:91
80. Labbaye C, Valtieri M, Barberi T, et al. J Clin Invest 1995;95:2346
81. Voltieri M, Venturelli D, Care A, et al. Blood 1991;77:1181
82. Soreq H, Ben-Aziz R, Prody CA, et al. Proc Nat Acad Sci USA 1990;87:9688

24 | The Cromer Blood Group System

In 1965, McCormick et al. (1) described an antibody made by a Black woman by the name of Cromer. Because Mrs. Cromer's red cells were Go(a+) and because her antibody, that detected an antigen of very high incidence, was non-reactive only with the red cells of her sister, that were also Go(a+), it was thought that the antibody might be anti-Go^b. However, once Go^a was shown to be an Rh system antigen (2,3) and once the Cromer antibody was shown (3) to react with Rh$_{null}$ red cells, it became apparent that the antibody could not be anti-Go^b. In 1975, Stroup and McCreary (4) described four additional examples of what were said in the abstract (but see below) to be the same antibody and suggested the name anti-Cr^a for the specificity. It was reported (4) that in addition to defining an antigen present on Rh$_{null}$ red cells, anti-Cr^a detected a determinant for which the controlling gene was not located at the *Rh* locus. All four antibody-makers described by Stroup and McCreary (4) were Black and all four had been transfused and/or pregnant. In a 1982 publication of Daniels et al. (5) some results attributed to Stroup and McCreary (4) were given. It was pointed out that the four antibodies described in 1975 did not have exactly the same specificity as the Cromer antibody. Indeed, the antibodies were shown as reacting with Cr(a-) red cells (presumably those of Mrs. Cromer) and each was shown as giving variable (weak or negative) reactions with the red cells of the other antibody-makers. The link between the four cell samples and the antibodies was that the sera failed to react with the cells of a patient listed as A.J., that were described as Cr(a-). As early as 1982 it was suspected that the red cells of A.J., who was dead, represented some sort of null phenotype. The antibody made by A.J. reacted with Cr(a-) red cells and with those of the four patients described by Stroup and McCreary (4). Daniels et al. (5) concluded that the patient they studied, Inab, a 27 year-old Japanese male who had received massive infusions of fresh frozen plasma, had red cells that were phenotypically the same as A.J. It was supposed (5) that Inab and A.J. were of a "null phenotype in the Cromer blood group complex". Thus the antibodies made by these two individuals were capable of reacting with Cr(a-) red cells because those cells lack Cr^a but not other closely related very common antigens. Reactions of the Inab and A.J. sera with the red cells of the four antibody-makers described by Stroup and McCreary (4) could be explained by similar reasoning. Those cells might carry Cr^a (some of them reacted with the Cromer serum, see above) and/or another high incidence Cromer

system antigen defined by the Inab and A.J. antibodies, but might lack a related high incidence antigen (or antigens) to which the antibody-makers had become immunized. Lack of the reaction of the Cromer (1) or other (4) antibodies with the Inab and A.J. red cells would be explained if those cells lacked a series of high incidence Cromer-related antigens, i.e. the Inab and A.J. cells were Cr$_{null}$. The explanations seemed to fit the observed serological reactions but Daniels et al. (5) pointed out that it could be argued that the phenotypes of Inab and A.J. were genetically independent of the Cromer complex and were perhaps of a null phenotype that affects more than one blood group system, just as Rh$_{null}$ cells are LW(a-b-) although the *CDE* and *LW* loci are independent. Although that possibility had to be regarded seriously in 1982, it has since been excluded. As described briefly later in this introduction and in more detail later in this chapter, serological and biochemical studies have shown, beyond doubt, that the Inab phenotype (of which two other examples (6,7) are now known) does indeed represent the Cr$_{null}$ situation. Inab phenotype red cells lack all ten Cromer system antigens, fail to react with an antibody that behaves as if it detects two of those antigens but cannot be divided into separable specificities, and lack or carry only trace amounts of the red cell membrane component, decay accelerating factor (DAF) on which the Cromer system antigens are carried (8-10).

In 1980, Laird-Fryer et al. (11) reported two examples of an antibody directed against a very common antigen. Both examples were made by Black women neither of whom had been transfused but both of whom had been pregnant. The antibody was called anti-Tc^a; the two examples were shown to react with Cr(a-) red cells. Another example was reported in 1981 (12) in a Black woman who had been transfused and pregnant. In 1983, Laird-Fryer et al. (13) published a full account of anti-Tc^a. By then the Tc(a-) phenotype had been found in four unrelated Black families. The link between Tc^a and Cr^a was that one of the first two patients who made what Laird-Fryer et al. (11,13) called anti-Tc^a, was one of the individuals described by Stroup and McCreary (4) as having made an anti-Cr^a-like specificity. That is not to say that the phenotype and the antibody were the same but that the same patient is described in the different reports (4,11,13). It is now apparent that different terms were used (see also 5) because the antibodies (anti-Cr^a and anti-Tc^a) define high incidence antigens, both of which are absent from Inab (Cr$_{null}$) red cells.

In 1982, Block et al. (14) described anti-Tc^b, an antibody to a low incidence antigen that seemed to be antithetical to Tc^a in Blacks, additional details were published later (15). Also in 1982, Law et al. (16) described anti-Tc^c that, like anti-Tc^b, defines a low incidence antigen. The antigen Tc^c seemed to be antithetical to Tc^a in Whites. Since the Tc(a-) phenotype is much more common in Blacks than in Whites, Tc^b is considerably more common than Tc^c. As of this writing (September 1996), Tc^b has not been reported in a White, Tc^c has not been reported in a Black.

Cromer achieved official recognition as an independent blood group system in 1991 (17). The promotion from collection to system status was based on the findings (9,10) that the antigens are carried on DAF (see above) and that the gene that encodes production of that PI-linked glycoprotein segregates independently of all other blood group loci (18). By the time independent system status was achieved, several other antigens had been added to the Cromer polymorphism. The high incidence antigens Dr^a and Es^a were both described in 1984 (19,20). In 1986, Daniels et al. (21) introduced the term IFC to describe the antigen defined by the antibody made by persons of the Inab phenotype. IFC is, of course, present in all Cromer system phenotypes except Cr$_{null}$ (Inab). In 1987, Sistonen et al. (22) described a low incidence antigen, first found in Finns, that they named WES and later in the same year, Daniels et al. (23) described an antibody that appeared to define the high incidence, antithetical partner to WES. The low incidence antigen is now called WES^a and its high incidence, probable antithetical partner, WES^b. The most recent addition to the system is the high incidence antigen UMC, described in 1989 by Daniels et al. (24).

During some of the early investigations that eventually resolved the relationships of various high incidence Cromer system antigens to each other, the terms Cr1, Cr2 and Cr3 were used (5,25). Those terms are now best forgotten. By the time the ISBT Working Party introduced (26) a numerical terminology for the system (then still a collection) the relationships were better understood. Thus the antigen Cr^a, that had also been called Cr1, became CROM1. However, the Tc^a antigen, that had also been called Cr3, became CROM2. Some of the early confusion reflected the fact that the antibody made by the Cr$_{null}$ individuals (now anti-IFC (21) see above, or anti-CROM7, see table 24-1) had not been recognized as having the specificity that is now apparent. Table 24-1 lists the conventional and ISBT terms for the Cromer system antigens, shows the year of their discovery and lists pertinent references. Details regarding the incidence of the antigens in various population groups are given in table 24-2.

The Antigen Cr^a and the Antibody That Defines It

As shown in table 24-2, Cr^a is of very high incidence. A number of individuals with Cr(a-) red cells, that

TABLE 24-1 Conventional and ISBT Terminology for the Cromer Blood Group System

Conventional Name: Cromer

Conventional Symbol: Cr

ISBT System Symbol: CROM

ISBT System Number: 021

Antigen Conventional Name	ISBT Antigen Number	ISBT Full Code Number	H=High L=Low Incidence	Year of Discovery	Pertinent References
Cr^a	CROM1	021001	H	1965	1, 4, 5
Tc^a	CROM2	021002	H	1980	5, 11-13
Tc^b	CROM3	021003	L	1982	14, 15
Tc^c	CROM4	021004	L	1982	16
Dr^a	CROM5	021005	H	1984	19
Es^a	CROM6	021006	H	1984	20
IFC	CROM7	021007	H	1986	21
WES^a	CROM8	021008	L	1987	22
WES^b	CROM9	021009	H	1987	23
UMC	CROM10	021010	H	1989	24

TABLE 24-2 Incidence of Some Cromer System Phenotypes in Different Population Groups

Phenotype	Incidence and Population Studied	Reference
Cr(a-)	0 in 4000 U.S. Blacks	1
	2 in 8858 U.S. Blacks in Detroit	27
Tc(a-)	1 in 950 U.S. Blacks	13
	0 in 5000 U.S. Whites	13
	0 in 5000 Japanese	13
Tc(b+)	19 in 358 (5.3%) U.S. Blacks	15
	0 in 304 U.S. Whites	15
Tc(c+)	Not found among random individuals, see text	
Dr(a-)	Not found among random individuals, see text	
Es(a-)	0 in 3400 mixed (largely White) U.S. Donors	20
IFC- (Cr$_{null}$)	Not found among random individuals, see text	
WES(a+)	61 in 10,982 (0.56%) Finns	22
	7 in 1460 (0.48%) U.S. Blacks	28
	5 in 245 (2.05%) North London (UK) Blacks	23
	2 in 1610 (0.12%) U.S. Whites	28
	0 in 1073 Hungarians, 1026 Somalis, 747 Poles	22
	0 in 707 Latvians, 500 Japanese, 210 Belgians	22
WES(b-)	0 in 270 English (mostly White)	23
	0 in 245 North London (UK) Blacks	23
UMC-	0 in 45,610 Japanese	24

were not of the Inab (Cr$_{null}$) phenotype, have been found (1,4,27,29-37) most often when the patient presented with anti-Cr^a in the serum. With the exception of one Spanish-American woman (30) all individuals known to have Cr(a-) red cells are Black. Both transfusion and pregnancy seem to be effective in stimulating production of anti-Cr^a. The Cr^a antigen survives treatment of red cells with trypsin, papain, ficin or neuraminidase but is denatured or removed when red cells are treated with alpha-chymotrypsin (38,39). The antigen is slightly weakened when red cells are treated with AET or DTT (39). Little seems to be known about the expression of Cr^a on the red cells of newborns, but, as described below, no case of HDN caused by anti-Cr^a has been reported. Since Cr^a, in common with other antigens of the Cromer system, is present on DAF, a PI-linked protein (see

below), the complement-sensitive PNH III population of red cells from patients with paroxysmal nocturnal hemoglobinuria, type as Cr(a-) or as very weakly positive for the antigen (9,10).

Anti-Cr^a is usually an IgG, red cell stimulated antibody, that is optimally reactive by IAT. Those examples that have been subclassed have been shown (32,33) to be largely IgG1 in composition although IgG2 and IgG4 components have been found. When they studied six examples of anti-Cr^a, Reid et al. (32) found that five of them could be recovered from Cr(a+) red cells only by the digitonin-acid elution method of Jenkins and Moore (40). Judd et al. (35) reported that one example of anti-Cr^a, that might have been of clinical significance in the patient involved, was regarded by the referring hospital as being a clinically benign, unidentified HTLA antibody when it was adsorbed by a commercially-supplied human platelet concentrate preparation. Those authors (35) showed that three other examples of anti-Cr^a were removed by a single adsorption with the platelet preparation and correctly pointed out that adsorption of an antibody in such a procedure does not equate with clinical insignificance of the antibody. Inhibition of anti-Cr^a (and other Cromer system antibodies) by human serum and concentrated urine is described in a later section.

In terms of clinical significance in transfusion therapy, it seems that each example of anti-Cr^a must be evaluated individually. In three patients with anti-Cr^a in the serum, in vivo ^{51}Cr survival studies were normal or close to normal and the patients were subsequently transfused with Cr(a+) blood (30,36,37). In each case the transfusions were well tolerated and appeared to effect expected increases in hematocrit. In another patient (31) similar close to normal in vivo survival of ^{51}Cr-labeled Cr(a+) red cells was demonstrated but the patient received only autologous transfusions. However, in at least three other patients (33-35) in vivo cell survival studies and/or monocyte monolayer assays suggested that Cr(a+) red cells would not be expected to survive normally. In one of these patients (34) transfusion was avoided, in a second (33) Cr(a-) blood was used and in the third (35) there was some evidence that accelerated clearance of Cr(a+) red cells had occurred before the anti-Cr^a was identified. Thus while many of the anti-Cr^a studied seem to have been clinically benign or capable of

clearing Cr(a+) red cells only at a clinically insignificant rate, exceptions may exist. As mentioned in many other places in this book, the decision to transfuse red cells that may not survive in a completely normal fashion in vivo but are highly unlikely to cause a catastrophic transfusion reaction, must be carefully weighted against the urgency of the need for transfusion. On a number of occasions, anti-Cr^a has failed to cause clinical HDN in an infant with Cr(a+) red cells born to a woman with anti-Cr^a in the serum. The possibility that Cromer system antibodies are adsorbed by placental tissue is discussed in a later section.

The most usual characteristics of Cromer system antibodies, including many that have not yet been described in this chapter, are shown in table 24-3.

The Antigens Tc^a, Tc^b and Tc^c and the Antibodies That Define Them

As described in the introduction of this chapter, Tc^a is an antigen of very high incidence (see table 24-2) that was initially associated with Cr^a and then the Cromer system because both Cr^a and Tc^a are missing from Inab (Cr_{null}) red cells. When Lacey et al. (14,15) found an antibody to a low incidence antigen, present in a serum that also contained anti-Go^a, they showed that it reacted with the red cells of 19 of 358 (5.3%) Go(a-) but otherwise unselected samples from Blacks. The antibody

TABLE 24-3 Usual Characteristics of Cromer System Antibodies

Antibody Specificity	Positive Reactions in In Vitro Tests				Usual Immuno-globulin		Ability to Bind Complement		Ability to Cause In Vitro Lysis		Implicated in		Usual Form of Stimulation		% of White Population Positive
	Sal	LISS	AHG	Enz*1	IgG	IgM	Yes	No	Yes	No	Transfusion Reaction	HDN	Red Cells	Other	
Anti-Cr^a			X		X			X		X	X	No	X		>99.9
Anti-Tc^a			X		X			X		X	X	No	X		>99.9
Anti-Tc^b			X		X			X		X		No	X		0
Anti-Tc^c			X		X			X		X		No			<0.1
Anti-Dr^a			X		X			X		X		No	X		>99.9
Anti-Es^a			X		X			X		X		No			>99.9
Anti-IFC			X		X			X		X	X	No			>99.9
Anti-WES^a			X		X			X		X		No	X		0.1*2
Anti-WES^b			X		X			X		X		No			>99.9
Anti-UMC			X		X			X		X		No			>99.9

*1   For variable reactions of different antigens with different enzymes see text.
*2   For variation in different White populations, see table 24-2.

reacted with all Tc(a-) samples and family studies were used to show that in Blacks, Tc^a and Tc^b are alleles. No Tc(b+) sample was found in tests on 5000 US Whites and 5000 Japanese (15).

In the same year in which anti-Tc^b was found, Law et al. (16) described an antibody to a low incidence antigen, that reacted with the Tc(a-b-) red cells of a White woman and those of her sister. The antibody was called anti-Tc^c and is presumed to define the antigen antithetical to Tc^a in Whites. The two women with Tc(a-b-) red cells did not have the Inab phenotype. In the family study (16) the parents of the proposita were shown both to have Tc(a+b-c+) red cells, three of their children were phenotypically Tc(a+b-c+), one was Tc(a+b-c-) and the proposita and her sister were Tc(a-b-c+). As described below, the woman with Tc(a-b-c+) red cells made an antibody best described as anti-Tc^{ab}; another example in a different White woman with Tc(a-b-) red cells has been reported (41).

Like Cr^a, the Tc^a, Tc^b and Tc^c antigens survive treatment of red cells with trypsin, papain, ficin or neuraminidase but are no longer detectable on red cells treated with alpha-chymotrypsin (38,39). Treatment of red cells with AET or DTT may weaken the expression of Tc^a, Tc^b and Tc^c (39). Like other Cromer system antigens Tc^a (and presumably Tc^b and Tc^c) is not detected or is present only in very low levels, on PNH III red cells (9,10).

Since anti-Tc^b and anti-Tc^c define antigens of low incidence, neither one of them is likely to pose a problem in transfusion therapy. Anti-Tc^a is, of course, a different matter since the Tc^a antigen is of very high incidence. Similarly, two women with Tc(a-b-c+) red cells formed an antibody that reacted with Tc(a+b-c-) and Tc(a-b+c-) but not with Tc(a-b-c+) red cells. The antibody was called (16,41) anti-Tc^{ab} and anti-Tc^{a}Tc^b since it could not be split into separable anti-Tc^a and anti-Tc^b components. Like anti-Cr^a, anti-Tc^a and anti-Tc^{ab} are usually IgG, red cell stimulated antibodies that react optimally by IAT. One example of anti-Tc^a was shown (42) to be composed of IgG1, IgG2 and IgG4, two years later only the IgG2 and IgG4 components could be detected. One example of anti-Tc^{ab} (41) and one example of anti-Tc^a (42) (tested when the IgG1 component was demonstrable, see above) gave results in ^{51}Cr in vivo red cell survival studies and MMAs that suggested that they would cause only slightly accelerated clearance of Tc(a+) red cells in vivo. Two other examples of anti-Tc^a (12,13) gave results in similar studies that suggested that they might be of greater clinical relevance. However, to the best of our knowledge that supposition was not put to the test since neither patient was transfused with Tc(a+) blood. The example of anti-Tc^a that gave a positive MMA when it contained IgG1, IgG2 and IgG4 components yielded an MMA result that suggested that Tc(a+) cells might survive near normally,

when the later sample, that lacked the IgG1 component was tested (42). No example of clinical HDN caused by antibodies to Tc^a, Tc^b or Tc^c has been reported. One White woman with Tc(a-b-c+) red cells had weak anti-Tc^a in her serum when her unaffected child was born. The infant's red cells were Tc(a+) and six months after the child was born, the woman's serum was found to contain anti-Tc^{ab} (16).

The Antigen Dr^a and the Antibody That Defines It

As indicated in tables 24-1 and 24-2 the Dr^a antigen is of very high incidence. The Dr(a-) phenotype was found in members of three apparently unrelated Jewish families living in Israel (19,44,45). All three families had moved to Israel from Uzbekistan, a country to the south of Russia. A fourth proposita with Dr(a-) red cells and anti-Dr^a in the serum was a Russian woman. For reasons that will become apparent from what is written below, the fourth example of Dr(a-) red cells was at first (46,47) thought to be of the Inab phenotype.

The Dr(a-) phenotype differs from all others in the Cromer system. In addition to the absence of the very common antigen Dr^a, those Cromer system antigens that are present are only weakly expressed (19,44,45). That is to say, on Dr(a-) red cells the antigens Cr^a, Tc^a, Tc^{ab}, Es^a, IFC, WES^b and UMC are all weak. As yet no Dr(a-) sample carrying Tc^b, Tc^c or WES^a has been found. In the numerical terminology, the phenotype can be written as CROM:w1,w2,-3,-4,-5,w6,w7,-8,w9,w10. Dr(a-) red cells also react only weakly with monoclonal antibodies to DAF. The low level of DAF and hence the weakened expression of all Cromer system antigens on Dr(a-) red cells has been explained at the molecular level (47,48 and see later in this chapter).

Questions have been raised as to whether inheritance of the Dr(a-) phenotype follows the usual Mendelian pattern for a recessive characteristic. In the first family described, the proposita had one sib with Dr(a-) and three with Dr(a+) red cells (19). In the second family, both sibs of the Dr(a-) proposita had Dr(a+) red cells but those of three of her four children were Dr(a-) (44). In the third family three of four sibs of the Dr(a-) proband also had Dr(a-) red cells (45). While these findings at least suggest the possibility of presence of a dominant suppressor, studies at the molecular genetic level (47,48) show that the difference between the presence and absence of Dr^a involves an amino acid change at one residue on the DAF glycoprotein. In other words, inheritance of the Dr(a-) phenotype represents the inheritance of the gene that fails to encode production of Dr^a, from each parent. Presumably, the second family mentioned above (44) represented the mating *DrDr* X *Dr^aDr*, where *Dr^a* is the gene that encodes production of Dr^a, and *Dr* is the gene that does not.

When Lublin et al. (48) investigated the Dr(a+)/Dr(a-) polymorphism at the molecular level they showed that the gene that fails to encode production of Dr^a differs from the gene that makes that antigen by a single nucleotide substitution. The *DAF* gene that makes Dr^a encodes a protein with serine at position 165, the *DAF* gene present on both chromosomes of persons with Dr(a-) red cells encodes production of a protein with leucine at position 165. The nucleotide substitution results in loss of a *Taq1* restriction site meaning that the two alleles can be differentiated. Lublin et al. (48) named the *DAF* allele that fails to encode production of the Dr^a antigen, *Dr^b*, and then described Dr^b as the first red cell antigen defined at the nucleotide level and not by an antibody. Daniels (49) pointed out that Dr^b cannot be used as an antigen name since an antigen is defined as a molecule that generates an immune response or as a molecule that reacts with antibodies or primed T cells (50). Since *Dr^b* represents a single nucleotide substitution, Dr^b would not qualify on either count. Until anti-Dr^b is found, there is no evidence that the altered structure on the DAF of Dr(a-) red cells is immunogenic. Later, Lewis and McAlpine (51) pointed out that there was no need to use *Dr^b* even as a gene symbol. The Guidelines for Human Gene Nomenclature (52) clearly had covered the situation arising from the delineation of the Dr(a+)/Dr(a-) polymorphism. Since the *DAF* gene that encodes production of Dr^a makes a protein with serine at position 165, it would be named DAF*165S. The allele, that in the homozygous state accounts for the Dr(a-) phenotype would be DAF*165L, since it encodes a protein with L (leucine) instead of S (serine) at residue 165. In responding to the comments of Daniels (49) and Lewis and McAlpine (51), Lublin and Telen (53,54) agreed that use of the term Dr^b for an antigen was premature since the altered structure on Dr(a-) red cells has not been defined by an antibody. They (54) defended the use of *Dr^b* as a gene term and believed that it would be as meaningful as the already accepted symbol *Dr^a*. However, it seems to us that herein lies the root of the problem. The term *Dr^a* is accepted because it describes a gene that encodes production of the Dr^a antigen that can, in turn, be identified by an antibody. The term *Dr^b* implies that the same is true. In fact, the altered portion of the protein has not yet been shown to be immunogenic, the term DAF*165L is more descriptive since it describes exactly the function of the allele and contrasts it to the DAF*165S that can, for the reasons given, justifiably also be called *Dr^a*.

Like other antigens of the Cromer system, Dr^a survives enzyme treatment of red cells with trypsin, papain,

ficin or neuraminidase but is not detectable on red cells treated with alpha-chymotrypsin and may be weakened by treatment of red cells with AET or DTT (38,39).

Anti-Dr^a seems usually to be an IgG, red cell stimulated antibody, best reactive by IAT (19,44). Nothing seems to have been published regarding the clinical significance or lack thereof, of the antibody. The role of Dr^a as a bacterial receptor is described in a later section.

The Antigen Es^a and the Antibody That Defines It

Only one example of anti-Es^a is known. It was made by a woman of Mexican extraction, the proposita whose parents were first cousins, and two of her sibs had Es(a-) red cells, those of one other sib were Es(a+) (20). Anti-Es^a was first seen to define a Cromer system antigen when it failed to react with red cells of the Inab (Cr_{null}) phenotype. Like other antigens of the Cromer system, Es^a is destroyed when red cells are treated with alpha-chymotrypsin but resists the actions of trypsin, papain, ficin and neuraminidase. Es(a-) red cells react less strongly with anti-WES^b than do Es(a+) cells and both examples of cells of the WES(a+b-) phenotype had to be tested in adsorption-elution studies before it could be shown that they are Es(a+) (23).

The Inab Phenotype and Anti-IFC

As mentioned several times already in this chapter, the Inab phenotype is the null phenotype of the Cromer system. That is to say, the Inab phenotype can be written as Cr(a-) Tc(a-b-c-) Dr(a-) Es(a-) IFC- WES(a-b-) UMC- or as CROM:-1,-2,-3,-4,-5,-6,-7,-8,-9,-10. Some of the early confusion regarding the relationship of Cr^a to Tc^a and to related antibodies and phenotypes, that is described in the introduction of this chapter, apparently arose because some red cells of the Inab Phenotype (A.J.) and perhaps one antibody made by an Inab individual were used, before the exact relationship of Inab to Cr^a and Tc^a and other Cromer system antigens was recognized.

Although A.J. may well have been the first studied person with Inab phenotype red cells that point will never be proved. A.J. was dead before Stroup and McCreary (4) linked the four anti-Cr^a-like sera to each other by virtue of their non-reactivity with the A.J. red cells. In 1982, Daniels et al. (5) described Inab, a Japanese male with apparently the same red cell phenotype as A.J. The patient had an ileocoecal tumor and a severe protein-losing enteropathy, his parents were cousins. The second established example of the Inab phenotype was found (6) in an American Jew with Crohn's disease, a form of protein losing enteropathy. The third example was found in an American White woman of Italian extraction (7). Neither the proposita nor her brother, who also had the Inab phenotype, had any history of intestinal disorder, the proposita was 86, her Inab phenotype brother was 70. As mentioned above a Russian woman who had a chronic intestinal disorder was at first thought (46) to have the Inab phenotype but was later shown (47) to have Dr(a-) red cells with the associated weakening of all other Cromer system antigens. Another probable example of the Inab phenotype was found by Daniels (29). The patient was a 12 year-old Black male with a protein-losing enteropathy. The antibody he made was apparently anti-IFC but his red cells were not tested with Cromer system antibodies.

Because of the association, mentioned above, of the Inab phenotype with protein losing disorders and other gastrointestinal diseases, Daniels and Levi (56) tested red cells from 13 patients with Crohn's disease and 11 with ulcerative colitis or similar disorders, none was of the Inab phenotype.

Before 1986, the Inab phenotype could be reasonably well described in written communications by virtue of the fact that it was becoming appreciated that it represents the Cr_{null} phenotype. It was much more difficult to describe the antibody made by Inab phenotype individuals since it seemed to define an antigen common to red cells of other Cromer system phenotypes, regardless of their actual Cromer antigen make-up. In 1986, Daniels and Walthers (21) learned that the parents of the Japanese patient, Inab (5), were first cousins. While this did not prove the point, it increased the likelihood that the Inab phenotype is inherited (a likelihood shown to be correct when the third example was found (7)). Based on this probability, Daniels and Walthers (21) did blood group serologists a considerable favor and named the antibody made by persons of the Inab phenotype, anti-IFC. Thus IFC became the name for the antigen expressed on all except Cr_{null} (Inab phenotype) red cells, regardless of the permutations of other Cromer system antigens on those red cells. In other words, IFC is to Cromer what Rh29 is to Rh (Chapter 12), Ku is to Kell (Chapter 18), Lu3 is to Lutheran (Chapter 20) and so on. No doubt, if IFC had been recognized for what it is, earlier than 1986, it would have become CROM2 (now Tc^a) or CROM3 (now Tc^b) and not CROM7.

Although few studies have been completed, the IgG, red cell stimulated, IAT-reactive, anti-IFC that have been studied, seem to have clinical significance. In one patient a probable anti-IFC (29) that is referred to as anti-Cr^a in the report (30) cleared all IFC+ red cells within 15 minutes of their injection. In another patient (6) anti-IFC cleared 62% of the injected test dose in the first 24 hours after injection.

The Antigens WES^a and WES^b and the Antibodies That Define Them

Sistonen et al. (22) described anti-WES (later called (23) anti-WES^a and described by that term hereinafter) in 1987 and performed extensive tests in different populations (see table 24-2). The antigen is of relatively low incidence in some populations and of very low incidence in others. In the same year that WES^a was reported, Daniels et al. (23) described an antibody, made by a woman with WES(a+) red cells, that appears to define the high incidence antithetical partner to WES^a. The antibody gave higher titer scores with WES(a-) red cells (presumably from *WES^b* homozygotes) than with incompatible WES(a+) samples (presumably from *WES^a/WES^b* heterozygotes). A Finnish woman with six WES(a+) and no WES(a-) children, had WES(a+) red cells that were non-reactive with the new antibody so were presumed to be WES(a+b-). One other WES(a+b-) sample was found (23).

Like other Cromer system antigens, WES^a and WES^b survive treatment of red cells with trypsin, papain, ficin or neuraminidase, but are no longer detectable on red cells treated with alpha-chymotrypsin (38,39). Daniels (39) reports that while Cr^a, Tc^a, Dr^a, Es^a, IFC and UMC survive pronase treatment of red cells, WES^b is no longer detectable on red cells treated with that enzyme. AET and DTT treatment of red cells may weaken but apparently do not totally denature WES^a and WES^b.

The Antigen UMC and the Antibody That Defines It

The UMC- phenotype was recognized (24) when a female Japanese blood donor was found to have an antibody directed against a very common antigen. The donor had borne three children but had never been transfused. That her antibody defined a Cromer system antigen became apparent when it was seen that it failed to react with Inab phenotype red cells, reacted only weakly with Dr(a-) red cells and was seen to detect an alpha-chymotrypsin sensitive antigen. The UMC- phenotype was seen to be an inherited characteristic when it was found that the red cells of one of the proposita's three sibs did not react with her antibody. In tests on samples from random donors in Japan, no other UMC- sample was found in tests on 45,610 bloods. The anti-UMC made by the proposita (24) is the only known example of that specificity. It was an IgG antibody optimally reactive by IAT. The antibody reacted strongly with UMC+ red cells treated with trypsin, papain, ficin or neuraminidase, its reactions were only marginally reduced when it was tested against AET or DTT-treated red cells.

A Possible Addition to the Cromer System

Cromer system antibodies are usually made as the result of exposure to foreign red cells via transfusion or pregnancy (96). What may be the first example of a non-red cell stimulated Cromer system antibody has been described in an abstract (97). The antibody was made by A.M., a never transfused male English blood donor. The antibody has been detectable in his serum over a period of six years. The A.M. red cells carry the high incidence Cromer system antigens Cr^a, Tc^a, Dr^a, IFC and UMC albeit perhaps in slightly weaker forms than normal red cells. The A.M. cells also react with MAb to DAF (anti-CD55). The A.M. serum reacts with all red cells except those of the Inab phenotype (Cr_{null}, IFC-), those that are Dr(a-) (Cr_{weak}) and his own. The abstract does not mention whether the antibody-maker's red cells have been tested for Es^a and WES^b, nor whether his antibody is adsorbed by Dr(a-) red cells that are not of the Inab phenotype.

Inhibition of Cromer System Antibodies

Daniels (57) realized, early in the studies that led to the association of the various Cromer system antibodies with each other, that they shared some common features. One of these was that they all reacted with trypsin, papain and ficin treated red cells, but failed to react with red cells treated with alpha-chymotrypsin. Another was that the antibodies could apparently be inhibited by plasma or urine. When Daniels (57) first noticed this phenomenon there were few controls, i.e. plasma from non-immunized individuals whose red cells lacked the high incidence antigen, available to confirm that inhibition by plasma from individuals with antigen positive red cells, was antigen specific. However, as more work was done and more samples became available for study, the observations of Daniels (57) were confirmed (7,13,22,23,44). It must be remembered that in hemagglutination inhibition studies such as this, controls are essential. If, for example, anti-Cr^a is inhibited using plasma from an individual with Cr(a+) red cells, a control showing that plasma from a person with Cr(a-) red cells does not cause similar inhibition, is necessary to show that the inhibition is antigen specific and not non-specific. Clearly, the plasma from the Cr(a-) person used as a negative control, must be from a Cr(a-) individual who has not made anti-Cr^a.

Daniels (60) and Daniels et al. (24) have also shown that antibodies to Cr^a, Tc^a, Dr^a, IFC and UMC can be inhibited by concentrated urine from persons with antigen positive red cells. It must be remembered that inhibition of Cromer system antibodies by plasma and urine was recognized (24,57,60) well before it was shown (9,10) that antigens of the system are carried on DAF.

Decay accelerating factor (DAF) is a widely distributed glycoprotein present on red cells, granulocytes, lymphocytes and platelets (see section on Cr^a for description of a case in which anti-Cr^a was adsorbed by a platelet preparation (35)) and tissue cells and is present in a soluble form in body fluids including plasma and urine.

Cromer System Antibodies, HDN and a Possible Defense Mechanism

As mentioned in the previous sections, no antibody in the Cromer system has ever caused clinical HDN. In 1989, Sacks and Garratty (91) described the outcomes of four pregnancies in a woman who had Cr(a-) red cells. The first pregnancy ended in an elective and the second in a spontaneous abortion. Anti-Cr^a was detected in the woman's serum during the second pregnancy. At 18 weeks gestation in the third pregnancy the anti-Cr^a had a titer of 512. Thereafter the titer of the antibody dropped and was no higher than 4 for the remainder of the pregnancy. At 39 weeks a healthy infant was delivered, the cord red blood cells were Cr(a+), DAT-negative and the infant had no symptoms of HDN. From ten to 25 weeks gestation in the woman's fourth pregnancy, the anti-Cr^a had a titer of 128, by 27 weeks it had dropped to 4 and remained at or below that level until term. The infant from this pregnancy also had Cr(a+), DAT-negative red cells and no signs of HDN. The authors (91) wondered if, during pregnancy, the anti-Cr^a had been adsorbed by white cells or platelets or neutralized by plasma, of the fetus.

A similar case was described by Dickson et al. (92) in 1995. A woman with Cr(a-) red cells and anti-Cr^a in the serum was followed through a pregnancy. The anti-Cr^a had a titer of 64 (score 59) early in the pregnancy but had declined to 16 (score 12) at delivery. As in the cases described above, the infant had Cr(a+), DAT-negative red cells and no HDN.

Most recently Reid et al. (93) have described two more cases of this type. In the first, a Black American woman was found to have an IgG1 anti-Cr^a with a titer of 128 early in her second pregnancy, the titer had diminished to 32 at 15 weeks gestation. The patient delivered a clinically normal infant at term. In her third pregnancy, when the authors (93) were able to follow her progress, her anti-Cr^a had a titer of 64 at ten weeks gestation. Serum samples collected at 20 and 21 weeks contained no detectable anti-Cr^a, the patient's red cells still typed as Cr(a-) thus ruling out sample mislabeling and probably excluding transient antigen depression. At term a healthy infant with no signs of HDN was delivered, the authors were unable to obtain a cord blood sample or a postpartum sample from the mother.

The second case (93) involved the fifth proband with

Dr(a-) red cells. The woman was a Russian Jew from the southeast area of Russia. She was first seen by the authors during her third pregnancy. At 12 weeks gestation, her serum contained an anti-Dr^a, with IgG1, IgG2 and IgG4 components, that had a titer of 256 by IAT. Repeat samples collected at 14 and 22 weeks contained anti-Dr^a with a titer of 512. A sample collected at 26 weeks (and repeat samples collected at 31 and 35 weeks and at delivery) contained no detectable anti-Dr^a. The woman's red cells continued to type as Dr(a-). The infant born at term had Dr(a+) red cells, a negative DAT and no signs of HDN. A sample collected from the mother five weeks after delivery, contained anti-Dr^a with a titer of 256 by IAT.

In considering partial or total disappearance of the high titered anti-Cr^a and anti-Dr^a by the end of the second trimester of pregnancy, antibody adsorption seems more likely than cessation of antibody production. In speculating on possible adsorption mechanisms, Reid et al. (93) point out that it is known (94,95) that DAF is preferentially expressed at the fetomaternal interface of the placenta and that there is a quantitative increase in the expression of DAF during placental development. Thus it seems entirely likely that as the placenta develops a sufficient amount of DAF is expressed that considerable or complete antibody adsorption can occur. Such a theory is supported by the observation that once the placenta is no longer present, detectable levels of antibody are again seen in the serum, i.e. start of the third pregnancy in case 1 and five weeks postpartum in case 2 (93). Unfortunately in none of the cases cited was the placenta saved, after the infant was born, for demonstration of bound antibody.

Monoclonal Antibodies in the Cromer System

A number of murine monoclonal antibodies have been described (8-10,58,67,72,85) that react with all red cells except those of the Inab phenotype. As expected these antibodies react less strongly with Dr(a-) than with other red cells. Whether one describes these MAb as anti-IFC or as anti-DAF depends on one's primary field of interest. Obviously use of these MAb facilitated identification (8) of the 70kD glycoprotein on which the Cromer system antigens are carried and recognition (9,10) of the fact that the glycoprotein is DAF.

Petty et al. (86) used a MAb to IFC/DAF in a monoclonal antibody immobilization of erythrocyte antigens (MAIEA, (90) and see Chapter 4) assay, to confirm the presence of the Cromer system antigens on DAF. As described in detail later in this chapter, the DAF molecule contains four short consensus repeat (SCR) segments. Because it was known that three of the MAb defined epitopes on different SCR (87), Petty et al. (86) used "blocking effect" in the MAIEA assay, to suggest which antigens were carried on which SCR. The results suggested that: Tc^a and Es^a are on SCR I; UMC on SCR II (but see the addendum); Dr^a on SCR III; and Cr^a, WES^a and WES^b on SCR IV or on the serine-threonine rich region between SCR IV and the PI anchor. Previous studies (48,88) had shown that: Tc^a is on SCR I, Dr^a on SCR III and Cr^a on SCR IV. In a study using transfectants expressing various DAF cDNA constructs, Telen et al. (89) showed that WES^b is on SCR 1 and not SCR IV as the blocking studies had suggested (in some instances the amino acid changes that comprise these polymorphisms are now known, see Chapter 46, the addendum).

Cromer System, DAF and Associations with Disease

As mentioned earlier in this chapter, two individuals with the Inab phenotype (5,6) and very likely a third (29) presented with abdominal disorders involving protein losing enteropathy. In the case of Inab himself (5) a hemicolectomy cured his clinical condition but did not alter the Inab phenotype of his red cells. A similar clinical condition was seen (47,48) in an individual with Dr(a-) red cells, a phenotype that involves the presence of a low level of DAF and marked depression of expression of all Cromer system antigens (see above). As described below, the absence of DAF (a complement activation regulatory protein) is compensated in many cells by the presence of other proteins that serve to control complement activation at different points in the activation pathways. It is also known (61) that DAF is present on the epithelial surface of cells of the gastrointestinal mucosa. In view of the above findings, it is tempting to speculate that in such cells, the absence of DAF is not compensated, so that the clinical condition described, results. However, such a speculative idea must also account for the 86 year-old lady, found to have the Inab phenotype when she was admitted to hospital after breaking her hip, and for her 70 year-old brother who also had the Inab phenotype, neither of whom had intestinal disorders (7). It is known in some other blood group systems (see Chapter 23) that genes can encode production of their proteins in a tissue specific manner. Thus it is possible that the two healthy individuals of the Inab phenotype (7) lacked DAF from their red cells but expressed that glycoprotein on the cells of their gastric mucosa, following tissue specific gene expression. It must now be added that such a suggestion is purely speculative and is not supported (nor excluded) by any findings reported in the case. As mentioned in an earlier section, a deliberate search (56) among patients with Crohn's disease and similar gastrointestinal disorders, failed to reveal any patient with the Inab phenotype.

As stated many times in this chapter, the Cromer system antigens are carried on DAF that is one of a number of glycoproteins attached to red (and sometimes other) cells via a phosphatidylinositol (PI) anchor (62-66). Red cells of the Inab phenotype lack DAF but express other PI-linked proteins normally (67,68,111). PNH III red cells (the complement sensitive population of red cells from patients with paroxysmal nocturnal hemoglobinuria) lack DAF and all other PI-linked proteins (59,65,66,69,111). In other words, the Inab phenotype results from the homozygous presence of a gene that fails to encode production of DAF. The clinical condition of PNH involves mutation in the *PIG-A* gene that normally encodes production of the phosphatidylinositol anchor (70).

As also stated above, the lack of DAF does not seriously compromise red cells in terms of susceptibility to complement-induced lysis. DAF serves as a complement regulatory protein in several ways (see Chapter 6). It interferes with the assembly of C3 and C5 convertases of the classical and alternative pathways and hastens their dissociation. When it was shown (59,71) that PNH red cells lack DAF, it was supposed that lack of that regulatory protein explained the sensitivity of the red cells to complement induced lysis. However, the limited role of DAF in the regulation of complement activation became clear when it was shown (67,72) that red cells of the Inab phenotype are only slightly more sensitive than normal red cells, to complement induced lysis. It is now appreciated (59,72-76) that lack of other proteins that serve as regulators of complement activation, explains the sensitivity of PNH red cells to complement induced lysis.

Well after the role of DAF as a complement activation regulatory protein was recognized, it was found (107) that DAF (CD55) also serves as a ligand for CD97, an activation-induced antigen on leukocytes (108-110). In view of the now recognized limited activity of DAF in the down regulation of activated complement, it is tempting to speculate that the glycoprotein has a different primary biological function. Clearly the interaction between CD97 and CD55 (DAF) has the potential to be important in cell-cell binding although the significance of the interaction is not yet known. Perhaps DAF is primarily concerned with cell adhesion and regulates C3 and C5 convertases only as a sideline.

The structure of DAF and the alterations in that protein that result in the various Cromer system phenotypes are described below. As will be seen while many of the Cromer antigens represent amino acid changes that do not affect the function of DAF, one phenotype, Dr(a-), involves both a qualitative and a quantitative alteration of

the protein (47,48,55). The Dr^a determinant also seems to be the receptor for the binding of some strains of *Escherichi coli* that are capable of causing urinary tract infections (77,99-103). The strains of *E. coli* involved bound to all except Dr(a-) and Inab (Cr$_{null}$) phenotype red cells; the Dr^a receptor is present on kidney cells. DAF is also the binding site for a variety of *Echoviruses* or *Picornaviridae* including *Echovirus 6, 7, 12, 13, 21, 29* and *33, Coxsackie* virus *A21, B1, B3* and *B5, Enterovirus 70* and *EV 7* (98,104-106,119).

The *Cromer* Locus in on Chromosome 1

The gene encoding production of DAF and hence the genes effecting the polymorphism recognized as the Cromer blood group system, is/are part of the cluster of genes known as the regulator of complement activation (*RCA*) linkage group. The *RCA* linkage group has been localized to the long arm of chromosome 1 at 1q32 (78-84).

Cromer Blood Group Antigens Are Carried on Decay-accelerating Factor (DAF, syn. CD55)

Identification of the molecule responsible for the Cromer blood group antigens was achieved through a project designed to identify and characterize red cell surface proteins using rodent monoclonal antibodies. When a series of murine monoclonal antibodies raised against intact red cells were screened for reactivity with a panel of rare red cell phenotypes, two were found which failed to react with cells of the Inab phenotype (8). Red cells of the rare Inab phenotype are characterized by lack of all Cromer blood group antigens (5). When these antibodies were used in immunoblotting experiments with the electrophoretically separated membrane components of normal red cells, a single band of apparent molecular weight 70,000 was observed if the experiments were carried out under non-reducing conditions. No bands were observed under reducing conditions (8). When membranes from red cells of the Inab phenotype were similarly treated no bands were observed under reducing or non-reducing conditions. Further studies showed that the 70kd band was present on membranes from trypsin-treated red cells but not on those from chymotrypsin-treated red cells and that the band showed a reduced apparent molecular weight in membranes from sialidase-treated red cells. When membranes from individuals with Tn syndrome (see Chapter 42) were studied a weak band of 70kd was observed together with an additional diffuse band of 50-55kd. Red cells from individuals with Tn syndrome frequently contain two populations of cells, one apparently normal and the other expressing the Tn antigen and so these results suggested that the lower diffuse band was representative of the Tn-affected component. Additional immunoblotting studies showed that human antibodies to Cr[a], Tc[a], Dr[a] and IFC also bound to a 70kd component under non-reducing conditions. Taken together these results indicated that the Cromer antigens are carried on a protein whose structure is maintained by one or more disulphide bonds and that contains a substantial content of O-glycans.

At the beginning of September 1987 a conference on complement attended by Tony Merry from the International Blood Group Reference Laboratory, was held in Chamonix, France where the structure of decay-accelerating factor (DAF) was reported. Tony noticed the similarity between the Cromer blood group protein described above and the structure of DAF. Immediately after the complement conference one of us (DJA) presented the work on identification of the Cromer blood group glycoprotein described above at the First Workshop on Monoclonal Antibodies to Red Cell Antigens held in Paris. Marilyn Telen was in the audience and also noticed the similarity between the Cromer glycoprotein and DAF. Proof that the two proteins were one and the same was obtained and reported independently by these workers and their colleagues in 1988 (9,10). These studies showed that: purified DAF reacted with monoclonal antibodies to Cromer glycoprotein and with antibodies to the Cromer antigens Cr[a] and Tc[a]; that anti-DAF failed to react with red cells of the Inab phenotype and that red cells from patients with paroxysmal nocturnal hemoglobinuria (PNH), which have a gross deficiency of DAF, are also deficient in Cromer glycoprotein. The study of Cromer thereafter became the study of DAF. DAF, at that time, was already a very well characterized and extensively studied molecule (see below). Nevertheless, the recognition that DAF carried Cromer antigens made an important contribution to the understanding of the biological importance of DAF because it drew attention to the Inab phenotype which was ipso facto a DAF-deficient phenotype and therefore an extremely valuable resource for obtaining information about the function of DAF (see below).

The Structure of Decay-accelerating Factor (DAF, syn. CD55)

The presence of a substance on human red cells which could inhibit complement-mediated lysis of antibody-coated sheep red cells was described by Hoffman (112). This substance was purified and shown to be a glycoprotein of 70kd by Nicholson-Weller et al. (113,114). The term decay accelerating factor derives from the protein's property of accelerating the decay of the complement component C3 convertase. DAF cDNAs were obtained in the conventional way. Synthetic oligonucleotide probes based on the amino terminal sequence of the purified protein were used to screen cDNA libraries constructed with mRNA from either the HeLa epithelial cell line or the HL-60 promyelocytic leukemia cell line (80,115). The amino acid sequence deduced from the isolated cDNAs predicts a protein of 381 amino acids including a signal peptide of 34 residues. At the amino terminus of the mature protein there are four units of 60 amino acids (short consensus repeats, SCRs). Each SCR contains four cysteine residues, a property consistent with two intrachain disulphide bonds in each SCR. Domains homologous to these SCRs are found in several other proteins involved in the regulation of complement components including CR1 which carries antigens of the Knops blood group system (see Chapter 28). The four SCRs are followed by a region of 76 amino acids which is rich in serine and threonine residues and ends with a hydrophobic stretch of 24 residues which is postranslationally cleaved and replaced by a glycosyl phosphatidyl inositol (GPI) tail which forms the membrane anchor (see figure 24-1). The presence of a GPI anchor was first shown by Davitz et al. (116) who reported that DAF could be released from peripheral blood cells by treatment with an enzyme (phosphatidylinositol-specific phospholipase C, PI-PLC) which cleaves such anchors.

DAF is extensively glycosylated, there is a single N-glycan of approximately 3kd between SCR1 and SCR2 and numerous O-glycans in the serine/threonine-rich region proximal to the lipid bilayer. Treatment of DAF with endo-alpha-N-acetylgalactosaminidase reduces the apparent Mr by approximately 26,000 (64). The presence of O-glycans is consistent with the observation that red cells from individuals with Tn syndrome have DAF of lower Mr than normal red cells (8).

Organization of the Cromer Blood Group (*DAF*) Gene

The organization of the *DAF* gene was determined by Post et al. (117), it spans approximately 40kb and comprises 11 exons. The first exon encodes the 5' untranslated region and the signal peptide. SCRs 1, 2 and 4 are encoded by single exons while SCR3 is encoded by two exons (4 and 5). The serine/threonine-rich domain is encoded by exons 7, 8 and 9. Exon 10 encodes an *Alu* family sequence (see Chapter 15 for a discussion of *Alu* sequences) which is found in a minor class of DAF cDNA (115). The significance of the protein product of this minor cDNA is unknown. Exon 11 which encodes the

FIGURE 24-1 Structure of CD55 (Decay Accelerating Factor) and Location of Blood Group Antigens of the Cromer Blood Group System

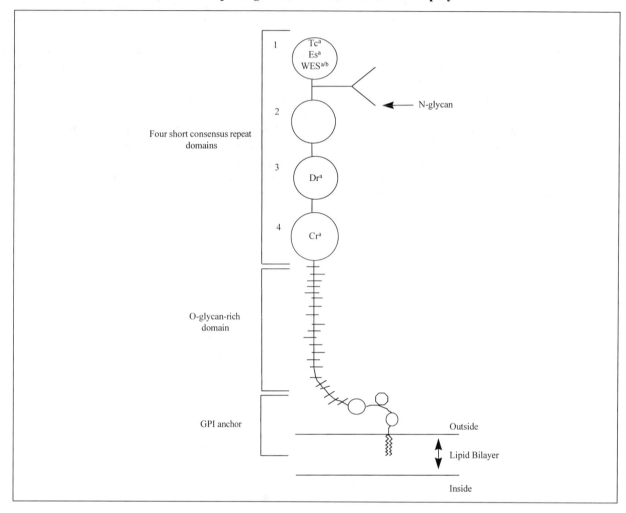

hydrophobic carboxy terminus and the 3' untranslated region is separated from exon 10 by a large intron (20kb). The *DAF* gene is located on chromosome 1q32 (78-84). Other genes which encode complement regulatory molecules are also found at this locus (*CR1, MCP, CR2, factor H, C4bp*). This group of genes is known as the regulation of complement activation (*RCA*) cluster (64).

The Molecular Basis of Cromer Blood Group Antigens

All the Cromer antigens that have been studied at the molecular level at the time of writing result from point mutations in the nucleotide sequence which result in single amino acid changes in the sequence of the protein (see figure 24-1). In the case of the antigens Tc[a]/Tc[b], Cr[a] and WES[b] the amino acid changes do not appear to be associated with any change in the level of expression of the pro-

tein. The absence of the Dr[a] antigen is very different. It results in very low levels of DAF expression. This means that the Dr(a-) phenotype usually comes to notice because of very low levels of all the high frequency Cromer system antigens. In fact the level of antigen expression is so low that the Dr(a-) phenotype is easily confused with the Inab phenotype and absorption/elution experiments may be required to make a correct interpretation.

A variety of approaches have been used to determine the molecular bases of these Cromer system antigens. One of the most powerful approaches has been to use domain-deletion mutants. Coyne et al. (87) used site-directed mutagenesis to prepare a set of mutants which lacked each of the SCRs of DAF and another mutant which lacked the serine/threonine rich region. The deletion mutants were expressed in Chinese hamster ovary (CHO) cells and used to map the epitopes recognized by 16 murine monoclonal anti-DAF. The results identified antibodies which recognized epitopes found on each of the SCRs and one which recognized an epitope in the serine/threonine-rich region of DAF. Petty et al. (86) used this information to carry out competitive binding assays (MAIEA) with monoclonal antibodies which recognized epitopes on SCR1, 2 and 3 and human antisera to Cromer antigens. In this way evidence was obtained that Tc[a] and Es[a] are located on SCR1 (only monoclonal anti-SCR1 was blocked by antibodies to these antigens), UMC was mapped to SCR2 and Dr[a] to SCR3. Antibodies to Cr[a], WES[a] and WES[b] did not block any of the antibodies tested and so could not be clearly assigned to particular regions of the protein. It was suggested that they may be on SCR4 or the serine/threonine rich region but antibodies to these regions were not used to test this hypothesis.

Nucleotide sequencing demonstrated that the Dr(a-) phenotype results from a single nucleotide substitution (C649 to T) which changes amino acid Ser165 to Leu in SCR3 (48). When anti-Cr[a] was tested with DAF-domain-deletion mutants expressed in CHO cells it reacted with all transfectants except those that lacked SCR4. Nucleotide sequencing of all the exons encoding SCR domains from an individual of the Cr(a-) phenotype revealed a single nucleotide change encoding a single amino acid change Ala193 to Pro in SCR4 (88). The validity of these data were confirmed by nucleotide sequencing the exon encoding SCR4 in two other Cr(a-) individuals and by using site-directed mutagenesis to convert Ala193 to Pro and by demonstrating that Cr[a] but not other Cromer system antigens were lost when the mutant DNA was transfected and expressed in CHO cells (88). A parallel analysis showed that anti-Tc[a] failed to react with domain-deletion mutants lacking SCR1 and that the Tc[a] antigen is lost as a result of a single nucleotide change which converts the codon Arg18 to a codon for Leu. When the WES[b] antigen was studied using the same approach the loss of the antigen in WES(b-) cells could be located to SCR1 (89). Since anti-WES[b] did not inhibit the binding of a monoclonal antibody to SCR1 whereas anti-Tc[a] did (86) it can be inferred that the mutation which gives rise to the WES[b] antigen is spatially distinct from that which defines Tc[a] on the three dimensional structure of this domain.

The Molecular Basis of DAF Deficiency in the Dr(a-) Phenotype

As discussed above, the Dr(a-) phenotype results (48) from a single nucleotide substitution which changes Ser165 to Leu but unlike single nucleotide changes responsible for other Cromer antigens examined to date the level of expression of DAF in the Dr(a-) phenotype is dramatically reduced. The explanation for this weak level of expression came in an unpredictable way. Reid et al. (46) reported a study of a patient, KZ, who was thought to have the Inab phenotype. Northern blots of mRNA from a lymphoblastoid cell line derived from the patient showed a dramatic reduction in the level of DAF mRNA in comparison with controls. KZ cDNA was prepared and when the PCR was performed in the presence of DAF specific primers a product of 247bp was obtained compared with a product of 291bp from control cDNA. The difference in size between the two products was shown to result from a 44bp deletion in KZ spanning nucleotides 644-687 of the normal product. The 44bp deletion changed the reading frame and would result in a termination codon six amino acids after the deletion. The resultant protein would lack a hydrophobic domain and it is therefore very unlikely that it could be posttranslationally modified so that the GPI membrane anchor could be added. The authors concluded that any translated product was likely to be secreted from the cell rather than become membrane-bound.

Since the defect in KZ involved a deletion of the region of the DAF cDNA that contains the single nucleotide which accounts for the Dr(a-) phenotype, the red cells of KZ were re-examined to see if any DAF expression could be found (47). When immunoblots of membranes from KZ red cells were carried out using a pool of monoclonal antibodies against the first three SCRs of normal DAF a faint band of Mr 70,000 could be demonstrated. Rigorous serological analysis also revealed evidence for very low levels of DAF expression. Furthermore, the antibody present in the serum of KZ reacted by flow cytometry with CHO cells expressing Dr(a+) but not those expressing Dr(a-) DAF. These results suggested that KZ was in fact Dr(a-) and not of the Inab phenotype but did not explain why cDNA from KZ contained a 44bp deletion while the Dr(a-) phenotype had previously been ascribed to a single nucleotide and resultant amino acid change in exon 5. PCR amplification of KZ cDNA was repeated using 35 cycles instead of the 30 cycles used in the previous study. Under these conditions the 247bp product was again obtained but an additional product of 291bp was also obtained. The fact that the 291bp product was not obtained with 30 cycles suggests that this mRNA is of low abundance compared with that giving rise to the 247bp product that was demonstrated. When the 291bp product amplified from KZ cDNA was sequenced it was found to contain a single nucleotide sequence change from wild type cDNA and this single change was identical to that found in the Dr(a-) phenotype (47). It follows from these studies that the single nucleotide change in exon 5 responsible for the Dr(a-) phenotype gives rise to two mRNAs, one of low abundance which differs from normal DAF by a single nucleotide and is expressed in the red cell membrane at low levels and another of higher abundance which contains a 44bp deletion and is not expressed on the red cell membrane. The most probable explanation for these two products arising from a single nucleotide change is that the mutation exposes an alternative cryptic splice site in exon 5 and alternative splicing of the resultant RNA leads to a reduction in synthesis of full-length DAF and hence reduced levels of DAF in the membrane (47). As Lublin et al. (47) point out, this study is of particular interest because it demonstrates that it may be necessary to investigate the molecular basis of blood group antigens at both the cDNA level and the genomic level in order to obtain a complete understanding of the molecular mechanisms involved.

Molecular Basis of the Inab Phenotype

The serological characteristics that define the Inab phenotype are described in a previous section. In essence, the phenotype is characterized by the complete absence of DAF on the red cells and the presence of anti-IFC in the serum. Tate et al. (68) studied a lymphoblastoid cell line derived from the lymphocytes of the original Inab propositus and found a gross reduction in the level of DAF mRNA in the absence of gross alterations in the DAF gene (as determined by Southern blotting). In a subsequent study (47) both mRNA and genomic DNA were extracted from this cell line and used for amplification of DAF by PCR. The entire coding region of DAF was sequenced from cDNA and from the gene. In the latter case the entire exons and at least 50bp of the surrounding introns were analyzed. The results revealed a single nucleotide change in exon 2 (G314 to A) which resulted in the conversion of Trp53 to a stop codon (47). This mutation prevents synthesis of DAF and explains the lack of expression of DAF in the membranes of this individual with the Inab phenotype. Lublin et al. (47) confirmed that this individual had the same mutation on both DAF alleles by exploiting the creation of a *Bcl* I restriction endonuclease site by the mutation and showing total cleavage of Inab DNA. Since the mutation is in the DAF gene itself these results mean that DAF cannot be expressed on any cells or tissues in this individual and that therefore lack of DAF is not incompatible with life. Uchikawa et al. (118) described another Japanese individual with the Inab phenotype. RFLP analysis suggested that the molecular mechanism giving rise to DAF deficiency in this individual is not the same as in the case studied by Lublin et al. (47).

References

1. McCormick EE, Francis BJ, Gelb AG. (abstract). Transfusion 1965;5:369 and supplemented by data presented but not included in the abstract
2. Lewis M, Chown B, Kaita H, et al. Transfusion 1967;7:440
3. Chown B, Lewis M, Kaita H, et al. Vox Sang 1968;15:264
4. Stroup M, McCreary J. (abstract). Transfusion 1975;15:522 and supplemented by data presented but not included in the abstract
5. Daniels GL, Tohyama H, Uchikawa M. Transfusion 1982;22:362
6. Walthers L, Salem M, Tessel J, et al. (abstract). Transfusion 1983;23:423
7. Lin RC, Herman J, Henry L, et al. Transfusion 1988;28:427
8. Spring FA, Judson PA, Daniels GL, et al. Immunology 1987;62:307
9. Telen MJ, Hall SE, Green AM, et al. J Exp Med 1988;167:93
10. Parsons SF, Spring FA, Merry AH, et al. (abstract). Book of Abstracts, 20th Cong ISBT, 1988:116
11. Laird-Fryer B, Dukes C, Walker EM Jr, et al. (abstract). Transfusion 1980;20:631
12. Gorman MI, Glidden HM, Behzad O. (Letter). Transfusion 1981;21:579
13. Laird-Fryer B, Dukes CV, Lawson J, et al. Transfusion 1983;23:124
14. Block U, Lacey P, Moulds J, et al. (abstract). Transfusion 1982;22:413
15. Lacey PA, Block UT, Laird-Fryer BJ, et al. Transfusion 1985;25:373
16. Law J, Judge A, Covert P, et al. (abstract). Transfusion 1982;22:413
17. Lewis M, Anstee DJ, Bird GWG, et al. Vox Sang 1991;61:158
18. Lewis M, Kaita H, Philipps S, et al. Vox Sang 1989;57:210
19. Levene C, Harel N, Lavie G, et al. Transfusion 1984;24:13
20. Tregallas WM. (abstract). Book of Abstracts, 18th Cong ISBT, 1984:163
21. Daniels G, Walthers L. (Letter). Transfusion 1986;26:117
22. Sistonen P, Nevanlinna HR, Virtaranta-Knowles K, et al. Vox Sang 1987;52:111
23. Daniels GL, Green CA, Darr FW, et al. Vox Sang 1987;53:235
24. Daniels GL, Okubo Y, Yamaguchi H, et al. Transfusion 1989;29:794
25. Issitt PD. Applied Blood Group Serology, 3rd Ed. Miami:Montgomery, 1985:402
26. Lewis M, Anstee DJ, Bird GWG, et al. Vox Sang 1990;58:152
27. Winkler MM, Hamilton JR. (abstract). Book of Abstracts, Joint Cong ISBT/AABB 1990:158
28. Copeland TR, Smith JH, Wheeling RM, et al. Immunohematology 1991;7:76
29. Daniels GL. PhD Thesis, Univ London, 1980
30. Smith KJ, Coonce LS, South SF, et al. Transfusion 1983;23:167
31. Ross DG, McCall L. (Letter). Transfusion 1985;25:84
32. Reid ME, Ellisor SS, Dean WD. Transfusion 1985;25:172
33. McSwain B, Robins C. (Letter). Transfusion 1988;28:289
34. Leatherbarrow MB, Ellisor SS, Collins PA, et al. Immunohematology 1988;4:71
35. Judd WJ, Steiner EA, Miske V. (Letter). Transfusion 1991;31:286
36. Whitsett CF, Oxendine SM. (Letter). Transfusion 1991;31:782
37. Chapman RL, Hare V, Oglesby SL. (abstract). Transfusion 1992;32 (Suppl 8S):23S
38. Daniels G. Vox Sang 1989;56:205
39. Daniels G. Immunohematology 1992;8:53
40. Jenkins DE, Moore WH. Transfusion 1977;17:110
41. Bell JA, Johnson ST, Moulds M, et al. (abstract). Transfusion

1989;29 (Suppl 7S):17S

42. Anderson G, Gray LS, Mintz PD. Am J Clin Pathol 1991;95:87
43. Udani MN, Anderson N, Rao N, et al. Immunohematology 1995;11:1
44. Levene C, Harel N, Kende G, et al. Transfusion 1987;27:64
45. Levene C, Kaufman S. Unpublished observations 1987 cited in Daniels G. Human Blood Groups. Oxford:Blackwell, 1995:568
46. Reid ME, Mallinson G, Sim RB, et al. Blood 1991;78:3291
47. Lublin DM, Mallinson G, Poole J, et al. Blood 1994;84:1276
48. Lublin DM, Thompson ES, Green AM, et al. J Clin Invest 1991;87:1945
49. Daniels G. (Letter). Transfusion 1992;32:492
50. Roitt I. Essential Immunology, 7th Ed. Oxford:Blackwell, 1991:65
51. Lewis M, McAlpine PJ. (Letter). Transfusion 1993;33:182
52. Shows TB, McAlpine PJ, Boucheix C, et al. Cytogenet Cell Genet 1987;46:11
53. Lublin DM, Telen MJ. (Letter). Transfusion 1992;32:493
54. Lublin DM, Telen MJ. (Letter). Transfusion 1993;33:182
55. Daniels G, Levene C. Vox Sang 1990;59:127
56. Daniels GL, Levi AJ. Unpublished observations 1984 cited in Daniels G. Human Blood Groups. Oxford:Blackwell, 1995:571
57. Daniels G. (abstract). Transfusion 1983;23:410
58. Ojcius DM, Jiang S, Young JD-E. Immunol Today 1990;11:47
59. Rosse WF. In: Clinical and Basic Science Aspects of Immunohematology. Arlington, VA:Am Assoc Blood Banks, 1991:13
60. Daniels GL. Unpublished observations 1984 cited in Daniels G. Human Blood Groups. Oxford:Blackwell, 1995:572
61. Medof ME, Walter EI, Rutgers JL, et al. J Exp Med 1987;165:848
62. Low MG. Biochem J 1987;244:1
63. Low MG, Saltiel AR. Science 1988;239:268
64. Lublin DM, Atkinson JP. Ann Rev Immunol 1989;7:35
65. Telen MJ, Rosse WF. Ballière's Clin Haematol 1991;4:849
66. Rosse WF. Sem Hematol 1993;30:219
67. Telen MJ, Green AM. Blood 1989;74:437
68. Tate CG, Uchikawa M, Tanner MJA, et al. Biochem J 1989;261:489
69. Yomtovian R, Prince GM, Medof ME. Transfusion 1993;33:852
70. Takeda J, Miyata T, Kawagoe K, et al. Cell 1994;73:703
71. Nicholson-Weller A, March JP, Rosenfield SI, et al. Proc Nat Acad Sci USA 1983;80:5066
72. Merry AH, Rawlinson VI, Uchikawa M, et al. Br J Haematol 1989;73:248
73. Holguin MH, Martin CB, Bernshaw NJ, et al. J Immunol 1992;148:498
74. Taguchi R, Funahashi Y, Ikezawa H, et al. FEBS Lett 1990;261:142
75. Yamashina M, Ueda K, Kinoshita T, et al. New Eng J Med 1990;323:1184
76. Fletcher A, Bryant JA, Gardner B, et al. Immunology 1992;75:507
77. Nowicki B, Moulds J, Hull R, et al. Infect Immun 1988;56:1057
78. Holers VM, Cole JL, Lublin DM, et al. Immunol Today 1985;6:188
79. Reid KBM, Bentley DR, Campbell RD, et al. Immunol Today 1986;7:230
80. Medof ME, Lublin DM, Holers VM, et al. Proc Nat Acad Sci USA 1987;84:2007

81. Lublin DM, Lemons RS, Le Beau MM, et al. J Exp Med 1987;165:1731
82. Rey-Campos J, Rubinstein P, de Cordoba SR. J Exp Med 1987;166:246
83. Rey-Campos J, Rubinstein P, de Cordoba SR. J Exp Med 1988;167:664
84. Carroll MC, Alicot EM, Katzman PJ, et al. J Exp Med 1988;167:1271
85. Daniels GL, Knowles R. Unpublished observations 1983 cited in Daniels G. Human Blood Groups. Oxford:Blackwell, 1995:571
86. Petty AC, Daniels GL, Anstee DJ, et al. Vox Sang 1993;65:309
87. Coyne KE, Hall SE, Thompson ES, et al. J Immunol 1992;149:2906
88. Telen MJ, Rao N, Udani M, et al. Blood 1994;84:3205
89. Telen MJ, Rao N, Lublin DM. (Letter). Transfusion 1995;35:278
90. Petty AC. J Immunol Meth 1993;161:95
91. Sacks DA, Garratty G. Am J Obstet Gynecol 1989;161:928
92. Dickson AC, Guest C, Jordan M, et al. Immunohematology 1995;11:14
93. Reid ME, Chandrasekaren V, Sausais L, et al. Vox Sang 1996;71:48
94. Holmes CH, Simpson KL, Wainwright SD, et al. J Immunol 1990;144:3099
95. Holmes CH, Simpson KL, Okada H, et al. Eur J Immunol 1992;22:1579
96. Storry JR. In: Blood Groups: Ch/Rg, Kn/McC/Yk, Cromer. Bethesda:Am Assoc Blood Banks, 1992:31
97. Poole J, Banks J, Jones J, et al. (abstract). Transf Med 1996;6 (Suppl 2):20
98. Bergelson JM, Mohanty JG, Crowell RL, et al. J Virol 1995;69:1903
99. Nowicki B, Truong L, Moulds J, et al. Am J Clin Pathol 1988;133:1
100. Nowicki B, Hull R, Moulds J. New Eng J Med 1988;319:1289
101. Nowicki B, Labigne A, Moseley S, et al. Infect Immun 1990;58:279
102. Nowicki B, Hart A, Coyne KE, et al. J Exp Med 1993;178:2115
103. Pham T, Kaul A, Hart A, et al. Infect Immun 1995;63:1163
104. Bergelson JM, Chan M, Solomon KR, et al. Proc Nat Acad Sci USA 1994;91:6245
105. Ward T, Pipkin PA, Clarkson NA, et al. EMBO J 1994;13:5070
106. Ward T. (abstract). Transf Med 1996;6 (Suppl 2):53
107. Hamman J, Vogel B, Schijndel GMW van, et al. J Exp Med 1996;184:1185
108. Hamman J, Eichler W, Hamman D, et al. J Immunol 1995;155:1942
109. Baud V, Chissoe SL, Viegas-Pequignot E, et al. Genomics 1995;26:334
110. Hamman J, Hartmann E, Lier RAW van. Genomics 1996;32:144
111. Telen MJ. In: Blood Groups Ch/Rg, Kn/McC/Yk, Cromer. Bethesda:Am Assoc Blood Banks, 1992:45
112. Hoffman EM. Immunochemistry 1969;6:405
113. Nicholson-Weller A, Burge J, Austen KF. J Immunol 1981;127:2035
114. Nicholson-Weller A, Burge J, Fearon DT, et al. J Immunol 1982;129:184
115. Caras IW, Davitz MA, Rhee L, et al. Nature 1987;235:545
116. Davitz MA, Low MG, Nussenzweig V. J Exp Med

1986;163:1150

117. Post TW, Arce MA, Liszewski MK, et al. Proc Nat Acad Sci
      USA 1990;144:740

118. Uchikawa M, Tsuneyama H, Wang L, et al. (abstract). Vox

Sang 1996;70 (Suppl 2):129

119. Shafren DR, Dorahy DJ, Ingram RA, et al. J Virol
      1997;71:4736

25 | The Xg Blood Group System

For more than 60 years after the ABO groups had been discovered, blood groupers searched for an antigen whose encoding gene was carried on a sex chromosome. The eagerly awaited event occurred in 1962 when Mann et al. (1) described Xg^a, an antigen encoded from a locus on the X chromosome. No antigen antithetical to Xg^a has been found so that the phenotypes are Xg(a+) and Xg(a-). The allele of Xg^a, i.e. the gene that does not make the antigen, is called Xg. In the ISBT terminology (the information does not justify a table), the system is called XG, the system number is 012, the Xg^a antigen is XG1 or, in its full code, 012001. Also in the ISBT terminology, Xg^a is $XG\ 1$, Xg is $XG\ 0$. Because the Xg locus is on the X chromosome, females (XX) can be homozygous for Xg^a or Xg (i.e. Xg^aXg^a or $XgXg$) or heterozygous for the two genes (i.e. Xg^aXg). Males (XY), on the other hand, can only be hemizygous for Xg^a or Xg, that is Xg^aY and XgY, respectively. The genotypes Xg^aXg^a, Xg^aXg and Xg^aY all result in the Xg(a+) phenotype, the genotypes $XgXg$ and XgY both lead to the Xg(a-) phenotype. Rare exceptions to these rules have been found but do not invalidate the statements above that apply to the overwhelming majority of individuals.

In 1981, Goodfellow and Tippett (2) used a monoclonal antibody, 12E7, produced following immunization of mice with cells from a human leukemia T cell line (3) to identify a quantitative polymorphism (CD99) associated with Xg^a. While all red cells carry the antigen defined, indirect antiglobulin tests and radioimmunoassays can be used to identify high expressors and low expressors of the antigen. Additional details about the antigen, its controlling genes and its relationship to Xg^a, are given below.

The Xg^a Antigen

Since females can be Xg^aXg^a or Xg^aXg and thus have Xg(a+) red cells, while all normal males with Xg(a+) red cells are genetically Xg^aY, it follows that Xg^a will be more common in women than in men. A number of studies (1,4-7) at the MRC Blood Group Unit in London were summarized by Race and Sanger (8). Samples from a total of 6784 unrelated individuals in Northern Europe had been tested. Among 3271 females, 88.7% had Xg(a+) red cells, among 3513 males the incidence of the antigen was 65.6%. In a large number of other series involving North Londoners (9), US Whites, Chinese from mainland China, Taiwan and Hakka, native

Taiwanese and US Navajo Indians (10), Canadians (11), Swiss (12), Austrians (13,14), Spaniards (15), Greeks (16), Sardinians (17), non-Ashkenazi Jews in Israel (18), US Blacks in New York and Jamaicans (19), Indians in Bombay (20), Indians, Malays and Chinese in Singapore (21,22), Thais (23), Japanese (24), Chinese in Hong Kong (25), Australian Aborigenes and Papua-New Guineans (26) the incidence of Xg^a has been seen to be relatively constant. The highest incidence of the Xg^a gene was reported (10,17,26) in New Guineans, Australian Aborigenes, Navajo Indians and Sardinians. The lowest incidence was seen (10,21,24,25) in native Taiwanese, Chinese in Singapore, Hong Kong, Taiwan and Hakka, and Malays in Singapore. While some of the differences in incidence may not be as marked as the studies suggest, since in some series the number of samples tested was relatively small, the higher incidence of the Xg(a-) phenotype in Orientals does seem to be reflected by the number of examples of anti-Xg^a found in some such population groups (see below).

Results of tests for Xg^a antigen dose are not in total agreement. Race and Sanger (8) described similar levels of Xg^a on the red cells of Xg^aY males and Xg^aXg^a females and noted that the antigen was sometimes weaker on the red cells of Xg^aXg females. Some five to 10% of females were seen to have weak expression of Xg^a, all of them were genetically Xg^aXg. Different findings were reported by Pavia et al. (27) who stated that Xg^aXg^a women have twice as much Xg^a antigen on their red cells as the amount on the red cells of their Xg^aY fathers and sons. Expected doses of Xg^a are not affected by the Lyon effect (X chromosome inactivation, see below) since the Xg^a locus is not subject to Lyonization. Szabo et al. (30) used radioimmunoassays to estimate that Xg(a+) red cells carry, on average, some 9000 available Xg^a binding sites.

The Xg^a antigen is detectable on cord blood red cells but is apparently not fully developed at birth. The antigen seems to develop fairly late in fetal life. Toivanan and Hirvonen (28) tested red cell samples from fetuses of 6 to 20 weeks gestation and found that only 19 of 54 were Xg(a+); based on the incidence of the antigen 41 Xg(a+) samples would have been expected. Other studies (6,29) have shown that cord blood red cells may react less strongly than those of adults, when tested with anti-Xg^a. It is possible (7) that some apparent upsets in the rules of X-linked inheritance represent failure to detect Xg^a on the red cells of infants. The Xg^a antigen apparently deteriorates, at least as defined by anti-Xg^a and measured in an indirect radioimmunoassay, as red cells age in vivo

(31). It was reported (30) that five to 10% of red cells from an Xg(a+) male had no detectable Xg^a antigen. We do not know if this difference in Xg^a level can be demonstrated at the serological level, using young and old red cells separated by the methods (32) that blood bankers normally use.

The Xg^a antigen is denatured or removed when red cells are treated with papain, ficin, bromelin, trypsin, chymotrypsin or pronase (24,33,34), it is not altered when red cells are treated with neuraminidase (33) or with AET (35,36).

Anti-Xg^a

The first example of anti-Xg^a was reported in 1961 (1), it was present in the serum of a man who had received many transfusions. The second example was described in print in 1963 (37), the third in 1964 (38), numerous other examples have been described since then (8,9,12,24,25, 34,39-43). The antibody is usually IgG in composition and has been found as both a red cell stimulated and as a non-red cell immune antibody. Even when anti-Xg^a presents as an agglutinin (8,12) it is usually made of IgG, one IAT-reactive example (9) was shown to contain IgG1 and IgG2 components. Several examples of the antibody have been shown (1,9,24,37) to activate complement, many other examples have not been tested for such ability.

Since the Xg(a-) phenotype is more common in men than in women, it would be expected that more examples of anti-Xg^a would be made by men than by women. The numbers are surprising in that the excess of males among individuals who make the antibody is greater than expected. Twelve of the first 14 examples of anti-Xg^a found were made by men (8). Similarly when Azar et al. (43) mentioned 13 examples found (44) in Japanese blood donors, they noted that 11 of them were made by men and all of five examples described by Mak et al. (25) were in males. In other words, among 32 examples of anti-Xg^a described (8,25,43,44) 28 (87.5%) were made by men although the incidence of the Xg(a-) phenotype is only 23% higher in men than in women. It is not known if the higher incidence of anti-Xg^a in males is, in any way, associated with expression of CD99. As described below, presence of CD99 represents a qualitative polymorphism. In females the Xg(a-) phenotype is always associated with low expression of CD99. However, among males with Xg(a-) red cells, some 74% are high expressors of CD99. We do not know if anyone has looked at level of expression of CD99 among males who have made anti-Xg^a.

As mentioned in the section dealing with the incidence of Xg^a in different population groups, it has been found (10,21-25) that the antigen is a little less common among Orientals than among other peoples. This seems to be par-

alleled by the large number of examples of anti-Xg^a found (25,43,44) in Chinese and Japanese people. As mentioned above, 13 examples of the antibody were found (44) in Japanese blood donors but the number tested during the time that those 13 examples were found is not given (43). Mak et al. (25) noted that of 325 bloods referred to them for antibody studies, four contained anti-Xg^a but that only one example was found in screening tests on the serum of 60,108 Hong Kong blood donors. Again this finding is a little surprising since, as mentioned above, anti-Xg^a has often been found in persons who have never been transfused or pregnant.

At the clinical level, anti-Xg^a seems to be benign in terms of the transfusion of red cells. No hemolytic transfusion reaction nor any case of HDN has ever been found that was caused by anti-Xg^a. One patient (37) with the antibody was transfused with six units of Xg(a+) blood with no ill effects (the patient was known to have made allo-anti-C and the six C-, Xg(a+) units were transfused before the presence of anti-Xg^a was established). A Black male with sickle cell disease who had formed anti-CD and anti-Xg^a was given (38) several small injections of ^{51}Cr-labeled Xg(a+) red cells. On each occasion in vivo red cell survival was normal and the strength of the anti-Xg^a being made did not increase. Azar et al. (43) described a male Japanese patient with anti-Xg^a who had a slight elevation of temperature and developed urticaria when transfused with Xg(a+) blood. The patient received Xg(a+) blood on three separate occasions (compatibility testing had been performed using a bromelin technique) but the authors found no evidence of antibody-mediated red cell destruction.

Auto-Anti-Xg^a

As far as we have been able to determine, only one example of auto-anti-Xg^a has been reported (45-47). The antibody was IgG and efficiently activated complement. It was described as causing severe hemolytic anemia in the patient (45,46). However, the patient was pregnant and when she delivered an infant with Xg(a+) red cells, the DAT on the infant's cells was positive but the infant was not anemic and had only a mild rise in bilirubin after birth (47). No information was provided regarding severity of the patient's hemolytic anemia after birth of the infant. As discussed in Chapter 37, warm antibody-induced hemolytic anemia can be markedly exacerbated during pregnancy.

Inheritance of Xg^a

On the overwhelming majority of occasions, the inheritance of Xg^a follows exactly the pattern expected of an X chromosome-borne characteristic (7,11,17, 18,24). That is to say, an X-borne paternal gene is passed to all daughters but no sons of a male who has the gene. If a female is heterozygous for the gene it will be passed to some (circa 50%) of her sons and daughters, if she is homozygous for the gene it will be passed to all her offspring. These patterns as applied to Xg^a and Xg^a are illustrated in table 25-1. Since Xg^a and *Xg* are co-dominant, Xg^a antigen will be made by all persons who have an Xg^a gene.

Exceptions to the inheritance patterns shown in table 25-1 are very rare but have been encountered. In five families (7,8,11,48,49) the matings Xg(a+) male by Xg(a-) female had produced 12 sons all of whom had Xg(a+) red cells. It was suggested (8) that these findings represented translocation of a small piece of the paternal X chromosome, including the Xg^a gene, on to the paternal Y chromosome. Since all twelve male offspring in the families had Xg(a+) red cells this seems the most logical explanation but as yet unexplained, was the finding (8) that one of the 12 males involved fathered an Xg(a-) son who must have inherited his father's Y chromosome but apparently did not get the translocated Xg^a gene. Other exceptions to the normal inheritance of the X and Y chromosomes have been seen in cases involving sex chromosome reversal (i.e. XX males and XY females) and in sex chromosome aneuploidy. Since descriptions of these complex situations are beyond the scope of this book and the understanding of at least one (PDI) of its authors, table 27-2 lists a number of conditions and gives references as to where details about the inheritance patterns can be found. Readers wishing to consult reviews about the invaluable contributions made by studies on the Xg^a antigen and the quantitative polymorphism described below to the study of unusual inheritance of X and Y, are referred to the excellent descriptions of Race and Sanger (8) and of Daniels (50).

Xg^a and the Lyon Effect

In 1961, Lyon (65-68) proposed that in females, one X chromosome is inactivated early in somatic cell development so that all products of X-borne genes in successive generations of the cell line involved, are representative of genes on the non-inactivated X chromosome. Inactivation of one of the two X chromosomes is random so that products of all genes on the two X chromosomes are found at the phenotypic level. It is supposed (68-70) that the biological function of Lyonization (as the inactivation process is often called) is to prevent excess formation of the products of X-chromosome-borne genes in females (XX) as compared to males (XY). It is clear that most X-borne genes do not have homologues on the Y chromosome (e.g. the gene that makes one ask for directions). It was originally supposed that inactivation involved an entire X chromosome of the pair in females. Over the years it has become necessary to modify the original hypothesis since it has become apparent (71-77,98,99) that some loci are subject to inactivation while others are not. At the level of the blood groups, determination as to whether the locus involved is subject to Lyonization can be made by looking for two populations of red cells in women heterozygous for the encoding gene providing, of course, that the antigen involved is not made elsewhere and adsorbed on to the red cells. In other words, if the Xg^a gene was subject to Lyonization and since inactivation is random, women shown by family study to be Xg^aXg heterozygotes should have two populations of red cells if Xg^a is carried on an intrinsic membrane structure. Those red cells descended from an ancestor cell in which the chromosome carrying Xg^a had been inactivated would be Xg(a-), those descended from a precursor cell in which the chromosome carrying *Xg* had been inactivated would be Xg(a+). Fortunately it is easy to recognize Xg^aXg heterozygotes. If a woman has chil-

TABLE 25-1 To Show the Usual Inheritance of Xg^a

Genotypic Mating	Phenotypic Mating			Sons			Daughters	
	Male		Female	Phenotype	Genotype		Phenotype	Genotype
$Xg^aY \times Xg^aXg^a$	Xg(a+)	X	Xg(a+)	Xg(a+)	Xg^aY		Xg(a+)	Xg^aXg^a
$Xg^aY \times Xg^aXg$	Xg(a+)	X	Xg(a+)	Xg(a+)	Xg^aY		Xg(a+)	Xg^aXg^a
				or Xg(a-)	XgY		or	Xg^aXg
$Xg^aY \times XgXg$	Xg(a+)	X	Xg(a-)	Xg(a-)	XgY		Xg(a+)	Xg^aXg
$XgY \times Xg^aXg^a$	Xg(a-)	X	Xg(a+)	Xg(a+)	Xg^aY		Xg(a+)	Xg^aXg
$XgY \times Xg^aXg$	Xg(a-)	X	Xg(a+)	Xg(a+)	Xg^aY		Xg(a+)	Xg^aXg
				or Xg(a-)	XgY	or	Xg(a-)	$XgXg$
$XgY \times XgXg$	Xg(a-)	X	Xg(a-)	Xg(a-)	XgY		Xg(a-)	$XgXg$

TABLE 25-2 References to Conditions That Result in the Unusual Inheritance of Xg^a

Condition	References
XX Males	51-55
XY Females	53
XXX Females	53
XXXX Females	56
Klinefelter's Syndrome	
XXY	53, 57
XXXY	8, 58, 59
XXXXY	8, 60, 61
XXYY	62, 63
Turner's Syndrome	
XO and XXp-	53
45X, Males	64

dren by a male who has Xg(a-) red cells and produces some children with Xg(a+) and some with Xg(a-) cells, it follows that she must be genetically Xg^aXg. Other pairings can lead to the same conclusion, see table 25-1. When the red cells of women genetically Xg^aXg are tested, it is seen that they all carry the Xg^a antigen. In other words, the *Xg* locus is not subject to Lyonization, indeed it was the first X chromosome locus shown (72,75) to escape inactivation. The *MIC2* gene that is described in the next section also escapes inactivation (100). The situation involving the *Xg* and *MIC2* loci is quite different from that involving *Xk*, the gene that encodes production of red cell Kx protein. As described in Chapter 18, women who are carriers of *Xk^o*, the gene responsible for the McLeod phenotype in *Xk^{o}Y* males, and are thus *XkXk^o* heterozygotes, have two populations of red cells. In numerous studies (see Chapter 18 for ten references) it has been shown that one population comprises acanthocytic, Kx-negative red cells (descendants of precursors in which the chromosome carrying *Xk* was inactivated) and the other, normocytic (biconcave discs) Kx+ red cells (descendants of precursors in which the chromosome carrying *Xk^o* was inactivated). In considering inactivation of genes on the X chromosome it is important to remember that the statements made above apply to the normal X chromosome. When that chromosome is structurally abnormal, genes, including *Xg^a* that normally escape inactivation, may be inactivated (101), while others that are normally inactivated may escape that fate (102).

That Xg^a is produced solely by red cells of the bone marrow (and is thus not adsorbed on to red cells like Le^a, Le^b (see Chapter 9) and Ch and Rg (see Chapter 27)) is also clear. Some natural chimeras, who have bone marrow

derived from two different individuals, have been shown (8,78,79) to have Xg(a+) and Xg(a-) red cells in their circulation. Further, bone marrow transplantation has been shown (80) to convert an Xg(a-) individual to Xg(a+).

The Monoclonal Antibody 12E7, the Antigen CD99, and the *Yg* and *MIC2* Loci

In 1979, Levy et al. (3) described a monoclonal antibody, 12E7, produced following the immunization of mice with leukocytes from a patient with T cell leukemia. The antigen defined, that is known as CD99, was shown (81) to be present on all tissue cells tested. On all except red cells, CD99 is expressed at the same level. On red cells there is a quantitative polymorphism of CD99 (2,82), both indirect antiglobulin tests and radioimmunoassay can be used to divide humans into high expressors and low expressors of CD99. Goodfellow and Tippett (2) showed that the quantitative polymorphism of CD99 is directly related to the presence or absence of Xg^a. All Xg(a+) females (whether genetically Xg^aXg^a or Xg^aXg) are high expressors of CD99. Xg(a-) females, i.e. genetically $XgXg$, are low expressors of CD99. In males, all Xg(a+) individuals were found to be high expressors of CD99. Among Xg(a-) males, some 74% were high expressors and some 26% low expressors of CD99 (82). To explain these observations (actually the explanation was advanced before all the observations were made) Goodfellow and Tippett (2) suggested that a number of different genes are involved. One gene, now known as *MIC2*, encodes production of CD99. In all individuals with *Xg^a*, the product of *MIC2*, CD99 is expressed in high levels on red cells (the Xg^aXg^a and Xg^aXg females and Xg^aY males, mentioned above). In males with no *Xg^a* gene (i.e. Xg(a-) red cells) the presence of *Yg^a* on the Y chromosome results in high expression of CD99, the presence of *Yg*, the allele of *Yg^a*, results (in *XgYg* males) in low expression of CD99. All females with Xg(a-) red cells are low expressors of CD99 because they lack *Xg^a* (i.e. genetically *XgXg*) and cannot have *Yg^a* because they have no Y chromosome. In considering this concept it is important to remember that *MIC2* encodes production of CD99 that is not polymorphic on tissue cells. *Xg^a*, *Xg*, *Yg^a* and *Yg* control the level of CD99 expressed on red cells. Since this concept was first advanced (2) additional findings (84-86) have supported its general applicability although it now seems possible (83) that another X chromosome-borne gene that controls the level of red cell Xg^a and CD99, may exist.

Like Xg^a, CD99 is carried on a red cell membrane sialoglycoprotein. Again like Xg^a, the CD99 antigen is denatured or removed when red cells are treated with trypsin, chymotrypsin, papain or pronase (81,87,88).

While CD99 usually resists treatment of red cells with neuraminidase (81,87) one monoclonal anti-CD99-like did not react with sialic acid-depleted red cells (88). While there seems no doubt that Xg^a and CD99 are located on different glycoproteins (89), there is evidence (84) that those glycoproteins are associated in situ, at least in red cells. It has been estimated (87) that the red cells of high expressors of CD99 carry about 1000 copies of that antigen per red cell while those of low expressors carry only about 100 copies per cell. In contrast, the same investigators (87) reported that there are some 29,000 CD99 sites per lymphocyte and 4000 per platelet. There is some evidence (82,83) that just as *Xg^a* can occasionally be translocated on to a Y chromosome, the *Yg^a* or *Yg* gene may occasionally be translocated on to the X chromosome.

Monoclonal Antibodies and the Xg System

As mentioned several times in the previous section, monoclonal antibodies to CD99 (3,88,103) have proved invaluable in recognition of that antigen and in establishing its relationship to Xg^a. A murine monoclonal anti-Xg^a was used (in conjunction with two anti-Xg^a raised by immunizing rabbits) to identify the structural gene encoding production of Xg^a (89 and see below).

Chromosomal Assignments of the *Xg*, *Yg* and *MIC2* Loci

As will by now be apparent, a custom of this book is to finish the portion of each chapter that deals with the serology and clinical significance of the blood group system with a brief description of the chromosomal location of the blood group locus. Clearly for this chapter the earlier sections indicate that the *Xg* locus is on the X chromosome and the *Yg* locus is on the Y chromosome. Indeed, it has now been shown (89,93) that the gene originally called (94-97) *PBDX* (pseudoautosomal boundary divided on X) is the *Xg^a* gene. As mentioned above, most genes on the X chromosome do not have homologues on the Y chromosome, most genes on Y do not have homologues on X. Indeed, if the X and Y chromosomes carried the same genes there would be no differences between males and females and life would be very dull! The *MIC2* locus is an exception to the above generalizations, that is, it is present on both the X and Y chromosomes (81,84,90-92) fortunately, it does not make life dull.

The Biochemical Nature of the Xg^a Antigen

The red cell membrane molecule expressing the Xg^a antigen was first identified in 1989. Herron and Smith (34) showed that when membranes from Xg(a+) red cells were subjected to immunoblotting with human anti-Xg^a (under reducing and non-reducing conditions) two diffuse bands of Mr 22,000 - 25,000 and 26,500 - 29,000 were observed. These results were confirmed by Petty and Tippett (104) who showed that immunoprecipitates obtained with human anti-Xg^a contain the same two bands. Immunoblotting or immunoprecipitation experiments with human anti-Xg^a and Xg(a-) red cells did not reveal any reactive components (34,104).

As mentioned above, the Xg^a antigen is destroyed by treatment of Xg(a+) red cells with bromelin, papain, chymotrypsin, trypsin or pronase. The antigen is not affected by sialidase treatment, although the apparent Mr of immunoblot reactive bands is reduced by approximately 1500 (34).

Cloning the *XG* Gene

The *XG* gene is found only on the X chromosome. There are, however, genes common to both the X and Y chromosomes. These are called pseudoautosomal genes. One such pseudoautosomal gene is *MIC2*. The regulation of *MIC2* and *XG* is linked. All Xg(a+) red cells have high levels of expression of the *MIC2* gene product (CD99), while many Xg(a-) red cells express CD99 at low levels (2).

The *XG* gene maps to the most distal part of the X-specific region of the X chromosome and is adjacent to the *MIC2* gene (see figure 25-1) (105,106). Ellis et al. (97) searched the boundary region between the *MIC2* gene and the X-specific region. Genomic sequences between the 3' end of the *MIC2* gene and a CpG-rich region proximal to the pseudoautosomal/X-specific boundary (pAB1X, see figure 25-1) were used to screen a bone marrow cDNA library and a clone of 820bp with an open reading frame of 540bp encoding a 180 amino acid polypeptide was obtained. The cDNA was located using a probe derived from a genomic sequence approximately 10Kb downstream of the last exon of the *MIC2* gene. The gene encoding the 180 amino acid protein was initially called *PBDX* (pseudoautosomal-boundary divided on the X chromosome) but it was soon proved to encode Xg^a and was renamed the *XG* gene (93). Northern blotting experiments showed that the *XG* gene has a restricted tissue expression. Only fibroblasts derived from a skin biopsy of a female gave a strong signal and bands of 1.1Kb and 2.4Kb were observed. Similar experiments with mRNA from numerous cell lines (HeLa, K562, HL60, PGF, NT2, X8/672, Y162.Ile, A23N), testis and fresh bone marrow failed to give a signal. Since the *XG* cDNA was isolated from a bone marrow library it can be concluded that the gene is expressed in this tissue but at a lower level than can be detected on Northern blots. These experiments leave open the possibility that the gene is expressed at similarly low levels in a wide variety of other tissues. Subsequent experiments employing RTC-PCR to look for RNA expression gave positive signals in cultured fibroblasts, fresh bone marrow, umbilical cord blood, fetal liver, fetal spleen, fetal thymus and fetal adrenal tissue but not in other tissues or the cell lines HeLa, K562, HL60, NT2 and lymphoblastoid cell lines (93).

Confirmation that the predicted protein product of the *PBDX (XG)* gene contains the Xg^a antigen was obtained by immunological methods. A synthetic peptide corresponding to the N-terminal 13 amino acids of the predicted protein product was used to raise polyclonal (rabbit) and monoclonal (mouse) antibodies. The polyclonal antibodies and one of the mouse monoclonal antibodies (NBL-1) agglutinated Xg(a+) but not Xg(a-) red cells regardless of their CD99 phenotype. Human anti-Xg^a did not block the binding of rabbit antisera or NBL-1 to red cells suggesting that the Xg^a antigenic determinant is not located at the extreme N-terminus of the protein. Confirmation that the rabbit antisera and NBL-1, react with different epitopes from those recognized by human anti-Xg^a was obtained using competitive binding assays (modified MAIEA when rabbit antisera was used). Immunoprecipitation experiments with antibodies to the N-terminal synthetic peptide gave bands of Mr 24,000 - 29,000 kD, a pattern indistinguishable from that obtained with human anti-Xg^a (93).

As discussed above, the antibodies raised to the N-terminal synthetic peptide of Xg^a protein do not react with Xg(a-) red cells but since they do not block the binding of two human anti-Xg^a they do not recognize the Xg^a antigen. This argument holds if all anti-Xg^a sera have the same specificity. If, as seems likely, the Xg(a-) phenotype

results from lack of expression of Xg^a protein, it is possible that other human anti-Xg^a will be found which do block the binding of the rabbit antisera and NBL-1. This is because the serological specificity of any human antibody failing to react with Xg(a-) red cells will be denoted anti-Xg^a. An analogy can be drawn with the MN system where antibodies failing to react with glycophorin A deficient cells (En(a-) red cells) were called anti-En^a but subsequent studies demonstrated that anti-En^a in fact describes antibody specificities against several different antigens located throughout the extracellular domain of GPA molecules (see Chapter 15 for further discussion).

Inspection of the predicted amino acid sequence of the Xg^a protein reveals a cleavable signal peptide sequence of 21 residues and an extracellular domain of about 117 residues with the remaining residues (about 42) comprising a single membrane spanning sequence and a short cytoplasmic domain. The predicted protein lacks any signal sequence motifs for N-glycosylation (97). Serine and threonine residues number 16, of which 11 would be predicted to be extracellular. The reduction in Mr of 1500 reported for sialidase treated Xg^a protein (34) suggests that some O-glycans are present on the Xg^a protein. The normal O-glycan structure found on red cell proteins is a sialotetrasaccharide containing two sialic acid residues and having a molecular weight of approximately 1000. Since both sialic acid residues are cleaved by *Clostridium perfringens* sialidase, a reduction of 1500 suggests about 3 O-glycans per Xg^a molecule.

Immunoblotting and immunoprecipitation studies have consistently demonstrated two Xg^a-bearing bands in red cell membranes (34,93,104). It is not yet clear whether these represent two different products of the *XG* gene resulting, for example, from alternative splicing. The two bands have the same N-terminus because antisera raised to a synthetic peptide identical to the N-termi-

FIGURE 25-1 Relative Locations of *XG* and *CD99* Genes on the X Chromosome (reference 97)

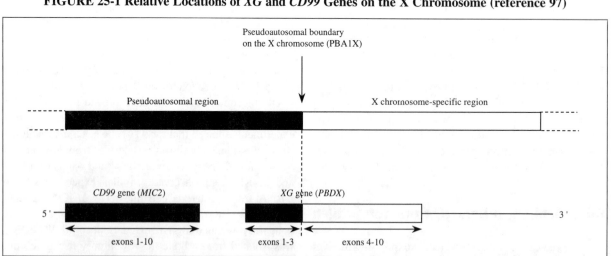

nal 13 amino acids react with both bands (93,104). The finding of two different mRNA species of 2.4Kb and 1.1Kb, respectively, in fibroblasts (97) might be consistent with alternative splicing. The 820bp cDNA clone isolated by Ellis et al. (97) is likely to correspond to the 1.1Kb mRNA species but it is not clear whether this 1.1Kb band corresponds to the 24 kD Xg^a protein or the 29 kD Xg^a protein. It seems unlikely that the 24 kD and 29 kD bands are the same protein with different glycosylation profiles since heterogeneity in glycosylation is usually reflected by diffuse staining of a single band. The occurrence of two discrete bands suggests differences in protein sequences.

Inspection of the amino acid sequence of the Xg^a protein cloned by Ellis et al. (97) reveals a number of interesting features. The extreme N-terminus is very hydrophilic and in particular, contains several aspartic acid residues. This is followed by a proline-rich segment. There are two further proline-rich segments in the sequence one of which is also preceded by an aspartic acid-rich sequence. Each of the proline-rich segments have sequences in which proline residues and basic residues (lysine (K) or arginine (R)) alternate (first proline-rich region YPKPKPPY, second region YPRPKPRPQP, third region YPPRPRPRPP). Six of the eleven potential O-glycosylation sites are found in the sequence between the last proline-rich region and the membrane spanning domain (see figure 25-2). Apart from the signal sequence (presumed to be cleaved from the mature protein) there is only one cysteine residue and this is in the predicted cytoplasmic domain of the molecule so there is no possibility of disulphide bonding involving the extracellular domain, a feature consistent with the fact that anti-Xg^a immunoblots the Xg^a proteins under reducing conditions (34). The function of the Xg^a protein molecule is not known. The occurrence of aspartic acid-rich sequences is reminiscent of members of the chemokine receptor family of which the Duffy protein is an example (see Chapter 14). The aspartic acid-rich sequences in the N-terminal region of the Duffy protein are thought to be important for chemokine binding (107). However, the Xg^a protein has only a single membrane spanning domain compared with the 7 membrane spanning domains found in proteins of the chemokine receptor family. Proline-rich sequences are known to be of considerable functional significance for signaling pathways when they occur in the cytoplasmic domains of proteins and there is extensive literature on this subject (108). One such proline-rich motif is found in the cytoplasmic domain of the Lutheran glycoprotein (see Chapter 20). Whether similar motifs occurring in extracellular domains are also involved in protein-protein interactions is unclear.

As discussed in a later section there is some evidence

that the related protein CD99 has a role in cell adhesion and a similar role for the Xg^a protein seems plausible. The alternating acidic and basic regions suggest a very simple and entirely speculative model for homotypic adhesion in which acidic regions on one molecule align with basic regions on another (see figure 25-2).

Structure of the *XG* Gene

The *XG* gene spans the boundary between the pseudoautosomal region and the X-specific region of the X chromosome. Exons 1-3 are located in the pseudoautosomal region and exons 4-10 in the X-specific region (97, see figure 25-1). The locations of exons 1-3 and 4-10 respectively were determined by Southern blotting. Genomic DNA from human lymphoblastoid cell lines from males and females and from somatic cell hybrids retaining either a human X chromosome or a human Y chromosome was digested with the restriction enzyme EcoRI and probed with the Xg^a cDNA clone (97).

Relationship Between Xg^a Protein and CD99, the Product of the *MIC2* Gene

CD99 was first identified using a murine monoclonal antibody (denoted 12E7) raised to human leukemia T cells (3). The epitope recognized by 12E7 has a wide tissue distribution being expressed on almost all human tissues (spermatozoa and granulocytes are exceptions (85,87,103)). Studies with human-rodent somatic cell hybrids demonstrated that the 12E7 epitope is only expressed by hybrids containing either the human X or the human Y chromosome (103). The genes encoding the 12E7 epitope were denoted *MIC2X* (X chromosome) and *MIC2Y* (Y chromosome) respectively. *MIC2X* and *MIC2Y* were subsequently shown to be identical (92).

Immunoblotting studies with 12E7 identified a component of Mr 32,500 in red cell membranes. Full length cDNA corresponding to the *MIC2* gene product predicts a protein of 184 amino acids which contains a cleavable signal sequence, has its N-terminus extracellular, contains a single membrane spanning domain and a cytoplasmic carboxy terminus. The predicted molecule lacks the signal motif for N-glycosylation but contains several serine/threonine residues which could be used as sites of O-glycan attachment. The *MIC2* gene comprises 10 exons (see figure 25-1). As discussed in the preceding section, a phenotypic relationship between the Xg^a antigen and 12E7 epitope expression on red cells described by Goodfellow and Tippett (2) led Ellis et al. (97) to look for the *XG* gene downstream of the *MIC2* gene. Comparison of the predicted amino acid sequences of the 12E7 protein

FIGURE 25-2 Structural Similarities Between the Xg^a and CD99 Protein

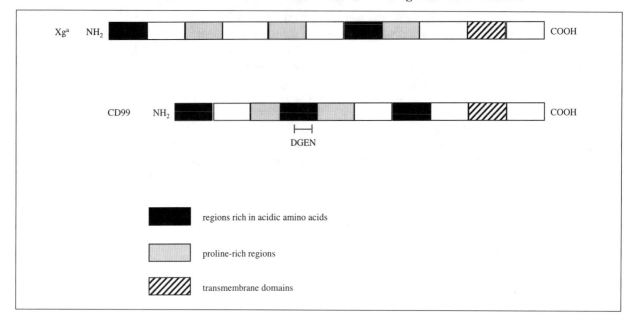

and Xg^a protein demonstrates that the proteins are homologous. When the sequences of 12E7 (CD99) and Xg^a proteins are aligned there is substantial homology between the extracellular and transmembrane domains of the mature proteins (48% when conservative amino acid changes are included, 37% when only identical amino acids are counted). Certain segments of the two proteins have higher homology. Both proteins have an N-terminal sequence rich in acidic amino acids followed by a proline-rich region containing basic amino acids (62% homology over 26 amino acids if conservative amino acid differences are included). 12E7 has a second region rich in acidic residues not found in the Xg^a protein followed by a proline-rich region and another acidic residues-rich region which shows 63% homology over 27 residues (conservative changes included). 12E7 lacks the third proline-rich region found in Xg^a but has 69% homology over the transmembrane domains and the region of 12E7 corresponding to the small cytoplasmic domain of Xg^a. The alignment of 12E7 and Xg^a is depicted in figure 25-2. CD99, like Xg^a, has eleven potential sites for O-glycosylation in its extracellular domain.

Several monoclonal antibodies to CD99 have been described, the epitope recognized by only one of these antibodies has been shown to be sialidase-sensitive (88). Banting et al. (84) showed that three monoclonal anti-CD99 recognize the peptide sequence DGEN (Asp-Gly-Glu-Asn). This sequence is located in the second region rich in acidic residues on CD99 and is not found in the Xg^a protein (see figure 25-2). Evidence that a partially purified preparation of 12E7-reactive glycoprotein isolated from Xg(a+) red cells inhibited a human anti-Xg^a suggests that the two proteins may be associated in the red cell membrane (87). More direct evidence for such an association was obtained by Petty and Tippett (104) who showed that a component of Mr 32,000 presumed to be CD99 is found in immunoprecipitates obtained with anti-Xg^a.

CD99 was first characterized with monoclonal antibody 12E7 but subsequently the same protein was described as E2-glycoprotein, a T cell surface adhesion molecule (109,110) and Hu Ly-m6 (111). Antibodies to the protein were clustered as CD99 at the Leucocyte Antigens Workshop in 1993 (112). Monoclonal antibodies to CD99 induce Mg⁺⁺-dependent homotypic aggregation of CD4⁺, CD8⁺ human thymocytes (113). At the time of writing, it is not known whether CD99 can adhere to itself and/or Xg^a proteins, through charge interactions of the type suggested above for Xg^a-Xg^a, interactions.

CD99 is a Blood Group-Active Molecule

In 1995, Uchikawa et al. (114) reported the detection of a human antibody to CD99 in 2 female, unrelated, healthy Japanese blood donors. The red cells of both donors were negative with monoclonal antibody 12E7. This is the first and at the time of writing, the only evidence that CD99 is a blood group-active molecule.

References

1. Mann JD, Cahan A, Gelb AG, et al. Lancet 1962;1:8
2. Goodfellow PN, Tippett P. Nature 1981;289:404
3. Levy R, Dilley J, Fox RI, et al. Proc Nat Acad Sci USA

1979;76:6552

4. Sanger R, Race RR, Tippett P, et al. Vox Sang 1962;7:571
5. Gavin J, Tippett P, Sanger R, et al. Vox Sang 1964;9:146
6. Noades J, Gavin J, Tippett P, et al. J Med Genet 1966;3:162
7. Sanger R, Tippett P, Gavin J. J Med Genet 1971;8:427
8. Race RR, Sanger R. Blood Groups in Man, 6th Ed. Oxford:Blackwell, 1975
9. Devenish A, Burslem MF, Morris R, et al. Transfusion 1986;26:426
10. Dewey WJ, Mann JD. J Med Genet 1967;4:12
11. Chown B, Lewis M, Kaita H. Canad J Genet Cytol 1964;6:431
12. Metaxas MN, Metaxas-Bühler M. Vox Sang 1970;19:527
13. Mayr WR. Schweiz Med Wschr 1969;99:1837
14. Herbich J, Meinhart K, Szilvassy J. Artzl Lab 1972;18:341
15. Valls A. Trab Inst Bernardino Sahagun Antrop Etnol 1973;16:261
16. Fraser GR, Steinberg AG, Defaranas B, et al. Am J Hum Genet 1969;21:46
17. Siniscalco M, Filippi G, Latte B, et al. Ann Hum Genet 1966;29:231
18. Adam A, Tippett P, Gavin J, et al. Ann Hum Genet 1967;30:211
19. Gavin J, Tippett P, Sanger R, et al. Nature 1963;200:82
20. Bhatia HM. Ind J Med Sci 1963;17:491
21. Saha N, Banerjee B. Vox Sang 1973;24:542
22. Boon WH, Noades J, Gavin J, et al. Nature 1964;204:1002
23. Rantanaubol K, Ratanasirivanich P. Nature 1971;229:430
24. Nakajima H, Murata S, Seno T. Transfusion 1979;19:480
25. Mak KH, Chua KM, Leong S, et al. (Letter). Transfusion 1993;33:443
26. Simmons RT. Nature 1970;227:1363
27. Pavia A, Rinaldi A, Melis A, et al. Cytogenet Cell Genet 1982;32:307
28. Toivanen P, Hirvonen T. Vox Sang 1973;24:372
29. Toivanen P, Hirvonen T. Scand J Haematol 1969;6:49
30. Szabo P, Campana T, Siniscalco M. Biochem Biophys Res Comm 1977;78:655
31. Campana T, Szabo P, Piomelli S, et al. Cytogenet Cell Genet 1978;22:524
32. Judd WJ. Methods in Immunohematology, 2nd Ed. Durham:Montgomery, 1994:119
33. Habibi P, Tippett P, Lebesnerais M, et al. Vox Sang 1979;36:367
34. Herron R, Smith GA. Biochem J 1989;262:369
35. Advani H, Zamor J, Judd WJ, et al. (abstract). Transfusion 1981;21:631
36. Advani H, Zamor J, Judd WJ, et al. Br J Haematol 1982;51:107
37. Cook IA, Polley MJ, Mollison PL. Lancet 1963;1:857
38. Sausais L, Krevans JR, Townes AS. (abstract). Transfusion 1964;4:312
39. Fisher N. Unpublished observations 1965 cited in Race RR, Sanger R. Blood Groups in Man, 6th Ed. Oxford:Blackwell, 1975
40. Allen FH Jr. Unpublished observations 1967 cited in Race RR, Sanger R. Blood Groups in Man, 6th Ed. Oxford:Blackwell, 1975
41. Shepherd LP, Feingold E, Shanbrom E. Vox Sang 1969;16:157
42. Konugres AA. Unpublished observations 1974 cited in Race RR, Sanger R. Blood Groups in Man, 6th Ed. Oxford:Blackwell, 1975
43. Azar PM, Saji H, Yamanaka R, et al. Transfusion 1982;22:340
44. Muramata S. Unpublished observations 1980 cited in Azar PM, Saji H, Yamanaka R, et al. Transfusion 1982;22:340
45. Yokoyama M, Eith DT, Bowman M. Hawaii Med J 1966;25:328
46. Yokoyama M, Eith DT, Bowman M. Vox Sang 1967;12:138
47. Yokoyama M, McCoy JE Jr. Vox Sang 1967;13:15
48. Sanger R, Race RR, Tippett P, et al. Lancet 1964;1:955
49. Tippett P. In: Human Genetics 1984: A Look at the Last Ten Years - and the Next Ten. Arlington, VA:Am Assoc Blood Banks, 1985:1
50. Daniels G. Human Blood Groups. Oxford:Blackwell, 1995:473
51. Ferguson-Smith MA. Lancet 1966;2:475
52. Sanger R, Tippett P, Gavin J. J Med Genet 1971;8:417
53. Sanger R, Tippett P, Gavin J, et al. J Med Genet 1977;14:210
54. Evans HJ, Buckton KE, Spowart G, et al. Hum Genet 1979;49:11
55. de la Chapelle A, Tippett PA, Wetterstrand G, et al. Nature 1984;307:170
56. de Grouchy J, Brissaud HE, Richardet JM, et al. Ann Génét 1968;11:120
57. Jacobs PA, Hassold TJ, Whittington E, et al. Ann Hum Genet 1988;52:93
58. Greenstein RM, Harris DJ, Luzzatti L, et al. Pediatrics 1970;45:677
59. Pfeiffer RA, Sanger R. J Med Genet 1973;10:142
60. Lewis FJW, Frøland A, Sanger R, et al. Lancet 1964;2:589
61. Murken J-D, Scholz W. Blut 1968;16:164
62. de la Chapelle A, Hortling H, Sanger R, et al. Cytogenetics 1964;3:334
63. Pfeiffer RA, Körver G, Sanger R, et al. Lancet 1966;1:1427
64. de la Chapelle A, Page DC, Brown L, et al. Am J Hum Genet 1986;38:330
65. Lyon MF. Nature 1961;190:372
66. Lyon MF. Lancet 1961;2:434
67. Lyon MF. Am J Hum Genet 1962;14:135
68. Lyon MF. Biol Rev 1972;47:1
69. Grant SG, Chapman VM. Ann Rev Genet 1988;22:199
70. Lyon MF. Prog Nucl Acid Res Mol Biol 1989;36:119
71. Gorman JG, di Re J, Treacy AM, et al. J Clin Lab Med 1963;61:642
72. Lawler SD, Sanger R. Lancet 1970;1:584
73. Fialkow PJ, Lisker R, Giblett ER, et al. Nature 1970;226:337
74. Fialkow PJ. Am J Hum Genet 1970;22:460
75. Race RR. Proc 4th Int Cong Hum Genet 1971:311
76. Davies K. Nature 1991;349:15
77. Brown CJ, Lafreniere RG, Powers VE, et al. Natue 1991;349:82
78. Klinger R, Miggiano VC, Tippett P, et al. Atti Acad Med Lomb 1968;23;1392
79. Ducos J, Marty Y, Sanger R, et al. Lancet 1971;2:219
80. Sparkes RS, Crist M, Sparkes MC. Vox Sang 1984;46:119
81. Goodfellow P. Differentiation 1983;23 (suppl):S35
82. Tippett P, Shaw M-A, Green CA, et al. Ann Hum Genet 1986;50:339
83. Goodfellow PJ, Pritchard C, Tippett P, et al. Ann Hum Genet 1987;51:161
84. Banting GS, Pym B, Goodfellow PN. EMBO J 1985;4:1967
85. Goodfellow PN, Pym B, Pritchard C, et al. Phil Trans Roy Soc London (Series B) 1988;322:145
86. Banting GS, Pym B, Darling SM, et al. Mol Immunol 1989;26:181
87. Latron F, Blanchard D, Cartron J-P. Biochem J 1987;247:757
88. Daniels G, Tippett P. (abstract). In: Proc 2nd Int Workshop on Monoclonal Antibodies Against Human Red Cells and Related Antigens. Paris:Arnette, 1990:127

89. Ellis N, Reid M, Banting G, et al. (abstract). Transfusion 1994;34 (Suppl 10S):60S

90. Goodfellow P, Banting G, Sheer D, et al. Nature 1983;302:346

91. Buckle V, Mondello C, Darling S, et al. Nature 1985;317:739

92. Darling SM, Banting GS, Pym B, et al. Proc Nat Acad Sci USA 1986;83:135

93. Ellis NA, Tippett P, Petty A, et al. Nature Genet 1994;8:285

94. Goodfellow PJ, Darling SM, Thomas NS, et al. Science 1986;234:740

95. Ellis N, Goodfellow PN. Trends Genet 1989;5:406

96. Rappold GA. Hum Genet 1993;92:315

97. Ellis NA, Ye T-Z, Patton S, et al. Nature Genet 1994;6:394

98. Shapiro LJ, Mohandas T, Weiss R, et al. Science 1979;204:1224

99. Mohandas T, Sparkes RS, Hellkuhl B, et al. Proc Nat Acad Sci USA 1980;77:6759

100. Goodfellow P, Pym B, Mohandas T, et al. Am J Hum Genet 1984;36:777

101. Polani PE, Angell R, Ginannelli F, et al. Nature 1970;227:613

102. Immken L, Mohandas T, Sparkes RS, et al. Am J Hum Genet 1984;36:979

103. Goodfellow P, Banting G, Levy R, et al. Somat Cell Genet 1980;6:777

104. Petty AC, Tippett P. Vox Sang 1995;69:231

105. Ferguson-Smith MA, Sanger R, Tippett P, et al. Cytogenet Cell Genet 1982;32:273

106. Yates JR, Goudie DR, Gillard EF, et al. Genomics 1987;1:52

107. Murphy PM. Ann Rev Immunol 1994;12:593

108. Sudol M. Trends Biochem Sci 1996;21:161

109. Aubrit F, Gelin C, Pham D, et al. Eur J Immunol 1989;19:1431

110. Gelin C, Aubrit F, Phalipon A, et al. EMBO J 1989;8:3253

111. Sandrin MS, Vaughan HA, Henning MM, et al. Immunogenetics 1992;35:283

112. Schlossman SF, Bounsell L, Gilks W, et al. Blood 1993;83:879

113. Bernard G, Zoccola D, Deckert M, et al. J Immunol 1995;154:26

114. Uchikawa M, Tsuneyama H, Tadokoro K, et al. (abstract). Transfusion 1995;35 (Suppl 10S):23S

26 | The Scianna Blood Group System

In 1962, Schmidt et al. (1) described an antibody, anti-Sm, directed against a very common antigen. Studies at that time suggested that Sm was not part of any known blood group system.

In 1963, Anderson et al. (2) described an antibody, anti-Bu^a, directed against an antigen of low incidence. Studies at that time suggested that Bu^a was not part of any known blood group system.

In 1964, Lewis et al. (3) reported studies with anti-Bu^a on blood samples from the family in which Schmidt et al. (1) had found Sm- members. They found that Sm-red cells behaved as if they carried a double dose of Bu^a and that Bu^a was present, in an apparent single dose, on the red cells of some members of the family who had Sm+ red cells. In 1967, Lewis et al. (4) presented additional evidence of an antithetical relationship between Sm and Bu^a. In a very large Mennonite kindred two Sm+ Bu(a-) X Sm- Bu(a+) matings were found. All five children resulting from the matings had Sm+ Bu(a+) red cells, i.e. as expected from *SmSm* X *Bu^{a}Bu^a* matings if *Sm* and *Bu^a* are alleles. In the same kindred three matings in which both parents had Sm+ Bu(a+) red cells, had produced, among them, 21 children. Of the children, three had Sm- Bu(a+), eleven Sm+ Bu(a+) and seven Sm+ Bu(a-) red cells. In other words, three children had inherited *Bu^a* from each parent, eleven *Bu^a* from one parent and *Sm* from the other and seven had inherited *Sm* from each parent. None of the children had failed to inherit *Bu^a* and/or *Sm*. In 1974, Lewis et al. (5) presented additional data on the genetic independence of *Bu^a* and *Sm* from other blood group loci and reported that they had obtained permission from the original family in which some individuals had Sm- red cells, to use the family name. Thus the blood group system was renamed Scianna, Sm became Sc1, Bu^a became Sc2, *Sm* became *Sc^1* and *Bu^a* became *Sc^2*. Findings made before 1974 have been translated into the Sc terminology in the remainder of this chapter. The original, conventional and ISBT terminology for the Scianna system are listed in table 26-1.

In 1973, McCreary et al. (6) reported a study of a highly inbred population living on Likiep Atoll in the Marshall Islands. The study was initiated when an antibody to a high incidence antigen was found in the serum of a woman whose red cells typed as Sc:-1,-2. However, as described below, it is possible that the proposita's red cells carried a very weak expression of Sc2. Again as described below, a more straightforward case of the Sc:-1,-2 phenotype was described by Nason et al. (7) in 1980. The

TABLE 26-1 Original, Conventional and ISBT Terminology for the Scianna Blood Group System

Conventional Name: Scianna			
Conventional Symbol: Sc			
ISBT System Symbol: SC			
ISBT System Number: 013			
Historical (now obsolete) Terms	Antigen Conventional Name	ISBT Antigen Number	ISBT Full Code Number
Sm	Sc1	SC1	013001
Bu^a	Sc2	SC2	013002
	Sc3	SC3	013003

propositus in that study had red cells that would neither react with nor adsorb anti-Sc1 or anti-Sc2. He had made an antibody to a high incidence antigen. The antibody was called anti-Sc3 and was shown not be a mixture of separable anti-Sc1 and anti-Sc2. Thus it appeared that: *Sc^1* encodes production of Sc1 and Sc3; *Sc^2* encodes production of Sc2 and Sc3; and that an apparently silent allele, *Sc*, exists that encodes no production of Sc1, Sc2 or Sc3. The possible absence of other very common antigens from Sc:-1,-2,-3 red cells is discussed below.

The Sc1 and Sc2 Antigens

Sc1 is a very common antigen. In tests on some 269,000 South London blood donors, only one individual with Sc:-1 red cells was found (8). No person lacking Sc1 was found in tests on 29,737 Welsh donors (9) nor in tests on samples from 1600 donors in the USA (1). The incidence of Sc2 is rather constant if studies on comparable populations are combined. The antigen was found on the red cells of 24 of 2560 Canadians (2,3,5) for an incidence of 1 in 107 (0.93%). Included in those studies were some samples from Mennonites, three of which were Sc:2 (see the introduction of this chapter for details about Sc2 in a large Mennonite family, not included in the above figures). The Canadian studies included at least 212 Blacks, none of whom had Sc:2 red cells. The Sc2 antigen was also found on the red cells of: 48 of 6345 individuals in Oxford and London (10,11) for an incidence of 1 in 132 (0.76%); 15 of 2015 donors in Berlin (12) for an incidence of 1 in 134 (0.74%); and 7 of 2100 Czech donors (13) for an incidence of 1 in 300

(0.33%). In smaller studies, Sc2 was not found on the red cells of 100 Manitoban Indians nor those of 75 Inuit (5) nor on those of 161 Taiwanese (3). If the above figures are combined (i.e. 102 Sc:2 samples in 14,381 tested) and the Sc:-1,-2 phenotype is considered too rare significantly to alter the figures, the antigen and phenotype frequencies given in table 26-2 can be calculated.

For detection in serological tests, the Sc1 antigen survives treatment of red cells with trypsin, chymotrypsin and papain; it is weakened on red cells treated with pronase or with a mixture of trypsin and chymotrypsin (26). Both Sc1 and Sc2 are slightly weakened when red cells are treated with dithiothreitol (DTT), they are much more markedly reduced on red cells treated with 2-aminoethylisothiouronium bromide (AET) (27).

Anti-Sc1 and Anti-Sc2 and Their Clinical Significance

Alloimmune anti-Sc1 is a very rare antibody since so few individuals have Sc:-1 red cells. What little is known about the clinical significance of the antibody comes mainly from studies on auto-anti-Sc1 (see below). Anti-Sc2 is a little more common than anti-Sc1 but is still rare. The first example described (2) was apparently made as a result of blood transfusions and was optimally reactive by IAT. Seyfried et al. (10) injected 14 persons who had Sc:-2 red cells with cells that were Sc:2, four of the 14 made anti-Sc2. Mollison (14) injected D+, Sc:2 red cells into 19 volunteers of the D-, Sc:-2 phenotype. Of the eight who formed anti-D, one also made anti-Sc2. Of the 11 who did not make anti-D, none made anti-Sc2.

Anti-Sc1 and anti-Sc2 seem most often to be IgG in nature (1,8,10,14,15), they are usually best detected in IATs. Although the antibodies are often said not to bind complement, some of the findings discussed below, particularly regarding autoantibodies of the system, show that some examples do bind complement. As far as we have been able to determine, neither anti-Sc1 nor anti-Sc2 has been reported to have caused a transfusion reaction. Anti-Sc1 has at least once caused a positive DAT in

TABLE 26-2 Approximate Antigen and Phenotype Frequencies in the Scianna Blood Group System

Phenotype	% Frequency	% of Bloods Reactive with	
		Anti-Sc1	Anti-Sc2
Sc:1,-2	99.28	} 99.9	
Sc:1,2	0.71		} 0.72
Sc:-1,2	0.01		

an infant with Sc:1,2 red cells born to a woman with IgG3 anti-Sc1 in the serum (8). However, the infant did not have clinical HDN and did not require treatment. It was noticed (8) that the antibody appeared to change, in terms of potential clinical significance, after delivery of the infant. That is to say, the percentage of lysis seen in an antibody-dependent cellular cytotoxicity assay (ADCC) ranged from 6% at 22 weeks of the patient's gestation to 11% at 39 weeks. Nine weeks after the infant's birth, the maternal antibody caused 44% lysis in an ADCC. This change was barely reflected by the titer of the antibody that was 16 throughout the pregnancy and 32 in the sample drawn at nine weeks postpartum.

DeMarco et al. (15) described a case in which anti-Sc2 apparently caused slow clearance of red cells in a newborn infant. The infant, with Sc:1,2 red cells was born to a woman with no previous history of pregnancy or transfusion, who had anti-Sc2 in the serum. At birth the infant had mild hyperbilirunemia and a hematocrit of 45%; the DAT was 2+ with anti-IgG. While the bilirubin level did not increase significantly, the hematocrit gradually dropped with no evidence of bleeding in the infant. On the twentieth day of life, the infant had a hematocrit of 17.3% and was transfused. Immediately after transfusion the infant's hematocrit was 43.8%, four months later it was 36.3%. An unusual finding in this case was that when the infant's blood was tested before transfusion, on day 20 of life, the DAT was 2+ with both anti-IgG and anti-C3. As mentioned above, Scianna system antibodies are often said not to bind complement.

Some characteristics of Scianna system antibodies, including anti-Sc3 that is described in more detail later in this chapter, are given in table 26-3.

Auto-Anti-Sc1

In 1979, Tregellas et al. (16) described an auto-anti-Sc1 that was clearly demonstrable when a healthy blood donor's serum was tested but which failed to react when the donor's plasma was used. The antibody-maker's red cells were Sc:1,-2 and the DAT was only weakly positive with small amounts of IgG and C3 being detected on the cells. The antibody was IgG3 in composition but, as might have been expected since it was active in serum but not plasma, appeared not to be causing in vivo red cell destruction. In 1982, a follow-up study on this antibody was reported (17). The IgG3 fraction of the donor's plasma was isolated and was treated with various endoproteases and exopeptidases. Trypsin and thrombin were the only enzymes tested that would cause the plasma to behave in the same way as the serum in terms of anti-Sc1 activity. The authors pointed out that both trypsin and thrombin are serine endoproteases specific for arginine-

TABLE 26-3 Usual Characteristics of Scianna System Antibodies

Antibody Specificity	Positive Reactions in In Vitro Tests				Usual Immunoglobulin		Ability to Bind Complement		Ability to Cause In Vitro Lysis		Implicated in		Usual Form of Stimulation		% of White Population Positive
	Sal	LISS	AHG	Enz	IgG	IgM	Yes	No	Yes	No	Transfusion Reaction	HDN	Red Cells	Other	
Anti-Sc1			Most	X	X		Some	Some		X	No	No	X		99.9
Anti-Sc2	Few		Most	X	X			Most		X	No	Mild	Most	Few	0.7
Anti-Sc3			Most	X	X		Few	Most		X	No		X		100

lysine bonds. Although they did not know the location of the bonds that were being cleaved, the authors suggested that the anti-Sc1 immunoglobulin molecules involved were not able to complex with their antigen until altered by one of the enzymes. It was supposed that the anti-Sc1 was demonstrable in serum since, in the coagulation process, thrombin is generated. It is not known if a similar mechanism is involved in those cases described by Garratty et al. (18) in which a number of patients with ulcerative colitis were found to have strongly positive DATs if tests were done on red cells from clotted samples but negative or only weakly positive DATs if red cells from anticoagulated samples were used (see also Chapter 37). Some of the patients with ulcerative colitis also appear to have potent autoantibodies of no recognizable specificity if tests are done with serum, but no autoantibodies if tests are done with plasma. In a later study on converted plasma from some of the patients with ulcerative colitis, that reacted as well with Sc:-1 as with Sc:1 red cells, Garratty (48) suggested that rather than the IgG3 immunoglobulin molecules being altered by serine proteases, the antibodies might be directed against those enzymes. It was suggested that perhaps the antibodies bound to the serine proteases and that the immune complexes generated then bound to red cells. Either theory, antibody molecule alteration or IgG3 antibody-serine protease immune complex formation, would explain the original reactivity of serum but not plasma since thrombin, generated in the coagulation process, is a serine protease. As far as we are aware, there is no evidence that any of these positive reactions were associated with an accelerated rate of red cell clearance in vivo.

In 1982, Steane et al. (19) described a patient with Evan's syndrome and a positive DAT. Thus it was impossible to be certain whether the anti-Sc1 in his serum was allo or autoimmune. From the results of adsorption studies we (20,21) thought that his red cells were probably Sc:-1. However, like others (1,6,22) we have experienced considerable difficulty in adsorbing anti-Sc1 with Sc:1 red cells. Because transfusion was essential and because no Sc:-1 blood was available, Steane et al. (19) used several plasma exchanges to lower the level of anti-Sc1 in the patient and then transfused incompatible blood. Although it seemed doubtful that the transfused cells survived normally, they remained in the patient's circulation long enough to get him through the acute medical emergency (reticulocytopenia caused by concurrent Legionnaire's disease) and eventually the patient went into complete remission. We were told (23) that once the patient was in remission, his red cells typed as Sc:1 and no anti-Sc1 could be detected in his serum. Thus it seems that like the situations in many other blood group systems, red cell Sc1 antigen production can be transiently suppressed with concurrent production of anti-Sc1. Clearly in the investigation of any individual with Sc:-1 red cells, the acquired and the genetic situations must be differentiated. Two cases in which auto-anti-Sc1 caused autoimmune hemolytic anemia have been documented (24,25). In one of them (24) it was noticed that the patient's red cells had a depressed expression of Sc1. In the other (25) the anti-Sc1 was identified by both serological tests and by immunoblotting, see later in this chapter for details of the red cell membrane structure that carries Scianna system antigens.

The Sc:-1,-2,-3 Phenotype and Anti-Sc3

As mentioned in the introduction of this chapter, in 1973, McCreary et al. (6) studied the red cells of a woman, who was a member of a highly inbred population living on Likiep Atoll in the Marshall Islands, whose serum contained an antibody to a very common antigen. The woman's red cells typed as Sc:-1,-2 and her serum reacted with all red cells except those of her cousin, that also typed as Sc:-1,-2. The red cells of other family members were Sc:1,-2. The proposita had been transfused, the cousin had been pregnant four times but her serum did not contain the antibody. The antibody was assumed to be anti-Sc1 plus anti-Sc2 in an inseparable form since it reacted equally with Sc:-1,2 and Sc:1,-2 red cells and could not be split into anti-Sc1 and anti-Sc2 by adsorption with such cells. However, the red cells of the antibody-maker and those of her compatible cousin were found to reduce the titer of anti-Sc2 in adsorption studies. No anti-Sc2 could be recovered by elution from the red cells used in the adsorptions. The cells did not reduce the titer of anti-Sc1 in parallel adsorption studies. Thus although red cell typing studies and the specificity of the antibody made suggested that the two women were phenotypically Sc:-1,-2 the possibility remained that they had some expression of Sc2 on their red cells. The red cells of other members of the nuclear family, that typed as Sc:1,-2, were not used in adsorption studies with anti-Sc2 (28) so that nothing further was learned about the possibility that a qualitatively or quantitatively different form of Sc2 might be present in the family.

In 1980, Nason et al. (7) described a previously transfused White male patient whose red cells typed as Sc:-1,-2 and whose serum contained an antibody to a high incidence antigen. The red cells of this patient did not reduce the titer of anti-Sc1 or anti-Sc2 in adsorption studies, the cells used in the adsorptions did not yield anti-Sc1 or anti-Sc2 on elution. The antibody in the patient's serum reacted with all red cells tested except those of the two women of Likiep Atoll that, as described above, also typed as Sc:-1,-2. In differential adsorption studies it was shown (7) that Sc:1,-2 and Sc:-1,2 red cells (that reacted equally with the antibody) adsorbed the antibody to exhaustion. Since no evidence was found to suggest that the patient's serum contained separable anti-Sc1 or anti-Sc2, the antibody present was called anti-Sc3 and Sc:-1,-2 red cells were classified as also being Sc:-3. A limited family study showed that the available relatives were all phenotypically Sc:1,-2. Titration studies were performed with anti-Sc1 and the red cells of the patient's mother and son, who would be obligate *Sc* heterozygotes if the patient's Sc:-1,-2,-3 phenotype represented the *ScSc* genotype (i.e. homozygous for a silent allele at the *Scianna* locus). Although Sc:1,2 red cells used as controls clearly showed presence of a single dose of Sc1 as compared to the Sc:1,-2 (double dose) control, the red cells of the mother and son reacted as if they carried a double dose of Sc1. While this does not exclude homozygosity of a silent allele as the explanation for the Sc:-1,-2,-3 phenotype, it fails to provide evidence in support of that interpretation.

A third proband with Sc:-1,-2,-3 red cells and anti-Sc3 in the serum was described by Woodfield et al. (29). The patient was a previously transfused 4 year-old child in Papua New Guinea. Investigations in this case showed that the patient's mother also had Sc:-1,-2,-3 red cells as did six of 29 family members and villagers from the child's home. It was believed that four of the six people with Sc:-1,-2,-3 red cells were related to the patient but

that the other two were not. All of a sudden these findings and those suggesting a double dose of Sc1 on the red cells of the mother and son of the Sc:-1,-2,-3 patient described by Nason et al. (7) seem to indicate that the simple explanation of a silent *Sc* allele at the *Scianna* locus may not apply or that more than one genetic background may be involved, see below.

Auto-Anti-Sc3

Peloquin et al. (30) presented brief details about two antibodies that were described as being autoimmune in nature and were thought to have anti-Sc3 specificity. In the first case the patient had lymphoma and marked anemia. The serum reacted moderately strongly with Sc:1,-2 red cells, weakly with Sc:-1,2 cells and was non-reactive with two Sc:-1,-2 and the patient's own cells. The expression of Sc1 and Sc3 on the patient's red cells was depressed. Presumably, the presence of some Sc3 on the patient's cells and the apparent specificity of the antibody led to the conclusion that the antibody was autoimmune in nature. The DAT was ± with anti-IgG and 1+^{s} with anti-C3d, eluates from the patient's cells were non-reactive. The patient was transfused with five units of incompatible blood with no apparent adverse effects. Within 70 days of transfusion the supposed anti-Sc3 was no longer demonstrable but the patient's red cells still had depressed expression of Sc1 and Sc3.

In the second case the patient had Hodgkin's disease, congestive heart failure and moderate anemia. The serum reacted to a strength of 2+ with Sc:1 red cells, less strongly with Sc:-1,2 and the patient's red cells and was non-reactive with Sc:-1,-2 cells. The DAT was 3+ with anti-C3d but negative with anti-IgG, an eluate made from the patient's red cells was non-reactive. The expression of Sc1 and Sc3 on the patient's red cells was described as slightly weakened. Six units of incompatible blood were transfused and the antibody became slightly weaker. No follow-up was possible.

Both cases resembled the situation described above in the section on auto-anti-Sc1. That is to say, both could have represented temporary suppression of Scianna system antigen production and concomitant transient production of a Scianna system antibody.

Do Sc:-1,-2,-3 Red Cells Lack Other Common Antigens?

In 1982, Skradski et al. (31) briefly described an antibody made by a patient with Sc:1,-2 red cells that reacted with all cells except those of the Sc:-1,-2 phenotype and those of the patient's brother, who like the patient was phenotypically Sc:1,-2. Additional details about this patient and about two others in whom the serological findings were similar, were reported by Devine et al. (32) in 1988. All three patients had Sc:1,-2 red cells. Each had made an IgG alloantibody, following blood transfusions, that was directed against a high incidence antigen. In each case the antibody was reactive with all red cells tested (for one exception see below) but was non-reactive with Sc:-1,-2 red cells. The one exception, as previously mentioned, is that one patient had a compatible sib, who was also of the Sc:1,-2 phenotype. The key finding in the study was that the antibody of each antibody-maker was reactive with the red cells of the other two. In other words, three different antigens seemed to be involved, each seemed to be missing from Sc:-1,-2 red cells. Although the patients' red cells were apparently not typed for Sc3, the remote possibility that the Sc:1,-2,-3 phenotype might exist, with persons of that phenotype able to make anti-Sc3, seems to be excluded since three different antigens, all missing from Sc:-1,-2 red cells seem to have been involved. Further, transient depression of Scianna antigen production with concomitant antibody production seems to have been excluded since in all three patients, Sc1 antigen expression appeared to be normal. In addition, the diagnoses were not of the type previously associated with depression of Scianna system antigen production. However, the diagnoses were similar, one patient had degenerative joint disease, the other two were scheduled for orthopedic surgery. Coincidence or a clue? Blood group serologists, you know where to look.

These findings may indicate that Sc:-1,-2,-3 red cells represent the null phenotype in the Scianna system and that such cells lack other high incidence antigens just as K_o red cells (see Chapter 18) and Rh_{null} red cells (see Chapter 12) lack a whole series of high (and low) incidence antigens in the Kell and Rh systems, respectively. Alternatively, if Sc:-1,-2,-3 red cells represent the Sc_{null} phenotype they may lack antigens of other systems, just as Rh_{null} red cells are LW(a-b-), Fy:-5. A third possibility is that the Sc:-1,-2 phenotype represents the presence of modifier or suppressor genes, that possibility is considered in the next section.

Is There an *In(Sc)* Gene Analogous to *In(Lu)* and *In(Jk)*?

Taken together, the findings described in the several previous sections indicate that the answer to the question that heads this section is a definite maybe! In the Sc:-1,-2 individuals described by McCreary et al. (6), there was evidence that Sc2 might be present in a small amount, just as Lu^b can be found on the red cells of persons with *In(Lu)* (see Chapter 20). In the Sc:-1,-2 individual described by Nason et al. (7) the mother and son of the Sc:-1,-2 propositus had a double dose of Sc1 on their red cells. Perhaps they were genetically Sc^1Sc^1 and perhaps the propositus inherited an unlinked dominant suppressor from his father, who was dead before the propositus' Sc:-1,-2 phenotype was discovered. In the family described by Woodfield et al. (29) the Sc:-1,-2 phenotype was seen in successive generations and in too many members of the family. Blood group serologists will not need to be reminded that the presence of *In(Lu)* results not only in suppression of expression of antigens of the Lutheran system but has a similar effect on some antigens encoded from genetically independent loci. Perhaps in the study of Devine et al. (32) the three antigens defined were suppressed like the high incidence antigens of the Lutheran system are affected by *In(Lu)* or perhaps they were independent of the Scianna system but affected by the same independent suppressor. For serologists who teach immunohematology this section can be used as an example as to how two plus two make five. On the other hand, if the suggestion turns out to be correct, please tell your students where you read it first.

The *Scianna* Locus is on Chromosome 1

As will be apparent by now, much of the serological work on the Scianna system was performed at the Rh Laboratory in Winnipeg. Thus it was fitting that the workers in Winnipeg should be the ones who first recognized that the locus for genes of the system is on chromosome 1. It is known that the *UMPK* (the locus for the polymorphic character uridine monophosphate kinase), *Rh* and *PGM₁* loci are linked and are carried on chromosome 1 (33-37). Family studies described by Lewis et al. (5,38-41) showed beyond doubt that the *Scianna* locus is linked to *UMPK*, *Rh* and *PGM₁* and must therefore be located on the short arm of chromosome 1. Independent confirmation of this finding has been provided by Noades et al. (11) who showed that *Scianna* is distal to *UMPK* on the short arm of chromosome 1. The locus is between 1p36.2 and 1p22.1

The Antigen Rd a.k.a. Rd^a

A rare antigen that was given the name Rd, was described by Rausen et al. (42) in 1967. Lundsgaard and Jensen (43) later suggested that the antigen be called Rd^a so that the active gene, *Rd^a*, could be distinguished from the locus, *Rd*. Since Rd (Rd^a) is still officially an independent antigen of low incidence, its characteristics and those of the antibody that define it, are described in

Chapter 32. The antigen is mentioned here because it may be part of the Scianna system. Lewis et al. (44,45) and Hilden et al. (47) showed that *Rd* is linked to *Rh* and is either a part of, or is very closely linked to the *Scianna* locus. One individual with Sc:1,2 Rd(a+) red cells was found (45) showing that *Rd*[^a] cannot be an allele of *Sc*[^1] and *Sc*[^2]. However, most of the blood group systems, e.g. Rh, MN, Kell, Lutheran are complex and *Rd*[^a] could be to *Sc*[^1] and *Sc*[^2] as, say, *Kp*[^a] is to *K* and to *k* (see Chapter 18). Whether Rd[^a] is antithetical to one of the antibodies described by Devine et al. (32) that reacted with all except Sc:-1,-2 red cells is not known. The red cells of one of the antibody-makers were Rd(a-), the cells of the other two were not typed for that antigen.

As described below, Spring et al. (27) have characterized the red cell membrane glycoprotein that carries Sc1 and Sc2. Spring (46) later showed that immunoblotting with anti-Rd identified a band of about the same size as the Scianna glycoprotein. However, Daniels (49) reports that the Scianna glycoprotein isolated with anti-Sc1 from Rd(a+) red cells was not stained by anti-Rd on a protein blot.

The Biochemical Nature of the Sc and Rd Antigens

Very little is known about the molecule which carries the Sc antigens. When anti-Sc1 and anti-Sc2 are used in immunoblotting experiments with the electrophoretically separated components of red cell membranes of appropriate Sc phenotype, a diffusely staining band of 60-68 kD is observed under non-reducing conditions (27). The band is a protein because the Sc antigens are destroyed by pronase although not by trypsin, chymotrypsin or papain. The protein is likely to be glycosylated because previous treatment of red cells with sialidase reduces the leading edge of the band by 1 kD and the trailing edge by 3 kD. The band observed when membranes from Tn red cells are examined is not markedly different from that on normal cells indicating that the Sc protein does not include a substantial content of O-glycans. When red cells were treated with a relatively crude preparation containing Endo F and N-peptidyl N-glycanase the band stained by anti-Sc2 was no longer observed. In contrast, the band stained by anti-Sc1 was of the same apparent molecular weight but was more weakly stained.

These results suggest that the Sc antigens are carried on a glycoprotein which contains one or more intrachain disulphide bonds. The results obtained with Endo F are difficult to interpret. If the glycoprotein contains one or more N-glycans a reduction in the apparent Mr of the protein would be expected. N-glycans are usually of the order of 3 kD or more. Such a reduction was not observed. The reactivity with anti-Sc1 was weakened and that with anti-Sc2 destroyed. The possibility that the Endo F preparation used in this study contained a contaminating protease was considered and when these experiments were repeated with a highly purified peptidyl N-glycanase a reactive band was obtained with antibodies to Sc1, Sc2 and Rd. In each case the reactive band had an Mr 2300 less than untreated control samples (Spring FA, unpublished observations). It appears, therefore, that the Sc glycoprotein probably contains a single N-glycan.

The Sc protein was retained in the pellet (with the red cell skeleton) when red cell membranes were extracted with Triton X-100 at a concentration of 10% (w/v). This result suggests that the Sc protein is tightly bound to the red cell skeleton. Immunoblotting studies with anti-Rd showed that the antibody bound to a component of similar size and characteristics to the Sc protein (46). The protein was only observed under non-reducing conditions and was destroyed by pronase-treatment. However, as pointed out by Daniels (49), formal proof that the Sc protein and the Rd protein are the same is not yet available.

References

1. Schmidt RP, Griffitts JJ, Northman FF. Transfusion 1962;2:338
2. Anderson C, Hunter J, Zipursky A, et al. Transfusion 1963;3:30
3. Lewis M, Chown B, Schmidt RP, et al. Am J Hum Genet 1964;16:254
4. Lewis M, Chown B, Kaita H. Transfusion 1967;7:92
5. Lewis M, Kaita H, Chown B. Vox Sang 1974;27:261
6. McCreary J, Vogler AL, Sabo B, et al. (abstract). Transfusion 1973;13:350
7. Nason SG, Vengelen-Tyler V, Cohen N, et al. Transfusion 1980;20:531
8. Kaye T, Williams EM, Garner SF, et al. Transfusion 1990;30:439
9. Gale SA, Rowe GP, Northfield FE. Vox Sang 1988;54:172
10. Seyfried H, Frankowska K, Giles GM. Vox Sang 1966;11:512
11. Noades JE, Corney G, Cook PJL, et al. Ann Hum Genet 1979;43:121
12. Fünfhausen G, Gremplewski K. Z Arztl Fortbild 1967;61:739
13. Calkovská Z. Folia Haematol 1974;101:661
14. Mollison PL. Blood Transfusion in Clinical Medicine, 7th Ed. Oxford:Blackwell, 1983:430
15. DeMarco M, Uhl L, Fields L, et al. Transfusion 1995;35:58
16. Tregellas WM, Holub MP, Moulds JJ, et al. (abstract). Transfusion 1979;19:650
17. Tregellas WM, Lavine KK. (abstract). Transfusion 1982;22:406
18. Garratty G, Davis J, Myers M, et al. (abstract). Transfusion 1980;20:646
19. Steane EA, Sheehan RG, Brooks BD, et al. In: Therapeutic Apheresis and Plasma Perfusion. New York:Liss, 1982:347
20. Boyd PA, Issitt PD. Unpublished observations 1980, cited in

[^a]: a
[^1]: 1
[^2]: 2

Issitt PD. Applied Blood Group Serology, 3rd Ed. Miami:Montgomery, 1985:389

21. Boyd PA. MS Thesis, Univ Cincinnati 1980

22. Cummings ER. Unpublished observations 1980, cited in Issitt PD. Applied Blood Group Serology, 3rd Ed. Miami:Montgomery, 1985:389

23. Steane EA. Personal communication 1983, cited in Issitt PD. Applied Blood Group Serology, 3rd Ed. Miami:Montgomery, 1985:389

24. McDowell MA, Stocker I, Nance S, et al. (abstract). Transfusion 1986;26:578

25. Owen I, Chowdhury V, Reid ME, et al. Transfusion 1992;32:173

26. Daniels G. Immunohematology 1992;8:53

27. Spring FA, Herron R, Rowe AG. Vox Sang 1990;58:122

28. Sabo B. Personal communication 1973, cited in Issitt PD, Issitt CH. Applied Blood Group Serology, 2nd Ed. Oxnard:Spectra, 1975:211

29. Woodfield DG, Giles C, Poole J, et al. (abstract). Book of Abstracts, 19th Cong ISBT, 1986:651

30. Peloquin P, Moulds M, Keenan J, et al. (abstract). Transfusion 1989;29(Suppl 7S):49S

31. Skradski KJ, McCreary J, Sabo B, et al. (abstract). Transfusion 1982;22:406

32. Devine P, Dawson FE, Motschman TL, et al. Transfusion 1988;28:346

33. van Cong N, Billardon C, Pickard JY, et al. Acad Sci Ser D Paris 1971;272:485

34. Ruddle FH, Riccoti F, McMorris FA, et al. Science 1972;176:1429

35. Marsh WL, Chaganti RSK, Garner FH, et al. Science 1974;183:966

36. Giblett ER, Anderson JE, Lewis M, et al. Birth Defects Orig Article Ser 1975;11:159

37. Mohr J, Eiberg H, Skude G. Birth Defects Orig Article Ser 1976;12:340

38. Lewis M, Kaita H, Chown B. Am J Hum Genet 1976;28:619

39. Lewis M, Kaita H, Cot GB, et al. Birth Defects Orig Article Ser 1976;12:322

40. Lewis M, Kaita H, Chown B, et al. Canad J Genet Cytol 1977;19:695

41. Lewis M, Kaita H, Giblett ER, et al. Birth Defects Orig Article Ser 1978;14:392

42. Rausen AR, Rosenfield RE, Alter AA, et al. Transfusion 1967;7:336

43. Lundsgaard A, Jensen KG. Vox Sang 1968;14:452

44. Lewis M, Kaita H. Vox Sang 1979;37:286

45. Lewis M, Kaita H, Philipps S, et al. Ann Hum Genet 1980;44:179

46. Spring FA. Transf Med 1993;3:167

47. Hildén J-O, Shaw M-A, Whitehouse DB, et al. (abstract). Cytogenet Cell Genet 1985;40:650

48. Garratty G. (abstract). Transfusion 1993;33(Suppl 9S):22S

49. Daniels G. Human Blood Groups. Oxford:Blackwell, 1995:498

27 | The Chido-Rodgers Blood Group System

In 1967, Harris et al. (1) described fourteen examples of anti-Chido "a nebulous antibody responsible for crossmatching difficulties". A better description could not have been applied. The antigen defined varied in strength on the red cells of different samples tested. Some cell samples reacted with the stronger but not with the weaker examples of the antibody, other cell samples gave equivocal reactions and even on repeat testing it was difficult to be certain whether or not the antigen was present. The antibodies seldom gave strong positive reactions even when titration studies gave high end points. In spite of these difficulties it appeared (1-3) that the antigen defined was present on the red cells of some 98% of random Whites. More recent studies, see below, have indicated that the incidence of the antigen is closer to 96%. During some of the early studies (1-6) the antigen defined was called, variously, Chido, Ch^a and Ch. For reasons that will become apparent later in this chapter, the term Ch for the antigen and anti-Ch for the antibody, will be used here. A major advance was made when Middleton (4) and Middleton and Crookston (5) demonstrated that Ch is present in soluble form in the plasma of persons with Ch+ red cells.

In 1976, Longster and Giles (7) described the first example of anti-Rg. Because the antibody gave reactions somewhat reminiscent of anti-Ch, these workers used plasma in hemagglutination inhibition studies and showed, right at the outset, that Rg is present in soluble form in the plasma of persons with Rg+ red cells. Like Ch, Rg was seen to be of high incidence, being found (7) on the red cells of some 97% of random Whites. While examples of anti-Rg often give reactions similar to those of anti-Ch in tests (agglutination and/or IAT) on red cells, the fact that it was known that plasma could be used in antibody-neutralization tests to determine the Rg phenotype (i.e. Rg+ or Rg-, see below for additional complexity) resulted in the Rg(a-) phenotype being recognized more easily than would otherwise have been the case. The terms Rodgers, Rg^a and Rg have all been used (7-10) for the antigen defined, here Rg will be used for the antigen and anti-Rg for the antibody.

The next step that led to Ch and Rg eventually achieving blood group system status was the finding (11) that the gene that encodes production of Ch is linked to the *HLA* locus. In turn, the *HLA* locus was shown (12) to be linked to the locus at which the genes encoding production of the fourth component of complement, C4, are located. Since it was known by then that Ch is present in soluble form in plasma and serum, it became logical to

look to see if Ch is a marker antigen on C4. The studies (13-15) showed that to be the case, subsequent investigations (16-18) showed that Ch is carried on the C4d portion (see Chapter 6) of C4. A similar story describes Rg. James et al. (9) showed that the phenotype HLA-A1,8 occurs more frequently in persons of the Rg- phenotype than would be expected by chance, then Giles et al. (8) demonstrated linkage between *Rg* and *HLA*. After *HLA* and *C4* had been shown (12) to be linked on chromosome 6 (19), the studies cited above (13-18) showed that like Ch, Rg is a determinant carried on C4.

In a later section of this chapter, the polymorphism of C4 that is represented by the determinants Ch1 to Ch6, Rg1 and Rg2, and WH will be described. However, in terms of practical blood banking it is convenient first to consider Ch and Rg as single entities since on most occasions in the blood bank, anti-Ch will present as an apparent single antibody made in an individual with Ch- red cells and anti-Rg will present as an apparent single antibody made by an individual with Rg- red cells. Thus the next two sections can be regarded as deliberate oversimplifications for practical purposes. The final section of this chapter includes a potential explanation, based on the molecular structure of C4, as to why anti-Ch is detected more often than anti-Rg when, based on frequencies of the negative phenotypes, the opposite might be expected.

The Antigen Ch and the Antibody That Defines It

As mentioned in the introduction, Ch is an antigen of high incidence. It is not carried on an intrinsic red cell structure but instead reaches the red cell membrane via the adsorption of C4 on to red cells. This fact no doubt explains, at least in part, the very considerable variation in expression (and hence detection) of Ch on Ch+ samples from different individuals. Indeed, phenotyping studies in which anti-Ch is used in direct tests on red cells are often difficult to interpret. Recognition (4,5) of the fact that Ch is present in plasma led to the use of hemagglutination inhibition studies as a far more reliable means to establish the Ch phenotype of an individual. In these tests (4,5,11,20-23) the most potent example of anti-Ch available is used in tests against red cells that have been treated, by the methods described below, so that they carry more C4 than do normal untreated red cells. Plasma or serum from the individual to be typed for Ch is then added to the anti-Ch. Saline is used as a control and is added to a separate aliquot of the anti-Ch in the same proportion as the plasma or serum under test. The mixtures are left for a brief period, 30 minutes at room temperature is usually sufficient, then the indicator red cells, coated with the increased amounts of C4 are added. If the plasma or serum under test prevents the anti-Ch from agglutinating the C4-coated red cells while the saline dilution-control is positive, it has been demonstrated that the plasma or serum under test contains Ch substance so comes from an individual of the Ch+ phenotype. In most instances, since Ch is of high incidence, total inhibition of the anti-Ch will be seen. Because Ch represents a polymorphism (see below) occasional samples from Ch+ persons will cause only partial inhibition. Plasma or serum from the 3 to 4% of random individuals who are of the Ch- phenotype, will not inhibit the anti-Ch.

Because the reaction between anti-Ch and Ch+ red cells is often weak, it is necessary to use, in the inhibition studies just described, indicator red cells to which additional C4, and hence Ch, has been bound. This is accomplished by mixing red cells with fresh ABO compatible plasma in a low ionic strength sucrose solution. C4 will bind to the red cells in the absence of an antigen-antibody reaction and the red cells can then be washed and used as indicator cells in the inhibition studies described. Since the treatment of C4-coated red cells with trypsin cleaves C4b and leaves C4d on the red cells (see Chapter 6) and since the Ch determinants are carried on C4d, the test can be made more sensitive by treating the indictor red cells with trypsin, before they are used (20). Exact details of the techniques used in these studies are given by Judd (24).

If sufficiently potent anti-Ch is available, the addition of homologous C4 to red cells can be used to enable direct typing of the cells for Ch phenotype. The principle is the same as that described above. Freshly drawn citrated whole blood from the individual to be tested is added to the low ionic strength sucrose solution. After the cells have been washed they can be tested directly or can be treated with trypsin and then tested. As discussed below in the section on the identification of anti-Ch, many examples of anti-Ch that react with untreated red cells only by IAT, will cause direct agglutination of C4-coated red cells (18,20).

When the inhibition or modified direct typing tests are used it is seen that Ch is present in some 96 to 98% of random Whites. While no large scale studies seem to have been reported, it appears that the incidence is similar in Blacks although there is one report (4) that most examples of anti-Ch are made by Whites, thus suggesting that the incidence of the antigen may be higher in Blacks. As mentioned already, Ch is polymorphic. There is apparently a higher incidence of the phenotype in

which the Ch2 determinant (see below) is absent in Japanese, than in Whites or Blacks.

Although the level of Ch on red cells varies widely when untreated red cells are tested with anti-Ch, the plasma or serum of individuals in whom red cell Ch is detected with difficulty, is as efficient as that of individuals in whom Ch is more readily detectable, when antibody inhibition studies are used. When untreated cord blood red cells are tested directly with anti-Ch it appears (2,3) that about 50% of them are Ch-. However, when cord blood plasma or serum is used in antibody inhibition studies it is seen (5,25,26) that the same percentage as seen in samples from adults, inhibit anti-Ch. This may simply be due to the fact that complement levels in newborns are lower than those in adults. The components C1q, C4 and C3 are present in about 50% of the levels seen in adults, in the sera of newborns (27,28). Thus it may be that too little C4 binds to the red cells of newborns for Ch to be detected on those cells while sufficient C4 is present in the plasma or serum to effect neutralization (inhibition) of anti-Ch.

Although the detection of Ch is enhanced when C4-coated red cells are treated with trypsin to cleave C4b into C4d, the same does not apply when untreated cells are exposed to proteases. It has been found (5,18,25,26,29) that trypsin, chymotrypsin, papain, ficin and pronase all denature Ch on red cells to which no additional C4 has been bound by the low ionic strength sucrose method described above. Giles et al. (29) used a monoclonal antibody to C4 to show that treatment of unmodified red cells with trypsin reduces the number of detectable C4 molecules by about a half.

The binding of C4 to red cells in a low ionic sucrose solution is dependent on the presence of sialic acid on those red cells. Wilfert et al. (30) showed that while sialidase did not remove C4 once that glycoprotein had been bound to red cells, C4 uptake did not occur when red cells previously treated with sialidase were used in the sucrose method. Somewhat similarly, Tippett et al. (31) found that En(a-) red cells and those from M^k homozygotes (both types have reduced levels of N-acetyl neuraminic acid on their membranes, see Chapter 15) react very weakly with antibodies that define determinants on C4. The small amount of C4 on untreated red cells is apparently covalently bound, it is not removed when red cells are treated with sulphydryl reagents or with chloroquine (32).

Most examples of anti-Ch are IgG in nature, in one study (33) it was found that IgG2 and IgG4 components predominate. In tests against unmodified red cells anti-Ch usually presents as an antibody reacting weakly, though sometimes to high titer, by IAT. Two useful modifications that aid in the identification of anti-Ch are based on findings described above. First, if red cells coated with C4 in a low ionic strength solution of sucrose are used, many examples of anti-Ch act as direct agglutinins in a saline system (18,20). Second, when identification of anti-Ch is in doubt, pooled plasma or serum can be used to inhibit the antibody (4,5). Although as already mentioned, Ch is polymorphic and although different anti-Ch may detect different epitopes, most random plasma or sera will contain all the different epitopes; the use of pooled plasma or serum in inhibition studies will virtually guarantee that all epitopes are represented.

In terms of red cell transfusions, anti-Ch is benign. Red cell survival studies, phagocytic cell assays and transfusions with antigen-positive red cells in many different cases (1,4,6,34-37) have produced unequivocal evidence that anti-Ch does not destroy Ch+ red cells in vivo. There is one report (38) in the literature of an IgG4 anti-Ch causing severe anaphylactic reactions in a patient transfused with platelets suspended in plasma and another (125) in which a 2 year-old child with IgG anti-Ch, the subclass of which could not be determined, had a less severe anaphylactic reaction when transfused with platelets. However, it seems that such reactions must be the exception not the rule. In virtually all transfusion services, once anti-Ch has been identified, random units that will almost all be Ch+, are transfused without being washed. Further, we know of no service that selects Ch- plasma products for patients with anti-Ch so that it seems that the antibody seldom creates any clinical problems.

The Antigen Rg and the Antibody That Defines It

Most of what has been written above, about Ch and anti-Ch, applies as well to Rg and anti-Rg. Like Ch, Rg is of high incidence being found in the plasma or serum, and hence by adsorption on the red cells, of some 97% of random Whites (7). Also like Ch, Rg is present on the C4d portion of the C4 component of complement (13-18). A later section of this chapter describes the usual presence of Ch and Rg on different portions of C4d that can be identified by the speed with which they migrate in electrophoresis in agarose gels (13,15) and the polymorphisms of the antigens. Because Rg reaches the red cell surface via adsorption of C4 on to the cell membrane, the same difficulties as described for Ch are encountered when direct typing tests for Rg are performed. Thus antibody inhibition studies and tests against red cells coated with additional amounts of C4 via use of the low ionic sucrose method, as described in the section on Ch, are appropriate. Again, although Rg is polymorphic, the use of pooled serum in antibody inhibition studies, ensures that the different epitopes of Rg will be present. Like Ch, Rg on unmodified red cells is subject to denaturation by trypsin, chymotrypsin, papain, ficin and pronase (7,18,25,26,29), it survives trypsin treatment of red cells

to which additional C4 has been bound in the low ionic sucrose method. The same comments made above about the relationship of Ch to membrane-bound sialic acid apply to Rg although the depression of Rg on En(a-) red cells and on those from M^k homozygotes was not always as marked as the depression of Ch (31).

Like anti-Ch, anti-Rg is usually IgG in nature, it is usually presumed from their lack of clinical relevance in red cell transfusions (see below) that the antibodies lack IgG1 and IgG3 components although this point does not seem to have been formally proved. Identification of anti-Rg is greatly enhanced if red cells coated with increased amount of C4 and/or antibody inhibition studies are used. Strohm and Molthan (39) described the successful transfusion of Rg+ blood to four patients with anti-Rg in the serum and it seems certain that many similar transfusions with antigen-positive blood have been performed but not reported in the literature since the successful outcomes were as expected. We are aware of phagocytic cell assays performed to determine the probable in vivo activities of different examples of anti-Rg that, similarly, were not described in print because the expected negative results were seen. There is one report (40) of a patient with anti-Rg in the serum suffering transfusion reactions to infusions of fresh frozen plasma and plasma prothrombin complex concentrate. For reasons discussed above, concerning the reactions to plasma in patients with anti-Ch (38,125), this type of reaction must be the exception rather than the rule.

The C4 Glycoprotein and the Polymorphisms of Ch and Rg

As described above, the plasma or serum of the majority of random individuals will totally inhibit anti-Ch and anti-Rg. However, some 2 to 3% of random plasmas effect only partial inhibition of anti-Rg (7) and perhaps fewer plasmas effect only partial inhibition of anti-Ch (10,41-45). While it at first appeared that partial inhibition represented quantitative variation in the levels of C4 and hence Rg and Ch in different plasmas, it is now appreciated that a different explanation obtains. Ch and Rg each comprise a number of different epitopes on C4d meaning that not every epitope is present in every plasma. Since different examples of anti-Ch and anti-Rg vary in complexing with different epitopes, partial inhibition can occur when the antibody contains specificities for two or more epitopes and the plasma used in the inhibition study lacks one or more of the epitopes to which the antibodies are directed.

The situation is highly complex and the details do not pertain to the situations normally encountered in the blood bank. Accordingly, a simplified explanation will be given, readers requiring additional information are referred to a number of excellent original papers and reviews (46-57). The glycoprotein C4 is synthesized by hepatocytes and macrophages (58) as a single protein of approximately 700 amino acids. That protein is known as pro-C4 and once made undergoes posttranslational cleavage so that the functional molecule comprises three polypeptide chains joined by disulphide bonds (59) (see figure 27-1). When activated by C1s (see Chapter 6) a small portion of the molecule, C4a, is cleaved. The remainder of the molecule, C4b, can attach to red cells. C4b is then further cleaved by factor I (again see Chapter 6), C3c is released while C4d remains membrane-bound (again see figure 27-1). The Ch and Rg epitopes are carried on C4d. Since complement activation and regulation (degradation) are dynamic processes, the above explains why Ch and Rg are found on normal red cells. Further, as already explained, additional C4 (and C3) attaches to red cells when whole blood (i.e. red cells and plasma) is put into a low ionic strength sucrose solution.

Production of C4 is controlled by genes at two closely linked loci on chromosome 6 (13-15,60,61). It is probable that the genes at these loci arose by duplication. When first proposing the two gene model with evidence in favor of two loci rather than two alleles at a single locus, O'Neill et al. (13,15) pointed out that much earlier studies (62) had demonstrated a structural polymorphism of the protein. Electrophoresis reveals dis-

tinct bands of C4, O'Neill et al. (13,15) designated these bands C4F (fast) and C4S (slow) based on their migratory patterns. A change in the nomenclature (63) has resulted in current use of the terms C4A (acidic) for C4F, and C4B (basic) for C4S. It should be noted that C4A and C4B apply to the form of C4 produced and do not equate to the terms C4a and C4b, as used above in the description of C4 activation.

O'Neill et al. (13) showed that plasma that contains C4A (C4F) and C4B(C4S) contains both Ch and Rg antigens. Plasma that contains C4A (C4F) but not C4B (C4S) is Ch-, Rg+; plasma that contains C4B (C4S) but not C4A (C4F) is Ch+, Rg-. In most studies completed since then, it has been found that the Ch determinants are carried on C4B (C4S) while the Rg determinants are carried on C4A (C4F). Rare exceptions have been found and are mentioned below. At this point the terms C4F and C4S will be abandoned and C4A and C4B will be used.

Based on eletrophoretic mobility it has been shown (64) that there are at least 19 alleles at the *C4A* locus and at least 22 at the *C4B* locus, those numbers include a silent allele at each locus. That does not mean that there are that many epitopes of Rg and Ch, respectively. Instead, many of the alleles encode production of proteins that carry the same Rg and Ch determinants. However, nucleotide substitutions within the encoding genes have resulted in some amino acid changes in the proteins encoded. In some instances the changes have resulted in

FIGURE 27-1 Structure of C4 (adapted from reference 91)

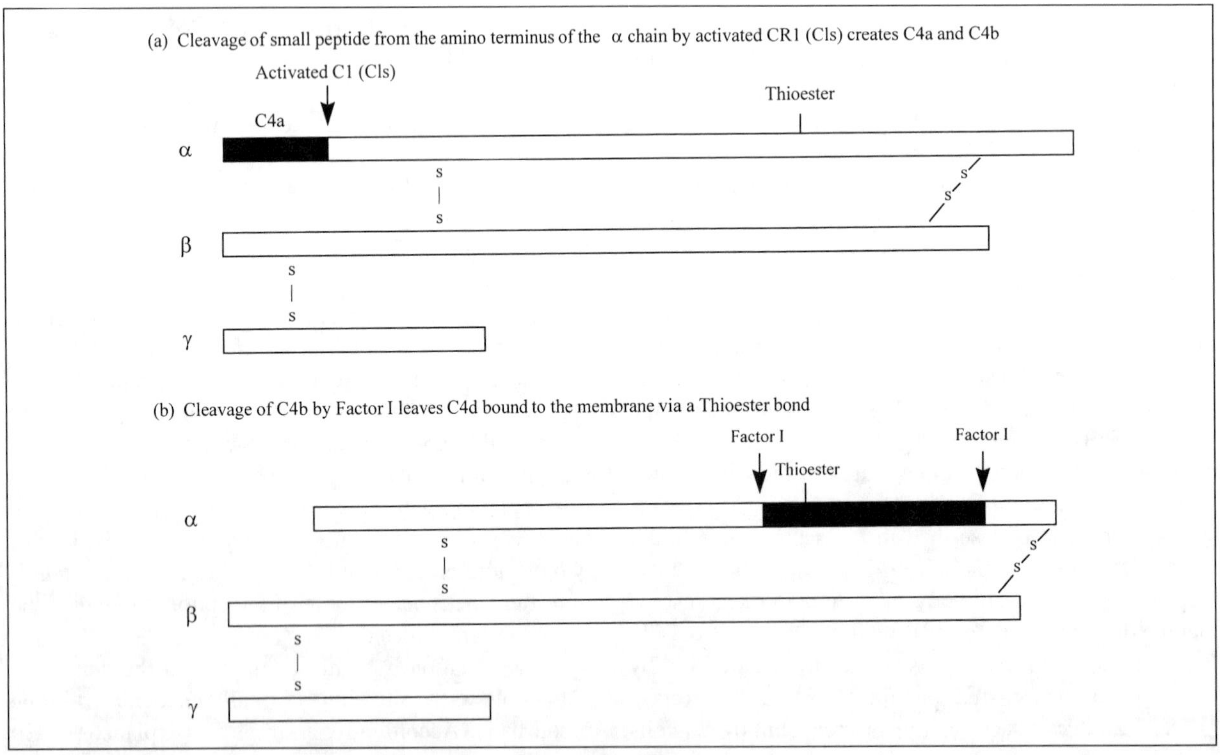

(a) Cleavage of small peptide from the amino terminus of the α chain by activated CR1 (C1s) creates C4a and C4b

(b) Cleavage of C4b by Factor I leaves C4d bound to the membrane via a Thioester bond

formation of immunogenic structures and antibodies directed against such structures have been recognized.

As shown in table 27-1, six antigens (epitopes) of Ch, Ch1 to Ch6, two of Rg, Rg1 and Rg2 and one inter-action product (WH) between Ch and Rg have been rec-ognized and named by the ISBT Working Party for Terminology of Red Cell Surface Antigens (65). The antigens Ch1 and Ch6 and Rg1 and Rg2 are all of high incidence. One or more of the Ch antigens are present in some 96%, and one or both of the Rg antigens in some 97%, of random Whites. The WH antigen has an inci-dence of about 15%. For some phenotype frequencies (42,48,112) see table 27-3. More complete details about Ch1, Ch2, Ch3, Rg1 and Rg2 will be found in Giles (44), about Ch4, Ch5 and Ch6 in Giles (66) and about WH in Giles and Jones (67). The six Ch and two Rg determi-nants and WH are not all simple linear structures on C4d. That is to say, each does represent a different to usual amino acid on the polypeptide. As shown in table 27-2, the Ch3 epitope is a configurational form that requires presence of both Ch1 and Ch6 for expression. Similarly, Ch2 is expressed only when Ch4 and Ch5 are present. Rg2 requires the presence of Rg1 and a hypothetical epi-tope Rg(3) to which no antibody has yet been identified. The WH epitope requires the presence of Rg1 on C4A and Ch6 on C4B, for its expression. The model depicted in table 27-2 is based on one devised by Yu et al. (50) and modified by Giles et al. (51). Presence of the various Rg and Ch epitopes is determined by the allotype of *C4A* or *C4B* present. Based on the antigenic determinants identi-fied and hypothesizing that Rg3 exists, Yu et al. (50) and Giles and Jones (67) predicted that 16 different C4 allo-types would eventually be recognized from serological tests. Serological evidence has thus far resulted in recog-nition of the existence of 13 of them (51).

Complex as the above situation may be, it does not tell the whole story. While in most individuals the Rg determinants are expressed on C4A and the Ch determi-nants on C4B, exceptions have been found. Both C4A variants expressing Ch epitopes and C4B variants expressing Rg determinants have been found (45,68,69). Gene conversion or unequal crossing over with the for-mation of hybrid *C4A/C4B* genes might explain these findings (45,52,68,70). In addition, duplicated *C4* genes seem to be quite common (10,71-74). Teisberg et al. (75) found that among 76 haplotypes studied, 58 had two *C4* genes, 12 had only one (see below for silent alleles), while six had three *C4* genes.

Silent Alleles at the *C4A* and *C4B* Loci

When it was originally recognized (13,15) that some individuals have only the fast moving bands and some

TABLE 27-1 Terminology for the Ch/Rg Blood Group System

Conventional Name: Chido/Rodgers
Conventional Symbol: Ch/Rg
ISBT System Symbol: CH/RG
ISBT System Number: 017

Antigen[1] Conventional Name	ISBT Antigen Number	ISBT[2] Full Code Number
Ch1	CH1	017001
Ch2	CH2	017002
Ch3	CH3	017003
Ch4	CH4	017004
Ch5	CH5	017005
Ch6	CH6	017006
WH	WH	017007
Rg1	RG1	017011
Rg2	RG2	017012

[1] As explained in the text, for practical purposes in transfu-sion therapy, Ch1 to Ch6 are called Ch, Rg1 and Rg2 are called Rg.

[2] The numbers 017008 to 017010 are reserved in case addi-tional Ch epitopes are recognized.

TABLE 27-2 To Show the Usual Relationships of the Ch and Rg Determinants to Each Other[1]

Epitope	C4A Protein	Amino Acid Residue (from NH$_2$ Terminus)	C4B Protein	Epitope		
	Asp	1054	Gly	Ch5		
	Pro	1101	Leu		} Ch4	} Ch2
	Cys	1102	Ser			
	Leu	1105	Ile			
	Asp	1106	His			
Rg2 { Rg3[2]	Asn	1157	Ser	Ch6		
Rg1 {	Val	1188	Ala		} Ch1	} Ch3
	Leu	1191	Arg			

[1] For examples of Ch determinants on C4A and Rg determi-nants on C4B, see text.

[2] Rg3 is a hypothetical determinant. No example of anti-Rg3 has been found.

The model is based on that proposed by Yu et al. (50) and mod-ified by Giles et al. (51).

The WH determinant (not shown) is dependent on the pres-ence of Rg1 and Ch6.

only the slow moving bands (on electrophoresis) of C4, it became apparent that genes that act as silent alleles at one of the loci, are not particularly uncommon. The genes are now known as *C4A*QO* and *C4B*QO* respectively, the *QO* designation implies "quantity zero" and merely indicates that the gene present fails to encode production of detectable product, without any implication as to the mechanism involved. It is now known (76,77) that about half the silent alleles represent a 28kb DNA deletion. *C4A*QO* also results from a two base pair insertion in exon 29 of *C4A* that causes a premature stop codon to arise in exon 30 (78). The importance of these observations in terms of blood group serology relates to the fact that most (but not all) persons who make anti-Ch are homozygous for *C4B*QO* but have genes that encode normal production of C4A, while most (but probably not all) persons who make anti-Rg are homozygous for *C4A*QO* but have genes that encode normal production of C4B. That is to say, most often the phenotype Ch-, Rg+ represents the genotype *C4A/C4A, C4B*QO/C4B*QO* while most often the phenotype Ch+, Rg- represents the genotype *C4A*QO/C4A*QO, C4B/C4B*. Only rarely is anti-Rg or anti-Ch encountered in an individual who has some but not all the epitopes of Rg or Ch, respectively, present.

The *C4* alleles are in linkage disequilibrium with *HLA*. In Whites, *C4A*QO* is most often associated with the HLA-A1, B8, DR3 phenotype, in Blacks it is associated with that phenotype and with the HLA-B44 and DR2 haplotypes (92,93,102). The Ch- phenotype (usually representing the homozygous state of *C4B*QO*) is seen with a higher frequency in the HLA-B12 and HLA-B5 phenotypes, than in others (11). No doubt linkage disequilibrium between the *C4* and *HLA* genes explains some of the reported associations between HLA phenotypes and disease susceptibilities.

On the Fine Specificities of Anti-Ch and Anti-Rg

As mentioned in the previous section, most examples of anti-Ch are made by persons with Ch-, Rg+ red cells, that is persons genetically *C4A/C4A, C4B*QO/C4B*QO*. Such persons are phenotypically Ch:-1,-2,-3,-4,-5,-6. Most anti-Ch are anti-Ch1 or contain that specificity (43,44), it is not unusual to find anti-Ch1 as the only antibody made. In those sera that contain additional specificities: 25% include anti-Ch2; 10% include anti-Ch3; 75% anti-Ch4; 16% anti-Ch5, while both anti-Ch6 and anti-WH are rare with only two examples of each having been found up to 1988 (48). Only on rare occasions are antibodies to the Ch determinants found in sera that lack anti-Ch1 (79).

Given the polymorphism of Ch it is clear that some

Ch+ persons will be able to make alloimmune anti-Ch and indeed this situation has been reported on a number of occasions. Giles et al. (79) identified anti-Ch2 and anti-Ch5 in a person of phenotype Ch:1,-2,3,4,-5,6; Fisher et al. (80) reported anti-Ch2 and anti-Ch4 made by person of phenotype Ch:1,-2,3,-4,5,6; and Poole et al. (69) described anti-Ch1 in a persons of phenotype Ch:-1,-2,-3,-4,5,6 and anti-Ch1, anti-Ch3 and anti-Ch4 in the serum of an individual of phenotype Ch:-1,-2,-3,-4,5. One of the ways in which a Ch+ individual can make alloimmune anti-Ch is when the Ch determinant(s) is (are) carried on C4A instead of C4B (see above and in more detail below).

At the level of the routine blood bank, most examples of anti-Ch will be seen in persons with Ch- red cells. That is to say, the most frequent event will be formation of (at least) anti-Ch1 by a person of phenotype Ch:-1,-2,-3,-4,-5,-6. Identification of anti-Ch in a patient with Ch+ red cells is a rare event and classification of the antibody's fine specificity and the exact Ch phenotype of the patient requires the assistance of a specialized laboratory with the appropriate reagents. The description of the polymorphism of Ch also explains the partial inhibition findings (10,41-45) described earlier. Obviously if the serum containing anti-Ch contains antibodies to several Ch determinants and the plasma used in the inhibition tests carries one or more and lacks one or more of those determinants, partial inhibition will occur. As mentioned above, total inhibition of anti-Ch, regardless of the fine specificity of the antibodies present, will invariably occur if pooled plasma (say from three or more individuals) is used. The chance that several random plasmas will all lack the same Ch epitope is essentially nil.

Anti-Rg has thus far been found (43,44) in the serum of individuals phenotypically Rg:-1,-2; all examples have contained anti-Rg1 and anti-Rg2. In other words, the polymorphism of Rg can be demonstrated, at the serological level, only by partial inhibition of anti-Rg1 plus anti-Rg2 with plasma from a person of phenotype Rg:1,-2. The Rg polymorphism can, of course, also be recognized by determination of the amino acid sequence of C4 allotypes (50,64,67).

The Ch and Rg phenotypes as determined in a limited number of English and Japanese donors are shown in table 27-3. By now it will be abundantly apparent why the terms Ch and Rg must be used in routine situations (where the full phenotypes are not known and do not need to be known) and why the terms Ch[a] and Rg[a] as previously used (81) are no longer suitable.

Monoclonal Anti-Ch, Anti-Rg and Anti-C4

Murine monoclonal antibodies to C4d have been

TABLE 27-3 Incidence of Some Ch and Rg
Phenotypes in English and
Japanese Donors (42,48,112)

Phenotype	Number and (%) Found in 309 English Donors	Number and (%) Found in 89 Japanese Donors
Ch:1,2,3	272 (88%)	67 (75%)
Ch:1,-2,3	15 (5%)	21 (24%)
Ch:1,2,-3	9 (3%)	0
Ch:1,-2,-3	Less than 1%	
Ch:-1,2,-3	Less than 1%	
Ch:-1,-2,-3	12 (4%)	1 (1%)
Rg:1,2	294 (95%)	89 (100%)
Rg:1,-2	9 (3%)	0
Rg:-1,-2	6 (2%)	0

produced and initially it appeared (82) that some of them defined C4A or C4B. However, tests (83,83) using red cells coated with C4 from individuals in whom Ch was carried on C4A instead of C4B and Rg was carried on C4B instead of C4A, showed that the monoclonal antibodies were apparently anti-Ch1 and anti-Rg1. Monoclonal anti-Ch3 has also been made (85). We are not aware of any studies on anti-C4, particularly anti-C4d, made in rabbits and goats, in terms of any relationship to anti-Ch and anti-Rg.

C4 Deficiency and Disease Associations

Total C4 deficiency is a genetically determined defect that is often associated with disease states such as systemic lupus erythematosus (SLE) or lupus-like syndromes (55,57,86-99). Of 18 patients with total C4 deficiency, 14 had SLE (113,114). The homozygous presence of *C4A*QO* or *C4B*QO* is sometimes associated with other diseases, e.g. Graves disease, systemic sclerosis, rheumatoid arthritis, Sjogren's syndrome, juvenile dermatomyositis, IgA neuropathy, subacute sclerosing panencephalities and increased susceptibility to bacterial meningitis. Full references to all these associations are given in Chapter 6. Presence of *C4B*QO* in individuals infected with HIV may be associated with the progression of ARC (AIDS related-complex) to AIDS (acquired immune deficiency syndrome) (100,101).

It would be expected that C4 deficient individuals would be of the Ch-, Rg- phenotype (i.e. Ch:-1,-2,-3,-4, -5,-6, Rg:-1,-2, WH-) and indeed in most instances this has proved to be the case (13,103-105) (several different C4-deficient individuals described in some of those publications). On a number of occasions (102,103,105) it ini-

tially appeared that C4-deficient individuals had Ch-, Rg-plasma but had Ch and/or Rg on the red cells. Giles and Swanson (105) believe that these apparently contradictory findings probably represented the presence of anti-Bg (anti-HLA, see Chapter 32) in the anti-Ch and anti-Rg reagents. The presence of anti-Bg and anti-Ch or anti-Rg in the same serum is a relatively common event (106).

The *C4* Locus is on Chromosome 6

With what has been written in this chapter about Ch and Rg being determinants carried on C4d and the linkage between *C4* and *HLA* it is hardly necessary to add that production of the determinants is encoded by genes on chromosome 6 (107). A number of excellent articles about *C4* and about chromosome 6 have been published (108-111).

The Structure and Function of C4

C4 is synthesized as a single polypeptide chain of approximately 1700 amino acids. This precursor polypeptide chain is then postranslationally modified by cleavage with a plasmin-like protease to yield the mature C4 molecule. The precursor polypeptide chain is folded and its structure defined by intrachain disulfide bonds. Proteolytic cleavage of the precursor chain at two sites creates three polypeptide chains (α, β, γ) (115, see figure 27-1). The α chain has a molecular weight of 94-96kDa and contains three N-glycans. The β chain has a molecular weight of 72-77kDa and contains a single N-linked high-mannose oligosaccharide. The γ chain has a molecular weight of 32-35kDa and is not glycosylated (116).

When complement is activated by the classical pathway (see Chapter 6) C1 binds to antigen-antibody complexes and becomes activated so that it can enzymatically cleave C4 and C2. C4 is cleaved into fragments known as $C\overline{4a}$ and $C\overline{4b}$. $C\overline{4a}$ is a small peptide released from the amino-terminus of the α chain. $C\overline{4b}$ has an intramolecular thioester located in the α chain which becomes accessible when $C\overline{4a}$ is released. This thioester can form covalent bonds with hydroxyl or amino groups on another surface and it is through such linkages that $C\overline{4b}$ becomes bound to red cells. The biological function of this thioester is to effect the binding of $C\overline{4b}$ to microorganisms and thereby mark them for destruction by the later components of complement. Bound $C\overline{4b}$ provides a site which triggers the formation of the membrane attack complex on the surface of the microorganism (117). $C\overline{4b}$ acts as an acceptor for the activated form of C2 ($C\overline{2b}$) and the complex of $C\overline{4b2b}$ comprises C3 convertase which cleaves C3 to activate $C\overline{3b}$ which also has a thioester and can covalently bind to microorganisms (and red cells) further facilitating their destruction by the later components of complement. CR1 on red cells recognizes C$\overline{4b}$ and C$\overline{3b}$ bound to immune complexes and effects their clearance from the circulation by transporting them to phagocytes in the liver (see Chapters 6 and 28 for further discussions of CR1).

Complex regulatory systems exist for degrading C$\overline{4b}$ and C$\overline{3b}$. A number of "cofactor" proteins (factor H, C4 binding protein (C4bp), CR1 and membrane cofactor protein (MCP)) (see also Chapter 6) can form a noncovalent complex with C$\overline{4b}$ or C$\overline{3b}$ and this complex formation facilitates further proteolytic cleavage of C$\overline{4b}$ and C$\overline{3b}$ by a protease known as factor I (118,119). Factor I cleaves C$\overline{4b}$ at two sites on the α chain leaving only a small peptide fragment (C$\overline{4d}$) bound through the thioester bond (see figure 27-1). The Chido and Rogers system antigens are located in the C$\overline{4d}$ fragment and it is the binding of C$\overline{4d}$ to red cells which has led to the inclusion of Ch/Rg in the world of blood groups.

There are two isotypes of C4 now known as C4A and C4B which can be distinguished by their electrophoretic mobility (62). Most people have both isotypes but about 5% lack either C4A or C4B (15,107). Family studies indicated that C4A and C4B derived from two closely linked genes (13,15).

Structure of the *C4A* and *C4B* Genes

The genes giving rise to C4A and C4B are about 10kb apart on chromosome 6. When cDNA sequences for *C4A* and *C4B* were first compared they were found to be remarkably homologous. There were only 14 nucleotide differences between the two cDNAs and 12 of these were found in the C4d fragment where they resulted in 9 amino acid differences (59). Subsequent studies on other cDNAs and genomic clones established the structural basis of the electrophoretic, serological and functional differences between the isotypes (120,121).

The structure of the *C4A* gene (specifically the *C4A3* allele) was elucidated by Yu (54) by sequencing almost all the gene in a cosmid clone (only the large intron 9 which comprises 6-7kb was not fully sequenced). The gene spans 21kb and comprises 41 exons (see figure 27-2). The coding sequences for the proteolytic cleavage sites at the β-α and α-γ chain junctions are located in the middle of exons 16 and 33 respectively. The β chain (656 residues) is encoded by exons 1-16. Exon 1 encodes a leader sequence of 19 residues and the first three residues of the precursor polypeptide. The single N-glycan (high-mannose) site found at residue 207 in the β chain is encoded by exon 6. The α chain (residues 661-1428) is encoded by exons 16-33. The three N-glycan sites found on this chain are from exon 20 (residue 843), exon 30

(residue 1309) and exon 32 (residue 1372) respectively. The γ chain (291 residues) is encoded by exons 33-41. Three tyrosine O-sulfation sites are encoded by exon 33. The C4A gene shows substantial homology with the genes giving rise to C3, C5 and α₂ macroglobulin suggesting that they have a common evolutionary origin.

The two cleavage sites for factor I are encoded by exons 23 and 30 respectively and it is this region of the gene that encodes C4d and contains: the polymorphic sites giving rise to Rogers determinants; the thioester site (formed by Cys994 and Gln997 from exon 24); and the residues that distinguish the C4A and C4B isotypes.

The Isotypic and Functional Differences Between C4A and C4B are Defined by Amino Acid Sequence Differences in C4d

Yu (54) notes that 20 polymorphic amino acid residues had been detected in C4 molecules by 1991. Fourteen of these polymorphic residues form a cluster C-terminal of the thioester site in the C4d fragment. C4B has a 3-4 fold greater hemolytic activity than C4A and this relates to the different efficiencies of C4B and C4A in covalently binding to red cells coated with antibody and C1 (122-124). C4A binds to a greater extent (3-fold higher than C4B) when C1 is on immune complexes (124). These functional differences between the isotypes are related to the nature of the amino acids in the polymorphic cluster C-terminal of the thioester site in C4d and in particular, residues 1101,1102, 1105 and 1106 (Pro, Cys, Leu, Asp in C4A; Leu, Ser, Ile, His in C4B) (121). Carroll et al. (124) constructed a series of chimeric C4A/C4B molecules and site-directed mutants to determine more precisely the functional importance of these residues. These authors found that Asp1106 was critical for C4A binding to immune complexes since by changing His1106 to Asp in C4B, the protein became as efficient as wild type C4A in performing this function. Somewhat surprisingly the mutation His1106 to Ala in C4B had the same functional activity as His1106 to Asp. When the binding to immune complexes was high the C4 bound covalently via an amide linkage. When binding to red cells was high the C4 bound covalently via an ester linkage (124). The results in relation to critical residues for hemolytic activity on red cells were less striking but suggested that both Cys1102 and His1106 contributed to the greater activity of C4B over C4A.

The Molecular Basis of Rg and Ch Antigens

A very fruitful collaboration involving the expert serological skills of Dr. Carolyn Giles formerly of the

FIGURE 27-2 The *C4A* gene and the C4A Precursor Polypeptide (adapted from reference 54)

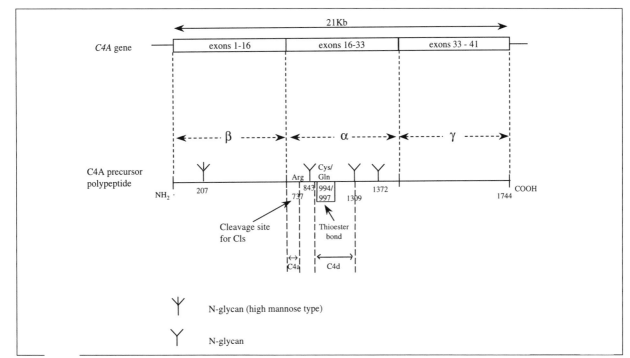

International Blood Group Reference Laboratory but then at the Hammersmith Hospital in London and the expert biochemical skills of Professor Rodney Porter's laboratory at the University of Oxford led to the elucidation of a model to account for the Rg and Ch antigens in the mid to late 1980s. The isotype-specific residues that define the functionality of C4A and C4B described in the previous section proved to be relevant to the structure of Rg and Ch antigens. Expression of the antigen Ch4 correlates with the C4B isotype-specific residues Leu1101, Ser1102, Ile1105, His1106. Ch2 also recognizes this sequence of residues but in addition, the C4B-specific residue Gly1054 is also required. Ch5 is defined by Gly1054.

Residues Val1188-Asp-Leu-Leu in C4A probably define the Rg1 antigen and the corresponding residues Ala1188-Asp-Leu-Arg in C4B define Ch1. Anti-Rg2 recognizes the same sequence as anti-Rg1 but also requires Asn1157 on the C4A molecule. The equivalent antigen to Rg2 on the C4B molecule is Ch3 which comprises the same sequence as Ch1 but requires in addition Ser1157. Ch6 is defined by Ser1157 on C4B (50,51, and see table 27-2).

It is obvious from the forgoing discussion that Ch antigens are generally found on C4B and Rg antigens on C4A. However, this is not always the case. C4A isotypes occasionally express Ch antigens and vice versa. Indeed, Ch+ Rg- C4A and Ch- Rg+ C4B allotypes were influential in defining the critical importance of residues 1101-1106 and 1188-1191 in defining Ch and Rg antigens.

Such hybrid *C4* genes may result from unequal cross-over events (48) or perhaps more likely, from gene conversion (54). Because C4B is more efficient than C4A in binding to red cells, it might be expected that, at the serological level, anti-Ch would be easier to detect than anti-Rg. That this indeed may be the case is reflected by the experience of most workers that anti-Ch is more common than anti-Rg. This in spite of the fact that some 3% of random individuals can make alloimmune anti-Rg (7) while only about 2% can make alloimmune anti-Ch (1).

References

1   Harris JP, Tegoli J, Swanson J, et al. Vox Sang 1967;12:140
2. Molthan L. (abstract). Book of Abstracts 13th Cong ISBT 1972:57
3. Humphreys J, Stout TD, Middleton J, et al. (abstract). Book of Abstracts 13th Cong ISBT 1972:57
4. Middleton J. Canad J Med Technol 1972;34:41
5. Middleton J, Crookston MC. Vox Sang 1972;23:256
6. Molthan L. Lab Med 1983;14:303
7. Longster G, Giles CM. Vox Sang 1976;30:175
8. Giles CM, Gedde-Dahl T, Robson EB, et al. Tissue Antigens 1976;8:143
9. James J, Stiles P, Boyce F, et al. Vox Sang 1976;30:214
10. Nordhagen R, Olaisen B, Teisberg P, et al. J Immunogenet 1981;8:485
11. Middleton J, Crookston MC, Falk JA, et al. Tissue Antigens 1974;4:366
12. Ochs HD, Rosenfeld SJ, Thomas ED, et al. New Eng J Med 1977;296:470

13. O'Neill GJ, Yang SY, Tegoli J, et al. Nature 1978;273:668
14. O'Neill GJ, Yang SY, Berger R, et al. Fed Proc 1978;37:1269
15. O'Neill GJ, Yang SY, Dupont B. Proc Nat Acad Sci USA 1978;75:5165
16. Tilley CA, Romans DG, Crookston MC. (abstract). Book of Abstracts 16th Cong ISBT 1978:685
17. Tilley CA, Romans DG, Crookston MC. (abstract). Transfusion 1978;18:622
18. Tilley CA, Romans DG, Crookston MC. Nature 1978;276:713
19. Weitkamp L, Francke U. Cytogenet Cell Genet 1978;22:92
20. Judd WJ, Kraemer K, Moulds JJ. Transfusion 1981;21:189
21. Ellisor SS, Shoemaker MM, Reid ME. Transfusion 1982;22:243
22. Lomas CG, Green CA, Atkins C, et al. Med Lab Sci 1983;40:65
23. Rittner C, Tippett P, Giles CM, et al. Vox Sang 1984;46:224
24. Judd WJ. Methods in Immunohematology, 2nd Ed. Durham:Montgomery, 1994
25. Nordhagen R, Heier Larsen AM, Beckers D. Vox Sang 1979;37:170
26. Atkins CJ. MSc Thesis, Brunel Univ 1985
27. Ewald RA, Williams JH, Bowden DH. Vox Sang 1961;6:312
28. Adinolfi M, Zenthon J. Rev Perinat Med 1984;5:61
29. Giles CM, Davies KA, Walport MJ. Transfusion 1991;31:222
30. Wilfert K, Atkins CJ, Tippett P. (abstract). Transf Med 1991;1 (Suppl 1):57
31. Tippett P, Storry JR, Walker PS, et al. (abstract). Transfusion 1994;34 (Suppl 10S):61S
32. Edwards JM, Moulds JJ, Judd WJ. Transfusion 1982;22:59
33. Szymanski IO, Huff SR, Delsignore R. Transfusion 1982;22:90
34. Moore HC, Issitt PD, Pavone BG. Transfusion 1975;15:266
35. Tilley CA, Crookston MC, Haddad SA, et al. Transfusion 1977;17:169
36. Silvergleid AJ, Wells RF, Hafleigh EB, et al. Transfusion 1978;18:8
37. Nordhagen R, Aas M. Vox Sang 1979;37:179
38. Westhoff CM, Sipherd BD, Wylie DE, et al. Transfusion 1992;32:576
39. Strohm PL, Molthan L. Vox Sang 1983;45:48
40. Lambin P, Le Pennec PY, Hauptmann G, et al. Vox Sang 1984;47:242
41. Nordhagen R, Olaisen B, Teisberg P, et al. J Immunogenet 1980;7:301
42. Giles CM. Vox Sang 1984;46:149
43. Giles CM. Vox Sang 1985;48:160
44. Giles CM. Vox Sang 1985;48:167
45. Giles CM, Batchelor JR, Dodi IA, et al. J Immunogenet 1984;11:305
46. Rittner CH, Giles CM, Roos MH, et al. Immunogenetics 1984;19:321
47. Yu CY, Campbell RD. Immunogenetics 1987;25:383
48. Giles CM. Exp Clin Immunogenet 1988;5:99
49. Atkinson JP, Chan AC, Karp DR, et al. Complement 1988;5:65
50. Yu CY, Campbell RD, Porter RR. Immunogenetics 1988;27:399
51. Giles CM, Uring-Lambert B, Goetz J, et al. Immunogenetics 1988;27:442
52. Braun L, Schneider PM, Giles CM, et al. J Exp Med 1990;171:129
53. Mauff G, Alper CA, Dawkins RL, et al. Compl Inflamm 1991;7:261
54. Yu CY. J Immunol 1991;146:1057
55. Moulds JM. In: Blood Groups: Ch/Rg, Kn/McC/Yk and Cr. Bethesda:Am Assoc Blood Banks, 1992:13
56. Barba GMR, Braun-Heimer L, Rittner C, et al. Eur J Immunogenet 1994;21:325
57. Moulds JM. In: Immunobiology of Transfusion Medicine. New York:Marcel Dekker 1994:273
58. Colten HR. In: Immunobiology of the Complement System. An Introduction for Research and Clinical Medicine. New York:Academic, 1986:174
59. Belt KT, Carroll MC, Porter RR. Cell 1984;36:907
60. Carroll MC, Belt KT, Palsdotirr A, et al. Immunol Rev 1985;87:39
61. Campbell RD, Carroll MC, Porter RR. Adv Immunol 1986;38:203
62. Rosenfeld SI, Ruddy S, Austen KF. J Clin Invest 1969;48:2283
63. Mauff G, Alper CA, Awdeh Z, et al. Immunobiology 1983;164:184
64. WHO-IUIS Nomenclature Subcommittee. Eur J Immunogenet 1993;20:301
65. Lewis M, Anstee DJ, Bird GWG, et al. Vox Sang 1990;58:152
66. Giles CM. Hum Immunol 1987;18:111
67. Giles CM, Jones JW. Immunogenetics 1987;26:392
68. Roos MH, Giles CM, Demant P, et al. J Immunol 1984;133:2634
69. Poole J, Moulds JM, Fisher B, et al. (abstract). Transfusion 1996;36 (Suppl 9S):55S
70. Palsdottir A, Arnason A, Fossdal R, et al. Hum Genet 1987;76:220
71. Bruun-Petersen G, Lamm LU, Jacobsen BK, et al. Hum Genet 1982;61:36
72. Raum D, Awdeh Z, Andersen J, et al. Am J Hum Genet 1984;36:72
73. Carroll MC, Belt KT, Palsdottir A, et al. Phil Trans Roy Soc London Series B 1984;306:379
74. Giles CM, Uring-Lambert B, Boksch W, et al. Hum Genet 1987;77:359
75. Teisberg P, Jonassen R, Mevag B, et al. Ann Hum Genet 1988;52:77
76. Carroll MC, Palsdottir A, Belt KT, et al. EMBO J 1985;4:2547
77. Schneider PM, Carroll MC, Alper CA, et al. J Clin Invest 1986;78:650
78. Barba G, Rittner C, Schneider PM. J Clin Invest 1993;91:1681
79. Giles CM, Hoffman M, Moulds M, et al. Vox Sang 1987;52:129
80. Fisher B, Laycock C, Poole J, et al. (abstract). Transf Med 1993;3 (Suppl 1):84
81. Issitt PD. Applied Blood Group Serology, 3rd Ed. Miami:Montgomery, 1985:420
82. O'Neill GJ, Nerl CW, Hauptmann G, et al. (abstract). Immunobiology 1986;173:466
83. Giles CM, Ford DS. Transfusion 1986;26:370
84. Giles CM, Fielder AHL, Lord DK, et al. Immunogenetics 1987;26:309
85. Chrispeels J, Grabbe J, Stradmann B, et al. Complement 1987;4:142
86. Hauptmann G, Grosshans E, Heid E, et al. Ann Derm Syph 1974;101:479
87. Schaller JG, Gilliland BG, Ochs HD, et al. Arthr Rheum 1977;20:1519
88. Ballow M, McLean RH, Yunis EJ, et al. Clin Immunobiol Immunopathol 1981;20:354
89. Urowitz MB, Gladman DD, Minta JO. J Rheumatol 1981;8:741

90. Kjellman M, Laurell AB, Löw B, et al. Clin Genet 1982;22:331
91. Porter RR. Mol Biol Med 1983;1:161
92. Fielder AHL, Walport MJ, Batchelor JR, et al. Br Med J 1983;286:425
93. Reveille JD, Arnett FC, Wilson RW, et al. Immunogenetics 1985;21:299
94. Dunckley H, Gatenby PA, Hawkins B, et al. J Immunogenet 1987;14:209
95. Kemp ME, Atkinson JP, Skanes VM, et al. Arthr Rheum 1987;30:1015
96. Goldstein R, Arnett FC, McLean RH, et al. Arthr Rheum 1988;31:736
97. Wilson WA, Perez MC, Michalski JP, et al. J Rheumatol 1988;15:1768
98. Kumar A, Kumar P, Schur PH. Clin Immunol Immunopathol 1991;60:55
99. Fan Q, Uring-Lambert B, Weill B, et al. Eur J Immunogenet1993;20:11
100. Cameron PU, Cobain TJ, Zhang WJ, et al. Br Med J 1988;296:1627
101. Plum G, Siebel E, Bendick C, et al. (abstract). Vox Sang 1990;59 (Suppl 1):15
102. O'Neill GJ, Berger R, Ballow M, et al. Transp Proc 1979;11:1941
103. O'Neill GJ. Sem Hematol 1981;18:32
104. Crookston MC, Tilley CA. In: Blood Groups and Other Red Cell Surface Markers in Health and Disease. New York:Masson, 1982:111
105. Giles CM, Swanson JL. Vox Sang 1984;46:291
106. Swanson JL. In: Recent Advances in Immunohematology. Washington, D.C.:Am Assoc Blood Banks, 1973:121
107. Teisberg P, Akesson I, Olaisen B, et al. Nature 1976;264:253
108. Alper CA, Raum D, Karp S, et al. Vox Sang 1983;45:62
109. Carroll MC, Campbell RD, Bentley DR, et al. Nature 1984;307:237
110. Carroll MC, Alper CA. Br Med Bull 1987;43:50
111. Ziegler A, Field LL, Sakaguchi AY. Cytogenet Cell Genet 1991;58:295
112. Giles CM, Tokunaga K, Zhang WJ, et al. J Immunogenet 1988;15:267
113. Hauptmann G, Goetz J, Uring-Lambert B, et al. Prog Allgy 1986;39:239
114. de Massias IJT, Reis A, Brenden M, et al. Compl Inflamm 1991;8:288
115. Schreiber RD, Müller-Eberhard HJ. J Exp Med 1974;140:1324
116. Chan AC, Atkinson JP. J Immunol 1985;134:1790
117. Kinoshita T. Immunol Today 1991;12:291
118. Reid KBM, Bentley DR, Campbell RD, et al. Immunol Today 1986;7:230
119. Campbell RD, Law SKA, Reid KBM, et al. Ann Rev Immunol 1988;6:161
120. Belt KT, Yu YC, Carroll MC, et al. Immunogenetics 1985;21:173
121. Yu CY, Belt KT, Giles CM, et al. EMBO J 1986;5:2873
122. Isenman DE, Young JR. J Immunol 1986;132:3019
123. Law SKA, Dodds AW, Porter RR. EMBO J 1984;3:1819
124. Carroll MC, Fathallah DM, Bergamaschini L, et al. Proc Nat Acad Sci USA 1990;87:6868
125. Wibaut B, Mannessier L, Horbez C, et al. (Letter). Vox Sang 1995;69:150

In 1970, Helgeson et al. (1) described an antibody that reacted with the red cells of all except four of 2091 unrelated donors. The antibody was called anti-Kn^a and the red cells of the antibody-maker's sib were found to be Kn(a+). However, during the investigation (1) it was found that the red cells of the first author of the report, Margaret Helgeson, and those of one of her four sibs, were Kn(a-). The senior author of the paper donated two units of blood that were transfused to the patient! It was clear from the outset that anti-Kn^a is not particularly uncommon, a total of seven examples are mentioned in the first paper. Since the original report it has become appreciated (see below) that a number of other high incidence antigens and perhaps some of low incidence that may be their antithetical partners, are associated with Kn^a. In serological studies, with many examples of these antibodies, the Helgeson cells give negative reactions. This has led to use of the term Helgeson phenotype to describe red cells that in many practical situations appear to be of the null phenotype in the system. In fact, as described in more detail below, non-reactivity of the Helgeson phenotype red cells results because of low antigen site numbers on those cells. Nevertheless, at the serological level, use of red cells of the Helgeson (nearly null) phenotype has been instrumental in expansion of the system.

In 1978, Molthan and Moulds (2) described another new antibody, that they named anti-McC^a, that defines a high incidence antigen, and showed that the antigen defined was somehow related to Kn^a. The relationship was seen via the incidence of the Kn(a-) McC(a-) phenotype. Although 98% of random bloods from US Whites and Blacks are Kn(a+) (1,3) and over 98% from US Whites and between 93 and 96% from US Blacks are McC(a+) (2,3) it was found (2) that among 90 persons with McC(a-) red cells, 48 (53%) had cells that were Kn(a-) as well. Had Kn^a and McC^a had nothing to do with each other, some two or three Kn(a-) samples would have been expected among the 90 that were McC(a-).

In 1980, another antibody defining a high incidence antigen that is related to Kn^a and McC^a was described. At the same meeting Lacey et al. (4) called the antibody anti-Sl^a while Molthan (5) called it anti-McC^c. Since the name anti-McC^c can be taken to suggest that McC^a and McC^c are the products of alleles, which they are not, the name Sl^a is preferred by most workers. The association between Sl^a, Kn^a and McC^a was based on the findings (4-8) that all Black individuals of the McC(a-) phenotype, regardless of their Kn(a+) or Kn(a-) status, are Sl(a-).

The Sl(a-) phenotype was not confined to those with McC(a-) red cells, some 45% of Blacks are phenotypically Kn(a+) McC(a+) Sl(a-). All Whites with Kn(a-) McC(a-) red cells were also found to be phenotypically Sl(a-) although the incidence of the Sl(a-) phenotype in Whites with Kn(a+) McC(a+) red cells is only about 1%. Thus by 1980 it had become apparent that the Helgeson phenotype appears, at the serological level, to be Kn(a-) McC(a-) Sl(a-).

In 1980, Mallan et al. (9) described an antibody that reacted with the red cells of some 4% of White Australian donors and with the red cells of White individuals of the Kn(a-) phenotype except when those cells were Kn(a-) McC(a-) i.e. of the Helgeson phenotype. Mallan et al. (9) suggested that the antibody defines Kn^b, the antithetical partner of Kn^a (that would be expected to be absent from red cells of the Helgeson, i.e. close to null phenotype). However, Molthan (7) reported that the Kn(a-) (non-Helgeson type) red cells of Blacks are Kn(b-) and suggested that in Blacks a different antigen might represent an antithetical partner to Kn^a. As far as we are aware, no other example of anti-Kn^b has been found. The Kn^b antigen has been assigned an ISBT number as part of the Knops system.

In 1983, Molthan (6) described an antibody that she called anti-McC^b, that was said to react with the Kn(a+) McC(a-) red cells of Blacks but not with those, of a similar phenotype, from Whites. Work with anti-McC^b has foundered in part because of scarcity of the antibody and in part because like the so-called anti-McC^d, anti-McC^e and anti-McC^f (6-8) results with anti-McC^b could not be duplicated by others. The antigen defined by the antibody that was called anti-McC^b has not been given an ISBT number.

When reporting anti-Sl^a, Lacey et al. (4) described a serum, Vil, that appeared to define an antigen antithetical to Sl^a, in Blacks. No Vil+ White person was found. We are not aware of any further report concerning the Vil serum or of any report describing an antigen antithetical to Sl^a in Whites. While pointing out that the antibody in the Vil serum might be defining an antigen antithetical to Sl^a, Lacey et al. (4), with due caution, avoided use of the term Sl^b for the antigen defined. For the sake of completeness that term is used, tentatively, in table 28-1. No ISBT term has been assigned to the antigen defined by the Vil antibody.

Some time before the antibodies to Kn^a, McC^a and Sl^a were found, two other antibodies to antigens of high incidence had been reported. Giles et al. (11) described an antibody, that they named anti-Cs^a, in the sera Copeland and Stirling, that reacted with the red cells of 98% of random White donors. The antibody was studied extensively by Giles (12). In 1969, four years after anti-Cs^a had been described, Molthan et al. (13) first described anti-Yk^a, a full report was published (14) in 1975. The Yk^a antigen was said to be present on the red cells of 92% of US Whites and 98% of US Blacks. In the paper on Yk^a (14) the frequency of Cs^a in US Whites and Blacks was reported. Of 626 US Whites, 25 (4%) had Cs(a-) red cells. Of 329 US Blacks, 4 (1.2%) had Cs(a-) red cells. Based on these antigen frequencies it can be calculated that the frequency of the phenotype Cs(a-), Yk(a-) should be about 1 in 213 (0.32%) in US Whites and 1 in 4166 (0.024%) in US Blacks if Cs^a and Yk^a are not associated with each other. The observed frequency (14) of the Cs(a-), Yk(a-) phenotype in US Whites was 1 in 52 (1.9%) and in US Blacks 1 in 165 (0.6%). Clearly, those figures strongly suggested an association between Cs^a and Yk^a. However, it was also reported (14) that in two of three informative families, *Cs^a* and *Yk^a* segregated independently. After these early combined studies, the authors presented data that were in conflict. Giles (15) continued to believe that one of the families demonstrated independent segregation even when the results with one of the anti-Yk^a had to be reinterpreted. Giles (15) attributed the discrepancies to heterogeneity of the anti-Yk^a that had been used. A serum Sieb was said to include the reactions of the original (York) anti-Yk^a but other examples of anti-Yk^a such as one investigated by Tilley and Crookston (16), were said to contain the Sieb type anti-Yk^a but to react with the red cells of the individual who made the York type anti-Yk^a. Giles (15) also reported that anti-Yk^a did not react with ficin-treated Yk(a+) red cells while the actions of anti-Cs^a were unaltered in tests against ficin-treated Cs(a+) red cells. Workers who were active during the early investigations of Cs^a and Yk^a will no doubt recall the difficulties that arose due to heterogeneity of anti-Cs^a and anti-Yk^a. The supposedly definitive Cs(a-), Yk(a+); Cs(a+), Yk(a-); and Cs(a-), Yk(a-) red cells samples gave various combinations of phenotypes, dependent on which anti-Cs^a and anti-Yk^a had been used to classify them.

Molthan (17) claimed that not only were Cs^a and Yk^a associated with each other, but that they were part of the same system to which Kn^a and McC^a belonged. Molthan (17) also believed that the family data had been misinterpreted and that none of the published families, nor any others that she had studied, denied linkage between *Cs^a* and *Yk^a*. Finally, Molthan (17) claimed that all of 19 anti-Yk^a that she studied reacted with ficin-treated Yk(a+) red cells. As described later in this section (where references are given) it is now known that Yk^a is part of the Knops system but Cs^a is not. At least some of

these early discrepancies can be attributed to the fact that the original red cells of the Helgeson phenotype (those of Margaret Helgeson herself (1)), that were often the only cells of that phenotype available during the early studies, type as Kn(a-) McC(a-) Sl(a-) Yk(a-) and Cs(a-). However, it has now been shown (18) that at least three other persons with the Helgeson phenotype have red cells that type as Kn(a-) McC(a-) Sl(a-) Yk(a-) but Cs(a+). Currently there is no explanation for the observed phenotypic association between Yk^a and Cs^a. Since Cs^a (and its supposed antithetical partner Cs^b (19)) are not part of the Knops system, their full description will be found in Chapter 30.

Antibodies to Kn^a, McC^a, Sl^a and Yk^a are difficult to study at the serological level. They often display characteristics of the so-called high titer, low avidity (HTLA, see Chapter 30) antibodies (20) although, as discussed below, the apparent low avidity almost certainly relates more to the paucity of antigen sites on red cells than to the avidity of the antibodies. Strong reactions with the antibodies, that usually react by IAT, are seldom seen, the reactions with weakly positive red cells are difficult to reproduce and, as discussed below, the near null type (Helgeson phenotype) is not truly null. In addition to antibodies to Kn^a, McC^a, Sl^a and Yk^a, most workers will have encountered antibodies that react weakly with all red cells except those of the antibody-maker and those of the Helgeson phenotype but cannot be shown to have specificity for one of the antigens listed. These antibodies are often called, in house, anti-Kn^a-like or anti-Kn/McC and do not get described in the literature because of the lack of definitive results. In a series of papers, that included many otherwise undocumented findings, published between 1980 and 1983, Molthan (3,5-8,21) extended her McC terminology. While McC^a, McC^b and McC^c, that have been mentioned above were included, the papers, among them, introduced McC^d, McC^e and McC^f. In retrospect it seems probable that at least some of the antibodies were what others (see above) have called anti-Kn^a-like or anti-Kn/McC. We are not aware of duplication of the described findings (3,5-8,21) by others although the reports mention that 16 examples of anti-McC^e and five examples of anti-McC^f were studied. One of us (PDI) had the opportunity to study some of the sera described in the various reports but was unable to obtain repeatable results (many of the antibodies gave equivocal reactions by IAT) and could not even approach duplication of the precision with which Molthan (6,7) documented antigen, phenotype and gene frequencies.

Some order was brought to the rather chaotic situation described above in 1991 when, following independent but simultaneous studies, Rao et al. (22) and Moulds et al. (23) reported that the Knops system antigens are carried on CR1 (complement receptor 1, CD35). As described in more detail below, Kn^a, McC^a, Sl^a and Yk^a were shown to be carried on CR1, Cs^a was not found to be similarly located. These observations showed that production of Kn^a, Kn^b, McC^a, Sl^a and Yk^a is encoded from a locus independent of those of all other blood group systems and resulted in recognition (24) of Knops as an independent blood group system. Before this, those five antigens together with Cs^a and Cs^b had been considered (25) to be part of a phenotypic collection (Collection 205, COST, for definition of a collection see Chapters 1 and 30). Table 28-1 lists the conventional and ISBT terminology for the Knops system, table 28-2 presents data from a large number of studies on the incidence of these antigens in Whites and Blacks.

As with some of the previous chapters, the next sections of this one describe the antigens of the Knops system as antithetical pairs, where such pairs exist, or as single entities. This is done to enable workers dealing with one particular antibody of the system to find pertinent information quickly. The antigens are considered as a whole in later sections.

The Antigens Kn^a and Kn^b and the Antibodies That Define Them

As shown in table 28-2, Kn^a is of high incidence, i.e. circa 98.8%, in both Whites and Blacks. Kn^b was found

TABLE 28-1 Conventional and ISBT Terminology for the Knops Blood Group System

Conventional Name: Knops
Conventional Symbol: Kn
ISBT System Symbol: KN
ISBT System Number: 022

Historical Name	Antigen Conventional Name	ISBT Antigen Number	ISBT Full Code Number
Knops	Kn^a	KN1	022001
Hall	Kn^b	KN2	022002
McCoy	McC^a	KN3	022003
	McC^b	*	*
Swain-Langley	Sl^a	KN4	022004
Vil	? Sl^b	*	*
York	Yk^a	KN5	022005

* Not recognized by the ISBT Working Party as antigens of the Knops System, no number assigned. For details, see text.

(9) to have an incidence between 4 and 5% in Australian and US Whites. Kn^a antigen strength on different Kn(a+) samples varies widely, the variations are apparently not related to the Kn^aKn^a and Kn^aKn^b genotypes (1,9). As discussed in the section on the Helgeson phenotype, the level of detectable Kn^a antigen does correlate with the number of copies of CR1 (18). Both Kn^a and Kn^b appear to be fully developed at birth (9,25) but neither anti-Kn^a nor anti-Kn^b has caused HDN. The only known example of anti-Kn^b was present in the serum of a woman who gave birth to an unaffected infant whose red cells were Kn(b+). The case (9) was unusual in that the red cells of the proposita's mother were Kn(a-). Presumably she could not have been Kn^bKn^b since her daughter had Kn(a+b-) red cells and made the only known example of anti-Kn^b. Perhaps the mother was heterozygous for the gene responsible for the Helgeson phenotype and passed that gene to her daughter.

Kn^a is denatured when red cells are treated with trypsin or chymotrypsin (26) but is usually detectable on red cells treated with papain or ficin (3,26). Some variation of this last characteristic is seen based on how the papain or ficin is used and on the individual example of the antibody. Kn^a is partially or wholly denatured (again somewhat dependent on the antibody used) when red cells are treated with 2-aminoethylisothiouronium bromide (AET) or with dithiothreitol (26-28). Marsh et al. (29) reported that even when AET-treated Kn(a+) red cells no longer react visibly with anti-Kn^a, they are capable of adsorbing the antibody. This is perhaps a little surprising since untreated Kn(a+) red cells are not usually very efficient at adsorbing anti-Kn^a.

Like other antibodies of the system, anti-Kn^a is not easy to work with in serological studies. Most examples react by IAT but often display the characteristics of HTLA antibodies (see later for information about paucity of antigen sites). While some anti-Kn^a clearly distinguish between Kn(a+) and Kn(a-) red cells, many others give reactions such that interpretation of the Kn^a status of a subset of red cells is difficult. Adsorption-elution studies are not of very much value since weakly reactive Kn(a+) red cells are relatively ineffective in adsorbing the antibody that can then not always be recovered by elution from the adsorbing red cells. These problems are magnified considerably when old or traveled red cells are tested.

There are few reports in the literature about subclass composition of anti-Kn^a. Of two "anti-Kn/McC-like" antibodies studied, one (32) was IgG4, another (33) contained IgG1, IgG3, IgG4 and IgA components. It has also been stated (34) that IgG anti-Kn^a do not activate complement. Anti-Kn^a does not seem often, if ever, to be of clinical significance in transfusion therapy. Transfusions with antigen-positive red cells, in vivo red cell survival studies and in vitro phagocytic cell assays have all been

TABLE 28-2 Incidence of the Knops System Antigens

Antigen	Population Tested	Number Tested	Number and (%) Negative	Number and (%) Positive	References
Kn[a]	US Whites	4553	55 (1.2%)		1, 3
Kn[a]	US Blacks	894	11 (1.2%)		3
Kn[b]	Australians	166		7 (4.2%)	9
Kn[b]	US Whites	63		3 (4.8%)	9
McC[a]	US Whites	3860	58 (1.5%)		2, 3
McC[a]	US Blacks	1539	78 (5.1%)		2, 3
McC[b]	US Blacks	371	168 (45.3%)	203 (54.7%)	6, 7, 10
Sl[a]	US Whites	833	18 (2.2%)		4, 6
Sl[a]	US Blacks	480	223 (46.5%)	257 (53.5%)	4, 6
? Sl[b]	US Blacks	*1		80%	25
Yk[a]	US Whites	4021	389 (9.7%)		3, 14
Yk[a]	US Blacks	1891	32 (1.7%)		3, 14

For high incidence antigens, the incidence of the negative, and for lower incidence antigens, the incidence of the positive phenotypes are shown.

When two references are shown, the numbers of samples and the findings represent pooled data.

*1 It is stated (25) that "the frequency of Vil+ was 80% in a small series" of randomly selected samples from Blacks.

used to demonstrate either that anti-Kn[a] allows normal in vivo survival of Kn(a+) red cells or that if any accelerated red cell clearance did occur it was of too small a degree to affect the clinical outcome of the transfusions (1,31-33,35,36). Like the anti-Kn[b] described above, an example of anti-Kn[a] failed to cause HDN in an infant with Kn(a+) red cells (37), see also the section on McC[a].

The Antigen McC[a] and the Antibody That Defines It and a Note on the Antibody Called Anti-McC[b]

As shown in table 28-2, the McC[a] antigen has an incidence of about 98.5% in US Whites and about 95% in US Blacks (2,3). The level of McC[a] on different McC(a+) red cells is variable. As with Kn[a] the variation is related to antigen copy number and is largely independent of gene dose. Again like Kn[a], McC[a] is destroyed when red cells are treated with trypsin or chymotrypsin (26), is denatured or weakened when red cells are treated with AET or DTT (26-28) but the antigen, as defined by most examples of anti-McC[a], appears to survive treatment of red cells with papain or ficin (2,3,5,26). Molthan (3) reported that two of 33 examples of anti-McC[a] failed to react with ficin-treated McC(a+) red cells. Given the heterogeneity of antibodies to Kn[a], McC[a], Sl[a], Yk[a] and Cs[a], as described in the introduction of this chapter, one

cannot help but wonder if the two antibodies that failed to react, were actually anti-McC[a].

Like anti-Kn[a], anti-McC[a] often displays characteristics of an HTLA antibody. Most examples are IgG, few subclassing studies have been reported. One anti-McC[a] in a pregnant woman was found (40) to contain IgG1, 2, 3 and 4 components. Like anti-Yk[a] (see below), some half of all examples of anti-McC[a] are found in sera that contain immune, non-Knops system antibodies.

There is no doubt that the numerous examples of anti-McC[a] that have been studied by in vivo red cell survival studies and in vitro phagocytic cell assays were clinically benign. In many of the cases studied (2,31,38,39) and many others known to one of us (PDI) but not published because the event is so expected, the patients with anti-McC[a] were transfused with McC(a+) blood with no indications that the survival of the transfused red cells was other than totally normal.

Ferguson et al. (40) described two cases in which women with anti-McC[a] in the serum delivered infants whose cord blood red cells typed as McC(a-). In one case at 5 months and in the other at 11 months, the children's red cells typed as McC(a+). At the time that the second infant was born, 18 randomly selected cord bloods were typed, all were McC(a+) and reacted to a degree that when compared to tests on the red cells of adults, suggested that McC[a] is fully developed at birth. When the second infant was tested at 11 months, 50 additional cord blood samples were tested. Forty-nine were McC(a+), the 50th came from an infant born to a mother with McC(a+) red cells and no anti-McC^a in the serum. That case appeared to represent a genetically determined McC(a-) infant. Based on these findings and the fact that in the second case, amniotic fluid collected during the pregnancy was found to contain anti-McC^a, the authors (40) speculated that the presence of maternal anti-McC^a in the two fetuses had somehow blocked development of McC^a on their red cells. While this phenomenon does not seem to have been reported in other blood group systems, it is of note that the infant described by Eska et al. (37) that was born to a woman with anti-Kn^a in the serum, was found to have Kn(a-) red cells at the time of its birth.

In spite of the data mentioned above about the clinically benign nature of anti-McC^a (and the descriptions in the previous section about the similarly benign nature of anti-Kn^a) Molthan (30) claimed that two examples of anti-McC^a and one each of anti-McC^d and anti-Kn^a caused transfusion reactions with extravascular red cell destruction. Most workers do not accept the conclusions of Molthan (30). Because other antibodies within and without the Knops system were similarly blamed by Molthan and her associates (41-44) for such atrocities in direct contradiction to the findings of others and because anti-Yk^a figure prominently in such discrepant observations, this topic is discussed in more detail in the section on Yk^a.

As mentioned in the introduction of this chapter, in 1983 Molthan (6) described an antibody that she called anti-McC^b, that was said to define the antigen antithetical to McC^a on the red cells of Blacks but not Whites, of the Kn(a+) McC(a-) phenotype (i.e. those of the Kn(a-) McC(a-) phenotype excluded). The incidence of McC^b in Blacks was said (6,7,10) to be about 45%, a figure that was close to the expected number based on the incidence of the McC(a-) phenotype in US Blacks (2,3 and see table 27-2). Unfortunately the findings reported by Molthan (6,7,10) were not duplicated by others.

The Antigen Sl^a and the Antibody That Defines It and a Note on the Serum Vil

As shown in table 28-2 the antigen Sl^a (4) (that was called McC^c by a different investigator (5)) is of high incidence, i.e. circa 98% in Whites, but of much lower incidence, i.e. circa 53.5% in Blacks (4,6). All Black persons with McC(a-) red cells are Sl(a-) regardless of whether they are also Kn(a-) (i.e. Helgeson phenotype) or Kn(a+). Since the incidence of both Kn^a and McC^a are high in Blacks, it follows that some 45% of Blacks have red cells that are phenotypically Kn(a+) McC(a+) Sl(a-). In Whites, those of the Helgeson phenotype have Kn(a-) McC(a-) Sl(a-) red cells, about another 1% are phenotypically Kn(a+) McC(a+) Sl(a-). The four White persons with Kn(a+) McC(a-) red cells found among 722 tested, had Sl(a+) red cells (6,7). Table 28-3 lists the Kn^a, McC^a, Sl^a phenotype frequencies found in Whites and Blacks. Like Kn^a and McC^a, Sl^a varies in strength on different Sl(a+) red cells.

Since it is a Knops system antigen, it would be expected that Sl^a would be denatured when red cells are treated with trypsin or chymotrypsin, denatured or weakened when red cells are treated with AET or DTT and remain largely unaltered when red cells are treated with papain or ficin. Save for the survival of Sl^a on ficin-treated red cells (4) the above assumptions do not seem to have been formally proved.

Relatively little has been written about anti-Sl^a. The antibody seems almost always to be IgG in nature, to be optimally reactive by IAT, and to be made by individuals who have been transfused and/or pregnant. Those examples of anti-Sl^a that have been mentioned in the literature (3-8,45,57) have all been made by Blacks, not a surpris-

TABLE 28-3 Knops System Phenotype Frequencies in Whites and Blacks (6,7)

Phenotype	Whites (722 tested)		Blacks (371 tested)	
	Number Found	Percent Incidence	Number Found	Percent Incidence
Kn(a+) McC(a+) Sl(a+)	695	96.3	189	50.9
Kn(a+) McC(a+) Sl(a-)	8	1.1	156	42
Kn(a+) McC(a-) Sl(a+)	4	0.6	0	-
Kn(a+) McC(a-) Sl(a-)	0	-	21	5.7
Kn(a-) McC(a+) Sl(a+)	6	0.8	2	0.5
Kn(a-) McC(a+) Sl(a-)	2	0.1	0	-
Kn(a-) McC(a-) Sl(a-)	7	1.0	3	0.8

The phenotype Kn(a-) McC(a-) Sl(a+) was not found in either group
The phenotype Kn(a-) McC(a-) Sl(a-) is the Helgeson phenotype

ing observation since some 46 to 48% of Blacks but only about 2% of Whites have Sl(a-) red cells. The antibody is not uncommon, in the first two abstracts documenting its existence, 20 examples were mentioned in one (4) and twelve in the other (5). At least one patient with anti-Sl[a] in the serum has been successfully transfused with Sl(a+) blood (46, there is a typographical error in the title of the letter whereby the units transfused are described as Sl(a-), the text of the letter reveals that they were actually Sl(a+)). An anti-Sl[a] in another patient caused no phagocytosis in an in vitro monocyte monolayer assay (47).

As mentioned in the introduction of this chapter, Lacey et al. (4) studied a serum Vil that behaved as if it contained an antibody that was detecting an antigen antithetical to Sl[a]. Some details were given in the abstract (4) others were included by Swanson (25) in a review. The antibody, that was made by a multiply transfused White man, reacted with all of 12 Sl(a-) samples from Blacks, that were not of the Helgeson phenotype. In tests on a small series of random Blacks (number tested not mentioned), 80% had red cells that reacted with the Vil serum. No Vil+ sample was found when bloods from 50 randomly selected Whites were tested. As also mentioned in the introduction, neither Lacey et al. (4) nor Swanson (25) used the term Sl[b]. That term has been used, with a qualifying question mark, in tables 28-1 and 28-2. Use of the term is merely for convenience and should not be taken to imply that an antithetical relationship to Sl[a] has been proved.

The Antigen Yk[a] and the Antibody That Defines It

Anti-Yk[a] was first described in an abstract (13) in 1969, additional details were published later (14-17). As mentioned in the introduction of this chapter, early examples of antibodies called anti-Yk[a] did not all have exactly the same specificity. As a result some confusion about the relationship of Yk[a] to Cs[a] (see introduction and Chapter 30) and to Kn[a] existed, such confusion was not totally resolved until 1991 when it was shown (22,23) that Yk[a] and Kn[a] are carried on CR1 while Cs[a] is not. As shown in table 28-2, Yk[a] is present on the red cells of some 90% of random Whites and over 98% of random Blacks. The figures in table 28-2 are taken from a 1975 publication of Molthan and Giles (14) and a 1983 publication of Molthan (3). It is not entirely clear whether the figures given in the 1983 publication include those listed in the 1975 report. In table 28-2 the figures from the two reports have been added together. If the 1983 report does include the 1975 figures, the numbers should show that 2598 of 2889 (89.9%) US Whites had Yk(a+) red cells while 1098 of 1117 (98.3%) of US Blacks were of the

Yk(a+) phenotype. As can be seen, the 1975 and 1983 reports are in close agreement as to the incidence of Yk[a] in US Whites and Blacks.

Like the high incidence antigens of the Knops system already described, Yk[a] varies greatly in strength on different Yk(a+) samples. The Yk[a] antigen appears to be fully developed on cord blood red cells (30) but no example of HDN caused by anti-Yk[a] has been reported. The Yk[a] antigen is denatured when red cells are treated with trypsin or chymotrypsin (26), denatured or weakened when red cells are treated with AET or DTT (26-28) but survives treatment of red cells with papain or ficin (3,26).

Anti-Yk[a] is usually made by persons who have been transfused and/or pregnant, is almost always IgG in nature and reacts best in IATs. Some half of all sera that contain anti-Yk[a] contain other antibodies to non-Knops system antigens. Everything that has been written about difficulties in working with other Knops system antibodies, applies also to anti-Yk[a].

Anti-Yk[a] is clinically benign with regard to the transfusion of red cells. Numerous transfusions with Yk(a+) red cells to persons with anti-Yk[a] in the serum, in vivo red cell survival studies, and in vitro phagocytic cell assays have shown that anti-Yk[a] does not cause appreciable acceleration of in vivo clearance of antigen positive red cells (14,36,39,48-52). In spite of these overwhelming data, Molthan and her colleagues (30,44) insisted that anti-Yk[a] is clinically significant. In one report (44) it is claimed that a patient with anti-Yk[a] plus anti-Cs[a] suffered a series of extravascular transfusion reactions, caused by those antibodies, that led eventually to oliguria and death of the patient. In reviewing this report and the claim that the anti-Yk[a] plus anti-Cs[a] caused in vivo destruction of the antigen-positive cells, Mollison (53) wrote "the evidence was rather slender and depended on differential agglutination carried out with relatively weak agglutinating sera". In another report, Molthan (30) describes what she claimed were nine cases involving extravascular clearance and one involving intravascular clearance of red cells, in patients who had transfusion reactions. The one in which intravascular clearance was said to have occurred was allegedly due to anti-Yk[a]; of the nine in which extravascular clearance was said to have occurred, three were allegedly due to anti-Yk[a], one to anti-Yk[a] plus anti-Cs[a], and four to less well characterized antibodies in the Kn/McC series. A review of the data presented shows that in most cases there are better explanations for the evidence that is taken by Molthan (30) to indicate antibody-mediated red cell destruction. Again, some of the evidence is based on failure to detect transfused red cells in tests on post-transfusion samples from the patients, using relatively weak agglutinins. The data that deal with post-transfusion increments in hemoglobin and hematocrit are impossible to interpret without knowing the age of the units that were used for transfusion and that information was not supplied.

Obviously, the data presented by Molthan (30) and Molthan et al. (44) are quite different from those presented by seven independent groups of investigators (36,39,48-52) each of which is in agreement with the others. One of us (PDI) now finds that he is not able to place much credence on data regarding transfusion reactions and in vivo cell destruction, published by the workers in Bethlehem, Pennsylvania. Lack of acceptance of the conclusions reached by those workers is not based solely on reports about anti-Yk^a and anti-Cs^a. As already mentioned, the only claim that anti-Kn/McC are clinically significant was made by Molthan (30). As described in earlier sections of this chapter, the universal experience of others (1,31-33,35,36,38,39,46,47) is that these antibodies do not cause transfusion reactions or clinically relevant increases in the rate of clearance of the transfused red cells. Along similar lines Molthan (41) described a hemolytic transfusion reaction presumed to be due to anti-Bg, while others (54,55) have found such antibodies to be benign in vivo. Strohm and Molthan (42) claimed that four of five patients with anti-P$_1$ suffered delayed transfusion reactions; the experience of others (56,57) is that such an event is so rare that it may not be encountered even once in large numbers of patients with anti-P$_1$ (58) or in those who have suffered delayed transfusion reactions (59,60). Molthan (43) also reported a case in which she claimed that an IgG non-complement binding anti-Mi^a plus anti-Vw caused intravascular hemolysis leading to death of the patient. As far as this author (PDI) is aware, no one knows of a mechanism by which an IgG non-complement binding antibody can cause intravascular lysis, nor did Molthan (61) propose any such mechanism when asked (62).

The point of this long discussion about the invalid claims regarding in vivo antibody-induced red cell destruction made by Molthan, is to reassure workers faced with the decision that they must use antigen-positive red cells to transfuse a patient with an antibody directed against Kn^a, McC^a, Sl^a, Yk^a, Cs^a, et al. Those antibodies are harmless and can be ignored in transfusion therapy. It is inconceivable that clinically significant examples of these antibodies would all be found in one laboratory, while other workers in at least 15 different centers (1,31-33,35-39,46-52) would encounter only benign forms.

Other Knops System Antibodies

As mentioned in the introduction to this chapter, not all antibodies in the Knops system fit a pattern such that they can be said to be anti-Kn^a, anti-McC^a, anti-Sl^a or anti-Yk^a. When an antibody fails to react with red cells of the Helgeson phenotype (see a later section) then gives variable reactions with samples that lack one of the antigens, Kn^a, McC^a, Sl^a or Yk^a a number of different explanations can be considered. First, it is possible that the antibody is of a strength such that it gives visibly positive reactions only with red cell samples on which the antigen recognized is well expressed. Second, when traveled red cells are used (often the case since Kn(a-), McC(a-), Sl(a-) and Yk(a-) samples are often shared via SCARF or other exchange programs) the difficulties may be compounded because of antigen deterioration during shipment. Third, since antibodies used to type the reference red cell samples are not often potent, the phenotype assigned to the cell sample may not be correct. Fourth, since the Knops antigens are known to be carried on CR1 (CD35) (see below) it is entirely possible that that glycoprotein may carry more polymorphisms than have currently been recognized. Fortunately none of this matters at the level of transfusion therapy. Once an antibody has been placed in the anti-Knops-like category it can be ignored and the blood banker can concentrate efforts to be sure that the presence of the anti-Kn/McC-like does not obscure detection of a simultaneously present clinically-significant antibody.

Useful information about the Knops system can still be transmitted via published reports without knowledge of exact antibody specificity. As examples, the reports of Eska et al. (37), Wells et al. (35), Ghandhi et al. (33) and Ballas et al. (32) all contributed significantly to the current pool of information about the clinically benign nature of Knops system antibodies although, in each case, the antibodies studied had been identified only as anti-Kn^a-like, anti-Kn/McC, etc. It is quite probable that the antigens tentatively called Kir, Oca and Mil (35), Winborne (63,64) and Minnie Pearl Davis (65) in the third edition of this book (66) were actually recognized by anti-Kn/McC-like specificities (2).

Some Other Notes about Kn^a, McC^a, Sl^a and Yk^a

As mentioned above, there is a currently unexplained higher than expected incidence of the Cs(a-) phenotype among samples that lack Yk^a and a less dramatic increase of Cs(a-) samples among those that lack Kn^a, McC^a or Sl^a. A useful method for differentiation between Knops system antibodies and anti-Cs^a involves the use of trypsin, chymotrypsin or AET treated red cells. While the two enzymes denature antigens of the Knops system and AET denatures or weakens them, Cs^a remains unaltered on such treated red cells (3,11,26-28).

It is relatively easy to mistake anti-Sl[a] for anti-Fy3. First, the reactions of both antibodies are often weak and difficult to reproduce. Second, the Sl(a-) phenotype has an incidence of 46% in Blacks but only 2% in Whites. Thus about half of the Fy(a-b-) samples used in antibody identification studies will be Sl(a-). Since both anti-Sl[a] and anti-Fy3 usually occur in the sera of patients with other antibodies, the number of Fy(a-b-) samples lacking other antigens to which the patient is immunized, that are used in antibody identification studies, may be quite small. Third, antibodies that appear to react with all except Fy(a-b-) cells may be seen in patients with sickle cell disease, in whom antibody identification is difficult anyway (see Chapter 35). Marion Reid (68) has told us that a number of samples said to contain anti-Fy3, in fact contain anti-Sl[a]. The ideal red cells for differentiation between anti-Sl[a] and anti-Fy3 are, of course, those of the phenotype Fy(a-b+), Sl(a-). For reasons discussed in Chapter 14, while Blacks with Fy(a-b-) red cells can occasionally form anti-Fy[a], most of them are not able to make anti-Fy[b]. Thus non-reactivity of an antibody with Fy(a-b+), Sl(a-) red cells will exclude anti-Fy3, since those cells are Fy:3.

Tests such as those involving the use of trypsin-treated red cells and tests against Fy(a-b+), Sl(a-) red cells, and similar, must often be used in the identification of Knops system antibodies. As mentioned earlier in this chapter, antibodies of the system cannot usually be adsorbed to exhaustion with antigen-positive red cells; eluates made from the red cells used in the adsorptions are often non-reactive. Very early in the study of anti-Yk[a], Swanson (95) reported that the antibody could be at least partially inhibited by plasma from persons with Yk(a+) red cells and could be adsorbed by leukocytes. Although most workers were unable to duplicate these observations, it is now known that CR1 is present on leukocytes (70,71) and that a soluble form is present in plasma (96).

Daniels et al. (69) reported that Kn[a], Kn[a]-like, McC[a], Sl[a], Yk[a] (and Cs[a]) are more weakly expressed on the red cells of persons with *In(Lu)* than on other cells. While the depression was not as marked as that involving the Lutheran system antigens and P[1] and while it was not demonstrable with all examples of the antibodies to the Knops system antigens, mean titration scores determined using many antibodies and red cells of many unrelated persons with *In(Lu)*, seemed to show that antigen expression is often weakened. Although it might have been a function of the antibodies used, it seemed that Yk[a] might be less affected than the other Knops system antigens. Telen (122) has suggested that the apparent effect of *In(Lu)* on Knops system antigens should be interpreted with caution since the experiments that appeared to show an effect on the antigens (69) and on CR1 (22), did

not include controls for CR1 regulatory genotypes (see below). Nevertheless, the number of samples tested by Daniels et al. (69) might have been sufficient to exclude any bias from CR1 regulatory genes.

The Helgeson Phenotype

As mentioned many times in this chapter, red cells of the Helgeson phenotype, of which many examples are now known (1,3,6,7) usually type as Kn(a-b-) McC(a-) Sl(a-) Yk(a-). Indeed, non-reactivity of a serum containing an antibody to an antigen of high incidence, with Helgeson phenotype red cells, is often the first clue that the antibody belongs to the Knops system. Over the years it was noticed (67) that the more potent antibodies of the system did react, albeit weakly, with some examples of red cells of the Helgeson phenotype. Thus it was known that although Helgeson phenotype red cells are useful at the serological level, where they often behave as if they are Kn[null], they are not truly devoid of all Knops system antigens. When CR1 was recognized as the red cell membrane glycoprotein that carries the Knops system antigens, it was shown (18,22,23) that red cells of the Helgeson phenotype carry only about 10% of the number of copies of CR1 as carried by normal red cells. Strength of the Knops system antigens as correlated with CR1 copy number per red cell, is discussed in the next section.

As shown in table 28-3, the incidence of the Helgeson phenotype is about 1% in Whites and perhaps the same or slightly lower in Blacks (6,7).

The Knops System Antigens and CR1

The complement regulatory glycoprotein, complement receptor 1 (CR1, CD35 and see Chapter 6) is a large structure present on red cells, granulocytes, monocytes, B lymphocytes, a subset of T cells and various other cells of the body, for reviews see 70 and 71. The most common form of the protein has a molecular weight of about 190kD (72). However, as mentioned briefly earlier, there is a size polymorphism of the protein and forms with apparent molecular weights of circa 190, 220, 160 and 250kD have been identified by SDS-PAGE under non-reducing conditions (73-79) and said to represent the allotypes A (common, the 190kD protein mentioned above (18)), B (less frequent), C (rare) and D (rare), respectively. Variation in size of the encoded proteins does not seem to be associated with any differences in function. In addition to the size polymorphism there is, as mentioned in the section on the Helgeson phenotype, variation in the number of copies of CR1 on red cells although other cells on which the protein is carried do not seem to show similar variation (70,76,77,79). Both size and copy number variations are described in more detail below.

By using immunoprecipitation with human and monoclonal antibodies Rao et al. (22) and Moulds et al. (23) independently showed that the Knops system antigens are carried on CR1. Similar conclusions were later reached by Petty (80) using the monoclonal antibody specific immobilization of erythrocyte antigens (MAIEA) method. Both immunoprecipitation and the MAIEA technique were used (23,80) to show that Cs^a is not on CR1. Moulds et al. (18) then showed that the variation in Knops system antigen levels on different red cell samples, as demonstrated by indirect antiglobulin tests, correlates closely with the number of copies of CR1 per red cell. When the red cells carry between 20 and 100 copies of CR1 per cell, they fail to react in indirect antiglobulin tests with Knops system antibodies. When the CR1 copy number is between 100 and 150 per cell, the red cells usually react weakly with the more potent antibodies and are non-reactive with the weaker ones. When the CR1 copy number per cell is greater than 200, the Knops system antigens can usually be detected in IATs with appropriate antibodies. The above figures are, of course, generalizations and some variation was seen. However, the correlation between strength of Knops system antigens and numbers of copies of CR1 was good. In tests on the red cells of four persons of the Helgeson phenotype (presumably unrelated although that fact is not stated), the number of copies of CR1 per red cell, were found (18) to be 20, 28, 55 and 66. In tests against different samples lacking one of the antigens Kn^a, McC^a, Sl^a or Yk^a, the CR1 copy numbers per red cell were found to be in the normal range. Thus it seems that the Helgeson phenotype is not truly a null phenotype but represents a very low number of antigens per red cell (i.e. not demonstrable by IAT using most Knops system antibodies). Quite differently lack of one of the antigens Kn^a, McC^a, Sl^a or Yk^a appears to represent a change in CR1 probably resulting from mutation in the original *CR1* gene.

Monoclonal Antibodies and the CR1 Glycoprotein

A number of reports, especially those describing the presence of the Knops system antigens on CR1 (18,22, 23,80,81) have mentioned use of various monoclonal antibodies to CR1. As far as we are aware, these antibodies have all been directed against determinants common to CR1 and none has yet been found that specifically identifies a Knops system antigen.

Knops System and Disease

CR1, that is also known as the C3b/C4b or immune adherence receptor, is thought (72,82-84) to play multiple roles in the immune response. One of these involves red cell born CR1 molecules. These receptors bind immune complexes present in the blood and transport them to the liver and spleen where phagocytic cells can remove them from circulation. In spite of this (and the other suggested roles for CR1 in the immune response) the Helgeson phenotype with its low number of copies on red cells, is not associated with a disease state. As mentioned above, in the situation where there are reduced numbers of copies of CR1 on red cells, normal numbers of copies are present on other cells. This may explain why low CR1 copy numbers on red cells is not associated with any disease state, i.e. sufficient copies of CR1 on other cells to allow normal T cell responses, activation of B cells and secretion of interleukin-1 by monocytes.

It has been suggested that low copy numbers of CR1 may result in deposition of immune complexes on blood vessel walls leading to damage during inflammation (85). Acquired deficiencies of CR1 have been described in patients with systemic lupus erythematosus (86), rheumatic diseases (87), AIDS (88), and malignant and inflammatory disorders (89). It will not escape the attention of blood bankers that many of the problems associated with the typing of red cells for Knops system antigens and the identification of Knops system antibodies, occur in patients afflicted with the clinical conditions listed.

The *Knops* Locus is on Chromosome 1

Like the *Cromer* locus (see Chapter 24) the *Knops* locus is part of the *RCA* (regulation of complement activation cluster) linkage group on chromosome 1q (90-93). The Cromer and Knops blood groups systems are independent because the *Cr (DAF)* genes encode production of decay accelerating factor (DAF) and the *Kn (CR1)* genes encode production of complement receptor 1 (CR1). DAF and CR1 are different proteins. Somatic cell hybridization and in situ hybridization have been used (94) to map the *Kn* locus to 1q32.

The Size Polymorphisms of CR1 (syn. CD35, C3b/C4b Receptor): Problems of Nomenclature

Human CR1 is a large glycoprotein which is unusual in that it occurs in four different polymorphic forms which vary in size. The molecular weights of these four allotypes on SDS-PAGE under reducing conditions are 250,000 (type A, also known as type F), 290,000 (type B, also known as type S), 330,000 (type D) and 210,000 (type C or F'). When SDS-PAGE is conducted under non-reducing conditions, type A has an apparent molecular weight of 190,000, type B 220,000, type C 160,000 and type D 250,000 (97). The commonest allotype is type A (frequency 0.82). Type B has a frequency of 0.18 while types C and D are rare (98). The differences in the sizes of these allotypes are not due to differences in post-translational modification like, for example, glycosylation, but relate directly to differences in the length of the polypeptide chain. Of course, individuals may be heterozygous for two of these allotypes. Inspection of the molecular size of each allotype reveals that the largest, type C is 40,000 more than type B which is 40,000 more than type A which is 40,000 more than type D suggesting that the allotypes differ in their utilization of a common structural unit or building block.

The literature relating to the different polymorphic forms of CR1 is confusing for several reasons. Different papers quote apparent molecular weights for the four polymorphic forms without explaining whether or not they refer to results obtained from SDS-PAGE carried out under reducing conditions or non-reducing conditions. Since, as will be seen in later sections, CR1 comprises numerous subunits all of which have intrachain disulphide bonds, the results obtained are very different depending on which of these conditions is chosen. However, the electrophoretic conditions chosen do not affect the relative sizes of the four polymorphic forms, the relationship D>B(or S)>A(or F)>C(or F') holds whether reducing or non-reducing conditions are used.

A second source of confusion concerns the nomenclature itself. The literature appears consistent with respect to the common alleles so that *B* always equals *S* and *A* always equals *F* but in at least one paper the largest allele is called *C* not *D* (98).

A third source of confusion concerns the nomenclature used for the common structural units or long homologous repeats (LHRs) from which the different CR1 proteins are assembled. These LHRs have been named A, B, C, D, etc.! It is hard to see how the scientists working in this field could have contrived to make things any more difficult for others to follow.

For the purposes of the following discussion this author (DJA) has adopted the terms *S*, *F* and *F'* for the alleles *B*, *A* and *C* respectively, *D* is assumed to refer to the largest allele that does not appear to have a name in the *S*, *F*, *F'* nomenclature - how about *ES* - assuming that *S*, *F* and *F'* stand for Slow, Fast and Faster (with respect to electrophoretic mobility on SDS-PAGE) then *ES* could stand for *Even Slower*! The adoption of this nomenclature allows the use of A, B, C, D, etc. for LHRs.

The Structure of CR1

A full length cDNA corresponding to the F allotype of CR1 was isolated and sequenced by Klickstein et al. (99,100). The predicted protein contains 2,039 amino acids. Inspection of the sequence revealed that it is composed of a series of 30 repeating units known as short consensus repeats or SCRs. The N-terminal 28 SCRs can be further subdivided into four sections each of 7 SCRs arranged in tandem. These four subsections are known as long homologous repeats or LHRs. Comparison of the sequences of LHRs revealed substantial sequence homology ranging from 60 to 90% suggesting that they arose by gene duplication (99,100). The cDNA predicts an extracellular domain comprising the 30 SCRs, a single membrane spanning domain (25 amino acids) and a short cytoplasmic domain (43 amino acids). Each SCR comprises 60 amino acids in a folded structure held in shape by two intrachain disulphide bonds (101). There are seven to ten N-glycans per molecule of CR1 which serve to stabilize the protein, but no O-glycans (71). CR1 is an extraordinarily long filamentous molecule which when fully extended could reach 114nm from the surface of the red cell - a fishing line waving above the glycocalyx of the cell hoping to get a 'bite' of an immune complex or a C3b-coated bacterium (see figure 28-1).

CR1 is a member of a large family of proteins known as the complement control protein (CCP) family. All members of the CCP family contain similar SCRs (102). CD55 which carries the Cromer blood group system antigens has four SCRs and is also a member of this superfamily (see Chapter 24).

The Structure of the *CR1* Gene

The structure of the gene giving rise to the type S form of CR1 was elucidated by Wong et al. (79). Restriction mapping of phage and cosmid genomic clones allowed the alignment of 25 overlapping clones encompassing 160kb which included the entire coding region of the *S* allele. Wong et al. (79) considered the gene to comprise 9 regions. The 5' non-coding region and signal sequence, five regions each containing exons encoding a LHR, a short region containing exons for the 2 SCRs not contained in LHRs, a segment containing exons encoding the transmembrane and cytoplasmic regions and a region containing a 3' untranslated sequence. The translated protein contains a cleavable signal sequence encoded within a single exon. The transmembrane and cytoplasmic regions are encoded by single exons. These authors (79) suggested that each LHR evolved as a 20-30kb genomic unit.

The S form of CR1 contains 5 LHRs whereas the F

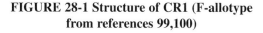

FIGURE 28-1 Structure of CR1 (F-allotype from references 99,100)

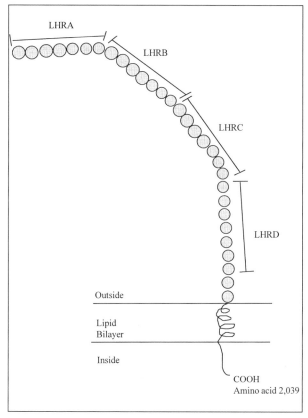

form contains 4 LHRs (see previous section) thereby explaining the difference in molecular size of the two proteins. The structure of the gene giving rise to the F protein was elucidated by Vik and Wong (103). The *F* allele comprises 39 exons arranged in four LHRs and spans 133kb. The *S* allele comprises 47 exons. Each LHR is encoded by 8 exons. Of the seven SCRs within each LHR, SCRs 1, 5 and 7 are each encoded by a separate exon, SCRs 2 and 6 are encoded by two exons and SCRs 3 and 4 are both encoded by the same exon (103).

The smallest form of CR1, F', is 40,000 smaller than type F and appears to have 3 LHRs (104) while the largest form (type D) has 6 LHRs (75). The different allotypes are most likely generated by non-homologous cross-over events at meiosis (79,103, and see figure 28-2) in a manner analogous to that which generates the Ls[a]-active glycophorin C/D molecules derived from duplicated exon 3 in the *GYPC* gene and the exon 2 and exon 3 deletions causative of different Ge-negative phenotypes (see Chapter 16). The smallest allotype F' is associated with systemic lupus erythematosus and Wong et al. (79) suggest that this may be related to impaired C3b binding capacity. These authors further point out that duplications of LHRs would have the dual advantage of introducing multivalent C3b-binding sites and thereby increased avid-

ity for C3b/C4b coated surfaces and the further extension of binding sites away from the cell surface.

The 4 LHRs of the F allotype are designated, LHR-A, B, C and D respectively with LHR-A being at the N-terminus. Examination of the C3b and/or C4b binding sites on the F allotype by deletion mutagenesis showed that three of the four LHR (A, B, C) bind C3b and/or C4b (100). Further studies have shown that LHR-A is specific for C4b whereas LHR-B and LHR-C primarily bind C3b. The specificity is contained within the first four SCRs of each LHR. The first two SCRs within each LHR confer specificity but SCRs 3 and 4 are also required to form the functional site (104-106,120).

The 5 LHRs of the S allotype are designated LHR-A, B/A, B, C and D (79). The second LHR is designated B/A because it shares sequence homology with the A and B LHRs of the F allotype and is thought to have arisen as a result of an unequal cross-over event between two *F* alleles (see figure 28-2).

Location of Knops System Antigens on CR1

The precise location of the Knops system antigens on the CR1 molecule is unknown at the time of writing. Moulds and Rowe (107) showed that a recombinant soluble form of the F allotype of CR1 inhibited antibodies to Kn[a], McC[a], Sl[a] and Yk[a]. Petty et al. (108) showed that Kn[a], McC[a] and Sl[a] were all expressed on CR1 from individuals homozygous genes encoding for the allotypes F, S and F'. The rare D allotype was not tested. These results are interesting and useful because the F' allotype is the smallest of the CR1 allotypes containing only 3 LHRs (104). Wong et al. (79,103) speculate that the F' allotype results from a non-homologous cross-over event between two *F* alleles. Such a crossover would generate one chromosome with an *S* allele and a second chromosome with an allele encoding three LHRs of structure A/B-C-D. It is the gene product on this second chromosome that appears to correspond to the *F'* gene (see figure 28-2). The repeating LHRs of the F allotype are known to have common epitopes recognized by certain monoclonal antibodies (100) and so it is possible that the Knops system antigens are expressed on more than one LHR in a given CR1 molecule. If this were so it might be expected that the strength of Knops system antigens would vary according to allotype because more than one antibody could bind to one CR1 molecule and the larger the number of LHRs the greater the number of antigen sites. However, this does not seem to be the case.

Deletion mutagenesis has been employed successfully to elucidate the location of C3b and C4b binding sites on CR1 (100,109). It would seem logical to employ the same approach to the elucidation of blood group anti-

**FIGURE 28-2 Generation of Different *CR1* Alleles by Unequal Cross-over at Meiosis
(adapted from reference 79)**

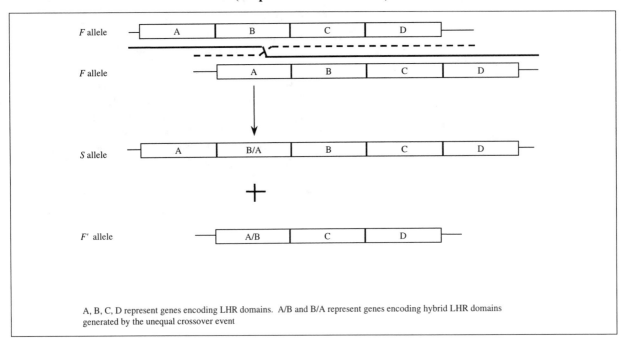

A, B, C, D represent genes encoding LHR domains. A/B and B/A represent genes encoding hybrid LHR domains generated by the unequal crossover event

gen structure. Recent evidence (121) suggesting that CR1, and the Sl[a] antigen in particular, can act as a receptor for blood cells infected with a laboratory strain of the malarial parasite *Plasmodium falciparum* provide the impetus for such a study.

The Quantitative Polymorphism of CR1

In addition to the occurrence of different allotypes of different sizes, CR1 also exhibits a quantitative polymorphism such that the number of molecules of CR1 varies from 20 to 800 copies/red cell between individuals (18). Petty et al. (108) suggest that this quantitative polymorphism is controlled by a gene genetically independent of the *CR1* locus because individuals who are heterozygous for *CR1* alleles have a reduction in the level of CR1 derived from both alleles when the red cell membranes are examined by immunoblotting. Others have linked the polymorphism to a *Hind* III RFLP which defines a single base change within an intron of the *CR1* gene (79).

The Functions of CR1

CR1 is found on a wide variety of cell surfaces (red cells, neutrophils, monocytes, B cells, some T cells, follicular dendritic cells and glomerular epithelial cells, astrocytes in the brain) and in soluble form in plasma (71,110). It plays a major role on phagocytic cells by binding to C3b (and to a lesser extent C4b) which is bound to the surface of microorganisms thereby effecting the destruction of the microorganisms (see Chapter 6 for a detailed discussion of the complement system). When complement activation effects cleavage of C3 and C4, an intramolecular thioester bond becomes accessible on C3b and C4b which allows these fragments to form a covalent bond with a hydroxyl or amino group on another surface. The bound C3b and/or C4b then acts as a target for CR1 on the surface of phagocytic cells (111). C3b targeting of microorganisms via the alternative pathway is thought to have evolved before an adaptive immune response (antibodies and Fc receptors) as a primitive host defense mechanism against infection, "However, this simple recognition mechanism cannot respond adaptively to poor stimulators, or memorize these adaptations to prevent recurrent infection. This is a severe limitation in an environment of opportunistic pathogens that are evolving much faster than their potential hosts" (112). Moulds et al. (113) quote a number of examples where pathogens have sought to turn this simple mechanism to their own advantage. One such example involves the causative agent of leprosy. *Mycoplasma leprae* expresses a major surface molecule, phenolic glycolipid-1, which binds C3 fragments. The organism uses the subsequent binding of macrophages through CR1 to invade the macrophages in which it lives and multiplies. It will be of considerable interest to investigate whether any of the Knops system antigens impart selective advantages to man in respect of any infectious diseases. It would be surprising if they do not. The possible selective advantage of the Sl(a-) phenotype in respect of *Plasmodium falciparum* malaria has already been alluded in an earlier section.

In red cells the main function of CR1 appears to be the binding of immune complexes. The red cell-bound complexes are thereby prevented from binding to the endothelial lining of blood vessels where they could otherwise mediate inflammation and tissue damage (98,114). The red cell-bound immune complexes are carried to the liver where the complexes are removed by macrophages and the red cells returned to the circulation (116,117). It has been argued that, despite the low numbers of CR1 molecules per red cell, immune complexes are bound efficiently because CR1 molecules on red cells are located in clusters (118,119). The fact that each of the first three LHRs (A, B, C) of the F protein can bind C3b and/or C4b (100,104-106 and discussed above) demonstrates that the multivalent binding potential of individual CR1 molecules may also be an important factor in this process. C3b dimers bind to red cell CR1 with 20-40-fold greater affinity than C3b monomers (106). C4b dimers bind to red cell CR1 with a 20-fold lower affinity than C3b dimers but more than 100-fold higher affinity than monomeric C4b (109). These results do not allow a distinction between the possibilities that the bivalent binding sites for C3b dimers and C4b dimers are on one CR1 molecule or are formed between two CR1 molecules. However, the binding affinity of C4b dimers for wild type CR1 and an artificial construct comprising the first four SCRs of LHR-A linked to LHR-D were the same suggesting that crosslinking of two CR1 molecules is most likely (109), a finding consistent with evidence that CR1 on red cells occurs in clusters (115-117). CR1 may also function by effecting the breakdown of C3bi into C3dg and C3c (see also Chapter 6). C3bi is deposited in normal tissue as a result of the incomplete clearance of immune complexes and tissue-bound C3bi can interact with CR3 on neutrophils with the result that tissue damage occurs (98).

References

1. Helgeson M, Swanson J, Polesky HF. Transfusion 1970;10:137
2. Molthan L, Moulds J. Transfusion 1978;18:566
3. Molthan L. Am J Med Technol 1983;49:49
4. Lacey P, Laird-Fryer B, Block U, et al. (abstract). Transfusin 1980;20:632
5. Molthan L. (abstract). Transfusion 1980;20:622
6. Molthan L. Med Lab Sci 1983;40:59
7. Molthan L. Med Lab Sci 1983;40:113
8. Molthan L, Moores P, Hartwell G. Med Lab Sci 1984;41:3
9. Mallan MT, Grimm W, Hindley L, et al. (abstract). Transfusion 1980;20:630
10. Moulds JJ, Moulds MK, Molthan L. Unpublished observations cited by Molthan L. Med Lab Sci 1983;40:59
11. Giles CM, Huth MC, Wilson TE, et al. Vox Sang 1965;10:405
12. Giles CM. PhD Thesis, Univ London 1968
13. Molthan L, Crawford MN, Giles CM, et al. (abstract). Transfusion 1969;9:281
14. Molthan L, Giles CM. Vox Sang 1975;29:145
15. Giles CM. In: Human Blood Groups. Basel:Karger, 1977:268
16. Tilley CA, Crookston MC. Unpublished observations 1977 cited in Giles CM. In: Human Blood Groups. Basel:Karger, 1977:268
17. Molthan L. (abstract). Transfusion 1978;18:622
18. Moulds JM, Moulds JJ, Brown M, et al. Vox Sang 1992;62:230
19. Molthan L, Paradis DJ. Med Lab Sci 1987;44:94
20. Rolih SD. Transf Med Rev 1989;3:128
21. Molthan L. Unpublished observations 1982 cited in Molthan L. Med Lab Sci 1983;40:113
22. Rao N, Ferguson DJ, Lee S-F, et al. J Immunol 1991;146:3502
23. Moulds JM, Nickells MW, Moulds JJ, et al. J Exp Med 1991;173:1159
24. Daniels GL, Anstee DJ, Cartron J-P, et al. Vox Sang 1995;69:265
25. Swanson J. In: Blood Groups Ch/Rg, Kn/McC/Yk and Cr. Bethesda:Am Assoc Blood Banks, 1992:1
26. Daniels GL. Immunohematology 1992;8:53
27. Moulds JJ, Moulds MK. (Letter). Transfusion 1983;23:274
28. Toy EM. Immunohematology 1986;2:57
29. Marsh WL, Johnson CL, Mueller KA. (Letter). Transfusion 1983;23:275
30. Molthan L. Rev Fr Transf Immunohematol 1982;25:127
31. Baldwin ML, Ness PM, Barrasso C, et al. Transfusion 1985;25:34
32. Ballas SK, Viggiano E, Draper EK. Transfusion 1984;24:22
33. Ghandi JG, Moulds JJ, Szymanski IO. Transfusion 1984;24:16
34. Moulds MK. Am J Med Technol 1981;47:789
35. Wells RF, Korn G, Hafleigh B, et al. Transfusion 1976;16:427
36. Schanfield MS, Stevens JO, Bauman D. Transfusion 1981;21:571
37. Eska P, Rosche ME, Grindon AJ. (Letter). Transfusion 1976;16:190
38. Valko DA, Silberstein EB, Greenwalt TJ, et al. (abstract). Transfusion 1981;21:603
39. Gutgsell NS, Issitt LA, Issitt PD. (abstract). Transfusion 1988;28 (Suppl 6S):32S
40. Ferguson SJ, Blajchman MA, Guzewski H, et al. Vox Sang 1982;43:82
41. Molthan L. (Letter). Transfusion 1979;19:609
42. Strohm PL, Molthan L. Canad J Med Technol 1981;41:153
43. Molthan L. Vox Sang 1981;40:105
44. Molthan L, Wick RW Jr, Gross BM. Blood Transf Immunohematol 1982;24:263
45. Wells J, Rise M, Moulds MK. (abstract). Prog Ann Mtg South Cent Assoc Blood Banks, 1981
46. Harpool DR. (Letter). Transfusion 1983;23:402
47. Wren MR, Issitt PD. (abstract). Transfusion 1986;26:548
48. Tilley CA, Crookston MC, Haddad SA, et al. Transfusion 1977;17:169
49. Shore GM, Steane EA. (abstract). Transfusion 1978;18:387
50. Ryden SE. (Letter). Transfusion 1981;21:130
51. Grove W, Peters B, Ellisor SS, et al. (abstract). Transfusion 1981;21:607
52. Lau PYL, Jewlachow V, Leahy MF. Vox Sang 1993;64:254
53. Mollison PL. Blood Transfusion in Clinical Medicine, 7th Ed. Oxford:Blackwell 1983

54. Silvergleid AJ, Wells RF, Hafleigh EB, et al. Transfusion 1978;18:8

55. Nordhagen R, Aas M. Vox Sang 1978;35:319

56. Ahrons S, Kissmeyer Nielsen F. Dan Med Bull 1968;15:259

57. Chandeysson PL, Flye MW, Simpkins SM, et al. Transfusion 1981;21:77

58. Cronin CA, Pohl BA, Miller WV. Transfusion 1978;18:728

59. Pineda AA, Brzica SM, Taswell HF. Mayo Clin Proc 1978;53:378

60. Moore SB, Taswell HF, Pineda AA, et al. Am J Clin Pathol 1980;74:94

61. Molthan L. (Letter). Vox Sang 1982;42:55

62. Avoy DR. (Letter). Vox Sang 1982;42:54

63. Haber JM. Unpublished observations 1965, cited in all three previous editions of this book

64. Allen FH Jr. Unpublished observations 1965, cited in all three previous editions of this book

65. Adebahr ME, Allen FH Jr. Unpublished observations 1965, cited in all three previous editions of this book

66. Issitt PD. Applied Blood Group Serology, 3rd Ed. Miami:Montgomery, 1985

67. Moulds MK. Unpublished observations cited in Moulds JM, Moulds JJ, Brown M, et al. Vox Sang 1992;62:230

68. Reid ME. Personal communication 1996

69. Daniels GL, Shaw MA, Lomas CG, et al. Transfusion 1986;26:171

70. Hourcade D, Holers VM, Atkinson JP. Adv Immunol 1989;45:381

71. Ahearn JM, Fearon DT. Adv Immunol 1989;46:183

72. Fearon D. J Exp Med 1980;152:20

73. Wong WW, Wilson JG, Fearon D. J Clin Invest 1983;72:685

74. Dykman TR, Cole JL, Iida K, et al. Proc Nat Acad Sci USA 1983;80:1698

75. Dykman TR, Hatch JA, Aqua MF, et al. J Immunol 1985;134:1787

76. Wilson JG, Murphy EE, Wong WW, et al. J Exp Med 1986;164:50

77. Wong WW, Kennedy CA, Bonaccio ET, et al. J Exp Med 1986;164:1531

78. Van Dyne S, Holers VM, Lublin DM, et al. Clin Exp Immunol 1987;68:570

79. Wong WW, Cahill JM, Rosen MD, et al. J Exp Med 1989;169:847

80. Petty AC. (abstract). Transf Med 1993;3 (Suppl 1):84

81. Holers VM., Seya T, Brown E, et al. Complement 1986;3:63

82. Bacle F, Haeffner-Cavaillon N, Laude M, et al. J Immunol 1991;144:147

83. Betz M, Filsinger S. Compl Inflamm 1991;8:128

84. Moulds JM. In: Immunobiology of Transfusion Medicine. New York:Marcel Dekker, 1994:283

85. Ng YC, Schifferli JA, Walport MJ. Clin Exp Immunol 1988;71:481

86. Iida K, Mornaghi R, Nussenzweig V. J Exp Med 1982;155:1427

87. Walport MJ, Lachmann PJ. Arthr Rheum 1988;31:153

88. Tausk FA, McCutchaan JA, Spechko P, et al. J Clin Invest 1986;78:977

89. Currie MS, Vala M, Pisetsky DS, et al. Blood 1990;75:1699

90. Holers VM, Cole JL, Lublin DM, et al. Immunol Today 1985;6:188

91. Reid KBM, Bentley DR, Campbell RD, et al. Immunol Today 1986;7:230

92. Rey-Campos J, Rubinstein P, de Cordoba DR. J Exp Med 1988;167:664

93. Carroll MC, Alicot EM, Katzman PJ, et al. J Exp Med 1988;167;1271

94. Weis JH, Morton CC, Bruns GAP, et al. J Immunol 1987;138:312

95. Swanson J. In: A Seminar on Recent Advances in Immunohematology. Arlington, VA:Am Assoc Blood Banks, 1973:121

96. Yoon SH, Fearon DT. J Immunol 1985;134:3332

97. Campbell RD, Law SKA, Reid KBM, et al. Ann Rev Immunol 1988;6:161

98. Ross GD. Curr Top Micro Immunol 1992;178:31

99. Klickstein LB, Wong WW, Smith GA, et al. J Exp Med 1987;165:1095

100. Klickstein LB, Bartow TJ, Miletic V, et al. J Exp Med 1988;168:1699

101. Janotova J, Reid KBM, Willis AC. Biochemistry 1989;28:4754

102. Reid KBM, Day AJ. Immunol Today 1989;10:177

103. Vik DP, Wong WW. J Immunol 1993;151:6214

104. Wong WW, Farell SA. J Immunol 1991;146:656

105. Krych M, Hourcade D, Atkinson JP. Proc Nat Acad Sci USA 1991;88:4353

106. Makrides SC, Scesney SM, Ford PA, et al. J Biol Chem 1992;267:24754

107. Moulds JM, Rowe KE. Transfusion 1996;36:517

108. Petty AC, Green CA, Poole J, et al. Transf Med 1997;7:55

109. Reilly BD, Makrides SC, Ford PJ, et al. J Biol Chem 1994;269:7696

110. Morgan BP, Gasque P. Immunol Today 1996;17:461

111. Kinoshita T. Immunol Today 1991;12:291

112. Farries TC, Atkinson JP. Immunol Today 1991;12:295

113. Moulds JM, Nowicki S, Moulds JJ, et al. Transfusion 1996;36:362

114. Beynon HLC, Davies KA, Haskard DO, et al. J Immunol 1994;153:3160

115. Cornacoff JB, Hebert LA, Smead WL, et al. J Clin Invest 1983;71:236

116. Schifferli JA, Ng YC, Peters DK. New Eng J Med 1986;315:488

117. Schifferli JA, Ng YC, Estreicher J, et al. J Immunol 1988;140:889

118. Chevalier J, Kazatchkine MD. J Immunol 1989;142:2031

119. Paccaud J-P, Carpentier J-L, Schifferli JA. Eur J Immunol 1990;20:283

120. Kalli KR, Hsu P, Bartow TJ, et al. J Exp Med 1991;174:1451

121. Rowe JA, Moulds JM, Newbold CI, et al. Nature 1997;388:292

122. Telen MJ. Personal communication to PDI, 1996

29 | The Indian Blood Group System and the Antigen AnWj

A serum Salis was first tested by Dr. Carolyn Giles at the Medical Research Council Blood Group Reference Laboratory in London in 1963. It was mentioned in reports from that laboratory over the years as an unsolved factor of common occurrence and was listed as an unpublished antigen of high incidence in Chapters 19 and 29 of the second edition of this book.

In 1973 and 1974, Badakere et al. (1,2) described a low incidence antigen, In^a, that was present on the red cells of some 3% of random donors in India.

Giles (3) astutely noted that the serum Salis was from a man from Pakistan and that of two patients with compatible (i.e. Salis-) red cells, one was from Pakistan and the other from India. When tested, all three Salis- samples reacted strongly with anti-In^a, another antithetical relationship between two blood group antigens had been found. Two other sera, Parra and Walls, both of which were also mentioned in Chapters 19 and 29 of the second edition of this book, were found (3) to be non-reactive with Salis- red cells. In neither case were red cells available for typing with anti- In^a.

Findings (4,5) that the In^a and In^b antigens are carried on the leukocyte homing receptor and cellular adhesion molecule, CD44; that CD44 production is encoded from a locus on chromosome 11 (6-11); and that no other blood group locus is known to be on that chromosome; resulted in the Indian system being formally recognized as an independent blood group system in 1995 (12). The conventional and ISBT terminology for the system is given in table 29-1. As described in detail later in this chapter, it is now known (31,60) that the In^a/In^b polymorphism represents an amino acid difference at position 46 of CD44. When the protein expresses In^b, the amino acid at position 46 is arginine, when the protein expresses In^a, proline occupies that position.

Between 1972 and 1982 a number of antibodies, with apparently the same specificity, that defined an antigen of very high incidence, were studied and became known as anti-Anton (13-15). Since the Lu(a-b-) red cells of persons who had inherited *In(Lu)* (see Chapter 20) were Anton-negative, the term Lu15 was reserved for the antigen. However, Poole and Giles (15) showed that the red cells of persons who inherit the genes that cause the recessive type of Lu(a-b-) (also see Chapter 20), express the Anton antigen normally. Since Anton is clearly not encoded by a gene at the *Lu* locus, the term Lu15 was never widely used and is now regarded as obsolete.

In 1983 the first report of anti-Wj, an autoantibody,

TABLE 29-1 Conventional and ISBT Terminology for the Indian System and the AnWj Antigen

Conventional Name: In

ISBT System Symbol: IN

ISBT System Number: 023

Historical (now obsolete) Name	Antigen Conventional Name	ISBT Antigen Number	ISBT Full Code Number
	In^a	IN1	023001
Salis	In^b	IN2	023002

Antigen in 901 series: High incidence antigens not assigned to systems or collections

Anton (Lu15)* Wj	AnWj	AnWj	901009

* The number Lu15 was provisionally assigned to the Anton antigen but was not widely used since it was rapidly appreciated that the antigen is not part of the Lutheran system, see text.

appeared (16). Additional studies (17-19) showed that anti-Anton and anti-Wj detect the same antigen. The antigen in question was renamed AnWj and although it is not formally a part of the Indian system, there is strong evidence (20) that it is carried on an isoform of CD44. Accordingly it is appropriate to describe AnWj in this chapter and to include it in table 29-1.

The In^a and In^b Antigens

The In^a antigen is of low incidence in India but is somewhat more frequent in some Arabs. As described later in this chapter, the inherited form of the AnWj- phenotype was first found in an Arab family (45). Results from several studies showing the incidence of In^a in certain population groups are listed in table 29-2. Based on the incidence of In^a, the In(a+b-) phenotype would be expected to be extremely rare in certain peoples. However, Joshi (23) found two of 700 Indian donors to have In(b-) red cells while Longster found two In(a+b-) persons among 251 Asian immigrants in England. As mentioned in the introduction to this chapter, five examples of what was eventually shown to be anti-In^b, were identified by Giles (3). This excess of people with In(b-) red cells might indicate that a silent allele, *In*, exists at the *In^{a}In^b* locus. That is to say, perhaps some of the In(b-)

samples represented the *In^aIn* or the *InIn* genotype. However, the evidence for the existence of a silent allele, *In*, is only circumstantial thus far. For example, Ferguson and Gaal (25) found the In(a+b-) phenotype in two generations of one family. As described below, when an individual with In(a-b-) red cells was found (24) it was not apparent whether the phenotype was genetically determined or related to the patient's hematological disorder.

In^a is apparently not fully developed at birth and its expression may be reduced on the red cells of pregnant women (26). Dumasia and Gupte (27) estimated that cord blood red cells carry about 25% of the number of In^a antigen sites seen on the red cells of adults and that during pregnancy there is about a 60% reduction of the number of In^a sites expressed. Normal expression of In^a was seen three to six months after delivery. In contrast, Longster and Robinson (22) did not find any reduction of expression of In^b on cord blood red cells. As discussed in detail later in this chapter, In^a and In^b are carried on the CD44 glycoprotein. Anstee et al. (38) estimated that there are between 6000 and 10,000 copies of that glycoprotein per red cell.

The expression of In^b is permanently reduced on the Lu(a-b-) red cells of persons who inherit *In(Lu)* (see Chapter 20). That the effect is on a membrane component genetically independent of the Lutheran system is clear from findings (4,25) that Lu(a-b-) red cells of the recessive and X-linked types (again see Chapter 20) express In^b normally. Presumably In^a would be seen to be affected similarly to In^b, if an individual with *In(Lu)* and In(a+) red cells was ever found.

Both In^a and In^b are denatured or removed when red cells are treated with trypsin, papain, chymotrypsin or pronase (2,3,22,28-30); a role for disulphide bonds in the antigens' structure is apparent from the findings (23,25, 28-30) that the antigens are denatured when red cells are treated with dithiothreitol (DTT) or 2-aminoethylisoth-iouronium bromide (AET). Sialic acid is apparently not involved in In^a or In^b structure, the antigens survive treatment of red cells with neuraminidase (28). As described in a later section, several amino acid substitutions have been found on CD44 (31,60). At present the Arg46Pro (In^b to In^a) change is the only one associated with a blood group antigen polymorphism (60).

The Phenotype In(a-b-)

In 1994, Parsons et al. (24) described a patient with a novel form of congenital dyserythropoietic anemia (CDA) that was associated with a deficiency of erythrocyte CD44. The red cells of that patient were highly unusual in terms of red cell antigens in that they typed as In(a-b-), AnWj-, Co(a-b-) and had a markedly reduced level of LW^ab. It was not clear whether the deficiency of CD44 was responsible for the CDA and the In(a-b-) phenotype or whether the patient had two *In* genes. A family study produced no conclusive evidence, the patient's parents and a sister had In(a-b+) red cells. Tests on the red cells of other patients with CDA did not reveal any abnormalities of the Indian, AnWj, Colton or LW blood groups but, as mentioned, the patient involved had a novel form of CDA.

Anti-In^a and Anti-In^b

These antibodies are not particularly uncommon, many examples of anti-In^a (2,3,26,32) and anti-In^b (3,22,23,25,33) have been documented in the literature. When 39 donors with D-, In(a-) red cells were injected with D+, In(a+) red cells in attempts to stimulate production of anti-D for use in the preparation of Rh immune globulin, 30 of them made anti-In^a in addition to anti-D (26). The antibody has also been formed following pregnancy (2,26) and transfusion (32). Anti-In^b has also been formed following transfusion and pregnancy, in one case the antibody was seen (25) during a first pregnancy in a woman who had not been transfused. While some examples of the antibodies present as agglutinins, most give stronger reactions in indirect antiglobulin tests. At least three examples of anti-In^b (22,25,33) have been shown to be, at least in part, IgG1.

One anti-In^b was said (23) to give a sufficient dosage effect as to be able to distinguish between In(a-b+) and In(a+b+) red cells. However, the titer scores reported showed only a very modest difference, i.e. 60 to 49, and in view of the complexities described in Chapter 3, would have to be interpreted with considerable caution. Some characteristics of the Indian system antibodies and anti-AnWj are given in table 29-3.

TABLE 29-2 Incidence of the In^a Antigen in Different Populations, from references 2, 21, and 22

Population Studied	Number Tested	Number In(a+)	Percent In(a+)
Indians in Bombay	1749	51	2.9%
Iranians	557	59	10.6%
Arabs in Bombay	246	29	11.8%
Asian Immigrants in Northern England	251	10	4.0%

Monoclonal Antibodies to CD44

As described in detail later in this chapter, a large number of monoclonal antibodies directed against CD44 have been produced (4,34-38,43,44). One murine monoclonal antibody with anti-In[b] specificity has been described.

Clinical Significance of Anti-In[a] and Anti-In[b]

As far as we are aware, anti-In[a] has not been incriminated as causative of a hemolytic transfusion reaction. However, since In[a] is of low incidence and since finding In(a-) blood is so easy, it is possible that no patient with anti-In[a] in the serum has ever been transfused with In(a+) blood. In vivo red cell survival studies of In(a+) red cells in two patients with anti-In[a] did show rapid clearance of the injected red cells (26).

An immediate hemolytic transfusion reaction after 50 ml of In(b+) blood had been transfused to a patient with anti-In[b] in the serum has been reported (23); a different example of the antibody was seen to cause accelerated clearance of a test dose of In(b+) red cells in an in vivo cell survival study (25).

Neither anti-In[a] nor anti-In[b] has ever caused HDN. Indeed, in a number of cases (22,25,33), infants born to women with IgG1 anti-In[b] in the serum had a negative DAT and no anti-In[b] was detectable in the infants' sera. This occurred in spite of the fact that the maternal anti-In[b] was sometimes used to show that the infants' red cells were In(b+). We do not know if this finding relates to the fact that CD44 is present in serum (40,41) and that In[b] can be detected in serum by hemagglutination inhibition (42). The possibility that anti-In[b] may have been adsorbed by placental or fetal tissue is discussed below.

The AnWj Antigen

In 1972, Boorman and Tippett (13) studied an antibody to a very common antigen, the antibody was made by a pregnant woman. A second example of the antibody, known as anti-Anton was described in 1980 (14). Since anti-Anton failed to react with the red cells of persons who had inherited *In(Lu)*, the term Lu15 was reserved for the antigen involved. However, when Poole and Giles (15) studied a further five examples of anti-Anton they found that the antigen was expressed normally on the Lu(a-b-) red cells of persons who had inherited two recessive *Lu* genes (see Chapter 20).

In 1983, Marsh et al. (16) described anti-Wj, an autoantibody, that reacted with all normal red cells and with those of the recessive Lu(a-b-) type but could be shown to react with the red cells of persons with *In(Lu)* only by adsorption-elution methods.

In 1985, Poole and Giles (17) suggested that anti-Anton and anti-Wj were likely detecting the same antigen. In 1986, Mannessier et al. (19) studied a patient with Hodgkin's disease in whom red cell Wj antigen production was depressed to the point of non-reactivity. Indeed, it was initially thought that the patient had Wj-negative red cells and had made allo-anti-Wj. When first studied the red cells of the patient failed to react with either anti-Wj or anti-Anton. The patient was induced into a remission from his disease and six months after the initial tests his red cells typed as Wj+, Anton+; he was no longer making anti-Wj. The antigen defined was renamed AnWj and it is now appreciated that the AnWj- phenotype most often represents an acquired condition that is frequently transient. That is to say, production of red cell AnWj antigen is depressed, often to the point of non-detection in serological tests and anti-AnWj is concomitantly made. In many instances red cell AnWj production later returns and production of anti-AnWj is curtailed.

In 1991, Poole et al. (45) described an Arab family in Israel in whom the AnWj- phenotype was seen to be inherited in a recessive manner. A consanguineous marriage had produced seven children, three of whom had AnWj- red cells and four of whom were of the AnWj+ phenotype. From the family study it was seen that *AnWj* is not at the *ABO, MNSs, Rh, Kell, Duffy, Kidd, Xg* or *Xk* loci and, most importantly, not at the *Lutheran* locus

TABLE 29-3 Characteristics of Indian System Antibodies and of Anti-AnWj

| Antibody Specificity | Positive Reactions in In Vitro Tests | | | | Usual Immuno-globulin | | Ability to Bind Complement | | Ability to Cause In Vitro Lysis | | Implicated in | | Usual Form of Stimulation | | % of White Population Positive |
	Sal	LISS	AHG	Enz	IgG	IgM	Yes	No	Yes	No	Transfusion Reaction	HDN	Red Cells	Other	
Anti-In[a]	Some		Most	No	X	?				X		No			<1
Anti-In[b]	Some		Most	No	X	?				X	X	No			>99.9
Anti-AnWj			X	Yes	X					X	X	No			>99.9

either. As shown in table 29-1, the high incidence *AnWj* antigen has been given the ISBT number 901009. Clearly the recessive AnWj- phenotype is rare. When Lukasavage (46) tested 2400 American group O donors (including 394 African Americans, 134 American Indians, 128 Asians, 178 Hispanics and 309 other donors of non-European White extraction) no AnWj- individual with normal Lutheran system antigens was found. The study did reveal three persons with *In(Lu)* whose red cells initially failed to react with anti-AnWj but could be shown to bind that antibody and yield it on elution.

The AnWj antigen, unlike In^a and In^b, is still demonstrable on red cells treated with trypsin, papain, chymotrypsin, pronase or AET, like In^a and In^b, the antigen is also present on red cells treated with neuraminidase (28).

Development and Loss of Red Cell AnWj Antigen

The AnWj antigen is not developed at birth and cord blood red cells usually fail to react with anti-AnWj; this finding provided an early clue in the recognition of auto-anti-Wj (16). Poole and Van Alphen (47) studied samples from 36 newborn infants. They noted that conversion from the AnWj- to the AnWj+ state occurs as early as 3 days to as late as 46 days of life. Extraordinarily, conversion was seen to take only one day to complete. In other words, red cells released from the marrow in the AnWj- state were converted to AnWj+ and were not simply replaced by newly released red cells. While such an observation clearly suggests an extrinsic cause for the change, no evidence for such a factor in serum could be found (47).

As mentioned above, the AnWj antigen can also be lost from red cells. This phenomenon is sometimes reversible as in the patient described above (19) whose original AnWj+ phenotype returned when his Hodgkin's disease was in remission. Loss of AnWj expression has been seen in several patients (19,47-49) (in whom Hodgkins and non-Hodgkins lymphoma seemed over represented) and in one healthy individual (50).

Clinical Significance of Anti-AnWj

In the first family in which the recessive type of AnWj- was recognized, both the proposita and her sister had anti-AnWj in their serum. Neither of the women had been transfused, both had been pregnant. Their brother with AnWj- red cells, who had never been transfused, did not have anti-AnWj in his serum. The proposita's anti-AnWj did not cause HDN in any of her children.

Severe hemolytic transfusion reactions have been

blamed on anti-AnWj. In one case (51) in which it was not possible to determine whether the AnWj- state was inherited or acquired (the patient had Waldenstrom's macroglobulinemia) three separate transfusion episodes resulted in hemolytic reactions. In another (49) the patient had non-Hodgkin's lymphoma and experienced a transfusion reaction after about 50 ml of AnWj+ blood had been transfused. In a third (54) both immune hemolytic anemia and a transfusion reaction were attributed to the auto-anti-AnWj in a patient with carcinoma of the ovary. In vivo red cell survival studies have also demonstrated (51-53) the ability of anti-AnWj, that based on the patients' diseases were probably made when red cell AnWj antigen expression was lost, to effect accelerated clearance of AnWj+ red cells. Whitsett et al. (55) described a patient with lymphoma and depression of expression of red cell AnWj antigen. In vivo survival studies using the patient's own red cells on which AnWj was depressed but not totally absent, were essentially normal. Similar studies using allogeneic AnWj+ red cells showed survival of 76% of the test dose at 24 hours and 55% at 7 days. In other words, a mildly elevated rate of in vivo red cell clearance. If they are available (they are not all that rare) red cells from an individual with *In(Lu)* might be expected to survive better in a patient with anti-AnWj, than random AnWj+ red cells.

Monoclonal Anti-AnWj

Immunization of mice with human T-cells from patients with acute lymphocytic leukemia and fusion of the mouse spleen cells with immunoglobulin secreting cells resulted in the production of two monoclonal anti-AnWj (56). Like human polyclonal anti-AnWj, these antibodies reacted (by IAT) with all red cells except those from persons with *In(Lu)*, those that were AnWj- and cord blood red cells. The monoclonal anti-AnWj showed considerable variation in strength with different AnWj+ red cell samples.

AnWj and *Haemophilus influenzae*

The AnWj receptor is apparently the binding site for fimbriae-bearing strains of *Haemophilus influenzae*. A culture of that organism agglutinated all red cells except those that were AnWj-, from individuals with *In(Lu)* or from cord blood samples. The organisms were non-reactive with AnWj- red cells of both the inherited and acquired types (57,58). When buccal epithelial cells were used in binding experiments with *H. influenzae*, the organisms bound to cells from one individual with the transient AnWj- red cell phenotype, from two individuals with *In(Lu)* and several newborns but not those of three persons from the same family, who had inherited the AnWj- phenotype (58,59). This suggests that perhaps in the *In(Lu)*, acquired AnWj- and newborn states, AnWj is poorly enough expressed not to be detectable on red cells but is present in sufficient amounts to allow bacterial binding to tissue cells. In the inherited AnWj- state, the antigen is apparently totally absent from both red cells and tissue cells.

Biochemistry of Indian Blood Group Antigens

Midway through the 1980s it became clear that the technique of immunoblotting could be a powerful tool for identifying molecules that carry blood group antigens in the red cell membrane. Spring et al. (4) used immunoblotting with eluates of human anti-In^a and anti-In^b to show that the In^a and In^b antigens were located on a molecule of apparent molecular weight 80kD in red cell membranes. In the same paper they showed that this molecule was identical to a glycoprotein known as CD44. CD44 had been defined by a cluster analysis of murine monoclonal antibodies at the Third Leucocyte Antigen Workshop (61). The first monoclonal anti-CD44 to be reported was F10.44.2, an antibody originally described as reactive with an antigen on human brain cells, granulocytes and T lymphocytes (43). Spring et al. (4) showed that CD44 purified using F10.44.2 would bind human anti-In^b. Since that time CD44 has been extensively studied and it is now established as a major adhesion molecule present on the surface of numerous different cell types (see below). The molecular basis of the In^a/In^b polymorphism was not established until 1996 when Telen et al. (60) reported that a single point mutation in the *CD44 gene* (G252 to C) resulted in a single amino acid substitution in the polypeptide chain of the CD44 molecule (Arg46 to Pro). The presence of Arg46 correlated with In^b antigen expression and Pro46 with In^a expression. Formal proof that Arg46 is the critical residue for the In^b antigen was obtained by expression studies. Jurkat cells were transfected with "wild type" cDNA having Arg46, cDNA from an In(a+b-) individual having Pro46 and "wild type" cDNA in which Arg46 was changed to Pro by site directed mutagenesis. The latter construct was necessary because the cDNA from the In(a+b-) individual showed five nucleotide sequences change from that of "wild type" and three of these predicted single amino acid differences (Arg46 to Pro, Tyr109 to Ser, and Glu239 to Gly). It was therefore necessary to examine the possible role of Arg46Pro in the absence of the other changes. When the transfected cells were tested with human anti-In^b by flow cytometry only the cells expressing the "wild

type" cDNA were reactive. These results establish that Arg46 is critical for In^b expression but since the transfected cells were not tested with anti-In^a, a role for the other amino acid changes (at residues 109 and 239) in the structure of the In^a antigen cannot formally be excluded. The tertiary structure of CD44 is not known but models of the protein deduced from available structural information suggest that residues 109 and 239 are likely to be distant from Pro46 and are therefore unlikely to be involved in In^a expression (see figure 29-1). As discussed in an earlier section, the In^a antigen is rare outside the indigenous peoples of India, Pakistan and the Middle East. If the "wild type" cDNA used in these studies was derived from an individual of a different ethnic group it is possible that some or all of the other amino acid sequence changes observed are a reflection of the different ethnic origins of the cDNAs.

Structure of CD44

After the original description of CD44 as an antigen recognized by monoclonal antibody F.10.44.2 (43) there followed a period of several years in which other researchers unknowingly described the same protein and gave it a different name. In 1981, Hughes et al. (62) found CD44 on mouse 3T3 cells and called it Pgp-1. Carter and Wayner (63) described a molecule of 90kD on human fibroblasts that bound collagen types I and VI and fibronectin and called the protein extracellular matrix receptor type III (E-III). Haynes et al. (64,86) and Telen et al. (40) described monoclonal antibodies that identified a protein of 80kD on red cells which they named p80. They further showed that red cells from individuals with the *In(Lu)* type of Lu(a-b-) gave very weak or negative reactions with monoclonal antibodies to p80. A series of monoclonal antibodies called Hermes 1, 2 and 3 are described by Jaklanen et al. (65,66) who showed that the antibodies inhibited the binding of lymphocytes to high endothelial venules. At the Third International Workshop on Leucocyte Differentiation Antigens in 1987 it was recognized (61) that several of the monoclonal antibodies against the various molecules described above were recognizing the same protein which was named CD44.

In 1989 three groups (67-69) reported the isolation of cDNA clones corresponding to CD44. Sequencing of the cDNA clone isolated by Stamenkovic et al. (67) revealed a protein sequence of 341 amino acid residues preceded by a signal peptide sequence of 20 residues (including the initiator methionine). It would be expected that the signal sequence would be cleaved in the mature protein but this has not been proved by sequencing the purified protein so that most publications number the amino acid residues from the initiator methionine. It is likely that the real amino terminus is glutamine 21. Inspection of the protein sequence predicted a large extracellular amino terminal domain of 268 residues, a single membrane spanning domain of 21 residues and a carboxy terminal cytoplasmic domain of 72 residues (see figure 29-1). The molecular weight of the polypeptide calculated from the amino acid sequence is 37kD. This contrasts with the apparent molecular weight of the protein on SDS-PAGE of red cell membranes (80kD) and is indicative of substantial post-translational modification of the protein that can be attributed to extensive glycosylation (see below).

The predicted extracellular domain has two distinct structural features. Distal from the membrane is a region with significant homology (30%) to the family of cartilage link proteins. Cartilage link proteins stabilize large aggregates of cartilage proteoglycan core proteins by binding to proteoglycan monomer or hyaluronic acid (66). This sequence homology gave the lead to studies which established CD44 as a hyaluronic acid binding protein (see below). The amino-terminal region of the molecule with homology to link proteins has six cysteine residues suggesting that it has a compact globular structure maintained by disulphide bonds. The presence of such a disulphide bonded domain would be entirely consistent with the serological observation that the In^a and In^b antigens are inactivated when red cells are treated with thiol reagents like AET and with evidence described above which identifies Arg46Pro within the link protein homology region, as the critical residue for defining the In^a/In^b polymorphism. There is however abundant additional evidence in support of a disulphide bonded domain. The majority of the many monoclonal antibodies made against CD44 react with CD44 on immunoblots run under non-reducing conditions but fail to react when reducing conditions are employed (38). The extracellular domain has seven potential sites of N-glycosylation (signal sequence, Asn-X-Ser/Thr) although at least one of these (Asn169) is unlikely to be utilized because in this case X is proline. Five of the remaining potential N-glycan sites are in the link protein homology region (see figure 29-1). There is no doubt that some of these sites are utilized in red cell CD44 because the apparent molecular weight of CD44 on SDS-PAGE is reduced after previous treatment of the cells with Endo F (4).

Proximal to the extracellular face of the membrane there is a stretch of approximately 130 residues that lack cysteine. This region is rich in threonine and serine residues which provide potential sites for O-glycans. It also contains Ser-Gly motifs that may provide potential sites for the attachment of glycosaminoglycans (67).

The cytoplasmic domain is rich in charged amino acids and contains one cysteine residue (Cys-295) positioned near the cytoplasmic face of the membrane in a sequence that contains three arginine residues and three lysine residues (see figure 29-1). Idzerda et al. (69) suggested that this cysteine may provide a site for attachment of fatty acid since a similar sequence is found in vesicular stomatitis virus G protein where the cysteine is acylated with palmitic acid. Guo et al. (70) showed that CD44 in normal human peripheral blood lymphocytes is palmitoylated. The presence of a cluster of basically charged amino acids near the cytoplasmic side of the membrane is a common feature of membrane proteins (see also Chapters 4, 15 and 16) and is thought to assist in anchoring the protein in the membrane. There is some evidence that CD44 binds to the cytoskeleton since it is retained with the red cell skeleton when red cell membranes are extracted with 10% (w/v) Triton X-100 (4) and associates with ankyrin in mouse T lymphoma cells (71). There is an additional cysteine residue (Cys-286) in the transmembrane domain of CD44 that Liu and Sy (72) suggest is critical for hyaluronan binding.

Organization of the *CD44* Gene

The *CD44* gene was mapped to the short arm of chromosome 11 (11p13) by Goodfellow et al. (6). The structure of the *CD44* gene was reported by Screaton et al. (73) in 1992. These investigators (73) obtained a genomic clone containing the *CD44* gene by PCR screening a yeast artificial chromosome (YAC) library. The clone was approximately 320kb in size and the *CD44* gene comprised 50-60kb. The gene comprised 19 exons. CD44 found on hematopoietic cells (CD44H) comprises the products of exons 1-5, 15-17 and 19 (see figure 29-2). Exons 6-14 are alternatively spliced in, to encode CD44 isoforms found on other cells. The exons encoding the distal link protein homology domain are conserved in all forms of the molecule. Tissue-specific variants are created by splicing in exons that enlarge the proximal extracellular domain (see figure 29-2). Alternative splicing of exons encoding the cytoplasmic domain has also been reported (68,73).

Function of CD44

CD44 has been implicated in a wide variety of normal cell functions: lymphocyte homing; leukocyte activation; extracellular matrix binding; and cell adhesion and migration (reviewed in 74). There is also evidence that abnormal expression or regulation of CD44 may have a role in some human cancers by enhancing tumor growth and/or the ability of tumor cells to metastasize (75).

Many studies of the function of CD44 have focused on the binding site for hyaluronic acid (synonyms hyaluro-

FIGURE 29-1 Structure of the Predominant Hematopoietic Form of CD44 and Location of the In^b Antigen

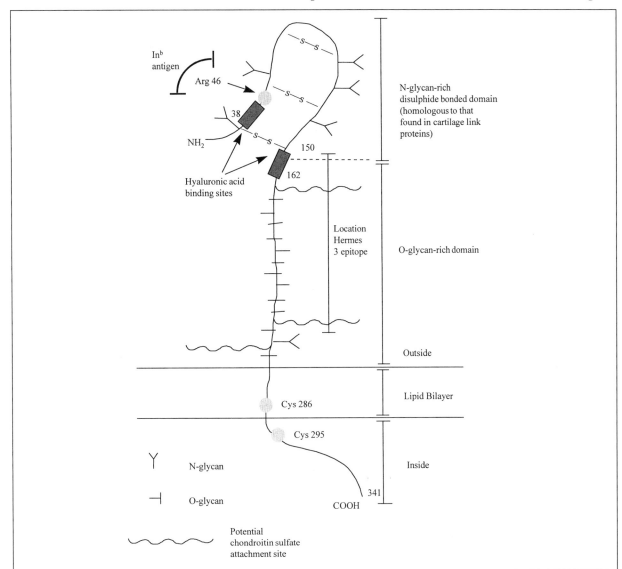

nan and HA). HA is the simplest of the glycosaminoglycans (GAGs) consisting of a long chain of up to 25,000 repeating disaccharide units comprising glucuronic acid and N-acetylglucosamine. The carboxyl group of glucuronic acid makes HA a highly negatively charged molecule and proteins whose function is to bind HA characteristically have a cluster of positively charged amino acid residues in the HA binding domain. HA is a highly extended polysaccharide that expands with water to occupy a large volume. It is thought (76) to play a major role in resisting compressive forces in tissues and joints.

HA is just one of many GAGs found in the extracellular matrix (ECM, the space between cells in tissues), others are chondroitin sulfate, dermatan sulfate, heparin sulfate, heparin and keratan sulfate. Also found in the ECM are structural proteins like collagen and elastin and

adhesive proteins like fibronectin and laminin. Interactions between cell surface proteins and proteins of the ECM are crucial to the many processes involving cell migration which are necessary for the development of an organism and the protection of that organism from microbial assault.

Given that CD44 is an HA binding protein it is not surprising to find it present on a wide variety of cells and tissues including brain, tongue, trachea, stomach, ileum, skin, spleen, liver and placenta to name but a few (38). Using site-directed mutagenesis and soluble chimeric proteins containing different portions of extracellular domain of CD44 linked to the C_H2 and C_H3 regions of human IgG1, Peach et al. (77) identified two regions of CD44 that contained clusters of basic amino acids important for HA binding. One region (residues 21-45) is near

FIGURE 29-2 Structure of the *CD44* Gene (from reference 73)

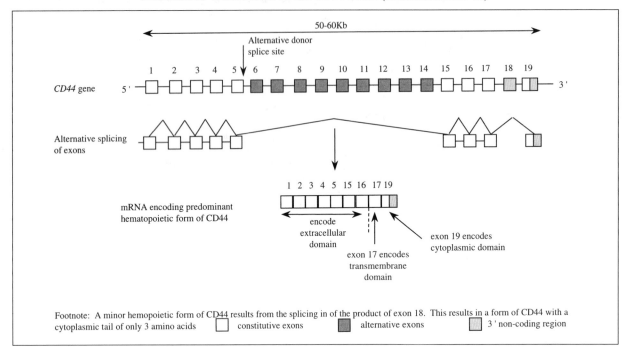

the amino terminus where Arg41 is critical and the other (residues 144-167) is outside the region of link protein homology and involves Lys158 and Arg162 (see figure 29-1). Liao et al. (78) came to similar conclusions using a different approach. They mapped the epitopes recognized by monoclonal antibodies capable of blocking HA binding to CD44. The observation that the critical residue for In[b] antigen activity (Arg46) is at the extreme C-terminus of the first site for HA binding led Telen et al. (60) to examine the binding of HA to "wild type" CD44 in which the Arg46 had been mutated to Pro, that is, to the residue found when In[a] antigen is present. Jurkat cells transfected with this mutant and exposed to phorbol 12-myristate 13 acetate (PMA) bound HA as effectively as PMA-treated Jurkat cells transfected with "wild type" CD44. Since individuals of phenotype In(a+b-) have normal health and since an inherited defect which adversely affected HA binding by CD44 in all the cells of the body where it is expressed, would be expected to have major pathological consequences, this result is not unexpected. Nevertheless it is interesting to note that such a dramatic change that would be expected to alter the structure of CD44 in this region does not compromise the function of the protein.

In an earlier section it is noted that neither anti-In[a] nor anti-In[b] has ever caused HDN. It seems possible that this is related to the presence of CD44 on many tissues in the body including the fetally-derived placenta. Anti-In[b] present in the serum of an In(a+b-) mother carrying an In(a+b+) fetus could be adsorbed by the placenta and/or other fetal tissues thereby obviating destruction of fetal

red cells. In this context it is interesting to note that anti-In[b] does not block HA binding in vitro when PMA-treated Jurkat transfectants are studied (60) suggesting that adsorption of the antibody by fetal tissues would not, of itself, have an adverse effect on this function of CD44.

It is important to note that the ability of CD44 to bind HA is highly regulated in a way that is not fully understood. Although many cell types express CD44 they do not all bind HA. A variety of factors have been identified as relevant to the regulation of this binding activity. They include cytoplasmic domain phosphorylation (79), clustering of CD44 molecules possibly through a mechanism requiring a cysteine residue in the transmembrane domain (72), interaction with cytoskeletal elements, particularly ankyrin (80) and the extent of glycosylation. Katoah et al. (81) and Lesley et al. (82) report that the degree of glycosylation has a marked effect on HA binding. Treatment of cells with tunicamycin, which inhibits N-glycosylation, converts them from non-binders to binders. The ligand binding capacity of purified CD44 is dramatically increased after sialidase treatment.

CD44 and the AnWj Antigen

In an earlier section the phenotypic association of AnWj with CD44 was described and it was noted that, unlike the In[a]/In[b] antigens, the AnWj antigen is resistant to protease digestion of intact red cells. The position of some protease cleavage sites on CD44 can be localized, approximately, from experiments with monoclonal anti-CD44. Most monoclonal anti-CD44 recognize epitopes that are lost on protease-treated red cells but there are a few which recognize protease-resistant epitopes (38,83). Five of 20 CD44 antibodies studied in the Fifth Workshop on Leukocyte Antigens held in Boston in 1993 gave positive agglutination reactions with chymotrypsin-treated and trypsin-treated red cells but failed to react with pronase-treated red cells (83). These five antibodies, unlike the other 15 antibodies in the Workshop, were reactive with AET-treated red cells suggesting that the relevant epitopes were not localized in the amino terminal disulphide bonded link protein homology domain (see figure 29-1). In immunoblotting studies carried out in reducing conditions, the five antibodies identified components of 51-56kD and 50-54kD in membranes from red cells pre-treated with chymotrypsin or trypsin respectively. One of these antibodies (Hermes 3) had previously been mapped to a region comprising amino acid residues 152 to 235 (68) suggesting that the trypsin and chymotrypsin sensitive sites are located between the amino terminal disulphide bonded domain and residues Thr152 to Thr235. Inspection of the amino acid sequence in this region of CD44 reveals the presence of several basic residues which might be sites for trypsin cleavage and several Tyr and Phe residues which might be sites for chymotrypsin cleavage. The AnWj antigen resists pronase digestion and so it cannot be located in the region recognized by monoclonal antibodies of the Hermes 3 type. Therefore, if AnWj is on CD44, it should be located between the Hermes 3 epitope and the lipid bilayer (see figure 29-1). This region of the protein contains several potential sites of posttranslation modification, an N-glycan site, several possible chondroitin sulphate attachment sites and several Ser and Thr residues that might be O-glycan attachment sites. Several observations suggest that AnWj is located on CD44 (lack of the antigen on CD44 deficient cells (Lu(a-b-) of the *InLu* type) and the novel form of CDA discussed below, and the appearance of the antigen on Jurkat cells transfected with "wild type" CD44 cDNA (20)). It is possible that the structure of the antigen depends upon posttranslational modification of the protein by a particular glycosylation. This possibility could be addressed by culturing cells transfected with CD44 cDNA in the presence of inhibitors of carbohydrate biosynthesis. It is also possible that the antigen is dependent on conformational change induced in this region of the protein by fatty acylation of cysteine in the transmembrane or cytoplasmic domain. This possibility could be addressed by site-directed mutagenesis of the relevant cysteines (already described by Liu and Sy (72)) and examining cells expressing the mutants for expression of AnWj. The most direct approach would be to sequence cDNA from

an individual who has inherited the AnWj- phenotype such as a member of the family described by Poole et al. (45) in the hope of finding a difference that would affect the protein sequence. Elucidation of the nature of the AnWj antigen is of considerable interest because the antigen is a receptor for *Haemophilus influenzae* (58) (see above), a major cause of respiratory tract infections.

Expression of CD44 on Blood Cells and the Significance of CD44 Deficiency in Hematopoietic Cells

Kansas et al. (84) examined the expression of CD44 during the normal development of monocytes, neutrophils and red cells in bone marrow using flow cytometry with selected monoclonal antibodies. They concluded that early committed erythroid cells have a high expression of CD44. High levels of CD44 expression were also found on a subset of cells that stained positively for glycophorin A. Intermediate levels of expression were found on a subset of glycophorin A positive, CD71 (transferrin receptor) positive cells. Glycophorin A positive, CD71 negative cells had low levels of CD44 similar to that found on normal circulating red cells. Normal red cells have between 5000 and 10,000 copies of CD44 per cell as determined in a quantitative binding assay using radioiodinated Fab fragments of monoclonal CD44 antibodies (38). Kansas et al. (84) also showed that myeloid cells committed to granulopoiesis underwent downregulation of CD44. Miyake et al. (85) found that some monoclonal anti-CD44 are able to inhibit the development of lymphoid and myeloid precursors when added to murine bone marrow cultures. These observations suggest that CD44 may play a role in the early maturation of hematopoietic cells through interaction with components of the ECM and/or stromal cells and/or homotypic interactions with other hematopoietic cells.

Individuals expressing the Lu(a-b-) phenotype as a consequence of the action of the dominant inhibitor gene *In(Lu)* have markedly reduced levels of CD44 on their red cells and on a subpopulation of monocytes (40). The Lutheran blood group system antigens are not located on CD44 but on a completely different molecule (87 and see Chapter 20) so that the name of this phenotype is particularly unfortunate. Individuals with this phenotype are not uncommon (1 in 3000, Shaw et al. (88)) and the phenotype is not associated with disease. Udden et al. (89), reported two related individuals with the phenotype who had acanthocytic red cells and the red cells of both individuals showed a slightly decreased osmotic fragility after incubation in autologous serum for 24 hours at 37°C that was accompanied by an increase in K⁺ efflux. It is not clear if these features are commonly associated with the phenotype (90). The CD44 deficiency observed in the *In(Lu)* form of the Lu(a-b-) phenotype is selective for erythroid/myeloid cells. The lymphocytes of affected individuals have normal levels of CD44 expression (86). A selective deficiency of CD44 from the erythroid cells of a patient with a novel form of CDA is described in a previous section. In this case a different disorder was involved because the Lutheran system antigens were expressed normally on the CD44 deficient red cells and the cells had the rare Co(a-b-) phenotype (24). The molecular mechanism giving rise to CD44 deficiency in these cases is unknown. In the case of the *In(Lu)* effect, an abnormality of regulation in hematopoietic cells that affects both CD44 and Lutheran antigens might result from the same abnormal transcription factor. A mutated erythroid transcription factor was suggested as a possible explanation of the CD44 deficient red cells of the patient with CDA (91). The lack of any disease associated with the inheritance of *In(Lu)* suggests that CD44 does not play a critical role in the late stages of erythroid/myeloid development, a feature consistent with downregulation of CD44 expression at these stages. It could also be argued that if the *In(Lu)* form of the Lu(a-b-) phenotype demonstrates that CD44 is not required at the later stages of erythroid development, then CD44 deficiency is not the critical defect giving rise to disease in the patient with a novel form of CDA.

References

1. Badakere SS, Joshi SR, Bhatia HM, et al. Ind J Med Res 1973;61:563
2. Badakere SS, Parab BB, Bhatia HM. Vox Sang 1974;26:400
3. Giles CM. Vox Sang 1975;29:73
4. Spring FA, Dalchau R, Daniels GL, et al. Immunology 1988;64:37
5. Telen MJ, Ferguson DJ. Vox Sang 1990;58:118
6. Goodfellow PN, Banting G, Wiles MV, et al. Eur J Immunol 1982;12:659
7. Francke U, Foellmer BE, Haynes BF. Somat Cell Genet 1983;9:333
8. Ala-Kapee M, Forsberg UH, Jalkanen S, et al. Cytogenet Cell Genet 1989;51:948
9. Forsberg UH, Jalkanen S, Schröder J. Immunogenetics 1989;29:405
10. Couillin P, Azoulay M, Henry I, et al. Hum Genet 1989;82:171
11. Couillin P, Azoulay M, Metezeau P, et al. Genomics 1989;4:7
12. Daniels GL, Anstee DJ, Cartron J-P, et al. Vox Sang 1995;69:265
13. Boorman KE, Tippett P. Unpublished observations 1972, cited in Race RR, Sanger R. Blood Groups in Man, 6th Ed. Oxford:Blackwell, 1975
14. Daniels GL. PhD Thesis, Univ Lond, 1980
15. Poole J, Giles CM. Vox Sang 1982;43:220
16. Marsh WL, Brown PJ, DiNapoli J, et al. Transfusion 1983;23:128
17. Poole J, Giles C. (Letter). Transfusion 1985;25:443
18. Marsh WL, Johnson CL. (Letter). Transfusion 1985;25:443
19. Mannessier L, Rouger P, Johnson CL, et al. Vox Sang 1986;50:240
20. Telen MJ, Rao N, Udani M, et al. (abstract). Transfusion 1993;33 (Suppl 9S):48S
21. Badakere SS, Vasantha K, Bhatia HM, et al. Hum Hered 1980;30:262
22. Longster GH, North DI, Robsinson EAE. Clin Lab Haematol 1981;3:351
23. Joshi SR. Vox Sang 1992;63:232
24. Parsons SF, Jones J, Anstee DJ, et al. Blood 1994;83:860
25. Ferguson DJ, Gaal HD. Transfusion 1988;28:479
26. Bhatia HM, Badakere SS, Mokashi SA, et al. Immunol Comm 1980;9:203
27. Dumasia AN, Gupte SC. Ind J Med Res 1990;92:50
28. Daniels GL. Immunohematology 1992;8:53
29. Joshi SR, Bhatia SM. Ind J Med Res 1987;85:420
30. Dahr W, Kruger J. Foren Sci Int 1983;23:49
31. Washington MK, Udani M, Rao N, et al. (abstract). Transfusion 1994;34 (Suppl 10S):62S
32. Joshi SR, Gupta D, Choudhury RK, et al. (Letter). Transfusion 1993;33:444
33. Sosler SD, Saporito C, Perkins JT, et al. (Letter). Transfusion 1989;29:465
34. Telen MJ, Palker TJ, Haynes BF. Blood 1984;54:599
35. Telen MJ, Shehata H, Haynes BF. Hum Immunol 1986;17:311
36. Telen MJ, Rogers I, Letarte M. Blood 1987;70:1475
37. Pickler LJ, de los Toyos J, Telen MJ, et al. J Immunol 1989;142:2046
38. Anstee DJ, Gardner B, Spring FA, et al. Immunology 1991;74:197
39. Stoll M, Dalchau R, Schmidt RE. In: Leukocyte Typing IV. Oxford:Oxford Univ Press, 1989:619
40. Telen MJ, Eisenbarth GS, Haynes BF. J Clin Invest 1983;71:1878
41. Lucas MG, Green AM, Telen MJ. Blood 1989;73:596
42. Kaye T. Unpublished observations 1978, cited by Daniels G, in Human Blood Groups. Oxford:Blackwell, 1995:599
43. Dalchau R, Kirkley J, Fabre JW. Eur J Immunol 1980;10:745
44. Flanagan BF, Dalchau R, Allen AK, et al. Immunology 1989;67:167
45. Poole J, Levene C, Bennett M, et al. Transf Med 1991;1:245
46. Lukasavage T. (Letter). Immunohematology 1993;9:112
47. Poole J, van Alphen L. (Letter). Transfusion 1988;28:289
48. Harris T, Steiert S, Marsh WL, et al. (Letter). Transfusion 1986;26:117
49. Magrin G, Harrison C. (abstract). Book of Abstracts Joint Cong ISBT/BBTS 1988:228
50. Poole J. Unpublished observations cited in Poole J, van Alphen L. (Letter). Transfusion 1988;28:289
51. de Man AJM, van Djik BA, Daniels GL. (Letter). Vox Sang 1992;63:238
52. Harrison CR, Heinz R, Chaudhuri TK. (abstract). Transfusion 1985;25:463
53. Davis K, Lucchesi G, Lyle B, et al. (abstract). Book of Abstracts, Joint Cong ISBT/AABB, 1990:153
54. Fitzsimmons J, Caggiano V. (abstract). Transfusion 1981;21;612
55. Whitsett CF, Hare VW, Oxendine SM, et al. Transfusion 1993;33:845
56. Knowles RW, Bai Y, Lomas C, et al. J Immunogenet 1982;9:353
57. van Alphen L, Poole J, Overbeeke M. FEMS Microbiol Lett 1986;37:69
58. van Alphen L, Levene C, Geelan-van der Broek L, et al.

Infect Immun 1990;58:3807

59. van Alphen L, Poole J, Geelan L, et al. Infect Immun 1987;55:2355
60. Telen MJ, Udani M, Washington MK, et al. J Biol Chem 1996;271:7147
61. Cobbold S, Hale G, Waldmann H. Leukocyte Typing III, Oxford:Oxford Univ Press 1987:788
62. Hughes EN, Colombatti A, August JT. J Biol Chem 1983;99:1613
63. Carter WG, Wayner EA. J Biol Chem 1988;263:4193
64. Haynes BF, Harden EA, Telen MJ. J Immunol 1983;131:1195
65. Jalkanen ST, Bargatze RF, Herron LR, et al. Eur J Immunol 1986;16:1195
66. Jalkanen ST, Jalkanen M, Bargatze R, et al. J Immunol 1988;141:1615
67. Stamenkovic I, Amiot M, Pesando JM, et al. Cell 1989;56:1057
68. Goldstein LA, Zhou DFH, Picker LJ, et al. Cell 1989;56:1063
69. Idzerda RL, Carter WG, Nottenburg C, et al. Proc Nat Acad Sci USA 1989;86:4659
70. Guo YJ, Lin S, Wang M, et al. Int Immunol 1994;6:213
71. Kalomiris EL, Bourguignon LYW. J Cell Biol 1988;106:319
72. Liu D, Sy M. J Exp Med 1996;183:1987
73. Screaton GR, Bell MV, Jackson DG, et al. Proc Nat Acad Sci USA 1992;89:12160
74. Lesley J, Hyman R, Kincase PW. Adv Immunol 1993;54:271
75. Bartolazzi A, Peach R, Aruffo A. J Exp Med 1994;180:53
76. Alberts B, Bray D, Lewis J, et al. The Molecular Biology of the Cell, 3rd Ed. New York:Garland, 1994:974
77. Peach RJ, Hollenbaugh E, Stamenkovic I, et al. J Cell Biol 1993;122:257
78. Liao H, Lee DM, Levesque MC, et al. J Immunol 1995;155:3938
79. Pure E, Camp RL, Peritt D, et al. J Exp Med 1995;181:55
80. Lokeshwar VB, Bouguignon LYW. J Biol Chem 1992;267:22073
81. Katoah S, Zheng Z, Oritani K, et al. J Exp Med 1995;182:419
82. Lesley J, English N, Perschl A, et al. J Exp Med 1995;182:431
83. Spring FA, Gardner B, Judson PA, et al. In: Leucocyte Typing V. Oxford:Oxford Univ Press, 1995:1738
84. Kansas GS, Muirhead MJ, Dailey MO. Blood 1990;76:2483
85. Miyake K, Medina KL, Hayashi S-L, et al. J Exp Med 1990;171:477
86. Haynes BF, Telen MJ, Hale LP, et al. Immunol Today 1989;10:423
87. Parsons SF, Mallinson G, Holmes CH, et al. Proc Nat Acad Sci USA 1995;92:5496
88. Shaw M-A, Leak MR, Daniels GL, et al. Ann Hum Genet 1984;48:229
89. Udden MM, Umeda M, Hirano Y, et al. Blood 1987;69:52
90. Telen MJ, Nelson J, Anderson N, et al. (abstract). Transfusion 1995;35 (Suppl 10S):60S
91. Agre P, Smith BL, Baumgarten R, et al. J Clin Invest 1994;94:1050

30 | Notes on the ISBT Collections of Antigens; the Antigens Cs^a and Cs^b; Er^a and Er^b; and Some Notes on HTLA Antibodies

At the 1988 meeting of the ISBT Working Party on Terminology for Red Cell Surface Antigens (1) assignments were made such that 19 independent blood group systems, that among them contained 157 antigens (some of which have subsequently been declared extinct), were recognized (for earlier deliberations see 2-5). These assignments left a large number of well studied antigens that had not been shown to be associated with a known blood group system, indeed several of them had been excluded from many, most or almost all of the known systems. Until 1988 these antigens had been assigned (2-5) to "holding series", that is the 700 series for antigens of low incidence and the 900 series for antigens of high incidence. In 1988, the Working Party concluded "that there is some merit in gathering together, into "Collections", specificities that have a serological, biochemical or genetic connection". It was decided that a serological connection could be based on dosage results supporting a genetic interpretation, on altered expression of some, or all, the antigens in a certain phenotype, or on absence of antigens from cells of an apparently null phenotype. A biochemical connection would be based on studies of epitope structures and a genetic connection might be indicated by family or population studies. Clearly, no matter the nature of the connections, they would fall short of proving that the antigens involved were encoded by genes at a locus independent of those of all known blood group systems. Indeed such evidence of an independent locus is the criterion for recognition of a blood group system. At the 1988 meeting nine collections: 201 Gerbich; 202 Cromer; 203 Indian; 204 Auberger; 205 Cost; 206 Gregory; 207 Ii; 208 Er; and 209 unnamed but including the antigens P, P^k and LKE, were established and among them included a total of 35 antigens. Movement of many high incidence antigens into Collections so decimated the 900 series that the series was abolished and the antigens left were reorganized into the 901 series (1). At the 1991 meeting of the Working Party (6) two additional collections were created: 210 unnamed but including the antigens Le^c and Le^d; and 211 Wright.

The decision to create Collections, that was not a unanimous one, can now be regarded as having been prophetic or as having been incorrect. The good news is that many of the Collections have subsequently graduated to full blood group system status or antigens from a single collection have moved en masse to the same blood group system (6-9). The other point of view is that had the antigens remained in the 700 and old 900 series, many of them could have been transferred into their permanent homes (systems) with relatively little delay, thus preventing an assortment of numbers (those of the now extinct collections) from being used and now being obsolete.

Table 30-1 lists the ISBT Collections still in existence (as of October 1996) and table 30-2 lists those now declared obsolete and gives reasons for their obsolescence. Other notes that pertain to tables 30-1 and 30-2 are that: 202 that was once called CROMER, became CROM; 209 that started with no name became GLOBO (for globoside) then GLOB when it was decided (9) that no more than four letters would be used in any name; and 210 that includes Le^c and Le^d (unaltered type 1 chain and type 1H, respectively, see Chapter 9) has defied the best efforts of the Working Party members to devise a name to describe it.

As will be apparent from table 30-1, antigens in some of the still existing Collections have already been described in this book. The I and i antigens (Collection 207) are in Chapter 10; the P, P^k and LKE antigens of the GLOB (209) Collection are in Chapter 11; and Le^c and Le^d of Collection 210 are in Chapter 9. Since all the antigens in table 30-2 now belong in independent blood group systems, they are described in the Chapter dealing with the blood group system itself. As will also be apparent from table 30-1, that leaves the Cs^a and Cs^b antigens of the COST (205) Collection and Er^a and Er^b antigens of the ER (208) Collection, to be described in this chapter.

The Antigens Cs^a and Cs^b and the Antibodies That Define Them

In 1965, Giles et al. (22) described three examples of a new antibody defining an antigen of high incidence. The two most fully studied examples were from the patients Copeland and Stirling, the authors named the antigen defined Cs^a, after the two patients. The term Cost, also derived from the names of the patients, was used to describe ISBT Collection 205 (see table 30-1). In the original study 354 of 363 (97.5%) samples from European Whites and 51 of 53 (96.2%) samples from US and African Blacks, were shown (22) to be Cs(a+).

TABLE 30-1 ISBT Collections as of October 1996

Collection Number	Conventional Name	Collection Symbol	Antigens Conventional Name	Antigens Full ISBT Code	Details in this Book
205	Cost	COST	Cs^a	205001	This Chapter
			Cs^b	205002	
207	Ii	I	I	207001	Chapter 10
			i	207002	
208	Er	ER	Er^a	208001	This Chapter
			Er^b	208002	
209		GLOB	P	209001	Chapter 11
			P^k	209002	
			LKE	209003	
210			Le^c	210001	Chapter 9
			Le^d	210002	

Similar figures emerged from a later study (23) in which it was found that 1931 of 2028 (95.2%) of US Whites and 883 of 894 (98.8%) US Blacks had Cs(a+) red cells. As discussed in Chapter 28, another study (24) revealed an unexpectedly high incidence of the phenotype Cs(a-), Yk(a-). Among 96 US Whites with Yk(a-) red cells, 12 were phenotypically Cs(a-). Among 13 Blacks with Yk(a-) red cells, one was also phenotypically Cs(a-). Based on the incidence of Cs^a (above) and Yk^a (see Chapter 28) in US Whites and Blacks, it would be expected that the Cs(a-), Yk(a-) phenotype would be seen in 1 in 213 Whites and 1 in 4166 Blacks. In the report

TABLE 30-2 Previously Recognized but now Obsolete ISBT Collections

Collection Number	Collection Symbol	Antigens Originally Included	Current Assignments of Antigens and Reason for Change
201	GE	Ge2, Ge3, Ge4, Wb, Ls^a	Became the Gerbich System (Chapter 16) and others added once seen to be encoded by *GYPC* that is independent of all other systems (10).
202	CROM	Cr^a, Tc^a, Tc^b, Tc^c, Dr^a, Es^a, IFC, WES^a, WES^b, UMC	Became the Cromer System (Chapter 24) once shown to be on DAF and *DAF* shown to be independent of all other systems (11).
203	IN	In^a, In^b	Became the Indian System (Chapter 29) when shown to be on CD44 and *CD44* shown to be independent of all other systems (12).
204	AU	Au^a, Au^b	Transferred to Lutheran System (Chapter 20) when shown to be encoded from the *LU* locus (13-15).
206	GY	Gy^a, Hy	Transferred to the Dombrock System (Chapter 21) when shown to be on the Dombrock glycoprotein (16,17).
211	WR	Wr^a, Wr^b	Transferred to the Diego System (Chapter 17) when shown to represent a polymorphism on band 3 (18).

Collection 205 (COST) originally included seven members. The antigens Yk^a,Kn^a,Kn^b,McC^a and Sl^a became the Knops System (Chapter 28) when they were shown to be carried on CRI and *CRI* was shown to be independent of all other systems (19,20). Cs^a and Cs^b are not on CRI (20,21) and remain in Collection 205 (see table 30-1)

cited above (24) and in others (23,26) the observed frequency of individuals with Cs(a-), Yk(a-) red cells was 1 in 52 in Whites and 1 in 165 in Blacks. Further, the red cells of Margaret Helgeson (also see Chapter 28) that type as Kn(a-) McC(a-) Sl(a-) Yk(a-) were found (23,25) also to be Cs(a-). In spite of the higher than expected (if Cs^a and Yk^a are not associated with each other) incidence of the Cs(a-), Yk(a-) phenotype, Cs^a, unlike Yk^a, is not an antigen of the Knops blood group system. First (24,26), *Cs^a* and *Yk^a* segregate independently. Second, while Kn^a, McC^a, Sl^a and Yk^a are carried on CR1 (19,20,27) Cs^a is not (20,21,27). Third, three additional red cell samples of the Helgeson phenotype (Kn(a-) McC(a-) Sl(a-) Yk(a-)) have been shown (21) to be Cs(a+). The different locations of Cs^a and Yk^a are further demonstrated by the facts that Cs^a survives treatment of red cells with trypsin and chymotrypsin and is not altered when red cells are treated with AET, while Yk^a is removed or denatured by the two enzymes listed and is at least partially degraded by AET (28).

In 1987, Molthan and Paradis (29) described an antibody, made by a woman who had received many transfusions, that reacted with 56 of 59 Cs(a-) samples. The antibody was said to define Cs^b, the antithetical partner of Cs^a. In tests on 175 Cs(a+) samples, 55 (31%) were said to be Cs(b+). Two somewhat discomforting findings in the study were first, that the antibody-maker had only a weak Cs^a antigen on her red cells. Second, if the antibody was truly anti-Cs^b, then three of the 59 Cs(a-) samples tested would have to have been Cs(a-b-). It is somewhat disturbing to find evidence for a third and/or a silent allele when an antithetical partner to a known antigen is first found. In the initial report (29) a family study supporting the existence of a third allele is described. However, such a finding would also be explained if the new antibody did not have anti-Cs^b specificity. We are not aware of another example of anti-Cs^b being found.

The Cs^a antigen is apparently developed at birth although the reactions of cord blood red cells with anti-Cs^a may be somewhat weaker than the reactions of red cells from adults (30); no case of HDN caused by anti-Cs^a or anti-Cs^b has been reported.

Anti-Cs^a is usually an IgG antibody that is optimally reactive by IAT, IgG subclassing studies do not seem to have been reported. Work with the antibody is difficult since most anti-Cs^a react only weakly and there is considerable variation in strength of the antigen defined, on different Cs(a+) samples. Although the reactions of anti-Cs^a are usually weak, some examples react at high dilutions (see the section on HTLA antibodies later in this chapter). Anti-Cs^a is a clinically insignificant antibody. Transfusions of Cs(a+) blood to patients with anti-Cs^a in the serum, in vivo red cell survival studies and in vitro phagocytic cell assays have all demonstrated that anti-

Cs^a does not bring about clinically relevant clearance of Cs(a+) red cells in vivo (22,26,31-34). We are aware of many other cases in which patients with anti-Cs^a in the serum have been uneventfully and successfully transfused with Cs(a+) blood. As with many of the antibodies described in Chapters 27 and 28, these events have not all been reported in the literature since the successful transfusions were exactly what was anticipated. Molthan et al. (35) and Molthan (30) have reported what they claimed were transfusion reactions caused by anti-Cs^a plus anti-Yk^a and by anti-Cs^a. There is a long discussion in the section on Yk^a in Chapter 28 explaining why we and the majority of other workers do not accept the validity of those reports. Those reasons need not be repeated here, suffice it to say that in spite of those reports we consider anti-Cs^a to be clinically benign.

The Antigens Er^a and Er^b and the Antibodies That Define Them

For many years before 1982, many workers tested serum samples from a patient by the name of Rosebush, that contained an antibody directed against an antigen of high incidence. In 1982, Daniels et al. (36) published the results of their study on three antibodies in the sera Ros (Rosebush), Min and Rod. They concluded first, that the sera contained the same antibody, that was named anti-Er^a, or antibodies of very similar specificities, and second, that Er^a differed from any other common antigen previously described. From the outset it was clear that heterogeneity exists among examples of anti-Er^a. In the Ros and Min families, the red cells of Er(a-) persons did not react with any of the three anti-Er^a. In the Rod family, the red cells of some apparently Er(a-) individuals gave unexpected findings. Two persons with supposedly Er(a-) red cells had cells that reacted weakly with the Rod serum but were non-reactive with the Ros serum while three others had cells that were non-reactive with the Rod serum but were weakly reactive with the Ros antibody. Since the Er(a-) phenotype was present in two successive generations in the Rod family, it seemed possible that dominant suppression of expression of Er^a in that family might explain the findings. In the Ros and Min families, inheritance of the Er(a-) phenotype fit the pattern of recessive inheritance of a rare allele not encoding production of Er^a. However, later findings (see below) showed that inheritance of the Er(a-) phenotype in the Rod family also appears to represent inheritance of recessive alleles.

Heterogeneity of anti-Er^a seems again to be involved in a Japanese family described by Naoki et al. (37). The proposita who had been both pregnant and transfused, made an antibody that reacted with all red cells except those known to be Er(a-b+) (for Er[b] see below), her own and those of two of her sibs. However, the red cells of the antibody-maker and her two compatible sibs while failing to react with five anti-Er[a] (including Ros) did react strongly with two other anti-Er[a] and weakly with a third. It is reported (38) that a number of other antibodies to high incidence antigens, that react only weakly with Er(a-) red cells, have been found and that cross-testing of the sera and red cells of the antibody-makers yields a complex pattern. Clearly, the term Er[a] describes a series of very similar but not identical antigens while some examples of so-called anti-Er[a] have slightly different specificities.

If the apparent heterogeneity of anti-Er[a] is ignored, which can be done for this purpose since the red cells of most random individuals react with all examples of anti-Er[a], it is seen that Er[a] is of very high incidence. In tests on the red cells of 63,762 donors, most of whom were White, no Er(a-) sample was found (36,39,40). Similarly, all of 13,521 random Japanese blood donors had Er(a+) red cells (37). Reported individuals with Er(a-) red cells that do not react with any anti-Er[a] have all been White (36,38,39,41,42). As described above, a phenotype in which the red cells reacted with three of eight anti-Er[a], was found in Japan.

In 1988, Hamilton et al. (43) described an antibody that gave many of the reactions expected of one that defines an antigen antithetical to Er[a]. The antibody was called anti-Er[b] and the antigen it defines has received an ISBT number, see table 30-1. The antibody reacted with most Er(a-) samples and with the red cells of four of 605 random White donors. Use of this antibody showed that the presence of the Er(a-) phenotype in two successive generations of the Rod family (see above) resulted from an Er(a-b+) X Er(a+b+) mating. Others (39,41,42) had also presented evidence that in different families, the Er(a-) phenotype represents a recessively inherited characteristic.

Good as the evidence was, that Er[b] is antithetical to Er[a], there were two disquieting findings. First, one known Er(a-) sample failed to react with the supposed anti-Er[b]. Second, an Er(a-b+) woman had borne a daughter whose red cells were Er(a+) but non-reactive with the supposed anti-Er[b]. Just as was the case with Cs[a] and the supposed anti-Cs[b] described above, it is somewhat disturbing to have to invoke existence of a third and/or silent allele, at the time the antibody defining an apparently antithetical antigen is first found. Clearly one of us (PDI) would have been very disturbed if the first example of anti-Fy[b] had been tested only against Fy(a+) and Fy(a-) red cells from Blacks. No further example of an antibody giving the same pattern as the supposed anti-Er[b] has been found.

If Er[a] and Er[b] are indeed encoded by alleles and if the silent gene *Er* (or a third allele) is very rare, it can be calculated (44) that the Er(a-) phenotype may have an incidence of only 1 in 100,000 Whites. If, as the data of Hamilton et al. (43) suggest, *Er* is not as rare as some other silent alleles, the incidence of the Er(a-) phenotype may be somewhat higher. That is, persons genetically *Er[b]Er* and *ErEr* would, like those genetically *Er[b]Er[b]*, have Er(a-) red cells.

Er[a] is fully developed on cord blood red cells. Both Er[a] (28,34,45) and Er[b] (43) survive the treatment of red cells with papain and ficin, additionally (28,34,43,45) Er[a] has been shown to survive treatment of red cells with trypsin, chymotrypsin, pronase, neuraminidase and AET, while Er[b] has been shown to survive treatment of red cells with DTT. Liew and Uchikawa (45) found that exposure of red cells to acid pH solutions, that are sometimes used in antibody elution procedures (46,47), resulted in denaturation of the Er[a] antigen. EDTA-glycine-HCl at pH 1.5 and pH 2.0 caused complete denaturation, glycine-HCl at pH 2.5 caused marked but not total denaturation while glycine-HCl at pH 3.0 and EDTA alone, had no measurable effect on the antigen.

Anti-Er[a] and the single example of anti-Er[b] are IgG antibodies that do not fix complement. All known examples of anti-Er[a] have been made by individuals who had been transfused, most of them had also been pregnant (36,37,39,41,42). The example of anti-Er[b] was made by a woman who had been pregnant five times but had never been transfused (43). Successful transfusions of Er(a+) red cells to patients with anti-Er[a] in the serum, in vivo red cell survival studies and in vitro phagocytic cell assays have all been used (36,39) to demonstrate that the anti-Er[a] involved were clinically benign. Both anti-Er[a] and anti-Er[b] have caused positive DATs on the red cells of infants born to immunized women, in no instance was clinical HDN seen.

Notes on HTLA Antibodies

In the 1960s and 1970s before some of the antigens listed in table 30-3 had been characterized, many workers encountered troublesome antibodies of poorly defined specificities. Characteristically, these antibodies gave variable and sometimes difficult to reproduce reactions with different antigen-positive red cell samples. Second, although the reactions of the antibodies were weak when undiluted serum was used in IATs, titrations of some of them showed the same weak reactions out to fairly high dilutions, i.e. 1 in 256 or 1 in 512. Third, most of the antigens defined seemed to be present on the red cells of most (i.e. 90 to 99%) random donors. Fourth, some but by no means all the antibodies could be neutralized with pooled human serum or plasma. Fifth, when patients with the antibodies were transfused with "least incompatible" blood as determined by serological studies, they did not have transfusion reactions, nor did the antibodies increase in strength after transfusion (i.e. no apparent secondary immune responses). Sixth, although some patients developed positive (mixed-field) DATs after transfusion and although the same antibody as present in the serum could sometimes be recovered by elution from the transfused red cells, there was no evidence of clinically relevant accelerated clearance of the transfused red cells. Seventh, some of the antibodies resisted attempts to remove them from sera even by multiple adsorptions with the most strongly reactive red cells. Eighth, all the serological difficulties described were magnified when traveled red cells (often the only supposed antigen-negative red cells available) were used. Early reviews on the difficulties caused by these antibodies in in vitro tests were published by Swanson (48), Giles (26), Vengelen-Tyler (49) and Moulds (50,51).

In order to describe some of the serological characteristics of these antibodies the term high-titer, low-avidity was introduced. Who first used the term, where and when, seems to be lost in the immunohematological mists of time. Given the disrepute in which the term is now held, it seems unlikely that a claim for its introduction will be made (if that is wrong and credit is claimed, please contact the authors through the publisher). The term high-titer was meant to explain the continued reactions of the antibodies at high dilutions (see above). While this description is still accurate for some of the antibodies, Rolih (52) in an excellent review, has pointed out that some antibodies of the specificities involved are,

in fact, of low titer. The term low-avidity was meant to explain the 1+ reactions with undiluted serum and the 1+ reactions of 1 in 256 or 1 in 512 dilutions of the same serum. There was never any real evidence that the antibodies had low avidity. Indeed, it is now generally believed (with a little more but far from complete evidence) that the equal strength reactions with undiluted and diluted sera represent a paucity of antigen sites on the red cells. That is to say that no matter how many antibody molecules are present in the serum, the antigen site density on red cells is low enough that when all, or most of the antigens bind antibody, there is still too little antibody bound to give greater than a 1+ or 2+ reaction in tests (IATs) with anti-IgG. As mentioned in other chapters of this book, while it is known that some antigens are present in only low copy numbers per red cell, the paucity of antigen sites is only an assumed explanation in others. Nevertheless, it is antigen site paucity versus low avidity that has caused the term HTLA to fall from favor. Those who wish to retain the term could claim that it stands for High Titer Low Antigen density.

Table 30-3 lists the antigens considered by Rolih (52) to be defined by antibodies regarded, in the past, to be of HTLA. A second portion of the table includes other antigens defined by antibodies often assumed to be of this type. A third portion of table 30-3 lists a series of antigens, the antibodies to which sometimes masquerade as HTLA. Therein lies the danger. Some antibodies that present in vitro with HTLA characteristics may, in fact, be of more clinical significance than those generally considered to be of the HTLA type. It must be added that while part 1 of table 30-3 is from Rolih (52), parts 2 and 3 represent the views of one of us (PDI).

Now that the antigens listed in the first part of table 30-3 have been better characterized, it is often possible to assign a specificity to an antibody that would previously have been described as one of HTLA. Most reference laboratories have red cell samples negative for the antigens listed. However, it is debatable as to whether the time, effort and expense necessary to identify such specificities are justified. Many workers, once convinced that the antibody falls into the group previously called HTLA, are prepared to issue serologically incompatible blood with the expectation that it will not cause a transfusion reaction and that the transfused red cells will survive normally in vivo. It is hard to argue with such logic and indeed the practice is followed in one of our (PDI) laboratories. However, two provisos need to be included. First, it should be shown that the reactions of the benign antibody are not masking the presence of a clinically more relevant antibody that is simultaneously present. Second, sufficient tests should be completed to show that the presumed clinically-insignificant antibody is not actually one of more clinical relevance that is presenting

---

TABLE 30-3 Antigens Defined by Antibodies That Often Have HTLA Characteristics

Part 1 Antigens defined by antibodies that usually have HTLA characteristics (after Rolih 52)

Cs^a Yk^a Kn^a Kn^b McC^a McC^b McC^c McC^d

McC^f Sl^a Sl^b Rg Ch JMH

Part 2 Antigens defined by antibodies that sometimes have HTLA characteristics

Gy^a Hy Jo^a(Jc^a)

Part 3 Antigens defined by antibodies, some of which have HTLA characteristics

Ge2 Ge3 Yt^a Lu^b para-Lu high incidence

para-Kell high incidence Cr system high incidence

Fy3 Co^a Di^b In^b Vel

with the characteristics of an HTLA antibody as outlined in the beginning of this section. Perhaps the greatest value in establishing specificity of an antibody as defining an antigen listed in the first part of table 30-3 is that it demonstrates that the antibody is not something else!

Three other points need to be added. First, while some antibodies previously said to be of HTLA will be recognizable as defining Cs^a, Yk^a, Ch, Rg, JMH, etc., many others will have similar but not exactly those specificities. Thus anti-Kn-like, anti-Cs^a-like, et al., will be seen due, presumably, to heterogeneity of the antibodies. Second, while antibodies to Ch, Rg and some other antibodies will be readily inhibited by plasma, in antibody neutralization studies, so too will some for which such inhibition is unexpected. One of us (PDI) has seen a fair number of antibodies, some of which failed to react with Cs(a-) and/or Yk(a-), etc. red cells, that were neutralized by serum but not by saline (i.e. the control). Perhaps the explanation is that Cs(a-), Yk(a-) and Kn-McC null-type red cells have a minor abnormality of the red cell membrane that results in structures other than Cs^a, Yk^a, Kn^a and McC^a being absent or difficult to detect. The inhibitable antibodies might thus have slightly different specificities from those that detect Cs^a, Yk^a, Kn^a, et al., but might still fail to react with red cells that lack one or more of the antigens listed. Whatever the explanation, one of us (PDI) continues to regard inhibition studies using pooled normal sera as a useful adjunct procedure in the recognition of antibodies to common antigens, that will not destroy antigen-positive red cells in vivo. Third, while assigning an antibody to the group with the characteristics listed of HTLA antibodies generally equates with clinical insignificance of the antibody, rare exceptions may be seen in that an antibody directed against an antigen in part 1 of table 30-3, has the ability to destroy antigen-positive red cells in vivo. This does not invalidate some of the serological criteria that correlate with clinical insignificance of an antibody. For example, the anti-JMH (see Chapter 31) that we studied (53,54) that

did destroy antigen-positive red cells in a ^{51}Cr red cell survival study, did not present with typical HTLA characteristics. The antibody gave progressively stronger reactions when tested by PEG-IAT, LISS-IAT and saline-IAT, exactly the opposite to what would be expected of an HTLA antibody. Table 30-4 shows the results most often seen with the antibodies described in this section. As will be appreciated from what is written in this section, patterns intermediate between those shown in table 30-4 will be encountered.

References

1. Lewis M, Anstee DJ, Bird GWG, et al. Vox Sang 1990;58:152
2. Allen FH Jr, Anstee DJ, Bird GWG, et al. Vox Sang 1982;42:164
3. Allen FH Jr. ISBT Newsletter, No 18, April 1983
4. Lewis M, Allen FH Jr, Anstee DJ, et al. Vox Sang 1985;49:171
5. Lewis M. ISBT Newsletter, No 34, April 1987
6. Lewis M, Anstee DJ, Bird GWG, et al. Vox Sang 1991;61:158
7. Daniels GL, Moulds JJ, Anstee DJ, et al. Vox Sang 1993;65:77
8. Daniels GL, Anstee DJ, Cartron J-P, et al. Vox Sang 1995;69:265
9. Daniels GL, Anstee DJ, Cartron J-P, et al. Vox Sang 1996;71:246
10. Zelinski T, Kaita H, Lewis M, et al. Vox Sang 1991;61:62
11. Lewis M, Kaita H, Philipps S, et al. Vox Sang 1989;57:210
12. Bruce LJ, Anstee DJ, Spring FA, et al. J Biol Chem 1994;269:16155
13. Daniels GL. Vox Sang 1990;58:56
14. Zelinski T, Kaita H, Johnson K, et al. Vox Sang 1990;58:126
15. Zelinski T, Kaita H, Coghlan G, et al. Vox Sang 1991;61:275
16. Banks JA, Parker N, Poole J. (abstract). Transf Med 1992;2 (Suppl 1):68
17. Spring FA, Reid ME, Nicholson G. Vox Sang 1994;66:72
18. Bruce LJ, Ring SM, Anstee DJ, et al. Blood 1995;85:541
19. Rao N, Ferguson DJ, Lee S-F, et al. Immunology 1991;146:3502
20. Moulds JM, Nickells MW, Moulds JJ, et al. J Exp Med 1991;173:1159
21. Moulds JM, Moulds JJ, Brown M, et al. Vox Sang

TABLE 30-4 Some Patterns in Titrations with Antibodies Often Called HTLA

	Serum Dilutions, 1 in									
	1	2	4	8	16	32	64	128	256	512
Common finding	1+	1+	1+	1+	$+^w$	$+^w$	$+^w$	$+^w$	$+^w$	$+^w$
Common finding	1+	1+	$+^w$	$+^w$	$+^w$	$+^w$	$+^w$	$+^w$	0	0
Less common finding	2+	2+	1+	1+	1+	1+	1+	$+^w$	$+^w$	$+^w$
Less common finding	$+^w$	$+^w$	$+^w$	$+^w$	$+^w$	0	0	0	0	0
Rare finding	$+^w$	$+^w$	$+^w$	$+^w$	$+^w$	$+^w$	$+^w$	$+^w$	$+^w$	0
Rare finding	1+	$+^w$	$+^w$	0	0	0	0	0	0	0
NOT an HTLA pattern	2+	1+	0	0	0	0	0	0	0	0

1992;62:230

22. Giles CM, Huth MC, Wilson TE, et al. Vox Sang 1965;10:405

23. Molthan L. Am J Med Technol 1983;49:49

24. Molthan L, Giles CM. Vox Sang 1975;29:145

25. Helgeson M, Swanson J, Polesky HF. Transfusion 1970;10:137

26. Giles CM. In: Human Blood Groups. Basel:Karger, 1977:268

27. Petty AC. (abstract). Transf Med 1993;3 (Suppl 1):84

28. Daniels G. Immunohematology 1992;8:53

29. Molthan L, Paradis DJ. Med Lab Sci 1987;44:94

30. Molthan L. Rev Fr Transf Immunohematol 1982;25:127

31. Shore GM, Steane EA. (abstract). Transfusion 1978;18:387

32. Valko DA, Silberstein EB, Greenwalt TJ, et al. (abstract). Transfusion 1981;21:603

33. Gutgsell NS, Issitt LA, Issitt PD. (abstract). Transfusion 1988;28 (Suppl 6S):32S

34. Issitt PD. Applied Blood Group Serology, 3rd Ed. Miami:Montgomery 1985

35. Molthan L, Wick RW Jr, Gross BM. Blood Transf Immunohematol 1981;24:263

36. Daniels GL, Judd WJ, Moore BPL, et al. Transfusion 1982;22:189

37. Naoki K, Okuma S, Uchiyama E, et al. (Letter). Transfusion 1991;31:572

38. Daniels GL, Poole J, Lacey P. Unpublished observations cited in Daniels G. Human Blood Groups. Oxford:Blackwell, 1995:627

39. Thompson HW, Skradski KJ, Thoreson JR, et al. Transfusion

40. Gale SA, Rowe GP, Northfield FE. Vox Sang 1988;54:172

41. Lylloff K, Georgsen J, Grunnet N, et al. (Letter). Transfusion 1987;27:118

42. Rowe GP. (Letter). Transfusion 1988;28:87

43. Hamilton JR, Beattie KM, Walker RH, et al. Transfusion 1988;28:268

44. Daniels G. Human Blood Groups. Oxford:Blackwell, 1995:626

45. Liew YW, Uchikawa M. (Letter). Transfusion 1987;27:442

46. Louie JE, Jiang AF, Zaroulis CG. (abstract). Transfusion 1986;26:550

47. Judd WJ. Methods in Immunohematology, 2nd Ed. Durham:Montgomery 1994

48. Swanson J. In: A Seminar on Recent Advances in Immunohematology. Washington, D.C.:Am Assoc Blood Banks, 1973:121

49. Vengelen-Tyler V. In: High-titer, Low-avidity Antibodies: Recognition and Resolution. Washington, D.C.:Am Assoc Blood Banks, 1980:21

50. Moulds MK. In: High-titer, Low-avidity Antibodies: Recognition and Resolution. Washington, D.C.:Am Assoc Blood Banks, 1980:33

51. Moulds MK. Am J Med Technol 1981;47:789

52. Rolih SD. Transf Med Rev 1989;3:128

53. Issitt PD, Combs MR, Mudad R, et al. (abstract). Transfusion 1995;35 (Suppl 10S):22S

54. Mudad R, Rao N, Issitt PD, et al. Transfusion 1995;35:925

1985;25:140

31 | Well Characterized Independent Antigens of High Incidence

As mentioned in Chapter 30, creation of antigen Collections by the ISBT Working Party on Terminology for Red Cell Surface Antigens (1) so decimated the 900 series that had previously (2) housed all independent antigens of high incidence, that a new series, 901, was created for those antigens of high incidence not assigned to a blood group system or to a collection. The antigens currently assigned to the 901 series are listed in table 31-1 and some details about them are provided in this chapter. As will be seen from table 31-1, the antigens of the 901 series are not numbered in sequence of discovery. As with the introduction of the term HTLA, the reasons that the 901 series is not in date sequence are lost in the mists of time.

The Vel Antigen

In 1952, Susman and Miller (3) described anti-Vel, an antibody that reacted with all except four of 10,000 samples tested. Many other examples of anti-Vel have been reported and the antibody has been used in a number of large scale surveys of Whites in Europe, the USA

and Australia (i.e. essentially from the same stock). If the results of surveys in the UK, Sweden, Norway, Finland, France, the USA and Australia (3,20-30) are summed, it is seen that 251,170 samples have been typed and 95 persons (i.e. 1 in 2644) with Vel- red cells have been found. However, more than half the Vel- individuals were found in one survey in Sweden where Cedergren et al. (27) found a much higher incidence of the phenotype in the north of that country than was found elsewhere. That is, in the Swedish study (27) 91,605 samples were typed and 52 were found to be Vel- for an incidence of 1 in 1762. If these tests are subtracted from those totaling 251,170 described above, it is seen that excluding Sweden, the incidence of the Vel- phenotype was 43 in 159,565 or 1 in 3711. There are some tantalizing data that suggest that the Vel- phenotype may be more frequent in other parts of the world. Chandanayingyong et al. (31) found that four of 328 Thais and Alfred et al. (32) that two of 160 Chilcotin Indians in Canada, had Vel- red cells.

When the early studies on the Vel- phenotype were performed there were some indications (24,33,34) that its inheritance might not be straightforward. However, in the majority of families studied (21,24,27,35-37) the pheno-

TABLE 31-1 Independent High Incidence Antigens

Historical Name	Conventional Symbol	ISBT Full Code Number	Incidence Among Random Whites	Original References	Year First Described
Vel	Vel	901001	>99.9	3	1952
Langereis	Lan	901002	>99.9	4	1961
Augustine	At^a	901003	>99.9	5	1967
Junior	Jr^a	901005	>99.9	6	1970
	Ok^a	901006	>99.9	7	1979
John Milton Hagen	JMH	901007	>99.9	8	1978
	Emm	901008	>99.9	9	1987
Anton	AnWj	901009	>99.9	10-13	1982
Raph	MER 2	901011	92	14	1987
Sid	Sd^a	901012	96	15, 16	1967
Duclos	Duclos	901013	>99.9	17	1978
	PEL	901014	>99.9	18	1980
	ABTI	901015	>99.9	19	1996

The numbers 901004 and 901010 were previously used for Jo^a and Wr^b, respectively. They became obsolete when Jo^a joined the Dombrock System as DO5 (014005), see Chapter 22, and Wr^b joined the Diego System as DI4 (010004), see Chapter 17.

type appears to represent a recessively inherited condition. Some phenotypic associations between the Vel- state and other blood group antigens are discussed below.

The strength of the Vel antigen varies considerably on the Vel+ red cells of different individuals. It is possible that some of the serological difficulties mentioned in this section and the next, relate to the difficulty of detection of the antigen when expressed in its weakest form. Variation in antigen strength does not always seem to be correlated with heterozygosity for the genes encoding and not encoding production of the antigen although the antigen may be difficult to detect on the red cells of infants born to Vel- women (i.e. infants heterozygous for the gene encoding production of Vel). The Vel antigen is not fully developed at the time of birth (22,38,39) although it has been detected on the red cells of fetuses at 12 to 28 weeks gestation (21,40). The antigen survives treatment of red cells with trypsin, chymotrypsin, papain, pronase, neuraminidase and AET (41). One case has been recorded (27) in which a patient with iron deficiency anemia was twice typed, at an interval of eight months, as Vel-. At the time of the second typing the woman was four months pregnant and two months later her red cells were seen to type as weakly positive for Vel. One month after that her red cells carried a normal expression of Vel that persisted to the time of her delivery and was still demonstrable when her red cells were typed six months later. No details are given of typings more than six months after the delivery.

Anti-Vel

Many examples of anti-Vel have been documented in the literature (3,20-24,27,35-38,42-45,47-49). The antibody seems always to be made by individuals who have been transfused (most examples) and/or pregnant. In many family studies it has been found that the never transfused, never pregnant Vel- sibs of the probands did not have anti-Vel in the serum. In spite of these findings anti-Vel is not uncommonly an IgM antibody capable of agglutinating untreated red cells in a saline system. IgM complement binding anti-Vel sometimes present as hemolysins (20-23,36,42,49), one of very few specificities outside the ABO system with this property. IgG anti-Vel also exist (45,47,56) two such examples were shown (47,56) to contain IgG1 and IgG3 components, another was shown (56) to be just IgG1.

Anti-Vel can be a difficult antibody with which to work in serological studies. As described above, while most red cell samples from random donors type as Vel+, a subset give only weak reactions. Attempts to confirm the Vel+ status of these samples may be difficult since anti-Vel do not often work well in adsorption-elution studies. It is

sometimes useful to run tests against papain or ficin-treated red cells since some examples of anti-Vel react more strongly with such cells than with untreated ones. In 1968, we (43) thought that we had found an explanation of some of these difficulties. We reported that most Vel- samples lacked two high incidence antigens and could thus be described as Vel:-1,-2. Persons of that phenotype were said to make anti-Vel 1,2 the common form of anti-Vel. We also said that the Vel:1,-2 phenotype existed and that persons with red cells of that phenotype could make anti-Vel 2. Adsorption-elution experiments appeared to confirm these findings and Vel:1,-2 red cells seemed to adsorb anti-Vel 1 and leave anti-Vel 2, when used to adsorb sera that contained both antibodies. We suspected that the weakly Vel+ samples mentioned above came from persons heterozygous for the genes that make and do not make Vel and from persons phenotypically Vel:1,-2. In spite of the clear cut results in our initial experiments (43) neither we (50) nor others were able to repeat them. Indeed, repeated adsorption of sera that supposedly contained anti-Vel 1 and anti-Vel 2 with red cells supposedly of the Vel:1,-2 phenotype, eventually removed all antibody. It appears (50) that the difference between what we (43) had called Vel 1 and Vel 2 is purely quantitative.

Anti-Vel can be a clinically-significant antibody. The first example found (3) and at least two other (23,33) alloimmune anti-Vel (for autoimmune examples see below) caused severe immediate hemolytic transfusion reactions. Another example (45) cleared 96% of a test dose of ^{51}Cr labeled Vel+ red cells in a little over an hour after their injection. An example described by Storry and Mallory (49) was overlooked when a prewarmed compatibility test was performed, the patient was transfused with two units of Vel+ blood and died some eight hours later. The abstract does not comment on the role (if any) of the anti-Vel in the patient's demise. When samples were referred to the authors' (49) laboratory, after the patient's death, the pretransfusion serum was shown to hemolyze Vel+ red cells when LISS and papain methods were used. Given the in vivo and in vitro activities of many examples of anti-Vel, most workers elect to transfuse only Vel- units to patients with the antibody. We had heard anecdotal reports about the successful use of Vel+ blood for transfusion to patients with weak anti-Vel in the serum and one such case is mentioned (51) briefly in the literature although few details are given. Accordingly, when we (52) encountered a patient with a rather weak anti-Vel (IAT no stronger than 1+ with any red cell sample tested) that did not cause hemolysis in vitro, we used a modified Ashby test (see Chapter 43) to demonstrate apparently normal survival of Vel+ red cells in the patient's circulation. Thus emboldened by the use of 200 ml Vel+ red cells in the Ashby test, we transfused the patient with another two units of Vel+ blood. There was neither an immediate nor a delayed transfusion reaction; the expected increase in hemoglobin was achieved and maintained; one week following the transfusions the level of anti-Vel in the patient's serum was the same as it had been before the transfusions. Two months later the patient required further transfusions, to relieve anemia caused by intensive chemotherapy, and was again successfully transfused with Vel+ blood.

In spite of the success in the case described in the previous paragraph, we would caution that most patients with anti-Vel must probably be transfused with Vel-blood. Vel+ blood should be used only if there is good evidence from carefully conducted tests, that the patient's antibody will not cause catastrophic in vivo destruction of antigen-positive red cells.

Anti-Vel has never been reported as causing severe HDN. No doubt the facts discussed above that the Vel antigen is not fully developed at birth and that many examples of anti-Vel are wholly or predominantly IgM in nature contribute to that finding. In one case (47) an infant with Vel+ red cells born to a mother with IgG anti-Vel in the serum, had a positive DAT at birth but the only treatment required was phototherapy.

Autoimmune Anti-Vel

Auto-anti-Vel has been reported a number of times (29,46,53,54) but the cases were not all straightforward. In the first documented case (53) the antibody would agglutinate and hemolyze Vel+ and the patient's own red cells, once the cells had been treated with bromelin. Although the antibody was active at 37°C there was no evidence that it was causing in vivo red cell destruction. Presumably the facts that the antibody was IgM and that it would agglutinate untreated Vel+ red cells only weakly and did not react with such cells by IAT, meant that it was more like a benign "enzyme-only" autoantibody than like those that cause WAIHA. In the second reported case (29) the auto-anti-Vel was present in a patient with severe anemia. Although the authors (29) concluded that the auto-anti-Vel was contributing to the patient's hemolytic anemia, they reported that Vel+ donor red cells had a reduced survival time in the patient's circulation but that the patient's own Vel+ red cells, that were coated with complement, survived normally. In the third case (46) it was concluded that the auto-anti-Vel was causing accelerated clearance of the patient's red cells. In the fourth case (54) the patient's red cells typed as Vel+ and the serum contained anti-Vel. The patient apparently had hemolytic anemia and also had a massive transfusion reaction when transfused, due to life-threatening complications, with Vel+ blood. In spite of these findings the DAT was consistently negative and no antibody could be recovered by

elution from the patient's red cells. Other findings in the case suggested that the auto-anti-Vel was IgM in nature. Although the patient, a nine week-old White girl, died from complications of the hemolytic process, complement was never detected on her own red cells.

Phenotypic Associations of Vel with Other Blood Group Antigens

Race and Sanger (39) pointed out that in vitro, anti-Vel and anti-Tj^a (see Chapter 11) are somewhat alike in that both can present as hemolysins. The antibodies differ, of course, in that anti-Vel is apparently only made following exposure of Vel- people to Vel+ red cells while anti-Tj^a is found in all persons with Tj(a-) red cells, including those who have never been transfused or pregnant. It was also pointed out (39) that there is an apparent excess of the P$_2$ phenotype (again see Chapter 11) among persons with Vel- red cells and that evidence for independent segregation of *Vel* from *P^1* was slow to emerge. As mentioned earlier, at one time it seemed possible that in some cases the Vel- phenotype arose due to inheritance of a dominant suppressor gene. As discussed in detail in Chapter 20, there is an excess of the P$_2$ phenotype (not a reduced incidence of the *P^1* gene) among persons who inherit the dominant suppressor, *In(Lu)*. When Cedergren et al. (27) conducted their large study in Sweden, they found six families in which it could be shown that Vel is not part of the P system. However, in those six families there was still an excess of the P$_2$ phenotype among persons with Vel- red cells.

In 1994, we (55) described a patient who had made an antibody to a high incidence antigen. Although his red cells failed to react with some anti-Vel, he was eventually shown to have Ge- red cells (see Chapter 16) and to have made anti-Ge. We then tested 14 anti-Vel against: eight Ge:-2,-3,4; one Ge:-2,3,4; and one Ge:-2,-3,-4 samples. Three of the anti-Vel failed to react with at least four of the Ge:-2,-3,4 samples while two others were non-reactive with some of these samples. The other nine anti-Vel reacted with all Ge:-2,-3,4 samples tested. Reactivity or lack thereof was not related to the strength of the anti-Vel and there was heterogeneity among the samples failing to react with some anti-Vel. All 14 anti-Vel reacted with the single examples of Ge:-2,3,4 and Ge:-2,-3,-4 samples available for testing. We are not aware of other investigations into this possible relationship between Vel and Gerbich. It was during this investigation that one of the technologists misheard that we were working on Gerbich and Vel and thought we were working on garbage from hell. In fact, some of the results were difficult to repeat.

When Schechter et al. (19) described the high incidence antigen ABTI (see table 31-1 and later in this chapter) they reported that among eight Vel- samples tested, six reacted only weakly and one did not react with anti-ABTI.

In considering the apparent associations between Vel and the P_2 phenotype, Vel and the Ge:-2,-3,4 phenotype and Vel and ABTI, it must be remembered that all occur at the phenotypic level. There is currently no evidence that any genetic relationships exist to explain the phenotypic observations.

The Antigen Lan and the Antibody That Defines It

In 1961, Hart et al. (4) described anti-Lan, an antibody detecting an antigen present on the red cells of all except one of 4000 random donors in the Netherlands. Additional tests (30,57-62) on blood samples, primarily from Whites, in the USA and Europe, revealed only one Lan- among 35,645 tested. Thus the incidence of Lan- in Whites is two in 39,645 or approximately 1 in 20,000. In one of the studies cited (59) the antigen was called Gn[a], in another (60) it was called So, see below. Okubo et al. (63) tested samples from 15,000 Japanese blood donors but found no Lan- sample. Family studies (4,58-64) have shown that the Lan- phenotype is inherited as a recessive condition. Similar inheritance explained (65) a phenotype in which the Lan antigen was only weakly expressed. The Lan antigen appears to be fully developed at birth. It survives treatment of red cells with trypsin, chymotrypsin, papain, pronase, neuraminidase and AET.

Anti-Lan is invariably IgG in nature, is best reactive in IATs and is made by persons who have been transfused and/or pregnant (4,57-63,66-70). In subclassing studies anti-Lan has most often been seen (56,63,67,70) to be a mixture of IgG1 and IgG3, although examples made only of IgG1 or IgG3 have been found (56) as have examples with an IgG4 component (67). It has been reported that some anti-Lan fix complement (4,58,63,68) while others apparently lack that ability (57,63). Other than three unrelated individuals in Japan (63) all persons who have made anti-Lan have been White, the Lan- phenotype has not yet been reported in a Black.

The first example of anti-Lan (4) caused an immediate transfusion reaction. While no other persons with anti-Lan in the serum seem to have been transfused with Lan+ red cells (save for one passively immunized newborn, see below) in vivo survival studies with ^{51}Cr labeled Lan+ red cells, and in vitro phagocytic cell assays, have indicated that many examples of the antibody have the potential to destroy antigen-positive red cells in vivo (61,66,68,71). It has also been shown (72) that the reactivity of anti-Lan in the in vitro monocyte monolayer assay is often enhanced when fresh serum is added to the anti-Lan at the time that red cells are coated with antibody in the test system.

Anti-Lan has not caused severe HDN. Three cases (58,62,69) are documented in which women with anti-Lan in the serum delivered infants in whom the DAT was positive. In two of the cases (62,69) anti-Lan was recovered by elution from the cord blood red cells, in the third (58) it was not. Two of the infants (62,69) were treated by phototherapy. In one of them (69) the mother's serum contained anti-c, anti-Jk[a] and anti-Lan, all three antibodies were recovered by elution from the cord blood red cells. The infant required top up transfusions of 16 ml on day 3 and 30 ml on day 29. Red cells phenotypically c-, Jk(a-), Lan+ were used for these transfusions, the infant was discharged from hospital on day 31 and did well.

One example of auto-anti-Lan has been reported (73). The patient was a 79 year-old female who had relatively mild hemolytic anemia. The DAT on her red cells was only weakly positive (1+) but anti-Lan was eluted from her red cells and was present in her serum where it gave 3+ reactions (IAT) with Lan+ red cells. The antibody was IgG3 and fixed complement. After chloroquine treatment (74) the patient's red cells typed as Lan+ but their reactions with anti-Lan were considerably weaker than those of control cells. It was concluded (73) that depression of expression of the Lan antigen on the patient's red cells explained the finding that the DAT was only 1+ while the serum anti-Lan gave 3+ reactions. The abstract does not mention whether the control cells to which the patient's cells were compared in the Lan typing studies, had also been treated with chloroquine (such treatment is known to cause depression of some red cell antigens). In a ^{51}Cr cell survival study, the patient was shown (73) to clear 60% of the test dose of Lan+ red cells within one hour of their injection. The patient was supported with transfusions of Lan- red cells until steroid therapy rendered her transfusion-independent.

As mentioned briefly above, two other antibodies that were originally described as detecting new antigens of high incidence, were later shown to be examples of anti-Lan. Anti-Gn[a], as originally described by Fox et al. (59) was shown by Nesbitt (75) to be anti-Lan, all red cell samples originally described as Gn(a-), were, of course, Lan-. Somewhat similarly an antibody originally called anti-So by Frank et al. (60) was shown by Walker (76) to be another example of anti-Lan. This latter finding was particularly fortuitous. As the original authors had pointed out in an earlier presentation (77) selection of the term So did not display forethought. Had the antithetical partner to So been found, So would have become So[a] meaning that its antithetical partner would have had an embarrassing name!

The Antigen At^a and the Antibody That Defines It

In 1967, Applewhaite et al. (5) described an antibody, anti-At^a, in the serum of a Black woman, that reacted with all of the 6600 random samples against which it was tested. The antigen was shown to be an inherited character since Mrs. Augustine, the original antibody-maker and her brother have At(a-) red cells, while those of her sister are At(a+). The At(a-) phenotype was shown to be uncommon in Blacks since Applewhaite et al. (5) estimated that at least 2200 of the 6600 random samples that they tested, were from New York Blacks. Because the Augustine family came from the West Indies, Applewhaite (78) went to the Caribbean island from whence their ancestors originated (population genetics research at its very best) and arranged to obtain samples from the population there. Although no other At(a-) sample was found the experiment was a success in that Frank got his trip to the island and the rest of us learned that the At(a-) phenotype is not common there, either.

In 1973, Gellerman et al. (79) described six additional examples of anti-At^a. Four of the antibodies had been studied and shown to be the same, but the antigen defined had not been given a name, before anti-At^a was reported (5). Since some of the sera had been extensively studied in other reference laboratories, it is worth mentioning that the sera involved were from the patients E.De, V.Ba, C.Br, L.Bu, O.Wa (Ola Ware, the serum also contains anti-D) and B.L.Ja. Sm. The At(a-) probands between them, had produced 31 children, all of whom had At(a+) red cells so that it seems safe to assume that the At(a-) phenotype arises by recessive inheritance.

The studies described above (5,60) and some (80,81) performed subsequently, showed that among random donors, one in about 16,400 US Blacks and none in about 7400 US Whites, have At(a-) red cells. In one of the studies cited (60) the anti-At^a was called anti-El (see below).

The At^a antigen appears to be fully developed at birth, it is not denatured when red cells are treated with trypsin, chymotrypsin, papain, pronase, neuraminidase or AET (41).

Anti-At^a has been reported many times (5,60,79,81-83), all antibody-makers have been Black and all have been either transfused or pregnant or both. Pregnancy seems to be a rather efficient method of stimulating production of the antibody, at least five of the antibody-makers had never been transfused but had been pregnant at least three times (5,60,79). Anti-At^a is usually IgG in nature and best reactive in IATs but at least one IgM anti-At^a that agglutinated saline-suspended red cells has been

reported (79). Two IgG anti-At^a have been subjected to subclassing studies (56), one was shown to be wholly IgG1, the other contained IgG1, IgG3 and IgG4 components. One example of the antibody was thought (79) to have caused a transfusion reaction, another (83) gave a result in a monocyte monolayer assay that suggested that it would cause at least some destruction of antigen-positive red cells in vivo. As mentioned above, pregnancy seems often to be the source of immunization to At^a. Among the various reports (5,60,79,81-83) nine women with anti-At^a in the serum have been described who, among them, had a total of 60 pregnancies. Although 15 of those pregnancies ended in miscarriages, anti-At^a has not been accused of being responsible. In spite of the numerous opportunities, i.e. at least 45 live births, anti-At^a seems only once (82) to have caused moderate HDN, even then the infant required only phototherapy.

As mentioned briefly above, the antibody originally called anti-El (60,77) was shown by Brown et al. (84) to be the same as anti-At^a. Ironically, the abstracts first describing At^a (85) and El (77) appear on the same page of a 1967 issue of *Transfusion*. It was not until 16 years later that they were shown (84) to be the same thing.

The Antigen Jr^a and the Antibody That Defines It

In 1970, Stroup and MacIlroy (6) described seven examples of an antibody, that they named anti-Jr^a, that defined an antigen of very high incidence. The antibodies were found in the sera of persons in six unrelated families, three of which were Japanese. The study was important in that it showed that the sera Fujikawa, Tamura, Tad, Souza, Powell and Jacobs, each of which had been studied by many different investigators, but in none of which had specificity for a previously reported antigen been found, all contained anti-Jr^a. By 1974, Gellerman and Stroup (86) had identified 18 examples of anti-Jr^a, seven of which had been made by Japanese people. Stroup and MacIlroy (6) originally wondered if Jr^a might be part of the P blood group system because six of the first makers of anti-Jr^a had P₁- red cells. However, it was also pointed out (86) that the incidence of the P₁-phenotype in Japanese was known (87) to be around 60%. By 1974, family studies performed by Gellerman and Stroup (86) had demonstrated independent segregation between *Jr^a* and *P¹*.

The original observation (6) that three of six families that included persons with Jr(a-) red cells, were Japanese, foretold the incidence of Jr^a in different populations. By pooling the results of the initial and subsequent screenings it is seen that no Jr(a-) blood was found in tests on the red cells of 11,682 (primarily White) donors in the USA, England and New Zealand (86,88-90) nor among samples from 1041 Asians and 75 Eskimos (86). In contrast, tests on red cell samples from 49,496 Japanese persons yielded 34 (1 in 1456) that were Jr(a-) (91-94). The incidence of the phenotype is variable within Japan. As examples, in the various population surveys Jr(a-) samples numbered: 8 in 460 (1 in 58) in Niigati (92); 7 in 1247 (1 in 178) in Fukuoka (94); 2 in 994 (1 in 497) and 3 in 5000 (1 in 1667) in Osaka (91 and 94 respectively); 3 in 2600 (1 in 867) in Kumagaya (94); 4 in 9060 (1 in 2265) in central Japan (94); 2 in 6174 (1 in 3087) in Hokkaido (94); and 0 in 4663 in Himeji (94). The Jr(a-) phenotype has also been seen in people of Northern European extraction (89,95), Bedouin Arabs (96), a Mexican American (97) and in a patient in Australia (98) whose ethnic background was not mentioned. All of those cases and some cited below came to light because the proband was found to have anti-Jr^a in the serum. In family studies that have been performed, no evidence has emerged to suggest that the Jr(a-) phenotype represents anything other than a recessively inherited condition.

The Jr^a antigen appears to be fully developed on cord blood red cells. The antigen survives treatment of red cells with trypsin, chymotrypsin, papain, pronase, neuraminidase and AET (41).

Production of anti-Jr^a seems often to be provoked by pregnancy (89,91,93,95-100), in two women who had never been transfused the antibody was detected in a first pregnancy (98,100). IgM anti-Jr^a was found (101) in two brothers, neither of whom had been transfused. Other examples of the antibody have been IgG (67,70,89,93,95-101,103), among the few that were subclassed (56,70,96,98,100) some were IgG1 and some were mixtures of IgG1 and IgG3. Production of some examples of IgG anti-Jr^a has occurred following transfusion. Some examples of anti-Jr^a (93,97,101) have been shown to activate complement, many others have not been tested for that ability.

One patient with anti-Jr^a in the serum is reported (102) to have developed rigors after 150 ml of serologically incompatible blood had been transfused. In the patient described by Kendall (95), the half-life of a small test dose of ^{51}Cr-labeled Jr(a+) red cells was said to be about 80 minutes. In contrast, a woman with what was eventually identified as anti-Jr^a in the serum, had to be transfused with three units of serologically incompatible blood in an emergency situation (98). No symptoms of either an immediate or a delayed transfusion reaction were seen and although the titer of the anti-Jr^a rose from 32 before transfusion to a peak of 2048 on the 20th day following transfusion, the Jr(a+) red cells were apparently cleared slowly over 35 days. On day 35 when the DAT

was negative, no anti-Jr^a could be eluted and no Jr(a+) red cells could be demonstrated in the patient's circulation, and the titer of the anti-Jr^a had fallen to 64 (98). The antibody was IgG1 in composition and the facts that it did not completely clear the antigen-positive red cells until well after the medical emergency and until the patient was making blood, clearly showed that the patient was much better served by being given serologically incompatible units than she would have been, by delaying transfusion in the life-threatening medical emergency. In a different patient with anti-Jr^a in the serum, Verska and Larson (103) used autologous blood to support the patient through open heart surgery, no mean feat since the year was 1973 when open heart procedures usually required more transfusion support than is currently the case and autologous transfusion was not as widely practiced as it is today.

No serious case of HDN caused by anti-Jr^a has been reported. In a number of instances (6,86,89,93,97-100) the DAT on the Jr(a+) red cells of an infant born to a mother with anti-Jr^a in the serum has been positive and anti-Jr^a has been recovered by elution from the cord blood red cells. However, there are no reports that any of the infants required transfusion. In one infant the bilirubin level reached 16 mg/dl on day 4 but the hemoglobin level remained high and the infant required only phototherapy (93); in another an increase in bilirubin was attributed to prematurity rather than to antibody-induced red cell destruction (100).

One IgG3 human monoclonal anti-Jr^a has been made following EBV-transformation of lymphocytes from a patient who was making anti-Jr^a and fusion of the transformed cells with mouse myeloma cells (94).

The Antigen Ok^a and the Antibody That Defines It

The first example of anti-Ok^a was found by Morel and Hamilton (7) in the serum of a Japanese woman who had been transfused but not pregnant. The proposita's parents, who were cousins, and one of her sibs had Ok(a+) red cells, those of two other sibs were Ok(a-). The proposita came from a small island in the Inland Sea off the coast of Onomichi, Honshu, Japan. Red cell samples from 400 persons from that island were all Ok(a+). In further studies, including use of anti-Ok^a in the AutoAnalyzer (104), no other example of Ok(a-) red cells was found as the result of testing samples from: 9053 US Whites; 1570 US Blacks; 3976 individuals in the USA who were thought to be of Oriental stock; 1378 US Mexicans; and 870 Japanese (7).

The Ok^a antigen is apparently well developed at birth. In terms of serological studies, e.g. IATs, treatment of red cells with trypsin, chymotrypsin, papain, pronase, neuraminidase and AET has no demonstrable effect on Ok^a. However, as described in more detail below, Ok^a expression is reduced when red cells are treated with chymotrypsin or pronase and then used in immunoblotting studies with anti-Ok^a (105).

The first example of human anti-Ok^a was IgG1 in composition (7). At least one other example of the antibody has been found in Japan (106). Anti-Ok^a was not present in Ok(a-) individuals who had not been pregnant or transfused (7,106).

That the original anti-Ok^a was of clinical importance was clearly shown in red cell survival studies (7). Ten ml of whole blood from a donor with Ok(a+) red cells was labeled with ^{51}Cr and injected into the antibody-maker. Three hours after the injection only 10% of the Ok(a+) red cells remained in the patient's circulation, at six hours only 2% were still present. An in vitro monocyte monolayer assay gave a result that was also indicative of the fact that the antibody would clear antigen-positive red cells in vivo.

It 1988, Williams et al. (107) described a monoclonal antibody that reacted by IAT, with all red cells tested except three samples known to be Ok(a-). The antibody, TRA-1-85 was made using spleen cells from a mouse immunized with a human teratocarcinoma cell line. As described in detail below, the glycoproteins on which Ok^a is carried are widely distributed in tissues. Another monoclonal antibody MA 103 (108) has been shown (109) to react (see also below) with the Ok^a-bearing glycoproteins, but does not have anti-Ok^a specificity (i.e. it reacts with Ok(a+) and Ok(a-) red cells). This, of course, shows that Ok(a+) and Ok(a-) red cells carry the glycoprotein and indicates that the difference between them represents a polymorphism (i.e. an amino acid change) on the glycoprotein.

As described below, the use of TRA-1-85 has enabled much to be learned about the glycoproteins that carry Ok^a, less is known about their function. Use of the monoclonal antibody in somatic cell hybridization techniques resulted in Williams et al. (107) being able to assign the *Ok* locus to chromosome 19, specifically in the region 19pter-p13.2.

The Structure of the Ok^a Glycoprotein (CD147) and the Molecular Basis of the Ok^a Antigen

The first studies on the biochemical nature of the Ok^a glycoprotein were carried out by Williams et al. (107). These authors used a murine monoclonal antibody (TRA-1-85) which failed to react with Ok(a-) red cells and human anti-Ok^a, in immunoblotting experiments, to show

that the antigen is located on a very diffusely staining band in human red cells, with an apparent molecular weight on SDS-PAGE of 35,000-68,000. Such a diffusely staining band would be expected to reflect substantial and heterogeneous glycosylation and direct evidence for this was obtained when it was shown that the apparent molecular weight of the Ok^a-reactive molecule was reduced by approximately 12,000 after treatment with an EndoF/peptidyl N-glycanase preparation (105). A second murine monoclonal antibody (MA103) was shown to react with the Ok^a glycoprotein by Frances Spring while working in the laboratory of one of us (DJA). MA103 does not however have anti-Ok^a specificity. It was noted that the pattern of staining obtained when red cell membranes were immunoblotted with MA103 was identical to that obtained with TRA-1-85 and human anti-Ok^a. It was proved that MA103 recognized an epitope on the Ok^a glycoprotein by purifying the MA103 glycoprotein (by immune precipitation from intact red cells) and showing that the purified glycoprotein reacted with human anti-Ok^a and TRA-1-85 by immunoblotting. Since red cells with the rare Ok(a-) phenotype were reactive with MA103 these results suggested that the Ok(a-) phenotype does not result from the absence of the Ok^a glycoprotein. Frances Spring went on to purify the Ok^a glycoprotein from detergent-solubilized human red cell membranes by immunoaffinity chromatography using MA103 cross-linked to Protein A-Sepharose. When the N-terminal amino acid sequence of the purified Ok^a glycoprotein was determined (29 residues) a search of protein and DNA sequence databases revealed that the sequence was identical with that of a previously characterized glycoprotein denoted M6 leukocyte activation antigen (200).

The M6 leukocyte activation antigen has also been cloned by other research groups and given other names, basigin (201), tumor cell-derived collagenase stimulatory factor (TCSF) and extracellular matrix metalloproteinase induction (EMMPRIN) (202). This information was used to obtain cDNA corresponding to the Ok^a glycoprotein from mRNA isolated from lymphoblastoid cell lines derived from donors of phenotype Ok(a+) and Ok(a-). Nucleotide sequencing of the cDNAs confirmed that the M6 leukocyte activation antigen is identical to the Ok^a glycoprotein and further showed that the cDNA sequence derived from three individuals with the Ok(a-) phenotype differed from that of Ok(a+) donors at a single nucleotide (G331A) which would change amino acid Glu92 to Lys (200). Transfection of these cDNAs in NS-0 cells confirmed that this sequence change defines the Ok(a-) phenotype (200).

The M6 leukocyte activation antigen and hence the Ok^a glycoprotein is a member of the immunoglobulin superfamily. The amino acid sequence predicts a protein with a large extracellular domain comprising two Ig domains, an N-terminal C2-set domain and a V-set domain, a single membrane spanning domain and a cytoplasmic domain. There are three potential N-glycosylation sites in the Ig domain (see figure 31-1). The amino acid sequence change which corresponds to the Ok(a-) phenotype is located in the N-terminal C2-set domain (also shown in figure 31-1).

Tissue Distribution and Function of Ok^a Glycoprotein (CD147)

The Ok^a glycoprotein has a very wide tissue distribution. It is found on most leukocyte populations and a wide variety of hematopoietic cell lines with strong expression on K562 cells and relatively weak expression on IM9 cells (107,200). These findings contrast with the distribution of M6 antigen which is reported to be restricted to resting monocytes and activated monocytes, granulocytes and T cells (203) suggesting that the M6 antigen itself is an activation-dependent epitope like the OX-47 antigen which is expressed by the rat homologue of the Ok^a glycoprotein (204). Strong reactivity is seen in adult epithelial tissues and in fetal epithelial and hematopoietic cells (107,200).

Homologues of M6/Ok^a glycoprotein are found in rat (OX-47 or CE9, 204-206), chicken (neurothelin or HT7, 207,208), rabbit (209) and mouse (gp42, basigin, 201,209,210). The gene giving rise to the mouse homologue, basigin, has been "knocked out" to create transgenic mice which are basigin-deficient. Most of the null mutant embryos died around the time of implantation but mice that survived were sterile indicating a role for basigin in development and reproduction (211). The mutant mice also had abnormal behavior in response to olfactory stimuli ("irritating odours") and a significantly enhanced mixed lymphocyte reaction (211). These results suggest a variety of important functional roles for basigin in the mouse and by analogy in man. However, the only well documented function of the Ok^a glycoprotein at the time of writing is its involvement in tumor cell invasion (212,213). There are no reports regarding red cell function in basigin "knock-out" mice at the time of writing.

Antibodies recognizing the Ok^a glycoprotein were clustered in CD147 at the VIth International Workshop and Conference on Human Leukocyte Differentiation Antigens, Kobe, Japan, November 1996.

The JMH Antigens and the Antibodies That Define Them

In 1975, in the second edition of this book (110), brief mention was made of an antigen or group of antigens called JMH (for John Milton Hagen). Numerous workers had seen examples of antibodies with the same or a closely related specificity and various nicknames were in use. One of these was "the over 60 group" because so many examples of the antibody were from older (now recognized as mature, wiser and experienced) patients. As mentioned below, the over 60 designation may well have been prophetic. Most of the antibodies were reactive only by IAT where they gave weak reactions and seemed to be defining a graded character. In 1978, Sabo et al. (8) brought a considerable amount of order to the situation when they described 49 examples of the antibody and used the term JMH to designate the antigen defined. The serum of Mr. Hagen contained one of the more widely studied early examples of anti-JMH. Many of the antibodies described (8) were of high titer in spite of the fact that, when undiluted, they reacted only weakly with red cells. Perhaps there are relatively few copies of the JMH determinant on each red cell. The JMH antigen was shown to be of high incidence and to be present on cord blood red cells. Later studies, see below, have suggested that the antigen is present but not fully developed at birth. Anti-JMH was invariably IgG in composition, was not inhibitable by serum and failed to react with trypsin or papain-treated red cells (8). Later, Daniels (18,41) showed that the antibody does not react with ficin or pronase-treated red cells either, that the antigen is denatured when red cells are treated with AET but that it survives treatment of red cells with neuraminidase.

Neither the JMH- phenotype nor its inheritance are straightforward. First, in the majority of patients who form anti-JMH, the red cell phenotype appears to represent total or near total cessation of expression of red cell JMH antigen (see below). Second, in the only family in which the JMH- phenotype was seen (111) to be directly inherited, it was present in three generations, thus suggesting dominant inheritance. It has often been assumed, and so stated in some papers on the system, that antigen loss or dominant inheritance are the only causes of the JMH- phenotype. Although not formally proved, it is entirely possible that the more usual genetic background associated with absence of a very common antigen, i.e. homozygosity for rare recessive alleles, may apply to JMH. Certainly and as described below, those situations in which individuals lack some but not all the epitopes of JMH from their red cells and can make alloimmune anti-JMH, appear to involve recessive inheritance of the JMH-variant phenotype.

To return to the most common situation, it has been noted (8,18,50,111-113) that many patients who form anti-JMH are older (i.e. 50 years of age or above) and that the JMH- phenotype is not seen among their younger sibs or other family members. Further, in some cases the DAT on the antibody-maker's red cells is weakly positive and anti-

FIGURE 31-1 Structure of the Okᵃ Glycoprotein and Location of the Okᵃ Antigen

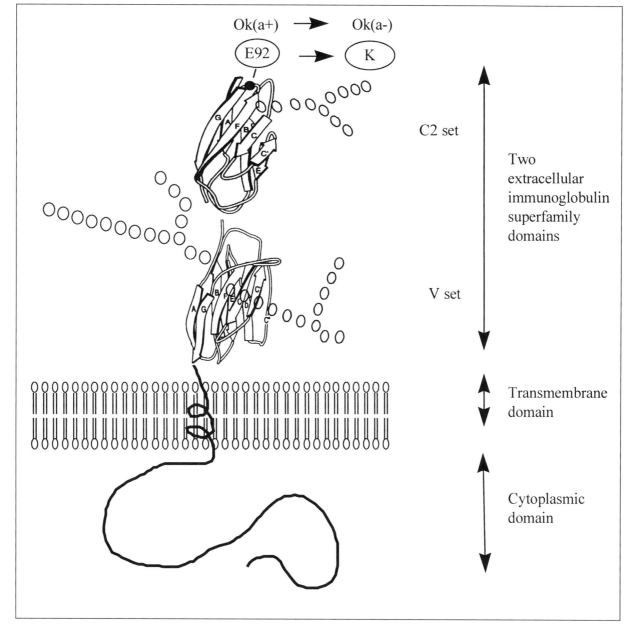

JMH can be found in eluates made from those red cells. In some other cases anti-JMH can be eluted from the patient's DAT negative red cells. Even when the DAT and eluate are negative but anti-JMH is present in the serum, it can be seen that the antibody-maker's red cells react weakly with other examples of anti-JMH. These observations have led to a widely accepted belief that during the later years of life, red cell levels of JMH decline, sometimes to the point of non-detection in serological tests. Once reduced expression of red cell JMH occurs, anti-JMH can be made. If the anti-JMH is made while some red cell JMH antigen is still detectable, the positive DATs and eluates, mentioned above,

are encountered. Three important points need to be made. First, this production of auto-anti-JMH and the positive DATs have never been associated with autoimmune red cell destruction. Second, although seen in hospital patients, the phenomenon does not seem to be associated with any one or a group of related disease states. We do not know if studies have been performed on healthy older people to see if the phenomenon occurs there too. Third, on some occasions the apparently acquired JMH- phenotype can be a transient condition. Daniels (18) described two children with different chromosomal disorders, whose red cells initially typed as JMH- but were later shown to be JMH+.

Bobolis and Telen (125) showed that when red cells were incubated at 37°C for 15 minutes a JMH-active protein (see below) was released into the supernatant. Release of the protein did not occur in the presence of protease inhibitors. When isolated red cell membranes were used, presence of the cytoplasmic contents of the red cells or of granulocytes was necessary for the release to occur. The authors (125) speculated that in vivo loss of JMH antigen, as described above, may involve the actions of a cellular protease.

The second type of JMH-, i.e. supposedly caused by inheritance of a gene dominant in effect, has been seen only in one family (111). The red cells of the JMH- persons in the family had a negative DAT and failed to react with any example of anti-JMH. None of the persons with JMH- red cells, all of whom were healthy, had anti-JMH in the serum. As mentioned above, the situation in which recessive inheritance is seen to be involved, most often seems to represent a polymorphism of the JMH-bearing membrane structure and is discussed below under the heading of JMH variants.

As mentioned above, although the JMH antigen may be detectable on cord blood red cells, it is often only weakly expressed and on occasion may not be detectable at all. Contreras and Daniels (114) studied one patient who had anti-JMH in the serum and who delivered twins. At birth, the red cells of both twins typed as JMH-, at ten months of age one twin had normal expression but the other only weak expression of JMH on the red cells. The case was further unusual in that the woman who made anti-JMH was only 26 years-old. No details as to whether a genetic (recessive) or an acquired situation was involved, are given.

Anti-JMH is most often IgG in composition (8,18,70,113,115-117) although the antibody is sometimes found (18,116,118) in the sera of individuals who have been neither pregnant nor transfused. In subclassing studies, anti-JMH have often been seen (56,70,115,116) to be IgG4 or mixtures of IgG4 and IgG2 in composition. However, at least two have been seen to be IgG1 only (56) and one has been seen to be IgG3 (117). Nothing seems to have been reported concerning the ability of anti-JMH to bind complement. One of us (PDI) has noticed that when anti-JMH causes a weakly positive DAT on the red cells of an individual with reduced expression of JMH (see above), the DAT is (weakly) positive with anti-IgG but negative with anti-C3.

Patients with anti-JMH, in whom reduction of expression of red cell JMH antigen is seen, seem to tolerate transfusion with JMH+ units without transfusion reactions and without any evidence of accelerated rates of clearance of the transfused red cells (8,113,115,116). One patient with anti-JMH received 20 units of JMH+ blood over a ten months period. His hemoglobin increased as expected (for the transfusion of compatible blood) and

there was no evidence of a secondary immune response to the JMH antigen. In two patients with anti-JMH, ^{51}Cr-labeled red cell survival studies were normal when JMH+ red cells were injected (8,113). The one example of anti-JMH that was shown (117) to be IgG3 in composition gave a result in a monocyte monolayer assay that suggested that it had the potential to cause accelerated clearance of antigen-positive red cells in vivo. However, since no transfusions were anticipated, no in vivo red cell survival study was performed nor, obviously, was any JMH+ blood transfused. In the next section it is pointed out that persons who have JMH+ red cells that appear to lack some epitopes of JMH, and who make anti-JMH to the portions of the antigen that their red cells lack, may make antibodies of more clinical significance than those described above. The patient with the IgG3 anti-JMH that gave a positive result in the MMA, is described (117) as having red cells that were non-reactive with five different examples of anti-JMH. Thus the patient involved may not have fit the group (described below) who can roughly be described as having partial JMH on their red cells.

The only opportunity that anti-JMH has had to cause HDN seems to be the case (114) described above in which the immunized mother produced twins, whose red cells typed as JMH- at birth.

Monoclonal Anti-JMH

In 1982 Daniels and Knowles (119) described a monoclonal antibody, H8, that failed to react only with JMH-red cells and the cells of R.M. (see below) that are known to carry a variant form of JMH. Additional details about this MAb were published a year later (120), at that time it was shown that H8 blocked the reaction of human anti-JMH with JMH+ red cells. The antibody was produced using spleen cells from a mouse immunized with lymphoid cells from a patient with lymphocytic leukemia. Use of H8 proved invaluable in two areas. First, it was used to help clarify the reactions of some red cells with variant JMH antigens (see next section) from patients who made alloimmune anti-JMH although their red cells were not truly JMH- (118,121,122). Second, the use of H8 resulted in identification (123-126) of the phosphatidylinositol-linked (PI-linked) protein on which the JMH antigens are carried, for additional details see below.

JMH Variants

As mentioned in the previous sections, rare individuals make an antibody that reacts with all except JMH-red cells, their own cells and those of compatible sibs, yet they (and their compatible sibs) have JMH+ red cells.

The fact that these individuals have compatible sibs suggests, of course, that these JMH variant phenotypes are inherited in an autosomal recessive fashion. Table 31-2 is reproduced from the previous edition of this book (50) but is expanded to include two cases (121,122) published since 1985. The sera V.G. and R.M. were described by Moulds et al. (118), the H8 monoclonal antibody was described by Daniels and Knowles (119,120). The results of tests on the V.G. and R.M. red cells are primarily from IATs. Results of tests on the G.P. and D.W. red cells are a combination of those obtained in IATs, radioimmunoassays and immunoblotting procedures. As indicated in the footnotes to table 31-2, we do not know if the two JMH- samples that reacted with the G.P. serum were of the reduced expression or variant JMH phenotype (we suspect the latter) nor do we know which of the anti-JMH used to test the G.P. and D.W. red cells were made by individuals with reduced expression of JMH and which by persons with a variant JMH phenotype. It is apparent, from table 31-2 that persons with a variant JMH phenotype are not all identical, nor are the anti-JMH-like specificities that they make the same. We have been told (127) that additional samples that would expand the heterogeneity shown in table 31-2 have been studied, but not described in print.

From findings (122) that the red cells of G.P., his one compatible sib, and D.W. carry JMH protein (see below) that is of the same molecular size as that on JMH+ red cells and is present in normal amounts, it appears that the variant JMH phenotypes represent changes (probably amino acid substitutions) in that protein. Such changes apparently result in loss of certain epitopes of JMH so that the individuals involved are able to make antibodies against the missing epitopes.

As already mentioned, persons with JMH variant phenotypes have been found to have compatible sibs (118,121,122) thus establishing the fact that lack of certain JMH epitopes is an inherited characteristic. Mrs. D.W., a White woman, was one of thirteen children, two of whom have red cells of the same JMH variant phenotype. Her blood was first studied in 1973, indeed she was one of the original 49 persons with anti-JMH, described by Sabo et al. (8). Studies by one of us (PDI) in 1973, 1978 and 1992 (121) showed that her red cell JMH phenotype did not change over the 19 year period, thus excluding temporary depression of red cell JMH antigen expression. The anti-JMH in her serum was of approximately the same strength in each example studied, she was not transfused with JMH+ blood other than her own. In 1978, she received all ten units that she had donated for frozen storage, following a gastrointestinal hemorrhage.

The patient G.P., a White male, had prosthetic aortic valve replacement eleven years before his anti-JMH was studied; two months before the antibody was found he was transfused with four units of packed red blood cells for a gastrointestinal hemorrhage. At that time no atypical antibodies were found in his serum and the transfusions were uneventful. When he presented for aortic valve replacement, at age 81, his serum was found (122) to contain an antibody, weakly-reactive (scores of 5 to 7), by PEG-IAT, with all red cells tested except his own. Because the antibody showed characteristics typical of an HTLA antibody, screening tests were repeated by LISS-IAT, with similar results. However, when the antibody was studied by saline-IAT (with no additives) it gave much stronger reactions, i.e. scores of 10 to 12. The titer of the antibody by saline-IAT was 512, the antibody was not inhibited by pooled human serum. Additional studies then revealed that his red cells were JMH+ while his serum contained an anti-JMH-like specificity.

TABLE 31-2 To Show the Reactions of Anti-JMH and Anti-JMH-like Antibodies (118-122)

Red Cells	Antibodies					
	Anti-JMH	V.G.	R.M.	G.P.	D.W.	H8
JMH+ (Common)	+	+	+	+	+	+
JMH- (Rare)	0	0	0	0/+[w*3]	0	0
V.G. and sibs	+	0	+			+
R.M. and sib	+	0	0			0
G.P. and sib	0/+[w*1]		+	0		+[w*4]
D.W. and sibs	0/+[w*2]		+		0	+

*1   The G.P. red cells were non-reactive with 3 and weakly reactive with 3 other anti-JMH.
*2   The D.W. red cells were non-reactive with 1 and weakly reactive with 8 anti-JMH.
*3   The G.P. antibody was non-reactive with 4 and weakly reactive with 2 JMH- samples.
*4   By RIA the red cells of G.P. and his brother bound less of the H8 antibody than did D.W. and random JMH+ red cells.
       The origins of the reactive and non-reactive anti-JMH and JMH- red cells are not known, see text.

Because of these findings, ^{51}Cr red cell survival studies, one with random JMH+ red cells and one with JMH+ red cells matched to the patient's phenotype for other antigens, were performed. In the first study, 54% of the test dose of red cells was cleared in the first 24 hours, in the second 33% of the test dose was cleared in 24 hours and 42% in 48 hours (121,122). The anti-JMH in his serum was IgG1; in addition to the ^{51}Cr red cell survival studies, an in vitro monocyte monolayer assay indicated that the antibody was likely to be clinically-significant. Mr. G.P. had two sibs, the red cells of his brother were serologically compatible, those of his sister were incompatible. In RIA using a human anti-JMH and the monoclonal antibody H8, the red cells of G.P. and his brother reacted similarly but gave different reactions to those of his sister and JMH+ red cells from a normal donor (122). In spite of his advanced age, G.P. was able to donate two units of blood, for autologous transfusion, in a four week period. Two units were also collected from his compatible brother. The surgery was successfully completed, the two autologous units were transfused, the two from his brother, who does not have anti-JMH in the serum, were not and remain in our collection of rare frozen units.

The finding of one example of clinically significant anti-JMH should not be taken to indicate that all patients with the antibody need to be transfused with JMH-blood. Indeed, as pointed out above, there are many reports (8,113,115,116) of successful transfusions of JMH+ red cells to patients with anti-JMH in the serum. We (122) suggested that perhaps in patients with reduced or lost expression of red cell JMH antigen, the anti-JMH made is clinically benign while perhaps, in some patients with JMH variant phenotypes, the antibody may be capable of clearing JMH+ red cells in vivo. In this respect it is a pity that it is not known whether the IgG3 anti-JMH that gave a positive reaction by MMA (117) was made by a person with a reduced or a variant JMH phenotype. In favor of reduced antigen expression was the fact that the patient's red cells were non-reactive with all of five examples of anti-JMH in contrast to the reactions of JMH variant red cells (see table 31-2). In favor of a variant phenotype, the patient was only 38 years-old. The family was non-informative, the red cells of the patient's parents, only sib tested and her three children were JMH+. In a different case, a 65 year-old Black female with IgG4 anti-JMH in the serum was described by Baldwin et al. (116). In a ^{51}Cr red cell survival study, normal survival was seen one hour after the injection of JMH+ red cells. The survival of the injected cells was followed for nine days and the results were extrapolated to calculate that half the ^{51}Cr dose would have been lost by 12 days (normal by this method (128) 25 to 31 days). However, the authors (116) pointed out first, that the T1/2 Cr was calculated not observed and second, that the

slow and limited clearance of the cells did not alter the therapeutic benefits of the transfusions (the patient received six units of blood immediately before the in vivo survival study). It is comforting that in the only case in which anti-JMH clearly reduced the in vivo survival of JMH red cells (122), the antibody indicated that is was unusual by its serological reactions, i.e. much stronger reactions by saline-IAT than by PEG or LISS-IATs.

The JMH-active Molecule (CDw 108)

JMH antisera and the murine monoclonal antibody, H8, failed to react with those red cells from patients with paroxysmal nocturnal hemoglobinuria (PNH) which have a complete deficiency of glycosylphosphoinositol-linked (GPI-linked) proteins suggesting that the JMH antigens are carried on a GPI-linked protein in the red cell membrane (123). Immune precipitation and immunoblotting experiments carried out with human and monoclonal anti-JMH identified a membrane component of 76kDa on normal red cells but absent from JMH-negative red cells (125). The apparent molecular weight of this molecule was the same under reducing and non-reducing conditions indicating that it does not exist as a disulphide-bonded homodimer or heterodimer. Evidence was obtained that a proportion of the JMH protein can be released from red cells by the action of PI-specific phospholipase C (PI-PLC), an enzyme known to cleave GPI-linked proteins (125). That the cleavage is partial rather than complete is not unexpected since there is evidence that the GPI anchor on other red cell GPI-linked proteins is modified by palmitoylation of the inositol ring (214) and that this impairs the action of the enzyme. Bobolis et al. (125) estimated the abundance of the JMH molecule on red cells at between 1000 and 3000 copies/red cell. The JMH protein appears to be a novel GPI-linked protein distinct from CD55 (see Chapter 24) which has a similar apparent molecular weight (125).

Mudad et al. (126) present evidence that the JMH protein is identical to CDw108. CDw108 describes a cluster of two monoclonal antibodies (MEM-121, MEM-150) raised against human lymphoblastic leukemia cells by Vaclav Horejsi at the Institute of Molecular Genetics in Prague. The antibodies recognize a GPI-linked protein of Mr 80,000 on activated lymphocytes (215). MEM-121 and MEM-150 react with JMH-positive but not with JMH-negative red cells and immunoblot a membrane component of Mr 76,000 on red cell membranes from JMH-positive cells (126). Competitive binding assays demonstrated that human anti-JMH and MEM-121/MEM-150 react with different epitopes on the same protein. JMH is expressed on a wide range of tissues, in addition to red cells and lymphocytes, including neurons and respiratory epithelium (126). Mudad et al. (122) provide evidence for the occurrence of variant JMH proteins. Further progress in the elucidation of the structure of this protein is likely to require successful cloning of the gene.

The Antigen Emm and the Antibody That Defines It

Although the antigen Emm has an ISBT number (see table 31-1) very little about it has appeared in print. The data below are from a 1987 report by Daniels et al. (9). The first example of the antibody now called anti-Emm was found in 1973 in the serum of a 29 year-old French man born in Madagascar. Four additional examples were described in the 1987 report: one in a 56 year-old White US woman; one in a Pakistani man, and two in brothers. Of the last two examples, one was found in a 61 year-old French-Canadian man and the other in his brother. In so far as red cell samples were available, mutual compatibility between the red cells and sera of the five antibody-makers, was demonstrated. The finding of brothers with Emm- red cells, who had seven sibs with Emm+ red cells, suggested that the Emm- phenotype is inherited.

In population studies using anti-Emm from the first propositus, all of 730 North London blood donors and all of 224 North London Black persons were found to have Emm+ red cells. The Emm antigen was not denatured when red cells were treated with trypsin, chymotrypsin, papain, ficin, pronase, neuraminidase or AET.

Of the five examples of anti-Emm studied, four were produced by males who had never been transfused. The authors (9) comment that if anti-Emm is always present in the sera of persons with Emm- red cells, as suggested by the above observation, the Emm- phenotype must be very rare since Emm- persons would draw attention to themselves when their sera reacted in antibody-screening tests. Of the five non-red cell stimulated anti-Emm, one was IgM and the others IgG. The IgM antibody was optimally reactive as an agglutinin in tests at 4°C, the four IgG examples reacted only in IATs. In the original study (9) anti-Emm was shown to react with an impressive collection of red cell samples that each lacked one or more high incidence antigens. The antigen has been mentioned in some other reports in which it was shown that the antibody being studied did not have the same specificity as anti-Emm. Emm- red cells were also shown to react with numerous antibodies to other high incidence antigens, they did not react with any of a large collection of antibodies to low incidence antigens, thus no antigen antithetical to Emm was identified.

In 1990, Telen et al. (123) showed that anti-Emm was non-reactive with the PNH III red cells of a patient whose PNH I red cells were Emm+. Since it is known

that PNH III red cells lack phosphatidylinositol-linked (PI-linked) proteins, for which the patients have the encoding genes, this finding indicates that Emm is probably carried on an as yet unidentified PI-linked protein. The antigen Emma, mentioned in table 20-3 of the third edition of this book (50) is the same as the antigen now called Emm.

The Antigen AnWj

This high incidence antigen was originally called Anton (hence An) (10,18,129) and Wj (11). When Anton and Wj were shown (12,13,130) to be the same thing, the name AnWj was applied. Because there is strong evidence (131) that AnWj is carried on an isoform of CD44, the glycoprotein known (133,134) to carry the antigens of the Indian blood group system, AnWj is described in detail in Chapter 29. Since the expression of CD44 and AnWj is down regulated on the red cells of persons who inherit *In(Lu)* (132,133) the AnWj antigen is also mentioned in Chapter 20.

The Antigen MER2 and the Antibody That Defines It

In 1987, Daniels et al. (14) described the first example of monoclonal antibodies that detected a hitherto unrecognized red cell blood group antigen. Properly to establish priority, it should be mentioned that the antibody had been described at a 1985 meeting, in the abstract (135) of that paper the antigen was called DEN. The two monoclonal antibodies 1D12 and 2F7 that recognize MER2, were produced following immunization of a mouse with human small cell carcinoma cells, they reacted with red cells in IATs using anti-mouse IgG. The strength of the MER2 antigen varied on different antigen positive red cells. In tests on samples from 1016 English blood donors, 934 (92%) were found to have MER2+ red cells (14). Family studies showed that MER2 is inherited in a normal manner, i.e. presence of *MER2* results in the MER2+ phenotype. The MER2 antigen was detected on cord blood red cells. The antigen was shown to be denatured when red cells are treated with trypsin, chymotrypsin, pronase or AET but it withstood treatment of red cells with papain and neuraminidase. In tests on the red cells of members of a large Sardinian family it was shown (136) that the nine family members who had inherited *In(Lu)* had a mean level of MER2 that was slightly less than the mean level on the red cells of the 12 members who had not inherited *In(Lu)*.

In 1988, Daniels et al. (137) reported the existence of human alloantibodies with anti-MER2 specificity.

Three examples were found in the sera of Jews from India who were living in Israel. Two of the antibody-makers were sibs, the third was unrelated, all three were patients being treated by renal dialysis (see below) and required repeated transfusions. All three of the anti-MER2 reacted in IATs read with anti-IgG but in two of the patients the antibodies had been made before dialysis started and before any transfusions had been given. At least two of the anti-MER2 were shown to be clinically benign. The two sibs with the antibody received many transfusions with serologically reactive blood but no transfusion reactions occurred nor were any indications of accelerated clearance of the transfused red cells seen. In blocking studies, convincing evidence was obtained (137) that the human and monoclonal anti-MER2 were detecting the same or a very closely related epitope.

Daniels et al. (14) used tests against somatic cell hybrids to demonstrate that the *MER2* locus is on chromosome 11 at 11p15. Since the gene that encodes production of CD44, the glycoprotein that carries the In^a and In^b antigens (133,134 and see Chapter 29) is also located on the short arm of chromosome 11, and since expression of In^b like that of MER2 (see above) is reduced on the red cells of persons with *In(Lu)*, it was necessary to show that MER2 is not on CD44. Daniels et al. (14) showed that monoclonal antibodies to CD44 reacted equally with MER2+ and MER2- red cells. Localization of the genes encoding production of MER2 and CD44 has shown (14,138-142) that the loci are different.

In discussing the fact that all three human anti-MER2 were made by Indian Jews with renal failure, Daniels (143) presents a most interesting speculation. He wonders if in the 8% of White people with MER2- red cells, the MER2 antigen is present on other (tissue) cells and thus prevents such persons from making anti-MER2. Further, perhaps in the three Indian Jews a mutation or a small chromosomal deletion results in their having no MER2 on red cells or tissue cells, so that they are able to make anti-MER2. Thus the MER2 antigen (or carrier protein) or the product of a very closely linked gene, deleted with *MER2*, might be essential for proper kidney function. While Daniels (143) points out that the idea is speculative, as he also says, the fact that the only three known makers of anti-MER2 have renal failure indicates that studies on the presence of MER2 on tissue cells, especially those of the renal system, are clearly in order.

The Antigen Sd^a on Red Cells

In 1967, in back to back papers, Macvie et al. (15) and Renton et al. (16) described a new antibody, anti-Sd^a. Initially it appeared that Sd^a had an incidence of about 91% in the predominantly White English population studied. However, as described in more detail below, it was later found (144) that among individuals whose red cells type as Sd(a-), a little over half secrete Sd^a substance in the urine, and in smaller amounts in the saliva. Thus, the true incidence of the Sd(a+) phenotype is around 96%. As far as we have been able to determine, no significant differences from that incidence have been found in other populations. Again, as discussed in more detail later, a small proportion of persons with Sd(a+) red cells (around 1% in the initial studies) have an exceptionally strong expression of the antigen on their cells. This phenotype is often written as Sd(a++) and in everyday parlance is called "super Sid". At one time it was believed (145) that the Sd(a++) and Cad+ phenotypes (see Chapter 42) were the same thing. Thus, "super Sid" appeared to be more common in Thailand than elsewhere (146,147). However, it is no longer certain that Sd^a and Cad are the same. The fact that the two share a common immunodominant structure may explain their close similarity at the serological level. While all individuals have a serum antibody that agglutinates Cad-polyagglutinable red cells it seems that anti-Sd^a, as demonstrable by conventional serological techniques, is made only by persons with Sd(a-) red cells whose saliva and urine lack Sd^a substance.

From the time it was first reported, it was clear that the Sd^a antigen is unusual in a number of respects. First, even when red cells with high expression of the antigen are tested, they give a mixed-field reaction with anti-Sd^a. The typical picture is a number of tight agglutinates superimposed on a field of unagglutinated red cells. However, if the agglutinates are removed and the previously unagglutinated red cells are exposed to the same anti-Sd^a, additional agglutinates are formed. Thus, it seems that all red cells of a person with the Sd(a+) phenotype carry the antigen; it has been suggested (16) that distribution of the antigen varies among the red cells. Such distribution is not related to red cell age; when young and older red cells are separated by centrifugation, both populations show the mixed-field reaction (16,39).

Second, there is great variation in strength of the Sd^a antigen on the red cells of different individuals. As mentioned, about 1% of persons have red cells that are so strongly agglutinated (albeit still with a mixed-field pattern) that they are called Sd(a++). In 80% of persons the antigen can be shown to be present but the positive reactions are weaker. In 10% of persons the antigen is detected with difficulty. In the next 5% of persons the red cells type as Sd(a-), even when potent anti-Sd^a is used, but Sd^a substance can be found in the urine. Because inhibition studies using urine have shown such individuals to be phenotypically Sd(a+), no attempts to adsorb and/or elute anti-Sd^a with such cells seem to have been reported. This leaves, of course, about 4% of persons who are

TABLE 31-3 The Sd^a Phenotypes

Reaction of RBCs with Anti-Sd^a	Sd^a in Saliva and Urine	Phenotype	Percent of Whites
4+	Yes	Sd(a++)	1
1+ to 3+^{*1}	Yes	Sd(a+)	80
±^{*2}	Yes	Sd(a+)	10
0	Yes	Sd(a+)	5
0	No	Sd(a-)^{*3}	4

*1   In the 80% of persons whose red cells give 1+ to 3+ reactions, more give 1+ than give 3+.

*2   In the 10% of persons whose red cells give ± reactions, presence of the antigen may be demonstrable only with potent anti-Sd^a.

*3   Anti-Sd^a in a form demonstrable by conventional serological techniques may be made only by persons who lack Sd^a from their red cells, saliva and urine.

truly Sd(a-) since their red cells, urine and saliva all lack the antigen. The findings described are summarized in table 31-3. Although it is convenient to divide persons as shown in the table, distribution of Sd^a on the red cells of different individuals actually represents a sliding scale from 4+ to negative.

Third, although some 96% of persons are genetically Sd(a+) there is a marked loss of antigen expression during pregnancy. In different studies, 75% (148), 48% (15) and 36% (149) of women at full term were found to have red cells that typed as Sd(a-). The differences may have been due in part to the abilities of different anti-Sd^a to react with red cells carrying low levels of the antigen. In their study, Morton and Pickles (148) found that the Sd(a-) phenotype persisted for at least 6 weeks after delivery in 25% of women. Spitalnik et al. (149) found that in the first trimester of pregnancy, 22 of 100 women had the Sd(a-) phenotype. Of 145 women tested at full term, 52 (36%) were Sd(a-). Thus, loss of Sd^a antigen expression seems to be progressive as pregnancy advances. In spite of the marked increase of the Sd(a-) phenotype in pregnancy, the incidence of anti-Sd^a was no different among pregnant and nonpregnant persons studied (149). As mentioned above, it seems that only those persons whose saliva and urine lack Sd^a form the antibody. Loss of Sd^a from the red cells during pregnancy is not accompanied by loss of Sd^a substance from saliva and urine.

Fourth, the Sd^a antigen is not developed on the red cells of newborn infants. Cord blood samples invariably type as Sd(a-); in infants who have inherited an *Sd^a* gene, red cell expression of the antigen is not usually readily detectable until about 10 weeks of age (148). This finding contrasts sharply with the presence of large amounts of Sd^a in the saliva of newborns (see below).

Fifth, it has been reported (150) that red cells agglutinated by anti-Sd^a characteristically appear as shiny orange clumps. While this phenomenon has been observed by several workers with whom we have discussed it, one of us (PDI) has never been able to see the color change, perhaps because of his difficulty in differentiation of the orange-red portion of the spectrum (he once wore an orange tie with a red shirt).

The Sd^a antigen has been shown (15,16,156,157) to survive treatment of red cells with trypsin, papain and AET.

Soluble Sd^a

As mentioned above, Morton and Pickles (144) showed that Sd^a is widely distributed in secretions, excretions and tissues of Sd(a+) persons. The largest amounts were found in urine but saliva, meconium and milk all contained enough Sd^a substance to effect some inhibition of anti-Sd^a. Serum from Sd(a+) persons was also found to contain Sd^a substance (144); much larger quantities were found in the sera of Sd(a++) persons (39). In using extracts from various tissues, evidence for the presence of Sd^a in the kidney, stomach, colon and lymph nodes was obtained; extracts made from the duodenum, jejunum, ileum, liver, spleen, muscles and brain were not inhibitory. In other species, Sd^a substance was found in the kidneys of guinea pigs, moles and hedgehogs but not in that of a lamb. Sd^a was not found in birds; chickens, turkeys, pheasants, wood pigeons and a tawny owl were tested.

These findings have led to a number of applications at the practical level. First, the most reliable way to determine an individual's phenotype when red cell typings give equivocal (or negative) reactions with anti-Sd^a, is to use the individual's urine in a hemagglutination inhibition study. Second, when an antibody is suspected of having anti-Sd^a specificity but the point has not been proved, inhibition studies with human or guinea pig urine can be used. Of the various secretions and tissue extracts listed above, guinea pig urine was shown (144) to contain the highest level of Sd^a substance. Details of methods used to perform Sd^a typing by urine inhibition, the use of urine to confirm the specificity of anti-Sd^a and the preparation of urine samples so that they do not cause nonspecific inhibition, are given by Judd (151,155). The findings that Sd^a was not present in the chicken explained an earlier observation (39) that a chicken, immunized with human red cells, made anti-Sd^a.

As described above, there is a marked depression of red cell expression of Sd^a in pregnancy and the red cells of newborns type as Sd(a-). Both observations relate only to red cells. The urine of pregnant women and that of newborns contains soluble Sd^a (providing, of course, that the women and newborns have *Sd^a*). The level of Sd^a in the saliva of newborns is some four times greater than that in the saliva of adults (144). Loss of red cell Sd^a antigen in pregnancy is reminiscent of the loss of red cell Le^b (see Chapter 9) and reduced production of *A* gene-specified transferase, in the same situation. As discussed below, the immundominant sugar of Sd^a is added by an N-acetylgalactosaminyl transferase. While Howell (152) showed that the level of Sd^a in an individual's plasma is directly proportional to the amount on the individual's red cells, incubation of Sd(a-) red cells in plasma from Sd(a+) and Sd(a++) persons did not result in the cells acquiring Sd^a (15,39).

Anti-Sd^a, Detection and Identification

There is no doubt that most examples of anti-Sd^a are of the non-red-cell-stimulated type. Of the 4% of persons who have Sd(a-) red cells and no Sd^a in the urine, about one quarter (16) to one half (144) have anti-Sd^a in the serum. That is to say, the antibody can be found in 1-2% of random individuals. However, the antibody is detected with this frequency only when Sd(a++) red cells are used in antibody screening tests. If Sd(a+) red cells of moderate strength are used in such tests, most examples of the antibody go undetected. This is, of course, a blessing. As described below, anti-Sd^a is a clinically insignificant antibody. Virtually all the early reported (15,16, 148) examples of anti-Sd^a (and many described since) were IgM in nature. Most of them presented as agglutinins, optimally reactive at around 20°C, although they were also detectable in IATs if anti-IgM was present in the antiglobulin reagent or if anti-C3 was present and the anti-Sd^a were tested in a system that allowed them to activate complement (148). As mentioned above, anti-Sd^a reacts with papain or trypsin-treated red cells and rare examples, when fresh, may cause in vitro hemolysis of such treated red cells (148,153). One of the more useful clues in the identification of anti-Sd^a is that it is one of relatively few antibodies to very common antigens that react by IAT but are non-reactive with cord blood red cells. As already described, urine inhibition is a useful method in confirming anti-Sd^a specificity.

Another factor that contributes to the paucity of examples of anti-Sd^a now detected is that currently used serological methods are not particularly favorable for its detection. The antibody usually reacts optimally at temperatures below 37°C. Even when it is detected in IATs, it is often found because the cell-serum mixtures converted to IATs were previously incubated, or left to stand, at room temperature. In methods such as LISS, PEG or Polybrene that are converted to IATs short (or

preferably no) incubation below 37°C is used (see Chapter 35). Further, many workers read such tests with anti-IgG so that anti-Sd^a will not be detected via the C3-anti-C3 reaction. Failure to detect such examples of anti-Sd^a is clearly an advantage. Again as discussed in detail below, anti-Sd^a is a clinically benign antibody. As with any antibody of that type, nondetection is an advantage since the work involved in antibody identification and possible delays in transfusion, while the antibody is being identified, are avoided.

As with most examples of cold-reactive, clinically-insignificant antibodies, the strength and immunoglobulin class of most examples of anti-Sd^a do not change in persons transfused with Sd(a+) blood. Although some exceptions are described below, even those have not been associated with immediate or delayed hemolytic transfusion reactions. In 1978, Silvergleid et al. (154) described three examples of anti-Sd^a that included IgM and IgG components and one that was solely IgG. The introduction of Sd(a+) red cells in the patients did not cause the anti-Sd^a to change in character or strength. In 1982, Spitalnick et al. (149) studied the sera of six patients with anti-Sd^a who had received Sd(a+) blood. In three of them no change in the strength of the antibody was associated with the transfusion. In the other three, the antibody titers did increase and much of the increase represented IgG anti-Sd^a. However, in none of the patients was there any evidence to suggest that the anti-Sd^a had caused accelerated clearance of the Sd(a+) red cells.

Anti-Sd^a, Usual Lack of Clinical Significance

As will be apparent from what has been written in the preceding section, anti-Sd^a is usually of no clinical significance. That is to say, it is usually incapable of bringing about accelerated in vivo clearance of Sd(a+) red cells. In the first two reports about the antibody, the authors (15,16) commented that since the antibody is relatively common and since 96% of random donors have the Sd(a+) phenotype, many persons with anti-Sd^a in the serum must have been transfused with Sd(a+) blood, even before those reports appeared. No patient in the studies, more than 37 examples of anti-Sd^a were mentioned (15,16), had a transfusion reaction. Although anti-Sd^a was identified in the sera of several pregnant women, no case of HDN caused by the antibody was seen, nor has any case been found since then.

In the patients studied by Silvergleid et al. (154) in vivo red cell survival studies using ^{51}Cr-labeled Sd(a+) red cells were performed. Although all four patients had at least some IgG anti-Sd^a, the 1-hour survival rate of the injected red cells was normal in each case. Three of the patients were subsequently transfused with a total of 13 Sd(a+) units among them. In all three, expected post-transfusion hematocrit levels were seen. In the fourth patient, who had IgM and IgG anti-Sd^a, the ^{51}Cr-labeled red cell survival study was done with Sd(a++) red cells. One hour following the injection, 92% of the injected red cells were still present in the patient's circulation.

Somewhat similarly, although they did not perform in vivo red cell survival studies, Spitalnik et al. (149) reported that in their six patients with anti-Sd^a who were transfused with Sd(a+) blood, the expected rises in post-transfusion hematocrit were seen and that neither clinical nor laboratory evidence of immune-mediated red cell destruction was found.

In 1973, Colledge et al. (158) described a case in which a patient with anti-Sd^a was transfused with 14 units of Sd(a+) blood during open-heart surgery. Red cell survival studies and careful posttransfusion evaluation indicated normal survival of the transfused red cells. In this case, the patient's IgM anti-Sd^a showed no change in immunoglobulin class or strength after the transfusions.

There must, by now, be hundreds of cases similar to those described above in which patients with anti-Sd^a have been transfused with Sd(a+) blood with an entirely satisfactory outcome. One of us (PDI) has personal experience of many and has heard anecdotal reports of many others. Because the benign nature of anti-Sd^a is so clearly established, such cases are no longer documented in the literature.

In spite of the numerous cases in which anti-Sd^a was clearly benign in vivo, there are two reports (159,160) in which the antibody is blamed for causing a hemolytic transfusion reaction. The patient described by Peetermans and Cole-Dergent (159) was given seven units of blood with no untoward reactions. Ten days later he was transfused again because of renewed gastric hemorrhage. This time he had an urticarial reaction to the first unit given and a hemolytic reaction to the fourth. His serum was found to contain an IgM anti-Sd^a; all the blood transfused was shown to have been Sd(a+). A ^{51}Cr-labeled red cell survival study, using Sd(a+) red cells that were not of the Sd(a++) phenotype, showed a two-component curve. Fifty percent of the small dose of injected cells was cleared with T1/2 of 2 days; the remaining cells survived normally (T1/2, 27 days). It was then shown that the donor's red cells that caused the reaction were of the Sd(a++) phenotype. The lesson from this case seems clear. Once identified, anti-Sd^a can be ignored for transfusion purposes providing that compatibility tests show only average reactivity indicating that the units to be used are of the Sd(a+) phenotype. In the rare event that a unit tested with the patient's serum shows strong reactivity, and may thus be of the Sd(a++) phenotype, that unit need not be given. This means that in patients with identified anti-Sd^a, only about one unit in 100 need be regarded as incompatible.

The patient described by Reznicek et al. (160) was thought to have had a hemolytic transfusion reaction caused by anti-Sd^a although the antibody in her serum was remarkably weak. The red cells of the unit that caused the reaction carried a greater than average level of Sd^a. The red cells of the unit were described as giving a 1+ macroscopic reaction with an anti-Sd^a that produced only microscopically positive reactions with other Sd(a+) red cells. Retrospective studies showed that the patient's pretransfusion serum reacted with red cells from the offending unit only microscopically by LISS-IAT. Thus, although there was no doubt that the patient had a transfusion reaction, considerable doubt that it was caused by anti-Sd^a remains. It must be remembered that there are a number of well-documented cases (161-166, for references to many cases reported before 1980, see 167) in which the patient clearly had a hemolytic transfusion reaction but in which heroic efforts at the serological level failed to demonstrate a causative antibody. If such a case occurred in a patient who had anti-Sd^a in the serum (the antibody is common, see above) the anti-Sd^a might be blamed for a hemolytic reaction caused by a different undetectable antibody, simultaneously present.

We experienced a situation in which exactly such blame could have been applied, but were able to show that the accelerated rate of clearance of red cells had nothing to do with the anti-Sd^a in the patient's serum. We (168) provided two units of packed red cells for a patient in whose serum no atypical antibodies were demonstrable. The units were well tolerated and effected the expected rise in hemoglobin. Nine days later the patient presented with all the clinical signs of a classic delayed transfusion reaction. On investigation we found anti-Sd^a now demonstrable in his serum. Because we did not want to believe that the anti-Sd^a was responsible for the delayed transfusion reaction, we undertook ^{51}Cr cell survival studies using Sd(a+) red cells and expecting a normal result. The half-time of the injected Sd(a+) red cells was markedly reduced! Because we had transfused Sd(a+) red cells to many patients with anti-Sd^a in the serum, at the time of transfusion, and had seen no evidence of accelerated in vivo red cell clearance in any of them, we still did not want to believe that the anti-Sd^a had caused the delayed transfusion reaction. Accordingly, we repeated the ^{51}Cr cell survival study using Sd(a-) cells. The half time of the Sd(a-) cells was identical to that of those that were Sd(a+). We were never able to detect the antibody responsible for the in vivo cell clearance in this patient but clearly, we absolved the anti-Sd^a from that role.

Some Other Findings About Sd^a

In one of the initial studies (15) on Sd^a, it was noted

that saliva samples from group A persons seemed to contain more Sd^a than those from persons of other ABO groups. Although secretors of ABH substances tended to have more Sd^a substance in the saliva than did nonsecretors, there was no correlation between the levels of A, B or H and Sd^a. Similarly, the level of Sd^a secreted was not correlated with the level of Le^b in saliva. In both initial studies (15,16) it was reported that *Sd^a* was genetically independent of the ABO system (and of many others) and that there was no disturbance in the incidence of the Sd(a+) and Sd(a-) phenotypes based on ABO groups. As discussed in detail in a later section of this chapter, the similarity between Sd^a and A in terms of the immunodominant structures, is now well established.

In 1973, Lewis et al. (169) described a family in which the gene responsible for the Sd(a++) phenotype and *Wr^a* were segregating. The count of six nonrecombinants to no recombinants was just short of statistical significance. As far as we have been able to determine, no further information about this hint of linkage has become available. However, given what is now known about the structure of Sd^a (see below) and the fact that the Wr^a/Wr^b polymorphism involves an amino acid difference on protein band 3 (see Chapter 17) association between Sd^a and Wr^a seems somewhat unlikely.

The Antigen Cad and the Biochemical Structure of Cad and Sd^a

In 1968, Cazal et al. (170) described the first example of polyagglutination of an inherited variety. The polyagglutinable red cells were said to carry the low-incidence antigen Cad that was inherited as a Mendelian dominant character and it was concluded that all normal sera contain some anti-Cad. Since that time, graded expressions of the Cad antigen on red cells that are not polyagglutinable have been found, leading to designations of the phenotypes Cad 1, 2, 3 and 4 (171,172) that are described in more detail in Chapter 42. As mentioned earlier, some workers (39,143,145) equate the Sd(a++) and Cad+ phenotypes. However, since Cad 1 red cells are polyagglutinable, that would mean that all Sd(a+) persons (but perhaps not those of the Sd(a++) phenotype) have anti-Sd^a in their sera. Since the structure of the Sd^a determinant has been determined primarily by studies on the Tamm-Horsfall (T-H) (174,175) urinary glycoprotein (176-186) while the Cad antigen has been characterized as representing a different to normal carbohydrate side chain on glycophorin A (i.e. the tetrasaccharide described in Chapter 15 that is converted to a pentasaccharide by the addition of a GalNAc residue, see Chapter 42) (187-191) we have elected to describe Cad in Chapter 42. Duffy and Marshall (192) have pointed out that in the Tamm-

Horsfall glycoprotein there are carbohydrate side chains in N-linkage to five asparagine residues and that at least two of these side chains are, or include, the Sd^a-active pentasaccharide (179,181). In contrast, on red cells the pentasaccharides that include the Cad determinant are O-linked to threonine or serine (188). However, it should be added that the exact structure of Sd^a on red cells, is not known. Serafini-Cessi et al. (184) isolated and purified a β-N-acetylgalactosaminyltransferase from the urine of individuals with Sd(a+) red cells. They found that the best acceptor for this enzyme, in its transfer of GalNAc in β(1→4) linkage to Gal, was a preparation of T-H glycoprotein isolated from the urine of an individual with Sd(a-) red cells. However, in a highly purified form (174-fold purification) the enzyme was also able to add GalNAc to the tetrasaccharides of native glycophorin A. The meaning of this observation is still not completely clear since Blanchard et al. (188) did not find the additional GalNAc residue in the oligosaccharide side chains attached to glycophorin A of Sd(a+), Cad- red cells. Thus, it remains possible that the *Sd^a*-specified transferase may have preferential catalytic activity for N-linked oligosaccharides and the *Cad*-specified transferase preferential catalytic activity for O-linked oligosaccharides. Dohi et al. (216) isolated cDNA encoding the Sd^a-galactosaminyltransferase from human gastric mucosa using RT-PCR with primers based on the sequence of a murine β(1→4) galactosaminyltransferase (217) that appeared to be the murine equivalent of the human *Sd^a* gene-specified transferase. The human enzyme showed 85-90% identity in nucleotide sequence with the mouse enzyme. These studies should enable analysis of the genetic basis of Sd^a expression on red cells and the relationship between Sd^a and Cad.

To summarize this long and somewhat tedious section, it will again be stated that the question of identity or nonidentity between Sd(a++) and Cad may not be resolved until the nature of the oligosaccharides that carry Sd^a on red cells is determined. While Sd^a and Cad on red cells may behave similarly in serological studies, with Sd(a++) and Cad appearing to be the same, that interpretation may or may not apply at the structural level. Figure 31-2 depicts the structure of the Sd^a-containing pentasaccharide on T-H urinary glycoprotein and the Cad-containing pentasaccharide on red cell glycophorin A. As can be seen, the immunodominant trisaccharides of the antigens are the same but the pentasaccharides are different and, as described above the differences may relate directly to their N or O linkage.

The Antigen Duclos and the Antibody That Defines It

In 1978, Habibi et al. (17) described an antibody in the

FIGURE 31-2 Structure of the Sd^a-containing Pentasaccharide on T-H Urinary Glycoprotein and the Cad-containing Pentasaccharide on Red Cell Glycophorin A

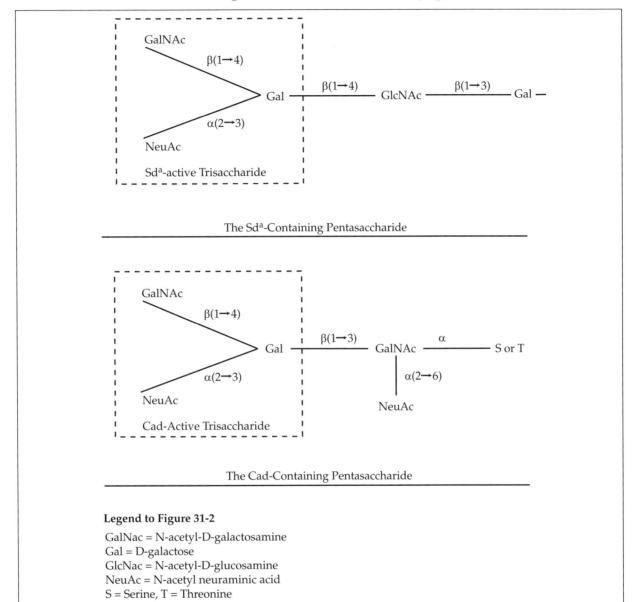

Legend to Figure 31-2

GalNac = N-acetyl-D-galactosamine
Gal = D-galactose
GlcNac = N-acetyl-D-glucosamine
NeuAc = N-acetyl neuraminic acid
S = Serine, T = Threonine

serum of a French lady, Madame Duclos, that defined an antigen of very high incidence. The Duclos antibody reacted strongly with red cells on which the Rh and U antigens were expressed normally. It reacted weakly with Rh_{null} red cells on which U could be detected and with U- red cells on which Rh antigens were expressed normally. Only trace amounts of the Duclos antigen seemed to be present on Rh_{null} red cells on which the U antigen was difficult to detect. Indeed, such red cells at first appeared to lack the Duclos antigen but were then shown to be capable of adsorbing anti-Duclos and yielding the antibody in eluates. The red cells of Madame Duclos were D+ C+ E- c+ e+ and

had apparently normal levels of Rh antigens. Her U antigen was slightly depressed in expression. Although the Duclos antigen was given the number Rh38 (193) the assignment was in error since production of the antigen is not encoded from the *Rh* locus. The term Rh38 has been declared obsolete and the Duclos antigen has been renumbered as shown in table 31-1.

A number of murine monoclonal antibodies have been shown (194-196) to be directed against Rh-associated glycoproteins (see Chapter 12). At least three of these antibodies, MB-2D10, LA-18.18 and LA-23.4 have specificities very close to that of the Duclos antibody. However, MB-

2D10 and the Duclos antibody are apparently not identical since MB-2D10 reacts with the red cells of Madame Duclos (197) and her antibody was alloimmune in nature. The MB-2D10 MAb was shown (196) to precipitate the Rh acylproteins, the Rh glycoproteins and, under some experimental conditions, glycophorin B. It was concluded that the epitope defined was part of the Rh complex that apparently exists on the red cell membrane (see Chapter 12). Mallinson et al. (195) then showed that MB-2D10 is directed against the Rh glycoproteins. Given the serological reactions of MB-2D10 and the Duclos antibody it would seem that glycophorin B must be involved in presentation of the antigen defined, in situ in red cells. Indeed, Mallinson et al. (195) suggested that the U antigen might represent a structure formed by interaction between the Rh glycoprotein(s) and glycophorin B. von dem Borne et al. (196) showed that the determinant defined by MB-2D10 is not expressed on erythroid progenitor cells but appears very early, at the proerythroblast stage in cell differentiation. The MB-2D10 defined determinant is detected earlier in cell differentiation than are the non-glycosylated Rh polypeptides. Since the determinant was also found in malignant erythroblastoid cell lines, these workers (196) suggested that it might be a useful differentiation marker in certain disease states involving malignant erythroid cell lines. The antigen defined by the monoclonal antibody MB-2D10, that has a specificity very similar to that of anti-Duclos, is present on cord blood red cells. The antigen survives the treatment of red cells with trypsin, papain, neuraminidase and AET; it is weakened when red cells are treated with chymotrypsin and denatured by the actions of pronase. It is possible, but not proved, that the Duclos antigen has similar characteristics.

Although quite different from MB-2D10 and the Duclos antibody, Le Pennec et al. (198) described a human alloantibody that reacted only with D+, S+ red cells. The antibody was made by a patient with D+, S- s+ red cells, whose Rh polypeptides and glycophorin B appeared grossly normal. The antibody reacted in the AutoAnalyzer. Not only did it react only with D+, S+ red cells, it was not adsorbed by: D+, S-; D-, S+; or D-, S- red cells. Clearly MB-2D10 and related MAbs, the Duclos antibody and the antibody reacting only with D+, S+ red cells are trying to send a message about the interactions between the non-glycosylated Rh polypeptides, the Rh glycoproteins and glycophorin B.

The Antigen PEL (and MTP) and the Antibody That Defines It

This high incidence antigen is defined by an antibody that was found (18) in 1980, in the serum of a French-Canadian woman during her second pregnancy. The patient had also been transfused. The antigen defined was not shown to be an inherited characteristic until another example of anti-PEL was found in 1994 (199). The second example of anti-PEL was also found in a French-Canadian woman, the proposita had been pregnant and transfused. The proposita had seven sibs, three of whom had PEL- red cells. The PEL antigen was shown to survive treatment of red cells with trypsin, chymotrypsin, papain, pronase, neuraminidase and AET. The PEL antigen is detectable on cord blood red cells but anti-PEL has not caused HDN. A ^{51}Cr-labeled red cell survival study showed normal survival of PEL+ red cells in one patient with anti-PEL.

When the second example of anti-PEL was reported (199) two additional antibodies were described. Both were made by French-Canadians and their specificity was very close to that of anti-PEL. The antibodies reacted with all red cells except those that were PEL- and those of the antibody-makers. However, the red cells of the antibody-makers were shown, in adsorption studies, to carry some PEL antigen. The antibodies were provisionally called anti-MTP as a working designation until such time as the nature of the relationship between PEL and MTP is established. Sibs with compatible red cells were found in the families of the probands who made anti-MTP. The antigen defined by the antibodies provisionally called anti-MTP survived treatment of red cells with trypsin, chymotrypsin, papain, pronase, neuraminidase and AET.

Like the two individuals who made anti-PEL, the two who made anti-MTP had been transfused. One of them had also been pregnant. Anti-MTP did not cause HDN but in a ^{51}Cr red cell survival study, 26% of a test dose of serologically reactive red cells was cleared in the first 24 hours after injection.

The Antigen ABTI and the Antibody That Defines It

As of this writing (November 1996) the high incidence antigen ABTI has been described only in one abstract (19). Three women in an inbred Israeli Arab family were found to have the same specificity antibody in their sera. All the antibody-makers had been pregnant, none of them had been transfused and none of their infants had HDN. The antibody was called anti-ABTI and three other individuals in the family were shown to have ABTI- red cells. In tests on random samples, 509 Jews, 121 Arabs and 70 persons attending a health clinic in the Arab village from whence came the proposita, were found to have ABTI+ red cells. The ABTI antigen survived treatment of red cells with trypsin, chymotrypsin, papain, ficin, neuraminidase and AET. In tests on eight Vel- samples, six reacted weakly and one did not react with anti-ABTI. Thus it is possible that a

TABLE 31-4 The Most Usual Characteristics of Antibodies Directed Against Antigens Described in this Chapter.

Antibody Specificity	Positive Reactions in In Vitro Tests				Usual Immuno-globulin		Ability to Bind Complement		Ability to Cause In Vitro Lysis		Implicated in		Usual Form of Stimulation		% of White Population Positive
	Sal	LISS	AHG	Enz	IgG	IgM	Yes	No	Yes	No	Trans-fusion Reaction	HDN	Red Cells	Other	
Anti-Vel	X	X	X	X	Some	Some	Some		Some		X	No	X		>99.9
Anti-Lan			X	X	X		Some	Some		X	X	Mild	X		>99.9
Anti-At^a			X	X	X	Rare				X	Poss	Mild	X		>99.9
Anti-Jr^a			X	X	X	Rare	Some			X	Poss	Mild	Most	Few	>99.9
Anti-Ok^a			X	X	X					X	X		X		>99.9
Anti-JMH	X	X	X	No	Most	Few		Most		X	V. rare	No			>99.9
Anti-Emm	X		X	X	Most	Rare				X				X	>99.9
Anti-MER2			X		X					X	No	No	Rare	Most	>99.9
Anti-Sd^a	X		X		Few	Most	Many			X	Most No	No		X	96.0
Anti-Duclos			X	X	X					X		No	X		>99.9
Anti-PEL			X	X	X					X	No	No	X		>99.9
Anti-ABTI			X	X	X					X		No	X		>99.9

relationship exists between Vel and ABTI.

The original example of anti-ABTI reacted in IATs, it was composed in part of IgG1 and in part of IgG3. The antibody had a titer of 2048.

Antibodies Directed Against Antigens Described in this Chapter

As will be appreciated, different examples of antibodies to the antigens described in this chapter, vary somewhat in their characteristics. Further, for some of the antigens, only a few examples of the definitive antibodies have been studied. In spite of these limitations, table 31-4 summarizes the most frequent findings about these antibodies.

References

1. Lewis M, Anstee DJ, Bird GWG, et al. Vox Sang 1990;58:152
2. Lewis M, Allen FH Jr, Anstee DJ, et al. Vox Sang 1985;49:171
3. Sussman LN, Miller EB. Rev Haematol 1952;7:368
4. Hart van der M, Moes M, Veer van der M, et al. Proc 8th Cong Eur Soc Haematol. Basel:Karger 1961
5. Applewhaite F, Ginsberg V, Cunningham CA, et al. Vox Sang 1967;13:444
6. Stroup M, MacIlroy M. (abstract). Prog 23rd Ann Mtg Am Assoc Blood Banks 1970 and supplemented by information presented but not included in the abstract
7. Morel PA, Hamilton HB. Vox Sang 1979;36:182
8. Sabo B, Moulds JJ, McCreary J. (abstract). Transfusion 1978;18:387
9. Daniels GL, Taliano V, Klein MT, et al. Transfusion 1987;27:319
10. Poole J, Giles CM. Vox Sang 1982;43:220
11. Marsh WL, Brown PJ, DiNapoli J, et al. Transfusion 1983;23:128
12. Poole J, Giles C. (Letter). Transfusion 1985;25:443
13. Marsh WL, Johnson CL. (Letter). Transfusion 1985;25:443
14. Daniels GL, Tippett P, Palmer DK, et al. Vox Sang 1987;52:107
15. Macvie SJ, Morton JA, Pickles MM. Vox Sang 1967;13:485
16. Renton PH, Howell P, Ikin EW, et al. Vox Sang 1967;13:493
17. Habibi B, Fouillade MT, Duedari N, et al. Vox Sang 1978;34:302
18. Daniels GL. PhD Thesis, Univ London, 1980
19. Schechter Y, Chezar J, Levene C, et al. (abstract). Transfusion 1996;36 (Suppl 9S):25S
20. Levine P, Robinson EA, Herrington LB, et al. Am J Clin Pathol 1955;25:751
21. Cleghorn TE. MD Thesis, Univ Sheffield 1961
22. Sussman LN. Transfusion 1962;2:163
23. Battaglini PF, Ranque J, Bridonneau C, et al. Proc 10th Cong ISBT 1964:309
24. Albrey JA, McCullough WJ, Simmons RT. Med J Austral 1965;2:662
25. Nevanlinna H. Unpublished observations 1966 cited in Race RR, Sanger R. Blood Groups in Man, 6th Ed. Oxford:Blackwell, 1975
26. Kornstad L. Unpublished observations 1970 cited in Race RR, Sanger R. Blood Groups in Man, 6th Ed. Oxford:Blackwell, 1975

27. Cedergren B, Giles CM, Ikin EW. Vox Sang 1976;31:344
28. Bowell P. Unpublished observations cited in Cedergren B, Giles CM, Ikin EW. Vox Sang 1976;31:344
29. Herron R, Hyde RD, Hillier SJ. Vox Sang 1979;36:179
30. Gale SA, Rowe GP, Northfield FE. Vox Sang 1988;54:172
31. Chandanayingyong D, Sasaki TT, Greenwalt TJ. Transfusion 1967;7:269
32. Alfred BM, Stout TD, Lee M, et al. Am J Phys Anthropol 1970;32:329
33. Levine P, White JA, Stroup M. Transfusion 1961;1:111
34. Leisen G. Unpublished observations 1970 cited in Race RR, Sanger R. Blood Groups in Man, 6th Ed. Oxford:Blackwell, 1975
35. Strickel P, Brown WG, Jack JA. (abstract). Prog 12th Ann Mtg Am Assoc Blood Banks 1959
36. Wiener AS, Gordon EB, Unger LJ. Bull Jewish Hosp Brooklyn 1961;3:46
37. White JA, Reinert I. Transfusion 1962;2:269
38. Drachmann O, Lundsgaard A. Scand J Haematol 1970;7:27
39. Race RR, Sanger R. Blood Groups in Man, 6th Ed. Oxford:Blackwell, 1975
40. Toivanen P, Hirvonen T. Scand J Haematol 1969;6:49
41. Daniels G. Immunohematology 1992;8:53
42. Brandish EB, Shields WF. Am J Clin Pathol 1959;31:104
43. Issitt PD, Øyen R, Reihart JK, et al. Vox Sang 1968;15:125
44. Sussman LN, Pretshold H. Haematologia 1972;6:129
45. Tilley CA, Crookston MC, Haddad SA, et al. Transfusion 1977;17:169
46. Ferrer Z, Cornwall S, Berger R, et al. Rev Fr Transf Immunohematol 1984;27:639
47. Williams CK, Williams B, Pearson J, et al. (abstract). Transfusion 1985;25:462
48. Stiller RJ, Lardas O, Haynes de Regt R. Am J Obstet Gynecol 1990;162:1071
49. Storry JR, Mallory DM. (abstract). Transfusion 1993;33 (Suppl 9S):17S
50. Issitt PD. Applied Blood Group Serology, 3rd Ed. Miami:Montgomery, 1985
51. Branch DR, Gallagher MT, Mison AP, et al. Br J Haematol 1984;56:19
52. Moore RE, Lenes BA, Brendel WL, et al. (abstract). Prog 38th Ann Mtg Florida Assoc Blood Banks 1984
53. Szaloky A, Hart van der M. Vox Sang 1971;20:376
54. Becton DL, Kinney TR. Vox Sang 1986;51:108
55. Issitt P, Combs M, Carawan H, et al. (abstract). Transfusion 1994;34 (Suppl 10S):60S
56. Garratty G, Arndt P, Nance S. (abstract). Transfusion 1996;36 (Suppl 9S):50S
57. Grindon AJ, McGinniss MH, Issitt PD, et al. Vox Sang 1968;15:293
58. Smith DS, Stratton F, Johnson T, et al. Br Med J 1969;3:90
59. Fox JA, Taswell HF. Transfusion 1969;9:265
60. Frank S, Schmidt RP, Baugh M. Transfusion 1970;10:254
61. Clancy M, Bonds S, Eys van J. Transfusion 1972;12:106
62. Page PL. Transfusion 1983;23:256
63. Okubo Y, Yamaguchi H, Seno T, et al. Transfusion 1984;24:534
64. Gerbal A, Daniels GL. Unpublished observations 1976 cited in Daniels G. Human Blood Groups. Oxford:Blackwell, 1995
65. Poole J, Rowe GP, Leak M. (abstract). Book of Abstracts. 20th Cong ISBT 1988:303
66. Lampe TL, Moore SB, Pineda AA. (abstract). Transfusion 1979;19:640
67. Vengelen-Tyler V, Morel PA. (abstract). Transfusion 1981;21:603

68. Judd WJ, Oberman HA, Silenieks A, et al. (Letter). Transfusion 1984;24:181
69. Shertz WT, Carty L, Wolford F. (Letter). Transfusion 1987;27:117
70. Pope J, Lubenko A, Lai WYY. (abstract). Transf Med 1991;1 (Suppl 2):58
71. Nance SJ, Arndt P, Garratty G. Transfusion 1987;27:449
72. Nance SJ, Arndt PA, Garratty G. (Letter). Transfusion 1988;28:398
73. Dzik W, Blank J, Getman E, et al. (abstract). Transfusion 1985;25:462
74. Edwards JM, Moulds JJ, Judd WJ. Transfusion 1982;22:59
75. Nesbitt R. (Letter). Transfusion 1979;19:354
76. Walker ME. Unpublished observations 1970 cited in an addendum to their paper by Frank S, Schmidt RP, Baugh M. Transfusion 1970;10:254
77. Schmidt RP, Frank S, Baugh M. (abstract). Transfusion 1967;7:386 and supplemented by comments made in the oral presentation but not included in the abstract.
78. Applewhaite F. Unpublished observations 1968 cited in Issitt PD, Issitt CH. Applied Blood Group Serology, 2nd Ed. Oxnard:Spectra Biologicals, 1975
79. Gellerman MM, McCreary J, Yedinak E, et al. Transfusion 1973;13:225
80. Vengelen-Tyler V. (abstract). Transfusion 1985;25:476
81. Winkler MM, Hamilton JR. (abstract). Book of Abstracts. Joint Cong ISBT/AABB 1990:158
82. Culver PL, Brubaker DB, Sheldon RE, et al. Transfusion 1987;27:468
83. Sweeney JD, Holme S, McCall L, et al. Transfusion 1995;35:63
84. Brown A, Harris P, Daniels GL, et al. Transfusion 1983;44:123
85. Ginsberg V, Applewhaite F, Gerena J, et al. (abstract). Transfusion 1967;7:386
86. Gellerman M, Stroup M. Unpublished observations 1974 cited in Race RR, Sanger R. Blood Groups in Man, 6th Ed. Oxford:Blackwell, 1975
87. Lewis M, Kaita H, Chown B. Am J Hum Genet 1957;9:274
88. Stavely JM. Unpublished observations 1974 cited in Race RR, Sanger R. Blood Groups in Man, 6th Ed. Oxford:Blackwell, 1975
89. Tritchler JE. Transfusion 1977;17:177
90. Contreras M. Unpublished observations 1982 cited in Daniels G. Human Blood Groups. Oxford:Blackwell, 1995
91. Yamaguchi H, Okubo Y, Seno T, et al. Proc Jpn Acad 1976;52:521
92. Yamada K, Nagashima S, Kishi M, et al. 1976 cited in Yamaguchi H, Okubo Y, Seno T, et al. Proc Jpn Acad 1976;52:521
93. Nakajima H, Iko K. Vox Sang 1978;35:265
94. Miyazaki T, Kwon KW, Yamamoto K, et al. Vox Sang 1994;66:51
95. Kendall AG. Transfusion 1976;16:646
96. Levene C, Sela R, Dvilansky A, et al. (Letter). Transfusion 1986;26:119
97. Vedo M, Reid ME. Transfusion 1978;18:569
98. Bacon J, Sherrin D, Wright RG. (Letter). Transfusion 1986;26:543
99. Orrick LR, Golde SH. Am J Obstet Gynecol 1980;137:135
100. Toy P, Reid M, Lewis T, et al. Vox Sang 1981;41:40
101. Armitage S. Unpublished observations 1980 cited in Daniels G. Human Blood Groups. Oxford:Blackwell, 1995
102. Jowitt S, Powell H, Shwe KH, et al. (abstract). Transf Med 1994;4 (Suppl 1):49

103. Verska JJ, Larson NL. Transfusion 1973;13:219
104. Biro V. Unpublished observations 1979 cited in Morel PA, Hamilton HB. Vox Sang 1979;36:182
105. Anstee DJ, Spring FA. Transf Med Rev 1989;3:13
106. Yamaguchi H, Okubo Y. Unpublished observations 1983 cited in Daniels G. Human Blood Groups. Oxford:Blackwell, 1995
107. Williams BP, Daniels GL, Pym B, et al. Immunogenetics 1988;27:322
108. Mattes MJ, Cairncross JG, Old LJ, et al. Hybridoma 1983;2:253
109. Spring F, Daniels GL. Unpublished observations 1991 cited in Daniels G. Human Blood Groups. Oxford:Blackwell, 1995
110. Issitt PD, Issitt CH. Applied Blood Group Serology, 2nd Ed. Oxnard:Spectra Biologicals, 1975:259
111. Kollmar MB, South SF, Tregellas WM. (abstract). Transfusion 1981;21:612
112. Daniels GL, Nordhagen R. Unpublished observations 1982 cited in Daniels G. Human Blood Groups. Oxford:Blackwell, 1995:651
113. Whitsett CF, Moulds M, Pierce JA, et al. Transfusion 1983;23:344
114. Contreras M, Daniels GL. Unpublished observations 1984 cited in Daniels G. Human Blood Groups. Oxford:Blackwell, 1995:652
115. Tregellas WM, Pierce SR, Hardman JT, et al. (abstract). Transfusion 1980;20:628
116. Baldwin ML, Ness PM, Barrasso C, et al. Transfusion 1985;25:34
117. Geisland J, Corgan M, Hillard B. Immunohematology 1990;6:9
118. Moulds JJ, Levene C, Zimmerman S. (abstract). Book of Abstracts. 17th Cong ISBT 1982:287
119. Daniels GL, Knowles RW. J Immunogenet 1982;9:57
120. Daniels GL, Knowles RW. J Immunogenet 1983;10:257
121. Issitt PD, Roy RB, Combs MR, et al. (abstract). Transfusion 1992;32 (Suppl 8S):55S
122. Mudad R, Rao N, Issitt PD, et al. Transfusion 1995;35:925
123. Telen MJ, Rosse WF, Parker CJ, et al. Blood 1990;75:1404
124. Bobolis KA, Telen MJ. (abstract). Transfusion 1991;31 (Suppl 8S):46S
125. Bobolis KA, Moulds JJ, Telen MJ. Blood 1992;79:1574
126. Mudad R, Rao N, Angelisova P, et al. Transfusion 1995;35:566
127. Moulds JJ. Personal communication, 1992
128. International Committee for Standardization in Haematology. Br J Haematol 1980;45:659
129. Boorman KE, Tippett P. Unpublished observations 1979 cited in Race RR, Sanger R. Blood Groups in Man, 6th Ed. Oxford:Blackwell, 1975
130. Mannessier L, Rouger P, Johnson CL, et al. Vox Sang 1986;50:240
131. Telen MJ, Rao N, Udani M, et al. (abstract). Transfusion 1993;33 (Suppl 9S):48S
132. Telen MJ, Eisenbarth GS, Haynes BF. J Clin Invest 1983;71:1878
133. Spring FA, Dalchau R, Daniels GL, et al. Immunology 1988;64:37
134. Telen MJ, Ferguson DJ. Vox Sang 1990;58:118
135. Daniels GL, Tippett P, Palmer DK, et al. (abstract). Transfusion 1985;25:482
136. Daniels G. In: Blood Group Systems: Duffy, Kidd and Lutheran. Arlington, VA:Am Assoc Blood Banks, 1988:119
137. Daniels GL, Levene C, Berrebi A, et al. Vox Sang 1988;55:161
138. Goodfellow PN, Banting G, Wiles MV, et al. Eur J Immunol 1982;12:659
139. Francke U, Foellmer BE, Haynes BF. Somat Cell Genet 1983;9:333
140. Ala-Kapee M, Forsberg UH, Jalkanen S, et al. Cytogenet Cell Genet 1989;51:948
141. Forsberg UH, Jalkanen S, Schröder J. Immunogenetics 1989;29:405
142. Couillin P, Azoulay M, Henry I, et al. Hum Genet 1989;82:171
143. Daniels G. Human Blood Groups. Oxford:Blackwell, 1995:655
144. Morton JA, Pickles MM, Terry AM. Vox Sang 1970;19:472
145. Sanger R, Gavin J, Tippett P, et al. Lancet 1971;1:1130
146. Sringarm S, Chupungart C, Giles CM. Vox Sang 1972;23:537
147. Sringarm S, Chiewsilp P, Tubrod T. Vox Sang 1974;26:462
148. Pickles MM, Morton JA. In: Human Blood Groups. Basel:Karger, 1977:277
149. Spitalnik S, Cox MT, Spennacchio J, et al. Vox Sang 1982;42:308
150. Moulds MK. In: Blood Groups: P, I, Sd^a, and Pr. Arlington, VA:Am Assoc Blood Banks, 1991:113
151. Judd WJ. Methods in Immunohematology. 2nd Ed. Durham:Montgomery, 1994
152. Howell P. MS Thesis, Univ Manchester, 1968
153. Mollison PL, Engelfriet CP, Contreras M. Blood Transfusion in Clinical Medicine, 8th Ed. Oxford:Blackwell 1987:400
154. Silvergleid AJ, Wells RF, Hafleigh EB, et al. Transfusion 1978;18:8
155. Judd WJ. (Letter). Transfusion 1983;23:404
156. Advani H, Zamor J, Judd WJ, et al. (abstract). Transfusion 1981;21:631
157. Advani H, Zamor J, Judd WJ, et al. Br J Haematol 1982;51:10
158. Colledge KI, Kaplan HS, Marsh WL. (abstract). Transfusion 1973;13:340
159. Peetermans ME, Cole-Dergent J. Vox Sang 1970;18:67
160. Reznicek MJ, Cordle DG, Strauss RG. Vox Sang 1992;62:173
161. Davey RJ, Gustafson M, Holland PV. Transfusion 1980;20:348
162. Halima D, Postoway N, Brunt D, et al. (abstract). Transfusion 1982;22:405
163. Garratty G, Vengelen-Tyler V, Postoway N, et al. (abstract). Transfusion 1982;22:429
164. Baldwin ML, Barrasso C, Ness PM, et al. Transfusion 1983;123:40
165. Harris CR, Hayes TC, Trow LL, et al. Vox Sang 1986;51:96
166. Garratty G, Arndt P, Postoway N, et al. (abstract). Transfusion 1996;36 (Suppl 9S):23S
167. Issitt PD, Gutgsell NS. In: Immune Destruction of Red Blood Cells. Arlington, VA:Am Assoc Blood Banks, 1989:77
168. Issitt CH, Muhlman AF Jr, Issitt PD. Unpublished observations 1976 cited in Issitt PD. Applied Blood Group Serology, 3rd Ed. Miami:Montgomery, 1985:428
169. Lewis M, Kaita H, Chown B, et al. Vox Sang 1973;25:336
170. Cazal P, Monis M, Caubel J, et al. Rev Fr Transf 1968;11:209
171. Cazal P, Monis M, Bizot M. Rev Fr Transf 1971;14:321
172. Cazal P, Monis M, Bizot M. Rev Fr Transf Immunohematol 1977;20:165
173. Tamm I, Horsfall FL. Proc Soc Exp Biol Med 1950;74:108
174. Tamm I, Horsfall FL. J Exp Med 1952;95:71
175. Morgan WTJ, Soh C, Watkins WM. In: Glycoconjugates. Stuttgart:Tieme, 1979:582
176. Soh CPC, Morgan WTJ, Watkins WM, et al. Biochem Biophys Res Comm 1980;93:1132
177. Morgan WTJ, Soh CPC, Donald ASR, et al. Blood Transf Immunohematol 1981;24:37

178. Donald ASR, Soh CPC, Watkins WM, et al. Biochem Biophys Res Comm 1982;104:58

179. Donald ASR, Yates AD, Soh CPC, et al. Biochem Biophys Res Comm 1983;115:625

180. Serafini-Cessi F, Dall'Olio F. Biochem J 1983;215:483

181. Williams J, Marshall RD, Van Halbeek H, et al. Carbohyd Res 1984;134:141

182. Donald ASR, Yates AD, Soh CPC, et al. Biochem Soc Transact 1984;12:596

183. Donald ASR, Feeney J. Biochem J 1986;236:821

184. Serafini-Cessi F, Malagolini N, Dall'Olio F. Arch Biochem Biophys 1988;266:573

185. Donald ASR, Soh CPC, Yates AD, et al. Biochem Soc Transact 1987;15:606

186. Piller F, Blanchard D, Huet M, et al. Carbohyd Res 1986;149:171

187. Cartron J-P, Blanchard D. Biochem J 1982;207:497

188. Blanchard D, Cartron J-P, Fournet B, et al. J Biol Chem 1983;258:7691

189. Herkt F, Parente JP, Leroy Y, et al. Eur J Biochem 1985;146:125

190. Catelani G, Marra M, Paquet F, et al. Carbohyd Res 1986;155:131

191. Marra A, Sinay P. Gazz Chim Ital 1987;117:563

192. Duffy FA, Marshall RD. Biochem Soc Transact 1985;13:1128

193. Issitt PD, Pavone BG, Shapiro M. Transfusion 1979;19:389

194. Avent N, Judson PA, Parsons SF, et al. Biochem J 1988;251:499

195. Mallinson G, Anstee DJ, Avent ND, et al. Transfusion 1990;30:222

196. von dem Borne AEGKr, Bos MJE, Lomas C, et al. Br J Haematol 1990;75:254

197. Le Pennec PY, Klein MT, Le Besnerais M, et al. Rev Fr Transf Immunohematol 1988;31:123

198. Le Pennec PY, Rouger P, Klein MT, et al. (abstract). Book of Abstracts. Joint Cong ISBT/AABB 1990:29

199. Daniels GL, Simard H, Goldman M, et al. (abstract). Transfusion 1994;34 (Suppl 10S):26S

200. Spring FA, Holmes CH, Simpson KL, et al. Eur J Immunol 1997;27:891

201. Miyauchi T, Kanekura T, Yamaoka A, et al. J Biochem (Tokyo) 1990;107:316

202. Biswas C, Zhang Y, DeCastro R, et al. Cancer Res 1995;55:434

203. Kasinrerk W, Fiebiger E, Stefanova I, et al. J Immunol 1992;149:847

204. Fossum S, Mallett S, Barclay AN. Eur J Immunol 1991;21:671

205. Paterson DJ, Jefferies WA, Green JR, et al. Mol Immunol 1987;24:1281

206. Nehme CL, Cesario MM, Myles DG, et al. J Cell Biol 1993;120:687

207. Seulberger H, Unger CM, Risau W. Neurosci Lett 1992;140:93

208. Seulberger H, Lottspeich F, Risau W. EMBO J 1990;9:2151

209. Schuster VL, Lu R, Kanai N, et al. Biochim Biophys Acta 1996;1311:13

210. Altruda F, Cervella P, Gaeta ML, et al. Gene 1989;85:445

211. Igakura T, Kadomatsu K, Taguchi O, et al. Biochem Biophys Res Comm 1996;224:33

212. Kataoka H, DeCastro R, Zucker S, et al. Cancer Res 1993;53:3154

213. Biswas C. Cancer Lett 1984;24:201

214. Roberts WL, Myher JJ, Kuksis A, et al. J Biol Chem 1988;263:18766

215. Schlossman SF, Boumsell L, Gilks W, et al. Blood 1994;83:879

216. Dohi T, Yuyama Y, Natori Y, et al. Int J Cancer 1996;67:626

217. Smith PL, Lowe JB. J Biol Chem 1994;269:15162

32 | Well Characterized Independent Antigens of Low Incidence

The 700 series in the ISBT terminology contains antigens of low incidence that have not been shown to belong to any blood group system or collection. In its 1995 publication (1) the ISBT Working Party on Terminology for Red Cell Surface Antigens listed 37 members of the 700 series. At its 1996 meeting (2) the Working Party transferred three of those antigens, Wd^a, Rb^a and WARR to the Diego blood group system (see Chapter 17). Since the official transfer of Wd^a, Rb^a and WARR has occurred, those antigens are not listed in table 32-1, the 700 series. At the 1996 meeting of the AABB, data were presented that will likely result in the transfer of a number of other antigens to the Diego system. First, Coghlan et al. (3) reported that the anion exchanger gene 1 (*AE1*) controls the expression of the low incidence antigens ELO and Wu. The *AE1* and *Di* locus are, of course, the same thing (4,5). Second, Jarolim et al. (6) reported that the antigens ELO, Vg^a, Wu, Bp^a, Mo^a and probably Hg^a, each represent an amino acid change at different positions on protein band 3, the *AE1* gene product. Third, in different reports Jarolim et al. (144,147) present evidence that Tr^a also represents an amino acid change on band 2. Fourth, at the 1997 AABB meeting, data were presented showing that Sw^a (145), NFLD (146) and Jn^a (150) also represent amino acid substitutions on "wild type" protein band 3. Earlier, Coghlan et al. (7) had presented evidence supporting the assignment of the *Sw* and *Fr* genes to chromosome 17q (*Fr* had previously been thought (8) perhaps to be on chromosome 13p). Given the known serological association (9) between the antigens Sw^a, SW1 and Fr^a, it seems possible that all three will eventually be shown to be part of the Diego system. Somewhat similarly, since the antigens Wu (previously known also as Hov and Haakestad) and NFLD are part of the Diego system, the serologically related (10) antigen BOW, may belong to the system as well. Because the antigens ELO, Wu, Vg^a, Bp^a, Mo^a, Hg^a, Tr^a, Sw^a, SW1, Fr^a, NFLD, Jn^a and BOW have not yet officially graduated the 700 series (the next meeting of the ISBT Working Party will be in Oslo in 1998) they are all listed in table 32-1. However, in anticipation of the happy events that some, most or all of them will eventually be called up to the majors (the Diego system) they are all described in the text of Chapter 17. With that lengthy preamble, that seems to say more about the Diego system than about the 700 series, the first three tables for this chapter can be introduced. Table 32-1 lists the current (November 1996) members of the 700 series. Table 32-2 lists former members for which the numbers are now obsolete and indicates where and why the antigen left. Table 32-3 lists low

incidence antigens that have not been given ISBT numbers but that we consider qualify for inclusion here, given the title of the chapter. With the exceptions noted above and in table 32-1, the antigens in tables 32-1 and 32-3 will now be described.

The Antigen By

Simmons et al. (11) found the first example of anti-By when it caused mild HDN. Cleghorn (75) tested the red cells of 31,522 English donors and found two By+ samples. Using those red cells to screen sera, Cleghorn (75) found six more examples of anti-By five of which were in the sera of patients with antibody-induced hemolytic anemia. Each serum containing anti-By also contained anti-Wr^a, several contained anti-Sw^a and some also contained antibodies to other low incidence antigens. Other examples of anti-By have been found, one (16) in a deliberate search using papain-treated By+ red cells to screen 7987 normal sera, and another (76) in a pregnant woman. Other than the two By+ samples found by Cleghorn (75) no other has been found by screening random individuals, the tests involved samples from 500 Whites and 24 Aborigines in Australia (11); 200 Copper Eskimos (77); 157 Blacks (78) and 78 Bostonians (79).

The Antigen Chr^a

This antigen was found on the red cells of one of 500 Danes (12). The first example of anti-Chr^a appeared to be non-red cell stimulated, a second example of the specificity was found (80) ten years after the first had been reported.

The Antigen Bi

Wadlington et al. (14) found anti-Bi in the serum of a pregnant woman. No Bi+ sample was found in tests on the red cells of 1610 random donors who were US Whites, Blacks and Indians. The anti-Bi caused mild HDN (14).

The Antigen Bx^a

This antigen was first detected in 1961, by the

TABLE 32-1 Current Members of the
ISBT 700 Series of Antigens

Historical Name	Symbol	ISBT Number	References	Observations
Batty	By	700002	11	
Christiansen	Chr^a	700003	12	
Swann	Sw^a	700004	13	Described in Chapter 17
Biles	Bi	700005	14	
Box	Bx^a	700006	15	
Traversu	Tr^a	700008	16	Described in Chapter 17
Bishop	Bp^a	700010	16	Described in Chapter 17, will become DI10
Wulfsberg	Wu	700013	17	Described in Chapter 17, will become DI9
Nunhart	Jn^a	700014	18	Described in Chapter 17
Radin	Rd or Rd^a	700015	19	May be in Scianna system (44-46), see Chapter 26
Torkildsen	To^a	700017	20	
Peters	Pt^a	700018	21	
Reid	Re^a	700019	22	
Jensen	Je^a	700021	23	
Moen	Mo^a	700022	24	Described in Chapter 17, will become DI11
Froese	Fr^a	700026	25	Described in Chapter 17
Livesey	Li^a	700028	26	Possibly part of the Lutheran System (26)
Van Vught	Vg^a	700029	27	Described in Chapter 17, will become DI13
Hughes	Hg^a	700034	28	Described in Chapter 17, will become DI12
Newfoundland	NFLD	700037	29	Described in Chapter 17
Milne		700039	30	
Rasmussen	RASM	700040	31	
	SW1	700041	9	Described in Chapter 17
Oldeide	Ol^a	700043	32	Mentioned in Chapter 12
	JFV	700044	33	
Katagiri	Kg	700045	34	
Bowyer	BOW	700046	35	Described in Chapter 17
Jones	Jones	700047	36	
	HJK	700049	37	
	HOFM	700050	38	Mentioned in Chapter 12
	ELO	700051	39, 40	Described in Chapter 17, will become DI8
Sarah	SARA	700052	41	
	LOCR	700053	42	Mentioned in Chapter 12
	REIT	700054	43	

Some of the antigens listed in this table have now been assigned Diego system numbers (149). In sequence from the table: Bp^a is DI10; Wu is DI9; Mo^a is DI11; Vg^a is DI13; Hg^a is DI12; and ELO is DI8.

TABLE 32-2 Former Members of the ISBT 700 Series of Antigens

Historical Name	Previous Symbol	Former ISBT Number	Current Designaton and Location
Wright	Wr^a	700001	Now Di3, Diego system, Chapter 17
	Ls^a	700007	Now Ge6, Gerbich system, Chapter 16
Webb	Wb	700009	Now Ge5, Gerbich system, Chapter 16
Orris	Or	700011	Now MNS31, MN system, Chapter 15
Griffiths	Gf	700012	Obsolete*
Heibel		700016	Obsolete*
Ahonen	An^a	700020	Now Ge7, Gerbich system, Chapter 16
Hey		700023	Obsolete*
Roselund	Rl^a	700024	Same as 700007, see above
Indian	In^a	700025	Now In1, Indian system, Chapter 29
Redelberger	Rb^a	700027	Now Di6, Diego system, Chapter 17
Waldner	Wd^a	700030	Now Di5, Diego system, Chapter 17
Duch	Dh^a	700031	Now Ge8, Gerbich system, Chapter 16
Pollio	POLL	700032	Obsolete*
	Os^a	700033	Now MNS38, MN system, Chapter 15
	Tc^b	700035	Now Cr3, Cromer system, Chapter 24
	Tc^c	700036	Now Cr4, Cromer system, Chapter 24
	Hov	700038	Same as 70013, see table 32-1
	WES^a	700042	Now Cr8, Cromer system, Chapter 24
	FPTT	700048	Now Rh50, Rh system, Chapter 12
Warrior	WARR	700055	Now Di7, Diego system, Chapter 17

* An antigen and its number are declared obsolete when no antibody remains to type red cells and no antigen-positive (for low incidence antigens) red cells remain to identify new examples of the antibody.

alloimmune anti-Bx^a in the serum of a patient with autoimmune hemolytic anemia (15). Tests on the red cells of 7445 English donors revealed (15,16) one addi-

TABLE 32-3 Aditional Low Incidence Antigens Described in This Chapter (some are also listed in table 32-2)

Historical Name	Current Symbol	References
Donna, Bennett, Goodspeed, Ho, Ot, Stobo	Bg^a, Bg^b, Bg^c	47-51
Griffiths	Gf	130
Heibel		131
Hey		132
Pollio	Poll	133
Jobbins		65
Becker		66
Ven		67
Romunde	Rm	68
Good		69
Skjelbred	Sk^a, Sk	20
Hunt	Ht^a	70
	Zd	71
	Pe	72
Tsunoi	Ts	73

tional Bx(a+) sample but tests on 8215 sera (6711 from blood donors, 1388 from pregnant women and 116 from hospital patients) did not identify another example of anti-Bx^a (81). Additional information was provided by Contreras et al. (82) in 1980. The original and a new family with members who had Bx(a+) red cells were investigated and independent segregation of *Bx^a* from the genes of several blood group systems was demonstrated. One additional example of anti-Bx^a was found (81,82) in tests on sera from 23,081 normal donors. The three examples of anti-Bx^a studied, (see below for the third example in a serum containing multiple antibodies) all seemed to be non-red cell stimulated, no anti-Bx^a was found in the sera of three women of the Bx(a-) phenotype who had given birth to infants with Bx(a+) red cells. Blood samples from 17,661 random North London blood donors were tested with a serum that contains antibodies to, at least: Wr^a, Sw^a, M^g, Bp^a, Or, Rb^a, Ri^a, Mi^a, Tr^a, Gf, Rh37, Go^a, Bg^a, Bg^b and Bx^a. Single examples were found of donors with Bx(a+), or Sw(a+), or Rh:37 red cells, while two others had Go(a+) cells.

The Antigen Rd (a.k.a. Rd^a)

In 1967, Rausen et al. (19) described the first five

examples of anti-Rd, each in a different family and each causing rather mild HDN. In two of the five families there was Ashkenazi Jewish ancestry, in the others the US Black and US Indian populations were represented. In tests on 7335 random blood samples, three were found to be Rd+. All three were among 559 White, New York Jews included in the 7335 random donors. None of 2443 random sera tested contained anti-Rd.

In 1968, Lundsgaard and Jensen (83) described another two examples of the antibody but used the name anti-Rd[a]. In tests using the two anti-Rd[a], 24 individuals with Rd(a+) red cells were found among 4933 Danes. Thus the incidence of Rd[a] in Denmark was very different from in the USA (19), i.e. 1 in 206 compared to 1 in 2445, respectively. In the Danish study only one of the 24 persons with Rd(a+) red cells was Jewish. Also in the Danish study (83) two additional examples of anti-Rd[a] were found in tests on approximately 30,000 sera from normal donors. In 1976, Winn et al. (84) reported the presence of an IgG anti-Rd in the serum of a man who had been transfused with one unit of Rd+ blood.

As mentioned in table 31-1, there are data (44-46,85,86) that suggest that Rd might be a part of the Scianna blood group system. Those findings are discussed in Chapter 26.

The Antigen To[a]

The first example of the antibody defining this antigen was found, by Kornstad et al. (20), in a serum that also contained antibodies to Wr[a], St[a] and Jn[a]. In screening tests with To(a+) red cells, 135 reactive sera were found among 5704 Norwegian donors. At least 66 of those sera contained anti-To[a], sometimes with and sometimes without other antibodies. The presence of anti-To[a] in at least 1 in 86 sera contrasted sharply with the fact that only one To(a+) sample was found among 6461 Norwegian bloods tested.

Gralnick et al. (87) found a donor with To(a+) red cells, by chance, when investigating an unexpected positive reaction in a compatibility test. The donor with To(a+) red cells had one daughter with To(a+) and one with To(a-) red cells. No other To(a+) sample was found in tests on 1092 random donors but like Kornstad et al. (20) Gralnick et al. (87) found anti-To[a] to be common; it was found in 284 of 2365 sera tested, i.e. 1 in 8. Examples of anti-To[a] ranged from cold-reactive, complement-binding, IgM forms to IgG antibodies reactive only in IATs.

A third family that included persons with To(a+) red cells was described by Crossland et al. (88). The anti-To[a] used in the study also contained antibodies to Wr[a], Mo[a] and Middel.

The Antigen Pt[a]

When Pinder et al. (21) first reported the Pt[a] antigen they described the presence of anti-Pt[a] in 14 sera. Six were found in screening tests on the sera of 460 pregnant women, each of the six sera also contained antibodies to other low incidence antigens. Six more anti-Pt[a] were found in sera known to contain anti-Wr[a] and two in sera known to contain anti-Vw. The original family studied included nine persons, spanning three generations, with Pt(a+) red cells. No other Pt(a+) sample was found among 14,500 New Zealand blood donors, most of whom were White and of European extraction but some of whom had Polynesian ancestry. Similarly, no Pt(a+) sample was found in tests on red cells from 21,825 Norwegians and 126 persons of Mongolian extraction (21,32).

A second family in which Pt[a] was present was investigated by Contreras et al. (89) after they found one Pt(a+) sample in tests on the red cells of 10,200 donors in England. This time ten family members, spanning four generations, were shown to have Pt(a+) red cells. No Pt(a+) sample was found in tests on the red cells of 313 non-White immigrants in England. A third unrelated proband with Pt(a+) red cells was reported by Young and Smith (90).

The Pt[a] antigen survives treatment of red cells with trypsin or neuraminidase but is denatured when red cells are treated with chymotrypsin, papain or pronase (100). Immunoblotting studies using anti-Pt[a] showed that the antigen is carried on a glycoprotein with a molecular weight of about 31.6 kD. Herron et al. (100) gave reasons for supposing that the Pt[a]-bearing structure is one that had not previously been described on red cells.

The Antigen Re[a]

In 1971, Guévin et al. (22) described anti-Re[a] that caused a positive DAT on the red cells of the infant born to the proposita, but did not cause clinical HDN. No Re(a+) sample was found in tests on the red cells of 10,000 Canadian donors, almost all of whom were White. In 1985, Rowe and Bowell (91) described two families in whom Re[a] was present. In the first, four persons spanning four generations were found to have Re(a+) red cells. In the second, seven persons, in three generations, had Re(a+) red cells. No Re(a+) sample was found in tests on the red cells of 4770 donors in Wales, one (the proposita in the second family studied) was found in tests on the red cells of 6635 donors in England. No other example of anti-Re[a] was found when papain-treated Re(a+) red cells were used to screen the sera of 2358 random donors in Wales, likewise no anti-Re[a] was detected in 132 sera containing antibodies to other low frequency antigens. Like the first example of anti-Re^a (22), the second (91) caused a positive DAT but no clinical HDN in the infant with Re(a+) red cells born to the mother with anti-Re^a in her serum. For use of the term Hol in the family with members with Re(a+) red cells (91) see the section below, on the antigen Jones.

The Antigen Je^a

Skov (23) discovered anti-Je^a in the serum of a once pregnant, once transfused woman when Je(a+) red cells were unknowingly used in antibody screening tests. The anti-Je^a was primarily IgM in nature. The Je^a antigen was found on the red cells of four members, spanning three generations, of the original family, but not on the cells of any of 1038 random Danes. The Je(a+) red cells had been used in antibody screening tests for some time and it was calculated that over 100,000 sera had been tested before the first example of anti-Je^a was found.

The Antigen Li^a

The antibody defining Li^a was described in 1980 (26) when three examples were reported. The antibodies were found in a three year period when each reacted with a cell sample used in antibody screening tests. Apparently anti-Li^a is a rare antibody since the red cells then recognized as being Li(a+) had been used in antibody identification studies for 20 years before the anti-Li^a were found. In the family of the proposita with Li(a+) red cells there is a hint that the antigen might be part of the Lutheran system. No other Li(a+) sample was found in tests on the red cells of 4046 random English donors. Later in 1980 an example of anti-Li^a was found (92) in the USA when it caused mild HDN. The second family in which the Li^a antigen was found originated in England.

Daniels (93) undertook immunoblotting studies with Li(a+) red cells to determine whether Li^a is carried on the Lutheran glycoproteins but no bands were seen.

The Antigen Milne

In 1984, Pinder et al. (30) described the antigen Milne. In the family in which the antigen was found four persons, spanning three generations, had Milne+ red cells. Part of the family resides in New Zealand, the other part resides in Scotland. In tests on samples from 2643 random White and Polynesian donors in New Zealand, no other Milne+ blood was found. No anti-Milne was present in the sera of two women of the Milne- phenotype who had borne children with Milne+ red cells.

However, anti-Milne was found in 58 of 1242 sera from mainly prenatal and fewer hospital patients and in several sera that contained antibodies to other low incidence antigens. All examples of anti-Milne tested were IgM, as determined by reduction cleavage by DTT. The majority of anti-Milne activated complement and hemolyzed protease-treated (enzyme used not specified in the report) Milne+ red cells.

The Antigen RASM

The antigen RASM was found, by Brown et al. (31) in four members, spanning three generations, of a White Canadian family of European extraction. The RASM antigen was still detectable on red cells treated with trypsin, papain or ficin but it was denatured when red cells were treated with AET or DTT. No association between RASM and the Kell system could be established (94). No other RASM+ sample was found in tests on 9541 (primarily White) Canadian and US donors. The anti-RASM was IgG in nature, it did not bind complement. The antibody caused a positive DAT but not clinical HDN in an infant with RASM+ red cells born to the woman who made anti-RASM. No other example of anti-RASM was found in tests of the sera of 543 random blood donors.

The Antigen Ol^a

The antibody that defines the Ol^a antigen was found by Kornstad (32), in the serum Kirk, that also contains, at least, antibodies to the low incidence antigens Jn^a, Bp^a, Pt^a, Rl^a (Ls^a), Wd^a, Wr^a, Wu, Rb^a, Tr^a, Vg^a, BOW, Jones (Holmes) and Donaldson. Anti-Ol^a was recognized when the Kirk serum reacted with a red cell sample that lacked all the antigens just listed. Anti-Ol^a could be separated from all the other antibodies in the Kirk serum by adsorption on to and elution from, the proposita's red cells. A study of the proposita's family revealed 10 other persons, spanning three generations, with Ol(a+) red cells. No other Ol(a+) sample was found in tests on the red cells of 7150 Norwegian blood donors. Anti-Ol^a was found in two other sera that contain multiple antibodies to low incidence antigens, one of them, serum Blo, contains antibodies to, at least, Bp^a, Gf, Jn^a, Mo^a, Or, Pt^a, Ri^a, Sw^a, Tr^a, Vg^a, Vw, Wr^a, BOW and Skjelbred. The two most potent anti-Ol^a (in the sera Kirk and Blo) reacted as saline active agglutinins at 18°C. Their reactions were enhanced in the presence of albumin, they were negative or only weakly reactive at 37°C and were nonreactive by IAT. The third serum, He, also reacted well in methods using albumin. Three additional examples of anti-Ol^a were found that reacted only with papain-treated Ol(a+) red cells.

Anti-Ol^a has been mentioned in Chapter 12 because in the family studied (32) the Ol(a+) red cells had depressed expression of some of their Rh antigens. When Ol(a+) and Ol(a-) red cells from family members with matched Rh phenotypes were compared, it was seen that depression of expression of C and E was marked, while expression of D was depressed but to a lesser degree. No consistent depression of c or e on the Ol(a+) red cells was observed but it was noted that different examples of antibodies to C, E and D varied in their ability to illustrate antigen depression. Thus it is possible that anti-c and anti-e that would have demonstrated depression of antigen expression, were not available. In spite of this intriguing phenotypic association between Ol^a and some Rh antigens, the family studied (32) showed that *Ol^a* is not at the *CDE* locus.

The Antigen JFV

In 1988, Kluge et al. (33) described two examples of a new antibody to a low incidence antigen. The antibodies were named anti-JFV, one of them had been reported briefly earlier (95) as anti-Jf and as anti-Jennifer. The JFV antigen was found on the red cells of seven persons in a three generation family of Dutch origin living in Canada and on those of another seven persons in a three generation German family. In the German family the first born child of the mother with anti-JFV in the serum suffered mild HDN (maximum bilirubin 10.8 mg/dl) and was treated with phototherapy and a transfusion of 50 ml of blood. In the Dutch family in Canada, the seventh born child of the mother with anti-JFV in the serum had a positive DAT at birth but did not have clinical HDN. Of the six previous pregnancies of the woman with anti-JFV, three had resulted in children with JFV+ and two, children with JFV- red cells, the sixth pregnancy resulted in a miscarriage. No other JFV+ sample was found in tests on the red cells of 1014 people in Germany, 200 in Canada and 60 Black North London donors. The JFV antigen survived treatment of red cells with papain, neuraminidase, AET and ZZAP (DTT plus papain) (96). One of the anti-JFV gave enhanced reactions in tests using papain-treated JFV+ red cells.

Both examples of anti-JFV were IgG in nature and reacted in IATs. As mentioned, the Dutch proposita in Canada had been pregnant seven times, the German proposita had never been transfused. The anti-JFV was present in her first pregnancy. No other antibodies to low incidence antigens were detected in the two sera that contained anti-JFV. Further, none of 256 sera containing multiple antibodies to low incidence antigens nor any of 534 sera from random donors was found to contain anti-JFV.

The Antigen Kg

This antigen was recognized by Ichikawa et al. (34) when the third child of a Japanese woman suffered HDN severe enough that an exchange transfusion was performed. The causative antibody was named anti-Kg and the red cells of the woman's husband and two previous children were shown to be Kg+, other relatives of the antibody-maker and her husband refused to provide samples for testing. No other Kg+ sample was found in tests on the red cells of more than 600 random Japanese donors. Treatment of Kg+ red cells with trypsin, papain and bromelin neither abolished nor enhanced their reaction with anti-Kg.

In tests to exclude identity of Kg with any other low incidence antigen and in a search for an antithetical partner to Kg a promising lead developed but could not be followed to completion. The red cells of a Mrs. J., a Mexican woman whose blood was studied in the Philip Levine Laboratories in Raritan, N.J., in 1979, were found to react with anti-Kg. Mrs. J. had produced an antibody to a high incidence antigen. Her antibody had reacted with all red cells tested except her own, no specificity had been assigned to the antibody. Unfortunately, proof that Mrs. J.'s antibody was detecting the high incidence antithetical partner to Kg was not forthcoming because of lack of suitable quantities of the relevant red cells and serum and current unavailability of additional samples from Mrs. J. and her family.

The anti-Kg that caused the HDN was an IgG antibody with a titer of 256 against the red cells of the antibody-maker's husband. The antibody did not bind complement.

The Antigen Jones

In 1989, Reid et al. (36) reported that two previously unpublished antigens of low incidence, Jones and Hol are the same thing, both were listed in table 20-1 of the third edition of this book (97) and both had been mentioned in numerous papers (for references see 97) when other low incidence antigens were shown not to be the same as Jones or Hol. The Jones antigen was first detected in 1974 when the red cells of the second infant born to the maker of anti-Jones were seen to have a positive DAT. The child did not have clinical HDN, its elder sib was shown to have red cells that reacted with the maternal antibody. In 1984, the antibody-maker's third child was found to have moderate HDN. The cord red blood cells had a strongly positive DAT, the hemoglobin at birth was 9 g/dl and although no exchange transfusion was necessary (phototherapy was used) the infant was transfused on the fourth day of life.

In 1982, the Hol antigen was recognized in similar circumstances. The antibody-maker had borne three children. The first had a strongly positive DAT at birth but no clinical HDN. The second and third infants both required exchange transfusion. When the antibodies in the Jones and Hol cases were shown to be the same, the name Jones, which had priority over Hol, was chosen for the antigen, the antibody thus became anti-Jones.

In the Hol family, 11 persons spanning four generations were found to have Jones+ red cells. In tests on samples from 6635 random donors in England, 8111 in Wales and over 2000 in California, only one Jones+ blood was found. The Jones antigen is clearly well developed at birth, see above, it is not denatured when red cells are treated with trypsin, chymotrypsin, papain, ficin, pronase or AET. The reactions of anti-Jones were enhanced in tests against papain or ficin-treated red cells, similar enhancement was not seen in tests against red cells treated with trypsin, chymotrypsin or pronase.

In both cases described above, anti-Jones was an IgG antibody reactive by IAT in saline, LISS and albumin systems. No further example of anti-Jones was found in tests on samples from over 2000 donors in California. Thirty-four sera containing multiple antibodies to low incidence antigens were tested, anti-Jones was found in only one, the Kirk serum that is described above in the section on the Ol^a antigen.

In a concluding comment in the paper the authors (36) point out that there is no evidence of recombination between *Jones* and *Rh* in the large Hol family. They further comment that there are some similarities between the Jones antigen and those of the Rh system and between anti-Jones and Rh system antibodies. We are not aware of any further evidence to associate Jones with Rh.

In a publication (91) on the Re^a antigen (see above) the anti-Re^a was said to be present in a serum Hol, and some members of the Hol family had Re(a+) red cells. In the paper on the Jones antigen (36) the Jones+ red cells are described as being present in members of the Hol family. The clinical situations with anti-Re^a and anti-Jones are similar (i.e. newborns with positive DAT but no clinical HDN) and the dates of the reports are such that the Hol family infants with Re(a+) or Jones+ red cells could have been born to the same mother. However, Re^a (700019) and Jones (700047) are not the same. Carole Green (148) has kindly sorted out our confusion by telling us that the anti-Re^a (Hol) serum is Hollister and the Jones+ (Hol) red cells are in members of the Holmes family. Workers who advocate the use of numbers for antigens will be excused for saying, "I told you so!"

The Antigen HJK

The only published report about anti-HJK (37) appeared in an obstetrics journal and was primarily concerned with the severe HDN caused by the antibody. However, the paper identifies three highly competent immunohematology reference laboratories in which work on the antibody was performed. Since the HJK antigen was not shown to have identity with any other low incidence antigen it was assigned an ISBT number in the 700 series (see table 32-1).

The woman who produced anti-HJK was 26 years old, her ethnic background and transfusion history are not mentioned in the paper. Her first pregnancy ended in a spontaneous abortion of a grossly normal fetus at 18 weeks. Her second pregnancy resulted in the delivery of a healthy infant in whom the DAT on the cord blood red cells was positive but for whom phototherapy was not required. At 27 weeks gestation in her third pregnancy a hydropic placenta and a grossly hydropic fetus were observed. A fetal blood sample obtained by funipuncture showed a hematocrit of 6%. The fetus was given intravascular transfusions at 27, 31 and 34 weeks. The infant was delivered at 35.5 weeks and did not require transfusion or phototherapy. On the 7th day of life a Kleihauer-Betke test suggested that about 88% of the infant's red cells were of donor (intrauterine transfusion) origin.

In a family study it was shown that the antibody-maker's husband, his mother, one of his two sibs and both of the couples' children had HJK+ red cells. Although as mentioned in a discussion at the end of this chapter, many antibodies to low incidence antigens cause positive DATs in newborns, relatively few of them cause severe HDN. Clearly in this case the antibody was one of the relatively few.

The Antigen HOFM

In 1990, Hoffman et al. (38) published a report describing a new antibody, anti-HOFM, to a low incidence antigen. The antibody was made by a woman of Dutch ancestry (Mrs. Hofman, the antibody is named for the proposita, not the senior author!) and caused HDN in her second child. The infant had a peak bilirubin of 14.7 mg/dl on the third day of life but responded to phototherapy and did not have to be transfused. In the family study six persons, spanning three generations, were found to have HOFM+ red cells (the six included the proposita's husband and both of their children). In tests on samples from 926 random Dutch blood donors, no further HOFM+ blood was found. The HOFM antigen survived treatment of red cells by papain, bromelin, AET and DTT. The titer of the anti-HOFM was: 16 by saline and albumin IAT; 8 by manual polybrene test; 32 against papain and bromelin treated red cells; and 64 by PEG IAT. The antibody was primarily IgG3 in composition, did not bind complement but was consistently weakened when the serum was treated with 2-ME or DTT. Tests on 66 sera containing antibodies to other antigens did not detect another example of anti-HOFM.

As discussed in Chapter 12, those members of the family who had HOFM+ red cells had depression of expression of C on their red cells as compared to C+ HOFM- red cells from members of the same family. No depression of expression of other Rh antigens was seen. The depression of C was demonstrated in three independent laboratories using many different anti-C.

The Antigen SARA

The antigen SARAH (abbreviated to SARA by the ISBT Working Party based on the four letter rule) was described in print by Stern et al. (41) in 1994. The antigen was found on the red cells of a regular donor who is homozygous for *K* and whose red cells are regularly used in antibody identification panels. Initially, two sera were found to react with the SARA+ red cells but not with any others. In a family study, four persons, covering two generations were shown to have SARA+ red cells. No studies were performed to determine the incidence of the SARA antigen in random donors. The SARA antigen was shown to survive treatment of red cells with papain and AET. SDS-PAGE and immunoblotting studies were uninformative as to location of the SARA antigen. Similarly, studies using DNA extracted from the white cells of the family members who had SARA+ red cells showed no association with the RFLP used.

In addition to the two anti-SARA originally studied, the authors (41) mention that they have been sent five other sera and have been informed of two more, that react with the SARA+ red cells. The Wilcox serum that contains antibodies to, at least, the antigens By, Sw^a, Tr^a, Bp^a, Wu, Jn^a, Pt^a, Rb^a, Vg^a, Hg^a, NFLD, BOW, SHIN, Vr, Mt^a, St^a, Ri^a, Dantu, Wr^a and five unpublished antigens, was also shown to react with SARA+ red cells. In tests on samples from 3150 Australian blood donors, one additional example of anti-SARA was found.

The Antigen LOCR

In 1994, Coghlan et al. (42) described two examples of an antibody, that they named anti-LOCR, that defines an antigen of low incidence. Both antibodies were made by wives of White propositi who had LOCR+ red cells and both caused mild HDN in the infants with LOCR+

red cells born to the women. A third and unrelated individual with the LOCR antigen was found when her red cells were studied because they carried an atypical c antigen. In order to determine the incidence of the LOCR antigen in the general population, red cells from 1826 pregnant women in Manitoba were typed. Of those women 1166 had D+ and 660 D- red cells. One sample was found to be LOCR+, the red cells of the woman involved were D- C- E+ c+ e+^{w}. In tests on the families of three of the four probands with LOCR+ red cells, 12 additional persons with the antigen on their red cells were found.

The LOCR antigen is apparently developed at birth since the first two examples of anti-LOCR caused HDN. The antigen was shown to survive the treatment of red cells with trypsin, papain, ficin or AET. Indeed, the reactions of anti-LOCR were enhanced in tests against protease-treated red cells. Fifty-one sera containing multiple antibodies to low incidence antigens were tested against LOCR+ red cells, none of them contained anti-LOCR.

As discussed in Chapter 12, a phenotypic association between LOCR and Rh was demonstrated. In the first two families studied and in the third proband, presence of the LOCR antigen is associated with a weakened expression of c. Indeed, the C- c+, LOCR+ red cells reacted similarly, in terms of expression of c, to C+ c+, LOCR- red cells. In the fourth family no alteration of c was seen but the proposita's red cells had a reduced expression of e. The weakening of e was not seen in the proposita's daughter who inherited the maternal *LOCR* gene. However, the proposita's red cells are E+ e+, LOCR+ while those of her daughter are E- e+, LOCR+. Perhaps the weakening of e can only be seen in a *Ee* heterozygote. In all three families studied, *LOCR* was transmitted with *r*.

The Antigen REIT

This low incidence antigen was assigned an ISBT number at the 1995 meeting of the ISBT Working Party (1). However, as of November 1996, nothing seems to have been published about the antigen. The 1995 report cites unpublished observations of Hamilton and Coghlan (43) and in a table states that the antigen has been excluded from the ABO, MN, Rh, Duffy, Xg and Xk systems. Daniels (98) also cited unpublished observations from Hamilton and Coghlan in reporting that anti-REIT caused severe HDN in an infant who had to be treated by exchange transfusion and that no REIT+ sample was found in tests on the red cells of 4086 random Canadian donors. If additional details about this antigen and its antibody become available, they will be included in Chapter 46, the addendum of this book.

The Antigen SHIN

This antigen does not yet have an ISBT number. However, a description of the antigen belongs here and not with those antigens described later in the chapter that may be extinct, since SHIN+ red cells and anti-SHIN are available. In the publication describing the SHIN antigen (74) it is stated that SHIN has been differentiated from all low incidence antigens except Rh35, Rh43, Kn[b] and Er[b]. Since the SHIN antigen is protease sensitive (see below) it appears not to be the same as any of those antigens.

The SHIN antigen was detected when the red cells of a donor reacted with the serum of a 55 year-old, never transfused Japanese male patient. In an investigation of the donor's family, ten persons covering two generations, were found to have SHIN+ red cells. In a survey of random donors in Tokyo, one with SHIN+ red cells was found among 3000 tested. The SHIN antigen was denatured when red cells were treated with trypsin, chymotrypsin, papain, ficin or bromelin; it was not altered when red cells were treated with AET.

The original anti-SHIN agglutinated red cells in a saline system in tests at room temperature and below. Its reactions were enhanced in tests to which bovine albumin was added. The antibody did not react by IATs in which anti-IgG and polyspecific AHG were used. As judged by reduction cleavage tests using 2-ME or DTT, the antibody was wholly IgM in nature. In tests on samples from 19,380 Tokyo blood donors and 800 pregnant women, no anti-SHIN was found. One example was detected when samples from 1662 hospital patients were screened. Like the first example, the other anti-SHIN behaved as a cold-reactive agglutinin. In tests on sera containing multiple antibodies to low incidence antigens, anti-SHIN was found in 11 of 104 in one reference laboratory and in 17 of 126 in another. Some of the sera were tested in both laboratories. No anti-SHIN was detected in the sera of two women from the original family, who had SHIN- red cells and had borne children with SHIN+ cells. Nothing is known about the clinical significance of anti-SHIN. Given the fact that the first two examples found were cold-reactive agglutinins, those examples at least would be expected to be clinically benign.

The original anti-SHIN contained anti-Rb[a], the original SHIN+ red cells were Rb(a-) and the anti-SHIN and anti-Rb[a] in the serum were separated by differential adsorption. The SHIN+ red cells of the first propositus were Di(a+). The anti-SHIN did not contain anti-Di[a]. This fact is discussed again in the next section.

Low Incidence Antigens and the Diego Blood Group System

As described in Chapter 17, the Diego blood group system already includes the low incidence antigens Di[a], Wr[a], Wd[a], Rb[a] and WARR. Further, there are data (3) that show that production of the low incidence antigens ELO and Wu is controlled by *AE1* (*Anion Exchanger 1*, the gene encoding production of protein band 3 on which the Diego system antigens are carried). The antigens ELO, Vg[a], Wu, Bp[a], Mo[a], Tr[a], Sw[a], NFLD, Jn[a] and probably Hg[a], represent amino acid changes on band 3 (6,144-147,150) so presumably also belong in the Diego system. There are serological findings (10) that show that Wu and NFLD (both Diego system antigens, see above), and BOW have some sort of association, at least at the phenotypic level. A similar relationship (9) seems to associate the antigens Sw[a], SW1 and Fr[a] with each other. The *Sw* locus is in tight linkage with the *D17S4* RFLP of chromosome 17 and no segregation between *Fr[a]* and *AE1* was seen (7,8). Thus it is perhaps more than coincidence that the first individuals found to have the low incidence antigens Kg (34) and SHIN (74) on their red cells, were also of the Di(a+) phenotype. While both individuals were Japanese and were thus more likely than Whites to have Di(a+) red cells and while anti-Kg and anti-SHIN clearly did not have anti-Di[a] specificity, the findings suggest that it might be worthwhile to look for associations between Kg and/or SHIN and some of the other antigens listed above. Perhaps findings like those involving Wu, NFLD and BOW, or those involving Sw[a], SW1 and Fr[a] are waiting to be made.

It is, of course, no surprise to find that protein band 3 is a home for many established and presumed Diego system antigens of low incidence. The protein is large, with a molecular weight of some 100 kD, is believed to cross the red cell membrane some 14 times and to have at least five (and perhaps seven) extracellular loops. A change in an amino acid, from the native or wild type configuration of the protein, in an extracellular loop (or perhaps elsewhere in the protein) could thus create a "different" blood group antigen. If the amino acid change did not compromise the function of band 3, presence of the new antigen would not represent selective disadvantage (nor advantage) so would be propagated. As discussed in Chapter 17 in the section dealing with structure of the *AE1* gene, there seem to be some regions within the gene that are hypersensitive to mutation.

As mentioned many times in the preceding sections of this chapter, many sera have been found to contain multiple antibodies to low incidence antigens. In a lot of these cases, antibodies to several established or presumed Diego system antigens are present in one serum. However, these findings may not equate to the antigen associations known and speculated above, since many of the sera also contain antibodies to antigens outside the Diego system, that is antibodies to antigens in the Rh, MN and Gerbich systems.

In concluding this section on the Diego system and antigens of low incidence it must again be stressed that some data provide more solid evidence than others. Thus Di^a, Wr^a, Wd^a, Rb^a and WARR are firmly established as Diego system antigens of low incidence. Genetic and biochemical evidence appears, beyond any reasonable doubt, to establish that ELO, Wu, Bp^a, Mo^a, Hg^a, Vg^a, Tr^a, Sw^a, NFLD and Jn^a are low incidence antigens in the system, indeed the first six antigens on that list have been assigned Diego system numbers (149). Fr^a seems very likely to join the system based on the location of the encoding Fr^a gene (7). The evidence that associates SW1 and BOW with Diego is currently less conclusive, being based primarily on serological findings (9,10). The suggestion that Kg and SHIN are part of the system is speculative as of this date (November 1996). A large part of the fun of being a blood group serologist is, of course, to speculate about the explanation of initial tentative clues.

The Bg Antigens and the Antibodies That Define Them

Between 1959 and 1963 a number of red cell antigens, that seemed in some obscure way to be related to each other, were reported. These antigens: Ot (48); Ho (49); Bennett-Goodspeed-Sturgeon or Donna (50,51) (later more commonly known as DBG) and Stobo (47); were all of low incidence. Of 7583 cell samples tested for one or more of the antigens (47-51) 49 were found to be positive. Early work on these antigens was beset with problems and some of the serological findings were difficult to reproduce. In addition, inheritance of the antigens did not always appear to be straightforward and in at least eleven families (47,49,51) one of the antigens was found on the red cells of apparently legitimate children of parents both of whom had red cells that lacked the antigen involved.

In 1967 Seaman et al. (52) studied the reactions of many of these antibodies in tests in the AutoAnalyzer. The antigens defined were renamed Bg^a, Bg^b and Bg^c, and reactive sera were classified as often being mixtures of antibodies against two or more of the antigens. Table 32-4 reproduces the conclusions of Seaman et al. (52). In addition, these workers showed that the antigens were not as uncommon as had previously been supposed. Indeed, in AutoAnalyzer tests it was shown that between 30% and 40% of random red cell samples carry one or more of the antigens.

In 1969 another advance was made when Morton et al. (53) reported that Bg(a+) red cells came almost exclusively from donors with HLA-7 (now HLA-B7) on their leukocytes. Two years earlier, Rosenfield et al. (102) had reported that some antibodies against leukocytes react with red cells when the AutoAnalyzer is used. In 1971, Morton et al. (54) reported correlations between Bg^b and the leukocyte antigen W17 or Te57 (now HLA-B17) and between Bg^c and W28, Ba and Da15 (now HLA-A28). Since there was already evidence (103,104) that HLA antigens can be detected on reticulocytes, it was assumed that during red cell maturation not all the HLA antigens are always totally lost. Later Nordhagen (109) showed that Bg^c can also sometimes be demonstrated on the red cells of persons of the HLA-A2 phenotype, it is known that antibodies to HLA-A28 and HLA-A2 cross-react. The detection of HLA antigens other than those listed above, on red cells, is discussed later in this chapter.

The Bg antigens are carried on HLA class 1 products, that is products of the *HLA-A, HLA-B* and *HLA-C* genes of the major histocompatibility locus on chromosome six. Class 1 HLA products are heterodimers in which the alpha chain, that has three extracellular domains, is non-covalently linked to a beta$_2$-microglobulin. When it was found (110) that chloroquine-treatment of red cells removes their HLA antigens and that hemagglutinins to HLA can be inhibited by plasma from appropriate phenotype individuals (109,111,129) it was suggested (110) that HLA antigens on red cells may get

TABLE 32-4 To Show the Relationship of Stobo, Ot, Ho and DBG to Bg^a, Bg^b and Bg^c from Seaman et al. (52)

Original Name of Antibody	Reaction with Red Cells of the Phenotypes			New Name of Antibody
	Bg(a+)	Bg(b+)	Bg(c+)	
Anti-DBG	+	+ or 0	+ or 0	Anti-Bg^a, Anti-Bg^a+Bg^b, Anti-Bg^a+Bg^c or Anti-Bg^a+Bg^b+Bg^c
Anti-Ho	+	+	0	Anti-Bg^a+Bg^b
Anti-Ot	+	0	+	Anti-Bg^a+Bg^c
Anti-Stobo	+	+ or 0	0	Anti-Bg^a or Anti-Bg^a+Bg^b

there via adsorption from the plasma. However, it is now known (see above) that the HLA antigens on red cells are remaining molecules from those present in more profusion on erythroid precursor cells (103,112). Giles et al. (63) showed that chloroquine treatment of red cells removes the beta$_2$-microglobulin but not the alpha chain of HLA molecules. Since the HLA antigens are carried on the alpha chain it follows that the beta$_2$-microglobulin must function by orienting the alpha chain in such a way that antibody-complexing with antigens occurs. Botto et al. (113) showed that as red cells age in vivo their expression of class 1 HLA molecules decreases. This, of course, is the opposite to what would be expected if red cells adsorbed their HLA antigens from plasma. As expected from what has been described above, monoclonal antibodies directed against a common structure on HLA class 1 molecules, bind to red cells (114).

The Bg^a, Bg^b and Bg^c antigens survive treatment of red cells with trypsin, chymotrypsin, papain, ficin, pronase, AET and DTT (63,109). In patients with systemic lupus erythematosus red cell HLA antigens are expressed more strongly than on the red cells of healthy individuals (62), increases are seen, but are less dramatic in patients with rheumatoid arthritis, leukemia and some other hematological disorders (62,123). Morton et al. (124) noticed that in patients with HLA-B7 on the leukocytes, HLA levels of red cells were dramatically increased if the patients had infectious mononucleosis and that the elevated red cell levels sometimes persisted for years. Rivera and Scornick (114) showed that if RIA and flow cytometry are used, some 50% of normal individuals can be shown to have HLA on their red cells. Earlier, Salama et al. (125) had shown that red cell HLA can be detected more readily in a test using radio-labeled anti-IgG than in conventional IATs. It is not clear that findings such as these equate directly to the detection of Bg^a, Bg^b and Bg^c on red cells.

Anti-Bg are not uncommon. The frequency with which they are detected is highly dependent on the method used. In conventional blood bank tests, anti-Bg^a was detected in some 1.5% of sera from normal individuals (55,126) and in the sera of more than 10% of multiply transfused patients (127).

In spite of the observations described above, the correlation between red cell Bg antigens and leukocyte HLA antigens is not straightforward. First, not all persons who have leukocytes that carry HLA-B7, B17 and A28, have red cells that carry serologically detectable Bg^a, Bg^b and Bg^c, respectively. Second, antibodies with a single anti-Bg specificity are comparatively rare. Third, the Bg status of red cells from a single donor is not always consistent over a period of time. A donor whose red cells have typed as say, Bg(a+), over a period of months or years, may eventually present with red cells that type as Bg(a-).

Similarly, a donor whose red cells have consistently typed as negative for all Bg antigens may suddenly be found to be positive for one of them (55). These findings no doubt explain why some children, with two parents whose red cells lack the antigens, have one or more of the antigens on their red cells. It seems that most of the discordant findings are related to the extreme variability of the strengths of Bg antigens on the red cells of different individuals, the variability of the strength of the Bg antigen on the red cells of a single individual over a period of time, and the extreme variability in the strengths of anti-Bg in different sera.

As an example, an anti-Bg may have been in use for a long time and may have behaved as if it is a potent single specificity antibody. If the serum involved is then found to react with a red cell sample thought to lack the Bg antigen that the serum defines, but thought to carry a strong expression of a different Bg antigen, a complex situation will exist. It will be extremely difficult to determine whether the serum contains a second anti-Bg that reacts only with cell samples having that Bg antigen very strongly expressed, or whether the cells concerned carry a weak expression of a second Bg antigen, detectable only by the most potent examples of the specificity involved. This considerable difficulty is compounded by the facts that it is exceedingly difficult to adsorb anti-Bg from sera and that the antibodies can seldom successfully be recovered in eluates made from the adsorbing red cells.

Some of the technical difficulties described were resolved, at least in part, when Crawford et al. (105) reported success in typing for the Bg antigens using a capillary tube method. The method was said to be more sensitive than tube tests when the same anti-Bg were used in parallel. The capillary tube method was used to confirm the Bg-HLA correlations reported by Morton et al. (53,54) and described above.

From the studies of Crawford et al. (105) and those of others (56-59,106,107) further explanations of the difficulties experienced in working with the Bg antibodies have become apparent. It is now clear that some sera contain anti-HLA cytotoxins and anti-Bg red cell antibodies of corresponding specificity. However, at least when conventional testing procedures are used, others appear to contain either anti-HLA cytotoxins or anti-Bg red cell antibodies, so that the HLA-Bg correlations are much more difficult to see. As well as this consideration it must be remembered that the presence of HLA (Bg) antigens on mature red cells is neither a consistent feature in different individuals, nor consistent in a single individual over time. Crawford and Pollack (60) used a microcytotoxicity test in conjunction with an antiglobulin reagent. They found that they could demonstrate anti-HLA cytotoxins in some sera that had previously appeared to contain predominantly, or almost exclusively, anti-Bg red cell antibodies. However, for reasons already discussed, the Bg-HLA correlations are much more difficult to demonstrate when conventional blood bank methods are used.

Red Cell Antibody Identification Panels and the Bg Antigens

When red blood cell antibody identification panel sheets show the results of Bg antigen typings some anti-Bg can be identified in a straightforward manner. If the anti-Bg in question has anti-Bg^a or anti-Bg^b specificity and is strong enough to react with all Bg(a+) or Bg(b+) samples, no difficulties will be encountered. However, for many of the reasons already discussed, listing the results of Bg antigen typings on the panel sheet sometimes creates more problems than it solves.

First, as described, anti-Bg vary greatly in strength, strong examples exist but are comparatively rare. Obviously in typing red cells that will be used in an antibody identification panel, the strongest available sera are used by the most sensitive technique. If the worker using the red cell panel then encounters a weaker example of anti-Bg, it may not react with all the samples marked as positive for the antigen it defines. For example, a potent example of anti-Bg^b was used in this author's laboratory (108) to identify ten Bg(b+) samples. Of several other examples of anti-Bg^b available, none gave positive reactions with all ten Bg(b+) samples. Some reacted with five or six of the Bg(b+) samples, others with only one or two. Thus, users of cell samples typed for the Bg antigens must constantly remember that weaker examples of the antibodies will react only with those cells carrying the strongest expression of the Bg antigen. It is a futile exercise to perform HLA antigen typing on leukocytes and then label the red cells of the donors for the Bg antigens. As mentioned above, some persons with HLA-B7, HLA-B17 and HLA-A28 (or HLA-A2) on their leukocytes will never express serologically detectable Bg^a, Bg^b and Bg^c, respectively, on their red cells (128).

Second, this problem of variation of Bg antigen strength is further compounded by mixed anti-Bg specificities in some sera. If among the panel cells in use, three are known to be Bg(a+), and two Bg(b+), with one example of each having a very strong expression of its Bg antigen, a serum containing relatively weak anti-Bg^a and anti-Bg^b might react with just the cell samples having very strong Bg antigens. Then, of five known Bg-positive samples, one Bg(a+) and one Bg(b+) will be seen to have reacted. Again, it must be remembered that not every anti-Bg will react with all red cells said to carry the antigen that it defines.

Third, there is no doubt that in testing red cells, the

techniques and the sera used can create too sensitive a test system. If the majority of panel cells are shown to react to a greater or lesser degree with at least one anti-Bg serum, then say eight of ten samples would be labeled as Bg+ (this has actually occurred with one commercial panel). Obviously, such labeling will be of little use to users of the panel who would be extremely unlikely to duplicate such results in routine tests on sera that contained one or more anti-Bg. To resolve this difficulty, the manufacturer of the cell panel may wish to label as Bg+ just those cell samples likely to react with moderate strength anti-Bg. This in turn creates a dilemma for the manufacturer, who may feel obligated to describe as Bg+, any sample that has given a positive reaction.

A fourth problem that besets a commercial manufacturer of red cell panels is what to do when a particular red cell sample, that types as Bg-negative with all the sera available to him is found to be reactive with a serum, that appears to contain anti-Bg, in a customer's blood bank. If, as is usually the case, the serum is not available in quantity (to enable the manufacturer to type all his panel cell donors) the manufacturer is left in a very real quandary. He knows that the sample may be Bg+, but cannot so label it because he does not have the appropriate serum, so is obliged to issue that cell sample without a Bg+ designation when it is used in subsequent panels. This although it may accompany other cell samples labeled as Bg+, that did not react with the serum in question. Unless the manufacturer is able to obtain the new, supposed anti-Bg-containing serum in large enough quantities to perform exhaustive tests, there also exists the danger that a cell sample positive for an unrelated low incidence antigen will be thought to be Bg+. Each serum used for Bg typing must be very thoroughly tested to show that it does not contain an antibody that defines a different antigen of low incidence.

A fifth problem has already been mentioned. Single specificity anti-Bg are comparatively rare. As table 32-4 shows, the antibody at first called anti-Ot is now known most often to be anti-Bg^a plus anti-Bg^c. Sera previously called anti-DBG may contain just anti-Bg^a, or anti-Bg^a plus anti-Bg^b, or anti-Bg^a with anti-Bg^c, or even all three of the anti-Bg. If a serum studied is thought to contain just anti-Bg^a, but is then found to react with a red cell sample, typed by all other available sera as Bg(a-), Bg(b+) it is extremely difficult to differentiate between two possible explanations. The serum in question may contain anti-Bg^a and a weak anti-Bg^b that reacts only with the strongest Bg(b+) samples. Alternatively, the red cell sample may be Bg(a+) Bg(b+) and not Bg(a-) as supposed with its Bg^a being detectable only by the most potent anti-Bg^a.

Sixth, the story does not end with Bg^a, Bg^b and Bg^c. As shown in table 32-5 there are other HLA antibodies that have been shown to react with some red cell samples. While the antigens defined have not been given names, it is clear that the antibodies against them will not fit a pattern expected of antibodies directed against Bg[a], Bg[b] and Bg[c].

Obviously, simply listing Bg typings on a panel sheet does not resolve all problems encountered with Bg antibodies. On occasion it may help, at other times it will obfuscate. A clear and present danger is that an antibody of real clinical significance (the Bg antibodies usually are not, see below) might be incorrectly identified as anti-Bg if it happens to fit the appropriate pattern on an antibody identification panel.

Lack of Clinical Significance of Bg Antibodies

Troublesome as they are in in vitro studies, the Bg antibodies seem usually to be benign in vivo. There are a few reports (115-117) that describe modest increases in the rate of clearance of ^{51}Cr-labeled Bg+ red cells in patients with anti-Bg. In several of the patients studied, two component curves were seen. That is, a small proportion of the injected red cells were cleared rapidly then the remainder showed essentially normal survival. Further, Mollison et al. (118) have pointed out that in the study of Panzer et al. (117) an inappropriate method was used to determine the $T_{50}Cr$. While Panzer et al. (117) interpreted their data as demonstrating accelerated clearance of labeled red cells in six patients with anti-Bg, Mollison et al. (118) believe that in four of the six patients the survival was, in fact, normal. Other investigators (119,120) have described the normal survival of Bg+ red cells in patients with anti-Bg when in vivo red cell survival studies were performed. As mentioned elsewhere in this book, it is impossible to accept the claim of Molthan (121) that an anti-Bg[a] was responsible for a transfusion reaction involving intravascular hemolysis and hemoglobinuria, particularly since the allegedly responsible unit was never typed for Bg[a].

In considering Bg antibodies in the transfusion setting one other pertinent point can be made. Because of the serological problems that anti-Bg create and because of general acceptance of the fact that anti-Bg are benign in vivo, most manufacturers of antibody-screening red cells go to considerable lengths to ensure that the red cell samples used will not detect anti-Bg. Thus it follows that most anti-Bg go undetected in antibody-screening tests. Given the incidence of anti-Bg and the incidence of Bg antigens on red cells (see earlier) it follows that when immediate spin compatibility tests (that do not usually detect Bg-anti-Bg reactions) are used, a considerable number of patients with anti-Bg in the serum must be transfused with Bg+ blood. If the antibodies caused

TABLE 32-5 Different Studies on Sera in Attempts to Correlate Their Cytotoxic and Red Cell Antibody Specificities

Study (Reference)	Specificity of Cytotoxins	Specificity of Red Cell Antibodies
56	Anti-HLA-A2	Anti-HLA-A28
	Anti-HLA-A8	Anti-HLA-A8, some donors
57	Anti-HLA-A2 Antibodies adsorbed by leukocytes and red cells of persons with HLA-A2 or HLA-A28	Anti-HLA-A28
58	Anti-HLA-A7 plus B27	Anti-HLA-A7
	Anti-HLA-A5 plus B5 plus B15	No specific pattern
59	Antibodies to HLA-A9, A10, B7, B12, B15	Corresponded to cytotoxins
	Anti-HLA-A28, Anti-HLA-B7	Corresponded to cytotoxins plus weak activity for HLA-B12
	Anti-HLA-A1, Anti-HLA-B13	No correspondence but anti-HLA-B7 in several
116	Anti-HLA-A28 plus others	Anti-HLA-A28
140	15 examples of Anti-HLA-A2	All Anti-HLA-28
141	Anti-HLA-A2, Anti-HLA-A28	Separable by adsorption but most reacted as Anti-HLA-A28
142	Anti-HLA-A2 plus A-28	Cross react with HLA-B17 when antigen is present on red cells
141, 143	Anti-HLA-B8	Anti-HLA-B8

Much of the HLA nomenclature in the table has been updated from the original reports e.g. W5 and W15 are shown as B5 and B15.

transfusion reactions it would be expected that by now, the problem would have surfaced, it has not.

Bg Antibodies in Typing Reagents

Obviously, if a typing reagent to be used by IAT contains an undetected anti-Bg the potential for error exists. FDA regulations require that anti-D reagents, to be used in IATs to detect weak D, be shown to be non-reactive with D-, Bg(a+) red cells. Most reagent manufacturers test far more thoroughly. Human source reagents to be used by IAT (where most anti-Bg react) are tested against the strongest reacting Bg(a+), Bg(b+) and Bg(c+) red cells, that lack the antigen that the reagent defines, available. The problem of contaminating anti-Bg in red cell typing reagents is far less acute than was the case in 1974 (108,122). However, when human source reagents are considered, no manufacturer (no matter what claims are made) can guarantee absolutely, that all his reagents are free of anti-Bg. For example, a reagent may have been used for years with entirely correct results but then a sample lacking the antigen that the reagent defines, but carrying a stronger expression of Bg^a, Bg^b or Bg^c than any previously encountered, may react with the reagent. For this reason and because it is impossible to test every commercially-prepared reagent against red cells positive for all low incidence antigens (Bg and others) a typing test that yields an unexpected or weaker than usual positive reaction should be repeated with a different source reagent. For similar reasons, many workers who perform blood typing tests in cases of disputed parentage use two different source examples of each antibody used. It is important to know the source of the antibody. Reagents made from human sera, by different manufacturers, often contain antibody from the same donor, the manufacturer must be contacted re source of the antibody. The problem described is becoming less acute. In addition to careful testing of human source reagents by manufacturers, their gradual replacement by monoclonal antibody-based reagents will end the problem.

Antigens of Low Incidence That may be Extinct

In an attempt to ensure that the 700 series of antigens of low incidence include just those antigens for which tests could still be performed, the ISBT Working Party surveyed its members about availability of red cells and antibodies. The numbers for those antigens for which no supply of the appropriate antibody, to identify new examples of antigen-positive red cells, and no red cells positive for the antigen, to identify new examples of the antibody, exist, were declared obsolete. Thus it is clear that for some of the antigens, briefly described below, no further studies can be performed. However, it is equally clear that the Working Party does not include representatives from every red cell serology reference laboratory in the world. Thus it is possible that red cells positive for, or antibodies directed against some of the antigens listed below do still exist, unbeknownst to the Working Party. Further, although monospecific antibodies may not be available, sera containing multiple antibodies to low incidence antigens have been described, in some fairly recent publications, as containing antibodies to some of these antigens. As examples, the serum Blo was said to include anti-Sk and the serum Wilcox to

include anti-Gf (101). When the antigen Kg was described (34) it was shown to differ from Gf, Hey, POLL, Good, Sk and Pe. Similarly the antigen Jones was differentiated from the antigens Gf, Hey, POLL, Good, Sk^a, Zd and Pe (36). In both cases exclusion was possible when red cells carrying the newly defined antigen, Kg and Jones respectively, were shown to be non-reactive with multispecific sera previously shown to contain antibodies to the antigens listed. As recently as 1993, SHIN+ red cells were described as being non-reactive with sera that included antibodies to Hey and POLL.

The Antigen Gf

This antigen was detected by an alloantibody present in the serum of a patient with hemolytic anemia. Cleghorn et al. (130) found two further examples of anti-Gf in screening tests on 2000 normal sera but no further Gf+ cell sample in tests on 6886 English donors.

The Antigen Heibel

The first example of the antibody detecting this antigen caused fairly severe HDN (131). The antigen was present in three generations of the family involved but in none of 500 random West Berlin donors.

The Antigen Hey

In 1974, Yvart et al. (132) described a low incidence antigen, Hey, that was present on the red cells of one of their panel donors. In tests on the cells of 8127 unrelated French donors, two more Hey+ samples were found. In screening tests on 7369 sera, three were found to contain anti-Hey. A family of European extraction, now living in the USA, was shown by Strohm (134) to have five members, in three generations, with Hey+ red cells. The mother of the propositus with Hey+ red cells had IgG anti-Hey in her serum but the antibody did not cause HDN. A daughter of the proposita, who had Hey- red cells and who had delivered a child with Hey+ red cells and four individuals who had Hey- red cells and had been transfused with Hey+ blood, did not have anti-Hey in the serum.

The Antigen POLL

The only example of anti-POLL described in print (133) caused fatal HDN in the antibody-maker's second pregnancy and severe HDN in her third. The infant from the third pregnancy was delivered following induction of labor at 33 weeks (analysis of amniotic fluid had indicated that the fetus was severely affected) and required two exchange transfusions. Recognition of the presence of a maternal antibody directed against an antigen on the husband's red cells resulted in the third pregnancy being carefully monitored and in its successful outcome. Four members of the Poll family, that originated in Capri, Italy, in three generations, were shown to have POLL+ red cells. No other POLL+ sample was found in tests on the red cells of 1500 donors in Northern Ireland.

The Antigens Jobbins, Becker, Ven and Rm

In each instance these antigens were defined by a single antibody, descriptions of which appeared in the literature (65-68) before 1955. Thus these four antigens may truly be extinct.

The Antigen Good

In 1960, Frumin et al. (69) found this antigen in two generations of a US Black family. Anti-Good was responsible for severe HDN in several infants in this family (69,135) that as far as we are aware remains the only one in which the antigen has been found. Molthan and Eichman (136) screened the sera of 2718 normal donors and found eight examples of anti-Good for an incidence of one in 340. Abelson and Rawson (137) reported that both IgM and IgG anti-Good acted as agglutinins and that the reactivity of the IgG antibody was not enhanced in IATs.

The "Antigen" Skjelbred

While investigating a serum that contained antibodies to To^a, Wr^a, Jn^a and St^a, Kornstad et al. (20) found that the serum also reacted with some red cells that carried none of those antigens. However, they pointed out that they had been unable to demonstrate inheritance of the additional factor that was called Skjelbred. In 1978, Kornstad et al. (138) reported that the Skjelbred factor is present in serum as well as on red cells and that the state of having the factor (both on red cells and in the serum) is transient and reversible. These observations were extended in 1980 by Chaves et al. (139) so that now, the Skjelbred factor (that has also been called Sk^a (138) and Sk (139)) is thought to be an acquired marker that can be present in serum and adsorbed on to red cells. While the exact nature of the marker is not known (a viral origin has been suggested (139)) the observation that the factor

can disappear from the red cells and serum of an individual in whom it was previously present, correlates with the findings (20,138,139) that it cannot be shown to be inherited.

The Antigen Ht^a

Jahn and Cleghorn (70) studied anti-Ht^a when it caused HDN. None of 453 random English blood donors tested had Ht(a+) red cells.

The Antigen Zd

In 1970, Svanda et al. (71) described an antibody, anti-Zd, that caused HDN. The affected infant was given a 750 ml exchange transfusion although the DAT was reported as being only weakly positive. No figures for hemoglobin or bilirubin levels were given. The Zd antigen was found in eight members of the original family, who represented three generations, but not in any of 270 Czech donors. No further example of anti-Zd was found in tests on sera from 447 donors with high titered ABO antibodies. As mentioned in Chapter 12, the facts that *Zd* traveled with *r* in the family studied, that anti-Zd reacted well with papain and ficin-treated red cells and that the antibody caused HDN, raised the possibility that Zd might be an Rh antigen. Even if that is the case, it seems that lack of suitable test materials will prevent it from ever being proved.

The Antigen Pe

In 1979, McPherson et al. (72) described Pe, a rare antigen that is not serologically demonstrable on red cells treated with proteases. Anti-Pe did not react with the red cells of any of 1500 random donors (primarily White), six Japanese, seven Chinese, 31 Mexican-Americans or 17 US Blacks. In an addendum to the paper it is mentioned that a second family with members with Pe+ red cells had been found. No report is given of tests on random sera for the presence of anti-Pe.

The Antigen Ts

As far as we are aware, nothing further has been published about this antigen since Nakajima et al. (73) described its presence on the red cells of two of 150 Japanese donors whose blood was tested. Anti-Ts was found in the serum of a patient with antibody-induced hemolytic anemia.

Recognition of an Antigen of Low Incidence

As will by now be abundantly apparent, many sera contain antibodies to different and often unrelated antigens of low incidence. This fact makes identification of already known and new rare antigens difficult. If a serum is seen to react with red cell samples from two unrelated individuals and to fail to react with the red cells of hundreds or thousands of others, it is tempting to suppose that the cells of the two unrelated individuals carry the same antigen of low incidence. However, an explanation that is perhaps more likely is that the serum in question contains antibodies to two (or more) different antigens. Adsorption-elution tests can be used in this situation. In order to show that the same antigen is present on each cell sample, each should be shown to be capable of adsorbing all antibody activity for the other sample, from the serum. Eluates made from the adsorbing red cells should be shown to react with the other cell sample. If the antigen involved has previously been recognized and named, the two cell samples should be shown to react with all available sera, known to contain the antibody in question. While such maneuvers will answer questions about identity or non-identity of the antigen on red cell samples from unrelated individuals if the antigens are the same or have no relationship to each other, difficulties will be encountered if the antigens are different but phenotypically related. Exactly such situations have been described in Chapter 17 regarding the antigens Wu, NFLD and BOW; and the antigens Sw^a, SW1 and Fr^a. Similar situations in the Rh system (Go^a, Rh32 and Evans; D^w and Rh32) are described in Chapter 12 where a speculative explanation for the findings is offered. When this difficulty is encountered, the use of different sera containing monospecific activity for one of the antigens and red cell samples known to carry only one of the antigens may resolve the situation. Such studies usually involve lengthy collaborative studies (i.e. over several years) by many reference laboratories.

Sera from Patients with Autoimmune Hemolytic Anemia

As mentioned several times in this chapter, sera from patients with antibody-induced hemolytic anemia are a rich source of antibodies directed against low incidence antigens. Such sera are particularly useful when they do not contain autoantibodies that react with all red cell samples. The antibodies to rare antigens in those sera are invariably alloimmune in nature and do not contribute to the accelerated rates of in vivo red cell clearance in the patients.

Another Immunological Consideration

The presence of multiple specificities within a single serum is of considerable interest at the immunological level. In the section of Chapter 17 that describes anti-Wr^a, it is pointed out that the frequency with which the antibody is detected gradually increases in individuals with increasing levels of activity of their immune systems and/or increasing levels in the rate of destruction of red cells. The same is true of many antibodies described in this chapter. Cleghorn (78) has suggested that perhaps most (or all) persons have all these antibodies present in levels that are not usually detectable in serological tests. Perhaps as the immune system becomes more active, some of these antibodies are made in detectable amounts. Those easily identified may simply be the ones being made in largest amounts.

HDN and Confusion with ABO HDN

Although the antibodies described in this chapter have not all been characterized by immunological methods, it is clear that many of them were at least in part IgG for they crossed the placenta and caused HDN. In cases such as those caused by antibodies of this type, the serological picture can be confusing if the investigator fails to appreciate the potential role of these antibodies. The red cells of the affected infant may have a positive DAT but no antibodies may be demonstrable in the maternal serum because the antibody screening cells do not carry the rare antigen involved. In investigating such cases it should be remembered that the red cells of the child's father will carry the antigen against which the maternal antibody is directed and should be tested against the maternal serum if ABO compatible (and, of course, compatible with any other recognized specificity antibodies in the maternal serum). Similarly, the red cells of previous children of the couple may carry the rare antigen and are a source of test cells. In other instances use of an eluate from the affected infant's red cells may be necessary to show reactivity of the maternal antibody with the paternal antigen. However, it must be remembered that ABO incompatibility may interfere here as well. If, for example, the mother is group O and the child and its father are group A, the eluate from the affected infant's cells may contain an antibody to a rare antigen and anti-A. To exclude the possibility that a positive reaction with the paternal cells is due to an ABO antibody eluted from the infant's cells, control cells of the same ABO type as the father should be tested. It is very highly unlikely that random ABO control cells will carry the same rare antigen, as is present on the father's red cells. One other clue in this respect is severity of the HDN. If the child is severely affected, ABO HDN is an unlikely explanation and further investigations, as described above, are indicated.

Low Incidence Antigens in New Homes or with Different Names

Since the third edition of this book was written in 1983 and 1984 and published in 1985, many new findings have been made about the antigens described in the chapters dealing with low incidence antigens, in that edition. Many that were in those chapters in the third edition, have been shown to belong to one of the blood group systems. Others have been shown to be the same as antigens described earlier so have taken the name that had priority. While many of these findings have been described in the chapters that precede this one, or in this chapter, table 32-6 has been constructed as a ready reference to new names and addresses.

References

1. Daniels GL, Anstee DJ, Cartron J-P, et al. Vox Sang 1995;69:265
2. Daniels GL, Anstee DJ, Cartron J-P, et al. Vox Sang 1996;71:246
3. Coghlan G, Punter F, Zelinksi T. (abstract). Transfusion 1996;36 (Suppl 9S):49S
4. Spring FA, Bruce LJ, Anstee DJ, et al. Biochem J 1992;288:713
5. Bruce LJ, Anstee DJ, Spring EA, et al. J Biol Chem 1994;269:16155
6. Jarolim P, Rubin HL, Reid M. (abstract). Transfusion 1996;36 (Suppl 9S):49S
7. Coghlan G, Philipps S, McAlpine PJ, et al. (abstract). Transfusion 1995;35 (Suppl 10S):59S
8. Zelinkski T, Kaita H, Phillips S, et al. (abstract). Book of Abstracts. 20th Cong ISBT 1988:301
9. Contreras M, Teesdale P, Moulds M, et al. Vox Sang 1987;52:115
10. Kaita H, Lubenko A, Moulds M, et al. Transfusion 1992;32:845
11. Simmons RT, Were SOM. Med J Austral 1955;2:55
12. Kissmeyer Nielsen F. Vox Sang (Old Series) 1955;5:102
13. Cleghorn TE. Nature 1959;184:1324
14. Wadlington WB, Moore WH, Hartmann RC. Am J Dis Childh 1961;101:623
15. Jenkins WJ, Marsh WL. Lancet 1961;2:16
16. Cleghorn TE. Unpublished observations 1962 to 1967 cited in Race RR, Sanger R. Blood Groups in Man, 6th Ed. Oxford:Blackwell, 1975
17. Kornstad L, Howell P, Jorgensen J, et al. Vox Sang 1976;31:337
18. Kornstad L, Kout M, Larsen AMH, et al. Vox Sang 1967;13:165
19. Rausen AR, Rosenfield RE, Alter AA, et al. Transfusion 1967;7:336
20. Kornstad L, Øyen R, Cleghorn TE. Vox Sang 1968;14;363
21. Pinder L, Staveley JM, Douglas R, et al. Vox Sang 1969;17:303
22. Guévin RM, Taliano V, Fiset D, et al. Rev Fr Transf 1971;14:455
23. Skov F. Vox Sang 1972;23:461
24. Kornstad L, Brocteur J. (abstract). Book of Abstracts. 13th Cong ISBT 1972:58
25. Lewis M, Kaita H, McAlpine PJ, et al. Vox Sang 1978;35:351
26. Riches RA, Laycock CM. Vox Sang 1980;38:305
27. Young S. Vox Sang 1981;41:48
28. Rowe GP, Hammond W. Vox Sang 1983;45:316
29. Lewis M, Kaita H, Allerdice PW, et al. Hum Genet 1984;67:270
30. Pinder LB, Farr DE, Woodfield DG. Vox Sang 1984;47:290
31. Brown A, Plantos M, Moore BPL, et al. Vox Sang 1986;51:133
32. Kornstad L. Vox Sang 1986;50:235
33. Kluge A, Roelcke D, Tanton E, et al. Vox Sang 1988;55:44
34. Ichikawa Y, Sato C, McCreary J, et al. Vox Sang 1989;56:98
35. Chaves MA, Leak MR, Poole J, et al. Vox Sang 1988;55:241
36. Reid M, Fischer ML, Green C, et al. Vox Sang 1989;57:77
37. Rouse D, Weiner C, Williamson R. Obstet Gynecol 1990;76:988
38. Hoffmann JJML, Overbeeke MAM, Kaita H, et al. Vox Sang 1990;59:240
39. Coghlan G, Kaita H, Zelinksi T. (abstract). Book of Abstracts. Joint Cong ISBT/AABB 1990:124
40. Coghlan G, Green C, Lubenko A, et al. Vox Sang 1993;64:240
41. Stern DA, Hawksworth DN, Watt JM, et al. Vox Sang 1994;67:64
42. Coghlan G, McCreary J, Underwood V, et al. Transfusion 1994;34:492
43. Hamilton JR, Coghlan G. Unpublished observations 1993 cited in Daniels GL, Anstee DJ, Cartron J-P, et al. Vox Sang 1995;69:265
44. Lewis M, Kaita H. Vox Sang 1979;37:286
45. Lewis M, Kaita H, Philipps S, et al. Ann Hum Genet 1980;44;179
46. Spring FA. Transf Med 1993;3:167
47. Wallace J, Milne GR. Proc 7th Cong ISBT 1959:587
48. Dorfmeier H, Hart van der M, Nijenhuis LE, et al. Proc 7th Cong ISBT 1959:608
49. Hart van der M, Moes M, Veer van der M, et al. Prog 8th Cong Eur Soc Hematol, 1961
50. Buchanan DI, Afaganis A. Vox Sang 1963;8:213
51. Chown B, Lewis M, Kaita H. Vox Sang 1963;8:281
52. Seaman MJ, Benson R, Jones MN, et al. Br J Haematol 1967;13:464
53. Morton JA, Pickles MM, Sutton L. Vox Sang 1969;17:536
54. Morton JA, Pickles MM, Sutton L, et al. Vox Sang 1971;21:141
55. Marshall JV. Canad J Med Technol 1973;35:26
56. Nordhagen R, Orjaseter H. Vox Sang 1974;26:97
57. Nordhagen R. Vox Sang 1974;27:124
58. Nordhagen R. Vox Sang 1975;29:23
59. Nordhagen R. Vox Sang 1977;32:82
60. Crawford MN, Pollack MS. Transfusion 1978;18:731
61. Issitt PD. Adv Immunohematol Vol 7, No 1, Sept 1979
62. Giles CM, Walport MJ, David J, et al. Clin Exp Immunol 1987;69:368
63. Giles CM, Darke C, Rowe GP, et al. Vox Sang 1989;56:254
64. Giles CM, Botto M, King MJ. Transfusion 1990;30:126
65. Gilbey BE. Nature 1947;160:362
66. Elbel H, Prokop O. Zf Hygiene 1951;132:120
67. Loghem van JJ, Hart van der M. Bull Cent Lab Ned Rode Kruis 1952;2:225

TABLE 32-6 New Names and Addresses for Some Low Incidence Antigens

Current Name	Previous Name(s) (Some Historical)	Current Address
Wr^a or Di3		Diego system, Chapter 17
Ls^a or Ge6	Rl^a, Lewis II	Gerbich system, Chapter 16
Wb or Ge5	Webb, Reiter	Gerbich system, Chapter 16
Or or MNS31	Orris	MN system, Chapter 15
An^a or Ge7	Ahonen	Gerbich system, Chapter 16
Dh^a or Ge8	Duch	Gerbich system, Chapter 16
Os^a or MNS38		MN system, Chapter 15
Wd^a or Di5	Waldner	Diego system, Chapter 17
Rb^a or Di6	Redelberger	Diego system, Chapter 17
WARR or Di7	Warrior	Diego system, Chapter 17
Sw^a	Swann	Diego system, Chapter 17
Bp^a or Di10	Bishop	Diego system, Chapter 17
Wu or DI9	Wulfsberg, Hov, Haakestad	Diego system, Chapter 17
Mo^a or Di11	Moen	Diego system, Chapter 17
Fr^a	Froese	Probably Diego system, Chapter 17
Vg^a or Di13	Van Vugt	Diego system, Chapter 17
Hg^a or Di12	Hughes, Tarp, Tarplee	Diego system, Chapter 17
NFLD	Newfoundland	Diego system, Chapter 17
SW1		Probably Diego system, Chapter 17
BOW	Bowyer	Possibly Diego system, Chapter 17
HOFM		Possibly Rh system, Chapter 12
ELO or Di8		Diego system, Chapter 17
LOCR		Possibly Rh system, Chapter 12
Far or MNS22	Kam, Kamhuber	MN system, Chapter 15
Jones	Hol, Holmes	This chapter
Tr^a	Traversu, Lanthios	Diego system, Chapter 17
Pe	Co, PeCo	This chapter
Jn^a	Nunhart	Diego system, Chapter 17

68. Hart van der M, Bosman H, Loghem van JJ. Vox Sang (Old Series) 1954;4:108
69. Frumin AM, Porter MM, Eichman MF. Blood 1960;15:681
70. Jahn EFW, Cleghorn TE. Unpublished observations 1962 cited in Race RR, Sanger R. Blood Groups in Man, 6th Ed. Oxford:Blackwell, 1975
71. Svanda M, Prochazka R, Kout M, et al. Vox Sang 1970;18:366
72. McPherson GE, Wells RF, Hafleigh EB, et al. Vox Sang 1979;36:252
73. Nakajima H, Kuniyuki M, Takahara N. Jpn J Hum Genet 1967;12:187
74. Nakajima H, Satoh H, Komatsu F, et al. Hum Hered 1993;43:69
75. Cleghorn TE. Vox Sang 1960;5:556
76. Jakobowicz R, Albrey JA, McCullough WJ. Med J Austral 1960;2:294
77. Chown B, Lewis M. Am J Phys Anthropol 1959;17:13
78. Cleghorn TE. MD Thesis, Univ Sheffield, 1961
79. Walker ME, Tippett JP, Roper JM, et al. Vox Sang 1961;6:357
80. Jorgensen J, Kissmeyer Nielsen F. Unpublished observations 1973 cited in Race RR, Sanger R. Blood Groups in Man, 6th Ed. Oxford:Blackwell, 1975
81. Cleghorn TE. Unpublished observations 1974 cited in Contreras M, Lubenko A, Armitage S, et al. Vox Sang 1980;39:225

82. Contreras M, Lubenko A, Armitage S, et al. Vox Sang 1980;39:225

83. Lundsgaard A, Jensen KG. Vox Sang 1968;14:452

84. Winn LC, Eska PL, Grindon AJ. Transfusion 1976;16:351

85. Hildén J-O, Shaw M-A, Whitehouse DB, et al. Cytogenet Cell Genet 1985;40:650

86. Spring FA, Herron R, Rowe AG. Vox Sang 1990;58:122

87. Gralnick MA, Sherwood GK, De Peralta F, et al. (abstract). Prog 24th Ann Mtg AABB, 1971:105 and supplemented by information presented but not included in the abstract

88. Crossland JD, Kornstad L, Giles CM. Vox Sang 1974;26:280

89. Contreras M, Stebbing B, Armitage SE, et al. Vox Sang 1978;35:181

90. Young DJ, Smith DA. Clin Lab Haematol 1983;5:307

91. Rowe GP, Bowell P. Vox Sang 1985;49:400

92. Brown M, Mathur G, Moulds J, et al. (abstract). Transfusion 1980;20:630

93. Daniels GL. Unpublished observations 1992 cited in Daniels G. Human Blood Groups. Oxford:Blackwell, 1995:638

94. Marsh WL. Unpublished observations 1983 cited in Brown A, Plantos M, Moore BPL, et al. Vox Sang 1986;51:133

95. Kluge A, Roelcke D, Tippett P. (abstract). Blut 1982;45:50

96. Branch DR, Petz LD. Am J Clin Pathol 1982;78:161

97. Issitt PD. Applied Blood Group Serology, 3rd Ed. Miami:Montgomery, 1985:441, 628 and 629

98. Daniels G. Human Blood Groups. Oxford:Blackwell, 1995:633

99. Kornstad L. Unpublished observations 1974 cited in Race RR, Sanger R. Blood Groups in Man, 6th Ed. Oxford:Blackwell, 1975

100. Herron R, Smith GA, Young D, et al. Vox Sang 1989;56:112

101. Kornstad L, Jerne D, Tippett P. Vox Sang 1987;52:120

102. Rosenfield RE, Rubinstein P, Lalazari P, et al. Vox Sang 1967;13:461

103. Harris R, Zervas JD. Nature 1969;221:1062

104. Silvestre D, Kourilsky FM, Niccolai MG, et al. Nature 1970;228:67

105. Crawford MN, Gottman FE, Rogers LC. Vox Sang 1976;30:144

106. Shaw JF. In: Transfusion With "Crossmatch-Incompatible" Blood. Washington, D.C.:Am Assoc Blood Banks, 1975:26

107. Frist S, Wenz B. Transfusion 1976;16:261

108. Wilkinson SL, Vaithianathan T, Issitt PD. Transfusion 1974;14:27

109. Nordhagen R. Vox Sang 1978;35:49

110. Swanson JL, Sastamoinen R. Transfusion 1985;25:439

111. Swanson JL. In: A Seminar on Recent Advances in Immunohematology. Arlington, VA:Am Assoc Blood Banks, 1973:121

112. Brown G, Biberfield P, Christensson B, et al. Eur J Immunol 1979;9:272

113. Botto M, So AKL, Giles CM, et al. Br J Haematol 1990;75:106

114. Rivera R, Scornik JC. Transfusion 1986;26:375

115. Hart van der M, Szaloky A, Berg-Loonen van der EM, et al. Nouv Rev Fr Hematol 1974;14:555

116. Nordhagen R, Aas M. Vox Sang 1978;35:319

117. Panzer S, Mueller-Eckhardt G, Salama A, et al. Transfusion 1984;24:486

118. Mollison PL, Engelfriet CP, Contreras M. Blood Transfusion in Clinical Medicine, 9th Ed. Oxford:Blackwell 1993:461

119. Perkins HA. In: Transfusion and Immunology. Plenary Session Lectures 14th Cong ISBT 1975:107

120. Silvergleid AJ, Wells RF, Hafleigh EB, et al. Transfusion 1978;18:8

121. Molthan L. (Letter). Transfusion 1979;19:609

122. Pavone BG, Issitt PD. Br J Haematol 1974;27:607

123. Morton JA, Pickles MM, Turner JE, et al. Immunol Comm 1980;9:173

124. Morton JA, Pickles MM, Darley JH. Vox Sang 1977;32:27

125. Salama A, Mueller-Eckhardt G, Strauss B-E, et al. Tissue Antigens 1982;19:183

126. Eska PL, Grindon AJ. Br J Haematol 1974;27:613

127. Contreras M. Unpublished observations cited in Mollison PL, Engelfriet CP, Contreras M. Blood Transfusion in Clinical Medicine, 9th Ed. Oxford:Blackwell 1993:281

128. Crawford MN. HLA and the Red Cell, a Monograph. Malvern, PA:Accugenics, 1983

129. Krangel MS. Hum Immunol 1987;20:155

130. Cleghorn TE, Grant J, Pickles MM. Unpublished observations 1966 cited in Race RR, Sanger R. Blood Groups in Man, 6th Ed. Oxford:Blackwell, 1975

131. Ballowitz L, Fielder H, Hoffman C, et al. Vox Sang 1968;14:307

132. Yvart J, Gerbal A, Salmon C. Vox Sang 1974;26:41

133. McClelland WM, McLaughlin KG, Poole J, et al. Clin Lab Haematol 1982;4:201

134. Strohm PL. Vox Sang 1982;43:31

135. Eskin BA, Laufer EV, Pettit MD. Am J Obstet Gynecol 1961;81:997

136. Molthan L, Eichman MF. Transfusion 1967;7:327

137. Abelson NM, Rawson AH. Transfusion 1967;7:330

138. Kornstad L, Chaves M, Giles CM, et al. (abstract). Transfusion 1978;18:375

139. Chaves MA, Poole J, Giles CM, et al. Vox Sang 1980;39:28

140. Nordhagen R. Vox Sang 1978;35:375

141. Nordhagen R. Vox Sang 1979;37:209

142. Nordhagen R. Unpublished observations cited in Mollison PL. Blood Transfusion in Clinical Medicine, 7th Ed. Oxford:Blackwell, 1983:437

143. Nordhagen R. Vox Sang 1978;35:58

144. Jarolim P, Murray J, Rubin H, et al. Transfusion 1997;37:607

145. Zelinski T, Rusnak A, McManus K, et al. (abstract). Transfusion 1997;37 (Suppl 9S):89S

146. Zelinski T, Pongoski J, Coghlan G. (abstract). Transfusion 1997;37 (Suppl 9S):90S

147. Jarolim P, Moulds JM, Moulds JJ, et al. (abstract). Blood 1996;88 (Suppl 1):182a

148. Green C. Personal communication 1996

149. Daniels G. BBTS Newsletter No 44, Spring 1987:14

150. Poole J, Hallewell H, Bruce L, et al. (abstract). Transfusion 1997;37 (Suppl 9S):90S

When antibody screening and compatibility tests are performed, occasional sera are found that clearly react with one red cell sample but not with any others. A natural reaction to this situation is to suppose that the serum contains an antibody to an antigen of low incidence and, by chance, has been tested against a red cell sample that carries that antigen. Indeed, many of the low incidence antigens in the blood group systems and many of the independent rare antigens described in Chapter 32, were first detected in exactly such a circumstance. As will be apparent from the large number of antigens of low incidence already described in this book, identification of the antigen and antibody involved is not straightforward. The serum in question may have to be tested against dozens of rare red cell samples, each of which carriers a different antigen of low incidence and the cells in question may have to be tested with dozens of sera that contain antibodies to such antigens. If the positive reaction represents an antigen and antibody that have not previously been recognized, the task of showing that they are new is daunting. Collaborative studies by many different reference laboratories, that sometimes take years to complete, are necessary before all previously encountered antigens of low incidence can be excluded. As a result, many reference laboratories have collections of sera thought to contain unreported antibodies to low incidence antigens and red cells thought to carry previously unreported antigens. The antigens presumed to be involved usually have local names, based on the name of the red cell donor or the antibody-maker. These names are sometimes used in publications. That is to say, when a new antigen is reported a list of local factors from which it has been differentiated, is provided. This chapter provides compilations of such names, culled from the literature over the years.

In considering the names listed in this chapter, a number of points must be borne in mind. First, it is not claimed that each name represents a different and distinct antigen. No doubt in some instances the same antigen is known by different names in different laboratories because duplication of the antigen has not yet been recognized. Second, in some instances inheritance of the supposed antigen has not been proved, thus the lists no doubt include some acquired or transient factors that are not blood group antigens in the usually accepted sense of that term. However, since such factors are defined by antibodies, a claim that they are antigens can still be made. Third, in some instances the supply of reactive red cells or serum containing the antibody is exhausted before the case is solved. Thus some of the names listed, particularly those cited in the older literature, represent extinct characters.

The value of preparing a catalog of these names, that is essentially what this chapter comprises, has been questioned by some workers. Obviously, we believe that there is some value in the exercise since the catalog is here provided. First, by listing these names a historical perspective of when an antigen was first defined is provided. Some of the antigens listed by name in this chapter will no doubt graduate to positions of greater importance than they currently enjoy, in blood group systems or as established independent antigens. In support of such a belief it can be pointed out that in the equivalent tables to those provided here, in the third edition of this book, a number of antigens were listed that do indeed, now enjoy a higher stature. As examples, table 20-1 in the third edition included the antigens: Allen J, now JAL or Rh48; Doughty, now known to be the same as Mit, MN24; Webb, now Wb or Ge5; Elo, BOW, Haakestad (now Wu), and Tarplee (now Hg[a]) all of which are apparently ready to join the Diego system; and Jones, Oldeide (Ol[a]), Hollister (now Jones), Pe Co (now Re[a]), each of which is now established as an independent antigen of low incidence (see Chapter 32).

Second, we believe that a catalog such as this can be of help when one of the factors listed is studied in more detail. The references provided, here and in Chapter 44, point investigators to publications in which the factor has been mentioned and to other workers who may have antigen-bearing red cells or antibodies available.

The names that we have culled from the literature are presented in the tables. Table 33-1 lists names that have been mentioned in publications appearing since 1985. Table 33-2 lists names mentioned in publications that appeared between 1975 and 1984, references to those publications are listed in Chapter 44. Table 33-3 lists names that do not seem to have been mentioned in the literature since 1975. Clearly, many of those factors must now be extinct. Table 33-1 does not include all factors studied since 1985. In some publications describing new low incidence antigens the authors choose (perhaps to prevent the compilation of lists such as those given here) to list the excluded antigens that are well established (i.e. those described in Chapter 32) and then add "and X unsolved antigens" (the X varies from 3 to 20 or more).

The Direct Antiglobulin Test: An Essential Control

When a serum is found to give an unexpected reaction with a single red cell sample and the presence of an

TABLE 33-1 Antigens or Factors of Low Incidence Mentioned in the Literature Since 1985*

Name Used	Mentioned in Reference	Name Used	Mentioned in Reference	Name Used	Mentioned in Reference
Askwith	3	Gnade/Vetterlein	5	Pellegran	5
Balkacemi	5	Heron	3	Ragus	5
Berrio	5	Hull	5	Rasmussen	5
Bio 5	3, 5	Joyce	5	Reiter[*5]	5
Braithwaite	3	Kannellis	5	Reynolds	5
Burrows	5	Korving	5	Sadler	3, 5
Cassidy	5	Krog	5	Shindler	5
Dickinson	3	Laviscount	5	Street	5
Donaldson	3, 5	Malvenda	3	Tofts	3, 5
L. Evans	3	Mans[*4]	3	Tollefsen-Oyen	3, 5
Fielding	5	Maurer	5	Visser	5
Finlay[*2]	5	Niemetz	4	Walker	5
Fleck	3	Norlander	5	Wells	5
Friedberg	5	Overwheel	5	Wiggins	5
Ga^a, Ga[*3]	1, 2, 4, 6	Palfruman	3	Young	5
Gambino[*3]	5	Paschal	5	Zt, Zt^a[*6]	1, 2, 4, 5
Gibson	5	Peacock[*4]	5		

*1   The references cited do not describe the antigens named but mention them while describing others.
*2   Finlay is the same as Burrett.
*3   Ga^a, Ga and Gambino may be the same.
*4   Mans may be the same as Mansfield, which is the same as Peacock.
*5   We do not know if Reiter is the same as Reit (see Chapter 32).
*6   Zt and Zt^a may be the same as Marriott.

antibody to an antigen of low incidence is suspected, the next step in the investigation should always be a DAT on the reactive red cell sample. Many antibodies to low incidence antigens react best by IAT. Some healthy individuals have red cells that have a positive DAT (see Chapter 39). Thus it is essential to show that the unexpected reaction represents antibody activity in the test serum and not a positive DAT on the test red cells. Use of this simple control can save many hours of investigation and the unnecessary use of rare red cells and serum, on a serum sample that does not contain an antibody to a low incidence antigen at all. If the unexpected reaction occurs in an agglutination test that does not involve the use of antiglobulin serum, it is worth performing an autocontrol using the same method by which the supposed antibody was found. Although a positive DAT explaining an apparent and unexpected positive IAT is more common in this setting, spontaneous agglutination of the test red cells can also initiate a fruitless search.

High Incidence Antigens

Some of the problems in recognizing the fact that an antibody to a low incidence antigen defines a previously unrecognized character, also apply to antibodies directed against very common antigens. That is to say, before the antigen defined can be said to be one not previously recognized, the serum involved must be shown to react with a collection of rare red cell samples that between them represent all known high incidence antigen-negative phenotypes. Since not all reference laboratories have all such red cell samples, the same situation as that described above, results. In other words, most reference laboratories have a collection of sera, usually identified by the name of the antibody-maker, that contain "unsolved" antibodies to antigens of high incidence. Some of these names are then mentioned in publications when the antigen defined by the serum is differentiated from others being described. The chance that an unsolved high incidence antigen will become extinct is rather greater than the

TABLE 33-2 Low Incidence Antigens or Factors Mentioned in the Literature Between 1975 and 1984*1

Alda	Allchurch	A.M.	Arun	A8306	Balkin
Banks	Bell	Binge	Bovet	Bregi	Bullock
B7358	B9208	B9724	BOA 3150	Cameron	Caw
Craig	Davis J	Donavieski	Don E.W.	Dropik	Dugstad
Duvall	Elder	Enriquez	Epi	Evelyn	Fare*2
Ghawiler*3	Gladding	Gomez	Gould	Greenlee	Hall(J)*4
Haven	Hildebrandt	Horn	Jacobs	Jordan	Joslin
Kemma	Kennedy*5	Knoebnchild	Kominiarek	Kuhn	LaFave
Lagay	Laine	LeProvost	Madden	Maliff	Manley
Marcus	Margaret	Mateen	McKenney	Mateja*6	Middel
Milano	Mitch	Morrison	Nielsen	Oliver	Paris
Payer	Peretz	Pillsbury	Raison	Rios	Ryan
R_2R_2-202*7	rr-35*7	Schor	Swend	Sharp	Stevenson
Stewart	Taur	Taylor	Teremok	Tg^a	Tichmeyer
Toms	vanBuggenhout	Walin	Webb*8	Welsh	Westerlund
Wetz	Wolfe	Yh^a*9	1123K		

*1 References to papers describing other low incidence antigens in which these names are mentioned are listed in previous editions of this book.

*2 Not the same as Far (MN22).

*3 Spelled Gahwiler in some publications.

*4 Hall and Hall J are listed in different publications. We do not know if they are the same.

*5 The serum Kennedy contains anti-Rh32. We do not know if the Kennedy antigen is Rh32 or a second antigen defined by another antibody in that serum.

*6 Spelled Meteja in some publications.

*7 Not Rh antigens.

*8 Not the same as Wb (Ge5).

*9 Also called Yahuda.

chance that a low incidence antigen will no longer be identifiable. This, because with the low incidence antigens, the red cells carrying the antigen are often from normal donors, or their family members, and additional samples can often be obtained. For the high incidence antigens, the antibody is usually from a hospital patient, may not be available in large quantity even when first studied and further supplies may not be available once the original sample has been used. Similarly it is more difficult to obtain and freeze in quantity, red cells from patients than from normal donors.

Sometimes during the investigation of a "new" antigen of high incidence, some sera containing previously unidentified antibodies can be shown to contain the same specificity. For example, when Stroup and MacIlroy (7) described anti-Jr^a, they reported that the sera Fujikawa, Jacobs, Powell, Souza, Tamura and Tad, each of which had been studied in many laboratories, all contained anti-Jr^a. Similarly, Sabo et al. (8,9) reported that the sera

Horowitz, Warren, Juneau, 157G, Lazicki and Baugh, again sera much studied by others, all contained anti-JMH. In describing In^b and its antithetical relationship to In^a, Giles (10) reported that the sera Salis, Parra and Walls, all contained anti-In^b. After Applewhaite et al. (11) had reported anti-At^a, Gellerman et al. (12) showed that the well known sera E.De, V.Ba, C.Br, L.Bu and Ola Ware were other examples of that antibody (in case anyone has a supply left, the Ola Ware serum also contains anti-D). Thus any time that a patient appears to have made an alloantibody to a new high incidence antigen, it is well worth testing all unsolved antibodies to common antigens, against the patient's red cells. Of particular note, Race and Sanger (13) showed that the famous serum Swarts was non-reactive with Co(a-b-) red cells when that phenotype was first recognized (14). Mrs. Swarts had died in 1964, three years before the Colton system was discovered (15) but the retrospective finding (13) showed that what was probably the first example

TABLE 33-3 Low Incidence Antigens or Factors That do not seem to Have Been Mentioned in Print Since 1975*1

E. Amos	Baltzer	Big	Black	Bonde	BR726750
Braden	Bridgewater	Carson	Charles	Coates	Cross
Dahl	Driver	Duck	D1276*2	French	Fuerhart
Gerhany	Gilbraithe	Gon*3	Green	Haase	Hands
Hartley	Hil*4	Lindsay	Lucy	Man*5	Marks
Martin*6	McAulay	McCall	Nijhuis	Noble	Powell
Pr^{a*7}	Rich	Rils	Rutherford	Simpson	John Smith
Suhany	Th^{a*8}	Terruno	Wade	Whittle	754

*1   References to papers describing other low incidence antigens in which these names are mentioned are listed in previous editions of this book.

*2   Not associated with the Rh system.

*3   Not the same as Go^a (Gonzales) of the Rh System.

*4   Not the same as Hil (MN20).

*5   We do not know if Man is the same as Manley of table 33-2 or Mansfield (Peacock) of table 33-1.

*6   Not the same as Mt^a (MN14).

*7   Also known as Pritchard, not one of the Pr antigens described in Chapter 34.

*8   Also known as Thomas.

of anti-Co3 had been studied for ten years before the Co(a-b-) Co:-3 phenotype was identified.

Many of the new high incidence antigens discovered since 1985 have been recognized, at the time of their discovery or soon thereafter, as belonging in one of the known blood group systems and are described (with references) in other chapters of this book. A few examples are: MAR or Rh51 (Rh): Ge4 (Gerbich); Lu20 (Lutheran); and UMC or Cr10 (Cromer). The new (since 1985) independent high incidence antigens Emm, MER2, PEL and ABTI, are described in Chapter 31. Thus tables 33-4 and 33-5, that list names of sera that contain unsolved antibodies to very common antigens, mentioned in the literature since and before 1975 respectively, are not much different to the equivalent tables published in the third edition of this book. Sera such as Emma and Pelletier, that define antigens now more fully characterized (and described elsewhere) that is, Emm and PEL respectively, have been deleted from table 33-4. Few additions have been made. Two of the antigens from table 33-4 about which a little more is known, are described, briefly, below.

The Antigen Schneider

Two examples of the antibody defining this antigen were described in a 1983 abstract (16). One was made by a 67 year-old White male and other by a 72 year-old woman. Both patients had been transfused. The antibody defines an antigen that is present on the red cells of about 80% of random donors and can be detected on cord blood red cells. The antibody gave weak reactions by IAT, those reactions were slightly enhanced when protease-treated red cells were tested. Four of six Lu(a-b-) samples failed to react with anti-Schneider. Although the IgG non-complement binding antibody made by the male patient gave only weak reactions in vitro, it was thought possibly to have caused a delayed transfusion reaction. As far as we are aware, nothing has been published about this antigen since 1983.

The Antigen Gill

A 1981 abstract (17) described the high incidence antigen Gill. The IgG1 anti-Gill caused a positive DAT on the red cells of the US antibody-maker's first child but did not cause HDN. The antibody-maker had not been transfused. Her second child had a negative DAT at birth although the cord blood red cells were shown, in vitro, to react with the maternal antibody. Tests on red cells from 2000 random donors and on those of the antibody-maker's family, including three sibs, did not disclose another Gill- sample. However, a female patient in France was found to have red cells that were non-reactive with anti-Gill and an antibody in her serum that reacted with all red cells except the US Gill- sample. As far as we are aware, nothing has been published about this antigen since 1981. The abstract (17) describing Gill holds the

TABLE 33-4 Antigens or Factors of High Incidence Mentioned in the Literature Since 1975[*1]

Austin	Barrett	Baumler[*2]	Bert	Block	Boil
Boldog	Boston	Bothrops	Buckalew	Chase	Covas
Dalman	Dautriche	Donati[*3]	Englund	Giaigue	Gill[*4]
Groslovis	L. Harris[*5]	Hoalzel	Holmes	Jan	Kumiya
Koopman	Kursteiner[*6]	Langer	Mackin	Mathison	McDermott
McKeever[*7]	Mineo	Much	Nuz	Neut	O'Connor
A. Owens[*8]	Pantaysh	Panzar	Pruitt	Ramskin	L. Reynolds[*9]
Ridd	Ritter	Savery	Schneider[*4]	Seymour[*10]	Shannon
Simon	Smith	Stiarwalt	Swietlik	Tajama[*11]	Terrell[*12]
Terry	Thompson	Towey	Tri W	Ull	Vennera
Vienna[*13]	V.K.	Weeks[*14]	Whittaker	Wiley	Wilson[*15]
Woit	Zaw	Zim			

[*1] References to papers describing other high incidence antigens in which these names are mentioned are listed in previous editions of this book.
[*2] Called Baum in some publications.
[*3] May be the same as the character called Don in some publications.
[*4] See text.
[*5] Also known as Lenore Harris and Harris.
[*6] May be the same as the character called Kur in some publications.
[*7] May be the same as the character called McKee in some publications.
[*8] Also known as Alonzo Owens and Owens.
[*9] Called Reynolds in some publications.
[*10] Called Seymour-Wilson in some publications.
[*11] Called Taj in some publications.
[*12] Called Ter in some publications.
[*13] Called Vienna 522877 in some publications.
[*14] No association with Wk^a, a low incidence antigen in the Kell System, that was originally called Weeks.
[*15] We do not know if Wilson and Seymour-Wilson (see footnote 10) are the same thing.

distinction of ending with the most dangled preposition one of us (PDI) has ever seen.

A New Serum: A Useful Control

Bacterially contaminated sera sometimes have the ability to react with all red cell samples. Thus when investigating a serum that appears to contain an antibody to a very common antigen, it is always worthwhile to obtain a new sample to show that an antibody really is present. A bacterially contaminated serum can be thought of as sometimes detecting the antithetical wild goose to a positive DAT masquerading as a low incidence antigen.

Can Low and High be Shown to be Antithetical and Live Happily Everafter?

Any time that a sample that appears to contain an antibody to a new high incidence antigen is studied, the red cells of the antibody-maker should be tested with all available antibodies to low incidence antigens. The red cells of the antibody-maker lack the antigen to which the antibody is directed so may well come from an individual homozygous for the gene that encodes the low incidence antithetical partner of the high incidence antigen. A second possibility is that the antibody-maker is heterozygous for the rare allele encoding production of the low incidence antithetical partner and the null gene of the complex.

Tests in the other direction are less likely to produce an exciting finding. That is, based on the rarity of the genes that encode production of low incidence antigens, most individuals with red cells that carry such an antigen will be heterozygous for the gene encoding production of the rare antigen and the gene encoding production of its high incidence antithetical partner (if such a gene and antigen actually exist). However, tests with an antibody to an antigen of very high incidence against red cells car-

TABLE 33-5 Antigens or Factors of High Incidence That do not Seem to Have Been Mentioned in Print Since 1975[*1]

Armstrong	Anuszewska	Begovick	Bryant	Bouteille	Bultar
Bruno	Bradford	Cartwright[*2]	Clements	Cooper	Cipriano
Davis	Frando	Fuller	Fedor	Fleming	Griffith
Gallner	Geslin	Hutchinson	Hamet	Henry	Kollogo
Kennedy	Kelly	Kosis	Lee	MZ443	Pearl
Paular	Perry	Robert	Ryan	Snyder	Sisson
Schuppenhauer	Savior	Santano	Sadler	Terschurr	Talbert
Truax	Tasich	Todd	Waldner[*3]	Wimberly	Wallin
Zwall					

[*1] References to papers describing other high incidence antigens in which these names are mentioned are listed in previous editions of this book.

[*2] Not the same as Yt^a.

[*3] No association with Wd^a, a low incidence antigen in the Diego system, which was originally called Waldner.

rying low incidence antigens can sometimes lead to suggestive findings. Some antibodies to high incidence antigens react less strongly with red cells from individuals heterozygous for the gene in question than with those from individuals homozygous for that gene.

The tests described in the last two paragraphs should not be restricted to red cells carrying rare or common antigens not previously characterized. As an example, an antibody to an unidentified low incidence antigen should be tested against red cells known to lack high incidence MN, Gerbich, Diego, Kell, Lutheran, etc., system antigens. This time as a single example, Judd et al. (18) tested an antibody to a low incidence antigen, in a serum Hof, against high incidence antigen negative red cells and showed that it reacted with all known examples of cells of the Lu:-8 phenotype. Not only did the finding result in the antibody being called anti-Lu14 right from the time of its discovery, the subsequent investigation resolved what, at that time, appeared to be contradictory evidence about an association between Sw^a and the Lutheran system (see Chapter 20).

Given the plethora of unsolved antigens of very low and very high incidence, as illustrated by the tables in this chapter, it is somewhat disappointing that relatively few antithetical partnerships have been revealed by tests such as those described in this section. Nevertheless, some dramatic successes have been achieved. As examples (with apologies to those investigators whose similar successes are not used as examples) Lewis et al. (19,20) showed that red cells that lacked the (then named) high incidence antigen Sm, were Bu(a+). Sm is now Sc1, Bu^a is Sc2 and the antigens are part of the Scianna system (Chapter 26). As described above, Judd et al. (18) showed that serum Hof contains anti-Lu14 that defines

the antithetical partner to Lu8. Although it took longer to prove the point (and convince skeptics) the antithetical relationship between Di3 (formerly Wr^a) and Di4 (formerly Wr^b) was first suggested when it was shown (21) that the lady who made the first alloimmune anti-Wr^b had Wr(a+) red cells and that those cells carried a double dose of Wr^a (22,23).

The Antigen Sf^a

The antigen Sf^a, that has also been called Sf and Stoltzfus, is not of low or high incidence, indeed the only example of anti-Sf^a ever described (24) was said to react with the red cells of 34% of random Whites. The antigen is described in this chapter since we believe that, like some others mentioned here, it is now extinct. While the *Sf* gene was said (25) to be on chromosome 4 and thus to be either linked to or syntenic with *MN* (26), no serological studies seem to have been performed since 1969 nor, apparently, has another example of anti-Sf^a been found. The antibody was said (24) to be IgA in composition, other workers did not have the same success in working with the antibody as did the original investigators.

References

1. Reid M, Fischer ML, Green C, et al. Vox Sang 1989;57:77
2. Ichikawa Y, Sato C, McCreary J, et al. Vox Sang 1989;56:98
3. Chaves MA, Leak MR, Poole J, et al. Vox Sang 1988;55:241
4. Kluge A, Roelcke D, Tanton E, et al. Vox Sang 1988;55:44
5. Kornstad L. Vox Sang 1986;50:235
6. Rowe GP, Boswell P. Vox Sang 1985;49:400
7. Stroup M, MacIlroy M. (abstract). Prog 23rd Ann Mtg Am

Assoc Blood Banks, 1970:86 and supplemented by information presented but not included in the abstract.

8. Sabo B, Moulds JJ, McCreary J. (abstract). Transfusion 1978;18:387
9. Sabo B. Unpublished observations 1978 cited in Issitt PD. Applied Blood Group Serology, 3rd Ed. Miami:Montgomery, 1985:440
10. Giles CM. Vox Sang 1975;29:73
11. Applewhaite F, Ginsberg V, Cunningham CA, et al. Vox Sang 1967;13:444
12. Gellerman MM, McCreary J, Yedinak E, et al. Transfusion 1973;13:225
13. Race RR, Sanger R. Blood Groups in Man, 6th Ed. Oxford:Blackwell, 1975:393
14. Rodgers MJ, Stiles PA, Wright J. (abstract). Transfusion 1974;14:508
15. Heisto H, Hart van der M, Madsen G, et al. Vox Sang 1967;12:18

16. Mougey R, Tippett P, Martin J, et al. (abstract). Red Cell Free Press 1983;8:25
17. Frederick J, Brendel W, Daniels G, et al. (abstract). Transfusion 1981;21:613
18. Judd WJ, Marsh WL, Øyen R, et al. Transfusion 1977;32:214
19. Lewis M, Chown B, Schmidt RP, et al. Am J Hum Genet 1964;16:254
20. Lewis M, Chown B, Kaita H. Transfusion 1967;7:92
21. Adams J, Broviac M, Brooks W, et al. Transfusion 1971;11:290
22. Issitt PD, Pavone BG, Wagstaff W, et al. Transfusion 1976;16:396
23. Wren MR, Issitt PD. Transfusion 1988;28:113
24. Bias WB, Light-Orr JK, Krevans JR, et al. Am J Hum Genet 1969;21:552
25. Bootsma D, McAlpine PJ. Human Gene Mapping 1979;5:21
26. Bias WB, Meyers DA. (abstract). Cytogenet Cell Genet 1982;32:524

34 | Antigens Defined by Cold-Reactive Autoantibodies

As described in Chapters 10 and 38, most cases of "cold" antibody-induced hemolytic anemia (also known as cold hemagglutinin disease (CHD) and as cold agglutinin disease) are caused by autoantibodies directed against I, i and related antigens. As described in Chapters 11 and 38, most cases of paroxysmal cold hemoglobinuria (PCH) are caused by auto-anti-P. However, many other cold-reactive autoantibodies with different specificities (and hence names) have been recognized. Often these antibodies were first studied because they caused (sometimes severe) CHD. In a few instances, after the specificities had been recognized and partially characterized, benign forms of the same specificity were found. This chapter describes these antibodies and the antigens they define. Because of the fact that almost all these autoantibodies were first found when they caused CHD, frequent mention of that fact will be made. However, it should be borne in mind that if all cases of CHD caused by other than I blood group collection antibodies are added together, they still comprise a small minority of the total cases.

The Pr Antigens: Discovery

In 1968, Marsh and Jenkins (1) described several examples of a cold-reactive autoantibody that caused severe CHD in some of the subjects studied. In tests on samples from thousands of normal donors, no nonreactive red cells were found. The antibodies clearly differed from those of the I blood group collection; red cells from adults and from newborns reacted to about the same degree (using undiluted sera and in titrations) and the antigen(s) defined was (were) denatured when red cells were treated with ficin. The authors pointed out that lack of a nonreactive blood sample meant that while they could describe the antibodies as similar and likely to be related, they could not be certain that all examples defined the same antigen. Such a conclusion was prophetic; as described below the fine specificities of these antibodies have resulted in recognition of a large number of antigens. Marsh and Jenkins (1) assigned the name anti-Sp_1 to the new antibody. The Sp was an abbreviation for species (since the red cells of all humans were reactive) and the subscript was used to characterize the first antibody; allowance was already being made for the many specificities now known. In fact, the terms Sp_2, Sp_3 etc., were not used; instead, the change in terminology described below took place.

At about the same time as work on Sp_1 was being done in England, autoantibodies of similar specificity were being studied in Germany. When they published their initial findings, Roelcke and Dorrow (2) called the antibody anti-HD, after Heidelberg, the city in which the study was performed. However, a comment was published (3) that the term HD might be taken to imply that the antigen was present only on red cells that carried both H and D. This led Roelcke and Uhlenbruck (4) to suggest that the terms Sp_1, HD_1 and HD_2 be replaced by Pr_1 and Pr_2. The Pr was derived from protease, since by then it was known (1,5-10) that more than one antigen was involved, that all the antigens were protease-sensitive and that at least some of them were destroyed (or removed) when red cells were treated with neuraminidase. The name Pr was said to be more suitable than Sp since it had also been shown (1,4-6,10) that the antigens were present on the red cells of many species in addition to man. At this point it should be added that while these antigens are denatured when human red cells are treated with proteases, the same is not true of red cells from other species. As discussed below, some Pr antibodies give markedly enhanced reactions when tested against protease-treated red cells from dogs.

Following these initial studies, an enormous amount of work was done at the serological and biochemical levels, on the Pr antigens and antibodies, most of it in the laboratories of Dr. Dieter Roelcke in Heidelberg. Brief synopses of many of the findings are given below. Extensive references are provided for those readers who wish to consult the original papers.

The Pr Antigens: Serology

Most (but not quite all, see below) antibodies to the Pr series of antigens, present as agglutinins optimally reactive close to 0°C. Clearly, those that are causative of CHD have a wide enough thermal amplitude that they can bind to red cells at body temperature (sometimes during exposure of the patient to cold, see Chapter 38). Most of the antibodies, again particularly the pathological forms, react well in tests at room temperature and are nearly as reactive at room temperature as at 4°C. The red cells of almost all humans react equally with anti-Pr of most specificities (see below for exceptions). The Pr antigens differ from I, i and some other antigens described later in this chapter, in that they are removed from red cells when those cells are treated with papain, ficin or bromelin. All Pr antigens except Pr_a (again see below) are denatured when red cells are treated with neuraminidase. Thus non-reactivity of a potent cold-reactive autoagglutinin with protease-treated and neuraminidase-treated red cells, virtually establishes that the antibody defines an antigen in the Pr series. However, as described in a later section, care is necessary to avoid interference by anti-T when tests against neuraminidase-treated red cells are performed.

The Pr antigens have been divided into those now called Pr_1, Pr_2, Pr_3, Pr_a, Pr^M (and probably Pr^N). The initial distinction between Pr_1 and Pr_2 was that the Pr_1 antigen, as defined by some antibodies, was found on human but not on canine red cells. Although other examples of anti-Pr_1 did react with canine red cells (for this subdivision see below) that reaction was abolished when the canine cells were treated with a protease. Anti-Pr_2 reacted strongly with untreated but not with protease-treated human red cells; it reacted with canine red cells, that reaction being enhanced when such cells were protease-treated (11). Pr_3 was differentiated from Pr_1 and Pr_2 when it was found on the red cells of cats and sheep; both species have red cells that lack Pr_1 and Pr_2 (12). Differences between Pr_1, Pr_2 and Pr_3 have also been found at the biochemical level (see below). Such findings have very clearly authenticated that different antigens are involved and have illustrated how perceptive were the conclusions drawn from the serological studies (11-15).

The antigens Pr_1 and Pr_3 have both been subdivided. Pr_{1h} and Pr_{3h} are found on human but not on canine red cells. Pr_{1d} and Pr_{3d} are found on both human and canine red cells (10-13,19). As mentioned above, all examples of anti-Pr_2 have reacted with canine red cells (13,16,17). With considerable industry, Roelcke (11) studied the Pr_{1d} and Pr_{3d} status of red cells from 13 different breeds of dogs. Humans and dogs are not the only species whose red cells carry Pr antigens. Various different publications (12,13,16-19) have described the presence of some of the antigens (see table 34-1) on the red cells of guinea pigs, rats, sheep and cats. Some of the antigens have also been found on the tissue cells of guinea pigs and rats (20).

In 1971, a new Pr series antigens, Pr_a, was described (21). When first studied, Pr_a was said to be denatured when red cells were treated with proteases but to survive when red cells were treated with neuraminidase. When the original antibody was reinvestigated (22) it was shown that it was anti-T in the serum that was responsible for the reaction with the neuraminidase-treated red cells. However, Habibi et al. (23) found an antibody in a newborn that fit the criteria established (21) for anti-Pr_a specificity. Thus Pr_a differs from Pr_1, Pr_2 and Pr_3 in that it is detectable on neuraminidase-treated red cells. As with all Pr antigens, Pr_a is denatured by protease treatment of red cells.

The first antibody said to have anti-Pr^M specificity was reported (24) in 1986. As described in some detail in the section below on biochemistry of the Pr antigens, those determinants are known to reside in some oligosaccharide side chains attached to the MN, Ss and other sialoglycoproteins. However, Pr_1, Pr_2, Pr_3 and Pr_a are not dependent on the presence of M or N for reactivity. In contrast, anti-Pr^M behaves much like other examples of anti-Pr in tests at low temperatures (i.e. it reacts equally well with M+ N- and M- N+ red cells) but shows a distinct preference for M+ red cells in tests at higher temperatures. In other words, the Pr^M determinant is influenced by the amino acid sequence of glycophorin A (see Chapter 15) and in that respect differs from Pr_1, Pr_2, Pr_3 and Pr_a. When describing anti-Pr^M, Roelcke et al. (24) pointed out that it was very probable that some antibodies described earlier (25-27) as having auto-anti-M specificity, were actually examples of anti-Pr^M. It seems that antibodies that at first appear to be auto-anti-M can be divided in to two specificities. Auto-anti-Pr^M (24-27) recognizes a Pr determinant, the orientation of which is affected by the amino acid sequence of the NH_2 terminal portion of *M* gene-specified glycophorin A. Auto-anti-M recognizes the M antigen and is specific for that antigen at all temperatures (28-36). At the serological level, probable differentiation can be made based on reactivity of the antibody at different temperatures. For example, the autoantibody seen retrospectively (24) to have anti-Pr^M specificity, that was described by Chapman et al. (27,37) reacted with M- N+ red cells to titers of 1,000,000 at 4°C; 512 at 15°C; and 64 at 20°C. Its preference for M+ red cells was seen only at higher temperatures. We (38) also pointed out that while anti-Pr^M always activates complement (and can cause severe CHD (27)) auto-anti-M only rarely has that capability (35,36,39). Having established the specificity of anti-Pr^M (24), Roelcke (17) also pointed out that an earlier described antibody (40) probably had anti-Pr^N specificity.

Given the differences between Pr_{1h}, Pr_{1d}, Pr_2, Pr_{3h} and Pr_{3d} as one group of antigens and Pr_a, Pr^M and Pr^N as another group, a case can be made (165) that the second group are not truly members of the Pr series. Such subtle differences aside, it is convenient still to consider them all together. Accordingly, table 34-1 summarizes the characteristics of the antigens as described in this section.

Tests on Neuraminidase-Treated Red Cells

As described above, all Pr antigens except Pr_a are denatured when red cells are adequately treated (41) with the enzyme neuraminidase. Thus anti-Pr can be identified in part by the use of such treated cells. However,

TABLE 34-1 Reactions of Anti-Pr[*1]

Red Cells		Pr_{1h}	Pr_{1d}	Pr_2	Pr_{3h}	Pr_{3d}	Pr_a	Pr^M	Pr^N
					Antibody to				
Adult I	Unttd	+	+	+	+	+	+	+[*2]	+[*2]
	Prot	0	0	0	0	0	0	0	0
	Nmdase	0	0	0	0	0	+	0	0
Adult i	Unttd	+	+	+	+	+	+	+	+
	Prot	0	0	0	0	0	0	0	0
	Nmdase	0	0	0	0	0	+	0	0
Cord i	Unttd	+	+	+	+	+	+	+	+
	Prot	0	0	0	0	0	0	0	0
	Nmdase	0	0	0	0	0	+	0	0
Canine	Unttd	0	+[*3]	+	0	+	0		
	Prot	0	V	E	0	0	0		
	Nmdase	0	0	0	0	0	0		
Rabbit[*4]		0	0	0		0			
Guinea Pig		V	V	+		E			
Rat		V	V	V		V			
Sheep		0	0	0	+	+			
Cat		0	0	0	+	+			

<u>Legend to table 34-1</u>

Unttd = Untreated; Prot = Protease-treated; Nmdase = Neuraminidase-treated

+ = Positive; 0 = Negative; V = Variable, positive with some sera, negative with others; E = Enhanced positive reactions.

[*1]   The most usual reactions are shown; for rare exceptions, see text.
[*2]   Preference for M+ or N+ red cells seen only at higher temperatures, see text.
[*3]   Some anti-Pr_{1d} react only weakly with canine red cells.
[*4]   Rabbit red cells can be used to adsorb anti-I (and anti-i) from sera and leave anti-Pr unadsorbed.

direct tests using sera from adults against neuraminidase-treated red cells are always positive. This, because neuraminidase-treatment of red cells removes N-acetyl-neuraminic acid (NeuAc) residues, exposes the T antigen and because all normal sera from adults contain anti-T (see Chapter 42, Polyagglutination). Thus in order to identify anti-Pr from their failure to react with neuraminidase-treated red cells, it is necessary to adsorb anti-T from the serum under test. This can be accomplished by adsorbing the serum with neuraminidase-treated red cells (for a method for preparation of such cells see Judd (42)) until it no longer reacts with such treated cells. If the serum contained anti-Pr, that antibody will not have been adsorbed and the serum will still react with untreated red cells. Since the I antigen is not denatured when red cells are treated with neuraminidase, the absorption method can be used to differentiate anti-Pr from anti-I. An alternative method is to adsorb the serum under test on to untreated red cells and make an eluate.

Such an eluate will not contain anti-T. However, as with many cold-reactive antibodies, it is not always easy to obtain large amounts of anti-Pr in an eluate.

Red Cells with Reduced Levels of Pr Antigens

As mentioned above and discussed in more detail below, the Pr determinants are carried in oligosaccharide side chains attached to red cell membrane-borne glycophorins. The majority of Pr sites appear to be located in tetrasaccharide side chains attached to glycophorin A between the NH_2 terminus and residue 26 (43). As expected, En(a-) red cells and those of M^k homozygotes, that lack glycophorin A (see Chapter 15), carry reduced levels of Pr antigens. Red cells, such as those from Mi^V homozygotes, that carry altered sialoglycoproteins, may behave similarly. Such is the difference between the number of copies of the Pr determinants on normal and En(a-) red cells that anti-Pr may fail to react visibly with En(a-) red cells and may be mistaken for anti-En^a (44). Differentiation between anti-Pr and anti-En^a can be made by the use of adsorption tests. En(a-) red cells will adsorb anti-Pr, they will not adsorb anti-En^a. The reason for this is that although the majority of Pr determinants are present in tetrasaccharides attached to glycophorin A, they are also expressed in oligosaccharide side chains attached to other red cell glycophorins and perhaps other structures. In other words, the difference in Pr status between normal red cells and those that lack or have altered forms of glycophorin A is quantitative not qualitative. A study (72) in which it was shown that many examples of anti-Pr reacted poorly with red cells with no or with altered MN SGP, clearly related to the number of copies of Pr determinants on the test red cells. Red cells that are S- s- U- have been shown (see Chapter 15) to lack glycophorin B, so carry fewer copies of the Pr determinants than do red cells that carry glycophorins A and B. However, such is the profusion of Pr determinants on glycophorin A, that is expressed normally on S- s- U- cells, that we (75) have not been able to demonstrate any weakening of Pr antigen expression on those cells. Homberg et al. (76) succeeded in making anti-Pr agglutinate En(a-) red cells by performing tests in a system adjusted to pH 6.2. As described in Chapter 15, individuals homozygous for M^k, whose red cells carry neither glycophorin A nor glycophorin B, may have anti-Pr in the serum (45). We do not know if experiments have been performed to determine whether the red cells of these individuals would adsorb their own anti-Pr, that is, do other membrane structures on red cells carry enough copies of the Pr antigens to effect adsorption of the antibody?

Anti-Pr: Serology

Autoantibodies directed against the Pr determinants may be IgM (1,13,16,17,24,46-55,59,60), IgG (21,44,55-58) or IgA (2,16,17,55,61-65) in composition. In reviewing reports about a large number of cold-reactive autoantibodies and in comparing the findings to those in his own laboratory, Roelcke (17) pointed out that among IgM autoantibodies with kappa light chains, all specificities are found but anti-I predominates. IgM autoantibodies with lambda light chains are more likely to have specificity outside the I blood group collection; Pr antibodies are often included. Roelcke (17) also pointed out that all published examples of pathological IgA cold agglutinins had Pr specificity and wondered if their apparently universal occurrence in this group indicates a restriction in the immune response mechanism. As discussed in more detail below, many of the Pr-specific

autoantibodies found (as with other specificity autoantibodies causative of CHD) have been monoclonal in nature. Also discussed below are possible mechanisms by which IgA anti-Pr might clear red cells in vivo.

The overwhelming majority of auto-anti-Pr, regardless of their immunolgobulin class, present as agglutinins optimally reactive at low temperatures. The antibodies agglutinate red cells suspended in saline at neutral pH although enhanced antibody activity is often seen in test systems with an acid pH (see below). In titration studies the antibodies often react with red cells of all Ii phenotypes at dilutions of 1 in 1000 or greater. Those examples causative of CHD activate complement and cause primarily intravascular hemolysis, often after the patient has been exposed to cold (see Chapter 38). Discussed below are a number of examples that had characteristics different from those just described. In reading these details it should be remembered that although the descriptions take more space than those describing the typical antibodies, the antibodies mentioned are exceptions to the more commonly encountered forms.

A patient described by McGinniss et al. (44) had a warm-reactive IgG auto-anti-Pr$_a$. The patient had a purine nucleoside phosphorylase deficiency and when the authors found a similar antibody in another patient with that disorder, they suggested that the two conditions might, in some way, be related. The patient described by Curtis et al. (58) had life-threatening hemolytic anemia and failed to respond to conventional drug therapy. His autoantibody was an IgG anti-Pr$_a$ and his hemolytic anemia was resolved by splenectomy. In classic paroxysmal cold hemoglobinuria (PCH) a biphasic hemolysin (the D-L or Donath-Landsteiner antibody) that almost always has anti-P specificity (66,67) causes sudden acute episodes of red cell hemolysis that lead to hemoglobinuria. Episodes of hemolysis are precipitated by exposure of the patient to cold temperatures. However, not all D-L biphasic hemolysins cause PCH. In some cases there is no hemoglobinuria and hemolysis is neither episodic nor precipitated by cold exposure. Such cases are most accurately described as D-L hemolytic anemia (68). At least one case has been seen (69) in which the biphasic hemolysin had some form of anti-Pr specificity. An IgM anti-Pr$_{1d}$ causative of CHD, in a patient described by Green et al. (59) was highly unusual in that it was inhibited in vitro by sodium citrate. Indeed, when unwashed red cells in preservatives were used for testing, the cold agglutinin appeared too weak to be of clinical significance. When it was titrated against washed red cells, its titer was greater than 2000.

Most examples of anti-Pr described in the literature were studied, then reported, because they were causative of CHD. However, some clinically benign forms have been found (18,19,23,60,70-74). In some hematologically normal individuals with auto-anti-Pr, C3 was found on the red cells when DATs were performed. In the patient described by Bell et al. (70) there was evidence that transfused red cells did not enjoy normal in vivo survival although no clinical signs of a transfusion reaction were noted when the patient was transfused with blood passed through a warming coil. Two patients described by O'Neill et al. (73) had anti-Pr_1 reactive only in tests performed at low ionic strength. Again, there was no evidence for CHD and transfusions were uneventful, but both patients had positive DATs with C3 on their red cells.

In some early descriptions of the specificities of the various anti-Pr some antibodies were mentioned that are now better classified. Two forms of anti-Pr_3 were originally described. It is now known that the anti-Pr_3 described by Roelcke et al. (12) was an example of anti-Pr_{3d}, while that described by Birgens et al. (18) was the first example of anti-Pr_{3h}. An antibody described by Roelcke et al. (19) that was listed as anti-Pr Ad in an earlier review (75) has been classified (17) as a somewhat atypical form of anti-Pr_{1d}. As already mentioned, some examples of anti-Pr_{1d} react only weakly with canine red cells.

False Positive Reactions in ABO Typing, Caused by Anti-Pr

As described in Chapter 8, currently used ABO typing reagents are often monoclonal antibodies made in vitro. Following some early findings (186-189) in which it was shown that an anti-B from one particular clone (ES4) gave positive reactions with red cells with acquired B (see Chapter 8) that were indistinguishable from those of true group B red cells, various steps were taken to resolve the problem. One of these steps involved use of the anti-B at a different pH. Since it was known (129) that the ES4 anti-B-acquired B reaction could be prevented or greatly weakened in a test system at pH 6.0, anti-B reagents based on ES4 were often adjusted to that pH. Although the unwanted detection of acquired B was largely prevented, a new problem occurred. Some individuals, including normal blood donors, have benign cold autoagglutinins in their sera that do not usually interfere in ABO grouping tests. However, the activity of some of those autoagglutinins is so enhanced at acid pH that when unwashed red cells are tested with a reagent at pH 6.0, agglutination occurs not because the antigen that the reagent defines is present on the red cells, but because the trace of autoantibody present in the unwashed red cell suspension causes autoagglutination (190,191). If this situation is suspected (i.e. discrepancy in forward and reverse ABO typing) it can be resolved either by repeating the red cell typing on well washed red

cells (providing that they do not have autoantibody irreversibly bound) or by the use of a human source ABO typing reagent in a test at neutral pH. Beck (60) and Kirkegaard et al. (192) have studied this phenomenon in some detail. They report that pH dependent cold autoagglutinins that can cause this problem are present in one person in about 500. In each case studied (60,192) the pH dependent cold agglutinin had anti-Pr_a specificity.

Biochemistry of the Pr_1, Pr_2 and Pr_3 Antigens

The early finding that protease-treated red cells do not react with anti-Pr clearly indicated that the antigens are carried on protease-sensitive components of the red cell membrane. The finding that most anti-Pr do not react with neuraminidase-treated red cells showed that neuraminic acid (NeuAc), that is specifically cleaved when red cells are treated with neuraminidase, must be an integral part of the antigens. Thus, it was not surprising to learn (16,135,199,200) that when extracts are made from red cell membranes in such a way that they include glycophorin A (the MN SGP), they have the ability to inhibit antibodies to Pr_1, Pr_2 and Pr_3. As discussed in detail in Chapter 15, glycophorin A carries multiple copies of O-linked glycans that include NeuAc. Many of those side chains are the tetrasaccharide described by Thomas and Winzler (201). That structure contains one NeuAc residue in $\alpha(2\rightarrow3)$ linkage to Gal, and another in $\alpha(2\rightarrow6)$ linkage to GalNAc (201,202) (see figure 15-3 in Chapter 15). It is now apparent (194) that NeuAc in both linkages contributes to Pr antigen structure. While each copy of glycophorin A carries 15 O-linked side chains, they are not all tetrasaccharides. Studies (136,165) have shown that while tetrasaccharides predominate on the outer or NH_2 portion of glycophorin A, the O-glycans bound to the glycophorin closer to the membrane, are often trisaccharides. The trisaccharides include NeuAc in $\alpha(2\rightarrow3)$ or $\alpha(2\rightarrow6)$ linkage, those NeuAc residues are also involved in Pr antigen structure. Lisowska et al. (136) have shown that on most red cells the ratio of tetrasaccharides to trisaccharides lacking the $\alpha(2\rightarrow6)$ linked NeuAc to trisaccharides lacking the $\alpha(2\rightarrow3)$ linked NeuAc, is 8:3:1. Dahr (203) first showed that glycophorin B (the Ss SGP) that also carries copies of the tetrasaccharides and trisaccharides, is Pr_1, Pr_2 and Pr_3-active.

As discussed below, Pr determinants are also present in side chains attached to minor red cell sialoglycoproteins and on some other membrane structures. In considering the Pr antigens on glycophorin A it is apparent that Pr_1, Pr_2 and Pr_3 are carried wholly within the O-glycans. That is to say, the MN polymorphism that results from different amino acids at positions one and five at the NH_2

terminal end of the protein backbone of the MN SGP (see Chapter 15), plays no role in the structure of these antigens. When the tetrasaccharides are isolated from the protein backbones of the SGPs, they retain Pr activity (204). For some time it appeared that the NeuAc residue in $\alpha(2{\rightarrow}3)$ linkage to Gal represented Pr antigen structure. As mentioned above, it is now known (194) that NeuAc in $\alpha(2{\rightarrow}3)$ linkage to Gal, and NeuAc in $\alpha(2{\rightarrow}6)$ linkage to GalNAc are both involved in Pr antigen structure. While the NeuAc in $\alpha(2{\rightarrow}3)$ linkage to Gal appears to play a major role, it must be remembered that more of the O-linked glycans include NeuAc in that linkage, than include NeuAc in $\alpha(2{\rightarrow}6)$ linkage to GalNAc. There are conflicting reports on the inhibition of Pr antibodies using NeuAc alone. Roelcke and Kreft (16) used NeuAc at concentrations of up to 20 mmol/L (6.2 mg/ml) but saw no inhibition of any anti-Pr in their collection. In contrast, Garratty and O'Neill (74) found five anti-Pr that were inhibited using NeuAc at concentrations from 1 to 10 mg/ml; the two LISS-dependent anti-Pr that those workers (73) reported were not inhibited.

Different inhibition and enhancement patterns, closely correlated to anti-Pr subspecificities, were seen when chemically modified preparations of isolated glycophorins that included tetrasaccharides were used. When such extracts are periodate-oxidized the trihydroxyside chain of NeuAc is shortened, creating a C7 NeuAc derivate (205). Carbodiimide treatment of the glycophorin extracts may produce an N-acyl-urea derivative of NeuAc, that is formed by rearrangement from an O-acyl-urea derivative of NeuAc after reaction with the carboxy group of NeuAc (206). Both periodate oxidation and carbodiimide treatment destroyed Pr_1 activity. For Pr_2, periodate oxidation increased activity some 100 to 200-fold; carbodiimide treatment destroyed it. For Pr_3 the effects were exactly the reverse of those on Pr_2. Periodate oxidation destroyed Pr_3 activity, while carbodiimide treatment increased it some 100 to 200-fold (12,135,207,208). As mentioned earlier, these findings at the biochemical level were a triumphant endorsement of the Pr_1, Pr_2 and Pr_3 subdivisions made earlier at the serological level. These findings, expressed in terms of enhancement or destruction of Pr antigen activity, are summarized in table 34-2.

As will by now be clear, distinct differences between Pr_1, Pr_2 and Pr_3 exist at the biochemical level. To these can be added the observation that of the three determinants, Pr_2 alone appears to be present on gangliosides and other lipids (128,209). As mentioned in the section on the serology of Pr, Pr_2 is still detectable on protease-treated canine red cells. These two observations have led Roelcke (17) to suggest that perhaps on canine red cells, Pr_2 is restricted to gangliosides. That the same is not true of human red cells is clear from the findings that Pr_2 is denatured when such red cells are treated with a protease and that glycophorin preparations from human red cells are Pr_2-active. Thus, it seems unlikely that ganglioside-borne Pr_2 contributes significantly to the reaction between human red cells and anti-Pr_2.

Some observations (43) suggest that the Pr determinants are largely confined to the O-glycans attached between residue 1 (NH_2 terminus) and residue 26 of glycophorin A. However, adsorption studies and some observations cited below seem to suggest that while the outer portions of the SGPs carry the number of copies of Pr determinants necessary for red cells to be agglutinat-

TABLE 34-2 Inhibition and Enhancement of Anti-Pr by Unaltered and Chemically Modified Glycophorin Extracts[*1]

Antibody	Unmodified Glycophorin Extract	Periodate-oxidized Glycophorin Extract	Carbodiimide-treated Glycophorin Extract
Anti-Pr_{1h}	+	0	0[*2]
Anti-Pr_{1d}	+	0	0[*2]
Anti-Pr_2	+	+↑	0
Anti-Pr_{3h}	+	0	+↑
Anti-Pr_{3d}	+	0	+↑
Anti-Pr_a	+		

Legend to table 34-2

[*1] Note that symbols are used oppositely to agglutination tests.
   + = Antibody neutralized—no longer acts as an agglutinin.
   0 = No antibody inhibition—antibody still agglutinates rbc.
   +↑ = Inhibitory effect of extract 100 to 200 fold greater than that of unmodified extract.
[*2] Some anti-Pr_1 partially inhibited.

ed by anti-Pr, a smaller number of copies may well be present in oligosaccharides attached to the more internal portions of glycophorins A and B. Dahr (165) has pointed out that the minor red cell sialoglycoproteins (glycophorins C, D, etc.) are also glycosylated and may well carry tetrasaccharides or similar structures that include Pr determinants.

At both the serological and biochemical levels, proving this point is difficult because of the paucity of copies of the minor SGPs as compared to glycophorins A and B. Indeed, similar considerations may well apply to nonglycophorin glycosylated red cell membrane components that may include structures that carry Pr. The finding that protease-treated red cells no longer react with anti-Pr does not contradict the suggestion that some Pr determinants may be present on red cell membrane components other than glycophorins A and B. Indeed, under some circumstances protease-treatment of red cells does not effect total cleavage of glycophorin B. Further, some protease-resistant minor red cell membrane structures may carry a few Pr determinants. The finding (210) mentioned above that En(a-) red cells, that lack glycophorin A, will adsorb anti-Pr to exhaustion certainly seems to confirm the observation (203) that Pr determinants are present on glycophorin B. Thus, the apparent conversion from the Pr+ to the Pr- state, by treatment of red cells with proteases, may simply reflect a quantitative difference in the number of available Pr receptors on red cells with glycophorin A present and those (protease-treated) from which most of that structure has been removed. Red cells from individuals homozygous for M^k lack glycophorins A and B (45). Thus the question as to whether red cell membrane components other than glycophorins A and B carry Pr determinants might be answered if such cells were shown capable or incapable of adsorbing anti-Pr to exhaustion. However, that experiment does not seem to have been performed.

Biochemistry of Pr_a, Pr^M and Pr^N

Based on serological observations, it would seem that Pr_a must have a fundamentally different biochemical structure to the Pr_1, Pr_2 and Pr_3 antigens. Anti-Pr_a fails to react with protease-treated human red cells; it does react with such cells treated with neuraminidase. Thus, while Pr_a (as with Pr_1, Pr_2 and Pr_3) would appear to be carried on a protease-sensitive red cell membrane component, it would seem not to require NeuAc for its structural integrity. However, Roelcke and Kreft (16) found that one anti-Pr_a in their collection was strongly inhibited with chemically modified glycophorin extracts while a second example was not. This finding would seem to suggest two possibilities. First, perhaps not all antibodies

called anti-Pr_a have exactly the same specificity. Second, since the modifications to the glycophorin preparations should have altered only sialyl groups, perhaps one form of anti-Pr_a defines a determinant that includes one or more neuraminidase-insensitive NeuAc residues on glycophorins. Given the already well-established subdivisions of Pr_1 and Pr_3, it would not be at all surprising to find that Pr_a can be subdivided.

Little need be added about Pr^M and Pr^N. As described in the section on serology of the antigens, the definitive antibodies behave as anti-Pr in tests at low temperatures but are influenced by the presence or absence of M and N when tests are performed at higher temperatures. Thus the antigens can be thought of as Pr determinants whose presentation (steric orientation) is influenced by amino acids at positions one and/or five of the NH_2 terminal portion of glycophorin A. An alternative view would be that the antigens are actually forms of M and N, influenced in presentation by the Pr determinants. Such an explanation seems less likely than the first since, in tests performed at refrigerator temperature, the definitive antibodies do not have anti-M or anti-N specificity. Inhibition studies also support the first explanation. While anti-Pr^M was preferentially inhibited by glycophorin extracts made from M+ N- red cells, it was also inhibited by similar extracts from M- N+ red cells (24).

Anti-Pr: Some Immunological Considerations

Cases in which auto-anti-Pr cause immune red cell destruction can be divided into two broad general categories. First are those hemolytic episodes that are short-lived and self-limiting that result from the transient production of auto-anti-Pr following infections (12,14,16, 17,21,57,58,63,64,69,197,198). Second are those cases of chronic CHD caused by the continued production of auto-anti-Pr (1,6,13,14,24,59,63,77,78). Transient production of auto-anti-Pr has been seen following infections with *Mycoplasma pneumoniae*, Epstein-Barr virus, rubella, varicella, cytomegalovirus and other agents including some that cause vague influenza-like illnesses. Infection with the rubella virus seems particularly to be associated with the transient production of auto-anti-Pr (17,55,96,197). In cases of chronic CHD, auto-anti-Pr is seen in patients with lymphoproliferative disorders, lymphoma and sometimes in patients without other discernible clinical abnormalities (40,46,47,50,52,53). This, of course, is no different from chronic CHD caused by autoantibodies other than anti-Pr. It is known (79) that the Pr determinants are present on T and B lymphocytes and on macrophages. It is not yet known how this observation relates to the transient or continued production of pathological auto-anti-Pr. Many of the pathological auto-anti-Pr that have been studied have been shown (13,16,17,24,50,52,53,56-58,64,77,78) to be monoclonal in nature. This finding applies to some auto-anti-Pr made following infection and some causative of chronic CHD.

As mentioned earlier, there are some indications that production of monoclonal, pathological cold-reactive autoantibodies is more likely to be a function of, or may be restricted to, certain clones of immunocytes. For example, most but not quite all, pathological auto-anti-I are IgM molecules with kappa light chains. Exceptions have been reported (48,49,211,212). While many auto-anti-i are IgM antibodies with kappa light chains, a higher proportion of anti-i than of anti-I are IgM with lambda light chains. In this respect auto-anti-Pr are somewhat heterogeneous. References are given above to reports describing auto-anti-Pr that were IgM, IgG and IgA. However, when 36 anti-Pr were studied in one laboratory (16), 31 were IgM, four IgA and one IgG. Among 19 of the antibodies typed for light chain type, 18 had kappa and one had lambda light chains. While auto-anti-Pr may be of any immunoglobulin type (with IgM predominating), IgA cold-reactive autoantibodies that actually cause CHD may all have anti-Pr specificity. Roelcke (17) has suggested that this may represent a restriction of pathological IgA cold autoantibodies to Pr specificities. While Ratkin et al. (71) and Hsu et al. (80) have presented evidence that many persons who make pathological IgM anti-I, make small amounts of IgG and IgA anti-I as well, the IgG and IgA antibodies in those patients may not have contributed to the immune red cell destruction. A case (81) in which a patient made IgM and IgA anti-I was unusual in that the patient had a biclonal gammopathy.

It is still not clear exactly how IgA cold-reactive autoagglutinins effect in vivo red cell destruction. Romer et al. (100) showed that, like other IgA antibodies, IgA anti-Pr do not activate complement. Although there are reports (101-104) of macrophages with IgA receptors and the binding of IgA by polymorphonuclear leukocytes (101,103-105) the role of those cells in clearing IgA-coated red cells in vivo is far from established. Salama et al. (106) believe that direct cold agglutinin-red cell contact may bring about non-complement dependent hemolysis on some occasions. While such direct lysis (the mechanism has not been suggested) has been said (107) to have been caused by IgM non-complement binding cold-reactive autoagglutinins in children and by IgM anti-I in an in vitro system in which complement activation was blocked by EDTA (106) there are, as yet, no claims of IgA cold autoagglutinins with this ability. In a different case, that involved a warm-reactive IgA autoantibody, the C5b-C9 terminal attack sequence of complement activation was mobilized in the absence of demonstrable C3 activation (108). Reactive lysis or the bystander mechanism (see Chapter 6) was thought to be involved.

Because monoclonal cold-reactive autoagglutinins have singular specificities, it might be hoped that some with the same specificity would share idiotypes. (For a definition and discussion of idiotypes see Chapter 2). Antibodies against idiotypes can be raised in animals (82,83) by using hybridoma technology (84) or by EBV transformation of B cells (85). However, the use of anti-idiotypes to study cold agglutinins is not as straightforward as the above, somewhat simplistic, suggestion might imply. For example, while some anti-idiotypes raised against Pr antibodies did define idiotypes shared by different examples of the antibodies (78,82) and some were shown (82,83) not to cross-react with anti-I or anti-i, others, raised against anti-I cold agglutinins, were shown (86,87) to react with some paraproteins that were not antibodies to red cell antigens. In other cases (88-90) anti-idiotypes have been quite individualistic and have reacted only with the antibody against which they were raised.

Silberstein et al. (91) used EBV transformation of B cells from a patient with a pathological anti-Pr$_2$ in the serum to produce a series of clones of cells secreting anti-Pr$_2$. Jefferies et al. (90) then used cells from those clones to immunize mice whose spleen cells were later fused with a mouse myeloma cell line and monoclonal anti-idiotype specificities were obtained. Two of the anti-idiotypes were IgG1, two were IgM and all four had kappa light chains. Inhibition experiments suggested that the four anti-idiotypes were directed against identical or neighboring idiotypes on the anti-Pr$_2$ molecules, both heavy and light chains of those molecules were necessary for idiotype integrity, but the anti-idiotypes did not combine with anti-Pr other than that of the original patient. The authors (90) pointed out that anti-idiotypes produced against B-cell lymphomas, in which no red cell autoantibodies were being made, also appeared to be tumor specific (92-94).

More progress has been made in studying anti-idiotype specificities directed against anti-I than in studying those directed against anti-Pr. Clearly, work on anti-idiotypes to cold agglutinins has two important objectives. First, their use may help to answer the question as to which clones produce monoclonal autoantibodies and provide information as to the nature of the defect that results in activation of those clones. Second, the anti-idiotypes may be of value in immunotherapy either by neutralizing the pathological cold agglutinins in vivo or by curtailing their production.

Monoclonal Antibodies to Pr, Made In Vitro

It must be remembered that monoclonal cold autoagglutinins that cause CHD were recognized as such (95) long before the technology was developed

(84,85) to produce monoclonal antibodies in vitro. In CHD, of course, the production of a monoclonal antibody represents a malfunction of the individual's immune system. A few monoclonal antibodies related to the Pr antigens have been made in vitro. The F11 MAb of Ochiai et al. (97) may well have anti-Pr$_a$ specificity. In addition, other MAbs that recognize NeuAc-containing epitopes in oligosaccharides attached to glycophorins A and B may be defining epitopes of the Pr antigens (97-99). More often than not, mouse MAbs directed against antigens carried on glycophorins A and B have had specificities against epitopes that include some of the protein backbone of the SGPs. Thus, as explained in detail in Chapter 15, those MAbs define MN system rather than Pr antigens. As will be seen, as far as the Pr determinants are concerned, the in vitro production of MAbs has been more fruitful in the area of anti-idiotypes to Pr antibodies than in the production of MAbs against the Pr antigens themselves.

Terminology for Some Other Antigens Defined by Cold-Reactive Autoagglutinins

Initial discoveries, that are described in more detail below, led to reports (references also given below) describing the antigens Gd, Sa, Fl, Lud, Vo, Li, Me, Om and Ju. As work on the biochemical nature of the antigens defined progressed, some relationships between the antigens became apparent. This, in turn, led to the introduction of some new names (109). The new terms that were introduced were Sia-l1, Sia-b1, Sia-lb1 and Sia-lb2. In each of those names the Sia indicates that the antigen defined is sialic acid-dependent. The l designation indicates that the antigen is carried on the l or linear (unbranched) form of type 2 chains (see also Chapters 8, 9 and 10) on red cells. The b designation indicates that the antigen is carried on b or branched type 2 chains. The lb designation indicates that the antigen is carried on both l or linear and b or branched type 2 chains. The numbers following l, b or lb indicate the number of determinants recognized. In other words, anti-Sia-lb1 recognizes one sialic acid-dependent antigen present on l, linear and on b, branched type 2 chains, while anti-Sia-lb2 recognizes a different antigen that is also sialic acid-dependent and is carried on l, linear and b, branched type 2 chains. The antibody now called anti-Sia-l1 was originally called anti-Vo, the one now called anti-Sia-b1 was originally anti-Fl, and the antibodies now called anti-Sia-lb1 and anti-Sia-lb2 were originally anti-Gd1 and anti-Gd2, respectively. Table 34-3 is a ready-reference list of the new and original names. Since readers may be more familiar with the older names than with the new ones, both are used in the sections below describing the antigens and their antibod-

ies. Although as table 34-3 indicates, four of the antigens have been renamed based on their biochemical structures, the antigens are described below, in the sequence of their discovery. Anti-j that defines a protease-resistant, neuraminidase-resistant structure related to I and i, that is present on both linear and branched type 2 chains (195), is described in Chapter 10.

The Gd (Sia-lb) Antigens

The first two examples of anti-Gd (now anti-Sia-lb) were reported in 1977 (110); further examples have been found (111-114). Some but not all of the known examples have caused CHD, most often of the type secondary to infection. As described below, the antigen defined was recognized as being glycolipid-dependent, hence choice of the name Gd. The Gd antigen is equally well-expressed on the red cells of adults (of the I and i phenotypes) and newborns. Protease-treated red cells retain Gd activity; the antigen is denatured when red cells are treated with neuraminidase.

One example of the antibody, anti-Gd(Kn), failed to react with ape and monkey red cells. A second example, anti-Gd(Hei), reacted strongly with those cells. Because of these findings and some made at the biochemical level, antibodies with the specificity of anti-Gd(Kn) were called anti-Gd1 (now anti-Sia-lb1); those with the specificity of anti-Gd(Hei) were called anti-Gd2 (now anti-Sia-lb2).

Konig et al. (114) tested 192 sera containing anti-I for the concomitant presence of anti-Gd and anti-Fl (see below). Three of the sera tested contained at least anti-I and anti-Gd. Since it has been shown (116-123) that the Gd (and Fl, see below) antigens are identical to structures identified as receptors for *M. pneumoniae*, Konig et al. (114) concluded that the production of anti-Gd (and of anti-Fl) following infection with *M. pneumoniae* represents production of antibodies directed against those receptors. It will be noted that in many of the papers dealing with the *M. pneumoniae* receptor, the I and i antigens are named. In fact, the Gd (and Fl) structures repre-

TABLE 34-3 New and Original Names for Some Antigens Recognized by Cold-Reactive Autoagglutinins (from 109)

New Name	Old Name
Sia-l1	Vo
Sia-b1	Fl
Sia-lb1	Gd1
Sia-lb2	Gd2

sent I- and i-bearing structures to which terminal NeuAc has been added. It seems that the terminal NeuAc is an essential component in the receptor recognized by *M. pneumoniae* (121).

Initial recognition of the fact that Gd is removed from red cells by treatment of those cells with neuraminidase, but that it is retained on protease-treated cells (110,115) meant that while NeuAc must be essential for Gd antigen structure, the antigen must be carried on other than protease-sensitive glycoproteins of the red cell membrane. Indeed, it is now known (124) that glycophorins are Gd-inactive. Studies on glycolipids that include terminal NeuAc residues have shown (115,125-128,196) that Gd1 (Sia-lb1) is represented by the immunodominant monosaccharide NeuAcα(2→3). While the monosaccharide is Gd1-active, alpha configuration is necessary. Gd2 (Sia-lb2) is more complex in that the terminal NeuAc must be linked to galactose, i.e., NeuAcα(2→3)Galβ1.... Such structures are present on many glycolipids of the red cell membrane, including those that carry I and i. Thus, as mentioned above, in some instances Gd1 (Sia-lb1) and Gd2 (Sia-lb2) are sialylated versions of I- and i-bearing chains. That the straight chain i structure is as suitable as the branched chain I structure as a carrier for Gd is evidenced by the fact that I adult, i adult and i cord cells carry equally well developed Gd antigens. Indeed, this point has been proved at the biochemical level since Gd has been shown (109) to be present in linear and branched type 2 chains.

Findings that: the antibody called anti-p (130-132) (see Chapter 11) does not recognize the structure postulated to be a precursor of P, but recognizes sialylneolactotetrasylceramide (sialylosylparagloboside), a product of an alternative pathway (133); that two of four anti-Gd showed enhanced reactions with Tj(a-) red cells (134); and that Tj(a-) red cells carry increased levels of the major Gd-active ganglioside (134); suggest that anti-Gd (anti-Sia-lb) would be a more appropriate name than anti-p for the antibody (126).

The Antigen Sa

In 1980, Roelcke et al. (124) gave the name anti-Sa to an IgM monoclonal cold agglutinin with kappa light chains, that was causative of CHD. The Sa determinant was found to be present in about equal amounts on the red cells of adults of phenotypes I and i and those of newborns. Unlike I and i but similar to Pr and Gd, the Sa determinant was no longer detectable on red cells treated with neuraminidase. Unlike Pr, the Sa determinant was not completely denatured when red cells were treated with proteases. However, anti-Sa reacted less strongly with protease-treated than with untreated red cells and

thus differed from anti-I and anti-i (whose reactions are enhanced) and anti-Gd (whose reactions are unchanged) when such cells are used.

These serological findings suggested that Sa might be present on both protease-sensitive glycoproteins (copies of antigens removed by proteases) and protease-resistant glycolipids (copies of antigens resistant to proteases). Such suggestions were then confirmed at the biochemical level. Glycophorin A was shown (124,135) to be Sa-active and the structure NeuAcα(2→3)Gal was found to be immunodominant. The studies of Dahr et al. (135) showed that the Sa determinants are included in oligosaccharides attached to the portion of glycophorin A that is fairly close to the red cell membrane. As discussed in Chapter 15 and above, it is known (136) that in that region some of the side chains are trisaccharides and not the tetrasaccharides that occur as side chains near the NH_2 terminus of glycophorin A. Thus, it seems entirely possible that the Pr antigens are present in the tetra- and trisaccharides, while on membrane glycoproteins, Sa is predominantly located in the trisaccharides. Most recently Kewitz et al. (194) have shown that while anti-Pr may recognize immunodominant α(2→3)- or α(2→6)-sialyl groups on glycophorins, with the former more often defined than the latter, anti-Sa seem to recognize only the α(2→3)-sialyl structures.

Unlike the Pr_1 and Pr_3 determinants that are confined to glycoproteins, Pr_2 and Sa are present on glycolipids as well (128). On such components the immunodominant grouping of Sa seems to be NeuAcα (2→3)Galβ(1→4)Glc (126). While Sa and Pr_2 are both optimally expressed on long chain gangliosides, Pr_2 is present on those of the neolacto and ganglio series, while Sa is restricted to the neolacto series (128). Kundu et al. (127) showed that the gangliosides that inhibited anti-Gd and anti-p (arguably the same antibody, see previous section) did not inhibit anti-Sa.

Pruzanski et al. (137) used anti-Sa in cytotoxicity studies and found that it killed B cells from normal individuals somewhat more efficiently than it killed T cells from those donors. Anti-Sa was almost as active as anti-I and more active than anti-i in killing B cells from patients with chronic lymphocytic leukemia. T-helper cells from such patients were also highly susceptible to the actions of anti-Sa. Dorken et al. (138) showed that similarly to Gd but unlike Pr_1, the Sa determinant is not cell-type associated in patients with leukemia.

The Antigen Fl (Sia-b1)

In 1981, Roelcke (139) described a new specificity cold agglutinin, to which he gave the name anti-Fl, in the serum of a 69 year-old woman who had an immunoblastoma. Other examples of the antibody, that reacts with untreated and protease-treated red cells, have since been found (114). The first example of anti-Fl reacted strongly (titer 2000) with I adult, weaker (titer 128) with i cord and weakest (titer <16) with i adult red cells. Thus, Fl (now Sia-b1) was clearly different from Pr, Gd and Sa, that are present in about the same amounts on red cells of all three Ii phenotypes. Anti-Fl closely resembled anti-I in its initial reactions but was shown to differ from that antibody when it was found (139) to be nonreactive with neuraminidase-treated red cells.

As discussed in Chapter 10, NeuAc, that is specifically cleaved by neuraminidase, plays no role in the structure of any Ii collection antigen. Biochemical characterization of the Fl (Sia-b1) determinant explained the serological findings. The antigen is present in membrane glycoproteins and glycolipids that carry I (126,140); its immunodominant carbohydrate is NeuAc. In other words, Fl, as with Gd, can be thought of as being on an I-bearing structure to which terminal NeuAcα (2→3) has been added. Unlike Gd, which is formed by sialylation of straight chain (i-active) and branched chain (I-active) glycolipids so is present on I adult and i adult red cells, Fl is formed only by sialylation of the branched chain I-active structures. This, of course, explains why anti-Fl closely resembles anti-I in its reactions with I adult, i adult and i cord cells. It also explains why Fl has been called Sia-b1 (first sialic acid-dependent antigen identified on branched chain glycolipids) and why Gd1 and Gd2 have been called Sia-lb1 and Sia-lb2 (first and second sialic acid-dependent antigens identified on linear and branched chain glycolipids) (109).

Many different glycolipids have been isolated from the red cell membrane. The one that carries the highest level of Fl (Sia-b1) has terminal NeuAcα(2→3) at the (1→3) branch and Fucα(1→2) at the (1→6) branch of the I-active branched structure (141). The NeuAc residue is essential for Fl antigen integrity (128) and the Fuc (fucose) residue is necessary for optimal binding of anti-Fl (141). Roelcke (54) reports that O_h (Bombay) red cells carry reduced levels of Fl (Sia-b1). The close similarities between the I-active branched structures (142) and Fl-active glycolipids (141) are thought perhaps to account for the presence of both anti-I and anti-Fl (anti-Sia-b1) in the sera of a number of patients (114,143,144).

The Antigen Lud

In 1981, Roelcke (145) reported yet another cold agglutinin with a specificity different from any previously described. He named the new antibody anti-Lud. Similarly to the Pr, Gd, Sa and Fl determinants but unlike those of the Ii antigen collection, Lud was denatured when red cells were treated with neuramindase. Unlike the Pr antigens that are not detectable on protease-treated red cells, or Gd and Fl that are unaffected by such treatment, Lud is partially denatured by proteases and in that respect resembles Sa. Anti-Lud differs from anti-Sa in that it reacts less strongly with cord blood red cells than with those of adults. It differs from anti-Fl in that it reacts about equally with the red cells of adults of the I and i phenotypes. Thus, in terms of strongest to weakest reactions, anti-Lud places red cells in the order I adult and i adult > i cord, while anti-Fl places them in the sequence I adult > i cord > i adult. Anti-Sa, of course, reacts about equally with red cells of all three phenotypes.

As discussed above, the Gd antigens (Sia-lb1 and Sia-lb2) are present on sialylated I- and i-bearing chains; Fl (Sia-b1) is on sialylated I-bearing chains and Vo and Li (see next section) are on sialylated i-bearing chains. Thus it is tempting to speculate that Lud may represent a sialylated form of the structure that carries an antigen originally called I^T (146-151). However, Pennington and Feizi (152) studied the agglutinating ability of type XIV pneumococcus antisera, that are somewhat similar to anti-Lud but do not require NeuAc in the structure(s) they recognize, and speculated that the antibodies might define a developmentally regulated increase of unsubstituted type 1 chains. Roelcke (17) suggests that the speculation could be taken one step further to propose that anti-Lud defines a structure on sialylated type 1 chains. This, at first, seems to negate the suggestion of a possible relationship between Lud and I^T. If the original interpretation (146,147) of I^T as a "transitional" step in the development of I from i is correct, I^T should be present on type 2, not type 1 chains. However, there are data (148,149 and see Chapter 10) that call into question such an interpretation. Thus, it seems possible that the antigen called I^T is actually carried on type 1 chains and is not truly related to the I and i of type 2 chains.

Kajii et al. (153) reported a second example of anti-Lud, this one in a patient with chronic CHD. The antibody was IgM with kappa light chains and was used, as an eluate, in an immunoblotting procedure against red cell membranes separated by SDS-PAGE. The anti-Lud reacted with a protein of molecular weight of about 43 kD. The requirement for NeuAc in the Lud determinant was confirmed when it was shown that anti-Lud failed to bind to membranes prepared from neuraminidase-treated red cells.

The Antigen Vo (Sia-l1)

Anti-Vo (now anti-Sia-l1) was described by Roelcke et al. (154) in 1984. The antibody, that caused CHD, was IgM with lambda light chains. The antigen defined is protease-resistant, NeuAc-dependent and is fully expressed only on i adult and i cord red cells. These findings explain, of course, why Vo is now called Sia-l1 (i.e., the first sialic acid-dependent antigen identified on linear glycolipids). Anti-Vo (anti-Sia-l1) initially resembles anti-i in serological studies but can be differentiated from that antibody in tests against protease and neuraminidase-treated red cells. The Vo (Sia-l1) antigen is not fully denatured when untreated red cells are treated with neuraminidase but total denaturation does occur when red cells are sequentially treated, first with a protease, then with neuraminidase (see also below).

The Antigen Li

In 1985, Roelcke (155) described anti-Li, another cold autoagglutinin that caused CHD. The reactions of anti-Li were similar to those of anti-Vo (anti-Sia-l1) in that anti-Li defined a protease-resistant, NeuAc-dependent determinant that was fully expressed only on i adult and i cord red cells. The Li determinant differed from Vo in that it was completely denatured when previously untreated red cells were treated with neuraminidase. The difference between the partial resistance of Vo (Sia-l1) to neuraminidase (see above) and lack of such resistance by Li, led Roelcke (17) to suggest that Li is probably carried on sialylated neolacto chains of common length while Vo (Sia-l1) may be restricted to shorter versions of such chains.

The Antigen Defined by the Antibody IgM^{woo}

Kabat et al. (156) described a human monoclonal IgM protein that complexed best with Galβ(1$\rightarrow$3) GlcNAcβ(1$\rightarrow$3)Galβ(1$\rightarrow$4)Glc and that was specific for Galβ(1$\rightarrow$3)GlcNAcβ(1$\rightarrow$3)Gal. Readers may recognize this structure as being part of the type 1 chain. The antibody, that recognized unsubstituted type 1 chains, did not react with type 2 chains that carry I and i. The antibody did not react with untreated or protease-treated human red cells but did react with such cells after they had been treated with neuraminidase. Picard et al. (157) then showed that IgM^{woo} is specific for type 1 chains but that its determinant on native chains is masked by NeuAc. In this latter study a hybridoma-produced monoclonal antibody, FC10.2, with apparently the same specificity as IgM^{woo}, was used. As blood group serologists will known, treatment of human red cells with neuraminidase exposes the T receptor so that the cells become polyagglutinable (see Chapter 42). That IgM^{woo} and FC10.2 were not anti-T was proved when it was shown (157) that both complex with the structure

Galβ(1$\rightarrow$3)GlcNAcβ(1$\rightarrow$3)Gal from type 1 chains but not with the structure Galβ(1$\rightarrow$3)GalNAc, that is the T receptor.

The patient who produced IgM^{woo} (156) had bronchogenic carcinoma and the monoclonal IgM was a Waldenstrom's macroglobulin.

The Antigen Me

In 1985, Salama et al. (158) named a new specificity cold-reactive autoagglutinin anti-Me because its reactions were enhanced in a test system to which human milk had been added (Me = milk enhanced). The name M^e had, of course, already been used (in 1961 (159)) for an MN system antigen (MN13, see Chapter 15). The Me defined by the cold-reactive autoagglutinin has no relationship to M^e of the MN system. The anti-Me described by Salama et al. (158) was an IgM cold agglutinin with kappa light chains, that caused CHD in a patient with Waldenstrom's macroglobulinemia. The antibody reacted equally well with the red cells of adults of the I phenotype and those of newborns. Since red cells of the i adult phenotype were not available for testing, HEMPAS cells, that are known (160,161) to have enhanced i, were used. The HEMPAS cells reacted similarly to those from I adults and newborns. Anti-Me was shown to differ from the cold agglutinins that define I, i, Pr, Gd, Sa, Lud, Fl, Vo and Li in part because of its equal reactions with the red cells of adults and newborns and in part because its reactions were enhanced in tests against protease and neuraminidase-treated red cells.

Anti-Me was unusual in a number of other respects. First, it had a high thermal range and was apparently able to activate complement at temperatures up to 40°C. Second, it was hemolytic in vitro and caused hemolysis of I adult and i cord red cells over a wide range from pH 5.0 to pH 9.0. Third, tests with added human milk from eight different women were performed since it is known (162) that such milk inhibits some examples of anti-I (see Chapter 10). Rather than causing inhibition, the addition of human milk markedly enhanced the reactivity of anti-Me. The enhancement was shown not to be due simply to the presence of glucose or galactose in the milk.

The Antigen Om

Anti-Om (163) was an IgM cold agglutinin with kappa light chains made by a 59 year-old man suffering from CHD. It differed from the antibodies that define I, i, Fl, Vo and Li in that it reacted equally with red cells from adults of the I phenotype and with those of newborns. It differed from the antibodies that define Pr, Gd,

Sa and Lud in that it gave enhanced reactions with protease and neuraminidase-treated red cells. In terms of previously recognized cold agglutinins, anti-Om was most like anti-Me. However, unlike anti-Me, anti-Om was markedly inhibited by human milk and by galactose. Thus, the antigen defined may be carried on a red cell membrane glycoplipid and may include galactose, but not NeuAc, in its immunodominant configuration.

The Antigen Ju

In 1990, Gottsche et al. (164) described a cold agglutinin in the serum of a 63 year-old man who had a one year history of mild CHD. The antibody was named anti-Ju after the patient and differed from the antibodies that define I, i, Fl, Vo and Li by reacting equally with red cells from adults and newborns. In titration studies, anti-Ju reacted equally with untreated, protease and neuraminidase-treated red cells at refrigerator temperatures. When the tests were done at 16° and 22°C, the antibody reacted best with untreated red cells, to lower titers with protease-treated and to its lowest titers with neuraminidase-treated red cells. Thus, Ju appeared to differ from Pr, Gd and Sa in being only partially denatured by neuraminidase. This conclusion was supported by the finding that neuraminidase-treated red cells were able, albeit slowly, to adsorb anti-Ju to exhaustion. Human milk and sialyllactose did not inhibit anti-Ju. Thus, anti-Ju differed from anti-Om, that is inhibited by human milk. Its difference from anti-Me was based on the fact that anti-Me gives enhanced reactions with neuraminidase-treated red cells.

A Brief Summary of the Antigens Pr, Gd1 (Sia-lb1), Gd2 (Sia-lb2), Sa, Fl (Sia-b1), Lud, Vo (Sia-l1), Li, IgM^woo, Me, Om and Ju

The reactions of the cold agglutinins described in this chapter thus far, at first appear to represent a bewildering array of specificities. However, Roelcke (17,55) has pointed out that there are certain recognizable interrelations between many of them. The antibodies that define the Pr and Sa determinants appear to recognize epitopes, carried within O-glycans, that are dependent on the presence of NeuAc for immunogenic structure. They differ in that the Pr determinants appear to be present only in the O-glycans of glycoproteins while the Sa determinants appear to be present in the O-glycans of both glycoproteins and glycolipids. Possible exceptions are Pr_a, Pr^M and (the putative) Pr^N. Indeed, Dahr (165) has expressed reservations about the propriety of including determinants that may include contributions from the

protein of glycophorins in their structure, with the Pr antigens.

The Gd, Fl, Lud, Vo and Li determinants appear to be glycolipid-borne. The I and i antigens are carried on lipid- and protein-linked branched and straight N-acetyl-lactosamine chains (see Chapter 10). These type 2 chains are the carrier molecules of ABH antigens; H specificity arises by fucosylation (see Chapter 8). An alternative substitution by sialylation may result in formation of the Gd, Fl, Vo and Li determinants. The specific sites (i.e., I-bearing, i-bearing or both) of the NeuAc-dependent antigens are discussed in the sections describing those antigens.

The Lud and IgM^woo determinants may be present on type 1 chains. Lud may be formed by the addition of NeuAc (sialylation) at specific sites on those chains. The determinant recognized by IgM^woo is known to be present but is apparently not accessible to its antibody until NeuAc is cleaved. Less can be said about the Me, Om and Ju antigens since little is known about them at the biochemical level. However, the determinants have some of the characteristics of glycolipid-borne antigens. The I and i determinants are found on both glycoproteins and glycolipids. While this chapter has stressed the probable glycolipid nature of the carriers of several of the other antigens, it should be borne in mind that future biochemical investigations may show the presence of copies of some of those antigens on glycoproteins as well.

To continue the summary, table 34-4 lists some of the serological characteristics of the antibodies that define these antigens and table 34-5 lists possible minimal structures of some of the determinants. Tables 34-4 and 34-5 perforce include some oversimplifications, the text about each determinant should be consulted for some data that cannot be included in tables. Table 34-6 lists some characteristics and possible membrane sites of the determinants.

A Note On Identifying Specificities of Cold-Reactive Autoantibodies

When an alloantibody to a high incidence blood group antigen is investigated, eventual recognition of its specificity usually involves tests of the antibody against antigen-negative red cells and recognition of the absence of a high-incidence antigen from the antibody-maker's red cells. When a "warm" autoantibody is investigated, resolution of the problem is more complex. The antibody-maker's red cells will be positive for the antigen that the autoantibody defines. However, even in this difficult circumstance it is sometimes possible (but by no means essential, see Chapters 37, 39 and 40) to determine specificity of the autoantibody. Some such antibodies have the same or similar specificities as alloantibodies and will fail

TABLE 34-4 Typical Reactions of Some Cold Agglutinins Described in This Chapter

Specificity	Test Red Cells				
	Unttd Adult I	Unttd Adult i	Unttd i cord	Prot-ttd	Nmdase-ttd
Anti-Gd1[*1] (Anti-Sia-lb1)	+	+	+	+	0
Anti-Gd2[*1] (Anti-Sia-lb2)	+	+	+	+	0
Anti-Sa	+	+	+	+↓	0
Anti-Fl (Anti-Sia-b1)	+	+↓↓	+↓	+	0
Anti-Lud	+	+	+↓	+↓	0
Anti-Vo (Anti-Sia-l1)	+↓↓	+	+	+	0[*2]
Anti-Li	+↓↓	+	+	+	0
IgM^woo	0	0	0	0	+
Anti-Me[*3]	+		+	+↑	+↑
Anti-Om[*4]	+		+	+↑	+↑
Anti-Ju[*5]	+		+	+	+

Legend to table 34-4

+ = Positive
0 = Negative
+↓ = Positive but weaker than +
+↓↓ = Positive but weaker than +↓
+↑ = Positive and stronger than +
Unttd = Untreated
Prot-ttd = Protease-treated
Nmdase-ttd = Neuraminidase-treated

[*1] Anti-Gd1 and anti-Gd2 differentiated by tests against ape and monkey red cells, see text.
[*2] Antigen denatured by neuraminidase only on red cells previously treated with a protease.
[*3] Antibody reactivity enhanced by human milk.
[*4] Antibody reactivity inhibited by human milk.
[*5] Tests at different temperatures show different enzyme sensitivity of antigen, see text.

to react with some red cell samples, e.g. Rh$_{null}$ or LW(a-b-) or Wr(b-), etc. In working with the cold autoagglutinins described in this chapter, similar aids to the recognition of specificity are not available. All the determinants described in this chapter are present on all red cells from humans. Accordingly, tests against enzyme (protease and neuraminidase) treated red cells, inhibition studies (using human milk, carbohydrates, etc.) and tests against animal red cells, must often be used. Even then assignment of specificity may not be possible without resorting to inhibition studies with purified carbohydrate complexes. Fortunately, at the clinical level, determination of the exact specificity of a cold-reactive autoagglutinin is not necessary to make a diagnosis of transient or chronic CHD, or to treat the patient. As discussed in more detail in Chapter 38, the thermal amplitude and strength of a cold autoagglutinin (the former more than the latter) are

correlated with the extent of CHD at the clinical level, autoantibody specificity is not. If transfusions must be given (they are not often necessary to correct the anemia of CHD) serologically incompatible blood must be used, there are no antigen-negative red cells (see Chapter 38 for use of a warming coil). Thus recognition of the nature of determinants recognized by cold-reactive autoagglutinins is of major importance for what it reveals about the structure of red cell membrane-borne glycolipids and glycoproteins. Hopefully such information will eventually lead to a better understanding of defects of the immune system that allow these antibodies to be made.

The Antigen Rx (formerly Sd^x)

The last named antigen to be described in this chap-

TABLE 34-5 Possible Minimal Structures for Some Determinants[*1]

Determinants	Possible Minimal Structures
Gd1 (Sia-lb1)	NeuAcα(2→3)....
Gd2 (Sia-lb2)	NeuAcα(2→3)Galβ1....(on glycoproteins) NeuAcα(2→3)Galβ(1→4)Glc....(on glycolipids)
Sa	NeuAcα(2→3)Galβ(1→4)Glc.... OR NeuAcα(2→3)Galβ(1→3)GalNAc....

Fl (Sia-b1)	NeuAcα(2→3)Galβ(1→4)GlcNAcβ1→3
	  ⟍
	   Galβ1....
	  ⟋
	Fucα(1→2)Galβ(1→4)GlcNAcβ1→6

Lud[*2]	NeuAcα(2→3)Galβ(1→3)GlcNAcβ1....
Vo[*2] (Sia-l1)	NeuAcα(2→3)Galβ(1→4)GlcNAcβ(1→3)....
Li[*2]	NeuAcα(2→3)Galβ(1→4)GlcNAcβ(1→3)....
IgM^woo[*3]	Galβ(1→3)GlcNAc....

Legend to table 34-5
NeuAc = N-acetylneuraminic acid (a sialic acid)
Gal = D-galactose
Glc = D-glucose
GalNAc = N-acetyl-D-galactosamine
GlcNAc = N-acetyl-D-glucosamine
Fuc = L-fucose

[*1] Minimal structures are shown. For additional structures necessary for optimal antibody binding and different linkages of minimal structures to glycoproteins and glycolipids, see text.
[*2] Postulated minimal structures.
[*3] Structure thought to be blocked by NeuAc on untreated red cells. IgM^woo did not react with Galβ(1→3)GalNAc, that is the T antigen.

ter is defined by an antibody that has characteristics somewhat different from those already described. In 1980, Marsh et al. (166) reported two examples of a complement-binding IgM autoagglutinin that reacted optimally at around 22°C. In one case the antibody clearly caused an acute but transient hemolytic episode; in the second case, in vivo destruction of red cells by the autoantibody seemed probable. The antibodies were unusual in two respects. First, they were more active over a temperature range of 12-22°C than at 4°C or 37°C. Second, the in vitro reactions of the antibodies were pH sensitive. Optimal reactions were seen in a saline system at pH 6.5; as the pH was raised, the antibodies lost activity and were only very weakly reactive at pH 8.0.

The antigen defined appeared to be present in about equal amounts on the red cells of adults of the I and i phe-notypes; it was less well developed on cord blood red cells. Unlike many other antigens described in this chapter, this one survived treatment of red cells with proteases and neuraminidase. In tests on 5000 samples from random donors, no nonreactive sample was found. The antibodies were partially inhibited by human saliva and milk and were strongly inhibited by urine from humans with Sd(a+) red cells and by urine from guinea pigs. No inhibition was seen with urine from persons with Sd(a-) red cells. The antibody was clearly not anti-Sd^a (see Chapter 31) since it reacted equally (in titrations) with Sd(a++) and Sd(a-) red cells, but appeared from the inhibition studies to have some sort of relationship to that antibody. Accordingly, the name anti-Sd^x was used.

After several other examples of this specificity had been studied (see below) the same investigators who first described the antibody showed (167) that it is not related to Sd^a at all. It was shown that in urine from Sd(a+) humans and from guinea pigs, there are charged molecules that had altered both the pH and salt concentration of the test system and had caused the antibody to become nonreactive. The urine from the Sd(a-) hospital patients had apparently not acted similarly. When urines from Sd(a+) persons were adjusted so that their conductivity was below the threshold at which nonspecific antibody inhibition occurred, they no longer had an inhibitory effect on the antibodies. In other words, inhibition of anti-Sd^x was not caused by presence of Sd^a on the T-H urinary glycoprotein (see Chapter 31) present in the urine of persons with Sd(a+) red cells.

The authors (167) renamed the antibody anti-Rx, after the first patient in whom it had been found. These observations illustrate that urine inhibition tests are not straightforward; the simple addition of urine to a sample can cause nonspecific inhibition of an antibody. A method suitable for the preparation of urine for use in inhibition studies is given by Judd (42,193).

There is no doubt that anti-Rx (described by its original name of anti-Sd^x in the early publications) can be a clinically important antibody. Later, in 1980, Marsh et al. (168) described four more cases of hemolytic anemia caused by the antibody; one of the patients died in an acute hemolytic episode. Among the first six patients in whom auto-anti-Rx was found (167,168) four had experienced a recent upper respiratory tract infection (URTI). Marsh et al. (168) wondered if a cause-and-effect relationship existed between URTI and the production of anti-Rx. An incomplete IgG anti-Rx that caused "warm" antibody-induced hemolytic anemia was described by Denegri et al. (169).

Unnamed Antigens Defined by Cold-Reactive Autoagglutinins

In spite of the numerous named antibodies

TABLE 34-6 Summary of Some Characteristics and Possible Sites of Determinants

Pr	NeuAc-dependent, protease-sensitive. Carried in O-linked tetra- and trisaccharides of at least glycophorins A and B. Pr_2 but not Pr_1 or Pr_3 also carried on glycolipids. May involve both $\alpha(2\rightarrow3)$ and $\alpha(2\rightarrow6)$ sialyl groups on glycophorins.
Gd (Sia-lb)	NeuAc-dependent, protease-resistant. Probably carried on both linear and branched Type 2 glycolipid chains. Gd1(Sia-lb1) is on human but not on ape and monkey red cells. Gd2 (Sia-lb2) is on human, ape and monkey red cells.
Sa	NeuAc-dependent, partially resistant to proteases. Carried in O-glycans (perhaps mainly trisaccharides) of glycophorins A and B (protease-sensitive) and on glycolipids (protease-resistant) that may not carry I or i.
Fl (Sia-b1)	NeuAc-dependent, protease-resistant. Probably carried on branched but not on linear, Type 2 glycolipids. Presence of fucose on the branched Type 2 glycolipid is necessary for antigen expression.
Lud	NeuAc-dependent, partially resistant to proteases. May be carried on Type 1 glycolipids that do not carry I or i. See text for a speculation that Lud may be related to I^T if that determinant is Type 1 chain-borne and not related to I and i.
Vo (Sia-l1)	NeuAc-dependent but neuraminidase cleaves NeuAc involved in Vo antigen structure only from red cells previously treated with a protease. Thus the NeuAc residues may not be accessible to neuraminidase on native red cells. Determinant is protease-resistant and present on linear but not on branched Type 2 glycolipids.
Li	NeuAc-dependent, protease-resistant. Present on linear but not on branched Type 2 glycolipids and apparently accessible to neuraminidase on native red cells.
IgM^{woo}	NeuAc-independent. May be present on Type 1 glycolipids and blocked by NeuAc on native red cells.
Me	NeuAc-independent, protease-resistant. May be glycolipid-borne.
Om	NeuAc-independent, protease-resistant. May be glycolipid-borne and may include galactose in its immunodominant structure.
Ju	Partially but not wholly NeuAc-dependent. Partially but not wholly protease resistant. Neuraminidase effects more denaturation of determinant than do proteases. May be glycolipid-borne with NeuAc contributing to tertiary structure (as reflected by antibody binding) but not being essential for antigen integrity.

described in this chapter it is possible that still more exist. There are a number of reports of cases in which such antibodies caused severe hemolytic anemia but were not identified in terms of known specificities. In rare cases, hemolytic anemia is seen to be caused by both IgM and IgG and/or both cold- and warm-reactive autoantibodies in the patient (150,170-176). Other papers give important information about CHD without necessarily naming the specificity of the causative autoantibody (177-182). While all sera contain relatively weak, polyclonal cold agglutinins with restricted thermal range and anti-I specificity (183,184), it is rare to find a high-titer cold agglutinin with a broad thermal range that is benign in vivo; one such antibody was described by Sniecinski et al. (185).

It is, of course, entirely possible that some of the unnamed cold agglutinins had one of the specificities described in this chapter but that the tests necessary for identification would have contributed nothing at the clinical level, so were not done. It is equally possible that some of the antibodies were studied before the specificities described herein were recognized and documented. A more sobering thought, that represents an equally plausible explanation, is that there remain new specificities, yet to be recognized and named.

References

1. Marsh WL, Jenkins WJ. Vox Sang 1968;15:177
2. Roelcke D, Dorrow W. Klin Wochenschr 1968;46:126
3. Bird GWG. (Letter). Vox Sang 1969;17:468
4. Roelcke D, Uhlenbruck G. (Letter). Vox Sang 1970;18:478
5. Marsh WL, Nichols ME. Vox Sang 1969;17:217
6. Roelcke D. Vox Sang 1969;16:76
7. Roelcke D, Uhlenbruck G. Z Immunforsch 1969;137:333
8. Roelcke D, Uhlenbruck G. Z Immunforsch 1969;138:273
9. Roelcke D, Uhlenbruck G. Z Med Mikrobiol Immunol 1969;155:156
10. Roelcke D, Uhlenbruck G, Bauer K. Scand J Haematol 1969;6:280
11. Roelcke D. Vox Sang 1973;24:354
12. Roelcke D, Ebert W, Geisen HP. Vox Sang 1976;30:122
13. Roelcke D. Clin Immunol Immunopathol 1974;2:266
14. Roelcke D, Ebert W, Anstee DJ. Vox Sang 1974;27:429
15. Geisen HP, Roelcke D, Rehn K, et al. Klin Wochenschr 1975;53:767
16. Roelcke D, Kreft H. Transfusion 1984;24:210
17. Roelcke D. Transf Med Rev 1989;3:140
18. Birgens HS, Dybkjaer E, Roelcke D. Scand J Haematol 1982;29:207
19. Roelcke D, Forbes IJ, Zalewski PD, et al. Blut 1982;45:109
20. Romer W, Seelig HP, Lenhard V, et al. Invest Cell Pathol 1979;2:157
21. Roelcke D, Anstee DJ, Jungfer H, et al. Vox Sang 1971;20:218

22. Mollison PL. Blood Transfusion in Clinical Medicine, 7th Ed. Oxford:Blackwell, 1983:322 and 448

23. Habibi B, Cregut R, Brossard Y, et al. Br J Haematol 1975;30:499

24. Roelcke D, Dahr W, Kalden JR. Vox Sang 1986;51:207

25. Bowes A. (abstract). Proc 8th Conf, Nat Blood Transf Serv (UK) 1976

26. Sangster JM, Kenwright MG, Walker MP, et al. J Clin Pathol 1979;32:154

27. Chapman J, Murphy MF, Waters AH. Vox Sang 1982;42:272

28. Boccardi V, Gaetano de G, Dolci G, et al. Haematol Lat 1962;5:191

29. Fletcher JL, Zmijewski CM. Int Arch Allgy App Immunol 1970;37:586

30. Tegoli J, Harris JP, Nichols ME, et al. Transfusion 1970;10:133

31. Howard PL, Picoff RC. Transfusion 1972;12:59

32. Hysell JK, Beck ML, Gray JM. Transfusion 1973;13:146

33. Lown JAG, Barr AL, Kelly A. Vox Sang 1980;38:301

34. Vale DR, Harris IM. Transfusion 1980;20:440

35. Branch DR, McBroom R, Jones GL. Blood Transf Immunohematol 1983;26:565

36. Combs MR, O'Rourke MM, Issitt PD, et al. Transfusion 1991;31:756

37. Chapman J, Murphy MF, Waters AH. (Letter). Transfusion 1992;32:391

38. Combs MR, Issitt PD, Telen MJ. (Letter). Transfusion 1992;32:391

39. Judd WJ, Steiner EA, Knafl P, et al. (abstract). Transfusion 1992;32 (Suppl 8S):22S

40. Hinz CF Jr, Boyer JT. New Eng J Med 1963;269:1329

41. Judd WJ, Issitt PD, Pavone BG. Transfusion 1979;19:7

42. Judd WJ. Methods in Immunohematology, 2nd Ed. Durham:Montgomery, 1994

43. Anstee DJ. In: Immunobiology of the Erythrocyte. New York:Liss, 1980:67

44. McGinniss MH, Wasniowska K, Dopf DA, et al. Transfusion 1985;25:131

45. Tokunaga E, Sasakawa S, Tamaka K, et al. J Immunogenet 1979;6:383

46. Macris NT, Capra JD, Frankel GJ, et al. Am J Med 1970;48:524

47. Seligmann M, Brouet JC. Sem Hematol 1973;10:163

48. Pruzanski W, Cowan DH, Parr DM. Clin Immunol Immunopathol 1974;2:234

49. Feizi T. Science 1976;156:1111

50. Isbister JP, Cooper DA, Blake HM, et al. Am J Med 1978;64:434

51. Kuenn JW, Weber R, Teague PO, et al. Cancer 1978;42:1826

52. Lee CH, Cherian R, Hughes WG, et al. Austral NZ J Med 1979;9:602

53. Pascali E, Pezzoli A, Melato M, et al. Acta Haematol 1980;64:94

54. Roelcke D. Unpublished observations cited in Roelcke D. Transf Med Rev 1989;3:140

55. Roelcke D. In: Immunobiology of Transfusion Medicine. New York:Marcel Dekker, 1994:69

56. Dellagi K, Brouet JC, Schenmetzler C, et al. Blood 1981;57:189

57. Northoff H, Martin A, Roelcke D. Eur J Haematol 1987;38:85

58. Curtis BR, Lamon J, Roelcke D, et al. Transfusion 1990;30:838

59. Green ED, Curtis BR, Issitt PD, et al. Transfusion 1990;30:267

60. Beck ML. In: Blood Groups: Refresher and Update. Bethesda:Am Assoc Blood Banks, 1995:18

61. Angevine CD, Anderson BR, Barnett EV. J Immunol 1966;96:578

62. Garratty G, Petz LD, Brodsky I, et al. Vox Sang 1973;25:32

63. Roelcke D. Eur J Immunol 1973;3:206

64. Tonthat H, Rochant H, Henry A, et al. Vox Sang 1976;30:464

65. Roelcke D, Hack H, Kreft H, et al. Transfusion 1993;33:472

66. Levine P, Celano MJ, Falkowski F. Transfusion 1963;3:278

67. Knapp T. Canad J Med Technol 1964;26:172

68. Wolach B, Heddle N, Barr RD, et al. Br J Haematol 1981;48:425

69. Judd WJ, Wilkinson SL, Issitt PD, et al. Transfusion 1986;26:423

70. Bell CA, Zwicker H, Spira S, et al. Vox Sang 1973;25:271

71. Ratkin GA, Osterland CK, Chaplin H Jr, et al. J Lab Clin Med 1978;82:67

72. Brunt DJ, Vengelen-Tyler V. (abstract). Transfusion 1981;21:615

73. O'Neill P, Shulman IA, Simpson RB, et al. Vox Sang 1986;50:107

74. Garratty G, O'Neill P. Unpublished observations 1986 cited in O'Neill P, Shulman IA, Simpson RB, et al. Vox Sang 1986;50:107

75. Issitt PD. Applied Blood Group Serology, 3rd Ed. Miami:Montgomery, 1985:451

76. Homberg J, Krulick M, Habibi B, et al. Nouv Rev Fr Hematol 1971;11:489

77. Rose VL, Kwaan HC. Am J Hematol 1985;19:419

78. Silberstein LE, Robertson GA, Hannam Harris AC, et al. Blood 1986;67:1705

79. Pruzanski W, Roelcke D, Armstrong M, et al. Clin Immunol Immunopathol 1980;15:631

80. Hsu TCS, Rosenfield RE, Burkart P, et al. Vox Sang 1974;26:305

81. Tschirhart D, Kunkel L, Shulman IA. Vox Sang 1990;59:222

82. Feizi T, Kunkel HG, Roelcke D. Clin Exp Immunol 1974;18:283

83. Lecomte J, Feizi T. Clin Exp Immunol 1975;20:287

84. Kohler G, Milstein C. Nature 1975;256:495

85. Steinitz M, Klein G, Koskimies S, et al. Nature 1977;269:420

86. Evans SW, Feizi T, Childs R, et al. Mol Immunol 1983;20:1127

87. Stevenson FK, Wrightham M, Glennie MJ, et al. Blood 1986;68:430

88. Pfreudschuh M, Dorken B, Roelcke D, et al. Blut 1983;46:111

89. Romer W, Roelcke D, Rautenberg E. Immunobiology 1983;164:380

90. Jefferies LC, Stevenson FK, Goldman J, et al. Transfusion 1990;30:495

91. Silberstein LE, Goldman J, Kant JA, et al. Arch Biochem Biophys 1988;264:244

92. Miller RA, Maloney DG, Warnke R, et al. New Eng J Med 1982;306:517

93. Thielemans K, Maloney DG, Meeker T, et al. J Immunol 1984;133:495

94. Meeker TC, Lowder J, Maloney DG, et al. Blood 1985;65:1349

95. Harboe M, Furth van R, Schubothe H, et al. Scand J Haematol 1965;2:259

96. König A, Börner CH, Braun RW, et al. (abstract). Immunobiology 1985;170:46

97. Ochiai Y, Furthmayr H, Marcus DM. J Immunol 1983;131:864

98. Anstee DJ, Edwards PAW. Eur J Immunol 1982;12:228

99.   Anstee DJ. In: Red Cell Membrane Glycoconjugates and Related Genetic Markers. Paris:Arnette, 1983:37

100. Romer W, Rother U, Roelcke D. Immunobiology 1980;157:41

101. Fanger MW, Goldstine SN, Shen L. Mol Immunol 1983;20:1019

102. Gauldie J, Richards C, Lamontagne L. Mol Immunol 1983;20:1029

103. Shen L, Maliszewski CR, Rigby WFC, et al. Mol Immunol 1986;23:611

104. Maliszewski CR, March CJ, Schoenborn MA, et al. J Exp Med 1990;172:1665

105. Yeaman GR, Kerr MA. Clin Exp Immunol 1987;68:200

106. Salama A, Gottsche B, Viadya V, et al. Vox Sang 1988;55:21

107. Salama A, Mueller-Eckhardt C. Br J Haematol 1987;65:67

108. Salama A, Bhakdi S, Mueller-Eckhardt C. Transfusion 1987;27:49

109. Roelcke D, Hengge U, Kirschfink N. Vox Sang 1990;59:235

110. Roelcke D, Riesen W, Geisen HP, et al. Vox Sang 1977;33:304

111. Weber RJ, Clem LW. J Immunol 1981;127:300

112. Staub CA. Transfusion 1985;24:414

113. Pruzanski W, Roelcke D, Donnelly E, et al. Acta Haematol 1986;75:171

114. König AL, Kreft H, Hengge U, et al. Vox Sang 1988;55:176

115. Roelcke D, Brossmer R. Prot Biol Fluids 1984;31:1075

116. Feizi T, Taylor-Robinson D, Shields MD, et al. Nature 1969;222:1253

117. Costea N, Yakulis VJ, Heller P. Proc Soc Exp Biol Med 1972;139:476

118. Lind K. Acta Path Microbiol Immunol Scand (B) 1973;81:487

119. Feizi T. Med Biol 1980;58:123

120. Tardieu M, Epstein RL, Weiner HL. Int Rev Cytol 1982;80:27

121. Loomes LM, Uemura K, Childs RA, et al. Nature 1984;307:560

122. Feizi T, Gooi HC, Loomes LM, et al. Biosci Rep 1984;4:743

123. Loomes LM, Uemura K, Feizi T. Infec Immun 1985;47:15

124. Roelcke D, Pruzanski W, Ebert W, et al. Blood 1980;55:677

125. Roelcke D, Brossmer R, Riesen W. Scand J Immunol 1978;8:179

126. Roelcke D, Brossmer R, Ebert W. Prot Biol Fluids 1981;29:619

127. Kundu SK, Marcus DM, Roelcke D. Immunol Lett 1982;4:263

128. Uemura K, Roelcke D, Nagai Y, et al. Biochem J 1984;219:865

129. Beck ML, Korth J, Judd WJ. (abstract). Transfusion 1992;32 (Suppl 8S):17S

130. Engelfriet CP, Beckers D, von dem Borne AEGKr, et al. Vox Sang 1972;23:176

131. Metaxas MN, Metaxas-Bühler M, Tippett PA. (abstract). Book of Abstracts. 14th Cong ISBT 1975:95

132. Issitt CH, Duckett JB, Osborne BM, et al. Br J Haematol 1976;34:19

133. Schwarting GA, Marcus DM, Metaxas M. Vox Sang 1977;32:257

134. Roelcke D. Vox Sang 1984;46:161

135. Dahr W, Lichthardt D, Roelcke D. Prot Biol Fluids 1981;29:365

136. Lisowska E, Duk M, Dahr W. Carbohydr Res 1980;79:103

137. Pruzanski W, Armstrong M, Roelcke D. Blut 1981;43:307

138. Dorken B, Roelcke D, Bohn B, et al. Prot Biol Fluids 1981;29:623

139. Roelcke D. Vox Sang 1981;41:98

140. Ebert W, Roelcke D, Weicker H. Eur J Biochem 1975;53:505

141. Kannagi R, Roelcke D, Peterson KA, et al. Carbohydr Res 1983;120:143

142. Feizi T, Childs RA, Watanabe K, et al. J Exp Med 1979;149:975

143. König AL, Kather H, Roelcke D. Blut 1984;49:363

144. Roelcke D, Weber MT. Vox Sang 1984;47:122

145. Roelcke D. Vox Sang 1981;41:316

146. Booth PB, Jenkins WJ, Marsh WL, Br J Haematol 1966;12:341

147. Booth PB. Vox Sang 1972;22:64

148. Garratty G, Hafleigh EB, Dalziel J, et al. Transfusion 1972;12:325

149. Garratty G, Petz LD, Wallerstein RD, et al. Transfusion 1974;14:226

150. Freedman J, Newlands M, Johnson CA. Vox Sang 1977;32:135

151. Hafleigh EB, Wells RF, Grumet FC. Transfusion 1978;18:592

152. Pennington J, Feizi T. Vox Sang 1982;43:253

153. Kajii E, Ikemoto S, Miura Y. (Letter). Vox Sang 1988;54:248

154. Roelcke D, Kreft H, Pfister AM. Vox Sang 1984;47:236

155. Roelcke D. Vox Sang 1985;48:181

156. Kabat EA, Liao J, Shyong J, et al. J Immunol 1982;128:540

157. Picard JK, Loveday D, Feizi T. Vox Sang 1985;48:26

158. Salama A, Pralle H, Mueller-Eckhardt C. Vox Sang 1985;49:277

159. Wiener AS, Rosenfield RE. J Immunol 1961;87:376

160. Crookston JH, Crookston MC, Burnie KL, et al. Br J Haematol 1969;17:11

161. Crookston JH, Crookston MC. In: Blood Groups and Other Red Cell Surface Markers in Health and Disease. New York:Masson, 1982:29

162. Marsh WL, Nichols ME, Allen FH Jr. Vox Sang 1970;18:149

163. Kajii E, Ikemoto S. Vox Sang 1989;56:104

164. Gottsche B, Salama A, Mueller-Eckhardt C. Transfusion 1990;30:261

165. Dahr W. In: Recent Advances in Blood Group Biochemistry. Arlington, VA:Am Assoc Blood Banks, 1986:23

166. Marsh WL, Johnson CL, Øyen R, et al. Transfusion 1980;20:1

167. Bass LS, Rao AH, Goldstein J, et al. Vox Sang 1983;44:191

168. Marsh WL, Johnson CL, DiNapoli J, et al. (abstract). Transfusion 1980;20:647

169. Denegri JF, Nanji AA, Sinclair M, et al. Acta Haematol 1983;69:19

170. Moore JA, Chaplin H Jr. Vox Sang 1973;24:236

171. Crookston JH. Arch Int Med 1975;135:1314

172. Freedman J, Newlands M. Vox Sang 1977;32:61

173. Sokol RJ, Hewitt S, Stamps BK. Br Med J 1981;1:2023

174. Sokol RJ, Hewitt S, Stamps BK. Acta Haematol 1983;69:266

175. Shulman IA, Branch DR, Nelson JM, et al. J Am Med Assoc 1985;253:1746

176. Silberstein LE, Shoenfeld Y, Schwartz RS, et al. Vox Sang 1985;48:105

177. Wortmann J, Rosse W, Logue G. Am J Hematol 1979;6:275

178. Crisp D, Pruzanski W. Am J Med 1982;72:915

179. Pruzanski W, Katz A. Clin Immunol Rev 1984;3:131

180. Sandhaus LM, Raska K, Wu HV. Am J Clin Pathol 1986;86:120

181. Silberstein LE, Berkman EM, Schreiber AD. Ann Int Med 1987;106:238

182. Pruzanski W, Jacobs H, Saito S, et al. Am J Hematol 1987;26:167

183. Jackson VA, Issitt PD, Francis BJ, et al. Vox Sang 1968;15:133

184. Issitt PD, Jackson VA. Vox Sang 1968;15:152

185. Sniecinski I, Margolin K, Shulman I, et al. Vox Sang 1988;55:26

186. Beck ML, Kowalski MA, Kirkegaard J, et al. (Letter). Immunohematology 1992;8:22
187. Beck ML, Kirkegaard J, Korth J, et al. (Letter). Transfusion 1993;33:623
188. Beck ML, Korth J, Kirkegaard J, et al. (Letter). Transfusion 1993;33:624
189. Garratty G, Arndt P, Co S, et al. (abstract). Transfusion 1993;33 (Suppl 9S):47S
190. Spruell P, Chen J, Cullen K. (abstract). Transfusion 1994;34 (Suppl 10S):22S
191. Kennedy MS, Waheed A, Moore J. (abstract). Transfusion 1994;34 (Suppl 10S):23S
192. Kirkegaard JR, Coon M, Beck ML. (Letter). Immunohematology 1995;11:9
193. Judd WJ. (Letter). Transfusion 1983;23:404
194. Kewitz S, Grob HJ, Kosa R, et al. Glycocon J 1995;12:714
195. Roelcke D, Kreft H, Hack H, et al. Vox Sang 1994;67:216
196. Herron B, Roelcke D, Orson G, et al. Vox Sang 1993;65:239
197. König AL, Keller HE, Braun RW, et al. Ann Hematol 1992;64:277
198. Herron B, Willison HJ, Veitch J, et al. Vox Sang 1994;67:58
199. Ebert W, Metz J, Weicker H, et al. Hoppe-Seyler's Z Physiol Chem 1971;352:1309
200. Roelcke D, Ebert W, Metz J, et al. Vox Sang 1971;21:352
201. Thomas DB, Winzler RJ. J Biol Chem 1969;244:5493
202. Adamany AM, Kathan RH. Biochem Biophys Res Comm 1969;37:171
203. Dahr W. Unpublished observations cited in Roelcke D. Transf Med Rev 1989;3:140
204. Ebert W, Fey J, Gartner CH, et al. Mol Immunol 1979;16:413
205. Suttajit M, Winzler RJ. J Biol Chem 1971;246:3398
206. Hoare DG, Koshland DE. J Biol Chem 1967;242:2447
207. Ebert W, Metz J, Roelcke D. Eur J Biochem 1972;27:470
208. Lisowska E, Roelcke D. Blut 1973;26:339
209. Tsai CM, Zopf DA, Wistar R Jr, et al. J Immunol 1976;117:717
210. Wilkinson SL, Issitt PD. Unpublished observations 1979 cited in Issitt PD. The MN Blood Group System. Cincinnati:Montgomery, 1981:206
211. Ambrus M, Bajtai G. Haematologia 1969;3:225
212. Roelcke D, Ebert W, Feizi T. Immunology 1974;27:879

35 | Antibody Detection and Identification and Compatibility Testing

The transfusion requirements of the vast majority of patients who need red cells could be met by supplying donor blood of the same ABO and D type as the patient. ABO-type identical or major side compatible blood (i.e. group A patient, group A or group O donor) is necessary because of the near-universal presence of ABO antibodies (see Chapter 8). Patients with D- red cells are normally given D- blood because of the high immunogenicity of D; patients with D+ red cells can be given D+ or D- blood (see Chapter 12). Although there are many additional red cells antigens (see Chapter 44) they can be ignored in most transfusions because relatively few people have serum antibodies directed against any of them.

The Incidence of Alloimmunization to Red Cell Blood Group Antigens

It should be noted that alloimmunization, as used in this chapter, refers only to the production of alloimmune antibodies to red cell blood group antigens. In fact, alloimmunization to antigens present on platelets and leukocytes, following the transfusion of allogeneic blood and as a result of pregnancy, is probably more common that alloimmunization to red cell blood group antigens but is beyond the scope of this chapter.

It is difficult to determine the actual rate of alloimmunization to red cell blood group antigens. Most attempts to determine the incidence have involved tests on samples from large numbers of patients admitted to hospital, in whom transfusion was considered a future possibility (i.e. tests on all samples submitted to the transfusion service). Such surveys suffer a number of disadvantages. First, the patients represent a highly heterogeneous population. That is, some have been transfused and pregnant, some pregnant but not transfused, and some have been neither transfused nor pregnant. Second, the patients include a few, such as those with sickle cell disease, thalassemia, etc., who have received multiple transfusions. There is evidence (see below) that the incidence of alloimmunization is much higher in such patients than in those who have received few or no transfusions. Third, the number of antibodies detected is directly related to the sensitivity of the antibody screening method used. There is no doubt that in 1996 a higher percentage of patients will be found to have red cell alloantibodies than was the case, say in 1966. Fourth, many patients who will make alloantibodies do so after their first series of transfusions. Since for many patients transfusion is a one time event, they will not be included in surveys of the type being described. There seems little doubt that if follow-up studies, i.e. tests on samples collected six months after transfusion, were performed on all patients who had been transfused, the incidence of alloimmunization caused by transfusion would be seen to be higher than the current numbers suggest. Fifth, if blood donors are included in the surveys, the incidence of alloimmunization will appear to be very low. Most such donors will not have been transfused and although a sizable number of them will have been pregnant, it is abundantly clear that alloimmunization (to red cell antigens) occurs far less frequently following pregnancy than following transfusion. Sixth, some surveys have counted all red cell antibodies detected, some only those antibodies considered to be red cell stimulated and still others, only those antibodies considered (on the basis of specificity) to be of potential clinical significance.

In spite of these difficulties and because there are few other data, the incidence of alloimmunization is usually calculated from the results of such surveys (1-12) nine of which were conducted more than 20 years ago. The figures most often cited are that between 0.5 and 1.5% of patients on whom antibody screening tests are performed, have antibodies to red cells in the serum.

Somewhat more recently Walker et al. (13) performed a retrospective analysis on samples tested in the blood transfusion service of a community hospital during an 18 year period (1970-1987). It was estimated that during the study period there were approximately 37,000 admissions, 5500 deliveries and 1000 blood donations each year. A breakdown of the samples tested indicated that approximately: 53% were from medical and surgical inpatients; 20% from obstetrics patients; 11% from patients to be admitted; 10% from patients in the emergency room; 4% from blood donors; and 2% from patients who would receive transfusions as outpatients. The antibody screening tests were designed to detect only warm (37°C) reactive antibodies. During the period 1970 to 1979 a saline-albumin enhanced IAT that started with a 67:1 serum:cell ratio was used. From 1980 onwards the method involved a LISS:IAT that started with a 100:1 serum:cell ratio. The survey concentrated on the incidence of newly formed antibodies, that were active at 37°C and were considered potentially to be of clinical significance. Such antibodies were found in the sera of 0.8% of patients (circa 1% if samples from blood donors were excluded from the calculation). The 0.8% or 1% number is probably higher than the 0.5 to 1.5% figure mentioned above since that figure may include all antibodies detected. Walker et al. (13) excluded 704 anti-Le[a], 284 anti-Le[b], 147 anti-Le[x], 18 anti-Lu[a] and 24 other antibodies of various specificities from their calculations because they correctly determined that those antibodies were of no clinical significance. Hoeltge et al. (14) performed a similar retrospective analysis on samples tested in the transfusion service of a tertiary care institution. The period covered was 1985 to 1993 and the method used for antibody screening was albumin/IAT read with polyspecific antiglobulin serum and used three red cell samples. Among 159,262 patients, 6996 antibodies were identified in the sera of 4700 patients. Thus it appeared that close to 3% of all patients studied were alloimmunized. However, there were some differences in the studies of Walker et al. (13) and Hoeltge et al. (14). As described, in the former study (13) only antibodies of potential clinical significance were considered in the calculations. Hoeltge et al. (14) report that they considered 4234 (the number 4235 is used in the abstract) of the 6996 antibodies detected to be of potential clinical significance. However, their list of 4234 potentially significant antibodies includes: 311 anti-Le[a]; 148 anti-P$_1$; 132 anti-Le[b]; 118 anti-M; 70 anti-A$_1$; 31 anti-N; and 14 miscellaneous antibodies including anti-Ch and anti-Sl[a]. If these antibodies are subtracted from the 4234 said to have clinical significance, so that the findings of Hoeltge et al. (14) can be compared with those of Walker et al. (13) it can be seen that of the 6996 antibodies found in the latter study (14) only about half are comparable with those found by Walker et al. (13). Although the 6996 antibodies were found in 4700 patients (14) the number of different patients making the 4234 antibodies considered by the authors to be of clinical significance, is not given. Nevertheless if the total incidence of alloimmunization was 3% (4700 of 159,262 patients) and half those antibodies were similar to those considered by Walker et al. (13) potentially to have clinical significance, the alloimmunization rates were probably not very different, i.e. circa 1% in the study of Walker et al. (13) circa 1.5% in the study of Hoeltge et al. (14). Another study was reported by Heddle et al. (244) in 1995, the data were collected during an evaluation of compatibility testing protocols that was described (245) in 1992. A total of 2490 patients were transfused 11,218 units of red cells, for follow-up one or more samples from the patient were tested for the presence of antibody within 7 days of transfusion. Among 2404 patients who had no antibody present at the time of transfusion, 2003 were followed, 51 of them (2.5%) became immunized. While this number appears to be higher than the 1 to 1.5% figures cited above, the list of antibodies detected

shows that all specificities were counted. If antibodies to A$_1$, I, Le[a], P$_1$, M, Lu[a], Sd[a], Yk[a] and Bg are excluded it is seen that some 60% of the antibodies detected had specificities such that most workers would regard them as having potential clinical significance. In other words, 60% of 51 antibodies in 2003 patients indicates an immunization rate of 1.5%. However, the study (244) was designed to detect posttransfusion alloimmunization in patients in whom the transfused red cells were still in the circulation and evaluate the role of such antibodies in causing delayed hemolytic and delayed serological (246 and see Chapter 36) transfusion reactions. No doubt the total rate of posttransfusion alloimmunization was higher than that detectable within 7 days of transfusion. Among the 86 patients in the study (244) who were alloimmunized before transfusion, 79 could be followed. Among those 79 patients, 7 (8.9%) made an additional antibody following the transfusions studied. As mentioned in many other places in this book, a patient who makes one antibody to a red cell antigen has a high likelihood of making others.

Thus based on the results of the many studies cited earlier (1-12) and the three more recent ones (13,14,244) it seems reasonable to conclude that among a general hospital population, some 1 to 1.5% of patients will present with one or more clinically significant antibodies in the serum while about an equal number will be seen to have non-red cell immune (naturally-occurring) antibodies.

The incidence of alloantibodies in healthy blood donors is very much lower than the incidence of such antibodies in hospital patients. In tests on samples from more than 200,000 blood donors in Seattle, between 1971 and 1975, Giblett (10) found that only 0.22% contained unexpected red cell alloantibodies. In London, in 1988, the incidence of unexpected alloantibodies in blood donors was 0.25% in 36,000 tested, in 1990 it was 0.16% in 35,000 tested (15).

Just as the incidence of alloimmunization in blood donors is lower than that in hospital patients, it is higher in patients who have received multiple transfusions. Many investigators (16-26) have studied patients with sickle cell disease who have received multiple transfusions. Immunization rates have varied from a low of 6% (22) to a high of over 35% (16,25) with an average of about 18%. In the largest study reported (26) the alloimmunization rate was 18.6%. Luban and Posey (18) studied the production of alloantibodies in multiply transfused patients with sickle cell disease. They reported that Blacks with one or both parents born outside the USA were more likely to form alloantibodies than those born to American Blacks. Perhaps this extraordinary observation represented chance since the number of patients in the non-American series was small. In some other disorders treated with multiple transfusions the alloimmunization rates have not been as high as in SSD, although they were still higher than the 1 to 1.5% incidence seen in general hospital patients. In four studies (17,27-29) on patients with thalassemia major, the incidence of alloimmunization varied from 2.7% (28) to 10% (17), in all, 85 of 1668 patients were alloimmunized for an average rate of 5.1%. In other reports, patients undergoing open heart surgery (30), some with chronic renal disease (31), some recipients of transplants and/or multiple platelet transfusions (32), and some with various other disorders (20), all of whom had received multiple transfusions, have been described. The rates of alloimmunization were similar in the various groups studied and ranged from 7% in patients with chronic renal disease (31) to 10% in those undergoing open heart surgery (30) at a time that far more blood was transfused than is now the case. In all, in the four series (20,30-32), 189 of 2167 (8.7%) of the patients were alloimmunized.

In several studies (16,22,24,26) it has been noticed that the rate of alloimmunization is directly proportional to the number of units transfused up to about 15-20 units. In other words, while alloimmunization rates increase during early transfusions, most patients who will make antibodies will have made at least the first one by the time they have received 15 to 20 units (20,22). Although it is customary to talk about alloimmunization rates in multiply transfused patients in terms of number of units given, it might perhaps be more accurate to speak of transfusion episodes. That is to say, patients given one unit of blood every month for 20 months (as in some with thalassemia major) are rather more likely to become alloimmunized than those given 20 units of blood in a period of hours during surgery or following trauma. The difference clearly relates to stimulation of primary and secondary immune responses (see Chapter 2) and the length of time that the transfused red cells remain in the recipient's circulation. In some other studies (17,20,27,31,210) the direct relationship between number of units transfused and the incidence of alloimmunization, was not seen. Some of those studies involved patients other than those with sickle cell disease or thalassemia. The rapid cessation of production of antibodies at a serologically detectable level, that is such a common feature in patients with sickle cell disease, is discussed below in the section on patients' records.

As also discussed in Chapter 2, some individuals are good responders to red cell blood group antigens (33-35). Blood bankers will already know that when such individuals receive multiple transfusions, they make multiple antibodies. Clearly the genetic ability to make antibodies and the role of the spleen in concentrating antigens of low immunogenicity (36) play major roles in such events. A contributing factor that is sometimes overlooked was demonstrated by Byrne and Howard (37). As

an example, when a patient with sickle cell disease forms say anti-C, anti-E and anti-Fy^a, blood selected for further transfusions will have to be C-, E-, Fy(a-). If the patient is D+ then C-, E-, Fy(a-) units from D+ donors should be used so as not to deplete the supply of D- blood. Most donors with the appropriate phenotype, i.e. R$_o$, Fy(a-) will be Black. Thus the patient transfused repeatedly with such blood will be exposed to the V, VS and Js^a antigens much more often than would be the case if random units were transfused. As a result antibodies to V, VS and Js^a are much more likely to be made (26,37).

A Note About Anti-D

Before the introduction of Rh immune globulin (RhIG) for the prevention of immunization to D during and following pregnancy, anti-D was by far the most commonly encountered immune antibody to a red cell antigen (1-6). Once RhIG became widely used, it was anticipated that the incidence of anti-D would decrease dramatically. Indeed under certain circumstances such a decrease can be seen. In tests on samples from about 21,000 patients in 1956 and 1957, Giblett (10) found that among 231 sera that contained antibodies, 162 (70%) were, or contained, anti-D. In similar tests on samples from about 43,000 patients, performed in 1974 and 1975 after RhIG had been introduced, among 704 sera that contained antibodies, 225 (32%) were, or contained, anti-D. In other words, although the incidence of patients found to have antibodies had increased from 1.1% in 1956-1957, to 1.6% in 1974-1975, the incidence of anti-D had dropped more than half. Tests on blood donor samples show a similar trend. Among 213,254 donors tested in Seattle in 1971, 1973 and 1975 (10) a time at which RhIG was already in use, the incidence of anti-D was 1 in 460 donors. In tests on 35,000 donors in London in 1990 (15) the incidence of anti-D was 1 in 636 donors. Clearly as more female donors who delivered infants before RhIG was available leave the donor pool and are replaced by D- women who were protected with RhIG, the incidence of the antibody will continue to fall. If studies on pregnant women are considered, the decrease in incidence of anti-D is even more dramatic. Before the introduction of RhIG, anti-D was found in approximately 1 in 170 pregnant White women in the US (38) and in England (39,40). In one survey in the US in 1988 the incidence had dropped to 1 in 963 (41) but was still 1 in 497 in one region in England (42).

Because of findings such as those described in the previous section, some workers have assumed that anti-D is no longer the most frequently encountered immune antibody to a red cell antigen. For workers testing only prenatal samples in a community in which adherence to the use of RhIG is good, that assumption will be seen to be correct. In some other circumstances exactly the reverse is true. As mentioned in Chapter 12, a procedure used to treat advanced breast cancer at Duke University Medical Center is to use high dose chemotherapy or irradiation to attempt to kill the tumor. Since the treatment causes total marrow ablation, bone marrow is collected before treatment begins and is used to reconstitute the marrow by autologous transplant once the chemotherapy or irradiation is completed. During the period between reinfusion of the marrow and hematological reconstitution, transfusion support, particularly with platelets, is required. The supply of platelets from D- donors is too small to enable all D- women on the regimen to be supported with such platelets. Accordingly, platelets from D+ donors are used. Such platelet preparations contain enough red cells that when platelet transfusions are given on a regular basis they constitute efficient stimuli for production of anti-D. Since the patients involved are either beyond child-bearing age or unlikely to become pregnant following irradiation, no attempts are made to prevent immunization to D with RhIG. Production of anti-D by these patients is not contraindicated for the usual reasons. The practice results in anti-D still being the most commonly encountered, newly formed immune red cell antibody in our service, we (43) see more examples now than were encountered before RhIG was introduced.

A Note About Anti-E

When surveys on the incidence of red cell antibodies are conducted, anti-E is always high on the list of number of examples found. In the study of Rosse et al. (26) it was the commonest specificity found. In the study of Hoeltge et al. (14) it was in second place, behind anti-K and ahead of anti-D, in the study of Walker et al. (13) it was in third place behind anti-D and anti-K. One of us (PDI) has noticed that when antibodies reactive by one technique but not by others are studied, anti-E figures prominently among those found. However, there are reasons to believe that many, perhaps a majority, of anti-E are not produced following exposure of the antibodymaker to foreign red cells. Several investigators (6,44-47) noted early that anti-E was often present in the sera of individuals with no known exposure to foreign red cells. Further, when we conducted retrospective tests (48) on the pretransfusion sera of patients who had already been transfused, we found 23 examples of anti-E that reacted in an IAT using ficin-treated red cells, that had not reacted by LISS/IAT in the original pretransfusion tests. Most examples of the 23 anti-E were also shown retrospectively to react by PEG/IAT or Polybrene IAT. Among the 23 patents, 17 had been transfused with

up to four units of E+ blood. None of those 17 patients showed any evidence of immediate or delayed transfusion reactions. Among the 17 patients who had received E+ blood, two showed an increase in anti-E level when studied later. However, among the six patients who had, by chance, received only E- blood, two also showed a post-transfusion increase in anti-E level. In other words, there was no evidence that the transfusion of E+ blood caused a secondary immune response in any of the patients. These findings, of course, argue strongly against the possibility that any of the 23 anti-E were red cell stimulated in origin. We (48) would like to believe, but cannot prove, that the antibodies were made against an immunogen other than E but have limited ability to cross-react with E. Certainly the finding that the transfusion of E+ red cells did not provoke any secondary immune responses suggests that the original immunogen was not red cell E antigen. Similar to the anti-E that we (48) found, Contreras (49) noted that among the antibodies found in blood donors in the 1988 and 1990 studies (15), about 30% had anti-E specificity.

The moral of this story seems to be that while anti-E is nearly always close to the top of lists of antibodies thought to be immune in nature and of probable clinical significance, when antibody-screening tests on patients and donors are reported, it is often (perhaps most often) there under false pretenses. At the level of practical transfusion therapy, this matters little. The incidence of E-donor blood is such that it is easier, and probably more cost effective, to provide E- units for transfusion to any patient in whom anti-E is found, than to conduct tests to determine which examples are clinically significant and which would be benign in vivo. At a different practical level these findings may mean that in the evaluation of a new antibody screening method or an automated antibody detection system, failure to detect an occasional example of anti-E, that is reactive only in sensitive in vitro tests, is not as serious a drawback as might at first be supposed.

Pretransfusion Testing - General Principles

In order to identify the small number of patients who have red cell antibodies other than anti-A and/or anti-B in the serum, it is conventional to test the sera of all prospective recipients of blood by several methods before transfusion. One series of tests, called antibody-screening, involves use of the patient's serum and specially selected red cell samples that between them carry the antigens against which the majority of atypical or irregular antibodies are directed. A second series, called compatibility tests, may involve a direct test between the potential recipient's serum or plasma and the potential donor's red cells. Alternatively, computer matching may be used to select units to be transfused to a patient. There has been considerable debate about the pros and cons of full testing, abbreviated testing and computer matching for the determination of compatibility between patient and donor. These considerations are discussed in detail, below. In the following sections, antibody-screening, identification and compatibility tests with the patient's serum are described. Although serum has traditionally been used for such tests, in some of the more recently introduced systems, plasma is as suitable as serum. This point is also discussed in more detail below.

Antibody-Screening

The way in which antibody-screening tests are commonly used today is rather different from what was intended when they were introduced in the early 1960s. The original intent was to test a patient's serum some weeks or days before blood was going to be needed. The advantages of such a program are:

1. The serum is tested against cells carefully selected to carry as many antigens as possible.
2. Early detection of antibodies prevents the postponement of surgery that may occur when antibodies are not detected until compatibility tests are done just before surgery.
3. Donor units can be typed where necessary, with potent antibodies as well as being tested with the patient's serum.
4. Those patients requiring rare blood (Kp(b-), Jk(a-b-), etc.) are recognized in time for transfusion services to seek aid from reference centers.
5. Screening tests on donor units identify those whose transfusion would result in the passive transfer of antibodies. While this will usually not harm the patient, the donor serum will (rarely) be better used as a typing reagent.

At present, at least in the USA, the majority of transfusion services perform antibody-screening and compatibility tests simultaneously and most often a short time before blood is required. Thus the advantage of early warning that an atypical antibody is present in a patient's serum, for which screening tests were originally introduced, is lost. The main advantage remaining is that screening tests sometimes detect an antibody present in a patient's serum, when that antibody fails to react in compatibility tests either because the red cells of the units tested lack the appropriate antigen, or because the antibody requires a double dose of its antigen on the test cells in order to give a visibly positive reaction. While

the first circumstance may not be too uncommon, the second occurs less frequently than opponents of antibody-screening to the exclusion of IAT compatibility tests seem to believe. If good techniques are used, antibodies that react only with red cells carrying a double dose of antigen are comparatively rare. Further, the advantage of knowing that a patient's serum contains anti-K when two K- units have been selected (by chance) for compatibility testing, is debatable. Again, these points are considered in more detail below.

In the second edition of this book (50) it was stated that "the object of screening tests is to detect all antibodies present so that tests using saline, albumin, enzymes, synthetic potentiating media and antiglobulin serum should all be used". That statement was as wrong then as it is now. What we should have said was that the object of screening tests is to detect clinically-significant antibodies so that relevant in vitro test methods should be used. If the object of antibody-screening and compatibility tests is to provide blood that will not cause a transfusion reaction when infused and will survive normally after infusion, there is no point in detecting (or identifying) antibodies that are benign in vivo. Good as currently used antibody-screening methods are, they do not detect all clinically significant antibodies. Very rarely a patient will destroy transfused red cells, apparently by an immune mediated mechanism, although all in vitro serological tests are negative. This subject is discussed in detail in Chapter 36.

Cold-Reactive Antibodies

There are some antibodies that are best not detected in antibody-screening (or compatibility) tests. There are abundant data (10,51-64) that antibodies such as those directed against the antigens A_1, H, I, IH, Le^a, Le^b, P_1, M, N, etc., that do not react at 37°C in vitro, do not effect the clearance of antigen-positive red cells in vivo. That statement should not be taken to mean that all antibodies of those specificities are clinically benign. It is the ability of an antibody to bind to red cells at 37°C, not its specificity, that is the critical factor. In other words, a patient who has formed one of the rare examples of anti-P_1 that is active at 37°C (51,65-67,100) should be transfused with P_1- blood. A patient who has anti-P_1 in the serum that is reactive in vitro only in tests at temperatures below 37°C, does not need P_1- blood. In such a patient, P_1+ blood will not cause a transfusion reaction nor will the P_1+ red cells be prematurely cleared. The determination as to whether an antibody is reactive at 37°C cannot be made from tests set up and/or incubated at room temperature and then transferred to 37°C for incubation. Many cold-reactive antibodies can bind to red cells very quickly. If the cells and serum are at room temperature when mixed and read in an immediate spin method, agglutination seen following 37°C incubation of the test will often merely represent carry-over of agglutination that occurred at a low temperature. When an antibody is detected in an immediate spin test and is still visibly reactive following 37°C incubation, a prewarmed test must be used to determine whether the antibody is truly active at 37°C. That is to say, the red cells and serum must be warmed to 37°C in separate tubes, the serum should be added to the cells using a warmed pipette and the tubes should preferably be centrifuged in a warm centrifuge. The tests should be read as quickly as possible to prevent cooling of their contents. If many tubes are involved they should be transferred to a 37°C incubator, water bath or heat block and be removed one at a time for reading. If the test is to be read with antiglobulin serum, the first two washes should be with saline warmed to 37°C. There is no need to warm the antiglobulin serum since the cold-reactive antibody will have been washed away before the antiglobulin serum is added. Reading the IATs with anti-IgG will avoid detection of any complement activated by the cold-reactive antibody. Clearly, from what is written above, there is no room in a modern transfusion service for routine antibody-screening or compatibility tests that involve incubation at room temperature or, for that matter, incubation at any temperature other than 37°C. By any temperature other than 37°C, we mean any other selected temperature such as 30°C or 22°C. There is no need to adhere slavishly to exactly 37°C. Garratty et al. (236) and Arndt and Garratty (237) have shown that variation of a couple of degrees in the water bath or heat block does not significantly alter the ability of clinically relevant antibodies to bind to red cells.

Because one of the traditions in blood banking has been to use antigen-negative blood for any patient with an antibody in the serum, some workers have been reluctant to abandon room temperature tests. Such workers should read the various reports cited above, that show that these antibodies are benign in vivo. First, there are numerous examples of cases in which antigen-positive units have been transfused. Transfusion reactions were not seen and expected increments in hematocrit and hemoglobin were attained and maintained showing that delayed transfusion reactions did not occur either. Second, in vivo cell survival studies, sometimes when the antibody was active at 30°C, have shown normal survival of the injected antigen-positive red cells. Because of reluctance to abandon a traditional test (room temperature incubation) some spurious reasons for retention of that test have been advanced. First has been an expressed fear that if a cold-reactive antibody is not detected, or is detected but ignored in the selection of blood, the introduction of antigen-positive red cells will result in a secondary immune response, widening of the antibody's thermal amplitude and a delayed transfusion reaction. There is no evidence that this occurs. If such events did take place, those transfusion services that changed to 37°C-only tests many years ago, would by now have seen more delayed transfusion reactions and would have encountered more 37°C-active antibodies of the specificities listed earlier, in patients requiring additional transfusions, than services that still honor cold-reactive antibodies. Neither of those events has happened. It seems that a secondary immune response or a widening of the antibody's thermal range following the introduction of antigen-positive blood, in a patient who had a cold-reactive antibody, is an extraordinarily rare event; its frequency was described as "almost never" by Mollison (68). For a number of years, one of us (PDI) studied cases to see if there was any evidence that some delayed transfusion reactions and some instances in which the production of 37°C-active antibodies occurs, could have been prevented by giving antigen-negative blood to patients with cold-reactive antibodies. There was no such evidence. There is no correlation between the presence of a cold-reactive antibody before transfusion and the occurrence of a delayed transfusion reaction or production of a 37°C-active antibody after transfusion. In other words, among patients who have delayed transfusion reactions or make a 37°C-active antibody after transfusion, between 0.5 and 1.5% had a cold-reactive antibody present before transfusion. Among patients in whom neither of those events occurred, between 0.5 and 1.5% had a cold-reactive antibody present before transfusion. Further, in those patients in whom a delayed transfusion reaction or production of a 37°C-active antibody occurred, the specificity of the antibody found after transfusion was different from that of the cold-reactive antibody present before transfusion.

A second spurious argument advanced for retention of room temperature tests is that rare examples of antibodies of specificities generally associated with clinical-significance are found. It is argued that while cold-reactive anti-A_1, anti-P_1, etc., can be ignored, rare examples of antibodies such as anti-K and anti-E are detected by the method. In fact, there is no evidence that such antibodies need to be detected. First, many services have used 37°C-only tests for many years meaning that some patients with cold-reactive anti-K must have been given K+ blood and more with cold-reactive anti-E must have received E+ red cells. There is no report of a transfusion reaction associated with such an event. Second, there is again no evidence that such patients undergo a secondary immune response. As discussed above (in the note about anti-E) there is now direct evidence (48) that weak examples of anti-E do not change characteristics in patients transfused with E+ blood. Third, if pretransfusion sera from patients who have had a delayed transfusion reaction caused by anti-E or anti-K are tested, cold-reactive anti-E and anti-K are not found (48).

In 1982, when questioned about the clinical significance of cold-reactive alloantibodies, one of us (69) conducted a survey. Data from five major institutions that had been performing antibody-screening and compatibility tests without incubation other than at 37°C, for periods ranging from 5 to 20 years, were reviewed. In all, a total of 1,500,000 units of whole blood or red cells had been transfused in that time. Since the average blood use per patient was 3.5 units, it could be seen that some 428,500 patients had received blood without their sera being tested by a room temperature method. If a figure of 1% (midway between the reported 0.5 to 1.5% incidence for cold-reactive antibodies) is used, it can be seen that some 4285 of those patients would have had a cold-reactive alloantibody in the serum. Again using the 3.5 units per patient average, those 4285 patients would have received about 15,000 units among them. Based on the frequency of A_1, P_1, Le^a, Le^b, etc., it can then be calculated that some 60%, or 9000 of the units, carried the antigen against which the patient's cold-reactive alloantibody was directed. In spite of the fact that some 9000 antigen-positive units must have been transfused to patients with cold-reactive alloantibodies in the serum, there was not one single report of a transfusion reaction (immediate or delayed) caused by such an antibody. This indirectly obtained evidence is exactly the same as that obtained directly by two groups of investigators. Cronin et al. (58) transfused blood compatible with the patient's serum, in in vitro tests at 37°C, to a series of patients with cold-reactive anti-P_1. Waheed et al. (61) did the same thing for patients with anti-Le^a and/or anti-Le^b. In both series it can be seen that the percentage of serologically non-reactive units was such that it must have included many that were antigen-positive but non-reactive with the patient's serum at 37°C. Neither group of investigators (58,61) was able to find any evidence that any of the patients had immediate or delayed transfusion reactions.

For many years it has been clear that antibody-screening and compatibility tests performed at temperatures below 37°C are not necessary in the provision of compatible blood for transfusion. In some ways it is fortunate that escalating costs of health care forced a reassessment of many medical practices including examination of the value of some tests traditionally performed in the transfusion service. It is expensive and time-consuming to detect and identify blood group antibodies. Because of pressures to contain costs and because the data show that cold-reactive antibodies are of no clinical significance, some workers abandoned such tests as a cost containment measure. In other words, economic pressure led directly to better science. As cost containment has become even more critical it has become unconscionable to waste patient care dollars by performing tests that add absolutely nothing to patient care. Unfortunately as late as 1996 one hears of transfusion services that still routinely perform room temperature tests. Clear as the message is, it has apparently not yet reached all those who should hear it.

Tests at 30°C

Because many of the early ^{51}Cr red cell survival studies were performed in patients with alloantibodies active below 30°C, some workers wondered if it might be prudent to use tests at 30°C to replace the room temperature tests that were being abandoned. Such tests were introduced at the NIH blood bank (70) but in more than two years of testing, only one antibody of dubious clinical-significance was detected at 30°C but not in other tests. Accordingly, it was decided that 30°C tests added nothing and those tests were abandoned in favor of ones performed at 37°C (71).

Cold-Reactive Antibodies and Hypothermia

A frequently asked question is whether a cold-reactive antibody becomes important in a patient whose body temperature will be reduced during a surgical procedure. Although data to answer the question are difficult to obtain, it seems that such antibodies are of no significance in this setting either. Mollison (72) described a patient in whom an anti-P_1 that was weakly reactive at 37°C, cleared a small amount of a test dose of red cells when they were injected. When the patient was subjected to hypothermia, no further destruction occurred. Kurtz et al. (73) described two patients with cold-reactive anti-M in whom M+ N- red cells survived normally during and after periods of hypothermia. These cases were particularly significant because the patients' body temperatures were reduced below the temperature at which the anti-M agglutinated M+ red cells in vitro and yet no red cell destruction was seen. In the survey mentioned above (69), it was determined that when the services were selecting blood for patients about to undergo hypothermia, antibody-screening and compatibility tests were still performed only at 37°C. There were no reports of adverse effects of transfusion in any of those patients although it can be assumed that some of them must have had antibodies present that would have reacted in tests at room temperature, had those tests been performed. Wertlake et al. (74) believed that an anti-IH, active in vitro at 15°C but not at 22°C, cleared A_2B but not A_1B

red cells in a patient subjected to hypothermia, in whom the body temperature was reduced to 29°C. The evidence presented did not seem to prove the point. First, the antibody was said to have bound to the red cells at 29°C (esophageal temperature) although it was active in vitro only up to 15°C. Second, as Mollison (72) pointed out, the IgM antibody would have been expected rapidly to elute from the red cells once the patient's body temperature returned to normal, yet hemoglobinuria continued for at least four days after the surgery. Klein et al. (75) performed an eight liter plasma exchange before surgery, in a patient who was to undergo hypothermia and who had anti-I in the serum that reacted with some I+ red cells at 30°C and with a few at 37°C. The authors commented that although they could not say that difficulties would have been encountered had the hypothermia been performed without plasma exchange, the procedure can be used when there is doubt about what an antibody might do in vivo. They (75) also pointed out that since so many cold-reactive autoantibodies are IgM in nature, they are present largely in the intravascular compartment so can be successfully removed by plasma exchange (76).

It is not easy to determine the fate of antigen-positive red cells in a patient with a cold-reactive antibody who is subjected to hypothermia. First, in many surgical procedures in which hypothermia is used there is considerable blood loss. Thus if a test dose of radio-labeled red cells is injected before surgery it must be estimated how many of those cells have been lost due to bleeding, before it can be seen whether any were lost because of immune destruction. Second and for the same reason, many such patients are transfused during surgery so that dilution of the test dose occurs. Third, in many of the procedures, an extracorporeal circulation system is used so that an estimate must also be made of the number of labeled cells lost because of physical trauma to those cells. One way around these problems is to label an aliquot of the patient's own cells in an attempt to determine how much of the label of the test cells has been lost because of bleeding, dilution and trauma to the red cells. However, even when the problem of using a double label is tackled, the levels of radio-activity representing the remaining test and control doses of red cells are sometimes too small, because of dilution and red cell loss not related to immune clearance, for reliable calculations to be made.

In view of the problems outlined above, the workers at the NIH Clinical Center tried to answer the question in a different manner. They divided patients subjected to hypothermia into two groups, namely those with no cold-reactive alloantibodies in the serum and those with such antibodies who received antigen-positive blood. The groups were compared in terms of amount of blood necessary during and after surgery, post-operative hemoglobin and bilirubin levels, bleeding complications requir-

ing platelet transfusions and any other parameters that might have suggested ill-effects in any of the patients because of immune red cell clearance. We understand (71) that the study did not produce any evidence of immune red cell clearance by the cold-reactive antibodies but that because of uncontrollable differences in different patients, the results were not totally conclusive.

Thus although no final answer to the question of the importance of these antibodies in patients to be cooled during surgery is available, the existing evidence seems to suggest that the antibodies are of no more significance in these patients than in any others. First, there are documented cases (72,73) in which three such antibodies did not clear antigen-positive red cells. Second, tests deliberately designed to avoid the detection of cold-reactive antibodies have been used for patients who are to be subjected to hypothermia and no difficulties have been encountered in those patients (69). Third, a comparative study (71) between patients with and without such antibodies has not yielded evidence that the antibodies clear significant numbers of antigen-positive red cells in vivo, during hypothermia.

We have heard anecdotal reports of difficulties resulting not from immune red cell destruction but from agglutinates that formed and blocked some of the tubing used in the extracorporeal equipment. Since such problems may occur because the patient has a potent cold-reactive autoantibody that agglutinates all red cells so cannot be avoided by the selection of appropriate donor units, the solution would seem to be to adjust the degree of hypothermia used.

Methods Using in Antibody-Screening

Because antibody-screening tests are performed only once on most samples sent to the transfusion service and because compatibility tests may have to be performed on many different donor units, some workers use a different series of tests for the two procedures. While we laud the aim of finding antibodies present in a patient's serum by the use of multiple techniques, we would also point out that the exercise loses meaning if the additional tests detect antibodies that are of no clinical significance. For example, there is no doubt that tests using protease pretreated red cells are more sensitive than those using untreated cells for the detection of Rh (and some other) antibodies and that some antibodies react only in tests using such treated cells (36,48,77-89). In spite of this, we continue to advise against the use of enzyme pretreated red cells for routine antibody screening. First, such cells are particularly sensitive for the detection of cold-reactive and other antibodies that are of no clinical significance. Second, we (48) have shown that antibodies detectable in tests against enzyme-treated red cells but not in LISS/IAT, do not clear antigen-positive red cells in vivo. Third, such antibodies do not increase in strength after antigen-positive red cells have been transfused. In other words, routine use of enzyme-pretreated red cells in screening tests greatly increases meaningless work: among 10,000 patients we (48) found 140 clinically irrelevant enzyme-only alloantibodies and 216 clinically irrelevant enzyme-only autoantibodies, but only one enzyme-only antibody that caused a delayed transfusion reaction; without significantly increasing transfusion safety.

A further disadvantage in using different methods for antibody-screening and compatibility tests is that an antibody may be found in one set of tests but not in the other. This will then entail repeat testing by alternative methods and will raise considerable doubt as to the meaning of the finding in terms of clinical significance of the antibody. It seems far preferable to select the most suitable method for the laboratory involved (see below) and to use that method for all routine tests. In antibody identification studies a much better case can be made for the use of multiple methods, this point is also discussed below.

In terms of selection of a method a number of points should be made. First, there is no (and probably never will be) one single method that detects all clinically significant antibodies (64,90,217). Second, for the most part, as the sensitivity of the methods increases so too does the detection of clinically-insignificant allo and autoimmune antibodies. Third, different methods yield different results when used by different workers. Thus selection of a method becomes a matter of individual choice based on two considerations. First, the method chosen must have sufficient sensitivity that it detects all, or almost all, antibodies that would cause frank transfusion reactions and/or accelerated in vivo clearance of transfused red cells. Second, the method must not result in the detection of so many clinically-insignificant antibodies that the workload of the laboratory becomes unmanageable and dilution of effort in working on antibodies that do matter, occurs. The method chosen will not be the same in all laboratories. We are well aware that the two objectives above are accomplished in different laboratories using any one of the methods: saline/IAT or albumin/IAT at normal ionic strength; LISS/IAT using LISS-suspended red cells or a LISS additive; PEG/IAT; Polybrene/IAT; solid phase methods; Gel tests; and probably some others that we have not remembered. Having made that statement we will add that we believe that saline/IAT and albumin/IAT methods achieve equivalence with the others only if higher serum:cell ratios and longer incubation times are used. Further, we are not convinced (91) that the use of albumin/IAT enhances results over a saline/IAT method although it clearly

results in a higher cost. Since Chapter 3 of this book now deals with the principles of serological methods and does not give details of the methods themselves, it will be added that details about performance of most of the tests described above are given by Judd (92).

Prewarmed Tests

Having discussed at (monotonous) length the inadvisability of detecting cold-reactive antibodies in routine tests, it will now be added that sometimes one has no choice. That is to say, some sera contain potent enough cold antibodies that positive reactions still occur in tests designed to avoid detection of such antibodies. This is particularly true in tests that use LISS, PEG or Polybrene, and in some others where cold agglutinins may interfere although in saline/IAT systems such antibodies would not react at 37°C. One method developed to avoid interference from these meaningless antibodies (both alloimmune and autoimmune cold agglutinins can interfere) is the prewarmed test that is described in the section on cold-reactive antibodies. In this setting, the objective of the test is to detect any 37°C-reactive antibodies whose reactions would otherwise be masked by those of the cold-reactive antibody.

Prewarmed tests have fairly recently been criticized by some (93,94,98) and defended by others (95,96,99). The major criticism of the prewarmed test is that its use can result in the non-detection of a clinically-significant, 37°C-antibody. There are two circumstances in which just such an event can occur. First, if the technologist performing the test is already convinced, before the prewarmed test is run, that the positive reactions seen in the initial screening tests were due to the actions of a cold-reactive antibody, then that technologist may read the prewarmed test in such a manner (e.g. shake the tubes a little harder) that the reactions of the 37°C-active antibody are missed. Clearly the criticism should be leveled at the technologist performing the test, not at the test itself (if an IAT gave a false negative result because the red cells were not washed before the anti-IgG was added, the tester not the test would be indicted for the failure). Second, some workers have used LISS or PEG, etc., for the initial screening test, then performed prewarmed tests in a saline system at normal ionic strength. Failure of the prewarmed test to detect the 37°C-active antibody then relates not to the fact that the test was prewarmed but to the fact that the additive needed to potentiate the reactions of the 37°C-active antibody was not used. This time execution of the test, not the test itself, was at fault. Perhaps the most important statement that can be made about prewarmed tests is that they must be identical, other than the prewarming, to the test that gave the positive reaction in the first place. In this respect the method given in the 12th Edition of the AABB Technical Manual (213, p635) is incorrect. The method listed uses red cells suspended in saline at normal ionic strength and the patient's serum. Although there is a cautionary statement that the test may reduce the sensitivity of detection of some clinically significant antibodies, it is clear that those that fail to react will do so because of lack of potentiation of antibody binding.

We continue to believe that if prewarmed tests are performed identically to the initial test, save for the prewarming, they provide a highly valuable and rapid means of avoiding interference by clinically-insignificant cold agglutinins. We (97) calculated that we use prewarmed tests in our transfusion service, on average, ten times each week and have done so since 1989. In the more than 4000 times that the test has been used, we are not aware of a single instance in which its use resulted in nondetection of an antibody that subsequently caused a transfusion reaction. Further, in order to keep interference by clinically meaningless cold agglutinins to a minimum, we routinely (in all antibody screening and identification tests) place the tube containing the patient's serum in a heat block or water bath at 37°C while we prepare the cell samples. Thus the serum is warm when it is added to the test red cells (known in our service as the warm test). We resort to a full prewarmed test (serum and cells prewarmed in separate tubes before mixing) only when the warm test fails to prevent interference by a cold agglutinin. It should be added that our high volume use of the warm and prewarmed tests is made necessary by our use of a PEG/IAT system for antibody-screening, antibody-detection and compatibility tests (in alloimmunized patients, see below). The PEG/IAT as used by us, detects many benign cold-reactive autoantibodies. Somewhat ironically, a major critic of prewarmed tests mentions use of the test in his book (92, p47) but (to be fair) specifies that it should be used only when the specificity of the cold agglutinin is known, while a major defender of the test has described (100) a transfusion reaction caused by an antibody that was overlooked when the test was performed differently to the original test (a 37°C reading in a LISS system was omitted in the prewarmed test) in the referring laboratory.

Should Antibody-Screening (and Compatibility) Tests be Read for Agglutination at 37°C?

When methods using saline, albumin, LISS, etc., were used for antibody-screening and compatibility tests it was customary to read the tests for agglutination and hemolysis before the red cells were washed and read by

IAT. Even when it became appreciated that reading for agglutination at room temperature caused more problems than it solved, a reading for agglutination following incubation of the tests at 37°C was retained. When newer methods such as PEG, solid phase and the gel test were introduced, for a variety of reasons a 37°C reading for agglutination could not be included. In 1992, Judd et al. (247) published a report describing 72 patients with alloantibodies whose specificities suggested that they might be of clinical significance, that reacted as agglutinins at 37°C in a LISS method but that were non-reactive when the LISS tests were read by IAT. Twenty-seven of the 75 antibodies (in the 72 patients three had two antibodies each) reacted by IAT in subsequently tested samples. The authors (247) concluded that some antibodies that are active as 37°C agglutinins but are non-reactive by IAT represent antibody produced early in an immune response (67 of the 72 patients had been transfused and/or pregnant) and will become IAT-reactive (and clinically important) as the immune response progresses. The report states that "Our data clearly indicate that some 37+ IAT- antibodies are clinically important..." and that "elimination of the 37°C reading for agglutination and hemolysis should not be undertaken lightly".

The report of Judd et al. (247) caused considerable confusion and consternation, at least in the USA. As one of us (PDI) continued to endorse use of a PEG/IAT method at various meetings and in lectures, a recurring question was "how can the method be used since it has no 37°C reading stage". Two aspects were described as causes for concern. First, the chance that an antibody that would then cause a delayed transfusion reaction would be missed. Second, the fear that elimination of the 37°C reading would place a blood bank in violation of regulations. For some time the answers to these concerns were based on lack of untoward consequences. At Duke University Medical Center we had stopped 37°C readings for agglutination in July 1991 when the PEG/IAT method was introduced. By May 1992 when the Judd et al. (247) report appeared, we had transfused some 34,000 units of blood without a 37°C agglutination reading in antibody-screening or compatibility tests, but had seen no delayed hemolytic transfusion reaction associated with a secondary immune response. To answer the regulatory issue we pointed out that the wording of the standard (219) was "methods of testing...shall be those that will demonstrate clinically significant antibodies. They shall include 37°C incubation preceding an antiglobulin test..."

Since that time we have supported our decision to eliminate the 37°C reading for agglutination with more solid data. First, we (248) took 100 antibodies that had reacted by PEG/IAT and repeated the test using saline instead of anti-IgG before the tests were read. Among the 100 antibodies, 40 gave positive reactions showing that when agglutination occurs in PEG at 37°C it is not dispersed in the washing stages of the IAT procedure but carries through to the reading stage. Second, we (248) took 189 PEG/IAT active antibodies and retested them in LISS. Among those antibodies 39 reacted as agglutinins at 37°C and by IAT, 144 reacted by IAT only while six failed to react at all in LISS. Rolih et al. (249) made similar findings using a solid phase method. Among 2460 samples containing antibodies, 11 were seen to react as 37°C agglutinins but were non-reactive by IAT. Among the 11 antibodies, eight were considered to be clinically-significant and all reacted by solid phase. Finally, Alkhashan (250) tested 5027 sera that were non-reactive by PEG/IAT in a LISS system for agglutination at 37°C. Nineteen of the 5027 sera contained 37°C agglutinins but only four of them were considered to be of potential clinical significance. Since this study (250) was performed at the same time as the one (248) that showed that six antibodies reactive by PEG/IAT were non-reactive in LISS, it was clear that eliminating the 37°C agglutination reading was a wiser choice than abandoning the PEG/IAT method. That is non-use of a 37°C agglutination reading resulted in non-detection of 4 antibodies among 5027 sera tested, non-use of the PEG/IAT (to enable a LISS 37°C reading for agglutination to be incorporated) would have resulted in non-detection of 6 antibodies among 189 tested.

Finally it should again be stressed that no example of an antibody that reacted as an agglutinin at 37°C but that failed to react by IAT has ever been seen to cause an immediate or a delayed transfusion reaction. We understand that in spite of their earlier publication (247), Judd et al. (251) have now also abandoned a 37°C reading for agglutination.

Red Cells Used in Antibody-Screening Tests

If the objective of antibody-screening tests is to detect as many clinically significant antibodies as possible, it follows that the red cells used in the tests should carry the antigens against which the most commonly encountered antibodies are detected. For many years most workers agreed that the sera of patients could be satisfactorily screened in tests against the red cells of two selected donors providing that the cells were not pooled. When type and screen and MSBOS procedures (see below) were introduced and when some workers began to advocate abandonment of the IAT portion of compatibility tests, it was apparent that antibody-screening tests would assume greater importance. Clearly, if a patient's serum was to be tested fully only once (antibody-screening test) before transfusion, any clinically significant antibodies present would have to be detected in that test. As a result many workers decided that it would be safer

to screen sera against three selected red cell samples than against two. As far as we are aware, a suggestion (101) that four samples be used did not gain much acceptance. If the compatibility test for all patients in a given transfusion service includes an IAT, then antibody-screening tests against two cell samples are perfectly adequate. If patients in whose sera no unexpected antibodies are found are to be given blood based on an immediate spin compatibility test, then perhaps a case can be made for the use of three cell samples. We say perhaps because we are aware that some large transfusion services still use two cell samples in antibody-screening and use immediate spin (or electronic) tests for compatibility and do not encounter problems as a result of the policy. The usual argument for the use of more than two red cells samples is that cells can then be used from individuals homozygous for genes such as c, E, S, s, Fy^a, Fy^b, Jk^a and Jk^b. It is, of course, almost impossible to find two donors who would represent such a state between them. The rationale for using red cells from homozygotes is, of course, that some antibodies will give observable positive reactions only with red cells carrying a double dose of the antigen they define. The case is probably over made. While it is true that if a very sensitive method, such as PEG/IAT, is used, rare antibodies to c, E, S, s, Fy^a and Fy^b that react only with red cells from individuals homozygous for the genes involved, will be found, the clinical significance of such antibodies is far from clear. The case with Jk^a and Jk^b is quite different. Examples of anti-Jk^a that react with Jk(a+b-) but not with Jk(a+b+) and of anti-Jk^b that react with Jk(a-b+) but not with Jk(a+b+) red cells can, and have caused immediate and delayed transfusion reactions when Jk(a+b+) red cells were transfused. If a two cell antibody-screening system is to be used, one sample must be Jk(a+b-) and the other Jk(a-b+).

One of the objectives of increasing the number of red cell samples used in antibody-screening tests is to increase the number of patients in whom full compatibility tests (including an IAT) need not be done so that the cost of pretransfusion tests can be reduced. Each service must do its own arithmetic rather carefully. If a third cell sample is included in all antibody-screening tests and the total number of full compatibility tests is not significantly reduced, the overall result can be an increase rather than a decrease in total costs. In performing the cost analysis it must be remembered that a proportion of samples are sent to the blood bank for ABO and Rh type and antibody-screening tests but that no blood for transfusion is ever requested. Thus the total number of full compatibility tests no longer performed on other patients' samples must compensate for the increase in work on those samples from patients for whom no blood is requested, before it begins to effect any savings. One factor that cannot be measured in terms of cost involves increased attention to critical samples. If the number of IAT compatibility tests that would give negative results (patients with no unexpected antibodies in the serum) can be reduced, more time can be spent in working on samples that do contain antibodies. It must be remembered that a patient in whom one antibody has been found is quite likely to have made other antibodies that will be detected only by further testing.

An Autocontrol Should Not be Part of Antibody-Screening Tests

At one time a control using the patient's red cells and serum (the autocontrol) was considered to be a necessary component of antibody-screening procedures. It's use gave the investigator an early indication as to whether a positive result in the screening test represented presence of an allo or autoantibody. However, since 97 to 98% of antibody-screening tests are negative, use of an autocontrol is a waste of effort and reagents most of the time and it should not be part of routine antibody-screening procedures (63,211). The argument that regular use of an autocontrol serves as a DAT on all samples and thereby identifies patients with unsuspected antibody-induced hemolytic anemia, has also been shown (211,212) to be spurious. The yield of useful information is too low to justify routine use of the test, the DAT is best performed at a physician's request and/or in cases of otherwise unexplained anemia. Most workers continue to include an autocontrol with each first antibody identification panel set up after the antibody-screening tests are positive. Although the test is of no value if the serum contains an easily identifiable alloantibody, it is of use if the patient has an antibody that reacts with all red cells on the panel or if the patient has autoantibody present in the serum. Thus it is probably more efficient to set up the autocontrol with each first panel (if negative it need not be repeated with extension panels performed using the same sample from the patient) than to go back and run the test separately on those occasions that it is needed.

Antibody-Screening Tests on Donor Blood

These tests need not be as sensitive as those used to screen the sera of patients because the passive transfer of donor antibody, directed against an antigen on the recipient's red cells, seldom effects red cell destruction. There are four major reasons for this. First, as the blood is transfused the donor antibody is diluted. In many patients who are anemic, the total blood volume is normal or close to normal, it is the red cell mass that is reduced, so that dilution of the donor antibody is consid-

erable. Second, as the donor antibody enters the patient's circulation and is diluted, it encounters a larger number of red cells, that carry the antigen against which it is directed, than when a smaller volume of donor cells is transfused to a patient with an antibody in the serum. As a result, the donor antibody invariably binds to the recipient's red cells in small numbers of molecules per red cell. As discussed in Chapter 6, one of the factors that affects the in vivo clearance of red cells is the amount of IgG bound, per red cell. Third, because of current methods of preparing red cell concentrates, only small amounts of donor plasma are transfused. Fourth, the passive transfer of donor antibody is usually a single event so that there is no danger of an increase in antibody level and a delayed transfusion reaction. Accumulation of ABO blood group antibodies can occur when blood components containing plasma are used. Problems that can result from such passive transfer of ABO antibodies are discussed in detail in Chapter 8.

For the reasons given above, many blood centers use pooled red cells from two individuals to test donor sera. Further, it is perfectly satisfactory to pool say five donor sera for a single test and read that test only by an automated method. The objective of the exercise is to detect those donor antibodies that are of high titer and are active at 37°C. Even this test may be more useful for the detection of donor antibodies that can be harvested and used as typing reagents than necessary for the protection of recipients (10,102). There are relatively few reports (103-110) of problems caused by the passive transfer of donor antibodies and the more serious ones described have involved destruction of transfused red cells, not the patient's own (see below). In those cases in which donor antibodies (other than ABO) have caused some destruction of the patient's red cells (103,108-110) the antibody involved has usually been of high titer, e.g. a 250 ml unit of fresh frozen plasma containing anti-D with a titer of 1000, that was given to a patient with D+ red cells (108). In some cases (104-107) the transfusion has involved inter-donor incompatibility. That is to say, the patient was transfused with one unit of blood containing an antibody (anti-K has most often been incriminated) to an antigen that the patient's red cells lacked. Then, by chance, the patient was given another unit with the antigen involved present on the donor's red cells. This time the situation described above in which few antibody molecules bind per red cell, does not exist. Instead, the passively immunized patient is placed in the same situation as an actively immunized patient transfused with incompatible red cells. As will be seen, reports of reactions of this type appeared between 1963 and 1978. It is probable that current methods of preparation of red cell concentrates, where so little donor plasma is infused, have negated the possibility of this type of reaction when only red cells are transfused. Such reactions might still be possible in patients transfused with plasma from one donor and red cells from another, if presence of the antibody in the plasma had not been noted.

Minor Compatibility Tests

A test using the donor's serum (or plasma) and the prospective recipient's red cells used to be part of pretransfusion tests for compatibility. It is highly doubtful if this test was ever necessary, antibody-screening tests on donor blood have made the minor compatibility test obsolete. We have often wondered how advocates of this test ever managed to transfuse patients who had a positive DAT!

Antibody Identification

Once an antibody with characteristics such that it can be considered to be of potential clinical significance has been detected, it should be identified. This is a straightforward procedure and is accomplished by the use of a panel of red cells, the full phenotype of each of which is known. Depending on which cells react with the serum and which do not, the antigen against which the antibody is directed can be recognized. Table 35-1 shows such a panel and the reactions of an unknown serum (the reactions in just the antiglobulin test are given for the sake of simplicity). Examination of the panel in table 35-1 shows that all samples reacting with the serum are S+ and that all non-reactive samples are S- so that the antibody is seen to be anti-S. Other possibilities can be excluded. For example, although cell samples 2, 4 and 10 are D+ and react with the antibody and cell samples 1, 5, 6, 7 and 8 are D- and fail to react, the antibody cannot be anti-D because cell samples 3 and 9 are D+ but do not react. By working through the antigens written along the top of the panel sheet, other antibodies can be similarly excluded. Using a ten cell panel such as the one shown, not all antibodies can be excluded. For example, the serum in question might contain anti-C^w as well as anti-S. The only cell sample on the panel that is C^w+ is number 2 and that sample has reacted because the cells are S+. Thus while anti-S has been shown to be present in the serum, anti-C^w has not been excluded from being present as well. Tests against C^w+, S- cells would be necessary to exclude or detect anti-C^w (and others, anti-C^w is simply used as an example). In practice, most workers would not attempt to exclude all other specificities from being present in the serum containing anti-S (unless the serum was to be used as a typing reagent). However, because of the known fact that patients who form one

blood group antibody often form others, S- units to be transfused to the patient should be tested in a full compatibility test that includes an IAT (or an equivalent test if one has been devised before this book is published). This applies in all services including those that use immediate spin (IS) compatibility tests for patients in whom antibody-screening tests were negative.

Identification of a single antibody in a serum is often as simple as the example in table 35-1. Knowledge of the reaction characteristics of each antibody, as given in the previous chapters, is of great help in antibody identification. For example, if all cells on a panel are I+ and Js(b+) and an antibody is found that reacts with all samples in immediate spin tests, but not at all in IATs, it is highly likely that the antibody is anti-I and highly unlikely that it is anti-Js[b]. Other clues are often helpful in the identification of single antibodies. For example, anti-M and anti-N often react more strongly with M+ N- and M- N+ cells, respectively, than with those that are M+ N+, i.e. double versus single doses of antigens present. Red cells vary somewhat in the amounts of some of the antigens they carry. By use of the same panel cells over a period of time, workers will soon learn which are the strong and which the weaker reactors for antigens such as P_1, I, C, Le[b] and others. This knowledge will often provide valuable clues in antibody identification. The antigen Sd[a] varies so much that the difference between one plus and two to three plus reactions of known Sd(a+) cells may be such that the presence of anti-Sd[a] can be deduced in the absence of Sd(a-) cells. Once such a deduction has been made confirmatory evidence, such as tests against known Sd(a-) cells and/or Sd[a] typing of the antibody-maker's red cells and/or urine inhibition of antibody reactivity, should be sought.

When a serum contains more than one antibody, various different ways can be used to recognize the specificities present. Table 35-2 shows the reactions of a serum containing anti-c and anti-Fy[b]. The anti-c reacts more strongly than does the anti-Fy[b] so that if the 4+ reactions are considered first, anti-c can be identified. The remaining, c- cell samples can be seen to react to a strength of 2+ or to be non-reactive and examination of the antigens on those cells reveals the presence of anti-Fy[b] (cell samples 2 and 3 react and are Fy(b+), cell samples 1 and 9 are non-reactive and are Fy(b-)). Confirmation of these specificities with more c+, Fy(b-); c-, Fy(b+); and c-, Fy(b-) cells samples (the last of which may detect another antibody present) is necessary as are c and Fy[b] typings on the antibody-maker's red cells.

In the serum illustrated in table 35-3, two antibodies are present that react with equal strength in the antiglobulin test so cannot be separated on the basis of strength of reactivity. However, in the tests against enzyme-treated red cells anti-C can be identified while the second

TABLE 35-1

Vial No.	Special Type	Rh Code	D	C	Cw	E	c	e	f	V	M	N	S	s	Lua	Lub	P1	Lea	Leb	K	k	Kpa	Kpb	Jsa	Jsb	Fya	Fyb	Jka	Jkb	Xga	Vial No.	IAT
1	U-	r'r'-2	0	+	0	0	0	+	0	0	+	+	0	0	0	+	+	0	0	0	+	0	+	0	+	0	0	+	+	+	1	0
2		R1R1^w-84	+	+	+	0	0	0	0	0	0	+	+	+	0	+	+	+	0	0	+	0	+	0	+	+	+	+	+	+	2	2+
3		R1R1-277	+	+	0	0	0	0	0	0	+	+	0	+	+	+	0	0	+	0	+	0	+	0	+	0	+	+	+	+	3	0
4		R2R2-93	+	0	0	+	+	+	0	0	+	0	0	0	0	+	+	0	+	+	+	0	+	0	+	+	0	+	+	0	4	3+
5		r''r''-2	0	0	0	+	+	+	0	0	0	+	0	+	0	+	+	0	0	+	0	+	0	+	0	+	+	0	+	+	5	0
6		rr-57	0	0	0	0	+	+	+	+	0	+	0	+	0	+	+	0	0	+	0	+	0	+	+	0	+	+	+	+	6	0
7		rr-167	0	0	0	0	+	+	+	0	+	+	0	+	0	+	0	+	0	+	0	+	0	+	+	0	0	0	+	+	7	0
8		rr-168	0	0	0	0	+	+	+	0	+	+	0	+	0	+	+	0	+	+	0	+	0	+	0	+	+	+	+	+	8	0
9		RzR1-4	+	+	0	+	0	0	0	0	+	0	0	+	0	+	+	0	+	0	+	0	+	+	0	0	+	0	+	+	9	0
10	Co(a-)	R1r-187	+	+	0	0	+	+	0	0	+	0	+	0	0	+	0	0	+	0	+	0	+	+	+	+	+	0	+	10	3+
Patient's Cells:	DAT	Neg.																															0

TABLE 35-2

Blood Group System			Rh								MN				Lutheran (Lu)		P	Lewis (Le)		Kell						Duffy (Fy)		Kidd (Jk)		Sex Link		
Vial No.	Special Type	Rh Code	D	C	C^w	E	c	e	f	V	M	N	S	s	Lu^a	Lu^b	P_1	Le^a	Le^b	K	k	Kp^a	Kp^b	Js^a	Js^b	Fy^a	Fy^b	Jk^a	Jk^b	Xg^a	Vial No.	IAT
1	U-	r'r-2	0	+	0	0	+	+	+	0	+	+	0	0	0	+	+	0	0	0	+	0	+	0	+	0	0	+	+	+	1	0
2		$R_1R_1^w$-84	+	+	+	0	0	+	0	0	0	+	+	+	0	+	+	+	0	0	+	0	+	0	+	+	+	+	+	+	2	2+
3		R_1R_1-277	+	+	0	0	0	+	0	0	+	+	0	+	+	+	0	0	+	0	+	0	+	0	+	0	+	+	+	+	3	2+
4		R_2R_2-93	+	0	0	+	+	0	0	0	+	0	+	0	0	+	+	0	+	+	+	0	+	0	+	+	0	+	+	0	4	4+
5		r''r''-2	0	0	0	+	+	0	0	0	+	0	0	+	0	+	+	0	+	0	+	0	+	0	+	0	+	0	+	+	5	4+
6		rr-57	0	0	0	0	+	+	+	+	0	+	0	+	0	+	+	0	0	0	+	0	+	0	+	+	0	+	0	+	6	4+
7		rr-167	0	0	0	0	+	+	+	0	+	+	0	+	0	+	+	+	0	0	+	0	+	0	+	+	0	+	+	+	7	4+
8		rr-168	0	0	0	0	+	+	+	0	+	+	0	+	0	+	+	0	+	+	+	0	+	0	+	0	+	+	+	+	8	4+
9		R_zR_1-4	+	+	0	+	+	+	0	0	+	0	0	+	0	+	+	0	+	0	+	0	+	0	+	0	0	+	+	+	9	0
10	Co(a-)	R_1r-187	+	+	0	0	+	+	+	0	0	+	0	0	0	+	0	0	+	0	+	0	+	0	+	+	+	+	0	+	10	4+
Patient's Cells:		DAT Neg.																														0

antibody fails to react. Since it is known that, at least, the antigens Fy^a, Fy^b, M, N and S are not detectable on protease-treated red cells, it is likely that the serum contains a second antibody directed against one of them. All the C- cells that react with the serum in the IAT can be seen to be Fy(a+), while the C-, Fy(a-) samples are all non-reactive. Again, the presence of anti-C and anti-Fy^a should be confirmed with additional C-, Fy(a+); C+, Fy(a-) and C-, Fy(a-) samples and the antibody-maker's red cells should be typed with appropriate antisera.

In the serum illustrated in table 35-4 three different antibodies can be identified because each reacts by a different method. By immediate spin, anti-M can be seen (showing dosage effect) while by antiglobulin test anti-E is apparent. The anti-M does not react in the antiglobulin test so that its presence does not obscure the specificity of the anti-E. In the enzyme tests the anti-E is, of course, enhanced but a third antibody, anti-c, is also seen. Thus, although only one cell sample (number 2) of the 10 cell panel is M-, E-, c- and therefore non-reactive with the serum, three different antibody specificities can be seen without difficulty. As previously, confirmatory tests are necessary.

Use of Enzyme-Treated Red Cells in Antibody Identification

Having decried the use of enzyme premodified red cells in routine antibody-screening tests, it will now be added that tests with such cells have a very real place in the transfusion service in antibody identification studies. When a patient's serum is shown to contain an antibody, two facts have been established. First, the patient has demonstrated a genetic ability to mount an immune response to a blood group antigen. Second, if one antibody has been made, others may be developing. Thus, in investigating sera already shown to contain one blood group antibody, the most sensitive methods available should be used to search for others. Other uses of enzyme-treated red cells are shown in tables 35-3 and 35-4. Antibody identification and differentiation was accomplished by the use of protease-modified red cells that gave enhanced reactions with some antibodies and were non-reactive with others.

Red Cell Typing in Antibody Identification

Part of the process of identifying an unexpected antibody should always be the demonstration that the antibody-maker's red cells lack the antigen against which the alloantibody is directed. Phenotyping studies on the antibody-maker's red cells can also be of great value during the investigation of sera containing multiple antibodies. By determining which antigens are lacking from the cells it will be apparent which alloantibodies could be made. This procedure is also valuable in obtaining new information about blood group antigens and antibodies. If the patient's cells are positive for the antigen against which the antibody is apparently directed, misidentification of the antibody or a false positive typing, are the most likely explanations. However, another possibility is that the antibody identification and the cell typing are both correct and that a previously undetected heterogeneity of the particular antigen has been uncovered.

Identification of Antibodies Directed Against High or Low Incidence Antigens

Identification of antibodies that define these antigens uses the same principle as described in this chapter for other antibodies but requires the use of rarer cells. Those cells that lack high incidence antigens or carry rare ones, have been described in the earlier chapters of this book. When an alloantibody against an antigen present on most red cell samples is encountered, typing tests on the antibody-maker's red cells to see which common antigen is lacking are particularly helpful. Because there are now so many known blood group antigens, many of which are of extremely high and many of extremely low incidence, antibody identification of the more unusual antibodies is best accomplished by reference laboratories that have collections of rare cells and uncommon antibodies.

The admonition given in Chapter 32 will be repeated here. When a serum is found to react, by IAT, with only one cell sample, the red cell sample must be shown to be DAT-negative, before tests to identify an antibody to a low incidence antigen are initiated.

Some antibodies to high incidence antigens would be better left undetected, some examples have been given in earlier chapters in this book. Another was that reported by Patten and Conti (214). The patient made anti-C, anti-E, anti-Jk^b and an antibody of "uncertain specificity" that reacted with an antigen of high incidence. The authors bled the patient's sister, said to be the only compatible donor, of 10 units in a 17 week period to provide blood to cover the patient's surgery. We (215) objected to subjecting the donor to such an extreme procedure particularly since no evidence was sought to show that the unidentified antibody was of any clinical significance. Indeed, from the original description (214) it sounded as if the antibody had HTLA characteristics (see Chapter 30) and might well have been benign in vivo. Obviously, had the antibody to the high incidence antigen been

TABLE 35-3

Vial No.	Special Type	Rh Code	D	C	Cw	E	e	c	f	V	M	N	S	s	Lua	Lub	P1	Lea	Leb	K	k	Kpa	Kpb	Jsa	Jsb	Fya	Fyb	Jka	Jkb	Xga	Vial No.	IAT	Enzyme Test
1	U−	r'r'-2	0	+	0	0	+	0	0	0	+	+	0	0	0	+	+	0	0	0	+	0	+	0	+	0	0	+	+	+	1	2+	4+
2		R₁R₁ʷ-84	+	+	+	0	+	0	0	0	0	+	+	+	0	+	+	+	0	0	+	0	+	0	+	+	+	+	+	+	2	2+	4+
3		R₁R₁-277	+	+	0	0	+	0	0	0	+	+	0	+	+	+	0	0	+	0	+	0	+	0	+	+	+	+	+	+	3	2+	4+
4		R₂R₂-93	+	0	0	+	0	+	0	0	+	0	0	0	0	+	+	0	+	+	+	0	+	0	+	+	0	+	+	0	4	2+	0
5		r''r'-2	0	+	0	+	+	+	0	0	0	+	0	0	0	+	+	0	+	0	+	0	+	0	+	0	+	0	+	+	5	0	0
6		rr-57	0	0	0	0	+	+	+	0	0	+	+	0	0	+	+	0	0	0	+	0	+	0	+	+	0	+	+	+	6	0	0
7		rr-167	0	0	0	0	+	+	+	0	+	+	0	+	0	+	0	+	0	+	0	+	0	+	+	0	0	0	+	7	2+	0
8		rr-168	0	0	0	0	+	+	+	0	+	+	0	+	0	+	+	0	+	+	+	0	+	0	+	0	+	+	+	+	8	0	0
9		R_ZR₁-4	+	+	0	+	+	0	0	0	+	0	0	+	0	+	+	0	+	0	+	0	+	0	+	+	0	0	+	+	9	2+	4+
10	Co(a−)	R₁r-187	+	+	0	0	+	+	+	0	+	0	0	0	0	+	0	0	+	0	+	0	+	0	+	0	+	+	0	+	10	2+	4+
Patient's Cells:	DAT	Neg.																														0	0

Blood Group System headers: Rh (D, C, Cw, E, e, c, f, V), MN (M, N, S, s), Lutheran (Lu) (Lua, Lub), P (P1), Lewis (Le) (Lea, Leb), Kell (K, k, Kpa, Kpb, Jsa, Jsb), Duffy (Fy) (Fya, Fyb), Kidd (Jk) (Jka, Jkb), Sex Link (Xga)

TABLE 35-4

Vial No.	Special Type	Rh Code	D	C	Cw	E	c	e	f	V	M	N	S	s	Lua	Lub	P1	Lea	Leb	K	k	Kpa	Kpb	Jsa	Jsb	Fya	Fyb	Jka	Jkb	Xga	Vial No.	IS	IAT	Enzyme Test
						Rh					MN				Lutheran (Lu)		P	Lewis (Le)		Kell						Duffy (Fy)		Kidd (Jk)		Sex Link				
1	U-	r'r'-2	0	+	0	0	0	+	0	0	+	+	0	0	0	+	+	0	0	0	+	0	+	0	+	0	0	+	+	+	1	2+	0	0
2		R1R1w-84	+	+	+	0	0	+	0	0	+	+	+	+	0	+	+	0	0	0	+	0	+	0	+	+	+	+	+	+	2	0	0	0
3		R1R1-277	+	+	0	0	0	+	0	0	+	+	0	+	+	+	0	+	0	0	+	0	+	0	+	0	+	+	+	+	3	2+	0	0
4		R2R2-93	+	0	0	+	+	0	0	0	+	0	+	0	0	+	+	0	+	+	+	0	+	0	+	0	0	+	+	0	4	3+	2+	4+
5		r'r''-2	0	0	0	+	+	+	0	0	+	0	0	+	0	+	+	0	0	0	+	0	+	0	+	0	+	0	+	+	5	3+	2+	4+
6		rr-57	0	0	0	0	+	+	+	0	+	+	0	+	0	+	+	0	+	0	+	0	+	0	+	0	0	+	0	+	6	0	0	2+
7		rr-167	0	0	0	0	+	+	+	0	0	+	0	+	0	+	0	0	0	0	+	0	+	0	+	+	0	0	+	+	7	2+	0	2+
8		rr-168	0	0	0	0	+	+	+	0	+	+	0	+	0	+	+	+	0	+	+	0	+	0	+	0	+	+	+	+	8	2+	0	2+
9		RzR1-4	+	+	0	+	0	+	0	0	+	0	0	+	0	+	+	0	+	0	+	0	+	0	+	+	0	0	+	+	9	3+	2+	4+
10	Co(a-)	R1r-187	+	+	0	0	+	+	+	0	+	0	0	+	0	+	0	0	+	0	+	0	+	0	+	0	+	+	0	+	10	3+	0	2+
Patient's Cells:	DAT Neg.																															0	0	0

shown to be benign, the provision of 10 units of C- E-, Jk(b-) blood would have been an easy problem to solve.

Use of Adsorption and Elution Methods in Antibody Identification

On some occasions these techniques may be useful. For example, a serum that contains say anti-Wr^b and has been made by an individual with D- red cells, needs to be tested to see if anti-D is present but masked by the anti-Wr^b. If insufficient D+, Wr(b-) cells samples are available to confirm or exclude anti-D, the serum can be adsorbed on to D-, Wr(b+) red cells. After a sufficient number of adsorptions (the number will be dependent on the strength and avidity of the antibody to be adsorbed) the serum (now free of anti-Wr^b) can be tested against D+ and D- samples. If anti-D is present, anti-Wr^b can be separated from that antibody by elution from the adsorbing D-, Wr(b+) red cells.

Sometimes, when a serum gives variable reactions with different red cell samples, but no clues as to antibody specificity, it may not be clear whether one or more antibodies are present. In such an instance it may be of value to run "blind" adsorption and elution tests using the most strongly and most weakly reactive red cell samples. In this way some specificity may be seen in one of the two eluates or in one of the two adsorbed aliquots of serum or it may become apparent, by virtue of the fact that both weakly reacting and strongly reacting red cells totally adsorb the antibody, that only one antibody is present.

Use of Phenotype Matched Transfusions to Prevent Alloimmunization

As discussed earlier in this chapter, patients who receive multiple transfusions often make multiple antibodies. While the incidence of immunization differs in the various groups of patients (see earlier), high rates of alloimmunization have been reported in multiply transfused patients with sickle cell disease (16-26), thalassemia major (17,27-29), and other conditions requiring continuing transfusion support (20,30-32).

While there is some disagreement as to how the transfusion needs of these patients should be met (see below), virtually all workers agree that the first step should be to perform as complete a phenotype as possible on the patient's blood. Ideally this is done when the patient is first seen and before any blood has been transfused. The phenotype determination should include, at least, typings for ABO, Rh, MNSs, Lewis, Kell, P$_1$, Duffy and Kidd system antigens; other typings e.g. in the Lutheran, Colton, Dombrock, etc. systems may prove

useful if they can be done. In the event that phenotyping must be performed after the patient has been transfused, it may be necessary to use one of the cell separation methods (111-114, details of methods in 92) that isolate reticulocyte-rich (i.e. the patient's own newly formed red cells) suspensions from post-transfusion blood samples. In patients with sickle cell disease, the method of Brown (115) that results in the lysis of transfused red cells (containing hemoglobin A) and the survival of the patient's own cells (containing hemoglobin S) is useful.

Since it is the most widely discussed condition in which frequent alloimmunization is seen, the transfusion of sickle cell disease (SSD) patients will be considered. However, the points raised can be applied to any group of patients receiving multiple transfusions.

There are currently at least four schools of thought regarding the selection of blood for SSD patients. First, some workers believe that these patients should receive phenotypically matched blood from the time of the first transfusion. It is argued that this maneuver will prevent alloimmunization and thus obviate later difficulties in finding compatible blood for the patient. If the sole object of this regimen is to prevent later problems it is obviously illogical. Indeed, by selecting phenotyped units from the start, the problem is simply introduced sooner, that is at the time of the first transfusion. Further, since it is not possible to forecast which patients will become alloimmunized and which will not, this system results in the considerable problem of finding phenotyped units for patients who would not have made antibodies. A simple example will illustrate the fallacious reasoning. Since almost all SSD patients are Black, some will have S- s- U- red cells. If U- blood is provided for all transfusions, scores of difficult to obtain U- units may be used to transfuse a patient who might never have made anti-U anyway.

A second school of thought, to which one of us (PDI) subscribed for many years is that SSD patients should receive random units of blood until alloimmunization occurs. Then, as for any other immunized patient, appropriate antigen-negative blood can be supplied. This regimen has the considerable advantage that no specially selected units are ever required for those SSD patients (the majority) who do not make alloantibodies. It is sometimes claimed that this system results in an increased incidence of delayed hemolytic transfusion reactions that can be extraordinarily difficult to differentiate from a sickle cell crisis in these patients. However, if careful antibody-screening tests are done most (if not all) alloantibodies can be detected early enough that delayed hemolytic transfusion reactions can be prevented. It is in the interpretation of these tests that knowledge of the patient's phenotype is extremely useful.

A third school of thought is that SSD patients should

be given unselected units from donors of the same ethnic group as the patient. It is argued that since the antigens C, E, S, K, Jk[b], Fy[a] and Fy[b] are more common in Whites than in Blacks, the transfusion of blood from Black donors to Black patients will result in a lower rate of exposure to these antigens. It is doubtful that the system is of very much value in practical terms. The incidence of these antigens in Black and White donors is such that with the exception of K and Fy[a] (the latter of which is not very immunogenic in Blacks anyway, see Chapter 14) multiple transfusions with units from Black donors will still result in the exposure of the patients to the antigens. While the system may (slightly) delay the onset of alloimmunization it will certainly not be preventive. In other words, at a practical level, essentially the same results could be achieved by typing the units involved for K and not using those that are K+.

The fourth school of thought is that SSD patients whose red cells lack C, E and/or K should be given blood that lacks the same antigen or antigens. The rationale for this reasoning is that in a small number of patients, alloimmunization is accompanied by the production of autoantibodies (243). In rare cases the autoantibody production has resulted in severe hemolytic anemia (207), even less frequently it has proved to be fatal (26). Thus the exposure of these patients to the antigens C, E and K, that are regarded as more likely to cause alloimmunization than others, is avoided not simply to prevent alloantibody production but to obviate the chance that such alloimmunization might result in concurrent serious autoimmunization. In those SSD patients who have already made a series of alloantibodies, blood is selected to lack other antigens that the patient lacks, to prevent further alloimmunization and possible simultaneous autoantibody production. If the practice of giving D+ C- E- K- blood to Black patients of that same phenotype is followed, the local blood supplier must be recruited to find units from R_0 donors. If the attempt to find C- E- units is made at the hospital transfusion service level, the danger (mentioned above) exists that Rh- (D- C- E-) blood will be unnecessarily used when D+ C- E- units cannot be found.

Clearly, requests made to the transfusion service for units to be used for patients in whom multiple transfusions are anticipated, will vary dependent on the beliefs of the physician treating the patients. However, automatic compliance with requests for fully phenotyped and matched units should not occur. Instead, the transfusion service medical director should establish the protocol to be followed by discussion with the physician ordering the blood. As can be seen from what is written above, those who belong to the first and third schools of thought outlined above, have based their decisions on flawed reasoning.

Compatibility Tests

For many years virtually all workers agreed that before a unit of blood was transfused, it was necessary to test the potential recipient's serum against the red cells of the donor. The object of the exercise was to determine whether the potential recipient's serum contained an antibody capable of reacting with and destroying the donor red cells when they were infused. A large number of different methods were used for compatibility tests; most services used one test or set of tests in routine circumstances and an abbreviated test or tests in emergency situations. Such was the importance attached to the tests that if a patient had the temerity to require transfusion before the tests could be completed, the patient's physician was required to sign a waiver stating that the urgency of the clinical situation was such that the transfusion service was absolved of all responsibility for the terrible things that we knew would happen to the patient. Times change; today many transfusion services do not do the test. This is a routine procedure in many institutions and the treating physicians are now told that very little, if any, danger exists for the patient.

Type and Screen (T and S) and Maximum Surgical Blood Order Schedules (MSBOS)

One of the problems with testing every unit of blood for compatibility with a patient's serum, before issue of that unit, was that a much larger number of compatibility tests were performed than units were transfused. If a surgeon ordered four units of blood to cover a procedure, then used only one, three-quarters of the work done in the transfusion service was wasted effort. Compatibility test to transfusion ratios (i.e. the number of units tested for each one transfused) in many services showed that a way to reduce the amount of wasted effort was much needed. Further, it was appreciated (116-119) that reserving blood for individual patients after compatibility tests had been completed, reduced the supply of blood available for other patients, resulted in aging of units reserved for but not used by individual patients and created very considerable problems in inventory control. A resolution of many of these problems was described by Friedman et al. (120) and by Mintz et al. (121) in 1976. These workers pointed out that there were many surgical procedures (e.g. cholecystectomy, dilation and curettage, partial thyroidectomy) for which blood was regularly ordered but almost never used. Further, for many other surgical procedures more units were regularly ordered than were used. For those procedures in which blood was hardly ever used, compatibility tests were replaced by typing and screening (T and S) of the patient's sample.

The maximum surgical blood order schedule (MSBOS) described, was a list of surgical procedures about which the transfusion service director and surgeons had agreed as to how much blood would be routinely tested for compatibility. For procedures in which the average use was two units of blood, only two were tested for compatibility. On those occasions when blood was needed quickly for patients whose samples had been tested only by T and S or when more than that tested was needed in another procedure, it became the transfusion service's responsibility to provide that blood with no delay. This meant that when necessary, the transfusion service must be prepared to issue blood of the same ABO and D type as the patient without performing a compatibility test other than immediate spin (IS). Obviously, negative antibody-screening tests had now to be relied on as indicating the absence of the most frequently formed alloantibodies and hence a very low possibility that the units not tested beyond IS would cause any ill-effects when transfused. The spate of reports that followed the publications of Friedman et al. (120) and Mintz et al. (121) left no doubt (12,122-160,239-242) that the T and S and MSBOS procedures work and work well.

There are a number of important considerations that relate to the introduction of the MSBOS. First, it is essential that the program be established as a joint venture between the surgeons who will use it and the blood bankers who will administer it. Attempts by blood bankers to impose MSBOS on surgeons will almost always result in failure. Second, it is generally better to start with too many units allocated to some procedures, than to antagonize the surgeons who will help make the program work, by insisting on more stringent allocations. Once the surgeons see that the program works well (they no longer have to remember to order blood, orders are filled automatically from a surgical schedule and the MSBOS allocations) they will be more amenable to reduction in some allocations. Third, the transfusion service must be prepared to issue units on which only IS compatibility tests have been done when the surgical emergency so dictates. If surgeons find that they must wait for additional units in emergency situations they will soon resort to overordering as an insurance that enough blood will be available on all occasions. Fourth and perhaps most important, the Medical Director of the transfusion service must assume responsibility (moral and legal) for units issued without full compatibility tests. Attempts to institute the system and still have the patient's physician sign a waiver for such units will tell the physician concerned that the transfusion service director does not have total faith that the system is safe. Having ascertained that fact the next and very reasonable request will be that the MSBOS be abandoned and that all orders again be filled with units on which full compatibility tests have been done. The transfusion service director is in a much more informed position than is the treating clinician in assessing

the safety of the program and must therefore convince the surgeons that the procedure is safe. Fifth, each program must have an override mechanism by which the surgeon can increase an order for a patient at high risk of complications.

The main reasons that T and S and MSBOS procedures work are that first, if the MSBOS is well prepared, the issue of a unit of blood not tested for compatibility by IAT will be a rare event. Second, even when this is done, the chance of issuing a unit for a patient in whom antibody-screening tests are negative and that unit being incompatible with an antibody in the patient's serum, is extremely small. Obviously, antibody-screening tests will not detect all antibodies. The red cells used cannot carry every known blood group antigen. However, many antibodies that go undetected will be directed against low incidence antigens such as Kp^a or Js^a and clearly, the possibility that a unit carrying such an antigen will be given to a patient with the corresponding antibody, by chance, is statistically small. It has been estimated (161) that based on the incidence of antigens such as C^w, Lu^a, Kp^a, Js^a, etc., and the frequency of antibodies directed against them, the chance that a patient will be given an incompatible unit is between one in 1600 and one in 10,000. Other authors (127,136) have concluded that the chance is even more remote but there are some other considerations not always included in such calculations (see next section).

Even in services that still use a full (IAT) compatibility test for all units issued, current rapid compatibility testing procedures are such that it is often possible to issue blood before completion of a full compatibility test, but still complete such a test before the unit is actually infused. As soon as the transfusion service is informed that a given patient is going to need blood, compatibility tests can be started. If a LISS, PEG or Polybrene method is used, there is a good possibility that the testing can be completed during the time that it takes to transport the unit from the transfusion service to the patient and set up the infusion. Thus while the issue of the unit must not be delayed (see above), its infusion can often be prevented if serological incompatibility is demonstrated before the actual transfusion begins. As discussed in more detail below, those patients with clinically-significant antibodies present in the serum must be given selected units, tested for compatibility, even when T and S and MSBOS or systems using abbreviated compatibility tests (see below) are used.

Can the IAT for Compatibility be Excluded When the Antibody-Screening Test is Negative?

Once T and S and MSBOS systems were shown to constitute an effective and safe way for the provision of blood for some patients in whom the antibody-screening tests were negative (120-125,127,128,130,132,133,135, 136,140,143,144,146-154,156,158,160,161) it was natural that another question would be asked. Since it was now accepted that when those systems were used, blood not tested for compatibility beyond an immediate spin method could be issued for patients in whom the antibody-screening tests were negative, could all patients with a negative antibody-screening test be treated similarly? In other words, if the system worked for some patients, could it be applied to all? Were there now any justifications for retention of the IAT in compatibility tests? The question prompted a debate among blood bankers in which virtually everyone had an opinion (not necessarily data, but always an opinion). In addition to the numerous reports about T and S and MSBOS, many of which address this question as well, there have been a number of other papers (162-174) that present arguments in favor of retaining the IAT in compatibility procedures or advocate abolition of the test (a few present both sides of the argument). In addition, some authors have pointed out that because suitable tests for compatibility can now be completed very rapidly (175-179), such tests can be retained and that blood can still be supplied quickly when needed. Use of these rapid tests and immediate release of units into available inventory once surgery is completed (they can be replaced by others tested in rapid methods for compatibility if needed later) can provide the same advantages in inventory management as T and S and MSBOS.

Before considering the various arguments that have been advanced in favor of discarding or retaining the IAT as part of compatibility testing methods, it should be stressed that the discussions have involved just that, discarding or retaining the IAT. With very few exceptions, persons involved in the debate have agreed that the immediate spin (or something equivalent) portion of the compatibility test should be retained. Patients who die as a result of the transfusion of incompatible blood, have invariably (180-189) received major-side ABO incompatible blood. Thus, it is essential that if a full compatibility test is not to be done, a test be retained, or a system devised, that will detect errors in patient or donor ABO grouping and mislabeling of, or selection of incorrect units. Listed below are a number of arguments that were advanced (216) in the debate about abolition or retention of the IAT in compatibility tests. No doubt there are other arguments that we have overlooked.

Arguments in Favor of Eliminating an IAT for Compatibility

1. Issuing blood tested only by immediate spin (or an

equivalent test) when the antibody-screening test is negative, is as safe as issuing blood fully tested for compatibility.
2. While number one above is not true, the risk involved is so small that it is acceptable.
3. Those incompatible transfusions that may occur (antibody to a rare antigen not detectable in screening tests) will not be severe or life-threatening.
4. Savings are effected in terms of time (blood is immediately available in a clinical emergency) labor and costs of pretransfusion tests.
5. Reduction of time spent testing samples from patients with no antibodies allows more time for work on samples that do contain antibodies.
6. Because units are not reserved for individual patients, more blood is available for all patients, better inventory control and a reduced level of outdating is achieved or outdating can be totally eliminated.
7. Based on number 6, above, most units of blood are used nearer to the date of collection, while more red cells are still viable.
8. Because so few clinically-significant antibodies are detected in IATs for compatibility that are missed in antibody-screening tests, the overall cost for detection on a per antibody basis is too high to justify retention of the test.
9. The lack of patient advocate argument (see below) is spurious because the patient does not have sufficient information to make an informed decision.

Arguments in Favor of Retaining an IAT for Compatibility

1. A few clinically-significant antibodies will be undetectable (antibody-screening cells lack the antigen) in screening tests but will be detected in IATs for compatibility.
2. A few clinically-significant antibodies will be undetected in screening tests (errors in test performance) but will be detected at a second attempt in IATs for compatibility.
3. Some transfusion reactions caused by undetectable (1, above) and undetected (2, above) antibodies may have serious consequences in a critically ill patient.
4. Savings effected in terms of time, labor and money, by elimination of the IAT for compatibility have been overestimated, or may not accrue in some services, or will not be passed on to the patient.
5. Existing systems result in appropriate amounts of time being dedicated to work on samples containing antibodies.

6. In some services, elimination of antibody-screening tests and retention of full compatibility tests would effect greater savings.

7. Equivalent time savings and improvements in inventory control can be accomplished using rapid methods (LISS, PEG, Polybrene, etc.) for IATs in compatibility tests.

8. The blood banker has no right to assume that the patient is willing to accept additional risk (albeit very small) of receiving incompatible blood when the patient has no advocate.

Obviously, from what is written above, good cases can be made for elimination or retention of the IAT in compatibility test procedures. Those workers who claim that its exclusion does not increase a patient's risk of receiving incompatible blood at all, simply do not understand red cell antigens and antibodies very well. Occasional patients with anti-Kp[a], anti-Js[a], anti-Go[a], etc. (the list is very long - see Chapter 44) will be transfused with incompatible blood. The fact that such an event did not occur in a given series (136) cannot be extrapolated to mean that it will never happen. It is not true that all antibodies to rare antigens occur in sera that contain other antibodies that will be detected in antibody-screening tests so that such patients will receive blood tested by IAT in the compatibility test. Again, the fact that they were present in such sera in a given series (190) cannot be extrapolated to mean that will always be the case. Those workers who argue that the IAT can be eliminated in compatibility tests because the risk to any given patient is minute and therefore acceptable are using good logic, unlike those who claim that there is no additional risk.

While the debate as to whether the IAT compatibility test should be discarded or retained was at its height various calculations were made regarding patient safety and risk, if the test was discontinued. Perforce, these calculations had to be based on the known incidences of antibodies directed against antigens not present on the screening cells and the incidences of the antigens in the donor population, i.e. what would be the incidence of a patient with the antibody receiving, by chance, a unit with the antigen. Fortunately, the figures calculated from theoretical considerations have now been replaced by actual data. One finding that has emerged from actual studies, for which no calculation could be made at the theoretical level, relates to the fact that antibody-screening tests are not infallible. That is to say, when antibody-screening tests are performed, an occasional antibody will go undetected because of test failure. If an IS test for compatibility is used with the serum in question and the missed antibody reacts only by IAT, the antibody will not be detected before the blood is transfused. If the serum in question is used in an IAT for compatibility, there will be a second

chance that the antibody will be detected so that the unit will not be issued. Thus antibodies that will be missed if the IAT for compatibility is discontinued fall in to two categories. First are those that are undetectable because the antigen defined is not present on the screening cells. Second are those that are undetected because an error was made in the screening tests. Table 35-5 lists results obtained in a number of large studies (12,126,139,140). Most of these studies were retrospective analyses of compatibility tests in which antibody-screening, immediate spin tests and IATs had all been done. When an antibody was found in the IAT for compatibility, that had not been found in the antibody-screening or IS test, a determination was made as to whether the antibody fell in to the undetectable or undetected category, as defined above. From the results in three of the studies (12,126,139) that are summarized in table 35-5, it can be seen that 24 undetectable antibodies had been found during 417,190 compatibility tests for an incidence of one in about 17,400. In the same 417,190 compatibility tests 35 undetected antibodies were found for an incidence of one in about 11,900. Thus the total number of undetectable and undetected antibodies was 59 in 417,190 tests for an incidence of one in about 7100. However, even with the T and S and MSBOS in use the compatibility testing:transfusion ratio remains at about 2:1. In other words, only about half the blood issued will actually be transfused so that the actual risk of transfusion of a serologically incompatible unit is around one in 14,200, not one in 7100. This figure can then be used as an argument for retaining the IAT for compatibility, the one in 14,200 can be avoided, or as an argument for its exclusion, the risk is small enough to be acceptable in view of the other advantages (see above) of eliminating the test.

The figures used above can be used in another calculation although some assumptions must be made. It is known that each year in the USA some 11 million units of red cells are transfused (191,235). For the sake of the calculation it will be assumed that, if the IS only compatibility test is used solely for patients with unanticipated needs following a T and S procedure, or to provide additional units when blood provided via a MSBOS system has been used, one million units will be issued following only an IS test for compatibility (the figure is probably an overestimate). Based on the figures calculated from the data in table 35-5 it would then follow that the potential existed for the transfusion of some 70 units (1 in 14,200 of one million) of serologically incompatible blood. If the IS only compatibility test is used for all patients in whom the antibody-screening tests are negative, the number of units issued following such a test will, of course, be very much higher. Again, for the sake of the calculation it will be assumed that 3 million of the 11 million units transfused will be given to patients

TABLE 35-5 Undetectable and Undetected Antibodies in IS Tests[*1]

Study and Reference	Number of Compatiblity Tests	Antibodies to LI Antigens	Antibodies Missed in Screening Tests
Oberman et al. (126)	82,647	6	9
Heisto (12)	73,407[*2]	5	3
Mayer (140)	480,000	see [*3]	4[*4]
Mintz et al. (139)	261,136	13	23

[*1]   Numbers not the same as originally reported. We have included only those antibodies that we consider to be of potential clinical significance.
[*2]   The antibody-screening tests used included the use of enzyme-treated red cells.
[*3]   No figure available, IATs for compatibility were not done when the antibody-screening tests were negative.
[*4]   Represents only transfusion reactions reported to the transfusion service. Thus the number is not directly comparable to those from other studies.

known to be alloimmunized and will thus be issued following an IAT for compatibility. Among the remaining 8 million units, issued following just an IS test for compatibility, the one in 14,200 figure forecasts that the potential would exist for 563 units of serologically incompatible blood to be used. Again the question becomes, is the total cost (that would probably be in the tens or hundreds of millions of dollars) justified to prevent 493 (or whatever the real number would be) incompatible transfusions? Again, the question can be answered in two ways. Some will say that the expenditure is justified because the total cost of all blood transfusions constitutes only a fragment of total health care costs and because there are many other areas (including some in the transfusion service) where costs could be reduced at no risk at all to the patient. Others will argue that the transfusion reactions that would occur would not, on their own, be likely to be fatal in any of the cases so that the expenditure is not justified.

How Has the Question been Answered?

Based on the data and arguments presented above, it is clear that some workers will eliminate the IAT portion of the compatibility test for patients in whom antibody-screening tests are negative, while others will decide that it is essential or desirable. Some who regard its retention as desirable but not necessarily essential believe that the advantages of its exclusion are less than the advantages of its retention. A survey conducted in 1987 (192) in the USA found that the IS compatibility test for patients in whom the antibody-screening tests were negative, was being used in 11% of the institutions surveyed. Another survey, in the USA conducted in 1990 (193) showed that the number of institutions using such a procedure had increased to about 33%. By 1995 the number (again in

the USA) was just over 50% (238). We believe that these figures may be somewhat misleading. In conversations with colleagues in the USA, we have found that the procedure has been adopted in many large transfusion services while many smaller ones have retained the IAT in compatibility tests. It seems likely that while only about a half of transfusion services have adopted the IS only test, the majority of blood (perhaps as much as 80 to 90%) issued for patients with negative antibody-screening tests is issued following such a test.

This division between services using or not using the IS only test may be based on perceived abilities and may, in fact, represent a desirable situation. In a very large transfusion service where the technologists work only in transfusion science, they rapidly gain considerable experience in all methods used. They perform large numbers of antibody-screening tests on a daily basis. In some smaller services the technologists rotate between the transfusion service, hematology and clinical chemistry laboratories, etc. and/or may only work in the transfusion service on an occasional or emergency basis. Thus in this setting there may be a distinct advantage in having the patient's serum tested twice by IAT, i.e. once in antibody-screening and again in compatibility tests. The above statement is not intended to denigrate the abilities of technologists working in small transfusion services. Clearly many of them will work at, at least the same level as their counterparts in large services. However, repeated large volume work is likely to increase the confidence of those who perform it. Some workers in smaller services may well appreciate what Mollison (72, p541) originally called a (desirable) "degree of redundancy" in performing the IAT twice.

There have been many reports of success when the IAT in compatibility tests was excluded for patients in whom the antibody-screening tests were negative. A few examples will be given (with apologies to those investigators whose reports are cited above but not described in detail here). Shulman et al. (144) as early as 1985, reported on an 8 month period during which 74,701 compatibility tests were ordered. In those patients in whom the antibody-screening tests were negative, the compatibility tests were not performed until the decision to transfuse had actually been made. This policy was possible since blood could be made available (by IS compatibility test) with an average time of 3.25 minutes, after the call for blood had been received. Among the 74,701 compatibility tests ordered 27,742 were actually performed (the number of IS only and IAT compatibility tests is not specified). The remaining 46,959 tests ordered were not performed since no requests for blood were received. It was calculated (144) that in the 8 month period, at least $49,300.00 in direct costs, was saved. During the same period, the incidence of units of blood outdating before use was reduced to 0.19%.

In 1992, Pinkerton et al. (158) described their eight year experience in using the IS only compatibility test for patients in whom the antibody-screening tests were negative. During that time 54,725 units of packed red cells or whole blood were transfused to 10,146 patients. Also during that time four clinically overt delayed transfusion reactions and 18 delayed serological reactions in which the patients did not manifest clinical signs, were found. In none of the 22 cases was there an antibody in the pretransfusion serum, detectable by IAT using untreated red cells. The authors (158) concluded that a compatibility test including an IAT on untreated donor red cells offered no advantage over their policy of using only the IS for compatibility when the antibody-screening tests were negative.

We have used the IS only compatibility test for patients with negative antibody-screening tests at Duke University Medical Center since 1983. Since introduction of that protocol, we have transfused about 600,000 units of red cells and estimate that some 540,000 of them were issued after IS only compatibility tests (i.e. the other 10% given to alloimmunized patients). During that time we have not seen a single example of a transfusion reaction caused by an antibody to a rare antigen that was not present on the antibody-screening cells. Clearly, some units carrying a low incidence antigen must have been transfused to patients with the corresponding antibody; based on the figures calculated above 16 such events would have been expected. The figure of 16 is based on the calculation that one IS only compatibility test in 17,400 will fail to detect an antibody to a low incidence antigen but that since only one unit in two is transfused the chance of the event occurring is actually one in 34,800. While we are able to calculate the expected incidence of undetectable antibodies, we cannot factor in undetected antibodies since we do not know how many (if any) are missed in our PEG/IAT antibody-screening

test. Thus the number of 16, represents one in 34,800 of 540,000. These data lend strong support to the contention, mentioned above, that such serological incompatibility rarely causes symptoms noticeable at the clinical level. However, we are careful not to say that such an event will not occur, simply because it did not occur in our series.

As described in a later section, some workers have now abandoned even the IS for compatibility in favor of computer matching of patients and donors.

The IS Compatibility Test and ABO Incompatibility

The major reason for retaining the IS portion of the compatibility test is to prevent the issue of ABO majorside incompatible blood. However, there have been a number of reports (194-198,201) of failure of the test to demonstrate such ABO incompatibility. In particular, the serum of group B patients may fail to react visibly with some A_2B red cells. Although Berry-Dortch et al. (195) reported an alarmingly high number of negative reactions, i.e. 204 of 531 in this setting, Pohl (199) pointed out that the 531 tests had been done using only a small number of group B sera and samples from A_2B donors. Park (200) pointed out that the figures reported (195) were misleading since they assumed that IS tests would be done without previous knowledge of the patients' and donors' ABO types. Park (200) used figures for the rate of ABO mistyping of patients and donors to calculate that at the incidence reported (195), the failure of an anti-B serum to react with A_2B cells would be seen in practice, where the patients and donors had been ABO typed, only once in more than two million tests. Clearly such an incidence is far smaller than the incidence of ABO transfusion reactions that result from mislabeled samples, clerical errors and transfusion of blood to the wrong patient.

A different cause of the same problem has been documented by others (202-205). If the IS test is set up but not spun immediately, potent ABO antibodies may not cause agglutination when the tests are spun after the delay. This is because such antibodies, some of which appear to prozone because of the same effect, rapidly fix complement and the C1 molecules bound prevent the cells coming into close enough contact for agglutination to occur (206).

The most frequently offered solution to the problem of weak antibodies and weak antigens failing to give positive reactions in IS tests is to verify the ABO groups of all patients' and donors' samples that will be used in the test. The solution to C1 blocking agglutination in such tests is to add EDTA to the saline being used to suspend the red cells, and thus prevent complement activation (203).

Frightening as the failure to detect ABO incompatibility in IS tests may appear at first, it is clear that the event is extraordinarily rare. As stated earlier, where numerous references are given, the test has been used before the issue of many millions of units blood and disasters have not been reported. The major reasons are, of course, those advanced by Park (200). First, for an error to occur either the patient or the donor will have had to be mistyped, the incidence of such an event is extraordinarily low. Second, superimposed on the mistyping, the antigen on the test cells or the antibody in the patient's serum will have to be much weaker than usual. The chance that the two events will occur in the same test is obviously extremely small, hence the reliability of the test almost every time it is used.

Compatibility Tests in Alloimmunized Patients

Virtually all workers agree that in alloimmunized patients, full compatibility tests including an IAT are essential. The IAT can be part of a saline, albumin, LISS, PEG, Polybrene, etc., protocol but must be included. The reason, as mentioned several times already, is that many patients who form one antibody, form others. Thus if a patient is known to have, say anti-Fy^a, and known Fy(a-) units are available, an IAT compatibility test is still necessary in case the patient has formed an antibody to an antigen on some of the Fy(a-) units. Similarly, for a patient known previously to have made an antibody but in whose serum the antibody is no longer demonstrable, antigen-negative units must be tested for compatibility in a system that includes an IAT.

Once an antibody of potential clinical significance has been unequivocally identified in a patient's serum, there is no point in performing identification tests for that antibody in subsequently received samples from the patient. However, many workers insist on doing exactly that. Again anti-Fy^a will be used as an example. When asked why identification studies are being performed to identify the anti-Fy^a shown previously to be present, the answer is usually, to confirm that the antibody is still there. The next question is what course will be followed if the anti-Fy^a is reconfirmed? The correct answer is that Fy(a-) blood will be issued. The third question is what course will be followed if the anti-Fy^a is no longer demonstrable? Again the correct answer is that Fy(a-) blood will be issued. The fourth question in the dialogue is then why does it matter if the anti-Fy^a is still active or no longer demonstrable? There is no sensible answer to that question.

In the situation described above, the correct course is to test Fy(a-) red cells to see if another antibody has

been made. Some workers elect to do this by testing selected (phenotyped) red cell samples that are Fy(a-) to rule out the presence of other antibodies. Others elect to proceed directly to IAT compatibility tests on known Fy(a-) units and to run selected (phenotyped) samples only if incompatibility with one or more of the Fy(a-) units is seen. The first course, use of phenotyped Fy(a-) samples, is said to be safer since samples from donors known to be homozygous for c, S, s, Jk^a, Jk^b, etc., can be used. In fact the second course seems to work just as well in practice. Some years ago one of us (PDI) elected to discontinue selected "rule out" panels. Now if the initial screening tests (done as a routine on all samples) fit the pattern of the previously identified antibody, we proceed directly to IAT compatibility tests on known antigen-negative units. The change was made when it was noticed that the yield from running selected "rule out" panels was small and that most of the new antibodies detected reacted strongly. The yield of new antibodies found following an unexpected positive reaction in a test for compatibility has been the same as that from "rule out" panels. We continue to use "rule out" panels when the original antibody has a specificity (e.g. anti-Le^a plus anti-Le^b) such that all the screening cells react.

Importance of Records

Workers who provide blood for transfusion to patients who have had multiple transfusions in the past will not need to be told that production of alloantibodies to red cell antigens is not a permanent feature of an individual's life. Patients with sickle cell disease are particularly difficult to manage in this respect although cessation of production of antibodies, in serologically detectable levels, is by no means confined to such patients. It is not particularly uncommon to identify one alloantibody in a patient's serum then to find, weeks, months or years later, when a new sample from the patient is tested, that the original antibody is no longer demonstrable and that a different specificity antibody is now being made. With sickle cell disease patients this can happen regularly so that after the patient has been seen repeatedly, over a period of many years, there is a long list of antibodies previously made, but not currently demonstrable. These events raise two important points. First, identification of each antibody needs to be certain. Once a specificity is listed in the patient's record, the patient must be given blood lacking the antigen involved, for the rest of his or her life. As mentioned in the section on patients who make multiple antibodies, phenotyping studies performed early in the course of the patient's treatment can be highly valuable in increasing the certainty of correct identification of an antibody. Second, it is important to keep accurate and readily accessible records on all patients who have been shown to be alloimmunized. Some workers advocate the use of cards, listing the patient's phenotype and the specificity of antibodies made. These cards are given to the patients who are instructed to present them if they return to hospital or, more importantly, if they are admitted to a different hospital. The experience of one of us (PDI) with the card system has been miserable. First, the patient usually gives the card to the admitting physician who, being unfamiliar with its significance, fails to forward the card to the transfusion service. Second, some patients apparently believe that possession of the card will result in their receiving preferential treatment. We have seen instances of the name being altered and the card being given to a brother, aunt or even a good friend, about to be admitted to hospital. Third, sometimes the card will carry incorrect information. We received one, issued by a reference laboratory with a good reputation, that described the patient as having A_2 red cells and anti-A_1 in the serum (why would anyone wish to convey such irrelevant data?). In our hands the patient was phenotypically A_1 and had anti-c in his serum. Thus now, when we are working on a sample from a patient who has been treated elsewhere, we call the transfusion service at the hospital involved and ask what records are in their computer. When we make that call, we also ask about the patient's transfusion history and details of pregnancies, if any (see below).

Patients who make multiple antibodies are not the only ones in whom antibody production falls below serologically detectable levels. Ramsey and Larson (208) tested samples from 160 patients who, among them, had made 209 antibodies, for periods of one to 60 months after the antibodies were first identified. In the time period covered, between 29 and 34% of the antibodies, that were of potential clinical significance, became undetectable in serological studies. In another study, Ramsey and Smietana (209) tested samples from 44 patients in whom antibodies had been detected, five and ten years after the antibodies had first been found. The rate of nondetection of these antibodies at five and ten years, were 42% and 48% respectively. In the studies described, approximately half the alloimmunized patients had sickle cell disease.

Patients' Histories

It is customary to obtain a history of any transfusions and/or pregnancies in patients in whom an antibody has been found. Such information is sometimes helpful in differentiation between antibodies that are almost always made following exposure of the individual to foreign red cells and those that occur without such exposure. While the information may sometimes be useful, it is not infallible. As described in the previous chapters of this book (where references are given) antibodies such as anti-D and anti-K, that are almost always red cell stimulated, have been found in never pregnant, never transfused individuals. Thus any given specificity may show up in unexpected circumstances. A further problem relates to the reliability of the information obtained. In some cases pregnancy may be denied for social reasons, or early miscarriage may not have been recognized as such and pregnancy may be denied. Similarly, some patients may not know or may have forgotten that they have been transfused. As an example, one patient was described (218) as having "naturally-occurring" antibodies to D, K and Fy^a in his serum. Many will suspect that the patient was unaware, or had forgotten, that he had been transfused earlier in his life.

Compatibility Tests and Massive Transfusions

Even those services that have retained a full compatibility test should not continue to run such tests for patients receiving huge volumes of blood. The current AABB Standards (219) specify that when a patient has received an amount of blood that approximates the total blood volume, within a 24 hour period, the compatibility test may be abbreviated. Some workers would continue to use the immediate spin compatibility test to ensure that an ABO incompatible unit was not issued, others would ensure simply that all blood issued, be ABO major-side compatible with the patient's blood. It must be remembered that in such massive transfusions, the plasma in the patient's circulation may be primarily that of the donors, not the patient. When group O blood is transfused to a non-group O patient (either in a dire emergency or in the massive transfusion setting) it is sometimes difficult to know when to revert to transfusions with blood of the patient's type. Most workers rely on antibody-screening tests. That is, when passively transferred anti-A and/or anti-B is no longer serologically demonstrable in a sample from the patient, it is apparently safe to transfuse blood of the patient's own type. Clearly in emergencies and/or massive transfusions it is highly desirable to ABO type the patient, whenever possible, before the first transfusion and supply blood of the patient's ABO type. Such a course not only avoids the question as to when it is safe to revert to the patient's type, just as importantly it avoids depletion of stocks of group O blood.

For alloimmunized patients requiring massive transfusions, it may be impossible to provide enough antigen-negative units to meet the need. A practical solution, when it is known that massive amounts of blood will be used, is to provide random units while the patient is bleeding heavily (the alloantibody will be rapidly diluted in the patient's circulation) and to reserve known antigen-negative units until the time that bleeding slows. By liaison with the physicians treating the patient it is sometimes possible to ensure that the last six or so units used are antigen-negative. In this way a delayed transfusion reaction, that may occur after the bleeding has stopped and as the patient begins to synthesize antibody, can often be minimized. A similar situation obtains in a D- patient in whom massive amounts of blood will be needed. For the initial transfusions D+ blood can be used, D- units can be reserved for the end of the procedure. Many workers elect, once transfusion with D+ blood in such a situation has been started, to continue to use D+ blood until such time as the patient makes anti-D. Certainly the supply of D- blood should not be exhausted by transfusing it to a patient who will lose most of the red cells via hemorrhage. In some instances no attempt need be made to prevent immunization to D, e.g. males and females beyond menopause. The clinical situation must also be taken into account. One of us (PDI) once had to talk an emergency room physician out of using huge quantities of D- blood for a 20 year-old D- woman. The reason that the use of D- blood was not justified was that during surgery following trauma, a hysterectomy was to be performed.

Compatibility Tests in Neonatal (Under Four Months of Age) Recipients

It is difficult to obtain blood samples from small infants. When blood is required for an exchange transfusion, compatibility tests can be performed with the mother's serum (see Chapter 41). The current AABB Standards (219) specify that neonates should receive only blood and blood components shown to lack antibodies reactive at 37°C. Further, if the initial tests on the infant's blood do not reveal the presence of atypical antibodies and if the infant has not been transfused with whole blood or plasma-containing components or derivatives, antibody-screening and compatibility tests need not be repeated during the first four months of the child's life. If only group O red cells of the same D type as the infant (or group O, D- cells) are transfused and the infant has not left the hospital, ABO and D typing need not be repeated during the first four months of life (219).

The reason that repeat antibody-screening tests are not mandated is that in a number of studies (220-226) no case of alloimmunization was seen in infants less than four months old, who had been transfused. However, there are exceptions. Anti-E was seen in one infant who

was 18 days old (227) and in another who was 11 weeks old (228). Anti-K was found (229) in a 12 week-old child who had received 28 red cell transfusions of 30 ml each and 23 transfusions, again 30 ml each, of fresh frozen plasma. As described in Chapter 18, anti-K was transiently produced by a 20 day-old infant with *E. coli* enterocolitis, who had not been transfused. It should be noted that the specificities seen are both also seen in never transfused, never pregnant individuals. In such circumstances anti-E is relatively common (see Chapter 12 and earlier in this chapter), while anti-K is rare (see Chapter 18) but not unknown. If, as suggested elsewhere, red cell E and K are not the original immunogens, it might be expected that an infant could be exposed to the actual immunogen, early in life. The findings (227-230) that occasional neonates make what react as alloantibodies has prompted some workers (228,229) to suggest that repeat antibody-screening tests in multiply transfused infants might be advisable.

Use of Serum or Plasma in Antibody Detection, Identification and in Compatibility Testing

In the original tests used for these purposes, red cells in saline at normal ionic strength (with or without the addition of bovine albumin) were incubated with the patient's serum. After various preliminary readings the tests were converted to IATs and read with polyspecific antiglobulin reagents that contained anti-IgG and anti-C3 (see Chapter 6). The use of serum and not plasma in such circumstances was (and still is if those tests are being used) important since in positive IATs part of the reaction was due to the detection of red cell bound IgG and part due to the detection of red cell bound C3. If plasma from anticoagulated samples is used in such tests, complement activation is prevented (again see Chapter 6) and the sensitivity of the test system is reduced.

When methods such as LISS, PEG and Polybrene IATs were introduced, it was found that unwanted (clinically meaningless) weakly positive IATs were seen if polyspecific antiglobulin serum was used. It was concluded that in such systems, benign cold-reactive autoantibodies often activate sufficient complement for it to be detected on red cells in IATs. Accordingly, most workers read IATs in such systems with anti-IgG. It is widely believed, although it does not seem to have been formally proved, that in such methods sufficient IgG is bound to the test red cells that clinically significant antibodies are detected without participation of the C3-anti-C3 reaction. If tests are to be read with anti-IgG, plasma is as suitable a test material as serum. However, the plasma should be from samples collected in to dry anticoagulants as the use of fluid anticoagulants could result in antibody dilution.

While one of us (PDI) has not experienced appreciable difficulties in reading LISS, PEG or Polybrene IATs with antiglobulin reagents that contain anti-C3, presence of that antibody apparently conveys no significant advantage, even when serum is used as the test material. Pereira and Alcorta (231) have claimed that the use of plasma instead of serum obviates the need for prewarmed tests. While it is true that the use of plasma will (largely) prevent the activation of complement by cold-reactive autoantibodies, it will not prevent those antibodies from causing agglutination that may then carry through to tests read at 37°C and/or to IATs read with anti-IgG.

Electronic Matching in Lieu of Compatibility Tests

Once it had become accepted that patients in whom antibody-screening tests were negative, could safely be transfused with units checked for ABO compatibility in an IS test, it was natural that workers would look for other ways to achieve the same objective. Some impetus for such studies were provided by the observations described above that while the IS test is highly reliable in the detection of ABO incompatibility, it is not infallible. In 1994, Butch et al. (232) described the use of a computer to match units of blood with patients, the units were then issued without further serological testing. While such an electronic matching system will vary in different institutions, dependent on the data processing equipment available, it is worth mentioning some critical features of the system described by Butch et al. (232,233).

For donor units

1. The bar code on the unit must allow computer entry of the unit number, component, ABO and D type and expiration date.
2. Results of confirmatory ABO and D typings on the unit must be entered directly in to the computer where they will be interpreted based on preestablished reaction patterns.
3. The computer must issue a warning if there is any discrepancy between the originally entered ABO and D type and the results of confirmatory tests or if only one set of typings has been entered.

For samples from patients

1. All patients must have a bar code wristband and all samples must be labeled at the bedside with a label generated from the bar code on the wristband.

2. Bar code entry of the sample accession number must be linked in the computer with details of patient identification.
3. Results of ABO and D typings on the samples must be entered directly in to the computer where they will be interpreted based on preestablished reaction patterns.
4. All patients must be typed twice for ABO and D. If a historical record exists in the computer, the current sample need be typed only once so long as the results are in concordance. If no historical record exists, the current sample must be typed twice.
5. At least one of the ABO and D typings must be on the current sample.
6. The computer must issue a warning if:
   a. There is any discrepancy between historical and current typings.
   b. There is any discrepancy between two current typings.
   c. Only one set of typings has been entered.
   d. If no typing on the current sample has been performed.
7. The computer must not display the historical ABO and D type until results of tests on the current sample have been entered.

The computer (repeats some of the above)

1. The computer must issue units based on bar code entry of the unit and bar code entry of patient's accession number.
2. The computer must block the issue of ABO incompatible units.
3. The computer must issue group O units in cases in which ABO discrepancies exist.
4. A computer warning must be issued if:
   a. Only one ABO and D type is on file.
   b. The current and historical ABO and D types differ.
   c. A D+ unit is selected for a D- patient.
   d. The patient is alloimmunized and requires an IAT for compatibility.
   e. The unit involved has not been retyped, has not been irradiated (when required), has outdated or has been quarantined for any reason.
5. The computer must generate a daily report of:
   a. Any reaction patterns that did not fit the predetermined criteria.
   b. Any instance in which a computer warning was followed by an override order.

Other

1. Staff must be trained in the IS test for compatibility for use during computer down time.

While using this system over a nine month period, Butch et al. (232) made 36,745 units available for issue, some 90% of them were computer matched. Among those units 22,771 were used with no known instance of ABO incompatibility. The requirement that two separate typings on each patient be recorded in the computer before a unit could be issued resulted in 3294 additional ABO and D typings. It was calculated that the cost of those typings was about one third of the cost that would have accrued if IS tests had been performed instead of computer matching. One advantage of computer matching not yet mentioned is that units to be issued can be selected, by the computer, based on their age. Clearly such automated selection has the potential to reduce outdating of units.

Cheng et al. (234) have described a system, for surgical patients, that is better described as computer listing than as computer matching. Each patient is typed for ABO. The computer then generates a list showing the patient's identification details and all units in inventory that are of the same ABO type as the patient. The units are stored in a refrigerator convenient to the operating rooms and as blood is needed, a nurse from the operating room simply picks one, by number, that is on the patient's list. Since each patient's list shows all suitable units, it does not matter if some have been used for other patients. From implementation of the system in 1995 until the report was written (234) 2154 patients had undergone surgery and 4861 units of blood had been transfused. About 40% of the blood transfused at the hospital was used for surgical patients. Since the incidence of the D- phenotype is less than 1% in the hospital in Hong Kong where the system was used, one presumes (the report did not specify) that patients with D- red cells were handled separately, as were non-surgical and alloimmunized patients. While this self-service system was well received by the surgical and nursing staffs, it is doubtful that many other transfusion services are yet ready to relinquish control as to which patient gets which unit of blood. One obvious addition that would be required in most transfusion services, would be highly accurate recording of which patient received which unit, for follow-up purposes as necessary.

A Final Note

Attentive readers may have noticed that in this long chapter, that includes much discussion about antibody detection and compatibility testing, the terms antibody-screen and crossmatch have not been used at all. One of us (PDI) continues to believe that the terms are slang for antibody-screening tests and compatibility tests, respectively. He clings to these beliefs in spite of the ridicule heaped upon him by colleagues, who should know better.

References

1. Vogel P. Bull NY Acad Med 1954;30:657
2. Kellner A. Obstet Gynecol 1955;5:499
3. Levine P, Robinson E, Stroup M, et al. Blood 1956;11:1097
4. Giblett ER. Transfusion 1961;1:233
5. Giblett ER. Clin Obstet Gynecol 1964;7:1044
6. Kissmeyer Nielsen F. Scand J Haematol 1965;2:331
7. Moore BPL, Humphreys P, Lovett-Moseley CA. Serological and Immunological Methods, 7th Ed. Toronto:Canadian Red Cross, 1972
8. Spielmann W, Seidl S. Vox Sang 1974;26:551
9. Stern K. Transfusion 1975;15:179
10. Giblett ER. Transfusion 1977;17:299
11. Issitt PD. In: Rh Problems in Clinical Practice. Groningen-Drenthe:Netherlands Red Cross, 1979:46
12. Heisto H. Transfusion 1979;19:761
13. Walker RH, Lin D-T, Hartrick MB. Arch Pathol Lab Med 1989;113:254
14. Hoeltge GA, Domen RE, Rybicki LA, et al. Arch Pathol Lab Med 1995;119:42
15. Knight R. Unpublished observations 1988 and 1990 cited in Mollison PL, Engelfriet CP, Contreras M. Blood Transfusion in Clinical Medicine, 9th Ed. Oxford:Blackwell 1993:111
16. Orlina AR, Unger PJ, Koshy M. Am J Hematol 1978;5:101
17. Coles SM, Klein HG, Holland PV. Transfusion 1981;21:462
18. Luban NLC, Posey L. (abstract). Transfusion 1982;22:413
19. Blumberg N, Peck K, Ross K, et al. Vox Sang 1983;44:212
20. Blumberg N, Ross K, Avila E, et al. Vox Sang 1984;47:205
21. Davies SC, McWilliam AC, Hewitt PE, et al. Br J Haematol 1986;63:241
22. Sarnaik S, Schornack J, Lusher JM. Transfusion 1986;26:249
23. Ambruso DR, Githens JH, Alcorn R, et al. Transfusion 1987;27:94
24. Reisner EG, Kostyu DD, Phillips G, et al. Tissue Antigens 1987;30:161
25. Patten ED, Patel SN, Soto B, et al. (abstract). Book of Abstracts, Sickle Cell Disease: Current Perspectives. NY Acad Sci, 1988
26. Rosse WF, Gallagher D, Kinney TR, et al. Blood 1990;76:1431
27. Blumberg BS, Alter HJ, Riddell M, et al. Vox Sang 1964;9:128
28. Economidou J, Constantoulakis M, Augoustaki O, et al. Vox Sang 1971;10:252
29. Sirchia G, Zanella A, Parravicini A, et al. Transfusion 1985;25:110
30. Lostumbo MM, Holland PV, Schmidt PJ. New Eng J Med 1966;275:141
31. Domen R, Ramirez G, Calero A. (abstract). Blood 1986;68 (Suppl 1):296a
32. Brantley SG, Ramsey G. Transfusion 1988;28:463
33. Issitt PD. Transfusion 1965;5:355
34. Archer GT, Cooke BR, Mitchell K, et al. Rev Fr Transf 1969;12:341
35. Issitt PD, McKeever BG, Moore VK, et al. Transfusion 1973;13:316
36. Mollison PL, Engelfriet CP, Contreras M. Blood Transfusion in Clinical Medicine, 9th Ed. Oxford:Blackwell 1993
37. Byrne PC, Howard JH. Immunohematology 1994;10:136
38. Walker RH. In: Hemolytic Disease of the Newborn.

Arlington, VA:Am Assoc Blood Banks, 1984:173

39. Walker W. Vox Sang 1958;3:225
40. Walker W. Vox Sang 1958;3:336
41. Walker RH. Unpublished observations 1991 cited in Mollison PL, Engelfriet CP, Contreras M. Blood Transfusion in Clinical Medicine, 9th Ed. Oxford:Blackwell 1993:111
42. Dovey GJ. Unpublished observations cited in Mollison PL, Engelfriet CP, Contreras M. Blood Transfusion in Clinical Medicine, 9th Ed. Oxford:Blackwell 1993:111
43. Combs MR, Issitt PD, Telen MJ. Unpublished observations 1989-1996
44. Malone RH, Dunsford I. Blood 1951;6:1135
45. Vogt E, Krystad E, Heisto H, et al. Vox Sang 1958;3:118
46. Dybkjaer E. Vox Sang 1967;13:446
47. Harrison J. Vox Sang 1970;19:123
48. Issitt PD, Combs MR, Bredehoeft SJ, et al. Transfusion 1993;33:284
49. Contreras M. Unpublished observations 1988 and 1990 cited in Mollison PL, Engelfriet CP, Contreras M. Blood Transfusion in Clinical Medicine, 9th Ed. Oxford:Blackwell 1993:111
50. Issitt PD, Issitt CH. Applied Blood Group Serology, 2nd Ed. Oxnard:Spectra Biologicals, 1975
51. Cutbush M, Mollison PL. Br J Haematol 1958;4:115
52. Mollison PL. Br Med J 1959;2:1035
53. Mollison PL. Br Med J 1959;2:1123
54. Mollison PL. Br Med Bull 1959;15:92
55. Mollison PL. Acta Haematol 1959;10:495
56. Mollison PL, Johnson CA, Prior DM. Vox Sang 1978;35:149
57. Morel PA, Garratty G, Perkins HA. Am J Med Technol 1978;44:122
58. Cronin CA, Pohl BA, Miller WV. Transfusion 1978;18:728
59. Issitt PD. In: Clinically Significant and Insignificant Antibodies. Washington, D.C.:Am Assoc Blood Banks, 1979:13
60. Garratty G. In: Clinically Significant and Insignificant Antibodies. Washington, D.C.:Am Assoc Blood Banks, 1979:29
61. Waheed A, Kennedy MS, Gerhan S, et al. Am J Clin Pathol 1981;76:294
62. Issitt PD. In: Advances in Pathology: Anatomic and Clinical, Part 1. Oxford:Pergamon, 1982:395
63. Judd WJ, Butch SH. J Med Technol 1984;1:485
64. Beck ML, Tilzer LL. Transf Med Rev 1996;10:118
65. Moureau P. Rev Belge Sci Med 1945;16:258
66. Issitt PD. Unpublished observations 1961 cited in previous editions of this book
67. Di Napoli JB, Nichols ME, Marsh WL, et al. (abstract). Transfusion 1978;18:383
68. Mollison PL. Verbal comments during a lecture on Immune Red Cell Destruction. Univ Miami, 1982
69. Issitt PD. Unpublished observations 1982 cited in Issitt PD. Applied Blood Group Serology, 3rd Ed. Miami:Montgomery, 1985:479
70. Davey RJ. In: Clinical and Serological Aspects of Transfusion Reactions. Washington, D.C.:Am Assoc Blood Banks, 1982:1
71. Davey RJ. Personal communication 1983 cited in Issitt PD. Applied Blood Group Serology, 3rd Ed. Miami:Montgomery, 1985:480
72. Mollison PL. Blood Transfusion in Clinical Medicine, 7th Ed. Oxford:Blackwell, 1983
73. Kurtz SR, Ouellet R, McMican A, et al. Transfusion 1983;23:37
74. Wertlake PT, McGinniss MH, Schmidt PJ. Transfusion 1969;9:70
75. Klein HG, Faltz LL, McIntosh CL, et al. Transfusion 1980;20:354
76. Taft EG, Propp RP, Sullivan SA. Transfusion 1977;17:173
77. Löw B. Vox Sang (Old Series) 1955;5:94
78. Haber G, Rosenfield RE. PH Andresen, Papers in Dedication of his 60th Birthday. Copenhagen:Munksgaard, 1957:45
79. Pirofsky B, Mangum MEJ. Proc Soc Exp Biol 1959;101:49
80. Dodd BE, Eeles DA. Immunology 1961;4:337
81. Dodd BE, Wilkinson PC. J Exp Med 1964;120:45
82. Holburn AM, Frame M, Hughes-Jones NC, et al. Immunology 1971;20:681
83. Casey FM, Dodd BE, Lincoln PJ. Vox Sang 1972;23:493
84. Heisto H, Fagerhol MK. Transfusion 1979;19:545
85. Contreras M, de Silva PM, Teesdale P, et al. Br J Haematol 1987;65:475
86. Garratty G. Med Lab Sci 1988;45:5
87. Van Djik BA. PhD Dissertation, Univ Leyden 1991
88. Pereira A, Mazzara A, Gelabert A, et al. Haematologica 1991;76:475
89. Van Djik BA. (Letter). Transfusion 1993;33:960
90. Issitt PD, Gutgsell NS. In: Immune Destruction of Red Cells. Arlington, VA:Am Assoc Blood Banks, 1989:77
91. Issitt PD. (Letter). J Am Med Assoc 1985;24:3423
92. Judd WJ. Methods in Immunohematology, 2nd Ed. Miami:Montgomery, 1994
93. Judd WJ. Transfusion 1995;35:271
94. Judd WJ. (Letter). Transfusion 1996;36:192
95. Mallory DM. Transfusion 1995;35:268
96. Garratty G. (Letter). Transfusion 1996;36:192
97. Combs MR, Issitt PD. Unpublished observations 1989 - 1996
98. Judd WJ, Steiner EA, Knafl P, et al. (abstract). Transfusion 1995;35 (Suppl 10S):68S
99. Champagne K, Spruell P, Chen J, et al. (abstract). Transfusion 1995; 35 (Suppl 10S):67S
100. Garratty G, Arndt P, Marfoe R, et al. (abstract). Transfusion 1995;35 (Suppl 10S):22S
101. Winn LC, Svoboda R, Hafleigh EB, et al. (abstract). Transfusion 1980;20:651
102. Silvergleid AJ. Transfusion 1980;20:729
103. Bowman HS, Brason FW, Mohn J, et al. Br J Haematol 1961;7:130
104. Zettner A, Bove JR. Transfusion 1963;3:48
105. Franciosi R, Awer E, Santana M. Transfusion 1967;7:297
106. Abbott D, Hussain S. Canad Med Assoc J 1970;103:752
107. Morse EE. Vox Sang 1978;35:215
108. Goldfinger D, Kleinman S, Connelly M, et al. (abstract). Transfusion 1979;19:639
109. Ballas SK, Bosch J, Miguel O. (Letter). Transfusion 1981;21:577
110. Mollison PL. In: Safety in Transfusion Practices. Skokie, IL:Coll Am Pathologists, 1982
111. Wallas CH, Tanley PC, Gorrell LP. Transfusion 1980;20:332
112. Reid ME, Toy P. Am J Clin Pathol 1983;79:364
113. Branch DR, Sy Siok Hian AL, Carlson F, et al. Am J Clin Pathol 1983;80:453
114. Mougey R. In: Micromethods in Blood Group Serology. Arlington, VA:Am Assoc Blood Banks, 1984:19
115. Brown D. Transfusion 1988;28:21
116. Jennings JB. Transfusion 1968;8:335
117. Katz AJ, Morse EE. Transfusion 1973;13:324
118. Devitt JE. Canad Med Assoc J 1973;109:120
119. Hospital Record Study 1975. Ambler
120. Friedman BA, Oberman HA, Chadwick AR, et al. Transfusion 1976;16:380
121. Mintz PD, Nordine RB, Henry JB, et al. NY State J Med

1976;76:532

122. Henry JB, Mintz P. J Am Med Assoc 1977;237:451
123. Boral LI, Henry JB. Transfusion 1977;17:163
124. Bear MR, Friedman BA. PAS Reporter 1977;15, No 11
125. Henry JB, Mintz P. Qual Rev Bull 1977;3:7
126. Oberman HA, Barnes BA, Friedman BA. Transfusion 1978;18:137
127. Rouault C, Gruenhagen J. Transfusion 1978;18:448
128. Mintz P, Lauenstein K, Hume J, et al. J Am Med Assoc 1978;239:623
129. Blumberg N, Bove JR. J Am Med Assoc 1978;240:2057
130. Boral LI, Hill SS, Apollon CJ, et al. Am J Clin Pathol 1979;71:578
131. Friedman BA. Transfusion 1979;19:268
132. Seshadri RS, Odell WR, Roxby D, et al. Med J Austral 1979;2:575
133. Lang GE, Drozda EA. Wisc Med J 1979;78:27
134. Friedman BA, Burns TL, Schork MA. Transfusion 1980;20:179
135. Lee K, Lachance V. Transfusion 1980;20:324
136. Rouault C. In: Pretransfusion Testing for the 80s. Washington, D.C.:Am Assoc Blood Banks, 1980:125
137. Huang ST, Lair J, Floyd DM, et al. Transfusion 1980;20:725
138. Ness PM, Rosche ME, Barrasso C, et al. Am J Obstet Gynecol 1981;41:661
139. Mintz PD, Haines AL, Sullivan MF. Transfusion 1982;22:107
140. Mayer K. In: Safety in Transfusion Practices. Skokie, IL:Coll Am Pathologists, 1982
141. Svoboda R. Lab World 1982;32:26
142. Garratty G. Transfusion 1982;22:169
143. Shulman IA, Nelson JM, Saxena S, et al. Am J Clin Pathol 1984;82:178
144. Shulman IA, Nelson JM, Kent DR, et al. J Am Med Assoc 1985;254:93
145. Dodsworth H, Dudley HAF. Br J Surg 1985;72:102
146. Mintz PD, Sullivan MF. Obstet Gynecol 1985;65:389
147. Shulman IA, Kiyabu M, Nelson JM, et al. Lab Med 1986;17:407
148. Perrault RA, Barr RA. In: Progress in Transfusion Med, Vol 1. Edinburgh:Churchill Livingstone, 1986:95
149. Shulman IA, Meyer EA, Lam H-T, et al. CBBS Today 1987;5:8
150. Soloway HB, McClausin M, Belliveau RR. Med Lab Obs 1988;20:27
151. Shulman IA, Kent D. Arch Pathol Lab Med 1989;113:270
152. Meyer EA, Shulman IA. Transfusion 1989;29:99
153. Shulman IA. In: Immune Destruction of Red Blood Cells. Arlington, VA:Am Assoc Blood Banks, 1989:171
154. Shulman IA. Arch Pathol Lab Med 1990;114:412
155. Napier JAF, Boulton FE, Cann R, et al. Clin Lab Haematol 1990;12:321
156. Cordle DG, Strauss RG, Snyder EL, et al. Am J Clin Pathol 1990;94:428
157. Oberman HA. Transfusion 1992;32:794
158. Pinkerton PH, Coovadia AS, Goldstein J. Transfusion 1992;32:814
159. Contreras M. In: The Association of Clinical Pathologists Yearbook. Ashford, UK:Assoc Clin Pathologists, 1994:60
160. Shulman IA, Petz LD. In: Clinical Practice of Transfusion Medicine, 3rd Ed. New York:Churchill Livingstone, 1996:199
161. Walker RH. In: Current Topics in Blood Banking. Ann Arbor:Univ Michigan, 1977
162. Spivack M. In: Pretransfusion Testing for the 80s. Washington, D.C.:Am Assoc Blood Banks, 1980:133
163. Walker RH. Pathologist 1981;35:543

164. Micklos D. Med Lab Obs 1981;13:71
165. Oberman HA. Transfusion 1981;21:645
166. Oberman HA, Barnes BA, Steiner EA. Transfusion 1982;22:12
167. Myhre B. Diag Med 1982;Sept-Oct:23
168. International Forum. Published opinions of eleven experts. Vox Sang 1982;43:151
169. Walker RH. In: Safety in Transfusion Practices. Skokie, IL:Coll Am Pathologists, 1982
170. Masouredis SP. Blood 1982;59;873
171. Moore BP. Canad Med Assoc J 1984;130:1421
172. Napier JAF, Biffin AH, Lay D. Br Med J 1985;291:799
173. Isbister JP. Pathology 1987;19:113
174. Napier JA. Br J Haematol 1991;78:1
175. Löw B, Messeter L. Vox Sang 1974;26:53
176. Moore HC, Mollison PL. Transfusion 1976;16:291
177. Wicker B, Wallas CH. Transfusion 1976;16:469
178. Rock G, Baxter A, Charron M, et al. Transfusion 1978;18:228
179. Owen IA, Blajchman MA, O'Hoski P, et al. Transfusion 1979;19:95
180. Honig CL, Bove JR. Transfusion 1980;20:653
181. Schmidt PJ. In: Immunobiology of the Erythrocyte. New York:Liss, 1980
182. Schmidt PJ. J Florida Med Assoc 1980;67:151
183. Myhre BA. J Am Med Assoc 1980;244:1333
184. Myhre BA, Bove JR, Schmidt PJ. Anesth Analg 1981;60:777
185. Edinger SE. Med Lab Obs 1985;April:41
186. Murphy WG, McClelland DB. Vox Sang 1989;57:59
187. Bacon J, Young IF. Pathology 1989;21:181
188. Sazama K. Transfusion 1990;30:583
189. Linden JV, Paul B, Dressler KP. Transfusion 1992;32:601
190. Henry J. Unpublished observations cited in Garratty G. Transfusion 1982;22:169
191. Wallace EL, Churchill WH, Surgenor DM, et al. Transfusion 1995;35:802
192. Harrison CR. In: Comprehensive Blood Bank 1987 survey, Set J-D. Chicago:Coll Am Pathologists, 1987
193. Schmidt PJ. In: Comprehensive Blood Bank 1990 Survey, Set J-A. Northfield, IL:Coll Am Pathologists, 1990
194. Shulman IA. (Letter). Transfusion 1981;21:469
195. Berry-Dortch S, Woodside CH, Boral LI. Transfusion 1985;25:176
196. Steane EA, Steane SM, Montgomery SB, et al. Transfusion 1985;25:540
197. Sererat S, Beatty J, Schifano JV, et al. (Letter). Transfusion 1985;25:589
198. Shulman IA, Nelson JM, Lam H-T, et al. (Letter). Transfusion 1985;25:589
199. Pohl BA. (Letter). Transfusion 1985;25:588
200. Park H. (Letter). Transfusion 1985;25:588
201. Trudeau LR, Judd WJ, Butch SH, et al. Transfusion 1983;23:237
202. Judd WJ, Steiner EA, O'Donnell DB, et al. Transfusion 1988;26:334
203. Judd WJ, Barnes BA. (Letter). Transfusion 1989;29:84
204. Judd WJ. Transfusion 1991;31:192
205. Shulman IA, Calderon C. Transfusion 1991;31:197
206. Voak D. Vox Sang 1972;22:408
207. Sosler SD, Perkins JT, Saporito C, et al. (abstract). Transfusion 1989;29 (Suppl 7S):49S
208. Ramsey G, Larsen P. Transfusion 1988;28:162
209. Ramsey G, Smietana SJ. Transfusion 1994;34:122
210. Domen RE, Ramirez G. Nephron 1988;48:284
211. Judd WJ, Barnes BA, Steiner EA, et al. Transfusion 1986;26:220

212. Kaplan HS, Garratty G. Diagnostic Med 1985;8:29
213. Vengelen-Tyler V. Ed. Technical Manual, 12th Ed. Bethesda:Am Assoc Blood Banks, 1996
214. Patten E, Conti V. J Am Med Assoc 1982;247:209
215. Issitt PD, Tomasulo PA. (Letter). J Am Med Assoc 1982;248:169
216. Issitt PD. La Trasf Sangue 1987;32:273
217. International Forum. Published opinions of eighteen experts. Vox Sang 1995;69:292
218. Algora M, Barbolla L, Contreras M. (Letter). Vox Sang 1991;61:141
219. Klein HG. Ed. Standards for Blood Banks and Transfusion Services, 17th Ed. Bethesda, MD:Am Assoc Blood Banks, 1996
220. Pass MA, Johnson JD, Shulman IA, et al. J Pediat 1976;89:646
221. Rawls WE, Wong CL, Blajchman M, et al. Clin Invest Med 1984;7:13
222. Floss AM, Strauss RG, Goeken N, et al. Transfusion 1986;26:419
223. Ludvigsen C, Swanson JL, Thompson TR, et al. Am J Clin Pathol 1987;87:250
224. Strauss RG. Am J Dis Childh 1991;145:904
225. Strauss RG. Transfusion 1993;33:352
226. Strauss RG. In: Scientific Basis of Transfusion Medicine. Philadelphia:Saunders, 1994:421
227. Smith MR, Storey CG. (Letter). Transfusion 1984;24:540
228. De Palma L, Criss VR, Roseff SD, et al. Transfusion 1992;32:177
229. Maniatis A, Theodoris H, Aravani K. (Letter). Transfusion 1993;33:90
230. Marsh WL, Nichols ME, Øyen R, et al. Transfusion 1978;18:149
231. Pereira A, Alcorta I. (Letter). Transfusion 1995;35:885
232. Butch SH, Judd WJ, Steiner EA, et al. Transfusion 1994;34:105
233. Butch SH, Judd WJ. (Letter). Transfusion 1994;34:187
234. Cheng G, Chiu DSM, Chung ASM, et al. Transfusion 1996;36:347
235. Devine P, Goldstein R, Linden JV, et al. Transfusion 1996;36:375
236. O'Neill P, Garratty G. (abstract). Transfusion 1983;23:407
237. Arndt P, Garratty G. Transfusion 1988;28:210
238. Maffei LM. In: Pretransfusion Testing: Routine to Complex. Bethesda:Am Assoc Blood Banks, 1995
239. Fisher GA. Transfusion 1983;23:151
240. Ferrer Z, Wright J, Moore BPL, et al. Transfusion 1985;25:145
241. Mintz PD, Anderson G. Transfusion 1987;27:134
242. Lown JAG, Ivy JG. J Clin Pathol 1987;8:7
243. Castellino S, Combs MR, Kinney TR, et al. (abstract). Blood 1997;90 (Suppl 1):128b
244. Heddle NM, Soutar RL, O'Hoski PL, et al. Br J Haematol 1995;91:1000
245. Heddle NM, O'Hoski P, Singer J, et al. Br J Haematol 1992;81:579
246. Ness PM, Shirey RS, Thomas SK, et al. Transfusion 1990;30:688
247. Judd WJ, Steiner EA, Oberman HA, et al. Transfusion 1992;32:304
248. Alkhashan AA, Combs MR, Issitt PD. (abstract). Transfusion 1997;37 (Suppl 9S):28S
249. Rolih SD, Fisher FS, Figueroa D, et al. (abstract). Transfusion 1994;34 (Suppl 10S):19S
250. Alkhashan AA. MHS Thesis, Duke Univ 1996
251. Judd WJ, Fullen DR, Steiner EA, et al. (abstract). Transfusion 1997;37 (Suppl 9S):65S

36 | Transfusion Reactions

The term transfusion reaction is used to describe any unfavorable response by a patient, to the infusion of blood or blood products. This means that not all transfusion reactions are associated with red cell destruction following in vivo formation of antigen-antibody complexes. However, transfusion reactions that are caused by such destruction are among the more serious that can occur. Because this book deals predominantly with red cell antigens and the antibodies directed against them, most of this chapter is devoted to a discussion of transfusion reactions that involve antibody-mediated red cell clearance. Some other unfavorable responses to transfusion are mentioned briefly; readers requiring more information about those subjects should consult Mollison et al. (1). The types of unfavorable responses discussed in this chapter are:

1. Hemolytic reactions involving intravascular red cell destruction
2. Hemolytic reactions involving extravascular red cell destruction
3. Delayed reactions involving red cell destruction
4. Delayed reactions not involving red cell destruction
5. Febrile reactions
6. Allergic reactions
7. Anaphylactic reactions
8. Reactions caused by circulatory overload
9. Reactions caused by contaminated blood
10. Reactions caused when drugs are added to blood
11. Reactions caused by toxic substances in the blood.

Hemolytic Transfusion Reactions Involving Intravascular Red Cell Destruction

This type of reaction is dramatic and severe and is the type most likely to be fatal. It occurs when transfused red cells are destroyed in the patient's circulation (that being the definition of intravascular hemolysis (2,3)) often at the site of infusion. The major symptoms are fever, chills, a burning sensation at the site of infusion, feeling of chest-restriction, shock (often severe and life-threatening), hypotension and joint or lower back pain. Although it hardly sounds like a clinical symptom, patients experiencing a transfusion reaction sometimes express "a feeling of impending doom". Such a comment should be taken seriously in a patient who is being or has recently been transfused. The major complications that follow intravascular red cell destruction

are disseminated intravascular coagulation (DIC) and renal failure (1,4-17) that, together with irreversible shock may result in death of the patient. Although it was believed for many years that renal failure following the transfusion of ABO incompatible blood occurred because free hemoglobin directly damaged cells of the kidney, it is now appreciated that the situation is very much more complex. The pathophysiology of incompatible transfusion is discussed below.

Clinical symptoms characteristic of a transfusion reaction involving intravascular red cell destruction may be seen after transfusion of relatively small volumes of blood and usually occur before a whole unit is infused although exceptions are seen. The antibodies responsible for this type of red cell destruction are those that cause rapid activation of large amounts of complement. Immediately the incompatible cells are infused, antigen-antibody complexes are formed and complement is activated. The complement activation sequence proceeds rapidly from EAC1 to the EAC9 stage (see Chapter 6) and hemolysis of the transfused cells occurs in the patient's circulation. As this brief description of intravascular hemolysis will show, the antibodies most often causative of this type of transfusion reaction are those of the ABO system. Any time that major-side ABO incompatible blood is transfused, the potential for intravascular hemolysis exists. In this context, major-side ABO incompatible means the transfusion of group A, B or AB blood into a group O recipient; A or AB blood into a group B; or B or AB blood into a group A recipient. It does not include less significant ABO incompatibility such as the transfusion of A_1 cells to an A_2 recipient with anti-A_1 in the plasma or transfusion of O cells to an A_1 or B patient with anti-H. The net effects of the transfusion of ABO major-side incompatible blood are quite variable in different patients and some major reasons for that variation are described in the following sections.

ABO Incompatible Transfusions: Effect of Antigen and Antibody Levels

In severe transfusion reactions resulting from ABO incompatibility there are two major factors that contribute to immediate intravascular hemolysis. First, the red cells carry large numbers of copies of A or B; circa 1 to 2 X 10^6 per red cell (18-22). Second, the recipient's plasma contains many IgG and IgM molecules of anti-A or anti-B. Both forms of these antibodies activate complement (23-25). However, once complement is activated at the site of an antigen-antibody complex, many of its components (see Chapter 6) must travel and bind to the red cell membrane in order to effect the lesion that represents hemolysis. Since activated complement components decay rapidly in the fluid phase, it is likely that those activated close to the membrane are the ones that effect hemolysis. Rosenfield (26) believed that in view of the large numbers of copies of ABO system antigens on red cells and of ABO antibody molecules in plasma, anti-A and anti-B must be considered relatively inefficient hemolysins. Further, he (26) believed that those antibody molecules that bind to antigens carried on short chains (27) (i.e. close to the membrane) are the ones that effect most of the lysis (those bound to antigens on long chains, i.e. distant from the membrane, activate complement but many of the components are inactive by the time they reach the membrane). These suggestions certainly fit some observed findings. First, if some A and B antigens are close to the membrane and others are more distant (27) it would be expected that the small IgG antibody molecules would be better able to approach and bind to the close-in sites than would the larger IgM molecules (steric arrangement of membrane components would result in better access for small than for large molecules). Second, in ABO antibody-mediated red cell destruction, IgG anti-A and anti-B seem to play a greater role than do IgM anti-A and anti-B (3,28,29).

Obviously, since both antibody and antigen concentration are important in terms of the amount and rate of intravascular red cell destruction due to ABO incompatibility, the most severe transfusion reactions will be seen when both are high. There are data that show that a reduction in either one results in less, or slower intravascular hemolysis. Mollison et al. (1) describe several cases in which the recipients of ABO incompatible red cells had reduced levels of anti-A or anti-B. Sometimes this was a function of agammaglobulinemia and on other occasions because the transfusions were to older patients in whom ABO antibody production had decreased in level. In each instance, the rate of removal of red cells was slower then in persons with more potent anti-A and anti-B.

In terms of antigen content, Wiener et al. (30) and Mollison (31,32) have shown that group A_2 red cells are cleared more slowly in persons of group O, than are A_1 cells. However, transfusion reactions due to ABO antibodies can still occur when the donor cells carry a very low level of antigen. Schmidt et al. (33) described a group O patient who experienced some symptoms of a transfusion reaction when given a unit of blood later shown to be of the A_x phenotype. The patient's pretransfusion serum was shown to have a titer of 1000 against A_1 cells and 8 against A_x cells. In contrast, when Boose et al. (34) studied a family in which a number of individuals had a very

weak B antigen (category 2 in table 8-10, Chapter 8) they found that one of them was a blood donor whose unit had been typed as group O, found compatible with a group O patient's serum and had been transfused with no ill effects. Retrospective analysis indicated that the red cells with weak B had apparently survived normally in the group O recipient. Hemolytic transfusion reactions can also occur in spite of a very low level of an ABO antibody in the recipient's serum. Garratty et al. (35) described a 92 year-old male who was actually group A_1 and had an acquired B antigen (see Chapter 8) but who was mistyped as group AB when a monoclonal anti-B reagent (now adjusted in terms of pH to prevent the problem) was used. The patient was given three units of group AB and one unit of group A blood (all compatible by an IS method at the referring hospital) without untoward reactions being seen. After a fourth unit of AB blood was transfused the patient had a severe transfusion reaction, developed renal failure and died 10 days later. When the pretransfusion serum was tested at the reference laboratory, weak anti-B, most clearly demonstrable by IAT, was detected. Thus while the general rule is that ABO antibody-induced intrava~~~~~~~~~~~~~~~~~~~~~~~~~~~~~gh A or B antigen sit~~~~~~~~~~~~~~~~~~~~~~~~~ anti-B, exceptions h~~~~~~~~~~~~~~~~~~~~~~~at the failure of anti-A~~~~~~~~~~~~~~~~~~~~~to clear A_1 red cells d~~~~~~~~~~~~~~~~~r antibody concentra~~~~~~~~~~~~~~~~n antibodies to bind t~~~~~~~~~~~~~~~also section on cold-r~~~~~~~~~

[handwritten note: Volume of Blood Transfused]

ABO Incompatible Transfusions: Effect of Amount of Blood Transfused

Another factor of importance in the consideration of ABO incompatibility is the amount of blood transfused. Although the severity of the immediate reaction may not appear to be greatly influenced by volume (severe reactions may be seen when small amounts of blood are transfused) the consequences of incompatible transfusion are generally more severe, the larger the volume of blood infused (1,38-43). For this reason, it is imperative that transfusion be stopped immediately signs of a transfusion reaction are noticed. The smallest amount of ABO incompatible blood reported to have caused a fatal transfusion reaction seems to be about 30 ml (39,43) but more often, in patients who suffer severe reactions, 200 ml or more has been transfused.

ABO Incompatible Transfusions: Mortality

Both Mollison (44) and Wallace (45) have estimat-

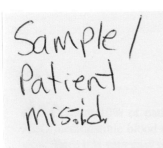

who receive major-side ... a result of the transfu- ... ermine the ABO types of both patients and donors, it would seem to be a comparatively straightforward task to avoid ABO incompatibility in transfusion. Indeed, those transfusion accidents that do occur, seldom result from mistakes in ABO typing. Instead they occur when samples are mislabeled or drawn from the wrong patient, or when a unit of blood intended for one patient is erroneously given to another. Honig and Bove (39) and Schmidt (41,46) reviewed all reported cases of transfusion related fatalities in the USA in 1976, 1977 and 1978. It was found (39) that of 70 patients who died, 44 had acute hemolytic transfusion reactions. Among those 44 patients, 38 had received ABO incompatible blood and in the 37 cases in which the error could be traced, 33 involved a clerical mistake. Lest blood bankers become too complacent and blame the errors on others (wrong sample submitted, blood given to wrong person, etc.) it should be added that 13 of the 33 clerical errors occurred in the blood bank. In 1990, Sazama (43) updated the numbers by reviewing all reported transfusion fatalities in the USA during the period 1976 to 1985. Among a total of 355 deaths, 99 were unrelated to transfusion or were due to hepatitis or AIDS. Among the remaining 256 reported deaths, 131 were said to involve acute hemolysis due to ABO incompatibility. Among those 131 cases, 124 involved the transfusion of major-side ABO incompatible red cells (the other seven deaths were reported to have resulted from the passive transfer of ABO antibodies in donor plasma or platelet preparations, a hard to accept conclusion, and will not be considered further, here). In those cases in which the error leading to the fatality could be identified some: 10% involved a sample drawn from the wrong patient or otherwise misidentified; 18% involved a clerical or management (system failure) error in the blood bank; 15% a technical error in the blood bank; and 57% transfusion of the unit to the wrong patient. Among units transfused to the wrong patient, only 29% of the errors occurred in operating rooms, thus dispelling another blood bankers' myth. As can be seen, the numbers have not changed, that is 38 avoidable deaths in 1976 to 1978 for an average of 12.6 per year, then 86 more from 1979 to 1985 for an average of 12.3 per year. When the absolute numbers are considered, the incidence of avoidable deaths caused by the transfusion of ABO incompatible units appears to be small. That is, between 1976 and 1985 some 110 million units would have been transfused to some 31 million patients. Thus 124 deaths represents a 1 in 250,000 chance of any given patient being killed by the transfusion. However, even this number is clearly unacceptable. If the death rate from an ABO incompatible trans-

fusion is 10% (44,45) then the chance that any given patient will be transfused with ABO major-side incompatible blood is 1 in 25,000, again an unacceptable number. Adding to this already grim picture, it is generally believed that transfusion fatalities are underreported. Since ABO typing is so straightforward and since numerous sophisticated positive identification systems for both people (patients) and units now exist, the only acceptable number would be zero. It is a rather sad commentary on the science of transfusion medicine that while we now have highly sensitive systems to detect very low levels of antibodies (some of which are clinically meaningless) and while we can clone the genes that encode production of most of the known blood group antigens, we have still not developed a foolproof system always to get the right blood to the right patient. This in spite of the fact that we have been aware of the importance of ABO compatibility for almost 100 years.

Another disturbing way of looking at the data is that as of January 1997, the risk of getting HIV from a transfusion is around 1 in 700,000 in the USA. As stated above, the risk of being killed by ABO incompatible blood is around 1 in 250,000, or almost three times higher than the risk of AIDS. Persons who elect to donate blood for autologous use are only aware of the smaller risk.

Intravascular Red Cell Destruction Caused by Other than ABO Antibodies

Antibodies other than those in the ABO system can cause intravascular destruction of red cells but the incidence of such reactions is very much lower than that caused by ABO antibodies. Antibodies, such as anti-Tj[a], anti-Vel and some examples of anti-Le[a] that act as hemolysins in vitro, can cause intravascular lysis in vivo. Anti-Le[a] does so only when active at 37°C and even then (for reasons discussed in detail in Chapters 6 and 9) is often capable of only limited in vivo red cell destruction.

Hemolytic Transfusion Reactions Involving Extravascular Red Cell Destruction

When blood incompatible with an antibody in the patient's plasma, that is unable to bind complement at all, or is able to bind complement only at relatively slow rates, is transfused, red cell destruction and a transfusion reaction may occur but generally the reaction will be less severe than that seen when intravascular destruction occurs. The symptoms of this type of reaction are similar to those seen in reactions involving intravascular destruction but again are generally less severe. Fever and chills are the most commonly reported symptoms but, unlike those seen in reactions involving intravascular red cell destruction, may not occur until some time after completion of the transfusion. It is important in the investigation of a transfusion reaction that all units of blood given to the patient be retested. For example, a patient who has received several units of blood may experience the symptoms of a transfusion reaction while receiving another unit. Demonstration, in the laboratory, that the unit being transfused at the time that the reaction occurred was compatible, does not by any means exclude a hemolytic transfusion reaction. A patient may develop the symptoms of a reaction while being transfused with a fourth unit of blood although actually reacting to one of the three units previously given. Because the destruction of red cells via an extravascular mechanism generally occurs more slowly than destruction via an intravascular mechanism, the resultant consequences are not usually as serious. It is difficult to determine the fatality rate that follows extravascular clearance of incompatible red cells; it is safe to say that it does not even vaguely approach the 10% associated with intravascular destruction. In reviewing the reported transfusion fatalities from 1976 to 1985, Sazama (43) lists 26 that were reported to involve non-ABO system antibodies. It should be pointed out that Sazama (43) used all data reported to the US Food and Drug Administration (FDA) and did not attempt to interpret some of them. Thus one of the deaths was reported (to the FDA) to have been caused by anti-Ch and another by an HTLA antibody. Clearly the list of 26 can immediately be reduced by two! Further, in 13 of the cases, death occurred nine or more (as long as 16) days after transfusion and in another eight the interval between transfusion and death could not be determined from the report to the FDA. Thus there must remain very considerable doubt that the transfusion was directly responsible for the patient's death in many of these cases.

Mollison (44) points out that disseminated intravascular coagulation following predominantly extravascular destruction of transfused red cells is also a rare event (6,47). He also notes that in extravascular red cell destruction most of the red cells are sequestered intact in organs of the body but that some escape from phagocytes and rupture in the circulation. This may be one explanation of the hemoglobinemia and hemoglobinuria sometimes seen following extravascular red cell destruction, other possibilities are considered below.

Renal failure following extravascular red cell destruction is a rare event and even when seen, is most frequent in patients who were at risk of renal failure had they not been transfused (1). There are, of course, two types of antibody that can cause extravascular red cell clearance. One type is non-complement binding (e.g. Rh antibodies) while the other type activates sub-lytic amounts of complement (e.g. Duffy and Kidd system antibodies). It seems that the latter type of antibody (i.e. one that can activate some complement) is often associated with somewhat more serious sequelae than the former, when extravascular red cell clearance occurs (1,44,48,49).

The mechanisms by which IgG-coated red cells are removed from circulation have been described in detail in Chapter 6. The major consequences of this type of red cell destruction are hemoglobinuria, an increase in bilirubin following the destruction of the incompatible red cells and failure to achieve or maintain the expected increase in hemoglobin. As would be expected (again see Chapter 6) the amount and rate of red cell destruction is directly related to the strength and binding constant of the causative antibody, i.e. the number of IgG molecules that bind per red cell and the number of copies of the antigen involved, on the transfused red cells (50,51). As also discussed in Chapter 6 and in detail by Garratty (51) numerous other factors serve sometimes to obscure this direct relationship.

Transfusion Reactions Caused by IgG Complement-binding Antibodies that do not Cause Lysis In Vitro

There are many IgG blood group antibodies that bind to red cells and cause the activation of complement at too low a level for the terminal attack sequence to be sufficiently activated for in vitro or in vivo hemolysis to occur (see Chapter 6). In vitro studies show that red cells that have such antibodies bound usually also have C3 attached but in too small an amount for appreciable activation of C5. These antibodies cause similar clinical effects to those that are IgG but do not bind complement, i.e. hemoglobinuria, elevated bilirubin levels and lack of increment of hemoglobin. Based on what is known of the role of C3 (again see Chapter 6) in augmenting macrophage-mediated clearance of IgG-coated red cells (1,66-71) it is not surprising to find that some IgG complement-binding antibodies, that appear relatively weak in in vitro tests, can cause fairly marked amounts of in vivo red cell clearance and hence fairly severe transfusion reactions (72-74). The findings described above, together with those discussed in the previous section, mean that an IAT using the serum of a patient who has made a clinically-significant antibody, sometimes provides a very poor forecast as to the amount and rate of red cell clearance that will occur in vivo.

Complement Activation In Vivo

Blood bankers are repeatedly told that complement

activation occurs in in vitro tests only when serum is used. Indeed, until fairly recently, AABB Standards specified that serum, not plasma, must be used for in vitro antibody detection and compatibility tests. As discussed in Chapter 35, in vitro test methods such as LISS/IAT or PEG/IAT that are read with anti-IgG, do not involve any detection of red cell-bound C3 so that plasma is suitable for use in such tests. Many anticoagulants used to prevent blood samples from clotting chelate calcium ions that are needed for coagulation and for complement activation. As a result, there is sometimes confusion as to how complement becomes activated in vivo since this occurs in the patient's plasma. The difference between in vivo and in vitro plasma is, of course, that in vitro plasma is created artificially by use of an anticoagulant. In vivo this added anticoagulant is not present so that C1 molecules do not lose their integrity. In vivo complement activation occurs as readily in plasma as in vitro complement activation occurs in serum.

Extravascular Red Cell Destruction and Delayed Hemolytic Transfusion Reactions are not the Same Thing

From talking to some blood bankers and from reading some recent publications, it has become apparent that there is considerable confusion about the two terms that head this section. While most cases of delayed hemolytic transfusion reactions (see below) involve extravascular clearance of the transfused red cells, the two terms are not synonymous.

When the antibody that will clear the transfused red cells is present in sufficient quantity to effect such clearance at the time of transfusion, a hemolytic transfusion reaction will occur. If the antibody activates sufficient amounts of complement that the terminal attack sequence is mobilized, the red cell destruction will be intravascular. If the transfused red cells become coated with IgG or IgG and C3, but the terminal attack sequence of complement is not mobilized, extravascular red cell destruction will follow. In some instances both types of clearance will be seen, one usually predominates over the other. In either case, the event is an acute and not a delayed hemolytic transfusion reaction. In cases involving intravascular red cell destruction, the symptoms of the reaction are usually seen while the transfusion is still in progress. In cases involving extravascular destruction the symptoms may not appear immediately but are usually seen within hours of the transfusion. Nevertheless, antibody-binding to the red cells occurs at the time of transfusion and red cell clearance begins shortly thereafter. The reaction is acute, not delayed.

By definition, delayed hemolytic transfusion reactions involve a situation in which the patient has undergone a primary immune response previously or has had primary and secondary immunizations but, at the time of transfusion, is not making antibody in sufficient amounts to effect in vivo red cell clearance. However, when transfused, the patient mounts a secondary (anamnestic) immune response. Once the antibody being made reaches a level at which it can clear antigen-positive red cells, it begins to clear those transfused red cells still present in the patient's circulation. The interval between transfusion and the start of in vivo red cell destruction is measured in days rather than hours. Classically, delayed hemolytic transfusion reactions are noticed some five to seven days after transfusion (52-65) although in exceptional cases hemolysis may be noticed as early as three or as late as 14 to 23 days after transfusion (58,61,63,135).

The distinction between extravascular and delayed extravascular hemolytic transfusion reactions is important at the practical level. Most often when extravascular clearance will begin during or soon after transfusion, the causative antibody is present in serologically demonstrable amounts in the patient's pretransfusion serum. Thus careful pretransfusion tests using appropriate methods (see Chapter 35) should prevent this type of reaction from occurring. In contrast, in true delayed extravascular hemolytic transfusion reactions, the antibody is not demonstrable by conventional techniques before transfusion (the patient has undergone only a primary immune response or is no longer producing antibody in serologically demonstrable amounts) so that unless records showing that an antibody was previously detected are available, the transfusion reaction may not be preventable.

The correlation between antibody present and detectable before an acute hemolytic transfusion reaction and present but not detectable before a delayed extravascular hemolytic transfusion reaction, is not absolute. As discussed in a later section (where references are given) there are rare but well documented cases in which the in vivo clearance of transfused cells began at the time of transfusion and some symptoms of a transfusion reaction were seen, although no antibody could be demonstrated in vitro, even when the most sensitive methods were used.

Pathophysiology of Transfusion Reactions

As already mentioned, the most severe clinical consequences that result from hemolytic transfusion reactions are: hypotension, that may cause irreversible shock; disseminated intravascular coagulation (DIC); and renal failure. While these consequences were recognized and documented more than 70 years ago (75-80) the exact mechanisms by which they occurred were not always well understood. The hypotension seen was usually attributed to the release of small polypeptides from native complement proteins during complement activation. Both C3a and C5a (see Chapter 6) stimulate degranulation of mast cells and basophils causing the release of histamine and other vasoactive substances. This in turn leads to increased vascular permeability and increased smooth muscle contraction. C5a also acts directly on the endothelial cells of capillaries and thus further induces vasodilation. Similarly the split components produced during complement activation were sometimes (81-83) described as interacting with components of the coagulation cascade to produce DIC. There was considerable debate as to the cause of renal failure following red cell destruction in vivo. Some of the data (84,85) suggest that free hemoglobin may directly damage renal cells while others (86,87) appear to indicate that such does not occur. In other studies (5) it appeared that kidney damage was caused by deposition of red cell stroma in the renal tubules. Thus it seems likely that the cause of renal failure in this setting is multifactoral, there seems little doubt that both hypotension (88) and DIC (8,13,89) are contributing factors.

Although the answers are not yet all in, a much clearer picture of the pathophysiology of the clinical sequelae that result from the in vivo destruction of transfused red cells has emerged from the pioneering studies of Davenport et al. (10,11,15-17,90,91). While some of the more significant observations are described briefly below, readers wishing to learn more about this fascinating subject are referred to the reviews of Davenport (92), Davenport and Kunkel (17) , Capon and Goldfinger (93) and Beauregard and Blajchman (65).

Davenport et al. devised in vitro systems to study the effects of ABO antibody-induced intravascular lysis (10,11) and IgG-mediated extravascular clearance of red cells (90). In the ABO model, washed ABO-incompatible red cells were added to freshly drawn whole blood collected in to heparin. The mixture was incubated at 37°C where hemolysis occurred. The plasma from the sample was then assayed for levels of various cytokines. It was found that maximum hemolysis occurred when about 6 ml of packed red cells were added per 1 ml of whole blood. The cytokine activity in the system representing ABO incompatibility was then compared to that in a normal control, that is whole blood from the same donor, to which washed ABO compatible red cells had been added. The model representing extravascular hemolysis involved the addition of IgG-coated red cells to freshly isolated peripheral blood mononuclear cells in culture medium. Phagocytosis of the IgG-coated red cells occurred and cytokine levels were determined in the culture medium. In addition to immunological and bioassays of cytokines, the expression of genes encoding cytokine production

was studied by Northern blot analysis of RNA extracted from buffy coats (intravascular model) or mononuclear cells (extravascular model). In order to determine the biological effects of the cytokines generated, other experiments involved incubation of endothelial cells with plasma (intravascular model) or culture medium (extravascular model) and assaying those cells for procoagulant activity, production of cytokines, expression of mRNA and of cell surface adhesion molecules.

Cytokines are protein hormones that are involved in cell to cell communication. They vary widely in their functions. For example, some are growth factors for various lines of hematopoiesis, some are interferons while others exert profound effects on the immune and inflammatory responses, including the coagulation cycle. It is now clear that many different cells make cytokines, often the same cytokine may be made by a variety of cells. Equally clear, most cytokines have multiple biological functions. Sometimes the most important function of a given cytokine is not the one that initially led to its recognition; sometimes the same cytokine will have different effects on different cells. In considering cytokine production and the effects of such production, it must be remembered that the new findings add to but do not negate some previously drawn conclusions. For example, when the intravascular model described above is set up using reconstituted whole blood in which the plasma has been heat inactivated, i.e. no complement action occurs, neither hemolysis nor cytokine production is seen (17).

In the ABO model of intravascular hemolysis, production of tumor necrosis factor (TNF) occurs rapidly after the incompatible red cells are added to the whole blood and reaches peak levels within two to four hours (11). Thereafter the production of TNF slows and returns approximately to baseline level by about 24 hours. The amount of TNF generated is directly related to the amount of hemolysis that occurs. The expression of the *TNF* gene in the buffy coat cells of the whole blood is upregulated in this model. Similarly *IL-1b* gene expression is seen in the buffy coat cells (94) but biologically active IL-1b is not demonstrable in the plasma. It is believed that IL-1 may remain cell associated or may bind to a carrier protein or may be inhibited by the anti-inflammatory cytokine IL-1ra (IL-1 receptor antagonist). The cytokines IL-8 and monocyte chemoattractant protein (MCP) are also generated in the ABO hemolysis model (10,15). Release of these cytokines is slower than the release of TNF, IL-8 is first detectable about four hours and MCP about six hours after the ABO incompatible red cells are added to the whole blood. Production of IL8 and MCP increases for at least 24 hours after hemolysis occurs. In addition to the in vitro model described above, one case has been reported (12) in which a group O patient was mistakenly transfused with 100 ml of group A blood. By chance, the patient was part of a study in which cytokine measurements were being made to determine physiological responses to cardiopulmonary bypass surgery. In this patient's plasma, TNF levels increased 14-fold and remained elevated for 48 hours; production of the enzyme neutrophil elastase increased over a 24 hour period. It is known (95,96) that IL-8 induces neutrophil degranulation that was presumably reflected by the gradual increase in neutrophil elastase levels. No other patient in the study (12) received incompatible blood and no other demonstrated a significant increase in TNF level.

When they developed their model to simulate IgG-mediated extravascular red cell destruction, Davenport et al. (90) found that high levels of IL-8, MCP and IL-ra (IL receptor antagonist) were generated in the first 24 hours after the IgG-coated red cells were mixed with the mononuclear cells. They also reported (90) lower levels of Il-1b, IL-6 and TNF. However, Hoffman (97) had earlier produced evidence that TNF but not IL-1 is produced by monocytes that have interacted with IgG-coated red cells. It is possible that different experimental conditions accounted for the difference, in one study (97) the monocytes were adhered to glass slides, in the other (90) they were in non-adherent chambers. It is known (98,99) that monocyte activity is affected by adherence to foreign surfaces. Davenport and Kunkel (17) point out that the difference may not be important in vivo since the biological activities of TNF and IL-1 are closely related and since each can stimulate the gene expression of the other in mononuclear phagocytes. Davenport and Kunkel (17) also suggest that the generation of both IL-1 and its receptor antagonist IL-1ra in IgG-mediated extravascular destruction, may account for the considerable variation in the amount of red cell destruction caused by different auto and alloantibodies. That is to say, in some situations the levels of IL-1 and IL-1ra may be more balanced than in others.

While the release of various cytokines and chemokines following the hemolysis of red cells or their phagocytosis by mononuclear cells in the in vitro systems have been well documented, it is more difficult to determine the exact roles of these substances in the clinical sequelae of transfusion reactions. Tables 36-1 to 36-4 include data from many of the publications cited above and list some of the functions and effects of various materials generated following red cell destruction or following red cell storage when leukocytes are present. Both IL-1 and IL-6 are potent pyrogens and are presumably involved in the fever that is characteristic of so many transfusion reactions (see also below in the section on non-hemolytic febrile reactions). IL-1 and TNF are powerful mediators of septic shock (100,101) and presumably act similarly following red cell destruc-

tion in hemolytic transfusion reactions. TNF has also been shown (102,103) to activate the extrinsic pathway of coagulation and its generation following red cell destruction may be one of several factors leading to DIC. Cytokines may also promote a hypercoagulable state via their interactions with endothelial cells (104-107). Davenport et al. (16,17,92,108) incubated cultured umbilical vein endothelial cells with plasma from their in vitro model of ABO incompatibility. A complex series of interactions was observed. First, the phago-cyte-derived TNF caused increased production of IL-8 and MCP by the endothelial cells. IL-8 and MCP are chemotactic factors for neutrophils and monocytes, respectively. Second, the TNF caused upregulation of gene action for thromboplastin and for the leukocyte adhesion molecules ICAM-1 (intercellular adhesion molecule-1) and ELAM-1 (endothelial cell adhesion molecule-1). Third, the TNF caused a measurable release of tissue factor procoagulants. These findings, of course, suggest that cytokine action on endothelial cells is intimately involved in both inflammation and thrombosis.

It is now also believed that alterations in the function of endothelial cells are a contributory factor in the renal failure sometimes seen following intravascular red cell destruction. Vascular resistance in the kidney, and hence renal perfusion, appears to be controlled by a balance between vasodilatory and vasoconstricting factors (109). The generation of abnormal levels of various cytokines can disrupt this balance and under extreme circumstances can lead to renal shutdown. Endothelial cells produce a variety of vasoactive mediators (110,111) including endothelin, the most powerful endogenous vasoconstrictor currently known (112). The release of endothelin from vascular tissue is induced by thrombin, bradykinin, epinephrine and IL-1 (113). Thus the generation of increased levels of thrombin in DIC, bradykinin in complement activation, epinephrine in shock and IL-1 following cytokine action may all contribute to vasoconstriction leading to parenchymal ischemia and reduced renal function or renal failure. It is also known (114) that inhibition of endothelial cell-derived nitric oxide can lead to enhanced adhesion of leukocytes to endothelium and subsequent invasion of vessel walls thus favoring thrombosis. However, the significance of this finding, in terms of renal damage following red cell destruction, is not known.

Clearly these better understandings of the pathophysiology of the events that follow intravascular or extravascular red cell destruction suggest alternative methods for the treatment of patients who have experienced transfusion reactions. Equally clear, a discussion of such treatment options is beyond the scope of this

TABLE 36-1 Hemolytic Transfusion Reactions:
Some Effector Molecules Generated and Consequences (from 17, 65)

Effector Molecules	Results	Consequences
Anaphylatoxins C3a, C4a, C5a	Release of histamine and serotonin from mast cells.	Vasodilation, hypotension. Leakage of plasma through endothelium. Smooth muscle contraction.
Immune complexes	Bradykinin generation via actions of kallikrein on kininogen and activation of Hageman factor.	Vasodilation, hypotension. Pain at infusion site and in lumbar and thoracic regions.
Immune complexes	Release of norepinephrine following Ag-Ab complex formation or secondary to shock and hypotension.	Vasoconstriction in kidneys and lungs. Tachycardia, nausea, vomiting.
Antibody-coated rbc	Upregulation mononuclear cell gene action and generation of cytokine release. (See tables 36-2 and 36-3)	Fever, capillary leakage, hypotension, shock.
Complement components C3b, C3dg, iC3b (see Chapter 6)	Bind to red cells, monocytes, neutrophils, platelets, T cells, B cells, NK cells.	Upregulation of immune and inflammatory responses. Enhanced phagocytosis and NK-cell activity.

book. Interested readers are referred to the publications of Capon and Goldfinger (13,93).

Hemoglobinemia and Hemoglobinuria

When intravascular red cell destruction occurs there is an immediate release of hemoglobin into the plasma. A useful way of determining that such a reaction has occurred is simply to collect a sample of blood from a site other than that of the transfusion and centrifuge the sample. Often the presence of free hemoglobin will be apparent. Sometimes spectroscopic examination of the serum for hemoglobin or one of its derivatives will be useful. Hemoglobin or one of its derivatives may also be demonstrable in the urine shortly after an acute episode of intravascular hemolysis. Once the transfused cells have been hemolyzed, bilirubin levels will increase as the breakdown products of the destroyed cells are cleared.

Since extravascular destruction often results in a rel-

TABLE 36-2 Hemolytic Transfuction Reactions:
Cytokine Generation and Some
Consequences (from 17, 65).

Cytokine Generated	Activity and Consequences
IL-1	Fever, hypotension, shock.
TNF	Mobilization of leukocytes from bone marrow. Activation T and B-cells. Induction adhesion molecules and procoagulants. Upregulation IL-1, IL-6, IL-8, TNF, MCP production.
IL-6	Fever. Upregulation B-cell antibody production. Activation T-cells.
IL-8	Chemotaxis of neutrophils and lymphocytes. Activation and degranulation neutrophils and basophils leading to protease and histamine release.
MCP	Chemotaxis of monocytes and neutrophils. Induction of respiratory burst. Generation of expression of adhesion molecules. Upregulation of IL-1 production.
IL-lra	Inhibition of IL-1 type 1 receptors.

TABLE 36-3 Hemolytic Transfusion Reactions:
Factors That May Lead to Disseminated
Intravascular Coagulation (DIC) (from 17, 65).

Effector	Activities
Activated complement components	Platelet activation and aggregation. Activation prothrombin and plasminogen. Release of tissue factor from leukocytes, red cells and endothelial cells. Inactivation factor XIIa by C1INH (see Chapter 6).
Immune complexes	Activation platelets and factor XII. Damage to endothelial cells leading to tissue factor release.
IL-1 and TNF	Downregulation thrombomodulin and upregulation tissue factor production by endothelial cells. Stimulation production plasminogen activation inhibitor. Hypotension resulting in vascular stasis and thrombosis. Leukocyte trapping in microcirculation via adhesion molecules generated on endothelial cells.
IL-8	Neutrophil chemotaxis and activation leading to protease release that causes endothelial cell damage and tissue factor release.

TABLE 36-4 Some Differences in Cytokine Generation as Illustrated by In Vitro Models of Intravascular and Extravascular Red Cell Destruction (from 17)

Intravascular Model	Extravascular Model
Rapid generation TNF	Relatively slow generation of high level of IL-8 and appreciable levels of IL-lra and MCP.
Slower generation IL-8	
Slightly delayed generation MCP	Rapid generation of lower level of IL-1 and slower generation of lower levels of IL-6 and TNF.
TNF then causes generation of (additional) IL-8 and MCP.	
TNF also causes generation of endothelial cell adhesion molecules ICAM-1 and ELAM-1 and causes release of tissue factor from endothelial cells.	

atively slow rate of red cell clearance, it might be expected that hemoglobinemia or hemoglobinuria would be uncommon following a transfusion reaction involving that type of red cell destruction. In fact, one or both are sometimes seen. There seem to be at least two reasons and perhaps a third, to account for this fact. First, as already mentioned, although IgG and IgG and C3-coated cells are predominantly phagocytosed in the spleen and the liver, some of them escape from tissue bound macrophages and re-enter the circulation. Those that are sufficiently badly damaged then rupture in the blood stream and release hemoglobin. Second, when the rate of hemoglobin release from red cells sequestered and destroyed in the spleen exceeds the capacity of that organ to process hemoglobin, some seems to be released into the circulation. Third, in vitro studies have shown that K cells (non-T, non-B lymphocytes) can effect destruction of some IgG-coated red cells without participation by complement (136-153). It is not yet clear how much (if any) K-cell lysis occurs in circulation so that it is not possible to calculate the contribution made via that mechanism, to the hemoglobin found in the patient's plasma when an antibody not capable of causing complement-mediated intravascular lysis causes red cell destruction in vivo.

For the reasons given, the finding of hemoglobinemia or hemoglobinuria following extravascular destruction of red cells in a reaction occurring at the time of, or soon after transfusion is perhaps not too surprising. Perhaps more surprising is the fact that a number of delayed transfusion reactions (see below) have been associated with hemoglobinuria (53,57,58,126,133). It would seem that when this occurs, either damaged red cells are released from macrophages and re-enter the cir-

culation (see above) or that the antibody level increases in such a way that the onset of hemolysis is so abrupt that the spleen cannot handle the full amount of released hemoglobin and some is excreted in the urine.

Red Cell Destruction by IgM Antibodies

Many IgM antibodies bind to red cells only at temperatures below 37°C. As discussed in detail in Chapter 35, such antibodies do not destroy antigen-positive red cells in vivo. Those IgM antibodies that bind to red cells at 37°C and activate complement at levels that do not effect mobilization of the terminal attack sequence (see Chapter 6) tend to clear red cells slowly and often in limited amounts. As discussed in Chapter 6, tissue bound macrophages do not carry receptors for IgM and the extravascular clearance of red cells coated with C3 but no IgG is rather inefficient. Studies using ^{51}Cr-labeled antigen-positive red cells in patients with 37°C-active IgM, complement binding antibodies, often show a two component curve (115-117). Initially there may be rapid destruction of a few of the red cells as the antibody binds and activates complement. Clearance represents those cells coated to the C3b stage and sequestered by macrophages before cleavage of C3b has occurred. Thereafter the rate of destruction may slow, often to the point of normal survival as in vivo cleavage of cell bound C3b, to the C3dg stage occurs (117 and again see Chapter 6).

IgM antibodies that do not bind complement do not bring about red cell destruction in vivo. Although some early reports (44,115,118) suggested that such antibodies could cause some in vivo red cell destruction, the data were later re-evaluated by Mollison (116). It was concluded that an anti-M previously studied, did, in fact, activate complement. The examples of non-complement binding IgM anti-D and anti-c that had apparently cleared red cells were thought both to contain small amounts of IgG antibody that had not been detected in the original immunoelectrophoretic studies on the sera (116).

Delayed Hemolytic Transfusion Reactions

Sometimes the transfusion of apparently well tolerated compatible blood is followed several days later by a drop in hemoglobin and a rise in bilirubin in the patient. This can occur when a patient has been previously exposed to an antigen but has no demonstrable antibody in the serum at the time of transfusion. The situation sometimes represents the fact that the patient has undergone primary immunization following an earlier transfusion or following pregnancy but has not yet made antibody in serologically detectable levels. On other occasions the patient may have previously made detectable antibody but the level has now dropped below the threshold detectable by in vitro tests. With the next transfusion, the red cells serve as a secondary immunogenic stimulus and antibody is produced while some transfused cells are still circulating. The patient thus has both antigen and antibody present and in vivo red cell destruction follows. The direct antiglobulin test is positive, with a mixed-field agglutination pattern, if performed before all the transfused cells have been destroyed. This type of reaction is obviously very difficult to prevent and some cases may not be preventable at all (i.e. no antibody demonstrable by any method when pretransfusion compatibility tests are performed). However, the incidence of delayed hemolytic transfusion reactions can certainly be reduced by the careful performance of pretransfusion tests using sensitive methods.

It would seem logical to expect that delayed transfusion reactions would be characterized by gradual onset, slow, extravascular clearance of red cells as the antibody being made gradually reached the level at which it could cause in vivo red cell clearance. Indeed, in many such reactions this is what is seen (52,54-56,58-65,119-125,134). However, there are some notable exceptions. In a number of cases (53,57,58,126-133) particularly five described by Pickles et al. (133) in which the antibody responsible for the delayed reactions was anti-C or anti-Ce, hemoglobinuria was noted. As mentioned above, it is not particularly easy to explain hemoglobinuria in cases in which slow clearance by an extravascular route was involved.

It is not absolutely clear that a delayed transfusion reaction per se, can cause renal failure. Although such occurrences have been reported (59,129,130), Mollison (1) has pointed out that none of the cases is straightforward. In the case described by Meltz et al. (130) in which the causative antibody was anti-U, no evidence that the renal damage was due to intravascular hemolysis was presented. The patient described by Holland and Wallerstein (129) had anti-Jk[b] and developed oliguria about two weeks after the transfusion of three units of Jk(b+) blood. However, an additional unit of Jk(b+) blood was transfused at about the time that the oliguria began. All of four patients described by Pineda et al. (59) as suffering renal failure had serious underlying disease.

There is also some doubt as to whether an antibody made in a primary immune response has ever caused a delayed hemolytic transfusion reaction. In the case described by Patten et al. (154), the authors claimed that a primary immune response to C caused red cell destruction some four weeks after transfusion of 12 units of blood. However, the patient was transfused for complications that arose following delivery of her child. While the infant's red cells were not typed, those of its father

were C+ c- meaning that the infant must have had C+ red cells. Thus it seems to one of us (PDI) that by far the most likely explanation of the case is that the woman underwent a primary immune response during pregnancy and that the transfusions represented secondary immunization. Thus the case seems to have involved a very delayed hemolytic transfusion reaction in a woman initially immunized by pregnancy. Taddie et al. (155) were more cautious in interpreting their case. The patient, a 42 year-old White woman, suffered a delayed hemolytic transfusion reaction caused by anti-Js[a] some 23 days after being transfused. The patient had been pregnant four times but had never been transfused, her husband had Js(a-) red cells. The authors (155) concluded that the findings suggested that the anti-Js[a] was the result of primary immunization despite its being made within 23 days of the transfusions. Given the facts that clinically-significant levels of an antibody made in a primary response are seldom made that quickly and that some individuals with no known exposure to foreign red cells make antibodies that, based on specificity, are usually expected to be red cell stimulated, it seems likely that no case of a delayed hemolytic transfusion reaction following primary immunization has been seen.

Delayed Serological Transfusion Reactions

Ness et al. (64) drew attention to a very important point that is often overlooked in considering the production of antibodies by patients who have recently been transfused. When the patient involved has clinical or laboratory evidence of antibody-mediated in vivo red cell destruction, it can justifiably be said that the patient has suffered (or is suffering) a delayed hemolytic transfusion reaction (DHTR). When the patient has a positive DAT and a newly formed antibody is found in the patient's serum or is eluted from the transfused red cells that are still circulating, but there is neither clinical nor laboratory evidence of hemolysis, the situation represents a delayed serological transfusion reaction (DSTR). In other words, antigen-antibody complexes may have formed in vivo but the event is clinically benign. In a 20 month period, 34 cases were found (64) in which a newly formed antibody had bound to the transfused red cells. However, in only six of the 34 cases was there evidence of an adverse clinical outcome. In other words, the incidence of a DSTR was 1 in 151 recipients whereas the incidence of a DHTR was only 1 in 854 patients. This very important distinction has not been made in all studies and in some of the series described below, the incidence figure actually represents the sum of DHTR and DSTR. Another finding of Ness et al. (64) regarding the persistence of antibody production in patients who have had a DHTR or a DSTR is considered in detail below.

DHTR and DSTR: Incidence

The incidence with which DHTR and DSTR are detected is directly related to the effort expended in looking for them. For example, during the period 1974 to 1978 at the Toronto General Hospital, 20,977 patients were transfused with 93,577 units of whole blood or packed red cells. Croucher (60) found 40 delayed reactions, that is 1 in 524 patients (0.19%) or 1 in 2339 transfusions (0.043%). Some of the reactions (DHTR) were detected when the patient became jaundiced or anemic, others were found when the DAT on a new sample from the patient, submitted because further transfusions were planned, was found to be positive (DSTR). At the Mayo Clinic from 1978 to 1980, 117,120 units were transfused and Taswell et al. (125) found evidence for 77 delayed reactions. That is an incidence of 1 in 1521 transfusions (0.066%) which is 1.5 times higher than the Toronto figure. The number of patients who received the 117,120 units in the Mayo Clinic series is not given but if it is assumed that the average number of units transfused per patient was the same at the Mayo Clinic as at the Toronto General Hospital, it can be calculated that the incidence of delayed reactions at the Mayo Clinic was 1 in 341 patients (0.29%), again a figure 1.5 times higher than in Toronto. The difference in the two studies was that at the Mayo Clinic, previous surveys (59,62,120) had prompted those investigators to undertake deliberate searches for evidence of delayed reactions (their figures from 1964 to 1977 were 60 delayed reactions in 416,000 transfusions or 1 in 6933 or 0.014%). In Toronto, the cases were found when the patient developed clinical symptoms or when the DAT on a subsequent sample was found to be positive. It is apparent that the Toronto approach is the more meaningful. There is no doubt that if deliberate searches are undertaken, additional cases of DSTR will be found. However, if the patient was given blood at surgery or in any other medical emergency and is now making a successful recovery, including the production of blood, the only reason for documenting the event is that blood lacking the antigen involved can be selected if transfusions are required in the future.

DHTR and DSTR: Antibody Specificities

Antibodies that cause DHTR and DSTR most often have the same specificities as those that cause acute reactions. In the many reports referenced in the previous sections, most warm-reactive alloantibodies that are known to cause in vivo red cell destruction are represented among those that have caused delayed reactions. Only on very rare occasions (59,156-159) has a cold-reactive antibody apparently broadened enough in thermal range, after the introduction of antigen-positive red cells, for a delayed transfusion reaction to result. Some of the few reports that claim that this event has taken place, do not contain very convincing evidence for antibody-induced red cell destruction by the previously cold-reactive antibody. Further, as discussed below, there are a number of well documented cases in which an antibody causative of immune-mediated in vivo red cell destruction could only be deduced to be present by indirect means. If such an antibody caused red cell destruction in a patient who, by chance, had a cold-reactive antibody present as well, the cold-reactive antibody could be blamed for the red cell destruction although it was actually quite benign.

Antibodies that seem most often to cause delayed hemolytic transfusion reactions are those of the Rh and Kidd systems. Among Rh antibodies, those directed against C, c and E have frequently been implicated. In reviewing all antibodies causative of reactions of this type, Mollison (1) found that 30% of them were anti-Jk^a or anti-Jk^b. Similarly, in reviewing the 40 cases seen at the Toronto General Hospital between 1974 and 1978, Croucher (60) found that eight patients had made anti-Jk^a and two, anti-Jk^b. In the experience of one of us (PDI), if just those delayed transfusion reactions that cause significant clinical effects (i.e. noticeable jaundice, appreciable anemia) are considered, the proportion caused by anti-Jk^a or anti-Jk^b is over 50%. This compares to a figure of about 3% for the incidence of Kidd system antibodies among all atypical antibodies detected and about 10% for Kidd system antibodies among clinically significant antibodies when anti-D, anti-CD and anti-CDE are excluded from the calculations (160). In the more recent study of Ness et al. (64), 24 (70%) of the 34 cases of DHTR and DSTR involved anti-E and/or anti-Jk^a. As discussed in more detail in Chapter 19, there are two principle reasons why Kidd system antibodies are so frequently causative of delayed hemolytic transfusion reactions. First, when present in low levels in a patient's serum, they are difficult to detect in serological tests. Second, many patients who become immunized to Jk^a or Jk^b make easily demonstrable (by serological tests) antibody for only short periods of time so that when compatibility tests are performed years after the primary and secondary immunizations, no serum antibody may be demonstrable, i.e. the prime setting for a delayed transfusion reaction if there are no records of the previously detected antibody.

DHTR and DSTR: Eluates

At one time, in many transfusion services, it was

standard practice to perform a DAT on all new samples received from patients transfused within about the previous 14 days (the time interval varied in different services). When the DAT was found to be positive, particularly if the pretransfusion DAT was known to have been negative, an eluate was made and tested for antibody specificity. The objective of the exercise was to identify those patients who had undergone a secondary immune response following transfusion and were now making a previously unrecognized antibody. In some services searching records to determine which patients had recently been transfused was more time consuming than performing a DAT so that the test was performed on all samples. In either system a lot of work was involved and little benefit accrued since the overwhelming majority of patients do not make new or additional antibodies soon after transfusion. The lack of value in performing DATs or autocontrols on all samples has been discussed in Chapter 35. In two large studies reported in 1986, the value of performing DATs on samples from recently transfused patients and making eluates when the DAT was positive, was called into question. Judd et al. (161) studied 65,049 samples from patients. In 3570 the DAT was positive and 778 of the samples, all from patients who had been transfused within the previous 14 days, were selected for further study. Among eluates made from those samples, 52 were shown to contain at least one alloantibody. However, the same antibodies were identified in the serum from 46 of the samples. In other words, among 778 samples only six contained an antibody identified solely in the eluate. Further, in three other samples an antibody was identified from tests on serum but not from tests on eluates. Stec et al. (162) made similar findings. Among 638 patients with a positive DAT, 23 had an alloantibody that could be identified in an eluate made from the DAT+ red cells. However, in 19 of those patients the same antibody was identified in the serum. Thus in the two series (161,162) 1416 samples with a positive DAT were evaluated, eluates from 75 of those samples contained an alloantibody but 65 of the antibodies were also identified in sera. Stec et al. (162) offer the sound advice that eluates should be performed, in this setting, only when hemolysis is suspected or a transfusion reaction is reported. Clearly if the patient is suffering immune red cell destruction an eluate is necessary to be sure that the antibody active in vivo and the one found in the serum, are the same.

For those workers concerned that in the studies described ten antibodies were found in eluates, that could not be identified in the serum, it should be added that in both studies (161,162) tests on the sera were by LISS/IAT. In our own service, over a two year period, we (163) identified 24 antibodies in eluates made from DAT+ red cells of recently (within 14 days) transfused patients.

By using PEG/IAT we were able to identify 23 of those antibodies in sera from the samples. We no longer perform DATs on recently transfused patients but instead rely on PEG/IAT testing of serum to detect new or additional antibodies. When such an antibody is found, we then perform a DAT and an eluate if the DAT is positive, to see if the antibody has bound to the transfused red cells in vivo. Even that information is of limited value to our clinicians since most events represent DSTR and not DHTR. Routine DATs on all samples are clearly not justified (164-166), abandoning such tests on all samples from recently transfused patients poses very little risk.

Persistence of Antibody Production after DHTR and DSTR

In 1984, Salama and Mueller-Eckhardt (167) described some unexpected findings in patients who had experienced delayed transfusion reactions. First, although many of the causative antibodies were of specificities usually associated with a lack of ability to bind complement, all of 26 patients were found to have appreciable amounts of C3 on their red cells. Second, the positive DATs (using anti-C3) were not of the mixed field type suggesting that C3 was bound to the patients' as well as to the transfused red cells. Third, C3 was detectable on the red cells of the patients for weeks or even months after the last transfusion. In five patients the DAT was still positive, with C3 on the red cells, for periods ranging from 130 to 163 days after transfusion, i.e. times at which transfused red cells would no longer be expected to be present. Fourth, in some patients IgG was also detected on the red cells at times when transfused red cells would no longer be expected to be circulating. Fifth, in some patients the antibody that was thought to have caused the delayed reaction was apparently recovered, by elution, again at a time when no transfused red cells would have been expected to be present in the patients' circulation. Among extreme examples, apparent anti-K was recovered from the K- red cells of two patients, one 108 days and the other 299 days after the last transfusion. Apparent anti-E was recovered from the E- red cells of a patient 183 days after the last transfusion and apparent anti-D and anti-E from the rr red cells of a patient 164 days after transfusion. When they published their important paper on the difference between delayed hemolytic and delayed serological transfusion reactions, Ness et al. (64) described similar but by no means identical findings. First, in long term follow-up studies after DHTR and DSTR, IgG was often found on the red cells but the active involvement of C3 seen in the earlier study (167) was not such a consistent finding. Second, in cases of both DHTR and DSTR many of the alloantibodies involved were apparently eluted from the patients' antigen-negative red cells at times when it would be expected that transfused red cells would no longer be present. Again anti-E was involved twice. In two patients with E- red cells, apparent anti-E was eluted, in one patient 109 days and in a second 168 days after transfusion. In a patient with Fy(a-) red cells, apparent anti-Fy^a was eluted 81 days after the last transfusion. Third and of considerable potential significance (see below), in four of the patients (two with DHTR and two with DSTR) the long-term persistence of a positive DAT and persistence of recovery of alloantibody by elution was associated with the eventual production of an autopanagglutinin. These autoantibodies were first seen 43, 54, 73 and 97 days after transfusion in the four patients. Fourth and also of potential significance (again see below), in all four patients who developed autopanagglutinins, apparent alloantibodies with Rh specificity were seen. In the patient who developed an autoantibody (eluate) at 43 days, anti-C and anti-e were found in the serum; in the one in whom autoantibody was eluted at 54 days, the serum contained anti-C and anti-G; in the one with autoantibody at 73 days anti-E and anti-K were in the serum; and in the one with autoantibody at 97 days, anti-E and anti-Jk^a were in the serum.

While there is as yet no proved explanation for the observations described above regarding the long term positive DATs and elution of apparent alloantibodies from the antigen-negative red cells of patients who have experienced DHTR and DSTR, there are a number of other documented findings that allow development of potential explanations. First, there are a number of reports (61,168-177,492) of positive DATs and the production of autoantibodies concurrent with alloimmunization. Second, in patients producing autoantibodies it is not unusual to find apparent alloantibodies bound to the patients' antigen-negative red cells. Extended adsorption studies show (178-182) that the apparent alloantibodies are in fact autoantibodies that mimic alloantibodies by showing preferential reactions with certain antigen-positive red cells. Third, the most common setting in which an autoantibody mimicking an alloantibody is seen, is when the patient has a true alloantibody of the specificity that the autoantibody mimics, in the serum (180,182). Fourth, mimicking autoantibodies frequently resemble alloantibodies of the Rh system in general and anti-E in particular (178,180,182). Thus it seems entirely likely that in a patient in whom a DHTR or a DSTR occurs, the immune system responds in a somewhat hysterical manner. The early antibody made may be of poor fit and may bind to both the patient's and the transfused red cells. If selection of antibody producing clones based on the goodness of fit of the antibody occurs, those immunocytes producing antibody of poor fit may die out with the result that only alloantibody of true specificity will

be produced in the long term. However, if the clones producing antibody of poor fit and those producing antibody of good fit are both propagated, the situations described (64,167) may be seen. That is, the patient's serum may contain a mixture of true specificity and mimicking antibody while the DAT may be positive with the mimicking antibody bound. Eluates from the patients' red cells may then appear to contain the same antibody as the one that caused the DHTR and DSTR although, in fact, the eluate really contains an autoantibody that mimics the alloantibody involved. There are a number of observations that support such an interpretation. First, many of the antibodies apparently recovered by elution in the long term studies appeared to have Rh specificity. Second, apparent anti-E, the most common mimicking specificity (178,180,182,183) was overrepresented in the two studies (64,167). Third, the situation described above of true specificity alloantibody in the serum and eluted antibody of apparently the same specificity (i.e. potentially the mimic) applied in almost every case described by Ness et al. (64) and by Salama and Mueller-Eckhardt (167). Fourth, in four of the patients described by Ness et al. (64) the eluate eventually contained a panagglutinating autoantibody. Clearly the next step in this story should be to test the apparent alloantibodies, eluted from a patient's red cells at a time when transfused red cells are no longer present, to see if those antibodies are eventually adsorbed to exhaustion by antigen-negative red cells and/or can be adsorbed on to and eluted from antigen-negative red cells other than those of the patient. There is some evidence from a somewhat parallel study (182) that this indeed occurs.

Hemolytic Transfusion Reactions when No Antibody is Detectable by Serological Tests

In spite of the (perhaps too) extreme sensitivity of currently used in vitro serological methods, rare patients have hemolytic transfusion reactions although no antibodies can be detected in their sera. There are a number of reports of such events in the literature. It is hard to evaluate the older reports (31,184-198) since the investigators describing the cases did not have the advantage of the use of the sensitive in vitro methods available today. In some of those older studies (185-187,193) tests with ^{51}Cr-labeled red cells were used to show that donor red cells were rapidly destroyed although no antibodies could be detected in in vitro tests.

Some more recently reported studies have used the same principle. Davey et al. (199) studied a patient who had experienced a delayed transfusion reaction, but in whom a wide variety of ultra sensitive methods failed to demonstrate an antibody. Because the patient's red cells lacked the c antigen, ^{51}Cr survival studies using c+ and c- red cells were done. In the test with c+ cells, only 1% survived for 24 hours; with c- red cells, survival was 80% at 24 hours. The patient was successfully transfused with eight units of c- blood. In a second patient studied by the same workers (199), antibodies to K, E, P$_1$ and Lu^a were demonstrable. However, because the patient's red cells were c- and because some (but not all) c+ samples showed equivocal reactions with the patient's serum, similar ^{51}Cr studies were used. Presence of anti-c in this patient was shown when 83% of the test dose of c+ red cells was destroyed in 48 hours. A somewhat similar case was described by Baldwin et al. (200). The patient experienced clinically severe hemolytic transfusion reactions but only anti-Bg^a could be found in her serum. Her red cells were e- and ^{51}Cr survival studies showed that 93% of a test dose of e+ red cells was cleared in 24 hours, while e- red cells survived normally. Transfusion of e- blood was successful. In a case described by Harrison et al. (201) intravascular destruction of red cells occurred in a patient in whom no antibodies could be found. The patient had C- red cells and a study using ^{99m}Tc-labeled C+ red cells showed that 71% of the test dose was destroyed in 4 hours. In contrast, two survival studies using C- red cells showed normal survival of those cells. Transfusion with C- cells was successful.

In considering the cases described above, a number of points should be borne in mind. First, since no serologically detectable antibodies were present, there was no indication as to what specificity antibody might be responsible for the red cell destruction. In each case cited, a useful clue was obtained by comparing the phenotype of the patient with those of the donors whose units had caused the reactions. For example, the first patient of Davey et al. (199) was found to have c- red cells while the donor units were c+. Tests on a sample from the patient after the delayed hemolytic transfusion reaction revealed that no c+ cells remained in circulation, hence the suspicion that anti-c might have cleared the transfused cells. Second, in another setting similar studies might help. Take for example a patient with c-, Jk(a-) red cells who had been transfused by chance, with two units of c+, Jk(a+) and two units of c+, Jk(a-) blood. If tests on the post-reaction sample revealed no c+ red cells present, it would be suspected that all four units had been cleared and that anti-c might be the culprit. If the post-reaction sample contained some c+ but no Jk(a+) red cells it would be suspected that the two c+, Jk(a+) units had been cleared but that the c+, Jk(a-) units had not, thus making anti-Jk^a a prime suspect. Clearly in some settings it will be necessary to perform in vivo survival studies with red cells of various phenotypes before a potential antibody can be suspected. The cases cited above have been simplified to illustrate the eventual successful outcome. Third, the antibodies involved were

not non-detectable because they were weak. The first patient described by Davey et al. (199) destroyed the remaining c+ red cells from four units of blood in the delayed transfusion reaction. The patient described by Baldwin et al. (200) destroyed two units of e+ blood in a delayed reaction and three units in an acute reaction, before the presence of anti-e was deduced. The patient described by Harrison et al. (201) destroyed four C+ units when transfused with six random units, the other two of which were, by chance, C-. Weak antibodies do not bring about such gross red cell destruction. Fourth and perhaps most intriguing of all, in spite of the fact that each of the patients had been transfused with four or more units of blood carrying the antigen against which the presumptive antibody was directed and had received more antigen-positive red cells in the cell survival studies, none of them made serologically demonstrable antibodies after the transfusion reactions. In the patient described by Baldwin et al. (200) a repeat red cell survival study with labeled e+ red cells, was performed two years after the initial study. Although there was still no serologically demonstrable anti-e in the patient's serum, the same accelerated clearance of e+ red cells was seen. Again, the antibodies in these patients were not weak. Instead, they were potent antibodies, capable of rapidly destroying large amounts of incompatible red cells, but were not demonstrable by any currently available serological technique.

It is not always possible to perform in vivo red cell survival studies in patients in whom unexplained hemolysis had occurred. If such patients must be transfused again, it is well worth phenotyping their red cells for antigens in the Rh, Ss, Kell, Duffy and Kidd systems (ABO compatibility is assumed) then transfusing blood lacking antigens that the patient's cells lack. For example, Halima et al. (202) encountered a patient in whom a delayed then two immediate, severe transfusion reactions occurred. Heroic efforts at the serological level failed to detect the responsible antibody (anti-K was found but most of the reactions involved K- units). Because the patient was C- and because no C+ cells could be found in post-transfusion samples, C- blood was transfused. No reaction occurred and the expected rise in hemoglobin was seen. We are aware of two unreported cases in which the Kidd system was similarly involved. In one, Jk(a-b+) and in the other Jk(a+b-) transfused cells survived normally although Jk(a+) and Jk(b+) cells respectively, had previously caused transfusion reactions. The two patients were followed, neither developed a serologically detectable Kidd system antibody.

Garratty et al. (203,204) have studied this problem in depth. In a ten year period, samples from 71 patients who had severe transfusion reactions but in whom no antibodies were detectable by standard methods, were referred to their laboratory. More than 70% of the patients had hemoglobinemia or hemoglobinuria during or following the transfusion. In spite of the use of a battery of ultra sensitive methods performed by a highly proficient team of workers, only a minority of the cases were solved. In 14 of the 71 patients an antibody was detected; the polybrene, PEG and 4% ficin capillary methods (205,206) proved of most value In another six patients successful transfusions were accomplished by the use of phenotype matched blood. Thus in 51 of 71 patients no explanation of the severe transfusion reaction was found.

The enzyme linked antiglobulin test (ELAT) was introduced in 1980 (207,208) and was used by several groups of investigators (51,209-216) to detect the increased level of IgG on the red cells of some patients with "warm" antibody-induced hemolytic anemia in whom the conventional DAT was negative. As described in more detail in Chapter 37, the ELAT will sometimes reveal the presence of low levels of IgG on red cells, that is to say enough IgG to mediate macrophage-induced clearance but not enough to give a positive reaction in the DAT read by agglutination. Given this success it was natural that the test would be used (203,204,217) in attempts to identify antibodies that had caused hemolytic transfusion reactions but were not detectable by any other serological method. Workers who have used the ELAT will know that this is not an easy proposition. The test itself must be run in triplicate to obtain accurate results, duplicate or triplicate hemolysis controls must be run on each cell sample to avoid reading minimal amounts of hemolysis as false positives, and a standard curve (again involving duplicate or triplicate tests and controls) using an antibody of known protein concentration must be used with each test series. We (217) found that in order to test a patient's serum against five different red cell samples, a minimum of 70 individual tests were necessary to obtain reliable results. We (217) studied one patient, in whose serum no atypical antibodies were detectable, who was transfused uneventfully with two units of blood. Ten days later she had hemoglobinuria and a drop in hemoglobin. Extensive antibody-screening tests, using ultra sensitive methods were negative. Two additional units of apparently compatible blood were transfused. Although the transfusions were well-tolerated, this time hemoglobinuria and a drop in hemoglobin occurred within 12 hours. Again, all serological investigations were negative. Phenotyping studies showed that the patient's red cells lacked only C, e and Fy^a of the antigens for which we typed. Accordingly the patient's serum was incubated with R_1R_1, Fy(a-) cells (to allow binding of anti-C and anti-e); rr, Fy(a-) cells (to allow binding of anti-e); R_2R_2, Fy(a+) cells (to allow binding of anti-Fy^a); R_2R_2, Fy(a-) cells (phenotype matched); and the patient's own cells, and the tests were read by

ELAT. To our dismay, all samples including the R_2R_2, Fy(a-) red cells, but not the patient's own cells, bound abnormal and equal amounts of IgG. In other words, the patient's serum appeared to contain an antibody, demonstrable only by ELAT, directed against an antigen of high incidence. When we tested serum from this patient using ficin-treated red cells (206,218) suspended in LISS (219-221), using the double incubation method (222) and reading the tests with a broad spectrum antiglobulin reagent, no antibody activity was demonstrable. Tests on the patient's red cells using all available antibodies to common antigens, did not reveal which one she lacks. Because the ELAT does not yield good results when thawed red cells are used (minimal amounts of hemolysis give false positive reactions) further studies were limited. Like other patients in whom hemolysis in the absence of demonstrable antibodies is seen, this lady was encouraged to donate units to be held frozen, once the medical emergency requiring transfusion had been resolved.

In a number of cases in which unexplained hemolysis of transfused red cells had been seen, tests have been undertaken (51,61,196,200,201,203,204,209,223) to see if a non-humoral event, such as cellular cytotoxicity, was involved. Although there is one report (224) of NK cell-induced destruction of autologous red cells in a patient with chronic lymphocytic leukemia, this mechanism has not been clearly implicated in alloantibody-induced destruction of transfused red cells.

Mention was made above regarding the value of phenotyping studies on the pretransfusion red cells of the patient, the donors and a posttransfusion sample from the patient. A second advantage of such studies is that they can sometimes be used to differentiate between alloimmune and autoimmune red cell destruction. Phenotypes of antigens in all systems, including those in which the antibodies are not clinically significant, are determined on the patient's and donors' red cells. If no pretransfusion sample from the patient is available the patient's cells can be separated from the transfused cells by harvesting the youngest cells from the posttransfusion sample (206,225-228). Once an antigen (or antigens) present on the donor's but not the patient's cells has (have) been identified, the posttransfusion sample is tested for that (those) antigen(s). The tests are read microscopically for mixed-field reactions. It is usually possible to calculate roughly what percentage of the cell mixture should be donors' red cells and to compare that estimate with one made from the mixed-field reaction (if any). If marked alloimmune red cell destruction has occurred, few or none of the transfused red cells will be found. If the expected percentage of transfused cells is seen, in the presence of unexplained hemolysis, autoimmune red cell destruction should be suspected. In this latter instance it

is, of course, necessary to exclude other causes of anemia, such as bleeding, that will result in equal loss of
autologous and transfused red cells.

Red Cell Destruction by Non-Immunological Mechanisms

In investigating cases in which unexplained
hemolysis occurred following a transfusion and in
which no causative antibody could be detected, it is
necessary to consider nonimmune causes of red cell
destruction. Table 36-5 presents a partial list of such
possibilities; it is highly probable that there are others
of which we have not thought. Mollison et al. (1) have
pointed out the value of examining segments or
remaining blood from the units in question for excessive hemolysis. Clearly, if such hemolysis is found
there is a high probability that the in vivo events were
not antibody-mediated. Diligent questioning may be
necessary to unearth evidence of some of the possibilities listed in table 36-5. One of us (PDI) well remembers spending a week running every test then known to
try to find a serological cause for hemolysis of two
units of blood in a patient without detectable antibodies. The entirely negative findings were eventually
explained when it was found that the blood had been
mixed with half-physiological-strength saline through
a Y set, in error. Extracting an admission of the error
from the nurse responsible was at least as difficult as
trying to find the causative antibody!

Transfusion Reactions that Do Not Involve Red Cell Destruction

Because this book is primarily about red cell antigens and the antibodies directed against them, the
lengthy descriptions about transfusion reactions already
presented describe either red cell destruction or secondary immune responses that result in the in vivo
uptake of antibodies by red cells. There are, of course,
many other types of transfusion reaction, some of which
are much more common than those involving red cell
destruction. Most (we hope) are mentioned briefly
below. Because of the nature of this book fewer details
about transfusion reactions not involving red cell
destruction than details about those in which that event
occurs, are given. Readers wishing to learn more about
the situations described below are referred to a number
of excellent publications about them (1,13,63,65,93,229-
234). Although less emphasis is placed, in this book, on
transfusion reactions that do not involve red cell destruction than on those that do, it should not be concluded that

TABLE 36-5 Some Examples of Causes of Non-Immune-Mediated Red Cell Hemolysis (includes data from 65)

Blood overheated (during storage, malfunctioning blood warmer, etc.) (470-478)

Blood frozen (accidentally, without cryoprotectants) (484)

Blood not completely deglycerolized after being thawed. (470,480) For a simple test to prevent this complication, see 481-483.

Blood mixed with non-physiological solutions, such as half-strength saline, 5% dextrose in 0.18% saline, etc. (485-488, 493-496)

Mechanical destruction of red cells by use of too small a bore needle, mechanical valves, incorrect use of cell salvage equipment, etc. (489-491, 497-500)

Mechanical push of red cells by pumps with or without use of micropore filters (501-503)

Transfusion of bacterially-contaminated blood products (for references, see text)

Variability of viability of red cells of different donors (see Mollison et al. [469] pages 141-143)

Reduced red cell survival associated with certain disease states (e.g., Rheumatoid arthritis, pernicious anemia, end-stage renal disease, fever, etc.) (See Mollison et al. [469] pages 112-113)

the former are trivial. Indeed while they are rare, anaphylactic reactions, the transfusion of bacterially contaminated blood or components, and transfusion related
acute lung injury (TRALI) can each prove fatal.

Febrile Non-Hemolytic Transfusion Reactions (FNHTR)

FNHTR are defined as involving a temperature
increase of 1°C or more in a transfused patient when
no other explanation exists for the fever. The definition
may specify the temperature increase during (238),
within 8 hours (239) or within 24 hours (240) of the
transfusion. In addition to fever, FNHTR may involve
any or all of the symptoms shaking chills, flushing,
shortness of breath, hypotension, headache, nausea and
vomiting and anxiety. Before the now fairly widespread use of leukocyte reduction filters, FNHTR were
seen in some 1 in 130 to 1 in 400 transfusions (240-
243). They are more common in women than in men by
a ratio of about 2:1 (244). This finding relates directly
to the role of anti-HLA in FNHTR (see below) and the
fact that anti-HLA are often made during or following
pregnancy. Multiple previous transfusions also
increase the chance that the patient will have a

FNHTR. The transfusion of platelets is a cause of FNHTR more often than is the transfusion of red cells (245). As explained in the following sections, the rise in temperature seen in FNHTR may be due to any one or more of a variety of causes.

FNHTR Caused by Pyrogens

Exogenous pyrogens (foreign substances including waste products of bacterial growth) present in transfusion sets, anticoagulant solutions or the like, cause an increase in temperature of the patient, if transfused. Pyrogenic febrile reactions were common when rubber and glass infusion sets and glass bottles were used. These pieces of apparatus were reusable and the exclusion of pyrogenic material was always a problem. Sterilization of glass and rubber sets and bottles does not inactivate pyrogens. Now that disposable plastic infusion sets and blood bags are in wide use the problems caused by externally produced pyrogens can largely be eliminated providing care is taken in the preparation of anticoagulant solutions and the like. That care is still necessary is clear from reports (235-237) of the presence of pyrogens in human albumin solutions prepared for intravenous infusion.

Although the introduction of exogenous pyrogens can now largely be prevented, febrile transfusion reactions caused by pyrogens are still seen. This because of the release of endogenous pyrogens following the in vivo interaction of antibodies with red cells, leukocytes, platelets, etc. The cytokines IL-1 (specifically IL-1a), IL-6 and TNF, are all endogenous pyrogens and their release from macrophages and endothelial cells following the in vivo formation of many different types of antigen-antibody complexes almost certainly contributes to fever (17,92,231,246-248). In addition, when blood components, particularly platelets, are stored in vitro, the leukocytes present release (at least) IL-1a, IL-6 and TNF so that these cytokines are passively transferred to the patient and may cause fever (249,250,268). It had earlier been reported (251,252) that there was an increase in the incidence of FNHTR that was directly associated with the length of time platelets had been stored in vitro, before being transfused. In spite of what initially appears to be an obvious cause, that is the increase in level of cytokine generation in stored blood products and fever (and other effects) in the recipient, there is still considerable debate as to the contributions made by passively transferred cytokines and those generated by the patients after transfusion (253-258). Clearly, this debate also involves selection of leukocyte reduction strategies. Filters used to remove leukocytes, remove those cells but not all soluble cytokines that the leukocytes may have already released. This subject is discussed again in the section on leukocyte removal at the time that the donor is bled,

in the laboratory immediately before the release of the blood, or at the time of transfusion at the bedside.

Role of Antibodies to Leukocytes in FNHTR

Transfusion reactions caused by antibodies directed against antigens present on leukocytes (some of which are also present on platelets) are not uncommon. At one time it was supposed that two major mechanisms were involved. First, the activation of complement following leukocyte-anti-leukocyte reactions was thought to be important because of the release of vasoactive substances, e.g. C3a and C5a, see earlier in this chapter. Second, the destruction of granulocytes in vivo was thought to be important because of the release of pyrogens from those cells. Although both of those facts are clearly important it is now apparent that they are not separate and distinct events. As pointed out in the previous section and in the earlier section on the pathophysiology of transfusion reactions, a complex series of interrelated events involving the immune and inflammatory responses and the coagulation cascade take place and cause various clinical changes.

Antibodies to the HLA-A, HLA-B and HLA-C series of antigens react with granulocytes, monocytes and lymphocytes. In addition, both granulocyte-specific and monocyte-specific antibodies exist. It is believed that in FNHTR caused by antibodies to leukocytes, anti-HLA are involved most often (242,259). There is evidence (260) that lymphocytes are only rarely involved. Since most patients who experience FNHTR because of the present of antibodies to leukocytes will tolerate further transfusions without similar reactions, an original recommendation (241,261) was that leukocyte reduced products not be used unless the patient experienced two or more such reactions to consecutive transfusions. With leukocyte reduction filters now so widely used, it is likely that most patients who experience one FNHTR and many who never have such a reaction, will now receive leukocyte-reduced blood products.

The much more serious transfusion reaction caused by antibodies to granulocytes, namely transfusion-related acute lung injury, is described in a later section.

Role of Antibodies to Platelets in FNHTR

Distinguishing between FNHTR caused by antibodies to platelets and those caused by antibodies to leukocytes is not easy. First, platelet concentrates usually contain leukocytes. Second, HLA antigens are present on both platelets and leukocytes. FNHTR are common in patients receiving platelet transfusions. The symptoms of these reactions are similar to those of other FNHTR and although anti-HLA are involved most of the time, some cases seem to have been caused by platelet-specific antibodies (259,262,263). It should be emphasized that FNHTR associated with the transfusion of platelets are different from the serious complication of refractoriness to platelet transfusions. Although that refractoriness is due to anti-HLA and/or platelet specific antibodies and although those antibodies destroy the transfused platelets, the patients involved do not necessarily have FNHTR at the time of transfusion. As with FNHTR caused by antibodies to leukocytes, the incidence of such reactions seen in patients receiving platelets can be reduced by the use of leukocyte-reduction filters. While a full discussion of the subject is beyond the scope of this chapter, it will be mentioned that the use of leukocyte-depleted products has already shown great promise in the prevention of alloimmunization that leads to platelet refractoriness (264-267,269,270).

Leukocyte Reduction by Filtration

As discussed several times in this chapter, soluble cytokines released by leukocytes during storage of blood and blood components can cause adverse effects when transfused to a patient. Thus it would seem that prestorage filtration (i.e. removal of leukocytes at the time that the donor is bled) would decrease such cytokine generation and result in a better transfusion product. Indeed, several studies (249,250,255,256,268) have shown lower levels of several cytokines in blood products made from units that were leukoreduced at the time of collection. In spite of this, logistical and cost considerations have resulted in many hospitals continuing to use poststorage (bedside) leukocyte reduction filters. Snyder et al. (258) performed a series of experiments using poststorage filters. They showed that the filters lowered the levels of the cytokines IL-8 and RANTES and of the activated complement component C3a. It was suggested that removal of these factors by the filters might involve ionic interactions between them and the filter medium. Use of the poststorage leukocyte depletion filters did not reduce the levels of IL-1b or of IL-6.

Leukocyte reduction of products to be transfused has many advantages in addition to lowering the levels of passively introduced cytokines. Removal of most of the white cells at the time of collection or at the time of transfusion has been shown to: reduce the incidence of immunization to HLA and hence platelet refractoriness (264-267, 269,270,285); at least in part ameliorate some of the immunomodulatory effects of transfusion (271-274); reduce the risk of reperfusion injury (275,276); largely prevent the transmission of CMV (277-280); and, of course,

reduce the incidence of FNHTR (253,254,282-284).

As inferred above, one of the advantages of poststorage (bedside) filtration is that the product can be made when needed. Leukocyte-depletion is relatively expensive and it is logistically easier to filter products at the time of infusion, just for the patients who need them, than to carry an inventory of prestorage filtered products, not all of which will be used for their intended purpose. On the other hand, Popovsky (257) has pointed out that the quality of prestorage filtered units can be better controlled than the quality of units filtered at the bedside (289). It has been found that persons using the filters at the bedside do not always use them correctly or in accordance with the manufacturer's instructions. Passing excessive amounts of blood or platelets through the same filter results in a rapid increase in the number of leukocytes passing the filter and entering the patient's circulation (281). Levels of IL-8 and RANTES return to prefiltration levels if the filters are used for more blood or platelets than intended (258). Further, both the temperature of the blood at the time of filtration (286,287) and the rate of flow of blood or platelets through the filter (288) are important in achieving maximum leukocyte reduction. Again, these variables are easier to control at the time of collection than at the time of transfusion. Nurses, with many other duties, may well overlook some of the requirements for correct use of the filters, some patients may not be able to tolerate transfusion at the rate the blood should flow through the filter to reduce the leukocyte numbers to the required level. There is also some evidence (264,290-295) that prestorage filtration may be better than poststorage filtration in ameliorating some of the immunomodulatory effects of allogeneic transfusion and in the prevention of alloimmunization to HLA that leads to platelet refractoriness. During prestorage filtration intact leukocytes are removed. When blood or platelets are stored without previous filtration, some of the leukocytes are degraded. During poststorage filtration most of the intact leukocytes are removed but fragments of the degraded ones pass the filter (296). It is presumed that these fragments carry sufficient HLA antigens for immunization to occur.

It will be interesting to see if the logistical and cost factors that result in the current widespread use of poststorage leukocyte reduction filters can be overcome and if the use of prestorage filtered products will increase.

Prevention and Treatment of FNHTR

As indicated in the previous section, most FNHTR caused by antibodies against leukocytes can be prevented if a sufficient level of leukocyte reduction is achieved. For many years it was accepted that units containing less than 0.5×10^9 leukocytes (i.e. removal of some 80% of the original number) were unlikely to induce leukocyte antibody-mediated FNHTR (377). Such leukocyte-poor units were prepared by various simple methods, such as removal of the buffy coat. Although Goldfinger (378-380) advocated the use of frozen-thawed units, that he and his colleagues (381-383) had shown reduced FNHTR caused by leukocyte antibodies by 50%, most workers (44,244,261,377,384-387) supported the type of approach outlined by Smith (389) in which washed red cells were used only when less expensive products (such as leukocyte-poor red cells) had caused repeated febrile reactions in an individual patient. The chief criticisms of the routine use of washed red blood cells were that the high costs were not justified by the benefits and that the loss of red cells during the washing procedure was unacceptable on a routine basis when less expensive procedures that resulted in no greater red cell loss, were equally effective. These older considerations, no longer apply. As indicated in the previous section, currently available leukocyte reduction filters, if used correctly, remove far more than 80% of the leukocytes from a bag of blood.

Some workers treat or attempt to prevent febrile reactions by the use of antihistamines. Mollison (44) has pointed out that experimental studies (390,391) have shown that those drugs are not effective in this role but that there is evidence (392,393) that antipyrexial drugs such as aspirin are effective. In severe cases, a low dose of corticosteroid may be of benefit (394). Antihistamines may be indicated in patients who suffer allergic reactions without fever and in whom the only sign is urticaria.

Mollison (44) also noted that two very easy to accomplish measures considerably reduce the severity of febrile reactions. First, the patient should be kept warm during the transfusion (395). Second, unless there is an urgent need for red cells, the transfusion should be given at a rate no greater than 500 ml of whole blood per hour (396). These two simple steps reduce the incidence of febrile reactions without any increase in the cost of transfusion.

Transfusion-Related Acute Lung Injury (TRALI)

TRALI (that is also called transfusion-related non-cardiogenic pulmonary edema) is a rare complication of transfusion being seen in about 1 in 10,000 transfusions (243). Acute respiratory distress that is clinically indistinguishable from adult respiratory distress syndrome (ARDS), occurs usually within two hours and almost always within four hours of transfusion (297). Because the symptoms, fever, hypotension, chills, cyanosis, nonproductive cough and dyspnea are usually severe and dramatic and because the outcome is sometimes fatal,

TRALI has received considerable attention in the literature (297-306). Although not formally proved, it is believed (297,305,307-310) that the etiology involves the interaction between granulocytes and granulocyte antibodies (or less frequently anti-HLA), complement activation, the interaction of activated complement and granulocytes with subsequent aggregation of the granulocytes that then block the pulmonary microvasculature. Unlike most transfusion reactions described in this chapter, TRALI most often involves antibodies to granulocytes that are present in the donor blood but exceptions, in which the antibody was present in the patient, have been seen. Because of the severity and sometimes fatal outcome of TRALI, it has been suggested (297) that those donors whose blood has been implicated in a case of TRALI should either be deferred or, if accepted, that their plasma be discarded and their red cells be used only as frozen-thawed or as washed red cell products.

Allergic Reactions

Patients with a history of allergy may develop urticaria during or following transfusion if the blood is from a donor recently exposed to the substance to which the patient is allergic. Pooled serum caused urticaria when infused in a series of individuals allergic to substances such as pollen, dust, milk and eggs (311). Michel and Sharon (312) described a transfusion reaction that was thought to be related to the presence of penicillin in a donor unit. They (313) then tested sera from 10,853 normal donors and found that 30 (0.27%) contained penicillin G in concentrations between 0.2 and 4.0mg/ml. Sharon et al. (314) then tested the sera of another 2,655 healthy donors and this time found that 158 (6%) contained aspirin in concentrations that ranged from 10 to 200mg/ml. One patient had an allergic reactions that may have been due to aspirin in the donor blood (314). Allergic reactions have also been reported (315,316) when the antibody to the allergen has been passively acquired by the patient from the donor, via the infusion of plasma. Workers who, like one of us (PDI), have long blamed all allergic reactions on IgE antibodies may be surprised to learn that in man, IgG antibodies also seem to have a role in urticarial responses (317). However, most often it seems that Fc receptors on mast cells and basophils bind IgE, that on contact with the allergen, are cross-linked and effect the release of histamine. The Fc receptors can also be cross-linked by IgG antibodies to IgE, by antibodies to idiotypes of IgE and by some lectins (318).

Anaphylactic Reactions

A particularly severe form of transfusion reaction

that does not involve any red cell destruction is associated with IgA deficiency. Some individuals have a genetic abnormality as a result of which they do not produce IgA. These people can form IgG, complement-binding anti-IgA that, because the antibody-makers are IgA deficient, is called class-specific. When transfused with blood or plasma that contains IgA, these individuals may experience a severe anaphylactic-type reaction. The symptoms of such reactions may include laryngeal edema, chills, fever, severe substernal pain, sweating, flushing, hypotension, shock and collapse. An almost invariable characteristic of anaphylactic reactions, caused by anti-IgA in IgA-deficient patients, is the speed with which the symptoms develop after the transfusion of small (10 to 15 ml) volumes of blood (319-328,339). Although rare (calculated incidence one in 20,000 to 50,000 transfusions (329)) these reactions are potentially lethal. They seem to be confined to individuals who have anti-IgA with a titer of 256 or more. Since the reactions occur because the blood being transfused contains IgA in the plasma, it would be expected that washed red cells would be well tolerated by these patients. In fact, it has been reported (322,324,325) that red cells washed twice, still cause some symptoms to develop. Frozen-thawed red cells (322) and units washed five times (325) have been transfused without the development of symptoms. At least two IgA-deficient patients suffered anaphylactic-type reactions although they had not previously been transfused or pregnant (320,323). In a case in which this type of reaction is suspected, immunodiffusion or other appropriate tests on the patient's serum for presence of the various immunoglobulins should be performed (338). A demonstrated absence of IgA strongly suggests that the patient is reacting to IgA transfused in blood or plasma. Such patients must then be transfused with washed or frozen-thawed red cells, as described above and with plasma products made from the blood of other IgA-deficient individuals. To this end, a number of workers have conducted large scale studies to identify IgA-deficient donors whose plasma or plasma-containing products (e.g. platelets) can be used for patients with anti-IgA class specific antibodies (330-338).

Materials other than whole blood or plasma (319,325,336,345) have also caused anaphylactic reactions when used to treat patients with class specific IgA deficiency who have made anti-IgA. These include: a gamma globulin product injected intramuscularly (319); IVIG (intravenous immune globulin) (340-343) and fibrin glue made from cryoprecipitated factor VIII (344). A number of methods for the detection of IgA deficiency have been published (338,346-349) as has one for the detection of anti-IgA (350).

While IgA deficiency was at first regarded as a somewhat benign condition, it is now appreciated that it is some-times, but not invariably, associated with autoimmune or infectious diseases and, less commonly, with malignancy (351-353). It is also now known that coexistent IgG2 and IgA deficiencies occur and may be associated with recurrent infections of the lungs, sinuses, ears and gastrointestinal tract (354-357). However, coexistent IgG2 and IgA deficiency has also been seen in persons with no abnormalities at the time the deficiencies were noted (358-360), including some (361) who were blood donors.

Because there are genetically determined differences in IgA molecules in man, anti-IgA can also be made by persons who have normal levels of that immunoglobulin. Such antibodies, usually called anti-IgA of limited specificity, have been incriminated as causative of some transfusion reactions (319,321,329,339,362-364) that were invariably less severe than those caused by the anti-IgA class specific antibodies described above. However, several groups of investigators (365-367) have studied large numbers of patients who experienced fairly mild anaphylactic reactions and have found that only about 8 to 10% of them had anti-IgA of limited specificity in the serum. Further, Ropars et al. (365) followed six patients who had anti-IgA of limited specificity and found that none of them had transfusion reactions. It seems that the majority of urticarial and anaphylactic reactions (excluding the severe ones caused by class specific anti-IgA) cannot be blamed on anti-IgA of limited specificity, nor does presence of that antibody mean that a transfusion reaction will always occur.

Although it is beyond the province of this book to give details about the clinical treatment of patients experiencing transfusion reactions, it will be added (in case somebody needs the information in a hurry at some time) that severe anaphylactic reactions caused by anti-IgA have been managed by stopping the transfusion and giving hydrocortisone intravenously (368).

Sandler et al. (328) point out that occasionally it is necessary to differentiate anti-IgA-induced anaphylactic reactions from generalized or anaphylactic reactions that have a different cause. Among those to be differentiated they list: TRALI (see above) and anaphylactic reactions caused by antibodies to HLA or platelet antigens (369); anti-C4 (370); and allergies to latex (371), food (372), drugs (373), anesthetic agents (374) and muscle relaxants (375). Shopnick et al. (376) described an anaphylactic reaction in a young hemophiliac treated with recombinant factor VIII. They were not able to identify any responsible agent in the factor VIII preparation thus making future treatment of the patient a daunting proposition.

Circulatory Overload

This type of transfusion reaction may occur when a

patient with a normal blood volume, but a reduced red cell mass, is transfused. Overloading the circulation may produce the symptoms of headache, tightness in the chest and dyspnea and an increase in central venous pressure may lead to pulmonary edema. This type of reaction can be fatal and if suspected, aggressive treatment (see Mollison (44)) should be instituted. To prevent this type of reaction, patients with normal blood volumes (some of whom may be severely anemic) should be transfused with packed red blood cells and the transfusion should proceed very slowly, i.e. over a four to six hour period. Further, in a patient with severe anemia but a normal or close to normal total blood volume, in whom there is no blood loss, transfusions should be given over a period of days. One or two units per day for two or three days is much less likely to cause circulatory overload than the infusion of five or six units in a single day. Particular care must be taken in oliguric patients in whom excretion of fluid is impaired.

Contaminated Blood

This type of transfusion reaction is severe, dramatic and sometimes fatal. It occurs when bacteria proliferate in units blood or blood products during storage. Endotoxins are produced and when the contaminated blood is transfused a severe reaction occurs. Patients transfused with contaminated blood may go into shock very rapidly and many such transfusion accidents have proved fatal (397-422). The introduction of plastic bags and closed systems used in component preparation have reduced the chance of bacterial contamination of blood and blood products. Nevertheless, considerable care must still be exercised during the collection of units of blood to prevent contamination by bacteria from the donor's skin. Some studies (399,423) have shown that as many as 2% of all units become bacterially contaminated during collection. However, there are a number of factors that mitigate this situation. First, most of the contaminating bacteria are unable to proliferate at 4°C and die when blood is stored at that temperature for one or two days. Second, when small numbers of bacteria are present, the donor's or patient's leukocytes are able to kill them. Third, the citrate present in the anticoagulant may also have a bacteriocidal or bacteriostatic effect. In spite of these factors, contamination of units by bacteria such as *Pseudomonas fluorescens, Pseudomonas putida, Yersinia enterocolitica, Eschericia freundii, Enterobacter cloacae,* etc., that are able to grow at 4°C, can still result in lethal transfusion reactions. In a review of 25 cases that was published in 1973, Habibi et al. (424) reported that more than half the patients involved had died. Similarly in 1984, Khabbaz et al. (409) described three patients transfused with contam-

inated blood, two of whom subsequently died, and in 1990, Tipple et al. (420) described five deaths from this cause. In her review of 355 transfusion-associated deaths in the USA in the period 1976 to 1985, Sazama (43) noted that at least 25 were attributable to the transfusion of bacterially contaminated red cells or platelets and one due to the transfusion of *Pseudomonas cepacia* contaminated cryoprecipitate. Because this type of reaction is so severe and so often fatal, treatment (see Mollison (44)) must be initiated quickly. Indeed if the situation is suspected, treatment may best be initiated before the cause of the reaction is confirmed. A gram stain on a smear of blood or (perhaps better) microscopic examination of a hanging drop of the blood will often rapidly reveal the presence of bacteria. Some workers (425) give huge doses of broad spectrum antibiotics immediately it is suspected that contaminated blood may have been transfused. Although such treatment will not counter the effects of transfused endotoxins, it may well prevent septicemia in those patients in whom the initial shock and hypotension are not fatal, if live bacteria have been introduced.

Although the use of closed systems for the collection of blood and the preparation of components have reduced the chance of bacterial contamination, they have by no means eliminated it. Indeed, the realization that transfused platelets function better in the recipient if they have been stored at 20° to 24°C than if they have been stored at 4°C, has resulted in an increase in the incidence of transfusion of bacterially contaminated platelet concentrates. Currently used preservative solutions prolong platelet life in vitro for seven days. However, platelet concentrates are assigned a five day not a seven day outdate because of the use of 20° to 24°C storage and the risk of bacterial growth in the products. Transfusion reactions, some of which had fatal outcomes, resulting from the transfusion of bacterially contaminated platelet concentrates have been reported both before and since the introduction of 20° to 24°C storage (426-435). A list of organisms involved is given by Goldman and Blajchman (422). The transfusion of contaminated plasma products has also been reported, in some cases the contaminating organisms were present in the water bath used to thaw the cryoprecipitate (436) or fresh frozen plasma (437), in other cases the source of contamination was not identified (438). A batch of albumin solution contaminated during manufacture resulted in the transfer of *P. cepacia* to a number of patients (439).

It is difficult and not always practical to include screening studies for bacterial contamination of blood products. Goldman and Blajchman (422) report that they use a sensitive radiometric technique (440) to monitor products such as platelets collected by apheresis, when the product is to be stored for more than 24 hours. Brecher et al. (504,505) have described the use of a chemiluminescence-linked bacterial ribosomal DNA probe. A visual check of all products containing red cells should be made at the time the unit is issued. Visible discoloration to a deeper than usual red, to a purple hue or to a brown appearance should alert the person making the inspection to the fact that some sort of test for bacterial contamination is necessary before the unit is used. Brecher and Taswell (421) observed that discoloration of the unit could be detected most easily by comparing the color of blood in the bag (contaminated and darker in color) with that of blood in the segments (distal segments often sterile). Kim et al. (441) published a series of photographs of contaminated units and thus illustrated how transfusion of some contaminated units could have been prevented had the unit/segment color comparison been made.

Addition of Drugs to Blood

There are many reasons why drugs should not be added to blood or to the infusion line through which blood is being given. Some drugs e.g., ethacrynic acid (44), cyclophosphamide (442), cause hemolysis of red cells and may cause a transfusion reaction by destroying some of the red cells before they are transfused. Other good reasons are that: some drugs are not stable when mixed with blood; the rate at which the drug is given is too slow and cannot be controlled if the drug is mixed with a unit of blood; and finally, addition of any material to a unit of blood introduces the risk of bacterial contamination.

A Situation Mimicking a Transfusion Reaction

There are at least two reports (443,444) of cases in which the intravenous administration of an iron-dextran solution caused a red-brown discoloration of plasma that, in patients transfused at about the same time, was at first thought to represent free hemoglobin. Simon et al. (444) describe a simple test using Gomori's iron stain, that can be used to show that the color change in the plasma is due to the presence of iron and not free hemoglobin.

Toxicity

The transfusion of large quantities of citrated blood in a short period of time introduces a risk of citrate toxicity in the patient. This toxicity can be overcome by giving injections of calcium chloride or calcium gluconate (445,446) although this procedure is not without hazard (447). Similarly, the transfusion of too much stored blood to a patient introduces some risk of potassium tox-

icity. Both citrate and potassium accumulation in the patient can be reduced by the use of blood from which the plasma is removed immediately before transfusion. Spear et al. (448) have suggested that the administration of large amounts of old stored blood, with increased ammonia levels, is undesirable for patients in liver failure. Many workers (449-453) now avoid the transfusion of excessive amounts of potassium or ammonia to neonates and small children. Excessive levels of potassium are also contraindicated in blood to be transfused to a fetus in utero (454).

There is no doubt that red cells that have been irradiated leak potassium into the plasma in which they are suspended at a faster rate than do non-irradiated red cells (455-459). This finding sparked a considerable debate about the use of red cells that have been irradiated then stored. While there seems to be no dispute that the levels of potassium in such products are of little moment for most adults, less agreement exists about their use in neonates. Some workers (456,457,460-462) believe that the amount of potassium present has the potential to cause harm in neonates while others (463-466) contend that the amounts are too small to be of any clinical consequence. Accordingly, some workers (457,462) believe that red cells that have been irradiated then stored, should be washed before being transfused to neonates, while another (466) does not believe this to be necessary on a routine basis. In selected cases where the patient's clinical condition may result in high potassium levels, washing the red cells immediately before transfusion may be advisable (466). Aside from the question of accumulation of potassium in the plasma of units that have been irradiated and then stored, there is evidence that irradiation damages the red cells so that once stored for long periods, their in vivo survival is impaired (467,468). Both groups of investigators reporting these findings recommend that once irradiated, units of red cells be stored for no longer than 28 days.

Other Untoward Effects of Transfusion

There are many other complications that can follow the transfusion of blood or components derived from blood. A partial list of these complications would include:

1. Transfusion transmitted diseases (viral)
    a) HIV-1, HIV-2
    b) Hepatitis, A, B, C and more
    c) HTLV-I, HTLV-II
    d) CMV
    e) EBV
    f) B19 (Parvovirus)

2. Transfusion transmitted diseases (non-viral)
   a) Bacteria (see earlier sections)
   b) Syphilis
   c) Malaria
   d) Chagas' disease (*T. cruzi*)
   e) Toxoplasmosis (*T. gondii*)
   f) Babesiosis (*B. microti*)
   g) Leishmaniasis (*L. donovani*)
   h) Microfilariae (*W. bancrofti, B. malayi, L. loa*)
   i) African trypanosomiasis
   j) ? Lyme disease (*B. burgdorferi*)
   k) ? Creutzfeld-Jacob disease, CJD
3. Transfusion of hemolyzed blood
   a) Following overheating
   b) Following accidental freezing
   c) Forced through fine bore needle
   d) Inadequately deglycerolized
4. Immune complications
   a) Graft versus host disease, GVHD
   b) Post-transfusion purpura, PTP
   c) Reactions to IgG
   d) Alloimmunization
5. Non-immune complications
   a) Transfusion hemosiderosis (iron overload)
   b) Hypothermia (rapid transfusion of cold blood)
   c) Air embolism
   d) Transfusion of extraneous matter (macroaggregates, microaggregates)
   e) Toxic substances from plastic
   f) Sensitivity to nickel

Investigation of a Suspected Transfusion Reaction

The full investigation of a suspected transfusion reaction is a time-consuming task. In order that it be done well it is important that it not be done too often. In other words, if every transfusion reaction reported to the blood bank is fully investigated, the workload will be too great and the methods used in the investigation will invariably be abridged so that sufficient time will be available to conduct the investigations. It is much better to match the extent of the investigation to the symptoms of the reaction, than to try to do a full work-up on each reported reaction. By having different protocols for the investigation of transfusion reactions it becomes possible fully to investigate those in which the clinical symptoms are such that the possibility of antibody-mediated in vivo red cell destruction exists. At the same time, a simple protocol can be used to investigate those reactions in which the clinical symptoms suggest that antibody-induced red cell destruction did not occur. Listed below are two suggested formats for the investigation of sus-

pected transfusion reactions. One is for use in cases when antibody-mediated red cell destruction is a possibility, the other for investigation of cases in which such an event is improbable. Obviously, the protocols can be modified to intermediate levels for cases with an intermediate likelihood of red cell destruction.

Symptoms that Suggest the Possibility that Antibody-induced Red cell Destruction Occurred so that a Full Investigation is Necessary

1. An increase in temperature of $\geq 1°C$ or $2°F$ or more, during or within two hours of completion of the transfusion, in an otherwise afebrile patient.
2. Shock, hypotension, severe back pain, burning sensation at the site of infusion.
3. Abnormal bleeding, particularly in an anesthetized patient.
4. Any obvious sign of red cell destruction, e.g. hemoglobinuria

Symptoms that Suggest that Antibody-induced Red Cell Destruction is Unlikely so that an Abridged Investigation can be Performed

1. Mild to moderate fever in the absence of other symptoms.
2. Urticaria (hives) and/or pruritis (itching) in the absence of other symptoms.
3. Signs of circulatory overload in the absence of other symptoms.

Suggested Protocol for Investigation of a Reaction that May Have Involved In Vivo Red Cell Destruction (not every test need be done in every case)

I. *In the patient's room.*
   1. Stop the transfusion, keep the i.v. line open
   2. Collect a venous blood sample at a site away from the site of infusion
   3. Collect the next sample of urine voided
   4. Document symptoms of reaction (chills, fever, rigor, urticaria, back pain, maximum temperature, etc.)
   5. Send remains of unit, new blood sample, urine sample and information to the transfusion service.

II. *In the transfusion service*

1. Check all paperwork and records
   a. Was the patient given the intended unit?
   b. Has the patient been correctly identified?
   c. Are there any discrepancies in the original test results?
2. Repeat ABO (mandatory) and D (optional) typing on:
   a. Patient's pretransfusion sample
   b. Patient's posttransfusion sample
   c. Cells from actual bag of blood
   d. Cells from pilot tube
3. Repeat major compatibility tests using:
   a. Patient's pretransfusion serum and cells from the bag of blood
   b. Patient's posttransfusion serum and cells from the bag of blood
4. Repeat antibody-screening tests on:
   a. Patient's pretransfusion serum
   b. Patient's posttransfusion serum
   c. Plasma from donor unit
   d. Plasma from donor unit using the patient's pretransfusion red cells in place of the antibody-screening cells
5. Direct antiglobulin test on:
   a. Patient's posttransfusion cells
      NOTE: If positive, test pretransfusion cells to see if positive DAT was preexistent.
   b. Donor cells from bag of blood
6. If the above tests are all negative and there is still a high suspicion of antibody-induced red cell destruction:
   a. Perform compatibility tests using patient's pretransfusion serum and cells from the bag of blood by different methods to those used in 3a (i.e. LISS, enzymes, polybrene).
   b. As in 6a using the patient's posttransfusion serum
   c. As in 6a using antibody-screening cells
   d. As in 6b using antibody-screening cells

III. *Other laboratory tests*
   1. Examination of patient's posttransfusion serum for hemoglobin
   2. Examination of patient's urine for hemoglobin and its derivatives
   3. Serial bilirubin level determinations on the patient
   4. Test of patient's posttransfusion blood for haptoglobin (see below)
   5. Examination of donor plasma for hemoglobin
   6. Blood culture on patient and bag of blood

IV. *Interpretation of II and III*

Obviously, the finding of any incompatibility caused by a clinically-significant antibody or a signifi-

cant ABO discrepancy explains the transfusion reaction. If in vivo antibody-binding to the transfused red cells occurred, the DAT will be positive and may give a mixed-field agglutination pattern (donor cells antibody-coated, patient's own cells not). In the event of a severe intravascular reaction this test may be negative since the transfused cells may have been eliminated before the postreaction sample was collected.

The tests involving detection of antibodies in the patient's serum or in the donor's plasma are also significant. Obviously the finding of say, a weak anti-Jk^a in the patient's serum, by sensitive methods, followed by demonstration that the donor cells are Jk(a+) may explain the reaction although the patient's serum may not have reacted with the donor's red cells in the compatibility testing methods used. Similarly the detection of an antibody in the donor's plasma may be of significance. For this reason the suggested protocol includes antibody detection tests on the donor's plasma using the patient's red cells. In this way, an antibody directed against a low incidence antigen may be found if the antigen that it detects is present on the patient's red cells but not on the antibody-screening cells.

The detection of an antibody in the donor's plasma that is directed against an antigen not present on the recipient's red cells may also be significant. In this situation other units transfused to the patient should be tested for the presence of the antigen against which the passively transferred antibody is directed (i.e. inter-donor incompatibility).

Use of the patient's pre and posttransfusion samples in antibody-screening and compatibility tests will sometimes show (potent antibody in the latter but none in the former) that the pretransfusion sample was collected from the wrong patient. This fact will not be apparent from repeat blood grouping studies if, by chance, the two patients were of the same ABO and D type.

The finding of hemoglobin or its derivatives in the patient's serum or urine is suggestive of abnormal red cell destruction but in the absence of confirmatory serological findings does not necessarily indicate that an antigen-antibody reaction occurred. Other possible explanations are poor storage of the blood (hemolyzed before transfusion which should be indicated by the tests suggested on the unit), the patient's clinical condition (WAIHA, etc.), or poor collection of the postreaction sample.

A plasma protein called haptoglobin binds free hemoglobin present in the circulation and the complex is then excreted. Low levels or an absence of haptoglobin may indicate that hemoglobin has recently been cleared from circulation. However, there are many other causes of reduced or absent haptoglobin so that finding alone by no means proves that in vivo red cell destruction occurred.

Suggested Protocol for the Investigation of Reactions in Which Antibody-induced Red Cell Clearance is Improbable

I. *In the patient's room*

Same as in the previous protocol. It is especially important to keep the i.v. line open since once the investigation has shown that no red cell incompatibility exists, the patient may be medicated (e.g. anti-pyrexial medication) and the transfusion continued. Indeed some workers stop the infusion of blood but leave the bag in place, pending the resumption of transfusion.

II. *In the transfusion service*

1. Centrifuge the posttransfusion sample from the patient and examine the serum or plasma for free hemoglobin. In the absence of severe symptoms (see above) absence of free hemoglobin can be taken to indicate that intravascular red cell destruction did not occur.
2. DAT on the posttransfusion sample from the patient. In the absence of severe symptoms (see above) a negative DAT can be taken to indicate that extravascular red cell destruction did not occur.
3. Check all paperwork and records (optional but not a bad idea since transfusion reactions due to clerical errors are much more common than those due to technical errors).
4. In the absence of severe symptoms, inform the patient's physician that an antibody-mediated cause of the transfusion reaction is unlikely.

Treatment of Patients Who Have Had Hemolytic Transfusion Reactions

A full description of treatment of such patients is obviously beyond the scope of this book. Physicians who may have to treat such patients should be thoroughly familiar with the procedures described by Mollison (44) and by Smith (389). Unfortunately, this is not always the case and a blood banker with little medical training may sometimes be asked to provide instant advice (particularly at 3 a.m.) to a physician or a nurse who has never before seen such a reaction. Accordingly, a brief synopsis of an appropriate course of action (culled from Mollison (44) and Smith (389)) is given below.

1. Unless the only adverse signs are urticaria and/or pruritis, stop the transfusion at once. Keep the intravenous line open (see also point 7, below).
2. If there is evidence of oliguria attempt to provoke a diuresis. Dopamine (infused at 3 - 5mg/kg per minute) produces selective renal vasodilation. Frusemide may be given in doses of up to 250mg, by infusion over a 4 hour period. If a diuresis occurs it should be maintained by giving further doses of frusemide if the urinary output falls below 30 ml per hour.
3. If a diuresis cannot be provoked, restrict fluid input to no more than the patient can excrete (circa 500 ml a day via the lungs, skin and feces). If renal failure appears probable, exclude electrolytes from the patient's fluid intake. A patient with renal failure is susceptible to overloading with fluid and subsequent development of pulmonary edema.
4. Control hypotension by maintenance of intravascular volume and blood pressure. Infuse colloids or crystalloids if a diuresis has been induced.
5. Monitor for DIC. Use heparin (if at all) only before significant DIC has occurred.
6. Begin to arrange for dialysis if renal shut down seems likely. The patient's clinical condition may worsen very rapidly and early dialysis is associated with a lower rate of mortality than is dialysis begun later.
7. If the *only* signs of a reaction are urticaria and/or pruritis the infusion of blood should be temporarily suspended and the i.v. line kept open with saline. The antihistamine diphenhydramine (50mg, intramuscularly) can be given and the transfusion can be continued once the urticaria and/or itching is (are) controlled.

References

1. Mollison PL, Engelfriet CP, Contreras M. Blood Transfusion in Clinical Medicine, 9th Ed. Oxford:Blackwell, 1993
2. Fairly NH. Br Med J 1940;2:213
3. Fairley NH. Quart J Med 1941;10:95
4. Barry KG, Crosby WH. Transfusion 1963;3:34
5. Schmidt PJ, Holland PV. Lancet 1967;2:1169
6. Rock RC, Bove JR, Nemerson Y. Transfusion 1969;9:57
7. Lopas H, Birndorf NI. Br J Haematol 1971;21:399
8. Goldfinger D. Transfusion 1977;17:85
9. Capon SM, Sacher RA. J Intens Care Med 1989;4:100
10. Davenport RD, Strieter RM, Standiford TJ, et al. Blood 1990;76:2439
11. Davenport RD, Strieter RM, Kunkel SL. Br J Haematol 1991;78:540
12. Butler J, Parker D, Pillai R, et al. Br J Haematol 1991;79:525
13. Capon SM, Goldfinger D. In: Alloimmunity: 1993 and Beyond. Bethesda:Am Assoc Blood Banks, 1993:141
14. Rappaport SI. West J Med 1993;158:153
15. Davenport RD, Burdick M, Strieter RM, et al. Transfusion 1994;34:16
16. Davenport RD, Polak TJ, Kunkel SL. Transfusion 1994;34:943
17. Davenport RD, Kunkel SL. Transf Med Rev 1994;8:157
18. Greebury CL, Moore DH. Immunology 1963;6:421

19. Economidou J, Hughes-Jones NC, Gardner B. Vox Sang 1967;12:321
20. Cartron J-P, Gerbal A, Hughes-Jones NC, et al. Immunology 1974;27:723
21. Anstee DJ. Vox Sang 1990;58:1
22. Anstee DJ. J Immunogenet 1990;17:219
23. Rawson AJ, Abelson NM. J Immunol 1960;85:636
24. Polley MJ, Adinolfi M, Mollison PL. Vox Sang 1963;8:385
25. Romano EL, Mollison PL. Br J Haematol 1975;29:121
26. Rosenfield RE. In: A Seminar on Performance Evaluation. Washington, D.C.:Am Assoc Blood Banks, 1976:93
27. Watkins WM. Proc Roy Soc Biol London, Series B 1978;202:31
28. Ervin DM, Young LE. Blood 1950;5;61
29. Ervin DM, Christian RM, Young LE. Blood 1950;5:553
30. Wiener AS, Samwich AA, Morrison H, et al. Exp Med Surg 1953;11:276
31. Mollison PL. Br Med J 1959;2:1123
32. Mollison PL. Br Med J 1959;2:1305
33. Schmidt PJ, Nancarrow JF, Morrison EG, et al. J Lab Clin Med 1959;54:38
34. Boose GM, Issitt CH, Issitt PD. Transfusion 1978;18:570
35. Garratty G, Arndt P, Co A, et al. Transfusion 1996;36:351
36. Jakobowicz R, Simmons RT, Carew JP. Vox Sang 1961;6:320
37. Mollison PL, Johnson CA, Prior DM. Vox Sang 1978;35:149
38. Tovey GH. Vox Sang 1963;8:257
39. Honig CL, Bove JR. Transfusion 1980;20:653
40. Myhre BA. J Am Med Assoc 1980;244:1333
41. Schmidt PJ. J Florida Med Assoc 1980;67:151
42. Edinger SE. Med Lab Obs April 1985:41
43. Sazama K. Transfusion 1990;30:583
44. Mollison PL. Blood Transfusion in Clinical Medicine, 7th Ed. Oxford:Blackwell, 1983
45. Wallace J. Blood Transfusion for Clinicians. Edinburgh:Churchill Livingstone, 1977
46. Schmidt PJ. In: Immunobiology of the Erythrocyte. New York:Liss, 1980:251
47. Wiener AS. NY State J Med 1954;54:3071
48. Bove JR. Connecticut Med 1968;32:36
49. Sherwood GK, Haynes BG, Rosse WF. Transfusion 1976;16:417
50. Mollison PL, Crome P, Hughes-Jones NC, et al. Br J Haematol 1965;11:461
51. Garratty G. In: Immune Destruction of Red Blood Cells. Arlington, VA:Am Assoc Blood Banks, 1989:109
52. Pinkerton FJ, Mermod LE, Liles BA, et al. Vox Sang 1959;4:155
53. Joseph JIJ, Awer E, Laulicht M, et al. Transfusion 1964;4:367
54. Stuckey MA, Osoba D, Thomas JW. Canad Med Assoc J 1964;90:739
55. Day D, Perkins HA, Sams B. Transfusion 1965;5:315
56. Morgan P, Wheeler CB, Bossom EL. Transfusion 1967;7:307
57. Rauner RA, Tanaka KR. New Eng J Med 1967;276:1486
58. Croucher BEE, Crookston MC, Crookston JH. Vox Sang 1967;12:32
59. Pineda AA, Taswell HF, Brzica SM. Transfusion 1978;18:1
60. Croucher BEE. In: A Seminar on Laboratory Management of Hemolysis. Washington, D.C.:Am Assoc Blood Banks, 1979:151
61. Petz LD, Garratty G. Acquired Immune Hemolytic Anemias. New York:Churchill Livingstone, 1980
62. Moore SB, Taswell HF, Pineda AA, et al. Am J Clin Pathol 1980;74:94
63. Popovsky MA. In: Immune Destruction of Red Cells. Arlington, VA:Am Assoc Blood Banks, 1989:201
64. Ness PM, Shirey RS, Thoman SK, et al. Transfusion 1990;30:688
65. Beauregard P, Blajchman MA. Transf Med Rev 1994;8:184
66. Mantovani B, Rabinovitch M, Nussenzweig V. J Exp Med 1972;135:780
67. Schreiber AD, Frank MM. J Clin Invest 1972;51:575
68. Schreiber AD, Frank MM. J Clin Invest 1972;51:583
69. Jaffe CJ, Atkinson JP, Frank MM. J Clin Invest 1976;58:942
70. Ehlenberger AG, Nussenzweig V. J Exp Med 1977;145:357
71. Gaither TA, Vargas I, Inada S, et al. Immunology 1987;62:405
72. Kronenberg H, Kooptzoff O, Walsh RJ. Austral Ann Med 1958;7:34
73. Degnan TJ, Rosenfield RE. Transfusion 1965;5:245
74. Maynard BA, Smith DS, Farrar RP, et al. Transfusion 1988;28:302
75. Ottenberg R. Ann Surg 1908;47:486
76. Crile GW. Hemorrhage and Transfusion: An Experimental and Clinical Research. New York:Appleton, 1909
77. Ottenberg R. J Exp Med 1911;13:425
78. Ottenberg R, Kaliski DJ. J Am Med Assoc 1913;61:2138
79. Ottenberg R, Thalheimer W. J Med Res 1915;33:213
80. Oehlecker F. Arch Klin Chir 1928;152:477
81. Zimmerman TS, Müller-Eberhard HJ. J Exp Med 1971;134:1601
82. Ghebrehiwet B, Silverberg M, Kaplan AP. J Exp Med 1981;153:665
83. Sundsmo JS, Fair DS. Springer Sem Immunopathol 1983;9:231
84. Savitsky JP, Doczi J, Black J, et al. Clin Pharacol Ther 1978;23:73
85. Dzik WH, Sherburne B. Transf Med Rev 1990;4:208
86. Birndorf NL, Lopas H. J Appl Physiol 1970;29:573
87. Rabiner SF, O'Brien K, Peskin GW, et al. Ann Surg 1970;171:615
88. Smith K, McClure Browne JC, Shackman R, et al. Lancet 1965;2:351
89. Lopas H, Birndorf NI, Robboy SJ. Transfusion 1971;11:196
90. Davenport RD, Burdick M, Moore SA, et al. Transfusion 1993;33:19
91. Davenport RD, Burdick MD, Strieter RM, et al. Transfusion 1994;34:297
92. Davenport RD. Immunol Invest 1995;24:319
93. Capon SM, Goldfinger D. Transfusion 1995;35:513
94. Davenport R. Unpublished observations 1990 cited in Davenport RD, Kunkel SL. Transf Med Rev 1994;8:157
95. Matsushima K, Oppenheim JJ. Cytokine 1989;1:2
96. White MV, Yoshimura T, Hook W, et al. Immunol Lett 1989;22:151
97. Hoffman M. Vox Sang 1991;60:184
98. Haskill S, Johnson C, Eierman D, et al. J Immunol 1988;140:1690
99. Kasahara K, Strieter RM, Chensue SW, et al. J Leuk Biol 1991;50:287
100. Beveler B, Milsark IW, Cerami AC. Science 1985;229:689
101. Tracey KJ, Beutler B, Lowry SF, et al. Science 1986;234:470
102. Conkling PR, Greenberg CS, Weinberg JB. Blood 1988;72:128
103. Van der Poll T, Buller HR, Ten Cate H, et al. New Eng J Med 1990;322:1622
104. Griffin JH, Mosher DF, Zimmerman TS, et al. Blood 1982;60:261
105. Nawroth PP, Handley DA, Esmon CT, et al. Proc Nat Acad Sci USA 1986;83:3460
106. Nawroth PP, Stern DM. J Exp Med 1986;163:740
107. Moore KL, Esmon CT, Esmon NL. Blood 1989;73:159

108. Davenport RD, Burdick M, Kunkel SL. (abstract). Transfusion 1992;32 (Suppl 8S):53S
109. Griendling KK, Lassegue BP, Taylor WR, et al. J Crit Illness 1993;8:355
110. Brenner BM, Troy JL, Ballermann BJ. J Clin Invest 1989;84:1373
111. Palmer RMJ, Ashton DS, Moncada S. Nature 1988;333:664
112. Yanagisawa M, Kurihara H, Kimura S, et al. Nature 1988;332:411
113. Kon V, Badr KF. Kidney Int 1991;40:1
114. Kubes P, Suzucki M, Granger DN. Proc Nat Acad Sci USA 1991;88:4651
115. Cutbush M, Mollison PL. Br J Haematol 1958;4:115
116. Mollison PL. Transfusion 1986;26:43
117. Mollison PL. Transfusion 1989;29:347
118. Burton MS, Mollison PL. Immunology 1968;14:861
119. Mollison PL, Newlands M. Vox Sang 1976;31:54
120. Pineda AA, Brzica SM, Taswell HF. Mayo Clin Proc 1978;53:378
121. Marsh WL, DiNapoli J, Øyen R, et al. Transfusion 1979;19:604
122. Boyd PA, Issitt PD, Tessel JA. (abstract). Book of Abstracts. 16th Cong ISBT 1980:285
123. Diamond WJ, Brown FL, Bitterman P, et al. Ann Int Med 1980;93:231
124. Reeves WB, Ballas SK. (Letter). Transfusion 1980;20:477
125. Taswell HF, Pineda AA, Moore SB. In: A Seminar on Immune-Mediated Cell Destruction. Washington, D.C.:Am Assoc Blood Banks, 1981:71
126. Roy RB, Lotto WN. Transfusion 1962;2:342
127. Giblett ER, Hillman RS, Brooks LE. Vox Sang 1965;10:448
128. Kurtides ES, Salkin MS, Widen AL. J Am Med Assoc 1966;197:816
129. Holland PV, Wallerstein RO. J Am Med Assoc 1968;204:1007
130. Meltz DJ, Bertles JF, David DS, et al. Lancet 1971;2:1348
131. Montcrieff RE, Thompson WP. Am J Clin Pathol 1975;64:251
132. Rothman IK, Alter HJ, Strewler GJ. Transfusion 1976;16:357
133. Pickles MM, Jones EM, Egan J, et al. Vox Sang 1978;35:32
134. Vichinsky EP, Earles A, Johnson RA, et al. New Eng J Med 1990;322:1617
135. Boyland IP, Mufti GF, Hamblin TJ. (Letter). Transfusion 1982;22:402
136. Urbaniak SJ. Br J Haematol 1976;33:409
137. Shore SL, Mellwicz FM, Gordon DS. J Immunol 1977;118:558
138. Fleer A, Schaik van MLJ, Borne von dem AEGKr, et al. Scand J Immunol 1978;8:515
139. Handwerger BS, Kay NW, Douglas SD. Vox Sang 1978;24:276
140. Milgrom H, Shore SL. Cellular Immunol 1978;39:178
141. Northoff H, Kluge A, Resch K. Z Immun Forsch 1978;154:15
142. Kurlander RJ, Rosse WF, Logue GL. J Clin Invest 1978;61:1309
143. Urbaniak SJ. Br J Haematol 1979;42:303
144. Urbaniak SJ. Br J Haematol 1979;42:315
145. Urbaniak SJ, Greiss MA. Br J Haematol 1980;46;447
146. Yust I, Goldsher N, Greenfeld R, et al. Israel J Med Sci 1980;16:174
147. Wiedermann G, Rumpold H, Stemberg H, et al. African J Clin Exp Immunol 1981;2:39
148. Yust I, Frisch B, Goldsher N. Am J Hematol 1982;13:53
149. Armstrong SS, Weiner E, Garner SF, et al. Br J Haematol 1987;66:257
150. Anderson CL. Clin Immunol Immunopathol 1989;53:S63
151. Kumpel BM, Leader KA, Merry AH, et al. Eur J Immunol 1989;19:2283
152. Kumpel BM, Wiener E, Urbaniak SJ, et al. Br J Haematol 1989;71:415
153. Kumpel BM, Hadley AG. Mol Immunol 1990;27:247
154. Patten E, Reddi CR, Riglin H, et al. Transfusion 1982;22:248
155. Taddie SJ, Barrasso C, Ness PM. Transfusion 1982;22:68
156. Boorman KE, Dodd BE, Loutit JF, et al. Br Med J 1946;1:751
157. Salmon C, Schwartzenberg L, Andre R. Sangre 1959;30:223
158. Perkins HA, Day D, Hill E. Proc 9th Cong ISBT. Basel:Karger, 1964:97
159. Lundberg WB, McGinniss MH. Transfusion 1975;15:1
160. Issitt PD. In: A Symposium on Rh Problems in Clinical Practice. Groningen:Netherlands Red Cross, 1979:46
161. Judd WJ, Barnes BA, Steiner EA, et al. Transfusion 1986;26:220
162. Stec N, Shirey RS, Smith B, et al. Transfusion 1986;26:225
163. Combs MR, Issitt PD, Telen MJ. Unpublished observations 1993
164. Judd WJ, Butch SH. In: Blood Banking in a Changing Environment. Arlington, VA:Am Assoc Blood Banks, 1984:15
165. Judd WJ, Butch SH. J Med Technol 1984;1:485
166. Garratty G. Transfusion 1986;26:217
167. Salama A, Mueller-Eckhardt C. Transfusion 1984;24:188
168. Polesky HF, Bove JR. Transfusion 1964;4:285
169. Mohn JF, Bowman HS, Lambert RM, et al. Prog 10th Cong ISBT, 1964
170. Beard MEJ, Pemberton J, Blagdon J, et al. J Med Genet 1971;8:317
171. Cook IA. Br J Haematol 1971;20:369
172. Lalezari P, Talleyrand NP, Wenz B, et al. Vox Sang 1975;28:19
173. Worlledge SM. Br J Haematol 1978;39:157
174. Issitt PD. Unpublished observations 1978 cited in Mollison PL, Engelfriet CP, Contreras M. Blood Transfusion in Clinical Medicine, 9th Ed. Oxford:Blackwell, 1993:119
175. Contreras M, Hazlehurst GR, Armitage SE. Br J Haematol 1983;55:657
176. Sosler SD, Perkins JT, Saporito C, et al. (abstract). Transfusion 1989;29 (Suppl 7S):49S
177. Rosse WF, Gallagher D, Kinney TR, et al. Blood 1990;76:1431
178. Issitt PD, Zellner DC, Rolih SD, et al. Transfusion 1977;17:531
179. Henry RA, Weber J, Pavone BG, et al. Transfusion 1977;17:539
180. Issitt PD, Pavone BG. Br J Haematol 1978;38:63
181. Weber J, Caceres VW, Pavone BG, et al. Transfusion 1979;19:216
182. Issitt PD, Combs MR, Bumgarner DJ, et al. Transfusion 1996;36:481
183. Fudenberg HH, Rosenfield RE, Wasserman LR. J Mt Sinai Hosp 1958;25:324
184. Fudenberg H, Allen FH Jr. New Eng J Med 1957;256:1180
185. Goudsmit R, Krijnen HW. Vox Sang 1957;2:357
186. Jandl JH, Greenberg MS. J Lab Clin Med 1957;49:233
187. Adner PL, Sjolin S. Scand J Clin Lab Invest 1957;9:265
188. Stewart JW, Mollison PL. Br Med J 1959;1:1274
189. Mollison PL. Blood Transfusion in Clinical Medicine, 1st Ed. Oxford:Blackwell, 1951:107
190. Heisto H, Myhre K, Vogt E, et al. Vox Sang 1960;5:538
191. Kissmeyer-Nielsen F, Jensen KB, Ersbak J. Br J Haematol 1961;7:36
192. Vullo C, Tunioli AM. Vox Sang 1961;6:583
193. Chaplin H, Cassell M. Transfusion 1962;2:375
194. Heisto H, Myhre K, Borresen W, et al. Vox Sang 1962;7:470

195. Adner PL, Foconi S, Sjolin S. Br J Haematol 1963;9:288
196. Hart van der M, Engelfriet CP, Prins HK, et al. Vox Sang 1963;8:363
197. Loghem van JJ, Hart van der M, Moes M, et al. Transfusion 1965;5:525
198. Mollison PL. Blood Transfusion in Clinical Medicine, 2nd Ed. Oxford:Blackwell, 1956:354
199. Davey RJ, Gustafson M, Holland PV. Transfusion 1980;20:348
200. Baldwin ML, Barrasso C, Ness PM, et al. Transfusion 1983;123:40
201. Harrison CR, Hayes TC, Trow LL, et al. Vox Sang 1986;51:96
202. Halima D, Postoway N, Brunt D, et al. (abstract). Transfusion 1982;22:405
203. Garratty G, Vengelen-Tyler V, Postoway N, et al. (abstract). Transfusion 1982;22:429
204. Garratty G, Arndt P, Postoway N, et al. (abstract). Transfusion 1996;36 (Suppl 9S):23S
205. Crawford MN. Transfusion 1978;18:598
206. Judd WJ. Methods in Immunohematology, 2nd Ed. Durham:Montgomery, 1994
207. Leikola J, Perkins HA. Transfusion 1980;20:138
208. Leikola J, Perkins HA. Transfusion 1980;20:224
209. Garratty G, Postoway N, Nance S, et al. (abstract). Transfusion 1982;22:430
210. Sokol RJ, Hewitt S, Booker DJ, et al. J Clin Pathol 1985;38:912
211. Postoway N, Nance SJ, Garratty G. Med Lab Sci 1985;42:11
212. Wilson L, Wren MR, Issitt PD. Med Lab Sci 1985;42:20
213. Sokol RJ, Hewitt S, Booker DJ, et al. J Clin Pathol 1987;40:254
214. Tomasulo PA, Issitt PD, Gutgsell NS, et al. (abstract). Book of Abstracts. 20th Cong ISBT 1988;121
215. Gutgsell NS, Issitt PD, Tomasulo PA, et al. (abstract). Transfusion 1988;28 (Suppl 6S):36S
216. Garratty G, Postoway N, Nance S, et al. (abstract). Book of Abstracts. Joint Cong ISBT/AABB 1990:87
217. Issitt PD, Gutgsell NA. In: Immune Destruction of Red Cells. Arlington, VA:Am Assoc Blood Banks, 1989:77
218. Issitt PD. Amtec Sci Pub Ser 1988;2:1
219. Löw B, Messeter L. Vox Sang 1974;26:53
220. Moore HC, Mollison PL. Transfusion 1976;16:291
221. Lincoln PJ, Dodd BE. Vox Sang 1978;34:221
222. Caren LD, Bellevance R, Grumet FC. Transfusion 1982;22:475
223. Garratty G. In: Autoimmune Disorders of Blood. Bethesda:Am Assoc Blood Banks, 1996:79
224. Gilsanz F, de la Serna FJ, Molto L, et al. Transfusion 1996;36:463
225. Wallas CH, Tanley PC, Gorrell LP. Transfusion 1980;20:332
226. Reid ME, Toy P. Am J Clin Pathol 1983;79:364
227. Branch DR, Sy Siok Hian AL, Carlson F, et al. Am J Clin Pathol 1983;80:453
228. Brown D. Transfusion 1988;28:21
229. Blajchman MA. Transfusion 1993;33:1
230. Jenner PW, Holland PV. In: Clinical Practice of Transfusion Medicine, 3rd Ed. New York:Churchill Livingstone, 1996:905
231. Boyle L, Moore SB. In Transfusion Reactions: Refresher and Update. Bethesda:Am Assoc Blood Banks, 1996:III-1
232. Herman JH. In: Transfusion Reactions: Refresher and Update. Bethesda:Am Assoc Blood Banks, 1996:IV-1
233. Julius CJ. In: Transfusion Reactions: Refresher and Update. Bethesda:Am Assoc Blood Banks, 1996:VI-1
234. Yomtovian R. In: Transfusion Reactions: Refresher and Update. Bethesda:Am Assoc Blood Banks, 1996:VII-1

235. Barker LF. In: Proc Workshop on Albumin. Bethesda:Div Blood Prod FDA, 1975:22
236. Hochstein HD, Seligmann EB Jr. Proc Workshop on Albumin. Bethesda:Div Blood Prod FDA, 1975:284
237. Steere AC, Rifaat MK, Seligmann EB Jr, et al. Transfusion 1978;18:102
238. Klein HG, Ed. Standards for Blood Banks and Transfusion Services, 17th Ed. Bethesda:Am Assoc Blood Banks, 1996
239. Wenz B. Transfusion 1983;23:95
240. Kasprisin DO, Yogore MG, Salmassi C, et al. Plasma Therap 1981;2:25
241. Menitove JE, McElligott MC, Aster RH. Vox Sang 1982;42:318
242. Decary F, Ferner P, Giavedoni L, et al. Vox Sang 1984;46:277
243. Walker RH. Am J Clin Pathol 1987;88:374
244. Thulstrup H. Vox Sang 1971;21:233
245. Heddle NM, Klama LN, Griffith L, et al. Transfusion 1993;33:794
246. Dinarello CA, Cannon JG, Wolff SM. Rev Infect Dis 1988;10:168
247. Snyder EL, Stack G. In: Principles of Transfusion Medicine. Baltimore:Williams and Wilkins 1991:641
248. Sacher RA, Boyle L, Freter CE. Transfusion 1993;33:962
249. Muylle L, Joos M, Wouters E, et al. Transfusion 1993;33:195
250. Stack G, Snyder EL. Transfusion 1994;34:20
251. Muylle L, Laekeman G, Herman AG, et al. Transfusion 1988;28:226
252. Muylle L, Wouters F, De Bock R, et al. Transf Med 1992;2:289
253. Mangano MM, Chambers LA, Kruskall MS. Am J Clin Pathol 1991;95:733
254. Heddle NM, Klama L, Singer J, et al. New Eng J Med 1994;331:625
255. Stack G, Baril L, Napychank P, et al. Transfusion 1995;35:199
256. Bubel S, Wilhelm D, Entelmann M, et al. Transfusion 1996;36:445
257. Popovsky MA. Transfusion 1996;36:470
258. Snyder EL, Mechanic S, Baril L, et al. Transfusion 1996;36:707
259. de Rie MA, Plas-van Dalen van der CM, Engelfriet CP, et al. Vox Sang 1985;49:126
260. Greenwalt TJ, Gajewski M, McKenna JL. Transfusion 1962;2:221
261. Kevy SV, Schmidt PJ, McGinniss MH, et al. Transfusion 1962;2:7
262. Marchal G, Dausset J, Colombani J. Prog 8th Cong ISBT, 1960
263. Cooper MR, Heise E, Richards F, et al. In: Leukocytes: Separation, Collection and Transfusion. New York:Academic Press, 1975
264. Rawal BD, Davis RE, Busch MP, et al. Transf Med Rev 1990;4 (Suppl 1):36
265. Blajchman MA. Semin Hematol 1991;28 (Suppl):14
266. Marwijk Kooy van M, Prooijen van HC, Moes M, et al. Blood 1991;77:201
267. Lane TA, Anderson KC, Goodnough LT, et al. Ann Int Med 1992;117:151
268. Muylle L, Peetermans ME. Vox Sang 1994;66:14
269. Sniecinski I, O'Donnell MR, Nowicki B, et al. Blood 1988;71:1402
270. Saarinen UM, Kekomäki R, Siimes MA, et al. Blood 1990;75:512
271. Klein HG. Blood 1992;80:1865
272. Blajchman MA, Bardossy L, Carmen R, et al. Blood

1993;81:1880

273. Nusbacher J. Transfusion 1994;34:1002
274. Freedman JJ, Blajchman MA, McCombie N. Transf Med Rev 1994;8:1
275. Breda MA, Drinkwater DC, Laks H, et al. J Thorac Cardiovasc Surg 1989;97:654
276. Pillai R, Bando K, Schueler S, et al. Ann Thorac Surg 1990;50:211
277. Gilbert GL, Hayes K, Hudson IL, et al. Lancet 1989;1:1228
278. Bowden RA, Slichter SL, Sayers MH, et al. Blood 1991;78:246
279. Goldman M, Delage G. Transf Med Rev 1995;9:9
280. Bowden RA, Slichter SJ, Sayers M, et al. Blood 1995;86:3599
281. Sprogøe-Jakobsen U, Saetre AM, Georgsen J. Transfusion 1995;35:421
282. Hughes AS, Brozovic B. Br J Haematol 1982;50:381
283. Schiffer CA, Patten E, Reilly J, et al. Transfusion 1987;27:162
284. Snyder EL. Transfusion 1989;29:568
285. Brand A, Claas FH, Voogt PJ, et al. Vox Sang 1988;54:160
286. Beaujean F, Segier JM, le Forestier C, et al. (Letter). Vox Sang 1992;62:242
287. Heaton WA, Holme S, Smith K, et al. Br J Haematol 1994;87:363
288. Ledent E, Berlin G, Transfusion 1994;34:765
289. Sirchia G, Rebulla P, Parravicini A, et al. Transfusion 1994;34:26
290. Blajchman MA, Bardossy L, Carmen RA, et al. Blood 1992;79:1371
291. Bordin JO, Heddle NM, Blajchman MA. Blood 1994;84:1703
292. Williamson LM, Wimperis JZ, Williamson P, et al. Blood 1994;83:3028
293. Blajchman MA, Bordin JO. Curr Opin Hematol 1994 Issues:457
294. Novotny VM, van Doorn R, Witvliet MD, et al. Blood 1995;85;1736
295. Federowicz I, Barrett BB, Anderson JW, et al. Transfusion 1996;36:21
296. Ramos RR, Curtis BR, Duffy BF, et al. Transfusion 1994;34:31
297. Popovsky MA, Moore SB. Transfusion 1985;25:573
298. Ward HN, Lipscomb TS, Cawley LP. Arch Intern Med 1968;122:362
299. Ward HN. Ann Intern Med 1970;73:689
300. Wolf CFW, Canale VC. Transfusion 1976;16:135
301. Campbell DA Jr, Swartz RD, Waskerwitz JA, et al. Transplantation 1982;34:300
302. Yomtovian R, Kline W, Press C, et al. Lancet 1984;1:244
303. Latson TW, Kickler TS, Baumgartner WA. Anesthesiology 1986;64:106
304. van Buren NL, Stroncek DF, Clay ME, et al. Transfusion 1990;30:42
305. Popovsky MA, Chaplin HC Jr, Moore SB. Transfusion 1992;32:589
306. Popovsky MA. (Letter). Transfusion 1995;35:180
307. Hammerschmidt DE, Weaver LJ, Hudson LD, et al. Lancet 1980;1:947
308. Henson PM, Larsen GL, Webster RO, et al. Ann NY Acad Sci 1982;384:287
309. Nordhagen R, Conradi M, Dromtorp SM. Vox Sang 1986;51:102
310. Seeger W, Schneider U, Kreusler B, et al. Blood 1990;76:1438
311. Maunsell K. Br Med J 1944;2:236

312. Michel J, Sharon R. Br Med J 1980;1:152
313. Michel J, Sharon R. Vox Sang 1980;38:19
314. Sharon R, Kidroni G, Michel J. Vox Sang 1980;38:284
315. Ramirez MA. J Am Med Assoc 1919;73:985
316. McGinniss MH, Goldfinger D. (abstract). Prog 24th Ann Mtg AABB, 1971:80
317. Parker CW. In: Textbook of Immunopathology, 2nd Ed. New York:Grune and Stratton, 1976
318. Roitt I, Brostoff J, Male D. Immunology, 2nd Ed. London:Gower, 1989
319. Vyas GN, Perkins HA, Fudenberg HH. Lancet 1968;2:312
320. Schmidt AP, Taswell F, Gleich GJ. New Eng J Med 1969;280:188
321. Vyas GN, Levin AS, Fudenberg HH. Nature 1970;225:275
322. Miller WV, Holland PV, Sugarboker E, et al. Am J Clin Pathol 1970;54:618
323. Bjerrum OJ, Jersild C. Vox Sang 1971;21:411
324. Ropars C, Gerbal A, Poncey C, et al. Rev Fr Transf 1971;14:401
325. Leikola J, Koistinen J, Lehtinen M, et al. Blood 1973;42:111
326. Nadorp JHS, Voss M, Buys WC, et al. Eur J Clin Invest 1973;3:317
327. Branigan EF, Stevenson MM, Charles D. Obstet Gynecol 1983;61 (Suppl):47S
328. Sandler SG, Mallory D, Malamut D, et al. Transf Med Rev 1995;9:1
329. Vyas GN, Perkins HA. (Letter). Transfusion 1976;16:289
330. Frommel D, Moullec J, Lambin P, et al. Vox Sang 1973;25:513
331. Holt PD, Tandy NP, Anstee DJ. J Clin Pathol 1977;30:1007
332. Wells JV, McNally MP, King MA. Austral NZ J Med 1980;10:410
333. Ropars C, Muller A, Paint N, et al. J Immunol Meth 1982;54:183
334. Sharon R, Amar A. (Letter). J Clin Pathol 1982;35:582
335. Clark JA, Callicoat PA, Brenner NA, et al. Am J Clin Pathol 1983;80:210
336. Laschinger C, Shepherd FA, Naylor DH. Canad Med Assoc J 1984;130:141
337. Kanoh T, Mizumoto T, Yasuda N, et al. Vox Sang 1986;50:81
338. Sandler SG, Eckrich R, Malamut D, et al. Blood 1994;84:2031
339. Pineda AA, Taswell HF. Transfusion 1975;15:10
340. Burks AW, Sampson HA, Buckley RH. New Eng J Med 1986;314:560
341. Ferreira A, Rodriguez MCC, Lopez-Trascasa M, et al. Clin Immunol Immunopathol 1988;47:199
342. McCluskey DR, Boyd NAM. Lanet 1990;1:874
343. Seligmann M, Aucoutuier P, Danon F, et al. Clin Exp Immunol 1991;84:23
344. Milde LN. Anesth Analg 1989;69:684
345. Wells JV, Buckley RH, Schanfield MS, et al. Clin Immunol Immunopathol 1977;8:265
346. Yap PL, Pryde EAD, McClelland DBL. Transfusion 1982;22:36
347. Schulenburg BJ, Plapp FV, Rachel JM. Transfusion 1991;31:633
348. Eckrich RJ, Mallory DM, Sandler SG. Transfusion 1993;33:1
349. Fox SM, Stavely-Haiber LM. Immunohematology 1988;4:5
350. Hunt AF, Read MI. Lancet 1990;336:1197
351. Petty RE, Palmer NR, Cassidy TJ, et al. Clin Exp Immunol 1979;37:83
352. Hong R, Ammann AJ. In: Immunologic Disorders in Infants and Children, 3rd Ed. Philadelphia:Saunders, 1989:329
353. Liblau RS, Bach JF. Int Arch Allgy Immunol 1992;99:16

354. Oxelius VA. Clin Exp Immunol 1974;17:19
355. Oxelius VA, Laurell AB, Lindquist B, et al. New Eng J Med 1981;304:1476
356. Cunningham-Rundles C, Oxelius VA, Good RA. Birth Defects Orig Article Ser 1983;19:173
357. Björkander J, Bake B, Oxelius VA, et al. New Eng J Med 1985;313:720
358. Plebani A, Monafo V, Avanzini MA, et al. Monogr Allgy 1986;20:171
359. Preud'homme JL, Hanson LA. Immunodef Rev 1990;2:129
360. Hanson LA, Söderström R, Nilssen DE, et al. Clin Immunol Immunopathol 1991;61:S70
361. Sandler SG, Trimble JT, Mallory DM. Transfusion 1996;36:256
362. Vyas GN, Holmdahl L, Perkins HA, et al. Blood 1969;34:573
363. Vyas GN, Perkins HA, Yang YM, et al. J Lab Clin Med 1975;85:838
364. Strauss RA, Gloster ES, Schanfield MS, et al. Clin Lab Haematol 1983;5:371
365. Ropars C, Caldera LH, Griscelli C, et al. Vox Sang 1974;27:294
366. Koistinen J, Leikola J. Vox Sang 1977;32:77
367. Homburger HA, Smith JR, Jacob JL, et al. Transfusion 1981;21:38
368. Vyas GN. In: Transfusion Problems. Washington, D.C.:Am Assoc Blood Banks, 1970
369. Hitoshi T, Tamura T, Sawamura M, et al. Br J Haematol 1993;83:673
370. Lambin P, Le Pennec PY, Hauptmann GY, et al.. Vox Sang 1984;47:242
371. Gold M, Swartz JS, Braude BM, et al. J Allgy Clin Immunol 1991;87:662
372. Sampson HA, Mendelson L, Rosen JP. New Eng J Med 1992;327:380
373. Dattwyler R, Kaplan AP, Austen KF. In: Allergy. New York:Churchill Livingstone, 1985:559
374. Levy JH. Anaphylactic Reactions in Anesthesia and Intensive Care, 2nd Ed. Boston:Butterworth Heinemann, 1992
375. Baldo BA, Fisher MM. Mol Immunol 1983;20:1393
376. Shopnick RI, Kazemi M, Brettler DB, et al. Transfusion 1996;36:358
377. Perkins HA, Payne R, Ferguson J, et al. Vox Sang 1966;11:578
378. Goldfinger D. In: Clinical and Serological Aspects of Transfusion Reactions. Washington, D.C.:Am Assoc Blood Banks, 1982:37
379. Goldfinger D. (Letter). Transfusion 1982;22:82
380. Goldfinger D. (Letter). Transfusion 1982;22:400
381. Goldfinger D, Solis RT, Meryman HT. Transfusion 1974;14:151
382. Goldfinger D, Lowe C. Transfusion 1981;21:227
383. Goldfinger D, Lowe C. In: Safety in Transfusion Practices. Skokie, IL:Coll Am Pathol, 1982
384. Westphal R. (Letter). Transfusion 1982;22:82
385. Lieden G, Hilden J-O. Vox Sang 1982;43:263
386. Chaplin H Jr. Blood 1982;59:1118
387. Goldman H. (Letter). Transfusion 1983;23:400
388. Frankel KA. (Letter). Transfusion 1982;22:82
389. Smith DM. In: Clinical and Serological Aspects of Transfusion Reactions. Washington, D.C.:Am Assoc Blood Banks, 1982:121
390. Wilhelm RE, Nutting HM, Devlin HB, et al. J Am Med Assoc 1955;158:529
391. Hobsley M. Lancet 1958;1:497
392. Dare JG, Mogey GA. J Pharm Pharmacol 1954;6:325
393. Jandl JH, Tomlinson AS. J Clin Invest 1958;37:1202
394. Leverenz S, Ihle R, Frick G. Dtsch Ges-Wesen 1975;30:1688
395. Altschule MD, Friedburg AS. Medicine 1945;24:403
396. Grant RT, Reeve EB. Special Report Series. London:Med Res Council, 1951:No 277
397. Mollison PL. Br Med J 1943;1:4
398. Borden CW, Hall WH. New Eng J Med 1951;245:760
399. Braude AI, Sanford JP, Bartlett JE, et al. J Lab Clin Med 1952;39:902
400. Pittman M. J Lab Clin Med 1953;42:273
401. Braude AI, Carey FJ, Siemienski J. J Clin Invest 1955;34;311
402. James JD, Stokes EJ. Br Med J 1957;2:1389
403. Braude AI. New Eng J Med 1958;258:1289
404. Thuillier M, Gandrille MC. Rev Fr Transf 1969;12:477
405. Sack RA. Am J Obstet Gynecol 1970;107:394
406. Pepersack F, Prigogyne T, Butzler JP, et al. (Letter). Lancet 1979;2:911
407. Stenhouse MAE, Milner LV. Transfusion 1982;22:396
408. Schmitt JL, Bataille P, Coevoert B, et al. Med Malad Infec 1982;13:197
409. Khabbaz RF, Arnow PM, Highsmith AK, et al. Am J Med 1984;76:62
410. Bjune G, Ruud TE, Eng J. Scand J Infect Dis 1984;16:411
411. Tabor E, Gerety RJ. (Letter). Lancet 1984;1:1403
412. Phillips P, Grayson L, Stockman K, et al. (Letter). Lancet 1984;2:879
413. Wright DC, Selss IF, Vinton KJ, et al. Arch Pathol Lab Med 1985;109:1040
414. Galloway SJ, Jones PD. (Letter). Austral NZ J Med 1986;16:248
415. Murray AE, Bartzokas CA, Shepherd AJN, et al. J Hosp Infect 1987;9:243
416. Scott J, Boulton FE, Govan JRW, et al. Vox Sang 1988;54:201
417. Bettigole R, Amsterdam D, Levin J. (abstract). Blood 1989;74 (Suppl 1):383a
418. Mollaret HH. Med Malad Infec 1989;4:186
419. Holland PV. In: Clinical Practice of Transfusion Medicine, 2nd Ed. New York:Churchill Livingstone, 1989:713
420. Tipple MA, Bland LA, Murphy MJ, et al. Transfusion 1990;30:207
421. Brecher ME, Taswell HF. In: Principles of Transfusion Medicine. Baltimore:Williams and Wilkins, 1991:619
422. Goldman M, Blajchman MA. Transf Med Rev 1991;5:73
423. Spooner ETC. Unpublished observations 1942 cited in Mollison PL. Blood Transfusion in Clinical Medicine, 7th Ed. Oxford:Blackwell, 1983:767
424. Habibi B, Kleinknecht D, Vachon F, et al. Rev Fr Transf 1973;16:41
425. Alexander JW. Unpublished observations 1978 cited in Issitt PD. Applied Blood Group Serology, 3rd Ed. Miami:Montgomery, 1985:505
426. Buchholz DH, Young VM, Friedman NR, et al. New Eng J Med 1971;285:429
427. Buchholz DH, Young VM, Friedman NR, et al. Transfusion 1973;13:268
428. Rhame FS, Root RK, MacLowry JD, et al. Ann Intern Med 1973;78:633
429. Blajchman MA, Thornley JH, Richardson H, et al. Transfusion 1979;19:39
430. Van Lierde S, Fleisher GR, Plotkin SA, et al. Pediat Infect Dis 1985;4:293
431. Anderson KC, Lew MA, Gorgone BC, et al. Am J Med 1986;81:405
432. Braine HG, Kickler TS, Charache P, et al. Transfusion 1986;26:391

433. Arnow PM, Weiss LM, Weil D, et al. Arch Int Med 1986;146:321
434. Heal JM, Jines ME, Forey J, et al. Transfusion 1987;27:2
435. Douglas D, Sorace JM, Kickler T. (abstract). Transfusion 1987;27:512
436. Rhame FS, McCullough JJ, Cameron S, et al. (abstract). Transfusion 1979;19:653
437. Casewell MW, Slater NGP, Cooper JE. J Hosp Infec 1981;2:237
438. Farmer JJ, Davis BR, Hickman FW. Lancet 1976;2:455
439. Steere AC, Terrey JH, Mackel DC, et al. J Infect Dis 1977;135:729
440. Ali AM, Elder D, Richardson H, et al. (abstract). Blood 1987;70 (Suppl 1):325a
441. Kim DM, Brecher ME, Bland LA, et al. Transfusion 1992;32:221
442. Wood L, Jacobs P. J Clin Apheresis 1985;2:250
443. Colburn WJ, Barnes A. Transfusion 1982;22:163
444. Simon SD, Kuriyan MA, Kim HC. Transfusion 1982;22:341
445. Ludbrook J, Wynn V. Br Med J 1958;2:523
446. Jennings ER, Beland AJ, Cope JA, et al. Surg Gynecol Obstet 1965;120:997
447. Howland WS, Jacobs RG, Goulet AH. Anesth Analg 1960;39:559
448. Spear PW, Sass M, Cincott JJ. J Lab Clin Med 1956;48:702
449. Scanlon JW, Krakaur R. J Pediat 1980;96:108
450. Shortland D, Trounce JQ, Levene MI. Arch Dis Child 1987;62:1139
451. Brown KA, Bissonnette B, MacDonald M, et al. Canad J Anesth 1990;37:401
452. Brown KA, Bissonnette B, McIntyre B. Canad J Anesth 1990;37:747
453. Hall TL, Barnes A, Miller JR, et al. Transfusion 1993;33:606
454. Galligan BR, Cairns R, Schifano JV, et al. Transfusion 1989;29:179
455. Moore GL. Ledford ME. Transfusion 1985;25:583
456. Ramirez AM, Woodfield DG, Scott R, et al. (Letter). Transfusion 1987;27:444
457. Rivet C, Baxter A, Rock G. (Letter). Transfusion 1989;29:185
458. Leitman SF, McCoy N, Sullivan J, et al. (abstract). Book of Abstracts. Joint Cong ISBT/AABB 1990:195
459. Anderson G, Mintz PD. (Letter). Transfusion 1991;31:476
460. Rock G, Shear JM. (Letter). Transfusion 1989;29:749
461. Rock GA. (Letter). Transfusion 1990;30:764
462. Questions and Answers. AABB News Briefs 1990;13:6
463. Ferguson DJ. (Letter). Transfusion 1989;29:749
464. Avoy DR. (Letter). Transfusion 1990;30:764
465. Benzinger J, Singaraju C, Friedman KD. (abstract). Book of Abstracts. Joint Cong ISBT/AABB 1990:117
466. Strauss RG. Transfusion 1990;30:675
467. Friedman KD, McDonough WC, Cimino DF. (abstract). Transfusion 1991;31 (Suppl 8S)50S
468. Davey RJ, McCoy NC, Yu M, et al. Transfusion 1992;32:525
469. Mollison PL, Engelfriet CP, Contreras M. Blood Transfusion in Clinical Medicine, 8th Ed. Oxford:Blackwell, 1987
470. Staples PJ, Griner PF. New Eng J Med 1971;285:317
471. McCullough J, Polesky HF, Nelson C, et al. Anesth Analg 1972;51:102
472. Coroneos NJ. (Letter). Anaesth Inten Care 1978;6:87
473. Linko K, Hynynen K. Acta Anaesth Scand 1979;23:320
474. Linko K, Hekali R. Acta Anaesth Scand 1980;24:46
475. Vaughan RL. Am J Dis Childh 1982;136:646
476. Inoue K, Reichelt W, Kleesiek K. Anesthesiologist 1987;36:180
477. Opitz JC, Baldauf MC, Kessler DL, et al. J Pediat 1988;112:111
478. Iserson KV, Huestis DW. Transfusion 1991;31:558
479. Bechdolt S, Schroeder LK, Samia C, et al. Arch Pathol Lab Med 1986;110:344
480. Cregan P, Donegan E, Gotelli G. Transfusion 1991;31:172
481. Silver H, Umlas J, Kenney P, et al. Transfusion 1982;22:254
482. Silver H, Umlas J, Anderson J. (Letter). Transfusion 1991;31:676
483. Cregan P. (Letter). Transfusion 1991;31:676
484. Lanore JJ, Quarre MC, Audibert JD, et al. Vox Sang 1989;56:293
485. Noble TC, Abbott J. Br Med J 1959;2:865
486. Jones JH, Kilpatrick GS, Franks EH. J Clin Pathol 1962;15:161
487. De Cesare WR, Bove JR, Ebaugh EG Jr. Transfusion 1964;4:237
488. Ryden SE, Oberman HA. Transfusion 1975;15:250
489. Macdonald WB, Berg RB. Pediatrics 1959;23:8
490. Howard JE, Perkins HA. J Am Med Assoc 1976;236:289
491. Bowman JM, Pollack JM. Lancet 1980;2:1190
492. Castellino S, Combs MR, Kinney TR, et al. (abstract). Blood 1997;90 (Suppl 1):128b
493. Easton DJ. (Letter). Transfusion 1985;25:85
494. Davey RJ, Lee BJ, Coles SM. Lab Med 1986;17:282
495. Whitelaw JP. (Letter). Transfusion 1990;30:78
496. Danielson C, Parker C, Watson M, et al. J Clin Apheresis 1991;6:161
497. Dhaene M, Gulbis B, Lieter N, et al. Clin Nephrol 1989;31:327
498. Martin R, McKenty S, Thisdale Y, et al. Cardiothor Anesth 1989;3:737
499. Hombrouckx RO, De Vos JY, Larno LA, et al. ASAIO Transact 1990;36:M335
500. El-Reshaid K, Kapoor M, Shuhaiber H. Nephron 1992;62:90
501. Schmidt WP III, Kim HC, Tomassini N, et al. J Am Med Assoc 1982;248:1629
502. Denison M, Paul U, Bell R, et al. Austral Phy Eng Sci Med 1991;14:39
503. Burch KJ, Phelps SJ, Constance TD. Am J Hosp Pharm 1991;48:92
504. Brecher ME, Boothe G, Kerr A. Transfusion 1993;33:450
505. Brecher ME, Hogan JJ, Boothe G, et al. Transfusion 1994;34:750

37 | "Warm" Antibody-Induced Hemolytic Anemia (WAIHA)

As discussed in Chapter 2, the immune system in man is normally regulated in such a way that foreign antigens are recognized as being different from host or self antigens. Thus antibodies against foreign antigens are produced as part of the normal immune response. The term alloantibody is used to describe an antibody directed against an antigen not present on the antibody-maker's cells. At the same time, the immune system is apparently programmed (1) in such a way that host or self antigens are recognized as being non-threatening so that antibodies against them are not made. Occasionally and for reasons that are discussed below but that are not yet understood in complete detail, the immune system malfunctions and an autoantibody is produced. An autoantibody may be defined as one directed against an antigen that is present on the antibody-maker's cells, though not necessarily the red cells. A whole range of clinical situations involving autoantibodies is seen in man. At worst, the autoantibodies destroy the red cells or tissue cells that carry the target antigen or antigens against which they are directed and cause disease, or death of the antibody-maker. At the opposite end of the scale, the autoantibody made may be benign in vivo so that no adverse consequences result from its production. Indeed, it seems that a few benign autoantibodies (such as cold-reactive anti-I in the sera of all individuals with I+ red cells (2), see Chapter 10) may be products of a normally functioning immune system.

Autoantibodies, An Overview

To the blood banker, the terms autoantibody and hemolytic anemia are closely correlated. In fact, hemolytic anemia is but one manifestation of autoimmune disease. Once the immune system malfunctions and a pathological autoantibody is made, the nature of the disease that results will be dictated by the specificity of the autoantibody formed and the site of the cells that carry the antigen against which it is directed. Table 37-1 lists a few diseases in which it is established that autoantibodies are causative in many cases. There are literally dozens of others that are currently believed to have an autoimmune basis but in which, for some of the reasons discussed below, the role of the autoantibody cannot always be firmly established. These include diseases of the kidney, liver, heart and lungs to mention but a few.

In many instances it is difficult to study the immune mechanism thought to be responsible for the autoimmune disorder. First, it may not be possible to identify the antigen carried on the tissue cells. Second, circulating antibody against the antigen may not be obtained in adequate amounts for detailed study. Because of these factors, autoimmune hemolytic anemia is probably the best understood of all autoimmune disorders. The cells carrying the antigens are red cells so are easy to obtain in large quantities. Similarly, the autoantibodies can be collected and studied. Often they are present in the sera of affected patients, alternatively, they can be recovered by elution from the patients' red cells. In this latter instance there can be no doubt about the autoimmune nature of the antibodies since they bound to the patients' red cells in vivo.

The Malfunction of the Immune System

Although not universally accepted, a widely held view is that production of autoantibodies represents loss of T cell regulation of B cells. It is supposed (1) that those B cells that would develop into clones of immunocytes producing autoantibodies, are normally restrained from proliferating by the actions of T suppressor cells. Apparently, in autoimmune disease, the T cell surveillance is impaired or lost so that forbidden clones of immunocytes proliferate and autoantibodies are made. In "warm" antibody-induced hemolytic anemia (see below) it seems that often several clones of immunocytes are involved because the autoantibodies are frequently polyclonal in nature (but see also below). In cold hemagglutinin disease (see Chapter 38) it seems that one clone of immunocytes is involved since in the idiopathic form of the disease, the causative autoantibody is usually monoclonal in nature.

There are numerous reports (for original reports and reviews, see 1, 3-19) that provide evidence to support the concept that the production of autoantibodies occurs when T cell surveillance of B cells is impaired or lost. In some instances (20-25) the number of T cells is reduced, in others T cell function is abnormal (4,26-31). However, the situation is by no means straightforward. For example, there may be a reduction in number of T cells in autoantibody-induced multiple sclerosis. However, the oligodendrocytes damaged by the autoantibody in that disease and T cells have certain epitopes in common. Thus it is not entirely clear whether the reduction in T cell number allows autoantibody to be made or whether the autoantibody is made first, against structures on the oligodendrocytes, and then causes a reduction in T cell

TABLE 37-1 Some Examples of Autoimmune Diseases in Man

Disease	Site of the antigens against which the autoantibodies are directed
Antibody-induced hemolytic anemia	Red blood cells
Rheumatoid arthritis	Immunoglobulin (IgG)
Pernicious anemia	Intrinsic factor responsible for B_{12} adsorption or cells of the gastric mucosa
Type 1 diabetes mellitus	Pancreatic islet beta cells
Multiple sclerosis	Central nervous system myelin cells
Ulcerative colitis	Cells of the colon
Hashimoto's Disease	
Primary myxedema	Various cells of the thyroid
Thyrotoxicosis	
Idiopathic thrombocytopenic purpura	Platelets
Goodpasture's syndrome	Glomerular basement membrane cells
Systemic lupus erythematosus	Nucleii of many cells (DNA)
Sjörgen's syndrome	Cells of the salivary ducts
Idiopathic adrenal atrophy	Adrenal cells
Myasthenia gravis	Muscle cells

numbers (5). In a review of self-tolerance and autoimmune disease, Schlomchick (19) points out that immunoregulatory failure can occur at a number of different steps in the development of B cells. First, T cell tolerance may be lost, second clonal deletion may occur, third anergy may block clonal expansion and fourth (and more speculative) clonal disability may block memory cell formation and/or antibody secretion by B cells. It is conceivable that T-helper or T-suppressor cell activities contribute at the first three of those steps.

Although autoimmune diseases are not restricted to the elderly, their frequency is considerably higher in the old than in the young. There is evidence (1,5,12,15-18,32-37) that with increasing age, the immune system becomes more prone to malfunction so that production of autoantibodies becomes more likely. However, again the situation is neither simple nor straightforward. There is also evidence that a genetic predisposition to lose the ability to continue to recognize host or self antigens exists (see below) so that autoimmune diseases are more likely in

some persons than in others. Further, external triggering factors, e.g. viral infections (particularly in children, see below), toxins, heavy metals and even blood transfusion, may play a role in the initiation of autoantibody production (1,5,12,15-18,38-54). Thus it seems that autoimmune diseases almost always have a multifactorial background. In oversimplified terms, in individuals genetically predisposed, external factors may prompt autoantibody production with failure of the immune system involving, at least, loss of T cell regulation of B cells.

A complicating factor in autoimmunity is that the loss of T cell regulation of B cells does not always seem to be a generalized phenomenon. As discussed in detail below, certain specificities (often in the Rh system) are regularly seen as autoantibodies in patients with "warm" antibody-induced hemolytic anemia. Others, such as those in the ABO system, are exceedingly rare. Dahr (55) has pointed out that if autoimmunity resulted from a generalized loss of T cell regulation of B cells, one might expect to see all blood group antibodies causing hemolytic anemia in roughly the same proportions as they occur as alloanti-bodies. As discussed later in this chapter, that is certain-ly not the case. There are other data that also suggest that if loss of T cell regulation of B cells results in the production of autoantibodies, only certain clones partic-ipate in the autoreactive response. Litwin et al. (56) studied six patients with warm-reactive autoantibodies and hemolytic anemia, all of whom had the Gm allotype Glm(a+f+). In three of the patients, the autoantibody eluted from the red cells contained only Glm(a), in the other three that antigen predominated. Similar findings with a high incidence of Glm(a) in warm-reactive autoantibodies were reported by Le Petit et al. (57). Leddy and Bakemeier (58) and Hsu et al. (59) have reported that many but not all warm-reactive autoanti-bodies contain only one type of light chain. Although some warm-reactive autoantibodies may be monoclonal in nature, it seems that many others are not. As described in a later section of this chapter, some patients who make warm-reactive autoantibodies have red cells coated (in vivo) with IgG and IgA and/or IgM. Further, when only IgG is found on the red cells, more than one subclass is usually present. These observations may mean that warm-reactive autoantibodies are more often polyclonal than monoclonal in nature but that there are restrictions as to which gene products are utilized in the synthesis of their heavy and light chain variable regions (see Chapter 2) (i.e. an oligoclonal response).

As mentioned above, the view that autoimmunity represents only loss of T cell regulation of B cells is not universally held. Some investigators believe that subtle alterations in antigen structure initiate the disorders. It is supposed that once a change in antigen structure has occurred (the mechanism leading to such a change is not known but may involve external factors) the antigen(s) is(are) no longer recognized as host or self and antibod-ies against them can be made. As far as antibody-induced hemolytic anemia is concerned, it can be said that if such antigen changes do occur they are too subtle to be recognized in serological tests. When the causative autoantibodies are studied in vitro, they react as well with normal red cells as with the cells of the patients. Although the above concept seems to represent a minor-ity view, there is evidence (60-66) from animal studies, that the affinity maturation and isotype switch in autoan-tibody production is antigen driven. This evidence is discussed in more detail below in the section describing autoantibodies that mimic a specificity that they do not actually possess. Further, in a most attractive model to explain autoimmunity (5), it is supposed that persons with an autoimmune disorder have inherited at least one abnormal immune response gene and at least one abnor-mal gene encoding a structural (antigen) product. This concept is discussed in the next section.

Genetics of Autoimmunity

None of the autoimmune disorders is inherited in a direct fashion. Although there are reports (67-77) of anti-body-induced hemolytic anemia in sibs or in the child of an affected person, such cases are exceptions and are not the general rule. However, as mentioned above, there is a tendency towards a familial incidence of autoimmune disorders (5,15,18,78-92). Different members of a single kindred may present with different diseases, some of which clearly have an autoimmune basis and others of which may well be autoimmune nature. Figure 37-1 shows such a kindred studied by one of us (PDI) (93). The proband's maternal grandmother and mother pre-sented with severe debilitating rheumatoid arthritis. The proband has pernicious anemia caused by an autoanti-body directed against the intrinsic factor responsible for B_{12} adsorption. The proband's cousin has insulin-depen-dent diabetes mellitus as does one of his daughters. The cousin's other daughter has chronic lymphocytic leukemia. As can be seen, while the inheritance pattern is not straightforward and while the diseases differ in nature, there is a definite propensity towards loss of recognition of host or self antigens, in the family. Also typical of the inheritance of this propensity, one branch of the family has no affected members while, in another branch, one generation is skipped. Clearly inheritance of an autoimmune disorder is multigenic. Shoenfeld and Schwartz (5) reviewed many data similar to those derived from the family shown in figure 37-1. A simpli-fied version of their model would suggest that persons who manifest an autoimmune disorder have defective genes at (at least) two genetically-independent loci. One of them can be thought of as an abnormal immune response (*IR*) gene, the presence of which allows the autoantibody to be made. The second can be thought of as a gene whose presence results in production of an abnormal structure on a particular cell line, for ease of communication that gene will here be described as the target antigen (*TA*) gene. The model is depicted in figure 37-2. I-2 in the family shown has autoantibody-mediated rheumatoid arthritis because he has an abnormal *IR* and an abnormal *TA* gene. His wife is homozygous for nor-mal genes at her *IR* and all *TA* loci. As a result neither II-1 who has an abnormal *TA* gene (from the father) but a normal *IR* gene from the mother, nor II-2 who has an abnormal *IR* gene (from the father) but a normal *TA* gene (from the mother) has an autoimmune disorder (each has one, neither has two, abnormal genes). II-3, the husband of II-2, is also disease free. Although he has an abnormal *TA* gene, his *IR* genes are normal so he has no autoim-mune disorder. III-1 on the other hand inherits an abnor-mal *IR* from her mother and the abnormal *TA* gene of her father and presents with juvenile onset type 1 diabetes

FIGURE 37-1 A Kindred in Which Different Autoimmune Disorders are Present

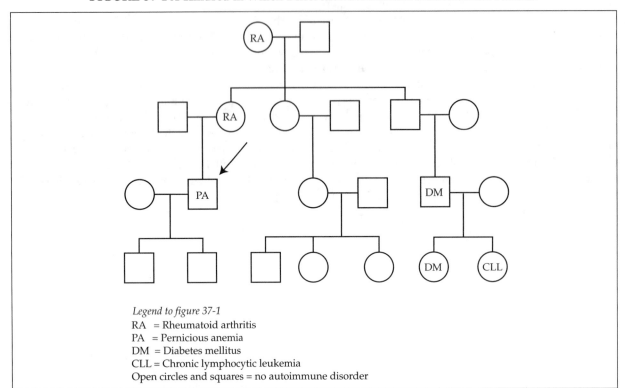

Legend to figure 37-1
RA = Rheumatoid arthritis
PA = Pernicious anemia
DM = Diabetes mellitus
CLL = Chronic lymphocytic leukemia
Open circles and squares = no autoimmune disorder

mellitus. III-2 inherits a normal *TA* gene from her mother and a normal *IR* gene from her father and is thus not only disease free, but will not have children with an autoimmune disease. The model fits two very common findings associated with familial autoimmune disease. First, a disorder occurs in generation I, skips generation II, and reappears in generation III. Second, the autoimmune disorder seen in I-2 is different from that seen in III-1. In I-2 the abnormal *TA* gene involved production of the target antigen of rheumatoid arthritis. In III-1, although the same abnormal *IR* gene is involved, a new abnormal *TA* gene has been introduced into the kindred by the unrelated II-3 husband of II-2. The new abnormal *TA* gene is one involved in production of the target antigen of diabetes mellitus. Clearly the kindred shown in figure 37-2 is a gross over simplification of a more complicated multigenic, environmentally susceptible condition. However, the model shown is useful in understanding the familial incidence of different autoimmune diseases and potential carrier states, in susceptible families. To the described model, three additional considerations must be added. First, since autoimmunity is seen more frequently in the elderly than in the young, it is possible that various forms of abnormal *IR* genes exist and that some fail early in life and others only as the individual ages. Alternatively, failure to continue to recognize host or self antigens later in life may indicate that the immune

system can fail (in terms of continuation of recognition of self) even if no abnormal *IR* gene has been inherited. Second, in view of the fact that a number of persons develop several different autoimmune disorders either concurrently or sequentially, failure of the immune system may lead to autoimmune disease in the absence of inheritance of abnormal *TA* genes. Third, it is possible that external factors (see above) can cause an autoimmune disorder to develop in the absence of abnormal *IR* and *TA* genes. With the points above borne in mind, it should come as no surprise that antibody-induced hemolytic anemia, that is one manifestation of an autoimmune disorder, is often seen as a secondary complication in individuals suffering from other forms of autoimmune disease. In other words, in genetically susceptible individuals, in whom the continued ability to recognize host or self antigens has become impaired or is lost, a number of different specificity autoantibodies may be made and different diseases (manifestations of the autoimmune state) may be seen simultaneously.

Hemolytic Anemia, Two Major Types

Since this chapter will present an in depth discussion of "warm" autoimmune or "warm" antibody-induced hemolytic anemia (WAIHA) it must be stressed that not

FIGURE 37-2 An Immune Response-Target Antigen Model for Autoimmunity

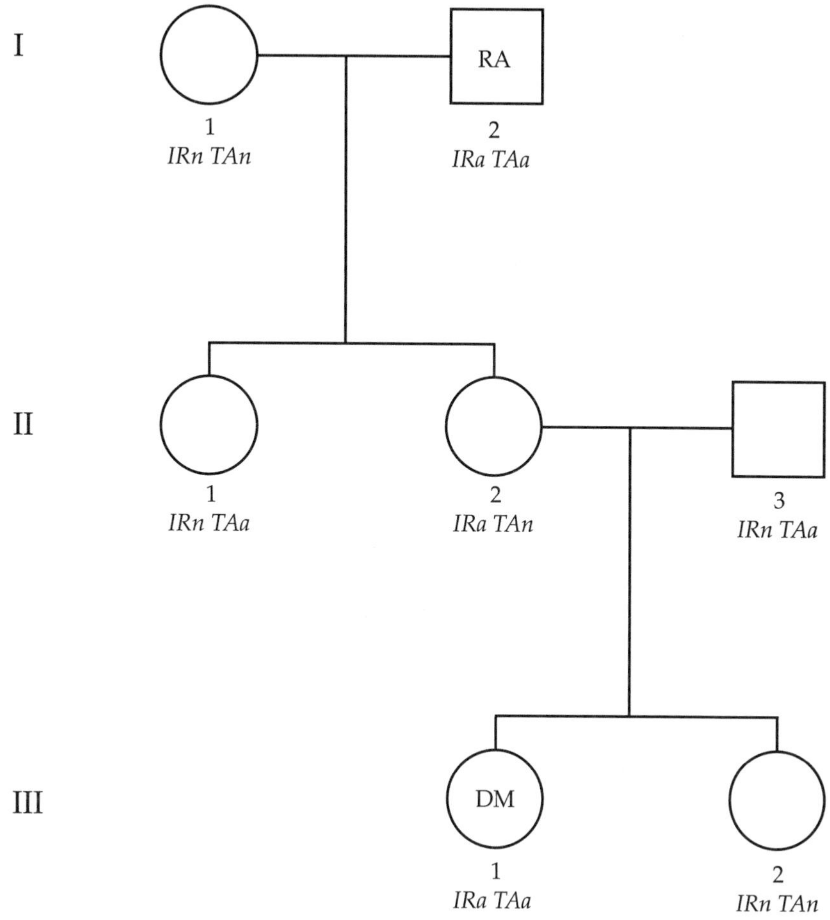

Legend to figure 37-2
IRn = Normal immune response gene
IRa = Abnormal immune response gene
TAn = Normal target antigen gene
TAa = Abnormal target antigen gene
RA = Rheumatoid arthritis
DM = Diabetes mellitus
Open circles and squares = no autoimmune disease

all cases of hemolytic anemia have this etiology. It is convenient to consider the hemolytic anemias as comprising two major types. In the autoimmune forms of the disorder, WAIHA (this chapter) and CHD and PCH (Chapter 38), the patient's red cells are normal in structure and function. However, because the patient makes an autoantibody that can combine with those red cells in vivo, the cells are prematurely cleared from the circulation (either intravascular or extravascular destruction (see Chapter 6) may be involved, see below). Once the rate of in vivo red cell destruction overtakes the rate at which the marrow can compensate by making new red cells, anemia develops. Because the cause of the anemia

is premature red cell destruction in vivo, the disease is called hemolytic anemia. Because the premature red cell destruction is caused by an autoantibody, the disease is called autoimmune hemolytic anemia (AIHA). In order to differentiate the disease from the type of anemia caused by a directly inherited abnormality, it is also often called acquired hemolytic anemia or acquired immune hemolytic anemia.

In the congenital forms of hemolytic anemia, the premature in vivo destruction of the red cells is not antibody-mediated. Instead, these disorders occur when the patients' red cells are abnormal. The abnormality may involve an essential red cell enzyme, hemoglobin structure, or an essential membrane or skeletal component. In such diseases, the abnormality results in the red cells failing to survive for a normal length of time in vivo. Again, as the rate at which red cell hemolysis occurs in vivo, overtakes the rate at which new (but defective) red cells can be produced by the marrow, anemia develops. Again, because the cause of the anemia is red cell destruction in vivo, the diseases are called hemolytic anemia. As the name implies, the congenital hemolytic anemias are inherited in a direct and recognizable manner. For example, patients with sickle cell disease have inherited a hemoglobin *S* gene from each parent. Hereditary spherocytosis (HS), a designation that has been applied to a heterogeneous group of disorders, represents malformation of the cytoskeleton of red cells. Most often this disease is caused by inheritance of a dominant gene (94) that is carried on chromosome 8 (95-97). As most blood bankers will know, the hemolytic anemias associated with the Rh_{null}, Rh_{mod} and McLeod phenotypes (99-106) represent the presence of red cells that do not survive normally in vivo. No autoantibody is involved in the destruction of those cells in the circulation. Accordingly, in this book, such disorders have been called (Chapters 4, 12 and 18) red cell deficiency or red cell abnormality hemolytic anemias. In fact, they are congenital hemolytic anemias since the Rh_{null}, Rh_{mod} and McLeod phenotypes are all inherited. However, those diseases, like some cases of hereditary spherocytosis, do not always manifest themselves at the clinical level until the individual involved reaches adult life. Because this book is about blood groups and the antibodies that define them, the rest of this chapter will deal with "warm" antibody-induced or autoimmune hemolytic anemia; the congenital forms of the disease will not be further described.

Autoimmune Hemolytic Anemias, Primary and Secondary

The disease now known to be antibody-induced hemolytic anemia was first recognized a very long time ago. In fact, the clinical syndrome was described long before the functions of the immune system and the existence of autoimmune disorders were recognized. If the literature of some sixty years ago is examined, it is found that some 70% of cases of WAIHA were described as primary or idiopathic. That is, the hemolytic anemia represented the patient's only clinical disorder. The other 30% of cases were regarded as secondary, that is the patient had another disease, the course of which was complicated by hemolytic anemia. If the current literature is examined, it will be found that the figures have been reversed so that some 70% of cases of hemolytic anemia are now

regarded as secondary and only some 30% as primary. Hemolytic anemia has not, of course, changed during those 60 years. What has changed are the methods used to diagnose disease. In other words, it is now possible to establish diagnoses of many diseases much earlier and much more accurately than was the case 60 years ago. As a result, another disorder can often now be recognized before a patient develops hemolytic anemia so that when the hemolytic anemia is seen, it appears to be secondary to the other disease. In fact, as stated in the sections above, WAIHA is but one manifestation of the autoimmune process so that it is not surprising that the disease is seen in many persons who have other autoimmune disorders. Use of the designations primary and secondary hemolytic anemia now, is largely a matter of convenience to describe the major complications of the patient's clinical state. There are many clinical conditions in which treatment of the underlying disease alleviates the hemolytic process.

Compensated Hemolytic Disorders

Not all patients who form autoantibodies capable of causing accelerated in vivo red cell destruction present with anemia. As mentioned above, anemia does not develop until the rate of in vivo red cell destruction exceeds the rate at which the marrow can compensate by increased production of red cells. Accordingly, particularly in the early stages of the disease, patients are encountered in whom the direct antiglobulin test is positive and in whom autoantibodies can be demonstrated, but in whom the hemoglobin level and hematocrit are normal. Some of these patients may present with other signs of the hemolytic process, e.g., splenomegaly, increased bilirubin levels, etc. If left untreated, many patients who have formed warm-reactive IgG autoantibodies, will proceed to an anemic state. A reliable way of documenting that an increased rate of in vivo red cell destruction is occurring in these patients is the reticulocyte count. Obviously, when the marrow is producing new red cells at a greatly increased rate so that the in vivo red cell destruction is fully compensated, the reticulocyte count will be high. Strictly speaking, this clinical condition is not hemolytic anemia since anemia is not yet present. However, the situation certainly represents a hemolytic disorder.

Antibody-Induced Hemolytic Anemia, Division by Type

In an earlier section of this chapter, the division of hemolytic anemia into two types, one caused by an autoantibody that is extrinsic to red cells and the other by an intrinsic red cell defect, was described. In a somewhat similar fashion, the autoantibody-mediated type of hemolytic anemia can be subdivided based on the nature of the causative autoantibody and its behavior in vitro. The most common form of the disease is called "warm" antibody-induced hemolytic anemia or WAIHA; the second type, cold hemagglutinin disease or CHD (also known as cold agglutinin disease or CAD); and the third form, paroxysmal cold hemoglobinuria or PCH. As the names imply, WAIHA is caused by an autoantibody optimally reactive at 37°C, while CHD and PCH are caused by autoantibodies optimally reactive at 0 to 4°C in vitro. Obviously, since the autoantibodies causative of CHD and PCH are able to cause in vivo destruction of the patient's red cells, they are active over a fairly wide thermal range that approaches and occasionally reaches 37°C. The autoantibody causative of WAIHA is most often but not quite always IgG in nature while the one causative of CHD is most often, but again not quite always IgM. By definition and based on the mechanism of in vivo red cell destruction, the autoantibody causative of PCH is an IgG biphasic hemolysin. These and other differences between the autoantibodies that cause WAIHA, CHD and PCH are listed in table 37-2. At first it may sound as if the different names used to describe antibody-induced hemolytic anemia are somewhat arbitrary and are applied because of the behavior of the causative autoantibodies in vitro. In fact, the three forms of the disease have some marked clinical differences as illustrated in table 37-3. Thus one of the more useful things that the immunohematologist can do, when a patient is suspected of having hemolytic anemia, is to perform appropriate tests (apparent from table 37-2) to distinguish between the autoantibodies that cause WAIHA,

CHD and PCH. These tests will usually indicate which of the three forms of the disease is present, will reveal what form of therapy is most likely to be effective and will give the clinician some idea of the patient's long term prognosis. As shown in table 37-3, WAIHA usually requires aggressive treatment. When corticosteroid therapy (see below) is effective when used on an intermittent basis, the prognosis is reasonably good and the patient can expect many years of good quality life. CHD is often a very mild disorder and then requires only conservative treatment (see Chapter 38) such as avoidance of exposure to cold to prevent hemolytic episodes. Idiopathic PCH is an extremely rare condition which is fortunate since there is no specific treatment. Most cases of PCH that are seen are secondary and transient (again see Chapter 38) so that the patient need only be managed through the acute episode, then total remission can be expected.

Incidence

AIHA is uncommon but not rare. New cases of WAIHA are seen with frequency of about one in 50,000 to one in 80,000 of a given population per year (107,108). Since studies on large numbers of patients (47,107,109-113) have shown that WAIHA comprises some 70 to 80% of all cases of AIHA, it can be calculated that the total incidence of the disorder is approximately one case in 60,000 of the population per year. Of the 20 to 30% of cases that are not WAIHA, almost all are CHD. The total incidence of PCH is probably less than 1% of all cases of AIHA. The above figures do not include cases of hemolytic anemia caused by drug-therapy. If such cases are included, they comprise some 10 to 15% of all cases seen (47). More than 70% of new

TABLE 37-2 Characteristics of Autoantibodies Causative of Three Types of Antibody-Induced Hemolytic Anemia

	WAIHA	CHD	PCH
Optimal in vitro reaction temperature	37°C	0-4°C	0-4°C Antibody-binding 37°C Hemolysis
Usual immunoglobulin type	IgG	IgM	IgG
Usual in vitro serological presentation	Incomplete (i.e., IAT reactive)	Agglutinin, sometimes a hemolysin	Biphasic hemolysin
Hemolysis of enzyme-treated red cells	Sometimes	Almost always	Almost always
Red cell antigens most often defined	Rh system, Kell system, LW, U, En[a], Wr[b]	I system, Pr series	P
Nature	Often polyclonal, sometimes monoclonal	Monoclonal in idiopathic CHD. Polyclonal in secondary hemolytic episodes	Polyclonal

TABLE 37-3 Some Differences Between WAIHA, CHD and PCH

	WAIHA	CHD	PCH
Most frequent nature of the disease	Usually permanent, often severe	Often clinically mild	Episodes of severe hemolysis
Clinical approach to treatment	Aggressive	Conservative	PCH often secondary. Treat underlying disease
Optimal forms of therapy	Corticosteroids and/or splenectomy. Less often other immunosuppresants	Avoid exposure to cold. Splenectomy sometimes helpful. In severe CHD, alkylating agents or sulphydryl compounds	No specific treatment for idiopathic PCH. Avoid exposure to cold in idiopathic and secondary PCH
Clinical improvement after splenectomy	Common	Occasional	Debatable
Red blood cell transfusions	Contraindicated. Use only to treat life-threatening anemia	Beneficial but seldom needed for anemia. Can be used to treat concurrent disorders.	Beneficial when needed.

cases of WAIHA are seen in persons over 40 years of age; the highest incidence of onset of the disorder is seen in persons between the ages of 60 and 70 (107). Some 55 to 60% of patients who develop WAIHA are female. However, it is not clear whether the disease is more common in women than in men or whether the difference simply reflects the fact that more women than men live beyond age 60.

Warm Antibody-Induced Hemolytic Anemia (WAIHA)

As indicated in table 37-2, WAIHA is most often caused by an IgG non-agglutinating autoantibody optimally reactive at 37°C. Once sufficient amounts of IgG autoantibody of certain subclasses (see below) become red cell-bound, the red cells are subject to sequestration and destruction by tissue bound macrophages that carry receptors for the Fc portion of IgG molecules. Cell destruction in WAIHA is predominantly extravascular in type, the mechanism for such red cell removal has been described in detail in Chapter 6. As with alloantibodies that are IgG in composition, the rate of removal of the patient's red cells is influenced by the amount of IgG on those red cells. While there are a number of other factors that influence the amount and rate of red cell destruction (114) the amount and IgG subclass of autoantibody bound to the red cells are of very considerable importance. As described below, one form of treating patients with WAIHA is to try to reduce the amount of autoantibody being made. Some patients with WAIHA present with thrombocytopenia; the condition is known as Evans' syndrome (115). The thrombocytopenia may be severe and may result in purpura (115-117). In patients

with severe idiopathic autoimmune thrombocytopenia, autoantibodies directed against red cells may be present (118). The occurrence of anemia and thrombocytopenia together may be less frequent than the occurrence of the two at different times in the same patient (107,109,117).

WAIHA and Red Cell Typing

Because autoantibody binds to red cells in vivo in patients with WAIHA, difficulties may be experienced in performing typing studies on the protein-coated red cells. Such cells may agglutinate spontaneously when mixed with typing reagents that contain potentiators of antigen-antibody reactions. The correct ABO type can usually be determined without difficulty because anti-A, anti-B and anti-A,B typing reagents are usually diluted in saline and because the autoantibodies in the patients' sera do not act as agglutinins so do not interfere with reverse ABO typing tests. If difficulties are encountered and if false positive reactions are suspected, the patient's red cells can be treated by one of the methods described below that attempt to free them of bound autoantibody. For workers who wish to control ABO typing tests on antibody-coated red cells, the cells can be tested with an AB serum known not to contain atypical blood group antibodies, in parallel with the ABO typing reagents. If that test is negative it is highly unlikely that any reactions with anti-A or anti-B represent false positives. Similarly, if the patient's serum is shown to be non-reactive with group O cells in reverse typing tests, it is highly probable that any reactions of the serum with A or B cells are due to the presence of anti-A or anti-B.

A real problem may arise when attempts are made to type red cells from patients with WAIHA for the D antigen. "Slide and rapid tube" Rh reagents contain potentiators and may cause spontaneous agglutination of antibody-coated red cells that are in fact D-negative. This problem was acute when such tests had to be controlled with ~30% bovine albumin (119). However, manufacturers of such reagents now usually make available Rh diluent controls that are supposed to be the same in composition as the typing reagent, except that no anti-D is present. In those instances in which the patient's red cells agglutinate in the diluent control, a positive typing for D is obviously invalid. One solution to the problem is to type the patient's red cells with saline-active anti-D. Another is to use an anti-D in which IgG molecules have been chemically reduced (120) so that they behave as agglutinins in the absence of high levels of potentiators. However, since either of these reagents may contain bovine albumin, it is still necessary to control the tests with a 6 or 10% solution of that medium. If this control is positive, it may be necessary to treat the red cells to remove autoantibody (see below) so that they can be typed for D. It is claimed that D typing reagents made from MAb do not cause spontaneous agglutination of antibody-coated red cells. The monoclonal anti-D are often IgM and react in saline systems. If the reagent based on MAb to D also contains some human polyclonal anti-D (see Chapter 12), some of the problems mentioned above are possible; the manufacturer of the reagent should be consulted.

The red cells of a patient with WAIHA and a positive DAT (that is 96 to 98% of such patients, see below) obviously cannot be typed using antisera that react only by the indirect antiglobulin test. Because the red cells are already coated with antibody, all such tests will be positive. There are now numerous methods that can be used to attempt to remove autoantibody from the cells so that they become suitable for use in typing tests using IAT-reactive reagents. These methods are also useful for preparing the patient's red cells for autoadsorption studies (see below in section dealing with transfusion in WAIHA). The methods most commonly used are those in which the red cells are treated with chloroquine diphosphate (121) or with the ZZAP (dithiothreitol and papain) reagent (122). Other methods for removing autoantibody from red cells that are left intact for use in typing or adsorption studies include use of: a variable pH/density gradient system (123); a cold acid method (124); a glycine-HCl-EDTA solution (125-127); and citric acid (128,129). Details of many of the above methods are given in Judd (130).

There are some points that must be remembered when typing tests on chloroquine or ZZAP-treated cells are undertaken. First, it has been reported (131-133) that red cells from which IgG has been removed by treatment with chloroquine may not react as strongly with anti-D

as do non-antibody coated red cells. The workers (121) who introduced the chloroquine-treatment method have pointed out (133) that untreated DAT+ red cells can often be satisfactorily typed with chemically reduced reagents if suitable controls are included. While these investigators (133) found that chloroquine-treated red cells reacted well when the IAT was used, others (131) saw some reduction in strengths of reaction by IAT. It has been found (131-133) that chloroquine-treated red cells may react less strongly than untreated cells in agglutination tests. It is not yet known if the mechanism that causes the weakened reactions affects only D or, as seems somewhat more likely, affects the ability of the treated cells to bind antibodies. If the latter explanation holds, chloroquine-treated cells may give weaker than expected and perhaps some false negative reactions, with other antibodies. Second, with some 20% of samples, chloroquine diphosphate does not effect total antibody dissociation (121). However, if the DAT has been reduced from 4+ to 1+, the cells may still be suitable for use in typing tests, the 1+ reaction can simply be subtracted as a "blank" from the results. Third, chloroquine diphosphate does not effect dissociation of C3 from red cells (121). Accordingly, if such treated cells are to be used in typing studies with IAT-reactive reagents and if the cells were known originally to be coated with C3, the typing tests must be read with anti-IgG and not with a polyspecific antiglobulin reagent. Fourth, the ZZAP reagent contains papain that denatures at least MN and Duffy system antigens and dithiothreitol that denatures those of the Kell, Cartwright, etc., systems (see individual chapters of this book). Thus while ZZAP-treated red cells may be suitable in autoadsorption procedures (but see below for a caution) there are considerable limits to their suitability for use in phenotyping studies.

Those workers who use chloroquine to effect in vitro dissociation of red cell-bound autoantibodies may be interested to learn that the first use of that compound in WAIHA was to treat patients (134-136). It seems that any benefits that accrued from that form of therapy may well have represented the ability of chloroquine to effect autoantibody dissociation in vivo as well as in vitro. Others (137-139) had earlier, described the effects of chloroquine diphosphate on red cells coated with IgG.

WAIHA and The Direct Antiglobulin Test

In this type of hemolytic anemia, the patient forms a, usually non-agglutinating, autoantibody directed against an antigen or antigens on the red cells. Thus, it is not surprising that in the majority of cases the direct antiglobulin test is positive, usually strongly so. The autoantibody binds to the patient's red cells in vivo and is detected in this test. Most workers use a polyspecific antiglobulin reagent, containing at least anti-IgG and anti-C3 to perform the initial DAT. Because red cells coated with complement in vivo usually have C3d but not C3c on the membrane, it is important that the reagent used contains anti-C3d (see Chapter 6). Once the initial DAT has been shown to be positive, the patient's red cells can be tested using antibodies to IgG, IgA, IgM and C3, to determine which abnormal proteins are present on those cells. It is now possible to purchase monospecific anti-IgG and anti-C3 (in the form of anti-C3c plus anti-C3dg or as anti-C3dg only) for use in DATs. Anti-IgM and anti-IgA are not so readily available. Some workers resolve this problem by making anti-IgM and anti-IgA in animals. Others purchase antibodies of those specificities that have been prepared for use in immunoprecipitation tests. While such reagents invariably contain hemagglutinating antibodies (that can be used to perform DATs) they often contain other antibodies (anti-A, anti-B, anti-species) that will interfere in DATs if the reagents are used in the undiluted form. Accordingly, the reagents must first be tested at a series of dilutions against normal washed red cells and red cells coated in vitro with IgM or IgA as appropriate (again, see Chapter 6). The dilution of the reagent that is suitable for use in a DAT is the lowest one that causes agglutination of the IgM or IgA-coated but not the normal red cells. As discussed in Chapter 6, the in vitro preparation of non-agglutinated IgM-coated red cells is not easy; the preparation of IgA-coated red cells is downright difficult. A potentially very useful solution to this problem is a gel card offered by DiaMed AG of Switzerland, that contains separate gels into which antibodies to IgG, IgA, IgM, C3c and C3d (plus a control) have been incorporated. As of this writing (January 1997) the gel card is available in Europe but not yet licensed for use in the USA.

Antibodies directed against IgG, IgM and IgA, that are to be used in DATs, must be heavy chain specific. A positive reaction between the test red cells and anti-IgG will be taken to mean that the red cells are coated with IgG. If the reagent contains only anti-gamma heavy chain that conclusion will be correct. If it contains say anti-kappa light chain and the antibody coating the red cells is IgM with kappa light chains, an erroneous conclusion could be reached (140).

Table 37-4 lists results obtained in several large studies (47,111,113) in which red cells from patients with WAIHA were tested with monospecific antiglobulin reagents to determine the nature of the proteins on those red cells. As can be seen, in the vast majority of cases in which IgA and/or IgM was found on the red cells, IgG and/or C3 was present as well. Accordingly, table 37-5 uses figures from the studies cited in table 37-4 and some from other studies (110,141-143) and shows the results

that would have been obtained if the patients' red cells had been tested with just anti-IgG and anti-C3. The figures in table 37-5 are useful on two counts. First, many workers perform DATs using only a polyspecific reagent, then monospecific anti-IgG and anti-C3. Second and the reason that is done, the most useful information for the clinician, that is obtained in DATs, is generated in tests that use only those three reagents (see below in section on in vivo red cell clearance in WAIHA). Those patients who present with apparently just IgA or with IgM and C3 on their red cells are discussed in later sections of this chapter. Table 37-6 shows the incidence of findings expected when DATs are performed on the red cells of patients with WAIHA, using the most readily available monospecific antiglobulin reagents. No doubt some of the variation in the series shown in tables 37-4 and 37-5 relates to the strengths of the antiglobulin sera used in the different studies.

WAIHA, the DAT and Subclasses of IgG

Since the red cells of the majority of patients with WAIHA are coated with IgG alone or with IgG and C3, it would seem that DATs using antibodies specific for IgG1, 2, 3 or 4 could be used to determine the subclass of the autoantibody. Indeed, several such studies have been reported (53,114,144-150) and it has been shown that the most common finding is that the red cells are coated with a mixture of IgG1 and IgG3. As discussed in the next section, the subclass of IgG of which the autoan-

TABLE 37-4 Proteins Detected in DATs on the Red Cells of Patients with WAIHA

	Percent of patients from number tested in the series of		
	Worlledge and Blajchman (111) (121 patients)	Issitt et al. (113) (87 patients)	Petz and Garratty (47) (104 patients)
IgG only	35.5	43.8	18.1
IgA only	2.5	0	1.7
C3 only	10.7	0	10.4
IgG and C3	43.0	47.1	46.0
IgM and C3	0	0	1.7
IgA and C3	0	0	1.7
IgG and IgA	3.3	1.1	2.7
IgG, IgA and C3	0	1.1	12.3
IgG, IgM and C3	5.0	4.6	3.7
IgG, IgA, IgM and C3	0	2.3	1.7

TABLE 37-5 Common Patterns of Red Cell Coating Seen in Patients with WAIHA

	Results expressed as a % of samples tested[*1]		
	Proteins detected on the red cells		
	IgG without C3	IgG and C3	C3 without IgG
Worlledge and Blajchman (111)[*2]	38	48	11
Issitt et al. (113)	45	55	0
Petz and Garratty (47)	21	64	14
Eyster and Jenkins (141)	24	31	45
Dacie and Worlledge (110)[*2]	56	31	13
Leddy and Bakemeier (142)	55	45	0
Miyazaki et al. (143)[*3]	41	41	18

[*1]   Figures do not total 100% in those series including cases in which IgA was found in the absence of IgG or C3.
[*2]   The two series may include some of the same patients.
[*3]   Series reports a study of 34 children with WAIHA. Other series describe primarily adult patients.

tibody is made has a direct bearing on the rate and amount of in vivo red cell destruction that will occur. However, subclass studies with monospecific antiglobulin reagents are more easily described than performed. It has proved rather difficult to make anti-IgG subclass antibodies in animals. It seems that determinants common to all four subclasses of IgG are more immunogenic than are the determinants that characterize the subclasses. As a result, an animal immunized with purified IgG of one subclass will often make an antibody that complexes with a determinant shared by all IgG molecules. Even when an animal makes an anti-IgG specific for one subclass, its serum may well contain antibodies to shared determinants as well. At present, the most widely used IgG subclassing reagents are those prepared by The Netherlands Red Cross Blood Center in Amsterdam. Because these reagents are expensive to prepare and because they are standardized for use in a sedimentation

TABLE 37-6 Expected Results in DATs Using Monospecific Antiglobulin Reagents and Red Cells of Patients with WAIHA

Proteins detected	Percent of patients
IgG without C3	40 to 50
IgG and C3	45 to 60
C3 without IgG	0 to 15

test that requires a fairly large volume of reagent in each test, some workers (151-154) have used them by modified techniques (i.e. in capillary tubes or microtiter plates). It then becomes difficult to control the tests so as to be sure that positive reactions represent the activity of the anti-subclass specificity and not the anti-shared determinant specificity that is present but not reactive in sedimentation tests. Indeed, there are conflicting reports (155,156) in the literature as to whether specificity of these reagents is maintained when techniques for their use are modified. However, it seems that the expertise developed and the careful controls performed by Garratty and his colleagues (53,114,150,155) show that alternatives to the sedimentation method can successfully be used with these reagents. A different problem encountered is that some of the subclassing reagents fail to yield positive results when red cells are coated with low levels of IgG. As described in the next section, this is unfortunate for it is those occasions on which low levels of red cell bound IgG cause in vivo red cell clearance, that knowledge of the subclass of the autoantibody present would be useful. No doubt the problems described will be resolved when monoclonal antibodies to IgG1, 2, 3 and 4, made in hybridomas, become available. The fact that such reagents have not yet appeared may well mean that difficulties similar to those described above in animals, apply to production of these antibodies in hybridomas that begin, of course, with animal immunization.

WAIHA and In Vivo Red Cell Destruction

The mechanisms by which antibodies cause red cell destruction in vivo have been described in detail in Chapter 6. Accordingly, this section will mention those mechanisms only as they pertain directly to red cell destruction in WAIHA. Intravascular red cell destruction in patients with WAIHA is seen (47,109,112,157-171) but fortunately is rare. When an IgM autoantibody is able to bind to red cells at 37°C, activate complement, and bring about intravascular hemolysis, an acute and extremely serious clinical situation will exist. That is to say, the patient will undergo continual intravascular red cell destruction, transfusion will not correct the problem and unless autoantibody production can be curtailed rapidly, a fatal outcome is probable. Indeed, in many of the cases referenced above the patient died, often within hours or a few days of the start of hemolysis. While the large number of references cited appears to give the lie to the statement that such intravascular hemolysis in WAIHA is rare, it is more likely that the cases are described in print because they are so dramatic and so unusual. In a patient presenting with such an autoantibody, plasmapheresis should be considered early in the patient's management.

If the antibody is IgM it will be predominantly in the intravascular compartment and thus amenable to removal by plasma exchange. If the plasma exchange procedure is delayed, the patient's physical condition may deteriorate so rapidly that he or she may no longer be able to withstand the rigors of the procedure.

Much more commonly, red cell destruction in WAIHA is via the extravascular mechanism of cell clearance. Red cells coated with IgG or IgG and C3 are sequestered, predominantly in the spleen and the liver, by tissue bound macrophages and are then subject to the actions of those cells, as described in Chapter 6.

The rate and amount of in vivo sequestration and destruction of red cells is directly affected by the type and amount of protein on their membranes. Red cells coated with IgG but not C3 are predominantly but not exclusively sequestered in the spleen. Those coated with IgG and C3 are subject to sequestration in the spleen and the liver (see below for a discussion of hepatic sequestration of red cells coated with high levels of IgG but no C3). Since it is known (see Chapter 6) that macrophages that carry receptor sites for C3c are not particularly efficient in clearing red cells coated with C3 but no immunoglobulin, it is currently believed that macrophages that trap red cells coated with IgG and C3, immobilize the red cells via the C3 receptor, until macrophages with IgG receptors can act. These explanations seem to fit very well with the known physiology of the spleen and the liver. It is known (172-183) that the receptor for the Fc portion of IgG on macrophages will bind free or cell-bound IgG. Thus in vivo, it might be expected that those receptors would not be very efficient at clearing IgG-coated red cells because they would already have bound plasma IgG (not necessarily autoantibody). However, in the spleen, the concentration of red cells is high and that of plasma is low (i.e. hematocrit circa 70 to 80%). In other words, relatively less plasma IgG is available for binding by tissue-bound macrophages so that the sequestration of IgG-coated red cells is efficient. In contrast, the hematocrit in the liver is lower (i.e. circa 45 to 50%) meaning that there is more plasma IgG to effect inhibition of macrophage action in the binding of IgG-coated red cells. However, the receptor for C3 on tissue bound macrophages does not recognize native C3 in its non-activated form, so will not bind plasma C3. That receptor recognizes the C3c piece of activated C3b, so effects trapping of red cells coated with IgG and C3 without interference from plasma proteins (184-198). Put in its most simple form, the presence of C3 on IgG-coated red cells augments the in vivo clearance of those cells. These concepts (and the clinical observations that support them) illustrate the importance of DATs using anti-IgG and anti-C3 on the red cells of patients with WAIHA. Although the C3 component

detected in the DAT is C3dg, while the component recognized by tissue-bound macrophages is C3c, the detection of C3dg in an in vitro test is taken to indicate that in vivo, other red cells (probably largely sequestered and destroyed before the sample for the DAT was collected) carried C3c. Many clinicians have found that when the DAT reveals the presence of IgG and C3 on red cells, the rate and amount of in vivo red cell clearance is greater than when just IgG is present. In other words, the laboratory findings correlate well with the clinical state of the patient. Not surprisingly, in view of what has been written above, many clinicians find that patients with IgG and C3 on the red cells require higher doses of steroids (see below) than do those who present with just IgG on the cells and that the steroid response may not be as good as when only IgG is membrane-bound.

When the red cells are coated with IgG but not with C3, the subclass of the IgG autoantibody directly affects the rate and amount of in vivo red cell destruction. When Engelfriet et al. (149) studied 273 persons with a positive DAT in whom only one subclass of IgG could be demonstrated on the red cells, they found that 259 of them had cells apparently coated only with IgG1. Of those 259 persons, about half had hemolytic anemia, the other half had a positive DAT but were not anemic. In contrast, all of eight patients in whom only IgG3 was demonstrable on the red cells had hemolytic anemia. Of the remaining six persons in the study, two had red cells on which only IgG2 and four only IgG4, could be demonstrated. None of those six patients had hemolytic anemia (but see below). Other patients who had made IgG4 autoantibodies that were benign in vivo have been described (53,112,114,199,200).

At one time it was supposed that the findings in persons with just IgG1 on the red cells might mean that two forms of that subclass existed with autoantibodies made of one type being pathological and those made of the other being benign. However, Meulen et al. (148) showed that this was not the case and that the difference between the presence of an IgG1 autoantibody on the red cells of patients with hemolytic anemia and on those with no anemia, is quantitative. These workers showed that below a certain level, IgG1 autoantibodies do not clear red cells in vivo but once the threshold for macrophage recognition (that varied relatively little among different individuals) is exceeded, in vivo red cell destruction begins. In later studies, Stratton et al. (201) concluded that macrophage-mediated red cell clearance occurs when more than 900 to 1000 molecules of IgG1 are bound, per red cell. This figure contrasts sharply with that for IgG3; Meulen et al. (148) had shown that significant in vivo red cell destruction can occur when only 100 molecules of IgG3 are bound per red cell. While they agreed that in general those patients with hemolytic anemia had higher levels of IgG on their red cells than those in whom the DAT was positive but there was no accelerated rate of in vivo red cell clearance, Nance and Garratty (553) and Garratty (114) did not see such a clear distinction between the two groups. That is to say, in a study that involved more cases than described by Meulen et al. (148) and Stratton et al. (201), the Los Angeles workers (114,553) noted considerable overlap in numbers of IgG molecules per red cell between patients with hemolytic anemia and those in whom the autoantibodies were benign. Garratty (114) concluded that there is no "magic number" below which hemolysis does not occur and above which it does, and that the onset of hemolysis will occur when different numbers of IgG molecules are bound to the red cells of different patients. From findings (149,199,200) that IgG2 and IgG4-coated red cells were not destroyed in vivo, it was supposed that macrophages with receptors for those subclasses might not exist. Similarly, it was thought that IgG3 autoantibodies might always cause hemolytic anemia. However, these rules are not inviolate. Nance et al. (202) and Roush et al. (302) have described cases of hemolytic anemia in which the causative autoantibodies appeared to be made entirely of IgG2. In the patient described by Roush et al. (302) the autoantibody had anti-U specificity (see below). Nance and Garratty (150) described six individuals with IgG3 on their red cells, none of whom had hemolytic anemia. Nance et al. (202) pointed out that previous studies on the abilities of macrophages to recognize and bind red cells coated with IgG of different subclasses, had mostly been performed using red cells to which purified proteins (e.g. myeloma proteins) had been passively coupled. They (202) wondered if macrophages might sometimes recognize individual autoantibodies via different Fc-borne determinants than those present on monoclonal myeloma proteins.

Garratty (53,114) studied the incidence of one or more than one subclass of IgG autoantibody on the red cells of 167 individuals with a positive DAT. Among the 167 individuals, 46 were patients with WAIHA, while 32 were patients and 89 blood donors, in whom the positive DAT was not associated with hemolytic anemia. The results are summarized in table 37-7. As can be seen, among the 46 patients with WAIHA, 58.8% had only one subclass of IgG on their red cells (in 50% of the 46 it was IgG1) while the remaining 41.2% had autoantibodies of two or more IgG subclasses on their red cells. In sharp contrast, among the 32 patients with a positive DAT but no hemolytic anemia, 84.6% presented with just one subclass autoantibody on the red cells, only 15.4% had autoantibodies of more than one subclass on the cells. Among the 89 blood donors with a positive DAT but no hemolytic anemia, 91.4% presented with just one subclass autoantibody on the red cells, only 8.6% had autoantibodies of more than one subclass on the cells. Clearly, WAIHA often represents a situation in which multiple clones of immunocytes are producing autoantibodies while a positive DAT in an individual who is not experiencing in vivo hemolysis much more often represents a situation in which a limited (perhaps sometimes monoclonal) clonal regulation failure has occurred.

Table 37-8 shows the currently accepted correlations between IgG subclass of the autoantibody and in vivo macrophage activity. As will be apparent from what has been written above, table 37-8 is a generalization and exceptions will be seen. It is noticeable that when C3 is present on red cells, the difference in the ability of IgG3

TABLE 37-7 Subclasses of IgG Autoantibodies in Patients with WAIHA and Patients and Donors with Benign Autoantibodies (from 114)

IgG subclass	Results expressed as a % of samples tested		
	Patients with WAIHA (n=46)	Patients with pos DAT, no WAIHA (n=32)	Blood Donors (n=89)
IgG1 alone	50.0	72.0	81.0
IgG2 alone	2.2	6.3	1.3
IgG3 alone	6.6	6.3	2.6
IgG4 alone	0	0	6.5
Percent with only one subclass	58.8	84.6	91.4
IgG1 with other(s)	37.0	12.5	7.9
IgG2 with other(s)	24.0	9.4	4.5
IgG3 with other(s)	22.0	6.3	4.5
IgG4 with other(s)	24.0	12.5	5.6
Percent with two or more subclasses	41.2	15.4	8.6

TABLE 37-8 Correlations Between Proteins on Red Cells and Macrophage Activity in Vivo

Proteins detected	Degree of red cell destruction mediated by macrophage action
IgG and C3	Maximal
IgG3	Usually high
IgG1	May be marked or none may occur, see text
IgG2 and IgG4	Usually none. See text for exceptions.
C3c	Some binding but limited red cell destruction
C3d	No red cell destruction

and IgG1 autoantibodies to bring about in vivo red cell destruction, largely disappears. This presumably relates to the augmentation of IgG antibody-mediated red cell binding to macrophages effected by activated C3, as described above.

Some other points must be borne in mind when in vivo red cell destruction in patients with WAIHA is considered. First, as discussed below, a primary form of treatment in this disorder is to suppress autoantibody production to a point where few enough molecules of IgG bind per red cell that in vivo red cell clearance either does not occur, or is within the range for which the marrow can compensate by increased red cell production. In patients in remission following this type of treatment, an exacerbation of hemolysis may be seen if the patient has an infection. It seems that when an infection occurs, macrophage activity is stimulated so that those phagocytes can clear red cells coated with levels of IgG that did not induce red cell sequestration before the infection. The mechanisms are relatively complex. There is evidence (203-208) that bacterially produced endotoxins and cytokines released during infections cause upregulation of the number of Fcγ and CR receptors on macrophages. However, the situation does not simply involve additional expression of Fc and CR receptors since other evidence (180,209,210) shows increased activity but not increased numbers of the receptors. Second, while it is known (211-213,246) that patients with WAIHA have increased numbers of Fc receptors on their macrophages, and that the numbers can be downregulated with corticosteroid therapy (212,246) it is not clear whether the increase represents cause or effect of the disease. Third, variation in macrophage activity in different individuals, in terms of the ability of those macrophages to sequester and destroy red cells coated with different amounts of IgG, has been little studied as yet. Fourth, as discussed in more detail below, the standard in vitro tests (DAT, IAT, autoantibody titration, etc.) are not very good for differentiation between the situations in which IgG autoantibodies cause

or fail to effect in vivo red cell destruction (see section below on quantitation of IgG on the red cells of patients with WAIHA).

It is not yet clear how in vivo red cell destruction occurs in patients who present with apparently only IgA on their red cells (47,53,111,114,214-223). Cells with receptors for that immunoglobulin have now been described (224-232) some of the reports document the presence of IgA receptors on monocytes or macrophages. However, a role for those receptors in immune red cell clearance does not seem to have been clearly demonstrated. IgA antibodies do not usually activate complement (233). As described in a later section of this chapter, a small number of patients with WAIHA (with active in vivo red cell clearance) present with a negative DAT. It is known that some of these patients have sufficient IgG autoantibody on their red cells to mediate in vivo clearance, but too little for detection in a standard DAT. Thus it is possible that some patients with WAIHA and apparently only IgA on their red cells, also have subdetectable (by standard methods) levels of IgG and that it is the low level of IgG and not the easily demonstrable IgA, that is responsible for the in vivo red cell clearance. Indeed, this has been proved in at least one case (47). The same concept can be invoked to explain those patients with active WAIHA who have only complement detectable on the red cells. As already described, macrophages do not efficiently clear red cells coated with C3 in the absence of immunoglobulin. Again, it is possible that the red cells that appear to be coated only with C3 carry low levels of IgG, not detectable in standard tests. The augmenting effect, in terms of in vivo red cell clearance, of C3 on red cells that also carry IgG, has been mentioned several times. It has been proposed (234,235) that IgA has a similar synergistic effect.

WAIHA, Complement Activation and Hemolysins

As shown in tables 37-4 and 37-5, more than half of all patients with WAIHA have C3 on their red cells. A majority of those patients have IgG but not IgM, cell-bound as well. Thus it would seem logical to assume that many IgG autoantibodies causative of WAIHA, activate complement after they have bound to red cells. In fact, this is not easy to demonstrate in vitro. If unbound autoantibodies from the patients' sera or autoantibodies recovered by elution from the patients' red cells, are tested against normal red cells in test systems to which fresh serum as a source of complement has been added, it is found that many, from patients who presented with both IgG and C3 on the red cells, do not activate complement in vitro. Borne et al. (158) reported that complement activation in these patients represents the presence of IgM hemolysins of the same specificity as the IgG autoantibodies in the patients. Indeed, some workers regard the detection of IgM on a patient's red cells in the DAT as a bad prognostic sign since it indicates the presence of an autohemolysin (this topic is discussed further, below). However when we (236) tested the sera of 60 patients with WAIHA, who presented with IgG and C3 on their red cells, we found only three (5%) that contained hemolysins. Somewhat similarly, Petz and Garratty (47) reported that when a sensitive method for the detection of hemolysins was used (i.e. acidified serum samples tested against protease-treated red cells) only 31 of 244 samples (12.7%) could be shown to contain hemolysins. Thus while a percentage of patients can be shown to have IgG-complement binding autoantibodies and/or autohemolysins, the total seems to fall far short of the some 60% of patients (table 37-5) who have C3 on the red cells, as detected in DATs. As described earlier, antibody-induced hemolytic anemia is one manifestation of autoimmune disease. A sizable number of patients with WAIHA present with a concurrent different autoimmune disorder. Thus it seems possible that in some of these patients immune complexes, not involving red cells, are present in the serum. If this is the case the immune complexes could have activated complement that then bound to the patients' red cells via the innocent bystander mechanism. While such a concept seems entirely possible, it remains poorly investigated. Although, for reasons given above, the presence of IgG and C3 on the red cells of a patient with WAIHA does not necessarily mean that the autoantibody present is capable of complement activation, the presence of C3 on a patient's red cells may be of considerable clinical significance. As discussed above, C3 on IgG-coated red cells augments the in vivo clearance of those cells, as discussed below, patients who present with IgG and C3 on the red cells are often more difficult to induce into remission than those who present with just IgG on the cells.

Other Notes on Red Cell-Bound Proteins in WAIHA

Previous sections have considered the relevance of the subclass of IgG, the presence or absence of IgM and the presence of IgA alone, on the red cells of patients with WAIHA. As mentioned above, the presence of IgM on the patient's red cells is believed by some (158) to indicate the presence of an autohemolysin. Patients with such autoantibodies are said to have a more severe form of WAIHA than those in whom the autoantibody is entirely IgG or IgA in composition. Certainly when an autoantibody capable of binding to red cells at 37°C and

bringing about intravascular hemolysis is present, the patient is desperately ill (47,109,112,157-171). However, the detection of IgM on the patient's red cells in a DAT, by no means indicates that massive intravascular hemolysis is occurring. Thus in the experience of one of us (113,236) the detection of IgM in the DAT is sometimes associated with severe disease but at other times is not associated with a condition any more acute than that seen in patients who present with just IgG on the red cells. Presumably the avidity, strength, thermal range and perhaps other variables of IgM autoantibodies result in variable consequences in the patient.

Ben-Izhak et al. (237) suggested that the presence of more than one type of immunoglobulin on the red cells of patients with WAIHA is associated with severity of disease. Among 25 patients with WAIHA, nine had IgM and/or IgA in addition to IgG on their red cells and were said to respond less well to steroid therapy than those patients who presented with IgG but no IgM or IgA on the red cells. Sokol et al. (238) used the enzyme-linked antiglobulin test to demonstrate the presence of IgM and/or IgA on the red cells in 37% of 218 samples from patients with WAIHA. When standard DATs were used, only 15% of the 218 samples could be shown to carry IgM and/or IgA in addition to IgG. The presence of IgM and/or IgA on the red cells of patients in this series (238) was associated with higher levels of IgG than those found on the red cells of patients who had IgG without IgM or IgA on the red cells. The two studies cited above (237,238) may, in fact, indicate that as clinical WAIHA progresses, additional clones of immunocytes producing autoantibody become activated. As mentioned several times above and as discussed in more detail in Chapter 39, production of "warm" reactive autoantibodies is not always associated with hemolytic anemia. It is entirely possible that the defects in the immune system that result in autoantibody production represent a sliding scale. Thus in some individuals benign IgG autoantibodies are seen, in those with severe hemolytic anemia, autoantibodies of many immunoglobulin types are made. The report of Sokol et al. (238) that associates production of autoantibodies of multiple immunoglobulin classes with severity of disease may be pertinent in this area. In previous publications, these authors (239-245) have described studies on very large numbers of patients with positive DATs caused by autoantibodies (i.e. 865 cases in one (239) report). However, in a number of the reports (239-241,244,245) it has seemed at least to one of us (PDI), that a positive DAT has been equated with hemolysis without supportive evidence that the autoantibody was pathological in vivo. Perhaps those patients with autoantibodies of multiple immunoglobulin classes represent a subset of the large series and are the patients with the most severe WAIHA.

Antibody-dependent Cell Cytolysis (ADCC) and K-cell Lysis

The term ADCC is sometimes used to described a situation in which non-T, non-B, K-cells (NK-cells or natural-killer lymphocytes) cause the destruction of antibody-coated red cells following cell-cell contact in a complement-independent system. George Garratty (247) has pointed out that although ADCC describes K-cell lysis, the term should not be restricted to that mechanism. When tissue-bound macrophages with IgG receptors bind to and eventually destroy red cells coated with IgG but not C3, the situation also represents ADCC. Accordingly, it seems better to call the actions of K cells in the peripheral blood, K-cell lysis (the mechanism is discussed in Chapters 6 and 36) and not ADCC, or at least to qualify K-cell lysis as being one form of ADCC. While there is no doubt that the lysis of IgG antibody-coated red cells by K cells can be demonstrated in vitro (146,248-272) and while more lysis occurs if K cells and antibody from the same individual are used than if the K cells are from one person and the antibody from another (262), it is not yet clear how much (if any) K cell lysis occurs in vivo. As described in Chapter 36, if IgG-coated, ^{51}Cr-labeled red cells are injected into a volunteer, sufficient counts over the spleen are recorded to account for sequestration of the test dose of cells in that organ. It is not known what happens when larger volumes of red cells are destroyed as in WAIHA or following the transfusion of incompatible red cells. Accordingly, it is not yet possible to state the extent (if any) of the role played by K-cells in in vivo red cell destruction in patients with WAIHA.

K-cell lysis may be more significant in certain clinical settings. Gilsanz et al. (456) described a patient with large granular lymphocytic leukemia and hemolytic anemia. The large granular lymphocytes isolated from the patient's blood were shown to cause lysis of her red cells but not of allogeneic red cells in vitro. The lysis was not antibody or complement dependent, nor was it enhanced in the presence of the patient's serum. The patient was treated with cyclophosphamide and went into remission. No cytotoxic activity of the lymphocytes was demonstrable once the patient was in remission. The authors cite other studies (457-463) on the cytotoxic activities of (particularly large) lymphocytes in certain settings.

WAIHA, Specificity of the Causative Auto-antibodies

For many years, the autoantibodies causative of WAIHA were regarded as being non-specific because they reacted with all red cells against which they were tested. In 1953, Weiner et al. (273) showed that a patient with e+ red cells had WAIHA caused by an auto-anti-e. As Dorner (274) described it, that publication "touched off an avalanche of reports which has yet to stop". In another report in 1953, Wiener and Gordon (275) suggested that autoantibodies causative of WAIHA might be directed against some nucleus or core material of Rh-Hr substance. As described below, that forecast proved to be extraordinarily accurate. Following the report of Weiner et al. (273) others appeared (116,276-281) that showed that specific autoantibodies were often present in patients with WAIHA, but were often accompanied by non-specific antibodies that had to be removed by adsorption before the identities of others could be recognized. In 1963, Weiner and Vos (282) published their classic paper showing that many of the so-called non-specific autoantibodies have specificities that can be seen in tests against certain rare red cells. They divided the previously called non-specific autoantibodies into three classes. The first specificity was called anti-nl, for anti-normal, because the antibody reacted with all red cells with a normal Rh phenotype (R_1R_1, R_1R_2, rr, etc.) but not with those that were partially deleted (D-- and Dc-) nor with those that were deleted (Rh_{null}). The second specificity was called anti-pdl, for anti-partially deleted, because the antibody reacted with all red cells of normal and partially deleted phenotypes (i.e. R_1R_1, R_1R_2, rr, D-- and Dc-) but not with those that were fully deleted (i.e. Rh_{null}). The third specificity was called anti-dl, for anti-deleted, because the antibody reacted with all cells, including those of phenotype Rh_{null}, that were fully deleted. Since anti-nl and anti-pdl fail to react with Rh-deletion and Rh_{null} and with Rh_{null} cells respectively, their specificities appear at least to be Rh system related. Table 37-9 shows the reaction patterns of anti-nl, -pdl and -dl and also lists some alloantibodies that give, ostensibly at least, the same reaction patterns. The antibodies listed in the bottom part of table 37-9 are alloimmune in nature. Thus, while they considerably complicate transfusion therapy in patients who have formed them, they do not cause antibody-induced hemolytic anemia.

About 50% of warm-reactive autoantibodies have Rh system specificity if anti-nl and anti-pdl are included in that category. We (113) conducted a detailed study of autoantibody specificity in 150 individuals with a positive DAT and a warm-reactive autoantibody in the serum or on the red cells. Not all the individuals studied had WAIHA. Of the 150 included in the study, 87 had WAIHA, 33 had formed autoantibodies while being treated with alpha-methyldopa (aldomet) and 30 were hematologically normal (for a more complete description of the latter groups see Chapters 40 and 39, respectively). We identified a total of 311 autoantibodies among the 150 patients, 157 (50.5%) of them had Rh system specificity. In this study (113), as in many others (111,283-286), Rh specificity of

TABLE 37-9 Reaction Patterns of Anti-nl, Anti-pdl and Anti-dl and Some Alloantibodies That Are Similar

Phenotype of test red cells	Reactions of autoantibodies		
	Anti-nl	Anti-pdl	Anti-dl
Normal Rh phenotype (i.e., R_1R_1, R_1R_2, r'r'', rr, etc.)	+	+	+
Rh-deletion (i.e., D--, Dc-, DC^w- and some cells such as those from R^{oHar} and $\bar{\bar{R}}^N$ homozygotes)	0	+	+
Rh$_{null}$	0	0	+
	Alloantibodies with similar reaction patterns		
	Anti-Hr	Anti-Rh29	Anti-En^a
	Anti-Hr$_0$	Anti-LW^a	Anti-Wr^b
	Anti-Rh34	Anti-LW^{ab}	Anti-Kp^b
		Anti-U	Anti-Di^b

the autoantibody was not always apparent from the initial tests. Often, the serum of a patient with WAIHA, or an eluate made from that person's red cells, will react with all red cell samples when first tested, i.e., anti-dl. If the serum or eluate is adsorbed with say Rh$_{null}$ cells until it no longer reacts with red cells of that phenotype (i.e. anti-dl removed) and is then retested, some specificity may be seen. The adsorbed serum or eluate may react with red cells of normal Rh phenotype but not with those that are deleted or partially deleted. In other words, adsorption has removed anti-dl and left unadsorbed anti-nl, that may have auto-anti-Hr or Hr$_0$ specificity. If the anti-nl is then adsorbed with say R$_2$R$_2$ red cells, the auto-anti-nl may be adsorbed and auto-anti-e may be left unadsorbed. In all the descriptions given below, on autoantibodies such as those that are directed against LW, U, Wr^b, etc., but with the possible exception of those in the Kell blood group system, specificities are more often seen following adsorption studies than when tests with unadsorbed sera or eluates are performed. In other words, while auto-anti-LW (286,287), auto-anti-U (288,289) or auto-anti-Wr^b (113,290), etc., see below, may be the only antibody present, mixtures of several different specificity Rh autoantibodies are more common. For example, in tests on the 150 persons mentioned above, we (113) found four examples of unadsorbed antibodies that failed to react with Wr(b-) red cells. When we adsorbed 110 examples of anti-dl with Wr(b-) red cells until the sera or eluates no longer reacted with those cells, we found that 42 of the anti-dl contained an anti-Wr^b component. In 15 of the cases studied, we (113)

found four or five autoantibodies by differential adsorption, in one we found autoantibodies directed against D, e, nl, pdl, dl and Wr^b. Table 37-10 lists the specificities of autoantibodies that have caused WAIHA and some that have caused a positive DAT but not hemolysis. As can be seen, autoantibodies directed against simple antigens such as D, C, c, E, e, rh$_i$, G, etc., have all been reported. Again, it is unusual to find such autoantibodies present without others. In our series of 150 persons, only four were found to have only simple specificity Rh autoantibodies; three had auto-anti-e only, one had auto-anti-c and auto-anti-E only. The total number of simple specificity Rh autoantibodies found was 60, meaning that 55 of them were present in sera or eluates that contained anti-nl, anti-pdl and/or anti-dl, as well. Textbooks and review articles often list Rh autoantibodies as the most common cause of WAIHA. That finding is only apparent if adsorption studies are done and if anti-dl and anti-pdl are considered to have Rh system specificities.

One Rh system antibody merits special mention here because it has thus far been found only in the autoimmune form. From the results of initial antibody identification tests, anti-Rh39 appears to have anti-C specificity (291). However, the antibody can be adsorbed to exhaustion by any C+ or C- red cells of normal Rh phenotype. Further, it differs from auto-anti-Hr and auto-anti-Hr$_0$ that mimic anti-E or anti-e (see below), in that it can also be adsorbed to exhaustion with D--/D-- red cells. Thus, unlike Hr, Hr$_0$ and Rh34, the Rh39 determinant is present on Rh-deletion red cells. Rh$_{null}$ red cells, of course, lack Hr, Hr$_0$, Rh34 and Rh39. Anti-Rh39 may, in fact, have been produced as an alloantibody. It is likely to be made as one antibody in a complex mixture, by a person who is phenotypically Rh$_{null}$ or has a very unusual Rh phenotype so that the red cells are Rh:-39 and (probably) lack other very common Rh antigens. Thus, allo-anti-Rh39 may have been encountered but not recognized. Auto-anti-Rh39 is not particularly uncommon in sera or eluates that contain anti-dl but its recognition requires that appropriate and reasonably complex adsorptions be performed.

In 1967, Celano and Levine (287) added anti-LW to the spectrum of autoantibodies causative of WAIHA. Vos et al. (286) found other examples of auto-anti-LW, usually after adsorption studies as described above had been performed. By reviewing the reports in retrospect it now seems likely that what would now (292-295) be called anti-LW^a and anti-LW^{ab} have both occurred as causative autoantibodies of WAIHA.

Nugent et al. (288) were astute enough to realize that an autoantibody that failed to react only with Rh$_{null}$ red cells (anti-pdl in table 37-9) might have anti-U specificity since Rh$_{null}$ cells fail to react with many examples of that antibody (296,297). They (288) described the first example of auto-anti-U, many others have subsequently been reported (74,113,286,289,298-304). Again, auto-anti-U may be a component of anti-dl and may not be recognizable until the serum or eluate involved has been adsorbed with U- red cells to remove the anti-dl component. Some examples of auto-anti-U were shown (300-303) to be pH sensitive, another (299) was made by a patient being treated with alpha-methyldopa (see Chapter 40) and a third was made (298) by a patient with myasthenia gravis who did not have hemolytic anemia. McGinniss et al. (304) reported that nine of 28 (32%) patients with AIDS severe enough that the patients were in hospital, had auto-anti-U that reacted only with enzyme-treated red cells, present in the serum. The propositus whose blood led to our study (305) on UPR and UPS (see Chapter 15) and whose serum contained the first recognized example of anti-UPS without anti-UPR, was also hospitalized with AIDS. We do not know if the apparently increased incidence of auto-anti-U in patients with AIDS (304) has been confirmed by others, nor whether the finding (if confirmed) has any significance.

Worlledge and Blajchman (111) and Leddy et al. (284) had already reported that about 30% of autoantibodies causative of WAIHA react with Rh_{null} red cells (more recent studies (47,113) have put the number higher) when Worlledge (306) showed that some of those autoantibodies do not react with cells that are En(a-). It was after the verbal report of Worlledge (306) that we (307,308) showed that En(a-) red cells are also Wr(a-b-). From these and subsequent studies (113,290,306,309) it became clear that both auto-anti-En^a and auto-anti-Wr^b can cause WAIHA. Recognition of the fact that the portion of MN SGP that remains on ficin-treated En(a+) red cells (310-316) contributes to the structure of the Wr^b antigen, correlated exactly with these findings. It is now abundantly clear that autoantibodies directed against En^aTS, En^aFS, En^aFR (318), En^aKT and Wr^b can and do cause WAIHA (113,162,166,169,171,290,306,307,309-311,313,317-319,321-324).

In 1972, Seyfried et al. (320) described a case of WAIHA caused by auto-anti-Kp^b. In addition to the unusual specificity of the autoantibody, it was shown that during the acute hemolytic episode, the Kell system antigens on the patient's red cells were markedly depressed. The hemolytic anemia in this patient was transient and following cessation of hemolysis, the expression of Kell system antigens on his red cells returned to normal. In 1979, Beck et al. (325) described another auto-anti-Kp^b formed by a patient whose red cell Kell system antigens were depressed; this time the autoantibody did not cause hemolytic anemia. In the same year, Marsh et al. (326) described an auto-anti-K13 that caused WAIHA and (327) an autoantibody to a hitherto unrecognized high incidence Kell system antigen and another example of auto-anti-

Kp^b, that did not. We (328) studied a case in which an auto-anti-Kp^b was made in a surgical patient whose red cell Kell system antigens were depressed. This autoantibody was apparently benign in vivo and was made by the patient only during a two week period. Once autoantibody production had ceased in our patient, her red cell Kell system antigen levels returned to normal. Other somewhat similar cases have been described (329-333) although in some of them further unexpected findings have been made. In two cases (329,330) benign autoantibodies that appeared to have anti-Kp^b specificity, were eluted from the patients' DAT+ Kp(b-) red cells. It is possible that the autoantibodies were directed against other high incidence Kell system antigens that were depressed in expression on the patients' red cells. In two other cases (332,333) patients with idiopathic thrombocytopenic purpura (ITP) were found to have antibodies to high incidence Kell system antigens in the serum and depressed expression of Kell system antigens on the red cells. In these patients the DAT was negative but when remissions of the ITP were achieved, production of the Kell system antibodies ceased and expression of the Kell system antigens on the red cells became normal. The second case (333) was further extraordinary in that during a later relapse, the patient's red cells showed marked depression of expression of their Lutheran system antigens.

Marsh et al. (326,327) suggested that one of two different mechanisms might be responsible for depression of expression of red cell Kell system antigens in patients who had made pathological or benign Kell system autoantibodies. First, it was suggested that an enzyme, possibly of bacterial or viral origin, might modify the antigens on the red cells in a manner that made them less able than usual to complex with antibodies. Second, it was considered possible that an unknown factor might inhibit the de novo production of Kell system antigens on the patients' red cells. In the case that we (328) studied and in at least one other (332), there was evidence that transfused as well as the patient's own cells underwent alteration of Kell system antigen expression. This finding would certainly support the first of the two concepts suggested above, better than the second. Further, our patient (328) and some of the others studied (325-327,332) were known to have or recently to have had, infections. While reduction of expression of red cell Kell system antigens in persons who form Kell system autoantibodies does not seem too uncommon, a similar phenomenon involving red cell Rh antigens seems to be very unusual (see below).

Autoantibodies of many other specificities have been described in the literature. While there are several reports of apparent auto-anti-K (116,279,334,351,352) it is known that in two (334,352) and suspected (353) that in a third (351) the autoantibody mimicked anti-K but could be adsorbed by K- red cells. Indeed, caution is now necessary in interpreting many early reports on autoantibody specificity in WAIHA. Those published before the mimicking nature of many autoantibodies was recognized, often described antibody identification but not adsorption studies. As described in detail in a later section, a high proportion of autoantibodies that appear to define a red cell antigen, mimic a specificity that they do not truly possess. Also in the Kell system, examples of auto-anti-Js^b have been described (335,354).

Reports on Kidd system autoantibodies (336-350,428) describe a wide variety of different situations. In some instances (341,344,345,347,350,428) an autoantibody to Jk^a, Jk^b or Jk3 caused frank WAIHA, in one case (347) caused by auto-anti-Jk^a, the patient was only eight months-old. Two other patients (348,349) had the hemolytic anemia and thrombocytopenia of Evan's syndrome, in one of them (349) the DAT was negative, in both cases auto-anti-Jk^a was present. One auto-anti-Jk^a said to be causing in vivo red cell destruction was seen (339) in a patient being treated with alpha-methyldopa (aldomet, see Chapter 40), another (346) caused acute hemolytic anemia in a patient being treated with chlorpropamide. In contrast, benign auto-anti-Jk^a has been reported in a blood donor (338) and in a healthy pregnant woman (340). Three benign examples of auto-anti-Jk^a were shown to react only in the presence of parabens and one (343) only in the presence of methyl esters of hydroxybenzoic acid (also a paraben). All four antibodies were initially detected in tests using commercially obtained LISS that contain parabens as preservatives.

Autoantibodies directed against S (355,356); Fy^b (357); Xg^a (358,359); Kx (360); Yt^{ab} (361,362); Co3 (363); Ge (76,222,364-367); Vel (368-371); Sc1 (372-374); Sc3 (375); AnWj (376-378); and Di^b (379) have been reported in addition to those already described in this section. Like virtually every specificity seen as an autoantibody, those listed above have sometimes been implicated as causative of WAIHA and sometimes have been found as benign autoantibodies in hematologically normal individuals. While not all examples of the specificity cause WAIHA, particularly severe cases of the disease have been caused by auto-anti-Ge (76,367) and auto-anti-Vel (371). Auto-anti-Di^b is discussed in more detail in a later section on the recognition of target antigens in WAIHA by the use of immunoprecipitation. Table 37-10 lists the specificities of "warm" reactive autoantibodies.

Depressed Expression of Rh (and Other) Antigens in WAIHA

As described in the previous section, depression of expression of red cell Kell system antigens in patients

TABLE 37-10 Target Antigens for Warm Reactive Autoantibodies

Blood Group System	Antigens against which autoantibodies have been directed *1
ABO	A, B
Rh	D, C, E, c, e, f, rh_i, G, etc. nl (Hr_0, Rh34), pdl (Rh29), Rh39
MN	M, N, S, U, En^aTS, En^aFS, En^aFR, En^aKT
Kell	Kp^b, K13, other Kell system antigens of high incidence
Duffy	Fy^b
Kidd	Jk^a, Jk^b, Jk3
LW	LW^a, LW^{ab}
Diego	Di^b, Wr^b
Scianna	Sc1, Sc3
Gerbich	Ge2, Ge3, Ge4
Others	Kx, Xg^a, Co3, Yt^{ab}, Vel, AnWj, dl
Still more*2	I^T, Pr, Rx

*1 Some of the autoantibodies have caused positive DATs but not in vivo hemolysis.
*2 More often targets for cold-reactive autoantibodies.

with WAIHA has been encountered a number of times. Apparently less often, a similar phenomenon affects antigens of the Rh system. Grabowska et al. (539) noticed this in an adult with WAIHA; exact details about their patient were not given. van't Veer et al. (540) described a young boy known to have WAIHA, in whom the autoantibodies were apparently directed against C and e. During a particularly severe hemolytic episode, the DAT on the child's red cells was negative and his red cells failed to react with autoantibodies directed against C and e (or perhaps with autoantibodies mimicking anti-C and anti-e). The depression of C and e on the child's red cells was not readily demonstrable using allo-anti-C and allo-anti-e. In spite of the negative DAT, very large amounts of autoantibody were present in the child's serum. We (541) encountered a somewhat similar case. This time a 22 month-old Black male presented with severe anemia (hemoglobin 3.2 g/100ml) of sudden onset and with clinical symptoms of WAIHA. The DAT was negative and the child's serum contained very strong antibodies, the specificity of which seemed most like anti-Hr and anti-hr^B in an inseparable form. Autoadsorption with the infant's DAT-negative red cells did not reduce the strength of the antibody even when ficin-treated autologous cells were used. In red cell phenotyping studies, the infant's cells appeared to carry normal amounts of c, a reduced expression of D and markedly reduced amounts of e, hr^S, hr^B, Hr and Hr_o. The reduced expressions of these antigens were equally well demonstrated in tests using allo and autoantibodies. Thus, in spite of the clinical picture and the presence of large numbers of spherocytes in the blood film, the case seemed to represent severe anemia of unknown etiology in an infant with a rare Rh phenotype in whom a complex specificity Rh alloantibody had been made. Two major observations were at variance with this conclusion. First, the infant was 22 months-old and had never been transfused so that no stimulus was known to explain the production of the potent IgG, apparent alloantibody. Second, a fairly extensive family study failed to produce any evidence for the presence of unusual *Rh* genes in the kindred. Because of the apparent alloimmunization, D--/D-- blood was transfused in the acute emergency and the infant made a good recovery. Ten months later, he again presented with anemia. This time the DAT was strongly positive and the antibodies previously detected were now shown to be autoimmune in nature. The child responded well to steroid therapy and when the DAT was reduced to 1+ it was possible to show (541) that the child's red cells would adsorb all antibody activity from a serum sample saved from the time of his first (DAT-negative) acute hemolytic episode. When the DAT eventually became negative, it was shown (542), using some of the sera used in the original tests, that his red cells carried normal amounts of D, e, hr^S, hr^B, Hr and Hr_o. It seems that on the first occasion that the infant had an acute hemolytic episode, his autoantibody had cleared most of his red cells and only those on which the Rh antigens were so reduced in expression that the autoantibody could not bind, had survived in vivo. The same can be said about the case of van't Veer et al. (540), the difference of reactivity of the red cells with allo and autoantibodies in the two cases may simply represent the sequence with which reduction of expression of Rh antigens occurs, i.e., Hr, Hr_o, etc., (nl) reduced first, C, e, etc., later. Thus, like the situation with the Kell system, reduction of expression of red cell Rh antigens may represent a protective mechanism in WAIHA. The mechanism responsible for reduced expression of Rh system antigens is not yet known.

As illustrated by the case of van't Veer et al. (540), this situation is readily recognizable in a patient already known to have WAIHA. As illustrated by our case (541,542), if red cell Rh antigen expression is so reduced in a patient's first hemolytic episode that the DAT is negative, confirmation of the autoimmune nature of the antibody may be impossible. Now that the situation has been recognized, WAIHA can be considered but it may be necessary to wait for red cell Rh antigen expression to revert to normal or near normal, before conclusive serological proof of that disease is obtained.

Vengelen-Tyler and Mogck (543) described two patients in whom red cell hr^B antigen levels were sufficiently depressed that the patients' autoantibodies at first appeared to be examples of allo-anti-hr^B. The cases differed from those described above in that although the DATs were negative, the autoantibodies were demonstrable in eluates made from the patients' red cells.

When the DAT is negative, WAIHA is suspected on clinical grounds, and the patient's serum contains what looks like an alloantibody to a high incidence antigen, a very real problem exists regarding selection of blood if the patient must be transfused. It is pointed out below, that when a patient with WAIHA must be transfused and no alloantibodies are present, blood incompatible with the autoantibody can be used. Thus the question was raised (544) as to whether searches for compatible units are necessary when the patient has an autoantibody in the serum, in spite of the negative DAT. The question is a good one since depression of e, hr^S, hr^B, etc., in patients who actually have autoantibodies, but appear to have alloantibodies, is probably more common than is generally appreciated (545). However, while blood incompatible with the autoantibody can be used in patients with WAIHA in whom no antigen depression has occurred, the situation may be rather different in the patients being described here. First, depression of antigen expression may result in the remaining red cells in the patient being protected from immune destruction by the autoantibody. Second, since the antigen is not expressed normally on the patient's red cells, but is on the cells of the donor, the transfusion of incompatible blood may well cause a transfusion reaction and/or clearance of the transfused red cells more quickly than would be the case if the patient's red cells carried the antigen and were able to compete in binding the antibody. Third, of course, if the DAT is negative and the patient's red cells will neither yield on elution, nor adsorb the antibody, it is not possible to be sure that the antibody is autoimmune and not alloimmune. As described above, such a determination can sometimes only be made with confidence months or years after the acute hemolytic episode, when expression of the antigen on the patient's red cells has returned to normal. Thus, somewhat regretfully, one of us (546) concluded that antibodies found in this setting must be regarded as being "temporarily alloimmune" and must be honored, whenever possible, by the transfusion of antigen-negative blood.

While the previous section considered depression of antigen expression in the Kell system and this one considers the phenomenon as it involves Rh system antigens, it can be added that similar depression has been seen to involve antigens of the LW (417,825); MN (162); Duffy (357,426); Kidd (344,349,427,428); Lutheran (333); Colton (363); Scianna (373); and Gerbich (222,365,366) systems as well.

In a later section of this chapter, WAIHA in other patients in whom the DAT is negative is described. In many of those cases the amount of autoantibody made is very small. It is for that reason that the cases described in the last two sections have been separated from others in which the DAT is negative. In the cases described in the above sections, the DAT was negative in spite of the presence of very large amounts of potent autoantibody in the patient's serum. In most of those described later, detection of the presence of any autoantibody was difficult.

WAIHA Caused by ABO System Autoantibodies

As mentioned in the introduction of this chapter, one of the current puzzles about WAIHA is why some autoantibodies (such as those with Rh system specificity) are seen so often, while others (such as those with ABO system specificity) are so rare. As would be expected, when an ABO autoantibody active at 37°C is formed, it causes very severe hemolytic anemia. The first such case reported seems to have been that documented by Szymanski et al. (380) in which an auto-anti-A that was either just IgG or was a mixture of IgG and IgM in nature, caused intravascular hemolysis in and rapid demise of a group A patient. A somewhat similar case described by Parker et al. (381), appeared to involve just IgM auto-anti-A. In some other cases (244,382-384) an ABO autoantibody was found to be reactive at 37°C but the dramatic hemolysis seen in the cases described above (380,381) was not seen. Perhaps these were actually more like cases of cold hemagglutinin disease (see Chapter 38) since the autoantibodies were optimally reactive at 0 to 4°C but apparently had a wide enough thermal range that some antibody binding occurred at 37°C. Similarly, in a series of cases of hemolytic anemia purportedly caused by ABO system autoantibodies described by Sokol et al. (245), it is not abundantly clear as to whether appreciable in vivo red cell destruction was occurring in all patients.

There are also a number of reports (385-392) describing hemolysis caused by ABO antibodies made by immunocytes from transplanted organs or bone marrow. This occurs when there is a minor side ABO incompatibility between the donor and the recipient. The situation does not represent true autoimmunization since donor-derived ABO antibodies directed against the patients' red cells are involved. However, the situation does represent true hemolytic anemia. Hemolysis most often begins five to eight days following transplantation and may persist for two weeks or a little longer. While this phenomenon is transient and resolves as the donor-derived immunocytes expire (solid organ transplants) or

the patient's red cells are cleared (bone marrow transplants), there is evidence (393,394) that red cell destruction involves more than simply the patient's own red cells. It seems that in the passenger lymphocyte syndrome, complement activation results in the destruction of some group O transfused red cells via bystander lysis. The phenomenon of excessive lysis in the passenger lymphocyte syndrome seems to be exacerbated when cyclosporine is used, it does not occur or is much milder if methotrexate but not cyclosporine is given (393,394). A case described by Contreras et al. (395) was unusual in that the anti-A_1 produced was apparently of the mimicking type (see below) and could be adsorbed to exhaustion with group O red cells.

WAIHA, Immunoprecipitation and Autoantibody Specificity Studies

In 1990, Victoria et al. (396) described the results of experiments in which they had used autoantibodies in immunoprecipitation studies in an attempt to identify the red cell membrane components that carry the target antigens for those autoantibodies. They concluded that those autoantibodies that cause hemolytic anemia are directed against epitopes on protein band 3 while those that cause positive DATs but no accelerated rate of in vivo red cell destruction (i.e. no hemolytic anemia) are directed against Rh polypeptides. In retrospect it seems that those conclusions were reached because too few autoantibodies were studied. First, as described in earlier sections of this chapter, serological studies have shown that autoantibodies directed against Rh antigens often cause WAIHA. Second, there is now direct evidence (see below) that some pathological warm-reactive autoantibodies precipitate Rh proteins but not band 3.

In 1992 Barker et al. (470) described studies in which they used autoantibodies causative of WAIHA in a non-radioisotypic immunoprecipitation method. Unlike Victoria et al. (396), Barker et al. (470) found that three pathological autoantibodies precipitated the Rh proteins while one precipitated an additional component. Further, serological studies on the autoantibodies showed complete correlation between antibody specificity and the components precipitated. In 1993, Leddy et al. (397) reported their results of immunoprecipitation studies using 20 warm-reactive autoantibodies, all of which were from patients with WAIHA. Nine of the 20 autoantibodies precipitated the Rh polypeptides, some of those autoantibodies also precipitated band 3, others did not. Five of the 20 autoantibodies precipitated band 3 alone while the remaining six coprecipitated band 3 and glycophorin A. Clearly, those autoantibodies that precipitated only the Rh polypeptides were similar to those described by Barker et al. (470) and would be expected to be ones (anti-dl or anti-pdl) that react with all except rare Rh-deletion and/or Rh_{null} red cells. A year after their original report, Leddy et al. (398) described specificity tests on the six autoantibodies that had coprecipitated band 3 and glycophorin A. As described in detail in Chapter 17, the Wr^b antigen requires both band 3 and a portion of glycophorin A to be present, for its expression. As described in an earlier section of this chapter, auto-anti-Wr^b sometimes occurs as the only antibody in an autoimmunized patient, much more frequently it is a component of autoantibodies that present as anti-dl. Thus, when Leddy et al. (398) ran serological tests on the six autoantibodies that coprecipitated band 3 and glycophorin A, they found that one was just anti-Wr^b, two were anti-Wr^b with at least one other component and a fourth probably contained an anti-Wr^b component. We (379) reasoned that since Di^b is also carried on protein band 3 (see Chapter 17) it would be likely that some autoantibodies that precipitate band 3 alone or coprecipitate band 3 and glycophorin A would be, or would contain auto-anti-Di^b. Lacking the facilities (and expertise) to perform immunoprecipitation studies, we approached the question from a serological direction. We tested 119 examples of anti-dl, some from patients with WAIHA and some from individuals in whom the anti-dl was benign, against Di(a+b-) red cells; all 119 reacted showing that no anti-dl was just anti-Di^b. We then adsorbed 74 of the 119 anti-dl with Di(a+b-) red cells until they no longer reacted with those cells and tested the adsorbed autoantibodies against Di(b+) red cells. Two of the 74 still reacted with the Di(b+) red cells thus showing that the original anti-dl from those patients contained a separable auto-anti-Di^b component. Of the two patients with auto-anti-Di^b, one had hemolytic anemia, the other did not.

It is noteworthy that of two very common antigens on band 3, one, Wr^b, is frequently a target of warm-reactive autoantibodies while the other, Di^b, only rarely fills that role. That is to say, in tests on 110 examples of anti-dl we (113) found that 4 (3.6%) were anti-Wr^b while 42 (38%) contained an anti-Wr^b component. In contrast (379) of 119 anti-dl, none was only anti-Di^b and only 2 of 74 (2.7%) tested by adsorption, contained anti-Di^b. While there is currently no explanation as to why Wr^b is a common and Di^b a rare target for autoantibodies, there are some known differences between the antigens. First, Wr^b represents an amino acid polymorphism on protein band 3 and an interaction of band 3 with a portion of glycophorin A. Di^b apparently represents only an amino acid polymorphism of band 3. There is ample evidence (see Chapter 12) that the other common targets for autoantibodies, the Rh epitopes, represent interaction products of several red cell membrane structures. Thus, perhaps "complex" structures (i.e. Rh and Wr^b) attract the attention of autoreactive clones of immunocytes

more readily than do "simple" structures (i.e. Di^b). Second, the Wr^a/Wr^b polymorphism on band 3 is located on the fourth extracellular loop of band 3 close to the attachment site of the single N-glycan of the protein (399-401). The Di^a/Di^b polymorphism is located on an external loop of the protein that is distal to the glycosylation site. Perhaps glycosylation is involved in the relative immunogenicity of autoantigens with the Rh-related glycoproteins (402-404) providing such glycosylation of Rh-associated autoantigens. Also awaiting an explanation is the very high incidence of alloimmune anti-Wr^a, that also defines an epitope on band 3, in the sera of patients with WAIHA (405-407).

WAIHA and Autoantibodies with Mimicking Specificities

As mentioned above, autoantibodies with simple specificity are the exception rather than the rule in WAIHA. Further, many autoantibodies that at first seem to have such simple specificity can be shown actually to have a specificity closer to anti-nl (see table 37-9) than to the specificity that seems apparent from initial antibody identification studies. We (408-412) studied 48 antibodies from persons with a positive DAT, not all of whom had WAIHA, that seemed to be directed against D, C, c, E, e, rh_i or G. In adsorption studies, we found that 34 of the 48 (71%) could be adsorbed (often to exhaustion) with red cells that were of normal Rh phenotype but that lacked the antigen against which the antibody was apparently directed. For example, an antibody might appear to have anti-c specificity in an initial panel study. In adsorption studies, that antibody could be adsorbed to exhaustion by one adsorption with rr (cde/cde) red cells *or* by three adsorptions with R_1R_1 (CDe/CDe) cells. Further, eluates made from the CDe/CDe cells used in the adsorption studies, contained what again appeared to be anti-c. We concluded that these antibodies with mimicking specificities were in fact, examples of anti-nl that had a preference for red cells carrying certain Rh antigens. In other words, the apparent anti-c reacted in IATs with c+ red cells either because those cells carry more of the antigen defined or have the antigen sterically arranged in such a manner that enough antibody can bind for the IAT to be positive. Red cells with a normal Rh phenotype, that lacked c, bound the antibody (as shown by the adsorption studies) but in too small an amount for the IAT to be positive. Of the 34 mimicking antibodies studied, 32 had anti-nl specificity as shown by the fact that red cells of any normal Rh phenotype would adsorb them, while Rh-deletion and Rh_{null} red cells would not (410). The other two had anti-Rh39 specificity (see above) and were completely adsorbed by cells of normal

Rh phenotype and by Rh-deletion, but not by Rh_{null} cells (291,410,411). All 32 examples of anti-nl, with mimicking specificity for other Rh antigens that we studied, were autoimmune in nature. We then learned that Rosenfield (413) had found similar mimicking specificities among examples of allo-anti-Hr and allo-anti-Hr_0 made by persons with rare Rh phenotypes. As shown in table 37-9, auto-anti-nl and allo-anti-Hr/Hr_0 have similar patterns of reactivity when tested against red cells with unusual Rh phenotypes.

When the autoantibody with a mimicking specificity is made by an individual whose red cells are positive for the antigen that appears to be defined, the fact that the antibody is of a mimicking and not a real specificity is not of great importance. As discussed above, the amount and rate of in vivo red cell destruction in a patient with WAIHA is largely related to the type and amount of IgG that binds to the red cells. In other words, an antibody that binds preferentially to c+ red cells will clear those red cells (if enough IgG of an appropriate subclass binds) regardless of whether the antibody is anti-c or anti-nl mimicking anti-c.

When the autoantibody with a mimicking specificity is made by an individual whose red cells lack the antigen that appears to be defined, a confusing serological picture will result unless the mimicking nature of the autoantibody is recognized. For example, if the patient's red cells are E- and the antibody appears to have anti-E specificity, it will appear that the antibody is allo and not autoimmune in nature. Demonstration that the apparent anti-E binds to, can be eluted from and can be adsorbed by the patient's or other E- red cells, will reveal the autoimmune status of the antibody. In our studies (291,408-410) 29 of 34 mimicking antibodies were in patients whose red cells carried the antigen against which the antibody at first appeared to be directed. In the other five cases, three involving antibodies that appeared to define E and one each of antibodies that appeared to define C and rh_i, the patient's red cells lacked the antigen that the antibody appeared to define so that adsorption studies were necessary to demonstrate the autoimmune nature of the antibody. In our studies, 16 of the 34 mimicking autoantibodies were in patients with WAIHA, 15 in patients who had formed autoantibodies while being treated with alpha-methyldopa (aldomet) and 3 in hematologically normal individuals with a positive DAT. Of the five autoantibodies made in persons whose red cells lacked the antigen apparently defined, three were in patients with WAIHA, one in a patient receiving aldomet and one in a hematologically normal individual with a positive DAT.

When we (410) tested eluates made from the red cells of patients who had formed autoantibodies with mimicking specificities, we found that all the recovered antibody was of the mimicking type. When we tested the sera of such patients we found that they often contained some mimicking and some real specificity antibody. In other words, when the eluate contained what appeared to be anti-e, but what was in fact a mimicking autoantibody, three adsorptions with e- red cells would invariably adsorb the apparent anti-e to exhaustion. When we tested the serum of such a patient, we found that after three adsorptions the titer of apparent anti-e might well have been reduced (i.e. mimicking antibody adsorbed) but that three subsequent adsorptions effected no further reduction in antibody strength (i.e. remaining serum antibody had real anti-e specificity and would not bind to e- red cells). We found this often to be the case when the antibody appeared to define an antigen not present on the patient's red cells. In studies completed after our data had been published, we (414) found that in some 75% of cases in which the antibody appeared to define an antigen not present on the patient's red cells, the eluate contained only a mimicking antibody while the serum contained part mimicking and part real specificity antibody. It seems that in some persons who become alloimmunized, an autoantibody of ostensibly similar but actually different specificity, is simultaneously produced. There are numerous examples in the literature (39,47,79,87,415-425) of allo and autoimmunization occurring concurrently. Further, there is evidence (60-66) that when an alloimmune response begins, the antibody made is of low affinity. Such an antibody may cross-react with the antibody-maker's red cells and may thus have the characteristics, described above, of an autoantibody that mimics an alloantibody. As the alloimmune response is refined, an antigen driven mechanism (66) appears to result in preferential selection of those clones of B cells making antibody of high affinity. In a normal immune response such selective pressures result in expansion of the clones making high affinity antibody (alloantibody in this example) to the exclusion of clones making antibody of low affinity (autoantibody mimicking an alloantibody in this example). However, if the immune response is defective, cessation of antibody production by the clones making antibody of low affinity may not occur and high affinity (alloantibody) and low affinity (mimicking specificity) antibody production may continue. In support of such a concept it can be pointed out that in many of the patients in whom mimicking antibodies are seen, the immune response is not normal, i.e. many of them have WAIHA. To summarize this section, the most common finding (412) is that the patient has a positive DAT, the eluate contains only mimicking specificity antibody while the serum contains mimicking antibody and real antibody of the specificity mimicked. While it is often assumed that mimicking specificities are seen only in persons whose red cells lack the antigen against which the mimicking antibody appears to be directed, this is not true. In other words, in some instances the antibody will appear to be an autoantibody and only adsorption tests with antigen-negative red cells, i.e., not from the antibody-maker, will reveal the mimicking nature of the antibody.

In addition to the interest they generate at the academic level, partially adsorbed autoantibodies that mimic alloantibodies are of considerable practical importance in transfusion therapy. Accordingly these antibodies are considered again, below, in the section dealing with selection of blood for transfusion to patients with WAIHA. Table 37-11 shows the apparent specificities of the mimicking antibodies that we studied (410). As can be seen, when an autoantibody appears to have anti-E or anti-e specificity, there is a high probability that it will be of the mimicking type. When an autoantibody appears to be anti-D, there is a higher probability that it will actually have anti-D specificity.

While the initial studies (408-414) were primarily concerned with autoantibodies that mimic Rh system alloantibodies, the phenomenon is by no means confined to the Rh system. Mimicking antibodies, often seen concurrently with depression of red cell antigen expression (see an earlier section of this chapter) have now been found in many blood group systems, i.e., at least: ABO (395); MN (162,429); Kell (329,330,352,429); Duffy (357,426); Kidd (341,427-429); Lutheran (429) and Colton (363).

WAIHA and Autoantibodies Directed Against Red Cells of Different Ages

As discussed in Chapter 38, cold-reactive autoantibodies sometimes react more strongly with older or stored red cells, than with younger or fresh ones. Some early studies (430-432), while describing cold-reactive autoantibodies with this characteristic, paved the way for the discovery of warm-reactive autoantibodies with a similar preference. First, several of the antibodies studied (431,432) had a wide enough thermal range that they had some ability to bind to red cells at 37°C. Second, some

of the patients (431) involved responded to corticosteroid therapy (see below), a finding more characteristic of WAIHA than of cold hemagglutinin disease.

In 1983, Gray et al. (433), while investigating the difference of some antigen levels on reticulocytes and mature red cells, found that four of five warm reactive IgG autoantibodies bound in greater quantities to mature red cells than to reticulocytes. In 1984, Branch et al. (434) reported their results from a study on autoantibodies made by 24 patients with WAIHA. It was shown that in 19 of the cases, the autoantibodies reacted exclusively or preferentially with older red cells in the patients' circulation. Indeed in seven of the cases, the DAT on a reticulocyte enriched preparation of the patient's red cells was negative. The autoantibody reacting exclusively or preferentially with older red cells was called type I. In the other five patients, the autoantibodies, that were called type II, reacted equally with young and old red cells. The type of autoantibody reacting equally with young and old red cells was associated (434) with more severe hemolytic anemia than the type reacting exclusively or preferentially with older red cells. It was suggested (434) that the type I autoantibody represented pathological over expression of the normal physiological autoantibody responsible for the clearance of senescent red cells. As discussed in Chapter 6, one of the postulated mechanisms for the clearance of red cells at the end of their in vivo life span is that a structure becomes exposed on band 3, that a physiological IgG antibody present at low levels in all individuals binds to that antigen, and that macrophage sequestration and destruction of the IgG-coated red cells follows (435). The structure exposed on aged red cells has been called the senescent cell antigen (SCA), the normal antibody present in low levels in all individuals has been called anti-SCA. Thus it was suggested (434) that the type I antibody might represent excess production of anti-SCA. In 1989, Arndt et al. (436) studied an autoantibody causative of WAIHA, that reacted preferentially with old cells. The autoantibody was inhibited by synthetic SCA (437) leading Arndt et al. (436) and Garratty (353) to conclude that the type I autoantibody of Branch et al. (434) and the anti-SCA of Kay (435,437) are the same thing, albeit present in different amounts in health and WAIHA. A little

TABLE 37-11 Incidence of Mimicking Specificity Autoantibodies Shown in Terms of Apparent Specificity (from 410)

	Apparent specificity based on initial antibody identification study						
	Anti-C	Anti-c	Anti-D	Anti-E	Anti-e	Anti-G	Anti-rh$_i$
Number tested	4	2	8	5	24	1	4
Number with mimicking specificity	3	2	3	4	20	0	2
Number with real specificity	1	0	5	1	4	1	2

earlier, Herron et al. (438) had described a patient with hemolytic anemia and a negative DAT, in whom an IgM auto-anti-e could be recovered by elution from the patient's red cells. The auto-anti-e had a marked preference for older e+ red cells and reacted poorly with the patient's cells. When the patient went into remission, the auto-anti-e reacted equally with the patient's and other e+ red cells. It was suggested that during the hemolytic episode the younger red cells in the patient's circulation survived better than the older ones, hence the weaker reaction of the auto-anti-e with the patient's cells at that time. This observation is somewhat more difficult to explain via the SCA, anti-SCA mechanism described above. Although Rh antigens may well be expressed in lower levels on erythroid precursor cells than on mature red cells (439,440), claims (433,441) that Rh antigen levels increase as red cells age and are higher on older cells than on reticulocytes, have not been unequivocally substantiated. Indeed, in a study in which reticulocyte enrichment of the "younger" red cell population was greater than that in the study of Ballas et al. (441) in which it was reported that Rh antigen levels increase as red cells age, Reeves (827) found no significant differences in Rh antigen levels between "young" and "old" red cells. Further, it would be difficult to implicate the SCA on band 3 if the auto-anti-e was causing the hemolysis (438).

Although in the study of Branch et al. (434) autoantibodies reacting preferentially with older red cells or reacting equally with old and young cells were described, it seems that on rare occasions an autoantibody is present that reacts exclusively or preferentially with erythroid precursor cells in the marrow. When a patient with WAIHA also has reticulocytopenia the clinical condition is very serious. That is to say, acute red cell hemolysis is occurring and far too few new red cells are being released from the marrow for even partial compensation of the anemia. The laboratory findings can be quite difficult to interpret. In some cases (442,826) autoantibodies directed against erythroid progenitor cells can be demonstrated but these are sometimes (442,443) accompanied by autoantibodies that react strongly with mature red cells. The autoantibody directed against mature red cells is easy to demonstrate in in vitro studies, the one directed against erythroid precursor cells is not. Hedge et al. (444) described three patients with immune hemolytic anemia and reticulocytopenia, in whom the DAT was negative. Further evidence that the autoantibody directed against the erythroid precursor cells and that directed against mature red cells are distinct, was provided by Mangan et al. (442). No matter whether the autoantibody directed against erythroid precursor cells can be demonstrated in vitro, red cell aplasia, as evidenced by reticulocytopenia, superimposed on WAIHA results in a medical emergency. As described in a later section, transfusion is best avoided in patients with WAIHA. In those patients with WAIHA and red cell aplasia, prompt trans-

fusion may be essential as a life-saving maneuver.

WAIHA and Autoantibodies Directed Against Phospholipids

Some of the antibodies causative of WAIHA that defy attempts made to establish blood group specificity (i.e. anti-dl in spite of extensive differential adsorptions) seem to be directed against negatively charged membrane phospholipids (445-449,767-770). Indeed, there is now evidence (445,448,450) that the positive DAT, sometimes associated with complement activation, and the hemolysis in some patients with systemic lupus erythematosus, may be caused by anti-phospholipids. Studies on autoantibodies in non-human species have often revealed that they are anti-phospholipid in nature (534-538).

Some Other Autoantibodies

Based on their observations that eluates from DAT+ red cells sometimes contain more IgG than the amount calculated to be present on the red cells from which the eluates were made, Masouredis et al. (451) suggested that some of the IgG eluted might be anti-idiotype or anti-Fab to the autoantibody. Additional studies (452) seemed to confirm this concept and it was suggested that the anti-idiotype (or anti-Fab) might be protective against macrophage-induced red cell clearance. In tests on a small number of subjects, those with hemolytic anemia had autoantibody but no anti-idiotype while those with a positive DAT but no anemia, had autoantibody and anti-idiotype.

Some autoantibodies described in the literature have been directed against components of the red cell cytoskeleton. Wiener et al. (453) found IgG anti-spectrin in eluates made from the red cells of patients with beta-thalassemia but not in eluates made from the red cells of patients with sickle cell disease nor those of normal donors. Wakui et al. (454) found anti-protein 4.1 in a patient with WAIHA. The meaning of these findings is not entirely clear since neither spectrin nor protein 4.1 is normally exposed on the red cell membrane. Of note, the patient with anti-protein 4.1 described by Wakui et al. (454) also had auto-anti-S and an autoantibody that resembled anti-En^a in his serum, while his brother, who did not have WAIHA, had anti-protein 4.1. Further, there are a number of reports (455,464,465,533) of what have been described as naturally-occurring antibodies to spectrin, actin and protein band 6 in normal healthy individuals.

While there are some claims of abnormalities of the red cell membrane in patients with WAIHA (466,467, 772,773), evidence for increased proteolysis of the red cells in vitro (468), and a suggestion that a mechanical factor may contribute to hemolysis (469), it is far from clear whether these effects contribute to hemolysis or are effects of autoantibody binding in vivo.

WAIHA, IATs and Eluates, Value of Determining Autoantibody Specificity

As has been mentioned above, the amount and rate of in vivo red cell destruction in patients with WAIHA is largely determined by the type and amount of IgG that becomes red cell bound. In this respect, autoantibody specificity is of little importance. There is not much correlation between specificity of the causative autoantibody and severity of disease in the patient. In spite of this, there are at least two good reasons for knowing something about the specificity of autoantibodies causative of WAIHA. First, it is hoped that by learning about the nature of the causative autoantibodies and the structure of antigens against which they are directed, something can be learned about the etiology of the disease so that better methods of treatment can be devised and so that eventually prevention of the disease will become possible. Along these lines some interesting findings have been made. While it has been thought that non-production of autoantibodies represents clonal deletion (15,18,22, 524,525,527) or anergy (15,18,528-530), it is also clear (471) that some potentially autoreactive B cells survive such processes and can be stimulated to produce autoantibodies. It has been shown (472,531,532) that both murine and human T-cells can be specifically stimulated, in vitro, by autologous red cells. Once auto-stimulated, the T-cells proliferate and secrete IL-2. Of considerable interest to immunohematologists, Barker and Elson (473) have shown that small synthetic Rh polypeptides representing sequences present on the red cells of subjects from whom the T-cells were isolated, stimulate immunologically ignorant T-cells in vitro. In other words, an early portion of an immune response to a host or self antigen was reproduced in an in vitro model.

The second reason for determining autoantibody specificity is more practical. When a clinician requests a DAT on the blood of a patient who may have WAIHA, an IAT is usually requested as well. In fact, the request for the IAT is a misnomer. As blood bankers know, the IAT will be positive if the patient has alloantibody or autoantibody present in the serum. It is the latter of these situations that is of interest to the clinician. As described below, one form of treatment of patients with WAIHA is to effect suppression of autoantibody production. The speed with which that goal can be accomplished is related to the total amount of autoantibody being made by the patient. If the DAT is positive and no autoantibody is demonstrable in the serum it follows that the amount of

autoantibody being made is somewhat limited because it has almost all bound to the patient's red cells in vivo. If the DAT is strongly positive and autoantibody is present in the serum, it is clear that more autoantibody is being made than when none is demonstrable in the serum. In other words, the patient's red cells are saturated with autoantibody and the excess is in the serum where it effects a positive IAT. Obviously, if the clinician wishes to know whether excess autoantibody is present in the serum and in fact none is there, but the IAT is positive because the patient also has an alloantibody, a report simply stating that the IAT is positive will mislead instead of help the clinician. This problem must be resolved in the blood bank. If the IAT is positive, serological studies are necessary to determine why the test is positive. The specificity of the antibody in the serum and that of the autoantibody eluted from the patient's red cells must be compared to determine whether the antibody in the serum is allo or autoimmune in nature. This does not mean that every autoantibody encountered in every patient with WAIHA must be tested with D--, Rh$_{null}$, LW(a-b-), U-, En(a-), K$_o$, etc., red cells to determine its exact specificity. If the eluted autoantibody and the antibody present in the serum, each react by IAT with all red cells on an antibody identification panel, each can be described as typical of the autoantibodies that cause WAIHA and the clinician's question as to whether excess autoantibody is present in the serum, can be answered. Most workers who regularly test the blood of patients with WAIHA, determine specificities such as those illustrated in tables 37-9 and 37-10, only when trying to answer a specific question, e.g., what is the incidence of auto-anti-Wr^b in WAIHA? In tests intended to confirm a clinical diagnosis of WAIHA, it is sufficient simply to establish that the autoantibody is typical of those causative of WAIHA, as described above. The chance that one patient will have auto-anti-dl on the red cells and say allo-anti-Yt^a in the serum (that will also react with all red cells on most panels so will look like anti-dl) is very small. Thus, in patients suspected of having WAIHA, whose sera contain antibody activity, simple comparative studies of the specificities of the eluted and serum antibodies are sufficient, exact specificity need not be determined in every case (the detection of alloantibodies in sera that contain autoantibodies is discussed below under the heading of transfusion in WAIHA).

In studies undertaken to determine the exact specificity of autoantibodies causative of WAIHA, it has been shown (47,110,111,113,115) that the autoantibody on the patient's red cells and that present in the serum are not always completely identical. It is not particularly unusual to find that an eluate contains, say anti-dl, while the serum contains anti-pdl. Presumably mixtures of autoantibodies of slightly different specificities (we

(113) found 191 autoantibodies in 87 patients with WAIHA and there were certainly others that could have been recognized if different red cells had been available for adsorption studies) include some with higher affinity than others, for antigens on the patient's red cells. Further, if the same patients are studied over a period of time, it is found (47,93,474-476) that in many, the specificities of the autoantibodies change. The most frequently seen pattern (47,93) is that the first autoantibody made has a relatively simple specificity (e.g. auto-anti-e) and that gradually the specificity broadens to say anti-nl and eventually to anti-dl. However, since many patients with WAIHA do not seek medical help until the disease is relatively advanced, a large proportion of patients will be found to have anti-nl, anti-pdl or anti-dl present, the first time a blood sample is studied. Since those and many other autoantibodies (see tables 37-9 and 37-10) causative of WAIHA react with all red cells on most antibody identification panels, the point made above, about comparing the specificities of the antibodies causing the positive DAT and the positive IAT, is not compromised.

Table 37-12 lists figures that show the frequencies with which autoantibodies were found in the sera of patients with WAIHA in two studies. It is important to appreciate that serum autoantibody detection in both series was via standard IATs. If more sensitive tests, such as those that use LISS, PEG, Polybrene or enzyme-treated red cells are used, the incidence figures for the presence of free autoantibody in the serum will be much higher, i.e. circa 90 to 100%. However, such data are of little value to a clinician accustomed to using the results of a DAT and an IAT as a rough guide to the total amount of autoantibody being made in an individual patient. The reason for the different incidence figures in table 37-12 is probably that in our series we (113) tested patients with long standing WAIHA while the series of Petz and Garratty (47) includes many patients seen early in the course of the disease.

Cold-reactive Autoagglutinins in Patients with WAIHA

A fair number of patients with WAIHA have cold-reactive autoagglutinins in the serum that have a thermal range that is wider and a titer that is higher than the majority of such autoantibodies in healthy individuals. Petz and Garratty (47) reported such findings in about 30% of their patients with WAIHA but said that in most instances the cold-reactive autoantibodies were not destroying red cells in vivo. They pointed out that if the serological findings of the WAIHA are not typical, there is a danger that the patient's condition may be misdiagnosed as CHD. We (477) noticed that the occurrence of

auto-anti-i is somewhat more frequent in persons with WAIHA than in persons who do not have hemolytic anemia, but that the auto-anti-i seem not to contribute to the in vivo red cell clearance.

Patients with Warm and Cold Antibody-Induced Hemolytic Anemia

Although as described in the previous section, the cold autoagglutinins in patients with WAIHA do not usually contribute to in vivo red cell destruction, there are some well documented cases (47,239,241,478-483) of patients with WAIHA and CHD. Since WAIHA is usually a polyclonal (perhaps more accurately an oligoclonal) disorder, while idiopathic CHD usually represents proliferation of one abnormal clone of immunocytes (so is perhaps closer to a liquid tumor, see Chapter 38) it can be presumed that in some of these patients, two pathological conditions existed. As yet there is no clearly documented single immune defect that would be expected to result in the production of polyclonal warm-reactive and monoclonal cold-reactive autoantibodies.

WAIHA, Treatment, Steroids and Splenectomy

Although a full description of treatment of patients with WAIHA is beyond the scope of this book, some details will be given since treatment often relates directly to laboratory findings in the disorder. As will be seen by comparing this section with the one on treatment in CHD in Chapter 38, one of the more valuable benefits of laboratory tests in patients with WAIHA and CHD is to differentiate between the causative autoantibodies because the diseases respond to different forms of treatment.

As mentioned already in this chapter, one of the prime forms of treatment in WAIHA is suppression of autoantibody production. The objective is to reduce the level of autoantibody being made to a point where too few

TABLE 37-12 To Show the Incidence of Serum Autoantibodies in Patients with WAIHA, as Detected in Saline IATs*

Series of	Number of Patients	Number with autoantibody in the serum	Percent with autoantibody in the serum
Issitt et al. (113)	87	68	78
Petz and Garratty (47)	244	139	57

* If more sensitive tests are used, the incidence is higher (see text).

molecules are bound per red cell for macrophage-induced sequestration and destruction to occur. Even if this goal cannot be achieved, it may be possible to reduce the rate of in vivo red cell destruction, by reducing the amount of autoantibody made and the level of IgG per red cell, to a point at which the marrow can compensate by making additional red cells, so that the anemia is corrected. The most usual way to attempt suppression of autoantibody production is to treat the patient with a corticosteroid (prednisone and prednisilone are most commonly used). Once the diagnosis of WAIHA is made and if there is severe anemia, high doses of steroids are given. As a hematological response is seen (i.e. patient's red cells surviving better in vivo so that anemia is being corrected) the dose of steroids is gradually reduced. If a complete remission is induced by steroid therapy, an attempt to taper and then withdraw the drug is made to avoid the side-effects of long term steroid therapy. In some patients, autoantibody production can be reduced to the point where steroids can be withdrawn and the remission may last for months or years. If autoantibody production gradually increases, after steroid therapy has been stopped, and again reaches the point where appreciable red cell destruction occurs, a further course of steroids is given. In other patients it may not be possible totally to withdraw steroids since such an action results in an increase of in vivo red cell destruction and anemia again develops. Some of those patients can be successfully treated with low dose steroid maintenance therapy. In patients in whom WAIHA is the only or major clinical condition, good responses are seen. Some 80 to 90% of patients have a response to steroids, in as many as two thirds of them a complete remission may be induced. In patients who have WAIHA secondary to another disorder, it is frequently necessary that the primary disease be controlled in order that the WAIHA be alleviated. Exacerbation of hemolysis in treated patients who become infected has been described earlier, in the section that deals with macrophage activity in in vivo red cell destruction. In those patients in whom steroid therapy is ineffectual, other forms of immunosuppression such as use of azathioprine or cyclophosphamide, may be necessary. With a severely anemic patient, the clinician must try to decide rapidly whether to continue with steroids and hope for a response or whether to substitute a different immunosuppressant. As discussed above, the presence or absence of serum autoantibody is of importance in this consideration. In a patient in whom the DAT is positive but no serum autoantibody is present (IAT-negative) an early response to steroids is expected. In one in whom the DAT is positive and excess autoantibody is present in the serum, the clinician may decide to persevere longer with steroids (more autoantibody to suppress) before concluding that the patient is a non-responder to that form of therapy. Clearly, a laboratory report that the IAT is positive when the antibody responsible is alloimmune in nature and is not contributing to the hemolytic process, can be misleading unless properly explained.

It is of considerable interest to blood bankers that when steroid therapy is efficient in suppressing autoantibody production, alloantibodies being simultaneously made are little affected. In other words, in a D- patient making allo-anti-D and auto-anti-nl (both of which are Rh antibodies) steroid therapy may suppress production of the anti-nl to the point that it is no longer demonstrable in serological tests, but the anti-D will usually be produced at about the same level as before initiation of therapy. It seems that while steroids act on immunocytes participating in an autoimmune response, they have little effect on cells participating in a normal one. Measurement of a response to steroids in a patient with WAIHA, by demonstrating that the amount of autoantibody being made is less, is discussed below in the section dealing with quantitation of IgG autoantibody levels.

Suppression of autoantibody production is not the only result of steroid therapy. There is evidence (211,484) that the ability of macrophages to bind IgG-coated red cells is reduced when steroids are used. This may well represent a steroid-induced reduction in number of Fc receptors on the macrophages (212). Further, when steroid therapy is first started, the amount of autoantibody on red cells may be reduced while the amount in the serum may increase, before the total amount produced is reduced. This finding suggests (485) that steroids may interfere with the ability of autoantibodies to bind to red cells. While both effects described above are helpful in the rapid alleviation of an acute hemolytic episode in a patient with WAIHA, it seems that the major long-term benefit of such therapy is suppression of autoantibody production as described above.

Another form of drug treatment for which success has been claimed (486-488,771) in patients with WAIHA, involves use of the vinca alkaloids (periwinkle alkaloids, vincristine and vinblastine). These compounds are known (489) to suppress both humoral and cellular immunity and appear to have a direct suppressive effect on macrophages (490-494). Since the vinca alkaloids are cleared rapidly from circulation in man (495,496), they must be infused slowly to ensure that therapeutic levels are attained (486,488), or can be attached to platelets that are also coated with IgG antibody, so that drugs are delivered directly to macrophages (via sequestration of the IgG-coated platelets) once they are infused (487). It seems that most clinicians treating patients with WAIHA prefer to use steroids than to use vinca alkaloids.

Another form of treatment that may be of benefit in patients with WAIHA, is splenectomy. As described earlier, the spleen is a major site of tissue-bound macrophages that carry IgG receptors. Thus removal of that organ removes the site at which many IgG-coated red cells are sequestered and destroyed. Some clinicians feel that splenectomy is of most benefit in patients with WAIHA who have IgG but no C3 on their red cells. As will be remembered, red cells coated with IgG and C3 are sequestered largely in the liver. However, other clinicians believe that this correlation does not hold and that patients who present with IgG and C3 on their red cells have as much chance of benefit from splenectomy as those whose red cells carry only IgG. Certainly there are many patients with WAIHA who have benefited from splenectomy regardless of which proteins were present on their red cells. The probable explanation of benefit from splenectomy, in patients with appreciable hepatic red cell sequestration and destruction, is that the spleen is involved in more than just red cell sequestration and destruction. It is one of the major sites of antigen processing and is involved in antibody production (15-18,497,498) so that its removal can be expected to help patients making warm-reactive autoantibodies.

It should now be pointed out that steroid therapy and splenectomy are not usually used independently. Typically, a patient who presents with WAIHA and is severely anemic, will not be in a suitable physical condition to undergo immediate splenectomy (although that is sometimes necessary in severe cases and is then undertaken with presurgical transfusion support and similar support at surgery). Thus in many patients, steroids will be used to induce a remission so that the anemia is at least partially corrected by longer survival of the patient's own red cells. Once the patient is in a more stable condition a splenectomy may be performed. This is sometimes the case even in patients who respond well to steroids, so that lower doses of steroids can be used post-splenectomy. After the splenectomy has been performed, it may still be necessary to treat the patient with steroids. If such drugs are not used, the level of autoantibody made may increase to the point at which a large amount is present. Red cells coated with high levels of IgG, in the absence of C3, may then be sequestered and destroyed in the liver so that the benefit of removal of the spleen, the previous major site of red cell sequestration and destruction, will be negated. On the other hand, some patients can have steroid therapy withdrawn following splenectomy and can be monitored to make sure that autoantibody production does not again approach dangerous levels.

As will be noticed, this discussion of treatment in WAIHA has seldom mentioned blood transfusion. Although the major clinical problems in WAIHA represent anemia due to a reduced red cell mass, the anemia is not simple and cannot be permanently corrected by blood transfusion. Some potential contraindications for transfusion are discussed in the next section.

WAIHA, Treatment, Transfusion

As discussed in the previous section, a major aim in treating patients who have WAIHA is to try to reduce the level of autoantibody being made. As discussed in the sections on autoantibody specificity, compatible blood is seldom available for transfusion to these patients since the autoantibodies react with all except very rare red cells. Units of such red cells must be reserved for alloimmunized patients so are not generally available for patients with WAIHA. The net result is that when a patient with WAIHA must be transfused, red cells incompatible with the autoantibody must be given. Many workers worry that this introduction of additional antigen will stimulate the production of more autoantibody and thus counter the effects of steroid therapy. Indeed, there is anecdotal evidence that transfusion too early in WAIHA worsens the long term prognosis of the patient. The effect (increase in level of autoantibody) is not immediate but may be noticed months or years later. Some clinicians believe that patients with WAIHA who have been transfused are more difficult to control with steroid therapy; require larger maintenance doses of the drug and are less likely to respond favorably. It is also felt that premature transfusion may cause a more rapid widening of specificity of the autoantibody made (say from auto-anti-e to auto-anti-dl) than occurs in patients, treated with steroids, who are not transfused. This widening of autoantibody specificity is often accompanied (284) by the change from IgG only to IgG and C3 on the patient's red cells. As discussed in the section on in vivo red cell destruction in WAIHA, red cells coated with IgG and C3 are often more rapidly cleared than those coated only with IgG.

The counter to this anecdotal evidence and a view held by other workers, is that early need for transfusion simply indicates that such patients had a more severe form of WAIHA than those in whom transfusion was not necessary. In other words, the patients who were transfused are more difficult to treat because they have severe WAIHA. One of us (PDI) subscribes to the first school of thought, that too early transfusion worsens the patient's long term prognosis. He has seen a series of patients treated by physicians who knew little about WAIHA and tried to correct the anemia with transfusions. Many of these patients were transfused when not particularly anemic, i.e. hemoglobin 9 or 10 g/dl and some others were given numerous transfusions before being referred to a clinician with expertise in treating WAIHA. Many of these patients then had stormy courses and it is difficult to accept that, by coincidence, they all had severe WAIHA and that their long term problems were not in some way related to the fact that they were transfused too soon. The author (PDI) has also seen patients with severe anemia, i.e. hemoglobin 3 or 4g/dl who were treated with steroids, bed rest and supportive oxygen so that transfusions could be avoided, who have later had prolonged steroid-induced remissions. It seems that some of those patients would have to be classified as having severe WAIHA and that they apparently benefited from the fact that transfusions were avoided. Mollison et al. (233) stipulate that transfusion is indicated only in special circumstances, e.g. severe anemia precipitating cardiac failure, neurological signs from or rapidly progressive anemia, preparation for splenectomy. To reduce the need for transfusion, measures such as bed rest and supportive oxygen are recommended while the hemoglobin level is monitored in anticipation of a steroid-induced response. Mollison et al. (233) also recommend that if transfusions must be given, packed red cells should be used only in sufficient quantities to raise the hemoglobin to a level that will permit other therapy to be used.

No matter whether or not one believes that premature transfusions are contraindicated in WAIHA, there are some patients with the disease in whom transfusion is unavoidable. However, the decision to transfuse must be made on clinical grounds and not be based on laboratory values. In other words, when cardiac complications develop and the anemia becomes life-threatening, the patient must be transfused regardless of the hemoglobin level. While it may be possible to manage one patient with a hemoglobin of 3g/dl with bed rest and supportive oxygen therapy while a steroid-induced remission is sought, it may be necessary to transfuse another, who has a higher level of hemoglobin, because of cardiac decompensation. Pirofsky (499) captured the essence of the situation when he wrote that, it is the patient not the hemoglobin level or the physician's apprehensions that must be transfused. Once the clinical decision to transfuse has been made, it is usually necessary to use incompatible blood. As already discussed, most autoantibodies causative of WAIHA react with all donor red cells. The fact that only incompatible blood is available should not be allowed to alter the decision to transfuse when such a course is essential. It is necessary to test the patient's serum in an attempt to identify any alloantibodies that are present but whose reactions may be masked by the autoantibody in the serum. Methods for accomplishing this very difficult task are discussed below in the section dealing with the selection of blood for transfusion in WAIHA. If clinically-significant alloantibodies are present, blood lacking the antigens against which they are directed, must be provided. If no alloantibodies are present, it may be possible to provide blood compatible with the patient's autoantibody. However, since only about 4% of patients with WAIHA make only simple specificity autoantibodies, this opportunity does not often arise (again, these points are discussed below in the section on

selection of blood for transfusion in WAIHA). Thus in the vast majority of patients with WAIHA, only blood incompatible with the autoantibody will be available. If the need for transfusion is real, such blood must be used. While the transfused red cells will not survive normally, they will usually be cleared no more rapidly than the patient's own red cells. Indeed, in many instances the transfused red cells may have a half-life of three or four days (233,500), a long enough period that the patient may be kept alive by the transfusions until a steroid-induced remission begins. The transfusion of blood compatible with any alloantibodies present but incompatible with the autoantibody, in a patient with WAIHA, does not cause an overt transfusion reaction. It must be remembered that since the patient's own red cells are (usually grossly) incompatible, he or she is already having a transfusion reaction, whether or not donor blood is infused. Once it becomes clear that incompatible blood must be transfused, there is no point in screening available units to select those that are "least incompatible". It is far better for the blood banker to conduct exhaustive tests to identify any alloantibodies that may be present than to spend time looking for the "least incompatible" units. Again, Pirofsky (499) has accurately described the situation. He has pointed out that as far as incompatibility with an autoantibody is concerned, the event is more significant than the degree, so that least incompatible (in this situation) can be likened to a little pregnant.

In concluding this section on transfusion in WAIHA, the two most important points bear repetition. First, blood should not be transfused until its use is clinically essential, for fear of worsening the patient's long term prognosis. Second, once transfusion is deemed essential to keep the patient alive, blood incompatible with the patient's autoantibody must almost always be used. The existence of incompatibility must not be allowed to prevent the transfusion, unfortunately some patients with WAIHA have died of anemia because the individuals treating them were not prepared to transfuse incompatible blood.

WAIHA, Treatment, Plasmapheresis and Use of IVIG

Since WAIHA is caused by an antibody in the patient's plasma, it may seem logical to try to treat the patient by plasma exchange. Indeed a number of attempts to achieve reduction in the level of circulating autoantibody by this method, have been described (for reviews see 501-505). The procedure is beset by at least two major difficulties. First, the causative autoantibodies of WAIHA are almost all IgG in composition. Almost 50% of the body's IgG is in the extravascular compartment (506) meaning that if IgG is removed from plasma, it is rapidly replaced from the extravascular compartment. Second, if the plasma removed is replaced with albumin, crystalloids or colloids there is a rebound effect in which IgG is rapidly synthesized. Thus soon after the plasma exchange is completed, the IgG autoantibody level may be higher than before the procedure. If the plasma removed is replaced with donor plasma to prevent the rebound effect, the patient is exposed to blood products from multiple donors and the risk that a transfusion-transmitted disease will follow, is increased. One solution to this second problem might be to return the patient's own plasma after it had been passed over an immunoadsorbent column of Staph protein A, to remove IgG (507-509). At least one group of investigators (510) have claimed success in such a procedure but the method does not seem to have been widely applied.

A different approach is to try to reduce the amount of immune red cell clearance in the patient by injecting large amounts of IVIG. There is some dispute as to the mechanism by which this form of therapy works. It is likely that splenic blockade (i.e. blocking Fc receptors on the patient's splenic macrophages with free IgG in the plasma) (726-734), the presence of anti-idiotype in the IVIG (735-740), interference with T-cell signals to B-cells (741-744), activation of T suppressor cells, and inhibition of B-cell maturation (745-750), may each play a role. There are numerous reports of success in treating WAIHA patients with IVIG (511-519,638,751-756) but in one study (520,757) the product was not found to be efficacious. Particular success has been reported (638,751,754-756) in patients with Evans syndrome in which there is autoantibody-induced destruction of both red cells and platelets. IVIG therapy has been seen to relieve both anemia and thrombocytopenia in these patients. The glowing reports of success must be tempered with some relevant points. First, IVIG can be used as a supplemental form of treatment, its use does not replace steroid therapy. Second, IVIG is most useful in treating patients in acute hemolytic episodes, to tide them over until corticosteroids start to work or in treating patients who have not responded to other forms of therapy. Third, in almost all patients treated with IVIG, corticosteroids and/or splenectomy have been used as well. It is not always easy to differentiate between the effects of different forms of therapy. For instance, if a patient has been on corticosteroid therapy for a time but has shown no appreciable clinical improvement, IVIG may be given. If, after several days of treatment with IVIG the patient's condition starts to improve, it is difficult to know whether the IVIG is responsible or if the patient is now responding to steroids. When IVIG therapy is instituted in such patients, corticosteroid therapy is not usually withdrawn. Fourth, for patients with WAIHA, IVIG must be used at high levels (i.e. 1 to >2 g/kg/day for 5 to 7 days) so is consequently an expensive

form of treatment. Thus it should be used only in those patients not responding to other forms of therapy or in acute emergencies. Flores et al. (521) compiled data on 36 patients with WAIHA treated with IVIG and compared the results with those seen in 37 patients described in the literature. They concluded that IVIG therapy "can be recommended only as an adjunctive therapy for selected cases of warm-antibody AIHA, given the limited response rate (40%) despite concomitant medication". After this largest study on the use of IVIG in WAIHA had been published, Hughes and Toogood (522) suggested that IVIG therapy is best used in patients who have already been treated by plasma exchange. Earlier, Hershko et al. (523) had suggested that a similar dramatic early response to that seen in IVIG therapy can be accomplished in some patients by the use of cyclosporine.

In discussing IVIG it should be mentioned that its use for other indications, in patients who do not have WAIHA, can cause a positive DAT. This occurs, of course, because IVIG preparations contain antibodies (e.g. anti-A, anti-B, sometimes anti-D and other antibodies (765,766)) that bind to the patient's red cells. While positive DATs in patients being treated with IVIG are not uncommon, immune red cell destruction by the passively transferred antibodies seems to be rare. Red cell destruction may be seen in bone marrow transplant recipients when a minor population of red cells produced by the graft, emerges from the marrow. That is, in a group O patient given a group A marrow, sufficient anti-A may be injected via continued use of IVIG that the first made A cells from the graft are destroyed.

Quantitation of IgG on the Red Cells of Patients with WAIHA

As described above, one form of treatment of patients with WAIHA involves suppression of production of the autoantibody. Obviously, it is desirable that a laboratory test be used to demonstrate such suppression, to show that the patient is indeed responding to treatment. Unfortunately, it is not easy to measure the change in red cell-bound autoantibody using commonly performed laboratory tests. Petz and Garratty (47) coated red cells in vitro with anti-D, carefully measured the amount of anti-D that had bound, then used those cells to correlate the strength of the antiglobulin test reaction with the number of molecules of IgG on the red cells. Their results are reproduced in table 37-13. As can be seen, the test reaches its maximum strength reaction (4+) when more than about 500 molecules of IgG are bound per red cell. Thus, in a patient with WAIHA with say 2000 molecules of IgG per red cell at the time of diagnosis, the DAT will be 4+. If say at one week and two weeks of steroid therapy, the number of IgG molecules per red cell is 1000 and 500 respectively, the DATs on those samples will still be 4+ although, in fact, the patient is responding well to steroids. To overcome this problem in demonstrating declining levels of IgG on red cells, titrations with anti-IgG can be performed and the results can be scored. As the number of molecules of IgG per red cell is reduced, the more dilute anti-IgG will fail to agglutinate the red cells. This method has all the disadvantages of a manual titration. It is affected by slight errors in preparation of the dilutions of anti-IgG so that accurate measurements (using volumetric pipettes) must be used. It is affected by lot to lot variation of anti-IgG, a problem that can be overcome by marking a vial of that reagent with the patient's name and using it only for subsequent titrations on that patient's red cells. The titrations are also affected by strength of the red cell suspensions used so those should also be prepared by accurate measurement. Finally, the test is affected by subjective readings, for which there is no cure other than consistency of the investigator. In spite of these drawbacks the method can be useful and if impeccable technique is used, results such as those shown in table 37-14 can be obtained. As can be seen, the conventional DAT (undiluted anti-IgG in the table) is 4+ on all three samples. However, the titer end points and titer scores (see Chapter 3) show that the level of IgG on the patient's red cells has been reduced during the two weeks of treatment. The use of commercially prepared antiglobulin serum in the titrations described represents one of very few instances in which it is appropriate to use such a reagent in dilutions. As indicated in Chapter 6, such reagents should almost always be used as supplied by the manufacturer.

When the enzyme-linked antiglobulin test (ELAT) was introduced (547,548) it was apparent that the method is highly suitable for following autoantibody levels in patients being treated for WAIHA. The quantitative test is read in an objective manner and variations in technique need not affect the final results since a series of dilutions of a serum containing a known amount of antibody can be used to prepare a standard curve, each time unknowns are tested. The ELAT procedure has been shown (549) to be very useful in following patients being treated for WAIHA, providing a number of variables are carefully controlled (550). However, when properly performed with a standard curve and all necessary controls (551) the test is labor-intensive and time consuming and thus expensive. For those laboratories with access to a flow cytometer, even more accurate measurements of IgG levels on red cells can be made (148,552-555). Studies using flow cytometry have led one group (148) to conclude that in vivo hemolysis or the lack thereof, correlates closely with the number of IgG molecules bound per red cell (see also the earlier section on in vivo clearance as related to

IgG1 or IgG3 subclass of the autoantibody). However, as mentioned earlier, from the results of a larger study Nance and Garratty (553) and Garratty (114) concluded that there is so much variation between individual patients that no "magic number" above which in vivo clearance will occur and below which it will not, exists.

Somewhat fortunately, since laboratory tests to measure the amount of IgG autoantibody on red cells can hardly be considered to be within the scope of a routine laboratory, other parameters, e.g. slowing of the rate of hemoglobin decline, stabilization of hemoglobin levels (even when low), an increase in the absolute number of reticulocytes, and improvement in the patient's general clinical condition (even allowing for the euphoric effects of steroid therapy), are rather reliable indications that the patient with WAIHA is responding to treatment.

WAIHA and Other Diseases

As indicated in the introduction of this chapter, WAIHA is one manifestation of autoimmune disease. Once loss of T-cell regulation of B-cells occurs, many different specificity autoantibodies may be made, for examples see table 37-1. Thus, it is not surprising that WAIHA is seen in patients with other autoimmune diseases. However, the disease is also seen in patients in

TABLE 37-13 Strength of Antiglobulin Test Reaction with Red Cells Carrying Measured Amounts of IgG, (From Petz and Garratty(47))

Strength of reaction of antiglobulin test	Number of molecules of IgG per test red cell
0	<25-120
± or 1/2+	120
1+	200
2+	300-500
3+ and 4+	>500

TABLE 37-14 Decrease of IgG on the Red Cells of a Patient with WAIHA as Shown in Titration Studies with Anti-IgG

Patient's sample	Dilutions of anti-IgG								Titer score
	1	2	4	8	16	32	64	128	
At diagnosis	4+	4+	4+	4+	3+	2+	1+	0	71
After 1 week of treatment	4+	4+	3+	3+	1+	0	0	0	49
After 2 weeks of treatment	4+	3+	2+	1+	0	0	0	0	35

whom the immune failure is less apparent. Following the classifications of Garratty and Petz (47) and Rosse (526) diseases with which WAIHA (when not the only disease) is most often associated can be listed as follows:

1. Diseases of Immune Dysfunction: systemic lupus erythematosus; rheumatoid arthritis; scleroderma; Sjogrens syndrome.
2. Neoplasms of the Immune System: chronic lymphocytic leukemia; non-Hodgkin's lymphoma; Hodgkin's disease; Waldenstrom's macroglobulinemia; multiple myeloma; thymomas.
3. Immune Deficiency States: hypogammaglobulinemia; dysgammaglobulinemias; Wiskott-Aldrich syndrome; other immune deficiencies.
4. During or Following Infections: post-viral syndrome (especially in children); infectious mononucleosis; cytomegalovirus infection; human immunodeficiency virus (HIV) infection.

In terms of disorders not listed above, there are a large number of reports (563-581,620,621) of warm-reactive red cell autoantibodies in patients with ulcerative colitis. Although some of these patients had full-blown WAIHA, many others had positive DATs and warm reactive IgG autoantibodies on the red cells (some also had unbound autoantibody in the serum) but no signs or symptoms of accelerated red cell clearance in vivo. The mechanism of the relationship between WAIHA and ulcerative colitis is not understood although, as mentioned earlier, ulcerative colitis is itself, sometimes at least in part, an autoimmune disorder. In 1980, Garratty et al. (579) made the fascinating observation that rarely, the red cells from a clotted sample of blood may be heavily coated with IgG, while red cells from the same patient collected into an anticoagulant have a negative or only a weakly positive DAT. This phenomenon was seen in eight patients with ulcerative colitis but in 30 others with that disease (four of whom had positive DATs) it was not seen. The IgG on the patients' red cells could be recovered by elution and would bind to normal red cells, no antibody specificity could be seen nor was there any evidence of immune red cell destruction in the patients involved. The authors (579) suggested that the patients might have an antibody directed against an activated coagulation factor and that during the coagulation process immune complexes might form and bind to the red cells. One year earlier, Tregellas et al. (372) had described an auto-anti-Sc1, in a normal blood donor, that was detectable when serum, but not when plasma samples, were tested. In 1982, Tregellas and Lavine (597) isolated the plasma component that contained the anti-Sc1 and showed that it could be "activated" (in terms of demonstrable serological activity) when

the plasma isolate was treated with the serine endoproteases trypsin and thrombin, that cleave arginine-lysine bonds. They (597) suggested that the donor's plasma contained a subpopulation of immunoglobulin molecules that were acted on, by thrombin, during the coagulation process, in such a way as to enable them to combine with antigen. While other examples of the antibody described above in patients with ulcerative colitis have been found, it is not clear (582) that their reactivity is the same as that postulated by Tregellas and Lavine (597).

It should be stressed that the phenomenon described above is not the same as that which results in a positive DAT, with C3 on the red cells, when clotted blood samples are tested, and a negative DAT when red cells from the same patient, that were collected into an anticoagulant, are tested. That situation results (see Chapter 6) because many sera contain complement-fixing, benign, cold-reactive autoantibodies. As the clotted sample cools, the cold-reactive autoantibody binds to the patient's red cells and activates complement in vitro. The activated C3 then binds to the red cells and can be detected in a DAT. The whole process is amplified if blood samples are refrigerated at 4°C before the DATs are performed. As discussed in Chapter 6, DATs should be performed on red cells collected into EDTA, that blocks in vitro complement activation.

There are also a number of reports (556-562) of WAIHA in patients with ovarian tumors. Although the relationship between the tumors, most of which have been benign although some malignant forms have been involved, and the WAIHA is not understood; removal of the tumor has several times resulted in correction of the hemolytic anemia.

While there is no evidence to suggest that cancer is frequently associated with the development of WAIHA, there are a fair number of cases in the literature (583-596) in which a patient with carcinoma suffered a relapse of previously well controlled WAIHA. As a single example, a woman with WAIHA who had experienced a complete steroid-induced remission of her WAIHA for seven years, presented with terminal steroid-resistant WAIHA, thrombocytopenia and gastric adenocarcinoma (593). It is probable, based on the separate incidences of cancer and WAIHA, that the number of patients who have both is no higher than would be expected from the incidence of each.

WAIHA and Pregnancy

There are many descriptions (47,107,109,598-619,819-824) of WAIHA in pregnant women. In some, WAIHA develops during a pregnancy then spontaneously disappears after the child is born. In women known to have WAIHA before they become pregnant, there may be an exacerbation of hemolysis during the pregnancy, or the disease may reappear in a patient previously in remission. In some women, increased doses of steroids may become necessary during the pregnancy; care must be taken to ensure that the level in the mother does not become high enough for the amount that crosses the placenta to harm the fetus. As might be expected, management of WAIHA in a pregnant woman can be difficult. In describing cases and reviewing the literature, Chaplin et al. (610) suggested that life-threatening anemia may occur in 40 to 50% of mothers and that stillbirth or severe anemia may occur in 35 to 40% of their infants. However, it is not clear that the problems in the infants actually represent hemolytic disease of the newborn caused by maternal autoantibody that has crossed the placenta. Indeed, in a number of infants with clinical problems, the DAT has been negative. It seems that a major contribution to the problems of the infants involves anemia of the mother. In a fairly high percentage of other cases the infants have been unaffected or have had only mild HDN. This may well relate to the fact that although the IAT is positive in many patients with WAIHA because unbound autoantibody is present in the serum, titration studies show that in most cases only moderate amounts of autoantibody are present. Thus the combination of low levels of autoantibody crossing the placenta, poor affinity constants of many autoantibodies and specificities that cause less severe HDN than does anti-D, may serve to spare the infants of women with WAIHA. In reviewing the many reports of WAIHA in pregnant women, one is left with the distinct impression that the mother may be more severely compromised at the clinical level, than is the infant.

In Chapter 39, hematologically normal individuals in whom the DAT is positive and in whom IgG warm-reactive autoantibodies are present, are described. Sokol et al. (240) studied a number of such women who became pregnant. During their pregnancies, the autoantibodies remained benign and their infants were not affected. In other words, the autoantibodies that were benign in the mothers were benign in their fetuses as well.

WAIHA in Children

As indicated in table 37-2, WAIHA in adults is usually a permanent condition that requires continued treatment and/or hematological monitoring. Happily, this is not necessarily the case in children. Indeed, from a review of the literature (41-44,46,49,143,622-630) it can be seen that in 75 to 80% of children who present with WAIHA, the disease is acute and transient. If the child can be managed through the acute episode, a full recov-

ery and reversion to a normal immune state can be anticipated. In children with the transient form of the disease, plasma exchange (631-635) (used in some children with secondary CHD, see Chapter 38) and IVIG (636,637, 732) therapy have proved rather more useful in managing the acute hemolytic episode than has been the case in adults with idiopathic WAIHA (see earlier section on treatment). It seems that a major difference between the 75 to 80% of children who make a complete recovery and the 20 to 25% who do not, is related to the cause of the WAIHA. In those children in whom the disorder is triggered by an external factor, such as a viral infection, the prognosis is good. In those in whom the WAIHA is associated with or secondary to an underlying disorder, such as lymphoma, SLE or congenital muscular dystrophy (41,42,143,623,638,639), the prognosis is not good. Even then, it is the underlying disorder and not the WAIHA that is usually responsible for the most serious medical problems of the child.

Hemolytic Anemia in Patients with Malaria

On a worldwide basis, malaria is by far the most common cause of hemolytic anemia. In most instances anemia results from intravascular hemolysis during the acute phase of the disease. Lysis represents the rupture of red cells that contain parasites. It is known (651-658) that some proteases produced by some malarial parasites, preferentially degrade cytoskeletal proteins that are present on the inner side of the red cell. However, children in particular and some adults with *P. falciparum* malaria have a positive DAT (659-665) and/or immune hemolytic anemia (758-764). It is not yet clear whether the proteins found on the red cells of these patients are related to the anemia. In some studies (659,662) no correlation between the degree of anemia and a positive DAT could be found; in addition, many of the positive DATs were due to just C3 on the red cells. In other studies (660,661,663) correlation between the degree of anemia and a positive DAT was noted. The finding (661) that the eluted IgG antibody reacted with malarial schizont antigens, suggested that perhaps an antibody was being made in an immune response to the malarial parasites. However, such a specificity would not prevent the antibody from clearing red cells if it could bind to such cells. Jeje et al. (663) found that the red cells of 26 children with *P. falciparum* malaria had from 215 to 1770 (mean 629) molecules of IgG bound per red cell, while the cells of a control group carried from 190 to 930 (mean 395) molecules per cell. Clearly, the possibility exists that in some cases of malaria an immune process contributes to the red cell destruction.

Autoantibodies in Patients with Parasitic Infections

Infections with *Babesia microti* (that can be transmitted by transfusion even when previously frozen blood is used (666)) may interfere with the functions of suppressor T cells (667) and autoimmune phenomena have been described in patients with babesiosis (668,669). Wolf et al. (670) described three such patients who made IgG autoantibodies. In one of the patients it was felt that the autoantibody contributed to in vivo red cell destruction although a delayed transfusion reaction caused by red cell alloantibodies was occurring at the same time. The autoantibodies made in patients with malaria and babesiosis seem to be different. As mentioned above, those in patients with malaria may be directed against parasite-borne antigens. Those studied by Wolf et al. (670) appeared to be directed against red cell antigens and reacted poorly or not at all with Rh_{null} red cells. Thus it is possible that babesia somehow affect the cells of the immune system and allow the production of true red cell autoantibodies, perhaps by a mechanism in some ways like that suggested for aldomet (alpha-methyldopa, see Chapter 40). Perhaps in some cases (668-672) one of the complications of babesiosis involves an autoantibody capable of reacting with red cells. There have, of course, been a number of reports (666,672-678) of transfusion-transmitted babesiosis. Positive DATs have also been seen (665) in patients infected with *Bartonella bacilliformis*.

WAIHA, Selection of Blood for Transfusion

As discussed in detail in the section dealing with treatment in WAIHA, many authorities believe that transfusion should be used in patients with the disorder only when essential for the maintenance of life and when no alternative form of therapy is working. Once that situation is reached, it is the responsibility of the blood bank to provide the most suitable blood possible for transfusion.

If the patient has a positive DAT, but no allo or autoantibody in the serum, the situation appears simple; it is not. First, although antibody-screening and compatibility tests are negative, the donor blood may not be compatible. The autoantibody bound to the patient's red cells is not permanently fixed there, some will elute from the red cells, and autoantibody production will continue after the donor red cells are transfused. In other words, if the autoantibody is directed against an antigen present on the donor red cells, some of it will become attached to those cells and effect their removal at a rate approximately equal to that at which the patient's cells are being destroyed. Second, although no allo or autoantibody may

be demonstrable in the patient's serum, it may still be possible to supply red cells for transfusion that are more compatible than the patient's own. An eluate should be made from the patient's antibody-coated red cells and tested for specificity. If the patient is say D+ with auto-anti-c on his or her c+ red cells, R₁R₁ (CDe/CDe) blood should be provided since it will survive longer in vivo than will the patient's own cells (the negligible risk of alloimmunization is discussed below).

If the patient's serum contains unbound autoantibody, particularly one that reacts with all cells on an antibody identification panel, it is much more difficult to determine whether an alloantibody or alloantibodies is/are simultaneously present. For a long time, immunohematologists used an adsorption procedure developed by Professor Dacie many years ago (i.e. at least the 1950s) that was taught to everyone who worked at the Royal Postgraduate Medical School in London but that may never have been published as an original method. Separate aliquots of the patient's serum are adsorbed with R₁R₁, R₂R₂ and rr red cells. The object of the exercise is as depicted in table 37-15, namely to adsorb the autoantibody present and leave alloantibodies unadsorbed so that they can be recognized in tests on the adsorbed serum aliquots. Although not shown in detail in table 37-15, an attempt was made to ensure that at least one of the cell samples used for adsorption was Fy(a-), another Fy(b-), one Jk(a-), another Jk(b-), etc., so that alloantibodies other than those in the Rh system could be detected in one or more of the adsorbed serum samples. The reason that allogeneic red cells were used in the adsorption studies was, of course, that the patient's red cells were usually saturated with autoantibody (i.e., DAT 4+) so would not remove serum autoantibodies if used for autoadsorption. This problem has now been overcome. First, Morel et al. (640) modified a technique devised by Stratton and Renton (641) in which the patient's red cells are subjected to partial heat elution at 56°C. The object of the exercise (for the method see Judd (130)) is to remove enough autoantibody that the patient's red cells can be used for autoadsorption. Second, Branch and Petz (122) developed the ZZAP reagent and Edwards et al. (121) used chloroquine diphosphate (both methods given in Judd (130)) while Hanfland (123) used a variable pH/density gradient method, to remove autoantibodies from cells while leaving the red cells intact and usable in autoadsorption procedures. Other methods that use: glycine-HCl; EDTA-glycine-HCl-TRIS (125); citric acid (128,129); or DMSO, have been devised to remove autoantibody and leave intact red cells available for use in autoadsorptions. None of these methods has been as widely applied as use of ZZAP or chloroquine diphosphate. Obviously, removal of the autoantibody by autoadsorption should leave any alloantibodies simultaneously present, in the serum so that they can be detected and identified. When using sera from which autoantibodies have been removed by adsorption for compatibility tests and antibody-screening, it may be necessary to change the method used. For example, we (429) routinely use PEG-IAT for those procedures. However, that method is so sensitive for the detection of warm-reactive autoantibodies that multiply adsorbed sera often still react, i.e. small amounts of autoantibody left unadsorbed. When such sera are tested by LISS-IAT they can be shown not to contain alloantibodies (429). Thus as a routine we test adsorbed sera that previously contained autoantibodies and sera from patients with a strongly positive DAT, by LISS-IAT in antibody-screening tests. We reason that the chance of a patient's serum containing both autoantibody and an alloantibody reactive by PEG-IAT that is not reactive by LISS-IAT is virtually nil. We are not alone (582).

Liew and Duncan (828) took advantage of the finding, mentioned above, that the use of PEG very markedly enhances the uptake of autoantibodies by red cells. These workers (828) cleverly added PEG to the red cell-serum mixture in adsorption studies and showed that the time of each adsorption and the number of adsorptions needed, totally to adsorb autoantibody could be reduced. Further, the adsorbed sera are ready to use, i.e. mixed with PEG, in potentiated tests when they are harvested from the adsorbing red cells. Although Champagne and Moulds (829) reported that they were not able to detect known alloantibodies following autoadsorption in PEG, neither Liew and Duncan (830) nor we (831) have experienced any such difficulties. Leger and Garratty (832) compared various methods for detecting alloantibodies in sera containing warm-reactive autoantibodies and con-

cluded that the PEG autoadsorption method is equal to or more efficient than adsorption with ZZAP-treated red cells and reduces adsorption time by 50%. We (831) have encountered autoantibodies that were autoadsorbed in PEG but not removed when other methods were used. It should be pointed out that in the original description of the method (828) no mention is made of modification of the adsorbing red cells. In answer to a question, Liew and Ducan (830) reported that they used papain-treated autologous red cells. In the study by Leger and Garratty (832) and in our own laboratory (831) untreated red cells were used. The use of untreated red cells removes one preparatory step and thus shortens the length of time required in the selection of blood for the patient without apparently reducing the efficiency of the method.

One advantage of the use of autologous instead of allogeneic red cells for adsorption of the autoantibodies is that an alloantibody to a very common antigen, e.g., anti-k, anti-Vel, would remain unadsorbed. Use of allogeneic R_1R_1, R_2R_2 and rr red cells, no matter how carefully they were selected, would almost always result in adsorption of such an alloantibody. However, the chance of such an antibody being present in the serum of a patient with WAIHA is small and even if such an antibody was present it would take a very astute blood banker to recognize its presence and not assume that its reactions were due to incompletely adsorbed autoantibody. Disadvantages of the use of autologous red cells for adsorption are first, that often they are not available in the quantities needed and second, that none of the methods mentioned (121-123,640) is likely to effect total removal of autoantibody. In other words, when the treated red cells are used in the autoadsorptions, some of their antigen sites are still blocked.

Some workers refuse to use autoadsorption procedures (for cold as well as warm-reactive autoantibodies) if the patient has recently been transfused. One of us (PDI) has never quite understood the rationale for the decision. Admittedly, if the patient has been transfused with red cells that carry an antigen to which an alloantibody is being made, that antibody may be removed if the adsorption is with a mixture of the patient's and transfused cells. However, if the patient has been transfused (by chance) with cells that lack the antigen against which the alloantibody is directed, a valuable finding can still be made. In other words, when adsorption with a mixture of the patient's and transfused cells suggests that no alloantibodies are present, an alternative method (such as adsorption with allogeneic red cells or one of the methods described below) may be necessary. When adsorption with the mixed cell population yields a positive result, such as revealing the presence of anti-Fy^a in a patient known (or shown) to have Fy(a-) red cells, the result is valid. As mentioned earlier in this chapter, cell

TABLE 37-15 Allogeneic Adsorption Studies on the Sera of Patients with WAIHA to Remove Autoantibodies and Leave Alloantibodies Unadsorbed

Adsorbing cells*	Antibodies that will be adsorbed	Specificities left in adsorbed serum
R_1R_1 (CDe/CDe)	Anti-C, Anti-D, Anti-e, Anti-nl, Anti-pdl, Anti-dl	Anti-c and Anti-E
R_2R_2 (cDE/cDE)	Anti-c, Anti-D, Anti-E, Anti-nl, Anti-pdl, Anti-dl	Anti-e and Anti-C
rr (ce/ce)	Anti-c, Anti-e, Anti-nl, Anti-pdl, Anti-dl	Anti-C, Anti-D and Anti-E

*　The cells used for adsorptions should be selected so that among them one sample lacks other antigens (e.g., K, Fy^a, Fy^b, Jk^a, Jk^b, etc.) to which the patient may be alloimmunized (see text).

typings to confirm the alloimmune nature of an antibody identified in adsorption studies will usually have to be performed on the patient's red cells from which autoantibody has been removed by one of the methods described (121-123). Reid and Toy (642) have pointed out that if it is known that a patient with autoantibodies present in the serum is going to require a series of transfusions over a period of time, autologous red cells can be collected before the first transfusion and used (following frozen storage if necessary) in autoadsoprtion studies on subsequent post-transfusion serum samples from the patient. While this solution sounds easy and eminently logical it may present a problem at the practical level. If the patient has say 3g/dl of hemoglobin before the first transfusion, it is unlikely that a sufficient quantity of autologous red cells will be available to be saved for later autoadsorptions.

When a patient's red cells are treated with ZZAP (a mixture of dithiothreitol (DTT) and papain (122)) to remove autoantibody, a number of blood group antigens on those red cells are denatured. When chloroquine-treated autologous (121) or allogeneic red cells are to be used in adsorption procedures, many workers pretreat them with a protease (e.g. papain, ficin). In the majority of cases, enzyme pretreated red cells have enhanced ability to bind autoantibody. The number of adsorptions necessary totally to remove autoantibody from a serum can often be reduced by the use of enzyme-treated red cells. However, it must be remembered that some antigens that are targets for autoantibodies are denatured by enzymes or DTT. As examples, some auto-anti-En^a will not be adsorbed by ZZAP-treated autologous or enzyme-treated autologous or allogeneic red cells (En^{a}TS and En^{a}FS (318) both denatured by papain, ficin, etc.). Autoantibodies directed against Kell system antigens (see an earlier section) will not be adsorbed by ZZAP-treated autologous red cells (all Kell system antigens denatured (122,680)). Accordingly before attempts to adsorb an autoantibody with ZZAP or enzyme-treated red cells are undertaken, the autoantibody should be shown to react with such treated cells. Sometimes when this simple test is forgotten, the fact that four adsorptions with ZZAP or enzyme-treated red cells have not reduced the strength of the antibody prompts the investigator to try adsorption with chloroquine-treated autologous or untreated allogeneic red cells. Chloroquine-treatment of red cells may slightly weaken some (131) but does not destroy any red cell antigens (121). Sometimes a single adsorption with unmodified red cells removes all autoantibody!

A problem with adsorption studies using autologous or allogeneic red cells is that they take a considerable amount of time that may simply not be available if the patient's clinical condition dictates immediate transfusion. A faster method is described by Petz and Garratty

(47). A titration is performed using the patient's serum and pooled antibody screening cells. This is read for total agglutination in IATs (i.e. mixed-field reactions are called negative) so that an idea of the titer of the unbound autoantibody can be obtained. If the autoantibody gives say, a 1+ reaction at a dilution of 1 in 8, the serum is diluted to 1 in 8 and is tested against a panel of red cells. If the Fy(a+) red cells on the panel give 3+ reactions and the Fy(a-) samples give 1+ reactions (i.e., they react with the autoantibody) it follows that anti-Fy^a is probably present and that the patient needs Fy(a-) blood. Obviously, this method works only if any alloantibody present is of higher titer than the autoantibody. However, this is not as much of a disadvantage as it might seem. As mentioned earlier, most patients with WAIHA who present with unbound autoantibody in the serum, have limited amounts of serum autoantibody. In most patients the autoantibody will be found to give only 1+ reactions at dilutions between 1 in 8 and 1 in 32. Many alloantibodies have higher titers than that, so can be recognized when the method is used.

On some occasions the patient's need for blood will be so urgent that there will be insufficient time even for tests with diluted serum. On such occasions, blood of the same Rh phenotype as the patient's can be issued. Obviously, there will not be enough time to treat the patient's red cells with chloroquine, ZZAP or by gradient/density centrifugation. Accordingly, tests with saline-active Rh reagents or MAbs have to be used to phenotype the patient's cells. Donor blood of the same phenotype is then issued. This will ensure that the patient is not transfused with blood carrying an Rh antigen against which an alloantibody is present in the serum. Obviously, this method will not safeguard against transfusion with blood incompatible with an alloantibody of another blood group system. Like the method that uses a dilution of the patient's serum, this one is better than it at first sounds. First, the majority of patients do not have clinically-significant antibodies in the serum. Second, of the minority who do, some 40% have an Rh system alloantibody (643). Third, limited as it is, this method is better than titrations with the patient's serum against random units to select those that are "least incompatible". Such titrations ignore the allo or autoimmune nature of any antibodies present. For example, if a patient's serum contains auto-anti-e with a titer of 32 and allo-anti-E with a titer of 16, and titrations are done with the patient's serum when the specificities of those antibodies have not been determined, an R$_1$R$_1$ (E- e+) unit will appear more incompatible than one that is R$_2$R$_2$ (E+ e-). In fact, the patient should be transfused with E- e+ red cells that (because they are of similar phenotype to the patient's) will not cause a transfusion reaction. Instead, the R$_2$R$_2$ unit will be selected as "least incompatible" and the allo-anti-E in the patient's serum may cause a transfusion reaction. Table 37-16 summarizes the methods that can be used to select blood for transfusion to patients who have autoantibodies in the serum. Working from the bottom of the table to the top, the methods gradually take longer to perform. However, working from the top of the table to the bottom, the methods gradually become less reliable.

The literature carries some fairly divergent figures about the incidence of alloantibodies in sera that contain autoantibodies. For example, Laine and Beattie (644) studied 109 sera that contained unbound warm-reactive autoantibodies, by adsorption, and concluded that 41 (37.6%) of them contained alloantibodies whose presence could be detected only following adsorption of the autoantibodies. Similarly, James et al. (645) found alloantibodies in 13 (31.7%) of 41, and Morel et al. (640) alloantibodies in eight (40%) of 20 sera, following removal of autoantibodies by adsorption. In marked contrast, in another large study, Wallhermfechtel et al. (646) found alloantibodies in only 19 (15.2%) of 125 sera after autoantibodies had been removed. Sokol et al. (244) reported detection of alloantibodies in 294 (13.7%) of 2149 individuals with autoantibodies. However, that series (244) included samples from individuals with warm-reactive and from individuals with cold-reactive autoantibodies present, the numbers for each type are not given so that it is impossible to compare that series with the others cited. Because our own experience suggested that the circa 15% incidence of Wallhermfechtel et al. (646) was closer to the true incidence than the 31.7 to 40% figure of the other series (640,644,645) we (429) undertook a large study. Mollison et al. (233) in commenting on the 37.6% incidence of Laine and Beattie (644) wrote that "this very high figure suggests that some of the "alloantibodies" may really have been autoantibodies with mimicking specificities". Accordingly, in our study (429) whenever we found what appeared to be an alloantibody, present in a serum from which some autoantibody had been adsorbed, we performed further adsorptions with antigen-negative red cells to differentiate between true alloantibodies (not removed by adsorption with antigen-negative red cells) and partially adsorbed autoantibodies mimicking alloantibody specificities (removed by adsorption with antigen-negative red cells). Among samples from 138 patients we found 59 (43%) that appeared to contain alloantibodies after the initial adsorptions, i.e., in agreement with the high incidence figures in the earlier series (640,644,645). However, continued adsorption with antigen-negative red cells showed that 47% of the apparent alloantibodies were partially adsorbed autoantibodies mimicking alloantibodies. After the continued adsorptions it was shown that among the 138 patients the true incidence of alloimmunization was 23%, i.e., in agreement with the

TABLE 37-16 Methods to Identify Alloantibodies and/or Find Suitable Blood When the Serum Contains Unbound Autoantibody

1. Autoadsorb serum with patient's red cells

    a) Treated with ZZAP[*1] (122)

    b) Treated with chloroquine diphosphate (121)

    c) Treated by variable pH/gradient centrifugation (123)

    d) Treated by partial heat elution at 56°C (640)

2. Alloadsorb separate aliquots of patient's serum with R_1R_1, R_2R_2 and rr red cells typed for other antigens

3. Identify alloantibodies in the patient's serum in tests with serum diluted to a point where the autoantibody reacts only weakly (47)

4. Issue blood of the same Rh phenotype as the patient

[*1] ZZAP treatment of red cells destroys some antigens so that autoantibodies against them will not be adsorbed, see text.

[*2] Blind titrations to select "least incompatible" units should not be used, see text.

lower incidence in the earlier series (646). We (429) also demonstrated the reason that different incidences had been reported in the earlier series. In the three studies (640,644,645) that suggested the 32 to 40% incidence of alloimmunization, autoadsorption was the exclusive (640,645) or primary (644) method of adsorption. In the study (646) that showed a 15% incidence of alloimmunization, allogeneic adsorption was used. In our study (429) initial autoadsorption left 16 apparent alloantibodies, 11 (69%) of which were, in fact, partially adsorbed autoantibodies. Initial allogeneic adsorption left 16 apparent alloantibodies of which only three (19%) were of the mimicking type. These latter findings are not surprising. First, autoadsorption must often be performed with limited quantities of red cells, particularly when the patient is grossly anemic. There are no limits to the amounts of cells (and hence antigen sites) that can be used in allogeneic adsorptions. Second, autoadsorption often involves the use of red cells from which autoantibody must first be removed. As discussed above, it is unlikely that total autoantibody dissociation ever occurs. In contrast, in allogeneic adsorption no antigen site blocking interferes in the adsorption of autoantibody.

These data are of significance in the provision of blood for patients with autoantibody in the serum. If the serum also contains a clinically-significant alloantibody, red cells lacking the antigen against which that alloantibody is directed must be provided. If the apparent alloantibody is, in fact, partially adsorbed autoantibody, antigen-negative blood is not necessary since it will be no more compatible than other units, with the unadsorbed autoantibody. If the serum contains only a mimicking antibody, the use of antigen-negative blood (i.e. negative for the antigen apparently but not actually involved) may be appropriate. That is, since there is appreciable correlation (114,233) between the amount of IgG that binds to red cells and the rate of in vivo red cell clearance, the use of red cells to which less IgG will bind, may be of benefit to the patient. Again this consideration does not apply when the mimic is part of the total autoantibody since, in vivo, the autoantibody will not have been adsorbed and will bind in approximately equal amounts to all red cells. When it is necessary to differentiate between true alloantibodies and partially adsorbed autoantibodies that mimic them, adsorption with antigen-negative red cells is required to exclude the close to 50% chance that an apparent alloantibody is not alloimmune at all.

On those occasions when a patient's serum has been shown, with a reasonable degree of confidence, to be devoid of alloantibodies, it is sometimes possible to avoid the autoantibody when the patient is transfused. For example, if the patient is R_1R_1 (CDe/CDe) and has formed auto-anti-e and no alloantibodies, R_2R_2 (cDE/cDE) blood will appear compatible. Opportunities to avoid autoantibodies in the selection of blood are rare since only about 4% of patients with WAIHA form only a simple specificity autoantibody (113). Further, such a finding is most often seen in the early stages of WAIHA when transfusion is less likely to be necessary. While the R_2R_2 blood, in the example given, will not actually be compatible if the patient has really made auto-anti-nl mimicking auto-anti-e, the R_2R_2 cells will survive longer in vivo than will cells that are e+ (423), as discussed above. When the opportunity to transfuse blood more compatible than the patient's own red cells does arise, there are two schools of thought about whether the opportunity should be taken. Some workers would not transfuse R_2R_2 blood to an R_1R_1 patient with auto-anti-e in the serum because it would involve the introduction of foreign Rh antigens (c and E in this instance). These workers are concerned that the patient might become alloimmunized and, as explained above, recognition of allo-anti-c and/or allo-anti-E in a patient who has gone on the make auto-anti-pdl or auto-anti-dl, is a difficult serological exercise. The second school of thought is that the benefits of transfusing red cells more compatible then the patient's own (i.e. E+ e- red cells for a patient with auto-anti-e) outweigh the risk of alloimmunization. First, alloimmunization may not occur. Second, if the patient responds to treatment, further transfusions may not be necessary. Third, even if alloimmunization occurs and further transfusions are needed, the alloantibodies can be identified and c- E- e+ blood can be used. Clearly one of us (PDI) has always belonged to this second school of thought but even he exempts D from this consideration. In other words, in a rr (cde/cde) patient making only auto-

anti-e, the author (PDI) would use rr not R_2R_2 blood for transfusion. This reasoning is based on the very high immunogenicity of D (see Chapter 12) in D- persons, as compared to the immunogenicity of any other blood group antigen in an individual lacking that antigen from the red cells. Not all workers think this way and some would use R_2R_2 blood for a rr patient with auto-anti-e. As already discussed, red cells that lack the antigen against which the autoantibody is directed, enjoy better in vivo survival than the patient's cells or donor cells that carry the antigen involved (278,423,500,647,648). In addition to alleviating the anemia for longer, use of such cells may also reduce the number of times that the patient must be transfused, obviously an advantage if one believes (see above) that transfusion in WAIHA is contraindicated anyway.

When the autoantibody in the patient's serum is directed against an antigen of very high incidence, the decision as to whether to use blood more compatible than the patient's own, is much more difficult. For example, D--/D--, Rh_{null}, U- and K_0 red cells are non-reactive with the sera of patients who have made auto-anti-nl, -pdl, -U and -K13, respectively. However, donor units of those phenotypes are much less common than are patients who form autoantibodies of the specificities listed. Accordingly, most workers are not prepared to release those units for transfusion to patients with WAIHA and believe, instead, that the units must be reserved for patients who make alloantibodies and cannot be transfused with antigen-positive red cells. Patients with autoantibodies can, of course, receive antigen-positive blood. Although such red cells may not survive normally in vivo, they will usually survive as long as the patient's own cells. There may be occasions when the policy of reserving ultra-rare units for alloimmunized patients has to be reevaluated. It has been claimed (327) that in patients who form Kell system autoantibodies, the in vivo survival of antigen-positive red cells may be so short as to make such transfusion meaningless and that K_0 red cells may have to be given for the patient to receive any benefit (K_0 cells survive normally in such patients). The situation usually seems different when the autoantibody has Rh specificity. For example, Mollison (423,500) showed that although e+ red cells were cleared more rapidly than e- red cells (that survived for a close to normal period) in a patient with auto-anti-e (that we (649) later showed was anti-nl mimicking anti-e), the mean survival of the e+ red cells was about seven days. Obviously, if the use of incompatible blood had been necessary in this patient, the transfused red cells could have helped prolong life until a steroid-induced remission was achieved.

As discussed above there is no point in using antigen-negative blood in a patient in whom simple autoantibody specificity is demonstrable only following adsorption studies. For example, in a patient in whom the serum autoantibody has anti-pdl or anti-dl specificity but is shown, by adsorption with R_2R_2 cells, to contain an auto-anti-e component, R_2R_2 cells cannot be expected to survive any longer than e+ red cells unless the anti-pdl or anti-dl is very weak and the auto-anti-e is very strong, in which case adsorption studies to permit recognition of the auto-anti-e would not have been necessary anyway! In other words, if the anti-pdl or anti-dl is strong enough to effect in vivo red cell destruction, e+ and e- cells will be removed at about the same rate. The decisions as to when antigen-negative or antigen-positive blood should be used (of necessity in the opinion of one of us (PDI)) are summarized in table 37-17.

Having written at such length about the selection of blood for transfusion to patients with WAIHA, we now feel obliged to repeat the admonition given earlier, that transfusion in these patients should not be undertaken lightly. On most occasions incompatible blood must be used. The effects of transfusion are usually palliative and short-lived. At worst, there is a danger that transfusion will adversely affect the patient's long term prognosis. Accordingly, transfusion in a patient with WAIHA should be used only when life-threatening consequences of anemia are present.

When transfusions must be used, packed red cells are the component of choice. There is no point in using washed red cells for a patient with WAIHA, unless the patient has a history of febrile transfusion reactions and/or is known to have a potent leukoagglutinin in the serum. Some physicians will request washed red cells for all patients with WAIHA but such requests should be questioned, like any others for that product. In those patients who must be transfused, the blood should be given slowly and in small amounts (650). Sometimes 100 ml of packed cells can be given on one day and a further 100 ml the next, if necessary. This practice serves several useful purposes. First, it reduces the chance of circulatory overload. Second, if an undetected alloantibody is present in the serum and the blood being given is incompatible with that alloantibody, the conse-

quences of the transfusion reactions will be less severe than if a whole unit of blood had been infused. Third, the patient may have a clinical response to the infusion of 100 ml of packed cells that is good enough that further transfusion is not necessary. If the introduction of donor red cells can stimulate the production of greater amounts of autoantibody, there are obvious benefits from transfusing as few donor red cells as possible.

WAIHA and Autoantibodies of Low Affinity

In a minority of patients with WAIHA the DAT may be only weakly positive in spite of fairly severe hemolysis in the patient. In some of these patients unbound autoantibody may be present in the serum although the patients' red cells are clearly not saturated with antibody. Garratty et al. (53,681) studied samples from a number of patients and made a series of pertinent observations. First, it was shown that in some cases in which the conventional DAT was negative or only weakly positive, stronger reactions were obtained when the red cells were washed in saline chilled to 4°C or in LISS or in LISS chilled to 4°C. The reactions were even weaker (or were negative) when the cells were washed in saline prewarmed to 37°C. In performing the DAT after cold washes it is essential to read a similarly washed control with 10% albumin to show that any agglutination seen is antiglobulin serum-mediated and not caused by a cold autoagglutinin bound to the patient's red cells. Second, when the red cells from these patients were washed and allowed to stand at room temperature for 20 to 160 minutes before the antiglobulin serum was added, the DATs were all much weaker or were negative. When 22 samples with positive DATs in conventional tests were similarly tested, the DATs and DAT titration scores were essentially the same as when the tests were read immediately after the red cells were washed. Third, some patients thought to have "DAT-negative WAIHA", see next section, could be shown to have positive DATs when

TABLE 37-17 Use of Blood "Compatible" with the Autoantibody in Patients with WAIHA, Some Examples

Phenotype of patient's red cells	Specificity of eluted or serum autoantibody	Phenotype of blood of choice for transfusion
R_1r	Auto-anti-e	R_2R_2
rr	Auto-anti-e	rr (Some workers would select R_2R_2, see text)
R_1r	Auto-anti-dl 4+, auto-anti-e, by adsorption	e-negative blood not indicated
D+, U+	Auto-anti-U, auto-anti-nl, etc.	U-negative, D--/D--, etc. not generally used, see text
Common Kell system phenotype	Autoantibody to a high incidence Kell system antigen	Antigen-negative or K_0 blood may be indicated, see text

the cold-wash systems were used. These findings were interpreted (53,681) as indicating that in some patients, autoantibodies of low affinity, that elute from the patients' red cells during the washing stage in conventional DATs (and IATs), are present. It has always been difficult to explain why some patients in whom these findings are made have fairly severe WAIHA since the low affinity autoantibodies would not be expected to effect efficient macrophage binding of red cells in vivo. Garratty (53) suggests that in such patients high affinity autoantibodies might also be present and may have bound to red cells in vivo, with subsequent clearance of those cells (and the attached autoantibody molecules) leaving only low affinity antibody-coated red cells in the patient's circulation.

Garratty (53) also points out that the cold-wash or LISS-wash modification may be useful as an adjunct procedure in the investigation of an apparent transfusion reaction in which no alloantibodies can be detected in conventional tests. Perhaps one of the ways in which systems using low ionic conditions (LISS-IAT, PEG, Polybrene) enhance the sensitivity of in vitro antigen-antibody tests is to slow the rate at which antibodies dissociate from red cells during the washing stages in IATs. Similarly, an advantage of the Gel test (682) may be that no washing is involved. Certainly the incidence of positive DATs is higher when the Gel test is used, unfortunately some of the positive reactions are clinically meaningless and create far more problems than they solve, e.g. waste of donor units that are perfectly suitable for transfusion (683).

WAIHA with a Negative DAT

The vast majority of patients with WAIHA present with a positive DAT. However, the fact that the DAT is negative does not automatically exclude the disorder and there are now many well documented cases of patients with the disease, in whom no red cell-bound autoantibody could be demonstrated by standard procedures (47,109,111,114,242,243,444,551,612,617,684-703). Evans and Weiser (684) found four such patients among 41 with WAIHA; Worlledge and Blajchman (111) 10 among 333 patients; while Chaplin (689) reported the incidence of a negative DAT in patients with WAIHA to be between 2 and 4%. One explanation for these apparently paradoxical findings seems to be that the number of IgG molecules per red cell necessary for accelerated in vivo destruction, is sometimes less than the number necessary for the DAT to be positive. While that relatively simple explanation seems to apply in many cases, there are exceptions as described below. As discussed earlier in this chapter, in vivo red cell destruction when low numbers of IgG molecules are bound per red cell seems, in

large part, to be related to the IgG subclass of the autoantibody. Based on quantitative studies (145,148,149,201) it would be expected that those cases of WAIHA caused by an autoantibody not detectable in a standard DAT would involve those made of IgG3. However, this theoretical assumption has not yet been shown to be a fact, primarily because of technical difficulties that arise when attempts are made to subclass IgG autoantibodies that are bound to red cells in very small amounts.

For some time, the diagnosis of WAIHA in a patient with a negative DAT was made by exclusion. In an anemic patient with the clinical symptoms of WAIHA and no evidence of red cell loss by bleeding, and in the presence of a high reticulocyte count, intrinsic (red cell defects) and extrinsic (serum or mechanical) factors were excluded and a tentative diagnosis of WAIHA was made. In such patients who then showed a good hematological and clinical response to steroid therapy (693) it was assumed that the diagnosis of WAIHA was correct. Clearly such empirical use of steroids was undesirable, particularly in view of their side effects in those patients who did not have WAIHA. There are now a number of laboratory tests and a number of observations that confirm that WAIHA with a negative DAT exists and that in some, but not all cases, the tests allow the correct diagnosis to be made before steroid therapy is initiated.

Gilliland et al. (685,686) used aliquots of the patient's and normal red cells to adsorb anti-IgG. The amount of anti-IgG left unadsorbed was then measured using a complement fixation assay. It was found (686) that the DAT- red cells of five of six patients suspected of having WAIHA had adsorbed more anti-IgG than had the normal cells. It was calculated (686) that normal red cells carry up to about 35 molecules of IgG per red cell (a similar figure was later reported by Merry et al. (704)) and that those of the patients carried more than the usual amount of that immunoglobulin. The range, in the five patients studied, was 70 to 434 molecules of IgG per red cell. This, in itself, did not prove that the patients had WAIHA for IgG and autoantibody are not synonymous. In other words, while the assay showed that an increased level of IgG had bound to the patients' red cells in vivo, it did not prove that the IgG was autoantibody. However, Gilliland et al. (686) were more than equal to the task. They then made eluates from large volumes (50 to 200 ml) of the patients' red cells and concentrated those eluates to a volume of circa 1 ml. The eluates were then shown to contain IgG autoantibodies with specificities typical of those seen in WAIHA. Similar studies that yielded similar results were described by Rosse (692) who found patients with between 50 and 450 molecules of IgG per red cell, in whom the DAT was negative. It is difficult to compare these findings with those of Idelson et al. (705) who reported that of 303 patients thought to have WAIHA, 133 (43.9%) had a negative DAT. One cannot help but wonder about the potency of the antiglobulin reagents and the techniques used in routine tests in that study. In spite of its obvious value, the technique described by Gilliland et al. (686) did not become widely used. Unfortunately, the assay procedure to determine how much anti-IgG has been adsorbed, is complicated. Simple serological assay (i.e., titration of the adsorbed aliquots of anti-IgG against antibody-coated red cells) is not sufficiently sensitive to be of use in demonstrating the difference in amount of anti-IgG adsorbed by the patients' and the normal red cells (706).

Direct antiglobulin tests performed in an Auto-Analyzer can be made very sensitive if PVP is used to augment the agglutination (59,707). Again this technique has not been widely applied first, because a dedicated manifold is necessary and second, because considerable expertise is necessary if false positive results are to be avoided. Attempts have also been made (708-710) to detect low levels of IgG on red cells by use of radio-labeled antiglobulin reagents. One problem that is encountered is that the background of bound isotope interferes with differentiation between normal and abnormal samples when the red cells of the abnormal samples carry only small amounts of IgG. Even when this problem is overcome (711) tests with radio-labeled anti-IgG are not appreciably more sensitive than are antiglobulin tests read by agglutination.

Fisher et al. (691), Garratty and Petz (687) and Petz and Garratty (47) have studied a number of patients with WAIHA, in whom the DAT was negative, but in whom autoantibodies could be demonstrated in the serum or in eluates made from the DAT-negative red cells. It seems particularly appropriate, when this situation is suspected, to test the patient's serum against enzyme-treated red cells (47,687). If an antibody is detected, its autoimmune status can be confirmed by tests against a sample of the patient's red cells that have been enzyme-treated and/or by antigen typing tests on the patient's cells if the antibody has recognizable specificity. On other occasions, eluates made from the patients' DAT-negative red cells have been shown to contain autoantibodies, sometimes when tested in a straightforward manner (694) and sometimes (47,695) after moderate concentration (i.e. by a factor of 2 to 5 times). In the cases cited above, the serum or eluted autoantibodies were relatively weak. Thus the cases seem to differ considerably from those described earlier, in the section on Rh antigen depression in WAIHA. In those cases the DAT was negative but very potent serum antibodies, giving 4+ reactions in saline to IAT, were present. No doubt some of the cases in which weak in vitro reactivity was seen involved autoantibodies of low affinity, as described in the previous section.

When the enzyme-linked antiglobulin test was first described (547,548) it was said to be more sensitive than the conventional manual test. Thus it was hoped that it could be used to demonstrate low levels of IgG on red cells. While the test has been used with considerable success in this respect it has not proved to be a panacea. It seems that while the ELAT method is highly suited for measuring IgG on red cells when those cells carry an appreciable amount of that immunoglobulin, it is not at its best when red cells carry small amounts of IgG. It seems that the normal range (i.e. the amount of IgG on red cells from different normal individuals) overlaps the range on the red cells of patients with WAIHA and a negative DAT. In other words, it is not always possible to tell the difference between normal and abnormal red cells when very low levels of IgG are bound. Garratty et al. (698) studied samples from 40 patients with hemolytic anemia of unknown origin, in whom an immune basis was suspected. In 12 of the 40 patients the ELAT method showed levels of red cell-bound IgG that were higher than those on the red cells of normal individuals run in parallel. Samples from some of the patients were also tested by the direct polybrene test (712), others by the direct bromelin test (713) and some in an in vitro system using a monolayer of monocytes. While it seemed that all tests will give an occasional positive result when all other tests are negative, Garratty et al. (698) felt that the direct polybrene test might eventually prove of most help in cases such as these. However, they also cautioned that the test is not specific and can give a positive reaction at times other than when the patient's red cells are coated with IgG autoantibody. For reasons that are far from clear but may simply have involved patient selection, we (551,699,700,703) found the ELAT of greater use in these patients. In a four year period we performed direct ELATs on the red cells of 40 anemic patients in whom cause of the anemia was not known at the time the test was done. In a few patients there were indications, such as elevated LDH and reduced haptoglobin levels, that suggested that immune-mediated hemolysis might be occurring. In many others the ELAT and other laboratory tests designed to reveal the cause of the anemia were performed simultaneously and soon after the anemia had been noted. In all 40 patients, conventional DATs using anti-IgG, anti-IgA and anti-IgM were negative. In nine of the 40 patients the ELAT was positive. In seven of those nine patients the anemia was corrected by steroid therapy and no cause for anemia, other than an autoimmune process was found. Thus those seven patients can reasonably be supposed to have had DAT-negative, IgG autoantibody-induced hemolytic anemia. Of the other two patients with a positive ELAT, whose anemia was not corrected by steroid therapy, one had a chronic viral illness and the other end-stage renal disease. Among the 31 patients with a negative ELAT, two were lost to follow-up. Among the other 29, a cause of the anemia other than WAIHA was eventually established in 27. In the other two, no explanation for the anemia other than WAIHA was found, both were treated with steroids and both responded. Thus in this study a positive ELAT was correlated with DAT-negative WAIHA in seven of nine patients, a negative ELAT was correlated with a different cause of anemia in 27 of 29 patients but two cases of DAT-negative WAIHA were not identified by ELAT.

Toy et al. (721) and Heddle et al. (722) have reported that the DAT may be positive in individuals with a high (not necessarily abnormal) level of IgG in the plasma. This occurs in some individuals in whom there is no increased rate of red cell destruction in vivo (see Chapter 39). The findings (721-723) that eluates made from the red cells of some of these persons are non-reactive, calls into question the significance of the finding of increased levels of IgG on the red cells of patients with supposed DAT-negative WAIHA. In other words, do patients with say a positive ELAT, as described above, simply have higher levels of IgG in their plasma (and non-specifically attached to their red cells) than those in whom the test is negative? Garratty and Arndt (724) answered this question by showing that there is no correlation between a positive ELAT and the level of IgG in the plasma, in these patients. Garratty (114,725) believes, and we agree entirely, that in this group of patients it is correct to conclude that a positive ELAT almost always indicates the presence of pathological IgG autoantibody on the patient's red cells.

As discussed in Chapter 36, the ELAT procedure is not one to be undertaken lightly. Including triplicate tests, hemolysis controls, a standard curve and hemolysis controls on the standard curve, testing a sample from one patient can involve the use of 40 or more tests (703,720).

Other methods that have been used in attempts to detect a low level of IgG on red cells include the use of Staph protein A labeled with ^{125}I (697,714) and use of fluorescein-conjugated with anti-IgG in a flow cytometer (701). Garratty (53) and Garratty et al. (701) report that in tests on large numbers of samples from patients suspected of having DAT-negative WAIHA, the flow cytometry method detected increased levels of red cell bound IgG in 15 of 70 (21%) while the ELAT detected increased levels in 32 of 201 (16%). Autoantibodies were detected in 15 of 162 (9%) concentrated eluates (not concentrated to the same degree as in the Gilliland et al. (686) study), the DAT was positive after cold saline washes in seven of 209 (3%) and the MMA was positive in four of 105 (4%) cases. The direct polybrene test was positive in 38 of 205 (19%) and the direct PEG test in 16 of 160 (10%) of cases. As mentioned above, some of these tests, particularly the last two, are not specific for the detection of red cell-bound IgG autoantibody. In all,

80 of 234 (34%) samples were positive in one or more tests. Table 37-18 lists tests that may be useful in this situation, as Garratty (53) points out, a battery of tests is of considerably more use than any single test.

As mentioned above, the most commonly advanced explanation of WAIHA in a patient in whom the DAT is negative is that the amount of IgG on the red cells, that is effecting in vivo red cell clearance, is below the threshold of detection in the DAT. However, this is clearly not always the case. As indicated in table 37-13, the DAT should be positive once more than about 100 to 150 (47,715) molecules of IgG per red cell are bound. In the studies of Gilliland et al. (686) up to 434 molecules; in those of Rosse (692) up to 450 molecules and in our study (699,700) up to 440 molecules of IgG per red cell were detected, yet the DATs were still negative. In tests on 27 patients with presumed DAT-negative WAIHA, Petz and Garratty (47) found that five of them had more than 400 molecules of IgG per red cell, the highest level was around 1400 molecules per red cell in one patient; in all five patients the DAT was negative. These findings show that in some cases the Fab portions of the IgG molecules bind to red cells but that cross-linking (agglutination) does not occur when the Fc pieces of those same IgG molecules bind anti-IgG (i.e. conventional DAT is negative). That anti-IgG does bind to the Fc pieces of the cell-bound IgG molecules is clear since detection of IgG in the ELAT and flow cytometer is dependent on anti-IgG binding to the red cell-bound IgG. Garratty (114) has used the same anti-IgG as is used in the ELAT and the flow cytometer, at the same dilution, in a form in which it is not coupled to an enzyme or to fluorescein and has found that it still fails to cause agglutination of the red cells to which it binds in the ELAT and flow cytometer. Further, that the Fc portions on the IgG molecules are functional is also demonstrated by the finding that the patients have hemolytic anemia. Obviously, in those patients, tissue-bound macrophages with receptors for IgG are able to recognize and bind to the Fc portions of the IgG molecules on the red cells.

A similar situation is seen with rare alloantibodies. As described in Chapter 36 there are a number of well documented cases (716-720) in which an alloantibody has cleared large numbers of antigen-positive transfused red cells but is not demonstrable in either pretransfusion or posttransfusion serum samples by any current in vitro method. Clearly there are rare, strong, IgG alloimmune and autoimmune antibodies capable of marked red cell destruction in vivo that defy all current attempts to detect them in vitro.

Hemolytic Anemia in Animals

In the third edition of this book, this section proved

TABLE 37-18 Methods That May be of Value for Detecting Autoantibodies in WAIHA When the DAT is Negative

Method	Details
Flow cytometry	Red cells tested with fluorescein-conjugated anti-IgG.
Enzyme-linked antiglobulin test	Anti-IgG coupled to an enzyme is bound to the test red cells and the bound enzyme is used to hydrolyze a substrate. The amount of substrate hydrolysis is directly proportional to the amount of IgG on the test red cells.
Adsorption of anti-IgG	Test and normal red cells are used to adsorb anti-IgG. The amount adsorbed is determined by assay of the unadsorbed anti-IgG.
DATS in the AutoAnalyzer	Red cells coated with low levels of immunoglobulin or complement are agglutinated in a system that uses PVP.
DATs with a radio-labeled antiglobulin	Red cells coated with low levels of immunoglobulin or complement are exposed to labeled reagents and the amount of label bound is measured.
Direct polybrene test	Red cells coated with low levels of protein are tested for agglutination in a system that uses polybrene.
Direct bromelin test	Red cells coated with low levels of protein are tested for agglutination in the presence of bromelin.
Concentrated eluate	An eluate is made from red cells and is concentrated then tested for autoantibody activity.
Serum tests	The patient's serum is tested by sensitive methods for the presence of autoantibody.
Monocyte/macrophage tests	The test red cells are exposed to monocytes or macrophages. Tests can be read by phagocytosis, rosetting or isotope release from labeled test red cells.

to be one of the more popular ones (who says blood bankers must be serious scientists all the time?). Accordingly, with apologies to those who have read some of the jokes before, the section is reproduced here, some new observations and comments have been added.

Hemolytic anemia continues to be a problem for black rhinoceroses (should that be rhinoceri?) (774-787). In these animals (*Diceros bicornis*) the disease may be secondary to leptospirosis, babesiosis, trypanosomiasis and unknown causes that temporarily respond to corticosteroid therapy (how does one calculate the prednisone dose for a rhinoceros?) Hemoglobinuria has also been reported (788) in the Indian rhinoceros (*Rhinoceros unicornis*) (one wonders if they had a giant dipstick) after ingestion of plants of the *Brassicae* family. Having written that section we hope that it is not politically incorrect to describe one animal as unicornis and the other as bicornis. At least in the black rhinoceros there seems to be a familial predisposition to fatal hemolytic anemia (785) obviously a serious problem for zoo authorities since these animals are very valuable. One death of a black rhinoceros was reported (775) in the *Journal of Small Animal Practice*, thus leaving the mind to boggle at what animals might be considered large!

Chaplin et al. (786) investigated the syndrome of acute intravascular hemolysis in the black rhinoceros. Six animals (presumably seen as outpatients) were tested: three were unrelated healthy animals, two had intravascular hemolysis and one had iron deficiency anemia. Rabbit anti-rhinoceros globulin was made using rhinoceros serum and purified rhinoceros IgG as the immunogens. The healthy animals and the one with iron deficiency were DAT-negative. One rhinoceros in whom the hemolysis was fatal had an increased level of C3 on the red cells. Let this be a lesson to those workers who, in the past, claimed (references excluded to spare their embarrassment) that anti-C3 was not a necessary component of antiglobulin reagents.

Hemolytic anemia has also been reported (789) in a horse, who was admitted to a hospital (for large animals). The hemolysis was thought to have been precipitated by ingestion of an unknown toxin. The report mentions that rectal examination revealed no enlargement of the spleen which should make readers who ever need to be examined for splenomegaly, glad they are not horses! It is well established in the equine literature (790-793) that dried-red-maple leaves are toxic and cause hemolytic anemia when eaten by horses.

Hemolytic anemia is also common in dogs (794-800,810,811) but seems to be less frequent in cats (799,810) suggesting (at least to one of us (PDI)) that the incidence of the disease in dogs and cats is inversely proportional to their intelligence. Afflicted dogs have included: Basenjis (801-804); an Alaskan Malamute (805); a Beagle (806); Poodles (807); and English Springer Spaniels (808,809). Given the intelligence level of the last breed mentioned, the hemolytic anemia-intelligence inverse ratio theory seems well supported.

In many dogs, hemolytic anemia is clearly antibody-induced. Serologists will be interested to learn that because of the rather poor activity of some anti-canine-IgG (812,813), the use of protease-treated dog red cells has been advocated (814-816) for detection of autoantibodies in dogs with WAIHA and a negative DAT. We found one paper (817) that described hemolytic anemia in a miniature Dachshund caused by the intake of large quantities of onions. While the revelation that dogs get antibody-induced hemolytic anemia was not too surprising, it was a distinct shock to learn that a Dachshund liked onions enough that he ate himself into a clinical syndrome and the world literature. The paper did not specify whether red cell sequestration in the unfortunate animal was hepatic thus removing the temptation to make a joke about liver and onions.

Finally, one report (818) describes antibody-induced hemolytic anemia in a five year-old domesticated raccoon (*Procyon lotor*). The animal was described as obese (by the veterinarians, other raccoons were apparently not consulted) and on admission complained (medical history presumably supplied by the owner not the patient) of listlessness and anorexia of two weeks duration. The raccoon was receiving phenobarbital for a chronic seizure disorder but the hemolytic anemia was not thought to be drug-induced because after steroid therapy had corrected the anemia, steroids were tapered and withdrawn, phenobarbital was continued at the original dosage and anemia did not recur. Because no anti-raccoon IgG or anti-raccoon complement were available, the diagnosis was based on spherocytosis and autoagglutination in the blood film and exclusion of other causes. The hemolytic episode was acute and apparently transient since the hematocrit remained normal eight months after steroid therapy was completed. For those still wondering how to calculate a steroid dose for a rhinoceros, the raccoon responded to a prednisolone dose of 2.2 mg/kg/day for two weeks then 1.1 mg/kg/day for five weeks, at which time the hemocrit reached a normal level. All that remains is to try to figure out how to weigh a rhinoceros!

References

1. Burnet FM . The Clonal Selection Theory of Acquired Immunity. London:Cambridge Univ Press, 1959
2. Issitt PD. Jackson VA. Vox Sang 1968;15:152
3. Schwartz RS, Costea N. Semin Hematol 1966;3:2
4. Fudenberg HH. In: Critical Factors in Cancer Immunology. New York:Academic, 1975
5. Shoenfeld Y, Schwartz RS. New Eng J Med 1984;311:1019
6. Souroujon M, White SM, Andreschwartz J, et al. J Immunol 1988;140:4173
7. Widmann FK. An Introduction to Clinical Immunology, Philadelphia:Davis, 1989
8. Nossal GJ. Curr Opin Immunol 1991;3:193
9. Lin RH, Mamula MJ, Hardin JA, et al. J Exp Med 1991;173:1433
10. Leanderson T, Kallberg E, Gray D. Immunol Rev 1992;126:47
11. Mamula MJ, Lin RH, Janeway CA Jr, et al. J Immunol 1992;149:789
12. Bona CA, Kaushik AK, eds. Molecular Immunobiology of Self-Reactivity. New York:Marcel Dekker, 1992
13. Weissman IL, Cooper MD. Sci Am 1993;269:65
14. Singer GG, Carrera AC, Marshak-Rothstein A, et al. Curr Opin Immunol 1994;6:913
15. Roitt IM. Essential Immunology, 8th Ed. Oxford:Blackwell, 1994
16. Kuby J. Immunology, 2nd Ed. New York:Freeman, 1994
17. Abbas AK, Lichtman AH, Pober JS, eds. Cellular and Molecular Immunology, 2nd Ed. Philadelphia:Saunders, 1994
18. Stites DP, Terr AI, Parslow TG, eds. Basic and Clinical Immunology, 8th Ed. Norwalk, CT:Appleton and Lange, 1994
19. Shlomchik MJ. In: Autoimmune Disorders of the Blood. Bethesda:Am Assoc Blood Banks, 1996:1
20. Krakauer RS, Waldmann TA, Struber W. J Exp Med 1976;144:644
21. Strelkaukas AJ, Callery RT, McDowell J, et al. Proc Nat Acad Sci USA 1978;75:5150
22. Kisielow P, Bluthmann H, Staerz UD, et al. Nature 1988;333:742
23. Kawabe Y, Ochi A. Nature 1991;349:245
24. Ucker DS, Meyers J, Obermiller PS. J Immunol 1992;149:1583
25. Orchansky PL, Teh HS. J Immunol 1994;153:615
26. Waldmann TA, Broder S, Blaese RM, et al. Lancet 1974;2:609
27. Broder S, Humphrey R, Durm M, et al. New Eng J Med 1975;293:887
28. Wofsky D, Hardy RR, Seaman W. J Immunol 1984;132:2686
29. Jenkins MK, Schwartz RS. J Exp Med 1987;165:302
30. Korthauer U, Graf D, Mages HW, et al. Nature 1993;361:539
31. Barcy S, Wettendorf M, Leo O, et al. Int Immunol 1995;7:179
32. Walford RL. The Immunologic Theory of Aging. Copenhagen:Munksgaard, 1970
33. Rodey GE, Good RA, Yunis EJ. Clin Exp Immunol 1971;9:305
34. Yu YV, Fernandes G, Greenburg LJ. J Am Geriat Soc 1976;24:258
35. Lange CF. In: Progress in Clinical Pathology VII. New York:Grune and Stratton, 1978:119
36. Kohout E, Dutz W. In: Progress in Clinical Pathology VII. New York:Grune and Stratton, 1978:197
37. Parkman R. Am J Pediat 1981;3:105
38. Fudenberg HH, Rosenfield RE, Wasserman LR. J Mt Sinai Hosp 1958;25:324
39. Meyer LM, Bertcher RW. Am J Med 1960;28:606
40. Polesky HF, Bove JR. Transfusion 1964;4:285
41. Zuelzer WW, Mastrangelo R, Stulberg CS, et al. Am J Med 1970;49:80
42. Habibi B, Homberg J-C, Schaison G, et al. Am J Med 1974;56:61
43. Buchanan GR, Boxer LA, Nathan DG. J Pediat 1976;88:780
44. Zupanska B, Lawkowicz W, Gorska B, et al. Br J Haematol 1976;34:511
45. Russo L, Russo AM, Viola M, et al. New Eng J Med 1976;295:623
46. Carapella de Luca E, Casadei AM, di Pietro G, et al. Vox

Sang 1979;36:13

47. Petz LD, Garratty G. Acquired Immune Hemolytic Anemias. New York:Churchill Livingstone, 1980

48. Tsai TF, Finn DR, Plikaytis BD, et al. Ann Int Med 1979;90:509

49. Haidas S, Ziva-Petropoulou M, Grafakos S, et al. Eur J Paediat 1983;140:83

50. Neu N, Craig SW, Rose NR, et al. Clin Exp Immunol 1987;69:566

51. Nepom BS, Nepom GT. In: Textbook of Rheumatology, Vol 1. Philadelphia:Saunders, 1993:89

52. Bigazzi PE. Lupus 1994;3:449

53. Garratty G. In: Immunobiology of Transfusion Medicine. New York:Marcel Dekker, 1994:493

54. Qasim FJ, Thiru S, Mathieson PW, et al. J Autoimmunity 1995;8:193

55. Dahr W. Cited in Issitt PD. Applied Blood Group Serology, 3rd Ed. Miami:Montgomery, 1985:515

56. Litwin SD. Balaban S, Eyster ME. Blood 1973;42:241

57. Le Petit JC, Rivat L, Francois N, et al. Vox Sang 1976;31:183

58. Leddy JP, Bakemeier RF. J Exp Med 1965;121:1

59. Hsu TCS, Rosenfield RE, Burkart P, et al. Vox Sang 1974;26:305

60. Caulfield MJ, Stanko D, Calkins C. Immunology 1989;66:233

61. Scott BB, Sadigh S, Stow M, et al. Immunology 1993;79:568

62. Scott BB, Sadigh S, Stow M, et al. Clin Exp Immunol 1993;93:26

63. Reininger L, Shibata S, Ozaki T, et al. Eur J Immunol 1990;20:771

64. Shibata T, Berney T, Reininger L, et al. Int Immunol 1990;2:1133

65. Caulfield M, Stanko D. J Immunol 1992;148:2068

66. Scott BB, Sadigh S, Andrew EM, et al. Scand J Immunol 1994;40:16

67. Kissmeyer-Nielsen F, Bent-Hansen K, Kieler J. Acta Med Scand 1952;144:35.

68. Dobbs CE. Arch Int Med 1965;116:273

69. Cordova MS, Baez-Villasenor J, Mendez JJ, et al. Arch Int Med 1966;117:692

70. Shapiro M. Transfusion 1967;7:281

71. Pirofsky B. Vox Sang 1968;14:334

72. Siep M, Harboe M, Cyvin K. Acta Pediat Scand 1969;58:275

73. Pollock JG, Fenton E, Barrett KE. Br J Haematol 1970;18:171

74. Blajchman MA, Hui YT, Jones TE. (abstract). Prog 24th Ann Mtg AABB, 1971:82

75. Toolis F, Parker AC, White A, et al. Br Med J 1977;1:1392

76. Reynolds MV, Vengelen-Tyler V, Morel PA. Vox Sang 1981;41:61

77. Ventura M, Urbano U, Rossi F, et al. Panmin Med 1984;26:69

78. Fialkow PJ, Fudenberg H, Epstein WV. Am J Med 1964;36:188

79. Beard MEJ, Pemberton J, Blagdon J, et al. J Med Genet 1971;8:317

80. McDevitt HO, Bodmer WF. Am J Med 1972;52:1

81. Gibofsky A, Winchester RJ, Patarroyo M, et al. J Exp Med 1978;148:1728

82. Stuart MJ, Tomar RH, Miller ML, et al. J Am Med Assoc 1978;239:939

83. Conley CL, Misiti J, Laster AJ. Medicine 1980;59:323

84. Russell AS. Sem Arth Rheum 1981;10:255

85. Conley CL. Johns Hopkins Med J 1981;149:101.

86. Lippmann SM, Arnet FC, Conley CL, et al. Am J Med 1982;73:827

87. Laster AJ, Conley CL, Kickler TS, et al. New Eng J Med

1982;307:1495

88. Rajewsky K, Takemori T. Ann Rev Immunol 1983;1:569

89. Moller G. Ed. Idiotypic Networks: Immunological Review. Copenhagen:Munksgaard, 1984

90. Paul WE. In: Fundamental Immunology. New York:Raven, 1984:439

91. Rodey GE. Prog Clin Biol Res 1984;149:235

92. Rodey GE, Scrivner DL. In: Immunology. Arlington, VA:Am Assoc Blood Banks, 1985:157

93. Issitt PD. In: Progress in Clinical Pathology VII. New York:Grune and Stratton, 1978:137

94. Morton NE, MacKinney AA, Kosower N, et al. Am J Hum Genet 1962;14:170

95. Kimberling WJ, Fulbeck T, Dixon L, et al. Am J Hum Genet 1975;27:586

96. Kimberling WJ, Taylor RA, Chapman RG, et al. Blood 1978;52:859

97. Bass EB, Smith SW Jr, Stevenson RE, et al. Ann Int Med 1983;99:192

98. Agre P, Orringer EP, Bennett V. New Eng J Med 1981;306:1155

99. Sturgeon P. Blood 1970;36:310

100. Hasekura H, Ishimori T, Furusawa S, et al. Proc Jpn Acad 1971;47:579

101. Chown B, Lewis M, Kaita H, et al. (Letter). Lancet 1971;1:396

102. Chown B, Lewis M, Kaita H, et al. Am J Hum Genet 1972;24:623

103. Mallory DM, Rosenfield RE, Wong KY, et al. Vox Sang 1976;30:430

104. Wimer BM, Marsh WL, Taswell HF, et al. Br J Haematol 1977;36:219

105. Symmans WA, Shepherd CS, Marsh WL, et al. Br J Haematol 1979;42:575

106. Issitt PD. Transf Med Rev 1993;7:139

107. Pirofsky B. Autoimmunization and the Autoimmune Hemolytic Anemias. Baltimore:Williams and Wilkins, 1969

108. Bottinger LE, Westerholm B. Acta Med Scand 1973;193:223

109. Dacie JV. The Haemolytic Anaemias, 2nd Ed, Part II. The Congenital and Acquired Haemolytic Anaemias. New York:Grune and Stratton, 1962

110. Dacie JV, Worlledge SM. Prog Hematol 1969;6:82

111. Worlledge SM, Blajchman SM. Br J Haematol 1972;23 (Suppl):61

112. Dacie JV. Arch Int Med 1976;135:1293

113. Issitt PD, Pavone BG, Goldfinger D, et al. Br J Haematol 1976;34:5

114. Garratty G. In: Immune Destruction of Red Blood Cells. Arlington, VA:Am Assoc Blood Banks, 1989:109

115. Evans RS, Duane RT. Blood 1949;4:1196

116. Dausset J, Colombani J. Blood 1959;14:1280

117. Allgood JW, Chaplin H Jr. Am J Med 1967;43:254

118. Zucker-Franklin D, Karpatkin S. New Eng J Med 1977;297:517

119. White WD, Issitt CH, McGuire DA. Transfusion 1974;14:67

120. Romans DG, Tilley CA, Crookston MC, et al. Proc Nat Acad Sci USA 1977;74:2531

121. Edwards JM, Moulds JJ, Judd WJ. Transfusion 1982;22:59

122. Branch DR, Petz LD. Am J Clin Pathol 1982;78:161

123. Hanfland P. Vox Sang 1982;43:310

124. Rekvig OP, Hannestad K. Vox Sang 1977;33:280

125. Louie J, Jiang A, Zaroulis C. (abstract). Transfusion 1986;26:550

126. Poole J, Liew YW, Banks J. Unpublished observations 1990 cited in Byrne PC. Immunohematology 1991;7:46

127. Byrne PC. Immunohematology 1991;7:46
128. Brown LA, Dease M. (abstract). Am J Clin Pathol 1982;78:267
129. Burich MA, AuBuchon JP, Anderson HJ. (Letter). Transfusion 1986;26:116
130. Judd WJ. Methods in Immunohematology, 2nd Ed. Durham, N.C.: Montgomery 1994
131. Prewitt PL, Steane EA, Steane SM. (abstract). Transfusion 1983;23:434
132. Sassetti R, Nichols D. (Letter). Transfusion 1982;22:538
133. Moulds JJ, Edwards JM, Judd WJ. (Letter). Transfusion 1982;22:538
134. Holtz G, Mantel W, Buck W. Z Immun Forsch Exp Ther 1973;146:145
135. Mantel W, Holtz G. Z Immun Forsch Exp Ther 1974;147:420
136. Mantel W, Holtz G. Vox Sang 1976;30:453
137. Domokos V, Aszody L. Haematol Hung 1964;4:179
138. Domokos V, Aszody L. Haematol Hung 1964;4:187
139. Szilagyi T, Kavai M. Acta Physiol Acad Sci Hung 1970;38:411
140. Shore SL, Phillips DJ, Reimer CB. Immunochemistry 1971;8:562
141. Eyster ME, Jenkins DE. Am J Med 1969;46:360
142. Leddy JP, Bakemeier RF. Proc Soc Exp Biol NY 1967;125:808
143. Miyazaki S, Nakayama K, Akabane T, et al. Acta Haematol Jpn 1983;46:6
144. Borne AEGKr von dem, Engelfriet CP. Br J Haematol 1977;36:467
145. Meulen FW van der, Hart M van der, Fleer A, et al. Br J Haematol 1978;38:541
146. Fleer A, Schaik MLJ van, Borne AEGKr von dem, et al. Scand J Immunol 1978;8:515
147. Fleer A, Meulen FW van der, Linthout E, et al. Br J Haematol 1978;39:425
148. Meulen FW van der, Bruin HG de, Goosen PCM, et al. Br J Haematol 1980;46:47
149. Engelfriet CP, Borne AEGKr von dem, Beckers D, et al. In: A Seminar on Immune-Mediated Cell Destruction. Washington, D.C.:Am Assoc Blood Banks, 1981:93
150. Nance S, Garratty G. (abstract). Transfusion 1983;23:413
151. Tregellas WM, Pierce SR, Hardman JT, et al. (abstract). Transfusion 1980;20:628
152. Hunt JS, Beck ML, Hardman JT, et al. Am J Clin Pathol 1980;74:259
153. Hardman JT, Beck ML. Transfusion 1981;21;343.
154. Vengelen-Tyler V, Morel PA. Transfusion 1983;23:114
155. Postoway N, Garratty G. (abstract). Transfusion 1982;22:410
156. Jakway JW, Schanfield MS. (abstract). Transfusion 1983;23:413
157. Dorner IM, Parker CW, Chaplin H Jr. Br J Haematol 1968;14:383
158. Borne AEGKr von dem, Engelfriet CP, Beckers D, et al. Clin Exp Immunol 1969;4:333
159. Freedman J, Newlands M, Johnson CA. Vox Sang 1977;32:135
160. Schanfield MS, Pisciotta A, Libnock J. (abstract). Transfusion 1978;18:623
161. Kennedy MS, Waheed A, Marsh WL. (abstract). Transfusion 1981;21:630
162. Garratty G, Brunt D, Greenfield B, et al.. (abstract). Transfusion 1983;23:408
163. Salama A, Mueller-Eckhardt C. Br J Haematol 1987;65:67
164. Shirey RS, Kickler TS, Bell W, et al. Vox Sang 1987;52:219
165. Freedman J, Wright J, Lim FC, et al. Transfusion 1987;27:464
166. Dankbar DT, Pierce SR, Issitt PD, et al. (abstract). Transfusion 1987;27:534
167. Wolf MW, Roelcke D. Clin Immunol Immunopathol 1989;51:55
168. Wolf MW, Roelcke D. Clin Immunol Immunopathol 1989;51:68
169. Garratty G, Arndt P, Clarke A, et al. (abstract). Book of Abstracts. Joint Cong ISBT/AABB 1990:154
170. Kuipers EJ, van Imhoff GW, Hazenberg CAM, et al. Br J Haematol 1991;78:283
171. Arndt P, Clarke A, Doman R, et al. (abstract). Transfusion 1991;31 (Suppl 8S):29S
172. Berken A, Benacerraf B. J Exp Med 1966;123:119
173. Lo Buglio AF, Cotran RS, Jandl JH. Science 1967;158:1582
174. Huber H, Fudenberg HH. Int Arch Allgy 1968;34:18
175. Huber H, Douglas SD, Fudenberg HH. Immunology 1969;17:7
176. Abramson N, Lo Buglio AF, Jandl JH, et al. J Exp Med 1970;132:1191
177. Abramson N, Gelfand WE, Jandl JH, et al. J Exp Med 1970;132:1207
178. Kurlander RJ, Batker J. J Clin Invest 1982;69:1
179. Unkless JC. J Clin Invest 1989;83:355
180. Fanger MW, Shen L, Graziano RF, et al. Immunol Today 1989;10:92
181. Ravetch JV, Anderson CL. In: Fc Receptors and the Action of Antibodies. Washington, D.C.:Am Soc Microbiol, 1990:211
182. Groom AC, Schmidt EE. In: The Spleen: Structure, Function and Clinical Significance. London:Chapman and Hall, 1990:45
183. van der Winkel JGJ, Anderson CL. J Leuk Biol 1991;49:511
184. Gigli J, Nelson RA. Exp Cell Res 1968;51:45
185. Pearlman DS, Ward PA, Becker HJ. J Exp Med 1969;130:745
186. Brown PL, Lachmann PJ, Dacie JV. Clin Exp Immunol 1970;7:401
187. Schreiber AD, Frank MM. J Clin Invest 1972;51:575
188. Schreiber AD, Frank MM. J Clin Invest 1972;51:583
189. Atkinson JP, Frank MM. J Clin Invest 1974;53:1742
190. Bianco C, Griffin EM, Silverstein SC. J Exp Med 1975;141:1278
191. Jaffe CJ, Atkinson JP, Frank MM. J Clin Invest 1976;58:942
192. Fearon DT. J Exp Med 1980;152:20
193. Wright SD, Rao PE, van Voorhis WC, et al. Proc Nat Acad Sci USA 1983;80:5699
194. Rothlein R, Springer TA. J Immunol 1985;135:2668
195. Klickstein LB, Wong WW, Smith JA, et al. J Exp Med 1987;165:1095
196. Klickstein LB, Bartow TJ, Miletic V, et al. J Exp Med 1988;168:1699
197. Graham IL, Gresham HD, Brown EJ. J Immunol 1989;142:2352
198. Wong WW. J Invest Dermatol 1990;6:64S
199. Gergely J, Fudenberg HH, Loghem E van. Immunochemistry 1970;7:1
200. Borne AEGKr von dem, Beckers D, Muelen W van der, et al. Br J Haematol 1977;37:137
201. Stratton F, Rawlinson VI, Merry AH, et al. Clin Lab Haematol 1983;5:17
202. Nance S, Bourdo S, Garratty G. (abstract). Transfusion 1983;23:413
203. Rosse WF. Prog Hematol 1973;8:51
204. Guyre PM, Morganelli J, Miller R. J Clin Invest 1983;72:393
205. Mannel DN, Falk W. Cell Immunol 1983;79:396
206. Perussia B, Dayton ET, Lazarus R, et al. J Exp Med 1983;158:1092

207. Shen L, Guyre PM, Fanger MW. J Immunol 1987;139:534
208. Guyre PM, Campbell AS, Kniffin W, et al. J Clin Invest 1990;86:1892
209. van der Winkel JGJ, van Ommen R, Huizinga TWJ, et al. J Immunol 1989;143:571
210. Erbe DV, Collins JE, Shen L, et al. Mol Immunol 1990;27:57
211. Kay NE, Douglas SD. Blood 1977;70:889
212. Fries LF, Hall RP, Lawley TJ, et al. J Immunol 1982;129:1041
213. Gallagher MT, Branch DR, Mison A, et al. Exp Hematol 1983;11:82
214. Wagner O, Haltia K, Rasauen JA, et al. Ann Clin Res 1971;3:76
215. Stratton F, Rawlinson VI, Chapman SA, et al. Transfusion 1972;12:157
216. Sturgeon P, Smith LE, Chun HMT, et al. Transfusion 1979;19:324
217. Suzuki S, Amano T, Mitsunaga M, et al. Clin Immunol Immunopathol 1981;21:247.
218. Wolf CFW, Wolf DJ, Peterson P, et al. Transfusion 1982;22:238
219. Clark DA, Dessypris EN, Jenkins DE, et al. Blood 1984;64:1000
220. Kowal-Vern A, Jacobsen P, Okuno T, et al. Am J Pediat Hematol Oncol 1986;8:349
221. Reusser P, Osterwalder B, Burri H, et al. Acta Haematol 1987;77:53
222. Göttsche B, Salama A, Mueller-Eckhardt C. Vox Sang 1990;58:211
223. Girelli G, Perrone MP, Adorno G, et al. Haematologica 1990;75:182
224. Lum LG, Muchmore AV, Keren D, et al. J Immunol 1979;122:65
225. Lum LG, Muchmore AV, O'Connor N, et al. J Immunol 1979;123:714
226. Fanger MW, Shen L, Pugh J, et al. Proc Nat Acad Sci USA 1980;77:3640
227. Fanger MW, Pugh J, Bernier G. Immunology 1981;60:324
228. Fanger MW, Goldstine SN, Shen L. Mol Immunol 1983;20:1019
229. Gauldie J, Richards C, Lamontagne L. Mol Immunol 1983;20:1029
230. Shen L, Maliszewski CR, Rigby WFC, et al. Mol Immunol 1986;23:611
231. Yeaman GR, Kerr MA. Clin Exp Immunol 1987;68:200
232. Maliszewski CR, March CJ, Schoenborn MA, et al. J Exp Med 1990;172:1665
233. Mollison PL, Engelfriet CP, Contreras M. Blood Transfusion in Clinical Medicine, 9th Ed. Oxford:Blackwell, 1993
234. Shen L, Fanger MW. Cell Immunol 1981;59:75
235. Panzer S, Niessner H, Lechner K, et al. Scand J Haematol 1986;37:97
236. Issitt PD, Tessel JA, Beiting CY. Unpublished observations 1978, cited in Issitt PD. Applied Blood Group Serology, 3rd Ed. Miami:Montgomery 1985:523
237. Ben-Izhak C, Shechter Y, Tatarsky I. Scand J Haematol 1985;35:102
238. Sokol RJ, Hewitt S, Booker DJ, et al. Transfusion 1990;30:714
239. Sokol RJ, Hewitt S, Stamps BK. Br Med J 1981;282:2023
240. Sokol RJ, Hewitt S, Stamps BK. Vox Sang 1982;43:169
241. Sokol RJ, Hewitt S, Stamps BK. Acta Haematol 1983;69:266
242. Sokol RJ, Hewitt S, Booker DJ, et al. J Clin Pathol 1985;38:912
243. Sokol RJ, Hewitt S, Booker DJ, et al. J Clin Pathol 1987;40:254
244. Sokol RJ, Hewitt S, Booker DJ, et al. Clin Lab Haematol 1988;10:257
245. Sokol RJ, Booker DJ, Stamps BK, et al. Haematologia 1995;26:121
246. Fries LF, Brickman CM, Frank MM. J Immunol 1983;131:1240
247. Garratty G. Personal communication 1981 cited in Issitt PD. Applied Blood Group Serology, 3rd Ed. Miami:Montgomery, 1985:523
248. Holm G. Int Arch Allgy App Immunol 1972;43:671
249. Yust I, Wunderlich JR, Mann DL, et al. J Immunol 1973;110:1672
250. Urbaniak SJ. Br J Haematol 1976;33:409
251. Yust I, Smith RW, Wunderlich JR, et al. J Immunol 1976;116:1170
252. Shore SL, Mellwicz FM, Gordon DS. J Immunol 1977;118:558
253. Kurlander RJ, Rosse WF, Logue GL. J Clin Invest 1978;61:1309
254. Handwerger BS, Kay NW, Douglas SD. Vox Sang 1978;34:276
255. Milgrom H, Shore SL. Cell Immunol 1978;39:178
256. Northoff H, Kluge A, Resch K. Z Immun Forsch 1978;154:15
257. Show GM, Levy PC, Lo Buglio AF. Blood 1978;52:696
258. Urbaniak SJ. Br J Haematol 1979;42:303
259. Urbaniak SJ. Br J Haematol 1979;42:315
260. Randazzo B, Hirschberg T, Hirschberg H. Scand J Immunol 1979;9:351
261. Kurlander R, Rosse WF. Blood 1979;54;1131
262. Urbaniak SJ, Greiss MA. Br J Haematol 1980;46;447
263. Yust I, Goldsher N, Greenfeld R, et al. Israel J Med Sci 1980;16:174
264. Sarmay G, Benczur M, Petranyi G, et al. Mol Immunol 1984;21:43
265. Sarmay G, Jefferis R, Klein E, et al. Eur J Immunol 1985;15:1037
266. Rozsnyay X, Sarmay G, Walker M, et al. Immunology 1989;66;491
267. Walker MR, Lund J, Thompson KM, et al. Biochem J 1989;259:347
268. Jefferis R, Lund J, Pound J. Mol Immunol 1990;27:1237
269. Leader KA, Kumpel BM, Hadley AG, et al. Immunology 1991;72:481
270. Hadley AG, Kumpel BM, Leader KA, et al. Br J Haematol 1991;77:221
271. Mollison PL. Vox Sang 1991;60:225
272. Hadley AG, Zupanska B, Kumpel B, et al. Immunology 1992;76:446
273. Weiner W, Battey DA, Cleghorn TE, et al. Br Med J 1953;2:125
274. Dorner I. In: A Seminar on Problems Encountered in Pretransfusion Tests. Washington, D.C.:Am Assoc Blood Banks, 1972:1
275. Wiener AS, Gordon EB. Am J Clin Pathol 1953;23:429
276. Dacie JV, Cutbush M. J Clin Pathol 1954;7:8
277. Loghem JJ van, Hart M van der. Vox Sang (Old Series) 1954;4:2
278. Hollander L. Vox Sang (Old Series) 1954;4:164
279. Fluckiger P, Ricci C, Usteri C. Acta Haematol 1955;13:53
280. Kissmeyer-Nielsen F. In. P.H. Andresen, papers in dedication of his 60th birthday. Munksgaard:Copenhagen, 1957
281. Dacie JV. Br Med Bull 1959;15:67
282. Weiner W, Vos GH. Blood 1963;22:606
283. Vos GH, Petz LD, Fudenberg HH. Br J Haematol 1970;19:57
284. Leddy JP, Peterson P, Yeaw MA, et al. J Immunol

1970;105:677

285. Vos GH, Petz LD, Fudenberg HH. J Immunol 1971;106:1172

286. Vos GH, Petz LD, Garratty G, et al. Blood 1973;42:445

287. Celano MJ, Levine P. Transfusion 1967;7:265

288. Nugent ME, Colledge KI, Marsh WL. Vox Sang 1971;20:519

289. Marsh WL, Reid ME, Scott P. Br J Haematol 1972;22:625

290. Goldfinger D, Zwicker H, Belkin GA, et al. Transfusion 1975;15:351

291. Issitt PD, Pavone BG, Shapiro M. Transfusion 1979;19:389

292. Sistonen P. Med Biol 1981;59:230

293. Sistonen P, Nevanlinna HR, Virtaranta-Knowles K, et al. Vox Sang 1981;40:352

294. Sistonen P, Tippett P. Vox Sang 1982;42:252

295. Sistonen P, Green CA, Lomas CG, et al. Ann Hum Genet 1983;47:277

296. Schmidt PJ, Lostumbo MM, English CT, et al. Transfusion 1967;7:33

297. Race RR, Sanger R. Blood Groups in Man, 6th Ed. Oxford:Blackwell, 1975

298. Beck ML, Butch SH, Armstrong WD, et al. Transfusion 1972;12:280

299. Kessey EC, Pierce S, Beck ML, et al. (abstract). Transfusion 1973;13:360

300. Bell CA, Zwicker H. Transfusion 1980;20:86

301. Sacher RA, McGinniss MM, Shashat GG, et al. Am J Clin Pathol 1982;77:356

302. Roush GR, Rosenthal NS, Gerson SL, et al. Transfusion 1996;36:575

303. Wojcicki RE, Hardman JT, Beck ML, et al. (abstract). Transfusion 1980;20:628

304. McGinniss MH, Macher AM, Rook AH, et al. Transfusion 1986;26:405

305. Issitt PD, Marsh WL, Wren MR, et al. Transfusion 1989;29:508

306. Worlledge SM. (abstract). Book of Abstracts. 13th Cong ISBT 1972:43. Note: The presentation included a report of the first examples of auto-anti-En^a but those data do not appear in the abstract

307. Issitt PD, Pavone BG, Goldfinger D, et al. Transfusion 1975;15:353

308. Issitt PD, Pavone BG, Goldfinger D, et al. Transfusion 1976;16:396

309. Bell CA, Zwicker H. Transfusion 1978;18:572

310. Dahr W, Wilkinson SL, Issitt PD, et al. Proc 10th Int Cong Soc Foren Hematogenet. Wurzburg:Schmidt and Meyer, 1983:135

311. Dahr W, Wilkinson SL, Issitt PD. (abstract). Transfusion 1983;23:424

312. Wren MR, Issitt PD, Dahr W. (abstract). Transfusion 1984;24:425

313. Dahr W, Muller T, Moulds J, et al. Hoppe-Seyler's Z Physiol Chem 1985;366:41

314. Dahr W, Wilkinson S, Issitt PD, et al. Biol Chem Hoppe-Seyler 1986;367:1033

315. Telen MJ, Chassis JA. Blood 1990;76:842

316. Bruce LJ, Ring SM, Anstee DJ, et al. Blood 1995;85:541

317. Pavone BG, Billman R, Bryant J, et al. Transfusion 1981;21:25

318. Issitt PD, Daniels GL, Tippett P. (Letter). Transfusion 1981;21:473

319. Postoway N, Anstee D, Wortman M, et al. (abstract). Transfusion 1982;22:412

320. Seyfried H, Gorska B, Maj S, et al. Vox Sang 1972;23:528

321. Laird-Fryer B, Moulds JJ, Dahr W, et al. (abstract). Transfusion 1983;23:434

322. Moulds MK, Lacey P, Bradford MF, et al. (abstract). Book of Abstracts. 19th Cong ISBT/AABB 1986:653

323. Ainsworth BM, Fraser ID, Poole GD. (abstract). Book of Abstracts. 20th Cong ISBT 1988:82

324. D'Orsogna DE, Heinz R, Wawryszczuk V, et al. (abstract). Transfusion 1991;31 (Suppl 8S):23S

325. Beck ML, Marsh WL, Pierce SR, et al. Transfusion 1979;19:197

326. Marsh WL, DiNapoli J, Øyen R. Vox Sang 1979;36:174.

327. Marsh WL, Øyen R, Alicea E, et al. Am J Hematol 1979;7:155

328. Brendel WL, Issitt PD, Moore RE, et al. Biotest Bull 1985;2:201

329. Manny N, Levene C, Sela R, et al. Vox Sang 1983;45:252

330. Puig N, Carbonell F, Marty ML. Vox Sang 1986;51:57

331. Rowe GP, Tozzo GG, Poole J, et al. Immunohematology 1989;5:79

332. Vengelen-Tyler V, Gonzalez B, Garratty G, et al. Br J Haematol 1987;65:231

333. Williamson LM, Poole J, Redman C, et al. Br J Haematol 1994;87:805

334. Hare V, Wilson MJ, Wilkinson S, et al. (abstract). Transfusion 1981;21:613

335. Waheed A, Kennedy MS. Transfusion 1982;22:161

336. Garratty G. Unpublished observations 1963 cited in Issitt PD. Applied Blood Group Serology, 1st Ed. Oxnard:Spectra, 1975:126

337. Issitt PD. Unpublished observations 1964 cited in Issitt PD. Applied Blood Group Serology, lst Ed. Oxnard:Spectra Biologicals 1970:126

338. Holmes LD, Pierce SR, Beck ML. (abstract). Transfusion 1976;16:521

339. Patten E, Beck C, Scholl C, et al. Transfusion 1977;17:517

340. Issitt PD, Pavone BG, Frohlich JA, et al. Transfusion 1980;20:733

341. Ellisor SS, Reid M, O'Day T, et al. (abstract). Transfusion 1981;21:631

342. Judd WJ, Steiner EA, Cochran RK. Transfusion 1982;22:31

343. Halima D, Garratty G, Bueno R. Transfusion 1982;22:521

344. Guillausseau PJ, Wautier JL, Biozard B, et al. Sem Hop Paris 1982;58:803

345. Strikas R, Seifert MR, Lentino JR. Ann Intern Med 1983;99:345

346. Sosler SD, Behzad O, Garratty G, et al. Transfusion 1984;24:206

347. Sander RP, Hardy NM, Van Meter SA. Transfusion 1987;27:58

348. Ciaffoni S, Ferro I, Potenza R, et al. Hematologica 1987;72:245

349. Ganly PS, Laffan MA, Owen I, et al. Br J Haematol 1988;69:537

350. Alpaugh K, Sysko-Stein L, Lusch C, et al. Lab Med 1989;20:682

351. Garratty G, Sattler MS, Petz LD, et al. Blood Transf Immunohematol 1979;22:529

352. Viggiano E, Clary NL, Ballas SK, Transfusion 1982;22:329

353. Garratty G. In: Clinical and Basic Science Aspects of Immunohematology. Arlington, VA:Am Assoc Blood Banks, 1991:33

354. Eveland D. (abstract). Book of Abstracts. ISBT/AABB Joint Cong, 1990:156

355. Johnson MH, Plett MH, Conant CD, et al. (abstract). Transfusion 1978;18:389

356. Allessandrino EP, Costamagna L, Pagani A, et al. (Letter). Transfusion 1984;24:369

357. van't Veer MB, van Leeuwen I, Haas FJLM, et al. Vox Sang 1984;47:88

358. Yokoyama M, Eith DT, Bowman M. Vox Sang 1967;12:138

359. Yokoyama M, McCoy JE. Vox Sang 1967;13:15

360. Sullivan CM, Klein WE, Rabin BI, et al. Transfusion 1987;27:322

361. Oxendine SM, Telen MJ, Rao N, et al. (abstract). Transfusion 1992;32 (Suppl 8S):18S

362. Rao N, Whitsett CF, Oxendine SM, et al. Blood 1993;81:815

363. Moulds M, Strohm P, McDowell MA, et al. (abstract). Transfusion 1988;28 (Suppl 6S):36S

364. Muller A, Andre-Liardet J, Garretta M, et al. Rev Fr Transf 1973;16:251

365. Beattie KM, Sigmund KE. Transfusion 1987;27:54

366. Poole J, Reid ME, Banks J, et al. Vox Sang 1990;58:287

367. Shulman IA, Vengelen-Tyler V, Thompson JC, et al. Vox Sang 1990;59:232

368. Szaloky A, Hart M van der. Vox Sang 1971;20:376

369. Herron R, Hyde RD, Hillier SJ. Vox Sang 1979;36:179

370. Ferrer Z, Cornwall S, Berger R, et al. Blood Transf Immunohematol 1984;27:639

371. Becton DL, Kinney TR. Vox Sang 1986;51:108

372. Tregellas WM, Holub MP, Moulds JJ, et al. (abstract). Transfusion 1979;19:650

373. McDowell MA, Stocker I, Nance S, et al. (abstract). Transfusion 1986;26:578

374. Owen I, Chowdhury V, Reid ME, et al. Transfusion 1992;32:173

375. Peloquin P, Moulds M, Keenan J, et al. (abstract). Transfusion 1989;29 (Suppl 7S):49S

376. Brown P, Wood M, Wojcicki R, et al. (abstract). Transfusion 1981;21:632

377. Marsh WL, Brown PJ, DiNapoli J, et al. Transfusion 1983;23:128

378. Ward JM, Caggiano V. (Letter). Transfusion 1983;23:174

379. Issitt PD, Combs MR, Allen J, et al. Transfusion 1996;36:802

380. Szymanski IO, Roberts PL, Rosenfield RE. New Eng J Med 1976;294:995

381. Parker AC, Willis G, Urbaniak SJ, et al. Br Med J 1978;1:26

382. Lopez M, Banopoulos H, Liberge G, et al. Vox Sang 1975;28:371

383. McClelland WM, Bradley A, Morris TCM, et al. Vox Sang 1981;41:231

384. Atichartakarn V, Chiewsilp P, Ratanasirivanich P, et al. Vox Sang 1985;49:301

385. Beck ML, Haines RF, Oberman HA. (abstract). Prog 24th Ann Mtg Am Assoc Blood Banks, 1971:98

386. Bird GWG, Wingham J. Immunol Comm 1980;9:155

387. Salamon DJ, Nusbacher J, Yang S, et al. (abstract). Transfusion 1983;23:408.

388. Rowley S, Braine H. (abstract). Blood 1982;60 (Suppl):171a

389. Hows J, Beddow K, Gordon-Smith E, et al. Blood 1986;67:177

390. Hazelhurst GR, Brenner MK, Wimperis JZ, et al. Scand J Haematol 1986;37:1

391. Ahmed KY, Nunn G, Brazier DM, et al. Transplantation 1987;43:163

392. Ramsey G. Transfusion 1991;31:76

393. Gajewski JL, Petz LD, Calhoun L, et al. (abstract). Blood 1990;76 (Suppl 1):398a

394. Petz LD. In: Clinical and Basic Science Aspects of Immunohematology. Arlington, VA:Am Assoc Blood Banks, 1991:73

395. Contreras M, Hazelhurst GR, Armitage SE. Br J Haematol 1983;55:657

396. Victoria EJ, Pierce SW, Branks MJ, et al. J Lab Clin Med 1990;115:74

397. Leddy JP, Falany JL, Kissel GE, et al. J Clin Invest 1993;91:1672

398. Leddy JP, Wilkinson SL, Kissel GE, et al. Blood 1994;84:650

399. Tanner MJA, Martin PG, High S. Biochem J 1988;256:703

400. Lux SE, John KM, Kopito RR, et al. Proc Nat Acad Sci USA 1989;86:9089

401. Tanner MJA. Sem Hematol 1993;30:34

402. Moore S, Green C. Biochem J 1987;244:735

403. Avent ND, Ridgwell K, Mawby WJ, et al. Biochem J 1988;256:1043

404. Anstee DJ, Tanner MJA. Bailliere's Clin Haematol 1993;6:401

405. Cleghorn TE. MD Thesis, Univ Sheffield, 1961

406. Greendyke RM, Banzhaf JC. Transfusion 1977;17:621

407. Issitt PD. Applied Blood Group Serology, 3rd Ed. Miami:Montgomery 1985

408. Issitt PD, Zellner DC, Rolih SD, et al. Transfusion 1977;17:531

409. Henry RA, Weber J, Pavone BG, et al. Transfusion 1977;17:539

410. Issitt PD, Pavone BG. Br J Haematol 1978;38:63

411. Weber J, Caceres VW, Pavone BG, et al. Transfusion 1979;19:216

412. Issitt PD. In: Red Cell Antigens and Antibodies. Arlington, VA:Am Assoc Blood Banks, 1986:99

413. Rosenfield RE. Unpublished manuscript 1961 cited in Issitt PD, Pavone BG. Br J Haematol 1978;38:63

414. Pavone BG, Issitt PD. Unpublished observations 1978-1979 cited in Issitt PD. Applied Blood Group Serology, 3rd Ed. Miami:Montgomery 1985:527

415. Dameshek W, Levine P. New Eng J Med 1943;228:641

416. Allen FH Jr. Proc 8th Cong ISBT. Basel:Karger, 1960:359

417. Chown B, Kaita H, Lowen B, et al. Transfusion 1971;11:220

418. Cook IA. Br J Haematol 1971;20:369

419. Lalezari P, Talleyrand NP, Wenz B, et al. Vox Sang 1975;28:19

420. Isbister JP, Ting A, Seeto KM. Vox Sang 1977;33:353

421. Worlledge SM. Br J Haematol 1978;39:157

422. Issitt PD. Unpublished observations 1979-1981 cited in Mollison PL. Blood Transfusion in Clinical Medicine, 7th Ed. Oxford:Blackwell, 1983

423. Mollison PL. Blood Transfusion in Clinical Medicine, 7th Ed. Oxford:Blackwell, 1983

424. Salama A, Mueller-Eckhardt C. Transfusion 1984;24:188

425. Ness PM, Shirey RS, Thomas SK, et al. Transfusion 1990;30:688

426. Harris T. Immunohematology 1990;6:87

427. Ellisor SS, Reid ME, O'Day T, et al. Vox Sang 1983;45:53

428. Issitt PD, Obarski G, Hartnett PL, et al. Transfusion 1990;30:46

429. Issitt PD, Combs MR, Bumgarner DJ, et al. Transfusion 1996;36:481

430. Stratton F, Renton PH, Rawlinson VI. Lancet 1960;1:1388

431. Jenkins WJ, Marsh WL. Lancet 1961;2:16

432. Ozer FL, Chaplin H Jr. J Clin Invest 1963;42:1735

433. Gray LS, Kleeman JE, Masouredis SP. Br J Haematol 1983;55:335

434. Branch DR, Shulman IA, Sy Siok Hian AL, et al. Blood 1984;6:177

435. Kay MMB. In: Immunobiology of Transfusion Medicine. New York:Marcel Dekker, 1994:173

436. Arndt P, O'Hoski P, McBride J, et al. (abstract). Transfusion 1989;29 (Suppl 7S):48S

437. Kay MMB. In: Red Cell Antigens and Antibodies. Arlington, VA:Am Assoc Blood Banks, 1986:35

438. Herron R, Clark M, Smith DS. Vox Sang 1987;52:71

439. Rearden A, Chiu PH. Blood 1983;61:525

440. Falkenburg JHF, Fibbe WE, Vaart-Duinkerken N van der, et al. Blood 1985;66:660

441. Ballas SK, Flynn JC, Pauline LA, et al. Am J Hematol 1986;23:19

442. Mangan KF, Besa EC, Shadduck RK, et al. Exp Hematol 1984;12:788

443. Conley CL, Lippman SM, Ness PM, et al. New Eng J Med 1982;306:281

444. Hedge UM, Gordon-Smith EC, Worlledge SM. Br Med J 1977;2:1444

445. Hazeltine M, Rauch Y, Danoff D, et al. J Rheumatol 1988;15:80

446. Sthoeger Z, Sthoeger D, Green L, et al. (abstract). Blood 1990;76 (Suppl):392a

447. Cabral AR, Cabiedes J, Alarcon-Segovia D. J Autoimmun 1990;3:773

448. Arvieux J, Schweizer B, Roussel B, et al. Vox Sang 1991;61:190

449. Out HJ, de Groot PG, Vleit M van, et al. Blood 1991;77:2655

450. Hammond A, Rudge AC, Loizou S, et al. Arth Rheumatol 1989;32:259

451. Masouredis SP, Branks MJ, Garratty G, et al. J Lab Clin Med 1987;110:308

452. Masouredis SP, Branks MJ, Victoria EJ. Blood 1987;70:710

453. Wiener E, Hughes-Jones NC, Irish WT, et al. Clin Exp Immunol 1986;63:680

454. Wakui H, Imai H, Kobayashi R, et al. Blood 1988;72:402

455. Lutz HU, Wipf G. J Immunol 1982;128:1695

456. Gilsanz F, de la Serna J, Molton L, et al. Transfusion 1996;36:463

457. Sheridan W, Winton EF, Chan WC, et al. Blood 1988;72:1701

458. Trinchieri G. Adv Immunol 1989;47:187

459. Suzucki N, Bianchi E, Bass H, et al. J Exp Med 1990;172:457

460. Moretta A, Bottino C, Pende D, et al. J Exp Med 1990;172:1589

461. Zambello R, Trentin L, Ciccone E, et al. Blood 1993;81:2381

462. Loughran TP Jr. Blood 1993;82:1

463. Tefferi A, Li CY, Witzig TE, et al. Blood 1994;84:2721

464. Lutz HU, Flepp R, Stammler P, et al. Clin Exp Immunol 1987;67:674

465. Lutz HU. Transf Med Rev 1992;6:201

466. De Angelis V, Pradella P, Biasinutto C, et al. Autoimmunity 1995;21:263

467. De Angelis V, De Matteis MC, Cozzi MR, et al. Br J Haematol 1996;95:273

468. De Matteis MC, De Angelis V, Sorrentino F, et al. Br J Haematol 1991;79:108

469. Delamarie M, Durand F, Grosbois B, et al. Br J Haematol 1992;80:91

470. Barker RN, Casswell KM, Reid ME, et al. Br J Haematol 1992;82:126

471. Elson CJ. Immunol Today 1980;1:42

472. Hooper DC. Immunol Today. 1987;8:327

473. Barker RN, Elson CJ. Eur J Immunol 1994;24:1578

474. Gerbal A, Homberg JC, Rochant H, et al. Nouv Rev Fr Hematol 1968;8:155

475. Beck ML, Dixon J, Oberman HA. Am J Clin Pathol 1971;56:475

476. Bird GWG, Wingham J. Vox Sang 1972;22:364

477. Pavone BG, Issitt PD. Unpublished observations 1976 cited in Issitt PD. Applied Blood Group Serology, 3rd Ed. Miami:Montgomery 1985:529

478. Crookston JH. Arch Int Med 1975;135:1314

479. Moake JL, Shultz DR. Am J Med 1975;58:431

480. Freedman J, Newlands M. Vox Sang 1977;32:61

481. Freedman J, Cheng LF, Murray D, et al. Am J Hematol 1983;14:175

482. Shulman IA, Branch DR, Nelson JM, et al. J Am Med Assoc 1985;253:1746

483. Kajii E, Miura Y, Ikemota S. Vox Sang 1991;60:45

484. Frank MM, Schreiber AD, Atkinson JP. In: Phagocytic Cells in Host Resistance. New York:Raven, 1975

485. Rosse WF. J Clin Invest 1971;50:734

486. Ahn YS, Harrington WJ. Adv Intern Med 1980;25:453

487. Ahn YS, Harrington WJ, Byrnes JJ, et al. J Am Med Assoc 1983;249:2189

488. Ahn YS, Harrington WJ, Mylvaganam R, et al. Ann Int Med 1984;100:192

489. Aisenberg AC, Wilkes B. J Clin Invest 1964;43:2394

490. Malawista SE. Blood 1971;37:519

491. Vassalli JD, Hamilton J, Reich E. Cell 1976;8:271

492. Atkinson JP, Michael JM, Chaplin H Jr. J Immunol 1977;118:1292

493. Wong P, Hiruma K, Endoh N, et al. Br J Haematol 1987;65:380

494. Bruggers CS, Kurtzberg J, Friedman HA. Am J Pediat Hematol Oncol 1991;13:300

495. Owellen RJ, Hartke CA, Hians FO. Cancer Res 1977;37:2597

496. Nelson RL, Dyke RW, Root MA. Cancer Tmt Rev 1980;7 (Suppl 1):17

497. Hosea SW, Burch CG, Brown EJ, et al. Lancet 1981;1:804

498. Ruben FL, Hankins WA, Zeigler Z, et al. Am J Med 1984;76:115

499. Pirofsky B. Sem Hematol 1976;13:251

500. Mollison PL. Br Med Bull 1959;15:59

501. Hamblin TJ. Apheresis Bull 1983;1:10

502. Shumak KH, Rock GA. New Eng J Med 1984;310:762

503. Urbaniak SJ. Clinics in Hematol 1984;13:217

504. Huestis DW. In: Progress in Transfusion Medicine. Vol 1. Edinburgh:Churchill Livingstone, 1986:78

505. Huestis DW. In: Therapeutic Hemapheresis. Milan:Wichtig, 1986:179

506. Wells JV. In: Basic and Clinical Immunology, 3rd Ed. Los Altos, CA:Lange, 1980:64

507. Sandor M, Langone JJ. Biochem Biophys Res Comm 1982;106:761

508. Verrier Jones J. Transf Sci 1990;11:153

509. Gjorstrup P, Watt RM. Transf Sci 1990;11:281

510. Besa EC, Ray PK, Swami VK, et al. Am J Med 1981;71:1035

511. MacIntyre EA, Linch DC, Macey MG, et al. Br J Haematol 1985;60:387

512. Bussell JB, Cunningham-Rundles C, Abraham C. Vox Sang 1986;51:264

513. Pocecco M, Ventura A, Tamaro P, et al. (Letter). J Pediat 1986;109:726

514. Newland AC, Macey MG, MacIntyre EA, et al. (abstract). Book of Abstracts. 21st Cong ISBT 1986:359

515. Hilgartner MW, Bussel J. Am J Med 1987;83 (Suppl 4A):25

516. Ritch PS, Anderson T. Cancer 1987;60:2637

517. Mitchell CA, Weyden MB van der, Firkin BG. Austral NZ J Med 1987;17:290

518. Besa EC. Am J Med 1988;84:691

519. Argiolu F, Diana G, Arnone M, et al. Acta Haematol 1990;83:65

520. Mueller-Eckhardt C, Salama A, Mahn I, et al. Scand J Haematol 1985;34:394

521. Flores G, Cunningham-Rundles C, Newland AC, et al. Am J Hematol 1993;44:237.

522. Hughes P, Toogood A. Acta Haematol 1994;91:166

523. Hershko C, Sonnenblik M, Ashkenazi J. Br J Haematol 1990;76:436

524. Kappler JW, Roehm N, Marrack P. Cell 1987;49:273

525. MacDonald HR, Pedrazzini T, Schneider R, et al. J Exp Med 1988;167:2005

526. Rosse WJ. Clinical Immunohematology: Basic Concepts and Clinical Applications. Boston:Blackwell, 1990:467

527. Nemazee DA, Bürki K. Nature 1989;337:562

528. Rammensee H-G, Korschewski R, Frangoulis B. Nature 1989;339:541

529. Goodnow CC, Crosbie J, Jorgenson H, et al. Nature 1989;342:385

530. Ramsdell F, Lantz T, Fowlkes BJ. Science 1989;246:1038

531. Hooper DC, Young JL, Elson CJ, et al. Cell Immunol 1987;106:53.

532. Plebanski M. PhD Thesis, Univ Bristol 1992, cited in Barker RN, Elson CJ. Eur J Immunol 1994;24:1578

533. Ballas SK. Br J Haematol 1989;71:137

534. Cox KO, Hardy SJ. Immunology 1985;55:263

535. Laing P, Parkar BA, Culbert EJ, et al. Scand J Immunol 1987;25:613

536. Kawaguchi S. Immunology 1987;62:11

537. Hardy SJ, Cox KO. Int Arch Allgy Appl Immunol 1990;91:108

538. Barker RN, Gruffydd-Jones TJ, Stokes CR, et al. Clin Exp Immunol 1991;85:33

539. Grabowska et al. of Warsaw, Poland. Cited by Koscielak J. in a report of a 1979 ISBT Meeting in Warsaw. Vox Sang 1980;39:291, no other details about authors given

540. van't Veer MB, van Wieringen PMV, van Leeuwen I, et al. Br J Haematol 1981;49:383

541. Issitt PD, Gruppo RA, Wilkinson SL, et al. Br J Haematol 1982;52:537

542. Issitt PD, Wilkinson SL, Gruppo RA. (Letter). Br J Haematol 1983;53:688

543. Vengelen-Tyler V, Mogck N. Transfusion 1991;31:254 543

544. Rolih S. (Letter). Immunohematology 1991;7:83

545. Issitt PD. Immunohematology 1991;7:29

546. Issitt PD. (Letter). Immunohematology 1991;7:83

547. Leikola J, Perkins HA. Transfusion 1980;20:138

548. Leikola J, Perkins HA. Transfusion 1980;20:224

549. Bodensteiner D, Brown P, Skikne B, et al. Am J Clin Pathol 1983;79:182

550. Postoway N, Nance SJ, Garratty G. Med Lab Sci 1985;42:11

551. Issitt PD, Gutgsell NS, Tomasulo PA, et al. In: Blood Bank Scientific News, Miami:Am Red Cross, 1988:1

552. de Bruin HG, Meulen FW van der, Aaig C. Flow Cytom 1980;4:233

553. Nance S, Garratty G. (abstract). Blood 1984;64 (Suppl 1):88a

554. Nance SJ, Garratty G. J Immunol Meth 1987;101:127

555. Nance ST. In: Progress in Immunohematology. Arlington, VA:Am Assoc Blood Banks, 1988:1

556. Singer K, Dameshek W. Ann Int Med 1941;15:544

557. Allibone EC, Collins DH. J Clin Pathol 1951;4:412

558. Barry KG, Crosby WH. Ann Int Med 1957;47:1002

559. Lewis SM, Szur L, Dacie JV. Br J Haematol 1960;6:122

560. Yam LT, Rudgke C, Busch S, et al. Am J Obstet Gynecol 1966;95:207

561. Dawson MA, Talbert W, Yarbro JW. Am J Med 1971;50:552

562. de Bruyere M, Sokol G, Devoitille JM, et al. Br J Haematol 1971;20:83.

563. Lorber M, Schwartz LI, Wasserman LR. Am J Med 1955;19:887

564. Balint JA, Hammak WJ, Patton JB. Am J Dig Dis 1963;8:537

565. Gastaldi F, Regazzini A, Chiappino G, et al. Riv Emot Immunoematol 1963;19:193

566. Fong S, Fudenberg H, Perlmann P. Vox Sang 1963;8:688

567. Molaro GL, Barillari B. Riv Emot Immunoematol 1964;11:43

568. Black AJ, Eisinger AJMF, Loehry CAEH, et al. Br Med J 1969;2:31

569. Bardana EJ, Pirofsky B. Int Arch Allgy 1970;37:325

570. Arner O, Brohult J, Engsted L, et al. Acta Med Scand 1971;189:275

571. Carcassonne Y. Med Chir Dig 1973;2:67

572. Thomas M, Homberg JC, Huguet C, et al. Clin Med Ther Paris Chir Dig 1973;2:73

573. Dmoszynska A. Pol Tyk Ledk 1973;28:1064

574. Goldstone AH. Br Med J 1974;8:556

575. Gorst DW, Leyland MJ, Delamore WI. Postgrad Med J 1975;51:409

576. Jacob J, Lance KP. Am J Gastroenterol 1976;65:324

577. Shashaty GG, Rath CE, Britt EJ. Am J Hematol 1977;3:199

578. Altman AR, Maltz C, Janowitz HD. Dig Dis Sci 1979;24:282

579. Garratty G. Davis J, Meyers M, et al. (abstract). Transfusion 1980;20:646

580. Fagiolo E, Carbonne D, Bianco A, et al. Ital J Gastroenterol 1982;14:34

581. Poulsen LO, Freund L, Lylloff K, et al. Acta Med Scand 1988;223:75

582. Garratty G. Personal communication, 1996

583. Jones E, Tillman C. J Am Med Assoc 1945;128:1225

584. Frumin AM, Mendel TH, Meranze GR. Gastroenterology 1954;27:183

585. Sohier JD, Juranies E, Aub JC. Cancer Res 1957;17:767

586. Zemak L, Strom L, Gordon G, et al. J Am Med Assoc 1964;187:232

587. Ellis LD, Westerman MP. J Am Med Assoc 1965;193:962

588. Sawitsky A, Ozaeta PB Jr. Bull NY Acad Med 1970;46:411

589. Miura AB, Shibata A, Akihama T, et al. Cancer 1974;33:111

590. Canale D, Feldman R, Rosen M, et al. Urology 1975;5:411

591. Gordon PA, Baylis PH, Bird GWG. Br Med J 1976;26:1569

592. Spira RYA, Lynch WG. Am J Med 1979;67:753

593. Inoue Y, Kaku K, Kaneko T, et al. Acta Haematol Jpn 1983;46:836

594. Johnson P, Gualtieri RJ, Mohler DN, et al. Southn Med J 1985;78:1129

595. Venzano C, De Micheli A, Cavallero GB. Haematologica 1985;70:166

596. Honan W, Balazs J, Jariwalla AG. Br J Clin Pract 1986;40:35

597. Tregellas WM, Lavine KK. (abstract). Transfusion 1982;22:406

598. Bromberg YM, Toaff R, Ehrenfeld E. J Obstet Gynaecol Br Emp 1948;55:325

599. Frumin AM, Smith EM, Taylor AG, et al. Am J Obstet Gynecol 1953;65:421

600. Craig GA, Turner RL. Br Med J 1955;1:1003

601. Burt RL, Pritchard RW. Obstet Gynecol 1957;90:444

602. Soderhjelm L. Acta Pediat 1959;48 (Suppl 117):34

603. Bateman DER, Hutt MSR, Norris PR. J Obstet Gynaecol Br Emp 1959;66:130

604. Seip M. Arch Dis Childh 1960;35:364

605. Swisher SN. Postgrad Med 1966;40:378

606. Silverstein MN, Aaro LA, Kempers RD. Am J Med Sci 1966;252:206

607. Letts HW, Kredenster B. Am J Clin Pathol 1968;49:481

608. Jankelowitz T, Eckerling B, Joshua H. S Afr Med J 1969;24:911

609. Blajchman MA, Gordon H. Transfusion 1972;12:276
610. Chaplin H, Cohen R, Bloomberg B, et al. Br J Haematol 1973;24:219
611. Baumann R, Rubin H. Blood 1973;41:293
612. Eldor A, Yatzin S, Hershko C. Br Med J 1975;4:625
613. Kageyama T, Iwakoshi K, Tsumoto S, et al. Bull Osaka Med Sch 1975;21:140
614. Hershko C, Berrebi A, Resnitzky P, et al. Scand J Haematol 1976;16:135
615. Jain S, Agarwal S, Dash SC, et al. J Assoc Phys Ind 1977;25:765
616. Goodall HB, Ho-Yen DO, Clark DM, et al. Scand J Haematol 1979;22:185
617. Yam P, Wilkinson L, Petz LD, et al. Am J Hematol 1980;8:23
618. Sacks DA, Platt LD, Johnson CS. Am J Obstet Gynecol 1981;140:942
619. Lawe JE. Transfusion 1982;22:66
620. Veloso T, Fraga J, Carvalho J, et al. J Clin Gastroenterol 1991;13:445
621. Yates P, Macht LM, Williams NA, et al. Br J Haematol 1992;82:753
622. Hitzig WH, Massimo L. Blood 1966;28:841
623. Zeulzer WW, Stulberg CS, Page RH, et al. Transfusion 1966;6:438
624. Johnson CA, Abildgaard CF. Acta Pediat Scand 1976;65:375
625. Greenberg J, Curtis-Cohen M, Gill FM, et al. J Pediat 1980;97:784
626. Burstein Y, Berns L, Ped Ann 1982;11:301
627. Heisel MA, Ortega JA. Am J Pediat Hematol Oncol 1983;5:147
628. Sokol RJ, Hewitt S, Stamps BK, et al. Acta Haematol 1984;72:245
629. Smith MA, Shah NS, Lobel JS. Am J Pediat Hematol Oncol 1989;11:167
630. Stellrecht KA, Vella AT. Immunol Lett 1992;31:273
631. Bernstein ML, Schneider BK, Naiman J. J Pediat 1981;98:774
632. Fosburg M, Dolan M, Propper R, et al. J Clin Apher 1983;1:215
633. Greuth M, Wagner HP, Pipczynski-Suter K, et al. Acta Pediat Scand 1986;75:1037
634. McConnell ME, Atchison JA, Kohaut E, et al. Am J Pediat Hematol Oncol 1987;9:158
635. Heidemann SM, Sarnaik SA, Sarnaik AP. Am J Pediat Hematol Oncol 1987;9:302
636. Leickly FE, Buckley RH. Am J Med 1987;82:159
637. Ware RE. Sem Ped Inf Dis 1992;3:179
638. Pui C-H, Wilimas J, Wang W. J Pediat 1980;97:754
639. Miller BA, Beardsley DS. J Pediatr 1983;103:877
640. Morel PA, Bergren MO, Frank BA. (abstract). Transfusion 1991;18:388
641. Stratton F, Renton PH. Practical Blood Grouping. Springfield, MO:Thomas, 1958
642. Reid ME, Toy PTCY. Vox Sang 1984;46:355
643. Issitt PD. In: A Symposium on Rh Problems in Clinical Practice. Groningen:Netherlands Red Cross, 1979:46
644. Laine ML, Beattie KM. Transfusion 1985;25:545
645. James P, Rowe GP, Tozzo GG. Vox Sang 1988;54:167
646. Wallhermfechtel BA, Pohl B, Chaplin H. Transfusion 1984;24:482
647. Ley AB, Mayer K, Harris JP. Proc 6th Cong ISBT. Basel:Karger, 1958
648. Hogman C, Killander J, Sjolin S. Acta Paediat 1960;49:270
649. Pavone BG, Issitt PD. Unpublished observations 1978 cited in Issitt PD. Applied Blood Group Serology, 3rd Ed. Miami:Montgomery 1985:535

650. Rosenfield RE, Jagathambal K. Sem Hematol 1976;13:311
651. Levy M, Siddiqui W, Chou S. Nature 1974;247:546
652. Chan V, Lee P. SE Asian J Trop Med Pub Health 1974;5:447
653. Kreger I, Urh I, Smith H, et al. In: Intracellular Protein Catabolism. New York:Plenum, 1977:250
654. Siegel D, Goodman S, Branton D. Biochim Biophys Acta 1980;598:517
655. Sherman IW, Tanigoshi L. In: Biochemistry of Parasites. New York:Pergamon, 1981:137
656. Gyang FN, Poole B, Trager W. Mol Biochem Parasitol 1982;5:263
657. Sherman IW, Tanigoshi L. Mol Biochem Parasitol 1983;8:207
658. Bruce-Chwatt LJ. Essential Malariology, 2nd Ed. New York:Wiley, 1985
659. Topley E, Knight R, Woodruff AW. Trans Roy Soc Trop Med Hyg 1973;67:51
660. Facer CA, Bray RA, Brown J. Clin Exp Immunol 1979;35:119
661. Facer CA. Clin Exp Immunol 1980;39:279
662. Abdalla S, Weatherall DJ. Br J Haematol 1982;51:415
663. Jeje OM, Kelton JG, Blajchman MA. Br J Haematol 1983;54:567
664. Brown KN, Berzins K, Jarra W, et al. Clin Immunol Allgy 1986;6:227
665. Petz LD, Catlett JP, Lessin LS. In: Textbook of Internal Medicine, 3rd Ed. Philadelphia:Lippincott-Raven, 1997:1467
666. Grabowski EF, Giardina PJV, Goldberg D. Ann Intern Med 1982;96:466
667. Desforges JF, Quimby F. New Eng J Med 1976;295:103
668. Grunwaldt E. NY State J Med 1977;77:1320
669. Cahill KM, Benach JL, Reich LM, et al. Transfusion 1981;21:193
670. Wolf CFW, Resnick G, Marsh WL, et al. (Letter). Transfusion 1982;22:538
671. Rosner F, Zarrabi MH, Benach JL, et al. Am J Med 1984;76:696
672. Anderson JF, Mintz ED, Gadbaw JJ, et al. J Clin Microbiol 1991;29:2779
673. Wittner M, Rowin KS, Tanovitz HB, et al.. Ann Int Med 1982;96:601
674. Smith RP, Evans AT, Popovsky MA, et al. J Am Med Assoc 1986;256:2726
675. Popovsky MA, Lindberg LE, Syrek AL, et al. Transfusion 1988;28:59
676. Popovsky MA. In: Emerging Global Patterns in Transfusion-Transmitted Infections. Arlington, VA:Am Assoc Blood Banks, 1990:45
677. Popovsky MA. Transfusion 1991;31:296
678. Mintz ED, Anderson JF, Cable RG, et al. Transfusion 1991;31:365
679. Nagl RL, Roth EF. Blood 1989;74:1213
680. Branch DR, Muensch HA, Sy Siok Hian S, et al. Br J Haematol 1983;54:573
681. Garratty G, Arndt P, Nance S, et al. (abstract). Book of Abstracts. ISBT/AABB Joint Cong 1990:87
682. Lapierre Y, Rigal D, Adam J, et al. Transfusion 1990;30:109
683. Boulton FE. (Letter). Br J Biomed Sci 1996;53:172
684. Evans RS, Weiser RS. Arch Int Med 1957;100:371
685. Gilliland BC, Leddy JP, Vaughan JH. J Clin Invest 1970;49:898
686. Gilliland BC, Baxter E, Evans RS. New Eng J Med 1971;285:252
687. Garratty G, Petz LD. (abstract). Prog 24th Ann Mtg AABB, 1971:83
688. Parker AC, Habeshaw J, Cleland JF. Scand J Haematol

1972;9:318

689. Chaplin H Jr. Prog Hematol 1973;7:25
690. Gilliland BC, Evans RS. In: A Seminar on Recent Advances in Immunohematology. Washington, D.C.:Am Assoc Blood Banks, 1973:31
691. Fischer J, Petz LD, Garratty G. Clin Red 1973;21:265
692. Rosse WF. Ser Hematol 1974;7:358
693. Gilliland BC. Sem Hematol 1976;13:267
694. Rand BP, Olson JD, Garratty G, et al. Transfusion 1978;18:174
695. Petz LD. In: Manual of Clinical Immunology, 2nd Ed. Chicago:Am Soc Microbiol, 1981
696. Schmitz N, Djibey I, Kretschmer V, et al. Vox Sang 1981;41:224
697. Yam P, Petz LD, Spath P. Am J Hematol 1982;12:337
698. Garratty G, Postoway N, Nance S, et al. (abstract). Transfusion 1982;22:430
699. Tomasulo PA, Issitt PD, Gutgsell NS, et al. (abstract). Book of Abstracts. 20th Cong ISBT 1988:121
700. Gutgsell NS, Issitt PD, Tomasulo PA, et al. (abstract). Transfusion 1988;28 (Suppl 6S):36S
701. Garratty G, Postoway N, Nance S, et al. (abstract). Book of Abstracts. Joint Cong ISBT/AABB 1990:87
702. Owen I, Hows J. Transfusion 1990;30:814
703. Issitt PD, Gutgsell NS. Gematol Transf 1992;37:29
704. Merry AH, Thomson EE, Rawlinson VI, et al. Clin Lab Haematol 1982;4:393
705. Idelson LL, Koyfman MM, Gorina LG, et al. Vox Sang 1976;31:401
706. Issitt PD, Pavone BG. Unpublished observations 1972 cited in Issitt PD. Applied Blood Group Serology, 3rd Ed. Miami:Montgomery 1985:537
707. Burkart P, Rosenfield RE, Hsu TCS, et al. Vox Sang 1974;26:289
708. Costea N, Schwartz R, Constantoulakis M, et al. Blood 1962;20:214
709. Rochna E, Hughes-Jones NC. Vox Sang 1965;10:675
710. McConahey PJ, Dixon FJ. Int Arch Allgy 1966;29:185
711. Jenkins DE Jr, Moore WH, Hawiger A. Transfusion 1977;17:16
712. Lalezari P, Jiang AF. Transfusion 1980;20:206
713. Pirofsky B. Br J Haematol 1960;6:395
714. Yam P, Petz LD, Spath P. (abstract). Transfusion 1980;20:642
715. Dupuy ME, Elliott M, Masouredis SP. Vox Sang 1964;9:40.
716. Davey RJ, Gustafson M, Holland PV. Transfusion 1980;20:348
717. Halima D, Postoway N, Brunt D, et al. (abstract). Transfusion 1982;22:405
718. Baldwin ML, Barrasso C, Ness PM, et al. Transfusion 1983;123:40
719. Harrison CR, Hayes TC, Trow LL, et al. Vox Sang 1986;51:96
720. Issitt PD, Gutgsell NS. In: Immune Destruction of Red Blood Cells. Arlington, VA:Am Assoc Blood Banks, 1989:77
721. Toy PTCY, Chin CA, Reid ME, et al. Vox Sang 1985;49:215
722. Heddle NM, Kelton JG, Turchyn KL, et al. Transfusion 1988;28:29
723. Garratty G. Gerontology 1991;37:68
724. Garratty G, Arndt P. (abstract). Transfusion 1987;27:545
725. Garratty G. In: Autoimmune Disorders of Blood. Bethesda:Am Assoc Blood Banks, 1996:79
726. Kimberley RP, Salmon JE, Bussel JB, et al. J Immunol 1984;132:745
727. Templeton JG, Cocker JE, Crawford RJ, et al. Lancet 1985;1:1337
728. Morfini M, Vannucchi AM, Grossi A, et al. (Letter). Thromb

Haemost 1985;54:554

729. Wordell CJ. Ann Pharmacother 1991;25:805
730. Collins PW, Newland AC. Sem Hematol 1992;29:64
731. Blanchette VS, Kirby MA, Turner C. Sem Hematol 1992;29 (Suppl 2):72
732. Nugent DJ. Clin Rev Allgy 1992;10:59
733. Todd AAM, Yap PL. Blood Rev 1992;6:105
734. Smiley JF, Talbert MG. Am J Med Sci 1995;309:295
735. Sultan Y, Kazatchkine MD, Maisonneuve P, et al. Lancet 1984;2:765
736. Rossi F, Kazatchkine MD. J Immunol 1989;143:4104
737. Berchtold P, Dale GL, Tani P, et al. Blood 1989;74:2414
738. Dietrich G, Kazatchkine MD. J Clin Invest 1990;85:620
739. Roux KH, Tankersley DL. J Immunol 1990;144:1387
740. Dietrich S, Kaveri SV, Kazatchkine MD. Clin Immunol Immunopathol 1992;62 (Supp 1):S73
741. Andersson JP, Andersson UG. Immunology 1990;71:372
742. Shimozato T, Iwata M, Kawada H, et al. Immunology 1991;72:497
743. Andersson UG, Björk L, Skansen-Saphir U, et al. Immunology 1993;79:211
744. Aukrust P, Froland SS, Liabakk NB, et al. Blood 1994;84:2136
745. Tsubakio T, Kurata Y, Katagiri S, et al. Clin Exp Immunol 1983;53:697
746. Delfraissy JF, Tchernia G, Laurian Y, et al. Br J Haematol 1985;60:315
747. Dammacco F, Iodice G, Campobasso N. Br J Haematol 1986;62:125
748. Macey MG, Newland AC. Br J Haematol 1990;76:513
749. Pogliani EM, Volpe AD, Casaroli I, et al. Allergol Immunopathol 1991;19:113
750. Dwyer JM. New Eng J Med 1992;236:107
751. Oda H, Honda A, Sugita K, et al. J Pediat 1985;107:744
752. Sasaki H, Akutagawa H, Kuwakado K, et al. Am J Hematol 1987;25:215
753. Basta M, Langlois PF, Marques M, et al. Blood 1989;74:326
754. Bolis S, Marozzi A, Rossini F, et al. Allergol Immunopathol 1991;19:186
755. Petrides PE, Hiller E. Clin Invest 1992;70:38
756. Roldan R, Roman J, Lopez D, et al. Scand J Rheumatol 1994;23:218
757. Salama A, Mahn I, Neuzner J, et al. Blut 1984;48:391
758. Barrett-Connor E. Am J Trop Med Hyg 1967;16:699
759. Adner MM, Altstatt LB, Conrad ME. Ann Intern Med 1968;68:33
760. Rosenberg EB, Strickland GT, Yang SL, et al. Am J Trop Med Hyg 1973;22:146
761. Abdalla S, Weatherall DJ, Wickramasinghe SN, et al.. Br J Haematol 1980;46:171
762. Facer CA, Brown J. Lancet 1981;1:897
763. Drouin J, Rock G, Jolly EE. Canad Med Assoc J 1985;132:265
764. Abdalla SH. Br J Haematol 1986;62:13
765. Pollack W, Gorman JG, Freda VJ. In: Progress in Hematology, Vol 6. New York:Grune and Stratton, 1968
766. Oberman HA, Beck ML. Transfusion 1971;11:382
767. Harris EN, Gharavi AE, Loizou S, et al. J Clin Lab Immunol 1985;16:1
768. Ross GD, Yount WJ, Walport MJ, et al. J Immunol 1985;135:2005
769. Galli M, Comfurius P, Maassen C, et al. Lancet 1990;335:1544
770. Mackworth-Young C. Immunol Today 1990;11:60
771. Ahn YS, Harrington WJ, Mylvaganam R, et al. Ann Int Med

1985;102:298

772. Kajii E, Miura Y, Ueki J, et al. Acta Haematol Jpn 1987;50:175

773. Kajii E, Ikemoto S, Ueki J, et al. Clin Exp Immunol 1988;73:406

774. Brocklesby DW. Vet Rec 1967;80:484

775. Chaffee PS. J Small Anim Pract 1968;9:133

776. McCulloch B, Achard PL. Int Zoo Year Book 1969;9:184

777. Hawkey CM. In: Comparative Mammalian Haematology. London:Heinemann, 1975:155

778. Schalm OW, Jain NC, Carroll EJ. Veterinary Hematology, 3rd Ed. Philadelphia:Lee and Febiger, 1975:642

779. Ettinger SJ. Textbook of Veterinary Internal Medicine. Philadelphia:Saunders, 1975:1616

780. Silberman MS, Fulton RB. J Zoo Anim Med 1979;10:6

781. Douglas EM, Plue RE, Cord CE. J Am Vet Med Assoc 1980;177:921

782. Mann PC, Brush M, Janssen DC. J Am Vet Med Assoc 1981;179:1123

783. Beggs T. Br Vet Zoo Soc Newslett and Summary, 1981:3

784. Klos D, Heinz G, Lang EM. Handbook of Zoo Medicine. New York:Von Nostrand Reinhold, 1982:194

785. Miller RE, Boever WJ. J Am Vet Med Assoc 1982;181:1228.

786. Chaplin H Jr, Malecek AC, Miller RE, et al. Am J Vet Res 1986;47:1313.

787. Paglia DE, Valentine WN, Miller RE, et al. Am J Vet Res 1986;47:1321

788. Jones DM. Int Zoo Year Book 1979;19:242

789. Warner AE. Compend Contin Educ Pract Vet 1984;6:S465

790. Tennant B, Dill SG, Glickman LT, et al. J Am Vet Med Assoc 1981;179:143

791. Koterba AM, Coffman JR. Compend Contin Educ Pract Vet 1981;3:S461

792. Divers TJ, George LW, George JW. J Am Vet Med Assoc 1982;180:300

793. George LW, Divers TJ, Mahaffey EA, et al. Vet Pathol 1982;19:521

794. Imapietro PF, Burr MJ, Fiorica V, et al. J Appl Physiol 1967;23:505

795. Schalm OW, Ling GV. Calif Vet 1969;23:19

796. Mackenzie CP. Vet Rec 1969;85:356

797. Avolt MD, Lund JF, Pickett JC. J Am Vet Med Assoc 1973;162:45

798. Schalm OW. Canine Prac 1975;2:37

799. Schalm OW. In: Manual of Feline and Canine Hematology. Santa Barbara:Veterinary Practice Publications, 1980:157

800. Giger U, Harvey JW, Yamaguchi RA, et al. Blood 1985;65:345

801. Tasker JB, Severin GA, Young S, et al. J Am Vet Med Assoc 1969;154:158

802. Ewing GO. J Am Vet Med Assoc 1969;154:503

803. Searcy GP, Miller DR, Tasker JB. Canad J Comp Med 1971;35:67

804. Brown RV, Teng Y. J Am Anim Hosp Assoc 1975;11:362

805. Fletch SM, Pinkerton PH, Brueckner PJ. J Am Anim Hosp Assoc 1975;11:353

806. Prasse KW, Crouser D, Beutler E, et al. J Am Vet Med Assoc 1975;166:1170

807. Randolph JF, Center SA, Kallfelz FA, et al. Am J Vet Res 1986;47:687

808. Giger U, Reilly MP, Asakura T, et al. Anim Genet 1986;17:15

809. Roudebush P, Easley JR, Harvey JW. J Small Anim Pract 1987;28:513

810. Werner LL. Compend Contin Educ Pract Vet 1980;2:96

811. Badylak SF. Compend Contin Educ Pract Vet 1980;2:685

812. Slapendel RJ. Vet Immunol Immunopathol 1979;1:49

813. Quimby FW, Smith C, Bushwein M, et al. Am J Vet Res 1980;41:1662

814. Jones DRE, Darke PGG. J Small Anim Pract 1975;16:273

815. Jones DRE. Med Lab Sci 1983;40:405

816. Jones DRE. Med Lab Sci 1984;41:63

817. Vanschous S. J South Afr Vet Assoc 1982;53:212

818. Noxon JO, Hill BL. J Am Vet Med Assoc 1984;185:1399

819. Issaragrisil S, Kruatrachue M. Scand J Haematol 1983;31:63

820. Ng S-C, Wong KK, Raman S, et al. Eur J Obstet Gynecol Reprod Biol 1990;37:83

821. Giacola GP, Azubuike K. Obstet Gynecol Surv 1991;46:723

822. Benraad CEM, Scheerder HAJM, Overbeeke MAM. Eur J Obstet Gynecol Reprod Biol 1994;55:209

823. Williamson TD, Liles LH, Blackall DP. Immunohematology 1997;13:6

824. Packman CH, Leddy JP. In: Hematology. New York:McGraw-Hill, 1995:677

825. Perkins HA, McIlroy M, Swanson J, et al. Vox Sang 1977;33:299

826. Hauke G, Fauser AA, Weber S, et al. Blut 1983;46:321

827. Reeves MR. MHS Thesis, Duke Univ 1994

828. Liew YW, Duncan N. (Letter). Transfusion 1995;35:713

829. Champagne K, Moulds MK. (Letter). Transfusion 1996;36:384

830. Liew YW, Duncan N. (Letter). Transfusion 1996;36:384

831. Combs MR, Issitt PD. Unpublished observations 1995-1997

832. Leger R, Garratty G. (abstract). Transfusion 1997;37 (Suppl 9S):65S

38 | Cold Hemagglutinin Disease and Paroxysmal Cold Hemoglobinuria

As indicated in table 37-2 of the previous chapter, there are a number of significant differences between cold hemagglutinin disease (CHD), (that is also known as cold agglutinin disease (CAD), cold agglutinin syndrome (CAS) and "cold" antibody-induced hemolytic anemia) and WAIHA. In CHD the autoantibody is optimally reactive at 0 to 4°C but, obviously, since in vivo red cell destruction occurs, is able to bind to red cells and activate complement at higher temperatures. In patients in whom the autoantibody is active up to about 30°C, the disease is usually very mild. In those in whom the antibody is active to about 34°C, more red cell destruction and hence anemia, may occur. As discussed below, while few autoantibodies causative of CHD act as agglutinins at 37°C, some of them are able to cause (often limited) complement activation at that temperature. That CHD is a somewhat distinct entity (but see below) that differs from WAIHA, was first clearly recognized by Schubothe (1).

CHD Mechanism

The causative autoantibody of CHD is almost (but not quite) always IgM in structure. At normal body temperature the antibody does not bind to red cells. When the patient is exposed to cold, the autoantibody binds to red cells, usually in the extremities such as the finger tips, toes, ears, tip of nose, etc., where the skin temperature is lower than in the central parts of the body. Being IgM, the autoantibody clears red cells in vivo only following the activation of complement. There are two major factors that limit the red cell destruction caused by autoantibodies of this type. First, complement activation occurs most efficiently at 37°C so is not immediately activated in large amounts in the colder body extremities where antibody binding to red cells has occurred. Second, being optimally reactive at low temperature many of the autoantibody molecules dissociate from red cells as the antibody-coated red cells re-enter the main circulation where the blood temperature is 37°C and where complement would be most efficiently activated. Thus in a patient with appreciable (at the clinical level) CHD, red cells may be destroyed by either of two mechanisms. That is, intravascular destruction if the terminal attack sequence of complement is mobilized and extravascular clearance of C3b-coated red cells (see Chapter 6). The in vivo clearance of red cells in this disorder is discussed in more detail below.

There are a number of observations that pertain directly to the mechanisms by which red cell destruction occurs in patients with CHD. First, the patient may relate the illness to exposure to cold when questioned. Sometimes the patient may report passing blood (hemoglobin)-stained urine after having been exposed to severe cold. More frequently the patient will report feeling "run-down" or lethargic in the winter but much healthier in the summer. The reason, of course, is that in cold weather the patient may experience a number of hemolytic episodes so may have a low grade anemia. In the summer, when the hemolytic episodes do not occur or are less frequent, the patient is not anemic. Second, the severity of the patient's disease is directly related to the highest temperature at which the autoantibody can bind to red cells. In a patient with an antibody active only as high as 30°C, episodes of hemolysis will be infrequent because the patient's body temperature will not often fall as low as 30°C. In a patient with an autoantibody active at 34°C, episodes of hemolysis will be more frequent since a reduction of body extremities to 34°C will not be too uncommon if the patient lives in a cold climate. Third, it is not necessary for the entire body temperature to be reduced for an episode of hemolysis to occur. As mentioned above, when exposed to cold weather, the extremities of the body (fingers, toes, tips of nose and ears, etc.) are invariably colder than the rest of the body. Clearly, patients with CHD should not live in areas that have cold winters. After moving to Florida, one of us (PDI) saw three to four times as many patients with CHD as he encountered in a similar time period in Ohio. Some of these individuals had moved to Florida at their own initiative simply because they felt better living in an area with a warm climate than when they lived in one with cold winters. They did not all know that they had CHD. In taking histories from patients with CHD one must take note of unusual events. For example, one of us (PDI) examined a blood sample from a patient in Ohio who had experienced an episode of hemolysis in the middle of a very hot and humid summer. Only prolonged questioning extracted the information that the patient, who was wearing shorts and a thin T shirt at the time, had met an old friend in a supermarket and had stood talking for a long time in front of an open freezer.

Rarely, patients with CHD in whom the autoantibody has become active over a wide thermal range, will be encountered. When the autoantibody can bind to red cells at 37°C and then cause intravascular hemolysis, the patient can be expected to be seriously ill. Fortunately such cases are extremely rare. One such case is described in the section below dealing with transfusion in CHD. Much more often, CHD is a relatively mild disorder and is characterized by only a moderate degree of, or no permanent anemia. Again as described below, many patients with CHD require treatment that is no more drastic than simple avoidance of exposure to cold. While there is ample evidence (2-16) that many of the target antigens against which cold-reactive autoantibodies are directed (see also Chapter 34) are present on platelets and leukocytes, thrombocytopenia and leukopenia are only rarely seen in patients with CHD.

Because agglutination occurs in the extremities of the body in CHD, some patients describe a situation that resembles Raynaud's phenomenon. Rosse (17) points out that true Raynaud's phenomenon represents vasoconstriction and that the observations of blue finger tips, etc., in CHD patients represent a different mechanism. In spite of this there are rare reports (18-20) of gangrene in the extremities of patients with CHD. However, there are reasons to believe (17,21) that the gangrene may have been a direct result of actions of the autoantibody and not caused by agglutination in the extremities.

Etiology of Idiopathic CHD

Idiopathic CHD is most often caused by a monoclonal IgM autoantibody. It seems that in the disorder, one pathological clone of immunocytes proliferates and produces the autoantibody. The etiology of secondary CHD is quite different and is described in a later section of this chapter. Proliferation of a single clone of immunocytes is not particularly uncommon, especially in older persons. In many cases the proliferation is harmless, as in benign monoclonal gammopathy, but it may range through various degrees of pathology, all the way to malignant lymphoma. That is to say, many persons have a monoclonal gammopathy but when the IgM molecules do not have antibody specificity for an antigen on red cells, CHD does not occur (22-30,40). Other problems, such as the hyperviscosity syndrome of Waldenstrom's macroglobulinemia may be seen and may be relieved by plasmapheresis (31-35) but red blood cell destruction is not involved. In other words, in some cases of CHD the primary defect represents a monoclonal gammopathy in which the IgM produced has blood group antibody activity. In such cases the disease is usually clinically mild. In other patients the autoantibody is produced by more malignant lymphocytes. Thus CHD may be seen (36-40) in patients with chronic lymphocytic leukemia, lymphoma, B-cell neoplasms, histiocytic lymphoma, etc. In a study reported in 1982, Crisp and

Pruzanski (40) gave details of 78 patients with persistent cold autoagglutinins in their sera. Among the patients studied 31 had lymphoma, 28 had chronic CHD, 13 had Waldenstrom's macroglobulinemia and six had chronic lymphocytic leukemia. Additional findings from this study are presented below in the section on immunoglobulin characteristics of cold autoagglutinins. There is direct evidence (41-46) that it is the malignant lymphocytes that produce the autoantibody although the amount of autoantibody made is not always directly related to the tumor load. Some of these patients have more severe CHD than those with a more benign gammopathy and, as would be expected, control of the hemolysis is achieved by controlling the primary tumor. In patients with idiopathic CHD, the synthesis of IgM may be five to ten times greater than in a normal individual (47). However, Rosse (17) reports that the excess monoclonal autoantibody is more readily seen on immunoelectrophoresis than in routine serum electrophoresis. As discussed below, one form of treatment in patients with severe CHD involves the use of drugs that reduce the mass of cells producing the autoantibody.

In Vivo Red Cell Destruction in CHD

Although there is no dispute as to the nature of the autoantibody and its thermal activities in CHD, there are different opinions regarding the contributions of intravascular and extravascular hemolysis to the anemia. If a patient with CHD is exposed to cold, antigen-antibody complexes form and sufficient amounts of complement are activated for the terminal attack sequence to be mobilized, an intravascular hemolytic episode can result. If the majority of red cells to which antibody and complement to the C3 stage have bound are acted on by factor I (C3b inhibitor, see Chapter 6) before the terminal attack sequence has been mobilized, intravascular hemolysis will not occur. Instead, macrophage recognition of the complement coated red cells will occur and extravascular clearance may follow. If the red cell encounters a macrophage while still carrying C3b, recognition via the macrophage CR1 receptor will follow (48). However, appreciable phagocytosis will not occur unless the red cells are heavily coated with C3b (49,50) and the macrophages are activated (51). C3b is rapidly downgraded to iC3b (52) by factor I and then binds poorly to CR1 but better to CR2 (48). However, such macrophage binding in the absence of cell-bound IgG, does not result in appreciable phagocytosis.

While most workers agree that both intravascular and extravascular red cell destruction can occur in CHD, as stated above there are different opinions regarding the frequencies of such events. Garratty (53,54) and Petz and

Garratty (55) point out that the conditions in patients with CHD are not optimal to lead to direct (intravascular) lysis of red cells. That is, antibody binding at low temperature is rapidly followed by antibody elution at the temperature at which complement activation is optimal. Petz and Garratty (55) write that while patients with CHD may experience hemoglobinuria (taken here as a sign that intravascular destruction occurred) "its incidence is difficult to determine and in many patients hemoglobinuria is never observed". Garratty (54) in discussing macrophage-mediated clearance of complement coated red cells, particularly in the liver, writes "this is probably the major mechanism for the hemolytic anemia in CAS (i.e. extravascular rather than intravascular destruction)". Rosse (17), on the other hand, writes that "intravascular hemolysis does occur in cold agglutinin disease and is often a presenting symptom". He believes that while the process is inefficient, sufficient complement is activated for hemolysis to occur. Rosse (17) also writes that "many if not most patients with cold agglutinin disease have a history of hemoglobinuria upon exposure to cold". Packman and Leddy (56) also subscribe to the view that intravascular hemolysis occurs in some patients with CHD. They write that "in some patients with cold agglutinin AHA, the clinical picture may be that of chronic hemolytic anemia with or without jaundice. In other patients, the principle feature is episodic, acute hemolysis with hemoglobinuria induced by chilling. Combinations of these clinical features may occur".

The experience of one of us (57,58) is that by far the most dramatic feature of CHD is the episode of acute intravascular hemolysis that may result in hemoglobinuria, that follows exposure to the cold. That is not to say that no extravascular red cell destruction occurs. Some patients in whom the diagnosis of CHD has been made carefully avoid exposure to cold. Some of them have low grade anemia and positive DATs, with C3 (actually residual C3dg) detectable on the red cells. However, the red cell destruction in these patients does not ever seem to be as dramatic or to occur to the same degree, as that seen in the episode of acute intravascular red cell destruction.

ABO, Rh and Other Typing Tests in Patients with CHD

These tests may be difficult to perform using blood samples that contain potent cold-reactive autoagglutinins. If the blood sample is allowed to cool after it has been collected, the patient's red cells may be strongly agglutinated before they are tested with ABO, Rh or other typing sera. Obviously, this can lead to incorrect interpretations. There are at least three methods that can be used to obtain a non-agglutinated sample of the patient's red cells for typing studies. First, a sample of the red cells in saline can be heated in an attempt to disrupt the agglutination. Dependent on the strength and thermal amplitude of the cold autoagglutinin involved, heating at 37, 45 or 56°C may be necessary. Once the agglutination is reversed, the cells must be washed in prewarmed saline (at the same temperature as that at which the agglutinates were dispersed) so that the autoantibody is removed before agglutination occurs again. Obviously, the use of incubation at 56°C must be for a short period (5 to 10 minutes) if intact red cells are to be recovered for typing tests. Second, when the agglutination cannot be reversed by heating the red cells, a sample of those cells in saline can be treated with 2-ME or DTT so that the IgM molecules holding the cells together are disrupted. Reid (59) devised this method (that is also listed in Judd (60)) that works extremely well when the autoagglutinin responsible for the agglutination is wholly IgM, that is, in the majority of cases. Third, because it is necessary (see below) also to have a serum sample from which no autoantibody has been lost by adsorption onto the patient's own red cells, warmed samples can be collected from the patient. A wide-mouth thermos vessel is filled with water heated to 40°C. Blood samples are collected from the patient into prewarmed well sealed tubes. These tubes are immediately immersed in the water in the thermos vessel and are allowed to remain there until the samples have clotted. A few red cells can then be transferred to a tube containing saline prewarmed to 37 to 40°C and can be washed several times in prewarmed saline in a heated (37°C) centrifuge. Such cells will not usually be agglutinated since they have never been in contact with the patient's serum at a temperature below 37°C. At the same time, the clotted blood samples can be spun in the heated centrifuge and the serum can be harvested before the samples cool. In this way, serum containing the same level of cold-reactive autoagglutinin as is present in the patient's circulation, can be obtained (see below for use of this serum in laboratory tests).

No matter which method is used to prepare an unagglutinated sample of the patient's red cells, several precautions must be taken when those cells are used in typing tests. First, the cells must be examined closely before the tests are started to make sure that no agglutinates are present. Second, when the cells are tested with ABO and Rh reagents, a control of AB serum known not to contain atypical antibodies must be run in parallel with the typing tests. Obviously, this control must be negative before any positive reactions in tests with the typing reagents can be considered valid and not due to spontaneous agglutination of the patient's cells in a high protein milieu. Further, for Rh typing, a suitable diluent control should be used in addition to the AB serum. Third, if the red cells are to be typed with antibodies reactive by IAT, those tests should be read with anti-IgG. This because a few cold-reactive autoantibodies that do not agglutinate red cells at 37°C will effect some complement activation at that temperature.

Reverse (serum) ABO typing on the blood of a patient with CHD presents a different problem because the autoagglutinin present will usually react with all red cell samples. Again, there are a number of different methods that can be used to resolve this problem. First, an attempt can be made to remove the autoantibody by adsorption with the patient's own red cells. While this method will usually be effective with samples that have non-pathological cold-reactive autoantibodies in the serum, it is less useful when the patient has CHD, because multiple adsorptions may not remove all the autoantibody. Second, an attempt can be made to perform reverse typing tests in a prewarmed (37°C) system. Sometimes the patient's autoagglutinin will be non-reactive while the ABO agglutinins present will still react at that temperature. Third, if the patient's serum is known to react with red cells from adults but not with those from cord blood samples, reverse typing may be possible using cord blood red cells previously shown to react with anti-A_1 and anti-B. Fourth, in some cases a sample of the patient's serum treated with 2-ME or DTT can be used if the cold autoagglutinin is entirely IgM in nature and the patient's serum contains IgG anti-A and/or anti-B agglutinins. This time, no matter which method is used, controls of group O red cells run in parallel with the tests are essential to show that any agglutination of the A or B cells was caused by anti-A or anti-B and not by the autoagglutinin.

The DAT in CHD

In most patients with CHD, the red cells will be coated with C3dg so will have a positive DAT if an appropriate antiglobulin reagent (see Chapter 6) is used. Most workers had assumed that the C3dg-coated red cells found in patients with CHD, represented those that had become complement-coated but not removed via intravascular or extravascular lysis at the time of the patient's last exposure to cold. However, Chaplin et al. (61) have shown that red cell-bound C3d is unstable in vivo and may not be detectable two or three days after it becomes attached to the cells. Thus in a patient who has been in hospital for several days and who has not been exposed to cold during that time, but in whom the red cells carry C3d, it must be supposed that a few antigen-antibody complexes are constantly forming and that complement is being activated at low levels. This is one of the findings that has led Garratty (53,54) to conclude that

extravascular red cell clearance occurs in some of these patients on a more regular basis than is sometimes supposed. The only difference in performing DATs on the red cells of patients with CHD and WAIHA is that in the CHD patients the precautions described above, to ensure that the red cells are not already agglutinated when the antiglobulin reagent is added, must be observed.

The IAT in CHD

Because the autoantibody most often causative of CHD is an IgM agglutinin that activates complement, results in IATs will vary dependent on how the tests are performed. If they are set up using serum and cells at room temperature and are read with a reagent that contains anti-C3, the tests will invariably be positive because complement will become red cell-bound. The amount of complement on the red cells and hence the strength of the positive IAT, will be dependent on the ability of the autoantibody to activate complement and the length of time that the tests are incubated at temperatures below 37°C. If the tests are set up using serum and cells prewarmed to 37°C, are not allowed to cool and if saline prewarmed to 37°C is used to wash the cells before the addition of the antiglobulin reagent, the IATs will usually be only weakly positive (limited complement activation at 37°C) or will be negative. If the IATs are read with anti-IgG, that is usually the case now that LISS, PEG, Polybrene, etc., methods are so widely used, they will usually be negative. The major use of the IAT in patients with CHD is detection and identification of any clinically-significant alloantibodies that are present in the patient's serum.

The Autoagglutinin in CHD

As will by now be apparent, the most useful information that can be obtained in the laboratory about patients with CHD, comes from the results of tests in which the autoantibody is allowed to act as an agglutinin (or as a hemolysin). For many years, it has been traditional to perform titration studies on the causative cold-reactive autoagglutinin and to try to correlate the strength of the antibody with clinical severity of the disease. Although such a test is of some value (most pathological cold-reactive autoantibodies have higher titers than those that are benign in vivo, see table 38-1) it does not correlate as well with the patient's clinical condition as a test that measures the thermal amplitude of the autoantibody. A review of the mechanism of in vivo red cell destruction in CHD, as described above, will reveal why this is the case. One patient may have an autoagglutinin with a titer of 4000 at 4°C and a thermal range such that the autoantibody is not active above 28°C. Another may have an autoagglutinin with a titer of 1000 at 4°C that is active up to 34°C. Clearly, the second patient with the weaker of two autoantibodies, will have more clinical symptoms because there is far more chance that exposure to cold will result in a lowering of temperature in the extremities to 34° than to 28°C. The principle of the thermal amplitude test is discussed in Chapter 3 under the heading Prewarmed tests and in the section on cold-reactive antibodies in Chapter 35. For this test and for the titrations, a sample of the patient's serum that has been harvested from blood collected and allowed to clot at 37°C, should be used. In determining the thermal amplitude and strength of the cold-reactive autoagglutinin it is important to use serum containing all that autoantibody, not serum from a sample allowed to cool to room temperature from which some of the autoantibody will have been removed by adsorption onto the patient's red cells. In studying the thermal amplitude of an autoantibody causative of CHD, the tests described to detect agglutination and complement activation at 37°C should first be performed. If one or both is/are negative, the test(s) should be repeated at a slightly lower temperature, say 35 to 34°C. Such tests should proceed at gradually lower temperatures until the highest temperatures at which the autoantibody can act as an agglutinin and can activate complement have been determined. As mentioned above, it will be found that some autoantibodies causative of CHD can initiate complement activation at a slightly higher temperature than that at which they can agglutinate red cells. As described below, in the section dealing with the differentiation between pathological and benign cold-reactive autoantibodies, the addition of bovine albumin to in vitro test systems often results in pathological autoantibodies being active at higher temperatures than was the case in test systems using saline.

Immunoglobulin Characteristics of Cold Autoagglutinins

As mentioned briefly above, most cold-reactive autoantibodies causative of idiopathic (as opposed to secondary) cold hemagglutinin disease are monoclonal in origin and IgM in composition. The monoclonal nature and the relatively high concentrations of these antibodies in the sera of some patients means that they are amenable to isolation and study at the physicochemical level. Many such studies have been reported. It has been shown (62-67) that when the mu heavy chains are coupled with kappa light chains, anti-I specificity predominates, when the antibody molecules have mu heavy and lambda light chains, anti-i and other specificities

(see below) are more frequent. In the study (40) on 78 cold agglutinins mentioned above, it was shown that among the 28 patients with chronic CHD, 93% of them had antibodies with mu heavy and kappa light chains and in 74% of the 28 patients the specificity of the autoantibody was anti-I. Among the 31 patients with lymphoma, 13 with Waldenstrom's macroglobulinemia and six with chronic lymphocytic leukemia, only 33% had pathological auto-anti-I, clearly anti-i and other specificities were more common. Among the 13 patients with Waldenstrom's macroglobulinemia, 71% had autoantibodies with mu heavy and kappa light chains; among the 31 with lymphoma, 71% had autoantibodies with mu heavy and lambda light chains. In the entire series (40), 58% of the autoantibodies that had mu heavy and kappa light chains were anti-I; 75% of the autoantibodies with mu heavy and lambda light chains had a specificity other than anti-I. This relatively simple correlation, that of course is not absolute, is depicted in table 38-1. Further complexities, beyond those shown in the table are described below.

There is ample evidence of restriction in the use of immunoglobulin genes in the production of pathological cold-reactive autoagglutinins. The restrictions have been seen to involve the genes on chromosome 14 that encode production of heavy chains (68); those on chromosome 2 that encode production of kappa (69-71) and those on chromosome 22 that encode production of lambda light chains (71) (references just given are to assignment of immunoglobulin genes to autosomes, not to restrictions in use of those genes in cold-reactive autoantibody synthesis).

Cooper et al. (66) studied 14 isolated IgM autoagglutinins and found a predominance of one form of mu chain among them. Williams (78) found some of the same determinants on mu heavy chains of both anti-I and anti-i molecules and showed that those determinants were not present on IgM molecules that were not cold agglutinins. Further, the anti-I and anti-i studied shared some features in their idiotype composition. Jacobson and Longstreth (79) then showed that some of these determinants were also present on IgM molecules in a polyclonal anti-I made by a patient with CHD secondary to *Mycoplasma pneumoniae* infection. This finding was of significance since the production of monoclonal anti-I in idiopathic CHD and the production of polyclonal anti-I following infections (see below in sections on secondary CHD) are thought to represent different mechanisms. Thus it seems that production of anti-I involves at least some of the same immunoglobulin restrictions whether the antibody is made in an abnormal autoimmune response or in what may represent a more normal immune response to infection. That the restrictions in immunoglobulin gene use are associated with antibody specificity seems apparent from the report of Gergely et

TABLE 38-1 Some Correlations Between Antibody Type and Disease

Type of CHD	Etiology	Clinical State	Autoantibody
Idiopathic or part of disease process.	Clonal disorder.	Chronic (mild) CHD. Benign monoclonal gammopathies.	Most often monoclonal anti-I with mu heavy and kappa light chains.
		Malignant lymphomas. Chronic lymphocytic leukemia.	More often monoclonal anti-i (or other than -I) with mu heavy and lambda light chains.
Secondary to infection.	Occurs during or following infection, most often viral.	PPLO-pneumonia. Infectious mononucleosis (IM). Transient self-limiting episodes of hemolysis.	Most often IgM polyclonal antibodies. Occasionally monoclonal. Anti-I common in PPLO, anti-i more common in IM. Anti-Fl and anti-Gd also seen.

al. (80) who studied four IgM anti-I and two IgM anti-Pr. While some of the anti-I shared determinants among them, those determinants were not present in the anti-Pr.

The variable regions of immunoglobulin heavy chains were originally (68,72-75) thought to be encoded by members of three families of genes, V_H1, V_H2 and V_H3 (V_HI, V_HII and V_HIII some publications). More recently additional families V_H4, V_H5 and V_H6 have been recognized (45,76,77). In several studies (45,77,81,82) it has been shown that the products of one gene in the V_H4 series, namely $V_H4.21$, predominate in both anti-I and anti-i, or that closely related gene products are involved. As described below, anti-I and anti-i often have the same V_H4 encoded mu chain and differ in terms of the product of variable light chain genes.

As described above, monoclonal cold-reactive autoagglutinins can have either kappa or lambda light chains. Since the antibodies are monoclonal in nature all the light chains will be identical kappa, or identical lambda, within one antibody population. It seems that there is more variation in use of variable light chain genes than in use of variable heavy chain genes in the synthesis of cold-reactive autoagglutinins. Variable *kappa I, II* and *III* gene products have been found (80-84) in cold autoagglutinins. However, Silverman et al. (81,82) showed that in 13 of 14 anti-I the light chain variable regions were products of the variable *kappa III* gene while in the anti-i studied the products of at least three families of variable region light chain genes were found.

Some other considerations apply to the findings described in this section. The V_H4 gene used in the production of so many anti-I and anti-i encodes a product that differs, in terms of the protein encoded, by only three amino acids from that expected of the $V_H4.21$ germ line gene. In contrast, the closest product of variable light chain genes differs by seven amino acids from the expected germ line gene product and, as stated above,

there is more variation in the use of variable light chain genes in the production of cold agglutinins so that often greater differences will be involved. Thus it has been suggested (45,81,82) that the production of auto-anti-I and auto-anti-i represents the propagation of immunocytes producing mu heavy chains via the activation of a fundamental V_H4 gene and that the difference between production of anti-I and anti-i may represent antigen-driven variation in the light chain variable gene used. It is suspected that close similarity between the I and i antigens (see Chapter 10) may be involved in use of the same heavy chain variable gene.

Roelcke (95) has suggested that the production of monoclonal cold autoagglutinins that cause chronic disease, may be a two-step procedure. In the first step, it is suggested that an infectious agent renders host or self antigens immunogenic. In the second step, production of the cold agglutinin may become chronic by a combined process of Ig isotype translocation and concomitant oncogene activation. It is, of course, entirely possible that what has here been called idiopathic CHD, results from a triggering event that has been long forgotten before the patient presents (much later in life) with CHD. Perhaps the difference between chronic CHD and the transient hemolytic episodes that follow recent infection (see later in this chapter) is that in the former, once autoantibody production is started and an oncogene becomes involved, antibody production cannot be regulated by the immune system. The pathologic clone of immunocytes proliferates and autoantibody production becomes permanent, thus causing chronic disease. Perhaps in the transient hemolytic episodes, the abnormal immunocytes can be regulated ("switched off") by the immune system, because no oncogene is involved, so that autoantibody production is transient and the episodes of hemolysis self-limiting; that is, they do not continue because autoantibody production is curtailed.

Although as already discussed, most cold autoagglutinins are IgM in composition, both IgG (85-96) and IgA (88,90,97-102) forms have been reported. As discussed in detail in Chapter 34, Roelcke (95) has suggested that restrictions in the use of certain immunoglobulin genes in the production of cold-reactive autoantibodies, similar to those described earlier in this section, may result in all IgA antibodies that actually cause CHD, having some form of anti-Pr specificity. In a few patients (85,91,92) both IgM and IgA cold autoagglutinins have been seen, in others (103,104) biclonal gammopathy was seen. In two patients described by Harboe (103) of the two monoclonal antibodies being made, only one was an antibody to a red cell antigen.

Autoantibody Specificity in CHD

A wide variety of different specificity autoantibodies have been incriminated as causative of CHD. However, auto-anti-I causes the disease much more frequently than all the other specificities added together. Just as in WAIHA, the specificity of the autoantibody causative of CHD is relatively unimportant in terms of the clinical disease. The maximum temperature at which the autoantibody can bind to red cells in vivo and to a lesser degree its strength, are the factors that determine the severity of clinical disease.

CHD was a well recognized clinical entity before it became apparent that the causative autoantibodies have blood group specificity. Indeed, because those autoantibodies usually react with all red cell samples against which they are tested, they were for many years called non-specific cold agglutinins. In 1956, Wiener et al. (105) tested the autoagglutinin of a patient with CHD against the red cells of some 22,000 random donors and found five samples that failed to react. They named the antibody anti-I and said that it divided red cell samples into two phenotypes, namely I+ that was very common and I- that was very rare. Once the so-called I- red cells became available for testing purposes, it became apparent that CHD is most often caused by auto-anti-I (55,106-110). Three years before the published report on the first named auto-anti-I, Wiener et al. (111) had suggested that the autoantibodies causative of CHD might be directed against a "nucleus" of ABO system antigens. As discussed in Chapter 10, it is now known that I (and i) are present on red cell membrane-borne structures that carry the A, B and H immunodominant carbohydrates at their termini. This remarkable forecast by Wiener et al. (111) was made in a paper that repeated their suggestion (112) that the autoantibodies causative of WAIHA might be directed against a "core" structure of Rh antigens. As discussed in Chapter 37, that forecast foreshadowed

much of what was later to be learned about autoantibody specificity in WAIHA.

In 1960, Marsh and Jenkins (113) described the first example of anti-i, an antibody subsequently shown (114) to behave in many ways as if it detects an antigen antithetical to I. Without repeating all that is written in Chapter 10, it is now known that phenotypes that could be called I+ i- and I- i+ do not exist. Instead, red cells that are for convenience sometimes called I+ i- carry a trace of i, while those that are called I- i+ (or adult i) carry a trace of I. Like anti-I, anti-i was shown to be capable of causing CHD (113,114), several of the early cases were seen in patients with diseases of the reticuloendothelial system.

After anti-I and anti-i had been described, it was found that related antibodies that can best be described as anti-IA, anti-IB, anti-IH, anti-iH, etc., exist. Identification of these antibodies (107,115,116) strengthened the idea put forth by Wiener et al. (111) that anti-I defines an antigen associated with the "nucleus" of ABO. Now that the I and i determinants are known to cohabit the membrane-borne structures that carry A, B and H, the reactions of these antibodies are better understood. Chapter 10 includes a more complete description of these antibodies and gives details as to how they can be differentiated at the serological level. Most of these antibodies are autoimmune in nature (e.g. anti-IH made by a person with A_1 red cells reacts most strongly with group O, I+ red cells but can be adsorbed by the antibody-maker's red cells) but many are benign in vivo. Most often their benign nature relates to their low thermal amplitude. One exception is anti-IH that may occur as the causative autoantibody of CHD but may not always be distinguished from anti-I, first because of the test cells used in antibody-identification (i.e. all group O) and second because differentiating anti-IH from anti-I in CHD is of no benefit to the patient. While most examples of autoantibodies with these specificities are benign in vivo (for references see Chapter 10), anti-IA (117,118) and anti-IB (119) have been reported rarely to cause CHD. Anti-I^T has also been incriminated as causative of CHD (120) and WAIHA (121,122). As discussed in Chapters 10 and 34, the relationship of I^T to I and i, is no longer clear. Other details about the Ii and related antigens and the antibodies that define them are given in Chapter 10 and need not be repeated here. It will be mentioned that since anti-I and anti-i causative of CHD are sometimes very potent antibodies, antibody identification by titration, as depicted in table 10-4 of Chapter 10, is often useful when working with the sera of patients with CHD. The newest member of the Ii collection, the antigen j, and the two examples of anti-j that caused CHD (123) are also described in Chapter 10.

In addition to autoantibodies in the Ii et al. series, there are a number of other cold-reactive autoagglutinins that have caused CHD although none of them is seen with a frequency that even approaches the incidence of auto-anti-I in the disorder. Details about the antigens involved and the antibodies that define them are given in Chapter 34. Table 38-2 lists those antigens that have been targets of cold-reactive autoagglutinins that have caused CHD. To avoid confusion it will be added that as far as we are aware there is only one report (126) of monoclonal auto-anti-P causing CHD although, of course, that specificity is seen in autoantibodies causative of PCH (see below). The auto-anti-P that caused CHD was a monoclonal IgM antibody with kappa light chains (126), it was made in a patient with immunoblastic non-Hodgkin's lymphoma.

Although defined by an antibody that does not completely fit the definition of a cold agglutinin, Rx (see Chapter 34) is included in table 38-2. Similarly, the table includes H_T. In 1952, Brendemoen (124) described an autoantibody that reacted only with stored red cells. Similar autoantibodies, that caused CHD, were reported in 1961 by Jenkins and Marsh (125). The autoantibodies were found to react with stored red cells and with red cells that had been heat or enzyme-treated. The name anti-H_T (for heat-treated) was applied to this specificity.

Differentiation Between Pathological and Benign Cold-Reactive Autoantibodies

It might be thought, because pathological cold-reactive autoantibodies cause CHD while the benign forms have no affect in vivo, that differentiation between them at both the clinical and serological level would be easy. In fact, this is not the case. Because CHD is often such a mild disorder, it is sometimes difficult to decide whether a patient with a low grade anemia and other clinical problems has CHD, or whether there is another cause that accounts for the anemia. In such circumstances, the physician may well ask the serologist to test the patient's blood with the object of including or excluding CHD. In some cases this task is relatively easy because the cold-reactive autoantibody present has all or none of the characteristics of a pathological autoantibody. On other occasions the task may be much more difficult because the autoantibody has some characteristics that suggest that it is pathological and others that suggest that it is benign. If the DAT is negative, the chance that the patient has CHD is probably small. Patients with CHD almost always have detectable C3dg on their red cells. However, the detection of a small amount of C3dg, on the red cells of a patient with a moderately active cold autoagglutinin present in the serum, is by no means diagnostic of CHD. Although the incidence of normal donors with C3dg on the red cells is low (probably less than 1% (55)) the incidence of that finding among hospital patients, in whom there is no evidence to support an assumption that in vivo red cell clearance is accelerated, is much higher, probably around 8% (55,110). Accordingly, there are occasions when it becomes necessary to test the cold-reactive autoagglutinin present to see if it seems likely to be causing in vivo red cell destruction. Table 38-3 summarizes some of the differences in behavior expected of pathological and benign cold-reactive autoantibodies. As will be seen, the specificity of the cold-reactive autoantibody is not listed as of being of any value in this differentiation. This is because most cases of CHD are caused by auto-anti-I, but a benign auto-anti-I can be found in all normal sera (127). Further, as discussed in Chapter 10, we have not found a useful correlation between pathological and benign anti-I, and the anti-I^F, anti-I^D (128) specificities.

As already mentioned, one of the more reliable guides to the autoantibody's probable in vivo activity is obtained from a thermal amplitude test. Expected results are shown in table 38-3. Also as mentioned, the titer of

TABLE 38-2 Antigens Defined by Autoantibodies that have caused CHD or PCH

Characteristics of Antigen	Blood Group System	Antigens Defined
Protease-resistant Neuraminidase-resistant	Ii and related P Others	I, i, IH, j, I^T, IA, IB P (PCH only) Me, Om, Ju, R_x, H_T
Protease-resistant Neuraminidase-sensitive		Gd1(Sia-lb1), Gd2(Sia-lb2) Sa*, Fl(Sia-b1), Lud*, Vo(Sia-l1), Li
Protease-sensitive Neuraminidase-resistant	Pr	Pr_a
Protease-sensitive Neuraminidase-sensitive	Pr	Pr_{1h}, Pr_{1d}, Pr_2, Pr_{3h}, Pr_{3d}, Pr^M, Pr^N

* Sa and Lud weakened but not denatured by protease-treatment. For other antigens, e.g., A, B, M, N, etc., see appropriate chapters.

TABLE 38-3 Some Differences Between Pathological and Benign Cold-Reactive Autoantibodies

	Pathological autoantibody in CHD	Benign autoantibody in hematologically normal persons
Highest temperature at which most autoantibodies act as agglutinins[*1]	30-34°C	Usually <25°C
Highest temperature at which most autoantibodies activate complement[*1]	30-37°C	Usually <25°C
Titer at 4°C[*1]	Often >500	Usually <64
Titer at 22°C[*1]	Often >128	Usually <16
Thermal range and titer increased in in vitro test systems in which bovine albumin is used	Usually yes	Usually no
Ability of autoantibody to hemolyze enzyme-treated red cells in an in vitro system using acidified serum	Almost 100%[*2]	Uncommon but not unknown
Nature of autoantibody	Monoclonal in idiopathic CHD, polyclonal in secondary hemolytic episodes	Polyclonal

[*1] In test systems using saline suspended red cells and serum dilutions made in saline
[*2] If the antigen defined is not denatured when red cells are treated with proteases

the autoantibody may be of some help in this differentiation but crossing-over between the headings and expected results in table 38-3 is seen; further, an autoantibody with a titer between 64 and 256 at 4°C and 16 and 64 at room temperature falls into a gray (a.k.a. grey) area. Sometimes an autoantibody from a patient who seems to have clinical CHD will be found to have too limited a thermal range and/or too low a titer for it to be classified as probably pathological. In such cases it is well worth repeating the thermal amplitude tests with red cells suspended in 30% bovine albumin and the titration using serum dilutions made and red cells suspended in, that medium. Haynes and Chaplin (130) described a pathological cold-reactive autoagglutinin with a titer at 4°C of 128 against saline-suspended but 131,000 against albumin-suspended red cells. Garratty et al. (131) found that in a number of patients with CHD the autoantibody agglutinated albumin-suspended but not saline suspended red cells at 30°C . Further (53,131) when an autoantibody agglutinated albumin-suspended red cells at 30°C or above the patient always had CHD, when it failed to cause agglutination in that test, the autoantibody was benign in vivo regardless of its titer. Thus some high titered cold autoagglutinins can be forecast to be benign in vivo by use of this simple test. As also shown in table 38-3, pathological cold-reactive autoantibodies that define antigens that are not denatured when red cells are treated with proteolytic enzymes, will usually act as hemolysins when enzyme-treated red cells are used in a test system adjusted to pH 6.5 to 6.8 (55). As already mentioned, autoantibodies causative of idiopathic CHD

are often monoclonal in nature. However, this feature is not particularly useful in distinguishing between pathological and benign cold-reactive autoantibodies since those that cause secondary episodes of intravascular hemolysis (see below) are polyclonal, and both monoclonal and polyclonal benign autoantibodies exist.

Correlations Between Laboratory Findings and Clinical Disease in CHD

As discussed in Chapter 37, the correlations between laboratory findings and severity of clinical disease in patients with WAIHA are rather good. The main correlation in CHD involves the thermal range over which the autoantibody is active. This is depicted diagrammatically in figure 38-1. As already described, the causative autoantibody is optimally reactive at 0°C and becomes less active as the temperature increases. In contrast, complement activation occurs optimally at 37°C and becomes less efficient as the temperature is reduced. Schubothe (1) has pointed out that the area of temperature overlap, where both autoantibody binding and complement activation can occur with a reasonable degree of efficiency, represents the "zone of hemolysis" as depicted in figure 38-1. If the range of antibody activity in the figure moves to the right in a patient with CHD, the overlap area of hemolysis will increase in size and a more severe clinical picture will be seen. Such a change (or a difference between two patients) can be measured in the laboratory by careful performance of thermal amplitude tests. If the line representing the range of complement activation is further to the left in one patient than in another, the same outcome will result and the hemolysis will be more severe. However, the ability to activate complement at different temperatures by different patients is not measured in any laboratory test routinely performed on patients with the disorder.

There are a number of other factors that are not routinely measured in laboratory tests that also affect the clinical severity of CHD in the patient. First, for reasons that will by now be obvious, the amount of red cell destruction that occurs will be directly related to the degree of exposure of the patient to cold. Second, since red cell destruction in CHD is via complement-dependent mechanisms, complement utilization and synthesis rates in different individuals may affect the amount of cell destruction that occurs. It is at least theoretically possible that the limiting factor in severe CHD could be the rate at which a depleted complement component was synthesized. Third, and again because red cell destruction is via complement-dependent mechanisms, a patient with a naturally high level of factor I (C3b INA) may experience less hemolysis than one in whom the level of that protein is lower. As discussed in detail in Chapter 6, the pivotal factor in complement-mediated red cell destruction is the amount of C3 activated and the rate at which it becomes available in the activated form. In a patient with a high level of factor I, activated C3 will be rapidly downgraded thus reducing the chance of intravascular (terminal attack sequence not activated) and extravascular (macrophages do not bind C3dg coated red cells) hemolysis. Fourth, if the patient's red cells

become heavily coated with C3dg but are not hemolyzed, they will be more resistant to complement-induced lysis than are uncoated red cells (132-136). This because the binding sites for the newly activated C3 (following another exposure of the patient to cold) are at least in part blocked by the C3dg that is already bound. When all these factors, that are listed in table 38-4 and many of which are not measured in laboratory tests, are considered in the various possible combinations and permutations, it is not surprising that the correlation between the results of laboratory tests and the clinical severity of disease in CHD is not as good as in WAIHA.

Treatment of Patients with CHD

As with treatment in WAIHA, a full description of treatment of patients with CHD is beyond the scope of this book. However, some forms of treatment relate directly to the actions of the causative autoantibodies so are of interest to blood bankers.

First, as already mentioned, many patients with mild CHD can be effectively managed simply by having them avoid exposure to cold. This simple step prevents episodes of hemolysis from occurring and thus prevents anemia. In those patients in whom the autoantibody is active over a wider thermal range, more aggressive therapy may be necessary. Since the cold-reactive autoantibody is often a product of malignant lymphocytes, alkylating agents (e.g. chlorambucil, cyclophosphamide, melphalan) can be used in an attempt to reduce the size of the liquid tumor, i.e. the number of immunocytes mak-

FIGURE 38-1 Degree of Hemolysis in Patients with CHD as Influenced by the Range of Autoantibody Activity and the Range over which Complement can be Activated.

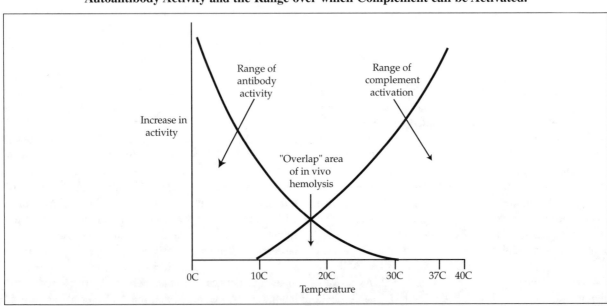

TABLE 38-4 Some Variables that Affect the Degree of Hemolysis in Different Patients with CHD

1.	Degree and duration of exposure to cold
2.	Thermal range of autoantibody activity
3.	Efficiency of complement activation at different temperatures
4.	Complement utilization and synthesis
5.	Level of factor I (C3b inactivator)
6.	Amount of C3dg on red cells still in circulation

ing autoantibody. However, Rosse (17) points out that each of the alkylating agents has the capability of inducing leukemia so that the agents should not be used unless "clear need is evident and clear response is seen". Rosse (17) also states that cell cycle active agents such as 6-mercaptopurine, methotrexate, cytosine arabinose, should not be used. The use of sulphydryl compounds (such as mercaptopyridoxin and penicillamine) has been suggested. It was proposed that these agents would denature IgM molecules in vivo (much as 2-ME and DTT do in vitro) and that the monomers of IgM would then be less able, or unable, to activate complement. This form of therapy has not become widely favored. Corticosteroids are useful in treating patients with CHD on those rare occasions that the causative autoantibody is IgG in composition. Corticosteroids seem to have little, or no effect, on the in vivo production of IgM autoantibodies.

As might be expected since IgM is confined to the intravascular space, plasmapheresis can be used to reduce the level of autoantibody in a patient with CHD. However, the procedure can hardly be considered a routine form of treatment. First, the whole procedure must be performed in a heated room using warm equipment. If blood passing through the pheresis equipment is allowed to cool, antigen-antibody complexes may form, complement may be activated and hemolysis may follow. Second, IgM is synthesized rapidly and although 80% of the IgM may be removed in a single plasmapheresis, close to half the removed antibody will be replaced within five days (137). Third, because of one and two above and because plasmapheresis is an expensive way to treat patients with CHD, its use should probably be reserved for those patients undergoing acute hemolysis, in whom chemotherapy is also being used. Plasmapheresis may keep those patients alive until the drugs being used start to effect reduction in production of autoantibody, but the treatment is not suitable for use on a chronic basis. Plasmapheresis may also be useful in removing autoantibody in a patient about to have surgery. When used in a technically sound manner and in appropriate clinical situations, plasmapheresis provides a useful adjunct form of treatment in CHD (138-152).

Selection of Blood for Transfusion to Patients with CHD

CHD is seldom severe enough that transfusion is necessary to relieve the anemia (but see below for an example of a rare exception). However, like other individuals, a number of persons with CHD will require transfusions at surgery or following accidents. There do not seem to be any contraindications to transfusion in this disorder. It seems that in these patients, the production of autoantibody proceeds independently of the further introduction of antigen so that the infusion of red cells incompatible with the autoantibody seems not to increase the amount of autoantibody being made. Thus the major concern before transfusion in a patient with CHD is to ensure that the cold-reactive autoagglutinin present in the serum does not mask the activity of any clinically-significant alloantibodies simultaneously present. There are several methods by which this objective can be attained. In many patients, prewarmed (37°C) compatibility tests can be used since at that temperature the autoagglutinin will not interfere. Such tests will not detect cold-reactive alloantibodies present in the patient's serum but as pointed out in several other places in this book, such antibodies do not clear antigen-positive red cells in vivo so that their non-detection is an advantage not a disadvantage. The autoantibodies in some patients with CHD will cause small amounts of complement to become red cell-bound even in tests performed strictly at 37°C. When this occurs, compatibility tests will all give weakly positive reactions when the IATs are read with a polyspecific antiglobulin reagent. Again as pointed out elsewhere, most IATs are now read with anti-IgG because they are part of tests that use LISS, PEG, Polybrene, etc., so that the problem now seldom occurs. However, the use of LISS, PEG, Polybrene, etc., will result in some cold-reactive autoantibodies agglutinating red cells at 37°C although they cannot agglutinate saline suspended cells at that temperature. Some workers elect to use autoadsorption to free a serum of the cold-reactive autoagglutinin before compatibility tests are undertaken. As described above, this is more easily accomplished when the autoantibody is of the benign type than when it is pathological in vivo. If it is known that the cold-reactive autoagglutinin complexes with an antigen that is still present on enzyme-treated red cells, the autoadsorption process can be made more efficient by treating the patient's cells with ficin or papain before they are used. However, initial tests are necessary since some antigens defined by cold-reactive autoagglutinins, e.g. those of the Pr series (see Chapter 34) are destroyed when red cells are protease-treated.

Other workers (153) used formaldehyde-treated rabbit red cells to adsorb anti-I from sera and a commercial product made with rabbit red cell stroma became widely used. However, there are some reports (154-158) that rabbit red cell stroma adsorb some alloantibodies, although not all investigators found this to be the case (153,159).

In 1970, Marsh et al. (160) reported that anti-I is sometimes partially and occasionally wholly inhibited by human milk. While it was subsequently suggested in a proficiency survey that the routine method for compatibility testing using sera that contain anti-I, should be neutralization of the anti-I by human milk so that the sera could be tested for the concomitant presence of alloantibodies, this is not possible. Indeed, Marsh et al. (160) reported that of 13 anti-I from patients with CHD, only one was totally inhibited and of the others, 11 still had a titer of 32 or more after the milk had caused partial inhibition. Similar studies on nine auto-anti-I from hematologically normal persons and two from individuals of the adult i phenotype showed more, but seldom complete inhibition. Of those 11 anti-I, one was totally inhibited, six others were still active at dilutions from 1 in 4 to 1 in 64 after the milk had caused partial inhibition.

It is seldom necessary to provide blood that lacks the antigen against which the autoantibody is directed, for transfusion to a patient with CHD. Indeed perusal of table 38-2 shows that such a maneuver would be impossible most of the time, anyway. As already discussed, adult i red cells are not totally devoid of I, nor do I+ red cells totally lack i. Similarly, antigens such as those of the Pr series, Gd, Sa, Lud, Fl, etc., are universally distributed on the red cells of humans. However, as already described, in CHD most of the autoantibodies cause red cell destruction only when the patient is exposed to cold. Obviously, such exposure can be prevented during and following a blood transfusion so that antigen-negative blood is not necessary. Equally obvious is the fact that the patient should not be transfused rapidly with a large volume of chilled blood. In spite of this, it is not always necessary to pass the blood through a warming coil on its way into the patient's circulation. On many occasions the unit of blood can be hung at room temperature and can be allowed to run at a rate such that its infusion is spread over two to four hours. At that rate of infusion, the blood is warmed as it enters the patient's circulation and does not affect significant reduction of the patient's blood temperature. In cases where the patient's autoantibody is active near 37°C, or when blood must be given more rapidly, use of a warming coil may be indicated. As described earlier, washed red blood cells are not indicated simply because a patient has WAIHA. However, in CHD that product may rarely be the one of choice. In a patient with severe CHD where the factor limiting the in vivo hemolysis is depletion of one or more of the complement components, those components should not be supplied via donor plasma. Although complement activation cannot take place in anticoagulated plasma

(because no free calcium ions are available) the complement components in the plasma are viable and can be used if transfused into a patient. This does not mean that routine use of washed red cells for patients with CHD is indicated. Indeed, for many years it was believed that washed red blood cells should be provided for CHD patients only when laboratory assays had documented complement depletion. However, methods for washing red cells have become ever easier while those for assaying specific complement components have not. Accordingly it is now easier to provide washed red cells even though demonstration of the strict need for such a product has not been made, than it is to insist that complement assays be performed.

Very rarely, it may be necessary to transfuse blood that is more compatible than the CHD patient's own. One of us (161) encountered a patient with an auto-anti-I that had a wide enough thermal range that it was causing intravascular hemolysis at 37°C. The patient was in an overheated hospital room and was covered with electric blankets. The room was so warm that the attending staff were grossly uncomfortable while there, but in spite of this the patient's hemolysis continued. We (161) transfused I+ blood, it was cleared from circulation as rapidly as the patient's own red cells. We then obtained and transfused three units of blood of the adult i phenotype. The patient was being treated with large doses of chlorambucil and the three units of adult i blood helped keep him alive long enough for the chlorambucil to begin to work. Three days after the adult i blood had been transfused, the level and thermal range of his auto-anti-I had been sufficiently reduced by the treatment, that I+ red cells were transfused and apparently survived well. The patient made a good recovery and was treated with maintenance doses of chlorambucil. For many years after the acute hemolytic episode, we (161) tested this patient's blood when he came to the hospital as an out-patient for follow-up visits. Eventually we were not able to demonstrate any difference between the cold-reactive autoagglutinin in his serum and those in the sera of normal individuals. It should be pointed out that patients such as the one described are encountered very rarely (162). Indeed, one of us (PDI) has not seen any other patient with auto-anti-I in whom the transfusion of adult i blood was necessary in more than 48 years of working in blood banks. Readers who have heard this author describe the above mentioned case in a lecture may remember that having admitted to more than 48 years of blood bank work, the author would now like everyone to believe that he was a child prodigy who began work at age five!

Secondary CHD Following Infections

The etiology of secondary CHD that occurs during

or following an infectious disease must differ from that of the idiopathic form of the disorder in which a pathological clone of immunocytes proliferates as the sole malfunction or as part of another disease process. In this secondary form of the disorder a cold autoagglutinin is produced either late in the course of an infection or during the convalescent stage following the disease. If sufficient cold autoantibody of wide enough thermal range is made, a hemolytic episode results. However, autoantibody production eventually stops and the patient makes a complete recovery. The diseases most often associated with secondary CHD are atypical pneumonia caused by the pleuro-pneumonia like organism, *Mycoplasma pneumoniae* (hereinafter PPLO-pneumonia) and infectious mononucleosis caused (often) by the Epstein-Barr virus (hereinafter IM). However, the same secondary disorder is sometimes seen, particularly in children, following a wide variety of viral disorders, e.g. mumps, measles, chicken-pox or even a vague influenza-like condition. Given the direct association between infection and subsequent transient production of an autoantibody, it would be hoped that the immunologic agent stimulating the autoimmune response would have been recognized, in fact this is not the case.

Many patients with PPLO-pneumonia make increased levels of cold-reactive autoagglutinins, relatively few of them experience hemolysis. Various studies (163-165) have shown elevated cold agglutinins in 30 to 50% of patients with the disease. Indeed, in cases in which bacterial cultures are negative, presence of an elevated cold agglutinin is a useful clue as to the cause of the pneumonia. The increased level of cold agglutinin and the hemolysis, if it occurs, are not usually seen until the second week of infection with the PPLO, or later. Although only a minority of patients with the disease experience hemolysis, PPLO-pneumonia is common enough that many cases have been studied (79,166-172). It was shown early (173) that the production of anti-I in patients infected with PPLO does not represent simple production of antibody to an antigen on the infecting organisms. Isolated organisms did not block the reaction of the cold agglutinin with red cells. In a series of publications (166-169,171) one group of investigators suggested that infection with PPLO somehow alters the structure of the host I antigen so that it is no longer recognized as self and an antibody against it is made. That antibody then has the ability to cross-react with normal I antigen that is present on the patient's red cells once the PPLO infection is resolved. Support for such a concept seems to be provided by the observation (174,175) that sialylated oligosaccharides of the Ii antigen type are erythrocyte receptors for *M. pneumoniae*. The fact that sialylated oligosaccharides are involved may explain the fact that although anti-I is by far the most common cold-reactive autoagglutinin

seen in patients with PPLO infections, autoantibodies to Fl and Gd have also been encountered (95,176). As explained in Chapter 34, Fl and Gd arise via sialylation of I-bearing chains. One report (177) of auto-anti-Pr in this setting is more difficult to explain.

Further support for the concept that the autoantibody made during or following PPLO infection is directed against an altered host or self antigen comes from the finding that most such antibodies include some molecules with kappa and some with lambda light chains. In other words, the autoantibodies are polyclonal and are in some ways like the products of a normal immune response, unlike the monoclonal autoantibodies causative of idiopathic CHD. It is not difficult to imagine that when a host or self antigen is altered in vivo, a normal immune response may occur. Unfortunately in instances like this it seems that the product of the normal immune response cross-reacts with the unaltered antigen and thus acts as an autoantibody. In spite of the polyclonal nature of the antibodies made, the same restrictions in the use of heavy chain immunoglobulin genes as described earlier in the description of production of monoclonal anti-I, seem to apply (79,178,179).

The occurrence of cold-reactive autoagglutinins during or following infectious mononucleosis somewhat parallels the situation seen with PPLO-pneumonia. Again production of increased levels of cold agglutinins is common, i.e. in up to 30% of patients, hemolysis is rare. Production of an increased level of the autoantibody usually begins in the second week of infection and persists for as few as three to as many as 12 weeks. Hemolysis, if it occurs at all, is usually seen during the third or fourth week when the autoantibody is being made at its highest level. Unlike PPLO-pneumonia, the cold-reactive autoantibody most often seen in IM, has anti-i specificity (180,181). While hemolysis is rare there are a number of reports (55,180-188) describing patients who produced auto-anti-i of wide enough thermal range that it caused in vivo red cell destruction or in whom a hemolytic episode occurred via a different mechanism (see below).

The auto-anti-i causative of the hemolytic episodes following IM is not the same as the heterophile antibody seen in patients with the disease; the two can be separated by adsorption (180,181). In some patients who suffer hemolytic episodes during or following the disease, the cause of the hemolysis is more obscure. There are two reports (189,190) of patients who formed IgG anti-i and also had IgM anti-IgG in the serum. It was supposed that the red cells became coated with IgG anti-i and were then cleared from circulation following the actions of the IgM anti-IgG. However, Petz and Garratty (55) point out that neither antibody was active at 37°C (the IgM anti-IgG reacted only at 4°C). Thus it was difficult to see how the antibodies working in concert would have caused in vivo red cell destruction. In spite of this, in a patient with cold reactive IgG anti-i and cold reactive rheumatoid factor (IgM anti-IgG) studied by Gronemeyer et al. (188) in whom IM was followed by hemolytic anemia, there was a good clinical response to steroid therapy. Since steroids are usually effective when the causative autoantibody is IgG, it was concluded (188) that in this patient the IgG anti-i was responsible for the hemolytic anemia. Wilkinson et al. (187) studied three patients who had episodes of hemolysis following IM. In one, a high thermal amplitude auto-anti-i was clearly implicated. In the other two, the auto-anti-i present was weak and was not active in vitro at 20°C. Although both patients had anti-IgG in the serum, no IgG auto-anti-i was demonstrated in either. Thus it seems that in some cases of hemolysis complicating IM, the red cell destruction may not be as straightforward as the initial tests may suggest. Rosse (17) reports that in some patients warm-reactive IgG autoantibodies may be made.

Clearly, the presence of auto-anti-i in the serum of a patient with IM, who is having a secondary hemolytic episode, should not be taken to represent cause and effect unless it can be shown that the autoantibody has a significantly wide thermal range, or other evidence can be obtained that the autoantibody is responsible for the in vivo red cell destruction. When antibody-induced red cell clearance is involved, production of the autoantibody is transient as with the production of auto-anti-I following PPLO-pneumonia. Management of the patient through the hemolytic episode can be expected to be followed by a complete return to normal (i.e. autoantibody no longer produced).

Less, perhaps that should read even less, is known about the stimulus for the production of auto-anti-i in IM, than about the stimulus for the production of auto-anti-I in PPLO-pneumonia. The seemingly logical guess that autoantibody production might be stimulated by increased levels of i on the atypical mononuclear cells seen in the disease proved to be wrong when it was found (193,194) that those cells will not adsorb the auto-anti-i. Similarly there is no evidence that auto-anti-i reacts with Epstein-Barr virus (EBV). It is known (191) that infection of B cells by EBV results in polyclonal proliferation of those cells and synthesis of antibody. Many other autoantibodies are made by patients with IM including ones against platelets, neutrophils, cardiolipin, etc. (192). What is not clear is why clones producing certain autoantibodies respond to EBV infection more readily than do others.

While production of increased levels of cold autoagglutinins and sometimes hemolytic anemia are more common in patients with PPLO-pneumonia and IM than in other patients, they are by no means confined to those

two conditions. As mentioned at the beginning of this section, cold-autoantibody-induced hemolytic episodes have been seen in children, and less frequently in adults, in association with mumps, rubella, measles, chickenpox, CMV infections, ornithosis, Legionnaire's disease, and vague virus-like illnesses that resemble influenza or infectious mononucleosis (94,95,182,195-199). It is difficult to determine whether the persistent cold agglutinins seen in patients with AIDS and related conditions are associated with HIV or concurrent infections in those patients (200). There are two unusual observations that relate to the topic of infection and CHD. First, when more potent than usual cold autoagglutinins are made in patients with rubella (german measles as opposed to measles) they invariably have anti-Pr specificity (95,196,201). While rubella infections seem to stimulate production of anti-Pr, production of that specificity is not confined to rubella infections. The reason that rubella stimulates anti-Pr is not known. Second, most of the viral diseases listed above can be followed and complicated by paroxysmal cold hemoglobinuria (PCH, see next section) instead of by CHD. Why, in these infections, the immune system sometimes makes an IgM antibody that causes CHD and at other times an IgG biphasic hemolysin that causes PCH, is not understood. The findings of different types of antibody and different specificities following infection with ostensibly the same virus, strongly suggest that the infecting virus somehow alters the immune mechanism rather than that the antibody is simply directed against an antigen on the virus.

Paroxysmal Cold Hemoglobinuria (PCH)

Because of its very dramatic clinical and serological presentation, PCH was one of the first types of antibody-induced hemolytic anemia to be recognized (202-204). The mechanism of in vivo red cell destruction is similar to that in CHD. The causative autoantibody binds to the patient's red cells in the extremities when the patient is exposed to cold, intravascular hemolysis occurs when the preformed antigen-antibody complexes return to the circulation at or near 37°C. PCH differs from CHD in that the causative autoantibody is IgG in nature. Perhaps because the autoantibody elutes from red cells less readily than does an IgM autoantibody, and perhaps because the antigen most often defined by the autoantibody causative of PCH is very close to the red cell membrane (see below), the disease is characterized by severe episodes of intravascular hemolysis.

The more usual laboratory tests are of somewhat limited value in working with samples from patients with PCH. First, although the disease is a form of cold-antibody-induced hemolytic anemia, the causative IgG autoantibody does not readily agglutinate red cells in in vitro tests at low temperatures. Second, because the cold-reactive IgG autoantibody elutes from red cells washed in saline at room temperature (see below) conventional DATs read with anti-IgG are negative. Third, although C3 can usually be demonstrated on the patients' red cells, those cells that bound large amounts of C3 may have been cleared (intravascular lysis) and those remaining may give a deceptively weak reaction, considering the degree of lysis and anemia, when the DAT is read with anti-C3. The more useful Donath-Landsteiner (D-L) test and modifications thereof, are described below.

PCH, Incidence

PCH as an idiopathic disorder is extremely rare and probably accounts for less than 1% of all cases of antibody-induced hemolytic anemia (205-207). That would suggest that it might be seen in 1 in 600,000 to 1 in 800,000 persons in a given population per year. If cases of secondary PCH (see below) are included, the disease is encountered more often than those figures indicate (i.e. 2 to 4% of all cases of antibody-induced hemolytic anemia (55,110,231)). PCH used to be seen among patients with advanced forms of syphilis. Now that syphilis can be successfully treated in its early stages, such cases are seldom encountered. The disease can also occur (but is still not common) as a secondary complication following various infectious states. As mentioned above, children, and less frequently adults, recovering from measles, mumps, chicken-pox, influenza, infectious mononucleosis, PPLO-pneumonia and even (very rarely) following small-pox vaccination, may present with secondary PCH (55,109,110,208-231). In studying 531 adults and 68 children with hemolytic anemia, over a four year period, Gottsche et al. (231) found 22 cases of PCH. All were in children and all were secondary to infections. In such cases, the hemoglobinuria may be more continual than paroxysmal and episodes of hemolysis may occur without the patient being exposed to cold. These findings prompted Wolach et al. (221) to suggest that some secondary episodes are more accurately described as transient Donath-Landsteiner hemolytic anemia than as secondary PCH. Since episodes of hemolysis can be extremely severe, early recognition of the secondary condition is essential so that exposure to cold by the patient can be avoided. Although hemolysis may occur in some patients not exposed to cold, it is invariably more severe following such exposure. Because the idiopathic form of the disease is so uncommon, it is relatively easy for a physician to forget PCH when considering various diagnoses in an anemic patient. Accordingly, it is worth the blood banker's time and effort to do the simple Donath-Landsteiner test (see below) whenever the blood of a patient (particularly a child) with severe unexplained anemia is tested. The test is particularly relevant if the patient (again special emphasis if the patient is a child) has recently had any form of viral illness. During his career, one of us (PDI) has six different times provided an explanation of severe anemia in a child by testing the child's serum in a D-L test and obtaining a positive result when, at the clinical level, no cause of the anemia had been determined.

It is entirely possible that acute episodes of intravascular hemolysis in recently infected children are more common than is generally realized. We have seen a number of cases in which we suspected but could not prove that hemolysis had occurred. A typical case involved a child who was recovering from a viral illness (a "flu-like" syndrome was common) and who was noticed, by a parent, to be pale, listless and lethargic. The child was then taken to a physician and marked anemia was found. Questioning often revealed a recent history of jaundice and on far fewer occasions, descriptions of what was probably hemoglobinuria. However, in these cases the D-L was negative and no serological evidence of a pathological cold-reactive autoantibody was found. Given the fact that production of the D-L antibody secondary to viral disease is transient and short-lived and the very similar clinical pictures of these children to those in whom a D-L antibody was detected, we suspect that in at least some children hemolysis occurs but that autoantibody production has stopped before the serological tests are done.

PCH, the Donath-Landsteiner (D-L) Test

The causative autoantibody of PCH is a biphasic hemolysin. That is to say, it binds to red cells optimally at 0 to 4°C and causes hemolysis optimally at 37°C. These facts are used in the D-L test that is diagnostic of PCH (203). Two samples of the patient's blood are collected into tubes that do not contain any anticoagulant. One is placed immediately at 37°C, the other is placed in a bath of melting ice for 30 minutes. The chilled sample is then incubated at 37°C for a further 30 minutes then both samples are centrifuged. Hemolysis in the tube placed at 0°C then 37°C, in the absence of hemolysis in the one maintained at 37°C, is indicative of the presence of the biphasic hemolysin of PCH. In other words, the in vivo activity of the causative autoantibody is duplicated in vitro.

When PCH is suspected but it is not practical to collect new samples from the patient for a direct D-L test, an indirect test can be performed. The patient's serum, to which fresh normal serum is added as a source of complement is tested, as described above for the clotted samples, against washed normal red cells. Again, detection of a biphasic hemolysin is indicative of PCH. This test is not as reliable as the direct test. When a sample from a patient with PCH is allowed to cool (even to room temperature) much of the autoantibody will bind to the patient's red cells so will not be present in the serum when the indirect D-L test is done. If PCH is suspected and only samples that have been standing at room temperature are available, it may help to place the clotted sample (with the serum returned to the clot if necessary) at 37°C for 30 to 60 minutes before centrifugation. The hope is that autoantibody may elute from the patient's cells and then be detectable in the patient's serum. Any complement activated while the sample was at room temperature must be replaced, hence the addition of fresh normal serum to the patient's serum in the indirect test. The indirect D-L test can be made more sensitive (17) by using red cells from a patient with paroxysmal nocturnal hemoglobinuria (PNH) in the test on serum from the patient suspected of having PCH. Red cells from patients with PNH are exquisitely sensitive to complement-induced lysis and will be hemolyzed in the presence of smaller amounts of activated complement than will normal red cells. However, if the modified indirect D-L test is used, controls with normal serum are necessary and need to be subtracted as background since most normal sera tested this way will cause some hemolysis of PNH red cells.

The antiglobulin test can be used in conjunction with the direct or indirect D-L test to demonstrate presence of the causative IgG autoantibody. After incubation of the test in the melting-ice bath for 30 minutes, enough red cells for an antiglobulin test are removed. Those cells are then washed four times in saline chilled to 0°C and the test is read with anti-IgG. Use of unchilled saline to wash the red cells nearly always results in spontaneous elution of the IgG autoantibody and a false negative result.

It is not always easy to distinguish between a biphasic hemolysin causing PCH and a potent monophasic hemolysin causing severe CHD. As the names imply, the biphasic hemolysin of PCH will cause hemolysis only when the two temperature test system is used. A potent monophasic hemolysin causative of severe CHD will cause hemolysis at a single temperature but may also give a positive reaction in the D-L test. One way to try to differentiate between the two is to study the immunoglobulin nature of the causative autoantibody. This can be done by treating the serum of the patient (harvested from a blood sample that was allowed to clot and was then centrifuged at 37°C) with 2-ME or DTT and then performing the indirect D-L test. An IgG autoantibody will still give a positive reaction, an IgM antibody will usually no longer act as a hemolysin. Alternatively, the antiglobulin test described above on red cells taken from the direct or indirect D-L test after incubation in the melting-ice bath, can be used. Since anti-IgG is used to read that test, it will obviously be negative if the autohemolysin is IgM in composition.

PCH, Autoantibody Specificity

Like so many other autoantibodies causative of hemolytic anemia, those that cause PCH were regarded for many years as being non-specific because they reacted with all red cell samples against which they were tested. In 1963, Levine et al. (232) showed that Tj(a-) (i.e. P_1- P- P^k-) red cells were non-reactive with the biphasic hemolysin that causes PCH; in an addendum in their paper, they (232) mentioned that P^k red cells were similarly non-reactive. Shortly thereafter, others (233,234) confirmed that PCH is most often caused by auto-anti-P. As mentioned above, the P antigen is known to be located close to the red cell membrane (235-243); this is one of the factors that make IgG auto-anti-P an extremely efficient hemolysin (244). The specificity of anti-P and the differences in reactivity between that antibody and anti-Tj^a (anti-P+P_1+P^k) and anti-P_1 are discussed in Chapter 11.

There is no doubt that in most cases of idiopathic and secondary PCH the causative autoantibody has anti-P specificity (55,213,217,222-226,228,230-234,245,246). Indeed some workers believe that PCH is caused only by a biphasic hemolysin with auto-anti-P specificity. Those clinical conditions caused by hemolysins of other specificities or by monophasic hemolysins, are considered to be cases of severe CHD. A more commonly held belief is that while PCH is, by definition, caused by a biphasic hemolysin, specificities other than anti-P are (rarely) seen as the causative autoantibody. Thus cases attributed to autoantibodies directed against: I (216,247); i (248); IH (249,250); H (251); and p (252) have been reported in the literature. In reading these reports, the difficulty described above, in distinguishing between a true biphasic hemolysin and a monophasic hemolysin that can cause a D-L test to be positive, must be borne in mind. For example, we (129) thought that we had seen a case of PCH caused by auto-anti-IH but, in retrospect, believe that the autoantibody was a monophasic hemolysin causing particularly severe CHD. Somewhat similarly, a case that we described (227) in which the autoantibody had specificity for one of the Pr antigens, was better described as D-L hemolytic anemia (see above) than as PCH.

PCH, Treatment

It is fortunate that idiopathic PCH is a rare disease

because no specific form of treatment has been unequivocally documented as being of benefit. Although the causative autoantibody is IgG, corticosteroid therapy does not often appear to cause appreciable suppression of autoantibody production. While some reports have claimed that splenectomy was beneficial, there are an equal number that report that it was not. In the absence of a specific form of treatment, strict avoidance of exposure to cold is the most efficient method of prevention of intravascular red cell destruction and anemia. As mentioned briefly above, the secondary episodes of PCH that are more common than the idiopathic form, are best handled by managing the patient through the acute phase by avoidance of cold and supportive transfusions if essential. Like secondary episodes of CHD, those that involve PCH are self-limiting and once the production of autoantibody stops, a reversion to the normal immune state can be expected. If transfusion is essential, there appears no doubt that P- blood (i.e. P^k or Tj(a-), see Chapter 10) survives better in a patient with auto-anti-P, than does P+ blood (253,254). However, in a life-saving situation, when no P- units are available, P+ blood should be used (17,55) and, as with any other form of hemolytic anemia, survival of the transfused red cells can be expected to approximate survival of the patient's own cells. It is particularly important in children that transfusion not be delayed or withheld because no compatible blood is available, when transfusion is necessary to prevent death from anemia.

Some Unusual Findings in PCH

Garratty (54) has pointed out that although typical reactions are found in many cases of PCH, several observations are not yet fully explained. First, in some cases of the disease, the IgG autoantibody does not bind to red cells, in vitro, at temperatures above about 16°C . Thus it is hard to imagine how in vivo antibody binding occurs although the considerable hemolysis that follows leaves little doubt that such binding did occur. Second, in some children with PCH, or at least with biphasic hemolysins, secondary to viral infections, hemolysis is not related to cold exposure (221,231). Again, it is difficult to explain continual, albeit acute and self-limited, hemolysis in these children. Garratty (54) points out that even if macrophages were highly activated in these patients, intravascular hemolysis would still not be explained and wonders if the viral infection plays a role in red cell destruction. Third, on rare occasions (213,226,255) the hemolysin of PCH has a much wider than usual thermal range. Indeed, in some patients in whom such a finding was made, the conventionally performed DAT detected the IgG autoantibody on the patients' red cells. We (265)

found one auto-anti-P that caused secondary PCH in a three-year old girl, that hemolyzed red cells in a PEG test system at 37°C. We did not find another biphasic hemolysin that had caused PCH that reacted similarly but the additional samples we tested were in sera that had been stored frozen for some time and/or had specificities other than anti-P. Finally, Garratty et al. (256) and Garratty (54,257) report that the C3-coated red cells of patients with PCH give (sometimes strong) positive reactions in in vitro monocyte monolayer assays (MMA) although red cells from patients with CHD, ostensibly coated with similar amounts of C3, are non-reactive in those tests. Since the causative autoantibody of PCH is IgG, while that of CHD is almost always IgM, it is tempting to suppose that the positive MMAs with PCH red cells, occur because the monocytes bind the IgG, not the C3, molecules on those red cells. However, the suggestion does not fit with the concept that IgG is removed when PCH red cells are washed (they were washed normally before the MMAs (256)) before DATs are read, nor could IgG be demonstrated on the red cells that were positive in the MMAs (54,256). Along similar lines, in vitro or in vivo engulfment of red cells by monocytes or neutrophils, in patients with PCH, has occasionally been seen (258-262).

Hemolytic Anemia Caused by Auto-Anti-Rx

This antibody cannot truly be called cold-reactive or warm-reactive since it reacts (at least in vitro) better at 22°C than at 4 or 37°C. Its activity and the hemolytic anemia that it caused (263,264) are described in Chapter 34.

References

1. Schubothe H. Semin Hematol 1966;3:27
2. Watkins SP, Shulman NR. Blood 1970;36:153
3. Shumak KH, Rachkewich RA, Crookston MC, et al. Nature (New Biol) 1971;231:148
4. Thomas DB. Eur J Immunol 1973;3:824
5. Shumak KH, Rachkewich RA, Greaves MF. Clin Immunol Immunopathol 1975;4:241
6. Pruzanski W, Farid N, Keystone E, et al. Clin Immunol Immunopathol 1975;4:248
7. Pruzanski W, Farid N, Keystone E, et al. Clin Immunol Immunopathol 1975;4:277
8. Crookston JH. Arch Int Med 1975;135:1314
9. Biberfeld G, Biberfeld P, Wigzell H. Scand J Immunol 1976;5:87
10. Pruzanski W, Delmage K. Clin Immunol Immunopathol 1977;7:130
11. Pruzanski W, Shumak KH. New Eng J Med 1977;297:538
12. Pruzanski W, Shumak KH. New Eng J Med 1977;297:583
13. Dunstan RA, Simpson MB, Rosse WF. Am J Clin Pathol 1984;82:74

14. Dunstan RA, Simpson MB. Br J Haematol 1985;61:603
15. Dunstan RA. Br J Haematol 1986;62:301
16. Grillot-Courvalin C, Brouet J-C, Piller F, et al. Eur J Immunol 1992;22:1781
17. Rosse WF. Clinical Immunohematology: Basic Concepts and Clinical Applications. Boston:Blackwell, 1990
18. Ferriman DG, Dacie JV, Keele KD, et al. Quart J Med 1951;20:275
19. Nelson MG, Marshall RJ. Br Med J 1953;2:314
20. Gaddy CG, Powell LW Jr. Arch Int Med 1958;102:468
21. Kuenn JW, Weber R, Teague PO, et al. Cancer 1978;42:1826
22. Waldenstrom J. Acta Med Scand 1944;117:216
23. Cohen RJ, Bohannon RA, Wallerstein RO. Am J Med 1966;41:274
24. Axelsson U, Bachmann R, Hallen J. Acta Med Scand 1966;201:235
25. Evans RS, Baxter E, Gilliland BC. Blood 1973;42:463
26. MacKenzie MR, Fudenberg HH. Blood 1974;39:874
27. Pruzanski W, Cowan DH, Parr DM. Clin Immunol Immunopathol 1974;2:234
28. Tubbs RR, Hoffman GC, Deodhar SD, et al. Cleveland Clin Quart 1976;43:21
29. Carter P, Koval JJ, Hobbs JR. Clin Exp Immunol 1977;28:241
30. Kyle RA. Am J Med 1978;64:814
31. Adams WS, Blahd WH, Bassott SH. Proc Soc Exp Biol Med 1952;80:377
32. Skoog WA, Adams WS. Clin Res 1959;7:96
33. Powles R, Smith C, Kohn J, et al. Br Med J 1971;3:664
34. Mc Grath MA, Penny R. J Clin Invest 1976;58:1155
35. Beck JR, Quinn BM, Meier FA, et al. Transfusion 1982;22:51
36. Isbister JP, Cooper DA, Blake HM, et al. Am J Med 1978;64:434
37. Dodds AJ, Klarkowski D, Cooper DA, et al. Am J Clin Pathol 1979;71:473
38. Pascali E, Pezzoli A, Melato M, et al. Acta Haematol 1980;66:299
39. Prchal JT, Crago SS, Mesteckly J, et al. Cancer 1981;47:2312
40. Crisp D, Pruzanski B. Am J Med 1982;72:915
41. Silberstein LE, Robertson GA, Hannam-Harris AC, et al. Blood 1986;67:1705
42. Silberstein LE, Goldman J, Kant JA, et al. Arch Biochem Biophys 1988;264:244
43. Silberstein LE, Litwin S, Carmack CE. J Exp Med 1989;169:1631
44. Stevenson F, Smith G, North J, et al. Br J Haematol 1989;72:9
45. Silberstein LE, Jefferies LC, Goldman J, et al. Blood 1991;73:2372
46. Friedman DF, Moore JS, Erikson J, et al. Blood 1992;80:2287
47. Brown DL, Cooper AG. Clin Sci 1970;38:175
48. Ross GD, Medof ME. Adv Immunol 1985;37:217
49. Mantovani B, Rabinovitch M, Nussenzweig V. J Exp Med 1972;135:790
50. Kurlander RJ, Rosse WF, Logue GL. J Clin Invest 1978;61:1309
51. Adams DO, Hamilton TA. Ann Rev Immunol 1984;2:283
52. Schreiber AD, Herskovitz BS, Goldwein M. New Eng J Med 1977;296:1490
53. Garratty G. In: Immune Destruction of Red Blood Cells. Arlington, VA:Am Assoc Blood Banks, 1989:109
54. Garratty G. In: Immunobiology of Transfusion Medicine. New York:Marcel Dekker, 1994:493
55. Petz LD, Garratty G. Acquired Immune Hemolytic Anemias. New York:Churchill Livingstone, 1980
56. Packman CH, Leddy JP. In: Hematology, 4th Ed. New York:McGraw Hill, 1990:675
57. Issitt PD. In: Progress in Clinical Pathology, Vol 7. New York:Grune and Stratton, 1978:137
58. Issitt PD. In: Immune Hemolytic Anemias. New York:Churchill Livingstone, 1985:1
59. Reid ME. Transfusion 1978;18:353
60. Judd WJ. Methods in Immunohematology, 2nd Ed. Durham:Montgomery 1994
61. Chaplin H, Coleman ME, Monroe MC. Blood 1983;62:965
62. Harboe M, Furth R van, Schubothe H, et al. Scand J Haematol 1965;2:259
63. Harboe M, Lind K. Scand J Haematol 1966;3:269
64. Cooper AG, Worlledge SM. Nature 1967;214:799
65. Feizi T. Science 1967;156:1111
66. Cooper AG, Chavin SI, Franklin FC. Immunochemistry 1970;7:479
67. Capra JP, Kehoe JM, Williams RC Jr, et al. Proc Nat Acad Sci Wash 1972;69:40
68. Croce CM, Shander M, Martinis J, et al. Proc Nat Acad Sci USA 1978;76:3416
69. Heiter PA, Max EE, Seidman JG, et al. Cell 1980;22:197
70. Malcolm S, Barton P, Murphy C, et al. Proc Nat Acad Sci USA 1981;79:4957
71. McBride OW, Heiter PA, Hollis GF, et al. J Exp Med 1982;155:1480
72. Early P, Huang H, Davis M, et al. Cell 1980;19:981
73. Kataoka T, Miyata T, Honjo T. Cell 1981;23:357
74. Rabbitts JS, Bently DL, Milstein CP. Immunol Rev 1981;59:69
75. Marcu KB, Lang RB, Stanton LW, et al. Nature 1982;298:87
76. Lee KH, Matsuda F, Kinashi T, et al. J Mol Biol 1987;195:761
77. Pascual V, Victor K, Lesz D, et al. J Immunol 1991;146:4386
78. Williams RC Jr. Ann NY Acad Sci 1971;190:330
79. Jacobson LB, Longstreth GF, Edgington TS. Am J Med 1973;54;514
80. Gergely J, Wang AC, Fudenberg HH. Vox Sang 1973;24:432
81. Silverman GJ, Goni F, Chen PP, et al. J Exp Med 1986;168:2361
82. Silverman GJ, Carson DA. Eur J Immunol 1990;20:351
83. Edman P, Cooper AG. Fed Eur Biochem Soc Lett 1968;2:33
84. Cohen S, Cooper AG. Immunology 1968;15:93
85. Goldberg LS, Barnett EV. J Immunol 1967;99:803
86. Ambrus M, Bajtai G. Haematologia 1969;3:225
87. Ratkin GA, Osterland CK, Chaplin H Jr. J Lab Clin Med 1973;82:67
88. Roelcke D. Clin Immunol Immunopathol 1974;2:266
89. Dellagi K, Brouet JC, Schenmetzler C, et al. Blood 1981;57:189
90. Roelcke D, Kreft H. Transfusion 1984;24:210
91. Silberstein LE, Shoenfeld Y, Schwartz RS, et al. Vox Sang 1985;48:105
92. Szymanski IO, Teno R, Rybak ME. Vox Sang 1986;51:112
93. Silberstein LE, Berkman EM, Schreiber AD. Ann Intern Med 1987;106:238
94. Northoff H, Martin A, Roelcke D. Eur J Haematol 1987;38:85
95   Roelcke D. Transf Med Rev 1989;3:140
96. Curtis BR, Lamon J, Roelcke D, et al. Transfusion 1990;30:838
97. Angevine CD, Bajtai G. J Immunol 1966;96:578
98. Roelcke D, Dorrow W. Klin Wochenschr 1968;46:126
99. Roelcke D. Eur J Immunol 1973;3:206
100. Garratty G, Petz LD, Brodsky I, et al. Vox Sang 1973;25:32
101. Tonthat H, Rochant H, Henry A, et al. Vox Sang 1976;30:464
102. Romer W, Rother U, Roelcke D. Immunobiology 1980;157:41
103. Harboe M. Vox Sang 1971;20:289

104. Tschirhart DL, Kunkel L, Shulman IA. Vox Sang 1990;59:222
105. Wiener AS, Unger LJ, Cohen L, et al. Ann Int Med 1956;44:221
106. Weiner W, Shinton NK, Gray IR. J Clin Pathol 1960;13:232
107. Tippett P, Noades J, Sanger R, et al. Vox Sang 1960;5:107
108. Jenkins WJ, Marsh WL, Noades J, et al. Vox Sang 1960;5:97
109. Dacie JV. The Haemolytic Anaemias, 2nd Ed. Part II. The Congenital and Acquired Haemolytic Anaemias. New York:Grune and Stratton, 1962
110. Dacie JV, Worlledge SM. Prog Hematol 1969;6:82
111. Wiener AS, Gordon EB, Gallop C. J Immunol 1953;71:58
112. Wiener AS, Gordon EB. Am J Clin Pathol 1953;23:429
113. Marsh WL, Jenkins WJ. Nature 1960;188:753
114. Marsh WL. Br J Haematol 1960;7:200
115. Rosenfield RE, Schroeder R, Ballard R, et al. Vox Sang 1964;9:415
116. Tegoli J, Harris JP, Issitt PD, et al. Vox Sang 1967;13;114
117. McGinniss MH, Binder RA, Kales AN, et al. Immunohematology 1987;3:20
118. McGinniss MH. Immunohematology 1987;3:23
119. Postoway N, Garratty G, Guerra-Zevallos M. (abstract). Book of Abstracts. Joint Cong ISBT/AABB 1990:27
120. Postoway N, Capon S, Smith L, et al. (abstract). Book of Abstracts. Joint Cong ISBT/AABB 1990:85
121. Garratty G, Petz LD, Wallerstein RO, et al. Transfusion 1974;14:226
122. Freedman J, Newlands M, Johnson CA. Vox Sang 1977;32:135
123. Roelcke D, Kreft H, Hack H, et al. Vox Sang 1994;67:216
124. Brendemoen OJ. Acta Path Microbiol Scand 1952;31:574
125. Jenkins WJ, Marsh WL. Lancet 1961;2:16
126. Borne AEGKr von dem, Mol JJ, Joustra-Maas, et al. Br J Haematol 1982;50:345
127. Issitt PD, Jackson VA. Vox Sang 1968;15:152
128. Marsh WL, Nichols ME, Reid ME. Vox Sang 1971;20:209
129. Geiger J, Issitt PD. Unpublished observations 1967 cited in Issitt PD. Applied Blood Group Serology, lst Ed. Oxnard:Spectra Biologicals 1970:128
130. Haynes CR, Chaplin H Jr. Vox Sang 1971;20:46
131. Garratty G, Petz LD, Hoops JK. Br J Haematol 1977;35:587
132. Boyer JT. Clin Exp Immunol 1967;2:241
133. Evans RS, Turner E, Bingham M. J Clin Invest 1967;46:1461
134. Engelfriet CP, Borne AEGKr von dem, Beckers D, et al. Clin Exp Immunol 1972;11:255
135. Rosse WF. Prog Hematol 1973;8:51
136. Rosse WF, De Boisfleury A, Bessis M. Blood Cells 1975;1:345
137. Waldmann TA, Strober W. Prog Allgy 1969;13:1
138. Logue GL, Rosse WF, Gockerman JP. J Clin Invest 1973;52:493
139. Rosenfield RE, Jagathambal K. Sem Hematol 1976;13:311
140. Taft EG, Propp RP, Sullivan SA. Transfusion 1977;17:173
141. Isbister JP, Biggs JC, Penny R. Austral NZ J Med 1978;8:154
142. Klein H, Faltz LL, McIntosh CL, et al. Transfusion 1980;20:354
143. Brooks BD, Steane EA, Sheehan RG, et al. Prog Clin Biol Res 1982;106:317
144. Frappaz D, Rigal D, Valla JS, et al. Pediatrie 1983;38:411
145. Hamblin TJ. Apheresis Bull 1983;1:10
146. Silberstein LE, Berkman EM. J Clin Apheresis 1983;1:238
147. Shumak KH, Rock GA. New Eng J Med 1984;310:672
148. Urbaniak SJ. Clin Haematol 1984;13:217
149. Huestis DW. In: Progress in Transfusion Medicine. Edinburgh:Churchill Livingstone, 1986:78
150. Urbaniak SJ, Robinson EA. In: ABC of Transfusion. London:BMJ Pub Group, 1992:53
151. Robinson EA. Vox Sang 1994;67 (Suppl 3):151
152. Borberg H. Vox Sang 1996;70 (Suppl 3):135
153. Marks MR, Reid ME, Ellisor SS. (abstract). Transfusion 1980;20:629
154. Waligora SK, Edwards JM. Transfusion 1983;23:328
155. Edwards-Moulds J, Waligora SK. (Letter). Transfusion 1984;24:369
156. Strauss RA, Gasich L, Gloster ES. Lab Med 1985;16:551
157. Orsini LA, Haase JE, Poling SR, et al. (abstract). Transfusion 1985;25:452
158. Dzik WH, Yang R, Blank J. (Letter). Transfusion 1986;26:303
159. Weiland DL. (Letter). Transfusion 1984;24:369
160. Marsh WL, Nichols ME, Allen FH Jr. Vox Sang 1970;18:149
161. Issitt CH, Issitt PD. Unpublished observations 1974-1980 cited in Issitt PD. Applied Blood Group Serology, 3rd Ed. Miami:Montgomery 1985:547
162. Woll JE, Smith CM, Nusbacher J. J Am Med Assoc 1974;229:1779
163. Finland M, Peterson OL, Allen HE, et al. J Clin Invest 1945;24:451
164. Florman AI, Weiss AB. J Lab Clin Med 1945;30:902
165. Finland M, Barnes MW. Arch Int Med 1954;101:462
166. McGinniss MH, Schmidt PJ, Carbone PP. Nature 1964;202:606
167. Schmidt PJ, Barile MF, McGinniss MH. Nature 1965;205:371
168. Schmidt PJ, McGinniss MH. Vox Sang 1965;10:109
169. Schmidt PJ, McGinniss MH. Nature 1967;214:1363
170. Feizi T. Ann NY Acad Sci 1967;143:801
171. Smith CB, McGinniss MH, Schmidt PJ. J Immunol 1967;99:333
172. Murray HW, Masur H, Senterfit LB, et al. Am J Med 1975;58:229
173. Feizi T, Darrell JH. Nature 1966;211:1156
174. Loomes LM, Uemura K, Childs RA, et al. Nature 1984;307:560
175. Loomes LM, Uemura K, Feizi T. Infect Immun 1985;47:15
176. König AL, Kreft H, Hengge U, et al. Vox Sang 1988;55:176
177. Schonitzer D, Kilga-Nogler S, Trenkwalder B, et al. Infus Klin Ern 1985;12:181
178. Feizi T, Lecomte J, Childs R. Clin Exp Immunol 1977;3:233
179. Evans WS, Feizi T, Childs R, et al. Mol Immunol 1983;20:1127
180. Jenkins WJ, Koster HG, Marsh WL, et al. Br J Haematol 1965;11:480
181. Rosenfield RE, Schmidt PJ, Calvo RC, et al. Vox Sang 1965;10:631
182. Horwitz CA, Moulds J, Henle W, et al. Blood 1977;50:195
183. Calvo R, Stein W, Kochwa S, et al. J Clin Invest 1965;44:1033
184. Wollheim FA, Williams RC. New Eng J Med 1966;274:61
185. Troxel DB, Innella F, Cochren RJ. Am J Clin Pathol 1966;46:625
186. Worlledge SM, Dacie JV. In: Infectious Mononucleosis. Oxford:Blackwell, 1969
187. Wilkinson LS, Petz LD, Garratty G. Br J Haematol 1973;25:715
188. Gronemeyer P, Chaplin H, Ghazarian V, et al. Transfusion 1981;21:715
189. Goldberg LS, Barnett EV. Ann NY Acad Sci 1969;168:122
190. Capra JD, Dowling P, Cook S, et al. Vox Sang 1969;16:10
191. Pattengale PK, Smith RW, Gerber P. Lancet 1973;2:93
192. Sutton RNP, Edmond RTD, Thomas DB, et al. Clin Exp Immunol 1974;17:427
193. Marsh WL. Unpublished observations 1972 cited in Issitt PD.

Applied Blood Group Serology, 3rd Ed. Miami:Montgomery 1985:548

194. White WD, Issitt PD. Unpublished observations 1973 cited in Issitt PD. Applied Blood Group Serology, 3rd Ed. Miami:Montgomery 1985:548

195. Costea N, Yakulis V, Heller P. Blood 1965;26:323

196. Geisen HP, Roelcke D, Rehn K, et al. Klin Wochenschr 1975;53:767

197. Vanherweghem JL, Dejonghe M, Geel P van. Nouv Presse Med 1977;6:851

198. King JW, Mayh JS. Arch Int Med 1980;140:1537

199. Horwitz CA, Skradski K, Reece E, et al. Scand J Haematol 1984;33:35

200. Pruzanski W, Roelcke D, Donnelly E, et al. Acta Haematol 1986;75:171

201. König AL, Börner CH, Braun RW, et al. (abstract). Immunobiology 1985;170:46

202. Donath J, Landsteiner K. Munch Med Wschr 1904;51:1590

203. Donath J, Landsteiner K. Abl Bakt (Abtl Orig) 1908;45:204

204. Donath J, Landsteiner K. Ergebn Hyg Bakt 1925;7:184

205. Pirofsky B. Autoimmunization and the Autoimmune Hemolytic Anemias. Baltimore:Williams and Wilkins, 1969

206. Howard CP, Mills ES, Townsend SR. Am J Med Sci 1938;196:792

207. Becker RM. Arch Int Med 1948;81:630

208. Kaiser AD, Bradford WL. Arch Pediat 1929;46:571

209. Ellis LB, Wallenman OJ, Stetson RP. Blood 1948;3:419

210. Green N, Goldenburg H. Arch Int Med 1960;105:108

211. Colley EW. Br Med J 1964;1:1552

212. O'Neill BJ, Marshall WS. Arch Dis Childh 1967;42:183

213. Reis CA, Garratty G, Petz LD, et al. Blood 1971;38:491

214. Bunch C, Schwartz FCM, Bird GWG. Arch Dis Childh 1972;47:299

215. Wishart MM, Davey MG. J Clin Pathol 1973;26:332

216. Bell CA, Zwicker H, Rosenbaum DL. Transfusion 1973;13:138

217. Bird GWG, Wingham J, Martin AJ, et al. J Clin Pathol 1976;29:215

218. Boccardi V, D'Annibali S, Di Natale G, et al. Blut 1977;34:211

219. Bird GWG. Br J Haematol 1977;37:167

220. Burkart PT, Hsu TCS. Transfusion 1979;19:535

221. Wolach B, Heddle N, Barr R, et al. Br J Haematol 1981;48:425

222. Sokol RJ, Hewitt S, Stamps BK. Acta Haematol 1982;68:268

223. Lau P, Sererat S, Moore V, et al. Vox Sang 1983;44:167

224. Nordhagen R, Stensvold K, Winsnes A, et al. Acta Pediat Scand 1984;73:258

225. Sokol RJ, Hewitt S, Stamps BK, et al. Acta Haematol 1984;72:245

226. Lindgren S, Zimmerman S, Gibbs F, et al. Transfusion 1985;25:142

227. Judd WJ, Wilkinson SL, Issitt PD, et al. Transfusion 1986;26:423

228. Lippmann SM, Winn L, Grumet FC, et al. Am J Med 1987;82:1065

229. Engelfriet CP, Ouwehand WH, van't Veer MB, et al. In: Clinical Immunology and Allergy. Alloimmune and Autoimmune Cytopenias. London: Baillière Tindall, 1987:252

230. Heddle NM. Transf Med Rev 1989;3:219

231. Göttsche B, Salama A, Mueller-Eckhardt C. Vox Sang 1990;58:281

232. Levine P, Celano MJ, Falkowski F. Transfusion 1963;3:278

233. Knapp T. Canad J Med Technol 1964;26:172

234. Worlledge SM, Rousso C. Vox Sang 1965;10:293

235. Naiki M, Marcus DM. Biochem Biophys Res Comm 1974;60:1105

236. Naiki M, Marcus DM. Biochemistry 1975;14:4837

237. Marcus DM, Naiki M, Kundu SK, et al. In: Human Blood Groups. Basel:Karger, 1977:206

238. Morgan WTJ. In: Human Blood Groups. Basel:Karger, 1977:216

239. Marcus DM. Immunol Ser 1989;43:701

240. Takeya A, Hosomi O, Shimoda N, et al. J Biochem 1992;112:389

241. Takeya A, Hosomi O, Yazawa S, et al. Jpn J Med Sci Biol 1993;46:1

242. Yang Z, Berström J, Karlsson KA. J Biol Chem 1994;269:14620

243. Spitalnik PF, Spitalnick SL. Transf Med Rev 1995;9:110

244. Rosenfield RE. In: A Seminar on Performance Evaluation. Washington, D.C.:Am Assoc Blood Banks, 1976:93

245. Vogel JM, Hellman M, Moloshok RE. J Pediat 1972;81:974

246. Johnsen HE, Brostrphom K, Madsen M. Scand J Haematol 1978;20:413

247. Engelfriet CP, Borne AEGKr von dem, Moes M, et al. Bibl Haematol 1968;29 part 2:473

248. Shirey RS, Park K, Ness PM, et al. Transfusion 1986;26:62

249. Weiner W, Gordon EG, Rowe D. Vox Sang 1964;9:684

250. Bell CA, Zwicker H. (abstract). Transfusion 1967;7:384

251. Ciruzzi J, Carreras-Vescio LA, Rey JA, et al. Sangre 1983;28:775

252. Engelfriet CP, Beckers D, Borne AEGKr von dem, et al. Vox Sang 1972;23:176

253. Rausen AR, LeVine R, Hsu TCS, et al. Pediatrics 1975;55:275

254. Sabio H, Jones D, McKie VS. Am J Hematol 1992;39:220

255. Nordhagen R. (Letter). Transfusion 1991;31:190

256. Garratty G, Nance S, Arndt P, et al. (abstract). Transfusion 1989;29 (Suppl 7S):49S

257. Garratty G. Transf Med Rev 1990;4:297

258. Ehrlich P. Z Klin Med 1881;3:383

259. Ehrlich P. Dtsch Med Wochenschr 1881;7:224

260. Eason J, Edin Med J 1907;21:440

261. Jordan WS Jr, Prouty RL, Heinle RW, et al. Blood 1952;7:387

262. Hernandez JA, Steane SM. Am J Clin Pathol 1984;81:787

263. Marsh WL, Johnson CL, Øyen R, et al. Transfusion 1980;20:1

264. Marsh WL, Johnson CL, DiNapoli J, et al. (abstract). Transfusion 1980;20:647

265. Combs MR, Issitt PD, Kirkland A. (abstract). Transfusion 1993;33 (Suppl 9S):21S

39 | Autoantibodies that are Benign In Vivo

Chapter 37 includes a discussion of "warm" antibody-induced hemolytic anemia (WAIHA) in patients in whom the DAT is negative. Just as a negative DAT does not exclude WAIHA, a positive DAT does not prove that the patient has hemolytic anemia. This chapter describes a number of situations in which the DAT is positive in hematologically normal individuals. In some of these situations, IgG autoantibody is involved and can be recovered by elution from the individual's red cells and less frequently can be detected in the person's serum. More often the DAT is positive because complement but no detectable immunoglobulin is present on the individual's red cells. While such findings often mean that there are no autoantibodies to red cells involved, it is convenient also to consider the benign finding of C3 and C4 on the red cells of a hematologically normal individual, in this Chapter.

As will quickly become apparent from what is written below, there is wide variation in the incidence figures reported for positive DATs in hematologically normal persons. However, the variation apparently relates more to the type of test performed and the type of data reported than to real differences in the populations studied. For example (references given below) if all positive reactions, i.e. ± upwards, seen when C3, C4 or IgG is detected on the red cells are considered, about 1 in 1000 blood donors has a positive DAT. If donors with strongly positive DATs, i.e. 3 to 4+ with anti-IgG, are counted, the incidence is between 1 in 10,000 and 1 in 25,000.

Positive DATs in Hematologically Normal Individuals: Incidence

Weiner (1) seems to have been the first investigator to publish details about hematologically normal individuals with strongly positive DATs. In a six year period in a population of about 60,000, a total of 21 normal blood donors were found to have a positive DAT. Among the 21, the DAT was: 3 to 4+ in 12; 2+ in five; 1+ in one; and weaker than 1+ in three. Thus the incidence of a positive DAT was about 1 in 3000, the incidence of a strongly positive (3+ or stronger) DAT was about 1 in 5000. In all cases except the three giving weak reactions, IgG was present on the red cells and autoantibodies could be recovered from those cells by elution. In four individuals in whom the DATs were among the strongest, small amounts of unbound autoantibody were detected in the serum. As discussed below, the autoantibodies in these persons have the same specificities as those causative of WAIHA.

In a study that covered about one million blood donations, Gorst et al. (2) estimated that the incidence of a positive DAT was about 1 in 14,000. However, the red cells of 43% of the donors in whom the DAT was positive carried C3d and C4d but no IgG. Thus the incidence of donors with a positive DAT due to IgG on the red cells was about 1 in 25,000. What at first appear to be very different figures emerged from the study of Allan and Garratty (3) on 1.3 million donors. The study was divided by the years over which it was performed and the incidence of a positive DAT among blood donors was seen to vary (very little) from 1 in 820 to 1 in 1270 in any given year, for an overall incidence of about 1 in 1000. While these figures look very different from those of Gorst et al. (2), only 4% of the positive reactions were 3+ or stronger so that the incidence of such a finding was 1 in 25,000. Further among all the positive reactions, 16% were due to IgG alone, 44% to IgG and complement and 40% to complement alone.

Another rather different study was that of Habibi et al. (4). These investigators found an incidence of 1 in 13,000 positive DATs in supposedly normal donors but found that in every case IgG (in 67) or IgM (in 2) was detectable on the red cells. The series differs from those described above in that some 25% of the donors with a positive DAT were being treated with alpha-methyldopa (see Chapter 40). In the other series, such donors were excluded. Further, Habibi et al. (4) claimed that in about half their donors, there was some evidence of an accelerated rate of in vivo red cell clearance. Although the evidence for hemolysis was meager in many of the cases, if the 50% are removed from the DAT-positive, hematologically normal group, the incidence of such individuals in this study (4) becomes 1 in 26,000 or the same as that reported by Gorst et al. (2) and by Allan and Garratty (3). A higher incidence of positive DATs in normal blood donors is seen if the Gel test (32) is used (33). This finding is discussed again in the section on lack of significance of these findings in blood donors.

The figures given above relate predominantly to normal blood donors. When hospital patients are considered some different findings are made. In several different series (5-9) it has been shown that 8% of hospital patients have a positive DAT but no evidence of hemolytic anemia. The series are extraordinary in that they represent studies at a number of different institutions but all agree on a figure of around 8%. Further, in each of the studies it has been found that the positive DATs are weak, i.e. most 1+ or less, and that some 80% or more of them represent the presence of complement without immunoglobulin on the red cells. In other studies (9-12) it has been shown that all normal red cells carry some C3dg and C4dg (see also the Ch and Rg determinants, Chapter 27) but that the amount is most often below the threshold of detection in conventional DATs. There are, of course, many clinical conditions in which there is an increase in the amount of complement activation over the low level that occurs in normal healthy subjects (see Chapter 6). Thus it is not surprising to find that far more hospital patients than normal donors, have positive DATs in the absence of hemolysis. In some of the studies (7,9) the presence of readily detectable C3 on the red cells has been associated with serious illness in the patients. There are fewer data about IgG than about C3 on the red cells of hospital patients who do not have hemolytic anemia. However, it follows that if 8% of such patients have positive DATs and that if in 80% of them the positive DAT represents the presence of just complement on the red cells, the remainder (i.e. 20% of 8%) must have IgG (with or without complement) on the red cells. This means that between 1 and 2% of hospital patients will have a positive DAT with IgG on the red cells (again mostly weak reactions) but no hemolytic anemia.

It has been reported (13-18) that hypergammaglobulinemia can result in a positive DAT without hemolysis. Huh et al. (13) found that 25 of 50 patients with high levels of IgG in the serum had positive DATs but no indication of increased red cell destruction. Eluates made from the red cells of these patients were non-reactive. Heddle et al. (14) studied 20 patients with high levels of serum IgG and positive DATs, none of the patients had hemolysis. Heddle et al. (14) then studied 44 patients with increased levels of IgG in the serum and found that the DAT was positive in the three with the highest levels of IgG. In the same study two patients who were treated with high doses of IVIG developed positive DATs. In all these cases the red cell eluates were non-reactive. It should be remembered (see Chapter 37) that IVIG sometimes contains red cell alloantibodies (e.g. anti-D, anti-K) so will occasionally cause a positive DAT due to the passive transfer of a red cell alloantibody. It is also worth mentioning at this point, that the increased levels of IgG found in tests such as ELAT, on the red cells of patients with DAT-negative, WAIHA, have been shown (19,20) to represent autoantibody and not simply the high levels of IgG of patients with hypergammaglobulinemia.

In spite of the variation in reported incidences and the difficulties in comparing studies that used different criteria to identify the donors and patients involved, table 39-1 attempts to summarize this section. It is hoped that the table will be of some use in indicating how often the phenomena described can be expected to be seen in a blood center and in a hospital transfusion service.

TABLE 39-1 Positive DATs in Blood Donors and Hospital Patients who do not have Hemolytic Anemia

Reagent	Strength of Positive Reaction	Blood Donors	Hospital Patients
Broad Spectrum anti-whole human serum	2 to 4+	1 in 25,000	1 in 100
	± to 1+	1 in 1,000	8 in 100
Anti-IgG	2 to 4+	1 in 25,000	not known
	± to 1+	1 in 1,700	2 in 100
Anti-C3dg	2 to 4+	not known	1 in 100
	± to 1+	1 in 1,200	8 in 100

Subclasses of Benign Autoantibodies

As discussed in Chapters 6 and 37, the in vivo clearance of IgG-coated red cells proceeds via macrophage recognition of the Fc portions of IgG molecules bound to the red cells. IgG3 and IgG1 are recognized by macrophages, with rare exceptions IgG2 and IgG4 do not mediate appreciable binding. Thus it might be expected that the benign IgG autoantibodies seen in patients who do not have hemolytic anemia would be predominantly IgG2 and IgG4 in composition. In fact this is not the case. Stratton et al. (21) studied 22 normal donors who had earlier been shown (2) to have IgG on their red cells. In 20 of the donors the IgG was solely IgG1, in the other two it was IgG4. Allan and Garratty (3) tested the red cells of 10 donors in their series in whom the DAT was strongly positive. Among those donors: five had only IgG1; one only IgG3; one IgG1 and IgG3; and three only IgG4 on the red cells. Similarly, in some other reports that were concerned primarily with WAIHA but included descriptions of some DAT-positive hematologically normal individuals, results of subclassing studies were given. Thus in many of these individuals the autoantibodies were shown to be IgG1 (22-24) or mixtures of IgG1 and IgG3 (24-26) although some that were solely IgG4 or IgG2 were also seen (24).

The findings described above raise some questions for which no complete answers are yet available. While there are certainly exceptions (20,27,28) there is some general correlation between the number of molecules of IgG bound per red cell and sequestration or lack thereof, of those red cells by macrophages (8,23,29-31). Recognizing that exceptions blur the boundaries, some published figures will be used for this discussion. Macrophage sequestration of IgG1-coated red cells has been said (23) to occur when about 1000 or more molecules of IgG1 are bound per red cell. Macrophage sequestration of IgG3-coated red cells has been said (21) to occur when about 100 or more molecules are bound per red cell. In the study of Stratton et al. (21) those donors with positive DATs but no hemolytic anemia in whom the autoantibodies were solely IgG1, were found to have between 110 and 950 molecules of IgG per red cell. This was used as an explanation for the lack of red cell destruction by the antibodies. However, the questions then become why do these persons continue to make autoantibodies at these levels and what prevents them from increasing the amount of autoantibody made to the point at which it destroys red cells in vivo? As discussed below, many of these donors have been followed for many years. While some of them eventually develop WAIHA and some others become DAT-negative, many of them continue to produce autoantibodies at apparently the same level for many years. Clearly an understanding as to how the immune system holds autoantibody production in check at a sublytic level, would have the potential to provide information useful in treating patients who do have WAIHA. A second question pertains to those donors in whom the autoantibody is IgG3. If red cells coated with 100 molecules of IgG3 per red cell are subject to macrophage sequestration and if 100 to 200 molecules of IgG per red cell are necessary for the DAT to give a 1+ reaction, how can lack of hemolysis be explained in those individuals who have strongly positive (3 to 4+) DATs and an IgG3 autoantibody? Clearly factors other than IgG subclass and quantity of IgG bound, are at play (20).

While it has sometimes been speculated that individuals with warm-reactive autoantibodies who do not have hemolytic anemia, have concurrent abnormalities in macrophage function that result in non-sequestration of the autoantibody-coated red cells, there is no evidence to support such an assumption. If these individuals had some malfunctions of macrophage activity, one might expect that, as a group, they would have a higher than usual rate of related clinical disorders and infections. Such findings have not been seen.

Specificity of Benign Autoantibodies

In addition to the studies already described and referenced, that concentrated on donors and patients with benign autoantibodies, there are many others in which such persons were included. For example we (34) performed tests on 150 consecutively received samples in which the DAT was positive and warm-reactive autoantibody was demonstrable in the serum and/or an eluate. Among the 150 samples, 87 were from patients with WAIHA, 33 were from patients being treated with alpha-methyldopa (aldomet, see Chapter 40), and 30 were from hematologically normal individuals. Among the hematologically normal individuals, five were patients with

other than an autoimmune disease and 25 were healthy blood donors. Most persons in this group had DATs that were 3 to 4+. Many other workers have included findings about such persons in their publications (35-41) but, as with our report (34) did not have the data to estimate incidence rates. However, these many additional reports have confirmed that the specificities of these benign autoantibodies are essentially the same as those that cause WAIHA. As a typical example of these findings, table 39-2 summarizes the specificities of autoantibodies found in the 150 individuals mentioned above, whom we studied (34). As indicated, 33 of the individuals had produced autoantibodies as a result of alpha-methyldopa therapy. In common with the majority of patients who form autoantibodies as a result of such therapy, none of our 33 had an accelerated rate of in vivo red cell destruction. As can be seen from table 39-2, when the incidence of the various antibodies is considered as a percentage of the patients studied, there are no differences between the three groups. For example, 21 of 30 (70%) normal donors, 22 of 33 (67%) aldomet-treated, and 62 of 87 (71%) WAIHA patients had made auto-anti-dl.

There are numerous other reports of benign autoantibodies in many blood group systems. Some typical examples are Rh (1,4,34,42-44), LW (45), MN (34,46,47), Kell (48-52), Kx (53), Kidd (54,55), Diego (34,56), Xg^a (57), Gerbich (58,59) and Vel (60,61). In some but by no means all the individuals with these autoantibodies, there was concurrent depression of antigen expression. In others there was no evidence of antigen depression and the DAT was strongly positive.

Significance of the Findings and Long-Term Follow-up Studies

As will be apparent from what has been written in this chapter thus far, the individuals described have (sometimes strongly) positive DATs and warm-reactive red cell autoantibodies, they do not have hemolytic anemia. Further, careful studies (1,2,34,62) have shown that they have normal levels of hemoglobin, haptoglobin, reticulocytes and bilirubin. Thus compensated WAIHA is excluded. As discussed in detail in Chapter 40, the most frequent finding in persons with drug-induced antibodies is that the DAT is positive, drug-dependent or drug-independent antibodies are present in the serum or in an eluate, but there is no evidence of an accelerated rate of in vivo red cell destruction; that is, no hemolytic anemia. If the role of alpha-methyldopa in causing autoantibodies to be made was not known, persons with such drug-induced autoantibodies would be included in the group of individuals being described in this chapter. However, when the DAT-positive hematologically normal persons

TABLE 39-2 To Show the Specificities of Benign and Pathological "Warm" Autoantibodies (from 34)

Autoantibody Specificity	Hematologically normal donors with a positive DAT (number 30)		Patients with alpha-methyldopa-induced autoantibodies (number 33)		Patients with WAIHA (number 87)	
	Only antibody present	Present with others	Only antibody present	Present with others	Only antibody present	Present with others
"Simple" anti-Rh*	0	7	1	15	4	33
Anti-nl	0	2	2	6	4	20
Anti-pdl	6	11	4	10	3	29
Anti-dl	9	12	7	15	13	49
Anti-Wr^b	2	6	0	4	2	32
Anti-U	0	0	0	1	1	1

* Anti-c, anti-e, anti-C, etc.

described here are questioned, no drug or combination of drugs being used by such persons emerges as a potential cause. When we investigated the 30 individuals of this type described in our study (34) we questioned them about over the counter as well as prescription drugs. Again no medication common to the group was found, Geritol was exonerated!

When a positive DAT and a warm-reactive autoantibody are found in a hospital patient, it is relatively easy to run tests to see if the patient has WAIHA. When the same findings are made in a blood donor, the decision as to what should be done is more difficult. First, if the donor is healthy and has passed all requirements for donation, it follows that he or she is not anemic. Second, since many individuals in this group remain DAT-positive and hematologically normal for very long periods (see below) there is a natural reluctance against alarming the donor by suggesting that a clinical problem may be present, while the autoantibody is and may remain benign. Third, in addition to not wishing to alarm the donor unnecessarily, is the consideration that physician and laboratory test fees may be incurred if consultation and testing to try to find the cause of the positive DAT are undertaken. Opposite to these concerns is the thought that if the donor is in the early stages of an autoimmune response, i.e. antibody not yet made at levels capable of clearing red cells in vivo, prompt intervention may ensure a better long term prognosis than if nothing is done. At very least it would seem prudent that the donor be monitored to see if anemia develops later. Many blood center physicians base the decision on what to do on the type of finding made. For example, if the DAT is 1+ or less and/or if C3 but no immunoglobulin is found on the red cells, most physicians feel that the donor need not be notified of the finding. This because such findings are relatively common (see table 39-1) and are not usually associated with later development of disease. If the DAT is 4+ and IgG is

detected on the red cells it seems that the donor should be notified and that, at very least, the hemoglobin level should be rechecked and a reticulocyte count should be performed. Even if these are normal, it would seem to be in the donor's best interests to have the values checked on a periodic but regular basis. When the DAT is between 1+ and 4+, the individual blood center physician must decide what course is to be followed. The difficult decision will be based in part on the donor's right to know about any abnormal finding and in part on what the blood center physician considers to be an abnormal finding. The significance of a positive DAT on the unit of blood and disposition of that unit are considered below.

A number of investigators have followed the donors described in this chapter for considerable periods of time (i.e. 10 or more years). The common experience (1,2,34,38,62) has been that a few of the donors (around 5 to 10%) eventually develop WAIHA. It becomes clear that they were first seen after autoantibody production had started but before in vivo red cell clearance began. Rather more, perhaps 20 to 25%, revert to the DAT-negative state and it is never learned why they started then stopped making autoantibody. Most persons in the group, i.e. 60 to 70% remain DAT-positive and hematologically normal. As mentioned above, learning how the immune system controls autoantibody production at subpathological levels or how autoantibody production is switched off in some donors, might provide valuable clues in the etiology and treatment of WAIHA.

Significance of a Positive DAT on a Donor Unit

The preceding section discussed the significance of a positive DAT in a hematologically normal individual in terms of that individual. A different question arises as to what should be done with the donor unit, after it has been found to have a positive DAT. Some years ago this was no problem. All units to be transfused were tested for compatibility, using the prospective recipient's serum in an IAT. If the red cells of the donor had a positive DAT, the unit was never found to be compatible and, eventually, was discarded. Whether the DAT-positive red cells, that clearly survived normally in the donor, would have survived equally well in the recipient, was never put to the test. When the type and screen, MSBOS and immediate spin (IS) compatibility tests were introduced (see Chapter 35) the question was still not answered, it was simply no longer asked. That is to say, because donor units are not tested by DAT and because autocontrols (a subterfuge way of doing a direct antiglobulin test) are performed only if the antibody-screening test on the unit is positive (it is not in the majority of cases when the DAT is positive), those units with a positive DAT were no longer detected because of use of IS compatibility tests. While such units are rare, it must be assumed that they are now unknowingly transfused. In the absence of reports to the contrary, it can be assumed that the DAT-positive red cells do indeed survive as well in the recipient as in the donor.

It should be stressed that the above discussion relates to units that give 3+ and 4+ reactions in DATs. Certainly it has never been suggested that red cells from those units in which the DAT is only weakly positive will enjoy anything but normal survival in the recipient. This makes more important the observation of Boulton (33) that when the Gel test (32) is used for compatibility tests, some apparent incompatibilities will be seen not because the patient's serum contains an alloantibody but because the donor red cells react weakly in a DAT and hence also in an IAT performed by this method. As Boulton (33) points out, these units are perfectly acceptable for transfusion and use of a sensitive in vitro method must not be allowed to result in their being discarded. Skeptics who worry about the transfusion of donor red cells on which the DAT is weakly positive should remember that, because of the test situations described above, many units with a 4+ DAT must now have been unwittingly transfused: that the event did not draw attention presumably indicates that the event, like the autoantibody, was benign.

Benign Cold-Reactive Autoantibodies

As discussed in detail in Chapter 38, all normal sera from adults contain benign cold-reactive autoantibodies (63,64). We (65) showed that if blood samples from adults were collected and kept at 37°C until the serum had been separated from the red cells, anti-I reactive as an agglutinin at 4°C could be detected in all sera. Since the differences between pathological and benign cold-reactive autoantibod-

ies have been discussed in detail in Chapter 38 they need not be repeated here. It will be mentioned that these benign autoantibodies are invariably polyclonal in nature and have auto-anti-I specificity. However, less frequently, different specificities and monoclonal antibodies are seen (66-71).

The "Normal Incomplete Cold Antibody"

This normal serum protein, first described by Dacie in 1950 (72) appears to have anti-H specificity (73) and is capable of causing complement activation at low temperatures (74). There is evidence first, that in spite of its apparent specificity, it is not an immunoglobulin (75-79) indeed it has some of the properties of properdin (77) and second, that unlike antibodies, it will not bind to red cells in the absence of complement (80). The major role played by this serum protein in serological studies is that red cells stored at 4°C in serum may become complement-coated because of the actions of the protein. However, it seems (81-83) that the amount of complement bound is so small as to be undetectable by most routinely used reagents.

Other Causes of Positive DATs of No Significance

Since this chapter deals with autoantibodies that are benign in vivo, it is convenient also to mention some causes of positive DATs, that do not necessarily represent the presence of an autoantibody, that are also of no clinical significance. Some of these events have been discussed in other chapters, as so indicated. Some points to consider follow.

1. Plasma versus serum, i.e. antibody demonstrable in serum but not in plasma, see Chapter 37.
2. Uptake of complement by red cells stored in serum at low temperatures. For cold-reactive autoantibodies see Chapters 6 and 38, for the "normal incomplete cold antibody" see above.
3. Drug-induced antibodies, i.e. the commonest cause of IgG or C3 binding to red cells in vivo, in patients who are not experiencing hemolysis, see Chapter 40.
4. There are occasional reports of "false" or meaningless positive DATs due to: T-activation (see Chapter 42); use of anti-lymphocyte globulin (see Chapter 6); presence of silicone gel in collection tubes (84); and inappropriate collection techniques (85).

References

1. Weiner W. Proc 10th Cong ISBT. Basel:Karger, 1965:35

2. Gorst DW, Rawlinson VI, Merry AH, et al. Vox Sang 1980;38:99

3. Allan J, Garratty G. (abstract). Book of Abstracts. Joint Cong ISH/ISBT 1980:150

4. Habibi B, Muller A, Lelong F, et al. Nouv Presse Med 1980;9:3253

5. Dacie JV, Worlledge SM. Prog Hematol 1969;6:82

6. Worlledge SM. Br J Haematol 1978;39:157

7. Freedman J. J Clin Pathol 1979;32:1014

8. Petz LD, Garratty G. Acquired Immune Hemolytic Anemias. New York:Churchill Livingstone, 1980

9. Chaplin H, Nasongkla M, Monroe MC. Br J Haematol 1981;48:69

10. Graham HA, Davies DM Jr, Tigner JA, et al. (abstract). Transfusion 1976;16:530

11. Graham HA, Davies DM Jr, Brower CE. In: The Nature and Significance of Complement Activation. Raritan, N.J.:Ortho Res Inst, 1977:107

12. Rosenfield RE, Jagathambal K. Transfusion 1978;18:517

13. Huh YO, Liu FJ, Rogge K, et al. Am J Clin Pathol 1988;90:179

14. Heddle NM, Kelton JG, Turchyn KL, et al. Transfusion 1988;28:29

15. Toy PT, Reid ME, Burns M. Am J Hematol 1985;19:145

16. Toy PT, Chin CA, Reid ME, et al. Vox Sang 1985;49:215

17. Huh YO, Lichtiger B. Am J Clin Pathol 1985;84:632

18. Kelton JG, Singer J, Rodger C, et al. Blood 1985;66:490

19. Garratty G, Arndt P. (abstract). Transfusion 1987;27:545

20. Garratty G. In: Immune Destruction of Red Blood Cells. Arlington, VA:Am Assoc Blood Banks, 1989:109

21. Stratton F, Rawlinson VI, Merry AH, et al. Clin Lab Haematol 1983;5:17

22. Meulen FW van der, Hart M van der, Fleer A, et al. Br J Haematol 1978;38:541

23. Meulen FW van der, Bruin HG de, Goosen PCM, et al. Br J Haematol 1980;46:47

24. Engelfriet CP, Borne AEGKr von dem, Beckers D, et al. In: A Seminar on Immune-Mediated Cell Destruction. Washington, D.C.:Am Assoc Blood Banks, 1981:93

25. Carbonelle F. Unpublished observations 1979 cited in Issitt PD. Applied Blood Group Serology, 3rd Ed. Miami:Montgomery 1985:539

26. Nance S, Garratty G. (abstract). Transfusion 1983;23:413

27. Constantoulakis M, Costea N, Schwartz RS, et al. J Clin Invest 1963;42:1790

28. Nance S, Garratty G. (abstract). Blood 1984;64 (Suppl):88a

29. Rosse WF. J Clin Invest 1971;50:734

30. Rosse WF. Prog Hematol 1973;8:51

31. Merry AH, Thomson EE. Biotest Bull 1985;2:137

32. Lapierre Y, Rigal D, Adam J, et al. Transfusion 1990;30:109

33. Boulton FE. (Letter). Br J Biomed Sci 1996;53:172

34. Issitt PD, Pavone BG, Goldfinger D, et al. Br J Haematol 1976;34:5

35. Mellarme J, Auzepy JF, Bercovici JA, et al. Nouv Rev Fr Hematol 1965;5:765

36. Gergely J, Fudenberg HH, Loghem E van. Immunochemistry 1970;7:1

37. Borne AEGKr von dem, Beckers D, Meulen W van der, et al. Br J Haematol 1977;37:137

38. Issitt PD. In: Progress in Clinical Pathology, Vol 7. New York:Grune and Stratton, 1978:137

39. Galili U, Flechner I, Knyszynski A, et al. Br J Haematol 1986;62:317

40. Garratty G. Transf Med Rev 1987;1:47

41. Garratty G. In: Current Applications and Interpretations of the Direct Antiglobulin Test. Arlington, VA:Am Assoc Blood Banks, 1988:1

42. Issitt PD, Zellner DC, Rolih SD, et al. Transfusion 1977;17:531

43. Henry RA, Weber J, Pavone BG, et al. Transfusion 1977;17:539

44. Issitt PD, Pavone BG. Br J Haematol 1978;38:63

45. Chown B, Kaita H, Lowen B, et al. Transfusion 1971;11:220

46. Beck ML, Butch SH, Armstrong WD, et al. Transfusion 1972;12:280

47. Sacher RA, Abbondanzo SL, Miller DK, et al. Am J Clin Pathol 1989;91:305

48. Beck ML, Marsh WL, Pierce SR, et al. Transfusion 1979;19:197

49. Marsh WL, DiNapoli J, Øyen R. Vox Sang 1979;36:174

50. Marsh WL, Øyen R, Alicea E, et al. Am J Hematol 1979;7:155

51. Brendel WL, Issitt PD, Moore RE, et al. Biotest Bull 1985;2:201

52. Eveland D. (abstract). Book of Abstracts. Joint Cong ISBT/AABB 1990:156

53. Sullivan CM, Kline WE, Rabin BI, et al. Transfusion 1987;27:322

54. Holmes LD, Pierce SR, Beck ML. (abstract). Transfusion 1976;16:521

55. Issitt PD, Pavone BG, Frohlich JA, et al. Transfusion 1980;20:733

56. Issitt PD, Combs MR, Allen J, et al. Transfusion 1996;36:802

57. Yokoyama M, McCoy JE Jr. Vox Sang 1967;13:15

58. Beattie KM, Sigmund KE. Transfusion 1987;27:54

59. Daniels GL, Reid ME, Anstee DJ, et al. Br J Haematol 1988;70:477

60. Szaloky A, Hart M van der. Vox Sang 1971;20:376

61. Herron R, Hyde RD, Hillier SJ. Vox Sang 1979;36:179

62. Bareford D, Longster G, Gilks L, et al. Scand J Haematol 1985;35:348

63. Landsteiner K. Munch Med Wschr 1903;50:1812

64. Landsteiner K, Levine P. J Immunol 1926;12:441

65. Issitt PD, Jackson VA. Vox Sang 1968;15:152

66. Booth PB, Jenkins WJ, Marsh WL. Br J Haematol 1966;12:341

67. Jackson VA, Issitt PD, Francis BJ, et al. Vox Sang 1968;15:133

68. Garratty G, Petz LD, Brodsky I, et al. Vox Sang 1973;25:32

69. Roelcke D, Kreft H. Transfusion 1984;24:210

70. O'Neill P, Shulman IA, Simpson RB, et al. Vox Sang 1986;50:107

71. Roelcke D. Transf Med Rev 1989;3:140

72. Dacie JV. Nature 1959;166:36

73. Crawford H, Cutbush M, Mollison PL. Lancet 1953;1:566

74. Dacie JV, Crookston JH, Christenson WN. Br J Haematol 1957;3:77

75. Polley MJ, Mollison PL, Soothill SF. Br J Haematol 1962;8:149

76. Adinolfi M, Daniels C, Mollison PL. Nature 1963;199:389

77. Adinolfi M. Immunology 1965;9:31

78. Adinolfi M. Immunology 1965;9:43

79. Adinolfi M. Immunology 1965;9:365

80. Polley MJ, Mollison PL. Transfusion 1961;1:9

81. Garratty G, Petz LD. Transfusion 1971;11:79

82. Issitt PD, Issitt CH, Wilkinson SL. Transfusion 1974;14:93

83. Issitt PD, Issitt CH, Wilkinson SL. Transfusion 1974;14:103

84. Geisland JR, Milam JD. Transfusion 1980;20:711

85. Grindon AJ, Wilson MJ. Transfusion 1981;21:313

40 | Drug-Induced Antibodies

Antibodies produced by patients being treated with various drugs are not necessarily autoimmune in nature although they usually react with the patient's red cells. For example, in a patient being treated with penicillin, the drug may bind to the patient's red cells and the patient may produce an antibody that reacts with penicillin-coated cells. The DAT will be positive and the patient may develop hemolytic anemia but, because penicillin is not normally present on the patient's cells and because the antibody is directed against an epitope on the penicillin molecules, the antibody is not truly autoimmune. In spite of this, it is convenient to consider drug-induced antibodies and drug-induced hemolytic anemia in a chapter that follows those on autoantibodies. The mechanisms of in vivo red cell destruction are the same in autoantibody and drug-induced immune hemolytic anemia. On many occasions laboratory tests are necessary to differentiate between the two types of hemolytic anemia. Further, in the hemolytic anemias caused by one group of drugs (see below), the causative antibodies are indistinguishable from those that cause WAIHA. That is to say, they are directed against red cell membrane-borne antigens and not against drugs or their metabolites. As described in more detail below, while drug-induced (or drug-stimulated) antibody production is not unusual, cases in which those antibodies actually cause hemolytic anemia are rather rare. Garratty (1) suggests that drug-induced immune hemolytic anemia affects one person per million, per year, in the population of the USA.

Drug-Induced Hemolytic Anemia

Some cases of drug-induced hemolytic anemia have nothing to do with antibodies. There are two major mechanisms by which drugs can cause an accelerated rate of in vivo red cell destruction. First, the drug or one of its metabolites may interfere with an essential metabolic pathway in the red cells thus causing premature death of those cells. Obviously, no antibody is involved in the red cell loss or resultant anemia. Second, the drug or one of its metabolites may cause production of an antibody that may then cause in vivo red cell destruction. The former of these two situations (i.e. non-immunologic) is more common than the latter (i.e. antibody-induced or immunologic). Because this book is about antibodies, the non-immunologic mechanisms will not be further described. As can be seen, the type of drug-induced hemolytic anemia to be described in

this chapter is most accurately described as drug-induced immune hemolytic anemia.

Drug-Induced Immune Hemolytic Anemia

The first case in which a drug was suspected of having caused hemolytic anemia seems to have been that reported by Snapper et al. (2) in 1953, in a patient being treated with mephenytoin. Three years later, in 1956, Harris (3) documented exact details of a case of hemolytic anemia in a patient receiving stibophen. Garratty (1) provides interesting data on the number of different drugs that have been incriminated as causing immune hemolytic anemia and/or a positive direct antiglobulin test. In reviews published in 1967 (4) and 1969 (5), 34 and 40 cases respectively, of hemolytic anemia caused by 15 different drugs, were described. By 1980 (6) some 32, by 1989 (7) over 50, and by 1994 (1) some 71 drugs had been incriminated. Those numbers apply to drugs for which there was reasonably good evidence of cause and effect. That is, the investigation showed some form of direct involvement of the drug in the hemolytic process and/or the antibody formation. There are very many other drugs that have been said to be implicated in antibody production or hemolytic anemia for which the evidence of their involvement is not as good: i.e. true (hemolytic anemia or positive DAT), true (drug-therapy) and unrelated, not excluded.

Drug-Induced Antibody Production

As mentioned above, many patients produce antibodies as a result of drug therapy and develop a positive DAT while relatively few progress to hemolytic anemia. Thus the most commonly encountered situation is one in which the DAT becomes positive, laboratory investigations are conducted to see if a drug is responsible, then the drug is withdrawn before antibody production reaches a high enough level for immune red cell clearance to occur. This means that blood bankers must be familiar with the mechanisms by which drug-induced antibodies act, in order to be able to perform the appropriate serological investigations. In those patients with hemolytic anemia, withdrawal of the drug usually reverses the process of red cell destruction so that often no therapy, other than such withdrawal of the drug, is necessary. Again, it is essential that the blood banker be aware of how the antibodies act in order to be able to show which (if any) drug is responsible.

Drugs are invariably small molecular weight substances and as such are not usually able to stimulate production of antibody unless bound to a carrier molecule. Such binding is often via covalent bonds (11,12) although exceptions have been seen (13,14). As described below, some drugs bind firmly to red cells and use those cells as carriers. Other drugs are unable to act similarly but use plasma proteins as carriers. When the drug is bound to a carrier molecule, the antibody that forms is often directed against a haptenic group on the drug. However, as discussed in more detail below, some antibody specificity may involve the carrier molecule itself. Indeed it is possible that some "drug-independent" antibodies are directed primarily against the carrier molecule, perhaps altered from "self" by the interaction with the drug.

For many years it was supposed that drug-induced antibodies and situations in which drug therapy resulted in a positive DAT, could be divided into a set of distinct categories based on the mechanism involved. It often appeared that in each case only one of the mechanisms was responsible for the findings. As discussed above, drugs of small molecular weights must bind to carriers in order to act as immunogens. Thus the mechanisms involved were thought to be:

1. Drug binds firmly to red cells (carriers) and stimulates production of antibody that then recognizes red cell-bound drug.
2. Drug does not bind to red cells but uses a plasma protein as a carrier. Antibody produced binds to drug plus carrier in circulation forming an immune complex. That complex or complement that it activates can then bind to red cells.
3. Drug alters membrane of red cells so that non-antibody-mediated binding of IgG and other plasma proteins occurs.
4. Drug modifies cells of the immune response in some manner that results in the production of true red cell autoantibodies.

More recently it has become apparent (1,7-10) that the above divisions do not represent distinct mechanisms of immune responses to drugs. Instead it is now appreciated that a single patient, responding to a single drug, may make antibodies with characteristics that blur the previous distinctions. For the remainder of this chapter, those antibodies that react with red cells to which drug has been bound and those that react with red cells only when the drug is present in the in vitro test system, will be called drug-dependent. Those antibodies whose production has been caused by drug therapy but that react with normal uncoated red cells in the absence of the drug, will be called drug-independent. Many patients (see later in this chapter) have now been seen to have made both drug-dependent and drug-independent antibodies. In some cases a single serum has been seen to contain antibody reacting with drug-coated red cells and antibody reacting with normal red cells in the presence of the drug. Sometimes the two types of drug-dependent antibodies have been present with drug-independent antibody. In some instances (again see later in this chapter) the structure to which the drug binds has been recognized, with both drug-dependent and drug-independent antibodies some of those structures have been seen to be red cell blood group antigens or their carrier molecules. In considering drug-dependent and drug-independent antibodies, it is important to remember that they are all believed to be drug-induced. As will become apparent, proving that point is not always easy but it is believed that production of all antibodies described in this chapter was induced by drug therapy.

In spite of the blurring of what were previously thought to be distinct mechanisms of drug-induced antibody production, it is still highly convenient to bear those mechanisms in mind when detecting and identifying the antibodies at the serological level. That is to say, while it is now believed that antibodies that behave in a variety of ways in vitro represent part of the same immune response to a drug, the methods used to characterize the antibodies have not changed. What must be remembered is that when a patient presents with either or both types of drug-dependent antibody, that patient may also have made drug-independent antibody. Thus what used to be regarded as distinct and separate mechanisms of drug-induced antibody production can now be used as useful guides for the in vitro investigation of drug-induced antibodies.

A Special Note on Drug-Induced Antibodies and Cephalosporins

For reasons given in the previous section, drug-induced antibodies will still be considered here on the basis of how they are recognized at the serological level. Such distinctions were made when it was believed that separate and independent mechanisms led to their production. Because of that, it is important to point out that the cephalosporin group of drugs can stimulate antibody production in many different ways. In the description of antibodies to drugs that bind firmly to red cells, anti-cephalothin is prominently featured. Indeed, most antibodies directed against first generation cephalosporins were of this type. However, antibodies made in patients treated with second and third generation cephalosporins are often rather different. While some of the antibodies bind to cephalosporin-coated red cells, others form immune-complexes with plasma proteins to which cephalosporin has bound in vivo, while still others are apparently drug-independent antibodies. Thus in the following sections, the anti-cephalothin described in patients treated with first generation cephalosporins, were often responsible for positive DATs and occasionally for rather slow onset drug-induced immune hemolytic anemia. The antibodies made in patients treated with second and third generation cephalosporins are often much more dangerous at the clinical level, indeed a number of fatalities associated with those antibodies have been reported. On the other side of the coin, first generation cephalosporins have also been seen to cause positive DATs when the red cells of patients being treated with the drugs bound plasma proteins nonspecifically, i.e. in the absence of antibody. The moral of this story is that when a patient being treated with a second or third generation cephalosporin is seen to have a positive DAT and/or is suspected of having immune-mediated hemolytic anemia, all different methods of investigation should be used in the laboratory. That is, the investigation must include tests against drug-coated red cells, tests against normal red cells in the presence of drug, and tests for the presence of a drug-independent antibody. Further, a positive finding in one series of tests must not result in the two other series not being performed. In some patients drug-dependent antibodies of both types and drug-independent antibodies have been found. Additional details (and references) are given in later sections of this chapter.

Drugs that Bind Firmly to Red Cells

As mentioned above, a number of drugs bind firmly to red cells and are not removed by multiple washing of the cells. Table 40-1 lists the drugs described by Garratty (1) as having this property. Once the haptenic group of the drug stimulates production of an antibody and if the patient is still being treated with the drug, both antigen and antibody will be present in the patient's circulation. As mentioned, while this will most often cause only a positive DAT, with IgG most frequently being detected on the red cells, it will occasionally result in accelerated in vivo clearance of red cells as well. When red cell destruction does occur it most often results from extravascular clearance of IgG-coated red cells (1,15-19) although on rare occasions, intravascular destruction has been seen (20-22). It has also been claimed (23-26) that K-cell lysis is involved in the red cell destruction, at least when antibodies directed against penicillin-coated red cells are involved. Some references to papers describing hemolytic anemia or positive DATs caused by antibodies directed against drugs that bind firmly to red cells, are given in table 40-1. It should be noted that most of the 67 papers cited describe cases in which the positive DAT or the hemolytic anemia, was caused by a drug-dependent antibody directed against the haptenic group of the drug bound to its carrier molecule. Several of the drugs listed in table 40-1 have now been associated with cases in which the patient made both drug-dependent and drug-independent antibody. Those cases are described in more detail in later sections of this chapter. Figure 40-1 is a simplified diagram of the mechanism by which drugs bind to red cells and stimulate antibody production.

Antibodies to Penicillin and Cephalothin

Since these two drugs stimulate antibody production more frequently than the others listed in table 40-1, some additional details about the antibodies will be given. Both drugs are thought to bind to red cells via a beta-lactam ring. They share a major haptenic grouping and most antibodies made by patients being treated with penicillin are directed against the benzyl-penicillol (BPO) group (29,31,40). Such antibodies react well with red cells coated with benzyl-penicillin G, prepared in the laboratory (6,38,47,82,83). Some patients being treated with some semi-synthetic penicillins (e.g. ampicillin, oxacillin, methicillin) also produce anti-penicillin that reacts with penicillin G-coated red cells (22,37,42). However, there are at least two reports (84,85) of patients being treated with the semi-synthetic penicillin, nafcillin, who made antibodies that reacted with nafcillin but not

TABLE 40-1 Some Drugs that Bind Firmly to Red Cells

Drug	References[*1]	Drug	References[*1]
Penicillin	15-43, 234, 377, 378	Cephalothin[*2]	44-52
Cephaloridine[*2]	53-55	Cephalexin[*2]	56-58
Cefamandole[*2]	59	Cefazolin[*2]	52
Cisplatin	60-64	Carbimazole	65
Carbromal	66	Cianidanol	67
Erythromycin	68, 233	Streptomycin	69-74
Tolbutamide	75, 76	Tetracycline	79-81

[*1] The papers referenced primarily describe cases in which only a drug-dependent antibody was involved. Some of these drugs have also been involved in provoking production of drug-independent antibodies (see text).

[*2] All cephalosporins.

[*3] For a review of antibodies associated with antibiotic therapy see Garratty (235).

**FIGURE 40-1 A Simplified Version of Drug-Dependent Antibody Production
When the Drug Binds Firmly to the Red Cell**

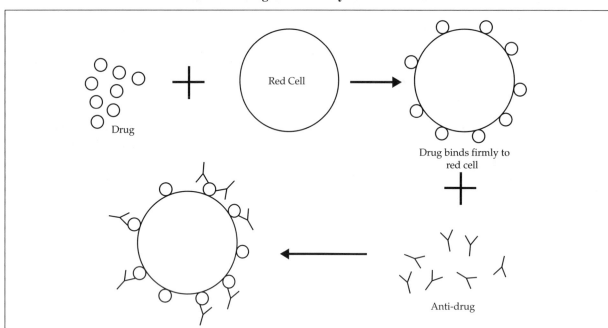

with penicillin G-coated cells.

If sera from normal healthy adults are tested, most can be shown to contain anti-penicillin, regardless of whether the individuals have ever been treated with that drug. For example, Levine et al. (33) found that 97% of sera from random individuals contained anti-penicillin. Among the reactive sera, 87% contained IgM and 13% IgM and IgG antibody. All the antibodies were directed against the BPO group and were inhibited by penicillin derivatives containing that grouping. The drug-induced forms of anti-penicillin that cause a positive direct DAT and sometimes hemolytic anemia are invariably IgG and are only partially inhibited by penicillin derivatives containing the BPO group. The pathological form of anti-penicillin is inhibited by benzylpenaldoyl propylamine (34).

The very high incidence of anti-penicillin, even among individuals never treated with that drug, no doubt relates to the widespread use of that drug for uses other than to kill infecting organisms. It is a rather sobering thought that, at least in affluent countries, simple acts like breathing air or eating one's cornflakes, exposes one to the haptenic group of penicillin.

Spath et al. (47) tested sera from a group of patients being treated with cephalothin, none of whom had drug-induced hemolytic anemia. They found anti-cephalothin in 88% of the sera. Of all sera tested, 63% contained just IgM, 10% just IgG and 15% IgM and IgG antibody. Antibodies to penicillin react with cephalothin-coated and antibodies to cephalothin with penicillin-coated red cells (379,380). Thus, the presence of these antibodies, in the sera of persons not suffering from drug-induced hemolytic anemia, is of great importance when laboratory tests are performed on the blood of a patient suspected of having such a hemolytic process. This point is discussed again below in the section dealing with laboratory identification of these antibodies.

Production of Antibodies in Patients Being Treated with Penicillin and Cephalothin

This section deals only with the production of antibodies of these specificities by patients in whom the DAT becomes positive or in whom hemolytic anemia occurs. In other words, it ignores the low levels of these antibodies found in the sera of healthy individuals and in the sera of patients being treated with the drugs in whom no sequalae are seen. About 3% of all patients receiving large doses of penicillin develop a positive DAT but only a minority of them suffer drug-induced hemolytic anemia (36,39). The development of a positive DAT and of hemolytic anemia is most likely in a patient receiving 10 million or more units of penicillin per day, for seven days or longer, via an intravenous route. Exceptions are seen in patients with impaired renal function (where excretion of the drug is inefficient and blood levels become higher than in patients with normal kidney function) and in children, in whom oral administration of penicillin has been shown to result in hemolytic anemia. However, in at least one child in whom this happened, the antibody made differed from those described above (41). In that case phenoxymethylpenicillin V was used to treat a three year-old. The anti-penicillin produced was IgM in nature and fixed complement.

It is known that allergy to penicillin and penicillin-induced hemolytic anemia are caused by different antibodies. The allergic reaction to the drug, that can involve life-threatening anaphylaxis, is caused by an IgE antibody. The hemolytic anemia is caused by an IgG antibody. While some workers (86,87) have suggested that patients allergic to penicillin are more likely than others to have IgG and/or IgM anti-penicillin as well, that observation has not generally been confirmed and most workers believe that the antibodies are formed independently of each other. This means that a patient with a known allergy to the drug should never be treated with penicillin again. On the other hand, a patient who has had penicillin-induced hemolytic anemia can receive the drug again but hematological and serological monitoring are in order in case the patient undergoes a secondary immune response and again makes clinically-significant levels of IgG anti-penicillin.

In early reports (44,45) it was said that between 40 and 75% of patients receiving cephalothin developed significant levels of IgG antibody to that drug. However, it seems that the early findings were on an unusual group of patients (many of whom had impaired renal function) and that many of the antibodies detected must have been similar to those in the sera of healthy individuals. Spath et al. (38,47) found that the incidence of a positive DAT in patients receiving the drug is around 4%. As with penicillin, the vast majority of these patients had a positive DAT but not hemolytic anemia and again the development of the positive DAT was directly related to the dose of the drug being given. As mentioned earlier, most of what has been written above applies to first generation cephalosporins. As discussed in detail below, second and third generation cephalosporins have a number of times been seen to stimulate production of drug-dependent and drug-independent antibodies. Such a situation can be far more serious than the production of drug-dependent antibodies directed against drug-coated red cells and some fatal cases have been reported (references given below). The other ways in which the cephalosporins can cause positive DATs are discussed below in the sections on immune complexes and on non-antibody-mediated uptake of proteins by red cells exposed to some drugs.

Laboratory Tests in Penicillin and Cephalothin–Induced Antibody Production

In most patients with a positive DAT or hemolytic anemia due to anti-penicillin or anti-cephalothin, the red cells are coated only with IgG (15,16,21,82,88,89). Less often IgM, IgA and/or IgD will be cell-bound as well (35). Rarely, complement will also be detected on the cells but even then, usually only in small amounts (20,88,90). Thus, the most common picture when antibodies to these drugs are involved, is that the patient's red cells react strongly with anti-IgG and not at all, or only weakly, with other antiglobulin reagents. The first useful clue to the presence of an antibody directed against a drug may be that an eluate made from the (often strongly) DAT+ red cells fails to react with normal red cells. If the patient is being treated with penicillin or cephalothin, the next step is to test the eluate against drug-coated red cells. In order to perform these tests it is necessary to coat separate aliquots of red cells with penicillin and cephalothin. Both drugs bind readily to red cells so that if a solution of the drug is mixed with red cells in saline, some drug will get on to the cells. However, unless optimal conditions are used, relatively small amounts of the drug will bind and the in vitro test reactions may not be very strong. To achieve maximum uptake of these drugs by red cells, the methods described by Spath et al. (38,47) and by Garratty (82), that are also listed by Judd (83), should be used. As mentioned above, most sera from healthy adults contain low levels of antibodies to penicillin and cephalothin. Accordingly, when the serum of a patient suspected of having hemolytic anemia due to one of these drugs is tested, titration studies must be performed using several normal sera as controls. It is difficult to list numbers for expected results of the titrations because the values will vary a great deal dependent on how much drug is bound to the test cells. For example if the most efficient methods (38,47,82) are used, normal sera may react to titers of about 8 or 16, while the patient's serum may have a titer in the thousands. If red cells in saline at a normal pH are used to prepare the drug-coated cells and smaller amounts of drug are bound, the patient's serum may have a titer around 32 to 64 while normal sera may have a titer of only 1 or 2. As already mentioned, anti-penicillin and anti-cephalothin may both react with penicillin and with cephalothin-coated red cells so that withdrawal of the appropriate drug to reverse the hemolytic anemia may be dependent on which and how much of the drug or drugs the patient is receiving.

There are a few other points that should be borne in mind when these tests are performed. First, the antibodies may react with the drug-coated red cells in agglutination tests at room temperature and 37°C and by IAT. In a patient with a positive DAT or hemolytic anemia due to an antibody against penicillin or cephalothin, in whom the serum or eluate reacts with red cells coated with either drug, the titers in the test may be informative in differentiating anti-penicillin from anti-cephalothin. The highest titer will usually be seen in the IAT. Second, it is important that the titrations measure anti-drug and not an alloantibody simultaneously present. Accordingly, the patient's serum should be shown to be non-reactive with a sample of untreated red cells from the donor whose cells were used to prepare the drug-coated cells. If the patient's serum contains an alloantibody, red cells that lack the antigen against which it is directed should be used when the drug-coated cells are prepared. Third, because normal sera contain anti-penicillin and anti-cephalothin, it is not always easy to be certain that one of those antibodies is responsible for hemolytic anemia in the patient. On some occasions more useful information will be obtained by working with an eluate from the patient's red cells. If anti-penicillin or anti-cephalothin is causing immune drug-mediated hemolytic anemia, the antibody should be identifiable in the eluate. Tests on eluates will, of course, not be as influenced by the normal levels of anti-drug, as will tests on serum.

Antibodies to Drugs that do not Bind Firmly to Red Cells: Immune Complex Formation

Some drugs, such as quinine, quinidine, stibophen, phenacetin, para-aminosalicylic acid and some sulfonamides, do not bind firmly to red cells but apparently (1,6,39,40,43,77,78,82,91-93) do bind to plasma proteins. Antibodies to the immunogenic portions of the drug may then be made by patients treated with the drugs. In other words, the haptenic grouping on the drug uses a serum protein instead of a red cell membrane structure as its carrier molecule. In a patient with an antibody to one of the drugs, immune complexes (antibody plus drug plus carrier protein) may form in the plasma. These complexes may then bind to red cells or (more often) activate complement that binds to red cells. If sufficient amounts of complement become red cell bound, an episode of intravascular hemolysis may occur. This type of drug-induced reaction may be dramatic and severe. In a patient in whom anti-drug is already present, administration of a small dose of the responsible drug may provoke marked hemolysis and/or profound thrombocytopenia and/or leukopenia. It has been found (1) that some 30 to 50% of patients in whom this form of drug-induced immune hemolytic anemia occurs have associated renal failure. Table 40-2 lists a large number of drugs that have been said to cause hemolytic anemia via this route. However, it must be remembered that in some instances the drug apparently involved has been incriminated in only one case, and in some of the reports involvement of the drug seemed likely but was not proved beyond all doubt. Table 40-2 includes references to typical cases, the list is not intended to be all-inclu-

sive. Figure 40-2 presents a simplified concept of how red cell coating (and eventually clearance) occurs when antibodies of this type are made. For the sake of simplicity, figure 40-2 shows only IgG antibodies, IgM forms that may agglutinate or bind to red cells are also known.

Laboratory Tests for Drug-Dependent Antibodies that Cause Immune Complexes to Form

In patients in whom a drug-dependent antibody has complexed with the haptenic group of the drug being carried by a plasma protein, the DAT is usually positive. In many cases complement but not immunoglobulin will be detected on the red cells in the DAT; there are several reasons. First, if the antigen-antibody immune complexes form in the plasma, complement may be activated and may bind to red cells via the innocent bystander mechanism. Indeed it is commonly believed that this is the mechanism that leads to the intravascular hemolysis seen with some drug-dependent antibodies of this type. Second, if the immune complexes themselves bind to the red cell (see figure 40-2 where IgG but not IgM is illustrated in the immune complexes) they may not be firmly attached and may be removed during the washing steps before the addition of antiglobulin serum. Third, those complexes that are not removed may be oriented on the red cell membrane in such a way that the Fc portions of the IgG or IgM molecules are not available to complex with the antiglobulin reagent.

When the sera of patients with antibodies of this type, or eluates made from their DAT+ red cells are tested, they are non-reactive with normal red cells. Further, because these drugs do not bind to red cells, tests like those described above for the detection of anti-penicillin and anti-cephalothin cannot be performed. Accordingly, an attempt must be made in vitro to reproduce the in vivo situation and thus detect the antibody. This can (sometimes) be accomplished as follows:

1. Prepare a buffered solution or suspension of the suspect drug so that the concentration is roughly the same (drug/ml) as that in the patient's plasma
2. Mix 1 volume of the patient's serum and 1 volume of antibody-free fresh normal serum (complement source) with 1 dry button of washed group O red cells and 1 volume of the drug solution
3. Incubate at room temperature for 30 minutes, then at 37°C for 30 minutes and read for agglutination, hemolysis and by IAT.

While the above procedure sounds relatively simple there are a number of points that must be considered.

TABLE 40-2 Some Drugs that do not Bind Firmly to Red Cells but are Believed to Stimulate Production of Drug-Dependent Antibodies that Participate in Immune Complex Formation

Drug	References	Drug	References	Drug	References
Acetaminophen	94	Dipyrone	113, 114	Quinidine	131-136, 157, 159
Aminopyrine	95	Doxepin	360	Quinine	137, 138, 157, 159
P-Aminosalicylic acid (PAS)	96, 97, 370, 371	Fluorouracil	10	Rifampicin	139-143
Antazoline	98	Hydralazine	93	Stibophen	89, 144-149, 373-375
Butizide	10	Hydrochlorothiazide	115, 116, 236	Streptomycin	70, 71, 150, 156
Carbimazole	10	9-Hydroxymethyl-ellipticinium	117	Sulfonamides	152, 242, 376
Cefotaxime	99	Ibuprofen	158	Teniposide (VM-26)	153
Cefotetan	100-104	Insulin	118	Tolmetin	155, 158
Cefoxitin	105	Isoniazid	119, 120	Triamterene	154
Ceftazidime	106	Melphalan	121	Zomax (Zomepirac sodium)	10
Ceftriaxone (Rocephin)	107	Methotrexate	122		
Cephalosporin	108, 109	Nalidixic Acid	10		
Chlorpromazine	110	Nomifensine	123-126, 151, 237-239		
Chlorpropamide	111, 112	Phenacetin	97, 127-129, 370, 372		
Cianidanol	67	Probenecid	130, 240, 241		

First, it may be necessary to consult with a pharmacist in an attempt to calculate the amount of drug likely to be present in the patient's plasma. The level will be based on factors such as dose of drug being used, frequency of dose, patient's size and blood volume, and catabolism rate for the drug. In the absence of better information, many workers use a 1mg/ml concentration of the drug. Second, it is very difficult to dissolve some drugs in saline. The problem can sometimes be resolved by visiting the pharmacy and obtaining a preparation of the drug prepared for intravenous injection. Third, if acidified or non-physiological solutions must be used to prepare the solution of the drug, adjustment to normal pH and a physiological system is necessary before the test is performed. No matter how the drug solution or suspension is obtained, i.e. made in house or obtained from the pharmacy, the pH of the test system must be checked and adjusted to neutral if necessary. Many drugs in solution are highly acidic or alkaline. Fourth, it is *essential* that the test be controlled by running several normal sera in parallel with that of the patient. Many drugs cause mechanical hemolysis or spontaneous aggregation of red cells. A positive finding with the patient's serum is valid *only* when normal sera are shown to be non-reactive in the same test system.

Drug Metabolites

An additional problem that can be added to the four described in the previous section is that the antibody may be directed against a metabolite of the drug and may not react with the drug in the form in which it is being given. Since most patients who form antibodies as a result of drug therapy are being treated with many drugs, it would be an enormous task to test a serum against every metabolite of each drug. As early as 1972, Eisner and Shahidi (254) solved this problem (in a patient with drug-induced immune thrombocytopenia) by running tests in the presence of serum and urine from an individual who had ingested the same drug as the patient. It was reasoned that between them, the serum and urine would contain all significant metabolites of the drug. The experiment was a success and the patient was shown to have an antibody to a metabolite of acetaminophen, although the antibody did not react with acetaminophen itself. In spite of this, tests for antibodies to drug metabolites were not widely used until after 1984 when Salama et al. (255) demonstrated metabolite-dependent antibodies in one patient being treated with nomifensine and one being treated with buthiazide. In 1985, Salama and Mueller-Eckhardt (151) described 19

FIGURE 40-2 A Simplified Version of Drug-Dependent Antibody Production and the Formation of Antibody-Drug-Carrier Immune Complexes in the Plasma

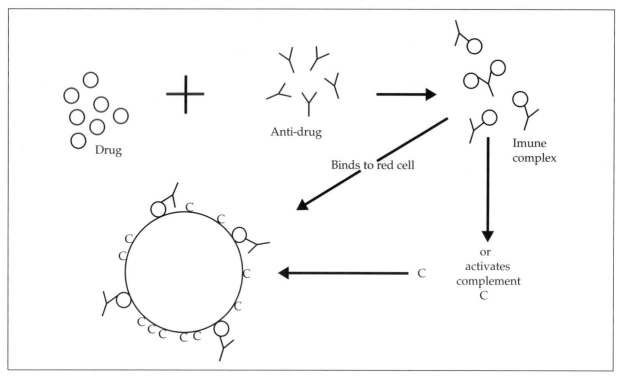

cases of immune hemolytic anemia in patients being treated with nomifensine. In all cases a metabolite-dependent antibody could be demonstrated in tests to which urine from a patient taking nomifensine was added. Six of the 19 antibodies were not detected in tests to which nomifensine had been added, three of those six also failed to react in tests in which chemically derived metabolites of nomifensine were used. Since the rediscovery (151,255,381) of the test originally devised by Eisner and Shahidi (254) the use of serum and urine in this setting has been widely applied and other metabolite-dependent antibodies have been described (9,67,160-162,256-258). Mueller-Eckhardt, Salama, and colleagues (160,162,259) have pointed out that if tests using drug metabolites are not included, cases of drug-induced immune hemolytic anemia (and other drug-induced cytopenias) will pass unproved. Most workers will have encountered cases of immune hemolytic anemia and positive DATs in which drug therapy was suspected as a cause, but confirmatory evidence could not be obtained. Clearly investigations for antibodies directed against drug metabolites are indicated. Providing the precautions outlined in Chapters 31 and 34 (sections on inhibition of anti-Sd[a] with urine) regarding pH, ionicity, conductivity, etc., are observed (methods in Judd (83)) tests using urine (and serum) from an individual who has ingested the drug involved, are a relatively straightforward way of accomplishing this.

Putative Modification of the Red Cell Membrane by Drugs

As well as stimulating antibody production, cephalothin can apparently modify the red cell membrane in such a manner that plasma proteins bind non-specifically to red cells. The exact method of modification is not known and while this alteration may result in a positive DAT (6,39,40,44,45,47,82,163) it has not usually been associated with hemolytic anemia (but see below). Further, while there is evidence for the non-immunological uptake of plasma proteins by the red cells of some patients being treated with cephalothin, it seems that in such patients production of anti-cephalothin with resultant immunological binding of antibody to the red cells is a more common cause of positive DATs when such tests give reactions of 1 to 2+ or greater (47).

While it has been suggested (44,45) that cephalosporin modifies the red cell membrane in such a manner that non-immunological uptake of plasma proteins by red cells occurs, there is not a lot of supporting evidence. It was found (47) that antiglobulin reagents that contained anti-albumin were more likely than ones that did not, to cause positive DATs in this setting. Certainly the binding of autologous albumin to red cells would seem to be non-immunologic in nature. Sirchia et al. (164) and Ferrone et al. (165) showed that red cells exposed to cephalothin behaved, in some ways, like red cells from patients with paroxysmal nocturnal hemoglobinuria (PNH). While PNH red cells have a number of abnormalities (see Chapter 4) they are not notable for any ability to bind proteins by non-immunologic means.

Jamin et al. reported that treatment with INOX (diglyaldehyde) (166) and Suramin (167) can also cause the patients' red cells to bind plasma proteins non-immunologically. It was suggested (166) that the uptake of protein occurs via the formation of Schiff's bases. While Cisplatin is included in table 40-1 as a drug that binds firmly to the red cell membrane, there is at least one suggestion (63) that treatment with Cisplatin instead results in the non-immunological uptake of plasma proteins and that in a patient being treated with the drug, the hemolytic anemia was coincidental, i.e. not caused by a drug-induced antibody.

The laboratory recognition of non-immunological uptake of proteins leading to a positive DAT is, at least in part, by exclusion of other causes. The DAT will be positive but neither the patient's serum nor an eluate made from the patient's red cells will react with normal or drug-coated cells (assuming, of course, that blood group alloantibody activity has been excluded). The reason for non-reactivity of the serum and eluate is, of course, that no antibody is involved. Useful tests for confirmation of the existence of this phenomenon can be performed if antibodies to other plasma proteins, that will bring about agglutination of coated red cells, are available. In DATs with such reagents any or all the plasma proteins IgG, IgM, IgA, C3, C4, albumin, fibrinogen, alpha$_1$-antitrypsin and alpha$_2$-macroglobulin may be demonstrable on the red cells. Cephalosporins other than cephalothin can also modify red cells so that those cells bind plasma proteins non-immunologically (39,54,55,57,168-171). A somewhat fanciful diagram to illustrate the non-immunological uptake of plasma proteins by red cells is presented as figure 40-3. Perhaps the thickening of the line that represents the red cell membrane represents Schiff's bases forming!

As mentioned above, for many years it appeared that the non-immunological uptake of proteins by the red cells of patients being treated with certain drugs could result in positive DATs but that hemolytic anemia did not follow. This may not always be the case. Certain drugs (e.g. Unasyn, Timentin, Augmentin, etc.) that contain beta-lactamase inhibitors such as sulbactam or clavulanate, appear to cause non-immunologic adsorption of proteins by red cells. Garratty and Arndt (382) studied one patient who was receiving Unasyn and two who were receiving Timentin. All three had hemolytic anemia and while the evidence for drug-induced hemolysis was not conclusive, it was highly suggestive. It was suggested (382) that the previously reported (352) high incidence of positive DATs in patients receiving Unasyn, is a result of the presence of sulbactam in that drug. In the vast majority of such patients the positive DAT is not associated with hemolytic anemia.

FIGURE 40-3 An Imaginary Version of Alteration of the Red Cell Membrane by a Drug and the Subsequent Non-Immunological Uptake of Plasma Proteins

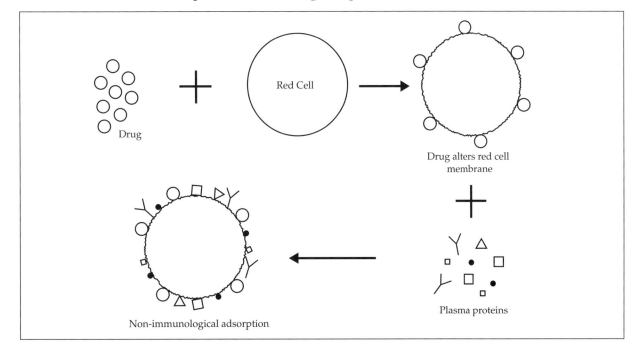

Modification of the Immune Response by Drugs

There are a number of drugs that appear to stimulate the production of autoantibodies without acting as the immunogen. It is commonly believed that treatment with these drugs in some way alters the immune response so that autoantibodies are made. While this belief is common, an understanding of how the immune response is modified is hazy at best.

There are two pieces of convincing evidence that the antibodies involved are not directed against the drug or one of its metabolites. First, the antibodies react with normal red cells that have not been exposed to the drug, in tests in which no drug has been added to the reaction mixture. At the serological level these autoantibodies are usually indistinguishable from those that cause WAIHA (see Chapter 37). Second, in the case of aldomet (alpha-methyldopa) that is probably the most comprehensively studied drug in this group, autoantibody production is not usually seen until the patient has been receiving the drug for about six months. If the drug is then withdrawn, autoantibody production gradually stops. If another course of the drug is then given, detectable autoantibody is not usually produced until after another six months of therapy. Clearly, if the drug was the immunogen, a secondary immune response would occur when the drug was reintroduced and serologically detectable autoantibody would be expected within days.

The first drug associated with the production of drug-independent autoantibodies and still the one for which most cases have been studied, was aldomet (alpha-methyldopa) (90,172). At the time that aldomet-induced hemolytic anemia was first recognized, aldomet was one of the most efficient antihypertensive drugs known; there were relatively few efficient alternatives. As a result the drug was widely used and many cases of autoantibody production by patients receiving the drug were documented (6,18,43,82,90,152,163,172-186). As described below, it was quickly appreciated that autoantibody production in patients receiving aldomet is dose-dependent. It is known that autoantibody production is infrequent and that hemolytic anemia is essentially not seen in patients receiving less than 1g aldomet per day. Nowadays there are many excellent alternative antihypertensives to aldomet so that if a dose of more than 1g/day of aldomet is required to control the blood pressure, an alternative antihypertensive is invariably prescribed. Thus cases of aldomet-induced autoantibody production and hemolytic anemia are now seen only rarely. Much of what is written below is of historical interest although some of the findings listed may eventually be shown to apply to other drugs that cause drug-independent antibodies to be made.

Table 40-3 lists a number of drugs that have been said to stimulate production of drug-independent antibodies. When a significant number of patients being treated with the same drug make autoantibodies, the production of which stops when the drug is withdrawn, it is reasonable to conclude a cause and effect relationship. Such findings have been made in the case of aldomet, levodopa, mefenamic acid (Ponstel) and procainamide. Far less certainty exists when only one or a few cases have been seen. One way to obtain proof of the role of the drug is to withdraw therapy with the drug, wait until autoantibody production stops, then challenge the patient again, with the drug. This is a somewhat difficult approach if an alternative drug has produced acceptable clinical results in the patient and may be a dangerous approach if acute hemolytic anemia previously occurred. If the patient cannot be challenged with the drug of suspicion, the possibility of the true (drug therapy), true (hemolytic anemia) and unrelated (idiopathic not drug-induced hemolytic anemia) phenomenon exists. As an example, cimetidine-induced hemolytic anemia had been reported (253) in two patients. However, in both patients the finding was that hemolytic anemia occurred concurrent with drug therapy. Petz et al. (208) found two more patients with hemolytic anemia who were also being treated with cimetidine, they withdrew the drug and treated the patients' hemolytic anemia. The patients were then given cimetidine again and were followed (one of them for 24 months). Neither developed hemolytic anemia and no autoantibody production occurred. Thus it was clear that in these patients (208), cimetidine had not caused autoantibody production and that hemolytic anemia in the patients receiving the drug was coincidental.

With the above findings in mind, table 40-3 should be regarded as a useful guide rather than as a definitive statement. While there is no doubt that aldomet, levodopa, mefenamic acid, procainamide and nomifensine have all caused drug-independent autoantibodies to be produced, there is much less certainty about the other drugs listed in that table. While aldomet, levodopa, mefenamic acid and procainamide seem to stimulate production of just drug-independent autoantibodies, nomifensine has stimulated production of drug-independent antibodies in some patients, drug-dependent antibodies in others, and both in still different patients (8,124,237,252,355). In addition to the drugs listed in table 40-3 there are others that have stimulated production of drug-independent antibodies but have most of the time stimulated production of drug-dependent antibodies as well. In most cases the drug-dependent antibodies appeared to be stronger than the drug-independent forms. Accordingly, those drugs are described in a later section of this chapter.

TABLE 40-3 Drugs Associated or Possibly Associated with Production of Drug-Independent Antibodies[*3]

Drug	References	Drug	References
Aldomet (alpha-methyldopa)	90, 172, 243 (many others, see text)	Nomifensine	124, 237, 252, 355
Levodopa	187-192	Diclofenac[*1,*2]	245
Mefenamic Acid (Ponstel)	158, 193-195	Azapropazone[*1,*2]	246
Procainamide	196-201, 244, 266 (For others, see text)	Ibuprofen[*1]	205-207
Catergen	1	Fenoprofen[*1]	247
Chaparral	202	Sulindac[*1]	248, 249, 356, 357
Cyclofenil	203, 204	Naporexen[*]	158
Diphenylhydantoin	353	Tolmetin[*1]	158
Glibenclamide	351	Zomepirac sodium[*1] (Zomax)	358
Methysergide	354		

[*1] For a general discussion about the role of these non-steroidal antiinflammatory drugs (NSAIDs) in stimulating autoantibody production, see references 158, 250 and 251.

[*2] The evidence that diclofenac and azapropazone are involved is better than that for the other NSAIDs listed.

[*3] Some of these drugs appear in other tables because they also have stimulated production of drug-dependent antibodies.

Concepts About Drug Modification of the Immune Response

Over the years many different theories that purport to explain how these drugs affect the immune system, have been advanced. Most of them relate to the supposed actions of aldomet, as mentioned above far more patients with aldomet-induced antibodies have been studied than persons in whom a different drug was involved.

In the initial studies on aldomet-induced autoantibody production it was suggested (90,152,172-177) that the drug might be incorporated into early red cell precursors in the marrow that then might give rise to red cells on which Rh and other antigens were altered enough that they were no longer recognized as self. There are a number of observations that are not explained by such a theory, some of them also provide strong evidence that neither aldomet nor one of its metabolites is the immunogen. First, if host or self antigens are altered in individuals treated with the drug, the alterations are not demonstrable in vitro at the serological level. Second, the autoantibodies made, react with normal red cells from persons never exposed to the drug. Third, modification of multiple antigens would have to be invoked since autoantibodies directed against (at least) antigens in the Rh, MN, Diego and Kidd systems, have been seen in treated patients (6,175,177,185,209,210). Fourth, the finding that patients being treated with aldomet often also make autoantibodies directed against other than red cells (i.e. antinuclear factor, rheumatoid factor, platelet antibodies and have

positive tests for lupus erythematosus (LE) cells) (174, 211-217,285-289,323) suggests that the alteration involves the immune system rather than individual antigens. Fifth, even given the maturation time of red cell precursors and the life-span of mature red cells (i.e. altered antigens not presented to cells of the immune system until senescence of the red cells) the intervals between initiation of treatment and/or reintroduction of drug, and autoantibody production, seem too long.

While these observations seem to exclude a role for aldomet as an immunogen, the concept of altered antigens should not be totally discarded. It has been suggested (7,224) that some drugs bind loosely to red cell antigens in vivo and that such binding may be difficult to demonstrate in vitro. Findings in support of this came from patients who had produced drug-dependent and drug-independent antibodies directed against the same red cell antigen. As discussed in more detail below, there are several other reports (8,9,67,160) of patients who have produced drug-dependent and drug-independent antibodies. A possible explanation (225) of these findings is that the drug-independent antibodies are made in response to subtle alterations of antigens (as has been demonstrated (226,227) in rabbits) and that the initiating event for the formation of both drug-dependent and drug-independent antibodies involves the formation of conjugates between the drug and the red cell membrane (7-9,160,162,224).

A totally different mechanism was suggested by others. It was claimed (218,219) that aldomet can be used to treat red cells in vitro and that the treated red cells react preferentially with the autoantibodies made by patients receiving the drug. However, other investigators (82,173,175,176) even when using the methods described, were not able to duplicate these findings and some (175) found that neither aldomet nor its derivatives would inhibit the reactions of the autoantibodies with red cells. The findings (175) that aldomet does not bind selectively to red cell membranes and that it combines poorly with plasma proteins seem to exclude a role for an aldomet hapten, as does the finding (174) discussed above, that reintroduction of the drug does not rapidly cause autoantibody production in a previously affected patient.

Aldomet oxidizes in the presence of air and light to form quinones that then polymerize to form pigmented aggregates (175). Vyas et al. (220) demonstrated that an aldomet polymer was immunogenic in rabbits if it was coupled to rabbit red cells or mixed with Freund's adjuvant. The polymer was not immunogenic when coupled to a protein carrier. The antibodies produced reacted with human IgG and other serum proteins, in spite of the fact that no human proteins had been injected. The significance of this finding is not clear since the autoantibodies made in patients treated with aldomet seem to be directed against red cell antigens and not against IgG or other serum proteins. However, the finding that pigmented aggregates are formed following the oxidization of aldomet and that the pigmented polymer is immunogenic (at least in animals) was fascinating. While the formation of antibodies in Whites treated with aldomet is relatively frequent (if high doses of the drug are used, see below) it is hardly ever seen (if seen at all) in Blacks and Orientals (216,221-223). One cannot help but wonder if the difference in level of melanin (pigment) in Whites, Blacks and Orientals, plays some role in the ability of those persons to mount or not mount an autoimmune response when treated with the drug. Even if pigment levels play a role the explanation cannot be simple. As noted in this section there are several lines of convincing evidence that neither aldomet nor its metabolites act as direct immunogens.

Other investigators have suggested that aldomet acts on lymphocytes that are involved in the immune response. Dameshek (228) suggested that aldomet or one of its metabolites might in some way disrupt the ability of those cells to recognize host or self antigens. Allison et al. (229) wondered if aldomet might "activate" a population of T cells that then instructed B cells to produce autoantibody that would not normally be made. The answers seemed finally to be at hand when Kirtland et al. (230-232) published their findings. These workers studied the effects of aldomet on lymphocytes both in vivo and in vitro. They worked with lymphocytes isolated from patients with aldomet-induced hemolytic anemia and with those of normal healthy donors, after the cells were exposed to aldomet in vitro. They reported that in both instances, the lymphocytes had a sustained increase of production of cellular cyclic AMP. Lymphocyte-derived AMP affects T cells in at least three ways. First, it inhibits their proliferation, second, it delays their maturation and third, it diminishes their degree of activation. Any one or any combination of these effects could have explained the production of autoantibodies by patients being treated with aldomet. The effects of the sustained high level of lymphocyte cyclic AMP might result in suppressor T cells no longer controlling clones of B cells that would then be able to produce autoantibodies. Certainly this concept fits with current ideas on the T suppressor cell control of B cells. It appears to provide an explanation as to how administration of a drug can induce the same change in the immune system that occurs via unknown causes in patients with autoimmune disorders, including WAIHA.

However, in spite of the reports of Kirtland et al. (230-232) the situation is still not understood. Kirtland et al. (232) used a method devised by Lipsky et al. (260) that measures the level of IgG generated by B cells and uses artificial manipulation to down regulate the synthesis of IgG. When the system used lymphocytes exposed to aldomet in vitro (232) the down regulation was abrogated and a significantly greater amount of IgG was generated. Similar results were obtained in studies using lymphocytes from patients being treated with aldomet. However, while Garratty et al. (261,262) confirmed the observations of Lipsky et al. (260) and could demonstrate a down regulation mechanism for B cell synthesis of IgG, they could not confirm that aldomet (or procainamide, see below) abrogated the down regulation or caused an increase in IgG synthesis. Both groups of workers (232,262) showed that aldomet depressed the proliferative response of mononuclear cells to mitogen stimulation.

Kirtland et al. (230,231) made another observation during their studies. They found that aldomet caused a sustained increase of production of cyclic AMP by monocytes as well as by lymphocytes. It is currently believed that high levels of monocyte-derived cyclic AMP have an inhibitory effect on tissue-bound macrophages that are themselves descendants of monocytes. This observation might explain the finding that while as many as 30% of patients being treated with aldomet make red cell autoantibodies, less than 1% of them develop hemolytic anemia. In other words, in spite of the presence of IgG autoantibody on the red cells, immune-mediated red cell clearance is uncommon because there is a concomitant decrease in macrophage activity in the patients. There is independent evidence (243 and see section on immune red cell clearance in patients with aldomet-induced autoantibodies) that the development of hemolytic anemia in these patients is directly related to the activity of their reticuloendothelial systems.

A different explanation for aldomet-induced hemolytic anemia was advanced by Branch et al. (263) and uses the concept of altered host or self antigens. These workers studied the interaction between autologous monocytes and IgG-coated red cells in two patients with aldomet-induced autoantibodies, first while the patients had active hemolytic anemia and then after the aldomet had been withdrawn and the patients were in hematological remission. In brief, they found that the IgG levels on the patients' red cells were similar throughout the periods of hemolysis and remission but that significant monocyte activity was seen only during the time that active hemolysis was taking place. To explain these observations, the authors (263) suggested that while aldomet was being given, an antigen on the patient's red cells was slightly altered so that when the antibody bound to the red cells, the Fc portions of the IgG antibody molecules were oriented in a manner that resulted in macrophage recognition and binding. It was further supposed that at some time after aldomet had been withdrawn, the alteration to the red cell antigen no longer occurred. Although the IgG antibody molecules could still bind to the red cells, in about the same numbers, it was suggested that because of the difference in antigen, the Fc portions of those IgG molecules were no longer suitably positioned for macrophage binding to occur. The authors (263) cited observations of Green et al. (264,265) in support of their contention that aldomet therapy can affect an alteration in antigen presentation on the red cell membrane. At what is perhaps too superficial a level, the observations of Branch et al. (263) seem to run counter to the suggestion (230,231) that therapy with aldomet reduced macrophage efficiency. That is, in the patients studied by Branch et al. (263) about the same level of IgG on red cells resulted in hemolysis when the patients were receiving the drug and no hemolysis once the drug was withdrawn.

Before leaving aldomet it should be mentioned that there are many reports (290-301) that treatment with the drug can cause liver damage resulting in hepatitis or, at worst, cirrhosis.

As shown in table 40-3 both levodopa (187-192) that is chemically similar to alpha-methyldopa (aldomet) and mefenamic acid (158,193-195) that is not, have caused production of drug-independent autoantibodies, some of which have caused immune hemolytic anemia. Both drugs (187,302,303) have also caused the production of non-red cell autoantibodies and clinical lupus-like conditions thus strengthening the concept that these drugs directly affect the immune system.

Although it was recognized (196-201,244,266,304)

as a cause of autoantibody production long after aldomet, there are as many theories as to how procainamide acts as advanced to explain the actions of aldomet. It has been suggested (197,267) that the drug interacts with protein in cell nucleii to form a new antigen or that it serves as an adjuvant in stimulating autoantibody producing clones (268). Alternatively, Cornacchia et al. (269) produced evidence that they believed showed that the drug inhibits T-cell DNA methylation that then induces T-cell autoreactivity. Several other groups of investigators (270-276) have produced evidence that procainamide interferes with immunoregulation. Many of the findings have been contradictory, some investigators felt that procainamide inhibits suppressor T-cell function, others that it enhances helper T-cell function and still others that the drug acts on B cells. It has also been claimed (200,304) that procainamide acts directly on red cell precursors and that either the drug has a toxic effect or the autoantibody inhibits red cell precursor maturation thus contributing to or causing the anemia seen in these patients. It seems unlikely that such a mechanism is the sole cause of the anemia since the clinical and laboratory findings point to a major immune-mediated, red cell destruction component.

Just as with aldomet therapy, treatment with procainamide results in the production of autoantibodies directed against other than red cells. Many of the papers cited above include descriptions of such autoantibodies, others describe procainamide-induced:granulocytopenia (259,304-314); a lupus-like condition (196,197,315-321); and thrombocytopenia (266,322).

From what is written in this section it is clear that while theories abound, the exact mechanism (or mechanisms if they differ) by which aldomet and procainamide cause autoantibody production is/are not known. This in spite of an enormous amount of work. Obviously there is great impetus to understand the mechanisms. In these drug-induced situations when immune hemolytic anemia or autoantibody production occurs, withdrawal of the drug results in total correction of the situation. That is, immune hemolysis stops very soon (i.e. days) after the drug is withdrawn. While autoantibody production may continue for longer (i.e. months or years), that too eventually stops. Clearly if the mechanism by which the immune system is repaired was understood, it would have the potential to suggest more effective ways of treating patients with idiopathic autoimmune disease.

Autoantibody Production as Related to Aldomet Dose

Of all patients treated with aldomet (or aldoril or

aldoclor that also contain alpha-methyldopa) between 20 and 30% develop a positive DAT but only about 1% suffer hemolytic anemia (6,39,40,82,90,152,172-186). There is a direct relationship between the dose of aldomet given and the likelihood that autoantibodies will be produced. In patients treated with more than 2g aldomet/day, some 30 to 36% develop a positive DAT. In those treated with between 1 and 2g/day, the incidence of a positive DAT is around 20% and in those treated with less than 1g/day, it is about 10%. Now that this correlation is known and suitable alternative drugs are available, cases of hemolytic anemia and autoantibody production due to aldomet therapy are seen much less frequently than was previously the case. Many physicians now use a different antihypertensive drug if the patient's blood pressure cannot be controlled with 1g or less of aldomet per day. A possible difference between patients who develop hemolytic anemia and those who do not, after autoantibody production is full blown, is discussed in the section dealing with in vivo red cell destruction in this setting.

Laboratory Findings in Patients with Aldomet-Induced Autoantibodies

In some 83% of patients who form autoantibodies due to aldomet therapy, the DAT is positive with only IgG being detectable on the red cells (6,152,185). While some 17% of patients have IgG and C3 on the red cells (1,6) it is often found that the amount of C3 bound is small and it is not always apparent that its presence on the red cells has anything to do with the aldomet-induced autoantibody. The IgG autoantibodies made are polyclonal (277) and may be IgG1 (278) and/or IgG3 (152). As mentioned above, eluates made from the patients' red cells or unbound autoantibodies present in the patients' sera, often react with all red cells (i.e. anti-dl, see Chapter 37) although, as discussed below, some with specificity for red cell antigens are seen.

The autoantibodies produced by patients being treated with aldomet have similar specificities to those made by patients with WAIHA. In our (185) series of 150 individuals with a positive DAT and warm-reactive autoantibodies, 87 had WAIHA and 33 had aldomet-induced autoantibodies (the other 30 were hematologically normal persons). None of the patients with aldomet-induced autoantibodies had hemolytic anemia. Autoantibodies with "simple" Rh specificity and ones directed against nl, pdl, dl, Wr[b] and U were seen in the WAIHA and aldomet-induced groups. In the 87 patients with WAIHA, 26 (30%) had apparently formed only one autoantibody. In the 33 patients with aldomet-induced autoantibodies, 14 (42%) had apparently made only one autoantibody. However, exactly half the patients with only one autoan-

tibody in the WAIHA and aldomet-induced groups, had just anti-dl. If these are excluded (anti-dl may well be a mixture of autoantibodies whose exact specificities have not been recognized, see Chapter 37) the incidence of patients with a single autoantibody becomes 13 of 87 (15%) in the WAIHA group and 7 of 33 (21%) in the aldomet-induced group, i.e. the same. Data from other studies are similar and those cited above have been used here simply to illustrate the fact that the same specificities are seen in patients with idiopathic WAIHA and aldomet-induced autoantibodies.

Sometimes a clinician will be treating a patient with aldomet and will ask the blood banker to determine whether the patient's hemolytic anemia is idiopathic or aldomet-induced. The task is formidable. One, sometimes useful clue from serological studies, is the presence of an appreciable amount of C3 on the patient's red cells. As discussed in Chapter 37, some 45 to 60% of patients with WAIHA have IgG and C3 on their red cells. As mentioned above, some 83% of patients with aldomet-induced autoantibodies have only IgG on their red cells, most of the other 17% have only small amounts of C3 on their red cells. Thus, if the DAT on the patient's red cells is more than weakly positive with anti-C3, it is unlikely that the patient's hemolytic anemia is due solely to the aldomet therapy. However, such a finding does not exclude the possibility that the aldomet therapy is contributing to the hemolytic process. In other words, the patient may have WAIHA *and* an aldomet-induced hemolytic process. When the patient's red cells are coated only with IgG, it is virtually impossible for the blood banker to know whether WAIHA or an aldomet-induced autoantibody is responsible. Again as discussed in Chapter 37, some 40 to 50% of patients with WAIHA present, like the 83% of patients with aldomet-induced autoantibodies, with only IgG detectable on their red cells. Petz and Garratty (6) mention another clue that they use to differentiate between patients with WAIHA and aldomet-induced autoantibodies. In their series, all patients with aldomet-induced hemolytic anemia presented with excess autoantibody in the serum so that the IAT was positive. In contrast, 43% of their patients with idiopathic WAIHA did not have IAT-detectable autoantibody in their serum. Thus in their series, hemolytic anemia in a patient with a negative IAT was never a result of aldomet therapy. At first, it looks as if our figures (185) are in disagreement with this observation. Of our 33 patients being treated with aldomet, 16 (48%) had no IAT-detectable autoantibody in the serum. However, none of our patients (185) with the aldomet-induced autoantibodies had hemolytic anemia; the 100% incidence of positive IATs described by Petz and Garratty (6) was in patients in whom the aldomet-induced autoantibodies were causing in vivo red cell destruction. In spite of this, the presence or absence of serum autoantibody would be of less use as a differentiation point in our series (185) than in that of Petz and Garratty (6). While 43% of their patients with WAIHA had a negative IAT, the incidence of that finding was only 28% in our series.

Often, the only way that the role of aldomet in the hemolytic process can be ascertained for sure is to withdraw the drug. The patient is then followed to see if the hemolytic process abates. Even then, before aldomet is incriminated unequivocally, it is prudent to challenge the patient with the drug again to see if autoantibody production recurs. This is not as dangerous as it may sound since serological evidence of repeat autoantibody production can be obtained and drug therapy can be stopped before hemolytic anemia occurs again.

In Vivo Red Cell Destruction in Patients with Aldomet-Induced Autoantibodies

Many workers assumed that the difference between patients with aldomet-induced autoantibodies who were suffering from hemolytic anemia and those who were not, was related to the amount (and perhaps the subclass) of IgG autoantibody on the red cells and some variation in macrophage recognition abilities in different persons. Indeed Meulen et al. (279) used a flow cytometer to measure the amount of IgG1 on the red cells of 29 patients with positive DATs. Among the 29 patients, 12 were receiving aldomet. Among those 12, seven had overt hemolysis while the other five had no hemolytic anemia. It was reported that a critical threshold of IgG per red cell existed above which hemolysis occurred and below which it did not. All seven aldomet treated patients with hemolytic anemia had an IgG/cell level above the threshold, all five with no hemolysis had a level below the threshold. However, when Garratty and Nance (280) undertook a flow cytometry study on the DAT+ red cells of 103 individuals some of whom had hemolytic anemia and some of whom did not, there was sufficient overlap in the amount of IgG/rbc between persons in the non-hemolyzing and hemolyzing groups, that they were unable to determine a cutoff threshold. While Garratty and Nance (280) agreed that the mean IgG/rbc number was higher in the hemolyzing than in the non-hemolyzing group, there was overlap in each of their three subsections, i.e. patients with idiopathic WAIHA, those with drug-induced immune hemolytic anemia, and infants with HDN. When the aldomet treated patients were analyzed separately: eight had hemolytic anemia; 17 did not; overlap was still seen, i.e. fluorescence per red cell 28-127, mean 57 in patients with hemolysis, 30-53, mean 40 in patients with no hemolysis.

A very different finding was reported by Lalezari et al. (281). These workers studied 11 patients with aldomet-induced autoantibodies, eight had hemolytic anemia, three did not. In the eight with hemolytic anemia, Lalezari et al. (281) reported the presence of IgG and IgM autoantibodies. In the three with no hemolysis, only IgG autoantibodies were found. The IgM autoantibodies, that were said to be responsible for the hemolytic anemia, were thought to be warm-reactive and largely confined to the patients' red cells (i.e. present in eluates but not in the patients' sera). Further, because they did not act as agglutinins, it was supposed that the IgM autoantibodies were monomeric. The IgM autoantibodies were said to activate C1q, C3 and C4 and Lalezari et al. (281) felt that it was these autoantibodies, not the IgG forms, that cause aldomet-induced hemolytic anemia. As far as we are aware, these observations have not been confirmed by others. However, it should be pointed out that Lalezari et al. (281) conducted their tests in a PVP-potentiated antiglobulin system in an AutoAnalyzer, a test system not widely used by others. If aldomet-induced hemolytic anemia is caused by an IgM complement-binding autoantibody, it is difficult to understand why other workers have found only IgG on the red cells of patients with the condition. DATs on very large numbers of patients with aldomet-induced hemolytic anemia must have been performed by now and as mentioned above some 83% of cases have involved only IgG on the red cells. In the absence of DATs performed with monospecific anti-IgM (i.e. not used by most workers) it is still noticeable that high levels of C3 have not regularly been found on the red cells of patients with aldomet-induced immune hemolytic anemia, as would be expected if IgM complement-binding antibodies are responsible for the red cell destruction.

In a study that seemed to confirm that the IgG form of the aldomet-induced autoantibody is responsible for the red cell clearance in vivo, Kelton (282) studied nine patients being treated with aldomet. Five patients had a positive DAT but only one had hemolytic anemia. In the four DAT+ patients who were not experiencing hemolysis significant impairment of reticuloendothelial red cell clearance (i.e. measured via injection of radiolabeled IgG-coated red cells) was demonstrated. In the patient with hemolytic anemia there was no impairment of the cell clearance mechanism. Kelton (282) suggested that the absence of hemolysis in many patients with aldomet-induced autoantibodies might represent a concomitant down regulation of the reticuloendothelial system. Further, as had been suggested by Kirtland et al. (230,231) the impairment of macrophage function was thought to be induced by the drug itself since abnormal reticuloendothelial cell function was demonstrated (282) in the patients being treated with aldomet, in whom the DAT was negative.

Treatment of Patients with Aldomet-Induced Hemolytic Anemia

Any form of drug-induced hemolytic anemia is obviously best treated by cessation of therapy with the responsible drug. In patients with aldomet-induced hemolytic anemia, the hemolysis usually stops within two to ten days (in the experience of one of us (PDI), cessation in two or three days is more frequent than in longer periods) and in most patients no other therapy is required. Rarely, in cases of severe anemia, a short course of corticosteroids may be beneficial, even less frequently transfusion may be required. Autoantibody production does not stop nearly as rapidly as the in vivo red cell destruction and the DAT may remain positive for periods that range from one month to two years (174). Second episodes of autoantibody production in these patients, who are again treated with aldomet, have been mentioned above.

Treatment of Patients with an Aldomet-Induced Positive DAT

When aldomet-induced hemolytic anemia occurs, aldomet therapy is almost always stopped. When a patient with an aldomet-induced autoantibody, in whom there is no evidence of hemolytic anemia is encountered, a decision must be made as to whether the aldomet will be withdrawn. Since the drug-induced hemolytic process is dose-dependent and apparently also related to the length of time over which the drug is given, some clinicians elect immediately to withdraw the drug. Since aldomet is an excellent antihypertensive, in the past others elected to continue therapy with the drug in spite of the positive DAT. Obviously, patients continued on the drug after the DAT became positive had to be monitored serologically and hematologically. The observation of Petz and Garratty (6) that aldomet-induced hemolytic anemia is always associated with a positive IAT is of value. In a patient on aldomet in whom the DAT is positive and the IAT negative, hemolytic anemia is improbable. In one in whom the DAT and IAT are both positive, the risk of hemolytic anemia is higher and closer hematological monitoring is indicated. As mentioned earlier in this chapter, the decision to withdraw aldomet therapy is easier now that other highly efficient antihypertensive drugs are available, than was the case in the mid and late sixties when aldomet-induced hemolytic anemia was first recognized.

Based on what is known about the role of aldomet in causing autoantibody production, a report by Habibi (283) came as a surprise. Ten patients with a positive DAT due to aldomet therapy, but with no evidence of hemolytic anemia, were continued on the drug. They were followed over a 12 to 30 month period. In eight of the 10 patients the serological picture did not change, none of them developed hemolytic anemia. In the other two patients, autoantibody production stopped and the DAT became negative, one at six and one at nine months after the study began. These findings may relate to the relatively small doses of aldomet being used. The patients were being treated with doses of 250 to 750 mg/aldomet/day and had been treated for periods between eight and 21 months before the DAT became positive. During the study the same 250 to 750 mg doses were used. In the two patients in whom autoantibody production stopped, the doses had been 250 and 500 mg/day for 15 and 18 months respectively before the DAT became positive. Autoantibody production stopped while each patient was receiving 500 mg/day. The autoantibody did not reappear in either patient, one was followed for 10 and the other for 22 months after the DAT became negative. Thus it is possible that whatever the mechanism that results in autoantibody production in patients being treated with aldomet, larger doses than those used in these patients are necessary for progression or continuation of that process.

Drug-Dependent and Drug-Independent Drug-Induced Antibodies in the Same Patient

As mentioned in the introduction to this chapter, it was originally believed that drug-induced antibodies could be divided into distinct types. Some were thought to react with red cells to which drug was firmly bound. Others were thought to complex with drugs bound to plasma proteins, to form immune complexes that then bound or caused complement to be bound to red cells. Antibodies of those two types were said to be drug-dependent since they reacted with red cells only when those cells were coated with the drug or when the drug was present in the test system. The third type of drug-induced antibody was said to be drug-independent. Although production of such antibodies was a direct result of drug therapy, the antibodies reacted with normal red cells in the absence of drug. These drug-independent antibodies were apparently identical to the autoantibodies made by patients with idiopathic "warm" antibody-induced hemolytic anemia. As more and more patients who have made antibodies as the result of drug therapy have been studied, it has become apparent that one or both types of drug-dependent and drug-independent antibodies can be made by the same patient in an immune response to, or initiated by, a particular drug. Such observations (for which references are given in table 40-4) led Mueller-Eckhardt and Salama (160) to propose a unifying concept to explain production of the antibodies that cause drug-induced immune cytopenias. With some modifications suggested, that concept has been embraced to greater or lesser degrees by others (1,9,10,19,224,225,235,284).

Our idea of the unifying concept, that is not necessarily the same as the original or the modified versions advanced by others, is shown diagrammatically in figure 40-4. The square box on the red cell membrane represents the receptor to which the drug in question binds. The square plus the triangle on the red cell membrane represents drug bound firmly to the red cell. The oblong plus the triangle represents the drug (triangle) bound to a plasma protein. Antibody A is the type that binds only to red cells previously coated with the drug. Its specificity is wholly for a haptenic group on the drug, most examples of anti-penicillin are of this type. Antibody B is similar to antibody A in being drug-dependent. It recognizes a haptenic grouping on the drug that is bound to a plasma protein. Antibody B is the type that participates in immune complex formation in the plasma. After the complexes are formed either they, or the complement components they have caused to be activated, bind to red cells. Antibody C has a specificity such that it recognizes part of the drug and part of the receptor to which the drug binds. An antibody of type C may thereby have the ability to bind to untreated cells but may give stronger reactions in tests in which the drug is present (i in figure 40-4; ii represents binding of the same antibody in the absence of drug). Antibody D is wholly drug-independent and binds to the cell receptor in the absence of drug, indeed in the absence of the red cell donor ever having been exposed to the drug. This type of antibody is typical of those made in response to therapy with aldomet, levodopa, mefenamic acid or procainamide.

As mentioned earlier, a number of cases have been described in which the same patient made drug-dependent and drug-independent antibodies. Table 40-4 gives some examples of these findings and divides the drug-dependent antibodies involved into type A (figure 40-4, drug bound firmly to red cell) and type B (figure 40-4 immune complex formation). As will be seen, many of the drugs listed in table 40-4 stimulate production of drug-independent antibodies. We agree with Garratty (1) that the mechanism by which drugs such as aldomet, levodopa, mefenamic acid and procainamide stimulate production of only drug-independent antibodies and the mechanism(s) by which the drugs listed in table 40-4 stimulate the production of drug-dependent and drug-independent antibodies, probably differ. That is to say, we believe that drugs that cause only drug-independent autoantibodies to be made, do so by interfering with the immune system of the antibody-maker. We believe that those drugs that cause drug-dependent and drug-independent antibodies to be made, stimulate production of

TABLE 40-4 Drugs Associated with Production of More Than One Type of Drug-Induced Antibody

Drug	Drug-Dependent Ab		Drug-Independent Antibody	References
	Type A*	Type B*		
Azapropazone	X		X	324
Carbimazole		X	X	65
Cefotaxime	X	X		99
Cefotetan	X	X	X	101-104, 325
Ceftazidime	X	X		106
Chlorinated hydrocarbons	X	X	X	127, 326
Cianidanol	X	X	X	67
Diclofenac		X	X	161
Galfenine		X	X	7
Latamoxef		X	X	7
Nomifensine		X	X	8
Phenacetin		X	X	327
Streptomycin	X		X	70, 71
Teniposide		X	X	7, 153
Tolmetin		X	X	328, 329

* For differentiation between drug-dependent antibodies type A and type B see figure 40-4 and text.

the latter by alteration of the membrane receptor to which they bind. If pressed, we would suggest that in figure 40-4, antibody D represents a true drug-independent (aldomet et al. type) autoantibody, while antibody C whose reactions are shown as ii in the figure, represents the drug-independent antibody made (often simultaneously) with a drug-dependent form (i.e. antibody C to structure i in figure 40-4).

Red Cell Blood Group Antigens as Receptors for Drugs

Given the fact that some drugs are capable of binding firmly to red cells and the current concept that even when such binding cannot be demonstrated it may well have occurred (7,330) (with the loose bonds broken and the drug released during washing stages preparatory for in vitro tests) it is perhaps not surprising that some of the sites to which some drugs bind are red cell blood group antigens. In 1977, Martinez et al. (70) described a streptomycin-dependent antibody that reacted with drug-coat-

FIGURE 40-4 One Interpretation of a Unifying Concept

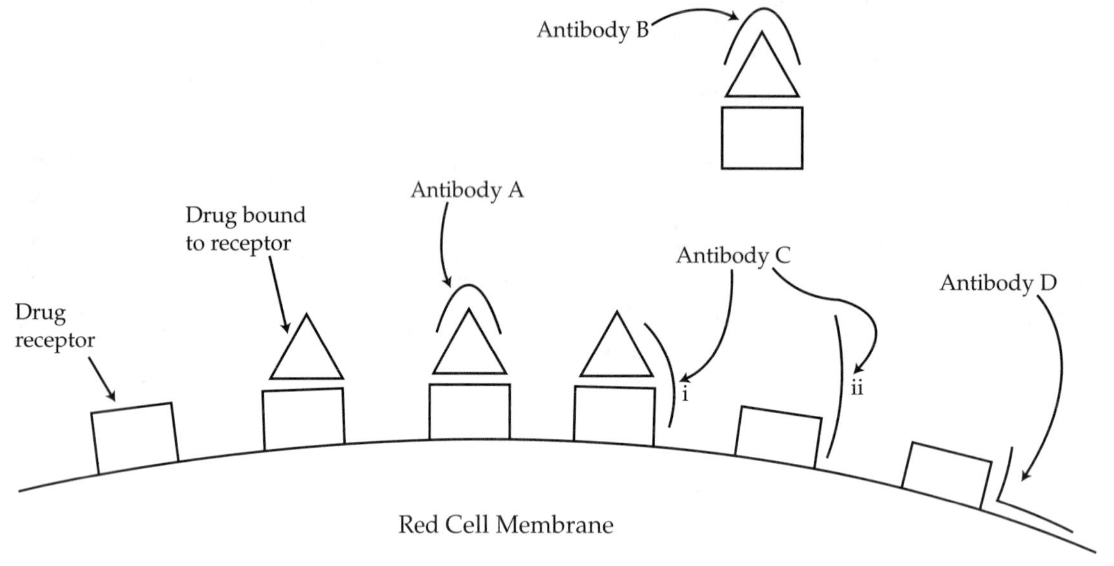

Antibody B

Antibody A

Drug bound
to receptor

Antibody C

Antibody D

Drug
receptor

i

ii

Red Cell Membrane

Footnote to figure 40-4

For specificities and reaction patterns of
antibodies A, B, C and D, see text

ed red cells in vitro, only when those cells were D-, M+. Duran-Suarez et al. (331) described five drug-dependent antibodies that would react with red cells only in the presence of rifampicin, nitrofurantoin or dexchlorphenyramine maleate and only if the red cells carried high levels of I. In these studies i cord and i adult cells were non-reactive. Somewhat similarly, Habibi et al. (332) described a thiopental-dependent, Salama and Mueller-Eckhardt (9) a nomifensine-dependent, and Pereira et al. (334) a rifampicin-dependent antibody that reacted with adult but not with cord blood red cells in the presence of the appropriate drug. Sandvei et al. (333) described a case of fluorouracil (5-FU)-induced hemolytic anemia caused by an antibody that reacted with the red cells of adults, of both the I and i phenotypes, but not with cord blood red cells. Habibi and Bretagne (335) then tested 19 antibodies from patients receiving, among them, 11 different drugs, against red cells lacking certain very common antigens. Six of the 19 antibodies reacted with all red cells, five failed to react with D--/D--, five failed to react with Lu(a-b-), two failed to react with P- and one failed to react with K_oK_o red cells. In tests on 30 antibodies made by patients being treated with nomifensine, Salama and Mueller-Eckhardt (9,355) found that 14 reacted with all cells tested, nine were non-reactive or reacted less strongly with Rh_{null} red cells while three did not react with cord red blood cells and could be neutralized with soluble I substance. The remaining four antibodies were non-reactive with some red cell samples but no specificity was recognized.

In reviewing the above data it should be borne in mind that when an antibody reacts with adult I but not with i cord or i adult red cells, or is neutralized by soluble I substance, anti-I specificity can be assigned with a reasonable degree of confidence. When an antibody reacts with the red cells of adults but not with cord blood red cells, it is not clear whether the antibody is anti-I or whether the reactions represent some other difference between the red cells of adults and those of newborns.

In 1984, Sosler et al. (112) described an auto-anti-Jk^a made by a patient being treated with chlorpropamide. Initially the antibody reacted with all Jk(a+) red cells but gave its strongest reactions in the presence of the drug. Once the drug was withdrawn (the patient had drug-induced immune hemolytic anemia) the antibody gradually became weaker and eventually reacted with Jk(a+) red cells only the presence of chlorpropamide. Of note, a number of benign auto-anti-Jk^a, reactive only in the presence of methyl esters of hydroxybenzoic acid have been reported (336,337).

As would be expected from what has been written above about drug-independent autoantibodies produced as the only antibody made and drug-independent antibodies made by patients who also make drug-dependent antibodies, we do not consider the specific antibodies made by patients being treated with aldomet or procainamide, as reflecting antibody production against an altered red cell membrane receptor. Thus we view the aldomet-induced autoantibodies that have Rh (175,177,277) specificity or are directed against Wr[b] (185), U (209) or Jk[a] (210) and those made by patients receiving procainamide, that have Rh specificity (201), in the same light as we view autoantibodies made by patients with idiopathic WAIHA (see Chapter 37). That is to say, we do not know why the immune system chooses to make autoantibody against one particular antigen, but we do not believe that the selection process is antigen-driven. Those autoantibodies described above (9,355), that were made by patients being treated with nomifensine and were directed against antigens associated with Rh, seem to fit the altered antigen concept better than the modified immune response concept because nomifensine is known (124,237,252) often to cause drug-dependent antibodies to be produced as well. However, we will admit that this distinction between altered antigen and modification of the immune system, for nomifensine, may actually reflect the fact that we have not wholly committed to the unifying concept.

The Second and Third Generation Cephalosporins Revisited

Although these drugs have been mentioned earlier, they are singled out here for further emphasis. The reason is that the first generation cephalosporins often caused positive DATs but seldom caused acute hemolytic anemia (6). Thus blood bankers can be excused for having come to regard therapy with the cephalosporins as somewhat innocuous. The story with the second and third generation cephalosporins is rather different (109,359). Between 1987 and 1992 ten cases of severe hemolytic anemia were reported (99-108,325,338) in association with these drugs. Five of the ten cases (100-103,338) involved cefotetan and in three cases, one each involving ceftriaxone (107), cefoxitin (105) and cefotetan (100,104) the outcome was fatal. The antibodies involved in the various cases covered the whole gamut of drug-induced antibodies. That is, antibodies reacting with cephalosporin-coated red cells, antibodies reacting by apparently forming immune complexes in the plasma, leading to complement activation and intravascular hemolysis, and drug-independent antibodies, were all seen.

One of the dangers of this type of drug-induced hemolytic anemia involves the use of these drugs in difficult to monitor situations. That is, with the way health care is now practiced, many women who have recently been delivered of infants are discharged from hospital within 24 or 48 hours of the infant's birth. A proportion of these women are treated prophylactically with third generation cephalosporins or, if a longer hospital stay was involved, are discharged at the time drug therapy is discontinued (325). Thus if hemolysis begins while the patient is not under close medical surveillance, a potentially life-threatening situation can develop in a healthy young female whose only medical history involves recent pregnancy. The danger is greatly magnified if red cell destruction occurs following the formation of immune complexes in vivo. Two of the common findings in this type of drug-induced immune hemolytic anemia are first, that hemolysis can occur following ingestion of a small dose of the drug, and second, that massive intravascular red cell destruction can occur rapidly. Clearly patients sent home with a supply of cephalosporin pills must be instructed on recognition of the symptoms of sudden onset anemia. Equally clear, if the situation is suspected, laboratory studies must involve tests against drug-coated red cells, tests in the presence of the drug, and tests for drug-independent antibodies. Table 40-5 lists first, second and third generation cephalosporins and some proprietary names under which they are marketed.

NSAIDs Revisited

Like the third generation cephalosporins, these drugs have been mentioned earlier. They are discussed again here because there are data (207,251) that suggest that at least some non-steroidal anti-inflammatory drugs (NSAIDs) can cause anemia in patients in whom there is no evidence of drug-induced antibody production or immune red cell destruction. That is to say, the clinical picture may be complex and may involve multisystem organ failure, shock, renal insufficiency, disseminated intravascular coagulation and anemia. In other words, negative findings in tests for drug-induced antibodies do not necessarily exclude the NSAID in question from a role in the patient's clinical problems. In one case that we (340) studied, in which we believe that NSAID therapy led to death of the patient, the only positive immunohematological finding was a dubious reaction in a Donath-Landsteiner test for which no specificity could be ascribed the putative biphasic hemolysin. As can be seen from table 40-3 there are many cases in which NSAIDs were thought perhaps to have altered the immune response, but few in which definitive evidence was obtained.

Drug-Induced Cytopenias not Involving Red Cells

As most readers will be aware, drug-induced

TABLE 40-5 Some Cephalosporins with Some Proprietory Names (expanded from 369)

First Generation		Second Generation	
Generic Name	**Proprietory Names**	**Generic Name**	**Proprietory Names**
Cefadroxil	Duricef	Cefaclor	Ceclor
Cefazolin sodium	Ancef, Kefzol	Cefamandole nafate	Mandol
Cephalexin	Keflex, Biocef	Cefmetazole	Zefazone
Cephalexin hydrochloride	Keftab	Cefonicid sodium	Monocid
Cephalothin	Keflin	Cefotetan disodium	Cefotan
Cephapirin	Cefadyl	Cefoxitin sodium	Mefoxin
Cephradine	Anspor, Velosef	Cefprozil	Cefzil
		Cefuroxime sodium	Zinadef, Kefurox
		Cefuroxime axetil	Ceftin

Third and Fourth Generations			
Generic Name	**Proprietory Names**	**Generic Name**	**Proprietory Names**
Cefixime	Suprax	Ceftibuten	Cedax
Cefoperazone sodium	Cefobid	Ceftizoxime sodium	Cefizox
Cefotaxime sodium	Claforan	Ceftriaxone sodium	Rocephin
Cefpodoxine proxetil	Vantin	Moxalactam	Moxam
Ceftazidime	Ceptaz, Fortaz, Pentacef, Tazicef, Tazidime	Cefepime hydrochloride (Fourth generation)	Maxpime

immune thrombocytopenia is probably more common than drug-induced immune hemolytic anemia. Clearly a discussion of that subject is beyond the scope of this book and even more clearly, beyond the scope of its authors. Interested readers are referred to a number of excellent reviews (160,162,284,341-349,362-368) about this topic. Similarly to drug-induced thrombocytopenia, drug-induced neutropenia is beyond the scope of this book. Appropriate references are 162,259,314,350 and 361.

References

1. Garratty G. In: Immunobiology of Transfusion Medicine. New York:Marcel Dekker, 1994:523
2. Snapper I, Marks D, Schwartz L, et al. Ann Intern Med 1953;39:619
3. Harris JW. J Lab Clin Med 1956;47:760
4. Dausset J, Contu L. Ann Rev Med 1967;18:55
5. Worlledge SM. Sem Hematol 1969;6:181
6. Petz LD, Garratty G. Acquired Immune Hemolytic Anemias. New York:Churchill Livingstone, 1980:267
7. Habibi B. Br J Haematol 1985;61:139
8. Salama A, Mueller-Eckhardt C. Br J Haematol 1986;64:613
9. Salama A, Mueller-Eckhardt C. Blood 1987;69:1006
10. Petz LD. In: Immune Destruction of Red Blood Cells. Arlington, VA:Am Assoc Blood Banks, 1989:53
11. Eisen HN, Carsten ME, Belman S. J Immunol 1954;73:296
12. Park BK, Coleman JW, Kitteringham NR. Biochem Pharmacol 1987;36:581
13. De Weck AL. In: The Antigens, Vol II. New York:Academic, 1974:142
14. Roitt IM. Essential Immunology, 8th Ed. Oxford:Blackwell, 1994
15. Petz LD, Fudenberg HH. New Eng J Med 1966;274:171
16. White JM, Brown DL, Hepner GW, et al. Br Med J 1968;3:26
17. Rossiter MA, Gray IR, Shinton NK. Br Med J 1968;3:28
18. Garratty G. Hum Pathol 1983;14:204
19. Garratty G. In: Immune Destruction of Red Blood Cells. Arlington,VA:Am Assoc Blood Banks, 1989:109
20. Kerr RO, Cardamone J, Dalmasso AP, et al. New Eng J Med 1972;287:1322
21. Ries CA, Rosenbaum TJ, Garratty G, et al. J Am Med Assoc 1975;233:432
22. Funicella T, Weinger RS, Moake JL, et al. Am J Hematol 1977;3:219
23. Yust I, Goldsher N, Greenfeld R, et al. Israel J Med Sci 1980;16:174
24. Yust I, Goldsher N. Br J Haematol 1981;47:443
25. Yust I, Frisch B, Goldsher N. Am J Hematol 1982;13:53
26. Yust I, Frisch B, Goldsher N, et al. Scand J Haematol 1982;28:408
27. Ley AB, Harris JP, Brinkley M, et al. Science 1958;127:1118
28. Watson KC, Joubert SM, Bennett MAE. Immunology 1960;3:1
29. Levine BB, Ovary Z. J Exp Med 1961;114:875
30. Strumia PV, Raymond FD. Arch Int Med 1962;109:603
31. Thiel JA, Mitchell S, Parker CW. J Allgy 1964;35:399
32. Van Arsdel PP, Gilliland BC. J Lab Clin Med 1965;65:277
33. Levine BB, Fellner MJ, Levytska V. J Immunol 1966;96:707
34. Levine BB, Redmond AP. J Clin Invest 1967;46:1085
35. Levine B. Int Arch Allgy Appl Immunol 1967;31:594
36. Abraham GN, Petz LD, Fudenberg HH. Clin Exp Immunol

1968;3:343

37. Nesmith LW, Davis JW. J Am Med Assoc 1968;203:81
38. Spath P, Garratty G, Petz L. J Immunol 1971;107:854
39. Petz LD. Postgrad Med J 1971;47 (Suppl):64
40. Garratty G, Petz LD. Am J Med 1975;58:398
41. Bird GWG, McEvoy MW, Wingham J. J Clin Pathol 1975;28:321
42. Seldon MR, Bain B, Johnson CA, et al. Scand J Haematol 1982;28:459
43. Petz LD, Branch DR. In: Immune Hemolytic Anemias. New York:Churchill Livingstone, 1985:47
44. Molthan L, Reidenberg MM, Eichman MF. New Eng J Med 1967;277:123
45. Gralnick HR, Wright LD, McGinniss MH. J Am Med Assoc 1967;199:725
46. Perkins RL, Mengel CE, Saslow S. Proc Soc Exp Biol Med 1968;129:397
47. Spath P, Garratty G, Petz L. J Immunol 1971;107:860
48. Gralnick HR, McGinniss MH, Elton W, et al. J Am Med Assoc 1971;217:68
49. Gralnick HR, McGinniss MH, Elton W, et al. J Am Med Assoc 1971;217:1193
50. Jeannet M, Bloch A, Dayer JM, et al. Acta Haematol 1976;55;109
51. Rubin RN, Burka ER. Ann Intern Med 1977;86:64
52. Moake JL, Butler CFR, Hewell GM, et al. Transfusion 1978;18:369
53. Kaplan K, Reisberg B, Weinstein L. Arch Int Med 1968;121:17
54. York PS, Landes RR, Seay LS. J Am Med Assoc 1968;206:1086
55. Fass RJ, Perkins RL, Saslow S. J Am Med Assoc 1970;213:121
56. Forbes CD, Craig JA, Mitchell R, et al. Postgrad Med J 1972;48:186
57. Schwarz S, Gabl F, Huber H, et al. Vox Sang 1975;29:59
58. Manoharan A, Kot T. Med J Austral 1987;147:202
59. Branch DR, Berkowitz LR, Becker RL, et al. Am J Hematol 1985;18:213
60. Getaz EP, Beckley S, Fitzpatrick J, et al. New Eng J Med 1980;302:334
61. Levi JA, Aroney RS, Dalley DN. Br Med J 1981;282:2003
62. Nguyen BV, Lichtiger B. Cancer Treat Rep 1981;65:1121
63. Zeger G, Smith L, McQuiston D, et al. Transfusion 1988;28:493
64. Cinollo G, Dini G, Franchini E, et al. Cancer Chemotherap Pharmacol 1988;21:85
65. Salama A, Northoff H, Burkhardt H, et al. Br J Haematol 1988;68:479
66. Stefanini M, Johnson NL. Am J Med Sci 1970;259:49
67. Salama A, Mueller-Eckhardt C. Br J Haematol 1987;66:263
68. Wong KY, Boose GM, Issitt CH. J Pediat 1981;98:647
69. Pla RP, Martin VC, Odriozola J, et al. Rev Fr Transf Immunohematol 1976;19:379
70. Martinez-L.Letona J, Barbolla L, Frieyo E, et al. Br J Haematol 1977;35;561
71. Florendo NT, MacFarland D, Painter M, et al. Transfusion 1980;20:662
72. Serrano J. Sangre 1980;25:850
73. Fernandez MN, Barbolla L. Sangre 1980;25:871
74. Fernandez MN, Barbolla L. (Letter). Transfusion 1982;22:344
75. Bird GWG, Eeles GH, Litchfield JA, et al. Br Med J 1972;1;728
76. Malacarne P, Castaldi G, Bertusi M, et al. Diabetes 1977;26:156

77. Miescher P, Cooper N. Vox Sang 1960;5:138
78. Miescher P, Straessle R. Vox Sang 1966;11:38
79. Takahashi R, Tsukada T, Hasegawa M. Keio J Med 1963;12:161
80. Wenz B, Klein RL, Lalezari P. Transfusion 1974;14:265
81. Simpson MB, Pryzbylik J, Innis B. New Eng J Med 1985;312:840
82. Garratty G. In: A Seminar on Problems Encountered in Pretransfusion Tests. Washington, D.C.:Am Assoc Blood Banks, 1972:33
83. Judd WJ. Methods in Immunohematology, 2nd Ed. Durham:Montgomery, 1993
84. Kroovand SW, Kirtland H, Issitt CH. (abstract). Transfusion 1977;17:682
85. Garratty G, Brunt D. (abstract). Transfusion 1983;23;409
86. De Weck AL, Blum G. Int Arch Allgy 1965;27:221
87. Levine BB, Redmond AP, Fellner MJ, et al. J Clin Invest 1966;45:1895
88. Swanson MA, Chanmougan D, Schwartz RS. New Eng J Med 1966;274:178
89. Croft JD Jr, Swisher SN, Gilliland BC, et al. Ann Int Med 1968;68:176
90. Carstairs KC, Breckenridge A, Dollery CT, et al. Lancet 1966;2:133
91. Shulman NR. Ann Intern Med 1964;60:506
92. Peterson BH, Graham J. J Lab Clin Med 1974;83;860.
93. Orenstein AA, Yakulis V, Eipe J, et al. (Letter). Ann Intern Med 1977;86:450
94. Manor E, Marmor A, Kaufman S, et al. J Am Med Assoc 1976;236:2777
95. Bernasconi C, Berarida G, Pollini G, et al. Haematologica 1961;46:697
96. MacGibbon BH, Loughridge LW, Hourihane DOB, et al. Lancet 1960;1;7
97. Loghem JJ van. Lancet 1960;1:434
98. Bengtsson U, Ahlstedt S,Aurell M, et al. Acta Med Scand 1975;198:223
99. Shulman IA, Arndt PA, McGehee W, et al. Transfusion 1990;30:263
100. Garratty G, Nance S, Domen R. (abstract). Book of Abstracts. Joint Cong ISBT/AABB 1990:32
101. Wojcicki RE, Larson CJ, Pope ME, et al. (abstract). Book of Abstracts. Joint Cong ISBT/AABB 1990:33
102. Gallagher NT, Schergen AK, Sokol-Anderson ML, et al. (abstract). Book of Abstracts. Joint Cong ISBT/AABB 1990:33
103. Weitekamp LA, Johnson ST, Fueger JT, et al. (abstract). Book of Abstracts. Joint Cong ISBT/AABB 1990:33
104. Garratty G, Nance SJ, Lloyd M, et al. Transfusion 1992;32:269
105. Toy E, Nesbitt R, Savastano G, et al. (abstract). Transfusion 1989;29 (Suppl 7S):51S
106. Chambers LA, Donovan LM, Kruskall MS. Am J Clin Pathol 1991;95:393
107. Garratty G, Postoway N, Schwellenbach J, et al. Transfusion 1991;31:176
108. Salama A, Göttsche B, Schleiffer T, et al. Transfusion 1987;27:460
109. Garratty G. Lancet 1991;338:119
110. Lindberg LG, Norden A. Acta Med Scand 1961;170:195
111. Logue GL, Boyd AE, Rosse WF. New Eng J Med 1970;283:900
112. Sosler SD, Behzad O, Garratty G, et al. Transfusion 1984;24:206
113. Lay WH. Vox Sang 1966;11:601

114. Ribera A, Monasterio J, Acebedo G, et al. Vox Sang 1981;41:32
115. Vila J, Blum L, Dosik H. J Am Med Assoc 1976;236:1723
116. Garratty G, Houston M, Petz LD, et al. Am J Clin Pathol 1981;76:73
117. Criel AM, Hidajat M, Clarysse A, et al. Br J Haematol 1980;46:549
118. Faulk WP, Tomsovic EJ, Fudenberg HH. Am J Med 1970;49:133
119. Robinson MG, Foadi M. J Am Med Assoc 1969;208:656
120. Freedman J, Lim FC. Vox Sang 1978;35;126
121. Eyster ME. Ann Int Med 1967;66:573
122. Wooley PV, Sacher RA, Priego VM, et al. Br J Haematol 1983;54:543
123. Bournerias F, Habibi B. Lancet 1979;20:95
124. Prescott LF, Illingworth RN, Critchley JAJH, et al. Br Med J 1980;281:1392
125. Habibi B, Cartron J-P, Bretagne M, et al. Vox Sang 1981;40:79
126. Lylloff K, Jersild C, Bacher T, et al. Lancet 1982;2:41
127. Muirhead EE, Halden ER, Groves M. Arch Int Med 1958;101:87
128. Dacie JV. Proc Roy Soc Med 1962;55:28
129. Dausset J, Contu L. Vox Sang 1964;9:599
130. Sosler SD, Behzad O, Garatty G, et al. (abstract). Transfusion 1979;19:640
131. Bolton FG. Blood 1956;11:547
132. Freedman AL, Barr PS, Brody EA. Am J Med 1956;20:806
133. Shulman NR. J Exp Med 1958;107:711
134. Bell CA, Zwicker H, Lee S, et al. Transfusion 1973;13:100
135. Ballas SK, Caro JF, Miguel O. Transfusion 1978;18:215
136. Zeigler Z, Shadduck RK, Winkelstein A, et al. Blood 1979;53:396
137. Steinkamp R, Moore CV, Doubek WG. J Lab Clin Med 1955;45:18
138. Kissmeyer-Nielsen F. Acta Med Scand 1956;154:289
139. Homberg JC, Pujet JC, Salmon C. Scand J Resp Dis 1973;84 (Suppl):36
140. Schubothe H, Weber S. Scand J Resp Dis 1973;84 (Suppl):53
141. Worlledge SM. Scand J Resp Dis 1973;84 (Suppl):60
142. Lakshminarayan S, Sahn SA, Judson LD. B Med J Clin Res 1973;2:282
143. Criel A, Vervilghen RL. Blut 1980;40:147
144. Ackroyd JF. Clin Sci 1949;7:249
145. Ackroyd JF. Clin Sci 1949;8:235
146. Ackroyd JF. Clin Sci 1949;8:269
147. Ackroyd JF. Clin Sci 1951;10:185
148. Ackroyd JF. Proc Roy Soc Med 1962;55:30
149. Ackroyd JF. In: Clinical Aspects of Immunology, 3rd Ed. Oxford:Blackwell, 1975
150. Nachman R, Javid D, Krauss S. Arch Int Med 1962;110:187
151. Salama A, Mueller-Eckhardt C. New Eng J Med 1985;313:469
152. Worlledge SM. Sem Hematol 1973;10:327
153. Habibi B, Lopez M, Serdaru M, et al. New Eng J Med 1982;306:1091
154. Takahashi H, Tsukada T. Scand J Haematol 1979;23:169
155. Jordan JV, Smith ME, Reid DM, et al. (abstract). Blood 1985;66 (Suppl):104a
156. Beris P, Miescher PA. Sem Hematol 1988;25:123
157. Christie DJ, Mullen PC, Aster RH. J Clin Invest 1985;75:310
158. Sanford-Driscoll M, Knodel J. Drug Intel Clin Pharm 1986;20:925
159. Smith ME, Jordan JV Jr, Reig DM, et al. J Clin Invest 1987;79:912
160. Mueller-Eckhardt C, Salama A. Transf Med Rev 1990;4:69
161. Salama A, Göttsche B, Mueller-Eckhardt C. Br J Haematol 1990;77:546
162. Salama A, Mueller-Eckhardt C. Sem Hematol 1992;29:54
163. Petz LD, Fudenberg HH. Prog Hematol 1975;9:185
164. Sirchia G, Murcuriali F, Ferrone S. Experienta 1968;24:495
165. Ferrone S, Zanella A, Mercuriali F, et al. Eur J Pharmacol 1968;4:211
166. Jamin D, Demers J, Shulman I, et al. Blood 1986;67:993
167. Jamin D, Shulman I, Lam HT, et al. Arch Pathol Lab Med 1988;112:898
168. Mine Y, Nishida M. J Antibiot 1970;23:575
169. Kosaki N, Miyakawa G. Postgrad Med J 1970;46:107
170. Kuwahara S, Mine Y, Nishida M. Antimicrob Ag Chemothpy 1970;10:374
171. De Torres OH. Drug Intell Clin Pharm 1983;17:816
172. Carstairs KC, Worlledge S, Dollery CT, et al. Lancet 1966;1:201
173. Worlledge SM, Carstairs KC, Dacie JV. Lancet 1966;2:135
174. Breckenridge A, Dollery CT, Worlledge SM, et al. Lancet 1967;2:1265
175. LoBuglio AF, Jandl JH. New Eng J Med 1967;276:658
176. Worlledge SM. Br J Haematol 1969;16:5
177. Worlledge SM. In: Blood Disorders Due to Drugs and Other Agents. Amsterdam:Excerpta Medica, 1973:11
178. Darnborough J. Lancet 1966;1:262
179. Hayes D. Lancet 1966;1:365
180. Schwartz M, Dige-Peterson H. Lancet 1966;1:434
181. Hamilton M, Jenkins GC, Turnbull AL. Lancet 1966;1:549
182. Ewing DJ, Hughes CJ, Wardle DR. Guy's Hosp Rev 1968;117:111
183. Dacie JV, Worlledge SM. Prog Hematol 1969;6:82
184. Dacie JV. Arch Int Med 1976;135:1293
185. Issitt PD, Pavone BG, Goldfinger D, et al. Br J Haematol 1976;34;5
186. Snyder EL, Spivak M. Transfusion 1979;19:313
187. Henry RE, Goldberg LS, Sturgeon P, et al. Vox Sang 1971;20:306
188. Joseph C. New Eng J Med 1972;286:1401
189. Gabor EP, Goldberg LS. Scand J Haematol 1973;2:201
190. Territo MC, Peters RW, Tanaka RT. J Am Med Assoc 1973;226:1347
191. Lindström FD, Lieden G, Engström MS. Ann Int Med 1977;86:298
192. Bernstein RM. Br Med J 1979;1:1461
193. Scott GL, Myles AB, Bacon PA. Br Med J 1968;2:534
194. Farid NR, Johnson RJ, Low WT. Lancet 1971;2:382
195. Robertson JH, Kennedy CC, Hill CM. Ire J Med Sci 1971;140:226
196. Beutler E. J Am Med Assoc 1964;189:143
197. Blomgren SE, Condemi JJ, Vaughan JH. Am J Med 1972;52:338
198. Jones GW, George TL, Bradley RD. Transfusion 1978;18:224
199. Kornberg A, Rachmilewitz E. Arch Int Med 1981;141:1388
200. Schifman RB, Garewal H, Shillington D. Am J Clin Pathol 1983;80:66
201. Kleinman S, Nelson R, Smith L, et al. New Eng J Med 1984;311:809
202. Tregellas WM, South SF. (abstract). Transfusion 1980;20:647
203. Micouin C, Bensa J-C, Schweitzer B. Nou Press Med 1978;43:3938
204. Russell ML, Schachter RK. Acta Med Scand 1981;210:431
205. Korsager S. Br Med J 1978;1:79
206. Law IP, Wickmann CJ, Harrison BR. South Med J 1979;72:707

207. Guidry JB, Ogburn CL, Griffin FM. J Am Med Assoc 1979;242:68
208. Petz LD, Gitlin N, Grant K, et al. J Clin Gastroenterol 1983;5:405
209. Kessey EC, Pierce S, Beck ML, et al. (abstract). Transfusion 1973;13:360
210. Patten E, Beck CE, Scholl C, et al. Transfusion 1977;17:517
211. Sherman JD, Love DE, Harrington JF. Arch Int Med 1967;120:321
212. Feltkamp TEW, Engelfriet CP, Loghem JJ van. (Letter). Lancet 1968;1:644
213. Harth M. Canad Med Assoc J 1968;99:277
214. Mackay IR, Cowling DC, Hurley TH. Med J Austral 1968;2:1047
215. Hunter E, Raik E, Gordon S, et al. Med J Austral 1971;2:810
216. Perry MH Jr, Chaplin H Jr, Carmody S, et al. J Lab Clin Med 1971;78:905
217. Devereux S, Fisher DM, Roter BLT, et al. Br J Haematol 1983;54:485
218. Wurzel HA, Silverman JL. Transfusion 1968;8:84
219. Gottlieb AJ, Wurzel HA. Blood 1974;43:85
220. Vyas GN, Sassetti RJ, Petz LD, et al. Br J Haematol 1969;16:137
221. Seedat YK, Vawada EI. Lancet 1968;1:427
222. Burns-Cox CJ. Lancet 1970;2:673
223. Chen BTM, Ooi BS. Lancet 1971;1;87
224. Habibi B. In: Alloimmune and Autoimmune Cytopenias. London:Baillière Tindall, 1987:343
225. Petz LD. Transf Med Rev 1993;7:242
226. Weigle WO. J Exp Med 1965;121:289
227. Weigle WO. Ann NY Acad Sci 1965;124:133
228. Dameshek W. New Eng J Med 1967;276:1382
229. Allison AC, Denman AM, Barnes RD. Lancet 1971;1:135
230. Kirtland HH, Mohler DN. Blood 1977;50:295
231. Kirtland HH, Horwitz DA, Mohler DN. Blood 1978;52:151
232. Kirtland HH, Mohler DN, Horwitz DA. New Eng J Med 1980;302:825
233. Nance SJ, Ladisch S, Williamson TL, et al. Vox Sang 1988;55:233
234. Gmus J, Walti M, Neftel KA. Acta Haematol 1985;74:230
235. Garratty G. Transf Med Rev 1993;7:255
236. Shirey RS, Bartholomew J, Bell W, et al. Transfusion 1988;28:70
237. Woodliff HJ, Wallace PF. (Letter). Med J Austral 1986;144:163
238. Fulton JD, Briggs JD, Dominiczak AF, et al. Scott Med J 1986;31:242
239. Bloomfield RJ, Wilson IF. Ann Intern Med 1986;105:807
240. Sosler SD, Behzad O, Garratty G, et al. Am J Clin Pathol 1985;84:391
241. Kickler TS, Buck S, Ness P, et al. J Rheumatol 1986;13:208
242. Kopicky JA, Packman CH. Am J Hematol 1986;23:283
243. Murphy WG, Kelton JG. Blood Rev 1988;2:36
244. van Bleek RJ, Bieger R, den Ottolander GJ. Scand J Haematol 1978;21:150
245. Kramer MR, Levene C, Hershko C. Scand J Haematol 1986;36:118
246. Chan-Lam D, Thorburn AW, Chalmers EA, et al. Br Med J 1986;293:1474
247. Shirey RS, Morton SJ, Lawton KB, et al. Am J Clin Pathol 1988;89:410
248. Johnson FP Jr, Hamilton HE, Liesch MR. Arch Int Med 1985;145:1515
249. Mintz PD, Anderson G, Clark S. Arch Int Med 1986;146:1639
250. Miescher PA, Pola W. Drugs 1986;32 (Suppl 4):90
251. Patmas MA, Willborn SL, Shankel SW. Arch Int Med 1984;144:519
252. Martlew VJ. J Clin Pathol 1986;39:1147
253. Rotoli B, Formisano S, Alfinito F. Lancet 1979;2:583
254. Eisner EV, Shahidi NT. New Eng J Med 1972;287:376
255. Salama A, Mueller-Eckhardt C, Kissel K, et al. Br J Haematol 1984;58:525
256. Kiefel V, Santoso S, Schmidt S, et al. Transfusion 1987;27:262
257. Salama A, Burger M, Mueller-Eckhardt C. Blut 1989;58:59
258. Christie DJ. Transf Med Rev 1993;7:230
259. Salama A, Schütz B, Kiefel V, et al. Br J Haematol 1989;72:127
260. Lipsky PE, Ginsburg WW, Finkelman FD, et al. J Immunol 1978;120:902
261. Garratty G, Arndt P, Prince H, et al. (abstract). Blood 1986;68 (Suppl):108a
262. Garratty G, Arndt P, Prince HE, et al. Br J Haematol 1993;84:310
263. Branch DR, Gallagher MT, Shulman IA, et al. Vox Sang 1983;45:278
264. Green FA, Jung CY, Rampal A, et al. Clin Exp Immunol 1980;40:554
265. Green FA, Jung CY, Hui H. Biochem Biophys Res Comm 1980;95:1037
266. Rubin RL. In: Autoimmunity and Toxicology. New York:Elsevier, 1989:119
267. Gold EF, Ben-Efraim S, Faivisewitz A, et al. Clin Immunol Immunopathol 1977;7:176
268. Schoen RT, Trentham DE. Am J Med 1981;71:5
269. Cornacchia E, Golbus J, Maybaum J, et al. J Immunol 1986;140:2197
270. Seeman P. Pharmacol Rev 1972;24:583
271. Bluestein HG, Weisman MH, Zvaifler N, et al. Lancet 1979;2:816
272. Bluestein HG, Redelman D, Zvaifler NJ. Arthr Rheum 1981;24:1019
273. Miller KB, Salem D. Am J Med 1982;73:487
274. Ochi T, Goldings EA, Lipsky PE, et al. J Clin Invest 1983;71;36
275. De Boccardo G, Drayer D, Rubin AL, et al. Clin Exp Immunol 1985;59:69
276. Yu C-L, Ziff M. Arthr Rheum 1985;28:276
277. Bakemeier RF, Leddy JP. Blood 1968;32:1
278. Meulen FW van der, Hart M van der, Fleer A, et al. Br J Haematol 1978;38:541
279. Meulen FW van der, Bruin HG de, Goosen PCM, et al. Br J Haematol 1980;46:47
280. Garratty G, Nance SJ. Transfusion 1990;30:617
281. Lalezari P, Louie JE, Fadlallah N. Blood 1982;59:61
282. Kelton JG. New Eng J Med 1985;313:596
283. Habibi B. (Letter). Br J Haematol 1983;54:493
284. Mueller-Eckhardt C. In: Alloimmune and Autoimmune Cytopenias. London:Baillière Tindall, 1987:369
285. de Gruchy GC. Drug-Induced Blood Disorders. Oxford:Blackwell, 1975
286. Marcus GJ, Stevenson M. Am J Clin Pathol 1975;64:113
287. Lundh B, Hasselgran KH. Acta Med Scand 1979;628 (Suppl):73
288. Manohitharaja S, Jenkins WJ, Roberts PD, et al. Br Med J 1979;1:494
289. Dupont A, Six R. Br Med J 1980;285:693
290. Goldstein GB, Lam KC, Mistilis SP. Dig Dis Sci 1973;18:177
291. Hoyumpa AM, Connell AM. Dig Dis Sci 1973;18:213
292. Toghill PJ, Smith PG, Benton P. Br Med J 1974;3:545

293. Schweitzer IL, Peters RL. Gastroenterology 1974;66:1203

294. Seggie J, Saunders SJ, Kirsch RE. Afr Med J 1974;55:75

295. Maddrey WC, Boitnott JK. Gastroenterology 1975;68:351

296. Rodman JS, Deutch DJ, Gutman SI. Am J Med 1976;60:941

297. Maddrey WC, Boitnott JK. Gastroenterology 1977;72:1348

298. Hyer SL, Knell AJ. Br Med J 1977;1:879

299. Zimmerman HJ. Drugs 1978;16:25

300. Sherlock S. Diseases of the Liver and Biliary System, 6th Ed. Oxford:Blackwell, 1981:305

301. Shalev O, Mosseri M, Ariel I, et al. Arch Int Med 1983;143:592

302. Costias GC, Papavasiliou PS. J Am Med Assoc 1969;207:1353

303. LoBuglio AF, Masouredis SP, Pisciotta AV, et al. Clin Res 1969;17:333

304. Beck RJJ van, Bieger R, Holander GJ den. Scand J Haematol 1978;21:150

305. Wang RIH, Schuller G. Am Heart J 1969;78:282

306. Kottinen YP, Tuominen L. Lancet 1971;2:925

307. Dubois EL. J Rheum 1975;2:204

308. Bluming AZ, Plotkin D, Rosen P, et al. J Am Med Assoc 1976;236:2520

309. Weitzman SA, Stossel TP, Desmond M. Lancet 1978;1:1068

310. Rothman IK, Arorose E. Arch Intern Med 1979;139:246

311. Rosenstein R, Kosfeld RE, Leight L, et al. Am J Hematol 1984;16:181

312. Yomtovian R, Kline W, Press C, et al. (abstract). Blood 1984;64 (Suppl):92a

313. International Granulocytosis and Aplastic Anemia Study. J Am Med Assoc 1986;256:1749

314. Stroncek D. Transf Med Rev 1993;7:268

315. Alarcon-Segovia D. Mayo Clin Proc 1969;44:664

316. Dubois EL. Medicine 1969;48:217

317. Tuffanelli DL. Arch Dermatol 1972;106:553

318. Blomgren SE. Sem Hematol 1973;10:345

319. Geltman EM, Gelfand ML. J Am Med Women Assoc 1975;30:343

320. Henningsen NC, Cederberg A, Hanson A, et al. Acta Med Scand 1975;198:475

321. Lee SL, Chase PH. Sem Arth Rheum 1975;5:83

322. Meisner DJ, Carlson RJ, Gottlieb AJ. Arch Int Med 1985;145:700

323. McFarland JG. Transf Med Rev 1993;7:275

324. Bird GWG, Wingham J, Babb RG, et al. Vox Sang 1984;46:336

325. Gallagher NT, Schergen AK, Sokol-Anderson ML, et al. Transfusion 1992;32:266

326. Muirhead EE, Groves M, Guy R, et al. Vox Sang 1959;4:277

327. Hart MN, Mesara BW. Am J Clin Pathol 1969;52:695

328. Squires JE, Mintz PD, Clark S. Transfusion 1985;25:410

329. Djik BA van, Rico PB, Hoitsma A, et al. Transfusion 1989;29:638

330. Kitigawa M, Yagi Y, Pressman D. J Immunol 1965;95:455

331. Duran-Suarez JR, Martin-Vega C, Argelagues E, et al. Vox Sang 1981;41:313

332. Habibi B, Basty R, Chodez S, et al. New Eng J Med 1985;312:353

333. Sandvei P, Nordhagen R, Michaelsen TE, et al. Br J Haematol 1987;65:357

334. Pereira A, Sanz C, Cervantes F, et al. Ann Hematol 1991;63:56

335. Habibi B, Bretagne Y. C R Acad Sci (D) Paris 1992;296:693

336. Judd WJ, Steiner EA, Cochran RK. Transfusion 1982;22:31

337. Halima D, Garratty G, Bueno R. Transfusion 1982;22:521

338. Eckrich RJ, Fox S, Mallory D. (abstract). Transfusion 1989:29

339. (Suppl 7S):17S

Tahan SR, Diamond JR, Blank JM, et al. Transfusion 1985;25:124

340. Lenes BA, Issitt PD, Ahn Y, et al. Unpublished observations 1986

341. Chong BH. Blood Rev 1988;2;108

342. Christie DJ, Lennon SS. Transfusion 1988;28:322

343. Aster RH, George JN. In: Hematology, 4th Ed. New York:McGraw Hill, 1990:1370

344. Warkentin TE, Kelton JG. Hematol-Oncol Clin North Am 1990;4:243

345. Christie DJ, van Buren N, Lennon SS, et al. Blood 1990;75:518

346. Visentin GP, Wolfmeyer K, Newmann PF, et al. Transfusion 1990;30:694

347. Chong BH. Platelets 1991;2:173

348. Nieminen U, Kekomaki R. Br J Haematol 1992;80:77

349. Anderson GP. Br J Haematol 1992;80:504

350. Pisciotta AV. Am J Hematol 1993;42:132

351. Nataas OB, Nesthus I. Br Med J 1987;295:366

352. Lutz P, Dzik W. (abstract). Transfusion 1992;32 (Suppl 8S):23S

353. Schwartz RS, Costea N. Sem Hematol 1966;3:2

354. Slugg PH, Kunkel RS. J Am Med Assoc 1970;213:297

355. Salama A, Mueller-Eckhardt C. Blood 1986;68:1285

356. Shirey RS, Kickler TS, Wiegman FL, et al. (abstract). Transfusion 1987;27:515

357. Weitekamp LA, Johnson ST, Fueger JT, et al. (abstract). Transfusion 1992;32 (Suppl 8S):54S

358. Schulenberg BJ, Beck ML, Pierce SR, et al. (abstract). Transfusion 1983;23:409

359. Petz LD, Mueller-Eckhardt C. Transfusion 1992;32;202

360. Wolf B, Conradty M, Grohmann R, et al. J Clin Psychiat 1989;50:99

361. Walz B, Zupnick J, Uden D, et al. West J Med 1988;149:460

362. Borne AEGKr von dem. In: Bailliere's Clinical Immunology and Allergy. London:Bailliere Tindal, 1987:269

363. Aster RH. In: Platelet Immunobiology. Philadelphia:Lippincott, 1989:387

364. Mueller-Eckhardt C. In: Transfusion Medicine in the 1990s. Arlington, VA:Am Assoc Blood Banks, 1990:63

365. Waters AH. Sem Hematol 1992;29:18

366. Shulman NR, Reid DM. In: Hemostasis and Thrombosis, 3rd Ed. Philadelphia:Lippincott, 1994:414

367. Lilleyman JS. In: Thrombocytopenia in Childhood. Basel:Editones Roche, 1994:141

368. Mueller-Eckhardt C. In: Autoimmune Disorders of Blood. Bethesda:Am Assoc Blood Banks, 1996:115

369. Vengelen-Tyler V. Ed. Technical Manual, 12th Ed. Bethesda:Am Assoc Blood Banks, 1996:404

370. Shinton NK, Wilson C. Lancet 1960;1:226

371. Dausset J, Bergerto-Blondel Y. Vox Sang 1961;6:91

372. Jacobson ES. Ann Int Med 1972;77:73

373. Harris JW. J Lab Clin Med 1954;44:809.

374. de Torregrosa MVV, Rosada Rodrigues AL, Montilla E. J Am Med Assoc 1963;186:598

375. Weiss HJ, Burger RE, Tice AD, et al. Am J Med Sci 1972;264:375

376. Tajima H. Acta Haematol Jpn 1960;23:188

377. Ley AB, Cahan A, Mayer K. Bibl Haematol 1959;10:539

378. Mickley H, Svensen PG. Scand J Haematol 1984;32:323

379. Gralnick HR, McGinniss MH. Nature 1967;215:1026

380. Petz LD. J Infect Dis 1978;137:S74

381. Mueller-Eckhardt C, Salama A. Dt Arzteblatt 1987;84:232

382. Garratty G, Arndt PA. Br J Haematol, in press 1998

41 | Hemolytic Disease of the Newborn

When a pregnant woman's serum contains a clinically significant IgG blood group antibody directed against an antigen on the red cells of her unborn child, some of that antibody may enter the fetal circulation via placental transfer and may cause destruction of fetal red cells. The resultant disease is called hemolytic disease of the newborn (HDN) or erythroblastosis fetalis. At worst, the anemia or consequences thereof, may result in death of the fetus in utero. Such infants are often grossly edematous and are said to have hydrops fetalis. Before Rh immune globulin was developed to prevent the formation of anti-D by D- women who deliver D+ infants (see below), HDN caused by anti-D was relatively common. It was estimated (1) that the rate of stillbirths due to HDN might be as high as 1% in women with anti-D in the serum. At the other extreme, red cell destruction may be limited enough that no treatment of the fetus in utero or the infant following birth may be necessary. Obviously, degrees of severity between these two extremes are seen. For reasons discussed below, treatment of severely affected infants must begin immediately after birth. Accordingly, an important role for the transfusion service is recognition of women at risk of producing infants with severe HDN and the provision of suitable blood for exchange transfusion as soon as the infant is born. On other occasions, the blood banker will have to provide suitable blood for in utero transfusion of a severely affected fetus (again see below).

The transfer of IgG antibody from mother to fetus is a normal physiological event and is essential as regards antibodies other than those directed against red cells. Mechanisms of immunoglobulin synthesis are not fully developed at birth (2-18) so that transferred maternal antibodies are necessary for protection against various infections for the first few weeks of the infant's life.

The mechanism of in vivo red cell clearance, when a blood group antibody causes HDN, is the extravascular one described in Chapter 6. Indeed HDN can be thought of as a form of warm antibody-induced hemolytic anemia, albeit one caused by an alloantibody not an autoantibody. That is to say, in HDN the antibody is made in the mother and red cell destruction occurs in the fetus. Thus the hemolysis in a newborn infant is limited. Following birth, no further supply of antibody will reach the infant's circulation so that management of the infant through the acute hemolytic episode will effect a total cure, if treatment is prompt and complete enough to prevent the complications that can result from gross red cell destruction in a newborn. Those complications are described more fully below.

History

Cases of what can in retrospect be seen to have been HDN, were described in the literature (19-23) long before the etiology of the disorder was understood. As reviewed by Zimmerman (24) the variety of clinical symptoms in infants with HDN delayed recognition of the fact that they have a common cause. In 1939, Levine and Stetson (25) first suggested that the disease is caused by a fetal-maternal blood group incompatibility. Although that suggestion might now appear to be the obvious one to make, in 1939 it was much more difficult to formulate as a hypothesis and very hard to support with serological findings. The reason was that in 1939, the only blood group antibodies that could be readily recognized were those that caused agglutination of red cells in saline. As is now known, HDN is caused by IgG antibodies, the majority of which do not act as saline-active agglutinins. In spite of this, in 1941 Levine et al. (26,27) described cases in which the mothers were shown to have serum antibodies that reacted with the infants' red cells and with those of the fathers of the infants. These observations provided support for the concept that the mother could become immunized to an antigen on the infant's red cells, that was present on those cells because of inheritance by the infant of a paternal gene. In retrospect it can be guessed that maternal IgM anti-D, that played no role in the hemolytic disease of the infants, was the antibody detected. Nevertheless, the IgM anti-D served as a marker in women immunized to D (both women studied undoubtedly had potent IgG anti-D as well but there was not yet a test for demonstration of that antibody) and thus provided support for the concept advanced. Again in retrospect, it can be seen that the theory advanced by Levine and Stetson (25) was remarkable for its extraordinary accuracy in forecasting the existence and actions of a large group of antibodies (IgG, non-agglutinins) before any in vitro method for their detection existed. Once methods were devised (28-33) that permitted the detection and identification of incomplete IgG antibodies, the theory of Levine and Stetson (25) about the cause of HDN, was seen to be entirely correct.

Maternal Immunization and HDN

Since HDN is caused by the placental transfer of maternal IgG antibody to the fetus, it follows that affected infants will be born of immunized women. At first, this would seem to suggest that ABO HDN would be very common. In fact, maternal IgG anti-A, anti-B and anti-A,B can be detected in the sera of most newborn infants but, for reasons discussed in more detail below, those antibodies only occasionally cause clinical HDN. When antibodies made in response to the introduction of foreign red cells are considered, it is found that HDN seldom occurs in the first pregnancy of women who have never received a blood transfusion. Although there is ample evidence (34-56) that fetal red cells enter the circulation of many pregnant women during pregnancy, immunization and the production of enough antibody that the first child has HDN is rare. The major contributing factor to this finding seems to be that the volumes of fetal red cells that enter the maternal circulation during pregnancy are usually too small to act as efficient immunizing doses. It is also possible that during pregnancy, the mother may have a degree of immunological tolerance towards antigens on the cells of her fetus. However, there is not much evidence to support this concept and if partial tolerance exists at all it is clear (see below) that it does extend beyond the time of delivery. Obviously, in women who have been transfused there is a greater chance that the first child will have HDN. In some 0.5 to 1% of transfused women, a blood group antibody will be formed and may cause HDN if the fetus's red cells carry the antigen against which it is directed. In others, the transfusion may have resulted in primary immunization to a blood group antigen so that although serologically detectable antibody may not be present, primed B cells may exist within the woman's immune system. While the small volumes of fetal cells that enter the maternal circulation during pregnancy seldom initiate a primary immune response, they may cause a secondary response and the production of detectable antibody in a woman in whom primary immunization had already occurred. When antibodies such as those directed against Rh antigens other than D, or against antigens of the Kell, Duffy and Kidd systems are found in the sera of pregnant women, a history of previous transfusion is common (57-63).

The above discussion illustrates clearly why women of child-bearing age and girls who will later reach child-bearing age, who are D-, must not be transfused with D+ blood. As discussed in Chapter 12, some 80% of D- persons who are transfused with one or more units of D+ blood, form anti-D. Since 85% of random males are D+, it follows that the chance of an immunized D- woman marrying a D+ male is high. Since potent anti-D can cause hydrops fetalis, it follows that a D- woman immunized to D by transfusion may, at worst, never be able to bear a live child. Most blood bankers are aware that when D- donor blood is in short supply, those units available must be reserved for female patients who might later bear children. This consid-

eration applies to transfusions with products other than red cells. For example, when platelets from D+ donors are transfused to a D- female who may later be capable of bearing children, the use of Rh immune globulin (RhIG) must be considered. The volume of red cells present in the platelet concentrates should be calculated so that an appropriate dose of RhIG can be used. If only RhIG suitable for intramuscular injection is available it should be given soon after the transfusion, when the platelet count is at its highest, so that the risk of bleeding into the tissues is reduced. If RhIG suitable for intravenous injection is available, its use is obviously preferable in this setting. RhIG can be used to prevent immunization by the D+ red cells, it will not interfere with the platelets infused since those cells do not carry D (64-68). There seems to be no danger of stimulating a primary immune response to D in D- persons transfused with plasma from D+ donors if that plasma has previously been frozen. As discussed in Chapter 12, previously frozen plasma from D+ donors may provoke a secondary immune response in a D- person already immunized to D (69) and unfrozen plasma may contain sufficient intact D+ red cells to initiate a primary response (70).

On those rare occasions that D+ blood is transfused by accident to a D- woman of child-bearing age, prevention of immunization to D can be accomplished by the use of large doses of RhIG (71-73). There are a number of points to consider. First, the amount of RhIG needed can be greatly reduced by performing a partial exchange transfusion with D- blood before the RhIG is injected. Second, the use of RhIG prepared for intravenous injection will result in the injection of less material and in less discomfort for the patient, than if the material prepared for intramuscular injection is used. Third, if a partial exchange transfusion is not feasible and if RhIG for intravenous use is not available, it may be desirable to divide the dose for intramuscular injection. The injections can then be given at different sites at the same time (71) or can be given over a period of two or three days. Fourth, if large volumes of D+ blood are to be destroyed in a previously anemic patient, supportive red cell transfusion may become necessary (obviously partial exchange transfusion before the RhIG is injected, is preferable). When RhIG is used to prevent immunization following the inadvertent transfusion of D+ blood to a D- woman, it seems that the primary mechanism involved is rapid clearance of the D+ red cells. This may be different to the way in which RhIG acts when injected into a D- woman who has just delivered a D+ child (see below). The use of RhIG following the accidental transfusion of D+ blood and indeed the use of D- blood for transfusion to women of child-bearing age should not be undertaken without thought. One of us (PDI) has encountered more than one physician who adamantly demanded D- blood for a non-immunized patient about to undergo hysterectomy! Obviously reason must prevail, prevention of immunization to D must be based on the female patient's age *and* her potential later to bear children.

The stress on prevention of immunization to D is based on two major considerations. First, as already discussed, the D antigen is highly immunogenic in D- individuals. Second, before RhIG was available, when immunization to D via pregnancy was common, it was found that anti-D was by far the most common cause of severe HDN. Of all infants with severe enough HDN that some form of transfusion was required, 90 to 95% were D+ infants born to women with potent anti-D (sometimes in the form of anti-CD or anti-CDE) in the serum (71,74,75). Further, when in utero death of the fetus occurred, anti-D was responsible over 99% of the time.

The volume of fetal red cells that enters the maternal circulation at the time of delivery is considerably greater than the volume that enters during the pregnancy (47,76-82). The physical act of delivery can result in a transplacental hemorrhage of fetal cells into the maternal circulation. Again before RhIG became available, the effects of the transfer of fetal cells to the mother were clearly demonstrable. In a few women, primary immunization presumably occurred during the pregnancy but serologically demonstrable antibody was not present at the time of delivery of the first infant. The larger volume of fetal cells, to which the mother was exposed at delivery, acted as a secondary immunizing dose and serologically demonstrable anti-D was found in the mother's blood some days or weeks after delivery of her first D+ child. Much more often, the larger volume of fetal cells that entered the maternal circulation at delivery resulted in primary immunization. In such women, anti-D was not made during the first pregnancy nor in the months following delivery. However, the antibody did appear during the second pregnancy with a D+ fetus. As already pointed out, the volumes of fetal cells that enter the maternal circulation during pregnancy are usually sufficient to cause a secondary but too small to cause a primary immune response. Thus it was apparent that primary immunization had occurred at the time of delivery of the first D+ child and that serologically demonstrable anti-D was made when the maternal immune system was challenged with D during the second pregnancy. As described below, it is the fact that in most women primary immunization to D occurs following delivery, that makes the postpartum use of RhIG so effective. However, as also discussed below, a minority of women become immunized during pregnancy. Accordingly, most obstetric services (at least in the USA) now use RhIG during pregnancy, in D- women, to prevent that immunization as well.

Immunization to D Via Pregnancy

As mentioned above and as discussed in more detail below, immunization to D in D- women who bear D+ infants can now largely be prevented by the injection of RhIG. Before this therapeutic agent was developed, fetal-maternal immunization resulted in the production of anti-D (or anti-CD or anti-CDE) far more often than in the production of any other antibody (75). For reasons discussed in the previous section, the appearance of serologically demonstrable anti-D during a first pregnancy in women who had never been transfused was an uncommon event and was seen (71,83) in less than 1% of women at risk (i.e., D- women carrying a D+ fetus). In D- women who delivered two or more D+ infants and in whom Rh immune globulin was not used, some 15 to 20% made anti-D (84-86). Again for reasons discussed in the previous section, some 50% of women who become immunized to D by pregnancy, form the antibody during their second D+ pregnancy (87). Although, as stated above, the incidence of detection of anti-D in never transfused D- women, during a first pregnancy was seen to be less than 1%, it was clearly demonstrated (88) that primary immunization to D occurs in between 1 and 2% of D- women carrying a D+ fetus during pregnancy, not after delivery. Again, this observation is discussed more fully below in the section on the prevention of immunization to D.

Unexpected Forms of Immunization

In the past, relatively small volumes of blood from one person, were injected into others in a practice known as heterohemotherapy (it was believed that immunity to disease could be passively transferred). Not surprisingly, cases of immunization and later, HDN, followed this practice (89,90). It might be expected that this form of immunization would no longer be seen. Unfortunately, other similar forms have taken its place. There are documented cases (91-95) in which the use of syringes, that have become contaminated with blood, for the injection of illegal drugs; "blood brotherhood" rituals; and the exchange of blood for "emotional-gratification" purposes, have resulted in immunization and subsequently in HDN. As mentioned in Chapter 12, other cases of immunization via these routes have been seen but not documented in the literature since the situations are now well recognized.

Prevention of Immunization to D

Levine (96,97) first noticed that immunization to D in D- women who deliver D+ infants is less common when the fetal red cells are incompatible with an ABO system antibody in the mother's plasma than when they are compatible. This observation was confirmed by others (98-100) although Vos (101) felt that the amount of anti-D made was more affected than the event. It was reasoned (102) that the protective effect of ABO incompatibility was related to the rate of clearance of the fetal red cells from the maternal circulation. When group A D+ fetal red cells enter the circulation of a group O D- woman, those cells are rapidly destroyed by the woman's anti-A. Thus they comprise a single immunogenic challenge. When group O D+ fetal red cells enter the circulation of a group O D- woman, whose serum does not contain anti-D, they survive normally. A few cells are removed from the woman's circulation each day as they reach the end of their normal life span. Thus the entry of a volume of group O D+ fetal cells into the circulation of the group O D- woman will result in a series of small immunizing doses (as a few cells are removed each day) over a period of months. As discussed in Chapter 2, a series of small immunizing doses is more likely to initiate antibody production than is a single dose. These observations are particularly important when it is remembered that predominant entry of fetal cells into the maternal circulation occurs, in terms of an appreciable volume of cells, as a single event at the time of delivery. Three groups of workers, two in the USA and one in England reasoned (103-105) that if anti-D was injected into D- women who had delivered D+ infants, soon after birth, it might act to clear the D+ fetal cells before they could initiate an immune response and thus provide protection against immunization in a similar manner to that apparently afforded by ABO antibodies. As workers now know, the protection afforded by anti-D (in the form of RhIG) is far more complete than that occasioned by ABO antibodies and the actual mechanism of action of the two is rather different (see below). Trials were initiated in D- male volunteers who were injected with D+ red cells. In one trial (106) some of the males were then given plasma containing anti-D while the controls were left untreated. In another (107) a concentrated form of IgG anti-D was used instead of plasma. It was found (106-108) that with remarkably few exceptions, the passive administration of anti-D prevented immunization to D. In the control series the expected numbers of males exposed to D+ red cells made antibody. Clinical trials were then undertaken in D- women who delivered D+ infants. From the numerous reports that have appeared (107,109-134) it is clear that immunization to D following delivery of a D+ child, can be prevented in 98 to 99% of women providing a suitable quantity of RhIG is injected relatively soon after delivery of the child. In the USA the standard dose comprises circa 250 to 300 μg IgG anti-D, that amount being sufficient to prevent immunization in women exposed to about 15 ml of fetal red cells (i.e., up to about 25 to 30 ml fetal whole blood). In

Europe the standard dose is often smaller, circa 100 to 150 μg IgG anti-D but is still largely efficient since the transfer of fetal red cells to the mother does not often exceed 5 ml (8 to 10 ml whole blood) in normal deliveries. In any service that provides Rh immune globulin for D- women, a method to detect the fact that a larger than usual fetal to maternal hemorrhage has occurred, must be used (see below). In such circumstances, an additional quantity of RhIG must be injected in order that immunization be prevented. Mollison et al. (71) point out that when RhIG is injected intramuscularly, a good rule of thumb is that 20 μg of anti-D should be given for each 1 ml of D+ red cells present. Although 20 μg of anti-D per 1 ml of D+ red cells appears to be sufficient to prevent immunization to D, it has been suggested (135) that 25 μg anti-D/1 ml D+ red cells be used to provide a safety margin. As most workers are aware, RhIG is IgG anti-D. The injection of IgM anti-D in the circumstances described, does not prevent immunization to D.

In the trials on male volunteers it was found that RhIG prevented immunization when given within 72 hours of exposure to the D+ red cells. As a result, it is now recommended that RhIG be given within 72 hours of delivery of the D+ child. There is no doubt that the time limit is somewhat arbitrary but since it has been shown that immunization can be prevented by such a regimen, it would seem wise to continue to observe the 72 hour requirement. On the other hand, RhIG should not be withheld simply because someone forgot to inject it within 72 hours of delivery. It is known (136) that there is some leeway and that immunization may still be prevented if RhIG is injected later. In this setting and in some others described below, such as cases in which there is doubt that cannot be immediately resolved, RhIG should be given and the doubts reviewed later. The rationale behind that statement is that the consequence of failure to give RhIG when it is needed, i.e. production of anti-D by a parous woman, is much more significant than the consequence of giving the RhIG when it is not actually needed, i.e. waste of product with no benefit.

Detection of Fetal Cells in the Maternal Circulation

D- women who do not have anti-D in the serum and who have delivered a D+ child, should receive RhIG regardless of whether tests to detect fetal red cells in the maternal circulation have been done. However, the simple use of one dose of RhIG for each D- woman cannot be applied as a routine. In some women the volume of fetal red cells that enters the maternal circulation is such that more than one dose of RhIG will be necessary if immunization is to be prevented. There are many different methods in use for the detection of a larger than usual fetal to maternal hemorrhage (FMH).

Since a 300 µg dose of RhIG protects against immunization to D in women in whom the FMH is 30 ml (i.e. 15 ml of red cells) or less, it follows that an initial screening test on blood from D- women who have delivered D+ infants should identify those in whom the FMH was 30 ml or more. At this point the screening test need give only a positive or negative result, it need not measure the size of the FMH other than less or more than 30 ml. This, of course, because in more than 99% of women the FMH is less than 30 ml. Once the few women in whom the FMH is 30 ml or greater have been identified, additional tests can be performed to measure the volume of the FMH so that the amount of RhIG needed can be calculated.

One of the earliest methods used to detect fetal red cells in the maternal circulation was described by Kleihauer and Betke (36,37,40). Blood films are made from a postpartum sample and are fixed with ethanol. After being washed in tap water and allowed to dry in air, the films are treated with a buffered citric acid solution at pH 3.3. This solution dissolves adult but not fetal hemoglobin. The films are then stained with hematoxylin and erythrosine and are examined microscopically. The maternal red cells appear as hemoglobin free ghosts while the fetal cells are darkly stained. Reading the stained films requires some skill. First, lymphocytes must not be mistaken for fetal red cells. Second, if the maternal blood contains many reticulocytes, precipitation of RNA with brilliant cresyl blue may be necessary before the films are treated with phosphate-citric acid buffer (152). Third, even experienced workers can overestimate the number of fetal cells present because the hemoglobin F (Hb F) level is higher in pregnant than in non-pregnant women (50,52,54,153). However, this is less of a problem than might be thought. The most marked increase in Hb F in pregnancy occurs between the tenth and thirty-second week of gestation so is declining at term. Further, it is far better to overestimate the number of fetal cells present and give too much RhIG than to underestimate the number and give too little. Some of the problems caused by the normal presence of some Hb F in the blood of adults are considered again below in the section on quantitation of the size of the FMH.

In part because staining blood films by the Kleihauer-Betke method and then reading them, is time consuming and in part because only rarely does the FMH exceed 30 ml so that most of the effort produces only negative findings, serological tests were devised in an attempt to use a rapid screening system. One of the original tests, that unfortunately is still used in some services, involves the use of anti-D and a red cell sample collected from the D- woman after delivery. The red cells are tested by IAT with the anti-D, the tests are read microscopically in a search for a mixed-field reaction, i.e. D+ fetal cells reactive, D- maternal cells non-reactive. The problem with the test and the reason that it should be replaced is that it lacks sensitivity. In a series of comparative trials (80,82,137,148) it was shown that samples representing FMH of 30 ml or more were missed about 15% of the time when the IAT method was used. To counter this problem other tests have been introduced.

The rosette test is based on one devised many years ago (39,138,139). Red cells from the D- woman are incubated with anti-D; any fetal D+ red cells present bind that antibody but agglutination is not seen since too few D+ cells are present. The red cell suspension is then washed to remove unbound anti-D and indicator D+ (usually R_2R_2) red cells are added. If fetal D+ red cells were originally present they will now be coated with anti-D and will bind the D+ indicator red cells via available Fab sites on the anti-D. When the preparation is examined microscopically, rosettes, of indicator cells attached around the fetal cells, will be seen. Sebring and Polesky (148) used enzyme-treated D+ indicator cells to make the test easier to read. Kebles et al. (149) used chemically modified anti-D and D+ indicator red cells suspended in albumin. When the rosette test is positive, most workers proceed to a quantitative method to estimate the size of the FMH (see below). As indicated above, the rosette test is a screening method to identify those women in whom the FMH was 30 ml or more. While it will accomplish this it will also identify a number of women in whom additional doses of RhIG are not required. The rosette test is usually positive when the FMH exceeds 2.5 ml (148-150). At first this sounds like a huge disadvantage, that is, a positive rosette test when the FMH exceeds 2.5 ml but additional RhIG not required until it exceeds 30 ml. However, the saving feature is the fact that in 96 to 98% of women the FMH at delivery is less than 2 ml (43,47,79,84,121,140-147). In other words, the number of cases in which the rosette test is positive but in which the FMH does not exceed 30 ml is small enough that the test is still useful for screening purposes. As indicated above, the rosette test is reliable in the detection of virtually all cases in which the FMH is 30 ml or more (149-151).

In addition to the methods for the detection of fetal red cells in a maternal circulation already described, many others have been devised. These include the use of fluorescein-labeled antibodies in manual methods (42,43,154); in the flow cytometer (155-160,278,279) and in a solid phase system (161). The enzyme-linked antiglobulin test has also been used (162-166) as have methods that measure α-fetoprotein in maternal serum (167-173) and some that use an antibody to Hb F (174,175).

Determination of the Size of the Fetal-Maternal Hemorrhage

A number of different methods based on some of the principles outlined above have been proposed to permit calculation of the amount of fetal blood that has entered the maternal circulation. The one most widely used seems to be that proposed by Kleihauer (152). Blood films are prepared and stained as described in the previous section. The fetal cells are counted and an estimate is made of the proportion of the total volume of the sample, that they comprise. In other words, the blood films must be prepared in such a way that it is known (or can be calculated) roughly how many total cells are present per viewed field. Once the percentage number of fetal cells has been estimated, the size of the FMH is calculated from the estimated red cell mass of the woman. Obviously, this method will not give exact results. Mollison et al. (71) point out that in the estimation a number of factors must be taken into account. First, the volume of a fetal red cell is about 22% greater than that of a red cell from an adult. Second, not all fetal cells stain darkly by the method used. Third, an arbitrary figure for the maternal red cell volume must be assumed. In spite of these difficulties the method and calculation seem to work. If it is accepted that one 300 µg vial of RhIG is protective against 15 ml of fetal D+ red cells (i.e. an FMH of 30 ml) and the calculation suggests that 20 ml are present (i.e. an FMH of 40 ml) two vials of RhIG should be used. If the calculation suggests that 30 ml of red cells (FMH 60 ml) are present, three vials should be used in case the real volume is greater than 30 ml. As mentioned above, Mollison et al. (71) suggest that 20 µg anti-D should be used for each 1 ml of D+ red cells present. Thus when 30 ml of D+ cells are present, 600 µg anti-D would be suggested. Since the dose per vial in the USA is between 250 and 300 µg, again three vials would be indicated. If more than one method for calculation is used and the number of vials indicated varies by one, the larger number should be used. Again, it is far better to give too much than too little RhIG.

Failure to Prevent Immunization to D and Use of Rh Immune Globulin During Pregnancy

As mentioned above, the postnatal use of RhIG prevents immunization to D in some 98 to 99% of D- women who deliver D+ infants. Some of the 1 to 2% of failures probably represent the use of too small a dose in women in whom there was a larger than usual FMH, or delay in the injection of the RhIG. Obviously, such failures can be prevented if careful tests are done to detect a higher than usual number of fetal red cells in the maternal circulation and by strict adherence to recommendations for use. Other failures undoubtedly represent cases in which primary immunization occurred during the pregnancy. While, as stated above, the appearance of serologically detectable anti-D during the first pregnancy of a D- woman who has never been exposed to D+ red cells is a rare event, production of anti-D by a number of women who had been protected with RhIG at the end of their pregnancies, clearly showed (88,176) that in some 1 to 2% of D- women carrying a D+ fetus, primary immunization occurs during the pregnancy and not following delivery. Once this fact had been established it became apparent that immunization to D could be prevented in this 1 to 2% of women by the injection of RhIG during pregnancy. While such a practice works (see below) and has become standard in many countries, there remain some in which prenatal protection with RhIG is not used. The two major arguments against the use of RhIG during pregnancy are first, that the practice protects too few women to be cost effective and second, that the supply of anti-D to make RhIG is inadequate for its use during pregnancy. Those who use RhIG during pregnancy counter that the number of cases of Rh HDN prevented by the practice, make its use effective both in terms of lives saved and in terms of cost (treatment avoided) and that by the time that the supply of human source anti-D becomes inadequate to meet the demand, suitable monoclonal anti-D will be available.

At first it might appear that the injection of anti-D into a pregnant woman would introduce the risk that antibody might cross the placenta and cause HDN. In fact, such fears are groundless (71). Hughes-Jones et al. (177) showed that at term, the amount of anti-D in an infant is only about 10% of the amount in the mother. Further, when anti-D is injected intramuscularly, only about 40% of the antibody appears in the plasma as compared to the amount that would be expected if the same dose was injected intravenously (71). Thus the injection of 300 µg IgG anti-D into a pregnant woman will result in only a small amount of antibody reaching the fetus. When RhIG for intravenous injection is used, the dose is reduced accordingly (178,179) so that the fetus is still not at risk.

Bowman et al. (88) conducted a large trial in which D- primiparae were injected with 300 µg of anti-D at 28 weeks gestation, another 300 µg at 34 weeks and 300 µg after delivery. Subsequent tests showed that none of 1004 D- mothers of D+ infants had anti-D in the serum six months after infants were born (tests could not be done at delivery because passively administered anti-D was present). Based on previous experience with women protected only postnatally, it could be forecast that some 15 of the women would have had serologically detectable anti-D present six months after they had delivered, if the antenatal injections of anti-D had not prevented primary immunization during the pregnancies. In other words, use of the correct amount of RhIG during and immediately following pregnancy can be expected almost always to prevent D- women becoming immunized to D. Other studies (55,124,125,180-183) have confirmed the above observations and in some it has been shown that a single 300 µg dose of RhIG given at 28 weeks gestation, or two 100 µg doses, one given at 28 and one at 34 weeks gestation, also prevent primary immunization during pregnancy. Mollison et al. (71) point out that these findings mean that both antenatal and postnatal care can be provided in countries that use 250 to 300 µg and in those that use 100 µg as the standard dose, without the confusion that might result from there being different size doses. Those workers who were active when RhIG was first introduced in the late 1960s will know that protection of D- women by the injection of RhIG during pregnancy reflects enormous credit on the determination of Dr. Jack Bowman of Winnipeg, Canada, who almost single handedly convinced the rest of the world of the need for antenatal use of the prophylactic.

A very important practical consideration is that accurate records must be kept when RhIG is used antenatally. Women who receive injections of anti-D at 28 and/or 34 weeks of gestation will have serologically demonstrable anti-D in the serum at term. It is critical that this anti-D be recognized as being residual RhIG and that it not be misidentified as anti-D made by an immunized D- woman who is then not a candidate for postnatal RhIG. The amount of injected anti-D still present at term is not protective against a moderate FMH meaning that the postnatal injection is essential. Serological tests to distinguish between passive and active immunization in this setting can be based only on strength of the anti-D present so are highly unreliable. The antenatal use of RhIG does more harm than good, if true candidates for postnatal RhIG do not receive that treatment because they are mistakenly thought to be immunized. As mentioned already, some 98% of women who make anti-D as a result of pregnancy, do so following the FMH that occurs at delivery. In cases in which there is doubt, D- women with low levels of anti-D demonstrable in the serum at delivery, must be given RhIG during the 72 hour postnatal period if there is any possibility that they received RhIG during the antenatal period.

The study of Bowman et al. (88) also showed that as expected, antenatal injection of RhIG is safe for the fetus. In the large study, 28% of ABO compatible infants had a weakly positive DAT but did not have clinical HDN (see below). The highest bilirubin level seen in any infant was 3.4 mg/dl (a level that can be exceeded in physiological jaundice) and no infant required even pho-

totherapy for jaundice. The injection of another full dose of RhIG in women who have not delivered by 40 weeks gestation and who have received RhIG at 28 and/or 34 weeks is discussed below following the sections dealing with augmentation of the immune response.

Use of RhIG in Women of the Weak D Phenotype

There is continuing debate as to whether RhIG should be given to women of the weak D phenotype who deliver D+ infants. When the American College of Obstetricians and Gynecologists issued a statement (184) that protection for such women was indicated, there was an immediate response by Konugres et al. (204) stating that the available data did not justify the use of RhIG in women of that phenotype. One of us (PDI) has never been convinced that consideration of the use of RhIG in women who are of the weak D phenotype should be summarily dismissed. A few women whose red cells type as weakly positive for D, lack portions of the D antigen from their cells (see Chapter 12) so can form anti-D. Obviously such women could be protected with an injection of RhIG. That statement shows that this author does not accept the suggestion that RhIG would bind to the woman's weak D cells and thus be non-protective. One problem, of course, is that many women of the weak D phenotype have red cells that carry all epitopes of D albeit in reduced amounts (again see Chapter 12), so cannot form anti-D and are not candidates for RhIG. Further, the red cells of many women in whom one or more epitopes of D is/are missing, type as D+ so that they are never recognized as candidates for RhIG. In spite of this, HDN caused by anti-D in women of the partial D phenotype has been reported, (71,185-192,198-200) in at least two cases (185,192) the outcome was fatal. In contrast, in the study of Mayne et al. (283) five women with partial D on their red cells and anti-D in their sera, produced among them eight D+ infants, none of whom had clinical HDN. Again, a major argument against the use of RhIG in women of the weak D phenotype is economic. An appreciable amount of RhIG would be used to protect very few women at risk. However, this argument is not very convincing to a woman with weak D who has just lost an infant to HDN. As far as she is concerned the incidence of immunization and fatal HDN is 100%. Perhaps a compromise would be a policy that this author followed for a number of years. Women of the weak D phenotype whose red cells were C+ were not considered candidates for RhIG because of the possibility that their weak D was of the *trans* position type (see Chapter 12). Those whose red cells typed as weakly positive for D and were C- were given RhIG in case their weak D was of the partial D phenotype. It should be added that when proposed (193) this suggestion was received with a quite spectacular lack of enthusiasm. A different idea was advanced by Soloway (194-197) who suggested that antenatal and postnatal use of RhIG could be justified in D- and weak D women if other tests such as the IAT for weak D (i.e. consider all women whose red cells type as D- in the initial test as D- without testing for weak D), antibody-screening, etc., were abandoned and all D-women were treated. It was claimed (194-197) that such a system would be more cost effective than identifying women with a large fetal-maternal hemorrhage and treating infants with Rh HDN. The flaw would seem to be that cases of Rh HDN would still be seen unless the regimen ensured no immunization to D, a situation that would seem difficult to achieve unless women exposed to large quantities of fetal D+ red cells were identified.

There is no danger that injection of RhIG to a woman of the weak D phenotype will result in in vivo destruction of her red cells. One of us (PDI) has heard of several cases in which the RhIG was injected into the D+ infant instead of the D- mother, because of lack of understanding on the part of persons administering the material. While the DAT became positive in these infants, no evidence of clinically significant in vivo red cell destruction was seen. In an instance known to one of us (PDI), the RhIG was injected into the D+ husband of a D-woman who had delivered a D+ child. One assumes that this was intended to teach him never to do it again!

Before closing this section on weak D it should be mentioned that a positive test for weak D in a recently delivered woman should be carefully investigated since it may, in fact, represent the presence of large numbers of D+ fetal red cells in the circulation of a D- woman. Obviously such a situation may require injection of more than a single dose of Rh immune globulin.

Use of RhIG in Women with Partial D on Their Red Cells

The previous section considered the use, or lack thereof, of RhIG in women in whom the D antigen was seen to be weakly expressed but in whom the distinction between quantitative and qualitative weakening of D had not been made. A somewhat different situation exists when epitope specific monoclonal anti-D are used for routine typing and some persons with partial D on their red cells are deliberately typed D- or D+. For example, one recommendation in the UK (201,202,370-372,374-376) was that two IgM monoclonal anti-D that react with all or most partial D samples except those of category VI, be used for routine D typing. In different publications (203,373) it was suggested that in order to

avoid the confusion that results when the two MAb to D give different results, a single, selected MAb be used in duplicate typings. By the use of such a reagent, pregnant category VI women would be typed as D- and would be given RhIG. Others (71,193,205,206) have similarly recommended the use of RhIG when it is known that the red cells of the women involved carry partial D. A problem, of course, is that most of the time the partial D status is not recognized until the individual involved makes anti-D. In the various publications discussing the use of RhIG for women with partial D on the red cells, it has been concluded that only those of category VI and types D^B and DBT are likely to be recognized and protected. In vitro studies were used with category VI and D^B red cells to show (205) that the anti-D of RhIG does not bind entirely to the partial D red cells suggesting that when injected into such persons, some remains available to bind to D+ fetal red cells and/or remains unbound to effect suppression of immunization to D (see below).

While the use of one or two MAb to D that type category VI red cells as D- is to be lauded in terms of prevention of immunization to D in women of category VI, the suggestion (202,203,373) that the same reagent or reagents are suitable for typing blood donors is highly debatable. The rationale seems to be that there is no evidence that category VI red cells stimulate production of anti-D in D- persons. However, it seems that there have been no opportunities for such evidence to be recognized if it does exist. For many years, manufacturers of human-source polyclonal anti-D typing reagents went to considerable trouble to ensure that the reagents recognized the partial D of all categories. Thus category VI blood donors were classed as D+ and the units of blood they donated were transfused to D+ patients. When a D-patient known to have been transfused with D+ blood made anti-D the event was expected, no attempt was made further to classify the D+ donor, i.e. frank D+ or D+ of category VI. Similarly, when a D- woman made anti-D following pregnancy either before RhIG was developed or because it was not given, if the red cells of her infant and those of its father typed as D+, again the event was expected and no attempt was made further to investigate the D+ status of the infant and its father. Thus it is entirely possible that partial D red cells of category VI have stimulated production of anti-D in D- persons but that the events have gone unrecognized because there were no reasons to suspect them. One case is described in the literature (335) in which the partial D, category V red cells of an infant stimulated production of anti-D in the infant's D- mother. Again if partial D, category VI red cells have been similarly immunogenic, such facts may not have come to light if the infant's red cells were typed as D+. Given the well established fact (71) that transfusion with D+ blood is very much more likely than a D+

pregnancy, to result in the production of anti-D by a D-individual, it would seem to be a highly dangerous exercise deliberately to type category VI donors as D-, without much better evidence that such red cells will not stimulate production of anti-D. It would be a calamity if the price paid for the protection of category VI women with RhIG, was production of anti-D in D- women transfused unwittingly with category VI red cells.

Anti-D, Anti-C, Anti-G and RhIG

As discussed in detail in Chapter 12, when standard antibody identification panels are performed, anti-G is usually not distinguished from a mixture of anti-D and anti-C. For practical transfusion purposes this hardly matters since compatibility tests will be performed against D- units, almost all of which will also be C- and G-. When an antibody that reacts as anti-CD is identified in a D- pregnant woman, the difference between anti-CD and anti-G becomes important. As described below, if the woman is immunized to D, RhIG injections are not indicated. If her antibody is actually anti-G or a mixture of anti-G and anti-C, RhIG is indicated to prevent immunization to D. HDN caused by anti-C and/or anti-G is invariably less severe than that caused by anti-D (71) so that prevention of immunization to D in a woman already making anti-C and/or anti-G remains important. While it is not a foolproof indicator, those sera that contain what appears to be anti-CD but in which the anti-C appears stronger than the anti-D are the first that should be suspected as potential anti-G or anti-G plus anti-C (291-293). Methods for differentiation among anti-D, anti-C and anti-G are described in Chapter 12.

Use of RhIG on Some Other Occasions

Earlier sections have considered prevention of immunization to D by the use of RhIG during normal pregnancies and following normal deliveries. In order that programs designed to eradicate HDN due to anti-D succeed, it is necessary that RhIG be used at other times as well. Such use is necessary following (primarily induced) abortion (55,207,208), amniocentesis (55,183,209-211), chorionic villus sampling (55,212-214) and any other procedure in which the possibility of an induced FMH exists. While it has been common practice in some countries to use a small dose of RhIG early in pregnancy, e.g. 50 µg in cases in which abortion occurs before 20 weeks gestation, there is no harm in using a standard dose, e.g. 300 µg, whenever the use of RhIG is indicated. An advantage of using one standard dose on all occasions is that confusion does not occur among those individuals who will admin-

ister the injections. Bowman (183) points out that before techniques for ultrasound placental location were available, FMH was common, i.e. documented in 10 to 11% of patients, following amniocentesis (215). With the use of ultrasound and restriction of the procedure to obstetricians skilled in performing amniocentesis, the incidence of FMH has been reduced. However, the procedure still carries sufficient risk of introducing fetal D+ red cells into the maternal circulation, that it should always be followed by the use of RhIG. Bowman (183) recommends that a full 300 µg dose of RhIG should be given at the time of amniocentesis and that the dose should be repeated at 12 week intervals until delivery. As indicated earlier, RhIG given during pregnancy does not harm a D+ fetus (88). Further, in any circumstance in which a FMH may occur after 20 weeks gestation, the tests described earlier for the detection of FMH of more than 30 ml (15 ml of red cells) must be used in case the use of more than 300 µg of RhIG is necessary to prevent immunization.

Does RhIG Turn Off or Down Regulate the Immune Response in Individuals in Whom Primary Immunization to D has Occurred?

When RhIG first became available, a natural question was whether it would prevent further production of anti-D in individuals in whom the primary immune response had already occurred? Indeed, there are some claims (216-219) that use of RhIG reversed immunization in women in whom weak anti-D had been detected and that in others it delayed the production of higher levels of anti-D than had first been detected. While there seems no logical explanation as to how RhIG could reverse immunization to D, its ability to slow development of production of anti-D was credited to its ability to block further immunization following delivery of a D+ infant in a D- woman. That is, it was supposed that its effect, when injected postnatally in a woman making a low level of anti-D, was similar to its effect in a non-immunized woman, i.e. reduction or abolition of immunogenicity of D+ fetal red cells that entered the maternal D- circulation at delivery. In spite of these claims most workers believe that RhIG cannot reverse immunization to D nor prevent the development of a progressive increase in antibody production. It is assumed that the delay in progression of production of anti-D in the women described (216-219) was coincidental and not related to the use of RhIG. Similar delays in expansion of anti-D production are seen in some women who have not been given RhIG. For example, Bowman et al. (281) followed 42 women making low levels of anti-D, through a subsequent pregnancy. In one third of them there was no increase in the amount of anti-D being made and it was shown that in these women, FMHs were too small to constitute secondary immunizing doses. Had these women been given RhIG (they were not (281)) it would have been easy to credit the RhIG for delaying expansion of anti-D production when, in fact, the actual reason was quite different.

Most workers agree with the conclusion of Bowman (183,282) and of Mollison et al. (71) that the use of RhIG in women in whom the primary immune response to D has occurred, is of no value. In addition to the study (281) described above, the results of others performed in Winnipeg (88,220,235) have supported the conclusion. First, in a series of D- women in whom anti-D could be detected only by the use of protease-treated red cells, injections of RhIG failed to alter the progression to production of higher levels of anti-D. Second, in other women in whom no anti-D could be detected by any serological method, injections of RhIG failed to prevent development of anti-D. Presumably these women had already undergone a primary immune response although serologically detectable anti-D was not yet being made. Elsewhere, DeSilva et al. (236) conducted a study on 14 women, who could no longer become pregnant, who had become immunized during pregnancies and who were making weak anti-D. Each woman was challenged by the injection of 0.28 ml of D+ red cells, seven of the 14 were given RhIG injections containing 500 µg anti-D. The secondary immune responses in the women who received RhIG and in the controls who did not, were the same. Again, it was concluded that RhIG cannot down regulate a secondary immune response in an individual already immunized to D, even when the amount of anti-D being made is small. As mentioned several times above, incompatibility of the infants' D+ red cells with the D- mother's ABO system antibodies, affords partial protection against immunization to D in the mother. Bowman (336) showed that just like RhIG, ABO incompatibility has no ameliorating effect on the production of anti-D once the primary immune response has occurred.

As the above observations illustrate, one reason for withholding RhIG is that the candidate is already making anti-D. However, as discussed in this chapter, if there is any doubt whatever about the specificity of the antibody being detected, or any possibility that the anti-D detected represents passively transferred antibody from the antenatal use of RhIG, then RhIG should be given. As mentioned above, the injection of RhIG can only help in cases in which its use is questionable, the sole contraindications of use when the product is not truly needed are cost to the patient and waste of a material that may be in short supply.

Mechanisms by Which RhIG Prevents Immunization to D

Readers may look at the sections about RhIG that proceed this one and suspect that their length is in part due to the fact that the author has been delaying the task of having to write this one. Such suspicions are well founded; although there is abundant evidence that RhIG always prevents immunization to D if used in sufficient quantity and at the right time, the mechanisms involved are not fully understood. Theories abound but the evidence to support them is sometimes conflicting.

Early attempts to suppress immunization to D by passive administration of antibody used IgM anti-D. There were two reasons for this. First, it was not yet appreciated that in the majority of women, immunization can be prevented by injecting antibody after delivery. In other words, it was assumed that the antibody would have to be given during pregnancy meaning that IgG anti-D was contraindicated since it would cross the placenta and enter the fetal circulation. It is now known, of course, that this does occur but that the amount of anti-D reaching the fetus does not cause red cell destruction. Second, the principle being tested was based on the ABO protective mechanism, described above, and it was assumed that IgM anti-A and anti-B afforded protection. In retrospect, one can see that IgM anti-D would not function like IgM anti-A and anti-B since it does not activate complement nor does it bring about intravascular destruction of antigen-positive red cells, both of which are characteristic of IgM anti-A and anti-B and may well explain the protective effects of those antibodies. Early trials with IgM anti-D showed that no protection against immunization to D was afforded (103,221); indeed in one series of experiments (221) there was a hint that IgM anti-D might have enhanced the immune response to D (see below). Although it was originally believed (225) that IgM anti-D could effect some clearance of D+ red cells in vivo, it was later concluded (226,227) that the IgM anti-D that was used contained enough IgG anti-D to produce the effect. The first clues that IgG anti-D might be protective were provided by the studies of Stern et al. (100,104) who showed that D+ red cells coated with IgG anti-D did not often stimulate production of anti-D when injected into D- volunteers. This observation, coupled with those (see above) that showed that most women become immunized to D when exposed to fetal D+ red cells at the time of delivery, prompted further work that led to the use of IgG anti-D in the immediate postnatal period. As discussed in detail above, it was found that passively administered IgG anti-D is far more protective than are anti-A or anti-B.

In spite of the principles that led to the development of RhIG, it is doubtful that it works by clearing fetal D+

red cells from the maternal circulation in a rapid manner. As judged by the amount of anti-D that is protective, it seems unlikely that the anti-D molecules can locate the few fetal D+ red cells in the maternal circulation and bind to them in sufficient numbers to effect immediate extravascular sequestration and destruction of those cells. Indeed, in four patients studied by Mollison (222) in whom the intravenous infusion of anti-D prevented immunization, the times of clearance of D+ cells varied from two to eight days. When RhIG is injected intramuscularly to a D- woman who has delivered a D+ child, it might be guessed that clearance of the fetal D+ cells takes even longer. Samson and Mollison (136) showed that in D- volunteers given 1 ml of D+ red cells, then injected with 100 μg IgG anti-D 13 days later, there was protection. Thus it seems that a different explanation than rapid destruction of the D+ red cells must be sought to explain the protective action of IgG anti-D.

While considering the clearance of red cells in vivo it should also be pointed out that the mechanisms by which anti-A and anti-B on one hand and anti-D on the other, clear red cells, have different implications in terms of the immune response. Following intravascular red cell destruction by anti-A and anti-B, red cell debris is cleared through the liver, an organ in which relatively few immunocytes are present. Red cells to which IgG anti-D has bound are eventually cleared predominantly through the spleen, an active site of immune responsiveness. However, as discussed below, the splenic macrophages that bind IgG coated red cells are not particularly efficient at antigen presentation.

Like rapid clearance of D+ red cells, blocking of D antigen sites cannot completely explain the protective mechanism of RhIG. Calculations of the number of IgG molecules in a dose of RhIG and the number of D sites on the number of red cells against which that dose is protective, show that not all D antigen sites are blocked (223).

In the so-called immunostat mechanism (224) it is supposed that the D antigen becomes trapped at the sites at which immune responses occur, i.e. the spleen and lymph nodes. When such antigen trapping occurs in the absence of antibody, T helper cells interact with naive B cells, via a series of secreted hormone-like signals, to initiate an immune response. In the presence of free antibody, i.e. after the RhIG has been injected, a negative feedback mechanism comes in to play, perhaps via participation of T suppressor cells and the signal from T helper cells is blocked. If the immunostat mechanism was the sole explanation of the efficiency of RhIG in preventing immunization to D, prevention of immunization should be antigen specific. Apparently it is not. Woodrow et al. (122) showed that when volunteers were injected with small amounts of D+, K+ red cells and with IgG anti-K, protection against immunization to D was achieved. This finding is not yet explained.

As mentioned above, D+ red cells coated with anti-D are removed from circulation predominantly in the spleen. Sequestration occurs when tissue bound macrophages bind the Fc piece of the antibody molecule. Further, it is known that the Fc piece is necessary for RhIG to be protective. First, F(ab)$_2$ preparations of IgG (i.e. Fc piece no longer present) are not protective (228), second, Fc is essential for the suppression of the primary immune response (229-232,674). This means that when they are cleared, the fetal D+ red cells coated with RhIG will be bound by macrophages. These macrophages have poor expression of class II HLA antigens and consequently are poor presenters of antigen to immunocytes (see Chapter 2). In contrast dendritic cells, that may be involved in the clearance of non-antibody coated red cells, have high expressions of class II HLA antigens and are essential for the presentation of antigens to immunocytes to initiate a primary immune response (233 and see Chapter 2). However, dendritic cells have no Fc receptors so will not bind the anti-D coated fetal red cells. This direction of the fetal red cells away from those cells (dendrocytes) most likely to initiate a primary immune response may be a key mechanism in the protection afforded by RhIG.

As with any complex situation, the mechanisms by which RhIG is protective may well be multifactoral and may involve all the situations described above. For example, in one splenectomized individual injected with D+ red cells and an amount of anti-D sufficient to effect protection, clearance of the D+ red cells was slow and the individual formed anti-D (234). Further, the in vivo survival of red cells is considerably longer than the in vivo survival of injected IgG. Thus in a D- woman exposed to ABO compatible D+ red cells via FMH, it would be expected that some of the D+ cells would be present (and thus immunogenic) after the injected anti-D had gone, if RhIG did not cause accelerated clearance of the D+ red cells. Thus it seems reasonable to conclude that even if RhIG does not act (like anti-A and anti-B) to effect immediate clearance of fetal D+ red cells, its ability to accelerate clearance of those cells is one of several contributory mechanisms in its immunosuppressive effect.

Can Small Amounts of Passively Administered Anti-D Augment the Immune Response to D?

As mentioned above, some early studies raised the possibility that IgM anti-D (221) might actually augment the immune response to D. This subject proved difficult to investigate since it seems that if augmentation does occur it involves the presence of a critical amount of anti-D, where the effective range is narrow, at a particular time that the individual is exposed to D. In some careful experiments, Contreras and Mollison (237) found that in subjects given 1 ml of D+ red cells and 5 µg of anti-D, there was some suppression but no enhancement of the immune response. In another series, the same investigators (238) found evidence that when 0.8 ml of red cells and 1 µg of anti-D were given there was evidence that some individuals who might otherwise not have responded to that dose of red cells, made anti-D. Thus although the evidence is not absolutely conclusive, there is a very real possibility that a low level of anti-D may augment the immune response to D in some individuals (239). The importance of this possibility is discussed in the next section.

Use of RhIG at Delivery in Women Given RhIG During Pregnancy

If the presence of a small amount of anti-D can augment the primary immune response to D, it may well be of very considerable practical importance. In women given RhIG at 28 weeks gestation, the amount still present at 40 weeks is small. Thus it may be that if a postnatal injection of RhIG is not given, the critical amount of anti-D that augments a primary response will be present at the precise time that the critical amount of fetal cells enters the maternal circulation. Obviously, the postnatal use of RhIG is necessary to prevent immunization; if not given, the net result may be that the woman has more chance of making anti-D than if RhIG had not been used at 28 weeks. The consideration also applies to pregnancies that go beyond 40 weeks. Bowman (183) who believes that augmentation can occur, points out that if RhIG was given at 28 weeks, by 40 weeks the amount remaining may be in the augmenting rather than the protecting range. He recommends that any woman who has not delivered within 12 weeks of the time that the antenatal dose of RhIG was given, be given another dose. If delivery occurs within three weeks of the second dose, a postpartum dose is recommended only when the FMH is greater than 0.1 ml.

Final Comments on the Use of Rh Immune Globulin in Pregnancy

As mentioned earlier, the only contraindications for the use of RhIG when it is not actually needed, are that it is a waste of money and of material that is in short supply in some countries. The material causes no clinical sequelae in D+ or phenotypically weak D individuals. On the other hand, failure to give RhIG when it is actually needed can have very serious consequences. Accordingly, as mentioned several times already, a good rule to follow when in doubt as to whether RhIG should be given is to give the injection first and seek advice later. Such considerations may apply but not be restricted to situations in which:

1. Miscarriage or abortion has occurred and the D type of the fetus is not known.
2. The woman may be phenotypically weak D or may have had a larger than usual fetal to maternal hemorrhage (perform tests to estimate the number of fetal cells present).
3. The infant is of the weak D phenotype.
4. The D type of the infant's red cells is not known and cannot quickly be determined (e.g., mother in one hospital, child in another).
5. There is doubt as to whether weak anti-D is present in the maternal serum, i.e. antibody activity detected but specificity not determined for sure.
6. There is weak anti-D in the maternal serum and doubt as to whether RhIG was injected during pregnancy.
7. There is weak anti-D in the maternal serum and a possibility that RhIG may have been injected during pregnancy.
8. In some (but not all) services, the woman is of the weak D phenotype.

Placental Transfer of Antibodies

As mentioned briefly above, the placental transfer of maternal antibodies to the fetus is an essential physiological event. Because the immune system of newborns is not fully functional, antibodies transferred from the mother serve to protect the infant from infections during the first few months of life. IgG molecules of all four subclasses cross the placenta and enter the fetal circulation, IgM and IgA molecules do not (177,240-268). At one time it was believed that the placenta acted as a simple sieve by allowing small but not large antibody molecules to enter the fetal circulation. However, it is now known (241,245-247,257-259,263,264) that cells of the placenta carry receptors for the Fc piece of IgG molecules and that there is an active transport system for antibodies to pass from the mother to the fetus.

When the maternal serum contains an IgG blood group antibody directed against an antigen present on fetal red cells, the transport mechanism works to the detriment of the fetus. It is known that during the first 12 weeks of gestation only small amounts of IgG enter the fetal circulation but when the mother has potent anti-D in the serum, the DAT may be positive as early as 6 to 10 weeks (242,269). At the 24th week of gestation, the level of IgG in the circulation of the fetus is about one seventh of that in the maternal blood (249) but then the rate of transfer increases so that at birth the IgG level in the infant may be equal to (266) or higher (247) than that in the mother. There is also evidence (254,256) that IgG1 crosses the placenta earlier in pregnancy and in greater amounts than does IgG3 and that the transfer of IgG2 occurs only to a limited degree (253). Pollock and Bowman (265) were able to follow the passage of IgG from mother to fetus but found no evidence that fetal IgG is transported into the maternal circulation.

In spite of there being a fairly good understanding of the transfer of IgG of different subclasses across the placenta, there is no general agreement as to which subclass is most often involved in clinical and/or severe (see next section) HDN. In terms of immunized pregnant women (most with anti-D but some with other antibodies) there is fairly good agreement (270-273) that about one third have only IgG1, about another one third IgG1 and IgG3 antibodies, with the remaining third having IgG3 alone or in mixtures with IgG1 and/or IgG2 and/or IgG4. However, when clinical and serious HDN is considered there is less agreement about the role of IgG antibodies of different subclasses. Schanfield (274) described a small series of affected infants. He concluded that anemia and bilirubinemia at the time of birth were higher in infants born to women with IgG1 anti-D but that bilirubin levels rose more quickly after birth in those born to women with IgG3 anti-D. These findings were attributed to the fact that IgG1 crosses the placenta early so has considerable time to effect clearance of fetal red cells while IgG3 crosses the placenta later but is more destructive than IgG1. It was also claimed (274) that among IgG1 antibodies, those carrying Glm(f) were more destructive than those carrying Glm(a). Among IgG3 antibodies those carrying G3m(b) or G3m(g) were said to be destructive.

Parineud et al. (272) also found that IgG1 antibodies were associated with higher bilirubin levels in neonates than were those made of IgG3; among the IgG1 antibodies, those of the Glm(4) allotype were associated with the most severe HDN. These workers (272) also reported that severe HDN was less common when the maternal antibody was made in part of IgG1 and in part of IgG3, it was suggested that IgG3 might somehow exert a protective effect. Cregut et al. (275), Nance et al. (277) and Iyer et al. (832) also reported that IgG1 antibodies caused more severe HDN than did those made of IgG3. However, other studies yielded quite different results. In a study much larger than that of Schanfield (274) and about equal in size to that of Parineud et al. (272), Frankowska et al. (270) were unable to find any correlation between IgG subclass of the maternal antibody and severity of HDN in the infants. Completely different from the other studies, Taslima et al. (276) found that clinical HDN occurred only when the maternal antibody was IgG3. Thomas et al. (686) described an ELISA method for determination of the percentage of each IgG subclass within a single IgG antibody. Lynen et al. (687) described a method for making such a determination by use of a flow cytometer. Both papers describe the measurement of subclasses within anti-D and other specificity antibodies present in the sera of pregnant women. In both studies (686,687) IgG1 was a little more prevalent than IgG3 in cases of moderate to severe HDN but in most cases both IgG1 and IgG3 were present. Clearly these disparities in the different studies show that when a pregnant woman with an IgG antibody in the serum is encountered, IgG subclassing of the antibody will not provide a totally reliable guide as to the severity of HDN to be expected. The role of IgG subclass composition of anti-A, anti-B and anti-A,B in causing ABO HDN is discussed below in the section dealing with ABO HDN.

Because IgM antibodies do not cross the placenta so do not cause HDN, laboratory tests with 2-ME and DTT (for methods see Judd (280)) can be useful when an antibody is found in the serum of a pregnant woman. In other words, it is sometimes possible to demonstrate that the infant is not at risk of HDN because the maternal antibody is IgM in composition.

Clinical and Subclinical HDN

Many women who are pregnant have in their sera, an IgG antibody directed against an antigen present on the red cells of the fetus. For example, based on the frequency of ABO phenotypes it can be calculated that some 15 to 20% of women have IgG anti-A or anti-B, or both in the serum and a group A or B infant in utero. In spite of this, clinical HDN is comparatively rare. It is important to realize that HDN cannot be diagnosed solely in the laboratory. The finding that the infant's red cells have a positive DAT and that maternal antibody can be recovered from the infant's cells by elution, does not establish the diagnosis. Indeed, many workers describe the situation in which the potential for HDN exists (i.e., maternal antibody on the infant's cells) but in which the infant has no clinical symptoms, as subclinical HDN. In fact, the situation is probably better described as maternal-fetal blood group incompatibility since that term does not include the word disease. Antibodies of systems other than ABO can cause a positive DAT but no disease in the newborn. On other occasions there may be a considerable amount of maternal antibody in the newborn's circulation but the antigen against which the antibody is directed may be poorly developed so that again, little red cell destruction occurs. The blood group literature contains many accounts of antibodies that caused a positive DAT in a newborn so were of interest to immunohematologists but caused no disease so were of no moment to the infant, its mother or their clinicians.

Clinical HDN is here defined as a condition in which the infant is anemic because of in vivo red cell destruction by the maternal antibody and/or has or develops an elevated bilirubin level because of the accumulation of breakdown products of the destroyed red cells. In some infants the anemia is sufficiently severe that red cell transfusion is necessary, often via exchange transfusion in which the infant's red cells coated with maternal antibody are replaced by appropriate antigen-negative cells. In many others the anemia is mild enough that no transfusion is necessary. In infants with hyperbilirubinemia, it is the rate with which the bilirubin level is increasing that determines whether intervention is necessary. In some infants exchange transfusions are indicated to control the bilirubin level, in many others simple phototherapy suffices or no treatment is needed. The anemia and hyperbilirubinemia of HDN are considered further below, in the sections dealing with treatment in the disorder.

Antibodies Causative of HDN

As mentioned earlier in this chapter, any IgG antibody directed against an antigen that is reasonably well developed on the red cells of the infant, while that infant is in utero, has the potential to cause HDN. In the chapter thus far, emphasis has been placed on anti-D (including anti-CD and anti-CDE), on its role in causing HDN and on prevention of its production. There are several reasons for this, most of which have already been mentioned. First, compared to other red cell antigens, D is very highly immunogenic so that production of anti-D is common unless preventive measures are used. Second, before development of RhIG, anti-D caused far more cases of severe HDN and hydrops fetalis than all other blood group antibodies added together. Third, any serologist who worked in the pre-RhIG era must have an indelible impression of the devastating effects of potent anti-D on the D+ infants of immunized D- mothers. Now that RhIG is widely used, younger workers may have difficulty in understanding the emphasis placed on anti-D in HDN, by their elders. Suffice it here to say that the earlier sections that deal with topics such as the history of HDN, maternal immunization and immunization via pregnancy and those that follow and deal with prenatal testing and the treatment of mothers and infants, can all be applied to other antibodies. However, the applications will be less frequent than they were to anti-D in the past

and with infrequent exceptions, cases of HDN caused by antibodies other than anti-D will be somewhat less severe. These points are well illustrated by the fact that there has been no need to develop an immune globulin to prevent immunization to any antigen other than D.

Rh Antibodies

In addition to anti-D, most other antibodies in the system have caused HDN. There is little point in listing all publications that have described HDN caused by an Rh antibody, the list might be longer than the chapter. Suffice it to say that any time a pregnant woman is found to have an IgG Rh antibody in her serum and tests on the red cells of her partner indicate the possibility that her fetus has the antigen to which her antibody is directed, the potential for HDN exists. In many cases, HDN caused by antibodies to c, e, Hr_o, Go^a, etc., is milder than that caused by anti-D. However, infrequent exceptions have been seen with perhaps anti-c being more likely than other non-anti-D Rh antibodies to cause severe HDN (61,62,123,284-290). Because anti-c sometimes causes severe HDN, it has been suggested (287,290) that girls and women of child-bearing age who are to be transfused, be typed for c and that those whose red cells lack the antigen be given c- blood. In Chapter 12 we have given our reasons for concluding that based on the rarity of severe HDN caused by anti-c (123,284), the number of c typings (on patients and donors) that would be necessary and the inventory problems that would be created, such a policy is not desirable and would not be cost effective. Similarly we have been told that in some countries Rh phenotype-matched blood is used for all, most or many transfusions to prevent immunization. Based on the incidence with which Rh antibodies other than anti-D are formed by recipients of blood transfusions, such a practice is not logical, it cannot possibly be cost-effective. Tables 41-1, 41-2 and 41-3 list antibodies that have caused HDN. Because so many examples of antibodies to C, c, E, e, rh_i, etc. have been reported, they are not listed individually in table 41-1. However, because of their interest to immunohematologists, antibodies to low incidence Rh antigens, that have caused HDN, are included in table 41-2, while those directed against high incidence Rh antigens, that have caused the disease are included in table 41-3. The importance of differentiating between anti-CD and anti-G or anti-G plus anti-C in a D-woman who is pregnant and thus a potential candidate for RhIG, is discussed above.

ABO Antibodies

Halbrecht (294) is credited as having been the first

to appreciate that ABO antibodies can cause the disease and Grumbach and Gasser (295) as being the first to document cases of severe HDN caused by such antibodies. Anti-A and anti-B are composed, most often, of a mixture of IgG and IgM. Since only the IgG antibody will cross the placenta, those women with a high level of that type of antibody will be the ones who will give birth to infants with HDN. The noted excess of group O mothers with affected infants (as compared to group A and B mothers) (71,296-303) was explained when it was shown (300,304) that while the so-called naturally-occurring anti-A and anti-B in O, B and A persons are primarily IgM, the immune response that follows exposure of those persons to immunization and vaccination with bacterial antigens, differs in persons of different ABO groups. Group A and group B persons produce primarily IgM anti-B and anti-A respectively; in some a lower level of IgG antibody is made. In contrast, group O persons injected with substances that contain A or B-like antigens tend to produce larger amounts of IgG anti-A, anti-B and anti-A,B. For many years it was believed that the excess of group O among women who produce infants affected with ABO HDN was also associated with specificity of the causative antibody. It was believed that group O women made more IgG anti-A,B than IgG anti-

A or anti-B and that anti-A,B most often caused the disease. However, when we (305) reviewed the results of tests on 70 infants with some evidence of ABO HDN, whom we had studied over a four year period, we found that while all had been born to group O women, the causative antibodies were anti-A in 28 (40%), anti-B in 26 (37%) and anti-A,B in only 16 (23%). Further, as judged by the degree of anemia at birth and the maximum bilirubin level recorded in the first few days of life, anti-A and anti-B tended to cause more severe HDN than did anti-A,B.

If ABO HDN is considered to have occurred when there is fetal-maternal incompatibility, jaundice of the infant and a slight degree of anemia, then the condition is as common as one in 30 (306) to one in 150 births (307-310). If the disease is considered to exist only when severe enough to warrant treatment, then it is as rare as one in 3000 births (71,296,311). In other words, subclinical disease is common whereas severe disease is rare. There are a few reports in the literature (354-357,859) that purport to describe hydrops fetalis, sometimes with death of the fetus, caused by an ABO system antibody. Bowman (183) points out that it is often difficult to exclude non-immune hydrops in such cases. Indeed, Castillo et al. (380) note that with the decline in number of women with potent anti-D in the serum, the most common form of hydrops now seen is the non-immune type. Of the various reports in the literature, Mollison et al. (71) describe two (355,357) as convincing.

From the results of a number of studies (312-315) it can be concluded that clinical ABO HDN is somewhat more common in Blacks and Arabs than in Whites and tends to be severe more often in Arabs.

TABLE 41-1 Antigens of Moderate Incidence Defined by Antibodies that have Caused HDN or a Positive DAT on the Red Cells of a Newborn

Antigen	References
Multiple[*1]	60, 61, 71, 183, 282, 285, 288, 289, 332, 333, 377-379, 399
Rh[*2]	59-62, 193, 284, 285, 289, 377-379, 399, 417-419
M	381-387, 420
N	388, 389, 420
S	390-394
s	395-398
K	60, 63, 71, 316-318, 320, 321, 338-340, 400-404, 995, 996, 1002
Jk^a	405-408, 789, 790
Jk^b	409-411
Fy^a	57, 58, 326, 412
Fy^b	413
Do^{a}[*3]	414-416

[*1] Papers referenced list many antibodies of various systems causative of HDN or of a positive DAT in a newborn.
[*2] Many of the papers listed in the "multiple antigen" category also describe Rh antibodies causative of HDN.
[*3] Has caused a positive DAT but (as yet) no clinical HDN.

Other Antibodies

Throughout the chapters of this book, tables about the antibodies of each system include information as to which have caused HDN. As will be seen (and as is expected) antibodies to antigens such as s, U, K, Fy^a, Jk^a, Jk^b, et al., have all caused the disease. Again, the frequency and severity of HDN caused by these antibodies is such that no steps to prevent maternal immunization need to be taken. When the world literature is reviewed it is noticeable that several antibodies with specificities other than anti-D have caused severe HDN including fatal cases. However, it should be remembered that severe and fatal cases are dramatic and exceptional so tend to be described in the literature out of proportion to their incidence. For example, if the results from three series (63,316,317) are combined, it is seen that 561 examples of anti-K were found in screening tests on the sera of some 517,000 pregnant women, i.e. anti-K found once in every 922 women. In one of the

TABLE 41-2 Antigens of Low Incidence Defined by Antibodies that have caused HDN or a Positive DAT on the Red Cells of a Newborn

Antigen	System	References	Antigen	System	References
C^w	Rh	421-424	Ul^a	Kell	475
C^x	Rh	425, 426	K23	Kell	476[*1]
E^w	Rh	427, 428	K24	Kell	477[*1]
D^w	Rh	429-431, 990	Di^a	Diego	478-487
Go^a	Rh	332, 432-434	Wr^a	Diego	488-491, 860, 861
Rh32	Rh	435-437	Fr^a	Diego	494, 495[*1]
Be^a	Rh	439-443	ELO	Diego	496, 497
Evans	Rh	438	Ls^a	Gerbich	498
Tar	Rh	444	Yt^b	Cartwright	612[*1]
Rh42	Rh	445	Sc2	Scianna	499
Riv	Rh	446	Rd(Rd^a)	?Scianna	500
JAL	Rh	447	Er^b	Er Collection	501[*1]
STEM	Rh	448	Bi	Ind[*3]	502
HOFM	?Rh	492	By	Ind	503[*1]
LOCR	?Rh	493	Good	Ind	504
Mi^a	MN	449	Heibel	Ind	505
Vw	MN	450-453, 1000	HJK	Ind	506
Mur	MN	454, 455, 1001	Ht^a	Ind	507
Mt^a	MN	456	JFV	Ind	508
MUT	MN	457, 458	Jones	Ind	509
Hil	MN	459	Joslin	Ind	510
Far	MN	460, 461	Kg	Ind	511
s^D	MN	462	Kuhn	Ind	512
Mit	MN	463, 464	Li^a	Ind	513, 514
Dantu	MN	465[*1]	Niemetz	Ind	515
ERIK	MN	466[*1]	RASM	Ind	516[*1]
M^V	MN	467	Re^a	Ind	517, 518[*1]
Lu^a	Lutheran	468, 469[*2]	Reiter	Ind	519, 520
Lu9	Lutheran	470[*1]	Sharp	Ind	521
Kp^a	Kell	471, 472	Zd	Ind	522
Js^a	Kell	473, 474			

[*1] Antibody has caused a positive DAT but not clinical HDN
[*2] Most Lutheran system antibodies cause a positive DAT but not clinical HDN
[*3] Ind = Antigen independent of known blood group systems

series (316) 102 of 127 (80%) infants born to women with anti-K in the serum, had K- red cells. In two other series (60,63) 80% and 88% respectively, of the women with anti-K in the serum had previously been transfused. Among the 517,000 women there were seven cases of severe or fatal HDN. By combining reports about births in England and Wales during the period 1977 to 1990,

Mollison et al. (71) noted that among approximately 9 million births there were 15 registered deaths from HDN in which the maternal serum contained anti-K. In 11 of the cases only anti-K was present, in the other four anti-c or anti-E were present as well. The above data are not included to trivialize the significance of fatal HDN due to antibodies other than anti-D. As mentioned elsewhere, to the

TABLE 41-3 Antigens of High Incidence Defined by Antibodies that have Caused HDN or a Positive DAT on the Red Cells of a Newborn

Antigen	System	References	Antigen	System	References
Hr_0	Rh	523-535, 991-994	PP_1P^k	P	572, 573[*3]
Rh29	Rh	536-540	Co^a	Colton	574-576
LW^{ab}	LW	541[*1]	Co3	Colton	577, 578
U	MN	364-367, 542, 543	Di^b	Diego	579-584, 903, 904
U^Z	MN	544[*1]	Wr^b	Diego	585
En^a	MN	545	Ge	Gerbich	586-589[*4]
Lu^b	Lutheran	546-550[*2]	Yt^a	Cartwright	590, 591, 919-921[*1]
k	Kell	321, 551-555, 571, 997-999	Gy^a/Hy	Dombrock	592, 593[*1]
Kp^b	Kell	556-559	Jo^a	Dombrock	594[*1]
Ku	Kell	561, 562	Cr^a/Tc^a	Cromer	595-597[*1]
Js^b	Kell	322-325	Er^a	Er Coll.	598, 599[*1]
K11	Kell	560	Vel	Ind[*5]	600
K22	Kell	563, 564	Lan	Ind	601-603
Jk3	Kidd	565-568	At^a	Ind	604, 605
Fy3	Duffy	569, 570	Jr^a	Ind	606-611

[*1] Antibody has caused a positive DAT but not clinical HDN
[*2] Most Lutheran system antibodies cause a positive DAT but not clinical HDN
[*3] For the role of antibodies to P and P^k in spontaneous abortion, see Chapter 11
[*4] HDN caused by antibodies to high incidence Gerbich system antigens is usually very mild
[*5] Ind = Antigen independent of known blood group systems

mother who has just lost an infant to the disease, the incidence is 100% no matter what the statistics. However, the figures do show that fatal HDN caused by an antibody other than anti-D is a less common occurrence than might be supposed from a cursory glance at the literature. It must also be remembered that after anti-D and anti-c, anti-K is the most common cause of severe HDN (71,183,288,337), cases caused by antibodies to antigens such as s, U, Fy^a, Jk^a, etc., will be even more uncommon.

There is at least one case reported in the literature (338) and two others (339,340) cited as personal communications by Mollison et al. (71) in which anti-K has appeared to suppress erythropoeisis in addition to clearing red cells in infants with HDN. It seems, from these findings, that anti-K may have a greater effect than anti-D in destroying or retarding maturation of erythroid precursor red cells. The net result is that anemia in the newborn may be considerably more severe at birth than had been forecast from measurement of bilirubin in amniotic fluid during pregnancy. That is, a decrease in red cell production contributes significantly to the anemia as opposed to anti-D HDN where the anemia is primarily caused by antibody-mediated destruction of red cells.

Because anti-K is encountered fairly frequently in pregnant women, attempts have been made to establish laboratory parameters that indicate the potential for severe HDN if the infant is K+. Strohm et al. (318) reviewed data on 103 anti-K found in screening tests on samples from 1215 immunized women in a 27 year period. Twelve women in whom anti-K was detected during pregnancy delivered infants with K+ red cells, two others also had K+ infants but the maternal anti-K was detected only at the time of delivery. Four of the twelve women with K+ infants had anti-K with a titer less than 32, none of their infants had clinical HDN. Among the eight women with an anti-K titer of 32 or more, two had infants who required both intrauterine and exchange transfusions, six had clinically unaffected infants. The most severely affected infant was born to the woman with the highest titer anti-K in the series, i.e. titer 256, after that there was overlap, i.e. titer of anti-K in the mother of the second affected infant 64, titers in women with unaffected infants 2 at 128, 2 at 64 and 2 at 32. From these observations the authors (318) concluded that when the anti-K titer is less than 32, no invasive procedure is necessary to assess potential HDN. Obviously this suggestion, even if correct, is of limited value since it applied in only four of 12 cases in this study. Further, there are reasons to believe that the limited recommendation made in 1991 (318), was not appropriate. In 1987, Mollison et al. (319) mentioned a case (320) in which anti-K with a titer of 2 during the 37th week of pregnancy caused hydrops fetalis. Similarly, in 1989, Bowman et al. (321) in a paper describing a case of severe HDN caused by anti-k, mentioned a woman with anti-K with a titer of 8 whose fetus was hydropic and required intrauterine transfusion. Differently to Strohm et al. (318), Bowman et al. (321) recommended that since it appears that severe HDN can be caused by anti-K or anti-k of low titer, investigative measures should be undertaken when the antibody titer, by IAT, is 8 or greater. This whole question of antibody titers in pregnant women is discussed again below.

In preparing tables 41-1, 41-2 and 41-3 initial attempts were made to indicate which antibodies had caused severe or fatal HDN and which had caused a positive DAT in a newborn but no clinical disease. The attempts were largely abandoned because so many antibodies have done both and have acted at levels intermediate between the two. As typical examples anti-Js^b has been seen to cause hydrops (322), to cause severe (323) and moderate (324) HDN, and to cause a positive DAT in an infant who required no treatment (325) although the maternal anti-Js^b had a titer of 64. Similarly, different examples of anti-Fy^a have caused cases of HDN that ranged from mild enough to need no treatment, to fatal (57,58,326). An attempt has been made, in the three tables, to indicate which antibodies have caused a positive DAT in a newborn but no clinical HDN. Even then it is entirely possible that we (and our computerized searches) have missed reports of an example of a particular antibody that did cause HDN. As mentioned earlier, any IgG antibody in the mother directed against an antigen on fetal red cells, when that antigen is reasonably well developed at birth, has the potential to cause HDN. For those specificities we have missed, reprints may be sent via the publisher (no irate letters please, we are doing our best).

As will be seen in table 41-1, the Rh system has been treated differently to others. The references given there are to large scale studies of HDN caused by Rh antibodies other than anti-D (e.g. a review of findings on infants born to 42 different women with anti-c in the serum (59)). One case has been reported in which it was claimed (327,328) that anti-Le^{bH} caused mild HDN. While it has been shown (329,330) that some portions of some anti-Le^a are IgG in nature, we are not aware of any report other than the one above (327) that makes a similar claim for

anti-Le^{bH}. Further, the Lewis antigens are known (see Chapter 9) to be present in only small amounts on the red cells of newborn infants. When they are demonstrable at all, Le^a appears first (regardless of the presence of *Se* with *Le*) and Le^{bH} is usually not detectable. Thus the claim of HDN caused by anti-Le^{bH} came as a very considerable surprise (331). If it existed one would have to suppose that the extraordinary combination of potent IgG anti-Le^{bH} in the maternal serum and very unusual development of Le^{bH} on the infant's red cells occurred. Mollison et al. (71) summarize the reported case (327) with the statement that "There was no clinical or haematological evidence of a haemolytic process".

HDN Caused by Antibodies to Rare Antigens

This situation is one that is particularly interesting at the serological level. When the maternal serum contains an antibody to a rare antigen, that antibody may not be detected in standard antibody-screening tests because the red cells used in those tests may not carry the low incidence antigen. Indeed, red cells used for such tests are best selected (see Chapter 35) for other properties, i.e., from persons homozygous for *Jk^a*, *Jk^b*, etc. Thus HDN caused by an antibody to a rare antigen may well occur unexpectedly, that is when a woman in whom no alloantibody has been detected, delivers a child. The most obvious laboratory sign that this has happened is that the DAT on the infant's red cells is positive. For this reason, a rather weak case can be made for the routine performance of DATs on the red cells of all newborns. However, most workers believe that the DAT should be performed only when there is evidence of clinical disease, i.e., anemia and/or an increased level of bilirubin and/or apparent jaundice. When the DAT is positive but the maternal serum is non-reactive in antibody screening tests, a number of additional tests should be performed. ABO HDN must be excluded. If the infant has red cells that are incompatible with ABO antibodies in the maternal serum, an eluate should be made from the infant's DAT+ red cells and should be tested for the presence of anti-A and/or anti-B (see also below). If ABO HDN can be excluded, or if anti-A and/or anti-B does not seem to be the sole cause of red cell destruction in the infant, further investigations are necessary. HDN caused by an antibody to a rare antigen occurs when the infant inherits a gene from the father, that results in the rare antigen being present on the infant's red cells and when the mother has made an IgG antibody to the antigen concerned. Thus a logical step is to test the maternal serum and an eluate from the infant's red cells against the red cells of the infant's father. However, a number of points must be borne in mind when such tests are undertaken.

First, the maternal serum may contain an ABO antibody directed against an antigen on the paternal red cells so that direct tests may not be possible. Second, the same may apply to the eluate made from the infant's red cells. If, for example, the mother is group O and the infant and the father are group A, the eluate may contain anti-A that may or may not be contributing to the in vivo red cell destruction, as well as an antibody to a rare antigen. When ABO incompatibility complicates the testing, anti-A and/or anti-B can be removed from the maternal serum and/or the eluate by adsorption with random group A or group B red cells. If an antibody to a rare antigen is causing the HDN, the chance of selecting random A or B cells that also carry that antigen is essentially non-existent if cells from unrelated persons are used. Even before ABO incompatibility (if it exists) has been overcome and the causative antibody in the maternal serum and the eluate from the infant's red cells has been shown to react with the paternal red cells, treatment of the infant presents no problems. If exchange transfusion is necessary, donor blood compatible with the maternal serum and/or the eluate from the infant's red cells, can be used. Such blood will be found very easily if the causative antibody is directed against a rare antigen. A third point to be considered is that the red cells of the infant's biological father are the ones that should be used to detect the causative antibody. If the maternal serum and the eluate from the infant's red cells fail to react with the red cells of the woman's husband, discrete inquiries may be indicated to determine whether there is a possibility that a different male could be the infant's father.

As can be seen, it is not necessary to identify the causative antibody in order to be able to transfuse the infant or the mother if she should need blood. Simple compatibility tests will suffice to identify suitable donors. However, most blood bankers who encounter such a case will be interested enough to want to identify the antibody or to have reference laboratories with large collections of red cells carrying rare antigens undertake such tests. From the point of view of adding knowledge about the human blood groups, such tests are well worthwhile. A number of antigens (e.g., Good, Rd^a, Ht^a, HJK) were first recognized when the corresponding antibody caused HDN. Others (such as Go^a and Be^a) were recognized as belonging to known blood group systems when family studies were conducted after a case of HDN had been encountered.

If severe or fatal HDN due to an antibody directed against a rare antigen is seen, genetic counseling of the couple involved is somewhat different to the situation in which anti-D causes severe or fatal disease. As mentioned below, among the husbands of women who have anti-D in the serum and produce affected infants, *D* homozygotes outnumber *D* heterozygotes by a ratio of

about 4 to 1. The chance that a male will be homozygous for a gene that encodes production of a very rare antigen is obviously very small. Thus in virtually all cases in which an antibody to a rare antigen causes severe HDN, there is a 50% chance that any subsequently conceived infant will be unaffected. Table 41-2 lists a number of rare antigens, some of which belong to established blood group systems and some of which appear to be genetically independent of all known systems, that are defined by antibodies that have caused (sometimes severe) HDN. Some of the data in table 41-2 are from Sabo (332) and some from Vengelen-Tyler (333).

HDN With Detectable Red Cell Bound IgG But No Identifiable Antibody

Marsh et al. (334) described a case in which a woman produced three infants in a ten year period (during which time she also had two abortions) each of whom had a positive DAT and of whom the first two became jaundiced. The protein on the red cells of the third child was IgG but neither the maternal serum nor an eluate from the child's red cells would react with antibody screening cells or with red cells from the father or either of the first two children. Non-paternity was apparently excluded since all three children had a positive DAT at birth. Red cells collected from the third child, when it was eight months old, would not react with the maternal serum or with an eluate made from that child's red cells at birth. The authors suggested that the children had probably inherited a paternal gene that encodes production of an antigen that is present on the surface of red cells only during fetal development.

Influence of Previous Pregnancies and Genotype of the Father of the Child: Rh HDN

As would be expected from what has been written above, once a woman is immunized to a blood group antigen, the level of antibody in her serum is likely to increase in subsequent pregnancies if the fetuses she carries have red cells positive for the antigen to which she is immunized and if some of those red cells enter the maternal circulation during the pregnancy. Although as mentioned above, FMHs during pregnancy most often involve volumes of red cells that are too small to initiate a primary immune response, they are sometimes large enough to constitute secondary or boosting doses in an already immunized woman. Thus in Rh HDN, the most commonly seen pattern (before the introduction of RhIG and the various intervention measures described below) was that among affected infants born to a woman with anti-D in the serum, the disease was progressively more severe in each infant born (1,71,341). Walker et al. (341) found that the risk of stillbirth in a woman who had previously produced an infant with mild HDN due to anti-D was around 2% whereas in a woman who had previously had a stillborn infant due to the antibody, it was around 70%. Obviously the *Rh* genotype of the father is of great importance in a woman who has made potent anti-D. If the father is homozygous for *D* all subsequently conceived infants will have D+ red cells and will be at risk of HDN. If the father is heterozygous for *D* there will be a 50% chance that each subsequently conceived child will have D- red cells. As blood bankers know, it is very difficult to determine zygosity of *D* in serological tests and interpretations of probable *Rh* genotype used to be made from phenotyping studies. Among fathers of infants who have had Rh HDN this is even more difficult because in situations involving severe clinical disease, fathers homozygous for *D* outnumber those heterozygous for that gene by about four to one. As discussed below, one way of attempting to forecast the severity of HDN in a woman who has anti-D in the serum and who is pregnant, is to measure antibody levels in serial maternal blood samples collected during the pregnancy. However, in a few women who are carrying a fetus with D- red cells, the anti-D level increases during pregnancy, e.g., four of 239 in the series of Hopkins (342) and 13 of 300 in the series of Fraser and Tovey (343). As also discussed below, there are now many other ways, some invasive and some non-invasive, of attempting to determine or forecast the severity of HDN in an individual case. There is, as yet, no complete agreement as to the most reliable non-invasive test.

Determination of the Blood Type of the Fetus While it is Still In Utero

As discussed in Chapter 12, the presence or absence of an antigen on the red cells of an unborn infant can be forecast by examination of the infant's DNA extracted from amniocytes present in amniotic fluid or extracted from cells following chorionic villus sampling. Clearly since anti-D is still the most common cause of severe HDN, prenatal determination of antigen type will, most often, involve D. However, as described below, forecasts of the presence or absence of other antigens can also be made.

While determining which genes are present (i.e. an actual genotype) will correlate with expressed phenotype (i.e. which antigens are present) on the vast majority of occasions, exceptions will be seen. That is to say, in some instances a gene may be present but for one of a variety of reasons, its product may not be expressed on red cells. On other occasions a hybrid gene may be present such that the portion (exon or intron) probed may be absent (the test will forecast absence of antigen) while other portions (exons) are present, that encode production of the antigen. The results of tests in these circumstances are sometimes called false positives and false negatives, respectively. In fact, the results are not false at all (assuming that the tests were correctly performed) since they are designed to detect the presence or absence of (pieces of) genes. The true explanation of contradictory findings is that presence or absence of a structural gene does not always correlate with presence or absence of antigen.

When it was first shown (941) that, in Whites, the phenotype D- most often represents the total absence of *D* genes, it was hoped that DNA from any fetus with D+ red cells could be identified by probes that detected a portion of the *D* gene. Bennett et al. (942) introduced the first method that probed for a portion of exon 10 of the *D* gene that differs from exon 10 of any *CE* allele. While in most D+ and D- individuals presence or absence of exon 10 of *D* correlates exactly with presence or absence of D, exceptions were soon found. As discussed in detail in Chapter 12, gene conversion between *D* and *CE* alleles can result in the formation of hybrid genes that will be recognized by probes for certain regions of *D*, but will not produce D antigen and others that will lack the portion of *D* probed but will carry exons that encode production of D. Many other investigations in these and related areas have been reported (943-964,987) and most workers now seem to agree that at a minimum, two probes for *D* be used, sometimes in a multiplex system, when tests on fetal DNA to forecast a D type are used (965,966). Some workers routinely use more than two sets of probes and test the DNA for presence/absence/differences in exon 10, exon 7, exon 4 and intron 4.

In addition to their application in prenatal studies, these methods have also been used to determine D type from a single cell in preimplantation, to prevent anti-D HDN (967). In spite of the great success achieved with these methods in forecasting the red cell D type of an unborn child, it is clear that they should be used only when the parents are White. Daniels et al. (968) reported that in tests on DNA from 25 South African Blacks, all of whom had D- red cells (confirmed as D- in adsorption-elution studies) they were able to find evidence for the presence of some portion of *D* in 22. Although some of the positive findings represented the presence of only exon 10 from *D* and could thus have been forecast not to be associated with expected presence of D, even the use of multiple probes would have led to an incorrect conclusion in 16 (64%) of the 25 persons studied. As the authors (968) pointed out, no PCR amplification test of fetal DNA from Black infants will be of value until the molecular background leading to the D- phenotype in the presence of the *D* gene is understood.

Although fewer women make antibodies to C, c, E and e than make anti-D, meaning that fewer infants are at risk of serious HDN, prenatal typings on fetal DNA to forecast which antigens will be made, have been described (969-972,988). Similarly, since the structure and organization of the *Kell* complex gene has been established (973-975) and the difference between *K* and *k* is known, methods have been described (976,977,986) for typing an unborn infant for K. The ability to distinguish between a fetus with K+ and one with K- red cells in a woman making anti-K may be of particular relevance in view of the suggestion (338) cited earlier, that anti-K may cause severe anemia in part because of its ability to suppress maturation of erythroid forming cells in the marrow.

Because the collection of fetal DNA involves an invasive procedure (amniocentesis or chorionic villus sampling) attempts have been made to isolate nucleated cells from the fetus, from the maternal circulation (978-981). At least one worker (982) in this field is skeptical that the efforts will succeed and, as pointed out in Chapter 12, attempts to forecast fetal blood types from such maneuvers have not approached the success rates achieved from fetal DNA isolation and characterization. Attempts have also been made (983) to obtain nucleated fetal cells from the cervical canal.

To conclude this section it will again be stressed that strenuous efforts are in order (e.g. use of multiple probes for as many portions of *D* as possible) whenever an attempt to forecast presence or absence of an antigen on the fetal red cells is made. A forecast that the antigen will not be made, when in fact the antigen is made, will clearly endanger the fetus. Appropriate monitoring may not be undertaken and intrauterine transfusion that may be the only means of keeping the fetus alive until delivery, may not be used. Though not as obvious, a forecast that the antigen will be made, when in fact it is not, will also have untoward consequences. Unnecessary invasive procedures may be used and may thus put the fetus at unnecessary risk. It should be remembered that however experienced the obstetrician, amniocentesis is not a totally benign procedure and carries a small, but measurable risk.

Influence of Previous Pregnancies and Genotype of the Father of the Child: ABO HDN

For reasons discussed above, ABO HDN is far more common when the mother is group O and the infant is A or B than in any other ABO incompatible situation.

Unlike Rh HDN, the severity of disease in previously born infants is not a reliable guide to expected severity in the next infant although occasionally a woman will be encountered in whom all infants are severely affected. Another difference between Rh and ABO HDN is that in the latter, the firstborn child may be as severely affected as any subsequently conceived infant. This relates, of course, to the fact that some women make high levels of immune ABO system antibodies following exposure to materials (e.g., smallpox and typhoid vaccines, tetanus toxoid (344-353)) other than red cells. As in Rh HDN, the genotype of the father will play a role. If the mother is group O and the father is genetically A^1A^1, all infants of the couple will be at risk. If the father is genetically A^1O there will be a 50% chance that the infant will be group O and therefore unaffected. Since ABO HDN is only rarely life-threatening (354-357, and see below) there is seldom any need to differentiate between the A^1A^1 and A^1O genotypes, that can only be accomplished at the molecular level anyway (358-363) in the fathers of potentially affected infants.

Influence of Previous Pregnancies and Genotype of the Father of the Child: HDN Due to Other Antibodies

As already mentioned, with the exception of a few antibodies to antigens of very low incidence, HDN caused by antibodies other than anti-D is seldom as severe as that caused by anti-D or anti-CD. The effects of previous pregnancies are similar to those discussed above for Rh HDN. Obviously if a woman has made say anti-Fy^a, the amount of that antibody in her serum is likely to increase if fetal Fy(a+) red cells enter her circulation. Similarly, if the father is genetically Fy^aFy^a all infants will be at risk whereas if he is Fy^aFy^b there will be a 50% chance that any subsequently conceived infant will have Fy(a-) red cells. Rare exceptions to the generally less severe cases of HDN caused by these antibodies will be seen. For example, anti-U has caused at least one stillbirth (364) and several cases (365-367) in which the infants were severely affected. However, the same specificity has caused mild HDN (368) and a sub-clinical condition in two successive infants born to one immunized woman (369). With an antibody directed against a high incidence antigen, such as U, the effects of previous pregnancies may be similar to those seen in successive cases caused by anti-D, but the chance that the father of the infant will be heterozygous for the gene encoding production of the antigen against which the maternal antibody is directed, will be negligible.

As would be expected, if the structure of the gene has been established and if the nucleotide difference in polymorphic genes is known (e.g. Fy^a or Fy^b (984,985), Di^a or Di^b (989)), tests on DNA from the fetus (as described above) can be used to forecast the infant's red cell phenotype.

Prenatal Testing: Antibodies Other Than ABO

Since HDN is caused by IgG antibodies produced by the mother, it is clear that most of those women at risk of delivering an affected infant can be identified by antibody-screening tests on their serum. In spite of that straightforward situation there is no international agreement as to who should be tested, when the tests should be done, nor what serological methods should be used. Once a maternal antibody with the potential to cause HDN is identified, there is even less agreement as to what should be done.

In the USA it is recommended (613,614) that all pregnant women be typed for ABO and D and that antibody-screening be done, during the first trimester, usually at the patient's first visit to the obstetrician. For those women who are D+ and in whom no antibodies are detected no further antibody-screening is recommended unless there is: a history of transfusion; evidence of HDN in a previous infant; or abdominal trauma during the pregnancy. For those women who are D- and in whom no antibodies are detected, it is recommended that repeat testing for antibodies be performed at 28 to 30 weeks gestation. It should be noted that the wording (614) is such that repeat testing of D+ women for the indications listed above is described as "should be considered". Repeat testing of D- women at 28 to 30 weeks is essential, it is at this visit that antenatal RhIG therapy should be started (71,180,183,615) in those in whom no anti-D was detected in the initial tests. In order that the woman does not have to visit twice, the sample for antibody-screening can be drawn, then the RhIG can be injected. In those few women in whom anti-D is detected in the sample collected before the injection of RhIG, observation throughout the rest of the pregnancy (see below) is necessary and RhIG administration is not indicated postnatally. Previously in the USA it was recommended (616) that repeat antibody-screening tests be performed on D+ and D- women at 28 to 30 weeks gestation. The change (613,614) by which repeat tests on D+ women were excluded was based on observations (60,289,617-620) on the paucity of formation of antibodies during pregnancy, whose presence necessitates some form of intervention. In other words, it was not disputed that some D+ women form antibodies during pregnancy and that those antibodies would not be found before delivery. However, it was concluded that the fact that presence of

such an antibody so rarely alters the way in which the woman's pregnancy is handled, that repeat screening of D+ women was not cost effective and that its abandonment would not place women, or their infants, in significant jeopardy. As discussed below, others do not agree with this conclusion.

For D- women with anti-D and for D+ and D- women with any antibody thought capable of causing HDN present, it was recommended (614) that from 20 weeks gestation onwards repeat antibody-screening, to see if additional antibodies had been made, and titration of identified antibodies, be performed at 2 to 4 week intervals. Titrations (that are discussed again below) were considered necessary only until such time as the antibody was considered strong enough that other means of fetal monitoring (amniocentesis, ultrasound, etc., see below) were begun. Again, it was felt that since the prime function of antibody titration is to indicate when other monitoring is necessary, there was nothing to be gained by further titrations, once such monitoring had begun (614,621). Thus repeat titrations in this setting were considered to fall outside the range of tests that produce data that aid in diagnosis or are used to modify patient care. In the current economic environment it is considered prudent, if not essential, to eliminate tests that fail to satisfy such criteria (622).

In some other countries the recommendation that antibody-screening tests be performed on serum from all D+ and D- women, once at 10 to 16 weeks and again at 28 to 36 weeks gestation, remains in effect (376,623). It is claimed (65,285,624) that detection and identification of an antibody developing late in pregnancy may indicate that intervention in care is necessary, and/or will enable compatible blood to be available at the time of the infant's birth in the event that the infant or the mother requires transfusion. While in an ideal world it would seem that knowledge of every antibody in every pregnancy would be desirable, it must be stated that in this instance (i.e. screening samples from every pregnant woman twice during the pregnancy) the amount and cost of the work involved seems enormous for the very limited (if any) benefit (i.e. change in the prenatal management of a pregnancy).

A similar argument to the above relates to the choice of tests to be used in antibody-screening of samples from pregnant women. While some workers (624,625) are adamant that the use of enzyme-treated red cells is essential if antibody-screening tests are to be done only once, at 10 to 16 weeks, and others (626,627) believe their use to be an advantage, many workers (376,614,619,621,622,628-633) do not agree. While it is claimed that detection and identification of an antibody early in pregnancy is an advantage, the counter is that if the management of the pregnancy is not altered as a result, no advantage accrues. There is no doubt that the use of enzyme-treated red cells in screening tests will result in the detection of a few Rh antibodies not yet reactive by any other method, in pregnant women. However, it has been shown (614,629-631,634) that women who reach term with an antibody detectable only in tests against enzyme-treated red cells, deliver infants who do not have clinical HDN. Further, in the majority of such infants, i.e. 15 of 19 (79%) the DAT at birth, is negative (629,630). Even in the case in which it was claimed (625) that it is important to monitor "enzyme-only" antibodies through pregnancy, the anti-E involved was detectable by IAT at 29 weeks gestation (it had reacted only with enzyme-treated red cells at 11 and 20 weeks) and had an IAT titer of 256 by 35 weeks. No intervention in the pregnancy was undertaken so that early knowledge of the anti-E was not of practical importance at that level, its high titer by 35 weeks clearly indicated the likelihood that the infant would require exchange transfusion (it did when born at 40 weeks) but provided ample time for such blood to be readied (and would still have done so if rare blood, not simply E-, had been needed).

Those who oppose the use of enzyme-treated red cells in prenatal antibody-screening do so on two major counts. First, as clearly indicated above, early knowledge of the antibody's presence does not provide any advantage to the mother or the infant. Second, the use of enzyme-pretreated red cells results in the detection of many clinically irrelevant alloimmune and autoimmune antibodies. The serological studies necessary to show that these antibodies are irrelevant are time-consuming, expensive and provide no benefit to anyone. In our study (628) on 10,000 sera known to be non-reactive in LISS/IAT antibody-screening tests, we found 28 clinically insignificant alloantibodies, 77 sera in which the antibody was too weak to identify, and 216 autoantibodies reactive only with ficin-treated red cells. Urbaniak (635) reviewed the results of some 45,000 enzyme antibody-screening tests on the sera of pregnant women. Among antibodies detected only by the use of enzyme pretreated red cells, 22 anti-E and 7 anti-C^w "remained enzyme-only" at term, none caused a positive DAT in the infant. Of two anti-D and one anti-c, one anti-D and the anti-c were detectable by IAT at 34 weeks gestation, both caused positive DATs but neither infant had clinical HDN. At the same time 77 of 14,925 maternal samples reacted only with enzyme-pretreated red cells, almost half the reactions were clinically irrelevant. The service recommended (635) stopping enzyme-screening tests since a second sample from each woman is tested between 28 and 34 weeks gestation. It is of note that in defending the follow-up of an antibody first detected in screening tests against enzyme-pretreated red cells through pregnancy, Garner et al. (624) report that their transfusion center and the transfusion service in the hospital where the patient was encountered "do not experience unwanted positive tests when using enzyme-treated cells for antibody detection". As

pointed out in Chapter 3, if red cells are correctly treated with proteases, i.e. suitably modified to ensure enhanced sensitivity of the test system, the detection of unwanted positives is unavoidable (71,628,636-639). It is also of note that in defending the follow-up of the antibody in question, Garner et al. (624) state that they do not claim that the use of enzyme-pretreated red cells is essential in prenatal antibody-screening. Indeed, the most recent guidelines from the UK (376) do not specify which methods should be used in such tests and mention that antibodies that have a significant IgG component are detectable by IAT. It is apparent from discussions (635,640-642) about the new recommendations, that abandonment of tests with enzyme pretreated red cells is considered appropriate only if samples from all pregnant women are tested a second time, at 28 to 34 weeks gestation. As indicated above, such tests are not considered necessary in the USA (613,614) since the incidence of severe HDN in a D+ woman with a negative IAT at 10 to 16 weeks gestation is minuscule.

If an unusual specificity antibody is found (e.g., anti-M, anti-Lu^a) tests using 2-ME or DTT (see Chapter 3) can be used to differentiate between IgM (no risk of HDN) and IgG (risk of HDN) antibodies. Further, the red cells of the child's father can be typed to see if the infant's red cells are likely to carry the antigen against which the woman is immunized.

Prenatal Testing: ABO Antibodies

Virtually all workers agree (376,613,614) that prenatal tests designed to identify which pregnant women will deliver infants affected with ABO HDN are pointless. The problem is that in any serological screening test, large numbers of women will be found to have ABO antibodies that have immune characteristics, yet only a tiny minority of them will deliver affected infants. Accordingly, a history is of more value than a laboratory test. Any woman who has had one child with ABO HDN should be considered to be potentially capable of having other affected infants. However, as mentioned above, a woman who has delivered one child with severe ABO HDN may later produce a child of the same ABO group that is only mildly affected. Amniocentesis (see below) to forecast severity of ABO HDN should probably only be used when the woman has a history of producing very severely affected infants.

Antibody Titrations and Severity of HDN

For many years the obstetrician's only guide to the severity of HDN that might be expected in a given infant was the strength of the maternal antibody. It was always accepted (758) that such an indicator was far from infallible. While there are now other means of forecasting the severity of the disease in an unborn infant and while the value of titrations in this setting is often decried, they are still widely used. There are a number of reasons for this. First, other methods, such as measurement of antibody in terms of µg/ml (676-678), are not readily available in many laboratories. Second, even when such figures can be generated they may not be much more reliable as forecasts of severity, than are titrations. Although Fraser and Tovey (343) found that among 490 women with more than 10 µg/ml anti-D in the serum, 68% gave birth to affected infants, results reported by Moreley et al. (643) did not show even that level of correlation. Hughes-Jones et al. (177) found that when low or high levels of anti-D were measured, mild and severe HDN respectively, could be forecast, but that the majority of women had intermediate levels of anti-D and then the measured level was not well correlated with severity. Third, while it is generally agreed that above a certain titer, titration end points do not correlate well with severity of disease, many workers believe that with some exceptions (see below) low titer values indicate that invasive procedures need not be undertaken. Fourth, some of the more reliable ways of forecasting the severity of HDN do involve invasive procedures. As such they introduce a risk to the fetus and/or the danger that an FMH will result. This, in turn, can serve as an additional immunizing dose and cause an increase in the maternal antibody level. Thus many workers continue to use titrations in an attempt to determine when invasive procedures should be undertaken although, as described below, their use in this manner has also been criticized.

The major problem with titration studies is that while most women with high titered antibodies will have affected infants and most women with low titered antibodies will not, there will be exceptions in both directions. That is to say, a woman with a high titer of antibody may produce an unaffected infant, or one whose red cells lack the antigen to which the maternal antibody is directed, or one in whom the disease is mild enough that phototherapy (see below) but no transfusion is required. Conversely, a woman with an antibody of low titer may produce a severely affected infant, a situation that may create an emergency if no preparations have been made in advance to treat such a case.

The limited value of using only titrations to forecast severity of HDN was illustrated in the study of Dijk et al. (644). Data from 359 women immunized to D were analyzed. Among the infants born to 40 women in whom the titer of anti-D was less than 16, 17 (43%) required no treatment, 15 (38%) required only phototherapy but 3 (8%) required simple transfusion for anemia while 5 (13%) required exchange transfusions. Among the 319

infants born to women in whom the anti-D titer was 16 or higher, 66 (21%) required no treatment, 101 (32%) required phototherapy, 24 (8%) required simple transfusion while 128 (40%) required exchange transfusions. Thus in 32 of 40 (80%) cases, a low titer of anti-D (i.e. below 16) was associated with mild disease (no treatment or only phototherapy) while in 152 of 319 (48%) a titer of 16 or greater was associated with a need for transfusion. Similar findings were made when data from 59 cases involving women immunized to antigens other than D were reviewed (644). Among the 59 women, 34 had anti-c, 19 anti-E and six anti-K. Among 26 infants born to women in whom the antibody titer was less than 16, 13 required no treatment, 12 required only phototherapy, and one required an exchange transfusion. Among 33 infants born to women in whom the antibody titer was 16 or higher, 5 required no treatment, 10 phototherapy only, 4 simple transfusion and 14 exchange transfusion. In other words, in 25 of 26 (96%) infants a low titer of the maternal antibody was associated with mild HDN while in 18 of 33 (55%) a titer of 16 or higher was associated with a need for transfusion. While the authors (644) and a commentator (645) concluded that the data listed above show that there is no critical titer that is associated with HDN severe enough to require transfusion and that titrations do not provide a reliable guide as to when invasive investigations should be undertaken, the data do show some correlation with disease severity. Titrations are clearly of more value when the antibody is weak than when it is strong. Of 66 women with an antibody with a titer of less than 16, only nine (14%) gave birth to an infant that required transfusion. Of 352 women with an antibody with a titer of 16 or higher, 182 (52%) gave birth to infants that required no treatment beyond phototherapy. Both Dijk et al. (644) and Clark (645) suggested that some of the in vitro cellular assays now being used might eventually prove to be more reliable than antibody titrations in forecasting severity of HDN. However, as described in more detail below, there is still debate as to which of the assays is most reliable, no single method stands out as clearly superior to the others. Further, since antibody titrations are performed in far more laboratories than are cellular assays, it is likely that titrations will continue in use in this setting for a number of years to come.

Presumably with the above considerations in mind a number of workers (616,646) have suggested that in women with anti-D, the critical level at which other investigations should be considered, is a titer of 16 (614). In a different set of recommendations (376) the titer value suggested as indicating a likelihood of HDN is given as 32. In the same recommendations the figures of Nicolaides and Rodeck (647) are used to forecast disease severity when anti-D levels have been measured in international units (iu). While it is noted that exceptions can occur, it is suggested that HDN is unlikely when the maternal anti-D level is less than 4 iu per ml, that there is a moderate risk of HDN at levels between 4 and 15 iu per ml, and that there is a high risk of hydrops fetalis when the anti-D level is greater than 15 iu per ml. Again the correlation of a low level of antibody with no disease or a mildly affected infant is better than correlations between higher levels of antibody and severity of clinical disease (177,647-649). In the recommendations regarding prenatal testing there is general agreement that antibody levels, as measured by titration or in terms of iu/ml, that correlate with disease severity when the antibody is other than anti-D, have not been reliably established. Judd et al. (614) suggest that when the titer is "low" and does not increase during pregnancy, invasive procedures can be avoided or delayed. While the authors (614) suggest that critical titers for antibodies other than anti-D have not been defined, the content of their paper suggests that a "low" titer is less than 16. In the BCSH guidelines (376) it is stated that significant titers (for antibodies other than anti-D) likely to cause HDN are 32 or greater except for Kell system antibodies that may affect the fetus even when the titer is low. As mentioned above, a critical titer of 32 for anti-K as suggested by Strohm et al. (318) seems far too high since there are a number of reports (318-321) of severe HDN caused by anti-K and other Kell system antibodies with considerably lower titers.

Since titrations are still widely used and, for reasons discussed above are likely to remain in use in prenatal serology, some other points about those tests should be considered. It is important that the titration method measures levels of IgG and not IgM antibody since the former but not the latter can cross the placenta and enter the fetal circulation. In this respect antiglobulin titrations are better than those using agglutination in albumin since they tend to measure IgG antibody while albumin methods measure both. From what has been written about critical titers of antibodies it is clear that the best suggestion is that the laboratory work closely with the obstetrical unit to build a meaningful clinical interpretation based on its own titration values. A rise in titer during pregnancy usually indicates that an affected infant will result but this is not without exception. A woman with a fairly high, unchanging level of antibody throughout pregnancy will sometimes give birth to a more severely affected infant that a woman who has maintained a low level of antibody throughout most of her pregnancy and has then had a sharp rise in titer at the end of the pregnancy. On the other hand, an unchanged antibody level throughout a pregnancy sometimes indicates that the woman is carrying a fetus, the red cells of which lack the antigen to which she is immunized.

Because of the reliance likely to be placed on titra-tion results, laboratory variables must be eliminated. The same red cell donor should be used for repeat titrations and cells should be collected regularly so that they are of about the same age at the time of each titration. A valuable control is to use the previous sample from the patient, that has been preserved frozen, in parallel when titrating the new sample. If the same value is not obtained with the previous sample as when it was originally tested, a testing variable has been introduced. If the same value is obtained, a rise or fall in titer of the new sample can be regarded as more likely to be significant. Similarly, changes in technique should not be introduced without full knowledge by the obstetricians. For example if, for years, titrations have been performed by a saline/IAT method the obstetricians will associate certain values with certain likelihoods of severity much of the time. If a change from saline/IAT to say PEG/IAT is made, an anti-D with a titer of 16 by the former method may have a titer of 256 by the latter. If the obstetrician is not informed of the change in method and its likely effect on titers reported, the results obtained by the new method will be far more misleading than helpful.

Other In Vitro Methods Used to Forecast the Severity of HDN

As described in more detail below, a major advance in forecasting the severity of HDN in any given case was made when it was shown (650) that measurement of total bile pigment in amniotic fluid provided a reliable guide to the degree of disease in the fetus. However, this advance did not exclude the potential value of a test on the maternal serum. The disadvantage of amniocentesis is that it is an invasive procedure. At worst the procedure can result in death of the fetus (651), a less dramatic but nevertheless serious problem is that amniocentesis can cause an FMH and hence an increase in maternal antibody level following exposure to additional antigen-positive fetal red cells. Because of this contraindication of amniocentesis (and other invasive procedures) attempts have been made to correlate the degree of severity of HDN with the results of various in vitro cellular assays (for reviews see 679-681). In reading the literature it is noticeable that the best correlation among the various assays described in any given report is often seen with the method developed or used predominantly in the reporting authors' laboratory. That statement is not intended to suggest that investigator bias affected the results but rather that the various assays are difficult enough to perform that the best results are likely to be obtained with the assay with which the investigators are most familiar. Bearing this point in mind, various reports describe success with the monocyte monolayer assay

(652,653), the ADCC (monocyte) assay (654,655), the ADCC (lymphocyte) assay (656) and the monocyte chemilumenescence (CL) test (657,682). In a collaborative study (658) nine laboratories in Europe tested 14 samples from 11 mothers immunized to D, using a variety of cellular assays. The results were considered "correct" when they forecast the degree of severity of HDN. In the study the ADCC (monocyte) test was "correct" in 60% of cases, the ADCC (lymphocyte) test in 57%, the CL test in 50%, the MMA using peripheral blood monocytes in 41% (but in 71% of the cases in one laboratory), and the MMA using U937 cells or cultured monocytes in 32%. It was suggested (658) that the low level of correct predictions might, at least in part, have been due to the fact that a number of the maternal samples were collected some time after delivery of the infants. It was also pointed out (658) that variation in test performance between the various laboratories means that the study does not show superiority of ADCC (monocyte) and ADCC (lymphocyte) tests in predicting disease severity. Perhaps the clearest indication of that fact is the observation the MMA (adherence and phagocytosis by peripheral blood monocytes) was correct overall only 41% of the time, but in 71% of the cases in a laboratory with particular expertise in that method. Once again, in this study (658) low level readings correlated with no clinical or only mild HDN, better than intermediate and high level positive results correlated with moderate and severe disease. In other comparative studies performed in various laboratories, Lucas et al. (683) suggested that the CL test might be less prone to positive reactions that are not associated with clinical HDN, than is the MMA while Hadley et al. (659) found the ADCC (monocyte) assay to be superior to the ADCC (lymphocyte) assay and the MMA using U937 cells or cultured monocytes, in correlating with severity of disease. Garner et al. (660) reported that in their hands the ADCC (monocyte) assay gave more meaningful results than did the MMA while Zupanska et al. (653), Zupanska (661) and Bromilow and Duguid (662) all reported good correlations between disease severity and results of MMAs. The MMA was superior to rosetting tests with monocytes or lymphocytes in two of the studies (653,661). In contrast to the above findings, Brown et al. (663) were unable to demonstrate any correlation between the results of MMAs and the severity of HDN. Garner et al. (684) used the ADCC (monocyte) and MMA assays in tests on 44 anti-D of which the subclass composition was determined. They found that both assays gave their most reliable results with anti-D that were mixtures of IgG1 and IgG3. The ADCC assay measured predominantly IgG1 while the MMA measured predominantly IgG3. The authors (684) concluded that these findings indicate that the ADCC assay yields superior predictions because IgG1 anti-D

levels are more closely correlated with severity of HDN than are IgG3 anti-D levels. Most of the work performed in attempts to forecast the severity of HDN by the use of cellular assays, has involved women with anti-D in the serum who have given birth to D+ infants. Garner and Devenish (685) used the ADCC(M) assay in cases in which the antibodies had different specificities. With eight sera: two anti-U and one example each of antibodies directed against Di[b], Wr[b], Sc1, In[b], Hy and Jr[a] the titers were low, the ADCC showed low activity and no HDN resulted. With two sera, one anti-Rh29 and one anti-En[a] the titers and ADCC activity were high, both antibodies caused severe HDN. With four other antibodies, two anti-U, one anti-Cr[a] and one anti-In[b], the ADCC forecast that HDN would occur but no significant disease was seen. It was supposed that the anti-Cr[a] and the anti-In[b] did not cause HDN because the Cr[a] and In[b] antigens are not fully developed at birth. There was no explanation of the failure of the two anti-U in this last group, to cause HDN. By reading the report (685) it is apparent that similar forecasts (both correct and incorrect) about the severity of HDN would have been made from the results of ADCC(M) assays and antibody titrations, before the infants were born.

Clearly several of the in vitro cellular assays have the potential to forecast the severity of HDN or at least to indicate when invasive procedures can be avoided. Equally clear, considerable technical expertise in the method of choice is necessary for reliable forecasts to be made. Bowman (183) concludes that in spite of their promise the cellular assays do not replace invasive measures such as amniocentesis and fetal blood sampling in differentiating between the fetus who requires treatment in utero and the one who does not. Since all the cellular assays (and other serological procedures) measure antibody activity, they cannot indicate that the fetus in utero has red cells that lack the antigen to which the antibody is involved so that HDN will not occur.

Maternal Antibodies that Block Fetal Fc Receptors

On some occasions mild or no clinical HDN occurs in an infant with D+ red cells born to a woman with potent anti-D in the serum. It is now known (655,905,906) that this situation sometimes, but not always, represents the presence of a maternal IgG antibody directed against the Fc receptor on fetal macrophages. The maternal IgG anti-Fc crosses the placenta and by blocking the Fc receptor, reduces or abolishes the ability of fetal macrophages to bind IgG anti-D-coated red cells. Among 13 infants who were unaffected or had only mild HDN in spite of the presence of potent maternal anti-D (ADCC(M) tests yielding more than 80% lysis) seven were born to women with Fc receptor-blocking antibodies in the serum (905,906). When sera from mothers of 14 infants with severe HDN were tested, none contained receptor-blocking antibodies. It has been reported (655) that Fc receptor blocking antibodies can be demonstrated in about 4% of women in their second or a subsequent pregnancy and that most of the antibodies have anti-HLA-DR specificity (905,906). In at least one other case (907) mildness of the HDN represented diminished transport of maternal IgG across the placenta, that may have been independent of Fc receptor blocking.

Non-Serological Methods Used to Forecast the Severity of HDN: Amniocentesis

As mentioned above, once maternal antibody levels reach a certain point, they become less reliable as a guide to the severity of HDN to be expected. As a result, examination of amniotic fluid can be used in selected cases. Early studies (664,665) showed that measurement of bilirubin in amniotic fluid is not useful, first because the levels are low and second, because the turbidity of the fluid interferes with the measurement. However, later work (650,666-670) showed that the total level of bile pigment in amniotic fluid, as measured by spectroscopic methods, does correlate with the degree of hemolysis occurring in the fetus. Measurements are made at a number of different wavelengths and an increase at some indicates the amount of red cell destruction that has occurred. Collection of the amniotic fluid in a careful manner is essential for several reasons. First, the presence of hemoglobin in the fluid is a cause of misleading results (671). Second, as mentioned above, one of the dangers of amniocentesis is that placental damage during collection of the fluid may cause a significant escape of fetal cells into the maternal circulation and a subsequent, highly undesirable rise in maternal antibody level (215,672,673). Indeed, it is generally agreed that when amniocentesis is performed (for reasons other than measurement of the degree of destruction of fetal red cells) in D- women who do not have anti-D in the serum, an injection of RhIG should be given to guard against immunization caused by the entry of fetal cells into the maternal circulation. As can be seen, the examination of amniotic fluid can provide valuable information about the state of the fetus in an immunized woman. However, the procedure is not benign; in addition to the danger of maternal immunization mentioned above, there have been cases in which the fetus has bled to death in utero following damage to one of its blood vessels during collection of the amniotic fluid (651). Accordingly, most workers believe that amniocentesis is not a procedure that should be undertaken lightly and suggest that its use be restricted to cases in which there are very real indications, such as a history of

severe HDN in a previous child. As described below, there are now some alternatives to amniocentesis. The fetus can be examined by ultrasonography, a non-invasive procedure, or fetal blood can actually be collected for direct examination, obviously the collection of such a sample is via an invasive procedure. Since ultrasound can be used to recognize severe HDN from about the eighteenth week of gestation while amniocentesis is not useful until about the twenty-eighth week, it has been suggested (675) that amniotic fluid analysis may have outlived its usefulness.

Non-Serological Methods Used to Forecast the Severity of HDN: Ultrasonography

Ultrasound imagining techniques are used in a number of ways in attempts to follow the fetus in utero (183,688). First, ultrasound allows an estimate to be made of placental and hepatic size and enables recognition of the presence of edema or ascites (689-693). Second, use of ultrasound reduces the incidence of damage to the placenta caused by amniocentesis. Third, it is used to guide the needle for both intraperitoneal and intravascular in utero transfusion of the fetus and allows observation of adsorption of the red cells from the peritoneal cavity (serial ultrasound) or of transfusion of red cells into the fetal circulation. Use of ultrasound and monitoring of the fetal heart rate is used to avoid unnecessary invasive procedures (692).

Percutaneous Umbilical Blood Sampling (PUBS)

PUBS involves the insertion of a needle percutaneously and guiding it, via the use of ultrasound monitoring, into the umbilical vein. Although the expertise to accomplish such collection of a sample from the fetus in utero was not developed until the mid-1980s (694) the procedure is now used on a regular basis in appropriate cases (695-699). Blood collected from the fetus can be tested to determine the degree of anemia, the level of bilirubin, the blood group of the fetus, a DAT can be performed and any other test that is indicated (e.g. when HDN is not involved but a different pathological state is suspected) can be done. In centers in which in utero transfusion of the fetus is performed, PUBS is used to measure the pretransfusion hemoglobin or hematocrit.

Treatment of the Mother When Severe HDN is Likely

In the most severe form of HDN, the fetus dies in utero before it is delivered. When such an outcome is a real possibility, there are several maneuvers that can be tried either to deliver a premature but live infant or to keep the infant alive in utero until nearer term. At one time such effort had to be directed towards the mother since the physician had no direct access to the fetus. As will be apparent from what has been written above, that situation has changed dramatically and it is now possible to treat the fetus in utero, such options are described below.

Induced Premature Delivery

Before any methods had been devised to treat the fetus in utero, one of very few options was to induce early delivery. It was shown (342,700,701,703) that of fetuses who died in utero, of HDN, some 50% died after 35 weeks gestation. Accordingly, induced premature delivery at 35 weeks was used. There was early reluctance to induce delivery before 35 weeks since, even in the absence of HDN, survival rates were not good. In the late 1950s the death rate among infants born at 30 weeks gestation was 60%, among those born at 34 weeks gestation it was 15%, again in the absence of HDN (704). As medical expertise in salvaging prematurely born infants developed, premature induction of delivery became a more viable option. However, in the absence of ways to treat the fetus in utero, premature induction often resulted in an infant with severe HDN superimposed on the complications of prematurity. Nevertheless premature delivery saved many infants who would otherwise have died before term. After methods for intrauterine transfusion of the fetus were developed, fetuses who would not otherwise have survived beyond 30 to 34 weeks gestation could be kept alive for premature delivery nearer term. Mollison (222) states that premature induction of delivery is not indicated in cases where only mild or moderate HDN is expected since the available data do not suggest that the hemolytic process will be much more severe at 40 weeks than at 36. By use of analysis of amniotic fluid or PUBS it is now possible to forecast with considerable accuracy when the HDN will be mild or moderate.

Plasmapheresis and Plasma Exchange

Since HDN is caused by an antibody in the maternal plasma that crosses the placenta and destroys the red cells of the fetus, it might appear that removal of the maternal antibody by plasmapheresis or plasma exchange could be used to prevent or ameliorate the disease. In fact, the immune system can synthesize immunoglobulin so rapidly that heroic efforts by both the pregnant woman and the plasma exchange team are necessary before any beneficial effect accrues for the fetus. There are a number of additional factors that must be borne in mind before this form of therapy is even contemplated. First, some 56 to 58% of the body's IgG is in the extravascular space (705,706). Thus as it is removed from circulation (the intravascular space) by plasmapheresis, it is rapidly replaced from the extravascular compartment. Second, if the plasma removed is replaced with albumin or other solutions that do not contain IgG, the maternal antibody level may increase as a result of the therapy. This is because depletion of maternal IgG levels results in a rebound effect with IgG (including the antibody) being synthesized at a greater rate following, than before the exchange. Third, if plasma containing normal levels of IgG, but no antibody, is used as the replacement fluid to prevent rebound, the risk of a transfusion-transmitted disease is introduced. Fourth, if plasma is used, it must be from D- donors (if the maternal antibody is anti-D). Plasma from D+ donors will contain some stroma from D+ red cells and while such material may be unable to initiate a primary response to D in a non-immunized individual, it can serve to cause an increase in the production of anti-D via a secondary immunization mechanism (69). Fifth, there is some evidence (69,707) that intensive plasma exchange may remove an (unknown) factor (perhaps antibody itself (708)) that normally serves to inhibit B cell proliferation. Thus, in some instances (69) intensive plasma exchange and replacement of IgG can cause an increase in production of maternal antibody, even in the absence of introduction of antigen. In other instances (707) removal of this factor has apparently allowed the production of autoantibody in addition to increased levels of maternal alloantibody that the procedure was designed to reduce. Sixth, intensive plasma exchange is not a benign procedure. Although occasional apheresis procedures, by which plasma, platelets or leukocytes are collected from normal donors for transfusion purposes are seldom associated with serious reactions, the same is not necessarily true for intensive plasma exchange. In rare individuals, who may not be readily identifiable by predonation medical or laboratory screening, severe complications and even death have occurred (709-716). We are aware of the death of one woman undergoing plasma exchange for no reason other than that she was pregnant and had a history of stillborn infants due to anti-D HDN, but do not know if a report of that case has appeared in the literature.

In spite of the many difficulties mentioned above, numerous women with a bad obstetrical history have been treated by plasma exchange (717-734). In some instances the procedures apparently helped for live-born infants were salvaged when the history suggested a high probability of hydrops. However, this does not necessarily mean that the treatment was a success since the delivery of a live-born child to a woman who has previously had stillborn infants is certainly not unknown among women not treated by plasma exchange. In other cases the plasma exchanges were apparently of no value. However, in some such cases, the problems outlined earlier in this section were identified, so that the failures were sometimes understood. Mollison (222) points out that the lack of a properly controlled clinical trial means that the benefits of extensive plasma exchange in this circumstance should be regarded as unproved and that the procedure cannot be recommended for routine use. However, Rock (735) noted that once some of the previously unrecognized problems (e.g., use of albumin or plasma from D+ donors as the replacement fluid) were resolved, success rates increased. Bowman (183) believes that plasma exchange should be reserved for the woman whose partner is homozygous for the gene encoding production of the antigen to which she is immunized and who has a previous history of hydrops at or before 24 to 26 weeks gestation. He believes that intensive plasma exchange should begin at 10 to 12 weeks of gestation and should continue until amniocentesis can be started at 18 weeks and/or fetal blood sampling, with intrauterine transfusion as necessary, at 19 to 22 weeks gestation.

Instances in which plasma exchange was believed to have removed enough antibody that a live infant was delivered to women who had previously suffered multiple miscarriages or had delivered stillborns have involved anti-P (910-913) and anti-M (383,387,914) and are described in Chapters 11 and 15 respectively. In the case of the anti-M, the plasma was passed over an immunoadsorbant column and was filtered before being returned to the patient (914,915). However, it has been pointed out (916) that such a procedure may be rather dangerous if the antibody causative of the severe HDN is anti-D. It is believed (916 and see Chapter 15) that material containing D antigen was released, from the adsorbing material and was infused when the adsorbed plasma was reinfused. This caused an increase in the level of anti-D being made (729).

IVIG Therapy During Pregnancy

IVIG can be used either during pregnancy, when it is injected into the mother or after delivery when it is injected into the newborn (see below). When injected into the mother the negative feedback mechanism created by the presence of very high levels of IgG can reduce the level of antibody being made by the mother by as much as 50% (736,737). An additional benefit (and see also section on treatment of the infant with IVIG) may accrue because some of the injected IgG molecules cross the placenta and block Fc receptors on the cells of the

infant's reticuloendothelial system (736-743). Again, Bowman (813) recommends that IVIG therapy be started at 10 to 12 weeks gestation, when maternal antibody is just starting to cross the placenta, and that the dose be 400 mg/kg maternal body weight for 5 days, repeated at three week intervals. As with the use of plasma exchange, amniocentesis at 18 weeks and/or fetal blood sampling at 19 to 22 weeks, with intrauterine transfusion if necessary, should always follow the early use of IVIG in this setting.

Maternal Treatments That Have Not Proved to be of Value

Attempts have been made either to desensitize women producing large amounts of anti-D or to use materials, including some made from D+ red cell membranes, to inhibit anti-D in vivo (744-746). In spite of claims of success by the original workers, others (747-749) have not been able to duplicate the results and the methods are considered by most authorities (71,183) to be of no value. Somewhat similarly, claims (750-752) that promethazine hydrochloride can be used to downregulate production of anti-D in pregnancy to such a degree that mortality can be reduced, have not been confirmed by others (183,303,753,754). Corticosteroids, that are of such benefit in downregulation of autoantibody production in WAIHA (see Chapter 37), have also been used to try to decrease production of alloantibodies in pregnant women. At doses up to those at which it was considered that transplacental passage of the steroids would put the fetus at risk, no alteration in levels of maternal antibody being made, were seen (755-757).

Treatment of the Fetus in Utero When Severe HDN is Probable

By analysis of amniotic fluid, ultrasonography and from the results of tests on samples collected by PUBS, it is now possible to determine with a high degree of accuracy which infants will be severely affected with HDN. When the above tests and the maternal history indicate that it is improbable that the fetus will survive until term or to a time when induction of premature delivery can be contemplated, the fetus can be transfused while still in utero.

Liley (702) first introduced intrauterine transfusion in 1963. In the procedure as originally practiced, blood was infused into the peritoneal cavity of the fetus from whence it was adsorbed into circulation. Early studies suggested that the best results were obtained if intrauterine transfusion could be delayed until after 31 weeks gestation, the procedure was associated with a mortality rate of around 40% in some studies (759,760). However, it should be remembered that if candidates for intrauterine transfusion are selected correctly, the mortality rate would be close to 100% without the treatment. Bowman et al. (761) and Walker and Ellis (762) then showed that the chance of a successful outcome in a fetus of less than 31 weeks gestation could be increased if the volume of blood infused was carefully matched to fetal size. Based on these two reports it seems that no more than 30-40 ml of blood should be transfused to a 23-25 week-old fetus and no more than 100 ml to a 30 week-old fetus. The major risks of intrauterine transfusion are trauma to the placenta and damage to the fetus by the transfusion needle. Clearly intrauterine transfusion will be safest when performed by experts with a great deal of experience in the method. Bowman and colleagues (55,183,288,303) have summarized the Winnipeg experience and have reported a success rate of over 70% with the procedure, some intrauterine transfusions were undertaken as early as 21.5 weeks although whenever possible the procedure was delayed until 24 to 25 weeks gestation.

The transfusion of red cells into the peritoneal cavity of the fetus while the fetus was still in utero represented a major advance in the prevention of death from HDN. However, problems remained. First, the procedure is of no value if the fetus is hydropic and is not breathing (763). Diaphragmatic movement is necessary for the absorption of red cells from the peritoneal cavity. Second, the adsorption of red cells from the peritoneal cavity takes from eight to ten days. Third, in the absence of PUBS, some fetus' who do not require intrauterine transfusion will be subject to the hazards of the procedure while a few others will not be recognized as needing such treatment and will die in utero.

In 1981, Rodeck et al. (764) described a procedure for intravascular transfusion of the fetus using the fetoscope. The procedure required considerable practical skill, fetoscopic visualization of the fetal blood vessels is not always possible. A number of infants with severe HDN received intravascular transfusions while still in utero, when this method was used (765). When ultrasound procedures were developed to allow fetal blood sampling from the umbilical vein (PUBS) it became possible to follow the sample collection, with intravenous (or rarely intraarterial (183)) transfusion. This method has now been used by many groups of workers (183,288,766-776) with outstanding success. From the many series it can be seen that the chance of saving a fetus who already has hydrops is at least 60 to 70% while the chance of saving one with severe HDN who is not hydropic, is even higher. That careful assessment of the degree of disease in the fetus is necessary before intravascular transfusion is undertaken is clear from the

finding (777) that even when performed by very experienced clinicians, a single intravascular transfusion has a mortality rate of 2%.

The selection of blood for transfusion while the fetus is in utero is based on straightforward principles. First, the red cells must be compatible with the maternal antibodies present in the fetal circulation. Second, since the ABO group of the fetus is not known, group O red cells should be transfused. Third, since maternal immunization to antigens on the red cells transfused to the fetus has been reported (see below), it is recommended (71) that K- blood be used (this suggestion is based on the high immunogenicity of K and the supposition that the maternal antibody is anti-D so that the blood being transfused will be rr, i.e. D- C- E-). Fourth, to ensure the longest possible survival of the transfused red cells, fresh blood should be used. Mollison et al. (71) recommend the use of blood no older than 72 hours. Fifth, the blood must be irradiated to exclude the possibility of transfusion-associated graft versus host disease. Sixth, in addition to being tested for other markers of infectious diseases that can be transmitted by transfusion, the blood should be CMV-negative. Seventh, the blood should be shown to be non-reactive in a test for HbS. As mentioned above, the amount of blood transfused will be based on the gestational age of the fetus, the hematocrit of the blood issued should be between 70 and 85% based on the request of the obstetrician who will infuse it.

Treatment of the fetus by intrauterine intravascular transfusion is associated with FMH in at least 40% of the cases (778). In one series the average size of the FMH was 2.4 ml whole blood. In those cases in which the FMH exceeded 1 ml following the first intravascular transfusion, the titer of the maternal anti-D rose by more than 150% within three weeks of the transfusion (778). While such an increase in maternal antibody level sounds alarming it should be remembered that if the cases are selected correctly, intrauterine transfusion is used only in those instances in which the maternal antibody is already at a level at which it is likely to cause death of the fetus. Nevertheless, this finding again emphasizes the fact that the decision to use intrauterine transfusion must be made carefully and that the procedure should be used only when essential.

When the FMH follows intrauterine transfusion, some of the donor's red cells as well as some of those of the fetus apparently enter the maternal circulation. Three cases have been reported (779,780) in which women carrying infants at risk of in utero death because of anti-D HDN, had those infants treated by intrauterine transfusion. Following amniocentesis and the transfusions, two women produced anti-Jk[a]. It was impossible to determine whether the Jk(a+) red cells of the donor of the blood used, or red cells of the fetus that had entered the maternal circulation at the time of the intrauterine transfusions, had stimulated production of the additional antibody. However, Contreras et al. (781) then described a case in which a woman with Fy(b-) red cells made anti-Fy^b in similar circumstances. The red cells of the woman's husband were Fy(a+b-), those of the infant could not be typed (strongly positive DAT; exchange transfusions were given before the infant died). Thus, unless the husband was not the father, the anti-Fy^b must have been produced following exposure of the woman to Fy(b+) red cells used for the intrauterine transfusion. Other similar cases have now been reported (782) and it is noticeable that among six women immunized via this route, four made anti-Jk^a and one made anti-Jk^b (some of the women made more than one antibody). Pratt et al. (783) studied this question and showed that the production of a new antibody during pregnancy is more likely if amniocentesis and intrauterine transfusions are used than if amniocentesis is done but no transfusion is given. Thus perhaps a case can be made for the use of phenotype matched (to the mother) blood for intrauterine transfusion (but see the addendum). It may seem incongruous that we, who pay little attention to the risk of immunization to any antigen other than D, should even suggest that there may be place for blood phenotypically matched to the mother's red cells (other than for ABO and D) for intrauterine transfusions. However, it must be remembered that some individuals are good responders to blood group antigens (784-787) and that among D- women who have produced anti-D, such good responders are well represented (784). Thus, while we do not believe that there is any risk of immunizing the fetus in utero (because it is immunologically incompetent: tolerance is more likely than immunization (788)) there does seem to be some risk of additional immunization in the mother. It should be remembered that these are women in whom the obstetrical course is already stormy because they already have a sufficient level of antibody (usually anti-D) that in utero death of the fetus is likely if intervention is not provided.

While intrauterine transfusion via an intravascular route has now largely superseded intrauterine transfusion via an intraperitoneal route, both Bowman (183) and Mollison et al. (71) indicate that it is essential that the skills needed to perform intrauterine intraperitoneal transfusions be retained. Bowman (183) points out that the intraperitoneal route must be used on those rare occasions when transfusion is needed before 20 to 21 weeks gestation when the cord blood vessels may be too small to use and on the more common occasions when transfusion is still needed after 30 weeks gestation and several successful intravenous transfusions, when increasing fetal size obscures a posterior cord vessel. Mollison et al. (71) point out that intravascular (imme-

diate addition of red cells to the fetal circulation) and intraperitoneal (slow adsorption of red cells into the fetal circulation) can be used together to increase the total volume of blood given to the fetus, thus prolonging the interval between transfusions (774,777).

Laboratory Diagnosis of HDN

Results of laboratory tests that are used in the diagnosis of this disease are not always closely correlated with clinical severity. This is particularly true of the direct antiglobulin test. This test is probably the most useful serological tool in diagnosis since in most cases severe enough to need treatment, the DAT will be strongly positive. The exceptions to this rule are usually cases involving antibodies in the ABO system that are described in more detail below. Since the anemia from which the newborn infant suffers is caused by red cell destruction due to maternal antibody that has crossed the placenta, it is not surprising that those cells remaining can be shown to be coated with IgG or IgG and complement. The DAT on cord blood red cells is so reliable an indicator of HDN that in an ABO compatible infant, a negative DAT almost always excludes significant HDN. The term almost always in the previous sentence, is used advisedly. In the only report of the event in the literature, Heddle et al. (980) described fatal and severe cases of HDN, caused by anti-C and anti-c, in which the DATs on the infants' red cells were negative. The strength of a positive DAT is not a reliable guide to severity of the disease. In infants severely affected with HDN, the DAT almost always gives a maximally strong positive result. However, equally strong positive tests are seen in infants suffering less severe forms of the disease. Indeed, some 40% of infants born with a positive DAT require no treatment (71). When a complement-binding antibody such as anti-Jk^a causes HDN, the major (or only) detectable protein on the cord blood red cells may be C3 (789,790). While it was reported (791) that 18 of 94 (19%) anti-D in women delivering infants with HDN activated C1q, the universal experience of Rh HDN is that complement is not involved in the red cell destruction. Even the authors describing the activation of C1q saw no correlation between that event and the severity of HDN.

Hemoglobin estimations are, of course, closely correlated with the severity of disease since the usual acute problem at birth is the anemia from which the affected infant suffers. However, the finding of a fairly high level of hemoglobin in the cord blood sample by no means excludes the disease since almost half of all affected infants have hemoglobin levels above 14.5g/100ml (792,793). Mollison et al. (71) point out that at birth, estimations of hemoglobin are more reliable if cord blood is used than if skin prick samples are collected. Infants who are born with no appreciable anemia do not always require immediate treatment.

The second serious complication of HDN is hyperbilirubinemia and the danger that this will result in kernicterus. This is discussed below but it should be mentioned here that some newborn non-anemic infants will require prompt treatment to alleviate high bilirubin levels while others will require treatment after a few hours or a few days of life.

In addition to the DAT and estimation of cord blood hemoglobin and bilirubin levels, there are other laboratory tests that can be used to assist in the diagnosis of HDN. In anemic infants, reticulocyte counts will be high and nucleated red cells may be seen in blood smears. Hemoglobin and methemalbumin will sometimes be found in the plasma. Microspherocytes in blood smears and increased osmotic fragility are two findings more common in HDN caused by ABO system antibodies than in Rh disease (295,794,795). As can be seen from the above, additional abnormal findings can be demonstrated. However, these are seldom necessary to establish a diagnosis of Rh HDN. The presence of anti-Rh (usually anti-D) in the maternal serum together with the findings of: a positive DAT on the cord blood red cells; a low cord blood hemoglobin and an elevated bilirubin are usually quite sufficient to establish the diagnosis beyond any reasonable doubt.

In most instances the causative antibody of HDN is readily identified. In a well run prenatal service the causative antibodies are mostly known before birth of the infant because of studies on the maternal serum. Many workers (614,621) are prepared to accept the presence of anti-D in the maternal serum and a positive DAT on a child who types as D+, as sufficient evidence that anti-D HDN has occurred. Other workers take the laboratory procedures one step further and prepare eluates from the cord blood red cells. This confirms the expected diagnosis when anti-D is demonstrated in the eluate. Eluates are useful when several antibodies are present in the maternal serum. For example, if a child is delivered to a woman who has both anti-D and anti-K in her serum, a positive DAT does not tell the investigator which of the antibodies is responsible for the HDN. Red cell typings (for D and K) may be useful but are not always easy in the presence of a positive DAT. Elution of the maternal antibody from the infant's cells, followed by tests to determine the specificity of the antibody (or antibodies) in the eluate may be of value. However, this particular procedure sometimes becomes a somewhat academic exercise. For one thing, blood for exchange transfusion must often be prepared before birth of the infant. If the maternal serum contains anti-D and anti-K; D-, K- blood will have been selected before the infant is born. The

compatibility test, before the infant's birth, is performed with maternal serum. Second, severity of disease will often give a clue as to which antibody is involved since anti-D HDN is so often more severe than that caused by other antibodies. Preparation of eluates from cord blood red cells may be of more help in establishing the specificity of the causative antibody in ABO HDN; indeed it is sometimes the most conclusive serological finding. Further considerations of compatibility tests with maternal serum, including the use of 2-ME, are discussed below in the section dealing with treatment.

The DAT in ABO HDN and Protective Mechanisms in that Disorder

In ABO HDN, the DAT is seldom as strongly positive as in cases caused by Rh and other antibodies. As a result, numerous other tests (35,296,309,795-798,800-812) that range from the identification of "immune" ABO antibodies via techniques such as inhibition with specific blood group substances or adsorption with pig red cells, to the spontaneous agglutination of the affected infant's red cells in an enzyme preparation, have been advocated. In general, these tests suffer a common major disadvantage in that they all detect ABO incompatibility between the maternal serum and the infant's red cells. The presence of maternal ABO antibody on the infant's red cells is very common, significant in vivo destruction of the infant's red cells by those antibodies and hence clinical HDN is rare (for incidence figures, see an earlier section on prenatal testing). For many years one of us (PDI) has used the following criteria for establishment of the diagnosis of ABO HDN.

1. Typing studies show that the maternal serum contains an ABO antibody directed against an antigen on the infant's red cells.
2. Clinical evidence of disease in the infant.
3. The maternal serum has been shown not to contain other antibodies.
4. An eluate from the cord red blood cells contains anti-A and/or anti-B.

Obviously, points 3 and 4 must be considered together. Sometimes antibody-screening tests will not detect maternal antibodies to antigens of low incidence and on other occasions an ABO system and another antibody may be contributing to the hemolytic process. When only an ABO antibody is involved, there is reasonably good correlation between the strength of the eluted antibody and existence of the disease (302,806,813). In our experience (305) the DAT has always been positive when the ABO HDN was severe enough that some form of treatment other than phototherapy was necessary. Graham (814) has reported that the DAT is stronger in ABO HDN if the infant's red cells are washed in saline to which 1% albumin has been added; presumably this reduces the dissociation rate of ABO antibodies during the steps before addition of the antiglobulin serum.

It had long been supposed that the weakly positive DAT in ABO HDN and the fact that the disease is usually clinically mild, had a common explanation. For example, one idea that was popular at one time was that the membrane of cord blood red cells had more crypts and valleys than did the membrane of red cells from adults. Thus it was supposed that when IgG anti-A or anti-B molecules were bound to antigen sites deep in a crypt or valley, the Fc pieces of those molecules could not complex either with macrophages (hence limited in vivo red cell clearance) or with anti-gamma heavy chain reagents (hence the weak DAT).

An alternative explanation was that since the A and B antigens are so poorly developed at birth, cord red cells can bind only small amounts of anti-A or anti-B, even when the antibody is present in large amounts. There are some data to support this concept. First, several groups of workers (815-821) have shown that under optimal conditions for antibody binding, cord red blood cells will take up only from one quarter to one third of the number of ABO antibody molecules bound by phenotype-matched red cells from adults. Second, it has been shown that in many cases of ABO HDN, the amount of IgG on the cord red blood cells is relatively low (822,823). These observations at first seem at variance with what is regularly seen in serological tests in ABO HDN. Even when the DAT on the cord blood red cells is only weakly positive, eluates made from those cells usually react strongly with appropriate ABO group red cells from adults. In view of the above mentioned data, it must be accepted that a low level of ABO antibody can produce strong reactions if enough copies of the appropriate antigen are present on the test cells, that is, red cells from adults. Several workers (822,824-828) have suggested that the elution procedure results in a considerable concentration of antibody molecules but if, as mentioned above, there are relatively few antibody molecules bound to begin with and if many of them dissociate when red cells are washed (more thoroughly before eluates are made than for the DAT) this explanation does not seem wholly satisfactory.

Romans et al. (829) advanced a somewhat different explanation for weakness of the DAT in ABO HDN. They suggested that in order that they become detectable by anti-IgG in the DAT, IgG anti-A and anti-B must bind both antibody combining sites to the red cell. The relatively low number of A and B antigen sites on cord red blood cells and particularly the deficiency of branched ABH-containing oligosaccharide chains on those cells, was believed to limit such binding. Thus it was supposed that in fact more molecules of anti-A or anti-B were bound than appeared to be the case from the result of the DAT or from studies designed to measure the amount of antibody bound when such studies depended on the recognition of bound IgG with anti-IgG. There are a number of findings that do not fit well with this concept. First, in order for the A or B antigen sites on cord blood cells all to be coated with antibody bound by only one combining site it would have to be supposed that cord sera contain high levels of anti-A or anti-B, in fact, they do not. Second, experimental data (830) suggest that anti-A and anti-B bind in a similar fashion to red cells from adults and those from cord bloods, albeit in different amounts. Third, if anti-A and anti-B had bound in greater profusion to cord blood red cells than the DATs appear to indicate, it might be expected that complement would be activated, in ABO HDN it is not (222,816, 831,840). Fourth, if a given anti-A is adsorbed with group A cord blood red cells, it is found (222) that those cells adsorb only about 11% of the amount of anti-A adsorbed by group A red cells of adults.

Another protective mechanism in ABO HDN involves the subclass of IgG of which the antibodies are made. Brouwers et al. (833) studied IgG anti-A and anti-B from pregnant women and showed that almost all contained an IgG2 component. It is known (258) that the Fc receptors on placental tissue cells bind IgG1 with a higher efficiency than they bind IgG2 and that IgG2 is transported across the placenta less readily than are IgG1 and IgG3 (252-254,268,834). Thus it is clear that those maternal sera that contain large amounts of IgG2 anti-A and anti-B will react to high titers in vitro but will not be the ones that cause clinical HDN. Ukita et al. (835) studied anti-A and anti-B bound to cord blood red cells. They showed that there was no association between clinical HDN and the presence of IgG2 on the cord blood red cells. It is, of course, known that IgG2 is a poor mediator of macrophage induced red cell clearance (228,836-838). Thus it seems that when the maternal anti-A or anti-B contains an appreciable IgG2 component, those antibody molecules have difficulty gaining access to the fetal circulation and those that do get there, cause little red cell destruction. When Brouwers et al. (839) studied ABO antibodies in an ADCC(M) assay they found that those associated with clinical ABO HDN, were IgG3 and that high levels of such antibodies were present. Moderate levels of reactivity in the ADCC test when weaker antibodies or those of other subclasses were studied, were not correlated with clinical HDN.

As already mentioned, ABO antibodies do not activate complement in the newborn even when they do cause HDN (222,816,831,840). Clearly if complement activation did occur, ABO HDN would be common (15% of White mothers are group O and have group A or group B children) and often fatal (if the complement activation resulted in intravascular hemolysis). The probable explanation for the lack of complement activation is the paucity of A and B antigen sites on cord blood red cells and their location on straight chain glycosphingolipids (841). That is to say, IgG molecules do not bind in close enough proximity for two of them to contribute Fc pieces to bind C1q (see Chapter 6). The facts that complement levels are lower in infants than in adults (842,843) and that complement is activated only poorly in newborns (844) probably play little role in this setting. The universal experience (887) has been that in ABO HDN, the DAT may be positive when anti-IgG is used (see above) but is negative when anti-C3 is used. A report of two exceptions to such findings (845) was challenged (846) on the basis that some newborns who do not have ABO HDN, have small amounts of C3 detectable on their red cells. In other words, most workers would regard the report (845) of complement activation in ABO HDN as true (the infants had red cells incompatible with the maternal ABO antibodies) true (the infants' red cells carried some C3) and unrelated.

Finally, in terms of protective effects that mitigate the severity of ABO HDN, it must be remembered that A and B substances present in the plasma, other fluids and on tissue cells, will cause at least some inhibition of maternal anti-A and anti-B that cross the placenta (847-850). As indicated above, the much believed concept that ABO HDN is almost always caused by anti-A,B in the plasma of group O women, has been shown (305) to be incorrect. While almost all women who produce infants affected with ABO HDN are group O, anti-A or anti-B in such plasmas cause the disease more often and perhaps in a more severe form, than does anti-A,B.

Red Cell Typings in Infants with HDN when the DAT is Strongly Positive

There are several difficulties that may be encountered when attempts are made to determine the D type of a newborn infant suffering from anti-D HDN. First, in severe disease, the D antigen sites on the infant's cells may be blocked with non-agglutinating anti-D so that the cells will not react with an agglutinating anti-D. Such blocking undoubtedly exists, indeed blocking tests were the first ones used to demonstrate (indirectly) the presence of non-agglutinating (incomplete) antibodies. However, the total blocking of D sites by IgG, leading to false negative typing tests when an IgM anti-D is used, is quite rare. When this section was written for the second

edition of this book (851), a survey in the authors' laboratory showed that among a group of workers with over 30 years experience between them, only four cases of false negative D-typings due to blocking anti-D had been encountered. The phenomenon is apparently more common in examination questions than in the laboratory!

A more commonly encountered problem involves false-positive reactions when DAT+ red cells are agglutinated by typing reagents to which potentiators have been added, although the red cells lack the antigen against which the antibody in the reagent is directed. This problem was more acute when an albumin solution was the only available control (852). While agglutinating anti-D may give occasional false negative reactions and reagents to which potentiators have been added may somewhat more often give false positive reactions, we have not yet heard of problems associated with the use of monoclonal anti-D. These reagents are now more and more often supplied as IgM antibodies so that at least the theoretical possibility of false negative reactions due to blocking exists. On the other side of this somewhat gloomy situation, many workers when testing red cells from a newborn whose mother has anti-D, whose DAT is strongly positive and from whose cells anti-D can be recovered by elution, accept that the infant has D+ red cells, without further tests (some do so without an eluate being included).

A somewhat different problem exists when the DAT is positive and only IAT-active reagents are available to type the red cells. Methods using chloroquine diphosphate (853), ZZAP reagent (854) and a combined pH-density gradient solution (855) to remove antibodies from red cells to permit typing tests, have been mentioned in Chapters 3 and 37. Again, in HDN, such procedures are scarcely necessary. For example, if the maternal serum is known to contain anti-Fy^a, the DAT on the cord blood red cells is positive and anti-Fy^a is present in an eluate made from those red cells, there seems no reason to doubt that the infant has Fy(a+) red cells.

As far as we are aware, the presence of IgG and/or complement on the red cells of an infant with HDN, has not been reported as interfering with correct determination of the ABO type of the infant.

ABO Typing Tests on the Red Cells of Infants with ABO HDN

As discussed earlier, A and B antigens are less well developed on cord blood red cells than on the red cells of adults. However, this does not prevent the correct ABO type from being determined. In terms of ABO HDN, we have never heard of a case in which the A or B antigen sites were sufficiently blocked with incomplete antibody to give a false-negative typing test. In addition to the general weakness of A and B antigens on cord cells, the antigens may be even less well developed on the cells of premature infants (856). Some workers (857) have suggested that group A infants with ABO HDN have better developed A antigens than do other group A newborn infants.

At birth, many infants who have inherited A^1, have red cells that fail to react or react only weakly, with anti-A_1 typing sera. The A_1 phenotype of such infants can be more reliably determined with *Dolichos biflorus* lectin than with human-source anti-A_1. However, the A_1 red cells of infants with ABO HDN may react less well with this lectin than do the red cells of unaffected A_1 infants (858). Tests to show an infant's true A_1 status may need to be done between six and 18 months after birth. Those infants of group A, affected with clinical HDN can invariably be shown (in retrospect if necessary (795)) to be of type A_1 (797) and it is entirely possible than an A_2 infant has such a weakly developed A antigen at birth that sufficient antibody attachment is not possible for the disease to occur.

Treatment of Infants Suffering from HDN: Exchange Transfusions

In severe forms of this disorder, the infants are seriously anemic and treatment must often be initiated immediately after the child is born. The number of red cells necessary to sustain life after the child is born may be more than the number necessary for it to survive in utero. Accordingly, when prenatal tests indicate that the birth of a severely affected infant can be anticipated, blood for use at an exchange transfusion (see below) must be available when the infant is born. That is, compatibility tests using the maternal serum must be used to select suitable donor blood before delivery of the infant. The section below, about exchange transfusion and the selection of suitable blood for that procedure, is written primarily in terms of HDN caused by anti-D. Much less often, cases in which the causative antibody has a different specificity (e.g., directed against c, K, Fy^a, etc.) will be encountered. Obviously, in such cases, selection of blood for the exchange transfusion must be based on the specificity of the antibody.

Although severe anemia may be the major reason for treatment of seriously affected infants, simple transfusions of packed cells can seldom be used. Because the infant will usually have (at least) a normal plasma (blood) volume, simple transfusion could result in circulatory overload leading to cardiac failure and death. Instead of simple transfusion, exchange transfusion (799) in which the fetal blood is gradually withdrawn

and is replaced with red cells compatible with the maternal antibody, is the treatment of choice (862,863). As is described more fully below, the second major complication of HDN, once the anemia has been corrected, is hyperbilirubinemia that can cause kernicterus and death. Exchange transfusion, immediately after birth, not only corrects anemia but also greatly reduces the chance that deep jaundice and kernicterus will occur. This because the infant's red cells present at birth are saturated with maternal antibody and will survive, in the infant's circulation, for only short period of time (864). At the time of the first exchange transfusion, very little bilirubin is removed but removal of a majority of the antibody-coated cells represents the removal of cells that would soon be destroyed and cause bilirubin levels to increase markedly. It has been calculated (865,866) that red cells with the potential, when destroyed, to create up to 500 mg of bilirubin can be removed at the time of an initial exchange transfusion.

When infants with anti-D HDN are considered, there are two schools of thought as to which ABO type of D- blood should be used. One set of workers claim that blood of the same ABO group as the infant should be used whenever possible. Such blood has the advantage that no ABO agglutinins, directed against an antigen present on the infant's cells are introduced in the plasma of the donor blood. The selection of such blood is easy in those situations where the maternal serum is ABO compatible with the infant's red cells. In other instances (e.g., O mother, A baby) the blood to be used will be group O (and not group A like the baby) otherwise compatibility with the maternal serum cannot be demonstrated in order that blood be available at the time of birth. Workers determined to perform exchange transfusions with blood of the same ABO group as the infant point out that if immediate exchange transfusion is not essential, blood can be tested for compatibility with the infant's serum and an eluate from the infant's antibody-coated red cells, after birth. In those cases in which immediate exchange transfusion is essential, blood of the infant's ABO group can be provided even if such blood is incompatible with maternal ABO agglutinins. If, for instance, a group O mother has only anti-D in her serum and produces a group A D+ child, group A, D- blood can be used for the exchange transfusion without compatibility tests being performed. This procedure is not dangerous if the most significant antibody has been correctly identified. If the unit used for the exchange transfusion is incompatible with a second, weaker antibody in the maternal serum, whose presence has been overlooked, much of that antibody will be removed at the time of exchange transfusion, if indeed it even reached the fetal circulation.

The second school of thought is that group O blood should be used for all infants regardless of their ABO group. Such blood can be used as partially packed (some plasma removed) or as packed red cells. Other workers use whole blood selected to have low titers of anti-A and anti-B while still others use whole group O non-selected units. One advantage of using group O blood is that compatibility tests can be completed in advance of delivery of the infant so that treatment can be instigated rapidly after birth. From many cases of exchange transfusion performed with group O partially packed red cells or whole blood, it is apparent that ABO agglutinins, introduced by transfusion of plasma in the unit, seldom cause appreciable destruction of the infant's A or B cells that remain following the exchange transfusion or that are subsequently released from the marrow. A popular resolution of the debate as to which ABO group red cells should be used is to use group O, washed or packed red cells, resuspended (most clinicians use blood with a hematocrit of about 60% for exchange transfusions) in AB fresh frozen plasma. However, this practice can be criticized on at least three counts. First, it may not be necessary, that is it may be designed to solve a problem that does not exist. Second, it exposes the fetus to blood products from two donors and thus doubles the risk of a transfusion-transmitted infection. Third, the use of blood products from two donors increases the cost of the treatment, unnecessarily if the first criticism is correct. One often overlooked advantage of using group O blood for all exchange transfusions is that if Rh and ABO HDN exist concurrently, both are treated by the use of group O, D- blood. The diagnosis of ABO HDN in the presence of Rh HDN may be no easy matter (801,867-869). It has been pointed out (869) that tests for ABO antibodies, on eluates made from the red cells of infants known to have anti-D HDN, can be useful in this respect.

Compatibility tests before birth can be performed even if blood of the same type as the baby is deemed necessary. If, for example, the mother is group A, two units, one A and one O, can be prepared and the appropriate one used once the infant is born and typed for ABO. A complication of using maternal serum, for compatibility tests to prepare units for exchange transfusion immediately after the infant is born, arises when the maternal serum contains several antibodies. A useful procedure in this situation is to perform the compatibility test with 2-ME (or DTT)-treated maternal serum (870). IgM agglutinins in the maternal serum are prevented from interfering in the compatibility tests and of course, this procedure is safe because IgM antibodies do not cross the placenta so do not participate in the hemolytic process, nor are they present in the cord blood plasma to complicate transfusions.

No matter what ABO group blood is used, it should be fairly fresh. In the past, many clinicians insisted on using blood less than 48 hours old, for exchange transfusions. With current requirements for testing donor blood

(871) it has become increasingly difficult to make fully tested blood available within that time. Fortunately, improvements in the anticoagulant/preservative solutions into which donor blood is now collected have resulted in blood collected from the donor within the previous five (71) to seven (623) days, being suitable for exchange transfusion. In addition to the usual tests for infectious agents, blood used for exchange transfusion should be tested for CMV and HbS. Ice cold blood should not be used for exchange transfusion (872,873).

Addition of Albumin to Donor Blood to be Used in Exchange Transfusions

Odell (874) showed that kernicterus and other complications of hyperbilirubinemia (see below) occur because excess bilirubin is not bound by albumin. Waters and Porter (875) added salt-poor human albumin to blood used in exchange transfusions and suggested that this procedure would reduce the risk of kernicterus. Diamond (876) maintained that the addition of albumin is not necessary unless the level of the infant's own plasma albumin is low, which occurs usually only in some premature infants. A controlled study (877) that compared the results in infants who received exchange transfusions with blood to which albumin had, or had not been added, found no differences in removal of bilirubin in the two groups of infants. Since the infusion of albumin causes an increase in the colloid osmotic pressure and an increase in intravascular fluid volume, its indiscriminate use in infants already in a critical clinical condition, is clearly contraindicated.

Prevention of Hyperbilirubinemia and Kernicterus

Most infants with severe HDN have relatively low bilirubin levels at birth. In utero, the bilirubin that is formed as a product of red cell breakdown, crosses the placenta from the infant to its mother and is excreted by her. Following birth the infant must obviously excrete its own bilirubin. In infants with anemia severe enough that immediate exchange transfusion is necessary, bilirubin levels may not rise to dangerous levels for several days after the initial exchange transfusion, or may not reach dangerous levels at all. As has been pointed out above, removal of antibody-coated red cells results in the removal of the major source from which bilirubin would be made. Infants with less anemia who do not require immediate exchange transfusion, may develop high bilirubin levels more quickly if fairly rapid red cell destruction occurs. In either case, the infants must be carefully observed for the development of jaundice and serial serum bilirubin level estimations are indicated. The danger, in untreated infants, is that high levels of unconjugated bilirubin will accumulate and that this bilirubin will cause irreversible damage to brain cells. This condition resulting in brain damage is known as kernicterus and dependent on the degree of damage, children affected will suffer from various degrees of permanent mental retardation.

Indications for treatment of infants with HDN but not serious anemia are therefore based primarily on bilirubin levels. As has been mentioned, unconjugated bilirubin is the dangerous factor and most authorities agree that the level of this pigment must not be permitted to go above 20mg/100ml (878) since above this level the risk of kernicterus is high. This does not mean that infants should be left untreated until the danger level is reached. Instead, most workers (879,880) suggest that serial bilirubin measurements be performed and when it becomes apparent, by extrapolation of the curve of the increasing bilirubin level, that dangerous levels are going to be reached, the infant be treated by exchange transfusion. In premature infants, exchange transfusion to relieve hyperbilirubinemia should be performed at lower levels of serum bilirubin than in full term infants since levels in premature infants are likely to increase for longer times than in full term infants and a higher proportion of the bilirubin is likely to be unconjugated (see below).

The excretion of bilirubin occurs only after the unconjugated lipid-soluble form is converted to a water-soluble gluceronide conjugate. Unconjugated bilirubin binds to albumin in the plasma and is transported to the liver where the enzyme uridine diphosphoglucuronyl (UDP) transferase effects conjugation of the bilirubin to gluceronic acid. In newborn infants the mechanism for production of UDP transferase is not fully developed. In full term infants, production of the enzyme usually reaches normal levels on the second or third day of life so that bilirubin excretion becomes efficient at that time. In premature infants the enzyme is often not produced in adequate amounts until the fifth or sixth day of life. Hence, as mentioned above, bilirubin levels in premature infants rise over longer time periods than in full term infants and exchange transfusion is indicated at a lower serum bilirubin level. It must also be remembered that in premature infants more bilirubin will be unconjugated than in full term infants. Thus in addition to poor excretion, more of the dangerous (in terms of kernicterus) type of bilirubin is present. It has been shown (881-883) that kernicterus can occur in premature infants with bilirubin levels as low as 10mg/100ml.

These factors must also be considered before labor is induced prematurely (see above). Although such a procedure may seem advisable based on the results of prenatal tests, it must be remembered that following premature delivery, the infant will have an inefficient bilirubin excretion mechanism so that the risk of kernicterus may extend over a longer period than if the infant had been born at term.

Infants treated by exchange transfusion at birth sometimes require additional exchange transfusions to counter the risk of kernicterus. There are several factors that can contribute to this need. First, following the initial exchange transfusion, bilirubin will enter the circulation from the extravascular compartment and the plasma concentration may again approach dangerous levels. Second, if the initial treatment does not remove enough antibody-coated red cells from the infant's circulation, the bilirubin level may increase as those cells are destroyed in vivo. Third, if the infant's marrow is active and maternal antibody remains in the infant's circulation after the first exchange transfusion, the newly made red cells may be cleared and another contribution to the total bilirubin level will be made.

Exchange Transfusion Using Rare or Incompatible Blood

On most occasions red cells compatible with the maternal antibody can be provided for exchange transfusion. Even when the antibody causative of the HDN is directed against a very common antigen, knowledge of the specificity of that antibody can be used to ensure that suitable blood is available when the infant is born. Red cells that have been stored in the frozen state are eminently suitable for exchange transfusion. The fact that the cells are washed after being thawed ensures that no excess sodium, potassium or ammonia is present; further this blood product does not contain ABO agglutinins.

When the maternal antibody is directed against an antigen of very high frequency and no compatible blood can be found among the mother's sibs or random donors, consideration should be given to using the mother as the donor (884-886). Obviously, her red cells will lack the antigen against which the causative alloantibody is directed. If maternal red cells are to be used, they should be washed before the exchange transfusion so that additional maternal antibody is not introduced into the infant's circulation. Further, when this course must be followed, early recognition of the possibility helps. Pregnant women may be able to donate partial units (the red cells from which can then be frozen) during their pregnancies, more easily and with less risk, than a whole unit immediately following delivery. While there is no requirement that blood to be used for an exchange transfusion after birth of the infant be irradiated (unlike blood used for intrauterine transfusion that must be irradiated) it follows that if maternal blood is to be used, it is from a first-degree relative so should be irradiated before being transfused (871,909). Because exchange or other transfusions must sometimes be used to treat premature or full-term infants soon after birth, some workers elect to irradiate blood products to be transfused to premature infants; others irradiate products to be transfused to all infants under a certain age (e.g. four months). The rationale for such procedures is that transfusions are sometimes given before immune deficiency in the infant is recognized. All immune deficient patients must, of course, receive irradiated blood products. Given the high fatality rate (between 90 and 100%) of transfusion-induced graft-versus-host disease (922-940) it is felt by some that irradiated products should be used until sufficient time has elapsed to be sure that an immune deficient state is not present.

On rare occasions, a woman who has not had prenatal care may deliver a child with HDN caused by an antibody to a high incidence antigen and compatible blood for an exchange transfusion may not be immediately available. If red cells from the mother are not available and if treatment of the infant with IVIG (see below) does not obviate the need for exchange transfusion, the clinician has two major choices. First, treatment can be delayed until blood is obtained through one of the rare donor files, assuming that blood of the appropriate phenotype is available. Second, an exchange transfusion using incompatible blood can be undertaken. The decision should be made in the light of the infant's clinical condition and the likelihood that it may suffer kernicterus. There is no doubt (367,884,888-890) that when the bilirubin level is increasing in a way that makes it apparent that a dangerous level will be reached, an exchange transfusion with incompatible blood is infinitely better than a wait for compatible blood, if that wait would introduce a real risk of kernicterus. When incompatible blood must be used, the exchange transfusion must usually be done with two or more units. It is necessary to achieve a better exchange than usual so that more of the maternal antibody is removed. Since the infant will have only incompatible red cells circulating after the exchange, any maternal antibody not removed will effect their destruction and the bilirubin level may increase rapidly. Rosenfield (890) advocates the use of three or four units of blood for the exchange when incompatible blood must be used and states that in his experience, most infants thus treated survive and if adequately handled, do not develop kernicterus. However, he also warns that the clinical course of such treated infants is stormy.

Use of IVIG to Treat the Infant

In an earlier section of this chapter, the use of IVIG in a pregnant woman to alleviate the degree of HDN in her fetus in utero, was described. As indicated, a number of successes have been reported (see earlier for references) particularly when the IVIG was used early in pregnancy, before intrauterine transfusion could be undertaken. IVIG has also been used to treat infants with HDN. A number of individual successes have been described (891-893) but the largest volume of data comes from a controlled trial, reported in brief by Rubo and Wahn (894). A total of 32 newborns with HDN were randomly assigned to treatment arms, one of which involved treatment only by phototherapy (see below) while the other involved phototherapy and the use of IVIG. In the infants treated only by phototherapy, 11 of 16 eventually required exchange transfusions to correct hyperbilirubinemia. In the infants treated by phototherapy and with IVIG, only two of 16 required exchange transfusions and in one of the two it was supposed (894) that the transfusion became necessary because treatment with IVIG was started too long after the infant's birth. In other words, it was concluded that treatment with IVIG helps to prevent hyperbilirubinemia but does not reverse it.

It would appear that IVIG must act differently in a pregnant woman and in a newborn infant. In the mother, the IVIG is believed to down regulate antibody production via a positive feedback mechanism, possibly to contain anti-idiotype that acts on immunocytes and/or to compete with the maternal antibody for active placental transfer to the fetus. In the fetus, the IVIG is presumed to compete with antibody-coated red cells for Fc receptors on macrophages and thus reduce the rate of red cell destruction. In the newborn the IVIG obviously cannot down regulate antibody production since the maternal antibody has already been made and is bound to the newborn's red cells. Similarly, no role for anti-idiotype or for interference with placental passage can be postulated when the IVIG is used to treat the newborn. Presumably then, the IVIG in this setting acts solely by splenic blockade. Apparently the excess of IgG results in the Fc receptors of macrophages binding free IgG from the plasma thus sparing IgG coated red cells. Presumably some of those cells are still bound by macrophages and cleared but apparently the rate of that event is so slowed that bilirubin accumulates more slowly and can be handled via the phototherapy and the natural (albeit not yet fully developed) clearance system (see above). While the use of IVIG is unlikely to alter the incidence of exchange transfusion necessary to correct anemia at birth, it may have a dramatic effect on the use of exchange transfusion to control hyperbilirubinemia.

Simple Transfusion

Some infants with relatively mild HDN can be treated with small amounts of packed red cells given as simple top-up transfusions. Obviously, careful calculations must be made before the transfusion to ensure that the volume of cells to be transfused is not large enough to introduce the risk of circulatory overload. Equally obvious, this form of therapy can be used to correct mild anemia but will not control an increasing level of bilirubin.

Phototherapy

We have been told but have not been able to find printed confirmation, that an astute nurse noticed that mildly jaundiced infants who slept in cribs on the side of the nursery exposed to sunlight, lost their jaundiced appearance more quickly than their counterparts who slept in cribs not exposed to the sun. Whether or not this story is true, it is now known that exposure to light, in the region of 420-480 nm (i.e. roughly equivalent to ultraviolet light in sunshine) converts bilirubin in to a non-toxic pigment biliverdin. Many infants with jaundice at levels such that no danger of kernicterus exists are now treated by phototherapy. This involves exposure of the infants to fluorescent light until the jaundice fades, obviously bilirubin measurements must be made if the jaundice increases or is slow to fade. Many infants with mild to moderate HDN can be treated by phototherapy so that the risks of exchange transfusion to relieve hyperbilirubinemia can be avoided (895-897). Phototherapy is often the only form of therapy needed in ABO HDN (898).

Physiological Jaundice

Because, as explained above, bilirubin excretion mechanisms are not fully developed at birth, some infants who do not have HDN will become jaundiced and in rare cases a dangerous level of bilirubin becomes potentially possible. In such rare cases, exchange transfusion may become necessary. As would be expected from what has been written above, in the section on prevention of kernicterus, an exchange transfusion in this circumstance is more likely to be necessary in a premature (899,900) than in a full term infant (901,902).

Concluding Comments

As mentioned above, most this chapter has dealt with HDN caused by anti-D or by antibodies of the ABO system. However, as shown in tables 41-1 to 41-3, many other antibodies have also caused the disease. Almost everything that has been written can be applied to other antibodies simply by substituting the appropriate name for the antigen and antibody involved. In most instances, cases of HDN caused by antibodies other than anti-D will be less severe than those noted in this chapter, exceptions to that generalization are seen.

Finally, HDN occurs in animals other than man. For example, its occurrence in thoroughbred horses bred for racing can be economically (and presumably for the mare, emotionally) serious when the disease is fatal. In animals, recognition of the presence of antibody can result in the avoidance of HDN by phenotyping and selective breeding. In man, other measures are employed. However, resolution of the problem is in sight. The draft of this chapter was finished in the same week as the successful Scottish sheep cloning was announced (917). Clearly HDN can now be avoided, if appropriate advice (918) is heeded, the fun need not be lost.

References

1. Walker W, Murray S. Br Med J 1956;1:187
2. Franklin EC, Kunkel HG. J Lab Clin Med 1958;52:724
3. Zak SJ, Good RA. J Clin Invest 1959;38:579
4. West CD, Hong R, Holland NH. J Clin Invest 1962;41:2054
5. Polley MJ, Mollison PL, Soothill JF. Br J Haematol 1962;8:149
6. Smith RT, Eitzman DV. Pediatrics 1964;33:163
7. Martensson L, Fudenberg HH. J Immunol 1965;94:514
8. Tosato G, Magrath IT, Koski IR, et al. J Clin Invest 1980;66:383
9. Maccario R, Nespoli L, Mingrat G, et al. J Immunol 1983;130:1129
10. Lucivero G, Osso AD, Iannone A, et al. Biol Neonate 1983;44:303
11. Solinger AM. Cell Immunol 1985;92:115
12. Andersson U. Acta Pediat Scand 1985;74:568
13. Burgio GR, Hanson LA, Ugazio AG. Immunology of the Neonate. Berlin:Springer-Verlag, 1987
14. Burgio GR, Ugazio AG, Notarangelo A. Curr Opin Immunol 1990;2:770
15. Durandy A, Thuillier L, Forveille M, et al. J Immunol 1990;144:60
16. Splawski JB, Jelinek DF, Lipsky PE. J Clin Invest 1991;87:545
17. Splawski JB, Lipsky PE. J Clin Invest 1991;88:967
18. Roilides E, Clerici M, DePalma L, et al. FASEB J 1991;5:A1699
19. Ferguson J. Am J Pathol 1931;7:277
20. Clifford S, Hertig A. New Eng J Med 1932;207:105
21. Blackfan K. New Eng J Med 1932;207:111
22. Diamond L, Blackfan K, Baty J. J Pediat 1932;1:269
23. Darrow R. Arch Pathol 1938;25:378
24. Zimmerman DR. Rh. The Intimate History of a Disease and its Conquest. New York:Macmillan, 1973:20
25. Levine P, Stetson R. J Am Med Assoc 1939;113:126
26. Levine P, Vogel P, Katzin EM, et al. Science 1941;94:374
27. Levine P, Katzin EM, Burnham L. J Am Med Assoc

1941;116:325
28. Wiener AS. Proc Soc Exp Biol NY 1944;56:173
29. Race RR. Nature 1944;153:771
30. Cameron JW, Diamond LK. J Clin Invest 1945;24:793
31. Diamond LK, Denton RL. J Clin Lab Med 1945;30:821
32. Coombs RRA, Mourant AE, Race RR. Lancet 1945;2:15
33. Coombs RRA, Mourant AE, Race RR. J Exp Pathol 1945;26:255
34. Chown B. Lancet 1954;1:1213
35. Gunson HH. Paediatrics 1957;20:3
36. Kleihauer E, Braun H, Betke K. Klin Wschr 1957;35:637
37. Betke K, Kleihauer E. Blut 1958;4:241
38. Hosoi T. Yokohama Med Bull 1958;9:61
39. Jones AR, Silver S. Blood 1958;13:763
40. Kleihauer E, Betke K. Internist 1960;1:292
41. Cohen F, Zuelzer WW, Evans MM. Blood 1960;15:884
42. Kevans JR, Woodrow JC, Nosenzo C, et al. Proc 10th Cong ISH, 1964
43. Cohen F, Zuelzer WW, Gustafson DC, et al. Blood 1964;23:621
44. Woodrow JC, Clarke CA, Donohoe WTA, et al. Br Med J 1965;1:279
45. Woodrow JC, Finn R. Br J Haematol 1966;12:297
46. Liedholm P. Acta Obstet Gynaecol Scand 1971;50:367
47. Poulain M, Huchet J. Rev Fr Trans 1971;14:219
48. Mollison PL. Br Med J 1972;3:31
49. Mollison PL. Br Med J 1972;3:115
50. Pembrey ME, Weatherall DJ, Clegg JB. Lancet 1973;1:1350
51. Wood WG, Stamatoyannopoulos G, Lim G, et al. Blood 1975;46:671
52. Boyer SH, Belding TK, Margolet L, et al. Johns Hopkins Med J 1975;137:105
53. Jørgensen J. MD Thesis, Univ Copenhagen, 1975
54. Popat N, Wood WG, Weatherall DJ. Lancet 1977;2:377
55. Bowman JM, Pollack JM. Transf Med Rev 1987;1:101
56. Huchet J, Defossez Y, Broussard Y. (Letter). Transfusion 1988;28:506
57. Greenwalt TJ, Sasaki T, Gajewski M. Vox Sang 1959;4:138
58. Weinstein L, Taylor ES. Am J Obstet Gynecol 1975;121:643
59. Astrup J, Kornstad L. Acta Obstet Gynaecol Scand 1977;56:185
60. Pepperell RJ, Barrie JU, Fleigner JR. Med J Austral 1977;2:453
61. Kornstad L. Acta Obstet Gynaecol Scand 1983;62:431
62. Bowell PJ, Brown SE, Dike AE, et al. Br J Obstet Gynaecol 1986;93:1044
63. Mayne KM, Bowell PJ, Pratt GA. Clin Lab Haematol 1990;12:379
64. Ashurst DE, Bedford D, Coombs RRA. Vox Sang 1956;1:235
65. Geruvitch J, Nelken D. Vox Sang 1957;2:342
66. Lawler SD, Shatwell HS. Vox Sang 1962;7:488
67. Dunstan RA, Simpson MB, Rosse WF. Transfusion 1984;24:243
68. Dunstan RA. Br J Haematol 1986;62:301
69. Barclay GR, Greiss MA, Urbaniak SJ. Br Med J 1980;2:1569
70. McBride JA, O'Hoski P, Blajchman MA, et al. (abstract). Transfusion 1978;18:626
71. Mollison PL, Engelfriet CP, Contreras M. Blood Transfusion in Clinical Medicine, 9th Ed. Oxford:Blackwell, 1993
72. Keith L, Cuva A, Houser K, et al. Transfusion 1970;10:142
73. Bowman HS, Mohn JF, Lambert RM. Vox Sang 1972;22:385
74. Loghem JJ van, Hart M van der, Borstel H. Vox Sang 1957;2:257
75. Giblett ER. Clin Obstet Gynecol 1964;7:1044
76. Weiner W, Norris V, Davidson S. Br Med J 1952;2:975

77. Clarke CA, Finn R, Lehane D, et al. Br Med J 1966;1:213
78. Kreiger VK. J Obstet Gynaecol Br Cwth 1966;73:99
79. Bartsch FK. Acta Obstet Gynaecol Scand 1972, Suppl 20:1
80. Sebring ES. In: Hemolytic Diseaseof the Newborn. Arlington, VA:Am Assoc Blood Banks, 1984;87
81. Ness PM, Baldwin ML, Niebyl JR. Am J Obstet Gynecol 1987;156:154
82. Sebring ES, Polesky HF. Transfusion 1990;30:344
83. Hartmann O, Brendemoen O. Acta Pediat 1953;42:20
84. Woodrow JC, Donohoe WTA. Br Med J 1968;4:139
85. Ascari WQ, Levine P, Pollack W. Br Med J 1969;1:399
86. Woodrow JC. Ser Haematol 1970;3:3
87. Nevanlinna HR, Vainio T. Proc 8th Cong ISBT, Basel:Karger, 1962;281
88. Bowman JM, Chown B, Lewis M, et al. Canad Med Assoc J 1978;118:623
89. Chown B. Canad Med Assoc J 1949;61;419
90. David MP, Milbauer B. Clin Pediat 1978;17:924
91. Aronsson S, Engelson G, Svenningsen NW. (Letter). Lancet 1965;2:847
92. Vontver LA. J Am Med Assoc 1973;226:469
93. Bichler A, Hetzel H. Geb Frauenh 1975;35:640
94. McVerry BA, O'Connor MC, Price A, et al. Br Med J 1977;1:1324
95. Wong LK, Smith LH, Jensen HM. Transfusion 1983;23:348
96. Levine P. J Hered 1943;34:71
97. Levine P. Hum Biol 1958;30:14
98. Nevanlinna HR, Vainio T. Vox Sang 1956;1:26
99. Clarke CA, Finn R, McConnell RB, et al. Int Arch Allgy 1958;13:380
100. Stern K, Berger M. Am J Clin Pathol 1961;35:520
101. Vos GH. Am J Hum Genet 1965;17:202
102. Race RR, Sanger R. Blood Groups in Man, 1st Ed. Oxford:Blackwell, 1950
103. Finn R. Lancet 1960;1:526
104. Stern K, Goodman HS, Berger M. J Immunol 1961;87:189
105. Freda VJ, Gorman JG. Bull Sloane Hosp Women 1962;8:147
106. Clarke CA, Donohoe WTA, McConnell RB, et al. Br Med J 1963;1:979
107. Freda VJ, Gorman JG, Pollack W. Transfusion 1964;4:26
108. Mollison PL, Hughes-Jones NC, Lindsay M, et al. Vox Sang 1969;16:421
109. Freda VJ, Gorman JG, Pollack W. Science 1966;151:828
110. Combined Study on Prevention of Rh HDN. Br Med J 1966;2:907
111. Chown B. Canad Med Assoc J 1967;97:1294
112. Leading Article. Prevention of Rh hemolytic disease. Med J Austral 1967;2:1035
113. Pollack W, Gorman JG, Hager HJ, et al. Transfusion 1968;8:134
114. Pollack W, Gorman JG, Freda VJ, et al. Transfusion 1968;8:151
115. Leading Article. Prevention of Rh hemolytic disease. Med J Austral 1969;1:1034
116. Clarke CA. Clin Genet 1970;1:183
117. Woodrow JC, Clarke CA, McConnell RB, et al. Br Med J 1971;2:610
118. Pollack W, Ascari WQ, Kochesky RJ, et al. Transfusion 1971;11:333
119. Pollack W, Ascari WQ, Crispen JF, et al. Transfusion 1971;11:340
120. Woodrow JC. Haematologia 1974;8:281
121. Report of MRC Anti-D Working Party. Br Med J 1974;2:75
122. Woodrow JC, Clarke CA, Donohoe WTA, et al. Br Med J 1975;2:57

123. Clarke CA, Whitfield AGW. Br Med J 1979;1:1665
124. Blajchman M, Zipursky A, Bartsch RR, et al. Vox Sang 1977;36:50
125. Tovey LAD, Murray J, Stevenson BJ, et al. Br Med J 1978;2:106
126. Davey MG, Zipursky A. Vox Sang 1979;36:5
127. Clarke CA, Whitfield AGW. Br Med J 1980;281:781
128. Clarke CA. Br J Haematol 1982;52:525
129. Thornton JG, Page C, Foote G, et al. Br Med J 1989;298:1671
130. Tovey LAD. Transf Med 1992;2;99
131. Clarke CA, Hussey RM. J Roy Coll Phys Lond 1994;28:310
132. Murphy WG, Ghosh S, Hughes RH, et al. (Letter). Br Med J 1994;309:806
133. Hughes RG, Craig JIO, Murphy WG, et al. Br J Obstet Gynaecol 1994;101:297
134. Howard HL, Martlew VJ, McFadyen IR, et al. Br J Obstet Gynaeol 1997;104:37
135. WHO. Technical Report Series, 1971:468
136. Samson D, Mollison PL. Immunology 1975;28:349
137. Polesky HF, Sebring ES. Transfusion 1971;11:162
138. Helderweirt G, Sokal G. Rev Belge Pathol Med Exp 1960;27:146
139. Helderweirt G. Ann Soc Belge Med Trop 1963;43:575
140. Fraser ID, Raper AB. Br Med J 1962;2:303
141. Sullivan JF, Jennings ER. Am J Clin Pathol 1966;46:36
142. Zipursky A, Israels LG. Canad Med Assoc J 1967;97:1245
143. Dudok C de Wit, Borst-Eilers E, Weerdt CMVD, et al. Br Med J 1968;4:477
144. Devi B, Jennison RF, Langley FA. J Obstet Gynaecol Br Cwth 1968;75:659
145. Bevan IDG, Truskett ID. Med J Austral 1969;1:551
146. Schneider J. Prog Immunobiol Stand 1970;4:284
147. Putte I van der, Renaer M, Vermylen C. Am J Obstet Gynecol 1972;114:850
148. Sebring ES, Polesky HF. Transfusion 1982;22:468
149. Kebles DB, Hall SJ, Graham HA. (abstract). Transfusion 1982;22:409
150. Baudin JC, Pederson BF, Cooper ES, et al. (abstract). Transfusion 1982;22:425
151. Taswell HF. Mayo Clin Proc 1983;58:342
152. Kleihauer E. Bieh Arch Kinderh 1966;53 (Suppl):10
153. Zago MA, Wood WG, Clegg JB, et al. Blood 1979;53:977
154. Cohen F, Zuelzer WW. Vox Sang 1964;9:75
155. Parks DR, Herzenberg LA. Meth Cell Biol 1982;25:277
156. Hensleigh PA. Am J Obstet Gynecol 1983;146:749
157. Medearis AL, Hensleigh PA, Parks DR, et al. Am J Obstet Gynecol 1984;148:290
158. Cupp JE, Leary JF, Cernichiari E, et al. Cytometry 1984;5:138
159. Nance S. In: Progress in Immunohematology. Arlington, VA:Am Assoc Blood Banks, 1988:1
160. Nance SJ, Nelson JM, Arndt PA, et al. Am J Clin Pathol 1989;91:288
161. Gemke RJBJ, Kanhai HHH, Overbeeke MAM, et al. Br J Haematol 1986;64:689
162. Salamon JL, Smith B, Riley JZ, et al. (abstract). Transfusion 1982;22:425
163. Riley JZ, Ness PM, Taddie SJ, et al. Transfusion 1982;22:472
164. Ness PM. Am J Obstet Gynecol 1982;143:788
165. Ness PM, Riley JZ. In: Rh Hemolytic Disease: New Strategy for Eradication. Boston:Hall, 1982:135
166. Salamon JL, Smith B, Ness PM. (abstract). Transfusion 1983;23:433
167. Seppälä M, Rouslahti E. Am J Obstet Gynecol 1972;112:208
168. Horacek I, Pepperell RJ, Hay DL, et al. Lancet 1976;2:200

169. Lachman E, Hingley SM, Bates G, et al. Br Med J 1977;1:1377
170. Caballero C, Vekemans M, Lopez del Campo JG, et al. Am J Obstet Gynecol 1977;127:384
171. Los FJ, de Wolf BTHM, Huisjes HJ. Lancet 1979;2:1210
172. Mennuti MT, Brummond W, Crombleholme WR, et al. Obstet Gynecol 1980;55:48
173. Chamberlain EM, Scott JR, Wu JT, et al. Am J Obstet Gynecol 1982;143:912
174. Tomada Y. Nature 1964;202;910
175. Hosoi T. Exp Cell Res 1965;37:680
176. Bowman JM. Obstet Gynecol 1978;52:385
177. Hughes-Jones NC, Ellis M, Ivona J, et al. Vox Sang 1971;21:135
178. Hoppe HH, Mester T, Hennig W, et al. Vox Sang 1973;25:308
179. Bowman JM, Friesen AD, Pollock JM, et al. Canad Med Assoc J 1980;123:1121
180. Bowman JM, Pollock JM. Canad Med Assoc J 1978;118:627
181. Clarke CA, Whitfield AGW. Br Med J 1980;280:903
182. Tovey LAD, Taverner JM. Lancet 1981;1:878
183. Bowman JM. In: Immunobiology of Transfusion Medicine. New York:Marcel Dekker, 1994:553
184. American College of Obstetricians and Gynecologists 1981;Tech Bull 61
185. Brandstadter W, Brandstadter M. Z Gynakol 1970;6:176
186. Wiener AS, Geiger J, Gordon EB. Exp Med Surg 1957;15:75
187. Unger LJ, Wiener AS. J Lab Clin Med 1959;54:835
188. Sacks HS, Wiener AS, Jahn EF, et al. Ann Intern Med 1959;51:740
189. Lowes BCR. Vox Sang 1969;16:231
190. Hill Z, Vacl J, Kalasova E, et al. Vox Sang 1974;27:92
191. Zaino EC, Applewhaite F. Transfusion 1975;15:256
192. Lacey PA, Caskey CR, Werner DJ, et al. Transfusion 1983;23:91
193. Issitt PD. Serology and Genetics of the Rh Blood Group System. Cincinnati:Montgomery, 1979:71
194. Soloway HB. Med Lab Obs 1981;13:21
195. Soloway HB. (abstract). Transfusion 1982;22:425
196. Soloway HB. Med Lab Obs 1982;14:21
197. Soloway HB. (Letter). Diag Med 1982;Sept-Oct:13
198. White CA, Stedman CM, Franks S. Am J Obstet Gynecol 1983;145:1069
199. Ostgard P, Fevang F, Kornstad L. Acta Pediat Scand 1986;75:175
200. Hedley G. BBTS, Blood Bank Technol Group Report 1993;Jan:4
201. BCSH Guidelines. Clin Lab Haematol 1987;9:333
202. Voak D, Waters A. (Letter). Clin Lab Haematol 1990;12:235
203. Jones J, Scott ML, Voak D. Transf Med 1995;5:171
204. Konugres AA, Polesky HF, Walker RH. Transfusion 1982;22:76
205. Lubenko A, Contreras M, Habash J. Br J Haematol 1989;72:429
206. Tippett P, Lomas-Francis C, Wallace M. Vox Sang 1996;70:123
207. Hocevar M, Glonar L. In: The Ljubljana Abortion Study. Bethesda, MD:NIH Cen Popn Res, 1974
208. Simonovits L, Timar I, Bajtai G. Vox Sang 1980;38:161
209. Medical Research Council Working Party. Br J Obstet Gynaecol 1978;85 (Suppl 2):1
210. Grant CJ, Hamblin TJ, Smith DS, et al. Int J Artific Organs 1983;6;83
211. Bowman JM, Pollock JM. Obstet Gynecol 1985;66:749
212. Kanhai HHH, Gravenhorst JB, van't Veer MB, et al. (Letter). Lancet 1984;2:157

213. Modell B. Lancet 1985;1:737
214. Warren RC, Butler J, Morsman JM, et al. Lancet 1985;1:691
215. Peddle LJ. Am J Obstet Gynecol 1968;100:567
216. Godel JC, Buchanan DI, Jarosch JM, et al. Br Med J 1968;4:479
217. Tovey LAD, Robinson AE. Br Med J 1975;4:320
218. Davey MG. Med J Austral 1975;2:263
219. Tovey LAD, Scott JS. Vox Sang 1980;39:149
220. Bowman JM, Pollock JM. Vox Sang 1984;47:209
221. Finn R, Clarke CA, Donohoe WTA, et al. Br Med J 1961;1:1486
222. Mollison PL. Blood Transfusion in Clinical Medicine, 7th Ed. Oxford:Blackwell, 1983
223. Pollack W. In: Hemolytic Disease of the Newborn. Arlington, VA:Am Assoc Blood Banks, 1984:53
224. Pollack W, Gorman JG. In: Rh Antibody Mediated Immunosuppression. Raritan, N.J.:Ortho Res Inst, 1976:115
225. Holburn AM, Frame M, Hughes-Jones NC, et al. Immunology 1971;20:681
226. Mollison PL. Transfusion 1986;26:43
227. Mollison PL. Transfusion 1989;29:347
228. Borne AEGKr von dem, Beckers D, Engelfriet CP. Br J Haematol 1977;36:485
229. St Sinclair NR. J Exp Med 1969;129:1183
230. Lee RK, St Sinclair NR. Immunology 1973;24:735
231. Chan PL, St Sinclair NR. Immunology 1973;24:289
232. Heyman B. Scand J Immunol 1990;31:601
233. Crowley M, Kayo I, Steinman RM. J Exp Med 1990;172:383
234. Weitzel H, Hunermann B, Stolp W, et al. In: Prophylaxe der Rhesus-Sensibiliserung. Frankfurt:Med Verlagsgesellschaft, 1974
235. Bowman JM. Am J Obstet Gynecol 1985;151:289
236. De Silva M, Contreras M, Mollison PL. Vox Sang 1985;48:178
237. Contreras M, Mollison PL. Br J Haematol 1981;49:371
238. Contreras M, Mollison PL. Br J Haematol 1983;53:153
239. Mollison PL, In: Rh Hemolytic Disease - New Strategy for Eradication. Boston:Hall, 1982:161
240. Vahlquist B, Lagercrutz R, Nordbring F. Lancet 1950;2:851
241. Hartley P. Proc Roy Soc Biol 1951;138:499
242. Chown B. Arch Dis Childh 1955;30:237
243. Du Pan RM, Wenger P, Koechli S, et al. Clin Chim Acta 1959;4:110
244. Brambell FWR, Hemmings WA, Oakley CL, et al. Proc Roy Soc Biol 1960;151:478
245. Gitlin D, Kumate J, Urrusti J, et al. Nature 1964;203:86
246. Gitlin D, Kumate J, Urrusti J, et al. J Clin Invest 1964;43:1938
247. Kohler PF, Farr RS. Nature 1966;210:1070
248. Brambell FWR. Lancet 1966;2:1087
249. Yeung CY, Hobbs JR. Lancet 1968;2:1167
250. Toivanen P, Mantyjarvi R, Hirvoven T. Immunology 1968;15:395
251. Mantyjarvi R, Hirvonen T, Toivanen P. Immunology 1970;18:449
252. Wang AC, Faulk WP, Stuckey MA, et al. Immunochemistry 1970;7:703
253. Hay FC, Hull MGR, Torrigiani G. Clin Exp Immunol 1971;9:355
254. Morell A, Skvaril F, Loghem E van, et al. Vox Sang 1971;21:481
255. Virella G, Nunes M, Amelia S, et al. Clin Exp Immunol 1972;10:475
256. Schur PJ, Alpert E, Alper C. Clin Immunol Immunopathol 1973;2:62
257. Matre R, Tonder O, Endresen C. Scand J Immunol 1975;4:741
258. McNabb T, Koh T-Y, Dorrington KJ, et al. J Immunol 1976;117:882
259. Balfour A, Jones EA. In: Maternofoetal Transmission of Immunoglobulins. Cambridge:Cambridge Univ Press, 1976
260. Brandon MR. In: Maternofoetal Transmission of Immunoglobulins. Cambridge:Cambridge Univ Press, 1976
261. Fukumoto T, Brandon MR. In: Immunological Influence on Human Fertility. Sydney:Academic, 1977
262. Loke YW. Immunology and Immunopathology of the Human Foetal-Maternal Interaction. Amsterdam:Elsevier, 1978
263. Pitcher-Wilmott RW, Hindocha P, Woods CBS. Clin Exp Immunol 1980;41:303
264. van der Meulen JA, McNabb TC, Haeffner-Cavaillon N, et al. J Immunol 1980;124:500
265. Pollock JM, Bowman JM. Vox Sang 1982;43:327
266. Lee SI, Heiner DC, Wara D. Monograph Allgy 1986;19:108
267. Hammerström L, Smith CIE. (Letter). Lancet 1986;1:681
268. Einhorn MS, Granoff DM, Nahm MH, et al. J Pediat 1987;111:783
269. Mollison PL, Blood Transfusion in Clinical Medicine, 1st Ed. Oxford:Blackwell, 1951
270. Frankowska K, Gorska B. Arch Immunol Ther Exp 1978;26:1095
271. Ouwehand WH, Engesser L, Huiskes E, et al. In: The Activity of IgG1 and IgG3 Antibodies in Immune Mediated Destruction of Red Cells. Amsterdam:Rodopi, 1984:44
272. Parinaud J, Blanc M, Grandjean H, et al.. Am J Obstet Gynecol 1985;151:1111
273. Garratty G. In: Immune Destruction of Red Blood Cells. Arlington, VA:Am Assoc Blood Banks, 1989:109
274. Schanfield MS. In: Blood Bank Immunology. Washington, D.C.:Am Assoc Blood Banks, 1977:97
275. Cregut R, Pinon F, Brossard Y. Nouv Presse Med 1973;29:1947
276. Taslimi MM, Sibai BM, Mason JM, et al. Am J Obstet Gynecol 1986;154:1327
277. Nance SJ, Arndt PA, Garratty G. (Letter). Transfusion 1990;30:381
278. Nance S, Nelson J, Garratty G. (abstract). Transfusion 1988;28 (Suppl 6S):9S
279. Garratty G, Arndt P. Transfusion 1995;35:157
280. Judd WJ. Methods in Immunohematology, 2nd Ed. Durham:Montgomery, 1994
281. Bowman JM, Pollock JM, Penston LE. Vox Sang 1986;51:117
282. Bowman JM. In: Antenatal and Neonatal Screening, 2nd Ed. Oxford:Oxford Univ Press, 1992
283. Mayne KM, Allen DL, Bowell PJ. Clin Lab Haematol 1991;13:239
284. Clarke CA, Mollison PL, Whitfield AGW. Br Med J 1985;291:17
285. Bowell PJ, Allen DL, Entwistle CC. Br J Obstet Gynaecol 1986;93:1038
286. Kornstad L. Ann NIPH 1987;10:3
287. Contreras M, Knight RC. Clin Lab Haematol 1989;11:317
288. Bowman JM. Transf Med Rev 1990;6:191
289. Walker RH, Hartrick MB. (abstract). Transfusion 1991;31 (Suppl 8S):52S
290. Contreras M, Knight RC. Transfusion 1991;31:270
291. Issitt PD, Tessel JA. Transfusion 1981;21:412
292. Shirey RS, Mirabella D, Lumadue JA, et al. (abstract). Transfusion 1996;36 (Suppl 9S):22S
293. Combs MR, Issitt PD. Unpublished observations 1996
294. Halbrecht I. Am J Dis Childh 1944;68:248

295. Grumbach A, Gasser C. Helv Pediat Acta 1948;3:447
296. Rosenfield RE. Blood 1955;10:17
297. Wiener AS, Unger LJ. Exp Med Surg 1955;13:204
298. Münk-Anderson G. Acta Path Microbiol Scand 1958;42:43
299. Wiener AS, Freda VJ, Wexler JB, et al. Am J Obstet Gynecol 1960;79:567
300. Kochwa S, Rosenfield RE, Tallal L, et al. J Clin Invest 1961;40:874
301. Voak D. Vox Sang 1968;14:271
302. Voak D. Vox Sang 1969;17:481
303. Bowman JM. In: Maternal-Fetal Medicine: Principles and Practice. Philadelphia:Saunders, 1989:652
304. Rawson AJ, Abelson NM. J Immunol 1960;85:640
305. Issitt PD, Combs MR. (abstract). Transfusion 1996;36 (Suppl 9S):23S
306. Rosenfield RE, Ohno G. Rev Hematol 1955;10:231
307. Halbrecht I. J Pediat 1951;39:185
308. Hsia DYY, Gellis SS. Pediatrics 1954;13:503
309. Valentine GH. Arch Dis Childh 1958;33:185
310. Desjardins L, Blajchman MA, Chintu C, et al. J Pediat 1979;95:447
311. Ames AC, Lloyd RS. Vox Sang 1964;9:712
312. Worlledge S, Ogiemudia SE, Thomas CO, et al. Ann Trop Med Parasitol 1974;68:249
313. Kirkman NN. J Pediat 1977;90:717
314. Peevy KJ, Wiseman HJ. Pediatrics 1978;61:475
315. Al-Jawad ST, Keenan P, Kholeif S. Saudi Med J 1985;7:41
316. Caine ME, Mueller-Heubach. Am J Obstet Gynecol 1986;154:85
317. Tovey LAD. Br J Obstet Gynaecol 1986;93:960
318. Strohm P, O'Shaughnessy R, Moore J, et al. Immunohematology 1991;7:40
319. Mollison PL, Engelfriet CP, Contreras M. Blood Transfusion in Clinical Medicine, 8th Ed. Oxford:Blackwell, 1987:685
320. McDonnell L. Unpublished observations cited in Mollison PL, Engelfriet CP, Contreras M. Blood Transfusion in Clinical Medicine, 8th Ed. Oxford:Blackwell, 1987:685
321. Bowman JM, Harman CR, Manning FA, et al. Vox Sang 1989;56:187
322. Ratcliff D, Fiorenza S, Culotta E, et al. (abstract). Transfusion 1987;27:534
323. Lowe RF, Musengezi AT, Moores P. Transfusion 1978;18:466
324. Purohit DM, Taylor HL, Spivey MA. Am J Obstet Gynecol 1978;131:755
325. Wake EJ, Issitt PD, Reihart JK, et al. Transfusion 1969;9:217
326. Baker JB, Grewar D, Lewis M, et al. Arch Dis Childh 1956;31:298
327. Bharucha ZS, Joshi SR, Bhatia HM. Vox Sang 1981;41:36
328. Bhatia HM. (Letter). Vox Sang 1982;42:278
329. Holburn AM. Br J Haematol 1974;27:489
330. Cheng MS. (Letter). Transfusion 1983;23:274
331. Reid ME, Ellisor SS. (Letter). Vox Sang 1982;42:278
332. Sabo BH. In: A Seminar on Perinatal Blood Banking. Washington, D.C.:Am Assoc Blood Banks, 1978:31
333. Vengelen-Tyler V. In: Hemolytic Disease of the Newborn. Arlington, VA:Am Assoc Blood Banks, 1984:145
334. Marsh WL, Mawby LJ, Mueller KA, et al. Transfusion 1984;24:19
335. Mayne K, Bowell P, Woodward T, et al. Br J Haematol 1990;76:537
336. Bowman JM. Vox Sang 1986;50:104
337. Filbey D, Hanson U, Wesstrom G. Acta Obstet Gynecol Scand 1995;74:687
338. Vaughan JI, Warwick RM, Letsky EA, et al. Am J Obstet Gynecol 1994;171:247
339. Bennebroeck-Gravenhort J. Unpublished observations cited in Mollison PL, Engelfriet CP, Contreras M. Blood Transfusion in Clinical Medicine, 9th Ed. Oxford:Blackwell, 1993:582
340. Frigoletto FD Jr. Unpublished observations cited in Mollison PL, Engelfriet CP, Contreras M. Blood Transfusion in Clinical Medicine, 9th Ed. Oxford:Blackwell, 1993:582
341. Walker W, Murray S, Russell JK. J Obstet Gynaecol Br Emp 1957;44:573
342. Hopkins DF. Am J Obstet Gynecol 1970;108:268
343. Fraser ID, Tovey GH. Clin Haematol 1976;5:149
344. Crawford H, Cutbush M, Falconer H, et al. Lancet 1952;2:219
345. Springer GF, Tritel H. J Am Med Assoc 1962;182:1341
346. Springer GF, Schuster R. Vox Sang 1964;9:589
347. Grundbacher FJ. Nature 1964;204:192
348. Grundbacher FJ. Z Immun Forsch 1967;134:317
349. Graham H, Morrison M, Casey E. Vox Sang 1974;27:363
350. Gupte SC, Bhatia HM. Ind J Med Res 1979;70:221
351. Grundbacher FJ. Transfusion 1976;16:48
352. Gupte SC, Bhatia HM. Vox Sang 1980;38:22
353. Grundbacher FJ. Transfusion 1980;20:563
354. Miller DF, Petrie SJ. Obstet Gynecol 1963;22:773
355. Gilja BK, Shah VP. Clin Pediat 1988;27:210
356. Cox MT, Shiels L, Masel D, et al. (abstract). Transfusion 1991;31 (Suppl 8S):29S
357. Sherer DM, Abramowicz JS, Ryan RM, et al. Obstet Gynecol 1991;78:897
358. Yamamoto F, Clausen H, White T, et al. Nature 1990;345:229
359. Chang J-G, Lee L-S, Chen P-H, et al. Blood 1992;79:2176
360. Ugozzoli L, Wallace RB. Genomics 1992;12:670
361. Johnson PH, Hopkinson DA. Hum Mol Genet 1992;1:341
362. O'Keefe DS, Dobrovic A. Hum Mutat 1993;2:67
363. Stroncek DJ, Konz R, Clay ME, et al. Transfusion 1995;35:231
364. Burki U, Degnan TJ, Rosenfield RE. Vox Sang 1964;9:209
365. Austin T, Finklestein J, Okada D, et al. J Pediat 1976;89:330
366. Dhandsa N, Williams M, Joss V, et al. Lancet 1981;2:1232
367. Gottschall J. (Letter). Transfusion 1981;21:230
368. Tuck S, Studd JWW. Br J Obstet Gynaecol 1982;89:91
369. Dopp SL, Isham BE. (Letter). Transfusion 1983;23:273
370. BCSH Guidelines. Clin Lab Haematol 1990;12:209
371. BCSH Guidelines. Clin Lab Haematol 1990;12:321
372. BSH/BBTS Guidelines. Clin Lab Haematol. 1990;12:437
373. Voak D, Scott M, Jones J, et al. (abstract). Vox Sang 1996;70 (Suppl 2):49
374. BCSH. Standard Haematology Practice. Oxford:Blackwell, 1991:150
375. BCSH Guidelines. Transf Med 1995;5:145
376. BCSH Guidelines. Transf Med 1996;6:71
377. Hardy J, Napier JAF. Br J Obstet Gynaecol 1981;88:91
378. Pinon F, Cregut R, Brossard Y. Rev Fr Transf Immunohematol 1981;24:483
379. Weinstein L. Clin Obstet Gynecol 1982;25:321
380. Castillo RA, Devoe LD, Hadi HA, et al. Am J Obstet Gynecol 1986;155:812
381. Bomchil G. Hematol Hemoterap 1951;3:104
382. Stone B, Marsh WL. Br J Haematol 1959;5:344
383. Simmons RT, Kreiger VI, Jacobowicz R. Med J Austral 1960;2:337
384. Freiesleben E, Jensen KG. Vox Sang 1961;6:328
385. MacPherson CR, Zartman ER. Am J Clin Pathol 1965;43:544
386. Yoshida Y, Yoshida H, Tatsumi K, et al. New Eng J Med 1981;305:460
387. Matsumoto H, Tamaki Y, Sato S, et al. Acta Obstet Gynaecol Jpn 1981;33:525
388. Giblett ER. Unpublished observations cited in Mollison PL.

Blood Transfusion in Clinical Medicine, 6th Ed. Oxford:Blackwell, 1979

389. Telischi M, Behzad O, Issitt PD, et al. Vox Sang 1976;31:109

390. Levine P, Ferraro LR, Koch E. Blood 1952;7:1030

391. Brizard CP, Selve A, Petit JC. Rev Fr Transf Immunohematol 1969;12:249

392. Feldman R, Luhby AL, Gromisch DS. J Pediat 1973;82:88

393. Griffith TK. Am J Obstet Gynecol 1980;137:174

394. Mayne KM, Bowell PJ, Green SJ, et al. Clin Lab Haematol 1990;12:105

395. Levine P, Kuhmichel AB, Wigod M, et al. Proc Soc Exp Biol NY 1951;78:218

396. Giblett E, Chase J, Crealock FW. Am J Clin Pathol 1958;29:254

397. Lusher JM, Zuelzer WW, Parsons PJ. Transfusion 1966;6:590

398. Drachmann O, Brogaard Hansen K. Scand J Haematol 1969;6:93

399. Issitt PD. Applied Blood Group Serology, 3rd Ed. Miami:Montgomery 1985

400. Coombs RRA, Mourant AE, Race RR. Lancet 1946;1:264

401. Race RR. Br Med Bull 1946;4:188

402. Wenk RE, Goldstein P, Felix JK. Obstet Gynecol 1985;66:473

403. Leggatt HM, Gibson JM, Barron SL, et al. Br J Obstet Gynaecol 1991;98:162

404. Bowman JM, Pollock JM, Manning FA, et al. Obstet Gynecol 1992;79:239

405. Greenwalt TJ, Sasaki T, Sneath J. Vox Sang 1956;1:157

406. Matson GA, Swanson J, Tobin JD. Vox Sang 1959;4:144

407. Geczy A, Matheson WA. Am J Obstet Gynecol 1965;82:576

408. Dorner I, Moore JA, Chaplin H. Transfusion 1974;14:212

409. Kornstad L, Halvorsen K. Vox Sang 1958;3:94

410. Geczy A, Leslie M. Transfusion 1961;1:125

411. Zodin V, Anderson RE. Pediatrics 1965;36:420

412. Geczy A. Vox Sang 1960;5:551

413. Carreras Vescio LA, Farinas D, Rogido M, et al. (Letter). Transfusion 1987;27:366

414. Polesky HF, Swanson J, Smith R. Vox Sang 1968;14:465

415. Moulds J, Futrell E, Fortez P, et al. (abstract). Transfusion 1978;18:375

416. Roxby DJ, Paris JM, Stern DA, et al. Vox Sang 1994;66:49

417. Bowell PJ, Inskip MJ, Jones MN. Clin Lab Haematol 1988;10:251

418. Clarke CA, Mollison PL. J Roy Coll Phys 1989;23:181

419. Montcharmont P, Juron-Dupraz F, Rigal M, et al. Haematologia 1990;23:97

420. Issitt PD. The MN Blood Group System. Cincinnati:Montgomery, 1981

421. Lawler SD, Loghem JJ van. Lancet 1947;2:545

422. Loghem JJ van, Klomp-Magnee W, Bakx CJA. Vox Sang (Old Series) 1953;3:130

423. Sacks MO, Schultz C, Dagovitz L, et al. Pediatrics 1958;21:443

424. Bowman JM, Pollock J. Vox Sang 1993;64:226

425. Stratton F, Renton PH. Br Med J 1954;1:962

426. Finney RD, Blue AM, Willoughby MLN. Vox Sang 1973;25:39

427. Greenwalt TJ, Sanger R. Br J Haematol 1955;1:52

428. Grobel RK, Cardy JD. Transfusion 1971;11:77

429. Chown B, Lewis M, Kaita H. Transfusion 1962;2:150

430. George S, Gidden M, LeNoir D. (abstract). Prog 23rd Ann Mtg South Cen Assoc Blood Banks, 1981

431. Spruell P. Personal communication, 1991

432. Alter AA, Gelb AG, Chown B, et al. Transfusion 1967;7:88

433. Lewis M, Chown B, Kaita H, et al. Transfusion 1967;7:440

434. Hossaini AA, Mirehandani I. (abstract). Book of Abstracts.

15th Cong ISBT 1978:192

435. Unger PJ, Feld J, Reddy RR, et al. (abstract). Transfusion 1978;18:379

436. Orlina AR, Unger PJ, Lacey PA. Rev Fr Transf Immunohematol 1984;27:613

437. Issitt PD, Gutgsell NS, Martin PA, et al. Transfusion 1991;31:63

438. Contreras M, Stebbing B, Blessing M, et al. Vox Sang 1978;34:208

439. Davidsohn I, Stern K, Strauser ER, et al. Blood 1953;8:747

440. Stern K, Davidsohn I, Jensen FG, et al. Vox Sang 1958;3:425

441. McCreary J, MacIlroy M, Courtenay DG, et al. Transfusion 1973;13:428

442. Ducos J, Marty Y, Ruffie J, et al. Unpublished observations cited in Race RR, Sanger R. Blood Groups in Man, 6th Ed. Oxford:Blackwell, 1975

443. Clark J, Yorek H, Schuler S, et al. (abstract). Book of Abstracts, Joint Cong ISBT/AABB, 1990:81

444. Levene C, Sela R, Grunberg L, et al. Clin Lab Haematol 1983;5:303

445. Moulds JJ, Case J, Thornton S, et al. (abstract). Transfusion 1980;20:631

446. Delehanty CL, Wilkinson SL, Issitt PD, et al. (abstract). Transfusion 1983;23:410

447. Lomas C, Poole J, Salaru N, et al. Vox Sang 1990;59:39

448. Marais I, Moores P, Smart E, et al. Transf Med 1993;3:35

449. Levine P, Stock AH, Kuhmichel AB, et al. Proc Soc Exp Biol NY 1951;77:402

450. Hart M van der, Bosman H, Logham JJ van. Vox Sang (Old Series) 1954;4:108

451. Alcalay D, Tanzer J. Rev Fr Transf Immunohaematol 1977;20:623

452. Taylor AM, Knighton GJ. Transfusion 1982;22:165

453. Rearden A, Frandson S, Carry JB. Vox Sang 1987;52:318

454. Cleghorn TE. MD Thesis, Univ Sheffield, 1961

455. Bergren MO, Morel PA. (abstract). Book of Abstracts. 15th Cong ISBT 1978:438

456. Field TE, Wilson TE, Dawes BJ, et al. Vox Sang 1972;22:432

457. Hart M van der. Unpublished observations 1971 cited in Race RR, Sanger R. Blood Groups in Man, 6th Ed. Oxford:Blackwell, 1975 :112

458. Sausais L, Mann J. Unpublished observations 1971 cited in Race RR, Sanger R. Blood Groups in Man, 6th Ed. Oxford:Blackwell, 1975:112

459. Worlledge SM, Giles CM, CleghornTE. Unpublished observations 1963 cited in Race RR, Sanger R. Blood Groups in Man, 6th Ed. Oxford:Blackwell, 1975:112

460. Cregut R, Lewin D, Lacomme M, et al. Rev Fr Transf 1968;11:139

461. Cregut R, Liberge G, Yvart Y, et al. Vox Sang 1974;26:194

462. Shapiro M, LeRoux ME. (abstract). Transfusion 1981;21:614

463. Battista N, Stout TD, Lewis M, et al. (abstract). Book of Abstracts. 14th Cong ISBT 1975:46

464. Battista N, Stout TD, Lewis M, et al. Vox Sang 1980;39:331

465. Contreras M, Green C, Humphreys J, et al. Vox Sang 1984;46:377

466. Daniels GL, Green CA, Poole J, et al. Transf Med 1993;3:129

467. Walsh TJ, Giles CM, Poole J. Clin Lab Haematol 1981;3:137

468. Francis BJ, Hatcher DE. Transfusion 1961;1:248

469. Inderbitzen PE, Windle B. (Letter). Transfusion 1982;22:542

470. Molthan L, Crawford MN, Marsh WL, et al. Vox Sang 1973;24:468

471. Jensen KG. Vox Sang 1962;7:476

472. Smoleniec J, Anderson N, Poole G. Arch Dis Childh 1994;71 (Suppl):F216

473. Donovan LM, Tripp KL, Zuckerman JE, et al. Transfusion 1973;13:153
474. Levene C, Rudolphson Y, Shechter Y. Transfusion 1980;20:714
475. Sakuma K, Suzuki H, Ohto H, et al. Vox Sang 1994;66:293
476. Marsh WL, Redman CM, Kessler LA, et al. Transfusion 1987;27:36
477. Eicher C, Kirkley K, Porter M, et al. (abstract). Transfusion 1985;25:448
478. Layrisse M, Arends T, Dominguez ER. Acta Med Venez 1955;3:132
479. Levine P, Robinson EA, Layrisse M, et al. Nature 1956;177:40
480. Levine P, Robinson EA. Blood 1957;12:448
481. Tatarsky J, Stroup M, Levine P, et al. Vox Sang 1959;4:152
482. Peenen HJ, Scudder J, Jack J, et al. Blood 1961;17:457
483. Graininger W. Vox Sang 1976;31:131
484. Alves de Lima LM, Berthier M, Sad WE, et al. Transfusion 1982;22:246
485. Riches RA, Laycock CM, Poole J. (abstract). Book of Abstracts. 20th Cong ISBT 1988:299
486. Zupanska B, Brojer E, McIntosh J, et al. Vox Sang 1990;58:276
487. Kusnierz-Alejska G, Bochenek S. Vox Sang 1992;62:124
488. Holman CA. Lancet 1953;2:119
489. Wiener AS, Brancato GJ. Am J Hum Genet 1953;5:350
490. Daw E. J Obstet Gynaecol 1971;78:377
491. Jørgensen J, Jacobsen J. Vox Sang 1974;27:478
492. Hoffman JJML, Overbeeke MAM, Kaita H, et al. Vox Sang 1990;59:240
493. Coghlan G, McCreary J, Underwood V, et al. Transfusion 1994;34:492
494. Lewis M, Kaita H, McAlpine PJ, et al. Vox Sang 1978;35:251
495. Harris PA, Vega MS de la, Clinton B, et al. Transfusion 1983;23:394
496. Ford DS, Stern DA, Hawksworth DN, et al. Vox Sang 1992;62:169
497. Better PJ, Ford DS, Frascarelli A, et al. Vox Sang 1993;65:70
498. Sistonen P. (abstract). Book of Abstracts. 19th Cong ISBT 1986:652
499. De Marco M, Uhl L, Fields L, et al. Transfusion 1995;35:58
500. Rausen AR, Rosenfield RE, Alter AA, et al. Transfusion 1967;7:336
501. Hamilton JR, Beattie KM, Walker RH, et al. Transfusion 1988;28:268
502. Wadlington WB, Moore WH, Hartmann RC. Am J Dis Childh 1961;101:623
503. Simmons RT, Were SO. Med J Austral 1955;2:55
504. Frumin AM, Porter MM, Eichman MF. Blood 1960;15:681
505. Ballowitz L, Fielder H, Hoffman C, et al. Vox Sang 1968;14:304
506. Rouse D, Weiner C, Williamson R. Obstet Gynecol 1990;76:988
507. Cleghorn TE. Unpublished observations 1962 cited in Race RR, Sanger R. Blood Groups in Man, 6th Ed. Oxford:Blackwell, 1975:433
508. Kluge A, Roelcke D, Tanton E, et al. Vox Sang 1988;55:44
509. Reid M, Fisher ML, Green C, et al. Vox Sang 1989;57:77
510. Feagans B. Unpublished observations cited in Sabo BH. In: A Seminar on Perinatal Blood Banking. Washington, D.C.:Am Assoc Blood Banks, 1978:31
511. Ichikawa Y, Sato C, McCreary J, et al. Vox Sang 1989;56:98
512. Stern R, Tregellas WM. Unpublished observations cited in Sabo BH. In: A Seminar on Perinatal Blood Banking. Washington, D.C.:Am Assoc Blood Banks, 1978:31
513. Riches RA, Laycock CM. Vox Sang 1980;38:305
514. Brown M, Mathur G, Moulds J, et al. (abstract). Transfusion 1980;20:630
515. Rosenfield RE. Unpublished observations cited in Sabo BH. In: A Seminar on Perinatal Blood Banking. Washington, D.C.:Am Assoc Blood Banks, 1978:31
516. Brown A, Plantos M, Moore BPL, et al. Vox Sang 1986;51:133
517. Guevin RM, Taliano V, Fiset D, et al. Rev Fr Transf 1971;14:455
518. Rowe GP, Bowell P. Vox Sang 1985;49:400
519. Beattie KM. Unpublished observations cited in Sabo BH. In: A Seminar on Perinatal Blood Banking. Washington, D.C.:Am Assoc Blood Banks, 1978:31
520. Hamilton JR, Coghlan G. Unpublished observations 1993 cited in Daniels G. Human Blood Groups. Oxford:Blackwell, 1995:637
521. Mumford B. Unpublished observations cited in Sabo BH. In: A Seminar on Perinatal Blood Banking, Washington, D.C.:Am Assoc Blood Banks, 1978:31
522. Svanda M, Prochazka R, Kout M, et al. Vox Sang 1970;18:366
523. Race RR, Sanger R, Selwyn JG. Br J Exp Pathol 1951;32:124
524. Buchanan DI. Am J Clin Pathol 1956;26:21
525. Gunson HH, Donohue WL. Vox Sang 1957;2:320
526. Tate H, Cunningham C, McDade MG, et al. Vox Sang 1960;5:398
527. Yokoyama M, Solomon JM, Kuniyuki M, et al. Transfusion 1961;1:273
528. De Torregrosa MV, Rullan MM, Cecile C, et al. Am J Obstet Gynecol 1961;82:1375
529. Salmon C, Gerbal A, Liberge G, et al. Rev Fr Transf 1969;12:239
530. Badakere SS, Bhatia HM. Vox Sang 1973;24:280
531. Reali G, Avanzi G, Ghinatti C, et al. Transf Sangue 1975;20:81
532. Sagisaka K, Tanaka H, Ohno T, et al. Acta Sch Med Univ Gifu 1978;26:403
533. Yuying D. (abstract). Book of Abstracts. 29th Cong ISBT 1988:295
534. Perez-Perez C, Taliano V, Mouro I, et al. Am J Hematol 1992;40:306
535. Cotorruelo C, Biondi C, Garcia Rosasco M, et al. (Letter). Transfusion 1996;36:191
536. Haber GV, Bastani A, Arpin PD, et al. (abstract). Transfusion 1967;7:389
537. Bar-Shany S, Bastani A, Cuttner J, et al. (abstract). Transfusion 1967;7:389
538. Gibbs BJ, Moores P. Vox Sang 1983;45:83
539. Gabra GS, Bruce M, Watt A, et al. Vox Sang 1987;53:143
540. Lubenko A, Contreras M, Portugal CL, et al. Vox Sang 1992;63:43
541. de Veber LL, Clark GW, Hunking M, et al. Transfusion 1971;11:33
542. Greenwalt TJ, Sasaki T, Sanger R, et al. Proc Nat Acad Sci USA 1954;40:1126
543. Alfonso JR, de Alvarez RR. Am J Obstet Gynecol 1961;81:45
544. Read SM, Taylor MM, Reid ME, et al. Immunohematology 1993;9:47
545. Leak M, Poole J, Kaye T, et al. (abstract). Book of Abstracts. Joint Cong ISBT/AABB, 1990:57
546. Kissmeyer-Nielsen F. Vox Sang 1960;5:532
547. Scheffer H, Tamaki HT. Transfusion 1966;6:497
548. Dube VE, Zoes CS. Transfusion 1982;22:251
549. Boulton FE. (Letter). Vox Sang 1990;59:61

550. Novotny VMJ, Kanhaii HHH, Overbeeke MAM, et al. Vox Sang 1992;62:49
551. Levine P, Backer M, Wigod M, et al. Science 1949;109:464
552. Kluge A, Jungfer H. Blut 1970;21:357
553. Rigal D, Juron-Dupraz F, Biggio B, et al. Rev Fr Transf Immunohematol 1982;25:101
554. Bowman JM, Harman CR, Manning FA, et al. Vox Sang 1990;58:139
555. Schultz MH. In: Blood Group Systems: Kell. Arlington, VA:Am Assoc Blood Banks, 1990:37
556. Anderson L, White JB, Liles BA, et al. Am J Med Technol 1959;25:184
557. Wright J, Cornwall SM, Matsina E. Vox Sang 1965;10:218
558. Dacus JV, Spinnato JA. Am J Obstet Gynecol 1984;150:888
559. Gorlin JB, Kelly L. Vox Sang 1994;66:46
560. Sabo B, McCreary J, Gellerman M, et al. Vox Sang 1975;29:450
561. Chown B, Lewis M, Kaita H. Nature 1957;180:711
562. Corcoran PA, Allen FH Jr, Lewis M, et al. Transfusion 1961;1:181
563. Manny N, Levene C, Harel N, et al. Vox Sang 1985;49:135
564. Levene C, Sela R, DaCosta Y, et al. (abstract). Book of Abstracts. 20th Cong ISBT 1988:295
565. Pierce SR, Hardman JT, Steele S, et al. Transfusion 1980;20:189
566. Kuczmarski CA, Bergren MO, Perkins HA. Vox Sang 1982;43:340
567. Woodfield DG, Douglas R, Smith J, et al. Transfusion 1982;22:276
568. Smart EA, Moores PP, Reddy R, et al. (abstract). Transf Med 1993;3 (Suppl 1):84
569. Albrey JA, Vincent EER, Hutchinson J, et al. Vox Sang 1971;20:29
570. Buchanan DI, Sinclair M, Sanger R, et al. Vox Sang 1976;30:114
571. Anderson NA, Tandy A, Westgate J, et al. (abstract). Transf Med 1990;1 (Suppl 1):58
572. Hayashida Y, Watanabe Y. Jpn J Legal Med 1968;22:10
573. Levene C, Sela R, Rudolphson Y, et al. Transfusion 1977;17:569
574. Simpson WK. S Afr Med J 1973;47:1302
575. McIntyre C, Finigan L, Larsen AL. Transfusion 1976;16:76
576. Beattie KM, Adams G, Sigmund KE, et al. (abstract). Transfusion 1978;18:379
577. Lacey PA, Robinson J, Collins ML, et al. Transfusion 1987;27:268
578. Savona-Ventura C, Grech ES, Zieba A. Obstet Gynecol 1989;73:870
579. Feller CW, Shenker L, Scott EP, et al. Transfusion 1970;10:279
580. Nakajima H, Hayakawa Z, Ito H. Vox Sang 1971;20:271
581. Gottlieb AM. Vox Sang 1971;21:79
582. Ishimori T, Fukumoto Y, Abe K, et al. Vox Sang 1976;31:61
583. Uchikawa M, Shibata Y, Tohyama H, et al. Vox Sang 1982;42:91
584. Habash J, Devenish A, Macdonald S, et al. Vox Sang 1991;61:77
585. Langley JW, Issitt PD, Anstee DJ, et al. Transfusion 1981;21:15
586. Rosenfield RE, Haber GV, Kissmeyer-Nielsen F, et al. Br J Haematol 1960;6:344
587. Peddle LJ, Josephson JE, Lawton A. Vox Sang 1970;18:547
588. Reid M, Rector D, Danneskiold T. Immunohematology 1984;1:7
589. Sacks DA, Johnson CS, Platt LD. Am J Perinatol 1985;2:208
590. Lavallee R, Lacobe M, Charron M, et al. Rev Fr Transf 1970;13:71
591. Gobel U, Drescher KH, Pottgen W, et al. Vox Sang 1974;27:171
592. Swanson J, Zweber M, Polesky HF. Transfusion 1967;7:304
593. Lacey P, Moulds M, Sobonya J. (abstract). Transfusion 1978;18:379
594. Jensen L, Scott EP, Marsh WL, et al. Transfusion 1972;12:322
595. Stroup M, McCreary J. (abstract). Transfusion 1975;15:522
596. Laird-Fryer B, Dukes C, Walker EM Jr, et al. (abstract). Transfusion 1980;20:631
597. Daniels GL, Tohyama H, Uchikawa M. Transfusion 1982;22:362
598. Lylloff K, Georgsen J, Grunnet N, et al. (Letter). Transfusion 1987;27:118
599. Rowe GP. (Letter). Transfusion 1988;28:87
600. Williams CK, Williams B, Pearson J, et al. (abstract). Transfusion 1985;25:462
601. Smith DS, Stratton F, Johnson T, et al. Br Med J 1969;3:90
602. Page PL. Transfusion 1983;23:256
603. Shertz WT, Carty L, Wolford F. (Letter). Transfusion 1987;27:117
604. Applewhaite F, Ginsberg V, Cunningham CA, et al. Vox Sang 1967;13:444
605. Culvery PL, Brubaker DB, Sheldon RE, et al. Transfusion 1987;27:468
606. Trichler JE. Transfusion 1977;17:177
607. Vedo M, Reid ME. Transfusion 1978;18:569
608. Nakajima H, Ito K. Vox Sang 1978;35:265
609. Orrick LR, Golde SH. Am J Obstet Gynecol 1980;137:135
610. Toy P, Reid M, Lewis T, et al. Vox Sang 1981;41:40
611. Bacon J, Sherrin D, Wright RG. (Letter). Transfusion 1986;26:543
612. Ferguson SJ, Boyce F, Blajchman M. Transfusion 1979;19:581
613. Technical Bulletin Number 148. Washington,D.C.:Am Coll Obstet Gynecol, 1990
614. Judd WJ, Luban NLC, Ness PM, et al. Transfusion 1990;30:175
615. Technical Bulletin Number 79. Washington,D.C.:Am Coll Obstet Gynecol, 1984
616. Technical Bulletin Number 90. Washington,D.C.:Am Coll Obstet Gynecol, 1986
617. Polesky H. Minn Med 1967;50:601
618. Smith BD, Haber JM, Queenan JT. Obstet Gynecol 1967;29:118
619. Solola A, Sibai B, Mason JM. Obstet Gynecol 1983;61:25
620. Walker RH. In: Hemolytic Disease of the Newborn. Arlington, VA:Am Assoc Blood Banks, 1984:173
621. Judd WJ, Steiner EA, Nugent CE. (Letter). Vox Sang 1992;63:293
622. Oberman HA, Judd WJ. In: Progress in Transfusion Medicine, Vol 3. Edinburgh:Churchill Livingstone, 1988:145
623. Contreras M, de Silva M. J Roy Soc Med 1994;87:256
624. Garner SF, Devenish A, Barber H, et al. Vox Sang 1992;63:295
625. Garner SF, Devenish A, Barber H, et al. Vox Sang 1991;61:219
626. Study Group of European Public Health Committee. Strasbourg:Council of Europe, 1986
627. Contreras M, Garner SF, de Silva M. Curr Opin Haematol 1996;3:480
628. Issitt PD, Combs MR, Bredehoeft SJ, et al. Transfusion 1993;33:284
629. Dijk BA van. Doctoral Thesis, Univ Leiden, 1991

630. Dijk BA van. (Letter). Transfusion 1993;33:960
631. Issitt PD. (Letter). Transfusion 1993;33:960
632. Pereira A, Mazzara R, Gelabert A, et al. Haematologica 1991;76:475
633. Pereira A, Mazzara R. (Letter). Transfusion 1993;33:884
634. Jemmolo G, Malferrari F, Tazzari PL, et al. (Letter). Vox Sang 1995;69:144
635. Urbaniak S. Br Blood Transf Soc Newsletter No 42, 1996:18
636. Dybkjaer E, Kissmeyer-Nielsen F. Vet Rec 1967;80:429
637. Mellbye OJ. Scand J Haematol 1969;6:166
638. Bell CA, Zwicker H, Nevius DB. Transfusion 1973;13:207
639. Randazzo P, Streeter B, Nusbacher J. (abstract). Transfusion 1973;13:345
640. De Silva M. Br Blood Transf Newsletter, No 42, 1996:18
641. Duguid J. Br Blood Transf Soc Newsletter, No 42, 1996:18
642. Webster R. Br Blood Transf Soc Newsletter No 42, 1996:18
643. Morley G, Gibson M, Eltringham D. Vox Sang 1977;32:90
644. Dijk VA van, Dooren MC, Overbeeke MAM. Transf Med 1995;5:199
645. Clark DA. Lancet 1996;347:485
646. Freda VJ. In: Hemolytic Disease of the Newborn. Arlington, VA:Am Assoc Blood Banks, 1984:33
647. Nicolaides KH, Rodeck CH. Br Med J 1992;304:1155
648. Bowell PJ, Wainscot JS, Peto TEA, et al. Br Med J 1982;285:327
649. Bowell PJ. Plasm Therap Transf Technol 1984;5:73
650. Liley AW. Am J Obstet Gynecol 1961;82:1359
651. Holman CA. Unpublished observations cited in Mollison PL. Blood Transfusion in Clinical Medicine, 7th Ed. Oxford:Blackwell, 1983:683
652. Nance S, Nelson J, Horenstein J, et al. Am J Clin Pathol 1989;92:89
653. Zupanska B, Brojer E, Richards Y, et al. Vox Sang 1989;56:247
654. Engelfriet CP, Brouwers HAA, Huiskes E, et al. (abstract). Book of Abstracts. 21st Cong ISH and 19th Cong ISBT 1986:162
655. Engelfriet CP, Ouwehand WH. Balliere's Clin Haematol 1990;3:321
656. Urbaniak S, Greiss MA, Crawford RJ, et al. Vox Sang 1984;46:323
657. Hadley AG, Kumpel BM, Merry AH. Clin Lab Haematol 1988;10:377
658. Mollison PL, reporting in behalf of nine collaborating laboratories. Vox Sang 1991;60:225
659. Hadley AG, Kumpel BM, Leader KA, et al. Br J Haematol 1991;77:221
660. Garner SF, Wiener E, Contreras M, et al. Br J Haematol 1992;80:97
661. Zupanska B. In: Immunobiology of Transfusion Medicine. New York:Marcel Dekker, 1994:465
662. Bromilow IM, Duguid JKM. Br J Haematol 1991;78:588
663. Brown SJ, Perkins JT, Sosler SD, et al. (abstract). Transfusion 1991;31 (Suppl 8S):53S
664. Bevis DCA. Lancet 1950;2:443
665. Mollison PL, Cutbush M. In: Recent Advances in Pediatrics. London:Churchill, 1954
666. Bevis DCA. J Obstet Gynaecol Br Emp 1956;63:68
667. Walker AHC. Br Med J 1957;2:376
668. Mackay EG. Austral NZ J Obstet Gynaecol 1961;1:78
669. Mayer M, Gueritat P, Ducos P, et al. Presse Med 1961;69:2493
670. Walker W, Fairweather DVI, Jones P. Br Med J 1964;2:140
671. Knox EG, Fairweather DVI, Walker W. Clin Sci 1965;28:147
672. Zipursky A, Pollock J, Chown B, et al. Lancet 1963;2:493

673. Fairweather DVI, Murray S, Parkin D, et al. Lancet 1963;2:1190
674. Gordon J, Murgita RA. Cell Immunol 1974;15:392
675. Nicolaides KH, Rodeck CH, Mibashan RS, et al. Am J Obstet Gynecol 1986;155:90
676. Judd WJ, Jenkins WJ. J Clin Pathol 1970;23:801
677. Austin EB, McIntosh Y, Hodson C, et al. Transf Med 1995;5:203
678. Hirvonen M, Tervonen S, Pirkola A, et al. Vox Sang 1995;69:341
679. Contreras M. Vox Sang 1994;67 (Suppl 3):207
680. Hadley AG. Transf Med Rev 1995;4:302
681. Filbey D, Garner SF, Hadley AG, et al. Acta Obstet Gynecol Scand 1996;75:102
682. Noble AL, Poole GD, Anderson N, et al. Br J Haematol 1995;90:718
683. Lucas GF, Hadley AG, Nance SJ, et al. Transfusion 1993;33:484
684. Garner SF, Gorick BD, Lai WYY, et al. Vox Sang 1995;68:169
685. Garner SF, Devenish A. Immunohematology 1996;12:20
686. Thomas NC, Shirey RS, Blakemore K, et al. Vox Sang 1995;69:120
687. Lynen R, Neuhaus R, Schwarz DWM, et al. Vox Sang 1995;69:126
688. Bowman JM. Curr Prob Obstet Gynecol 1983;7:4
689. Nicolaides KH, Rodeck CH. Br J Hosp Med 1985;34:141
690. Nicolaides KH, Rodeck CH, Millar DS, et al. Br Med J 1985;290:661
691. Nicolaides KH, Warenski JC, Rodeck CH. Am J Obstet Gynecol 1985;152:341
692. Frigoletto FD, Greene MF, Benaceraff BR, et al. New Eng J Med 1986;315:430
693. Chitkara U, Wilkins I, Lynch L, et al. Obstet Gynecol 1988;71;393
694. Daffos F, Capella-Pavlovsky M, Forestier F. Am J Obstet Gynecol 1985;153:655
695. Millar DS, Davis LR, Rodeck CH, et al. Prenat Diag 1985;5:367
696. Forestier F, Daffos F, Galacteaos F, et al. Pediat Res 1986;20:342
697. Pollock JM, Bowman JM, Manning FA, et al. Vox Sang 1987;53:139
698. Nicolaides KH, Soothill PW, Clewell WH, et al. Lancet 1988;1:1073
699. King JC, Sacher RA. In: Contemporary Issues in Pediatric Transfusion Medicine. Arlington, VA:Am Assoc Blood Banks, 1989:33
700. Armitage P, Mollison PL. J Obstet Gynaecol Br Emp 1953;60:605
701. Allen FH Jr. Quart Rev Pediat 1957;12:1
702. Liley AW. Br Med J 1963;2:1107
703. Chown B, Bowman WD. Pediat Clin North Am 1958;May:279
704. Carey HM, Liley AW. N Z Med J 1959;58:460
705. Cohen S, Freeman T. Biochem J 1960;76:475
706. Solomon A, Waldmann JA, Fahey FL. J Lab Clin Med 1963;62:1
707. Isbister PJ, Ting A, Seeto KM. Vox Sang 1977;33:353
708. Bystryn JC, Graf MW, Uhr JW. J Exp Med 1970;132:1279
709. Hammerschmidt DE, Craddock PR, McCullough J, et al. Blood 1978;51:721
710. Hammerschmidt DE, Weaver LJ, Hudson LH, et al. Lancet 1980;1:947
711. Marley PB, Gibco CM. Transfusion 1981;21:320

712. Huestis DW. Lancet 1983;1:1043
713. Rubenstein MD, Wall RT, Wood GS, et al. Am J Med 1983;75:171
714. Shumak KH, Rock GA. New Eng J Med 1984;310:762
715. Huestis DW. Arch Pathol Lab Med 1989;113:273
716. Robinson A. Transf Sci 1990;11:305
717. Bowman JM, Peddle L, Anderson C. Vox Sang 1968;15:272
718. Powell LC Jr. Am J Obstet Gynecol 1968;101:153
719. Clarke CA, Bradley J, Elson CJ, et al. Lancet 1970;1:794
720. Clarke CA, Elson CJ, Bradley J, et al. Lancet 1970;2:793
721. Graham-Pole JR, Donald I, Barr W, et al. Lancet 1974;1:1459
722. Fraser ID, Bennett MO, Bothamley JE. Br J Haematol 1974;28:147
723. Fraser ID, Bennett MO, Bothamley JE, et al. Lancet 1976;1:6
724. Bowman JM. Lancet 1976;1:421
725. Graham-Pole J, Barr W, Willoughby MLN. Br Med J 1977;1:1185
726. Tilz GP, Weiss PAM, Teubl I, et al. Lancet 1977;2:203
727. Woyton J, Partyka T, Gajewska E, et al. Arch Immunol Ther Exp Warsaw 1978;26:1139
728. James V, Weston J, Scott IV, et al. Vox Sang 1979;37:290
729. Robinson AE, Tovey LAD. Br J Haematol 1980;45:621
730. Veer-Korthof ET van't, Niterink JSG, Nieuwkoop JA, et al. Vox Sang 1981;41:207
731. Rock G, Lafreniere I, Chan L, et al. Transfusion 1981;21:546
732. Hauth JC, Brekken AL, Pollack W. Obstet Gynecol 1981;57:132
733. Rubinstein P. In: Rh Hemolytic Disease: New Strategy for Eradication. Boston:Hall, 1982
734. Robinson AE. Plasma Therap 1984;5:7
735. Rock GA. Plasma Therap 1982;2:211
736. Berlin G, Selbing A, Ryden G. (Letter). Lancet 1985;1:1153
737. Margulies M, Voto LS, Mathet E, et al. Vox Sang 1991;61:181
738. Rewald E. Lancet 1985;2:208
739. Smith CIE, Hammarströhm L.Obstet Gynecol 1985;66:39S
740. Carreras LO, Perez GN, Ruda-Vega H, et al. Lancet 1988;2:393
741. Barbui T, Finnazi G, Falanga A, et al. Lancet 1988;2:969
742. De la Camara C, Arrieta R, Gonzales A, et al. New Eng J Med 1988;318:519
743. Scott JR, Branch DW, Kochenour NK, et al. Am J Obstet Gynecol 1988;159:1055
744. Carter BB. Am J Clin Pathol 1947;17:646
745. Bierme SJ, Blanc M, Abbal M, et al. Lancet 1979;1:604
746. Bierme SJ, Blanc M, Fournie A, et al. In: Rh Hemolytic Disease: New Strategy for Eradication. Boston:Hall, 1982:249
747. Gold WR Jr, Queenan JT, Woody J, et al. Am J Obstet Gynecol 1983;146:980
748. Klarkowski DB. (abstract). Proc Austral Inst Med Lab Sci Mtg, 1983
749. Barnes RMR, Duguid JKM, Roberts FM, et al. Clin Exp Immunol 1987;67:220
750. Bierme-Alie-Enjalbert S. PhD Thesis, Toulouse 1967
751. Gudson JP Jr, Moore VL, Myrik QN, et al. J Immunol 1978;108:1340
752. Gudson JP Jr. J Reprod Med 1981;26:454
753. Stenchever MA. Am J Obstet Gynecol 1978;130:665
754. Bowman JM. Transf Med Rev 1988;2:129
755. Walker W. Vox Sang 1958;3:225
756. Walker W. Vox Sang 1958;3:336
757. Warrell DW, Taylor R. Lancet 1968;1:117
758. Bowman JM, Pollock JM. Pediatrics 1965;35:815
759. Palmer A, Gordon RR. Br J Obstet Gynaecol 1976;83:688
760. Robertson EG, Brown A, Ellis MI, et al. Br J Obstet Gynaecol 1976;83:694

761. Bowman JM, Friesen RF, Bowman WD, et al. J Am Med Assoc 1969;207:1101
762. Walker W, Ellis MI. Br Med J 1970;2:223
763. Menticoglou SM, Harman CR, Manning FA, et al. Fetal Therap 1987;2:154
764. Rodeck CH, Holman CA, Karnicki J, et al. Lancet 1981;1:625
765. Rodeck CH, Nicolaides KH, Warshof SL, et al. Am J Obstet Gynecol 1984;150:769
766. De Crespigny LC, Robinson HP, Quinn M, et al. Obstet Gynecol 1985;66:529
767. Grannum PA, Copel JA, Plaxe SC, et al. New Eng J Med 1986;314:1431
768. Seeds JW, Bowes WA. Am J Obstet Gynecol 1986;154:1105
769. Berkowitz RL, Chitkara U, Goldberg JD, et al. Am J Obstet Gynecol 1986;155:574
770. Nicolaides KH, Soothill PW, Clewell W, et al. Fetal Therap 1986;1:185
771. Grannum PAT, Copel JA. Sem Perinatol 1988;12:324
772. Berkowitz RL, Chitkara U, Wilkins I, et al. Am J Obstet Gynecol 1988;158:783
773. Grannum PAT, Copel JA, Moya FR, et al. Am J Obstet Gynecol 1988;158:914
774. Nicolini U, Rodeck CH. J Obstet Gynecol 1988;9:162
775. Harman CR, Bowman JR, Manning FA, et al. Am J Obstet Gynecol 1990;162:1053
776. Tannirandorn Y, Rodeck CH. Balliere's Clin Haematol 1990;3:289
777. Rodeck CH, Letsky E. Br J Obstet Gynaecol 1989;96:759
778. Nicolini U, Kochenour NK, Greco P, et al. Br Med J 1988;297:1379
779. Simpson MB, Pryzbylik JA, Denham JA, et al. Obstet Gynecol 1978;52:616
780. Harrison KL, Popper EI. Transfusion 1981;21:90
781. Contreras M, Gordon H, Tidmarsh E. (Letter). Br J Haematol 1983;53:355
782. Barrie JV, Quinn MA. (Letter). Lancet 1985;1:1327
783. Pratt GA, Bowell PJ, MacKenzie IZ, et al. Clin Lab Haematol 1989;11:241
784. Issitt PD. Transfusion 1965;5:355
785. Archer GT, Cooke BR, Mitchell K, et al. Rev Fr Transf 1969;12:341
786. Cook IA. Br J Haematol 1971;20:369
787. Issitt PD, McKeever BG, Moore VK, et al. Transfusion 1973;13:316
788. Parkman R, Mosier D, Umansky I, et al.. New Eng J Med 1974;290:359
789. Stratton F, Gunson HH, Rawlinson V. Transfusion 1965;5:216
790. Stratton F, Smith DA, RawlinsonVI. Clin Exp Immunol 1968;3:582
791. Poorkhorsandi ME, Gupte SC. Ind J Med Res 1996;104:208
792. Walker W, Neligan GA. Br Med J 1955;1:681
793. Mollison PL. Blood Transfusion in Clinical Medicine, 2nd Ed. Oxford:Blackwell, 1956
794. Robinson GC, Phillips RM, Prystowsky M. Pediatrics 1951;7:164
795. Crawford H, Cutbush M, Mollison PL. Blood 1953;8:620
796. Witebsky E, Rubin MI, Engasser LM, et al. J Lab Clin Med 1947;32:1339
797. Zuelzer WW, Kaplan E. Am J Dis Childh 1954;88:319
798. Shumway CN Jr, Miller GE, Young LE. Pediatrics 1955;15:54
799. Wallerstein H. Science 1946;103:583
800. Winstanley DP, Konugres A, Coombs RRA. Br J Haematol 1957;3:341
801. Gunson HH. Am J Clin Pathol 1957;27:35
802. Stern K. Am J Obstet Gynecol 1958;75:369

803. Lockyer JW. J Med Lab Technol 1959;16:42
804. Pirofsky B, Mangum MEJ. Proc Soc Exp Biol NY 1959;101:49
805. Lewi S, Clarke TK. Lancet 1960;2:456
806. Haberman S, Krafft CJ, Luecke PE, et al. J Pediat 1960;56:471
807. Pirofsky B. Br J Haematol 1960;6:395
808. Polley MJ, Adinolfi M, Mollison PL. Vox Sang 1963;8:385
809. Carapella de Luca E, Pacioni C, Tonelli C. Vox Sang 1976;30:200
810. Semberg R, Mazzi F, MacDonald MG, et al. Arch Dis Child 1977;52:219
811. Chan-Shu SA, Blair O. Am J Clin Pathol 1979;71:677
812. Kiruba R, Ong R, Han P. Pathology 1988;20:147
813. Yunis E, Bridges R. Am J Clin Pathol 1964;41:1
814. Graham HA. Unpublished observations 1982 cited in Mollison PL. Blood Transfusion in Clinical Medicine, 7th Ed. Oxford:Blackwell, 1983
815. Greenbury CL, Moore DH, Nunn LAC. Immunology 1963;6:421
816. Economidou J, Hughes-Jones NC, Gardner B Vox Sang 1967;12:321
817. Cartron JP, Gerbal A, Hughes-Jones NC, et al. Immunology 1974;27:723
818. Romano EL, Zabner-Oziel P, Soyano A, et al. Vox Sang 1983;45:378
819. Merry AH, Thomson EE, Anstee DJ, et al. Immunology 1984;51:793
820. Anstee DJ. Vox Sang 1990;58:1
821. Anstee DJ. J Immunogenet 1990;17:219
822. Romano EL, Hughes-Jones NC, Mollison PL., Br Med J 1973;1:524
823. Hsu TCS, Rosenfield RE, Rubinstein P. Vox Sang 1974;26:326
824. Voak D, Bowley CC. Vox Sang 1969;17:321
825. Voak D, Williams MA. Br J Haematol 1971;20:9
826. van Oss CJ, Beckers D, Engelfriet CP, et al. Vox Sang 1981;40:367
827. Absolom DR, van Oss CJ. Crit Rev Immunol 1986;6:1
828. van Oss CJ. In: Immunobiology of Transfusion Medicine. New York:Marcel Dekker, 1994:327
829. Romans DG, Tilley CA, Dorrington KJ. J Immunol 1980;124:2807
830. Economidou J. PhD Thesis, Univ London, 1966
831. Brouwers HAA, Overbeeke MAM, Huiskes E, et al. Br J Haematol 1988;68:363
832. Iyer YS, Kulkarni SV, Gupte SC. Acta Haematol 1992;88:78
833. Brouwers HAA, Overbeeke MAM, Gemke RJBJ, et al. Br J Haematol 1987;66:267
834. Loghem E van. In: Handbook of Experimental Immunology, 3rd Ed. Oxford:Blackwell, 1978
835. Ukita M, Takahashi A, Nunotani T, et al. Vox Sang 1989;56:181
836. Meulen FW van der, Hart M van der, Fleer A, et al. Br J Haematol 1978;38:541
837. Fleer A, Meulen FW van der, Linthout E, et al. Br J Haematol 1978;39:425
838. Engelfriet CP, Borne AEGKr von dem, Beckers D, et al. In: A Seminar on Immune-Mediated Cell Destruction. Washington, D.C.:Am Assoc Blood Banks, 1981:93
839. Brouwers HA, Overbeeke MA, Ouwehand WH, et al. Br J Haematol 1988;70:465
840. Carreras L, Castro R. Vox Sang 1990;58:231
841. Hakomori S. Semin Hematol 1981;18:39
842. Ewald RA, Williams JH, Bowden DH. Vox Sang 1961;6:312
843. Adinolfi M, Zenthon J. Rev Perinat Med 1984;5:61
844. Edwards MS, Buffone GJ, Fuselier PA, et al. Pediat Res 1983;17:685
845. Pujol M, Ribera A, Abella E, et al. Vox Sang 1991;61:76
846. Garratty G. (Letter). Vox Sang 1992;63:240
847. Tovey GH. J Path Bact 1945;57:295
848. Wiener AS, Wexler LB, Hurst JG. Blood 1949;4:1014
849. Hostrup H. Vox Sang 1963;8:567
850. Brouwers HAA, Overbeeke MAM, Ertbruggen I van, et al. Lancet 1988;2:641
851. Issitt PD, Issitt CH. Applied Blood Group Serology, 2nd Ed. Oxnard:Spectra Biologicals, 1975
852. White WD, Issitt CH, McGuire DA. Transfusion 1974;14:67
853. Edwards JM, Moulds JJ, Judd WJ. Transfusion 1982;22:59
854. Branch DR, Petz LD. Am J Clin Pathol 1982;78:161
855. Hanfland P. Vox Sang 1982;43:310
856. Schellong G. Proc 10th Cong ISBT. Basel:Karger, 1965:878
857. Ducos J, Ohayon E, Marty Y. Rev Fr Transf 1969;13 (Suppl):37
858. Gerlini G, Ottaviano S, Sbraccia C, et al. Hematologica 1968;53 (Suppl):1019
859. Boineau FG, Hallock JA. Clin Pediat 1971;10:180
860. Arriaga F, Palau J, Lopez F, et al. (Letter). Transfusion 1991;31:381
861. Lubenko A, Contreras M. (Letter). Transfusion 1992;32:88
862. Allen FH Jr, Diamond LK, Vaughan VC. Am J Dis Childh 1950;80:779
863. Mollison PL, Walker W. Lancet 1952;1:429
864. Mollison PL. Arch Dis Childh 1943;18:161
865. Mollison PL. Blood Transfusion in Clinical Medicine, 5th Ed. Oxford:Blackwell, 1972
866. With TK. Acta Med Scand 1949;Suppl:234
867. Ducos J. Lancet 1963;2:1170
868. Hamrick L. Transfusion 1964;4:382
869. Lowes BCR. J Med Lab Technol 1970;27:475
870. Decary F, Maniatis A, Scott PE, et al. (abstract). Book of Abstracts. 13th Cong ISBT 1972:66
871. Klein HG, Ed. Standards for Blood Banks and Transfusion Services, 17th Ed. Bethesda:Am Assoc Blood Banks, 1996
872. Shapiro M. Proc 10th Cong ISBT. Basel:Karger, 1965:883
873. Hey EN, Kohlinksy S, O'Connell B. Lancet 1969;1:335
874. Odell GB. J Pediat 1959;55:268
875. Waters WJ, Porter E. Pediatrics 1964;33:749
876. Diamond L. Pediatrics 1966;38:539
877. Chan G, Schoff D. J Pediat 1976;88:609
878. Mollison PL, Cutbush M. Blood 1951;6:777
879. Zuelzer WW, Cohen F. Pediat Clin N Am 1957;4:405
880. Allen FH Jr, Diamond LK. Erythroblastosis Fetalis. Boston:Little Brown, 1958
881. Gartner LM, Snyder RN, Chabron RS, et al. Pediatrics 1970;45:906
882. Ackerman BD, Dyer GF, Leydorf MM. Pediatrics 1970;45:968
883. Maisels JF. In: Neonatology: Pathophysiology and Management of the Newborn. Philadelphia:Lippincott, 1994:630
884. Allen FH Jr. Transfusion 1966;6:101
885. Schmidt PJ. (Letter). Transfusion 1981;21:231
886. Huestis DW. (Letter). Transfusion 1981;21:231
887. Garratty G. In: Pediatrics and Blood Transfusion. The Hague:Nijhoff, 1980:4
888. Giblett ER. (Letter). Transfusion 1981;21:231
889. Allen FH Jr. (Letter). Transfusion 1981;21:231
890. Rosenfield RE. (Letter). Transfusion 1981;21:232
891. Rubo J, Wahn V. Monatsschr Kinderheilkd 1990;138:216

892. Besalduch J, Forteza A, Duran MA, et al. (Letter). Transfusion 1991;31:380

893. Kubo S, Agira T, Tsuneta H, et al. Eur J Pediat 1991;150:507

894. Rubo J, Wahn V. (Letter). Lancet 1991;337:914

895. Cremer RJ, Perryman P, Richards DH. Lancet 1958;1:1094

896. Costa Ferreira H, Cardim WH, Mellone O. J de Pediat 1960;25:347

897. Tabb PA, Inglis J, Savage DCL, et al. Lancet 1972;2:1211

898. Osborn LM, Lenarsky C, Oakes RC, et al. Pediatrics 1984;74:371

899. Aidin R, Corner B, Tovey G. Lancet 1950;1:1153

900. Zuelzer WW, Mudgett RT. Pediatrics 1960;6:452

901. Killander A, Müller-Eberhard U, Sjolin S. Acta Pediat 1965;52:481

902. Trolle D. Lancet 1968;2:705

903. Lin-Chu M, Broadberry RE, Chang FC, et al. (abstract). Book of Abstracts. 2nd Reg Cong, West Pacif Reg ISBT 1991:32

904. Lin CK, Mak KH, Chan CMY, et al. Immunohematology 1997;13:17

905. Dooren MC, Kuijpers RWAM, Joekes EC, et al. Lancet 1992;339:1067

906. Dooren MC, Kamp IL van, Kanhai HHH, et al. Vox Sang 1993;65:55

907. Dooren MC, Engelfriet CP. Vox Sang 1993;65:59

908. Heddle NM, Wentworth P, Anderson DR, et al. Transf Med 1995;5:113

909. Vengelen-Tyler V. Ed, Technical Manual, 12th Ed. Bethesda:Am Assoc Blood Banks, 1996:472

910. Yoshida H, Ito K, Emi N, et al. Vox Sang 1984;47:216

911. Shirey RS, Ness PM, Kickler T, et al. Transfusion 1987;27:189

912. Shechter Y, Timor-Tritsche IE, Lewit N, et al. Vox Sang 1987;53:135

913. Cedergren B. Unpublished observations cited in Rydberg L, Cedergren B, Breimer ME, et al. Mol Immunol 1992;29:1273

914. Yoshida Y, Yoshida H, Tatsumi K, et al. Vox Sang 1982;43:35

915. Yoshida Y, Yoshida H, Tatsumi K, et al. (Letter). Vox Sang 1983;44:327

916. Robinson AE. (Letter). Vox Sang 1983;44:326

917. Wilmut I, Schnieke AE, McWhir A, et al. Nature 1997;385:810

918. Huxley A. Brave New World. London:McMillan, 1932

919. Lewis M, Chown B, Kaita H. Am J Hum Genet 1963;15:203

920. Bergvalds H, Stock A, McClure PD. Vox Sang 1965;10:627

921. Dobbs JV, Prutting DL, Adebahr ME, et al. Vox Sang 1968;15:216

922. Hathaway WE, Fulginti VA, Pierce CW, et al. J Am Med Assoc 1967;201:139

923. Burns LJ, Westberg MW, Burns CP, et al. Acta Haematol 1984;71:270

924. Kessenger A, Armitage JO, Klassen LW, et al. J Surg Oncol 1987;36:206

925. Arsura EL, Bertelle A, Minkowitz S, et al. Arch Int Med 1988;148:1941

926. Thaler M, Shamriss A, Orgad S, et al. New Eng J Med 1989;321:25

927. Jui T, Takahashi K, Shibata Y, et al. New Eng J Med 1989;321:56

928. Holland PV. Arch Pathol Lab Med 1989;113:285

929. Avoy DR. Transfusion 1990;30:849

930. Anderson KC, Weinstein HJ. New Eng J Med 1990;323:315

931. Ferrara JLM, Burakoff HJ. In: Graft-vs.-Host Disease. New York:Marcel Dekker, 1990:3

932. Capon SM, DePond WD, Tyan DB, et al. Ann Int Med 1991;114:1025

933. Anderson KC. Transf Sci 1991;12:277

934. Suzuki K, Akiyama H, Takamoto S, et al. Transfusion 1992;32:358

935. Moroff G, Luban NLC. Transfusion 1992;32:102

936. Linden JV, Pisciotto PT. Transf Med Rev 1992;6:116

937. Lo Y-MD, Bowell PJ, Selinger M, et al. (Letter). Lancet 1993;341:1148

938. Sazama K, Holland PV. In: Immunobiology of Transfusion Medicine. New York:Marcel Dekker, 1994:631

939. Kernan NA. In: Bone Marrow Transplantation. Boston:Blackwell, 1994:124

940. Shivdasani RA, Anderson KC. In: Clinical Practice of Transfusion Medicine, 3rd Ed. New York:Churchill Livingstone, 1996:931

941. Colin Y, Cherif-Zahar B, Le Van Kim C, et al. Blood 1991;78:2747

942. Bennett PH, Le Van Kim C, Colin Y, et al. New Eng J Med 1993;329:607

943. Wolter LC, Hyland CA, Saul A. (Letter). Blood 1993;82:1682

944. Warwick R, Bennett P. (Letter). Blood 1994;83:1156

945. Simsek S, Bleeker PMM, Borne von dem AEGKr. (Letter). New Eng J Med 1994;330:795

946. Bennett P, Warwick R, Cartron J-P. (Letter). New Eng J Med 1994;330:795

947. Fisk NM, Bennett P, Warwick RM, et al. Am J Obstet Gynecol 1994;171:50

948. Rossiter JP, Blakemore KJ, Kickler TS, et al. Am J Obstet Gynecol 1994;171:1047

949. Carritt B, Steers FJ, Avent D. (Letter). Lancet 1994;344:205

950. Arce MA, Thompson ES, Wagner S, et al. Blood 1993;82:651

951. Lo Y-MD, Noakes L, Bowell PJ, et al. Br J Haematol 1994;87:658

952. Hyland CA, Wolter LC, Saul A. Blood 1994;84:321

953. Blunt T, Daniels GL, Carritt B. Vox Sang 1994;67:397

954. Spence WC, Maddalena A, Demers BB, et al. Obstet Gynecol 1995;85:296

955. Bennett PR, Overton TG, Lighten AD, et al. Lancet 1995;345:661

956. Simsek S, Faas BHW, Bleeker PMM, et al. Blood 1995;85:2975

957. Yankowitz J, Li S, Murray JC. Obstet Gynecol 1995;86:214

958. Pope J, Navarette C, Warwick R, et al. (Letter). Lancet 1995;346:375

959. Lighten AD, Overton TG, Sepulveda W, et al. Am J Obstet Gynecol 1995;173:1182

960. Avent ND, Martin PG, Carritt B. (abstract). Transf Med 1995;5 (Suppl 1):20

961. Legler TJ, Maas JH, Lynen R, et al. (abstract) Vox Sang 1996;70 (Suppl 2):73

962. Muller TH, Gran S, Lammers I, et al. (abstract). Vox Sang 1996;70 (Suppl 2):99

963. Stoerker J, Hurwitz C, Rose NC, et al. Clin Chem 1996;44:356

964. Hyland CA, Wolter LC, Lieu YW, et al. Blood 1994:83:566

965. Avent ND, Martin PG, Armstrong-Fisher SS, et al. Blood 1997;89:2568

966. Aubin JT, Kim CL, Mouro I, et al. Br J Haematol 1997;98:356

967. Van den Veyver IB, Chong SS, Cota J, et al. Am J Obstet Gynecol 1995;172:533

968. Daniels G, Green C, Smart E. (Letter). Lancet 1997;350:862

969. Wolter LC, Hyland CA, Saul A. (Letter). Blood 1994;84:985

970. Le Van Kim C, Mouro I, Brossard Y, et al. Br J Haematol 1994;88:193

971. Faas BHW, Simsek S, Bleeker PMM, et al. Blood

1995;85:829

972. Fukumori Y, Ohnoki S, Shibata H, et al. (abstract). Vox Sang 1996;70 (Suppl 2):99

973. Lee S, Zambas ED, Marsh WL, et al. Proc Nat Acad Sci USA 1991;88:6353

974. Lee S, Wu X, Reid M, et al. Blood 1995;85:912

975. Lee S, Zambas E, Green ED, et al. Blood 1995;85:1364

976. Lee S, Bennett PR, Overton T, et al. Am J Obstet Gynecol 1996;175:455

977. Hessner MJ, McFarland JG, Endean DJ. Transfusion 1996;36:495

978. Thomas MR, Williamson R, Craft I, et al. Ann NY Acad Sci 1994;731:217

979. Lo Y-MD, Bowell JP, Selinger M, et al. Ann NY Acad Sci 1994;731:229

980. Liou JD, Hsieh T, Pao C. Ann NY Acad Sci 1994;731:237

981. Miele L, Peri A, Cordella-Miele E, et al. Ann NY Acad Sci 1994;731:246

982. Brambati B. Ann NY Acad Sci 1994;731:248

983. Adinolfi M, Sherlock J, Kemp T, et al. Lancet 1995;345:318

984. Olsson ML, Hansson C, Åkesson IE, et al. (abstract). Transfusion 1997;37 (Suppl 9S):102S

985. Rios M, Reid ME, Naime D, et al. (abstract). Transfusion 1997;37 (Suppl 9S):101S

986. Faas BHW, Christiaens GCML, Maaskant PA, et al. (abstract). Transfusion 1997;37 (Suppl 9S):100S

987. Legler TJ, Blaschke V, Bustami N, et al. (abstract).

Transfusion 1997;37 (Suppl 9S):100S

988. Gassner C, Muller TH, Wagner FF, et al. (abstract). Transfusion 1997;37 (Suppl 9S):101S

989. Kim DA, Kim TY, Choi TY. (abstract). Transfusion 1997;37 (Suppl 9S):33S

990. Spruell P, Lacey P, Bradford MF, et al. (abstract). Transfusion 1997;37 (Suppl 9S):43S

991. Kitao M, Aihara Y, Kamazawa I, et al. Nippon San Fuj Gak Zass 1972;24:14

992. Bunuel C, Aztaran E, Marzo L, et al. Sangre 1977;22:492

993. Kim HC, Joo KW, Hahn KS, et al. (abstract). Vox Sang 1996;70 (Suppl 2):74

994. Han KS, Kim HC, Han KS, et al. Am J Perinatol 1997;14:495

995. Berkowitz RL, Beyth Y, Sadovsky E. Obstet Gynecol 1982;60:746

996. Coppel JA, Scioscia A, Grannum PA, et al. Obstet Gynecol 1986;67:285

997. Kulich V. Cest Paediat 1967;22:823

998. Duguid JKM, Bromilow IM. Vox Sang 1990;58:69

999. Montcharmont P, Juron-Dupraz F, Doillon M, et al. Acta Haematol 1991;85:45

1000. Gorlin JB, Beaton M, Poortenga M, et al. (Letter). Transfusion 1996;36:938

1001. Lin CK, Mak KH, Yuen CMY, et al. Immunohematology 1996;12:115

1002. Constantine G, Fitzgibbon N, Weave JB. Br J Obstet Gynecol 1991;98:943

42 | Polyagglutination

Polyagglutination is a state in which red cells are agglutinated by all or most normal sera from adults. The phenomenon involves a change in red cells by which a cryptic, latent or hidden receptor is exposed or where red cells are released from the marrow with such a receptor accessible. The red cells are agglutinated because most normal human sera from adults contain a series of different specificity, IgM agglutinins directed against the receptors. The red cells are described as polyagglutinable and the sera are said to contain polyagglutinins. Sometimes in vivo or in vitro exposure of the receptors recognized by polyagglutinins is such that the red cells are agglutinated by all normal sera from adults. On other occasions it seems that fewer receptors become exposed so that only those sera with the highest level of polyagglutinins agglutinate the red cells.

Polyagglutination is not the same as panagglutination and care should be taken in differentiation between the two phenomena and use of the terms (1,2). As indicated, polyagglutination involves an abnormality of red cells in which those cells are agglutinated by normal sera. Panagglutination involves an abnormal serum factor, that can be but is not necessarily an antibody, that causes the serum to agglutinate all normal red cells.

Obviously, polyagglutinable red cells have the potential to cause incorrect interpretations to be made in blood grouping studies. When ABO and D typings were performed with reagents made using human polyclonal antibodies as the source material, positive reactions sometimes represented the actions of polyagglutinins in those reagents and not the antibody for which the reagent was being used. Such reactions sometimes came to light when a discrepancy was seen between red cell (forward) and serum (reverse) ABO typing. The problems were somewhat compounded because methods that could be used to determine the correct ABO and D type of polyagglutinable red cells varied slightly, dependent on what type of polyagglutination (see below) was involved. The acute problems caused by polyagglutinable red cells, namely difficulty in determination of the correct ABO and D type have largely disappeared now that monoclonal antibodies are widely used for ABO and D typing. This, of course, because the MAbs do not contain the polyagglutinins present in normal human sera. The reaction of Tn-activated red cells with some examples of anti-A and the reaction of certain monoclonal anti-B with red cells with an acquired B antigen, some of which are polyagglutinable, are discussed below. While polyagglutination was most often detected in the past via an

ABO typing discrepancy, it is now usually necessary to mount a deliberate search to find cases (3).

In view of the change in incidence with which polyagglutination is now detected at the routine level and the resultant lessening of the problems at the practical level, this chapter will deal predominantly with the mechanisms that lead to the various forms of polyagglutination. However, for those workers not yet able to use MAbs for routine ABO and D typing, some other aspects of polyagglutination will first be considered.

Recognition of the Polyagglutinable State

As mentioned, polyagglutination is most often first suspected when a discrepancy in ABO typing in tests using human-source polyclonal reagents, is seen. However, the phenomenon may first be noticed via any unexpected positive reaction, for example when donor red cells react with the sera of more than one patient in immediate spin compatibility tests.

Once polyagglutination is suspected there are several lines of investigation that can be used. Since most normal sera from adults contain the antibodies that cause polyagglutination, the red cells involved can be tested with several AB sera that are known not to contain unusual blood group antibodies. Saline tests at room temperature, for periods between five minutes and one hour, will usually be positive if the red cells are polyagglutinable. In cases of marked red cell alterations the test will usually be strongly positive after being left for just five minutes. Tests with sera from cord bloods will also be useful. Lind and MacArthur (4) first showed that most cord sera contain none (or only very low levels) of most of the antibodies that cause polyagglutination. Accordingly, red cells that react with sera from adults but not with those from cord blood samples should be suspected of being polyagglutinable. It should be remembered that cord sera contain ABO agglutinins (even if the infant has not formed its own ABO antibodies, IgG anti-A, anti-B and anti-A,B cross the placenta from the maternal circulation and are often found in cord sera) so that ABO compatible cord sera must be used. This may not be as simple as it sounds since, as has been mentioned, at the time that polyagglutination is first detected it may be difficult to determine the true ABO group of the polyagglutinable cells. It has been reported (39) that some cord blood sera can be shown to contain IgG anti-T (see below), presumably of maternal origin, if RIA tests against purified T

1097

substance are used. The anti-T detected did not agglutinate T-activated red cells in a saline system and caused only weak agglutination in a system potentiated with PEG and gelatin.

Another useful clue in the recognition of polyagglutination is the fact that the auto-control is most often negative. As discussed in more detail below, the sera of persons with polyagglutinable red cells often (but not quite always) lack serologically demonstrable levels of the particular agglutinin that reacts with the type of polyagglutinable red cells involved. When unexplained agglutination is due to a panagglutinin in the serum, the auto-control will usually be positive. If the panagglutinin causes agglutination of the patient's own cells before ABO typings and other tests are performed, the situation may be more difficult than usual to differentiate from polyagglutination. Here, a useful clue will be that the patient's serum will almost always agglutinate normal red cells from other persons, sera from patients with polyagglutinable red cells usually will not.

There is another test that is sometimes of use in the recognition of polyagglutinable red cells. Normal red cells are known (5) to carry a negative charge at and near the red cell surface. It has been shown (6,7) that when such cells are mixed with positively charged substances, such as polybrene, the negative charge is overcome and the red cells aggregate. Many polyagglutinable cells carry less of a negative charge because of a reduction of sialic acid at the membrane (see later in this chapter) and fail to aggregate in polybrene (8) or protamine (9). However, it should be added that there are several disadvantages to this test. First, red cells that are only slightly modified may aggregate in polybrene although they are polyagglutinable to some degree. Second, some polyagglutinable conditions involve mixed-cell populations with only a proportion of the red cells polyagglutinable. If the polyagglutinable red cell population that fails to aggregate in polybrene comprises only a small proportion of the cells and the non-polyagglutinable cells aggregate, the test may be misinterpreted. Third, it is now known that red cells of several different phenotypes are also deficient in sialic acid. For example, red cells from persons homozygous or heterozygous for *En*, M^k or Mi^V may fail to aggregate normally in polybrene (for details and references see Chapter 15) although none of them are polyagglutinable. A method of using the polybrene aggregation test for the detection of polyagglutination (10-12) and variant MN blood group system phenotypes (13) is given by Judd (14).

While there are many ways of detecting polyagglutination, the use of three or four fresh serum samples from group AB donors provides a rapid and reliable method for the initial recognition of the polyagglutinable state. Several sera must be used because the levels of

polyagglutinins in normal sera vary (15).

Most workers do not perform routine tests for polyagglutination and investigate such cases only when the phenomenon is recognized during other tests. However, a few workers routinely test all blood samples with either normal antibody-free AB serum or one of the lectins (see below) that reveal the most common types of polyagglutination. The polyagglutinable states are rare and it is hard for us to accept that such measures are cost effective. The state of having polyagglutinable red cells is a little more common in infants and children with severe bacterial infections, than in other patients. We have heard that in transfusion services in some childrens' hospitals, this state of affairs has led to reintroduction of the minor compatibility test. Even if necessary (the majority of workers believe that it is not) a single test for polyagglutination would be better than six such tests in a child for whom six units of blood were ordered. As a compromise to routine testing for polyagglutination, Bird (145) has suggested that since the condition is more frequent in newborns than in others (see sections later in this chapter on neonatal necrotizing enterocolitis and hemolytic uremic syndrome) tests with selected lectins (again see later in this chapter) be performed on the red cells of any newborn who types as group AB. Clearly the use of the AB phenotype as a possible first indicator of polyagglutination does not apply when monoclonal antibodies are used for ABO typing.

If the polyagglutinable red cells are from a blood donor (a rather rare occurrence) they are likely to be recognized as such even if the situation is not detected during ABO and D typing. The donor cells will, of course, react with sera from all or most patients when compatibility tests are performed. The fact that the immediate spin compatibility test will detect polyagglutination in a blood donor while an electronic compatibility test will not, can hardly be regarded as a disadvantage of the latter procedure. The event, i.e. a donor with unrecognized polyagglutinable red cells, will be extraordinarily rare.

In concluding this section, it can be said that the overwhelming majority of workers are prepared to rely on routine tests for detection of the polyagglutinable state. If those tests raise the suspicion that the red cells involved may be polyagglutinable (i.e. a positive or mixed-field positive reaction for which no cause is immediately apparent) the tests described in the next sections are used.

ABO (and other) Typing Tests on Polyagglutinable Red Cells

Two points mentioned earlier must now be reconsidered. First, the use of monoclonal based typing reagents usually obviates any difficulties encountered in typing polyagglutinable red cells. Indeed, use of such reagents is listed below as the method of choice in typing such red cells. Second, because the various types of polyagglutination have different characteristics, no one method solves problems in typing studies caused by all forms of polyagglutination. In spite of these observations, this section lists some modifications that are useful in this respect. The modifications are described briefly and are included for the benefit of workers who do not always have access to monoclonal reagents. Test modifications include:

1. Typing studies with monoclonal-based reagents that lack polyagglutinins. It was reported (73) that of three monoclonal anti-Le^a, one reacted strongly (i.e. more strongly than it reacted with non-polyagglutinable Le(a+) red cells) while two reacted very weakly, with polyagglutinable (T-activated, see below) Le(a-b+) red cells. While false positive reactions thus seemed possible, it is not likely that polyagglutinable red cells will often be typed for Le^a.
2. Typing studies with 2-ME or DTT-treated sera (for methods see 14). The polyagglutinins in normal human sera are invariably IgM and are no longer active as agglutinins in sera treated with either of these reducing agents. The method works, of course, only if the antibody in the typing reagent is IgG and is thus not inactivated. Most anti-A and anti-B contain sufficient levels of IgG agglutinins (see Chapter 8) that the modification can be used.
3. Typing studies with adsorbed sera. If suitable phenotype polyagglutinable red cells are available (group O red cells can be T-activated very easily, see below) the polyagglutinins can be removed by adsorption. Not very practical for those rarer forms of polyagglutination where the cells to be typed may be the only ones available. Easy to use to remove anti-T but seldom necessary for ABO typing as some of the other methods are easier.
4. Tests with cord sera shown to contain the required antibodies. As mentioned above, maternal IgG anti-A, anti-B, etc., cross the placenta and are present in selected samples of cord sera. Those sera usually lack IgM polyagglutinins since such antibodies do not cross the placenta and are not usually made by newborns.
5. Tests with old, stored sera. It is believed that on prolonged storage, IgM agglutinins deteriorate in sera. While such sera may still contain enough reactive anti-T to agglutinate strongly T-activated red cells, they may fail to agglutinate red cells with other forms of polyagglutination. As discussed below, controls must be used with all methods, they

are particularly critical if this modification is used.
6. Tests at 37°C. Some polyagglutinins may fail to react at 37°C, IgG anti-A and anti-B usually agglutinate red cells at that temperature. Again controls are critical if this modification is used.
7. Typing tests on protease-treated red cells. Efficient if the receptor recognized by the polyagglutinin is denatured or removed when red cells are treated with a protease. Quite variable as some receptors are readily denatured while others survive (see sections on the various forms of polyagglutination that follow). Obviously of no use if the antigen for which the red cells are to be typed is denatured or removed by proteases (e.g. M, N, Fy^a, Fy^b).

Whichever of the above modification(s) is (are) used, it is important that it/they be controlled as completely as possible although this is not always easy (and sometimes not even possible). The controls should be of two types. One should use non-polyagglutinable red cells that carry the antigen that the typing serum is intended to detect. This control is easy and should give a positive result to show that the antibody is active in the serum or treated serum. The second control should use red cells with the same form of polyagglutination as the test cells, that lack the antigen that the typing serum is intended to detect. This control should give a negative reaction to show that any positive reaction with the unknown cells represents the action of the antibody for which the serum is being used, and not a polyagglutinin in that serum. This control is the more difficult of the two to obtain. As described in the following sections, some forms of polyagglutinable red cells can be made in vitro. For example, it is very easy to T-activate red cells so that T-activated polyagglutinable antigen-negative control cells can be made. Some other forms of polyagglutination cannot be replicated in vitro so that polyagglutinable antigen-negative control cells may be available only from previously studied cases. As described in more detail in later sections of this chapter, some forms of polyagglutination involve structures in which N-acetyl-D-galactosamine is immunodominant. Accordingly, positive reactions of a sample only with sera that contain anti-A should arouse suspicion and prompt further investigation.

Different Types of Polyagglutination

Red cells may become polyagglutinable by any one of a variety of different mechanisms. Some of these are well understood and result in a serological pattern that is easily recognizable. In other instances different types of polyagglutinable red cells share some serological characteristics. However, if the appropriate reagents are available and if the appropriate tests are done, each type of polyagglutination can be differentiated from the others. The rest of this chapter describes different types of polyagglutination.

T-Activation

The first type of polyagglutination to be recognized was described in the literature as early as 1925 (16). Further observations were soon published (17,18) and the condition became known as the Huebner-Thomsen-Friedenreich phenomenon after the early workers. It became apparent that red cells could be altered either in vivo or in vitro so that they became polyagglutinable by this mechanism. Over the years this type of polyagglutination has become known simply as T-activation. The mechanism by which red cells become T-activated in vivo is that bacteria or viruses infecting the individual produce neuraminidase. That enzyme specifically cleaves terminal N-acetyl-neuraminic acid (NeuAc) residues from red cell membrane-borne structures. In many instances the subterminal carbohydrate of those structures is galactose. When NeuAc is removed and galactose residues are exposed, they comprise the recep-

tors (19) with which the normal anti-T in all sera from adults combines. As described below, an identical situation can be created in vitro. It is not difficult to understand that different degrees of T-activation occur in vivo in different patients. When a large amount of neuraminidase is produced, much of the red cell membrane-associated NeuAc will be removed. The red cells will then be strongly T-activated and will be agglutinated by all sera from adults, even those that contain only weak anti-T. When less neuraminidase is made, fewer NeuAc residues will be removed so that fewer T receptors will be exposed. The red cells may then be agglutinated only by those sera that contain potent anti-T.

As would be expected from these findings, T-activated red cells have reduced levels of membrane-associated sialic acid and react with the lectins *Glycine max* (syn *Glycine soja*) and *Sophora japonica* (12,20-24) that, while they may not be specific for sialic acid depleted red cells (25), do agglutinate most such cells (see also final section of this chapter, on lectins). Similarly and for the same reason, the cells do not aggregate normally in polybrene or protamine (6-9) and have reduced electrophoretic mobility (20,26).

The statement that exposed galactose residues comprise the T receptor should not be taken to mean that T is

FIGURE 42-1 The Usual Tetrasaccharide (32) of Red Blood Cell Sialoglycoproteins and the Modified Structures When T (19) and Tn (206,207) are Exposed

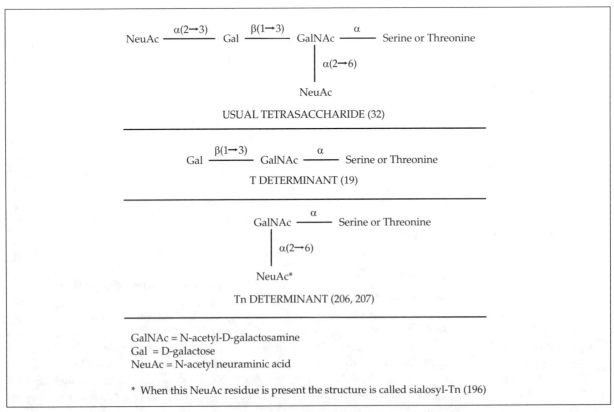

simply galactose. While that carbohydrate is immunodominant (19) it must be in the correct steric configuration (three dimensional shape) to be able to complex with anti-T (27). The steric configuration of the immunodominant galactose residue is probably determined by proximal carbohydrates and/or amino acids and/or linkage of the galactose to the next residue (see also the section on IgM^woo in Chapter 34, particularly table 34-5).

Because there are about one million copies of MN SGP on each red cell (28-30) and because each of those structures carries about fifteen copies (31) of a side chain in which a galactose residue is subterminal to NeuAc (32), it follows that much of the cryptic T antigen on red cells is carried on MN SGP. Figure 42-1 depicts a normal unaltered tetrasaccharide side chain, that structure with NeuAc removed so that T is exposed and that structure as it exists on Tn-activated red cells. Tn polyagglutination is described in a later section of this chapter but the Tn structure is shown in figure 42-1 for the sake of completeness. Although the MN SGP is a major site of cryptic T on red cells, it is by no means the only site. First, the Ss SGP carries tetrasaccharides, many of which are identical to those on MN SGP (33-35). Second, similar structures are probably present on minor SGPs of red cells. Clearly, when neuraminidase is present, it can cleave NeuAc and expose T (galactose) on those structures as well. In other words, En(a-) red cells that lack MN SGP and those that carry hybrid forms of the glycoprotein can be T-activated in vitro, using neuraminidase. Careful tests using human sera that contain anti-T (the lectin *Arachis hypogea*, see below, may be too potent to reveal the difference) have shown that, as expected, some of these cell samples carry less cryptic T antigen than do cells with normal amounts of MN and Ss SGP (36,37). Third, membrane structures other than MN, Ss and minor SGPs also carry oligosaccharide side chains in which galactose is subterminal to NeuAc. Anstee (38) has pointed out that cryptic T is carried on, at least, gangliosides in addition to SGPs.

Since in vivo red cell T-activation can occur in individuals infected with bacteria or viruses that produce neuraminidase, it is not surprising that many such cases have been described in the literature (40-73). T-activation is somewhat more common in infants and children than in adults. Seger et al. (69) reported its presence in nine of 26 newborns with necrotizing enterocolitis and later (74) in 16 pediatric surgical patients between the ages of three days and 14 years when those patients had severe anaerobic infections. Obeid et al. (61) described two children with bowel disorders; in one of them T-activation persisted for 12 and in the other for seven months. These cases were unusual, in most children and adults in whom in vivo T-activation occurs, the red cell change is transient and reversible. Normally, once the bacterial or viral infection is controlled, T-activation abates. In many but not quite all the cases cited above, the infection in the patient was apparent. The fact that this was not the case in a few of them suggests that neuraminidase-producing organisms can sometimes be present without causing obvious disease. The significance of T-activation in transfusion therapy and the highly questionable role of anti-T in causing in vivo red cell destruction in patients in whom red cell T-activation has occurred, are discussed below. Similarly, later sections describe concomitant T-activation and the presence of another form of polyagglutination in some of the cases cited above.

A Serum Factor That Inhibits In Vivo T-Activation

Francis (75) and Marsh (76) each reported the presence, in normal human sera, of inhibitors of T-activating bacterial filtrates that contain neuraminidase. These apparently normal inhibitors may prevent some cases of in vivo T-activation for in vitro studies (76) showed that powerful T-activating filtrates are necessary to overcome the effects of the inhibitors. The inhibitors play no role in preventing in vitro T-activation of red cells when washed cells are used. Because of the existence of these inhibitors, Gunson et al. (77) questioned the postulated mechanism of in vivo T-activation. However, there is a very close correlation between bacterial infections, in vivo T-activation and the ability of the microorganisms involved to produce neuraminidase. Kline and Issitt (78) have shown that when serum is treated with neuraminidase, the ability of that serum to inhibit anti-T is increased. These findings suggest first, that serum contains some structures than can complex with anti-T and second, that serum contains molecules that, like red cells, carry cryptic T antigens. In other words, the inhibitors of neuraminidase in normal sera may be structures that carry latent T antigens and in vivo, it may be necessary that neuraminidase first activates the serum structures before it is able to act on red cells to cause T-activation.

Anti-T in Normal Sera

Since very few humans are exposed to T-activated red cells and since virtually all sera from adults contain anti-T, the antibody is often said to be "naturally-occurring". Since one of us (PDI) has still not seen a satisfactory explanation as to how the immune system in man can produce an antibody without introduction of an immunogen, he was delighted to see the results of experiments performed by Springer and Tegtmeyer (79). These workers showed that many gram-negative bacteria and some vaccines contain a substance that is either identical or very similar to T. Infants and animals exposed to these substances made anti-T and thus showed the source of the immunogen against which the antibody is made. As mentioned above, most anti-T in human serum is IgM in nature and acts as an agglutinin in tests performed in saline at room temperature. As also mentioned, some sera also contain IgG anti-T that agglutinates red cells only in the presence of PEG and gelatin (39). Boccardi et al. (233) claimed that anti-T of higher titer than those seen in normal individuals, are seen in patients with cirrhosis of the liver and that (234) antibiotics that depress the normal intestinal flora cause reduced levels of anti-T to be made. We do not know if other workers have looked at anti-T levels in these circumstances.

T, Anti-T and Cancer

Springer and his associates (80-109) and many other groups of investigators (110-130) have studied the relationship between the T antigen and carcinoma. This topic is now so vast that it essentially needs a book of its own to do justice to the findings made. There are 51 papers cited above and many more cited below in the section on Tn. To summarize and greatly oversimplify the findings, it is apparent that the T and Tn antigens (for Tn see figure 42-1 and some sections below) are exposed on malignant cells in many different types of cancer, i.e. breast, prostate, bladder, colon, rectum, to name but a few. Detection of these antigens, often by immunofluorescence, is used in diagnosis and in establishing prognosis. Measurement of cellular (cytotoxic) and humoral responses to T and Tn can be used similarly and it is possible that manipulation and amplification of those responses may provide a means to control tumor growth. Clearly a full discussion of this topic is beyond the scope of this book, interested readers are referred to a number of excellent reviews (104,108,109).

T on Leukocytes and Platelets

As would be expected, since leukocytes and platelets have glycoproteins that extend from their membranes, those cells can be T-activated. In vitro treatment with neuraminidase resulted in T-activation of leukocytes and platelets (131), lymphocytes (132) and monocytes (133). Hysell et al. (134) showed that T-activation of leukocytes and platelets can also occur in vivo. Since leukocytes and platelets lack MN and Ss SGPs (135,136) the finding that they can be T-activated supplies another piece of evidence of the wide distribution of structures that have galactose subterminal to NeuAc on glycosylat-

ed membrane components. The net clinical effects that result from the in vivo T-activation of leukocytes and platelets are not entirely clear. Hysell et al. (134) found that the activation did not result in leukopenia or thrombocytopenia. However, the role of T-activation of platelets in some cases of hemolytic uremic syndrome (see later) is less well understood.

Specific Recognition of T-Activation

Although virtually all normal sera from adults contain anti-T, they also contain antibodies that cause the agglutination of other types of polyagglutinable red cells. Adsorption studies can be used specifically to recognize T-activation but this method is time consuming and dependent on the availability of other types of polyagglutinable cells. A better way of recognizing T-activation is by the use of lectins. Bird (137) showed that a lectin made from *Arachis hypogea* (peanuts to Americans, ground nuts to the English) contains potent anti-T. Although that lectin is now known to agglutinate other forms of polyagglutinable red cells (see table 42-3) most cases encountered, in which red cells are agglutinated by *Arachis hypogea* extract, represent T-activation. Further, as shown in table 42-3, various types of polyagglutination can be differentiated by use of a battery of lectins. A method for preparation of *Arachis hypogea* lectin is given by Judd (14).

As discussed in more detail below, a common finding in a patient who has T-activated red cells, is that the serum does not contain demonstrable anti-T. Since production of other agglutinins for polyagglutinable red cells is not usually impaired, lack of demonstrable anti-T in the presence of other polyagglutinins can be a useful clue as to the nature of the type of polyagglutination present. Possible reasons for the usual lack of anti-T in the sera of persons with T-activated red cells are discussed below, in the section on T-activation and intravascular red cell destruction.

Red Cell Typing in the Presence of T-Activation

Methods for ABO and D typing polyagglutinable red cells have been mentioned above. Those modifications that use MAb, 2-ME or DTT-treated reagents, adsorbed reagents or cord sera known to contain anti-A or anti-B, work well with T-activated red cells. In terms of enzyme-treatment of T-activated red cells, Gunson et al. (77) reported that protease-treated red cells no longer reacted with anti-T. However, the situation is not straightforward. It seems that in mild T-activation, removal of MN SGP (as occurs when red cells are treated with proteases) results in loss of sufficient copies of T that the red cells no longer react with anti-T. However, when red cells are strongly T-activated, it may be necessary (15) to treat them with 3 or 4% papain or ficin, to render them non-reactive with anti-T. Clearly, such harsh treatment makes the cells very susceptible to agglutination by other antibodies (such as anti-I in a typing reagent) so that incorrect ABO and D typing might still result. Judd (20) found that a cysteine-activated papain solution or one to which EDTA had been added, but not others, would depress but not abolish the reactivity of T-activated red cells with *Arachis hypogea*.

In addition to human sera, those of some animals contain anti-T. Thus such reagents should be tested (using T-activated red cells prepared in vivo) before being used to perform DATs or phenotyping tests via IAT, on T-activated red cells.

In Vitro T-Activation of Red Cells

There are a number of occasions in blood group serology when it is informative to test neuraminidase-treated red cells. Such tests have provided much information about certain MN system antigens (138-141 and see Chapter 15) and those of the Pr series (142,143 and see Chapter 34). However, if red cells are simply treated with neuraminidase and then tested, they will react with virtually all sera since they are T-activated. Fortunately there is a simple solution to this problem. Appropriate phenotype red cells can be T-activated in vitro and then used to adsorb anti-T from the serum that is to be tested, for other activity, against neuraminidase-treated red cells. Two organisms, *Vibrio cholera* and *Pneumococcus pneumoniae*, produce neuraminidase that efficiently T-activates red cells. While bacterial free filtrates of cultures of these organisms can be prepared and used, most workers now purchase purified neuraminidase solutions. Beck (144) has found that neuraminidase from *V. cholera* is the more efficient of the two for the in vitro preparation of strongly T-activated red cells. A method for T-activating red cells with bacterially produced neuraminidase is given by Judd (14). Once such cells have been prepared, they will totally adsorb anti-T from sera, often in a single adsorption (10,138-140).

Transfusion and T-Activation

It is highly unlikely that T-activated red cells would ever be transfused to a patient. First, since in vivo T-activation occurs in persons with infections it is unlikely that a person with T-activated red cells would present for blood donation or pass the medical screening in the event that

one did. Second, if donor red cells were T-activated (which could conceivably happen in an infected unit of blood after collection) they would be reactive with virtually all sera in immediate spin compatibility tests.

When the patient has T-activated red cells a different consideration applies, namely will the passive transfer of anti-T cause red cells destruction in the recipient? Based on two early reports in the literature (45,48) many workers have assumed that the passive transfer of anti-T must be avoided. Both reports described children with T-activated red cells and in both severe transfusion reactions were attributed to the introduction of anti-T in the donor plasma of the units transfused. Accordingly, several groups of workers (61,69,72,74,145,146) have used or have advocated the use of washed red cells for transfusion to patients with T-activated red cells. We (15) often wondered what we would do if a patient with T-activated red cells needed to be transfused with plasma. We ran titration studies on the plasma of normal blood donors using T-activated red cells. Although we did not find a sample that lacked anti-T, we found several in which the antibody was weak, i.e. titer of 2, 4 or 8. We assumed that if we had to transfuse plasma in the circumstance described, we would select those units with the lowest level of anti-T. An opportunity to test the theory in practice never arose. It now seems that use of washed red cells and the proposed use of plasma with low levels of anti-T may have been unnecessary. Heddle et al. (62) described three premature infants all of whom had necrotizing enterocolitis and T-activated red cells. All three were transfused with blood products containing anti-T, none of them had any signs of transfusion reactions or in vivo hemolysis. As discussed below, there is now considerable doubt that the intravascular hemolysis seen in some patients with hemolytic uremic syndrome and/or T-activated red cells, is caused by the anti-T in the patient's plasma. Alternative possible causes are discussed below.

In retrospect it seems that the suggestions of Heddle et al. (62) are more logical than the supposition that passively transferred anti-T will destroy a patient's T-activated red cells. The anti-T in question are invariably cold-reactive, IgM agglutinins. When antibodies with such characteristics, e.g., anti-P$_1$, anti-Le^b, are found in the sera of patients, they are ignored (or better yet not detected) for transfusion purposes. There seem no reasons to assume that anti-T are any more significant than such alloantibodies. However, it is clear that T-activation occurs somewhat more frequently in newborn infants who have neonatal necrotizing enterocolitis or hemolytic uremic syndrome than in others. Such infants are often very seriously ill and some workers may be unwilling to take even the smallest risk of further worsening the clinical condition by the passive transfer of anti-T, particularly since it is now so easy to wash red cells.

T-Activation and Intravascular Red Cell Destruction

In most patients in whom in vivo T-activation occurs, anti-T cannot be demonstrated in the plasma. Although that statement describes the most commonly encountered situation, the reason is by no means clear. There are at least three different theories that purport to explain the observation. First, it is thought that perhaps in the presence of overwhelming exposure of T, immune paralysis occurs and anti-T is no longer made. Such a theory does not fit well with observations on autoantibody production in immune hemolytic anemia (see Chapters 37 and 38). Second, it is possible that the patient's anti-T binds to his own T-activated red cells. However, there are essentially no serological observations to support such a supposition, we are not aware that anti-T is regularly detected on or eluted from such cells. Third, it is possible that the anti-T complexes with T-activated substances in the patient's plasma (78 and see above) and is thus neutralized. While this third possibility may seem the most likely, we do not know if anyone has looked for T-anti-T immune complexes in the sera of affected patients.

In some individuals, red cell T-activation and intravascular hemolysis of red cells have been seen concurrently (47,50,53,56,70,72,146). Bird (146) believed that the clinically significant hemolysis is due to the anti-T and cited the observation (147) that anti-T fixes complement, to support this supposition. However, there are a number of points that suggest that such a cause and effect relationship may not exist. First, the hemolysis seen has often been intravascular. Since IgG anti-T cannot be demonstrated in sera by conventional methods (it was found (39) to be present by a radioimmunoassay method, see above), it seems unlikely that there is enough of that antibody present to cause intravascular hemolysis. Second, the IgM anti-T present is often limited in thermal range and does not usually cause agglutination or readily demonstrable complement-activation in tests performed at 37°C. Third, in most cases neither imunoglobulin nor very much complement can be demonstrated on the patient's red cells in a DAT. Fourth, in those cases in which T-activation and hemolysis occurred, there was marked sepsis thus suggesting that perhaps the products of the infecting bacteria caused both T-activation and direct red cell hemolysis with no participation by anti-T. Judd et al. (70) described a case in which fatal intravascular hemolysis occurred in a patient in whom the red cells were T-activated. However, they could find no direct evidence that anti-T was responsible for the red cell destruction and concluded that although a Clostridial infection was not proved absolutely (the postmortem blood contained antitoxins to

Clostridium perfringens) it was more likely that bacterially produced lecithinases caused the hemolysis than it was that anti-T was responsible. Indeed, from a review of the cases cited above, the evidence seems to lean in the direction that toxins, enzymes or other products of the infecting organisms caused the hemolysis (and T-activation) without participation by anti-T.

T-Activation, Neonatal Necrotizing Enterocolitis (NNE), Hemolytic Uremic Syndrome (HUS) and Thrombotic Thrombocytopenic Purpura (TTP)

Neonatal necrotizing enterocolitis is a rare but often fatal disease in premature infants who have undergone stress, particularly hypoxia. While the exact etiology is not known, bacterial infection would appear to play some role since red cell T-activation has been seen (62,69) in affected newborns. Similarly it is now clear that bacterial infections are involved in the etiology of hemolytic uremic syndrome (HUS). The disease is most often seen in infants following episodes of bacterial gastroenteritis caused by *Escherichia coli*, 015:H7 that produces a veracytotoxin (VTEC) (148-150). Veracytotoxins are potent protein endotoxins that can cause irreversible cytopathic damage in certain cells, particularly those of the endothelium. The toxin appears to bind specifically to glycoproteins on endothelial vascular cells of renal tissue causing inactivation of ribosomes and cell death. HUS is also seen in adults where it shares many of the clinical features of thrombotic thrombocytopenic purpura (TTP, see below). In adults, HUS has been associated with infections with VTEC-producing organisms and with some involving *Shigella, Salmonella typhi, Campylobacter, Yersinia, Streptococcus pneumoniae, Legionella*, rickettsia, viruses and fungi. HUS is also strongly associated with the use of mitomycin C as a treatment for cancer. While the association of HUS and bacterial infections (60,67,151-154) has prompted some suggestions that bacterially produced neuraminidase causes red cell T-activation leading to hemolytic anemia, T-activation of platelets leading to their destruction and hence thrombocytopenia, and T-activation of kidney cells and hence renal damage, all attributable to anti-T, it seems much more likely that all three events are the direct result of VTEC activity (148-150,155). There is evidence (155) that in HUS, the anemia is microangiopathic and not immune in nature. Although anti-T may not cause the clinical complications of HUS, both Bird (146) and Beck (167) have pointed out that detection of red cell T-activation may be a useful early indicator of the condition.

The clinical condition known as thrombotic thrombocytopenic purpura (TTP) is remarkably similar to HUS and may represent one manifestation of a spectrum of related disorders. As in HUS, the triad of anemia, thrombocytopenia and renal dysfunction is seen. The anemia is microangiopathic in nature, the thrombocytopenia results from the consumption of platelets in thrombotic lesions (156,157) and temporary dialysis may be necessary while the patient is in renal failure. In spite of the acute thrombocytopenia, platelet transfusions may worsen the patient's clinical condition (presumably via increased endothelial cell damage) and probably should not be used unless there is life-threatening, thrombocytopenic-related bleeding (158-160). In both HUS and TTP, plasma exchange has been found (161-166) to be an effective form of therapy. Indeed in a patient with TTP and rapid onset of severe symptoms, an emergency plasma exchange may be the only life saving treatment available. While plasma exchange procedures seldom differ in efficacy based on the replacement fluid used, TTP provides a notable exception. Fresh frozen plasma or cryoprecipitate-poor plasma are clearly indicated (163,164), it is believed that a labile inhibitor of platelet aggregation is replaced in the patient, when either of these fluids is used. While the point is not proved it would seem reasonable to suppose, at least in HUS and in cases of TTP associated with infection, that one of the primary effects of plasma exchange in providing clinical benefit, is removal of VTEC that appears to be causative of the clinical complications.

Tn Polyagglutination

A form of polyagglutination, in which the red cells involved reacted with all or most human sera from adults, but not with the anti-T component of those sera, was first described by Moreau et al. (168). The unusual determinant on the polyagglutinable cells was named Tn and the antibody, found in most normal sera, was named anti-Tn. Later Dausset et al. (169) showed that the patient with Tn-activated red cells had hemolytic anemia. Since then it has been found that Tn polyagglutination involves a series of clinical abnormalities that are described below under the heading Tn syndrome. Many additional cases of Tn-activation have been described (77,170-199) as have some other cases of polyagglutination (200-205) that can be seen in retrospect to have been Tn although they were not described as such in the original publications.

One of the most common features of Tn-polyagglutination is that mixed-field agglutination is almost always seen. As explained below, this feature relates directly to the clonal nature of the phenomenon. In different cases as few as 30% or as many as 90% (or very

rarely 100%) of the red cells have been seen to be polyagglutinable. Not surprisingly in view of the association of Tn-polyagglutination with disease, the percentage of the polyagglutinable red cells in any given individual, varies over time. The one case of polyagglutination (203) that was named Tcr (205) was almost certainly a case of Tn-polyagglutination that differed from most of the others (see below) in that virtually 100% of the patient's red cells were polyagglutinable.

Mechanism of Tn-Polyagglutination and Biochemical Nature of the Determinant

Unlike T-activation, Tn-polyagglutination is not a result of direct action of a bacterial or viral enzyme. Instead, it seems that a somatic mutation occurs that results in some progenitor cells losing the ability fully to synthesize certain oligosaccharide side chains. As a result, descendant cells (that may be red cells, leukocytes or platelets, see below) of those progenitors enter the blood stream in the Tn-polyagglutinable state. Since the mutation does not usually affect all progenitors (presumably it occurs after cell differentiation in the blood forming organs has begun) the most common finding is that not all the circulating cells are polyagglutinable. Further, since the situation appears to be the result of a mutation, it is usually a permanent condition. Indeed, in several of the early reports the condition was described as permanent mixed-field polyagglutination. In spite of the fact that Tn-polyagglutination is not caused by a bacterially or virally-produced enzyme, many persons with Tn-polyagglutination give a history of infection.

Dahr et al. (206,207) studied the biochemical nature of the Tn determinant and concluded that one place in which it is present is the oligosaccharides (32) that are attached to the MN (and Ss and minor) SGPs (31). As shown in figure 42-1, the immunodominant carbohydrate of the Tn determinant was shown to be the N-acetyl-D-galactosamine (GalNAc) residue of the tetrasaccharide, to which no D-galactose (Gal) had been added. Subsequent studies have shown that anti-Tn and the lectins that have that specificity (see below) do not simply define GalNAc (if they did, they would have anti-A specificity). Two possibilities exist. First, the Tn-determinant may represent GalNAc in alpha linkage to serine or threonine and the presence of one of those amino acids may be necessary for total Tn structure. Alternatively, Tn may represent GalNAc in a three dimensional configuration (perhaps affected by serine or threonine and its linkage to that amino acid) that differs from the configuration of other antigens (such as A) in which GalNAc is immunodominant. Both Springer and Desai (208) and Murphy (209) have shown that anti-Tn lectins precipitate neuraminidase-treated ovine submaxillary mucin that before being treated has the structure NeuAc-α-(2-6)-D-GalNAc-α-serine or threonine. These concepts are similar to those discussed earlier regarding the three dimensional presentation of D-galactose in the T determinant.

The findings of Dahr et al. (206,207) showed that two other features of Tn should be expected. First, although the Tn and A antigens are not the same, they do have the same immunodominant carbohydrate. Thus it would be expected that some sera containing anti-A would cross-react with Tn. In fact, Gunson et al. (77) and Berman et al. (171) had already shown this to be exactly the case and had described the affinity of Tn-polyagglutinable red cells for anti-A. That observation was subsequently confirmed by others (172,176). Since then, Laird et al. (182) have reported that Tn-polyagglutinable red cells can have a pseudo B antigen that differs from the acquired B antigen (described in Chapter 8 and, in association with polyagglutination, below) in that it is denatured by proteases and fails to react with *Bandeiraea* (now *Griffonia*) *simplicifolia II* lectin (see also below). The second expectation from the findings of Dahr et al. (206,207) was that the mutation that leads to the Tn-polyagglutinable state would be shown to result in non-production of the transferase enzyme that adds D-galactose to GalNAc in the oligosaccharide (again see figure 42-1). Since there was no evidence that the Gal or NeuAc residues of the tetrasaccharide were being removed to expose Tn (GalNAc) it followed that the likely explanation was that, at least the Gal, was never added. This concept was shown to be correct when, in 1978, Cartron et al. (178,179) and Berger and Kozdrowski (180) showed that the Tn-polyagglutinable state results from a deficiency of 3-β-D-galactosyl transferase (T-transferase). Thus the situation could indeed be explained by a single mutation in which the ability to synthesize normal T-transferase is lost in some but not all progenitor cells. The data cited above showed the structure of T and Tn to be as depicted diagrammatically in figure 42-1, thus confirming the earlier forecast by Springer and Desai (208). In spite of the clear demonstrations (178-180) of a defect in production of T-transferase in the Tn-polyagglutinable state, Blumenfeld et al. (198) believe that the deficiency is not absolute. This conclusion is based on their finding that some Tn-activated red cells carry some copies of the full tetrasaccharide of Thomas and Winzler (32 and see figure 42-1). King et al. (259) have characterized two different defects of T-transferase in individuals in whom Tn is exposed.

Vainchenker et al. (187) cultured red and white cells from the marrow of two patients with Tn-polyagglutination. Those cultured from host progenitor cells that had Tn exposed, all had demonstrable Tn sites. Those cultured from progenitors on which Tn was not exposed, failed to

react with the fluorescently-labeled *Helix pomatia* extract used. These findings seem to confirm that Tn-polyagglutination arises by mutation and that clones of cells derived from progenitors descended from the stem cell in which the mutation occurred have Tn exposed, while those descended from an unaffected stem cell do not.

There are three reports in the literature (186,189,190) that describe Tn-polyagglutination in newborn infants. No polyagglutination was detected in any of the parents so that inheritance of the condition from a person in whom mutation had occurred was excluded. Further, in each case the condition was transient, the polyagglutination disappeared as the child grew older. Thus, mutation in the infants themselves was probably not the cause. In two of the cases (188,189) the authors noted that the mother had an infection during the pregnancy (a flu-like illness in one, gastric flu and an upper respiratory tract infection in the other) and wondered if Tn-exposure was the result of the action of bacterial enzymes in utero. In the other case, in which the child's red cells had both Tn and Th (see below) exposed, the authors (190) suggested that the condition might have represented temporary deficiency in production of β-3-galactosyl transferase. Further, from their finding that Tn-activation disappeared before Th-activation, they (190) wondered if Tn might be an intermediate product in the biosynthetic pathway. At least for exposure of Tn, production of a transferase at a lower level than in adults seems more likely than infection. There is essentially no evidence that in vivo Tn-polyagglutination ever represents enzymatic degradation of red cell membrane-borne structures.

Exposure of the Tn-Receptor In Vitro

Springer and Desai (208) reported that treatment of extracted T-substance with β-galactosidase removes the galactose residues and exposes Tn (see figure 42-1). As far as we are aware, this represents the only successful attempt to expose Tn in vitro. The amount of enzyme needed and the length of time required to convert T to Tn, precluded this method from becoming one that could be applied in the immunohematology laboratory for the preparation of Tn-polyagglutinable red cells, although such cells would be very useful for adsorption studies in the identification of in vivo Tn-exposure.

Specific Recognition of Tn-Polyagglutination

The above description of the mechanism by which cells with exposed Tn antigens are produced, will have indicated some of the serological findings to be expected when those cells are tested. First, because the situation

TABLE 42-1 Lectins Useful for the Recognition of Tn-Polyagglutinable Red Cells (from references 216 to 219 and 221 to 223)

(S=Salvia; L=Lamium; M=Marrubium; C=Cytisus; V=Vicia; Sp=Spartium)

ANTI-Tn

S. aethiopsis, S. argentea, S. aurea, S. candelabrum, S. forskohlei, S. grandiflora, S. haematodes, S. nemerosa[1], *S. pratensis*[1], *S. sclarea, S. sclarea turkestanica, S. sclareoides, S. superba*[1], *S. tarasacifolia, S. transylvanica, S. verbenaca, L. amplexicaule* L., *L. hybridum* Vill., *L. purpureum* L., *M. candidissimum.*

ANTI-Tn PLUS ANTI-Cad

S. farinacea, S. horminum

ANTI-Tn PLUS ANTI-T

C. scoparius, L. maculatum (anti-T activity weak)

ANTI-Tn PLUS ANTI-T PLUS ANTI-Cad

S. japonica (anti-Cad activity weak), *S. nicotica* (anti-T and anti-Cad both weak), *S. verticillata* (Anti-T and Anti-Cad both weak), *V. villosa, Sp. junceum.*

---

[1]   May be the same variety

represents mutation, Tn-polyagglutination is usually (but not always, see below) a permanent state, unlike T-activation that is transient and reversible. Second and for the same reason, Tn- polyagglutination may not be associated with a current or even a recent infection. Third, as discussed, not all the cells will be Tn-polyagglutinable so that mixed-field reactions will usually be seen when human sera or lectins are used. Fourth, like T-activated red cells, those that are Tn-polyagglutinable have reduced levels of sialic acid (NeuAc). Fifth, again for reasons discussed, Tn-polyagglutinable red cells react preferentially with sera that contain anti-A. None of these findings permits the positive identification of the Tn-polyagglutinable state and the certain exclusion of other forms of the phenomena described in this chapter.

In spite of the statement made above, about Tn-polyagglutination usually being a permanent state, there are a few cases in which the situation has reverted to one in which no polyagglutinable red cells are produced. When this happens in a patient receiving chemotherapy (175,181,185) the reversal can perhaps be understood (see section below dealing with Tn and leukemia). When it happens spontaneously (175) it is less easily understood.

Many other features of Tn-polyagglutinable red cells, some of which help in their recognition, are known. First, the cells are agglutinated by ABO compatible sera from adults, from which other polyagglutinins such as anti-T, have been removed by adsorption. Second, the sera of other persons with proved Tn-polyagglutination, lack anti-Tn. Third, Tn-polyagglutinable red cells are agglutinated by *Dolichos biflorus* lectin, even when they are group O or group B (77,171). Fourth, the cells are agglutinated by BS

I but not by BS II isolectin from *Bandeiraea* (now *Griffonia*) *simplicifolia* seeds (210-215).

A much easier method for the positive identification of Tn-polyagglutination became available in 1973 when Bird and Wingham (216) showed that a lectin made from *Salvia sclarea* seeds contains specific anti-Tn activity. Since then, the same authors have tested other varieties of *Salvia* seeds (217-219) and have found many useful lectins (see table 42-1). In 1977, Lockyer et al. (220) showed that separable anti-Tn and anti-Cad (see below) are present in the serum of the non-poisonous snake *Python sebae*. In 1980, Bird and Wingham (221) showed that lectins from *Vicia villosa* and *Spartium junceum* agglutinated T, Tn and Cad polyagglutinable red cells while that from *Cytisus scoparius* (syn *Sarothamnus scoparius*) agglutinated T and Tn but not Cad polyagglutinable cells. In 1981, Bird and Wingham (222) added the lectins *Lamium purpureum* L., *Lamium hybridum* Vill., and *Lamium amplexicaule* L. to those that agglutinate Tn but not T, Cad, Tk or Th (see below) polyagglutinable cells. A lectin from *Lamium maculatum* L. was shown (222) to agglutinate Tn-polyagglutinable cells strongly and those that were T-activated, only weakly. Another lectin specific for Tn was found, again by Bird and Wingham (223) in the seeds of *Marrubium candidissimum*. Yang et al. (224) described a lectin from *Hibiscus sabdariffa* seeds as containing an agglutinin for T, Th and Tn-polyagglutinable cells but added that Bird (225) had been able to confirm only agglutination of the first two of those types. Since this section sounds like a seed catalog we will, for relief, quote directly from Yang et al. (224) who confirmed that "the fleshy red petals and sepals which enclose the mature fruit of *Hibiscus sabdariffa* may be used to prepare a pleasant cordial, particularly if flavored with nutmeg, ginger and sugar". One presumes that the addition of vodka, rum or an alternative is at the choice of the investigator! The use of various lectins for the classification of polyagglutinable red cells is described more fully in table 42-3, but table 42-1 provides a summary of the lectin specificities described here.

Red Cell Typing Studies on Tn-Polyagglutinable Red Cells

We (171) found that once treated with standard strength preparations of papain or ficin that are used in blood group serology, Tn-polyagglutinable red cells were no longer polyagglutinable so could be typed for ABO and D with routine reagents. As far as we are aware, others have had similar experiences so that the typing difficulties associated with this form of polyagglutination are easily resolved. This finding probably does not mean that Tn receptors are confined to the MN

SGP that is removed when red cells are treated with proteases. It seems somewhat more likely that Tn sites exist elsewhere on red cells (such as on the Ss SGP) but that too few copies of the antigen remain on protease-treated red cells for them to create serious difficulties in ABO and D typing tests.

Transfusion in the Presence of Tn-Polyagglutination

Relatively little has been published about the effects of passive transfer of donor anti-Tn to a patient with Tn-polyagglutinable red cells. However, since a number of persons with this phenomenon have leukemia and other diseases in which transfusion therapy is common (see below) it seems reasonable to assume that many of them have been transfused. Since there are no reports to the contrary, it may also be safe to assume (this is known in one case (171)) that the transfusion of packed red cells can be tolerated by the patient because only a small quantity of plasma and hence anti-Tn, is infused. Haynes et al. (203) showed that, as expected, normal red cells do not become Tn-polyagglutinable when transfused to a patient with Tn-polyagglutination.

Although as described below, Tn-polyagglutination is often associated with disease, some healthy individuals with red cells of this type have been encountered (174,177,204,205,226). Myllylä et al. (204) showed that the survival of autologous red cells in a patient with Tn-activation was normal but presumably that patient had no anti-Tn in the serum. When a small dose of Tn-polyagglutinable red cells was injected into a normal individual, the cells were rapidly destroyed (204). In the event that a blood donor had Tn-polyagglutinable red cells, those cells would appear incompatible with the sera of all patients and would probably not be transfused.

Tn Receptors on Leukocytes and Platelets

In several of the early cases of Tn-polyagglutination (169,170,177) it was noticed that the phenomenon was associated with leukopenia and/or thrombocytopenia. In 1977, Beck et al. (177) examined the leukocytes and platelets of six persons with Tn-polyagglutination. Of these individuals, three were leukopenic (wbc counts 2700 to 3000 per mm^3) and thrombocytopenic (platelet counts 42,000 to 90,000 per mm^3). The other three did not have similar values although two had white cell counts in the low normal range (4000 and 4800 per mm^3, respectively), the third had a white cell count of 8300 per mm^3. In the latter three, the platelet counts were normal (131,000 to 215,500 per mm^3). In all six cases, the leuko-

cytes and platelets adsorbed *Salvia sclarea* lectin, the white cells and platelets of normal control donors did not. In two cases where sample size permitted cell separation, the granulocytes and lymphocytes of patients with Tn-polyagglutination adsorbed anti-Tn. Beck et al. (177) concluded that although Tn is exposed on leukocytes and platelets (a finding later explained by the discovery of lack of T-transferase and the clonal nature of Tn exposed and non-exposed cells (178,179,187)) that fact alone does not explain the leukopenia and thrombocytopenia associated with Tn-polyagglutination because three of their subjects were deficient in numbers of leukocytes and platelets, but the other three were not. As described in the next section, the difference may relate to the development of disease in some but by no means all persons with Tn-polyagglutinable cells.

Tn, Leukemia and the Tn Syndrome

In 1976, Bird et al. (175) described a patient with acute myelocytic leukemia and Tn-polyagglutinable red cells. It was not known whether the Tn-polyagglutination preceded or followed development of the leukemia. When the patient was treated with cytotoxic drugs the Tn-polyagglutinable red cells disappeared, it was presumed that the abnormal clones of cells had been destroyed. When two more patients with acute myelomonocytic leukemia and Tn-polyagglutinable red cells were reported in 1979 (181,183), Ness et al. (181) suggested that Tn-polyagglutination might be a marker of a preleukemic state. In the patient described (181) Tn-polyagglutination had been conclusively identified long before the leukemia developed. The patient had first experienced hematological problems (leukopenia and thrombocytopenia) in 1966. In 1972, he was found to have an enlarged spleen and again to be leukopenic and thrombocytopenic. In 1974, he required a splenectomy because of life-threatening thrombocytopenia. At the time that the splenectomy was undertaken, red cell polyagglutination due to Tn-exposure was demonstrated. In 1976, the patient presented with acute myelogenous leukemia. Chemotherapy resulted in a clinical remission of the leukemia and disappearance of the Tn-polyagglutinable red cells. A year later the patient suffered a relapse of the acute leukemia and died, no Tn-polyagglutinable red cells were detectable during the clinical relapse. In 1973, Jiji et al. (173) described a patient with Tn-polyagglutinable red cells and pancytopenia. The pancytopenia was successfully treated and the Tn-polyagglutination disappeared. In 1979, following the publication of the descriptions of Tn-polyagglutination as a possible preleukemic sign, Jiji (185) reported that the patient described in 1973 (173) had died of acute myeloid leukemia in 1975. An association between Tn and leukemia was described again in 1987 when Roxby et al. (227) described the detection of exposed Tn on leukemic cells, using a monoclonal antibody and immunohistochemical methods. The same group of investigators (199) extended these observations in 1992. They tested 725 abnormal marrow aspirates and detected Tn-activated red cells in five of them. Among the five, two patients had newly diagnosed acute leukemia and in two others the disease process terminated in acute leukemia. Of note, exposure of the Tn receptor on marrow cells was detectable, in the patients, between eight and 12 months, in different cases, before red cell Tn-polyagglutination was seen.

Clearly the mutation that results in some progenitors giving rise to clones of cells (at least red cells, leukocytes and platelets) in which there is incomplete oligosaccharide chain synthesis resulting in Tn being exposed, is often associated with acute myeloid leukemia. However, not quite all clinically affected individuals with Tn-polyagglutinable red cells have leukemia. In at least two (192,197) Tn-activation was associated with myelodysplasia but not leukemia, in others mild hemolytic anemia and/or leukopenia and/or thrombocytopenia have been seen (169,170,188,201) while Tn has at least once been associated with lymphoma (199). These findings have led to use of the term Tn-syndrome (188) to describe patients who are ill, have Tn-polyagglutinable cells but do not have leukemia. It is, of course, tempting to suppose that the Tn-syndrome is, indeed, a preleukemic condition.

Tn-Polyagglutination in Healthy Individuals

In direct contrast to the patients described in the previous section, there are several individuals (including at least one who wishes to be a blood donor but whose blood cannot be used) who are known to have had Tn-polyagglutinable red cells for a number of years but in whom there is no evidence of disease (174,177,204,205,226). Clearly, in view of the findings described above, these individuals should be followed on a regular basis so that early intervention can be initiated if signs that leukemia (or any other serious disorder) is developing are seen.

Tn, Anti-Tn and Cancer

As described in an earlier section, a great deal of work has been performed to demonstrate the exposure of T on malignant cells. Such studies have been proposed as being useful in diagnosis, prognosis and perhaps treatment. Soon after the involvement of T in this

setting was recognized, it became apparent that on many of the malignant cells, Tn is exposed as well. Indeed many of the publications referenced in the section on T, anti-T and cancer, also describe similar findings about Tn. Over the years, Tn has, perhaps, come to be regarded as a more reliable marker than T in this setting and some of the newer studies (104,108,109,191,193-196,227) stress the value of detection of the Tn receptor. Again, the topic is one that warrants a textbook of its own, readers wishing to learn more about the subject could begin with published reviews (104,108,109).

Monoclonal Antibodies to T and Tn

A large number of monoclonal antibodies to these determinants have been described, much of the work in establishing the biochemical structure of the antigens and the detection of the receptors on malignant cells have been performed using such monoclonal antibodies (105,106,125,191,193,195,196,199,227). In addition to the papers describing use of the MAb as listed above, other descriptions of MAb to T (228,229) and Tn (230-232) have appeared.

Cad Polyagglutination

In 1968, Cazal et al. (235) described the low incidence antigen Cad that was inherited as a Mendelian dominant character. The rare antigen differed from any other previously described in that in the original family the red cells of persons who had the Cad antigen were polyagglutinable. Thus Cad polyagglutination represented the first inherited form of the phenomenon. Later, Cazal et al. (236) found that the Cad antigen can be present on the red cells of unrelated persons in different amounts and that only when the highest quantity is present are the red cells polyagglutinable. Sringarm et al. (237,238) and Yamaguchi et al. (239) showed that Cad is somewhat more common in Orientals than in other population groups. Lopez et al. (240) studied 50 examples of Cad+ red cells found in French donors and confirmed the earlier reports that the amount of Cad antigen can vary in quantity on the cells of members of the same family. These workers (240) also found that some sera would agglutinate almost all Cad+ red cells in tests at 4°C, although the same sera did not react with Cad- cells at that temperature and that many of the Cad+ red cells were not polyagglutinable when tested with those and other sera at 22°C . There are many other reports (241-250,263) that describe Cad+ red cells. In the early recognition of Cad it was noticed (235,236) that group O and group B, Cad+ red cells reacted with *Dolichos biflorus* at a dilution at which that lectin was being used as an anti-A_1 reagent. Variation in the reactions of Cad+ red cells with anti-Cad polyaggglutinin, animal anti-Cad, human and snail anti-A, anti-Sd^a (see below) and *Dolichos biflorus* have led to a classification system in which Cad+ red cells are classed as Cad 1, Cad 2, Cad 3 or Cad 4 (236,247). The classification system is illustrated in table 42-2 but should not be taken too literally. As described below, the biochemical structure of the Cad antigen has been determined and it is apparent that to some degree at least, the Cad 1, 2, 3 and 4 phenotypes represent points on a sliding scale of antigen level somewhat analogous to A_1, A_2 to A_x, rather than distinct entities. As examples, Ellisor et al. (248) described one sample that appeared to be intermediate between Cad 1 and Cad 2 while Leger et al. (249,250) studied a sample that was polyagglutinable with 50 to 70% of normal sera and strongly reactive with anti-Sd^a (i.e. characteristic of Cad 1) but was not agglutinated by *Dolichos biflorus* or by three other lectins that agglutinate Cad 1, 2, 3 and 4 red cells. Clearly in spite of the sliding scale, the difference between various Cad+ cells is not wholly explained by quantitative variation of antigen expression. While table 42-2 attempts to illustrate some differences between the Cad 1, 2, 3 and 4 phenotypes that can be demonstrated easily and quickly in direct tests, it should be added that perhaps more reliable differentiation can be achieved by the use of adsorption

studies (247). Cad 1, 2, 3 and 4 red cells are progressively less efficient in adsorbing *Dolichos biflorus*, *Helix pomatia* and human anti-A. Also shown in table 42-2 are the percentage of group O and group B, Cad+ red cells, that are expected to be agglutinated by *Dolichos biflorus*. For comparative purposes the reactions of A_1 and A_2, Cad- red cells are shown (247).

In 1971, Sanger et al. (251) showed that Cad+ red cells react very strongly when tested with anti-Sd^a. This was taken to indicate that Cad represents the strongest known expression of Sd^a and that the antigens are the same. As discussed in Chapter 31, the immunodominant sugar of Sd^a is N-acetyl-D-galactosamine. Since the presence of the Cad antigen was often revealed in a test using *Dolichos biflorus*, a lectin known (244,252-258) to complex with N-acetyl-D-galactosamine, it followed that the same sugar was probably immunodominant in Cad as well. As discussed in detail below, while it is now known that Sd^a and Cad have the same immunodominant sugar and that antibodies that complex with N-acetyl-D-galactosamine combine with the Sd^a and Cad receptors, it is not certain that the two are completely identical.

Specific Recognition of Cad-Polyagglutination

Cad-polyagglutinable red cells do not react with

TABLE 42-2 Some Characteristics of the Cad Phenotypes (236, 247, 261-263)

Phenotype[*1]	*Dolichos biflorus*[*2]	Percent red cells agglutinated by *D. biflorus*	Human Anti-A[*3]	Human serum lacking Anti-A[*4]	*Helix pomatia*	*Salvia*[*5] *horminum*	*Leonurus*[*5] *cardiaca*
Cad 1	3+	80 to 100%	2+	2-3+	2+	+	+
Cad 2	2+	50 to 80%	1+	0[*6]	2+	+	+
Cad 3[*7]	1+	30 to 50%	1+	0[*6]	3+	(+)	
Cad4[*7]	(+)	<30%				(+)	(+)
Cad$_{Ber}$[*8]	0	0		2+		0	0
A_1, Cad-	2+	50-80%	3+	0	1+	0	0
A_2, Cad-	0	0	3+	0	3+	0	0

[*1]   All Cad + phenotypes shown are group O or group B. Reactions of A_1 and A_2, Cad- red cells shown for comparative purposes.
[*2]   At a dilution at which the lectin agglutinates A_1 but not A_2 red cells. See comparative reactions, diluted to give a 2+ reaction with A_1, Cad- red cells.
[*3]   Diluted to give 3+ reactions with A_1 and A_2, Cad- red cells.
[*4]   Anti-Cad polyagglutinin.
[*5]   Reported only as positive or negative, i.e., strength of reaction not described.
[*6]   According to Salmon et al. (409) these red cells are polyagglutinable when tested by "sensitive techniques." Such tests presumably involve low temperatures although that is not stated.
[*7]   Better differentiated by adsorption techniques (247).
[*8]   Atypical polyagglutination related to Cad, described by Leger et al. (250). The name Cad$_{Ber}$ (for Bermuda the home of the propositus) was suggested. Not shown in Table 42-2, Cad$_{Ber}$ cells were reactive with *Glycine soja*.

Arachis hypogea or *Salvia sclarea* lectins. They are agglutinated by *Dolichos biflorus* and by undiluted unadsorbed *Salvia horminum* (see table 42-3 for other lectins that agglutinate T and/or Tn and/or Cad-polyagglutinable red cells). The anti-Tn and anti-Cad agglutinins in *Salvia horminum* and *Salvia farinacea* can be separated by adsorption (1,146,217). Further, Bird and Wingham (260) have shown that a lectin made from *Leonurus cardiaca* seeds contains a potent anti-Cad agglutinin but reacts only weakly with neuraminidase-treated red cells and even less well with those that are Tn-polyagglutinable. The lectin does not react at all with Tk or Th-polyagglutinable red cells (see below). For further details on the recognition of Cad-polyagglutination see table 42-3.

Red Cell Typing in the Presence of Cad-Polyagglutination

Cad-polyagglutinable red cells are still polyagglutinable after they have been treated with proteases so that the simple method used to render Tn-polyagglutinable red cells suitable for testing with ABO and D typing reagents cannot be used. Although relatively little has been written, it seems (235,236) that anti-Cad in typing sera may be a separable agglutinin that can be removed by adsorption if group O, Cad-polyagglutinable red cells are available. Presumably anti-A, anti-B and anti-A,B could be diluted to a point at which the ABO agglutinins were still active but the anti-Cad was not. We were unable to find documentation as to the presence or absence of anti-Cad in the sera of newborn infants that contain maternal IgG anti-A or anti-B. Presumably, sera that contained IgG anti-A, anti-B and anti-D and only IgM anti-Cad, could be treated with 2-ME or DTT and then used as reagents to type Cad-polyagglutinable red cells.

Biochemical Structure of the Cad Determinant

As mentioned above, the finding (251) that Cad+ red cells are very strongly reactive with anti-Sd^a led to the suggestion that the two determinants might be the same thing. However, in a series of studies (261-263) in which various lectins, extracts of different snails and a natural antibody present in chicken serum were used, it was found that Cad and Sd^a gave different reaction patterns. Cartron and Blanchard (264) found that the major red cell sialoglycoprotein (the MN SGP) isolated from Cad+ red cells had a higher molecular weight than the one isolated from Cad- cells. The difference seemed to represent increased glycosylation of the SGP on Cad+ cells. Blanchard et al. (265) then studied the carbohydrate-con-

taining side chains attached to the MN SGP of Cad+ and Cad- red cells. They found that in the Cad+ cells, the side chain is often a pentasaccharide with an N-acetyl-D-galatosamine residue bound to the same galactose residue that carries NeuAc in the tetrasaccharide of the MN SGP of Cad- red cells. The GalNAc residue found on Cad+ red cells is additional to, not a replacement of the NeuAc residue of the usual tetrasaccharide. The two structures are depicted diagrammatically in figure 42-2. For comparative purposes, figure 31-2 in Chapter 31 shows the Sd^a antigen on Tamm and Horsfall urinary glycoprotein. From the finding that the MW of the MN SGP of Cad+ red cells is some 3000 daltons higher than that of the MN SGP of Cad- red cells (264), it was concluded (265) that most of the 15 alkali-labile side chains of the MN SGP on the Cad+ cells must carry the extra GalNAc residue. However, there was also evidence (265) that a few of the side chains of the Cad+ cells might be trisaccharides or tetrasaccharides. From a later study using nuclear magnetic resonance, Herkt et al. (266) concluded that the pentasaccharide is present instead of the tetrasaccharide at about 70 to 75% of the oligosaccharide attachment sites on MN and Ss SGPs.

As an aside to the description of the structure of the Cad antigen it can be added that Cartron et al. (267) have shown that presence of the pentasaccharide instead of the usual tetrasaccharide on Cad+ cells, affords some protection for those red cells against invasion by merozoites of *Plasmodium falciparum*, the parasite that causes the most severe form of malaria in man. That it is the usual tetrasaccharide to which the merozoites normally bind is also shown by the findings that Tn cells, that have side chains that lack the terminal NeuAc and Gal residues (see figure 42-1 and earlier text) and En(a-) red cells, that lack MN SGP altogether and thus have drastically reduced numbers of side chains (i.e. just those on Ss SGP and minor membrane components) are also more resistant to invasion than are normal (i.e. En(a+), Cad-, Tn-) red cells (267,268).

Are Cad and Sd^a the Same Antigen?

Clearly, at the serological level, antigens that have GalNAc as their terminal immunodominant carbohydrate will have similarities. This is well illustrated by the use of lectins. The *Dolichos biflorus* lectin recognizes both N-acetyl-alpha and beta-D-galactosamine (256). It agglutinates red cells that carry A and group O and B cells that carry Tn, Cad or "super" Sd^a (see Chapter 31). However, the specificity of a carbohydrate antigen is not wholly dependent on the terminal sugar residue. Serological studies can be used to differentiate between antibodies to A, P, Tn and Sd^a in each of which galac-

FIGURE 42-2 The Usual Tetrasaccharide (32) of Red Blood Cell Sialoglycoproteins and the Modified Structure on Cad-polyagglutinable Red Cells (264,265)

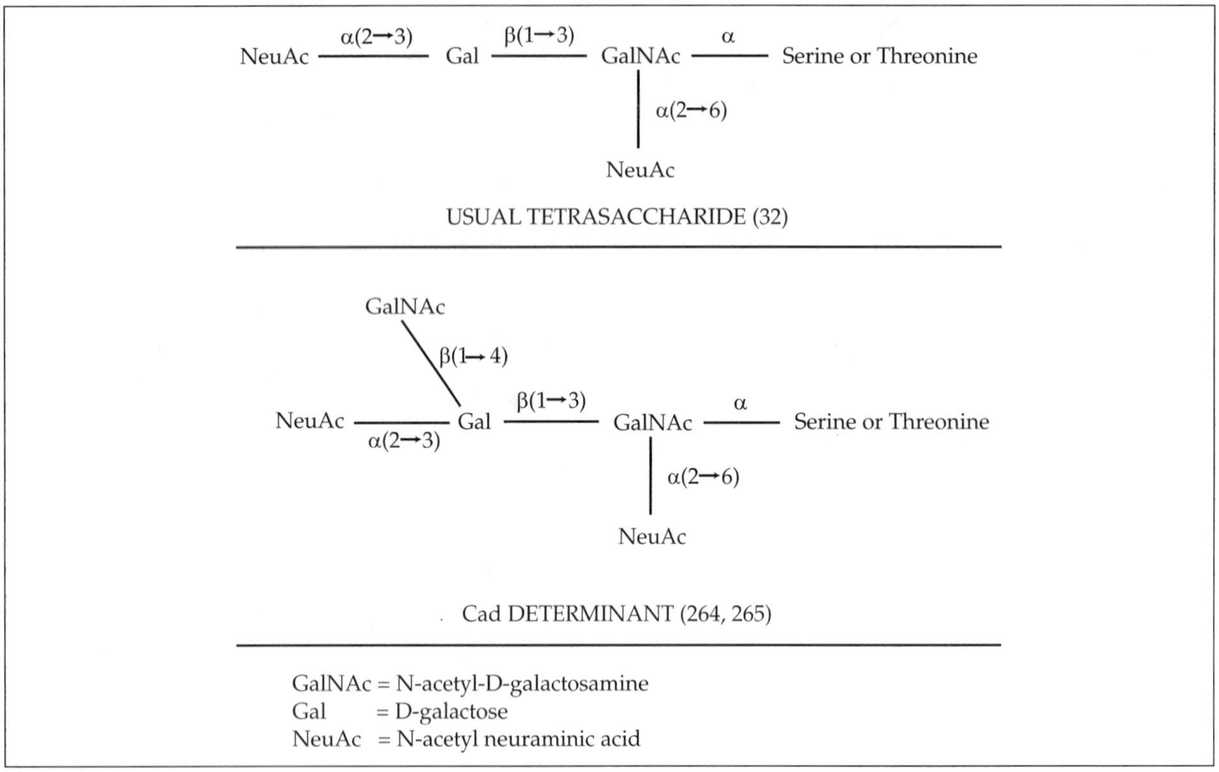

NeuAc $\xrightarrow{\alpha(2\rightarrow3)}$ Gal $\xrightarrow{\beta(1\rightarrow3)}$ GalNAc $\xrightarrow{\alpha}$ Serine or Threonine

$\Big| \alpha(2\rightarrow6)$

NeuAc

USUAL TETRASACCHARIDE (32)

GalNAc

$\diagdown \beta(1\rightarrow4)$

NeuAc $\xrightarrow[\alpha(2\rightarrow3)]{}$ Gal $\xrightarrow{\beta(1\rightarrow3)}$ GalNAc $\xrightarrow{\alpha}$ Serine or Threonine

$\Big| \alpha(2\rightarrow6)$

NeuAc

Cad DETERMINANT (264, 265)

GalNAc = N-acetyl-D-galactosamine
Gal   = D-galactose
NeuAc = N-acetyl neuraminic acid

tosamine is immunodominant. The same is not true for antibodies that react with Cad and Sd^a. In serological studies, *Dolichos biflorus* agglutinates all group A (i.e. the undiluted lectin agglutinates A$_2$ red cells) and those group O and group B cells that are Cad+ or Sd(a++). Cad+ red cells react strongly with anti-Sd^a, that is, those that are Cad 1 and some that are Cad 2, behave as if they are Sd(a++). What is not clear is whether these serological findings represent identity between Cad and Sd^a as suggested (251) or the presence of GalNAc in similar but not identical configuration in two slightly different antigens. If Cad and Sd^a are the same it would have to be supposed that *Sd^a* genes vary in quantitative expression (they do, see table 31-3 in Chapter 31). That is, some would make enough antigen to effect the Cad+, Sd(a++) phenotype while most would encode antigen levels as seen in the Cad-, Sd(a+) phenotype. Since *Sd^a* presumably encodes production of a galactosaminyltransferase, such an explanation would seem entirely tenable.

Identity between the two antigens appears less likely on some other grounds. If Cad and Sd^a are the same thing, almost all persons of the Sd(a+) phenotype would have to be thought of as making anti-Sd^a in order to explain the polyagglutinable nature of Cad 1 red cells. While the serological findings do not suggest that all sera from persons with Sd(a+) red cells contain anti-Sd^a it has been

claimed (269) that the sera from persons with Sd(a++) red cells do not agglutinate Cad 1 polyagglutinable red cells.

If Cad and Sd^a are different antigens, it would have to be supposed that *Cad* and *Sd^a* encode production of galactosaminyltransferases with slightly different specificities. If that is the case, the presence of anti-Cad (the polyagglutinin) in the sera of Sd(a+) and Sd(a-) persons would require no unusual explanation. The polyagglutinin would be thought of as being of universal incidence, like anti-T, anti-Tn, anti-Tk, etc.

Recognition of the biochemical structures of Cad and Sd^a does not provide an unequivocal answer as to identity or non-identity between Cad and Sd^a. While the structure of Cad (see figure 42-2) has been determined on red cells (264-266,278,283) the structure of Sd^a has been determined thus far only on the Tamm and Horsfall (T-H) urinary glycoprotein (270-278). Duffy and Marshall (279) have pointed out that in the T-H glycoprotein there are carbohydrate side chains in N-linkage to five asparagine residues; at least two of these side chains are or include the Sd^a-containing pentasaccharide (273,274). In contrast, on red cells the pentasaccharides that include the Cad determinant are O-linked to threonine or serine (265). There is only one N-linked (to asparagine) oligosaccharide on the MN SGP (280). The trisaccharides of Cad and Sd^a (figure 31-2 in Chapter 31) are the same. However, in the Cad-containing pentasaccharide, the trisaccharide is in $\alpha(1\rightarrow3)$ linkage to GalNAc. In the Sd^a-containing pentasaccharide, the trisaccharide is in $\alpha(1\rightarrow4)$ linkage to GalNAc. However, again it must be remembered that the Sd^a-active structure represents Sd^a in the urine. It is not known to what or how the Sd^a-active trisaccharide is linked on red cells. The structure that represents Cad on red cells was not found on red cells with average levels of Sd^a, i.e. Sd(a+) (264,265).

A different way in which the question about the identity or non-identify of Cad and Sd^a might be answered would be to study the galactosaminyltransferases encoded by the *Cad* and *Sd^a* genes. Serafini-Cessi et al. (281,307) isolated and purified the α-N-acetylgalactosaminyltransferase from the urine of individuals with Sd(a+) red cells. They found that the best acceptor for this enzyme, in its transfer of GalNAc in $\alpha(1\rightarrow3)$ linkage to Gal, was a preparation of T-H glycoprotein isolated from the urine of an individual with Sd(a-) red cells. However, in a 174 times purified form, the enzyme was able to add GalNAc to the tetrasaccharides of native MN SGP. The meaning of this observation is not entirely clear since, as mentioned above, Blanchard et al. (265) did not find the additional GalNAc residue in the oligosaccharide side chains attached to MN SGP of Sd(a+), Cad- red cells. It appears that the *Cad*-specified transferase may have preferential catalytic activity for O-linked oligosaccharides while the *Sd^a*-specified transferase may have preferential activity for N-linked oligosaccharides. Complex as the enzyme actions and biochemistry may be, the phenotypes involved can be differentiated at the serological level. By definition, Cad 1 red cells are polyagglutinable, Sd(a++) cells are not.

Tk-Polyagglutination

In 1972, Bird and Wingham (283) described a new form of polyagglutination that they called Tk. The condition was shown to be different from T, Tn or Cad-polyagglutination by differential adsorption of sera that contained anti-T, anti-Tn, anti-Cad and anti-Tk. Tk-polyagglutination was found to be transient and reversible and in this respect resembled T-activation. In addition, Tk-polyagglutinable red cells were agglutinated by an *Arachis hypogea* (anti-T) extract. The authors (283) considered the possibility that Tk-polyagglutination might represent mild, early or fading T-activation. In addition to the fact that the Tk-activated cells reacted with *Arachis*, it was found that they aggregated normally in polybrene and had a normal sialic acid level. These features are also seen when red cells are only mildly T-

activated. However, there were some differences between Tk and mildly T-activated red cells. First, the Tk cells were agglutinated by human sera from which anti-T had been removed by adsorption. Second, *Erythrina indica* lectin agglutinated Tk cells weakly and T-activated cells strongly. Third, elderberry juice agglutinated Tk and normal cells weakly but T-activated cells strongly. For these reasons, the authors (283) concluded that T and Tk-activation differed and that, like T-activation, Tk antigen exposure probably occurs following the action of a bacterially (or virally)-produced enzyme. Subsequent studies, described below, showed that both of these conclusions were correct.

Many other cases of Tk-activation have now been reported (55,63,284-294) and the mechanism by which the cryptic or latent Tk receptor is exposed is understood. Certain organisms such as *Bacteroides fragilis*, *Bacteroides thetaiotaomicron*, *Flavobacterium keratolycus*, *Serratis marcescens*, *Escherichia coli*, *Escherichia freundii*, *Aspergillus niger* and probably many others, produce endo or exo-beta galactosidases that, in vivo or in vitro, act on red cell membrane structures so that Tk becomes exposed. Not unexpectedly since it is caused by bacterial or virally produced enzymes, Tk-polyagglutination is seen in patients with infections and in newborns with neonatal necrotizing enterocolitis or hemolytic uremic syndrome. While a number of different types of polyagglutination have been seen in conjunction with an acquired B antigen, Tk is perhaps more common than any other type. This topic is described in more detail below.

Biochemical Structure of Tk

Doinel et al. (291) realized that the enzymes responsible for Tk-activation of red cells had already been shown (295-302) to degrade the red cell membrane-borne structure that carries H, I, i and P system determinants. Further, in several cases of in vivo Tk-activation, it had been reported (287-290) that the polyagglutinable red cells had depressed H and/or I and i antigens. In a series of in vitro experiments, Doinel et al. (291) showed that when bacterial endo-beta-galactosidases removed terminal galactose residues so that subterminal N-acetylglucosamine residues became exposed, the cryptantigen Tk became detectable. Judd (292) then showed that exo-beta-galactosidases have the same ability. Again, this does not mean that Tk is simply exposed N-acetyl-glucosamine. As with T and Tn, the immunodominant sugar (in this case N-acetyl-glucosamine) in a certain steric orientation (three dimensional shape) represents the antigen. Again, it is likely that proximal residues and linkage of the immunodominant sugar to the next structure on the chain, contribute greatly to the Tk determinant. Figure

42-3 depicts the proposed structure of Tk (145,291). Workers familiar with the biochemical composition of certain red cell membrane-borne structures will recognize the similarity between Tk and paragloboside, a structure that is part of the chain that carries H (and hence A and/or B if they are present) and P₁ (303,304, see also Chapter 11).

As mentioned above, Judd (292) showed that like endo-beta-galactosidases, some exo-beta-galactosidases also act to expose the Tk. Figure 42-4 was prepared by John Judd (305) to demonstrate the sites on various membrane-borne structures at which endo and exo-beta-galactosidases act. Judd (292) has also shown that some bacteria that produce enzymes that effect Tk-activation, also produce a different enzyme, beta-N-acetyl-glucosaminidase. Tk-polyagglutinable red cells react with both *Arachis hypogea* and GSII lectin (formerly BSII, see below). When Tk-polyagglutinable red cells are treated in vitro with beta-N-acetyl-glucosaminidase, their reaction with *Arachis* is enhanced, their reaction with GSII remains unchanged. From this observation, Judd (292) concluded that *Arachis hypogea* and GSII react with different determinants on the Tk-polyagglutinable red cells.

Specific Recognition of Tk-Polyagglutination

Although T, Tk and Th-activated (for Th, see below) red cells all react with *Arachis hypogea* lectin, the three conditions can be differentiated with relative ease. T-activated but not Tk or Th-activated red cells are agglutinated by *Glycine soja*. Tk, but not T or Th-activated red cells are agglutinated by a lectin now called GSII (*Griffonia simplicifolia* lectin II) that was previously known as BSII (*Bandeiraea simplicifolia* lectin II) (211,214,215). A lectin made from *Vicia hyrcanica* seeds is useful since it contains separable anti-T and anti-Tk (306). In other words, since T-activated cells can be made in vitro, so easily, the *Vicia hyrcanica* lectin can be adsorbed free of anti-T and a specific anti-Tk lectin can be made. Th-polyagglutination mentioned briefly above is described in more detail below and the use of lectins to identify the Tk (and other) polyagglutinable states is depicted in table 42-3.

Red Cell Typing in the Presence of Tk-Polyagglutination

Again, very little seems to have been written about determination of the ABO and D types of red cells that are Tk-polyagglutinable. We presume that if group O Tk-activated red cells are made in vitro using endo-beta-galactosidase isolated from *Escherichia freundii* or *Flavobacterium keratolycus* (291,292,305) they can be used to adsorb anti-Tk from sera that contain anti-A, anti-B and anti-D. Another approach, if anti-Tk is always (or predominantly) IgM in nature would be to use ABO and D typing reagents that had been treated with 2-ME or DTT. Again, we have not been able to find publications that answer the question as to whether anti-Tk is present in cord blood sera that contain IgG maternal anti-A or anti-B. Just like the situation with anti-Cad, we presume that typing sera could be diluted to a point where

FIGURE 42-3 To Show the Proposed Structure of Tk Compared to That of Paragloboside (145,291)

GlcNAc —— β(1→3) —— Gal —— β(1→3) —— Glc ———— Cer

Lacto-*N*-triosylceramide
The proposed structure of Tk

Gal —— β(1→4) —— GlcNAc —— β(1→3) —— Gal —— β(1→3) —— Glc ——— Cer

Paragloboside

Gal   = Galactose
GlcNAc = *N*-acetyl-D-glucosamine
Glc   = Glucose
Cer   = Ceramide (*N*-acetylsphingosine)

As can be seen, when the terminal galactose is enzymatically cleaved from paragloboside by a beta-galactosidase, the subterminal *N*-acetyl-D-glucosamine (the immunodominant carbohydrate of Tk) is exposed.

FIGURE 42-4 To Show the Sites of Action of Endo and Exo-beta-galactosidases on Some Red Cell Membrane-borne Structures (figure supplied by W. John Judd (305))

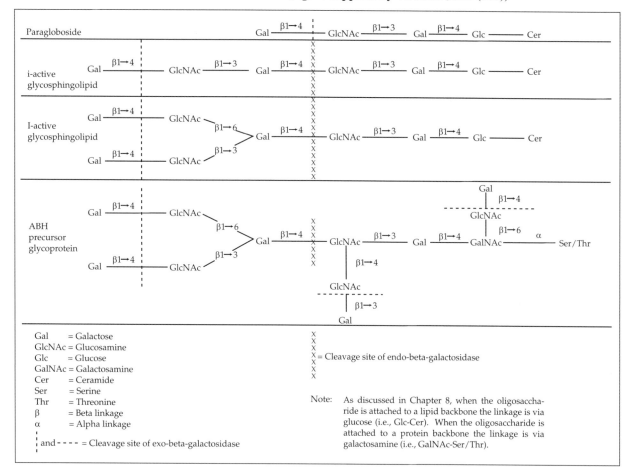

Gal = Galactose
GlcNAc = Glucosamine
Glc = Glucose
GalNAc = Galactosamine
Cer = Ceramide
Ser = Serine
Thr = Threonine
β = Beta linkage
α = Alpha linkage
and ---- = Cleavage site of exo-beta-galactosidase

X = Cleavage site of endo-beta-galactosidase

Note: As discussed in Chapter 8, when the oligosaccharide is attached to a lipid backbone the linkage is via glucose (i.e., Glc-Cer). When the oligosaccharide is attached to a protein backbone the linkage is via galactosamine (i.e., GalNAc-Ser/Thr).

anti-Tk is not active, but where the necessary antibodies, anti-A, anti-B and anti-D, will still react.

VA-Polyagglutination

In 1977, Graninger et al. (308) described a new form of polyagglutination that they called VA (that being an abbreviation for Vienna). The index case involved a 20 year-old male who was said to have suffered intermittent episodes of hemolytic anemia since the age of 5 months. In addition to being weakly agglutinated by almost all normal sera from adults, the red cells of the propositus had a reduced expression of H. The VA-polyagglutinable red cells did not react with *Arachis hypogea* or *Dolichos biflorus* so that T, Tn, Tk and Cad polyagglutination were apparently excluded. In addition, the VA red cells aggregated normally in polybrene and their MN determinants were normally expressed. In a companion study (309) the VA red cells were found to give a stippled pattern in immunofluorescence tests using anti-A$_{HP}$ from *Helix*

pomatia (with which the cells reacted directly but in a mixed-field pattern (308)). In the case described, no difficulties in ABO and D typing were encountered since the polyagglutination was so weak.

In a paper in which two patients with concomitant Tk and VA polyagglutination were described (288), it was concluded that both the Tk and VA receptors had been exposed on the red cells following the actions of bacterial enzymes. The reduction of H was suspected as being due to the presence of a bacterially produced α-fucosidase. Bird (145) suggested that VA might represent one end of a "Tk spectrum" that might begin with VA, include the atypical Tk-polyagglutination case of Mullard et al. (310) and end with clear cut Tk-activation. At the time that VA was first studied (308) the authors did not have GSII (BSII) lectin (the best reagent available for the classification of Tk-polyagglutination) available. However, Bird (145) pointed out that if VA is a form of early Tk-polyagglutination, the stippled appearance of the VA cells in fluorescence tests with anti-A$_{HP}$ would remain unexplained. If the hemolytic anemia of the first patient with VA polyagglutination (308,309, see above) was associated with the polyagglutinable state, it would be hard to explain the hemolysis in terms of Tk-polyagglutination.

Th-Polyagglutination (Low Level T-Activation)

In 1978, Bird et al. (24) described what was thought to be a new form of polyagglutination, the term Th was applied. Like T and Tk-activated red cells, those on which Th was exposed were agglutinated by *Arachis hypogea* lectin. However, Th appeared to differ from T and Tk in that the Th-polyagglutinable red cells were not agglutinated by *Glycine soja*, as are T-activated cells, nor by GSII (BSII) lectin, as are Tk-activated cells. It seemed likely that Th-activation represented the actions of bacterially produced enzymes. In the original cases (24,145,288) Th-activation was seen in different individuals who, among them, had infections with *Eschericia coli*, *Bacteroides melaninogenicus* and various strains of *Clostridia*, *Proteus* and other *Bacteroides*. Bird (145) reported that among ten additional cases of Th-activation that he had seen, two were associated with weak Tk-activation and one with Tn-polyagglutination. In two of the cases Th-activation was weak and the DAT was positive, in the others Th-activation was stronger and the DATs were negative. The Th-polyagglutinable state is either reversed or greatly weakened when the red cells are treated with standard solutions (as used in blood group serology) of papain or ficin.

Although the early studies (24,145,288) suggested that an enzyme made by an invading organism causes Th-activation, such an explanation was questioned. Veneziano et al. (311) described a three year-old child with a yolk-sac tumor of the vagina. The child had a hysterectomy and *Proteus mirabilis* and *Eschericia coli* were cultured from the urine. The child's red cells were Th-activated but so (to a lesser degree) were those of her mother. The authors (311) suggested that Th-polyagglutination might be an inherited condition. In another case Th-polyagglutination was seen (312) in a patient with congenital hypoplastic anemia, leading to the suggestion (313) that Th-activation is not representative of desialylation of red cell membrane sialoglycoproteins. Somewhat similarly in other cases (190,314) the red cells of newborns, who had no evidence of infection, have been seen to be Th-activated. These findings plus those in cases in which concomitant Th and Tn polyagglutination were seen (145,197) led to consideration of the possibility that Th-activation might, like Tn-exposure, arise from incomplete biosynthesis of alkali-labile tetrasaccharides or other similar structures (12).

In spite of the findings described above, it is now known that Th-activation can indeed result from the actions of neuraminidase made by infecting bacteria or viruses. Sondag-Thull et al. (315) studied a neuraminidase made by *Corynebacterium acquaticum*. That organism had previously been shown (316) to cause Th-activation in a contaminated stored blood sample. It was shown that when this enzyme and the neuraminidase made by *Vibrio cholera* (the classic T-activating enzyme) were used to treat red cells in a way that resulted in release of only small amounts of NeuAc, Th-polyagglutination resulted. When the same neuraminidases were used to remove larger amounts of NeuAc from the red cells, T-activation resulted. When less than 20 μg of NeuAc per 10^{10} red cells was removed, Th-polyagglutination was seen, when more than 20 μg of NeuAc per 10^{10} red cells was hydrolyzed, T-polyagglutination was seen. The finding that Th-activation represents early and mild T-activation made many of the features of Th-polyagglutination more understandable. As a single example, at the stage of activation called Th exposure (24) the red cells are reactive with *Arachis hypogea* but not yet sufficiently depleted in NeuAc to react with *Glycine soja*.

Recognition of the Th-Polyagglutination Stage of T-Activation

For those workers who wish still to differentiate between early T (Th) and more advanced T-activation, the findings mentioned above provide such a means. Th-polyagglutinable red cells are agglutinated by *Arachis hypogea* but not by *Glycine soja* or by GS II (*Griffonia simplicifolia* lectin II, formerly BSII) that agglutinate (fully) T and Tk-activated cells, respectively. Bird and Wingham (317) reported that the lectin from *Vicia cretica* seeds strongly agglutinates T and Th-activated red cells but not those that are Tk-activated or polyagglutinable due to any other mechanism described in this chapter.

Red Cell Typing in the Presence of Th-Polyagglutination

As mentioned above, Th-polyagglutination represents T-activation at a point at which the red cells can be made non-polyagglutinable by treatment with papain or ficin. Thus once treated they can be typed for ABO and D. If difficulties are encountered it would seem that the cells are intermediate between what are called the Th and T-activation states. Since Th-activation is now known (315) to represent early T-activation, the modifications described above, for ABO and D typing T-activated red cells can be used.

Tx-Polyagglutination

In 1982, Bird et al. (318) described another new form of polyagglutination that they called Tx. The investigators studied the red cells of children with pneumococcal infections and the effects of treating normal red cells with supernatants from cultures of the pneumococci isolated from those children. Many examples of T and Tk and some of Th-activation were seen. In four cases Tx-activation was seen, three times alone and once concomitantly with Tk-activation. Tx-polyagglutinable red cells were, like T, Tk and Th-activated cells, agglutinated by *Arachis hypogea*. However, the four exposed cryptantigens could be differentiated by the use of selected lectins. T-activated cells reacted with *Arachis hypogea*, *Glycine soja* and *Vicia cretica*. Tk-activated red cells reacted with *Arachis hypogea* and GSII (BSII). Th-activated red cells reacted with *Arachis hypogea* and *Vicia cretica*. Tx-activated red cells reacted only with *Arachis hypogea*. In a later publication, Bird and Wingham (319) reported that like *Vicia cretica*, lectins from *Medicago disciformis* and *Medicago turbinata* seeds, agglutinate T and Th but not Tk or Tx-activated red cells. Wolach et al. (320) described Tx polyagglutination in three young children in one family, it was presumed that all three had the same viral or bacterial infection.

Clearly, Tx-polyagglutination joins T, Tk, Th, acquired B-associated polyagglutination (see below, if that is different from T, Tk and Th) and perhaps VA-polyagglutination as arising from the in vivo or in vitro activity of bacterial or viral enzymes. Like T, Tx is only slightly weakened when red cells are treated with standard concentrations of proteases. Indeed T and Tx can be differentiated only by the use of *Vicia cretica*, *Medicago disciformis* and *Glycine soja* lectins.

NOR-Polyagglutination

Cad and HEMPAS (see below) can be considered to be inherited forms of polyagglutination. Another inherited type was described in 1982 by Harris et al. (321). Five members in two generations of a family had a character called NOR on their red cells, that were agglutinated by about 75% of ABO compatible sera from adults. The NOR character was inherited in a Mendelian dominant fashion.

The NOR-polyagglutinable red cells did not react with *Arachis hypogea*, *Salvia sclarea*, GSII (BSII), *Glycine soja*, *Dolichos biflorus*, *Salvia horminum* or *Helix pomatia*. Further, adsorption studies showed that anti-NOR was dif-

ferent from the antibodies that define T, Tn, Tk, Th, VA and Cad. Protease-treatment of NOR+ red cells enhanced their reactions with human sera. A possible clue to the site of NOR on the red cell membrane was the finding that anti-NOR was neutralized by hydatid cyst fluid and P_1-containing substances of avian origin. However, we are not aware of any further association between NOR and P_1 nor any other studies on the NOR antigen (but see the addendum).

Hyde Park Polyagglutination

Bird (A.R. not G.W.G) et al. (322) described a highly unusual form of polyagglutination in a large South African family of mixed ethnic background. Among 35 family members tested, 12 had a variant methemoglobin, hemoglobin M-Hyde Park and polyagglutinable red cells. The other 23 did not have hemoglobin M-Hyde Park and their red cells were not polyagglutinable. Previous reports (323,324) of individuals with hemoglobin M-Hyde Park did not associate its presence with polyagglutination.

Group O, N+ red cells from an individual with hemoglobin M-Hyde Park were agglutinated by seven of 40 normal human sera, gave enhanced reactions with *Vicia graminea* and *Ulex europaeus* lectins and with human anti-I and anti-i but showed no enhanced reactions with monoclonal or rabbit anti-N. The red cells were agglutinated by monoclonal anti-Tn but were non-reactive with *Salvia sclarea* lectin that is specific for Tn. The red cells were agglutinated by *Glycine soja*, *Sophora japonica* and *Vicia hyrcanica* but reacted only weakly with *Arachis hypogea* and GSII (BSII) (322,325). Between them, the serological and biochemical studies revealed two abnormalities of the membranes of these red cells. First, NeuAc is apparently not present in all the tetrasaccharides attached to MN and Ss SGP. Second, there is apparently incomplete biosynthesis of N-linked branched lactosaminoglycans, that normally (326) contain multiple Gal→β1→4 GlcNac linkages. These lactosaminoglycans are attached to red cell membrane band 3 and band 4.5 and in hemoglobin-M Hyde Park polyagglutinable red cells, the GlcNAc residues are left exposed. The absence of NeuAc probably accounts for the strong reactivity of the cells with *Vicia graminea* and *Glycine soja*, the terminally exposed GlcNAc residues probably account for the cells' strong reactivity with GSII. As yet there is no known relationship between the glycosylation changes and presence of the abnormal hemoglobin.

Polyagglutination Associated with the Acquired B Antigen

The acquired B antigen has been described in detail

in Chapter 8. Briefly, the situation most often represents the actions of bacterially-produced enzymes that effect deacetylation of the A antigen in such a way that anti-B is able to bind to the altered structure (327-329). In studying red cells with the acquired B antigen, Marsh (76) noticed that some of them were polyagglutinable and suggested that the same enzyme, or enzymes produced by the same bacteria, might cause acquisition of a B-like structure and T-activation. At that time it was not known if the acquired B phenomenon represented an enzymatic change of red cell surface structures or simple adsorption of a bacterial product (330). Later, Beck et al. (331) and Garratty et al. (332) described patients whose red cells had acquired a B-like structure and were polyagglutinable, but were either not T-activated (331) or had a cryptic antigen in addition to T, exposed (332). In 1977, Judd et al. (214) described a study in which a number of samples with acquired B were found to be Tk-activated. These workers (214) produced evidence that suggested that different bacterial enzymes were responsible for the deacetylation of A (leading to acquired B) and for the exposure of Tk. It was this study (214) that showed that a second isolectin isolated from *Griffonia simplicifolia* (*Bandeiraea simplicifolia*) seeds (the first one has anti-B specificity (210-212,333)) contains potent anti-Tk. In light of various reports (63,76,214,287,290,310,331,332,334) about the polyagglutinable state of some samples that have an acquired B antigen and/or a depressed expression of H, there seems little doubt that an assortment of bacterial enzymes effect changes in red cell surface structures and that sometimes T, sometimes Tk, sometimes Th, and perhaps sometimes VA (12,288,336) become exposed. As indicated in earlier sections of this chapter, each of those receptors can be exposed on red cells that do not have an acquired B antigen. Indeed, polyagglutination involving T, Tk, Th and VA is more common in the absence of acquired B than its presence.

Exposure of T, Tk, Th or VA on red cells with an acquired B antigen by no means explains all cases in which red cells with acquired B are polyagglutinable. Janvier et al. (337) studied eight such samples and found that three had Tk exposed while the other five did not. When the acquired B antigen was reacetylated, those five samples were no longer polyagglutinable. Reacetylation of acquired B does not reverse Tk-polyagglutination. Further, Gerbal et al. (328) showed that selected group AB sera from which anti-T, anti-Tk, etc., had been removed by adsorption, would still agglutinate the acquired B red cells on which polyagglutination seemed to be a function of deacetylation. Finally, group O red cells, that (obviously) cannot acquire a B antigen via deacetylation of A, can be rendered polyagglutinable by the same deacetylating enzymes (12). Taken together these findings clearly show that there is a form of

polyagglutination, that differs from all others, that is seen most often in association with the acquired B phenomenon. This form of polyagglutination has no name other than "associated with acquired B". Finally, in considering this type of polyagglutination, it must be remembered that there are a number of reports in the older literature (338-345) that describe the adsorption of bacteria, particularly the polysaccharides of those bacteria, on to red cells. Perhaps some of these relate to a situation in which a B-like structure might be adsorbed by red cells on which no deacetylation of A has occurred.

Red Cells with Mixed Forms of Polyagglutination

As mentioned a few times above, it is not uncommon to find more than one type of polyagglutination extant when a polyagglutinable blood sample is studied. Given the role of bacterially and virally produced enzymes in causing polyagglutination it is not at all surprising that one organism can produce more than one activating enzyme or that persons with infections have more than one type of organism present. Some typical examples of mixed forms of polyagglutination are: T and Tk (55); T, Tk and acquired B (63,332); T, Th and acquired B (294); Tk and acquired B (214,286,289,331,337); Tk and VA (288); Th and Tn (190,197). References to papers that deal with the specificity of enzymes made by various bacteria and viruses and the structures that some of those enzymes hydrolyse are 295-302,346-349.

Polyagglutination: A Classification

In a 1971 publication (331) a classification for various forms of polyagglutination was proposed. Although the classification has not been widely used and has not been expanded as new forms of polyagglutination have been described, it is used in a number of papers cited in this chapter. Accordingly, it will be mentioned that in the classification: type I polyagglutination is T-activation; type II is Tn-polyagglutination; type III is polyagglutination associated with acquired B but was later (214) used to describe Tk-activation; and type IV is Cad-polyagglutination.

Hereditary Erythroblastic Multinuclearity with a Positive Acidified Serum Lysis Test (HEMPAS)

As its name implies, HEMPAS is an inherited disorder of erythropoiesis, it is also known as congenital dyserythropoietic anemia, type II or CDA II. The reason for including HEMPAS in this chapter is that the red cells of patients with the disorder are agglutinated at 22°C and/or lysed at 37°C by about one third of normal sera.

After the initial descriptions of the clinical disorder (350-356) appeared, other cases were soon described (357-362). At first it seemed that HEMPAS red cells have enhanced expression of both I and i and reduced expression of H. However, it eventually became apparent that while the i of HEMPAS red cells is much increased, the apparent increase in I represents efficiency of the red cells in binding antibody and efficiency of the bound antibody in activating complement (353,373). It is now accepted (363) that while the i antigen of HEMPAS red cells is more strongly expressed than in the i adult and i cord phenotypes, there is no depression of I as is seen on i adult and i cord red cells. The depression of H has been confirmed (358).

As mentioned, some 30% of sera from adults agglutinate or hemolyze HEMPAS red cells. At first it was not clear whether this reactivity represented the actions of more potent than usual anti-i and/or anti-I in some sera, or what could be regarded as a polyagglutinin. That the latter explanation obtains is now apparent from two major lines of investigation. First, the antibody that has been called anti-HEMPAS (352) can be adsorbed by HEMPAS cells but not by normal cells (that would, of course, adsorb anti-I and anti-i) (355). Second, anti-HEMPAS is found in about one third of normal sera but never in the serum of a patient with HEMPAS. It is the presence of anti-HEMPAS in about one third of normal sera that results in HEMPAS red cells being regarded as being polyagglutinable (364). Because sera that lack anti-HEMPAS (at least in serologically-detectable levels) can be found, this type of polyagglutination does not cause such acute blood typing problems as those that arise when some of the other forms of polyagglutination described in this chapter are encountered.

Many studies (357,365-368) have been performed in attempts to identify the membrane abnormality of HEMPAS red cells. Mawby et al. (369) produced evidence for incomplete glycosylation of, at least, the membrane associated sialoglycoproteins (MN and Ss SGPs, et al.) and the anion transport protein (band 3), similar findings were reported by Fukuda et al. (370,374). More recently Fukuda et al. (375,376) and Fukuda (371) have described decreased activity of an N-acetylglucosaminyl-transferase that normally serves to effect branching in complex N-glycans of glycoproteins. Like Mawby et al. (370), Fukuda (371) pointed out that the structures most affected were those N-glycans attached to band 3 and 4.5 that contain repeating N-acetyllactosamine structures. It was concluded (371) that the reduced amount of branching resulted in an increase of i because of the increase of linear N-acetyl-

lactosaminylceramides and exposure of a cryptantigen recognized by the polyagglutinin that has been called anti-HEMPAS. Fukuda et al. (372) also found a HEMPAS patient who had a defect in a gene that encodes production of an alpha-mannosidase. It was suggested that HEMPAS may represent a heterogeneous collection of abnormalities of glycosylation of red cell membrane components.

Lectins

As will be abundantly clear by now, a very large number of different lectins are of use in the rapid identification of some types of polyagglutination. However, Bird (146) has warned against the exclusive use of these reagents in identification of the type of polyagglutination extant. He has pointed out that detailed serological comparisons with known examples of various polyagglutinable red cells are also necessary. As an example, Bird (146) mentioned that red cells coated with group C streptococci (or another bacterial polysaccharide of similar structure) are agglutinated by *Salvia sclarea* lectin so can be mistaken for Tn-polyagglutinable cells. Somewhat similarly, Bird (145) pointed out elsewhere that because polyagglutination can occur as a result of the adsorption of bacterial products by red cells and the presence in many sera of antibodies directed against bacteria, misclassification could occur if lectins alone or perhaps if sera alone were used in the tests.

Garratty et al. (377) identified another problem that can occur when lectins are used. They studied a case of strong in vitro T-activation in a contaminated sample (and confirmed their observations by using red cells deliberately T-activated in vitro) in which the red cells initially reacted with *Arachis hypogea*, *Glycine soja*, *Salvia sclarea* and *Salvia horminum*. They were able to show that the two *Salvia* lectins reacted not because the red cells had Tn or Cad antigens exposed but because the lectins had been prepared in a solution that included Tween and bovine serum albumin as potentiators. When the red cells were tested with non-commercially prepared *Salvia* lectins, that were made in phosphate buffered saline without potentiators, they were non-reactive. Clearly the use of potentiators to enhance agglutination by lectins introduces the danger that the lectins will no longer react with the expected specificity.

As will have been noticed, the lectin *Glycine soja* (*G. max*) is useful as a screening reagent when certain types of polyagglutination are suspected. As mentioned earlier in this chapter, the usefulness of this lectin stems from the fact that it agglutinates red cells that have a reduced level of sialic acid. However, Judd (20,25) has pointed out that the actions of the lectin are not quite that simple. *G. soja* agglutinates T and Tn-polyagglutinable and protease-treated red cells, all of which have reduced levels of sialic acid. It does not agglutinate M^g+ red cells that also have a reduced sialic acid level (see Chapter 15) perhaps because the reduction is too small. However, the lectin does agglutinate Cad+ red cells, on which the sialic acid level is almost normal (269). *G. soja* also agglutinates HEMPAS red cells (25).

Several workers have pointed out that it is sometimes difficult to compare results obtained with lectins in different laboratories and that some sort of standardization would be helpful. Bird (145) has commented that such standardization is not easy since different batches of seeds yield different levels of activity. Further, different extraction methods exist as well as different methods of using the lectins. In this same thoughtful discussion, Bird (145) pointed out that highly concentrated lectins are more likely to cross-react than are dilute preparations and that during storage, lectins may become stronger because the extraction process continues.

Judd (25) has described methods for the preparation of purified lectins and has discussed the advantages of using those preparations instead of crude saline extracts of seeds. Since albumin and Tween 20 are used in the diluent, it is again important that the lectin specificity be carefully established in titration studies and that an appropriate dilution be used to ensure the required reactivity (25,145,335).

Warnings of pitfalls that can arise when lectins are used are intended to enhance the usefulness of those reagents and should not be construed in any way as discouragement for the use of lectins. Because of the enormous value of these reagents in the study of polyagglutination, regular reviews about them are published. Reviews by Bird (23,145,146,154,397), Bird and Wingham (255) and by Judd (12,20,25,66) that have been cited many times in this chapter provide valuable information. Data about some other lectins will be found in the papers listed as references 378 to 395. It has been postulated (396) that the production of lectins by plants is under genetic control.

Table 42-3 lists the reactions of some lectins with polyagglutinable red cells of various types. Obviously, the table is not all inclusive. Those lectins whose reactions are shown are useful in the differentiation of one type of polyagglutination from others. In many instances a different lectin could be substituted and would be just as useful. In many other instances, additional information could be obtained by the use of still more lectins. In table 42-3, the various types of polyagglutination are listed in a sequence that reflects their causative mechanism. First are those caused by microbial enzymes, i.e., T, Tk, Th, Tx, VA and acquired B; then Tn as representing incomplete biosynthesis of an oligosaccharide following somatic mutation and finally the inherited forms, i.e., Cad, NOR, HbM-Hyde Park and HEMPAS. Lectins are grouped by seed source, as

will be seen botanical relationships are not necessarily reflected by reaction specificities, see particularly the three *Vicia* lectins. Their cousin, *Vicia graminea*, is so different again that it appears in Chapter 15 but not in table 42-3.

Animal Bites

One of the themes in this Chapter has been the effect of enzymes produced by bacteria in infected individuals. It may not be widely appreciated by blood bankers but a major source of infections are from wounds caused by animal bites (398). In a report on one patient bitten by a lion and another bitten by a tiger, Burdge et al. (399) point out that *Pasteurella* species are commensals of feline mouths. Some workers may remember that *Yersinia pestis* was previously *Pasteurella pestis*, we wonder if anyone had the good fortune to survive a tiger bite only to have the misfortune to develop bubonic plague? While *Pasteurella multocida* wound infections occur frequently following dog and domestic cat bites (398,400-405) they have also been reported following lion (399,406,407), tiger (399), lynx (400) and panther (408) bites. Burdge et al. (399) comment that the low number of reports of *P. multocida* infections following encounters with large cats probably reflects the infrequency of survival following such encounters. While *P. multocida*, *E. coli*, *Staphylococcus aureus*, *Staphylococcus epidermis*, other *Pasteurella* and *Ancinetobacter* species have all been found to infect animal bite wounds, we were not able to find an account of one causing polyagglutination (it could have happened!). Thus this section joins this chapter as a fine example of poetic license; after all, the chapter was rather long and somewhat dull.

References

1. Bird GWG. Blut 1970;21:336
2. Bird GWG. Nouv Rev Fr Hematol 1971;11:885
3. Buskila D, Levene C, Bird GWG, et al. Vox Sang 1987;52:99
4. Lind PE, MacArthur NR. Austral J Exp Biol Med Sci 1947;25:247
5. Klenk E. Angewandte Chemie 1956;68:349
6. Lalezari P, Spaet TH. J Lab Clin Med 1961;57:868
7. Lalezari P. Transfusion 1968;8:372
8. Greenwalt TJ, Pepper DS, Etoh N, et al. Transfusion 1969;9:289
9. Khan MY, Zinneman HH. Am J Clin Pathol 1970;54;715
10. Issitt PD. In: A Seminar on Problems Encountered in Pretransfusion Tests. Washington, D.C.:Am Assoc Blood Banks, 1972:81
11. Moulds JJ. In: Polyagglutination. Washington, D.C.:Am Assoc Blood Banks, 1980:1
12. Judd WJ. Immunohematology 1992;8:58
13. Metaxas MN, Metaxas-Bühler M, Ikin EW. Vox Sang 1968;15:102

TABLE 42-3 Reactions of Polyagglutinable Red Cells with Lectins and Other Reagents

Reagent[1,2]	T	Tk	Th	Tx	VA	AcqB	Tn	Cad	NOR	HbM[3]	HEMPAS	Group 0 Control
Human serum[4]	+	+	+	+	+[5]	+	+	+	+[5]	+	+[6]	0
A. hypogea	+	+[7]	+	+	0	0	0	0	0	(+)	0	0
A. hypogea PFTC[8]	+	+↑	+↓	+	0	0	0	0	0		0	0
G. soja (*G. max*)[9]	+	0	0	0	0	0	+	+	0	(+)	+	0[9]
S. sclarea	0	0	0	0	0	0	+[10]	0	0	0	0	0
S. horminum	0	0	0	0	0	0	+	+	0	(+)	0	0
D. biflorus[11]	0	0[12]	0	0	0	[12]	+	+	0	0	0	0[11]
H. pomatia[11]	+	0[12]	+		+	[12]	+	+	0	+	+	0[11]
G. simplicifolia I[13,14]	0	0	0	0	0	+	+	0	0	0	0	0
G. simplicifolia II[15]	0	+	0	0	0	0	0	0	0	+	0	0
V. cretica	+	0	+	0	0	0	0	0	0	(+)	0	0
V. villosa	+	0	0				+	+		+		0
V. hyrcanica	+	+	+				0	0		+		0
M. disciformis	+	0	+	0			0			+		0
M. candidissium[16]	0	0	0				+	0				0
L. cardiaca	0[17]	0	0	0	0	0	0[17]	+	0	0	0	0
C. scoparius	+	0	0				+	0				0
P. lunatus[18]	0	0	0	0	0	+	0	0	0		0	0

Blank spaces in the table indicate that the information has not been reported.

[1] Not all samples need to be tested with all reagents. Selected reagents should be used based on initial findings.

[2] For full names of reagents see text.

[3] Hemoglobin M Hyde Park (see text).

[4] From adults, ABO compatible, non-reactive in antibody-screening tests.

[5] A high percentage of normal sera will react weaker or not at all, than with other forms of polyagglutinable red cells.

[6] Only about one-third will react.

[7] In one report (317) *A. hypogea* was said to react with red cells Tk-activated with a *B. fragilis*-derived enzyme but not with those Tk-activated with an *E. freundii*-derived enzyme.

[8] Reactions of *A. hypogea* after test red cells have been treated with papain or ficin (standard solutions). +↑= enhanced reactivity, +↓= decreased reactivity, + = unchanged reactivity.

[9] Reactive with protease-treated red cells including those that are not polyagglutinable. *Glycine soja* is also known as soybean lectin.

[10] Non-reactive after red cells have been treated with a protease.

[11] Reactions shown are for group 0 and group B red cells when lectin is used at a dilution at which it behaves as anti-A$_1$.

[12] May be reactive with red cells on which deacetylation of A has occurred.

[13] *Griffonia simplicifolia* lectin I, previously *Bandeiraea simplicifolia* lectin I.

[14] Reactions with group A and group 0 cells shown, lectin agglutinates group B cells.

[15] *Griffonia simplicifolia* lectin II, previously *Bandeiraea simplicifolia* lectin II.

[16] Apparently a good substitute for *S. sclarea*.

[17] Undiluted lectin reacts weakly with T and Tn-activated red cells. When diluted appropriately, lectin behaves as anti-Cad.

[18] *Phaseolus lunatus* is also known as lima bean lectin.

14. Judd WJ. Methods in Immunohematology, 2nd Ed. Durham:Montgomery, 1994
15. Issitt PD, Issitt CH, Moulds J, et al. Transfusion 1972;12:217
16. Huebner G. Z Immun Forsch 1925;45:223
17. Thomsen O. Z Immun Forsch 1927;52:85
18. Friedenreich V. The Thomsen Haemagglutination Phenomenon. Copenhagen:Munksgaard, 1930
19. Uhlenbruck G, Pardoe GI, Bird GWG. Z Immun Forsch 1969;138:423
20. Judd WJ. In: Critical Reviews in Clinical Laboratory Sciences, Vol 12. Boca Raton:CRC Press, 1980:171
21. Beck ML. Unpublished observations 1979 cited in Judd WJ. In: Critical Reviews in Clinical Laboratory Sciences, Vol 12. Boca Raton:CRC Press, 1980:171
22. Levene C, Levene NA, Buskila D, et al. Transf Med Rev 1988;2:176
23. Bird GWG. Transf Med Rev 1989;3:55
24. Bird GWG, Wingham J, Beck ML, et al. Lancet 1978;1:1215
25. Judd WJ. Transfusion 1979;19:768
26. Bangham AD, Flemans R, Heard DH, et al. Nature 1958;183:642
27. Lotan R, Skutelsky E, Danon D, et al. J Biol Chem 1975;250:8518
28. Anstee DJ, Spring FA. Transf Med Rev 1989;3:13
29. Anstee DJ. Vox Sang 1990;58:1
30. Anstee DJ. J Immunogenet 1990;17:219
31. Tomita M, Marschesi VT. Proc Nat Acad Sci USA 1975;72:2964
32. Thomas DB, Winzler RJ. J Biol Chem 1969;244:5493
33. Furthmayr H. Nature 1978;271:519
34. Dahr W, Gielen W, Beyreuther K, et al. Hoppe-Seyler's Z Physiol Chem 1980;361:145
35. Dahr W, Beyreuther K, Steinbach H, et al. Hoppe-Seyler's Z Physiol Chem 1980;361:895
36. Vengelen-Tyler V, Anstee DJ, Issitt PD, et al. Transfusion 1981;21:1
37. Langley JW, Issitt PD, Anstee DJ, et al. Transfusion 1981;21:15
38. Anstee DJ. In: Immunobiology of the Erythrocyte. New York:Liss, 1980:67
39. Kim YD. Vox Sang 1980;39:162
40. Boorman KE, Loutit JF, Steabben DB. Nature 1946;158:446
41. Loghem JJ van, Hart M van der, Heier AM. Bull Cen Lab Bledtr Ned Rode Kruis 1951;1:43
42. Reepmaker J. J Clin Pathol 1952;5:266
43. Stratton F. Vox Sang (Old Series) 1954;4:58
44. Hendry PIA, Simmons RT. Med J Austral 1955;1:720
45. Loghem JJ van, Hart M van der, Land ME. Vox Sang (Old Series) 1955;5:125
46. Stratton F, Renton PH. Practical Blood Grouping. Oxford:Blackwell, 1958
47. Chorpenning FW, Hayes JC. Vox Sang 1959;4:210
48. Jorgensen JR. Vox Sang 1967;13:225
49. Beck ML. Transfusion 1968;8:109
50. Rickard KA, Robinson RJ, Worlledge SM. Arch Dis Childh 1969;44:102
51. Beck ML, Marsh WL. Vox Sang 1970;19:91
52. Beck ML. Med Lab Technol 1972;29:55
53. Gray JM, Beck ML, Oberman HA. Vox Sang 1972;22:379
54. Bird T, Stephenson J. J Clin Pathol 1973;26:868
55. Inglis G, Bird GWG, Mitchell AAB, et al. Vox Sang 1975;28:314
56. Moores P, Pudifin D, Patel PL. Transfusion 1975;15:329
57. Marsh S. Canad J Med Technol 1975;37:129
58. Tanaka H, Okubo Y, Yamaguchi H, et al. Ann Paediat Jpn 1977;23:48
59. Wilson J. Am J Med Technol 1977;43:147
60. Klein PJ, Bulla M, Newman RA, et al. Lancet 1977;2:1024
61. Obeid D, Bird GWG, Wingham J. J Clin Pathol 1977;30:953
62. Heddle NM, Blajchman MA, Bonder N, et al. (abstract). Transfusion 1977;176:686
63. Judd WJ, McGuire-Mallory D, Anderson KM, et al. Transfusion 1979;19:293
64. Poschmann A, Fisher K. Lancet 1979;1:824
65. Perkash A, Carlson A, Ellisor S. Transfusion 1980;20:301
66. Judd WJ. In: Polyagglutination. Washington, D.C.:Am Assoc Blood Banks, 1980:23
67. Seger R, Joller P, Baerlocher K, et al. Helv Pediat Acta 1980;35:359
68. Mullard GW, Thompson IH, Lee D, et al. Clin Lab Haematol 1981;3:357
69. Seger R, Joller P, Bird GWG, et al. Helv Pediat Acta 1980;35:121
70. Judd WJ, Oberman HA, Flynn S. (Letter). Transfusion 1982;22:345
71. Rawlinson VI, Stratton F. Vox Sang 1984;46:306
72. Levene C, Sela R, Blat J, et al. Transfusion 1986;26:243
73. Pisacka M, Stambergova M. Vox Sang 1994;66:300
74. Seger R, Kenny A, Bird GWG, et al. J Pediat Surg 1981;16:905
75. Francis T Jr. J Exp Med 1947;85:1
76. Marsh WL. Vox Sang 1960;5:387
77. Gunson HH, Stratton F, Mullard GW. Br J Haematol 1970;18:309
78. Kline WE, Issitt CH. (abstract). Transfusion 1976;16:527
79. Springer GF, Tegtmeyer H. Br J Haematol 1981;47:453
80. Springer GF, Codington JF, Jeanloz RW. J Nat Cancer Inst 1972;49:1469
81. Springer GF, Desai PR. Ann Clin Lab Sci 1974;4:294
82. Springer GF, Desai PR, Banatwala I. Naturwissenschaften 1974;61:457
83. Springer GF, Desai PR, Banatwala I. J Nat Cancer Inst 1975;54:335
84. Springer GF, Desai PR. Naturwissenschaften 1975;62:587
85. Springer GF, Murthy MS, Desai PR, et al. In: Proceedings of the Third International Symposium on the Detection and Prevention of Cancer. New York:Dekker, 1976
86. Springer GF, Desai PR, Scanlon EF. Cancer 1976;37:169
87. Springer GF, Murthy MS, Desai PR, et al. Naturwissenschaften 1976;63:300
88. Springer GF, Desai PR, Yang HJ, et al. In: Human Blood Groups. Karger:Basel, 1977:179
89. Springer GF, Desai PR, Yang HJ, et al. Clin Immunol Immunopathol 1977;7:426
90. Desai PR, Springer GF, McNeil C. Fed Proc 1977;36:1254
91. Springer GF, Desai PR, Murthy MS, et al. Prog Allgy 1979;26:42
92. Springer GF, Murthy MS, Desai PR, et al. Prot Biol Fluids 1979;27 Coll:211
93. Springer GF, Desai PR, Murthy MS, et al. Transfusion 1979;19:233
94. Springer GF, Desai PR, Murthy MS. In: Comprehensive Assays in the Immunodiagnosis of Human Cancer. Netherlands:Elsevier, 1979:97
95. Springer GF, Murthy MS, Desai PR. In: Comprehensive Assays in the Immunodiagnosis of Human Cancer. Netherlands:Elsevier, 1979:457
96. Springer GF, Desai PR, Murthy MS, et al. In: Comprehensive Assays in the Immunodiagnosis of Human Cancer. Netherlands:Elsevier, 1979:467

97. Springer GF, Desai PR, Scanlon EF. Glycocon Res 1979;2:941

98. Springer GF, Desai PR, Murthy MS, et al. Klin Woch 1979;57:961

99. Springer GF, Desai PR, Murthy MS, et al. J Surg Oncol 1979;11:95

100. Springer GF, Tegtmeyer H. Naturwissenschaften 1980;67:317

101. Springer GF, Yang HJ, Mbawa E. Naturwissenschaften 1980;67:473

102. Springer GF, Murthy MS, Desai PR, et al. Breast 1981;7:24

103. Springer GF, Desai PR, Fry WA, et al. In: Cellular Oncology, Vol 1. New York:Praeger, 1983:99

104. Springer GF, Science 1984;224:1198

105. Metcalfe S, Springer GF, Svvennsen RJ, et al. Prot Biol Fluids 1985;32:765

106. Clausen H, Stroud M, Parker J, et al. Mol Immunol 1988;25:199

107. Schlepper-Schäfer J, Springer GF. Biochim Biophys Acta 1989;89:266

108. Barr N, Taylor CR, Young T, et al. Cancer 1989;64:834

109. Springer GF, Desai PR, Wise W, et al. In: Immunodiagnosis of Cancer, 2nd Ed. New York:Marcel Dekker, 1990:587

110. Howard DR, Taylor CR. Cancer 1979;43:2279

111. Howard DR, Taylor CR. Oncology 1980;37:142

112. Cooper HS, Reuter VE. Lab Invest 1983;49:655

113. Holt S, Wilkinson A, Suresh MR, et al. Cancer Lett 1984;25:55

114. Böker W, Kalubert A, Bahnsen J, et al. Virchows Arch (Pathol Anat) 1984;403:149

115. Altavilla G, Lanza G Jr, Rossi S, et al. Tumori 1984;70:539

116. Seitz SC, Fisher K, Stegner HE, et al. Cancer 1984;54:830

117. Ghazizadeh M, Kagawa S, Izumi K, et al. J Urol 1984;132:1127

118. Ohoka H, Shinomiya H, Yokoyama M, et al. Urol Res 1985;13:47

119. Ørntoft TF, Mors NPO, Eriksen G, et al. Cancer Res 1985;45:447

120. Ghazizadeh M, Kagawa S, Kurokawa K. J Urol 1985;133:762

121. Schneider AW, Fisher K, Stegner HE, et al. Tumor Diag Ther 1986;7:78

122. Yuan M, Itzkowitz SH, Boland CR, et al. Cancer Res 1986;46:4841

123. Weinstein RS, Schwartz D, Coon JS. In: New Concepts in Neoplasia as Applied to Diagnostic Pathology (Int Acad Pathol Monograph 27) Baltimore:Williams and Wilkins, 1986:255

124. Kellokumpu I, Kellokumpu S, Andersson LC. Br J Cancer 1987;55:361

125. Longenecker BM, Williams DJ, MacLean GD, et al. J Nat Cancer Inst 1987;78:489

126. Yokoyama M, Ohoka H, Oda H, et al. Acta Urol Jpn 1988;34:255

127. Blasco E, Torrado J, Belloso L, et al. Cancer 1988;61:1091

128. Stein R, Chen S, Grossman W, et al. Cancer Res 1989;49:32

129. Itzkowitz SH, Yuan M, Montgomery CK, et al. Cancer Res 1989;49:197

130. Ghazizadeh M, Oguro T, Sasaki Y, et al. Am J Clin Pathol 1990;93:315

131. Hicklin BL, Beck ML. (abstract). Transfusion 1974;14:508

132. Novogrodsky A, Lotan R, Ravid A, et al. J Immunol 1975;115:1243

133. Winchester RJ, Fu SM, Kunkel HG. J Immunol 1975;114:410

134. Hysell JK, Hysell JW, Nichols ME, et al. Vox Sang 1976;31 (Suppl 1):9

135. Judson PA, Anstee DJ. Prot Biol Fluids 1979;27th Coll:871

136. Dunstan RA, Simpson MB, Nichols M, et al. (abstract). Transfusion 1983;23;416

137. Bird GWG. Vox Sang 1964;9:748

138. Judd WJ, Issitt PD, Pavone BG. Transfusion 1979;19:7

139. Judd WJ, Issitt PD, Pavone BG, et al. Transfusion 1979;19:12

140. Issitt PD, Wilkinson SL. Transfusion 1981;21:493

141. Issitt PD, Wilkinson SL. Transfusion 1983;23:117

142. Roelcke D. Transf Med Rev 1989;3:140

143. Roelcke D. In: Immunobiology of Transfusion Medicine. New York:Marcel Dekker, 1994:69

144. Beck ML. Unpublished observations 1971 cited in Issitt PD. In: A Seminar on Problems Encountered in Pretransfusion Tests. Washington, D.C.:Am Assoc Blood Banks, 1972:81

145. Bird GWG. In: Polyagglutination. Washington, D.C.:Am Assoc Blood Banks, 1980:71

146. Bird GWG. In: Plenary Session Lectures, 27th Cong ISH, 15th Cong ISBT. Paris:Arnette, 1978:97

147. Lauf PK. In: Human Blood Groups. Karger:Basel, 1977:383

148. Havens PL, O'Rouke PP, Hahn J, et al. Am J Dis Childh 1988;142:961

149. Cleary TG, Lopez EL. Pediat Infect Dis J 1989;8:720

150. Milford DV, Taylor CM, Guttridge B, et al. Arch Dis Childh 1990;65:716

151. Fischer K, Poschmann A. Monat Kinderheilkd 1971;119:2

152. Fischer K, Poschmann A, Vongjirad A. Proc 16th Cong Dtsch Ges Hamat, Bad Neuheim, 1972

153. Poschmann A, Fisher K. Med Klin 1974;69:1821

154. Bird GWG. In: Blood Groups and Other Red Cell Surface Markers in Health and Disease. New York:Masson, 1982:55

155. Hamilton DV, Black AJ, Darnborough J, et al. Clin Lab Haematol 1983;5:109

156. Lerner RG, Rapaport SI, Meltzer J. Ann Intern Med 1967;66:1180

157. Berkowitz LR, Dalldorf FG, Blatt PM. J Am Med Assoc 1979;241:1709

158. Berberich FR, Cuene SA, Chard RL, et al. J Pediat 1974;84:503

159. Gottschall JL, Pisciotta AV, Darin J, et al. Sem Thromb Hemost 1981;7:25

160. Harkness DR, Byrnes JJ, Lian ELY, et al. J Am Med Assoc 1981;246:1931

161. Shepard KV, Bukowski RM. Sem Hematol 1987;24:178

162. Byrnes JJ, Moake JL, Klug P, et al. Am J Hematol 1990;34:169

163. Rock GA, Shumak KH, Buskard NA, et al. New Eng J Med 1991;325:393

164. Bell WR, Braine HG, Ness PM, et al. New Eng J Med 1991;325:398

165. Obrador GT, Zeigler ZR, Shadduck RK, et al. Am J Hematol 1993;42:217

166. Hayward CPM, Sutton DMC, Carter JR, et al. Arch Int Med 1994;154:982

167. Beck ML. In: Blood Group Antigens and Disease. Arlington, VA:Am Assoc Blood Banks, 1983:45

168. Moreau R, Dausset J, Bernard J, et al. Bull Soc Med Hop Paris 1957;73:569

169. Dausset J, Moullec J, Bernard J. Blood 1959;14:1079

170. Chorpenning FW, Dodd MC. Vox Sang 1965;10:460

171. Berman HJ, Smarto J, Issitt CH, et al. Transfusion 1971;12:35

172. Bird GWG, Shinton NK, Wingham J. Br J Haematol 1971;21:443

173. Jiji RM, Jahn EFW, Bilenki LA. (abstract). Transfusion 1973;13:359

174. Moore BPL, Marsh S, Laschinger C, et al. Transfusion 1975;15:54

175. Bird GWG, Wingham J, Pippard MJ, et al. Br J Haematol 1976;33:289
176. Kourteva BT, Manolova VR, Mitova DK. Transfusion 1977;12:272
177. Beck ML, Hicklin BL, Pierce SR, et al. Med Lab Sci 1977;34:325
178. Cartron JP, Cartron J, Andreu G, et al. Lancet 1978;1:856
179. Cartron JP, Andreu G, Cartron J, et al. Eur J Biochem 1978;92:111
180. Berger EG, Kozdrowski I. FEBS Lett 1978;93:105
181. Ness PM, Garratty G, Morel PA, et al. Blood 1979;54:30
182. Laird B, Moulds JJ, Werner D, et al. (abstract). Transfusion 1979;19:642
183. Baldwin ML, Barrasso C, Ridolfi RL. Am J Clin Pathol 1979;72:1024
184. Cartron JP, Nurden AT. Nature 1979;282:621
185. Jiji RM. (Letter). Blood 1979;54:1451
186. Wilson MJ, Cott ME, Sotus PC. (abstract). Transfusion 1980;20:622
187. Vainchenker W, Testa U, Deschamps JF, et al. J Clin Invest 1982;69:1081
188. Cartron JP, Blanchard D, Nurden A, et al. In: Blood Groups and Other Red Cell Surface Markers in Health and Disease. New York:Masson, 1982:39
189. Rose RR, Skradski KJ, Polesky HF, et al. (abstract). Transfusion 1983;23:422
190. Schultz M, Fortes P, Brewer L, et al. (abstract). Transfusion 1983;23:422
191. Hirohashi S, Clausen H, Yamada T, et al. Proc Nat Acad Sci USA 1985;82:7039
192. Bird GWG, Wingham J, Richardson SGN. Haematologia Comm 1985;18:99
193. Roxby DJ, Skinner JM, Morley AA, et al. Br J Cancer 1987;56:734
194. Springer GF, Chandrasekaran EV, Desai PR, et al. Carbohyd Res 1988;178:271
195. Takahashi HK, Metoki R, Hakomori S. Cancer Res 1988;48:4361
196. Kjeldsten T, Hakomori S, Springer GF, et al. Vox Sang 1989;57:81
197. Janvier D, Guignier F, Reviron M, et al. Vox Sang 1991;61:142
198. Blumenfeld OO, Lalezari P, Khorshidi M, et al. Blood 1992;80:2388
199. Roxby DJ, Pfeiffer MB, Morley AA, et al. Transfusion 1992;32:834
200. Freiesleben E, Jensen KG, Knudsen EE. Proc 8th Cong Eur Soc Hematol, part 2. Basel:Karger, 1961:506
201. Sturgeon PD, McQuiston T, Sparkes R, et al. Blood 1969;33:507
202. Sanger R, Race RR, Nevanlinna H, et al. (Letter). Blood 1970;35:883
203. Haynes CR, Dorner I, Leonard GL, et al. Transfusion 1970;10:43
204. Myllylä G, Furuhjelm U, Nordling S, et al. Vox Sang 1971;20:7
205. Lalezari P, Al-Mondhiry H. Br J Haematol 1973;25:399
206. Dahr W, Uhlenbruck G, Bird GWG. Vox Sang 1974;27:29
207. Dahr W, Uhlenbruck G, Gunson HH, et al. Vox Sang 1975;28:249
208. Springer GF, Desai PR. Carbohyd Res 1975;40:183
209. Murphy LA. Unpublished observations 1977 cited in Judd WJ. Critical Reviews in Clinical Laboratory Sciences, Vol 12. Boca Raton:CRC Press, 1980:171
210. Hayes CE, Goldstein IJ. J Biol Chem 1974;249:1904
211. Judd WJ, Steiner EA, Friedman BA, et al. Vox Sang 1976;30:261
212. Iyer PN, Wilkinson KD, Goldstein IJ. Arch Biochem Biophys 1976;177:330
213. Murphy LA, Goldstein IJ. J Biol Chem 1977;252:4739
214. Judd WJ, Beck ML, Hicklin BL, et al. Vox Sang 1977;33:246
215. Judd WJ, Murphy LA, Goldstein IJ, et al. Transfusion 1978;18:274
216. Bird GWG, Wingham J. Lancet 1973;1:677
217. Bird GWG, Wingham J. Vox Sang 1974;26:163
218. Bird GWG, Wingham J. Vox Sang 1976;30:217
219. Bird GWG, Wingham J. Vox Sang 1977;32:121
220. Lockyer WJ, Gold ER, Bird GWG. Med Lab Sci 1977;34:311
221. Bird GWG, Wingham J. Clin Lab Haematol 1980;2:21
222. Bird GWG, Wingham J. Clin Lab Haematol 1981;3:169
223. Bird GWG, Wingham J. (Letter). Blood Transf Immunohematol 1981;24:347
224. Yang EKL, Spence LR, Harding RY, et al. Transfusion 1982;22:338
225. Bird GWG. Unpublished observations 1981 cited in Yang EKL, Spence LR, Harding RY, et al. Transfusion 1982;22:338
226. Bird GWG, Wingham J, Chester GH, et al. Br J Haematol 1976;33:295
227. Roxby DJ, Morley AA, Burpee M. Br J Haematol 1987;67:153
228. Rahman AFR, Longenecker BM. J Immunol 1982;129:2021
229. Seitz R, Fischer K, Poschmann A. Rev Fr Transf Immunohematol 1983;26:420
230. Bigbee WL, Langlois RG, Stanker LH, et al. Cytometry 1990;11:261
231. Numata Y, Nakada H, Fukui S, et al. Biochem Biophys Res Comm 1990;170:981
232. King MJ, Parsons SF, Wu AM, et al. Transfusion 1991;31:142
233. Boccardi V, Attina D, Bigliocchi S, et al. Vox Sang 1974;26:83
234. Boccardi V, Attina D, Girelli G. Vox Sang 1974;27:268
235. Cazal P, Monis M, Caubel J, et al. Rev Fr Transf 1968;11:209
236. Cazel P, Monis M, Bizot M. Rev Fr Transf 1971;14:321
237. Sringarm S, Chupungart C, Giles CM. Vox Sang 1972;23:537
238. Sringarm S, Chiewsilp P, Tubrod J. Vox Sang 1974;26:462
239. Yamaguchi H, Okubo Y, Ogawa Y, et al. Vox Sang 1973;25:361
240. Lopez M, Gerbal A, Bony V, et al. Vox Sang 1975;28:305
241. Bird GWG, Wingham J. Vox Sang 1971;20:55
242. Uhlenbruck G, Sprenger I, Heggen M, et al. Z Immun Forsch 1971;141:209
243. Bird GWG, Wingham J. Vox Sang 1972;22:362
244. Bird GWG, Wingham J. J Immunogenet 1976;3:297
245. Lopez M, Gerbal A, Girard-Debord M, et al. Rev Fr Transf Immunohematol 1977;20:457
246. Gerbal A, Lopez M, Chassaign M, et al. Rev Fr Transf 1976;19:415
247. Cazel P, Monis M, Bizot M. Rev Fr Transf Immunohematol 1977;20:165
248. Ellisor SS, Sugasawara E, Dean WD, et al. (abstract). Transfusion 1981;21:626
249. Leger R, Garratty G, Lines E, et al. (abstract). Transfusion 1994;34 (Suppl 10S):23S
250. Leger R, Lines E, Cunningham K, et al. Immunohematology 1996;12:69
251. Sanger R, Gavin J, Tippett P, et al. Lancet 1971;1:1130
252. Bird GWG. Curr Sci 1951;20:298
253. Morgan WTJ, Watkins WM. Br J Exp Pathol 1953;34:94
254. Williams MA, Voak D. Br J Haematol 1972;23:427
255. Bird GWG, Wingham J. In: Techniques in Clinical

Immunology. Oxford:Blackwell, 1977:43

256. Hammarstrom D, Murphy LA, Goldstein IJ, et al. Biochemistry 1977;16:2750

257. Etzler ME. Glycocon J 1994;11:395

258. Imberty A, Casset F, Gregg CV, et al. Glycocon J 1994;11:400

259. King MJ, Chan A, Roe R, et al. Glycobiol 1994;4:267

260. Bird GWG, Wingham J. Clin Lab Haematol 1979;1:57

261. Bizot M, Cayla JP. Rev Fr Transf 1972;15:195

262. Bizot M. Rev Fr Transf 1972;15:371

263. Gerbal A, Lopez M, Maslet C, et al. Haematologia 1976;10:383

264. Cartron J-P, Blanchard D. Biochem J 1982;207:497

265. Blanchard D, Cartron J-P, Fournet B, et al. J Biol Chem 1983;258:7691

266. Herkt F, Parente JP, Leroy Y, et al. Eur J Biochem 1985;146:125

267. Cartron JP, Prou O, Luilier M, et al. Br J Haematol 1983;55:639

268. Pasvol G, Wainscoat JS, Weatherall DJ. Nature 1982;297:64

269. Race RR, Sanger R. Blood Groups in Man, 6th Ed. Oxford:Blackwell, 1975:395

270. Morgan WTJ, Soh CPC, Donald ASR, et al. Blood Transf Immunohematol 1981;24:37

271. Soh CPC, Morgan WTJ, Watkins WM, et al. Biochem Biophys Res Comm 1980;93:1132

272. Donald ASR, Soh CPC, Watkins WM, et al. Biochem Biophys Res Comm 1982;104:58

273. Donald ASR, Yates AD, Soh CPC, et al. Biochem Biophys Res Comm 1983;115:625

274. Williams J, Marshall RD, Halbeek H van, et al. Carbohydr Res 1984;134:141

275. Donald ASR, Yates AD, Soh CPC, et al. Biochem Soc Transact 1984;12:596

276. Donald ASR, Feeney J. Biochem J 1986;236:821

277. Donald ASR, Soh CPC, Yates AD, et al. Biochem Soc Transact 1987;15:606

278. Watkins W. In: Blood Cell Biochemistry, Vol 6. New York:Plenum, 1995

279. Duffy FA, Marshall RD. Biochem Soc Transact 1985;13:1128

280. Marshesi VT, Furthmayr H, Tomita M. Ann Rev Biochem 1976;45:667

281. Serafini-Cessi F, Malagolini N, Dall'Olio F. Arch Biochem Biophys 1988;266:573

282. Marra A, Sinay P. Gaz Chim Ital 1987;117:563

283. Bird GWG, Wingham J. Br J Haematol 1972;23:759

284. Bird GWG, Wingham J, Inglis G, et al. Lancet 1975;1:286

285. Inglis G, Bird GWG, Mitchell AAB, et al. J Clin Pathol 1975;28:964

286. Judd WJ, Beck ML. (abstract). Transfusion 1976;16:527

287. Inglis G, Bird GWG, Mitchell AAB, et al. Vox Sang 1978;35:370

288. Beck ML, Myers MA, Moulds J, et al. Transfusion 1978;18:680

289. Byrne V, Brown A, Ropars C, et al. Vox Sang 1979;36:208

290. Andreu G, Doinel C, Cartron J-P, et al. Rev Fr Transf Immunohematol 1979;22:551

291. Doinel C, Andreu G, Cartron J-P, et al. Vox Sang 1980;38:94

292. Judd WJ. (abstract). Transfusion 1980;20:622

293. Liew YW, Bird GWG, King MJ. Rev Fr Transf Immunohematol 1982;25:639

294. Klarkowski DB, Ford DS. Transfusion 1983;23:59

295. Fukuda MN, Matsumura G. J Biol Chem 1976;251:6218

296. Childs RA, Feizi T, Fukuda M, et al. Biochem J 1978;173:333

297. Fukuda MN, Fukuda M, Watanabe K, et al. Fed Proc 1978;37:1601

298. Niemann H, Watanabe K, Hakomori S, et al. Biochem Biophys Res Comm 1978;81:1286

299. Fukuda MN, Watanabe K, Hakomori S. J Biol Chem 1978;253:6814

300. Watanabe K, Hakomori S, Childs RA, et al. J Biol Chem 1979;254:3221

301. Fukuda M, Fukuda MN, Hakomori S. J Biol Chem 1979;254:3700

302. Fukuda MN, Fukuda M, Hakomori S. J Biol Chem 1979;254:5458

303. Marcus DM, Naiki M, Kundu SK, et al. In: Human Blood Groups. Karger:Basel, 1977:206

304. Morgan WTJ. In: Human Blood Groups. Basel:Karger, 1977:216

305. Judd WJ. Figure 42-4 1982, first published in Issitt PD. Applied Blood Group Serology, 3rd Ed. Miami:Montgomery, 1985:469

306. Liew YW, Bird GWG. Vox Sang 1988;54:226

307. Serafini-Cessi F. Trends in Glycosci Glycotechnol 1996;8:279

308. Graninger W, Rameis H, Fischer K, et al. Vox Sang 1977;32:195

309. Graninger W, Poschmann A, Fischer K, et al. Vox Sang 1977;32:201

310. Mullard GW, Haworth C, Lee D. Br J Haematol 1978;40:571

311. Veneziano G, Rasore-Quartino A, Sansone G. Lancet 1978;2:483

312. Herman JH, Shirey RS, Smith B, et al. Transfusion 1987;27:253

313. Herman JH, Whiteheart W, Shirey RS, et al. Br J Haematol 1987;65:205

314. Wahl CM, Herman JH, Shirey RS, et al. Transfusion 1989;29:635

315. Sondag-Thull D, Levene NA, Levene C, et al. Vox Sang 1989;57:193

316. Levene NA. MD Thesis, Hadassah Med Sch, Hebrew Univ, 1984

317. Bird GWG, Wingham J. J Clin Pathol 1981;34:69

318. Bird GWG, Wingham J, Seger R, et al. Blood Transf Immunohematol 1982;25:215

319. Bird GWG, Wingham J. J Clin Pathol 1983;36:195

320. Wolach B, Sadan N, Bird GWG, et al. Acta Haematol 1987;78:45

321. Harris PA, Romans GK, Moulds JJ, et al. Vox Sang 1982;42:134

322. Bird AR, Kent P, Moores PP, et al. Br J Haematol 1988;68:459

323. Becroft DM, Douglas R, Carrell RW, et al. NZ Med J 1968;68:72

324. Efremov GD, Huisman THJ, Stanulovic M, et al. Scand J Haematol 1974;13:48

325. King MJ, Liew YW, Moores PP, et al. Transfusion 1988;28:549

326. Fukuda M, Dell A, Oates JE, et al. J Biol Chem 1984;259:2860

327. Gerbal A, Liberge AGG, Lopez M, et al. Rev Fr Transf 1970;13:61

328. Gerbal A, Maslet C, Salmon C. Vox Sang 1975;28:398

329. Gerbal A, Ropars C, Gerbal R, et al. Vox Sang 1976;31:64

330. Stratton F, Renton PH. Br Med J 1959;2:244

331. Beck ML, Walker RH, Oberman HA. Transfusion 1971;11:296

332. Garratty G, Willbanks E, Petz LD. Vox Sang 1971;21:45

333. Mäkelä O, Mäkelä P. Ann Med Exp Biol Fenn 1956;34:402

334. Janot C, Andreu G, Schooneman F, et al. Rev Fr Transf 1979;22:375

335. Steane EA. (Letter). Transfusion 1983;23:403
336. Beck ML, Myers M, Moulds J. (abstract). Transfusion 1976;16:527
337. Janvier D, Reviron M, Reviron J. (abstract). Transfusion 1983;23:412
338. Springer GF, Ansell NJ. Proc Nat Acad Sci Wash DC 1958;44:182
339. Muschel LH, Osana E. Proc Soc Exp Biol Med 1959;101:614
340. Springer GF, Williamson P, Brandes WC. J Exp Med 1961;113:1077
341. Young VM, Gillen HC, Akeroyd IH. J Pediat 1962;60:172
342. Springer GF, Horton RE. J Gen Physiol 1964;47:1229
343. Springer GF, Horton RE. J Clin Invest 1969;48:1280
344. Decker GP, Chorpenning FW, Frederick GT. J Immunol 1972;108:214
345. Chorpenning FW, Stamper HB. Immunochemistry 1973;10:15
346. Yamoto H, Iseki S. Proc Jpn Acad 1968;44:263
347. Muller HE, Werner H. Z Med Microbiol Immunol 1970;156:98
348. Mitchell AAB. J Clin Pathol 1973;26:738
349. Rudek W, Haque R. J Clin Microbiol 1976;4:458
350. Heimpel H, Wendt F. Helv Med Acta 1968;34:103
351. Crookston JH, Crookston MC, Rosse WF. (abstract). Blood 1969;34 (Suppl):844
352. Crookston JH, Crookston MC, Burnie KL, et al. Br J Haematol 1969;17:11
353. Lewis SM, Grammaticos JP, Dacie JV. Br J Haematol 1970;18:465
354. Enquist RW, Gockerman JP, Ennis EH, et al. Ann Int Med 1972;77:371
355. Crookston JH, Crookston MC, Rosse WF. Br J Haematol 1972;23 (Suppl 1):83
356. Verwilghen RL, Lewis SM, Dacie JV, et al. Quart J Med (New Series) 1973;166:257
357. Gockerman JP, Durocher JR, Conrad ME. Br J Haematol 1975;30:383
358. Bird GWG, Wingham J. Acta Haematol 1976;55:174
359. Worlledge SM. In: Dyserythropoiesis. New York:Academic Press, 1977
360. Barosi G, Gazzola M, Stefanelli M, et al. Br J Haematol 1979;43:243
361. Lowenthal RM, Marsden KA, Dewar CL. Br J Haematol 1980;44:211
362. Crookston JH, Crookston MC. In: Blood Groups and Other Red Cell Surface Markers in Health and Disease. New York:Masson, 1982
363. Rosse WF. In: Clinical Immunohematology. Basic Concepts and Clinical Applications. Boston:Blackwell, 1990:649
364. Rochant H, Gerbal A. Rev Fr Transf 1976;19:239
365. Joseph KC, Gockerman JP. Biochem Biophys Res Comm 1975;65:146
366. Anselsletter V, Horstmann HF, Heimpel H. Br J Haematol 1977;35:209
367. Harlow RWH, Lowenthal RM. Br J Haematol 1982;50:35
368. Baines AJ, Banga JPS, Gratzer WB, et al. Br J Haematol 1982;50:563
369. Mawby WJ, Tanner MJA, Anstee DJ, et al. Br J Haematol 1983;55:357
370. Fukuda MN, Papayannopoulou T, Gordon-Smith EC, et al. Br J Haematol 1984;56:55
371. Fukuda MN. Glycobiology 1990;1:9
372. Fukuda MN, Masri KA, Dell A, et al. Proc Nat Acad Sci USA 1990;87:7443
373. Rosse WF, Logue GL, Adams J, et al. J Clin Invest 1974;53:31
374. Fukuda MN, Klier B, Yu J, et al. Blood 1986;68:521
375. Fukuda MN, Bothner B, Scartezzini P, et al. Chem Phys Lipids 1986;42:185
376. Fukuda MN, Dell A, Scartezzini P. J Biol Chem 1987;262:7195
377. Garratty G, Brunt DJ, Postoway N. (abstract). Transfusion 1981;21:623
378. Bird GWG. Nature 1959;184:109
379. Bird GWG, Wingham J. Vox Sang 1970;18:235
380. Bird GWG, Wingham J. Experientia 1970;26:1257
381. Beck ML. In: Investigation of Typing and Compatibility Problems Caused by Red Blood Cells. Washington, D.C.:Am Assoc Blood Banks, 1977:1
382. Bird GWG. In: Handbook Series in Clinical Laboratory Science, Sec D, Vol 1. Cleveland:CRC Press, 1977:443
383. Bird GWG. Rev Fr Transf 1978;21:103
384. Bird GWG. Prot Biol Fluids 1979;27 Coll:515
385. Hardman JT, Beck ML, Owensby CE. (abstract). Transfusion 1981;21:623
386. Hardman JT, Hale ME, Beck ML, et al. (abstract). Transfusion 1983;23:412
387. Briseno AM, Beck ML. (abstract). Transfusion 1983;23:413
388. Miller RL, Collawn JF Jr, Fish WW. J Biol Chem 1980;257:7574
389. Tollefsen SE, Kornfeld R. J Biol Chem 1983;258:1572
390. Tollefsen SE, Kornfeld R. Biochem Biophys Res Comm 1984;123:1099
391. Spohr U, Hindsgaul O, Lemieux RU. Canad J Chem 1985;63:2644
392. Hiemstra PS, Gorter A, Stuurman MC, et al. Scand J Immunol 1987;26:111
393. Saxon A, Tsui F, Martinez-Mazo O. Cell Immunol 1987;104:134
394. Autcouturier P, Mihaesco E, Mihaesco C, et al. Mol Immunol 1987;24:503
395. Krishna Sastry MV, Banarjee P, Patanjali SR, et al. J Biol Chem 1987;261:11726
396. Khanna AK, Sehajpal PK. Vox Sang 1980;39:44
397. Bird GWG. In: Methods in Haematology, Vol 17, Blood Transfusion. Edinburgh:Churchill Livingstone, 1988:125
398. Weber DJ, Wolfson JS, Swartz MN, et al. Medicine 1984;63:133
399. Burdge DR, Scheifele D, Speert DP. J Am Med Assoc 1985;253:3296
400. Owen CR, Bucker EO, Bell JF, et al. Rocky Mt Med J 1968;65:45
401. Hawkins LG. J Bone Joint Surg Am 1969;51:363
402. Goldstein EJC, Citron DM, Wield B, et al. J Clin Microbiol 1978;8:667
403. Jaffe AC. Pediat Clin North Am 1983;30:405
404. Elenbaas RM, McNabney WK, Robinson WA. Ann Emerg Med 1984;13:155
405. Goldstein EJC, Citron DM, Finegold SM. Rev Infec Dis 1984;6 (Suppl 1):S177
406. McGeachie J. J Pathol Bacteriol 1958;75:467
407. Hubbert WT, Rosen MN. Am J Public Hlth 1970;60:1103
408. Rivoalen A. Bull Soc Pathol Exot Filiales 1936;29:709
409. Salmon C, Cartron J-P, Rouger P. The Human Blood Groups. New York:Masson, 1984:292

43 | Miscellaneous Conditions that may Affect Results in the Blood Transfusion Laboratory

For those who watch Seinfeld, this is a chapter about nothing. Gathered here are descriptions of a number of situations, most of which affect serological tests, about which the blood banker must be aware. While few of these phenomena apply directly to a particular blood group system, some of them can result in difficult to explain findings or in outright mistakes, if they are not recognized. When necessary and when one exists, a practical solution to the problem is suggested. The first half of the chapter describes phenomena that relate primarily to antibodies or sera, the second half those that relate primarily to antigens or red cells.

Spurious Agglutination Due to External Factors

This heading is used to describe those situations in which agglutination occurs independently of the antigen-antibody reaction that the test was designed to reveal. For example, Beattie et al. (1,2) have described antibodies against acriflavin, a dye commonly used to color anti-B typing serum. In each instance, the antibody in the patient's serum combined with acriflavin in the anti-B reagent and spontaneous agglutination of the red cells present occurred. The net result was that the patient's red cells appeared to carry the B antigen, but reverse typing tests revealed the presence of an apparent alloimmune anti-B. When washed red cells from the patients were tested, they were not agglutinated by anti-B because the antibody in the patient's serum was no longer present to complex with the acriflavin. Similarly, the patients' red cells were not agglutinated by sera containing anti-B that did not contain acriflavin.

There seem to be several mechanisms by which phenomena such as this can occur. First, an antibody in the patient's serum can combine with a dye, drug or chemical in the test serum to form antigen-antibody complexes. In the presence of these complexes, red cells may be aggregated or agglutinated. Second, the dye, drug or chemical may bind to the test red cells that are then agglutinated by an antibody directed against the adsorbed substance. Third, in the presence of some substances, agglutination or aggregation of red cells may be potentiated although no antigen-antibody reaction has taken place. Fourth, it is possible, but as far as we are aware not yet proved, that some substances modify the red cell membrane so that spontaneous agglutination or aggregation occurs. There are many materials that have resulted in spurious agglutination of this type. Table 43-1 lists them and gives references to publications describing the phenomena. In some but not all instances, the mode of action of the material causing the agglutination is known. Those substances listed in table 43-1 seem to have caused agglutination that is unrelated to antibodies with blood group specificity. In a later section, somewhat similar findings, but ones in which some blood group specificity was seen, are described.

When a serum under test reacts in such a way that the presence of an antibody dependent on one of the materials listed in table 43-1 is suspected, a great deal of work may be necessary to identify the cause of the reaction. If, for example, a serum reacts with all red cells of a commercially-supplied panel but not with donor cells used in compatibility tests, it is possible that one of the constituents in the preservative solution, in which the panel cells are suspended, is responsible. The investigator must then use a series of test systems each of which includes one ingredient of the preservative solution. If the drug or chemical causing the agglutination is not identified by this means, it may be necessary then to test various combinations and permutations of the ingredients. Several of the materials listed in table 43-1 were identified in exactly this manner.

Some of the findings referenced in table 43-1 merit some expansion here. When Bird and Roy (23) tested sera for the presence of antibodies capable of agglutinating melibiose-treated red cells, they examined 1000 of those sera from normal donors and hospital patients for their ability to agglutinate red cells exposed to other carbohydrates. Their (23) results are listed below; first the name of carbohydrate to which the red cells were exposed is given, then the figure refers to the number of reactive sera among the 1000 tested. Dextran (MW 40,000) 8; lactose 6; mannose 6; D-galactose 5; D-glucose 3; D-fructose 1. None of the sera agglutinated red cells exposed to maltose, sucrose, trehalose, cellobiose, raffinose, sorbitol, starch or dextrans of MWs 70,000, 90,000, 150,000 and 275,000. In tests with red cells exposed to melibiose, 712 of 1480 sera (48%) gave positive reactions. The other positive findings in this study have not been added to table 43-1 since that table refers primarily to cases in which the antibodies interfered in typing tests and not to deliberate screening studies.

The antibody that agglutinated red cells exposed to glucose, that was initially described by Lewis et al. (15)

TABLE 43-1 Some Substances that have Supported Non-blood Group Specific Agglutination

Material	References
Acriflavin	1, 2
Carboxylic acids	3
Chloramphenicol	4, 5
Citrate	6
Corticosteroids	7-9
EDTA	10-13
Gentamicin	14
Glucose	15, 16
Inosine	17, 272
Lactose	18
Lactate	19
LISS	20-22
Melibiose	23
Neomycin	24
Oxalate	6
Phenol	25
Saccharose	26
Saline	27-30
Tartrazine	31
Thimerosal	32
Thrombin (bovine)	33
Vancomycin	34, 35

was later tested (16) against and found to agglutinate the red cells of patients with diabetes mellitus although those cells had not been exposed to glucose in vitro. The authors (16) concluded that patients with that disorder have red cells that undergo a reversible change in vivo that is similar to the one induced when red cells from healthy donors are incubated in vitro with glucose.

The antibody that agglutinates red cells that have just been washed in saline was first described by Freiesleben and Jensen (27) in 1959. Several other examples have been reported since then (28-30). Allan et al. (29) studied four examples of the antibody and found that red cells that were washed in saline then allowed to stand at room temperature, gradually lost their ability to be agglutinated by the sera. The times with which the ability was lost varied between five minutes and four hours. The antibodies were most active when tested against red cells washed three times in saline, the age of the cells before washing made no difference to the strength of the reactions. Red cells washed in ACD or

Alsever's solution were not agglutinated by the antibodies. Very surprisingly, Davey et al. (30) found that an example of this antibody, that apparently activated complement, destroyed red cells in vivo. When donor red cells and the patient's own cells were labeled with ^{51}Cr and injected as saline suspensions, the one hour survivals were 32 and 46% respectively. When similar tests were done with red cells suspended in ACD the 1 hour survival of donor cells was 77% and that of the patient's own cells, 93%. It was supposed (30) that the 77% 1 hour survival figure for ACD-suspended donor red cells reflected alteration to those cells caused by excess washing in ACD during the labeling step, because the patient was subsequently transfused with 15 units of ACD whole blood and packed red cells with no evidence of any ill effects. Thus in spite of some positive results from in vivo tests it seems that this phenomenon can be ignored for practical purposes.

Blood Group Specific, Externally Supported Reactions

As mentioned earlier, the positive findings discussed in the preceding section were not associated with blood group specific reactions. However, a number of antibodies with blood group specificity have been described that reacted only, or much more strongly, in the presence of one of the materials in table 43-1, or a somewhat similar substance. A list of these antibodies is given in table 43-2.

Because the antibodies listed in table 43-2 had blood group specificity, many of them have already been described in appropriate chapters of this book. As will be seen, table 43-2 lists auto-anti-P reactive only in LISS (40). Table 43-1 includes two autoantibodies of no known specificity, also reactive only in LISS. It does not seem that either of those autoantibodies was tested against P- or Tj(a-) red cells (20,21) so that it is possible that they too had auto-anti-P specificity. Most, but perhaps not all the autoantibodies in table 43-2 were benign in vivo.

Agglutinins Active in the Presence of EDTA

As shown in table 43-1, some agglutinins have been said to be dependent on the presence of EDTA (10,11). In studying such an agglutinin, that had anti-H specificity, Gunson (47) concluded that the antibody was inhibited by ionized calcium. Now it seems that agglutinins that initially appear to be active only in the presence of EDTA can represent either of these backgrounds. In the cases described by Beck et al. (11,48) and by Howe et al. (3) agglutination was supported by unbound excess EDTA

TABLE 43-2 Some Substances that have Supported Blood Group Specific Reactions

Material	Antibody Specificity	Reference
Fatty acids (as in stabilized albumin)	Anti-c	36
Paraben (as in LISS)	Anti-Jk^a	37
Methyl esters of hydroxybenzoic acid (as in LISS)	Anti-Jk^a	38
Glucose	Anti-M and anti-N	39
LISS	Auto-anti-P	40
LISS	Auto-anti-U	41
Chlorpropamide	Auto-anti-Jk^a	42
Chloramphenicol	Auto-anti-A$_1$	43
Thimerosal	Auto-anti-I	44
Thimerosal	Anti-e Anti-rh$_i$	273[*1]

[*1]   The antibodies gave enhanced reactions in the presence of thimerosal but were not completely dependent on its presence. They reacted against ficin-treated red cells and by the polybrene method in the absence of thimerosal.

In addition to the above, there are two reports (45, 46) that describe anti-D as a contaminant of bovine thrombin used to make blood clot in vitro. It is not clear how anti-D got into the bovine thrombin preparations.

or carboxylic groups (polycarboxylic or monocarboxylic acids). In contrast, the auto-anti-H studied by Gunson (47) and an auto-anti-B studied by Yasuda et al. (49) were reactive only in the absence (or presence of a low level) of ionized calcium. A similar pair of backgrounds have been described (50) in studies on antibodies to platelets.

Resolution of the Problems

As mentioned, the antibodies described in the preceding subsections are not usually of any clinical significance. The problems that they cause in typing tests, antibody detection or identification studies, or compatibility tests, can be resolved by repeating the tests in the absence of the dye, drug or chemical that supports the reaction. It is not always necessary to know which agent is precipitating the unwanted agglutination. Tests using well washed red cells and sera from individual donors to which no external agents have been added, usually resolve the difficulties. If red cells have been modified

during storage (as with glucose) it may be necessary to collect new samples in anticoagulants that do not contain the dye, drug or chemical involved.

Autoagglutinins Reactive Only in the Presence of Albumin

Weiner et al. (53) seem to have been the first to report that some sera contain an autoagglutinin that is reactive only in the presence of albumin. The antibody is fairly common and since the original report, numerous others (54-77) have followed. Some of the antibodies described were IgM, others were IgG. Many reacted simply as agglutinins (at 22°C or 37°C) in the presence of albumin, others reacted in those tests and by IAT. Some failed to agglutinate red cells in the presence of albumin but caused positive IATs. A few examples caused complement activation and at least one acted as an in vitro hemolysin. In other words, these antibodies have run the whole gamut of serological reactions.

There has been some disagreement as to the precise mechanism by which these antibodies cause positive reactions. Some workers (60,65,67,71) believe that their reactivity is dependent on the presence of short chain fatty acids, that is fatty acid salts with aliphatic chains between three and eight carbons in length. Others (62,64) have suggested that when sodium caprylate is added to albumin as a stabilizing agent, there is an alteration of the native serum albumin so that it develops the property of supporting agglutination. Certainly, most of these antibodies will react in the presence of albumin that has been stabilized with sodium caprylate, but not in the presence of albumin free of that chemical. The final answer seems to have been supplied by Beck et al. (71) who showed that these agglutinins are active in albumin-free systems to which sodium caprylate has been added. In other words, while caprylate or a structurally similar chemical must be present for these antibodies to react, albumin itself plays no role. In view of these findings, Beck et al. (71) suggested that the name fatty acid dependent antibodies (FADA) is more suitable than albumin autoagglutinins or similar terms that imply that albumin is the key factor in the reactions. As far as we are aware, only two of the many FADA studied displayed blood group specificity. One reacted as anti-c (36) and the other as anti-e (75).

In terms of FADA that do not display blood group specificity, none seems to have been of any clinical significance. They cause problems in antibody-screening and compatibility tests when albumin is used, when blood selected by in vitro methods that do not use albumin is transfused, it survives normally in vivo. At least one volunteer with this type of antibody in the serum was given

50 ml of sodium caprylate-stabilized human albumin and suffered no ill-effects (76).

Resolution of the Problem

If an antibody of this type is encountered, the unwanted reactions that it causes can be avoided either by performing tests that do not use albumin or by substituting a sodium caprylate-free albumin solution for the stabilized one. The first solution is by far the better of the two. As discussed in Chapters 3 and 35, the uptake of antibody by red cells proceeds at the same rate in albumin and saline test systems (78) so that albumin to IAT is no more sensitive a method than is saline to IAT. While albumin may be useful in antibody identification studies when dealing with sera that contain several antibodies (i.e., one acts as an agglutinin in albumin, the others only by IAT) it plays no useful role in antibody detection or compatibility tests.

Problems Caused by Unexpected Antibodies in Sera

When typing sera are prepared for use, ABO agglutinins present must often be removed so that the sera can be used to test red cells of any ABO group. One common way that this is accomplished is by adsorbing the anti-A and/or anti-B with A and/or B cells that lack the antigen against which the useful antibody in the serum is directed. Another is to add A and/or B soluble substances (79,80) so that the ABO antibodies present are neutralized. When either of these procedures is used, some antigen-antibody complexes remain in the serum in a soluble form. Following adsorption with red cells, relatively few complexes are present, after neutralization virtually all the antibody is there in a bound form. When sera thus prepared are stored, some of the antigen-antibody complexes may dissociate and free anti-A and/or anti-B may reappear. Obviously, incorrect typing results can then result when A or B cells are tested.

Resolution of the Problem

When this problem is suspected, careful controls using A and/or B cells known to lack the antigen against which the antibody in the typing serum is directed, should be performed. Simple agglutination tests may not be sufficient as controls (unless the suspected incorrect result has been obtained by that method) since anti-A and anti-B reactive by IAT are the ones most likely to appear first in a serum when immune complex dissociation occurs. If

anti-A and/or anti-B are shown to be present and another serum of the same specificity is not available, the original serum can be adsorbed again. If suitable red cells are not available for such adsorptions, one of the methods mentioned later can be used. Elution of the required antibody after it has been adsorbed on to group O, antigen-positive red cells, is a particularly useful way of obtaining the antibody in a form free of anti-A and anti-B. Eventually this problem will disappear when all specificities are available as monoclonal antibodies.

Incorrect Use of Typing Reagents

Great care must be exercised if a typing reagent prepared for use by one method is used by a different one. For example, an anti-C prepared for use as a slide or rapid tube reagent may give a weak reaction with a test cell sample. In an attempt to determine whether the test cells are C+ or C-, the serologist may choose to use the anti-C by IAT or in a test against enzyme-treated red cells. A strongly positive reaction will not necessarily mean that the test cells are C+. The anti-C reagent may contain another antibody, such as anti-K or anti-Kp[a], that does not interfere when the anti-C is used by slide or rapid tube methods but that is active by another method. While it might be supposed that the use of monoclonal antibodies would obviate this problem, such reagents must still be used with some care. Some are particularly sensitive to changes in pH so that the use of incorrect methods might result in false negative reactions. Further, it has been demonstrated (51,52,81-84) that some monoclonal antibodies cross-react with various tissues. As far as we know, such cross-reactivity has not resulted in false positive reactions in blood group phenotyping tests but clearly it is at least as important with MAb-based reagents as with human polyclonal antibody-based ones, to follow the manufacturers directions for use with exactitude.

Resolution of the Problem

The test serum (the polyclonal anti-C in the example given above) can be used in adsorption-elution studies with the test cells. If the cells are C+, they will reduce the strength of the reagent if used in successive adsorptions, that reduction will best be demonstrated by titration studies using unadsorbed and adsorbed aliquots of the anti-C. It is, of course, essential that such adsorption studies be controlled by similar adsorptions with antigen-negative red cells. Similarly, if the test cells are C+, an eluate made from the cells used for the first adsorption should contain demonstrable anti-C. If only very weak anti-C reactivity is recovered, the Matuhasi-Ogata minimus condition that is described below, should be remembered. The direction circulars that accompany commercially-prepared typing reagents, specify by which techniques the reagents are specific. It is at least theoretically possible that MAb may be less suitable than human polyclonal antibodies for use in elution tests in the setting described. That is to say, if the MAb involved defines an epitope shared by more than one red cell antigen, a false positive reaction could be possible.

Other Ways of Preparing Typing Sera

Occasionally a valuable antibody will be found but no red cells will be available to remove unwanted ABO agglutinins. For example, anti-Lan made by a group O patient can be used to test group O cells to find others that are Lan-, it cannot be used in family studies to investigate inheritance of the antigen if the family members are other than group O. Øyen et al. (85) showed that killed suspensions of the organism *Escherichia coli* O_{86}:B7 effectively adsorb anti-A and anti-B from sera and leave most other antibodies unadsorbed (we do not know if anti-Lan remains unadsorbed so a small-size trial adsorption would be in order before a large volume of serum was committed!) Other investigators (86-88) have reported that autoclaved A and B red cells that are then treated with formalin, can be used similarly. If the useful antibody in the serum reacts with an antigen that is denatured when red cells are treated with proteolytic enzymes (for a list see table 3-3 in Chapter 3) such treated A and B cells can be used without regard to their other phenotypes (89).

When red cell samples are to be typed and the only available serum is ABO incompatible, the typings can be performed with an eluate. For example, anti-Lan from a group O patient can be adsorbed on to group O, Lan+ red cells. An eluate can then be made and can be used to type red cells of any ABO group since it will contain anti-Lan but no anti-A or anti-B. This method has to be used when suitable red cells for adsorption do not exist or cannot be used. The lady who made the first and still by far the most potent example of human anti-Wr^b, is D- and her serum contains weak anti-D in addition to the anti-Wr^b (90). The only D+, Wr(b-) red cells known are En(a-) so are obviously far too valuable to be used for adsorption. For many years we (90-93) have performed tests with anti-Wr^b purified by adsorption on to and elution from group O, rr, Wr(a-b+) red cells.

Once an antibody such as anti-Lan or anti-Kp^b has been rendered suitable for use in typing tests on other than group O cells, those tests should be restricted to family studies or other research investigations. Screening for

rare blood, e.g. Lan-, Kp(b-), etc., should be restricted to group O donors since their red cells can be transfused to persons of any ABO group.

Bacterially Contaminated Sera

Sera contaminated with certain bacteria will agglutinate all red cell samples. Davidsohn and Toharsky (94) called the agglutinin produced anti-h and assumed that all red cell samples carry the h antigen. It should be added that the symbol h, as used here, has no relationship to the genes *H* and *h* (see Chapter 8).

Concentration of Antibodies

This may be accomplished, in serum or in eluates, by pressure dialysis or dialysis against carbowax (both methods described by Mollison (95)) or by use of Minicon filters (Amicon Corp, Lexington, MA). A method in which serum is allowed to thaw while standing undisturbed and in which the uppermost aqueous layer is pipetted off leaving the lower protein-rich layer, is quick and easy but is less reliable (antibody is sometimes lost) than the other methods listed.

Anti-A, Anti-B and Other Antibodies in Therapeutic Concentrates

Several groups of workers (96-107) have pointed out that products such as immune serum globulin (IVIG), tetanus immune globulin, Rh immune globulin and factor VIII and IX concentrates may contain blood group antibodies. Sometimes, use of one of these therapeutics results in the presence of unexpected anti-A and/or anti-B in the recipient's plasma. If enough passively transferred antibody is present, the DAT may become positive. In hemophiliacs who are group A or group B, enough antibody can be transferred via factor VIII concentrate that in vivo hemolysis of the patient's own red cells may occur (96,102,103,107). The problem is not restricted to anti-A and anti-B. As early as 1971, Oberman and Beck (97) described a positive DAT in a newborn in whom anti-D was inadvertently injected when present in IVIG. Now that high dose IVIG therapy is relatively common, most workers will have encountered cases in which antibodies to D, C, K, etc., have been passively transferred in IVIG. Indeed, one of the early questions that should be asked when an unexpected serological finding is made is now, is the patient receiving IVIG? Such a question is particularly appropriate when a D+ patient presents with a positive DAT and anti-D is eluted from the red cells.

Resolution of the Problem

This is primarily a matter of recognition. Once it is appreciated from whence came the unexpected antibody, the serological results can be understood. In hemophiliacs in whom hemolysis is occurring because of the passive transfer of anti-A or anti-B in factor VIII concentrate, an alternative form of therapy must be instituted. One resolution is to continue therapy with ABO type-specific cryoprecipitate until such time as the level of passively transferred anti-A or anti-B falls sufficiently that hemolysis stops.

Problems Caused by Therapeutic Antiglobulins

Patients who receive allografts are sometimes treated with anti-lymphoblast or anti-thymocyte globulin that are immunosuppressive agents designed to modify the immune response in the transplant recipient and thus reduce the chance of graft rejection. Use of these therapeutics can cause problems in the transfusion service because they are made in animals and often contain antibodies that will agglutinate or coat human red cells. Swanson et al. (108) described in vitro testing problems that were resolved as described below. Lapinid et al. (244) reported positive direct antiglobulin tests in patients being treated with anti-lymphocyte globulin. Draper et al. (109) reported similar problems but claimed that in a few patients the antibodies caused in vivo red cell destruction. Andersen et al. (110) described the presence of what they called anti-Lu^{var} in anti-lymphocyte globulin (ALG). However, the relationship of the antibody to the Lutheran system was not established since the antibody failed to react only with 75% of Lu(a-b-) red cells tested. If the donors of those cells had *In(Lu)* (see Chapter 20) it is entirely possible (111,112) that the antibody in the ALG was directed against a non-Lutheran system antigen whose expression is depressed or prevented by *In(Lu)*.

Resolution of the Problem

Swanson et al. (113) showed that when therapeutics such as those listed above are made in horses, the recipient's red cells may become coated with horse globulin and will then be agglutinated by anti-human globulin reagents made in rabbits. The problem can be resolved by adsorbing the anti-human globulin with red cells coated with the therapeutic involved. Such adsorption removes the component in the anti-human globulin that reacts with the horse globulin but leaves unadsorbed, antibody that reacts with human globulin.

The Matuhasi-Ogata Phenomenon

Matuhasi-Ogata Minimus Condition

While conducting studies designed to answer the much asked question as to whether group O serum contains a mixture of anti-A and anti-B, or a single antibody with anti-A,B specificity, Matuhasi et al. (114-117) made some observations that were later applied to other blood group antibodies. When an antibody is mixed with red cells that carry the antigen against which the antibody is directed, specific antigen-antibody complexes form. Some findings (116-119) suggested that in the presence of those specific antigen-antibody complexes, a second antibody present in the same serum, the antigen for which was not present on the red cells, could also bind to the cells. When an eluate was subsequently made, it contained a large amount of the expected antibody (i.e. the one for which the cells were antigen-positive) and might also contain demonstrable levels of the unexpected or wrong antibody (i.e. the one not expected to bind to the red cells used). This suggestion was apparently confirmed in tests using antibodies other than anti-A and anti-B (119) and was used retrospectively as an explanation in several cases in which the red cells of a patient yielded an unexpected antibody when eluates were made. However, later studies by Bove et al. (120) showed that uptake of the wrong antibody by red cells was not enhanced in the presence of specific antigen-antibody complex formation. Indeed, in tests using radiolabeled antibodies, it was shown that the findings probably represented no more than the non-specific uptake of some IgG by red cells, a phenomenon that had been clearly documented in earlier studies (121-127). These findings left unexplained the serological observation (119) that there was a greater chance of eluting an unexpected antibody, if the cells from which the eluate was made had bound another antibody specifically, than if the cells did not carry antigens for any of the antibodies in the test sera. It may be that the difference relates to the amount of protein in the eluate. If the eluate is made from antibody-coated red cells it will contain some protein (i.e. the antibody that had bound specifically). If it also contains a low level of an unexpected antibody, the total protein content may be sufficient that the unexpected antibody can be detected in serological tests. Protein levels are known to affect the visible serological reactions of some antibodies. If on the other hand, the eluate is made from red cells that have not bound an antibody specifically, its protein content will be considerably lower. Thus, although such an eluate may contain the same amount of unexpected antibody as the one described above, it may be impossible to demonstrate the presence of that antibody in serological tests.

No matter what the true explanation of the Matuhasi-Ogata phenomenon, workers should be aware that it may occasionally interfere in serological studies. That is, some eluates may contain low levels of an antibody with a specificity such that it did not bind to the red cells from which the eluate was made, via formation of specific antigen-antibody complexes. One of us (PDI) renamed this situation the Matuhasi-Ogata minimus condition in the second edition of this book.

Resolution of the Problem

The Matuhasi-Ogata minimus condition is usually recognizable at the serological level without difficulty. The amount of unexpected antibody in the eluate is usually small and gives only weak reactions. If the problem is suspected and if the particular conditions permit, repeat adsorption-elution tests using the unexpected antibody in pure form, so that specific antigen-antibody complex formation will not occur, can be tried.

Matuhasi-Ogata Maximus Condition

Occasionally an eluate made from a patient's red cells will contain a strongly reactive antibody with what seems to be an unexplainable specificity. For example, the E- red cells of a patient with WAIHA may yield, on elution, an antibody that gives 4+ reactions with E+ and negative or very weak reactions with E- red cells. This finding was at one time thought to represent the Matuhasi-Ogata phenomenon; one of us (PDI) now believes that it has a quite different explanation. As described in detail in Chapter 37, some autoantibodies mimic a specificity that they do not actually possess (128-142). When such an antibody is bound to the patient's red cells in vivo, it will have an apparently wrong specificity when isolated by elution.

Resolution of the Problem

Laboratory studies can be used if the situation is suspected. To continue the example from above, if the eluted apparent anti-E can be adsorbed onto and eluted from, or adsorbed to exhaustion by other E- red cells (often the case) it follows that the antibody does not really have anti-E specificity. Confusion can arise since in many cases the antibody eluted from the patient's red cells will be of the mimicking type, while the patient's serum will contain a mixture of the mimicking antibody and a true alloantibody of the specificity mimicked by the autoantibody. Thus while antibody activity in the eluate will be adsorbed to exhaustion with antigen-negative red cells, that in the serum will be partially adsorbed, i.e. mimicking antibody adsorbed but then no further adsorption will occur because only true specificity alloantibody remains. In most instances, mimicking specificity autoantibodies actually have anti-nl specificity (131) although anti-pdl is sometimes seen (133, for a discussion of anti-nl and anti-pdl, see Chapter 37).

As can be seen, although these antibodies have been mentioned in the section dealing with the Matuhasi-Ogata phenomenon, the explanation of their behavior is quite different from the non-specific uptake of IgG that apparently explains the minimus condition. While mimicking specificity antibodies are most often encountered when eluates from the red cells of patients with WAIHA are tested, they can be seen in other situations. First, recovery of the wrong antibody by elution from other than the patient's cells can occur once the antibody has been isolated. Second, such antibodies are sometimes recovered from the DAT+ red cells of persons who are hematologically normal. Third, on rare occasions (143) such antibodies may be seen in eluates made from the DAT-negative red cells of patients with the clinical signs and symptoms of WAIHA. Fourth, on perhaps even rarer occasions, recognition of the true specificity of an alloantibody may be complicated by this phenomenon. On such occasions the antibody may not have bound to the patient's red cells in vivo, but will sometimes do so in serological tests performed in vitro.

Another Cause of Unexpected Antibodies in Eluates

Leger et al. (144) noticed that when using commercially supplied kits to perform acid elution they found anti-D in eluates made from D- red cells previously incubated with anti-D. Such findings were not made using heat, xylene or ether elution methods. In the subsequent investigation it was shown that the false positive eluates were caused by the low ionic strength wash solutions supplied in the kits. When phosphate buffered saline at normal ionic strength was used instead of the low ionic strength wash solution, no unexpected antibodies were eluted. When 10% sucrose was used instead of the supplied wash solution, even stronger expressions of the unexpected antibodies were found in the eluates. The authors (144) pointed out that while the use of a low ionic strength wash solution results in superior eluates on most occasions, in the presence of potent serum antibodies false positive eluates may result.

Placental Eluates

An often overlooked source of a large amount of

very useful antibody is the placenta of an immunized woman who has just given birth. Moulds et al. (145) reported recovery of liter quantities of anti-Rh17 and anti-Lan by making eluates at pH 3.0 from such tissue. Competition between blood bankers and workers using cord blood instead of bone marrow for transplantation seems unlikely since the latter group would probably not want to use cells coated with a blood group antibody.

Lectins that Agglutinate Lymphocytes

Numerous examples of lectins with specificity for red cell blood group antigens have been described in this book. There are now a number of reports (146-158) that describe lectins that agglutinate leukocytes. Such lectins may prove useful in the preparation of cell samples where cross contamination with other types of cells must be avoided.

Rouleaux Formation

Classic rouleaux formation is a condition, controlled by a property of serum, in which red cells are mechanically situated next to each other in a columnar fashion giving a typical microscopic appearance that has been likened to a stack of coins or, by younger workers, as being like Pringles. The condition is not agglutination and has no serological significance, but may be mistaken for agglutination by inexperienced workers. This is particularly true when rouleaux is marked, for in such a circumstance the classic columnar aggregation may be replaced by aggregates that look more like true agglutinates.

Rouleaux formation can be caused by an alteration of charge at the red cell surface (159). Further, when there is an alteration of the normal albumin:globulin ratio in a patient's plasma, rouleaux formation may be seen. Gralnick (160) pointed out that rouleaux may be associated with the following conditions: multiple myeloma (increased levels of IgM and/or IgA); macroglobulinemia (increased levels of IgM); cryoglobulinemia (increased levels of IgG and/or IgM); Boeck's sacroid and cirrhosis (both of which result in a generally increased globulin level) and hyperfibrinogenemia in infections (increased levels of fibrinogen). Mollison (95) notes that fibrinogen molecules, that are large and asymmetrical, are especially likely to induce rouleaux formation.

Rouleaux Formation Following Infusions

Infusions of dextran or PVP can cause marked rouleaux-forming properties to develop in a patient's serum. This is a particularly serious consideration since the type of rouleaux induced is highly atypical and often closely resembles agglutination so that even experienced workers may encounter difficulties in differentiation. While high molecular weight dextrans can be particularly troublesome in this regard (161) lower molecular weight dextrans can also create problems if given in sufficient quantity (162,163). Once rouleaux formation has been induced by the infusion of dextran or PVP it may persist as a function of the patient's plasma for 24 to 36 hours after the infusions (160). While it has been reported (162-165) that low molecular weight dextrans, infused in modest amounts, do not cause subsequently collected samples of serum to induce rouleaux formation of untreated red cells, the common experience (162,166-168) has been that such sera cause (sometimes marked) rouleaux formation when used in tests against enzyme-treated red cells. Physicians should be made aware of these difficulties and should be asked, when dextran or PVP infusions are to be used in appreciable amounts, to collect a blood sample for serological tests before the infusion is started, even if transfusion of blood is not immediately contemplated. Relatively easy to recognize rouleaux, that is readily dispersed by the addition of saline (see below) may be caused by sera from persons who have been given hydroxyethyl starch in leukapheresis or other procedures (169).

Typing Tests on the Red Cells of Patients with Multiple Myeloma

Red cells from patients with multiple myeloma may be difficult to type because of the presence of large amounts of proteins that cause atypical rouleaux formation or aggregation of the red cells. If not carefully handled, typing tests on these cells may all appear to be positive because the cells were agglomerated before the typing serum was added. Cell suspensions must be thoroughly washed before being used and careful control of the tests with an inert serum is necessary to show that any agglutination produced is specific and not due to the condition of the patient's red cells. If reverse grouping is deemed necessary, the patient's serum should be diluted to a point where its rouleaux-producing properties are no longer troublesome but where its ABO agglutinins are still active. Compatibility tests are difficult because serum should not be diluted for these tests. Accordingly, care in differentiating agglutination from rouleaux formation is necessary. These situations are compounded on occasion since some patients with multiple myeloma also have potent cold-agglutinins in their sera. As discussed in Chapters 3 and 38, it may be necessary to remove such cold-agglutinins by autoadsorption before the sera are tested.

Great care is also necessary in performing direct antiglobulin tests on the red cells of patients with multiple myeloma. The cells usually have to be washed many times so that they are not already aggregated before the antiglobulin serum is added. When the test is read, a control using saline in place of antiglobulin serum should be included and must give a negative reaction before a positive test with antiglobulin serum can be regarded as valid.

Resolution of Problems Caused by Rouleaux

There are four principal methods of differentiating between rouleaux and true agglutination. The easiest is to add one drop of saline to the cell-serum mixture on a glass slide, after the test has been read microscopically and when rouleaux is suspected. The serum-cell-saline mixture is rocked gently and re-examined under the microscope. Rouleaux formation will disperse, true agglutination will not (170). Although this method is very useful, it does not always disperse strong rouleaux, especially if the rouleaux is atypical. The second method avoids the problem by using dilutions of serum (171). Although, as pointed out above this method may be useful for the detection of anti-A and anti-B in reverse typing, it cannot be recommended for antibody-screening or compatibility testing since alloantibodies as well as rouleaux forming properties may be diluted to the point of non-reactivity. The third solution, that is better than the second, was originally suggested by Schmidt and Kevy (172). In this method, once rouleaux formation is suspected at the reading stage of a test, the test is centrifuged then the serum is removed and replaced with saline. Sometimes examination of the red cells to which the saline has been added will show that the rouleaux formation has gone. On other occasions the cells and saline must very gently mixed, respun and reread. Providing that this test is performed carefully, rouleaux formation but not true agglutination can be dispersed. The fourth solution is particularly useful when additional tests must be performed using a serum already known to cause rouleaux formation. Norris et al. (274) showed that if red cells are first treated with a dilute solution of 4,4′-diisothiocyanatostilbene-2,2′-disulfonic acid (DIDS) they resist induction of rouleaux formation by plasma or sera that have that inducing property and by sera to which dextran has been added. DIDS is thought to act by binding to protein band 3 thus blocking the sites to which the macromolecules that cause rouleaux formation would otherwise bind (275). In serological tests, the amount of DIDS required to block rouleaux was shown not to alter A, B or any of 19 other red cell antigens tested.

Wharton's Jelly and Spontaneous Agglutination

Wharton's jelly is an intercellular substance comprised of primitive connective tissue of the umbilical cord. It is rich in hyaluronic acid. If a cord blood sample is collected by cutting the cord and allowing blood to drain into a tube, the sample may become contaminated with Wharton's jelly and the red cells of the sample may agglomerate spontaneously (269). As little as one part in 1000 of Wharton's jelly may cause agglomeration (270) and washing the red cells in saline may not reverse the clumping.

Resolution of the Problem

The problem can be prevented by collecting the cord blood sample from the umbilical vein with a syringe and needle. If the sample has been collected incorrectly and has become contaminated, the clumping can be reversed by washing the red cells in a dilute solution of hyluronidase (271). Details of the method are given by Judd (178).

The LOX Antigen

In 1980 and 1981, Bruce et al. (173,174) described four antibodies that define an antigen that the authors named LOX. Production of the antigen is not genetically controlled; instead the antigen represents an acquired change on red cells stored in plastic blood bags that have recently been sterilized with the lower oxirane (hence LOX), ethylene oxide. Red cells treated with alpha chymotrypsin no longer react with anti-LOX, but treatment of LOX+ red cells with trypsin or papain does not abolish their reactivity. Other examples of anti-LOX and red cells converted to the LOX+ state have been found (175); none of the antibodies has been of clinical significance.

Separation of Red Cells of Different Ages

It is sometimes useful to be able to separate young and old red cells from a sample of blood. For example, if a patient has recently been transfused and there are reasons for wishing to know the patient's phenotype but the pretransfusion sample has been used or discarded, a newly collected sample may not be suitable since it will contain a mixture of the patient's and the transfused red cells. However, if the youngest population of red cells can be separated it can be anticipated that most of those cells will be the patient's, that have been released from the marrow since the transfusion. Most of the early methods for the separation of young and old cells were based on an observation by Stephens (176) that young cells are less dense than old ones so can be collected from the top of a column of centrifuged red cells. At first, red cells in saline were centrifuged (245), later red cells suspended in albumin were found (246-248) to give better separation. Reid and Toy (177) showed that for many purposes in immunohematology, simple centrifugation provides suitable separation. Red cells from a sample usually collected three or more days after transfusion (but see also below) are washed three times. Care must be taken not to remove the top layer of red cells during the washing steps since that layer contains many of the young cells. The washed cells are then used to fill microhematocrit tubes that are sealed and spun in a microhematocrit centrifuge at 13,500 x g for 15 minutes. The tubes are then cut so that the top 5mm of the column of red cells, containing the young cells, can be harvested. Judd (178) reports that this method works well and is worth trying before the phthalate ester method (179,180) that is more time consuming, is used. It must be remembered that the centrifugation methods, with or without phthalate esters, will produce a mixture of largely young but some old red cells. Thus phenotyping tests may yield mixed-field reactions and the investigator may have to decide (based on efficiency of the cell separation) whether it is the patient's or the donors' red cells that are reactive (or non-reactive).

Other methods of cell separation on density gradients have been tried (249,250). Percoll was used to separate reticulocytes (251,252) and bone marrow cells (253) and Renografin was used (254) to separate reticulocytes. The two were then combined (182-185) and the Percoll-Renografin method was used in the studies (181) on autoantibodies causative of WAIHA that react with old, or with young and old, red cells (see Chapter 37). While this method is considerably more complicated than simple centrifugation, the yield of reticulocytes in the separated young cell population may not be particularly high; figures between 2 and 20% have been reported (181,255,256). Thus the same mixed-field reactions as described above may be seen in phenotyping tests on red cells separated by this method. While reticulocyte-enrichment of the separated population of less dense red cells is not always numerically impressive, the method will be better than it may appear if most of the non-reticulocytes separated in the less dense population are, in fact, young red cells.

As would be expected, use of the flow cytometer to identify reticulocytes via fluorescent dyes or fluorescent-tagged antibodies, has provided impressive results (257-265). Since most transfusion services do not have full access to a flow cytometer (this book is taking so long to write that the statement may be out of date by the time book is published) those methods will not be discussed further.

In 1990, Brun et al. (186) described a novel method for the isolation of reticulocytes. A monoclonal antibody to the transferrin receptor, CD71, was coupled to magnetic beads. Once reticulocytes had bound the MAb via their transferrin receptor, they were separated from other cells via magnetic force. Since serum and plasma contain free transferrin receptors (266-268), mixing the antibody-bound reticulocytes with plasma or serum results in the eventual release of the reticulocytes from the MAb and blocking of the antibody combining sites with plasma or serum transferrin receptors (i.e. competitive replacement or inhibition). It was reported (186) that cell populations separated by this method contained 98 to 100% reticulocytes. In a later study (187) reticulocytes separated in this manner, from samples from recently transfused patients, were phenotyped with red cell antibodies to Rh, Kell, Duffy, Kidd, MN, Lutheran and Lewis system antigens, and the results were compared to typing tests on pretransfusion samples from the patients. It was shown (187) that reliable results could be obtained 8 to 10 hours after transfusion in patients transfused with as many as 15 units of blood. It appears that the MAb-magnetic bead method (186,187) is extremely useful when a pure preparation of reticulocytes is needed.

Mixed-field Agglutination Patterns and Minor Red Cell Populations

Sometimes when serological tests are read, it is noticed that agglutinates are present simultaneously with large numbers of unagglutinated cells. Although this is a typical finding with some antibodies (e.g., anti-Lu[a] (188), anti-Sd[a] (189,190)) it may also represent one of the alternative conditions listed below.

1. Recently transfused cells.
    The transfused cells may carry antigens lacking from the recipient's cells or vice versa.
2. Fetal-maternal hemorrhage.
    Fetal cells may be present in the circulation of a pregnant woman, thus comprising a minor cell population.
3. Intrauterine transfusion.
    When an infant has been transfused in utero, it is hoped that large numbers of the transfused cells (usually D- in a D+ infant) will be present at the time of birth.
4. Chimeras.
    Rarely, twins exchange blood-forming tissue in utero, resulting in two populations of cells that may have differing blood groups and that continue to be

produced throughout the lives of the individuals. The situation can be difficult to recognize when only one twin survives, especially if existence of the second was not suspected. The serological findings can be quite complex, excellent reviews have been published by Race and Sanger (239), Watkins et al. (240), Tippett (241) and Daniels (242).

5. Another possibility.
    Since natural chimeras are comparatively rare, the finding of a minor cell population in an adult, non-transfused, non-pregnant person should first be confirmed on repeat blood samples from the subject. Cross-contamination of one blood sample with another in the laboratory is more common than the chimeric state.

6. Chimeras created by bone marrow transplantation.
    Any time that a bone marrow transplant from other than an identical twin is given, there is a possibility that some of the patient's and some of the donor's progenitor cells will give rise to circulating cells of different phenotypes, thus creating a permanent artificial chimera (191-197). There is one report (198) of permanent chimerism resulting from intrauterine blood transfusion (see Chapter 41).

The principles of methods designed to separate two populations of red cells that differ in blood group phenotype have been discussed in Chapter 3, some details of methods are given by Judd (178). If one of the cell populations carries an antigen, e.g. D, C, E, K, etc., that the other lacks, a method that we described (199) is particularly efficient. The antigen-positive red cells in the cell mixture are coated with a potent IgG antibody. The red cells are then washed and are passed over a staph protein A column. The antigen-positive red cells, coated with IgG, bind to the staph protein A, the antigen-negative red cells pass through the column and can be collected. The column is then rinsed (to clear any remaining trapped antigen-negative red cells) then the antigen-positive cell population is recovered by elution from the column. The method produces essentially 100% pure separated cell populations in any desired quantity. For easy recognition of a mixed cell population, the gel test (243) is useful. With an appropriate antibody the antigen-positive red cells will be seen at the top of the gel, the antigen-negative cells will form a button in the bottom of the tube.

Estimation of the Survival of Transfused Red Cells by a Differential Agglutination Method

The need to forecast the in vivo survival of red cells that are reactive in vitro with an alloantibody thought not to be of clinical significance, arises frequently. When the blood transfusion service involved has the capability to label red cells with ^{51}Cr or a different isotope, in vivo survival can be forecast following the injection of small quantities (1 or 2 ml) of red cells (200-215). When in vivo red cell survival studies cannot be performed, the monocyte monolayer assay (MMA) can be used (215-222). This test has developed an impressive record in correlating in vitro and in vivo findings (221-223). When neither in vivo red cell survival studies nor the MMA is available an "in house" test based on differential agglutination can be used. Donohue et al. (224) modified a method originally devised by Greenwalt et al. (225) for this purpose. Since a relatively large volume of red cells (circa 100 to 200 ml) must be infused, the method can only be used when rapid in vivo destruction of the antigen-positive red cells is unlikely. Since the method, that can be of considerable value, does not seem to have been described in detail elsewhere, it is repeated, from the third edition of this book, below.

1. Calculate how many red cells must be infused to constitute a readily detectable percentage (e.g. 5 to 15%) of the patient's post transfusion total red cell mass. This is done by estimating the patient's red cell mass based on height, weight and/or surface area, sex and hematocrit (211).

2. Select and infuse an appropriate volume of red cells that can later be differentiated from the patient's own cells by serological means. Ideally and for the rest of this example, group O cells are transfused to say, a group A individual.

3. At 1, 24 and 48 hours and again at one week following infusion, collect an anticoagulated blood sample from the patient.

4. Mix 50µl of washed, tightly packed, patient's post transfusion red cells with 50 ml of physiological saline.

5. Place four 9 ml aliquots of this cell suspension in separate tubes.

6. To each of two of the 9 ml aliquots (test) add 3 ml anti-A typing serum diluted 1 in 10 in saline.

7. To the other two 9 ml aliquots (control) add 3 ml saline.

8. Place the tubes on a rotor and mix at RT for 3 hours.

9. Centrifuge the tubes at 1000 rcf for five minutes.

10. Return the tubes to the rotor for 5 minutes, gently to resuspend the unagglutinated red cells.

11. Place the tubes upright for exactly two minutes to allow the agglutinates to settle.

12. At two minutes, transfer the top 10 ml from each tube to a clean tube.

13. Prepare a 1 in 50 dilution of the unagglutinated

separated red cells and count in a cell counter.
Count each sample twice.

14. Calculate the mean cell count of the control and the mean cell count of the test from the four readings from each.

15. Express the number of unagglutinated cells in the test samples (transfused group O red cells) as a percentage of the total cell count (patient's own plus transfused cells) in the control samples.

A number of points need to be made about this method.

1. The percentages of transfused cells surviving at 1, 24 and 48 hours and at one week are compared. The method provides a comparison of survival of those cells over seven days, it does not give an exact rate of cell survival since some of the patient's own cells will remain unagglutinated.

2. Since the numbers are to be compared to each other, accurate measurement of each volume at each step of the test is essential.

3. If the patient is group O and a different antibody must be used to agglutinate the patient's cells (e.g. anti-M if M- N+ cells are infused in an M+ N- patient), less agglutination in steps 6-11 is likely. Accordingly, it may be necessary to estimate the percentage of the patient's cells that remain unagglutinated, using a sample drawn before the test dose is infused and to subtract this blank from the test results.

4. There is relatively little danger that rapid destruction of some of the transfused red cells in the first hour and relatively normal survival of the remainder will create the impression of normal survival of the whole test dose. As described in step one of the method, it can be calculated roughly what percentage of unagglutinated cells should be seen in the 1 hour sample if there is 100% survival of the test dose. A percentage significantly below the expected figure should alert the investigator to the possibility that some immediate red cell destruction may have occurred.

5. There is little value in collecting a sample before one hour after the infusion. Total in vivo mixing of the transfused and patient's own cells may not occur in less than an hour because of the relatively large test dose of red cells used.

6. If a test dose that comprises 12 to 15% of the total posttransfusion red cell mass can be used, the results are likely to be more reliable than if the transfused cells comprise say only 5% of the total red cell mass (i.e., small technical errors less significant if the percentage represented by the test dose is high).

7. As mentioned, a disadvantage of this method is that a relatively large test dose of cells must be infused. A huge advantage is that if the patient bleeds during the study, the results will still be valid. After the initial one hour mixing period following infusion, any blood loss by the patient will involve autologous and transfused cells in a ratio representing their concentrations. In other words, even if the total red cell volume is reduced by hemorrhage, the same percentage of unagglutinated (transfused) cells will be present after the hemorrhage if those cells are surviving normally. In this respect the method is better than the one using ^{51}Cr, for a hemorrhage during that test will result in loss of some of the label with no way to calculate how much was lost by hemorrhage and how much by antibody-induced red cell destruction.

We (226,227) were impressed with the utility of this method. In our experience the one hour figure was usually very close (i.e., plus or minus 1%) to the calculated expected number. Using the method we (226) showed that Vel+ red cells could be expected to survive normally in a patient with a weak anti-Vel in the serum; that expectation was realized when four units of Vel+ blood were subsequently transfused with no untoward effects and caused the expected increases in hemoglobin and hematocrit. We (227) also saw an anti-Gy^a that appeared benign in vivo in this test although that conclusion was neither confirmed nor refuted because the patient was not subsequently transfused. In another case (227) an unidentified antibody that defined an antigen of high incidence and that had all the serological characteristics of an antibody that could be expected to be benign in vivo, proved that the method works when in vivo red cell destruction does occur. The 24 hour figure showed that about 20% and the 48 hour figure that about 45% of the 100 ml test dose of red cells had been cleared, so that transfusion with serologically incompatible red cells was avoided. Although the method described lacks some of the advantages of survival studies with radiolabeled red cells, it is clearly much better than the biological test in which 50 ml of red cells are infused and a blood sample collected one hour later from the other arm, is examined for hemolysis. Indeed, such a test will forecast nothing other than the likelihood or lack thereof, that the antibody involved will cause immediate intravascular hemolysis.

The quantitative estimation of red cell survival by means of differential agglutination can be coupled with other tests for mixed-field reactions. For example, when we used the method to estimate the survival of Vel+ red cells in the patient with anti-Vel (226), we infused group O, D-, Vel+ red cells into a group A, D+, Vel- patient. Tests with anti-A, anti-D and anti-Vel on the 1, 24 and 48 hour and 1 week samples gave about the same strength mixed-field reactions, again suggesting normal survival of the serologically incompatible red cells.

Red Cell Stroma

When red cells are hemolyzed, the solid materials that can be separated from the hemoglobin and fluid contents of the cells and that are comprised primarily of the cell membranes, are called stroma. Since red cell stroma (that ironically are white when washed free of hemoglobin) carry most of the red cell antigens, they can be used for adsorption (228) and as immunogens although, in general, stroma are less efficient at stimulating antibody production than are intact red cells (229-231). At one time it became popular to use outdated platelet concentrates to adsorb sera that contained troublesome antibodies, such as those described as HTLA antibodies in Chapter 30. The objective was to adsorb the HTLA or similar antibody and leave clinically-significant antibodies unadsorbed. Because platelet concentrates invariably contain red cell stroma, and some contain intact red cells although that fact may not be obvious to the naked eye, the procedure was somewhat risky and the danger existed that significant antibodies to red cells might be adsorbed. While it was unlikely that a potent antibody capable of causing a frank transfusion reaction would be adsorbed, the danger that a weak antibody such as anti-Jk^a or anti-Jk^b, that could cause a delayed hemolytic reaction would be removed in the adsorption, was real. Fortunately the procedure seems no longer to be widely used.

Antigen Loss on Traveled Red Cells

Booth (232) noticed that traveled red cell samples sometimes fail to react with red cell antibodies that define antigens believed to be present on red cells in low numbers of copies. For example, a serum giving weak and variable IAT reactions with all panel and donor red cell samples might fail to react with one example each of red cells of the phenotypes Cs(a-), Kn(a-), JMH-, recovered from frozen storage. Reactions of other examples of cells of those phenotypes might exclude specificity of the antibody for Cs^a, Kn^a or JMH. Often the cell samples in question were comparatively old when shipped and had spent much time traveling under non-refrigerated conditions. Peter Booth (232) made the observation while working in Papua, New Guinea so had many such traveled red cells available for study. This observation should be borne in mind when unexpected negative reactions are seen. Red cells from the sample in question can then be tested for level of the appropriate antigen, using more potent examples of the appropriate antibody.

Substances in Donor Blood

Sharon et al. (233) tested samples from 2,655 units of blood collected from voluntary donors in Jerusalem and showed that 6% of them contained aspirin in concentrations ranging from 10 to 200 µg/ml. In a later study, the incidence was 7.7% (234). It is possible (233,235) but does not seem to have been conclusively proved, that the presence of aspirin might have a detrimental effect on the recipient of the blood. In another study, Sharon et al. (236) found acetaminophen in levels ranging from 10 to 58 µg/ml in 6.1% of samples from 1,176 units of blood collected in Jerusalem. Again, adverse effects of transfusing blood containing acetaminophen are somewhat more theoretical than proved (237).

Age is Relative

Moore (238) has pointed out that 40 year-old patients (and by extrapolation similarly aged blood bankers) should not be considered old or even middle-aged. He has suggested the following code:

Age	Interpretation
20-30	Young
30-40	Youthful
40-50	Mature
50-60	Prime-of-Life
60-65	Middle-aged
65-70	Elderly
70-75	Venerable
75 and on	Old

Alas, by the time this book is published, one of us (guess which) will have reached the Elderly classification meaning that if a fifth edition of this book is ever written, he will not be one of its authors. Now the only question that remains, see the first sentence of this chapter, is why a chapter about nothing, required 275 references?

References

1. Beattie KM, Zuelzer WW. Transfusion 1968;8:254
2. Beattie KM, Seymour DS, Scott A. Transfusion 1971;11:107
3. Howe SE, Sciotto CG, Berkner D. Transfusion 1982;22:111
4. Watson KC, Joubert SM. Nature 1960;188:505
5. Beattie KM, Ferguson SJ, Burnie KL, et al. Transfusion 1976;16:174
6. Parish HJ, MacFarlane RG. Lancet 1941;2:477
7. Mann JM. (abstract). Transfusion 1973;13:346
8. Pierce SR, Moore A, Hardman J, et al. (abstract). Transfusion 1979;19:641
9. Williams L, Lebeck L. (Letter). Transfusion 1981;21:288
10. Gillund TD, Howard PL, Isham B. Vox Sang 1972;23:369
11. Henry R, Freihaut BH, Pierce SR, et al. (abstract). Transfusion 1973;13:345
12. Reid ME, Battenfield LK, Toy PTCY, et al. Am J Clin Pathol 1985;83:534

13. Tobar M. Immunohematology 1987;3:40
14. Peloquin PM. (abstract). Prog 37th Ann Mtg Florida Assoc Blood Banks, 1983
15. Lewis T, Reid M, Ellisor S, et al. Vox Sang 1980;39:205
16. Avoy DR, Toy P, Reid ME, et al. (abstract). Transfusion 1980;20:629
17. Vengelen-Tyler V, Dearolf SJ, Haley SA. Transfusion 1981;21:315
18. Gray MP. Vox Sang 1964;9:608
19. Mougey R, Pierce S, Levy S, et al. (abstract). Transfusion 1980;20:628
20. Pfister M, Ellisor SS, Reid M. (abstract). Transfusion 1979;19:647
21. Morel PA, Tyler VV. (abstract). Transfusion 1979;19:647
22. Reid ME, Danneskiold T. Immunohematology 1984;1:9
23. Bird GWG, Roy TCF. Vox Sang 1980;38:169
24. Hysell JK, Gray JM, Hysell JW, et al. Transfusion 1975;15:16
25. Schulenburg BJ, Wadhams DL, Kowalski MA, et al. (abstract). Book of Abstracts. 16th Cong ISBT, 1980:264
26. Halhuber KJ, Linss W, Geyer G. Acta Biol Med Germ 1977;36:885
27. Freiesleben E, Jensen KG. (abstract). Prog 7th Cong Eur Soc Haematol, 1959:(abstract 330)
28. Harboe M, Reinskou T, Heisto H, et al. Vox Sang 1961;6:409
29. Allan CJ, Lawrence RD, Shih SC, et al. Transfusion 1972;12:306
30. Davey RJ, O'Gara C, McGinniss MH. Vox Sang 1979;36:301
31. Jones TE, Ayrton AS, Blajchman MA. Transfusion 1973;13:150
32. Shulman IA, Hasz LA, Simpson RB. Transfusion 1983;23:241
33. Shirey RS, Ciappi AB, Kickler TS, et al. Immunohematology 1993;9:19
34. Williams L, Domen RE. Transfusion 1989;29:23
35. Gilbert DM, Domen RE. Immunohematology 1989;5:119
36. Beck ML, McGuire D, Richardson C. (abstract). Book of Abstracts, 13th Cong ISBT, 1972:6
37. Judd WJ, Steiner EA, Cochran RK. Transfusion 1982;22:31
38. Halima D, Garratty G, Bueno R. Transfusion 1982;22:521
39. Morel PA, Bergren MO, Hill V, et al. Transfusion 1981;21:652
40. Judd WJ, Steiner EA, Capps RD. Transfusion 1982;22:185
41. Chiofolo JT, Reid ME, Charles-Pierre D. Immunohematology 1995;11:18
42. Sosler SD, Behzad O, Garratty G, et al. (abstract). Transfusion 1979;19:641
43. Hegarty JS, Dolphin E, Leonard WR. (abstract). Transfusion 1982;22:411
44. Shirey S, Harris J, Moore L. (abstract). Transfusion 1979;19:642
45. Dolor MC. Lab Med 1985;16:660
46. Bliznik AM. Lab Med 1985;16:695
47. Gunson HH. Vox Sang 1969;17:514
48. Beck ML, Freihaut B, Henry R, et al. Br J Haematol 1975;29;149
49. Yasuda H, Ohto H, Motoki R, et al. Transfusion 1997;37:1131
50. Onder O, Weinstein A, Hoyer LW. Blood 1980;56:177
51. Thorpe SJ. Br J Haematol 1989;73:527
52. Thorpe SJ. Br J Haematol 1990;76:116
53. Weiner W, Tovey GH, Gillespie EM, et al. Vox Sang 1956;1:279
54. Weiner W, Hallum JL. Vox Sang 1957;2:38
55. Moore BPL, Linins I, McIntyre J. Blood 1958;14:364
56. Crowley LV, Hyland YR. Am J Clin Pathol 1962;37:244
57. Powell DEB, Reese C. J Clin Pathol 1965;18:212
58. Hossaini AA, Burkhart CR, Hooper GS. Transfusion 1965;5:461
59. Yokoyama M, Park HS, Mermod L. Vox Sang 1968;14:67
60. Lovett CA, Moore BPL. Immunology 1968;14:357
61. Hedlund PA, Olson C, Polesky H. (abstract). Transfusion 1968;8:320
62. Golde DW, McGinniss MH, Holland PV. Vox Sang 1969;16:465
63. Smith DS, Howell P, Riches R. Vox Sang 1969;16:505
64. Golde DW, McGinniss MH, Holland PV. Am J Clin Pathol 1971;55:655
65. Spence L, Jones D, Moore BPL. Transfusion 1971;11:193
66. Golde DW, Greipp PR, McGinniss MH. Transfusion 1973;13:1
67. Beck ML, Pierce SR, Freihaut BH, et al. (abstract). Transfusion 1973;13:347
68. Hossaini AA, Kerhulas J, Dabbs D. (abstract). Fed Proc 1973;32:840
69. Reid ME, Ellisor SS, Frank BA. Transfusion 1975;15:485
70. Hossaini AA. (abstract). Fed Proc 1975;34:837
71. Beck ML, Edwards RL, Pierce SR, et al. Transfusion 1976;16:434
72. Case J. Vox Sang 1976;30:441
73. Hossaini AA, Wasserman AJ, Vennart GP. Am J Clin Pathol 1976;65:519
74. Hossaini AA, Hazeghi K, Amiri P. Transfusion 1977;17:54
75. Dube VE, Zoes C. Vox Sang 1977;33:359
76. Hossaini AA. In: Progress in Clinical Pathology, Vol 7. New York:Grune and Stratton, 1978:178
77. Kriesel DH, Reynolds MV, Behzad O. Transfusion 1982;22:406
78. Leikola J, Perkins HA. Transfusion 1980;20:224
79. Witebsky E, Klendshoj NC, McNeil C. Proc Soc Exp Biol NY 1944;55:167
80. Witebsky E. Ann NY Acad Sci 1946;46:887
81. Thorpe SJ, Bailey SW, Gooi HC, et al. Transf Med 1992;2:151
82. Thompson KM, Sutherland J, Barden G, et al. Immunology 1992;76:146
83. Thorpe SJ, Bailey SW. Br J Haematol 1993;83:311
84. Thorpe SJ, Boult CE, Bailey SW, et al. Appl Immunohistochem 1996;4:190
85. Øyen R, Colledge KI, Marsh WL, et al. Transfusion 1972;12:98
86. Lockyer JW, Darke C, Webb AJ. Vox Sang 1967;12:75
87. Wright J. Unpublished observations cited in Mollison PL. Blood Transfusion in Clinical Medicine, 5th Ed. Oxford:Blackwell, 1972
88. Gottleib AM. Unpublished observations 1971 cited in Issitt PD, Issitt CH. Applied Blood Group Serology, 2nd Ed. Oxnard:Spectra Biologicals, 1975
89. Issitt PD, Jerez GC. Transfusion 1966;6:155
90. Issitt PD, Pavone BG, Wagstaff W, et al. Transfusion 1976;16:396
91. Pavone BG, Pirkola A, Nevanlinna HR, et al. Transfusion 1978;18:155
92. Dahr W, Wilkinson SL, Issitt PD, et al. Biol Chem Hoppe-Seyler 1986;367:1033
93. Wren MR, Issitt PD. Transfusion 1988;28:113
94. Davidsohn I, Toharsky B. J Infect Dis 1940;67:25
95. Mollison PL. Blood Transfusion in Clinical Medicine, 5th Ed. Oxford:Blackwell, 1972
96. Rosati LA, Barnes B, Oberman HA, et al. Transfusion 1970;10:139

97. Oberman HA, Beck ML. Transfusion 1971;11:382
98. Niosi P, Lundberg J, McCullough J, et al. New Eng J Med 1971;285:1435
99. Case J, Schiff P, Walsh J. New Eng J Med 1972;287:359
100. Lang GE, Veldhuis B. Am J Clin Pathol 1973;60:205
101. Seeler RA, Telischi M, Langehennig PL, et al. J Pediat 1976;89:87
102. Seeler RA. In: Unsolved Therapeutic Problems in Hemophilia. Washington, D.C.: US Gov Printing Office, DHEW Publication No (NIH)77-1089, 1977:113
103. Glueck H, Issitt CH, Issitt PD. Unpublished observations 1977 cited in Issitt PD. Applied Blood Group Serology, 3rd Ed. Miami:Montgomery 1985:602
104. Glassy EF, Myhre BA, Nakasako Y, et al. Transfusion 1978;18:125
105. Wright J, Freedman J, Lim FC, et al. Canad Med Assoc J 1979;120:1235
106. Gordon JM, Cohen P, Finlayson JS. Transfusion 1980;20:90
107. Ryden SE. (abstract). Prog 37th Ann Mtg Florida Assoc Blood Banks, 1983
108. Swanson JL, Mann EW, Condie RM, et al. (abstract). Transfusion 1982;22:415
109. Draper EK, Dignam CM, Yang S, et al. (abstract). Transfusion 1982;22:415
110. Anderson HJ, Meisenhelder J, Stevens J. (abstract). Transfusion 1983;23:436 Note: The data cited in this chapter are from the verbal presentation of the report and differ significantly from those given in the abstract.
111. Postoway N, Garratty G. (abstract). Transfusion 1984;24:427
112. Anderson HJ, Aubuchon JP, Draper EK, et al. Transfusion 1985;25:47
113. Swanson JL, Issitt CH, Mann EW, et al. Transfusion 1984;24:141
114. Ogata T, Matuhasi T. Proc 9th Cong ISBT. Basel:Karger, 1964:528
115. Ogata T, Matuhasi T. Proc 8th Cong ISBT. Basel:Karger, 1962:208
116. Matuhasi T, Kumazawa H, Usui M. J Jpn Soc Blood Transf 1960;6:295
117. Matuhasi T. Proc 15th Gen Assembly Jpn Med Cong 1959;4:80
118. Svardal JM, Yarbro J, Yunis EJ. Vox Sang 1967;13:472
119. Allen FH Jr, Issitt PD, Degnan TJ, et al. Vox Sang 1969;16:47
120. Bove JR, Holburn AM, Mollison PL. J Immunol 1973;25:793
121. Boursnell JC, Coombs RRA, Rizk V. Biochem J 1953;55:745
122. Masouredis SP. J Clin Invest 1959;38:279
123. Hughes-Jones NC, Gardner B. Biochem J 1962;83:404
124. Pirofsky B, Cordova MS, Imel TL. Vox Sang 1962;7:334
125. Masouredis SP. Transfusion 1964;4:69
126. Gergely J, Arky J, Medgyesi GA. Vox Sang 1967;12:252
127. Victoria EJ, Mahan LC, Masouredis SP. Br J Haematol 1982;50:101
128. Fudenberg HH, Rosenfield RE, Wassermann LR. J Mt Sinai Hosp 1958;25:324
129. Issitt PD, Zellner DC, Rolih SD, et al. Transfusion 1977;17:539
130. Henry RA, Weber J, Pavone BG, et al. Transfusion 1977;17:547
131. Issitt PD, Pavone BG. Br J Haematol 1978;38:63
132. Weber J, Caceres VW, Pavone BG, et al. Transfusion 1979;19:216
133. Issitt PD, Pavone BG, Shapiro M. Transfusion 1979;19:389
134. Garratty G, Sattler MS, Petz LD, et al. Rev Fr Transf Immunohematol 1979;22:524
135. Viggiano E, Clary NL, Ballas SK. Transfusion 1982;22:329
136. Ellisor SS, Reid ME, O'Day T, et al. Vox Sang 1983;45:53
137. Manny N, Levene C, Sela R, et al. Vox Sang 1983;45:252
138. Van't Veer MB, Leeuwen I van, Haas FJ, et al. Vox Sang 1984;47:88
139. Puig N, Carbonell F, Marty ML. Vox Sang 1986;51:57
140. Moulds M, Strohm P, McDowell MA, et al. (abstract). Transfusion 1988;28 (Suppl 6S):36S
141. Harris T. Immunohematology 1990;6:87
142. Issitt PD, Combs MR, Bumgarner DJ, et al. Transfusion 1996;36:481
143. Rand BP, Olson JD, Garratty G, et al. Transfusion 1978;18:174
144. Leger R, Ciesielski D, Garratty G, et al. (abstract). Transfusion 1995;35 (Suppl 10S):67S
145. Moulds J, Mallory D, Zodin V. (abstract). Transfusion 1978;18:388
146. Young NM, Leon MA, Takahashi T, et al. J Biol Chem 1971;246:1596
147. Reisner Y, Biniaminov M, Rosenthal E, et al. Proc Nat Acad Sci USA 1979;76:447
148. Basu PS, Ray MK, Datta TK. J Exp Biol 1980;18:931
149. Barzilay M, Monsigny M, Sharon N. In: Lectins-Biology, Biochemistry and Clinical Biochemistry, Vol 2. Berlin:de Gruyter, 1981:67
150. Sandhu RS, Reen RS, Singh S, et al. In: Lectins-Biology, Biochemistry and Clinical Biochemistry, Vol 2. Berlin:de Gruyter, 1981:679
151. Sandhu RS, Kamboj SS, Reen RS, et al. Vox Sang 1982;43:345
152. Elias L, Epps E van. Blood 1984;63:1285
153. Hogeman PHG, Veerman AJP, Zantwijk CH van, et al. (Letter). Br J Haematol 1985;59:392
154. Krishna Sastry MV, Banarjee P, Patanjali SR, et al. J Biol Chem 1987;261:11726
155. Autcouturier P, Mihaesco E, Mihaesco C, et al. Mol Immunol 1987;24:503
156. Saxon A, Tsui F, Martinez-Mazo O. Cell Immunol 1987;104:134
157. Siena S, Villa S, Bonadonna G, et al. Transp Proc 1987;19:2735
158. Bird GWG. Transf Med Rev 1989;3:55
159. Wintrobe MM. Clinical Hematology, 6th Ed. Philadelphia:Lea and Febiger, 1967:357
160. Gralnick MA. In: A Seminar on Problems Encountered in Pretransfusion Tests. Washington, D.C.:Am Assoc Blood Banks, 1972:71
161. Bull JP, Ricketts C, Squire JR, et al. Lancet 1949;1:134
162. Selwyn JG, Seright W, Donald J, et al. Lancet 1968;2:1032
163. Chien S, Kung-Ming J. Microvasc Res 1973;5:155
164. Rutherford R, Gordon S. Med J Austral 1977;1:830
165. Bartholomew JR, Bell WR, Kickler T, et al. Transfusion 1986;26:431
166. Perkins HA, Rolfs MR, McBride A, et al. Transfusion 1964;4:10
167. Murray S, Dewar PJ. Transfusion 1971;11:378
168. Godwin G. (Letter). Transfusion 1987;27:366
169. Daniels MJ, Strauss RG, Smith-Floss AM. Transfusion 1982;22:226
170. Moore BPL, Humphreys P, Lovett-Moseley CA. Serological and Immunological Methods, 7th Ed. Toronto:Canadian Red Cross, 1972
171. Technical Methods and Procedures of the American Association of Blood Banks, 5th Ed. Chicago:Am Assoc Blood Banks, 1960
172. Schmidt PJ, Kevy SV. Transfusion 1963;3:198

173. Bruce M, Crawford RJ, Mitchell R, et al. Med Lab Sci 1980;37:171
174. Bruce M, Mitchell R. Med Lab Sci 1981;38:177
175. Cross RA. Austral J Med Technol 1979;10:169
176. Stephens JG. J Physiol 1940;99:30
177. Reid ME, Toy PTCY. Am J Clin Pathol 1983;79:364
178. Judd WJ. Methods in Immunohematology, 2nd Ed. Durham:Montgomery, 1994
179. Wallas CH, Tanley PC, Gorrell LP. Transfusion 1980;20:332
180. Wallas CH, Tanley PC, Gorrell LP. Transfusion 1982;22:26
181. Branch DR, Shulman IA, Sy Siok Hian AL, et al. Blood 1984;63:177
182. Vettore L, DeMatteis MC, Zampini P. Am J Hematol 1980;8:291
183. Branch DR, Sy Siok Hian AL, Carlson F, et al. Am J Clin Pathol 1983;80:453
184. Rennie CM, Thompson S, Parker AC, et al. Clin Chim Acta 1979;98:119
185. Lutz HU, Stammler P, Fasler S, et al. Biochim Biophys Acta 1992;1116:1
186. Brun A, Gaudernack G, Sandberg S. Blood 1990;76:2397
187. Brun A, Skadberg Ø, Hervig TA, et al. Transfusion 1994;34:162
188. Callender S, Race RR, Paycock ZV. Br Med J 1945;2:83
189. Macvie SJ, Morton JA, Pickles MM. Vox Sang 1967;13:485
190. Renton PH, Howell P, Ikin EW, et al. Vox Sang 1967;13:493
191. Branch DR, Gallagher MT, Forman SJ, et al. Transplantation 1982;34:226
192. Petz LD, Branch DR, Stock AD, et al. Transplant Proc 1985;17:432
193. Petz LD, Yam PY, Wallace RB, et al. Blood 1987;70:1331
194. Yam PY, Petz LD, Ali S, et al. Am J Hum Genet 1987;41:867
195. Yam PY, Petz LD, Knowlton RG, et al. Transplantation 1987;43:399
196. Ugozzoli L, Yam P, Petz LD, et al. Blood 1991;77:1607
197. Petz LD. In: Clinical and Basic Science Aspects of Immunohematology. Arlington, VA:Am Assoc Blood Banks, 1991:73
198. Naiman JL, Punnett HH, Destiné ML, et al. Lancet 1966;2:590
199. Issitt PD, Combs MR, Sammons TD, et al. (abstract). Transfusion 1992;32 (Suppl 8S):55S
200. Ebaugh FG Jr, Emerson CP, Ross JF. J Clin Invest 1953;32:1260
201. Read RC. New Eng J Med 1954;250:1021
202. Mollison PL, Veall N. Br J Haematol 1955;1:62
203. Donohue DM, Motulsky AG, Giblett ER, et al. Br J Haematol 1955;1:249
204. Mollison PL. Clin Sci 1961;21:21
205. Szymanski IO, Valeri CR. Br J Haematol 1970;19:397
206. Garby L, Mollison PL. Br J Haematol 1971;20:527
207. International Committee for Standardization in Haematology. Br J Haematol 1971;21:241
208. Bentley SA, Glass HI, Lewis SM, et al. Br J Haematol 1974;26:179
209. International Committee for Standardization in Haematology. Br J Haematol 1980;45:659
210. Mollison PL. In: A Seminar on Immune-Mediated Cell Destruction. Washington, D.C.:Am Assoc Blood Banks, 1981:45
211. Mollison PL. Blood Transfusion in Clinical Medicine, 7th Ed. Oxford:Blackwell, 1983
212. Baldwin ML, Ness PM, Barrasso C, et al. Transfusion 1985;25:34
213. Esty SS, Wahl T, Zawisza J, et al. Immunohematology 1987;3:6
214. Davey RJ. In: Diagnostic and Investigational Uses of Radiolabeled Blood Elements. Arlington, VA:Am Assoc Blood Banks, 1987:39
215. Davey RJ, Esty SS, Chin JF, et al. Immunohematology 1994;10:90
216. Schanfield MS, Stevens JO, Bauman D. Transfusion 1981;21:571
217. Hunt JS, Beck ML, Tegtmeier G, et al. Transfusion 1982;22:355
218. Branch DR, Gallagher MT, Mison AP, et al. Br J Haematol 1984;56:19
219. Douglas R, Rowthorne NV, Schneider JV. Transfusion 1985;25;535
220. Wren MR, Issitt PD. (abstract). Transfusion 1986;26:548
221. Nance SJ, Arndt P, Garratty G. Transfusion 1987;27:449
222. Gutgsell NS, Issitt LA, Issitt PD. (abstract). Transfusion 1988;28 (Suppl 6S):32S
223. Garratty G. In: Immune Destruction of Red Blood Cells. Arlington, VA:Am Assoc Blood Banks, 1989:109
224. Donohue C, Steane EA, Steane SM. Unpublished observations 1982 and 1983 cited by Issitt PD. Applied Blood Group Serology, 3rd Ed. Miami:Montgomery 1985:606
225. Greenwalt TJ, Myhre B, Steane EA. J Immunol 1965;94:272
226. Moore RE, Kraemer HJ, Lenes BA, et al. (abstract). Prog 37th Ann Mtg Florida Assoc Blood Banks, 1984
227. Moore RE, McCollister LS, Brendel WL, et al. Unpublished observations 1983 and 1984 cited in Issitt PD. Applied Blood Group Serology, 3rd Ed. Miami:Montgomery 1985:607
228. Milgrom F, Layrisse M. Nature 1958;182:189
229. Schneider J, Preisler O. Blut 1966;12:1
230. Mollison PL. Blood Transfusion in Clinical Medicine, 4th Ed. Oxford:Blackwell, 1967:203
231. Pollack W, Gorman JG, Hager HJ, et al. Transfusion 1968;8:134
232. Booth PB. Unpublished observations 1976 cited in Issitt PD. Applied Blood Group Serology, 3rd Ed. Miami:Montgomery 1985:607
233. Sharon R, Kidroni G, Michel J. Vox Sang 1980;38:284
234. Sharon R, Frutkoff I, Kidroni G, et al. J Clin Pathol 1982;35:59
235. Weltman JK, Szard RP, Settipane GA. Allergy 1978;34:273
236. Sharon R, Menczel J, Kidroni G. Vox Sang 1982;43:138
237. Shoenfeld Y, Shaklai M, Livini E, et al. New Eng J Med 1980;303:47
238. Moore BPL. (Letter). Transfusion 1982;22:83
239. Race RR, Sanger R. Blood Groups in Man, 6th Ed. Oxford:Blackwell, 1975:511
240. Watkins WM, Greenwell P, Yates AD. Rev Fr Transf Immunohematol 1980;23:531
241. Tippett P. Vox Sang 1983;44:333
242. Daniels G. Human Blood Groups. Oxford:Blackwell, 1995:684
243. Lapierre Y, Rigal D, Adam J, et al. Transfusion 1990;30:109
244. Lapinid IM, Steib MD, Noto TA. Am J Clin Pathol 1984;81:514
245. Kimura E, Suzucki T, Kinoshita Y. Nature 1960;188:1201
246. Danon D, Marikovsky Y. J Lab Clin Med 1964;64:668
247. Leif RC, Vinegrad J. Proc Nat Acad Sci USA 1964;51:520
248. Bishop C, Prentice TC. J Cell Compatibility Physiol 1966;67:197
249. Piomelli S, Lurinsky G, Wassermann LR. J Lab Clin Med 1967;69:659
250. Corash LM, Piomelli S, Chen HC, et al. J Lab Clin Med 1974;84;147

251. Pertoft H, Laurent H, Lass T, et al. Ann Biochem 1978;88:271

252. Segal AW, Fortunato A, Herd T. J Immunol Meth 1980;32:209

253. Olofsson T, Gärtner I, Olsson I. Scand J Haematol 1980;24:254

254. Desimone J, Kleve L, Schaeffer J. J Lab Clin Med 1974;84:517

255. Ballas SK, Flynn JC Jr, Pauline LA, et al. Am J Hematol 1986;23:19

256. Reeves MR. MHS Thesis, Duke Univ 1994

257. Tanke HJ, Nieuwenhuis IAB, Koper GJM, et al. Cytometry 1980;1:313

258. Tanke H, Rothbart P, Vossen J, et al. Blood 1983;61:1091

259. Sage BH Jr, O'Connell JP, Mercolino TJ. Cytometry 1983;4:222

260. Jaccobberger JW, Horan PK, Hare JD. Cytometry 1984;5:589

261. Lee LG, Chen C-H, Chiu LA. Cytometry 1986;7:508

262. van Hove L, Goossens W, Duppen V van, et al. Clin Lab Haematol 1990;12:287

263. Chin-Yee I, Keeney M, Lohmann C. Clin Lab Haematol 1991;13:177

264. Serke S, Huhn D. Br J Haematol 1992;81:432

265. Serke S, Huhn D. Clin Lab Haematol 1993;15:33

266. Kohgo Y, Nishisato T, Kondo H, et al. Br J Haematol 1986;64:277

267. Johnstone RM, Bianchini A, Teng K. Blood 1989;74:1844

268. Flowers CH, Skikne BS, Covell AM, et al. J Lab Clin Med 1989;114:368

269. Wiener AS. Blood Groups and Transfusion. Springfield, IL:Thomas, 1943:49

270. Flanagan CJ, Mitoma TF. Am J Clin Pathol 1958;29:337

271. Killpack S. (Letter). Lancet 1950;2:827

272. Voll V, Kanada Y, Namiki H, et al. (abstract). Transfusion 1996;36 (Suppl 9S):24S

273. Arndt P, Hunt P, Garratty G, et al. (abstract). Transfusion 1997;37 (Suppl 9S):34S

274. Norris SS, Allen DD, Neff TP, et al. Transfusion 1996;36:109

275. Janas T, Bjerrum PJ, Brahm J, et al. Am J Physiol 1989;257:C601

44 | In the Beginning There Was A and B . . . Now There are 434 Named Factors on Red Cells (and see the Addendum for Still More)

In spite of the optimistic title of this chapter, it is impossible to be certain, at any given time, exactly how many different red cell antigens have been detected. With so many immunohematologists working around the world, some duplication is bound to occur. In addition, the same name is sometimes used to describe two or more antigens that are not shown to be different from each other until years after the original name was assigned. Further, the title of this chapter has been liberally interpreted (our prerogative since the title was invented for this book!). Purists will find factors listed here that are not antigens. In general, antigens detected by specific antibodies, distinct phenotypic expressions (sometimes defined by different strength reactions with the same antibody e.g., A_3, A_x) and other factors that can be differentiated at the bench, are listed. We accept that some of the characters and factors are not antigens since they do not elicit production of an antibody specific only unto themselves. However, in determining the 434 total of antigens, phenotypes have not been counted. For example, in the ABO and H systems there are 11 entries but only three antigens (A, B and H) made it to the 434 total. In order to make this list as complete as possible, some rules have been stretched or bent (or both, i.e. euphemisms for broken!) No claim is made that every character listed is inherited. Indeed, in some instances far too little work has been completed for such a claim to be made.

Readers will notice that unlike the first three editions of this book where the total of red cell factors increased with each edition, i.e. 260, 408 and 641 respectively, the total in this edition is lower than in the last. There are a number of reasons. First, some reduction represents recognition that the same antigen was given different names in different investigations (see the last section of this chapter). Second, we have not included in the count, those antigens in recognized blood group systems that have been declared obsolete because antibodies and/or red cells for their recognition no longer exist. In some instances we have listed those antigens for historical reasons. Third and most significant in terms of reduction of the total number, when listing independent antigens of low or high incidence we have included only those described in their own right or in a blood grouping paper published since 1985. Names that were included in the lists in the third edition that are not

included here will be found in the appropriately labeled tables in Chapter 33.

Tempting as it was to consider each epitope of a given antigen as a separate factor (each can be recognized and differentiated if suitable epitope specificity antibodies are available) we did not do so in the total count. Thus the D antigen counts as one in the 434 total although MAb to D differentiate between nine (2) or far more (3,4) epitopes of that antigen. The whole question as to how an antigen count should be made can now be debated. The count of 434 in this chapter essentially represents the ability of man to make antibodies to the factors listed. If biochemical means to determine recognizable factors are used, the numbers become very different. The HLA system provides a classic example. As recently as 1992, serological methods had been used to identify 102 HLA antigens with 25 encoded from the *HLA-A* locus, 32 from the *B* locus, 11 from the *C* locus and 34 from the *DR* locus (41,42). Once DNA sequences had been recognized following PCR amplification (see Chapters 4 and 5) it became apparent that the HLA polymorphism is even more complex. By January of 1997 it was recognized (43) that there are at least 83 *HLA-A*, 186 *HLA-B*, 42 *HLA-C*, and 220 *HLA-DR* alleles for a potential total of 531 isoforms. In other words, new technology has resulted in a 520% increase in recognizable factors in a five year period.

In addition to listing antigen (and a few phenotype) names and frequencies, this chapter provides references to papers that first documented existence of the characters listed. In a few instances references are also given to publications that assigned an already known antigen to a blood group system when previously that antigen was thought to be independent of all others. For the sake of simplicity only the senior author's name is listed in each reference so that et al. sometimes means and one other, instead of, and others. Some of the references (particularly when unpublished antigens of low or high incidence are listed) refer to papers in which the antigen is mentioned but not necessarily described in any detail. For the sake of interest, a number of historical names have been given in the tables. Readers are reminded of the admonition (1) that such terms should be used only in an historical review. In scientific literature (papers, letters, reports, etc.) and in conversation, the antigen name should always be used.

In addition to the 434 named characters, there are a number of weakened forms of some of those antigens to which names have been applied (e.g., D^u, G^u, Fy^x). Again for the sake of completeness the names are listed but the phenotypes are not included as antigens in the total count. The percentage frequency figures listed in this chapter refer to Whites. Antigen frequencies in Blacks, where known, are given in appropriate chapters earlier in this book.

Readers may wonder why we list 434 factors while in the most recent publications (39,40) from the ISBT Working Party on Terminology for Red Cell Surface Antigens, only 259 are named. The major reason is that we list any character that can be recognized on red cells by use of an antibody. The ISBT Working Party requires that in order to qualify for a name (number) each antigen must also be shown to be inherited and to be genetically independent of all others. Thus as examples, antigens in the Pr series and others defined by cold-reactive autoantibodies (20 distinct entries in this chapter) are automatically excluded from the ISBT terminology. Since they are all present on the red cells of all persons, they cannot be shown to be inherited. Paradoxically both I and i have ISBT numbers. Similarly, many independent antigens of low and high incidence are known to exist for long periods before evidence of their inheritance and genetic independence emerges. Our philosophy is based on the fact that this book will be used predominantly by people who work at the bench. When working there and using known antibodies and/or sera currently being investigated, antigens such as IA, M_1, Bg, T (to name only four of some 175 that do not have ISBT numbers) will be detected and recognized. We rationalize that if the antigen can be found, it needs a name so that it can be described.

Finally, for the sake of completeness, some characters known to be the same as others are mentioned in the tables. Such characters have been counted only once in determining the total. In other instances one antigen that might be the same as another in the lists, has been shown. In determining the total we used our own information and (more often) intuition, to decide whether such a character should be counted once or twice. Thus it is unlikely that any reader who counted the antigens listed would arrive at the same 434 total (whoever would want even to try?).

TABLE 44-1 ABO and H Systems

Antigen or Phenotype	% Frequency	Reference
A	45	Landsteiner et al. Klin Woch 1901;14:1132
A_2	7	Dungern et al. Z Immun Forsch 1911;8:526
A_3	0.1	Freidenreich, Z Immun Forsch 1936;89:409
A_x	<0.1	Fisher et al. Z Immun Forsch 1935;84:177
A_m	<0.1	Gammelgaard, Hos Mennesket Copenhagen 1942
B	14	Landsteiner, Zbl Bakt 1900;27:357
B_3	<0.1	Moullec et al. Rev Hematol 1955;10:574
B_m	<0.1	Mäkelä et al. Med Exp Fenn 1955;33:35
B_w	<0.1	Yokoyama et al. Vox Sang 1957;2:348
H	>99.9	Boorman et al. Ann Eugen 1948;14:201
C	55	Landsteiner et al. J Immunol 1926;11:221

TABLE 44-2 Lewis System and
Some Related Antigens

Antigen	Historical or Alternative Name	% Frequency	Reference
Le^a		22	Mourant, Nature 1946;158:237
Le^b		72	Andresen, Acta Path Microbiol Scand 1946;24:616
Le^x	Le^{ab}	94	Andresen, Acta Path Microbiol Scand 1949;26:636
Le^c	Type 1 PS	1.2	Iseki et al. Proc Imp Soc Jpn 1957;33:492
Le^d	Type 1 H	4.8	Potapov, Prob Haematol Moscow 1970;15:45
Le^{bH}		32	Grubb, Acta Path Microbiol Scand 1951;28:61
Le^{bL}		72	Brendemoen, Acta Path Microbiol Scand 1952;31:579
A_1Le^b	Siedler	32	Seaman et al. Vox Sang 1968;15:25
BLe^b	Magard	10	Crookston et al. Lancet 1970;2:1110
A_1Le^d	Type 1 H,A	2.7	Andersen, Vox Sang 1958;3:251
BLe^d	Type 1 H,B	0.6	Tilley et al. Vox Sang 1975;28;25
Le^s	$Le^b + Le^d$	76.8	Potapov, Prob Haematol Moscow 1970;15:45
Le^{ns}	$Le^a + Le^c$	23.2	Potapov, Prob Haematol Moscow 1970;15:45
ILe^{bH}		32	Tegoli et al. Vox Sang 1971;21:397

TABLE 44-3 Ii Collection and
Some Related Antigens

Antigen	Alternative Name	% Frequency	Reference
I		>99.9	Wiener et al. Ann Intern Med 1956;44:221
I^F		>99.9	Marsh et al. Vox Sang 1971;20:209
I^D		>99.9	Marsh et al. Vox Sang 1971;20:209
i		>99.9	Marsh et al. Nature 1960;188:753
j		>99.9	Roelcke et al. Vox Sang 1994;67:216
IH	HI, IO	>99.9	Rosenfield et al. Vox Sang 1964;9:415
IA	AI	45	Tippett et al. Vox Sang 1960;5:107
IB	BI	14	Tegoli et al. Vox Sang 1967;13:144
iH	Hi, iO	>99.9	Giles et al. Vox Sang 1964;9:153
I^T		>99.9	Booth et al. Br J Haematol 1966;12:341
IP_1		79	Issitt et al. Vox Sang 1968;14:1
iP_1		79	McGinniss et al. Transfusion 1969;9:40
I^TP_1		79	Booth, Vox Sang 1970;19:85
IP		>99.9	Allen et al. Vox Sang 1974;27;442
IBH		14	Baird et al. Transfusion 1975;15:526
IAB		56	Doinel et al. Vox Sang 1974;27:515
I^s		>99.9	Dzierzkowa-Borodej et al. Vox Sang 1975;28:110

TABLE 44-4 P System and GLOB Collection

Antigen	% Frequency	Reference
P_1	79	Landsteiner et al. Proc Soc Exp Biol NY 1927;24:941
P	>99.9	Levine et al. Proc Soc Exp Biol NY 1951;77:403
P^k	<0.1	Matson et al. Am J Hum Genet 1959;11:26
LKE (Luke)	98	Tippett et al. Vox Sang 1965;10:269
p	<0.1	Engelfriet et al. Vox Sang 1971;23:176

TABLE 44-5 Rh System

Antigen	Historical or Alternative Name	% Frequency	Reference
D	Rh_o, Rh1	85	Described but not named by Levine et al. J Am Med Assoc 1939;113:126 Named by Landsteiner et al. Proc Soc Exp Biol NY 1940;43:223
C	rh', Rh2	70	Wiener, Arch Pathol 1941;32:227
E	rh'' Rh3	30	Wiener et al. Immunol 1943;47:461 Race et al. Nature 1943;152:563
c	hr', Rh4	80	Levine et al. J Obstet Gynecol 1941;42:925
e	hr'', Rh5	98	Mourant, Nature 1945;155:542
f	ce, hr, Rh6	64	Rosenfield et al. Br Med J 1953;1:975
Ce	rh_i, Rh7	71	Rosenfield et al. Am J Hum Genet 1958;10:474
C^w	rh^{w1}, Rh8	1	Callender et al. Ann Eugen 1946;13:102
C^x	rh^x, Rh9	<0.1	Stratton et al. Br Med J 1954;1:962
V	hr^v, Rh10	<1	DeNatale et al. J Am Med Assoc 1955;159:247
E^w	rh^{w2}, Rh11	<0.1	Greenwalt et al. Br J Haematol 1955;1:52
G	rh^G, Rh12	86	Allen et al. Vox Sang 1958;3:32
Hr_o	Rh17	>99	Mentioned but not named by Race et al. Nature 1950;166:520. Named by Allen et al. Proc 9th Ann Mtg AABB 1958
Hr	Hr^S, Rh18	>99	Shapiro, J Foren Med 1960;7:96
hr^S	Rh19	98	Shapiro, J Foren Med 1960;7:96
VS	e^s, Rh20	<1	Sanger et al. Nature 1960;186:171
C^G	Rh21	69	Levine et al. Am J Hum Genet 1961;13:299
CE	Rh22	<1	Dunsford, Proc 8th Cong Eur Soc Haematol 1961 p 491
D^w	Wiel, Rh23	<0.1	Lewis et al. Transfusion 1962;2:150
Rh26	c-like	80	Huestis et al. Transfusion 1964;4:414
cE	Rh27	30	Gold et al. Vox Sang 1961;6:157
hr^H	Rh28	<1	Shapiro, J Foren Med 1964;11:52
Rh29	rh_m, RH	>99	Haber et al. Transfusion 1967;7:389 (Abstract)
Go^a	D^{Cor}, Rh30	<0.1	Rosenfield et al. Proc 6th Cong ISBT, Basel:Karger, 1958:49
hr^B	Rh31	98	Shapiro et al. Haematologia 1972;6:121
Rh32		<0.1	Chown et al. Vox Sang 1971;21:385
Rh33		<0.1	Giles et al. Vox Sang 1971;21:289

TABLE 44-5 Rh System Continued

Antigen	Historical or Alternative Name	% Frequency	Reference
Rh34	Hr^B	>99	Shapiro et al. Haematologia 1972;6:121
Rh35		<1	Giles et al. Vox Sang 1971;20:328
Be^a	Rh36	<0.1	Davidsohn et al. Blood 1953;8:747. Shown to be part of the Rh system by Race and Sanger, Blood Groups in Man 6th Ed. 1975, Blackwell, Oxford
Rh37	Evans	<0.1	Contreras et al. Vox Sang 1978;34:208
Rh39		>99	Issitt et al. Transfusion 1979;19:389
Rh40	Tar	<1	Humphreys et al. Abstracts 14th Cong ISBT, 1975 p 46. Shown to be part of the Rh system by Lewis et al. Am J Hum Genet 1979;31:630
Rh41	rh$_i$-like	70	Svoboda et al. Transfusion 1981;21:150
Rh42	Ce^s	<1	Moulds et al. Transfusion 1980;20:631 (Abstract)
Rh43	Craw	<1	Cobb, Transfusion 1980;20:631 (Abstract)
Rh44	Nou	>99	Habibi et al. Blood Transf Immunohematol 1981;24:117
Rh45	Riv	<0.1	Delehanty et al. Transfusion 1983;23:410 (Abstract)
Rh46	Sec	>99	LePennec et al. Transfusion 1989;29:798
Rh47	Dav	>99	Daniels, Blood Transf Immunohematol 1982;24:185
Rh48	JAL	<0.1	Lomas et al. Vox Sang 1990;59:39 Poole et al. Vox Sang 1990;59:44
Rh49	STEM	<0.1	Marais et al. Transf Med 1993;3:35
Rh50	FPTT	<0.1	Bizot et al. Transfusion 1988;28:342 Lomas et al. Transfusion 1994;34:612
Rh51	MAR	>99	Sistonen et al. Vox Sang 1994;66:287
Rh52	BARC	<1	Green et al. Transf Med 1996;6 (Suppl 2):26 (Abstract)

Antigens that may be part of the Rh System

HOFM		<0.1	Hoffman et al. Vox Sang 1990;59:240
LOCR		<0.1	Coghlan et al. Transfusion 1994;34:492

TABLE 44-6 Weakened and Obsolete Rh Antigens

The following are weakened forms of Rh system antigens already listed in this table. They do not represent different antigens.

Weakened Form	Normal Antigen	Reference
D^u	D	Stratton, Nature 1946;158:25
C^u	C	Race et al. Nature 1948;161:316 and Vox Sang 1960;5:334
c^v	C	Race et al. Nature 1948;161:316 and Vox Sang 1960;5:334
E^u	E	Ceppellini et al. Boll 1st Sero Milan 1950;29:123
e^i	e	Layrisse et al. Nature 1961;191:503
V^u	V	Rosenfield, 2nd Int Mtg Foren Path Med 1961 (Abstract) and mentioned briefly in Transfusion 1962;2:287
G^u	G	Beattie et al. Transfusion 1971;11:152

The following antigens were formerly part of the Rh system but are now considered to be obsolete.

Antigen	Retired Rh number	Reference
Rh^A	Rh13	Wiener et al. Exp Med Surg 1957;15:75
Rh^B	Rh14	Unger et al. J Am Med Assoc 1959;170:1380
Rh^C	Rh15	Unger et al. J Lab Clin Med 1959;54:835
Rh^D	Rh16	Sacks et al. Ann Int Med 1959;51:740
E^T	Rh24	Vos et al. Vox Sang 1962;7:22

Epitopes of D

As discussed in Chapter 12, multiple epitopes of the antigen D have been recognized. Since each can be defined by an antibody, a case could be made for thinking of D as nine (2) or more (3,4) antigens or immunogens. In this chapter, D is counted as one antigen.

Transferred Rh Antigens

The antigen formerly known as Rh25 is now part of the LW system, see later. The antigen formerly known as Rh38 (Duclos) is now included in unrelated antigens of high incidence, see even later.

TABLE 44-7 LW System

Antigen	Old Name	% Frequency	Reference
LW^a	LW, Rh25	>99	Levine et al. Science 1961;133:332
LW^b	Ne^a	<1	Sistonen et al. Vox Sang 1981;40:352, see also reference for LW^{ab}
LW^{ab}	LW$_1$, LW$_2$, LW$_3$	>99	Sistonen et al. Vox Sang 1982;42:252

TABLE 44-8 Duffy System

Antigen	% Frequency	Reference
Fy^a	65	Cutbush et al. Nature 1950;165:188
Fy^b	80	Ikin et al. Nature 1951;168:1077
Fy3	>99	Albrey et al. Vox Sang 1971;20:29
Fy4	<0.1	Behzad et al. Vox Sang 1973;24:337
Fy5	>99	Colledge et al. Vox Sang 1973;24:193
Fy6	>99	Nichols et al. J Exp Med 1987;166:776

The term Fy^x has been used to describe a weakened form of Fy^b. The phenotype Fy(x+) has an incidence of about 1% in Whites. Chown et al. Am J Hum Genet 1965;17:384

TABLE 44-9 MN System

Antigen	Historical or Alternative Name*	% Frequency	Reference
M		78	Landsteiner et al. Proc Soc Exp Biol NY 1927;24:600
N		72	Landsteiner et al. Proc Soc Exp Biol NY 1927;24:600
Hu	Hunter	<1	Landsteiner et al. J Immunol 1934;27:469
S		57	Walsh et al. Nature 1947;160:504. Relationship to MN system shown by Sanger et al. Nature 1947;160:505
s		88	Levine et al. Proc Soc Exp Biol NY 1951;78:218
He	Henshaw	0.8	Ikin et al. Br Med J 1951;1:456
Mi^a	Miltenberger	<1	Levine et al. Proc Soc Exp Biol NY 1951;77:402
U		>99.9	Wiener et al. J Am Med Assoc 1953;153:1444
M^c		<0.1	Dunsford et al. Nature 1953;172:688
Vw	Verweyst, Gr, Graydon	<1	Hart et al. Vox Sang (O.S.) 1954;4:108
M^g	Gilfeather	<0.01	Allen et al. Vox Sang 1958;3:81
Vr	Vr^a, Verdegoal	<0.1	Hart et al. Vox Sang 1958;3:261
M_1		4	Jack et al. Nature 1960;186:642
Mur	Murrell	<0.1	Cleghorn, MD Thesis, Univ Sheffield, 1961
M^e		78	Wiener et al. J Immunol 1961;87:376
Mt^a	Martin	0.25	Swanson et al. Vox Sang 1962;7:585
St^a	Stones	<0.1	Cleghorn, Nature 1962;195:297
Ri^a	Ridley	<0.1	Cleghorn, Nature 1962;195:297
Cl^a	Caldwell	<0.1	Wallace et al. Nature 1963;200:689
Ny^a	Nyberg	<0.1	Ørjasaeter et al. Nature 1964;201:832
Or	Orris	<0.1	Bacon et al. Vox Sang 1987;52:330
Tm	Sheerin	25	Issitt et al. Vox Sang 1965;10:742
Hut	Hutchinson	<0.1	Cleghorn, Vox Sang 1966;11:219
Hil	Hill	<0.1	Cleghorn, Vox Sang 1966;11:219
M^v	Armstrong	0.6	Gershowitz et al. Am J Hum Genet 1966;18:264 Crossland et al. Vox Sang 1970;18:407
M^A		78	Konugres et al. Vox Sang 1966;11:189
Sul	Sullivan	<0.1	Konugres et al. Vox Sang 1967;12:221
Sj	Stenbar-James	2	Issitt et al. Vox Sang 1968;15:1
M'		9	Metaxas et al. Vox Sang 1968;15:102
Far	Kam, Kamhuber	<0.1	Kam was reported by Speiser et al. Vox Sang 1966;11:113. Far was reported by Cregut et al. Rev Fr Transf 1968;11:139. The two were shown to be the same thing by Giles, Vox Sang 1977;32:269

TABLE 44-9 MN System Continued

Antigen	Historical or Alternative Name*	% Frequency	Reference
En^{a}TS		>99.9	Taliano et al. Vox Sang 1980;38:87
En^{a}FS		>99.9	Darborough et al. Vox Sang 1969;17:241
En^{a}FR		>99.9	Furuhjelm et al. Vox Sang 1969;17:256

En^{a}TS, En^{a}FS and En^{a}FR were all originally called En^a. The expanded terminology was proposed by Issitt et al. (5).

Antigen	Historical or Alternative Name*	% Frequency	Reference
Shier		20	Beck ML. Unpublished 1969
N^A		72	Booth, Vox Sang 1971;21:522
U^z		>99.9	Booth, Vox Sang 1972;22:524. Originally named Z, name changed to U^z by Booth, Vox Sang 1978;34:212
'N'	N quotes	>99.9	Furthmayr, Nature 1978;271:519 Dahr et al. In: Human Blood Groups, Basel:Karger, 1977:197
Hop	Anek	<0.1	Chandanayingyong et al. Vox Sang 1977;32:272
Nob	Raddon/Lane	<0.1	Giles et al. Vox Sang 1977;32:277 Webb et al. Vox Sang 1977;32:274
U^x		>99.9	Booth, Vox Sang 1978;34:212
s^D	Dryer	<0.1	Shapiro et al. Transfusion 1981;21:614 (Abstract)
Can	Canner	27	Judd et al. Transfusion 1979;19:7
Mit	Mitchell	0.12	Battista et al. Vox Sang 1980;39:331
Dantu		<0.1	Unger et al. Transfusion 1981;21:614 (Abstract), (abstract describes Dantu+ cells but does not use that name)
Os^a		<0.1	Seno et al. Vox Sang 1983;45:60, shown to be part of MN by Daniels et al. Transf Med 1993;3 (Suppl 1):85
En^{a}KT		>99.9	Laird-Fryer et al. Transfusion 1986;26:51
UPS		>99.9	Issitt et al. Transfusion 1989;29:508
UPR		>99.9	Issitt et al. Transfusion 1989;29:508
DANE		<0.1	Skov et al. Vox Sang 1991;61:130
SAT		<0.1	Daniels et al. Transf Med 1991;1:39
TSEN		<0.1	Reid et al. Vox Sang 1992;63:122
MINY		<0.1	Reid et al. Vox Sang 1992;63:129
MUT		<0.1	Tippett et al. Transf Med Rev 1992;6:170 Reid et al. Immunohematology 1993;9:91
AVIS		>99.9	Moulds et al. Transfusion 1992;32 (Suppl 8S):55S (Abstract) Jarolim et al. Blood 1996;88 (Suppl 1):182a (Abstract)
MARS		<0.1	Moulds et al. Transfusion 1992;32 (Suppl 8S):55S (Abstract) Jarolim et al. Blood 1996;88 (Suppl 1):182a (Abstract)
ERIK		<0.1	Daniels et al. Transf Med 1993;3:129
ENEH		>99.9	Huang et al. Blood 1992;80:257 Spruell et al. Transfusion 1993;33:848
ENEP		>99.9	Poole et al. Transfusion 1995;35 (Suppl 10S):40S (Abstract)
HAG		<0.1	Poole et al. Transfusion 1995;35 (Suppl 10S):40S (Abstract)

TABLE 44-9 MN System Continued

The following are weakened forms of MN system antigens already listed in this table. They do not represent different antigens.

Weakened Form	Normal Antigen	Reference
M_2	M	Friedenreich et al. Acta Path Microbiol Scand, suppl 1938
N_2	N	Crome, Ztschr Gerichtl Med 1935;24:167
S_2	S	Hurd et al. Vox Sang 1964;9:487

* For MN system antigens that have ISBT numbers, see Chapter 15.

TABLE 44-10 Gerbich System

Antigen	Historical or Alternative Name	% Frequency	Reference
Ge1		>99.9	Booth et al. Vox Sang 1972;22:73
Ge2	Yussef	>99.9	Cleghorn, M.D. Thesis, Univ Sheffield 1961
Ge3	Gerbich	>99.9	Rosenfield et al. Br J Haematol 1960;6:344
Ge4	Gero	>99.9	Daniels et al. J Immunogenet 1983;10:103 Anstee et al. Biochem J 1984;218:615
Wb	Ge5, Webb	<0.1	First described by Simmons et al. Med J Austral 1963;1:8, shown to be a Gerbich system antigen by Reid et al. Biochem J 1985;232:289 and by Macdonald et al. Vox Sang 1986;50:112
Ls^a	Ge6, Lewis II, Rl^a	<0.1	First described by Cleghorn, Unpublished observations cited by Race RR, Sanger R. Blood Groups in Man, 6th Ed. Oxford:Blackwell, 1975. Shown to be a Gerbich system antigen by Macdonald et al. Vox Sang 1990;58:300. Ls^a and Rl^a are known to be the same, see Chapter 16.
An^a	Ge7, Ahonen	<0.1	First described by Furuhjelm et al. J Med Genet 1972;9:385, shown to be a Gerbich system antigen by Daniels et al. Blood 1993;10:3198
Dh^a	Ge8, Duch	<0.1	First described by Jørgensen et al. Hum Hered 1982;32:73, shown to be a Gerbich system antigen by Spring, Vox Sang 1991;61:65

TABLE 44-11 Diego System

Antigen	Historical or Alternative Name*	% Frequency	Reference
Di^a	Diego	<0.1	Layrisse et al. Acta Med Venez 1955;3:132
Di^b	Luebano	>99.9	Thompson et al. Vox Sang 1967;13:314
Wr^a	Wright	<0.1	Holman. Lancet 1953;2:119. Shown to be a Diego system antigen by Bruce et al. Blood 1995;85:541
Wr^b	Fritz	>99.9	Adams et al. Transfusion 1971;11:290. Shown to be a Diego system antigen by Bruce et al. Blood 1995;85:541
Wd^a	Waldner	<0.1	Lewis et al. Am J Hum Genet 1981;33:418. Shown to be a Diego system antigen by Bruce et al. Transfusion 1995;35 (Suppl 10S):52S (Abstract)
Rb^a	Redelberger	<0.1	Contreras et al. Vox Sang 1978;35:397. Shown to be a Diego system antigen by Jarolim et al. Blood 1995;86 (Suppl 1):445A (Abstract)
WARR	Warrior	<0.1	Crow et al. Transfusion 1991;31 (Suppl 8S):52S (Abstract). Shown to be a Diego system antigen by Jarolim et al. Transfusion 1996;36 (Suppl 9S):49S (Abstract)
ELO		<0.1	Coghlan et al. Vox Sang 1993;64:240. For association with Diego system see Coghlan et al. and Jarolim et al. both abstracts in Transfusion 1996;36 (Suppl 9S):49S
Wu	Wulfsberg Same as Hov and Haakestad	<0.1	Kornstad et al. Vox Sang 1976;31:337. For association with Diego system see Coghlan et al. and Jarolim et al. both abstracts in Transfusion 1996;36 (Suppl 9S):49S
Bp^a	Bishop	<0.1	Ørjasaeter et al. Vox Sang 1966;11:726. For association with Diego system see Jarolim et al. Transfusion 1996;36 (Suppl 9S):49S (Abstract)
Mo^a	Moen	<0.1	Kornstad et al. Book of Abstracts, 13th Cong ISBT, 1972;58. For association with Diego system see Jarolim et al. Transfusion 1996;36 (Suppl 9S):49S (Abstract)
Hg^a	Hughes Same as Tarplee, Tarp	<0.1	Rowe et al. Vox Sang 1983;45:316. For association with Diego system see Jarolim et al. Transfusion 1996;36 (Suppl 9S):49S (Abstract)
Vg^a	Van Vugt	<0.1	Young, Vox Sang 1981;41:48. For association with Diego system see Jarolim et al. Transfusion 1996;36 (Suppl 9S):49S (Abstract)
Sw^a	Swann	<0.1	Cleghorn, Nature 1959;184:1324. For association with Diego system see Zelinski et al. Transfusion 1996;36:419 and Zelinski et al. Transfusion 1997;37 (Suppl 9S):89S (Abstract)
Tr^a	Traversu, Lanthois	<0.1	Cleghorn, mentioned in reference 18. For association with Diego system see Jarolim et al. Transfusion 1997;37:607
NFLD	Newfoundland	<0.1	Lewis et al. Hum Genet 1984;67:270. For association with Diego system see Zelinski et al. Transfusion 1997;37 (Suppl 9S):90S (Abstract)
Jn^a	Nunhart, JN	<0.1	Kornstad et al. Vox Sang 1967;13:165. For association with Diego system see Poole et al. Transfusion 1997;37 (Suppl 9S):90S (Abstract)

Antigens that may be part of the Diego System. For associations see Chapter 17.

BOW	Bowyer	<0.1	Chaves et al. Vox Sang 1988;55:241
Fr^a	Froese	<0.1	Lewis et al. Vox Sang 1978;35:251
SW1		<0.1	Contreras et al. Vox Sang 1987;52:115

*For ISBT numbers not listed here, see Chapter 17.

TABLE 44-12 Kell System

Antigen	Historical or Alternative Name*	% Frequency	Reference
K	Kell	9	Coombs et al. Lancet 1946;1:264
k	Cellano	99.8	Levine et al. Science 1949;109:464
Kp^a	Penny	2	Allen et al. Vox Sang 1957;2:81
Kp^b	Rautenberg	99.9	Allen et al. Vox Sang 1958;3:1
Kp^c	Levay	<0.1	Callender et al. Br Med J 1945;2:83 Shown to be part of Kell system by Yamaguchi et al. Vox Sang 1979;36:29 and Gavin et al. Vox Sang 1979;36:31
Ku	Peltz	>99.9	Corcoran et al. Transfusion 1961;1:181
Js^a	Sutter	<0.1	Giblett, Nature 1958;181:1221
Js^b	Matthews	>99.9	Walker et al. Transfusion 1963;3:94. Js^a and Js^b were shown to be Kell system antigens by Morton et al. Vox Sang 1965;10:608 and by Stroup et al. Transfusion 1965;5:309
Ul^a	Karhula	<1	Furuhjelm et al. Vox Sang 1968;15:118. Ul^a was shown to be a Kell system antigen by Furuhjelm et al. Vox Sang 1969;16:496
K11	Côté	>99.9	Guévin et al. Vox Sang 1976;31 (Suppl 1):96
K12	Boc	>99.9	Marsh et al. Vox Sang 1973;24:200
K13	Sgro	>99.9	Marsh et al. Vox Sang 1974;26:34
K14	Santini	>99.9	Heisto et al. Vox Sang 1973;24:179 Wallace et al. Vox Sang 1976;30:300
K16	k-like	99.8	Marsh, Adv Immunohematol 1976, Vol 4, No 2
Wk^a	Weeks	0.3	Strange et al. Vox Sang 1974;27:81
K18	V.M.	>99.9	Barrasso et al. Vox Sang 1975;29:124
K19	Sub	>99.9	Sabo et al. Vox Sang 1979;36:97
K20	Km	>99.9	Marsh, Vox Sang 1979;36:375 (Letter)
K22	N.I.	>99.9	Bar Shany et al. Vox Sang 1982;42:87
K23	Centauro	<0.1	Marsh et al. Transfusion 1987;27:36
K24	Cls, Callois	<0.1	Eicher et al. Transfusion 1985;25:448 (Abstract)
K25	VLAN	<0.1	Jongerius et al. Vox Sang 1996;71:43
K26	TOU	>99.9	Jones et al. Transf Med 1994;4 (Suppl 1):45 (Abstract)

For details about which antigens are known to be encoded from the *Kell* complex locus, see Chapter 18

Antigen with a phenotypic relationship to the Kell system that is produced by a gene that is on the X chromosome

Kx	K15	>99.9	Marsh et al. Br J Haematol 1975;29:247

For full details about the antigens previously called K^w or K8 and KL or K9, see Chapter 18. In brief, K^w is now considered extinct, the antibody called anti-KL is now regarded (6,7) as a separable mixture of anti-Km and anti-Kx.

Antigen that might be part of the Kell System

RAZ		>99.9	Daniels et al. Transfusion 1994;34:818

* For ISBT numbers not listed here, see Chapter 18

TABLE 44-13 Kidd System

Antigen	Alternative Name	% Frequency	Reference
Jk^a		77	Allen et al. Nature 1951;167:482
Jk^b		73	Plaut et al. Nature 1953;171:431
Jk3	Jk^{ab}	>99.9	Pinkerton et al. Vox Sang 1959;4:155

TABLE 44-14 Lutheran System

Antigen	Historical or Alternative Name	% Frequency	Reference
Lu^a		8	Callender et al. Br Med J 1945;2:83
Lu^b		99.8	Cutbush et al. Nature 1956;178:855
Lu6	Jan	>99.9	Marsh et al. Transfusion 1972;12:27
Lu8	M.T.	>99.9	MacIlroy et al. Vox Sang 1972;23:455
Lu9	Mull	2	Molthan et al. Vox Sang 1973;24:468
Lu14	Hof	2.4	Judd et al. Vox Sang 1977;32:214
Au^a	Auberger	80-90	Salmon et al. Nouv Rev Fr Haematol 1961;1:649
Au^b	Pren	51	Frandson et al. Vox Sang 1989;56:54 Au^a and Au^b were shown to be Lutheran system antigens by Daniels, Vox Sang 1990;58:56, Daniels et al. Vox Sang 1991;60:191 and Zelinski et al. Vox Sang 1991;61:275

Antigens that may be part of the Lutheran System

Antigen	Historical or Alternative Name	% Frequency	Reference
Lu3	Lu^{ab}	>99.9	Darnborough et al. Nature 1963;198:796
Lu4	Ba	>99.9	Bove et al. Vox Sang 1971;21:302
Lu5	Be and Fo	>99.9	Marsh et al. Transfusion 1972;12:27
Lu7	Ga	>99.9	Marsh et al. Transfusion 1972;12:27
Lu11	Re	>99.9	Gralnick et al. Vox Sang 1974;27:52
Lu12	Much	>99.9	Sinclair et al. Vox Sang 1973;25:156
Lu13	Hughes	>99.9	Marsh et al. Transfusion 1983;23:128
Lu16		>99.9	Sabo et al. Transfusion 1980;20:630 (Abstract)
Lu17	Petaracchia	>99.9	Turner, Canad J Med Tech 1979;41:43
Lu20		>99.9	Levene et al. Rev Paulista Med 1992;110:1H-13 (Abstract)

The number Lu10 was reserved, but not used, for a low incidence antigen Singleton, that was later shown (8) not to be part of the Lutheran system. The number Lu15 was assigned to a high incidence antigen Anton that was shown (9) not be part of the Lutheran system and to be the same (10,11) an another high incidence antigen Wj (12). Production of AnWj is not encoded from the *Lutheran* locus (13) and the antigen is listed below with other unrelated antigens of high incidence. For ISBT numbers not shown, see Chapter 20.

TABLE 44-15 Colton System

Antigen	Historical or Alternative Name	% Frequency	Reference
Co^a	Colton	99.7	Heisto et al. Vox Sang 1967;12:18
Co^b		9.7	Giles et al. Br J Haematol 1970;19:267
Co3	Co^{ab}	>99.9	Rodgers et al. Transfusion 1974;14:508

TABLE 44-16 Dombrock System

Antigen	Historical or Alternative Name	% Frequency	Reference
Do^a	Dombrock	66.7	Swanson et al. Nature 1965;206:313
Do^b		82.8	Molthan et al. Vox Sang 1973;24:382
Gy^a	Gregory	>99.9	Swanson et al. Transfusion 1967;7:304
Hy	Holley	>99.9	Frank et al. Transfusion 1970;10:254
Jo^a	Joseph	>99.9	Jensen et al. Transfusion 1972;12:332

Weaver et al. (14) showed that Jo^a and Jc^a (15) are the same thing. Banks et al. (16,17) showed that the antigens Gy^a, Hy and Jo^a are all part of the Dombrock system.

TABLE 44-17 Cartwright System

Antigen	Historical or Alternative Name	% Frequency	Reference
Yt^a	Cartwright	99.6	Eaton et al. Br J Haematol 1956;2:333
Yt^b		8	Giles et al. Nature 1964;202:1122

TABLE 44-18 Cromer System

Antigen	Historical or Alternative Name	% Frequency	Reference
Cr^a	Cromer	>99.9	McCormick et al. Transfusion 1965;5:369 (Abstract) and Stroup et al. Transfusion 1975;15:522 (Abstract)
Tc^a		>99.9	Laird-Fryer et al. Transfusion 1980;20:631 (Abstract)
Tc^b		<0.1	Block et al. Transfusion 1982;22:413 (Abstract)
Tc^c		<0.1	Law et al. Transfusion 1982;22:413 (Abstract)
Dr^a		>99.9	Levene et al. Transfusion 1984;24:13
Es^a		>99.9	Daniels, Transfusion 1983;23:410 (Abstract)
IFC	Inab	>99.9	Daniels et al. Transfusion 1986;26:117 (Letter)
WES^a		<0.1	Sistonen et al. Vox Sang 1987;52:111
WES^b		>99.9	Daniels et al. Vox Sang 1987;53:235
UMC		>99.9	Daniels et al. Transfusion 1989;29:794

An antigen that may belong in the Cromer System

AM		>99.9	Poole et al. Transf Med 1996;6 (Suppl 2):20 (Abstract)

TABLE 44-19 Xg System and a Related Antigen

Antigen	Historical or Alternative Name	% Frequency	Reference
Xg^a		89 Females 66 Males	Mann et al. Lancet 1962;1:8
Yg^a	12E7, CD99	Varies based on Xg^a type. See Chapter 25	Goodfellow et al. Nature 1981;289:404

TABLE 44-20 Scianna System

Antigen	Historical or Alternative Name	% Frequency	Reference
Sc1	Sm, Scianna	>99	Schmidt et al. Transfusion 1962;2:338
Sc2	Bu^a, Bullee	0.3	Anderson et al. Transfusion 1963;3:30
Sc3		>99.9	McCreary et al. Transfusion 1973;13:350(Abstract) / Nason et al. Transfusion 1980;20:531
Not named	R.S.	>99.9	Skradski et al. Transfusion 1982;22:406 (Abstract). Also described (Case 3) Devine et al. Transfusion 1988;28:346
Not named	Case 1	>99.9	Both Devine et al. Transfusion 1988;28:346
Not named	Case 2	>99.9	

TABLE 44-21 Chido-Rodgers System

Antigen	Historical or Alternative Name	% Frequency	Reference
Ch	Chido, Ch^a	96	Harris et al. Vox Sang 1967;12:140
Ch1		96	Giles, Vox Sang 1985;48:167
Ch2		96	Giles, Vox Sang 1985;48:167
Ch3		96	Giles, Vox Sang 1985;48:167
Ch4		96	Giles, Hum Immunol 1987;18:111
Ch5		96	Giles, Hum Immunol 1987;18:111
Ch6		96	Giles, Hum Immunol 1987;18:111
WH		15	Giles et al. Immunogenetics 1987;26:392
Rg	Rodgers, Rg^a	97	Longster et al. Vox Sang 1976;30:175
Rg1		97	Giles, Vox Sang 1985;48:167
Rg2		97	Giles, Vox Sang 1985;48:167

TABLE 44-22 Knops System

Antigen	Historical or Alternative Name	% Frequency	Reference
Kn^a	Knops	98	Helgeson et al. Transfusion 1970;10:137
Kn^b	Hall	<0.1	Mallan et al. Transfusion 1980;20:630 (Abstract)
McC^a	McCoy	98.5	Molthan et al. Transfusion 1978;18:566
McC^b		<0.1	Molthan, Med Lab Sci 1983;40:59
Sl^a	Swain-Langley, McC^c	97-99	Lacey et al. Transfusion 1980;20:632 (Abstract) Molthan, Med Lab Sci 1983;40:59
Vil	?Sl^b	<0.1	Lacey et al. Transfusion 1980;20:632 (Abstract)
Yk^a	York	92	Molthan et al. Vox Sang 1975;29:145
Not named	Sieb	92	Giles, In: Human Blood Groups. Basel:Karger, 1977:268

Antigens said by some to be part of the Knops System, claims not accepted by others.

Antigen	Historical or Alternative Name	% Frequency	Reference
McC^d		94.6	Molthan, Med Lab Sci 1983;40:59
McC^e		0.1	Molthan, Med Lab Sci 1983;40:113
McC^f		31.6	Molthan, Med Lab Sci 1983;40:113

Other antigens that may be part of the Knops System

Antigen	Historical or Alternative Name	% Frequency	Reference
Win	Winbourne, may be the same as McC^a	99	Haber, Unpublished 1965
MPD	Minnie Pearl Davis, may be the same as Kn^a	99	Adebahr et al. Unpublished 1965

For Kir, Mil and Oca, all Kn^a-like, see list of unrelated antigens of high incidence.

TABLE 44-23 Indian System

Antigen	Historical or Alternative Name	% Frequency	Reference
In^a	Indian	<0.1	Badakere et al. Ind J Med Res 1973;61:563
In^b	Salis	>99.9	Giles, Vox Sang 1975;29:73

TABLE 44-24 Cost Collection

Antigen	Historical or Alternative Name	% Frequency	Reference
Cs^a	Cost-Stirling	97.5	Giles et al. Vox Sang 1965;10:405
Cs^b		31	Molthan et al. Med Lab Sci 1987;44:94

TABLE 44-25 Er Collection

Antigen	Historical or Alternative Name	% Frequency	Reference
Er^a	Rosebush	>99	Daniels et al. Transfusion 1982;22:189
Not named Er^a-like	Rod	>99	Daniels et al. Transfusion 1982;22:189
Not named Er^a-like	Min	>99	Daniels et al. Transfusion 1982;22:189
Er^b		<1	Hamilton et al. Transfusion 1988;28:268

TABLE 44-26 High Incidence Antigens of the ISBT 901 Series (See Chapters 31 and 33)

Antigen	Historical or Alternative Name	% Frequency	Reference
Vel		>99.9	Sussman et al. Rev Hematol 1953;7:368
Lan	Langereis. Same as So and Gn^a (Gonsowski)	>99.9	Hart et al. Proc 8th Cong Eur Soc Hematol Basel:Karger, 1962:493
At^a	Augustine. Same as Ola Ware, El (Eldridge), E.De., V.Ba., C.Br., L.Bu. and B.L.Ja.Sm.	>99.9	Applewhaite et al. Vox Sang 1967;13:444
Jr^a	Junior. Same as Fujikawa, Tamura, Tad, Souza, Powell and Jacobs	>99.9	Stroup et al. Prog 23rd Ann Mtg AABB 1970;86 (Abstract). Many data presented but not included in the abstract
Ok^a		>99.9	Morel et al. Vox Sang 1979;36:182
JMH	John Milton Hagen. Same as Baugh, Horowitz, Juneau, Lazicki, Warren and 157G	>99.9	Sabo et al. Transfusion 1978;18:387 (Abstract)
Emm		>99.9	Daniels et al. Tranfusion 1987;27:319
AnWj	Anton	>99.9	Poole et al. Vox Sang 1982;43:220 Marsh et al. Transfusion 1983;23:128
MER2	Raph	92	Daniels et al. Vox Sang 1987;52:107
Sd^a	Sid	96	Macvie et al. Vox Sang 1967;13:485 Renton et al. Vox Sang 1967;13:493
Duclos		>99.9	Habibi et al. Vox Sang 1978;34:302
PEL		>99.9	Daniels, PhD Thesis, Univ London, 1980
ABTI		>99.9	Schechter et al. Transfusion 1996;36 (Suppl 9S):25S (Abstract)

Determinants that do not have an ISBT number but that may be related to antigens in the 901 series

Not named but possibly related to JMH

V.G.		>99.9	Both Moulds et al. Book of Abstracts, 19th
R.M.		>99.9	Cong ISBT, 1982:287
G.P.		>99.9	Both Mudad et al. Transfusion 1995;35:925
D.W.		>99.9	

Possibly related to PEL

MTP		>99.9	Daniels et al. Transfusion 1994;34 (Suppl 10S):26S (Abstract)

TABLE 44-27 Low Incidence Antigens of the ISBT 700 Series (See Chapter 32)

Antigen	Historical or Alternative Name	% Frequency	Reference
By	Batty	<0.1	Simmons et al. Med J Austral 1955;2:55
Chr^a	Christiansen	<0.1	Kissmeyer-Nielsen, Vox Sang (O.S.) 1955;5:102
Bi	Biles	<0.1	Wadlington et al. Am J Dis Childh 1961;101:623
Bx^a	Box	<0.1	Jenkins et al. Lancet 1961;2:16
Rd	Rd^a, Radin	<0.1	Rausen et al. Transfusion 1967;7:336
To^a	Torkildsen	<0.1	Kornstad et al. Vox Sang 1968;14:363
Pt^a	Peters	<0.1	Pinder et al. Vox Sang 1969;17:303
Re^a	Reid	<0.1	Guévin et al. Rev Fr Transf 1971;14:455
Je^a	Jensen	<0.1	Skov, Vox Sang 1972;23:461
Li^a	Livesey	<0.1	Riches et al. Vox Sang 1980;38:305
Milne		<0.1	Pinder et al. Vox Sang 1984;47:290
RASM	Rasmussen	<0.1	Brown et al. Vox Sang 1986;51:133
Ol^a	Oldeide	<0.1	Kornstad, Vox Sang 1986;50:235
JFV		<0.1	Kluge et al. Vox Sang 1988;55:44
Kg	Katagiri	<0.1	Ichikawa et al. Vox Sang 1989;56:98
Jones		<0.1	Reid et al. Vox Sang 1989;57:77
HJK		<0.1	Rouse et al. Obstet Gynecol 1990;76:988
SARA	Sarah	<0.1	Stern et al. Vox Sang 1994;67:64
REIT		<0.1	Hamilton et al. Unpublished observations cited in Daniels et al. Vox Sang 1995;69:265
SHIN		<0.1	Nakajima et al. Hum Hered 1993;43:69

TABLE 44-28 The Bg and Related Series of Antigens

Antigen	Historical or Alternative Name	% Frequency	Reference
Bg^a	DBG, Ho, Ot, Stobo, HLA-B7	Combined frequency circa 30-40	All in Seaman et al. Br J Haematol 1967;13:464
Bg^b	DBG, Ho, Stobo, HLA-B17		
Bg^c	DBG, Ot, HLA-A28		
For original reports on DBG, Ho, Ot and Stobo see:			Wallace et al. Proc 7th Cong ISBT 1959, p 587 Dorfmeier et al. Proc 7th Cong ISBT 1959, p 608 Hart et al. Proc 8th Cong Eur Soc Hematol 1961 Buchanan et al. Vox Sang 1963;8:213 Chown et al. Vox Sang 1963;8:281
For relationship of Bg antigens to HLA see:			Morton et al. Vox Sang 1969;17:536 Morton et al. Vox Sang 1971;21:141 Nordhagen, Vox Sang 1978;35:58 Nordhagen, Vox Sang 1979;37:209

TABLE 44-29 Some Other HLA Antigens that can be Detected on Some Red Cells

Antigen	Historical or Alternative Name	Reference
Not named	HLA-B8	Nordhagen, Vox Sang 1978;35:58
Not named	HLA-A8	Nordhagen et al. Vox Sang 1974;26:97
Not named	HLA-A9	Morton et al. Vox Sang 1971;21:141
Not named	HLA-A10	Nordhagen, Vox Sang 1977;32:82
Not named	HLA-B12	Nordhagen, Vox Sang 1979;37:209
Not named	HLA-B15	Nordhagen, Unpublished 1983 cited in reference 19
Not named	HLA-A7	Nordhagen, Vox Sang 1975;29:23

TABLE 44-30 The Pr Series of Antigens

Antigen	Historical or Alternative Name	% Frequency	Reference
Pr_{1h}	Sp_1	>99.9	Marsh et al. Vox Sang 1968;15:177 Roelcke et al. Klin Wschr 1968;46:126
Pr_{1d}		>99.9	Roelcke, Eur J Immunol 1973;3:206
Pr_2		>99.9	Roelcke, Vox Sang 1969;16:76
Pr_{3h}		>99.9	Roelcke et al. Vox Sang 1976;30:122 Birgens et al. Scand J Haematol 1982;29:207
Pr_{3d}		>99.9	Roelcke et al. Vox Sang 1976;30:122 Roelcke et al. Blut 1982;45:109
Pr_a		>99.9	Roelcke et al. Vox Sang 1971;20:218 Habibi et al. Br J Haematol 1975;30:499
Pr^M			Roelcke et al. Vox Sang 1986;51:207
Pr^N			Hinz et al. New Eng J Med 1963;269:1329 Roelcke et al. Transf Med Rev 1989;3:140

TABLE 44-31 Other Antigens Defined by Cold-Reactive Autoagglutinins

Antigen	Historical or Alternative Name	% Frequency	Reference
Gd1	Sia-lb1	>99.9	Roelcke et al. Vox Sang 1977;33:304
Gd2	Sia-lb2	>99.9	Roelcke et al. Prot Biol Fluids 1984;31:1075
Sa		>99.9	Roelcke et al. Blood 1980;55:677
Fl	Sia-bl	>99.9	Roelcke, Vox Sang 1981;41:98
Lud		>99.9	Roelcke, Vox Sang 1981;41:316
Vo	Sia-l1	>99.9	Roelcke, Vox Sang 1984;47:236`
Li		>99.9	Roelcke, Vox Sang 1985;48:181
Me		>99.9	Salama et al. Vox Sang 1985;49:277
Om		>99.9	Kajii et al. Vox Sang 1989;56:104
Ju		>99.9	Gottsche et al. Transfusion 1990;30:261
H_T		>99.9	Jenkins et al. Lancet 1961;2:16
Rx	Sd^x	>99.9	Marsh et al. Transfusion 1980;20:1

For the Sia-1b, 1 and b terminology, see Roelcke et al. (20), for the change from Sd^x to Rx, see Bass et al. (21).

TABLE 44-32 Antigens Exposed on Polyagglutinable Red Cells

Antigen	Historical or Alternative Name	Reference
T	Thomsen, Huebner, Freidenreich	Huebner, Z Immun Forsch 1925;45:223
Tk		Bird et al. Br J Haematol 1972;23:759
Th		Bird et al. Lancet 1978;1:1215
Tx		Bird et al. Blood Transf Immunohematol 1982;25:215
VA		Graninger et al. Vox Sang 1977;32:195
Not named	On red cells that have an acquired B antigen	{ Beck et al. Transfusion 1971;11:296 Garratty et al. Vox Sang 1971;21:45
Tn		Moreau et al. Bull Med Hop Paris 1957;73:569
Cad		Cazal et al. Rev Fr Transf 1968;11:209
HEMPAS		Crookston et al. Br J Haematol 1969;17:11
NOR		Harris et al. Vox Sang 1982;42:134
HbM	Hyde Park	Bird et al. Br J Haematol 1988;68:459

TABLE 44-33 Antigens of Low Incidence Currently Thought to be Independent of all Others

Notes: List includes only antigens mentioned in the literature since 1985. When a full publication exists it is referenced regardless of date, when no full published description exists, the most recent mentions in the literature are referenced. For additional but older references that mention the antigens in the list, see the third edition of this book.

Antigen	Historical or Alternative Name	Reference
Askwith		Mentioned in 22
Balkacemi		Mentioned in 23
Berrio		Savarese, mentioned in 23 and 24
Becker	Bec	Elbel et al. Zf Hygiene 1951;132:120
Bio 5		Mentioned in 22 and 23
Braithwaite		Mentioned in 22
Burrett	Finlay	See Finlay
Burrows		Mentioned in 23
Cassidy		Mentioned in 23
Dickinson		Mentioned in 22
Donaldson		Mentioned in 22 and 23
L.Evans		Mentioned in 22
Fielding		Mentioned in 23
Finlay	Fin, Burrett	Mentioned in 23
Fleck		Mentioned in 22
Friedberg		Mentioned in 23
Ga	Ga^a	Gellerman et al. Read by title, 27th AABB Ann Mtg 1974, mentioned since 1985 in 25 to 28
Gambino	May be the same as Ga	Mentioned in 23
Gf	Griffiths	Cleghorn, Unpublished 1966, cited in reference 18
Gibson		Mentioned in 23
Good		Frumin et al. Blood 1960;15:681
Gnade	Vetterlein	Mentioned in 23
Heibel		Ballowitz et al. Vox Sang 1968;14:307
Heron		Mentioned in 22
Hey		Yvart et al. Vox Sang 1974;26:41
Ht^a	Hunt	Jahn et al. Unpublished, mentioned in reference 18
Hull		Mentioned in 23
Jobbins	Job	Gilbey, Nature 1967;160:362
Joyce		Mentioned in 23
Kannellis	Kan	Mentioned in 23
Korving		Mentioned in 23
Krog		Mentioned in 23
Laviscount		Mentioned in 23
Maluenda		Mentioned in 22

TABLE 44-33 Antigens of Low Incidence Currently Thought to be Independent of all Others Continued

Antigen	Historical or Alternative Name	Reference
Mans	May be the same as Mansfield which is the same as Peacock	Mentioned in 22
Mauer		Mentioned in 23
Niemetz	Niemitz	Mentioned in 26
Norlander		Mentioned in 23
Overwheel		Mentioned in 23
Palframan		Mentioned in 22
Paschal		Mentioned in 23
Pe		McPherson et al. Vox Sang 1979;36:252
Peacock	Mansfield	See Mans
Pellegran		Mentioned in 23
Poll	Pollio	McClelland et al. Clin Lab Haematol 1982;4:201
Ragus		Mentioned in 23
Rasmussen		Mentioned in 23
Reiter	We do not know if this the same as REIT (see ISBT 700 Series listing)	Mentioned in 23
Reynolds		Mentioned in 23
Rm	Romunde	Hart et al. Vox Sang (O.S.) 1954;4:108
Sadler		Mentioned in 22 and 23
Sf^a	Stolzfus	Bias et al. Am J Hum Genet 1969;21:552 Said to have an incidence of 34% in Whites but no data have been published since 1969
Shindler		Mentioned in 23
Sk^a	Sk, Skjelbred	Kornstad et al. Transfusion 1978;18:375 (Abstract) and Chaves et al. Vox Sang 1980;39:28. An acquired not an inherited character.
Street		Mentioned in 23
Tofts		Mentioned in 22 and 23
Tollefsen-Oyen		Mentioned in 22 and 23
Ts	Tsunoi	Nakajima et al. Jpn J Hum Genet 1967;12:187
Ven		Loghem et al. Bull Cen Lab Ned Rod Kruis 1952;2:225
Visser		Mentioned in 23
Walker		Mentioned in 23
Wells		Mentioned in 23
Wiggins		Mentioned in 23
Young		Mentioned in 23
Zd		Svanda et al. Vox Sang 1970;18:366
Zt^a	Zt, Marriott may be the same as Zt^a	Mentioned in 23 and 26 to 28

TABLE 44-34 Antigens of High Incidence Currently Thought to be Independent of all Others

Notes: Most antigens that fit the above description are members of the ISBT 901 series and are included in that listing. Of the 144 antigens listed in the above named category in the third edition of this book, very few have been mentioned in print since 1985. Accordingly, those antigens listed below are ones known to the authors to have been reasonably well studied and/or known still to be extant. More complete listings of names that have been used are given in tables 33-4 and 33-5 in Chapter 33. Since most of those antigens must be extinct, references are not given. Details as to where the antigens have been mentioned in print are given in Chapter 28 of the third edition of this book.

Antigen	Historical or Alternative Name	Reference
Baumler		Mentioned in references 29 and 30
Buckalew		Mentioned in references 29, 31 and 32
Gill		Frederick et al. Transfusion 1981;21:613 (Abstract)
Groslouis	Groslovis	Mentioned in reference 29
h		Davidsohn et al. J Infect Dis 1940;67:25
Holmes		Mentioned in references 30 and 32
Kir	Kur	Wells et al. Transfusion 1976;16:427
Mil		Wells et al. Transfusion 1976;16:427
Mineo		Mentioned in reference 32
Oca		Wells et al. Transfusion 1976;16:427
L. Reynolds	Reynolds	Mentioned in references 31 and 32
Ritter	Rit	Mentioned in reference 30
Schneider		Mougey et al. Red Cell Free Press 1983;8:25 (Abstract)

Antigens That have Duplicated Others

Throughout this book we have made note of antigens given a name when found, that have later been shown to duplicate others named earlier. Since this chapter is essentially a dictionary of antigens, an alphabetically arranged list of these antigens is given below for ready reference. Antigens that now have additional names but that are likely still to be known by their original names are not included. As an example, although Au^a and Au^b have been shown (33-35) to be antigens of the Lutheran blood group system and have been assigned the terms Lu18 and Lu19 respectively (36), they will continue to be called Au^a and Au^b in a manner analogous to that in which the terms Js^a and Js^b are still used although the antigens concerned are part of the Kell blood group system (37,38). Accordingly, antigens such as Wb, Ls^a, An^a and Dh^a each of which now has a Gerbich system number (36,39 and see Chapter 16) and Wr^a, Wr^b, Wd^a, Rb^a, WARR and many others each of which now has a Diego system number (39,40 and see Chapter 17) are not listed except when another antigen with a different alphabetical name, duplicated one of them. In the listing below, the name of the blood group system of which the antigen is a part, is shown where known. The terms LI (low incidence) and HI (high incidence) are used for those antigens currently thought to be independent of known blood group systems.

Antigen	System	Duplicated by
At^a	HI	Multiple, see 901 listing in this chapter
Co3	Colton	Swarts
Far	MN	Kam
Finlay	LI	Burrett
Hg^a	Diego	Tarplee, Tarp
In^b	Indian	Salis, Parra, Walls
JFV	LI	Jf
JMH	HI	Multiple, see 901 listing in this chapter
Jo^a	Dombrock	Jc^a
Jones	LI	Hol (Holmes)
Jr^a	HI	Multiple, see 901 listing in this chapter
Kp^c	Kell	Levay
K14	Kell	Dp
Lan	HI	So, Gn^a
Ls^a	Gerbich	Rl^a
LW^b	LW	Ne^a
Mansfield	LI	Peacock
Mit	MN	Doughty
Re^a	LI	Hol (Hollister), PeCo
Rx	HI	Sd^x
Sl^a	Knops	McC^c
Tr^a	Diego	Lanthois
Wu	Diego	Hov, Haakestad
Zt^a	LI	Marriott

References

1. Issitt PD, Crookston MC. Transfusion 1984;24:2
2. Lomas C, Tippett P, Thompson KM, et al. Vox Sang 1989;57:261
3. Jones J, Scott ML, Voak D. Transf Med 1995;5:171 and see 5:304 for corrections
4. Tippett P, Lomas-Francis C, Wallace M. Vox Sang 1996;70:123
5. Issitt PD, Daniels G, Tippett P. (Letter). Transfusion 1981;21:473
6. Marsh WL, Øyen R, Nichols ME, et al. Br J Haematol 1975;29:247
7. Marsh WL. (Letter). Vox Sang 1979;36:375
8. Crawford MN. Personal communication 1983, cited in Issitt PD. Applied Blood Group Serology, 3rd Ed. Miami:Montgomery 1985:381
9. Poole J, Giles CM. Vox Sang 1982;43:220
10. Poole J, Giles CM. Transfusion 1985;25:443
11. Mannessier L, Rouger P, Johnson CL, et al. Vox Sang 1986;50:240
12. Marsh WL, Brown PJ, DiNapoli J, et al. Transfusion 1983;23:128
13. Poole J, Levene C, Bennett M, et al. Transf Med 1991;1:245
14. Weaver T, Lacey P, Carty L. (abstract). Transfusion 1986;26:561
15. Laird-Fryer B, Moulds MK, Moulds JJ, et al. (abstract). Transfusion 1981;21:633
16. Banks JA, Parker N, Poole J. (abstract). Transf Med 1992;2 (Suppl 1):68
17. Banks JA, Hemming N, Poole J. Vox Sang 1995;68:177
18. Race RR, Sanger R. Blood Groups in Man, 6th Ed. Oxford:Blackwell, 1975
19. Mollison PL. Blood Transfusion in Clinical Medicine, 7th Ed. Oxford:Blackwell, 1983:437
20. Roelcke D, Hengge U, Kirschfink N. Vox Sang 1990;59:235
21. Bass LS, Rao AH, Goldstein J, et al. Vox Sang 1983;44;191
22. Chaves MA, Leak MR, Poole J, et al. Vox Sang 1988;55:241
23. Kornstad L. Vox Sang 1986;50:235
24. Riches RA, Laycock CM. Vox Sang 1980;38:305
25. Rowe GP, Boswell P. Vox Sang 1985;49:400
26. Kluge A, Roekcke D, Tanton E, et al. Vox Sang 1988;55:44
27. Ichikawa Y, Sato C, McCreary J, et al. Vox Sang 1989;56:98
28. Reid M, Fischer ML, Green C, et al. Vox Sang 1989;57:77
29. Habibi B, Fouillade MT, Duedari N, et al. Vox Sang 1978;34:302
30. Morel PA, Hamilton HB. Vox Sang 1979;36:182
31. Gellerman MM, McCreary J, Yedinak E, et al. Transfusion 1973;13:225
32. Giles CM. Vox Sang 1975;29:73
33. Daniels G. Vox Sang 1990;58:56
34. Daniels GL, Le Pennec PY, Rouger P, et al. Vox Sang 1991;60:191
35. Zelinski T, Kaita H, Coghlan G, et al. Vox Sang 1991;61:275
36. Lewis M, Anstee DJ, Bird GWG, et al. Vox Sang 1991;61:158
37. Stroup M, MacIlroy M, Walker RH, et al. Transfusion 1965;5:309
38. Morton NE, Krieger H, Steinberg AG, et al. Vox Sang 1965;10:608
39. Daniels GL, Anstee DJ, Cartron J-P, et al. Vox Sang 1995;69:265
40. Daniels GL, Anstee DJ, Cartron J-P, et al. Vox Sang 1996;71:246
41. Bodmer JG, Marsh SGE, Albert ED, et al. Tissue Antigens 1992;39:161
42. Tsuji K, Aizawa M, Sasazuki T. HLA 1991. Oxford:Oxford Univ Press, 1992
43. Middleton D. Biologist 1997;44:322

45 | Glossary

Some terms used in blood banking are applied in a manner different from the way in which they are used in classical genetics and sometimes differently from the definition given in a standard dictionary (1,2). Listed below are a number of terms used in this book and explanations of what we and some but not all others mean by them. In addition to definitions a few frequently used abbreviations are included as are some terms not used in this book, that show which term we used instead.

ADCC(L), ADCC(M): Terms used to describe in vitro bioassays that measure the reactivity of mononuclear leukocytes with antibody-coated red cells. The terms refer to antibody-dependent cell-mediated cytotoxicity assays using lymphocytes (L) or monocytes (M).

Adsorption: The process by which an antibody is removed from serum. That is, a serum rendered free of antibody is said to have been adsorbed. Red cells that have bound an antibody from a serum are said to have adsorbed that antibody. In other words, because he never knew when to use absorb and when to use adsorb, one of us (PDI) followed the excellent advice of Rosenfield (3) and dropped the word absorb from his vocabulary.

Allele, Allelomorph or Allelic Gene: An alternative form of a series of genes that can occupy a single locus on either of a pair of homologous chromosomes. Normally the gene products (expressed in terms of red cell antigens) are antithetical. As an example, Fy^a and Fy^b are a pair of allelic genes and the antigens, Fy^a and Fy^b whose production the genes encode are antithetical.

Allogeneic: The correct word to describe blood, marrow, tissue, etc., from members of the same species who are not genetically identical. Formerly the word homologous was used but Walker (4) and Mollison (5) pointed out that allogeneic is more accurate and was used by others (6,7) before blood bankers made the appropriate change.

Alloimmune: Used to describe an immune response or an antibody directed against an antigen lacking from the cells of the antibody-maker.

Amorph: A gene that fails to encode production of a detectable character. In immunohematology it is difficult to differentiate (at the serological level) between a number of possible explanations. First, the gene may fail to encode production of the carrier molecule. Second, the gene may encode production of an enzyme for which no substrate is present so that although the gene is functional, the end product with which it is associated, is not made. Third, the gene may encode production of an antigen whose presence is not recognized because no antibody against it is available. For all these reasons, the term silent allele (see below) is now preferred.

Anamnestic response: Now used synonymously with secondary immune response in an individual previously immunized and now exposed to the same antigen. Originally used to include all antibodies made in a secondary immune response, i.e. those directed against the antigen reintroduced and those produced as a result of increased activity of the immune system and directed against (an) antigen(s) other than that prompting the secondary response. Now always almost used to describe a specific secondary immune response.

Antibody: A serum protein (i.e. an immunoglobulin with specific combining sites), produced as a result of the introduction of a foreign antigen, that has the ability to combine with (and in many instances destroy) the cells carrying the antigen that stimulated its production. For a more complete explanation see Chapter 2 on the immune response. As mentioned in that Chapter, blood group antibodies made by persons who have never been exposed to foreign red cells via transfusion, pregnancy or injection, are made in response to the introduction of structurally similar antigens on substances other than red cells. Note that in naming antibodies the prefix anti and the name of the antigen detected, such as A or Fy^a are always joined with a hyphen. Anti is a prefix not a word. The name of an antibody is always a word thus the antibody reacting with the A antigen is anti-A and that reacting with the Fy^a antigen, anti-Fy^a. Use of terms such as anti A and anti Fy^a, without the hyphens, is grammatically and serologically incorrect.

Antigen: A substance that when introduced into the circulation of a subject lacking that antigen, can stimulate the production of a specific antibody. For a more complete explanation see Chapter 2 on the immune response. As mentioned above, some blood group antibodies are produced in response to the introduction of antigens on molecules other than those carried by red cells. In many instances the antigen and the gene that encodes its production share the same name, e.g., K antigen, K gene. For correct terminology to differentiate between antigens and genes, see Chapter 1.

Antigenic determinant: Often used to describe the portion of the antigen-bearing structure with which the antibody combines. However, if the definition of an antigen is that it can stimulate the production of a specific antibody, there can be no difference between an antigen and an antigenic determinant. In the past, the term antigenic determinant has sometimes been used to describe what is now called an epitope. Since the term epitope is more specific than antigenic determinant, it should not be used loosely (see below).

Association: In terms of antigen-antibody reactions the term relates to the uptake of antibody by antigen.

Autogeneic: Blood, marrow, etc., from one's self, i.e. one's own genes.

Autoimmune: Used to describe an immune response or an antibody directed against an antigen on the cells of the antibody-maker.

Autologous: Blood, marrow, etc., from one's self, i.e. one's own.

Autosome: Any chromosome other than X and Y.

Bilirubin: A breakdown product that accumulates following red cell destruction. Normally present in small amounts following the removal of senescent red cells. Bilirubin levels in plasma often increase in patients with accelerated in vivo red cell destruction but there are many other causes of hyperbilirubinemia.

Bioassay: In immunohematology, an in vitro test performed using live cells, e.g. ADCC(L), ADCC(M), MMA.

Blocking antibody: An antibody that has the ability to combine with its antigen on the red cell surface but that is unable to cause agglutination in a saline system. Named because of its ability to engage all (or most) receptor sites on the red cell surface and thus prevent agglutination of the cells if they are subsequently tested with a saline agglutinating antibody of the same specificity. Now more often called an incomplete antibody. Blocking antibodies are now sometimes used in studies with red cells or isolated membrane components in competitive inhibition studies designed to identify antigen location sites.

Cellular bioassay: See bioassay.

Chimera: An organism (a human for the purposes of this book) whose cells represent the presence of two or more zygotes. This situation differs from mosaicism (see below) in which somatic mutation results in two cell lines in a person representing a single zygote. Most natural human chimeras represent twins, i.e., in utero exchange of genetic material, or dispermy, i.e., fertilization of two maternal nuclei by two sperm with subsequent fusion of the zygotes and development of one person with two cell lineages. Artificial human chimeras may be formed following intra-uterine transfusion or bone marrow transplantation.

Chromosome: The structures, located within the cell nucleus, that carry genes. In humans, nucleated cells carry 23 pairs of chromosomes. At the time of mitosis 23 like pairs of chromosomes are produced for the new cell. At meiosis the 23 pairs of chromosomes divide so that each sex cell formed carries one of each pair, or 23 single chromosomes.

Cis: See position effect.

Clone: A set of cells descended from a common precursor cell. In a normal immune response many different clones of immunocytes produce antibody molecules with similar but not identical characteristics. In a pathological immune response a single clone of immunocytes may proliferate and produce identical antibody molecules.

Cluster of Differentiation (CD) Markers: Markers, largely on leukocytes, identified with monoclonal antibodies. CD markers are extremely useful in the differentiation of developmental and functional characters of T and B cells (see Chapter 2). The carrier molecule that bears the markers is usually described in CD terms. Many CD proteins are now known to be present on red cells. These include but are not limited to: CD35, CR1 the receptor for C3b (8) and carrier of the Knops system antigens (42,43) (see Chapter 28); CD44, the carrier of In^a and In^b (9-11) (see Chapter 29); CD47, the integrin-associated protein that is apparently part of the Rh cluster (12-15) (see Chapter 12); CD55, decay-accelerating factor, the carrier of the Cromer system antigens (16,17) (see Chapter 24); CD59, MIRL or membrane inhibitor of reactive lysis (18) (see Chapter 6); and CD99, the carrier of 12E7 (19,20) (see Chapter 25).

Coating antibody: Same as an incomplete antibody.

Cordocentesis: A technique for obtaining blood from the umbilical cord vein.

Complete antibody: An antibody capable of causing agglutination in a simple saline system.

Complement: A series of alpha, beta and gamma globulins present in all normal sera. Some antibodies activate complement once they have complexed with antigen. Activation of the complement pathway serves as the effector mechanism by which some antibodies destroy the structures carrying the antigens against which they are directed.

Consanguineous: Descended from a common ancestor. Thus a consanguineous mating is one between two persons sharing a common (blood) ancestor. The presence of two rare genes, in an individual born of a consanguineous mating, often represents passage of the same gene through two branches of the family.

Crossing-over: The transfer of genetic information from one chromosome to its homologous partner that sometimes occurs at mitosis or meiosis. See also unequal crossing-over.

Crossmatch: A slang term used to describe a compatibility test.

Crossreacting antibody: An antibody that can combine with an antigen apparently different from the one that elicited its production because the two antigens share structures that are similar in shape and charge.

Cytokine: A protein, usually secreted by a leukocyte, that regulates a biological function. Over 100 cytokines are known in man, many play key roles in the immune and inflammatory responses. Examples of cytokines are: interleukins; interferons; tumor necrosis factors; erythropoietin; and colony stimulating factors.

Cytoskeleton: The internal structural framework of a cell. In red cells, spectrin, actin, proteins 4.1, 4.2 and 2.1 are critical. Some transmembrane proteins, e.g. band 3 and glycophorin C, are attached to the cytoskeleton.

Deletion: A term often applied at the genetic level to suggest that absence of an expected character (e.g. an antigen) at the phenotypic level represents deletion of the encoding gene. It is now well established that the situation can represent absence (deletion) or presence of a (sometimes structurally normal) gene that fails to encode production of a recognizable characteristic. Thus at the genetic level, deletion can mean absence or absence of function of a gene. At the phenotypic level, the term indicates absence of antigen, e.g. Rh-deletion usually means presence of D and absence of E and e, or of C, c, E and e (see Chapter 12).

DIC: Disseminated intravascular coagulation.

Diploid number: The number of chromosomes found in a tissue (non-sex) cell. The diploid number varies in different species; in man it is 46, i.e. 22 pairs of autosomes plus XX (female) and XY (male).

Dissociation: In terms of antigen-antibody reactions the term relates to the (usually) spontaneous elution of antibody from antigen. The non-word dissassociation is often used in error, one cannot diss-ass (21).

Dominant gene: A gene that is expressed, in terms of antigen production, when present in double or single dose.

Dosage effect: The difference in amount of antigen made when two like genes are present compared to the amount made when two dissimilar genes are present. Recognized by the reactions of some antibodies that are dependent on the amount of antigen present for the strength of their reaction. In serological tests, titration studies or quantitative methods such as the enzyme-linked antiglobulin test are usually necessary for convincing evidence of dosage effect. Some spectacular results showing dosage effect have been obtained in tests using a flow cytometer (22-24).

ELAT: Enzyme-linked antiglobulin test.

Eluate: Antibody, recovered by a process called elution following the binding of that antibody to its antigen. In blood banking, eluates are most often made, from red cells that have bound antibody, by a process that destroys the bonds between antigen and antibody. In many elution procedures the red cells are destroyed although this is not an essential step in the recovery of bound antibody.

Epitope: That portion of an antigen with which a specific single population of antibody molecules combines. A single antigen, e.g., D, will contain may epitopes. Polyclonal anti-D as made by an immunized D- individual will contain a series of specificities recognizing different epitopes. A monoclonal anti-D will contain antibody molecules all recognizing the same epitope. Now that monoclonal antibodies directed against most red cell antigens are available, it will be possible to characterize the multiple epitopes of certain antigens. Such characterization of the epitopes of D is well advanced (25-27) (see Chapter 12). Now that epitopes can be clearly identified using monoclonal antibodies it becomes important that the term epitope not be misused, i.e. when antigen is intended.

Exon: That portion of the gene that is translated in terms of part of the protein that represents the whole gene product. Many genes are composed of multiple exons that are separated, at the DNA level, by introns that are not translated (see below). The final gene product can be regarded as the protein encoded by all the exons in the DNA that were translated. For more information see Chapter 5.

Exon-skipping: A process by which a different to usual gene product is made because the exons used in production of the usual gene product were not all used. That is to say, the protein encoded lacks a portion or portions normally made by the exon or exons not used in production of the variant protein. For more information see Chapter 5.

Family antigen: A term sometimes used to describe a rare, or low incidence antigen. A poor description since most rare antigens are eventually detected on the red cells of unrelated persons.

FMH: Fetal to maternal hemorrhage.

Gene: The basic unit of inheritance that encodes production of a protein. Although in immunohematology the presence of an antigen often equates with the presence of a gene, i.e. Fy^a is made when Fy^a is present, it is now appreciated that some genes encode the production of proteins that carry more than one serologically recognizable antigen. For example, M encodes production of a form of glycophorin A that carries, at least, M and the En^a series of antigens. S and s encode production of forms of glycophorin B that carry, at least, ′N′, S and U, and ′N′, s and U, respectively (see Chapter 15). When the protein encoded by the gene is an enzyme, the red cell antigen present is an indirect product, e.g. A and B are made by the actions of A and B gene-specified transferases (see Chapter 8).

Gene conversion: A process by which a portion of a gene (a part, one or more exons, a part, one or more introns or a mixture of those structures) is inserted, sometimes as a reciprocal replacement, into another gene. If the converted gene is functional it encodes production of a hybrid protein (see particularly Chapters 12 and 15). Not all gene conversion events involve reciprocal exchanges.

Gene deletion: See deletion.

Genotype: A list of genes thought, from the results of typing tests, to be present in an individual. Very often a genotype represents interpretation of which genes appear to be present, based on observed serological findings (phenotype). A common mistake is to state that red cells can be or have been genotyped. Red cells can be phenotyped and an interpretation of the genotype of the individual from whom the red cells came, can be made. A genotype can be determined by analysis of DNA if the

structure of the gene of interest is known. However, as pointed out in several chapters in this book (particularly Chapter 41) the presence of a gene does not always correlate exactly with the production of expected antigen.

Growth factors: A cytokine capable of stimulating growth of a particular cell line or lines. Often called colony stimulating factors.

Haploid number: The number of chromosomes found in a normal sex cell. The haploid number varies in different species; in man it is 23.

Haplotype: Genes, residing on one of the pair of homologous chromosomes, that usually travel together. In an individual with red cells that type as D+ C+ E- c+ e+ the most likely haplotypes would be *DCe* and *ce*. However, the haplotypes could be *Dce* and *Ce*. As discussed in Chapter 12, while *DCe* and *Dce* are haplotypes, i.e. *D* and *Ce* and *D* and *ce* alleles respectively, *ce* and *Ce* are actually genes since in most White persons with D- red cells, *D* is deleted (28).

Hemizygote: An individual with a gene on one chromosome, when a paired chromosome is not present. For example, since males have one X and one Y chromosome, they can be hemizygous for Xg^a or Xg. They cannot be homozygous or heterozygous for either gene. Since females have two X chromosomes they can be homozygous for Xg^a or Xg or Xg^aXg heterozygotes. They cannot be hemizygous for either gene.

Hemoglobinemia: The presence of free hemoglobin or one of its derivatives in the plasma.

Hemoglobinuria: The presence of free hemoglobin or one of its derivative in the urine.

Hemolysin: An antibody capable of destroying red cells in the presence of complement.

Heterozygote: An individual with dissimilar alleles at a given locus on homologous chromosomes. Note that a person can be heterozygous, red cells cannot. Red cells can be from a heterozygote.

High incidence antigen: A common antigen found on the red cells of most random donors.

Homologous: See allogeneic that is the correct term to describe blood, marrow, tissue, etc., from members of the same species who are not genetically identical. The word homologous is used to describe, for example, a pair of chromosomes that are alike or similar but not identical.

Homozygote: An individual with identical alleles at a given locus on homologous chromosomes. A person can be homozygous, red cells cannot. Red cells can be from a homozygote, e.g., Jk(a+b-) red cells usually carry a double dose of Jk^a and come from a person homozygous for *Jk^a* who can also be described as a *Jk^a* homozygote.

Hybridoma: A cell culture originating from an artificial fusion of two cell types. Often used to produce monoclonal antibodies by fusing an antibody-producing cell (immunocyte) from one animal or individual with an immunoglobulin secreting cell from another. The immunoglobulin secreting cell used in the fusion should be one that secretes that material without antibody specificity. The specificity can then be dictated by the immunocyte used in the fusion.

Hyperbilirubinemia: An elevated level of bilirubin in the plasma.

Hypothermia: Exposure to cold. Induced hypothermia is used in some surgical procedures but does not alter compatibility testing considerations (see Chapter 35).

Idiotype: The specific configuration of the antigen-combining site of an antibody molecule. Anti-idiotypes can be raised since the arrangement of amino acids in the specific antigen-combining site (the idiotype) can be immunogenic.

Immunized individual: A person making an antibody.

Immunocyte: A cell with the ability to synthesize antibody.

Immunogen: A description of an antigen or an epitope in its role of stimulating antibody production.

Immunoglobulin: Protein, or more specifically gamma globulin, of which antibodies are made. Major types involved in the production of blood group antibodies are IgG, IgM and, to a lesser degree, IgA. Others, IgD and IgE, may be involved in the production of non-blood group antibodies.

Independent segregation: The passage of genes from parents to children in a manner that demonstrates that the inheritance is on a random basis and that the genes involved are not linked. For example, a group AB, Fy(a+b+) parent may pass *A* and *Fy^a* to one child, *A* and *Fy^b* to another, *B* and *Fy^a* to a third and so on. The *ABO* and *Duffy* system genes would then be said to segregate independently. The situation is also called random assortment.

Inhibition: The process of preventing an antibody from reacting by adding, to the serum containing the antibody, a substance capable of combining with (and hence neutralizing) the antibody.

Inseparable antibody: An antibody with characteristics that suggest that it reacts with more than one antigen (such as anti-Jk^{ab} formed by a Jk(a-b-) person) that cannot be split into separable components by adsorption. May be an antibody reacting with a common determinant present on Jk(a+b-) and Jk(a-b+) red cells, in this case Jk3, that would then be said to be a product of both *Jk^a* and *Jk^b*.

Intron: That portion of a gene that is situated between exons and is edited out between the pRNA and mRNA stage. Introns do not encode production of the final gene product but differences between introns of genes that display considerable homology can be useful in gene recognition. For example, *D* and *CE* (*Ce, cE, ce* and *CE* alleles) are homologous over much of their lengths. In DNA studies *D* can be distinguished from *CE* because intron 4 of *D* comprises 600 base pairs while intron 4 of *CE* comprises 1200 (44,45) (see also Chapters 5, 12 and 41).

In vitro: Outside the body, in the blood bank often in a test tube.

In vivo: Within the body.

Incomplete antibody: An antibody that attaches to its specific antigen on the red cell surface but that is unable to cause agglutination in a saline system.

Kernicterus: Damage to brain cells. Can be caused by abnormally high levels of plasma bilirubin.

Laked: Hemolyzed.

Lectin: An extract, often made from seeds, that has the ability to react with red cells. Lectins commonly used in blood group serology have specificity for known red cell antigens. Many others are known that agglutinate all red cells.

Linkage disequilibrium: The situation in which some haplotypes are more common than others because of unequal distribution of certain alleles, with others that are at closely linked loci. For example, the haplotype *Ns* is more common than *NS* and the difference is greater than would be expected from the individual frequencies of *N, S* and *s*. Genes at the *MN* and *Ss* loci are thus said to be in linkage disequilibrium.

Linked genes: Genes that travel together from parent to offspring. In some systems linkage is absolute. For example, a parent with K+ k+ Kp(a+b+) red cells will transmit *KKp^b* or *kKp^a* to all offspring. While this situation is called linkage it actually represents the fact that one gene encodes production of a glycoprotein that carries K and Kp^b, while the other encodes production of a glycoprotein that carries k and Kp^a. An individual with M+ N+ S+ s+ red cells, who is genetically *MS/Ns* will transmit *MS* or *Ns* almost all the time. However, because linkage between the *MN* and *Ss* loci is not absolute, the *MS/Ns* parent may have a cross-over between the loci and transmit *Ms* or *NS*. The incidence of crossing-over between the genes of different blood group systems (e.g., *Rh* and *Sc* (29,30)) is used to determine the distance between the loci.

LISS: Low ionic strength solution.

Locus (plural loci): The site of a gene on a chromosome.

Low incidence antigen: A rare antigen found on the red cells of very few random donors.

Lymphokine: A cytokine produced by a lymphocyte.

MAIEA: Monoclonal antibody-specific immobilization of erythrocyte antigens.

Meiosis: The process of cell division by which the sex cells are formed. For chromosome content of ova and sperms, see chromosome.

Mimicking antibody: An antibody (often autoimmune in nature) that appears to have one specificity, based on conventional antibody identification procedures, but that can be shown to have a different specificity by use of adsorption studies. The antibody can be adsorbed to exhaustion by red cells with which it does not react in a visible manner in conventional tests (31,32) (see Chapters 37 and 43).

Mitosis: The process of cell division by which all new cells except sex cells are formed. For chromosome content of cells, see chromosome.

Mixed-field reaction: An agglutination pattern in which some but not all cells are agglutinated. Differentiated from a weak positive reaction by virtue of tight agglutinates of the reactive cells. Often an indication of two cell populations (see Chapter 43).

MMA: Monocyte monolayer assay.

Modifying gene: A gene, often at a locus independent of the blood group gene that is apparently affected, that in some way alters the expression of that gene or its normal product. For example, the dominant modifying gene *In(Lu)* is not at the *Lutheran* locus but its presence prevents *Lu^a*, *Lu^b*, etc., from expressing themselves in terms of normal antigen production. The recessive modifying gene *X^o r* is not at the *Rh* locus but in double dose results in the Rh_null phenotype in spite of the presence of normal *Rh* genes (see Chapter 12). In many instances the mechanisms by which modifying genes act are not known. However, it has now been shown (33) that *X^o r* is a mutant form of the gene that normally encodes production of an Rh glycoprotein (34,35) that is a necessary component of the Rh cluster (again see Chapter 12). In the past, modifying genes were often called suppressor genes. The term modifier or regulator gene is much better. For example, in the genotype *hh*, no red cell A or B antigens are made although *A* and/or *B* may be present. However, *h* does not suppress *A* or *B* since those genes, if present, make the expected transferase enzymes (36,37) (see Chapter 8). In effect, *hh* results in no production of H so that the *A* and *B*-specified transferases have no substrate to which they can add A or B immunodominant carbohydrates. In most other blood group systems, the actions of the modifying genes are less well understood. Accordingly, it is much safer to use the term modifier or modifying gene than suppressor or suppressor gene.

Monoclonal antibody: An antibody in which all molecules are identical since they have been produced by immunocytes belonging to a single clone. Monoclonal antibodies are made in some pathological conditions (such as CHD, see Chapter 38) and can now be made in vitro (46). Each antibody molecule complexes with the same epitope of the antigen.

Monokine: A cytokine produced by a macrophage or a monocyte.

Mosaic: This term was previously used to describe an antigen made of multiple parts, e.g. D. More recently lack of some epitopes of the antigen has been described as resulting in a partial antigen (e.g. partial D) (38-40) being present. It is to be hoped that the designation of partial antigens will replace the term mosaic antigen. In people, the term mosaic describes the presence of cells of two different phenotypes derived from a single zygote (i.e. not a chimera). In immunohematology the somatic mutation that leads to Tn-polyagglutination (see Chapter 42) leads to mosaicism.

Mutation: A change in genetic material recognizable by

the appearance of a new character or the loss of one previously present. Although blood group polymorphisms probably arose by mutation (plus unequal crossing over, gene conversion, exon-skipping, etc.) it is very unusual to find evidence of de novo mutation when family studies are performed.

Non-specific: In immunohematology this term is usually used to describe the joining of two substances (such as red cells and a serum protein) in the absence of a specific reaction (such as an antigen-antibody reaction). Cells exposed to cephalosporin are said to adsorb serum proteins non-specifically. Some serum proteins (including small amounts of IgG) can bind non-specifically to normal red cells. When an antigen and antibody combine, the reaction always has specificity. This is true even if the specificity of the antibody cannot be recognized from its reaction pattern. A non-specific antigen-antibody reaction cannot occur since all antibodies have specificity (they were produced by immunocytes in response to exposure to an antigen). A so-called non-specific antibody is actually an antibody of undetermined specificity.

Non-specific antibody: A contradiction of terms, see above.

Non-specific cold agglutinin: A contradiction of terms applied to an antibody optimally reactive at low temperatures, see above. Non-specificity is in the eye of the beholder.

Partial antigen: A situation in which one or more but not all epitopes of a given antigen is/are present. If red cells are involved they will give variable (i.e. some positive, some negative) reactions with antibodies of ostensibly the same specificity. The reactions will be dependent on the epitope specificities of the antibodies. Persons with a partial antigen on the red cells can mount an alloimmune response to those epitopes that their red cells lack. At the serological level it will then appear that the individual is antigen positive but has made an alloantibody to the antigen involved. The most fully studied example of this phenomenon involves partial D (25-27,38-40).

PEG: Polyethylene glycol.

Phenotype: A list of antigens, shown by test to be present on an individual's red cells. Can be used to infer the probable genotype of the individual. Red cells can be phenotyped, they cannot be genotyped. First, they do not have genes. Second, typing studies usually reveal the phenotypic expressions of the genes present in the individual from whom the red cells were collected.

Polyclonal antibody: The type of antibody made in a normal alloimmune and sometimes in an autoimmune response. Made by several different clones of immunocytes so that it is a mixture of slightly different antibody molecules. This type of antibody usually appears to be monospecific and to be made of only one type of immunoglobulin, e.g., IgG anti-K. In fact such an antibody will be a mixture of many different anti-K. These will vary in terms of binding constants and affinity and sometimes in terms of specificity since the different molecules may combine with different epitopes of the K antigen.

Polymorphism: The existence, in a population, of more than one phenotype for any character or set of characters.

Position effect: An effect (usually noticed by the amount of antigen serologically demonstrable) exerted on one gene by another gene (or genes) simultaneously present on the same, or opposite member of a pair of homologous chromosomes. Note: *cis* position involves a gene or genes present on the same chromosome as the one whose product is affected. *Trans* position involves a gene or genes present on the other chromosome of the pair.

Post-translation-modification: A change in the protein gene product that occurs after the protein has been made by translation of the mRNA at the ribosome. See Chapter 5.

Primary immune response: The initial response to antigen in which immunocytes are programmed to make a specific antibody and in which memory cells, that will recognize the same antigen if it is introduced again later, are created. In immunohematology, the primary immune response may result in the production of such a low level of antibody that it is not demonstrable in in vitro tests. That a primary immune response had occurred is often apparent when appreciable amounts of demonstrable antibody are made within days of (re)exposure to antigen.

Private antigen: A term sometimes used to describe an antigen of very low incidence. Not a good term since most such antigens are eventually found on the red cells of unrelated individuals.

Proband: The first studied member of a family. The person whose unusual blood type initiated a study of the blood of the pedigree members. Plural is probands.

Proposita: A female proband. Plural is propositae.

Propositus: A male proband. Plural is propositi.

Protease: An enzyme, the substrate for which is protein. The enzymes papain, ficin, bromelin, trypsin and pronase, all commonly used in immunohematology, are proteases.

Prozone: A situation in which an antibody reacts more strongly when diluted than when used in the undiluted (raw) state.

Public antigen: A term sometimes used to describe an antigen of very high incidence. Not a good term since some members of the public will eventually be found to have red cells that lack the antigen.

PUBS: Percutaneous umbilical vein blood sampling.

Receptor or receptor site: The portion of the antigen to which the antibody binds. Essentially the epitope but the term was in use before epitopes could be precisely defined.

Recessive genes: Genes whose presence is recognizable from random tests on individuals, only in homozygotes. The situation usually involves the absence of an otherwise expected antigen.

Ribosome: The site in the cell at which mRNA is transcribed and protein is assembled.

Secondary immune response: The activation of memory cells and the rapid production of detectable levels of antibody in individuals in whom exposure to and recognition of the antigen, i.e. the primary immune response, had already occurred. In spite of the second in its name, multiple secondary responses following second, third, fourth, to nth exposure to antigen, can occur.

Senescent red cells: Red cells at the end of their normal in vivo life span that are removed from circulation as a normal physiological event.

Sensitized red cells: Red cells coated with but not agglutinated by an antibody.

Sensitized individual: An incorrect way of describing an immunized individual.

Sibling or sib: A brother or sister of the proband, proposita or propositus.

Silent allele: A gene that does not encode for production of a serologically recognizable character. For a more complete discussion, see amorph, although, in fact, silent allele is a better term than amorph.

Specificity: The property of an antibody that enables it to combine with one but not other antigens. Specificity depends on shape and goodness of fit (21).

Suppressor gene: Previously used to describe a gene thought to prevent another gene from functioning. For reasons given above, the term modifying gene is preferable, see entry under modifying gene.

Syngeneic: Same gene, as in identical twin or same strain of highly inbred animal.

Synteny: The presence of genes on the same chromosome when such genes are located far enough apart that linkage, by conventional family studies, cannot be demonstrated. In other words, the rate of crossing-over between the loci is sufficiently high that the genes appear to segregate independently. Such loci or genes are said to be syntenic.

Tanned red cells: Red cells treated with tannic acid. Such cells can be used as carriers to which an antigen is passively coupled.

Thermal amplitude: The temperature range over which an antibody is active. See particularly Chapter 38.

Titer: A measure of the strength of an antibody. Serial dilutions of the antibody are tested against appropriate red cells and a titer value is assigned based on the highest dilution of the antibody still capable of causing a 1+ macroscopically positive reaction. The titer is correctly expressed as a reciprocal of the serum dilution. That is, if the highest dilution giving the 1+ reaction is 1 in 64, the titer is 64. To determine a titer, the antibody is titrated, it cannot be titered since there is no verb, to titer (41).

Titer score: The sum of all positive reactions (graded for strength) from an antibody titration. For numerical values assigned to each reaction strength see Chapter 3. It is sometimes easier to see dosage effects from titer scores than from titer end points.

Trans: See position effect.

Translocation: The transfer of genetic material from one chromosome to another. Different from crossing-over since homologous chromosomes are not always involved and the translocated material, removed from its usual site, often becomes non-functional. Often associated with a pathological condition.

Unequal crossing-over: Crossing-over within a gene as opposed to crossing-over of intact genes between chromosomes (see crossing-over, above). Unequal crossing-over results in the formation of new genes composed of material that was previously present in separate genes or in the removal of material that was previously present in separate genes (see Chapter 15).

Xenogeneic: Involving different species.

References

1. American Heritage Dictionary of the English Language, 3rd Ed. Soukhanov AH, Exec Ed. Boston:Houghton Mifflin, 1992
2. The Concise Oxford Dictionary, 5th Ed. Fowler HW, Fowler FG Eds. Oxford:Clarendon, 1964
3. Rosenfield RE. Personal communications 1967 to 1971 cited in Issitt PD. Applied Blood Group Serology, 3rd Ed. Miami:Montgomery 1985:636
4. Walker RH. Transfusion 1992;32:397
5. Mollison PL. (Letter). Transfusion 1992;32:494
6. Barrett JT. Textbook of Immunology, 4th Ed. St Louis:Mosby, 1983:224
7. Roitt IM. Essential Immunology, 8th Ed. Oxford:Blackwell, 1994
8. Ahearn JM, Fearon DT. Adv Immunol 1989;46:183
9. Spring FA, Dalchau R, Daniels GL, et al. Immunology 1988;64:37
10. Picker LJ, de los Toyos J, Telen MJ, et al. J Immunol 1989;142:2046
11. Parsons SF, Jones J, Anstee DJ, et al. Blood 1994;83:860
12. Miller YE, Daniels GL, Jones C, et al. Am J Hum Genet 1987;41:1061
13. Avent N, Judson PA, Parsons SF, et al. Biochem J 1988;251:499
14. Poss MT, Swanson JL, Telen MJ, et al. Vox Sang 1993;64:231
15. Lindberg FP, Lublin DM, Telen MJ, et al. J Biol Chem 1994;269:1567
16 Spring FA, Judson PA, Daniels GL, et al. Immunology 1987;62:307
17. Telen MJ, Hall SE, Green AM, et al. J Exp Med 1988;167:93
18. Fletcher A, Bryant JA, Gardner B, et al. Immunology 1992;75:507
19. Goodfellow P. Differentiation 1983;23 (Suppl):S35
20. Tippett P, Shaw M-A, Green CA, et al. Ann Hum Genet 1986;50:339
21. Steane EA. Personal communication, 1965
22. Oien L, Nance S, Garratty G. (abstract). Transfusion 1985;25:474
23. Nelson J, Choy C, Vengelen-Tyler V, et al. Immunohematology 1985;2:38
24. Nance ST. In: Progress in Immunohematology. Arlington, VA:Am Assoc Blood Banks, 1988:1
25. Lomas C, Tippett P, Thompson KM, et al. Vox Sang 1989;57:261
26. Jones J, Scott ML, Voak D. Transf Med 1995;5:171 and see 5:304 for corrections
27. Tippett P, Lomas-Francis C, Wallace M. Vox Sang 1996;70:123
28. Colin Y, Chérif-Zahar B, Le Van Kim C, et al. Blood 1991;78:2747
29. Lewis M, Kaita H, Chown B. Am J Hum Genet 1976;28:619
30. Noades JE, Corney G, Cook PJL, et al. Ann Hum Genet 1979;43:121
31. Issitt PD, Pavone BG. Br J Haematol 1978;38:63
32. Issitt PD, Combs MR, Bumgarner DJ, et al. Transfusion 1996;36:481
33. Chérif-Zahar B, Raynal V, Gane P, et al. Nature Genetics 1996;12:168
34. Ridgwell K, Spurr NK, Laguda B, et al. Biochem J 1992;287:223
35. Ridgwell K, Eyers SAC, Mawby WJ, et al. J Biol Chem 1994;269:6410
36. Race C, Watkins WM. FEBS Letts 1972;27:125
37. Mulet C, Cartron J-P, Badet J, et al. FEBS Letts 1977;84:74
38. Salmon C, Cartron J-P, Rouger P. The Human Blood Groups. New York:Masson, 1984:220
39. Tippett P. In: Blood Group Systems:Rh. Arlington, VA:Am Assoc Blood Banks, 1987:25
40. Tippett P. Med Lab Sci 1988;45:88
41. Issitt PD, Crookston MC. Transfusion 1984;24:2
42. Rao N, Ferguson DJ, Lee S-F, et al. J Immunol 1991;146:3502
43. Moulds JM, Nickells MW, Moulds JJ, et al. J Exp Med 1991;173:1159
44. Arce MA, Thompson ES, Wagner S, et al. Blood 1993;82:651
45. Simsek S, Faas BHW, Bleeker PMM, et al. Blood 1995;85:2975
46. Köhler G, Milstein C. Nature 1975;256:495

46 | Addenda

During the more than two years that it has taken to write this book, numerous new findings have been made and described in print. In many instances it has proved possible to incorporate the new findings in appropriate chapters. As an example, the first draft of Chapter 17, on the Diego system, included descriptions of seven antigens; the current version includes descriptions of 20. On other occasions a new finding was reported when the relevant chapter was too near final form for an addition to be made. Even with the above example, an additional Diego system antigen is described in this chapter. Accordingly, this chapter lists some new findings, arranged in the sequence of chapters of this book, that could not be included in the appropriate chapter. Perforce, some of these observations are described in less detail than their significance warrants. When that is clearly the case, readers are urged to read the paper cited.

Chapter 1 Terminology

Yet more attempts to persuade blood bankers to use correct terminology for blood group antigens, phenotypes and genes have been made by Issitt (228, the smart one!) and by Kitchen (229). In spite of all efforts, terminological atrocities continue. The abstracts of papers presented at the 1997 Annual Meeting of the American Association of Blood Banks include ones that describe Rh32+, Rh32-, Rh33+, Es^a+ and Es^a- red cells (references not given, the responsible authors are friends) when Rh:32, Rh:-32, Rh:33, Es(a+) and Es(a-) would have been correct. Those of us who try (230), find that the battle seems to be against an increasingly steep incline, see also page 611, "Anti-Kell does not exist".

Chapter 2 Immunology

Mendez et al. (231) constructed two megabase-sized YACs containing approximately 66 variable heavy and 132 variable kappa human immunoglobulin genes in nearly germline configuration. When the YACs were introduced into mice in which Ig genes had been inactivated, high affinity human antibodies to a variety of antigens, including some of human origin, could be generated. These results represent a major breakthrough and herald a new era of diagnostic and therapeutic antibodies.

Siegel et al. (1) have published additional details about the use of magnetically-activated cell sorting in the

isolation of antibodies using the phage display technology (2-4). Using peripheral blood lymphocytes from a single alloimmunized individual they isolated dozens of monoclonal IgG1 anti-D, some with kappa and some with lambda light chains. Studies of this type are, of course, contributing greatly to an understanding of gene usage in initial antibody production and subsequent refinement of specificity by somatic mutation (2-7). A study (8) using anti-D made using phage display and red cells carrying partial D, led to the proposal of an alternative explanation of the topology of the epitopes of D. This topic is discussed in the addendum to Chapter 12.

Use of the V_H4.21 heavy chain variable segment in the production of pathological auto-anti-I and auto-anti-i, and in human IgM monoclonal Rh antibodies is also discussed in the addendum to Chapter 12.

Chapter 3 Serological Methods

The increase in detection of positive DATs among hematologically normal blood donors, that Boulton (9) showed was associated with use of the gel test, has been confirmed by others (10-13). Essentially all column technologies have been associated with an increased incidence of meaningless positive reactions and Rushton et al. (12) found that other factors, e.g. better reagents to detect IgG autoantibodies of low affinity, played only a minor role. The increase is not insignificant, i.e. five times higher in 1996 than in 1990 in one study (12). It is highly undesirable in that the positive results are meaningless in terms of the donor's health; create extra unnecessary work in investigation of the findings; and have the potential to result in discard of perfectly acceptable units of blood. The high rate of positive reactions in hematologically normal individuals calls into question the claim (14) that the increased sensitivity of these methods in the DAT is an advantage.

Palfi and Hildén (207) have reported encouraging results from use of the gel test to determine the IgG subclass of antibodies. Additional observations about the gel test are given in the addenda to Chapters 8 and 35.

Chapter 4 Red Cell Membrane

Several groups of workers are studying the effects of covalently linking polyethylene glycol (PEG) to red cells in an attempt to block specific antibody binding by those cells. The hope is that such modified cells, that apparently survive and function normally, at least in mice, could be transfused in the face of incompatibility of the same cells before treatment. While Murad et al. (15) reported that the treatment abolished agglutination of the red cells by specific antibodies, they also found, by use of a flow cytometer, that antibody binding was reduced but not abolished. Similarly, Fisher et al. (16) showed that while antibody-specific agglutination was abrogated, antibody binding was demonstrable using IATs or flow cytometry. Garratty et al. (17) found that the PEG-treated red cells would also bind IgG and IgM non-specifically when incubated in antibody-free serum and gave strongly positive reactions in in vitro monocyte monolayer assays. It was suggested (17) that the results might indicate that the good survival of PEG-treated red cells in mice, might not be paralleled in man. Blood bankers are likely to find it somewhat ironic that PEG, that so enhances antibody uptake when used in solution (18), is capable of partial antigen masking and reduction of antibody binding, when covalently linked to the red cell membrane.

Griffiths et al. (232) reported the cloning of a human nucleoside transporter from a human placental cDNA library. The placental cDNA encodes a 456 residue protein of molecular weight 50,249 which is predicted to possess 11 membrane-spanning regions. Information derived from determining the amino-terminal protein sequence of the human red cell nucleoside transporter was used to isolate the cDNA. The authors (232) designated the protein product of this cDNA hENT1 (human equilibrative nucleoside transporter 1). The protein has three potential N-glycosylation sites of which only the first (on the first extracellular loop) is likely to be utilized. A nucleoside transporter is required for nucleoside synthesis via salvage pathways in red cells.

Chapter 6 Antiglobulin Tests

In Chapter 6 it is pointed out that when methods such as those using PEG or Polybrene were introduced for antibody-screening and compatibility testing, anti-IgG replaced broad spectrum antiglobulin reagents. While it was commonly assumed that the IgG, complement-binding antibodies previously detected best or only via the C3-anti-C3 portion of IATs, would be detected via increased uptake of IgG, little evidence for that assumption existed. Accordingly, we (19) tested pretransfusion samples from patients in whom an antibody with the potential to activate complement was detected within 16 days of transfusion, when no antibody had been detected by PEG/IAT (read with anti-IgG) before the transfusions. Tests on the pretransfusion sera were such that any complement activated by an antibody would have been detected. In a 17 month period, 23 antibodies (4 -K, 3 -Fy^a, 12 -Jk^a, 4 -Jk^b) were found in the post transfusion sera of 22 patients at times that varied from 2 to 16 days after transfusion. A total of 28 pretransfusion samples from the 22 patients were tested but in no instance did the use of a broad spectrum antiglobulin reagent result in unequivocal detection of an antibody in a pretransfusion sample. It seems that most IgG antibodies best detected by the C3-anti-C3 reaction in saline or albumin IATs are indeed detected with anti-IgG when PEG, Polybrene, etc., are used to potentiate antibody uptake.

Chapter 7 Antibodies

In the production of murine monoclonal antibodies the first step, i.e. immunizing mice with human red cells, results in the mice being exposed to a wide variety of red cell antigens. Chu et al. (197) have modified this approach by using transfected cells that do not normally carry human red cell blood group antigens, that have been engineered to express a high level of the antigen (carrier protein) of interest. Thus MEL cells transfected to produce the Kell glycoprotein were used successfully to raise murine monoclonal antibodies to k, Kp^b, Js^b and Ku. Murine monoclonal anti-Js^b had not previously been made. Clearly, the method has potential application for any situation in which the gene of interest can be transfected and is expressed.

Chapter 8 ABO and H Systems

Cheng et al. (20) reported that tests on the sera of six para-Bombay individuals failed to detect anti-H when the gel test was used but that the antibody was detectable by IAT in all six sera. No details are given regarding the type of IAT used, i.e. which potentiators (if any) were used in the antibody uptake portion of the tests.

Recent evidence (233-235) suggests that crossover or gene conversion events can give rise to hybrid genes in the ABO system. Suzuki et al. (234) described a case of disputed paternity in a Japanese family. A phenotypically A$_1$ child was born to a group B mother and a group O father. Analysis revealed that a hybrid allele in the child arose from a de novo recombination event in the germline of the mother. The crossover point occurred between exon 6 of a *B* and exon 7 of an *O^1* allele. The product of this hybrid gene would be predicted to have A$_1$ transferase activity, thus explaining the A$_1$ phenotype of the child. Olsson et al. (235) reported analysis of *ABO* genotypes in 138 group O Brazilians from three different ethnic backgrounds (Whites, Blacks and Amerindians). About one third of the samples (mostly from Blacks) did not represent the presence of previously described *O* alleles. The authors (235) pointed out that problems can arise when DNA-based typing methods developed and validated in one ethnic group are applied to another. As documented in Chapter 12 and in the addendum to that chapter (below) similar problems arise when DNA-based methods of typing for D, developed from tests on Whites, are used in Blacks and Orientals. Olsson et al. (235,236) provide data that indicate that crossover events giving rise to hybrid *ABO* alleles have occurred in Brazilians. In one example four samples from unrelated Blacks had genotypes that suggested a hybrid *O^{lv}-B* allele. (*O^{lv}* is a variant form of the *O^{1}* gene.) The crossover point was between exon 6 of the *O^{lv}* and exon 7 of a *B* allele. These data, taken together with those of Susuki et al. (234), suggest that the region between exons 6 and 7 in the *ABO* gene, may be a hotspot for recombination.

Chapter 10 The Ii Collection

Arndt et al. (21) described two examples of clinically significant anti-IH (called anti-HI in the abstract). One was in a patient who was group A, the antibody acted as an agglutinin and a hemolysin at 37°C in vitro. The transfusion of group A_2 red cells resulted in hemoglobinemia and hemoglobinuria, the transfusion of group A_1 red cells did not. The second patient was group B and her anti-IH was active at 35°C in vitro. Transfusion with two units of group O red cells resulted in no rise in hemoglobin. Both patients had greatly increased levels of i on their red cells, one had a reduced amount of I. Thus the cases could have represented a genetic state, i.e. patient of the adult i or similar phenotype with anti-IH rather than anti-I in the serum. Alternatively, the increased level of i on the red cells could have been associated with the patients' disease states, the first had myelofibrosis, the second thalassemia. The cases provide a good example of a statement made in other places in this book that, on occasion, thermal range of an antibody is more important than its specificity, in terms of clinical significance.

The anti-I and anti-i reactivities of human monoclonal IgM Rh antibodies are discussed in the addendum to Chapter 12.

Chapter 11 P_1 and Related Antigens

Sudakevitz et al. (22) reported that PA-I, a lectin made from *Pseudomonas aeruginosa*, can be of use in the recognition of various P-related phenotypes. In agglutination tests against papain-treated red cells and in adsorption studies, the PA-I lectin was found to place red cells in the sequence $P^k > P_1 > P_2 > p$. The difference could be demonstrated using red cells of any ABO group. The soybean lectin (*Glycine max*) can be used in conjunction with PA-I since it places the phenotypes in the reverse order, i.e. $p > P_2 > P_1 > P^k$.

Chapter 12 Rh System

In Chapter 12 considerable detail is given about partial D category VI. When those sections (on serology and on molecular structure) were written, two types of category VI were known to exist. In category VI, type I, exons 4 and 5 of *cE* replace those of *D*. In category VI, type II, exons 4, 5 and 6 of *Ce* replace those of *D* (see Chapter 12 for references). Flegel et al. (23) have now shown that a third type exists. In category VI, type III, exons 3, 4, 5 and 6 of *D* are replaced by those of *Ce*. In estimates of D antigen site density it was found (23) that: D^{VI} type I cells averaged 500; D^{VI} type II cells 2400; and D^{VI} type III cells 12,000; D sites per red cell. That is to say, D^{VI} type III red cells carry a near normal (for D+ cells) number of D sites. Both type I and type III D^{VI} red cells are BARC+ (i.e. Rh:52), type II, D^{VI} are Rh:-52 (24). Partial D category VI red cells are further unusual in that when the monoclonal anti-D, LOR-15C9, that is the first known MAb to D to give positive reactions in immunoblotting studies (25,26), is used, D^{VI} cells show an extra band. That is, when other D+ red cells are used, LOR-15C9 precipitates a 33kD protein, when D^{VI} cells are used, that band plus another of 21kD are precipitated (24-26).

Jones et al. (27) have described a new partial D phenotype to which they have given the name, DHR. The phenotype represents a single point mutation (G686 to A) in exon 5 of the *D* gene, that results in an arginine 229 to lysine change in what is predicted to be the fourth exofacial loop of the D polypeptide. The amino acid change results in lack of epD1, epD2, epD12 and epD20 of the 30 epitope model (28-30 and see Chapter 12). As discussed in Chapter 12, gene conversion is the most common mechanism by which partial D phenotypes arise. However, there are several instances, e.g. D^{VII}, Leu110 to Pro (31), D^{II}, Ala354 to Asp (32), DNU, Gly353 to Arg (32) and DHMi, Thr285 to Ile (33,34) and now DHR, Arg229 to Lys (27) in which point mutation is responsible. Full details of the DBT phenotype of partial D, in which Rh32 is expressed, have been published by Wallace et al. (222).

The mechanisms by which different genetic events, leading to the production of unusual Rh polypeptides, can effect production of the same low incidence Rh antigen, are described in Chapter 12. Another example of this phenomenon is provided by a study of Reid et al. (35). Anti-D^w is a rare antibody that defines a low incidence antigen on partial D red cells of category Va. Some anti-D^w contain an inseparable component that reacts weakly with Rh:32 red cells. The authors (35) described two sera that reacted strongly with D^w+ Rh:-32 and D^w-Rh:32 red cells but in which no separable anti-D^w or anti-Rh32 was present. It was pointed out that the genes that encode production of partial D category Va and partial D category DBT (that are Rh:32) and the $\bar{\bar{R}}^N$ gene (that encodes Rh32) all have a junction of exon 4 of *D* to exon 5 of *CE* (36-39). It appears that the amino acids at that junction comprise the antigen defined by these sera that were said to have anti-D^w/Rh32 specificity.

In Chapter 12 brief mention is made of HDN caused by anti-D^w. Some of the case reports are in difficult to obtain journals but now Spruell et al. (40) have summarized four cases known to them. In three cases, all involving Black parents, the infants had positive DATs but required no treatment. In an infant whose parents were Spanish, two exchange transfusions were given. Of the four anti-D^w listed (40) one is described as anti-D^w plus anti-Rh32 (see above).

Faas et al. (41) have reported that the c+ Rh:-26 phenotype results from presence of a *ce* gene in which a G→A point mutation at nucleotide 286 has occurred. This mutation is forecast to result in production of a ce polypeptide in which glycine replaces serine at position 96. Apparently other polymorphic sites are involved as well because Rh26 is expressed only on the c-bearing polypeptide, whereas glycine is expressed at position 96 on other Rh polypeptides. It is supposed that the Gly96 Ser change affects c as well since all c+ Rh:-26 red cells expressed c less strongly than c+ Rh:26 samples.

As would have been expected, the transplant of a kidney from a donor with anti-E in the serum, failed to cause hemolysis in the recipient who had E+ red cells (224).

The extreme heterogeneity of the e antigen, described in detail in Chapter 12, was also seen in tests using a series of monoclonal anti-e. Powell et al. (42) used seven such antibodies in tests against e variant, r^G, Be(a+), Rh:33, Rh:48 and so called e+ hr^S-, e+ hr^B-, and e+ hr^S- hr^B- samples. The seven MAb gave different patterns of reactivity and it was not possible to recognize a series of categories of partial e from the results.

In 1995, Green et al. (43) described a low incidence antigen, JAHK, defined by an antibody present in several multispecific sera (i.e. sera containing multiple antibodies to rare antigens, see Chapter 32). While JAHK is not officially part of the Rh system, it seems rather likely that its production is encoded by the rare gene, r^G. In the original description (43) JAHK was said to be produced by members of three unrelated families, who inherited r^G. Reid and Lomas (44) list JAHK as an antigen for which family studies support but have not yet proved the supposition that it is an Rh antigen. Daniels (45) points out that the r^G gene comprises a *ce* allele in which part of exon 2 appears to be derived from the

equivalent section of *D* (46). He (45) suggests that the unique amino acid sequence encoded by the r^G allele is responsible for the JAHK antigen and further, that the antigen is likely to reside in the second extracellular loop of the Rh polypeptide.

The English Rh_null (*X^orX^or* type) mentioned briefly in Chapter 12, has now been described in a full report (47). The patient had a weak anti-Rh29 in her serum and was transfused with four units of D- blood. No untoward effects resulted from the transfusions but the anti-Rh29 was made in greater amounts following the transfusions.

Matassi et al. (48) have pointed out that several gene conversion events that lead to the formation of *D-CE-D* hybrid genes involve certain portions of introns and describe a hot spot for such events.

Huang et al. (49) have reported that partial D, category IIIa red cells carry a protein that is associated with multiple dispersed amino acid changes from wild type D. The cDNA from category IIIa donors was found to contain four nucleotide substitutions scattered in three exons: A to C, nt 455, exon 3; C to G, nt 602, exon 4; C to G, nt 654, exon 5; and T to G, nt 667, exon 5. These substitutions would effect the amino acid changes: Asn152 to Thr; Thr201 to Arg; Ile218 to Met; and Phe223 to Val. Since the four changes identified in the *D* gene that encodes partial D category IIIa, all represent nucleotides/amino acids present in *CE* and CE protein, by far the most likely explanation seems to be templated micro-conversion of *D* by *CE*. It was also concluded that a C to G, nt 736 mutation, leading to Val245 might result in the expression of VS (see also Chapter 12 and later in this addendum).

Liu et al. (50) have used site directed mutagenesis and retroviral transduction of K562 cells (51) with the mutant constructs, to demonstrate that epD3 and epD9 of D require the amino acids encoded by *D*, at positions 350, 353 and 354 in the sixth external domain of the D polypeptide, for expression. Studies such as these together with serological studies (52, 53 and see Chapter 12 for earlier references) using epitope specific monoclonal anti-D and red cells with partial D antigens, have led to the proposal of models to explain the positions of various D epitopes on the D polypeptide (29,55-59) and some supposed interactions between amino acids on different exofacial loops of that polypeptide in the composition of some epitopes.

As mentioned in the addendum to Chapter 2, Chang and Siegel (8) used anti-D produced by the phage display technology in tests against red cells with partial D antigens. A study on 83 randomly selected clones produced from the peripheral blood lymphocytes of an individual immunized to D, resulted in the recognition of 28 unique gamma 1 heavy chain and 41 unique light change segments. The heavy and light chains were paired in a manner that resulted in 53 unique Fab pieces that among them defined at least half the epitopes of D. In spite of the diversity of the Fabs only 4 closely-related heavy chain germline genes were used. Similarly 15 of 18 kappa chains used the same germline gene and 22 of 23 lambda light chains used the same J gene. From the results of tests against partial D red cells, it was concluded (8) that the epitope specificity of an anti-D can change via somatic mutation during the course of continued antibody production. As discussed in Chapter 12, some individuals with partial D on their red cells initially make anti-D that reacts with all D+ red cells including their own, then make an epitope specific alloimmune anti-D as the immune response is refined. The change in epitope specificity of the anti-D, as described above, was thought perhaps to be the explanation of such observations.

Based on the development of the anti-D and the change in epitope specificity via somatic mutation, Chang and Siegel (8) suggested that the epitopes of D as defined by monoclonal anti-D may not be distinct entities but instead may reflect the abilities of different anti-D to combine with a particular structure.

Monoclonal IgM Rh system antibodies frequently use the V_{4-34} ($V_H4.21$) heavy chain variable gene segment (215,216). The same gene segment is mandatory for the production of pathological cold-reactive anti-I and anti-i (217-219). Thorpe et al. (220) tested 54 human IgM monoclonal Rh antibodies by immunohistochemical methods (195) for their ability to bind to tissue I and i antigens and for their ability to agglutinate adult I and cord i red cells that lacked the Rh antigen to which the MAb was directed. Among the 54 MAb, 32 had been produced using the V_{4-34} gene segment. Among those 32 antibodies five agglutinated untreated I adult and 14 agglutinated untreated i cord red cells in tests at 4°C. When papain-treated red cells were used, 27 agglutinated adult I and 30 agglutinated i cord red cells, again in tests at 4°C. None of the MAbs made using gene segments other than V_{4-34} agglutinated adult I or cord i red cells that lacked the appropriate Rh antigen. That the I and i antigens are involved was confirmed when it was shown that the MAbs did not agglutinate endo-beta-galactosidase-treated (Ii structures cleaved) red cells. While we are not aware of any false positive Rh typings caused by this situation, the potential for such might exist if red cells with particularly strong expressions of I or i were Rh typed with these antibodies. Perhaps more likely, it is possible that misleading results could be obtained in elution studies. That is to say, perhaps a MAb to D might bind to the I or i antigen on D- red cells and the recovered (eluted) antibody might be seen to have anti-D specificity in subsequent sensitive tests. It must be remembered that since these are monoclonal antibodies, the same antibody is responsible for the reactions, i.e.

apparently anti-I or anti-i at 4°C, anti-D at higher temperatures. Perhaps a saving grace is that IgM antibodies are not often used in elution procedures.

Scott et al. (60) tested cytoskeletal extracts from triton X-100 treated red cell membrane preparations and confirmed an earlier observation (61) that D is associated with the membrane skeleton. In addition, the extracts were shown to inhibit antibodies to C, c and e.

As has been pointed out several times in Chapters 12 and 41, most Whites with D- red cells represent a genetic state in which *D* is deleted. As indicated in Chapter 41 in the section dealing with methods to forecast the D status of an infant while the infant is still in utero, the same does not apply in Blacks (54). That is to say, in Blacks, DNA studies often show the presence of at least some portions of the *D* gene in individuals with D- red cells. The situation in the Japanese is similar to that in Blacks. In other words, cDNA studies reveal the presence of *D* in many persons whose red cells type as D- (85). Fukumori et al. (221) studied samples from 306 Japanese blood donors whose red cells typed as D-. Among the donors, 102 had red cells that would adsorb anti-D and yield that antibody on elution, i.e. donors with the D_{el} phenotype (see Chapter 12). All 102 donors of that phenotype were shown to have some expression of exons 4, 7 and 10 of *D* when PCR was used with sequence specific primers. No portion of *D* was found in any of the 204 donors of the D-, non-D_{el} phenotype. As mentioned elsewhere in this book, there is as yet no explanation as to why the D_{el} donors do not express D at the phenotypic level.

For many years it was believed (62-64) that an extracellular cysteine residue (more recently (65-67) identified as the exofacial Cys285) is essential for expression of the D and C antigens. The cysteine residue at position 285 is exofacial on both the D and CE polypeptides and its presence was believed to be essential for expression of D, C and c (62,63,67,68) and perhaps for expression of E and e although it was accepted (67,68) that a different exofacial cysteine might be involved in expression of E and e. Suyama et al. (69) challenged this concept and suggested that Cys285 is not essential for the integrity of expression of D. They believed that their findings differed from those of others because they (69) used intact red cells in their experiments whereas others (62-64) had used isolated red cell membranes. Smythe and Anstee (70) seem now to have resolved the argument and have shown that Cys285 is not essential for expression of D. These workers (70) used the retroviral gene transfer method to express Rh antigens on K562 cells (51). Some K562 cells were transfected with normal *D* cDNA, others were transfected with a mutated *D* cDNA that encodes alanine instead of cysteine at position 285. The transfected cells expressed the same level of D whether they had cysteine or alanine at position 285.

Daniels et al. (71) have extended their studies, described in Chapter 12, on the molecular basis of the V and VS polymorphisms. They report that, at least in South African and Dutch Black individuals, the VS+ V+ phenotype is associated with valine at position 245 of the ce polypeptide. The VS+ V- phenotype was found to be associated with valine 245, cysteine 336 and usually with a *D-CE* hybrid exon 3.

As described in Chapter 12, Chérif-Zahar et al. (72) have shown that the X^or and X^Q genes that, in double dose, cause the modifier Rh$_{null}$ and Rh$_{mod}$ phenotypes, respectively, are in fact a series of mutated forms of the genes that normally encode production of the Rh glycoproteins. In the original report (72), in different individuals, frameshift, nucleotide mutations and failure of amplification, were all seen. Huang et al. (73) have also described an Rh$_{mod}$ individual in whom the mutation involves the translation initiator (i.e. failure to amplify) of the Rh glycoprotein gene.

Mayer et al. (74) described a somewhat unexpected apparent association between the D- phenotype and gastric cancer. The incidence of D- persons among patients with gastric carcinoma was the same as that in the general population thus ruling out any predisposition of D- persons to the disease. However, the D- phenotype was said to be an independent predictor of poor prognosis and overall survival in these patients. This applied among the whole group of patients and among a selected cohort whose cancer was curatively resected. The association involved increased tumor recurrence and shortened long term survival; further, in multivariate analysis the D- phenotype was said to be the most important independent prognostic marker in the resected patients. In attempting to explain these findings, Mayer et al. (74) made two suggestions. First, since the function of the Rh polypeptides is not yet known, it was suggested that one role might involve cell growth and differentiation and that lack of the D polypeptide might compromise such a function. Alternatively, it was noted that there is a putative gastric carcinoma, tumor-suppressor gene, located on chromosome 1 in the same region as the *Rh* locus (75,76). It was suggested that when the *D* gene is lost (as in most White persons of the D- phenotype, see Chapter 12) the tumor suppressor gene might also be deleted. In other forms of cancer the D- phenotype has supposedly been: associated with tumor progression in oral squamous cell carcinoma (77,78); a favorable tumor stage in colorectal cancer (79); but had no association with prognosis in urogenital carcinoma (80-82). In small cell cancer of the lung no association between the D- phenotype and survival has been seen but it has been suggested (83,84) that the D- phenotype is associated with predisposition to the tumor.

Although Sandler et al. (20) showed that serological reactivity of a patient's red cells with WinRho (the preparation of IgG anti-D suitable for intravenous use) does not correlate with the Rh phenotype of the patient and thus does not forecast which D+ patients with ITP will respond to therapy with the immunoglobulin, we (201) obtained slightly different results. In our study (201), the amount of anti-D that bound to the patient's red cells was correlated with clinical response, i.e. the greater the amount of anti-D bound, the greater the chance of a response in terms of increase of the platelet count. The discrepant findings almost certainly represent the fact that there is overlap in the number of D sites on the red cells of individuals of different phenotypes. That is to say, it appears that the clinical response correlates with the amount of anti-D that binds and that the amount that binds varies among patients of the same Rh phenotype and overlaps among patients of different phenotypes. While the expected clinical response cannot be forecast from the Rh phenotype, it can (in part) be forecast by measurement of antibody uptake, using the flow cytometer (201).

As discussed in Chapter 12, the Rh polypeptide and Rh glycoproteins have structures that suggest that they function as membrane transporters. One commonly used approach to elucidate the function of a protein is to search protein and DNA sequence databases for molecules of known function that have significant sequence homology with the protein of interest. Progress in determining the structure of genes is currently so rapid that the number of gene sequences in databases is constantly increasing. Regular searches are necessary so that new and informative similarities are found. Marini et al. (237) have reported the results of a search for Rh polypeptide and Rh glycoprotein homologs that revealed significant homology between those proteins and a family of NH$_4^+$ transporters. Members of this family of proteins (Mep/Amt family) have been found in plants, yeast, bacteria and the nematode *Caenorhabditis elegans*. The sequence similarity is greater for the Rh glycoprotein than for the Rh polypeptides. NH$_4^+$ transporters have not yet been described in animals and it does not automatically follow that the Rh glycoprotein and/or the Rh polypeptides have such a function. Nevertheless this observation may provide clues that eventually lead to recognition of the function of those proteins.

Chapter 14 Duffy System

Tzeng et al. (86) used the monoclonal antibody specific immobilization of erythrocyte antigens (MAIEA) assay to produce evidence that Fy3 is carried on the same molecule as Fy6.

Chapter 15 MN System

Reid et al. (87) studied three monoclonal anti-S (MS-

93, MS-94 and MS-95) with regard to the structures defined. Only one of the three, MS-95, reacted with TSEN+ red cells that carry partial S on their GPA-B hybrid glycophorin. MS-93 and MS-95 reacted with neuraminidase-treated red cells and thus define sialic acid independent epitopes; MS-94 was non-reactive with sialidase-treated red cells. MS-94 but not MS-93 or MS-95 reacted with red cells treated with sodium hypochlorite. Differences in epitope specificity of monoclonal anti-S were not unexpected. Human polyclonal anti-S all require methionine at position 29 of glycophorin B but vary in their requirements for threonine 25 (or the attached tetrasaccharide), glutamic acid 28, glutamic acid 31, histidine 34 and arginine 35 (88,89).

Rasamoelisolo et al. (209) used agglutination, immunoblotting, inhibition with chemically-modified peptides derived from glycophorin A, and binding to synthetic peptides, to characterize seven new monoclonal antibodies directed against glycophorins. One antibody defined the N-terminal portion of glycophorin A when N was present and the same portion of glycophorin B (i.e. when 'N' was made). A second antibody recognized a homologous portion of glycophorins A and B corresponding to amino acids 6 to 26. A third determinant, recognized by three of the MAbs, comprised the portion of glycophorin A from amino acid 38 to 45. The fourth specificity, represented by the two remaining MAbs, was for amino acids 119 to 124 on the intracellular portion of glycophorin A. These findings correlated very well with the heterogeneity of human anti-En[a] that is described in Chapter 15.

As described in Chapter 15, the high frequency antigen AVIS and the low frequency antigen MARS represent an antithetical polymorphism of glycophorin A. Jarolim et al. (90) have shown that when glycophorin A carries AVIS, glutamine is present at residue 63. The CAA to AAA nucleotide substitution in the *GYPA* gene that encodes production of MARS, results in the presence of lysine at position 63. Residue 63 is within the region of glycophorin A that interacts with protein band 3 with the result that MARS+ red cells have a weakened expression of Wr[b] (see Chapters 15 and 17). The authors (90) propose that wild type glycophorin A folds on band 3 and interacts with the C-terminal end of the fourth ectoplasmic loop of that protein. Moulds et al. (91) performed population studies of the MARS and AVIS antigens. It appeared that the polymorphism is not a marker of Oriental populations, the low incidence antigen MARS was found on the red cells of 26 of 174 (15%) unrelated Choctaw Indians and, in this study, was found only in that population.

As discussed in Chapter 15, the *Mi[V]* gene encodes production of a GPA-B hybrid glycophorin that lacks the portion of glycophorin A that combines with protein band 3, to form Wr[b]. Poole et al. (92) have described a second *Mi[V]* homozygote who made anti-Wr[b].

Three autoantibodies against different determinants (i.e. En[a], Wr[b] and Pr) carried on glycophorin A, that were documented in abstracts cited in Chapter 15, have now been described in a full report (208). In each case the autoantibody was IgM and was active at 37°C, in two of the three patients the hemolysis was fatal. Additional details are given in the addendum to Chapter 37.

Chapter 16 Gerbich System

It is pointed out in Chapter 16 that the Ls(a+) phenotype in the Gerbich system represents the presence of normal and of larger than normal glycophorin C and D molecules, production of the latter being encoded by a *GYPC* gene in which exon 3 is duplicated (93). Uchikawa et al. (94) have now described an individual with Ls(a+) red cells in whom exon 3 of *GYPC* is triplicated. The abnormal glycophorin C and D molecules of the individual's red cells were some 5500 to 6000 kD larger than those of other persons with Ls(a+) red cells, those molecules are, in turn, 5500 to 6000 kD larger than those on Ls(a-) red cells. The individual with triplicated exon 3 of *GYPC* had two exon 3-exon 3 junctions that produce the Ls[a] antigen.

King et al. (214) described a novel phenotype in the Gerbich system. The proposita had been pregnant three times but did not make any unexpected antibodies until after she had been transfused with two units of red cells. The antibody she then made was alloimmune in nature and behaved serologically as anti-Ge2. However, the red cells of the proposita were reactive with all of 20 allo-anti-Ge2, one auto-anti-Ge2, three allo-anti-Ge3 and one allo-anti-Ge4 that were human polyclonal antibodies, and with mouse and rat monoclonal antibodies specific for glycophorins C and D. With the human antibodies, the red cells of the proposita and those of her four compatible sibs, reacted to lower titers than did control Ge+ red cells. No weakening of the antigens on the proposita's red cells or those of her compatible sibs was seen in tests with the monoclonal anti-glycophorin C/D. The explanation was that the proposita was heterozygous for the *GYPC* gene that makes the Ge-type glycophorin (i.e. Ge:-2,-3,4) and for a *GYPC* gene in which an A to T mutation had occurred at nucleotide 173 of exon 3 resulting in an Asp58 to Val change in the encoded glycophorin. In other words, one *GYPC* gene made the Ge-type glycophorin, the other made glycophorins C and D in which the amino acid change resulted in loss of the epitope recognized by the proposita's antibody. Such an epitope is missing from Ge:-2 red cells hence the anti-Ge-2 specificity of the proposita's antibody. The glycophorins C and D of the proposita's red cells carried other portions of the structure recognized by anti-Ge2, hence her Ge:2 status. The same findings were made in tests on the red cells and cDNA of the proposita's four compatible sibs but not on those of four other sibs whose red cells were incompatible with the proposita's antibody. A year after the anti-Ge2 had been found, the proposita required transfusion for a condition unrelated to the first that had required transfusion. Because of the presence of the anti-Ge2, the group O, D-proposita was transfused with group O, D+ red cells from a compatible (with the anti-Ge2) brother. As expected, she then made anti-D.

Chapter 17 Diego System

In presenting the data that show that Sw^a is a Diego system antigen, Zelinski et al. (95) mentioned that SW1 has the same mutation that leads to the Arg646→Gln change on band 3 of Sw(a+) red cells, but that the molecular difference between Sw^a and SW1 has not yet been determined. In Chapter 17 the Diego system antigens from DI1 to DI13 are listed. We understand (96) that Sw^a will become DI14 although, in fact, Tr^a, that does not yet have a Diego system number, was described in a full publication (97) as being a Diego system antigen, some time before the abstract (95) about Sw^a, appeared.

In describing the band 3 change that results in the presence of NFLD, Zelinski et al. (98) pointed out that the low incidence antigen BOW has a serological relationship with Wu and NFLD, both of which are now known to be part of the Diego system. However, the place (if any) of BOW in the system is not yet firmly established.

In their abstract showing that Jn^a is a Diego system antigen, Poole et al. (99) described two different mutations, C to T and C to G, at nucleotide 1696 of *AE1* (the band 3 gene). These lead to a proline to serine and a proline to alanine change, respectively, at residue 566 in the third exofacial loop of band 3. In Chapter 17 it was supposed that one of these changes would be represented by Jn^a and the second by a different low incidence antigen. Although details are not included in the abstract (99), Joyce Poole reported in the presentation that the Pro566 to Ser change is associated with Jn^a and the Pro566 to Ala change with an antigen to be called KREP. Among 12 multispecific sera tested, 11 contained anti-Jn^a and anti-KREP, one contained anti-KREP without anti-Jn^a (data from presentation, not the abstract).

Chapter 18 Kell System

Chapter 18 includes information about the molecular bases of the Kell system antigens K, k, Kp^a, Kp^b, Kp^c,

Js^a, Js^b, Ul^a, Wk^a and K11 (Côté). Lee et al. (100) have now identified the molecular basis of the fifth antithetical pair of Kell system antigens K24 (Cls, low incidence) and K14 (San, high incidence). When the Kell glycoprotein carries K14, arginine occupies position 180. In the K:-14,24 individual a G659 to C mutation in exon 6 of the *Kell* complex gene, resulted in proline replacing arginine at residue 180. Lee et al. (212) have also provided data about additional high incidence Kell system antigens. The K:-12 phenotype represents an A1763 to G nucleotide substitution that will change His548 to Arg, in the Kell glycoprotein. K:-19 involves a G1595 to A nucleotide substitution that will change Arg492 to Gln in the glycoprotein. K:-22 involves a C1085 to T mutation that will result in an Ala332 to Val amino acid change while K:-26 (TOU-) involves a G1337 to A nucleotide substitution that will effect an Arg409 to Gln change in the glycoprotein. Most of the above changes were seen in two or more unrelated persons of the same phenotype. In unrelated individuals with K:-18 red cells, two different mutations were seen. One involved a nucleotide substitution of C508 to T and the other, in the same codon, G509 to A. These mutations would result in Arg130 to Trp and Arg130 to Gln changes, respectively, in the Kell glycoprotein. While definite proof that these point mutations are responsible for the antigen changes will require expression of the mutated cDNA and identification of the antigen expressed (see below) it is very highly probable that the point mutations and antigen changes are directly correlated. First, as mentioned above, the nucleotide substitutions were found in unrelated individuals of the same (high incidence antigen-negative) phenotypes. Second, individuals of the same phenotype were often from different ethnic backgrounds. Third, the mutations seen in the persons with K:-12, K:-18, K:-19, K:-22 and K:-26 red cells were not seen in the exons of many other persons whose red cells carried the antigens involved (100-103), see also below.

The fact that a TOU- proband (104) had a son with TOU+ red cells, in whom the G1337A mutation was found (i.e. heterozygous for the gene that fails to encode production of TOU) showed that the antigen (TOU or K26) is an inherited character. In the paper describing the newly found point mutations (100) it is mentioned that a Gln382 to Arg change has been found in a person with K:23 red cells. K23 is a low incidence antigen first shown (105) to be part of the Kell system in biochemical studies. For the sake of completeness, table 46-1 lists the bases of all the Kell system polymorphisms currently known.

Yazdanbakhsh et al. (199) described studies in which they used transfected CHO cells to confirm that the nucleotide substitutions apparently responsible for the K/k, Kp^a/Kp^b and Js^a/Js^b polymorphisms do indeed

TABLE 46-1 To Show the Molecular Bases of the Kell System Antigens (from references 100-103, 212, 213)

Antigen/Phenotype	Nucleotide (bp)	Exon	Amino Acid and Position
K	T698	6	Met 193
k	C698	6	Thr 193
Kp^a	T961	8	Trp 281
Kp^b	C961, G962	8	Arg 281
Kp^c	A962	8	Gln 281
Js^a	C1910	17	Pro 597
Js^b	T1910	17	Leu 597
Ul(a+)	T1601	13	Val 494
Ul(a-)	A1601	13	Glu 494
K11 (Côté)	T1025	8	Val 302
Wk^a (K17)	C1025	8	Ala 302
K14 (San)`	G659	6	Arg 180
K24 (Cls)	C659	6	Pro 180
K:-12	G1763	15	Arg 548
K:12	A1763	15	His 548
K:-18	T508	4	Trp 130
K:-18	A509	4	Gln 130
K:18	C508, G509	4	Arg 130
K:-19	A1595	13	Gln 492
K:19	G1595	13	Arg 492
K:-22	T1085	9	Val 322
K:22	C1085	9	Ala 322
K:-26	A1337	11	Gln 406
K:26	G1337	11	Arg 406
K:-5, Ku-	In one *K^{o}K^o* person, whose red cells are K:-5, there was a C502T nucleotide substitution that changed codon 128 for arginine to a stop codon (213).		

correlate directly with production of those antigens. Of particular note, it was shown that more than one of the low incidence antigens could be expressed in the same transfection experiment. This led the authors (199) to conclude that "failure to detect more than one low incidence antigen is a consequence of statistical probability and not due to physical constraints". Such a conclusion is a considerable surprise to one of us (PDI). As stated in Chapter 18 he would have expected, if there are no constraints, that one gene producing any two of the antigens K, Kp^a, Kp^c, Js^a, Ul^a, Wk^a, K23 and K24, would have been found by now.

Øyen et al. (225) have published a comprehensive and useful review on conditions that result in weak expression of Kell system antigens.

Chapter 19 Kidd System

In the same study in which they showed that triton X-100 extracted red cell membranes will inhibit Rh antibodies, Scott et al. (60) showed that the extracts would inhibit anti-Jk^a and anti-Jk^b, specifically, i.e. dependent on the phenotypes of the red cells from which the extracts were made. These findings provided the first evidence that the urea transport protein, that carries the Kidd system antigens, is associated with the membrane skeleton.

An example of anti-Jk3 that caused a 1+ positive DAT on the cord blood red cells of an infant (Kidd type not given) born to the immunized mother, but caused no clinical HDN, was described by Hunter and Ziebol (223). The anti-Jk3 involved was apparently in large part

IgM although some IgG anti-Jk3 crossed the placenta and was eluted from the infant's red cells.

Chapter 20 Lutheran System

The study to determine the molecular background in the recessive (*LuLu*) type of Lu(a-b-), mentioned briefly in Chapter 20, has now been reported in an abstract. Mallinson et al. (106) showed that the Japanese propositus is homozygous for a C→A substitution at nucleotide 733 in exon 2 of the *Lutheran* gene. This mutation changes the codon TGC, that normally encodes Cys237 in the first domain of the Lutheran glycoprotein, to TGA, a stop codon. This finding presumably indicates that the propositus has no Lutheran glycoprotein on any of his blood or tissue cells. In spite of this, no pathology appears to be associated with the genotype.

Chapter 22 Dombrock System

Although in Chapters 22 and 44 reference is made to studies (107) that purported to show that the high incidence Dombrock system antigens Jo[a] and Jc[a] are the same thing, that conclusion has now been questioned. Reid (108) speculated that the states of being Jo(a-) and Jc(a-) might be correlated with differences in Dombrock system phenotypes, e.g. Do(a+b-) versus Do(a-b+).

Strupp et al. (109) described three examples of anti-Do[a] in patients with sickle cell disease, in each case the antibody was thought to have contributed to a delayed hemolytic transfusion reaction. Shirey et al. (110) described an example of anti-Do[b] that did cause a delayed hemolytic transfusion reaction. The clinical significance of the antibody was confirmed in a ^{51}Cr in vivo survival study and in an in vitro MMA.

Chapter 24 Cromer System

Although most Cromer system antibodies have proved to be benign in vivo, Kowalski et al. (111) described a complement-binding anti-Tc[a] that caused two delayed hemolytic transfusion reactions, involving six units of blood, before it became serologically demonstrable. That primary immunization to Tc[a] had occurred was apparent when it was found that the patient's records indicated that the antibody had been demonstrable 14 years previously. At that time the patient delivered a healthy infant whose Tc(a+) red cells were DAT-negative.

Rare phenotypes in the Cromer blood group system seem to be a little more common in Japan than elsewhere. Daniels et al. (112) described one new propositus

TABLE 46-2 To Show the Molecular Bases and Locations of the Cromer System Antigens (from references 113-121)

Antigen or Phenotype Change	Nucleotide Change and Position	Amino Acid Change and Position	Antigen Carried on SCR
Cr(a+) to Cr(a-)	G→C nt 679	Cr(a+) Ala 193	4
		Cr(a-) Pro 193	
Tc[a]	G nt 155 (CGT)	Tc(a+) Arg 18	1
Tc[b]	T nt 155 (CTT)	Tc(b+) Leu 18	1
Tc[c]	C nt 155 (CCT)	Tc(c+) Pro 18	1
Dr(a+) to Dr(a-)	C nt 649	Dr(a+) Ser 165	3
	T nt 596	Dr(a-) Leu 165	
	(44 bp deletion in Dr(a-))		
Es(a+) to Es(a-)	T→A nt 239	Es(a+) Ile 46	1
	(ATC→AAC)	Es(a-) Asn 46	
IFC+ to IFC-	G→A nt 261	IFC+ Trp 53	
	(TGG→TGA)	TGA is stop codon in Inab	
WES[a]	T nt 245 (CTT)	WES(a+) Arg 48	1
WES[b]	G nt 245 (CGT)	WES(b+) Leu 48	1
UMC+ to UMC-	C→T	UMC+ Thr 216	4
	(ACG→ATG)	UMC- Met 216	

with the Inab phenotype, caused by a mutation leading to a premature stop codon in the *DAF* gene that was identical to that seen in the original Inab propositus, and a new propositus with Dr(a-) red cells, in whom the causative mutation was probably the same as that previously reported. For the molecular bases of the Inab and Dr(a-) phenotypes, see Chapter 24 and below (table 46-2).

Lublin et al. (113) used PCR amplification of DNA from individuals of known Cromer system phenotypes and Daniels et al. (114) performed inhibition studies with whole soluble recombinant DAF, three deletion mutants, and used the MAIEA assay, further to establish the molecular structure and location of the Cromer system antigens. For the sake of completeness the new findings from these studies (113,114) are added to previously reported (115-121) data and table 46-2 lists what is now known about the structure and location of these antigens.

In addition to the data shown in table 46-2, the study of Lublin et al. (113) showed that the UMC antigen is located on short concensus repeat (SCR) domain 4 and not on domain 2 as had previously been suspected (117). The MAIEA assays of Daniels et al. (114) suggested that Tc^a and WES^b are located on opposite faces of SCR1, that the Cr^a antigen on SCR4 may be close to SCR3, and also showed that UMC is on SCR4. It seems likely that the determinant(s) recognized by anti-IFC (the antibody made by immunized individuals of the Inab phenotype) is (are) carried on more than one SCR domain (114).

Chapter 31 High Incidence Antigens

An example of anti-At^a described by Cash et al. (122) was of clinical significance. The patient, who had been pregnant three times but had not previously been transfused, was given nine units of blood at a time that her serum was found to be non-reactive in antibody-screening tests. The patient suffered a delayed hemolytic transfusion reaction and developed symptomatic anemia. Because the antibody now demonstrable in her serum was thought to be an autoimmune panagglutinin, the patient was transfused with two units of serologically incompatible red cells. These units also caused a transfusion reaction and anti-At^a was then identified in her serum and in an eluate. Further transfusion was avoided.

The suggestion (123) made in Chapter 31, that anti-JMH might be clinically significant only when recognizing a polymorphism (i.e. red cells of antibody-maker JMH+, antibody alloimmune in nature) is perhaps supported by the results in a case described by Powell et al. (124). The patient was a 75 year-old male with anti-JMH that had a titer of 2048 by IAT. His red cells typed as JMH-. Although in vitro chemiluminescence tests gave positive reactions with eight JMH+ samples and the

patient's surgery was covered by autologous donation, in vivo ^{51}Cr survival studies, performed after the surgery, showed that JMH+ red cells survived normally in the patient. Thus the case seems to represent another in which anti-JMH was benign in a patient with JMH- red cells.

In 1993, Anderson et al. (125) described a patient, M.A.M. whose serum contained an antibody that included IgG1, IgG2 and IgG3 components and that reacted with all red cells tested except her own. Further, the antibody was shown to bind to platelets, lymphocytes and monocytes. M.A.M.'s third infant had a positive DAT at birth, did not have clinical HDN, but was thrombocytopenic and was treated with platelet transfusions. In 1997, Montgomery et al. (126) described another patient with an antibody to multiple cell lines that failed to react only with the antibody-maker's and M.A.M.'s red cells. Various studies showed that the antibody made by M.A.M. and by A.N. (the second patient (126)) are the same. The antibody of A.N. caused severe HDN. In the study on M.A.M. (125) evidence was obtained that the antigen defined might be carried on the alpha subunit of vitronectin. We understand that the antigen defined by the antibody in the M.A.M. and A.N. sera is to be called MAM and will be given (96) ISBT number 901016.

Chapter 32 Antigens of Low Incidence

Lubenko et al. (128) have confirmed that red cells carry HLA antigens in addition to those represented by Bg^a, Bg^b and Bg^c. In Chapter 32 some correlations between antibodies that react with red cells and HLA phenotypes are given in table 32-5. The new study (128) showed that, in addition, some sera with broad specificity for HLA determinants react with most or all red cells. The abstract claims that some of these antibodies might cause febrile transfusion reactions and that on occasion red cell hemolysis might occur via an innocent bystander mechanism once complement is activated. However, no evidence is offered to support this latter, somewhat controversial supposition.

Chapter 34 Cold Agglutinins

An IgM warm-reactive auto-anti-Pr that caused severe hemolytic anemia (208) is described in more detail in the addendum to Chapter 37.

Chapter 35 Antibody Detection

A 1992 publication by Judd et al. (129) that described the detection of antibodies that acted as agglutinins at 37°C in LISS but that were non-reactive by LISS-IAT, caused considerable consternation among U.S. blood bankers. This, because methods such as PEG/IAT, gel and solid phase do not include a reading for agglutination at 37°C. However, we (130) showed that of 100 antibodies detected by PEG/IAT, 40 were reactive when saline was substituted for anti-IgG. Clearly, agglutination in PEG at 37°C survives the washing preparatory for IATs. Rolih et al. (131) showed that the solid phase method is also efficient in the detection of antibodies that act as agglutinins at 37°C in LISS. Alkhashan (132) tested 189 known PEG/IAT reactive antibodies and 5027 sera that had given negative reactions in PEG/IAT antibody-screening tests, no evidence was found to suggest that omission of a 37°C agglutination reading compromised transfusion safety for any patient. At the same meeting that we (130) reported that 37°C agglutinins can be detected by other means, Judd et al. (133) concluded that the risk of eliminating a 37°C reading is minimal and that the test is not cost-effective anyway. The conclusion that exclusion of the test for agglutinins active at 37°C in LISS does not compromise patient safety is repeated in a full published report (134).

In a series of studies we compared the gel test and a solid phase method to PEG/IAT for antibody-screening (135,136); used PEG in the gel test (137) and used the solid phase method in an attempt to resolve equivocal serological findings (138). The inescapable conclusion from these studies and others referenced in Chapter 35, is that use of any one of the PEG, Polybrene, gel, solid phase, enzyme or LISS methods results in the detection of some antibodies that are not detectable by any or all of the others. Based on their specificities it might be thought that some of these "only" antibodies (i.e. detected only in PEG, only in Polybrene, etc.) would be of clinical significance. Since most transfusion services use only one of the methods listed, it is clear that ALL services, miss SOME antibodies. In spite of this, frank and delayed hemolytic transfusion reactions due to missed antibodies are rare events. Thus it is clear that currently used methods are more sensitive than necessary and create additional meaningless work in the investigation of benign antibodies. Until there is a rapid, reliable and inexpensive way of determining the in vivo clinical significance of an antibody, from in vitro test results, this situation of overkill will continue (one cannot currently pick out which few of many weak antibodies will cause red cell clearance). However, it is clear that the next major advance in serological tests for antibody detection and compatibility will increase the relevance not the sensitivity of the test(s).

Garratty et al. (196) have pointed out that a belief, apparently held in some reference laboratories, that most antibodies directed against certain high incidence antigens, i.e. LW, Ge, Di[b], Lu[b], Lu3, Lu8, Lu12, Co[a], Gy[a], Hy, Jo[a], Yt[a], Cr[a], Es[a], Sc1, In[b], AnWj, JMH, Vel, Lan, At[a] and Jr[a], are clinically insignificant, is not true. In MMAs using a total of 166 such antibodies, 115 (69%) yielded results that suggested that they might be capable of in vivo clearance of antigen-positive red cells. The authors believe that antibodies of these specificities should be regarded as being of potential clinical significance unless proved otherwise. It is also pointed out (196) that clinical significance may involve only shortened in vivo red cell survival, not an obvious hemolytic transfusion reaction. In other words, it may be in the patient's best interests to receive red cells that will have an acceptable but not normal in vivo lifespan. As mentioned elsewhere in this book, if the patient requires surgery or blood replacement following trauma, a completely normal in vivo lifespan of the transfused red cells is not an absolute requirement. For example, at surgery, the use of red cells that will have an in vivo half life of say 14 days, rather than the normal 28 to 30 days, may satisfy the patient's needs. By the time an appreciable number of the transfused red cells are cleared, the patient will be making blood and will replace the transfused cells with his own. More harm may accrue by delaying necessary surgery while "compatible" blood is found than by using red cells that will have a sub-normal but acceptable survival, in vivo.

The same principle as that described in the addendum to Chapter 7, i.e. high expression of selected red cell antigens on cells that do not normally carry red cell antigens, used in the production of murine monoclonal antibodies (197), has been applied at the serological level. MEL cells transfected with genes that encode production of k, Kp[b], Js[b], Ku, Fy[a] or Fy[b] were used in antibody identification and adsorption studies (198). The technique is particularly suitable in studies on sera containing multiple antibodies since transfection can result in the production of cell lines carrying only one of the antigens to which the serum contains antibodies.

In the U.S.A. it has long been believed (139-142) that to obtain a significant p value to support the validity of antibody identification, a minimum of three positive and three negative reactions with red cells of appropriate phenotype is necessary. When the Blood Transfusion Task Force of the British Committee for Standards in Haematology decreed (143) that two positive and two negative samples were sufficient to provide statistical support that the antibody identification was correct, various parties debated the issue. Kanter et al. (144) suggest that the p value is misused in this setting, that a p value of 0.05 is often overemphasized, that confounding variables may not be considered, that discrepant serological results are not considered and that other observations (i.e. temperature of antibody reaction, nature of antibody as IgG or IgM, ability of antibody to activate complement) most importantly the antigen type of the antibody-maker, are not sufficiently considered in the use of what the authors (144) believe is a flawed statistical method anyway. In direct contradiction, Judd and Davenport (145) vehemently defend the "3+/3-" rule and purport to show its greater reliability than a "2+/2-" rule. Those readers confused with the debate about statistics (144,145) should read the well balanced and down to earth editorial by Case (146) that accompanies the two publications cited above. The editorial considers more than just the statistical aspects of the situation and points out that there are many ways more likely than those disclosed by statistical analysis, in which antibodies can be misidentified. After reading the editorial it is hard to place much credence of the claim of Judd and Davenport (145) that a change from the "3+/3-" to the "2+/2-" rule would have a "high probability" of being "detrimental to patient care". Kanter et al. (147) have replied to the criticisms of Judd and Robertson (145), again their observations are that the "3+/3-" rule does not function (statistically) as claimed and if used, should be recognized for what it really achieves.

On a lighter note concerning statistics, Widmann (148) has pointed that in his initial experiments, Landsteiner had a low probability of discovering the ABO groups. This, because of the distribution of those groups in Austria and the fact that he tested blood from only six individuals. Widmann (148) wonders whether the discovery represents a non-chance event with divine providence perhaps involved.

Chapter 36 Transfusion Reactions

Better to study the pathophysiology of hemolytic transfusion reactions, Davenport and Kunkel (149) have devised an experimental model using mice. The effects of transfusing human red cells to previously immunized mice were similar, in terms of cytokine generation, to the results seen in in vitro models developed by this same research team and described in detail in Chapter 36.

Using the in vitro model of an ABO hemolytic transfusion reaction developed earlier (150-152), Udani et al. (153) confirmed downregulation of CD14 and increased binding of hyaluronic acid reflecting monocyte activation as a result of red cell hemolysis. No evidence of lymphocyte activation was found.

Chapter 37 WAIHA

In Chapter 37 mention is made of the studies of Barker et al. (154,155) and Elson et al. (156) that, among other findings, have shown that in vitro, naive T cells can be shown to respond to stimuli comprising synthetic Rh peptides that represent "self" antigens. These workers have now extended their studies (157) and have shown that in patients with WAIHA, activated T-cells that mount secondary immune responses when challenged with self antigens, are present. In other words, WAIHA does not involve only primary responses to host or self antigens, instead memory cells are involved in the same autoimmune response. The authors (157) believe that the recognition of helper T-cell epitopes on Rh proteins may be a step towards peptide immunotherapy in patients with WAIHA. On a more mundane level, the presence of memory cells as part of the autoimmune response could perhaps be used to support the concept that transfusion in this disease is contraindicated unless it is necessary to relieve life-threatening anemia. As discussed in Chapter 37, one of us (PDI) has long believed that premature transfusion (involving introduction of more antigen) in WAIHA worsens the patient's long term prognosis. Perhaps the existence of memory cells that can make antibody against the additional antigen load (transfused red cells) plays a role in this situation.

An unusual autoantibody that caused hemolytic anemia was described by Arndt et al. (158). The antibody reacted preferentially with e+ red cells, was predominantly IgM in composition and appeared to activate complement both in vivo and in vitro. The patient's hemolytic anemia did not respond to steroid or IVIG therapy but the patient responded to splenectomy.

As described in Chapter 37, patients who have IgM autohemolysins active at, or near, 37°C are often seriously ill. Obviously, if intravascular hemolysis is caused by an autoantibody that can bind to red cells at normal body temperature, severe acute anemia is likely. Three such IgM autohemolysins were described in abstracts that are cited as references 162, 169 and 171 in Chapter 37. Garratty et al. (208) have now published full details of those cases. Patient 1 made auto-anti-En[a]; patient 2, auto-anti-Wr[b]; and patient 3, auto-anti-Pr. Both the auto-anti-En[a] and auto-anti-Wr[b] gave enhanced reactions in tests at pH 6.5 compared to those in tests at pH 7.3, both were enhanced in tests to which bovine albumin had been added. Red cells from the patients with autoantibodies to En[a] and Pr agglutinated spontaneously in saline (1+ reactions) and more strongly in 6% bovine albumin (3+ reactions). The auto-anti-En[a] had a titer of 16 at 37°C, of 32 at 30°C and 20°C, and 16 at 4°C. The auto-anti-Pr had a titer of 16 at 37°C, of 64 at 30°C and 20°C, and 32 at 4°C. The auto-anti-Wr[b] had a titer of 16 at 37°C, 8 at 30°C, 4 at 20°C and was non-reactive at 4°C. The patient with auto-anti-En[a] died in the emergency room in spite of multiple transfusions, the patient with auto-anti-Wr[b] died six days after the onset of acute symptoms, again in spite of transfusions, the patient with auto-anti-Pr was a 15 year-old male who was treated with erythromycin, predisone, IVIG and with supportive and exchange transfusions and eventually recovered. As will be apparent from the above descriptions, the autoantibodies in cases such as these do not always behave typically in in vitro tests. Tests for autoagglutination (in saline and 6% albumin), at different pH levels, on DAT and chloroquine-treated red cells, at different temperatures and using the patient's sera and rare red cells, may all be informative.

Chapter 39 Benign Autoantibodies

Win et al. (210) found that antibodies to phospholipids occasionally explain the positive DAT seen in some normal healthy blood donors. However, the finding seems to represent the cause of the positive DAT in only a small minority of cases. In tests on 474,545 samples, 42 were found to have a positive DAT. Elevated levels of antibodies to phospholipids were subsequently found in three of the donors.

Chapter 40 Drug-Induced Antibodies

Further to the warnings in Chapter 40 about the danger of drug-induced hemolytic anemia associated with therapy with non-steroidal anti-inflammatory drugs (NSAIDs), Madoz et al. (159) describe a fatal case apparently related to Aceclofenac. The antibody appeared to be part IgM part IgG in composition and seemed to cause hemolysis via an immune complex mechanism.

Chapter 41 HDN

Yet another study (168) this time on some 75,000 samples from pregnant women, found 450 "enzyme only" antibodies but not a single case in which one of them caused HDN.

In addition to the examples listed in tables 41-1, 41-2 and 41-3 of Chapter 41, cases of HDN caused by anti-D^W (40) anti-MAM (126 and see addendum to Chapter 31), anti-S (160), anti-Ce and anti-s (161), anti-K (162) and anti-Kp^a (226) have been described. In many cases anti-G, when present without anti-D, causes a positive DAT but no or only mild HDN (163-165) however, exceptions may be seen (166-167). The observation that differentiation between anti-CD and anti-G is important in a pregnant woman but of little moment in a patient to be transfused, is discussed in Chapter 41. Briefly, in a woman of the D- phenotype, in whom the fetus is D+, and in whom immunization to D has occurred, RhIG is not indicated. However, if the woman has actually made anti-G or anti-C plus anti-G, RhIG should be used during pregnancy and following delivery to prevent immunization to D. As stated, HDN caused by anti-D is nearly

always more severe than that caused by anti-G or anti-G plus anti-C. The study that brought this observation to light is referenced as an abstract in Chapter 41, a full report has now been published (164). In a transfusion recipient, rr (i.e. D- C- G-) blood will be used regardless of whether the antibody is anti-CD or anti-G (or any mixture thereof). However, Mosley et al. (227) have pointed out that failure to distinguish between anti-CD and anti-G in a previously transfused D- patient, may lead some persons not aware of the serology of G, to conclude that D+ blood was transfused in error.

In an attempt to learn more about the transfer of IgG from mother to fetus, Armstrong-Fisher et al. (169) used an in vitro placenta model (170) to study the passage of IgG in polyclonal antibodies and monoclonal IgG1 and IgG3. In spite of the many claims for differences cited in Chapter 41, these investigators (169) found no evidence for the preferential transfer of IgG1 and suggested that IgG3 might be transferred more rapidly than IgG1.

As described in Chapter 41, intrauterine transfusion of the fetus, in cases in which HDN will be severe, is sometimes followed by the production of additional (i.e. different specificity) antibodies in the mother (171-175). These observations have led to suggestions that red cells to be used for this purpose, be phenotype matched to those of the mother. In a balanced discussion of this topic, Todd (176) has pointed out that the introduction of an increasingly restrictive transfusion regimen introduces the risk of causing unacceptable delay in a situation in which the fetus needs red cells in an emergency setting. Such concern is appropriate when the limited benefits that accrue from the use of phenotype matched blood are considered. In what is by far the largest study documented in the literature, Viëtor et al. (177) described their findings after 91 women had received, among them, 280 ultrasound-guided intrauterine transfusions. Among the 91 women, 24 (26%) made an antibody that was not demonstrable before the intrauterine transfusion. However, in the 14 women in whom the source of immunization could be definitively identified (i.e. by comparing antibody specificity and presence or absence of the relevant antigen on the fetus' or transfused red cells) 11 had produced an antibody against an antigen on their infant's red cells. In other words, only three made an antibody (one of the three made two antibodies) because of the introduction of a foreign antigen on the transfused red cells. There seems to be some agreement that blood to be used for intrauterine transfusion should (obviously) lack the antigen(s) to which the antibody(ies) that will cause the HDN are directed and should be K- (unless, of course, the maternal antibody is anti-k). Attempts to avoid additional immunization to K seem justified since, as described in Chapter 41, anti-K seems capable of suppressing red cell production in the fetus as well as capable of causing red cell destruction. Attempts to prevent immunization to other antigens, by extensive phenotyping of the red cells to be transfused, may not be indicated. Sesok-Pizzini et al. (206) have provided additional evidence that a primary cause of anemia in infants with HDN caused by Kell system antibodies involves destruction or non-maturation of erythroid precursor cells.

In order to improve the reliability of forecasting the D phenotype from amplification of fetal DNA, several groups of workers (178-183,211) have used multiple probes against various regions of the *D* gene. Some of these studies (181,182,184) have included tests to forecast the presence of C, c, E or e, as well. Faas et al. (182) pointed out that forecasts about the presence of absence of C are not reliable in other than White populations. As described in some detail in Chapter 41, Daniels et al. (54) have shown that forecasts of the D type in Blacks, via amplification of DNA, is highly unreliable and will remain so until the mechanism that results in lack of expression of D antigen in many Blacks with (at least some parts of) *D* genes, is understood. Somewhat similarly, Okuda et al. (85) performed PCR amplification of DNA from 130 Japanese individuals who had D- red cells. They showed that 36 (28%) of them had both intron 4 and exon 10 of *D* while two others had exon 10 without intron 4. The presence of any portion of *D* was often associated with the C+ D- red cell phenotype, no individual with C- red cells was seen to have any portion of *D*.

As predicted in Chapter 41, if the genetic basis of the polymorphism is known, PCR amplification of fetal DNA can be used to identify a fetus at risk of HDN or neonatal alloimmune thrombocytopenia. Various studies have been performed to forecast the presence or absence of antigens in the Kell, Kidd, Duffy and Diego red cell systems (185-193) and the PLA antigens of platelets (191).

Win et al. (202) have presented data that suggest that the additional potassium present in red cell concentrates that have been irradiated, is rapidly excreted by the fetus following intrauterine transfusion. They (202) concur with recommendations (203) that state that it is safe to transfuse red cells less than five days old and within 24 hours of irradiation (25 Gy). However, they caution that when intracardiac (intrauterine) transfusion is necessary because of failed umbilical cord transfusions (204,205) special precautions may be necessary to avoid the introduction of excess potassium.

Chapter 43 Miscellany

Listed in table 43-2 of Chapter 43 are an anti-e and an anti-Ce, formed by an R_2R_2 patient, whose reactions were considerably enhanced in the presence of thimerosal (194). Previous examples of thimerosal-enhanced or dependent antibodies (for references see table 43-1 in Chapter 43) had not been seen to have blood group specificity. The Rh antibodies were enhanced but not dependent on thimerosal, that is they reacted with ficin-treated red cells and by a polybrene method, in the absence of thimerosal.

Chapter 44 Antigen Catalog

Already mentioned in this chapter are three antigens that can now be added to the 434 listed in Chapter 44. The newcomers are:

JAHK, an antigen of low incidence that may be an Rh antigen, i.e. a product of r^G (43);

KREP, another low incidence antigen that is almost certainly part of the Diego system (99);

MAM (901016), a high incidence antigen that at present seems to be independent of known blood group systems (96,125,126).

Further, as described in the addendum to Chapter 22, Jc^a that was equated with Jo^a (107) may yet rise, phoenix-like, in its own right.

References

1. Siegel DL, Chang TY, Russell SL, et al. J Immunol Meth 1997;206:73
2. Siegel DL, Silberstein LE. Blood 1994;83:2334
3. Burton DR, Barbas CF. Adv Immunol 1994;57:191
4. Marks C, Marks JD. New Eng J Med 1996;335:730
5. Dörner T, Brezinschek H-P, Bresinschek R, et al. J Immunol 1997;158:2779
6. Boucher G, Broly H, Lemieux R. Blood 1997;89:3277
7. Siegel DL. In: Applications of Molecular Biology to Blood Transfusion Medicine. Bethesda:Am Assoc Blood Banks, 1997:73
8. Chang TY, Siegel DL. Blood, in press 1998
9. Boulton FE. (Letter). Br J Biomed Sci 1996;53:172
10. Pirkola A. Vox Sang 1995;69:299
11. Engelfriet CP, Reesink HW. Vox Sang 1995;69:292
12. Rushton L, Booker DJ, Stamps R, et al. (abstract). Transf Med 1997;7 (Suppl 1):22
13. Moulds JM, Diekman L, Wells TD, et al. (abstract). Transfusion 1997;37 (Suppl 9S):30S
14. Sajur J, Fournier Y, Sheridan B, et al. (abstract). Transfusion 1997;37 (Suppl 9S):27S
15. Murad KL, Mahany KL, Brugnara C, et al. (abstract). Transfusion 1997;37 (Suppl 9S):2S
16. Fisher TC, Armstrong JK, Meiselman HJ, et al. (abstract). Transfusion 1997;37 (Suppl 9S):88S
17. Garratty G, Leger R, Arndt P, et al. (abstract). Blood 1997;90 (Suppl 1, part 1):473a
18. Nance SJ, Garratty G. Am J Clin Pathol 1987;87:633
19. Allen J, Issitt PD, Combs MR. (abstract). Transfusion 1997;37

(Suppl 9S):28S

20. Cheng G, Choi F, Wong L. (Letter). Clin Lab Haematol 1996;18:64

21. Arndt P, Garratty G, Haverty D, et al. (abstract). Blood 1997;90 (Suppl 1, part 1):472a

22. Sudakevitz D, Levene C, Sela R, et al. Transfusion 1996;36:113

23. Flegel WA, Müller TH, Schunter F, et al. (abstract). Transfusion 1997;37 (Suppl 9S):101S

24. Halverson GR, Reid ME, Blancher A. (abstract). Transfusion 1997;37 (Suppl 9S):91S

25. Halverson G, Reid ME, Apoil PA, et al. (abstract). Transfusion 1996;36 (Suppl 9S):53S

26. Apoil PA, Reid ME, Halverson G, et al. Br J Haematol 1997;98:365

27. Jones JW, Finning K, Mattock R, et al. Vox Sang 1997;73:252

28. Jones J, Scott ML, Voak D. Transf Med 1995;5:171 and see 5:304 for corrections

29. Scott ML, Voak D, Jones JW, et al. Transf Clin Biol 1996;6:391

30. Scott ML, Voak D, Jones JW, et al. Biotest Bull 1997;5:459

31. Rouillac C, Le Van Kim C, Blancher A, et al. Am J Hematol 1995;49:87

32. Avent ND, Jones JW, Liu W, et al. Br J Haematol 1997;97:366

33. Jones J. Vox Sang 1995;69:236

34. Liu W, Jones JW, Scott ML, et al. (abstract). Transf Med 1996;6 (Suppl 2):21

35. Reid ME, Sausais L, Zaroulis CG, et al. (abstract). Transfusion 1997;37 (Suppl 9S):35S

36. Rouillac C, Colin Y, Hughes-Jones NC, et al. Blood 1995;85:2937

37. Beckers EAM, Faas BHW, von dem Borne AEGKr, et al. Br J Haematol 1996;92:751

38. Rouillac C, Gane P, Cartron J, et al. Blood 1996;87:4853

39. Beckers EAM, Faas BHW, Simsek S, et al. Br J Haematol 1996;93:720

40. Spruell P, Lacey P, Bradford MF, et al. (abstract). Transfusion 1997;37 (Suppl 9S):43S

41. Faas BHW, Ligthart PC, Lomas-Francis C, et al. Transfusion 1997;37:1123

42. Powell VI, Reid ME, Rhodes M. (abstract). Transfusion 1997;37 (Suppl 9S):35S

43. Green CA, Lomas-Francis C, Wallace M, et al. (abstract). Transf Med 1995;5 (Suppl 1):19

44. Reid ME, Lomas-Francis C. The Blood Group Antigen Facts Book. San Diego:Academic, 1997:96

45. Daniels GL. Biotest Bull 1997;5:399

46. Mouro I, Colin Y, Gane P, et al. Br J Haematol 1996;93:472

47. Snowden JA, Poole J, Bates AJ, et al. Clin Lab Haematol 1997;19:143

48. Matassi G, Chérif-Zahar B, Mouro I, et al. Am J Hum Genet 1997;60:808

49. Huang C-H, Chen Y, Reid M. Am J Hematol 1997;55:139

50. Liu W, Smythe J, Jones JW, et al. (abstract). Transf Clin Biol 1996;3 (Suppl):35S

51. Smythe JS, Avent ND, Judson PA, et al. Blood 1996;87:2968

52. Overbeeke MAM, Rhenen van DJ, Ligthart PC, et al. Transf Clin Biol 1996;6:397

53. Le Pennec PY, Noizat-Pirenne F, Klein MT, et al. Transf Clin Biol 1996;6:401

54. Daniels G, Green C, Smart E. (Letter). Lancet 1997;350:862

55. Cartron J-P, Rouillac C, Le Van Kim C, et al. Transf Clin Biol 1996;6:497

56. Avent ND. Biotest Bull 1997;5:415

57. Faas BHW, Beckers EAM, Maaskant-van Wijk PA, et al. Biotest Bull 1997;5:439

58. Smythe J, Anstee DJ. Biotest Bull 1997;5:467

59. Sonneborn HH, Ernst M, Voak D, et al. Biotest Bull 1997;5:475

60. Scott ML, Guest AG, Rodkey LS. (abstract). Transf Med 1997;7 (Suppl 1):29

61. Paradis G, Bazin R, Lemieux R. J Immunol 1986;137:240

62. Green FA. Immunochemistry 1967;4:247

63. Abbott RE, Schachter D. J Biol Chem 1976;251:7176

64. Green FA. Mol Immunol 1983;20:769

65. Le Van Kim C, Mouro I, Chérif-Zahar B, et al. Proc Nat Acad Sci USA 1992;89:10925

66. Arce MA, Thompson ES, Wagner S, et al. Blood 1993;82:651

67. Dahr W, Schmitz G, Ernst M, et al. Biotest Bull 1997;5:451

68. Schmitz G, Sonneborn HH, Ernst M, et al. Vox Sang 1996;70:34

69. Suyama K, Lunn R, Goldstein J. Transfusion 1995;35:653

70. Smythe JS, Anstee DJ. (abstract). Transf Med 1997;7 (Suppl 1):29

71. Daniels GL, Green CA, Avent ND, et al. (abstract). Transfusion 1997;37 (Suppl 9S):101S

72. Chérif-Zahar B, Raynal V, Gane P, et al. Nature Genetics 1996;12:168

73. Huang CH, Cheng GJ, Liu Z, et al. (abstract). Blood 1997;90 (Suppl 1, part 1):22a

74. Mayer B, Schraut W, Funke I, et al. Br J Cancer 1997;75:1291

75. Sano T, Tsujino T, Yoshida K, et al. Cancer Res 1991;51:2926

76. Ezaki T, Yanagisawa A, Ohta K, et al. Br J Cancer 1996;73:424

77. Bryne M, Eide GE, Lilleng R, et al. Cancer 1991;68:1994

78. Bryne M, Thrane PS, Lilleng R, et al. Cancer 1991;68:2213

79. Halvorsen TB. Scand J Gastroenterol 1986;21:979

80. Kvist E, Krogh J, Rye B. Scand J Urol Nephrol 1990;24:253

81. Kvist E, Krogh J, Hjortberg P. Int Urol Nephrol 1992;24:417

82. Raitanen MP, Tammela TLJ. Scand J Urol Nephrol 1993;27:343

83. Cerny T, Blair V, Anderson H, et al. Int J Cancer 1987;36:146

84. Cerny T, Fey MF, Oppliger R, et al. Int J Cancer 1992;54:504

85. Okuda H, Kawano M, Iwamoto S, et al. J Clin Invest 1997;100:373

86. Tzeng J, Dodd R, Mallory D. (abstract). Transfusion 1997;37 (Suppl 9S):32S

87. Reid ME, Halverson GR, Sutherland J, et al. (abstract). Transfusion 1997;37 (Suppl 9S):89S

88. Dahr W, Gielen W, Beyreuther K, et al. Hoppe-Seyler's Z Physiol Chem 1980;361:145

89. Dahr W, Beyreuther K, Bause E, et al. Prot Biol Fluids 1982;29:57

90. Jarolim P, Moulds JM, Moulds JJ, et al. (abstract). Transfusion 1997;37 (Suppl 9S):90S

91. Moulds JM, Reveille JD, Arnett FC, et al. (abstract). Transfusion 1997;37 (Suppl 9S):32S

92. Poole J, Banks J, Kjeldsen-Kragh J, et al. (abstract). Transf Med 1997;7 (Suppl 1):27

93. High S, Tanner MJA, Macdonald EB, et al. Biochem J 1989;262:47

94. Uchikawa M, Tsuneyama H, Nakajima K, et al. (abstract). Transfusion 1997;37 (Suppl 9S):4S

95. Zelinski T, Rusnak A, McManus K, et al. (abstract). Transfusion 1997;37 (Suppl 9S):89S

96. Daniels GL. Communication to the ISBT Working Party on Terminology for Red Cell Surface Antigens, October, 1997

97. Jarolim P, Murray JL, Rubin HL, et al. Transfusion

1997;37:607

98. Zelinski T, Pongoski J, Coghlan G. (abstract). Transfusion 1997;37 (Suppl 9S):90S

99. Poole J, Hallewell H, Bruce L, et al. (abstract). Transfusion 1997;37 (Suppl 9S):90S

100. Lee S, Naime D, Reid M, et al. Transfusion 1997;37:1035

101. Lee S, Wu X, Reid M, et al. Blood 1995;85:912

102. Lee S, Wu X, Reid M, et al. Transfusion 1995;35:822

103. Lee S, Wu X, Son S, et al. Transfusion 1996;36:490

104. Jones J, Reid ME, Øyen R, et al. Vox Sang 1995;69:53

105. Marsh WL, Redman CM, Kessler LA, et al. Transfusion 1987;27:36

106. Mallinson G, Green CA, Okubo Y, et al. (abstract). Transf Med 1997;7 (Suppl 1):18

107. Weaver T, Lacey P, Carty L. (abstract). Transfusion 1986;26:561

108. Reid ME. Remarks (not printed) during a presentation on the Dombrock System in Short Topic No 309, AABB Ann Mtg, 1997

109. Strupp A, Cash K, Uehlinger J. (abstract). Transfusion 1997;37 (Suppl 9S):33S

110. Shirey RS, Boyd JS, King KE, et al. (abstract). Transfusion 1997;37 (Suppl 9S):34S

111. Kowalski MA, Pierce S, Edwards RL, et al. (abstract). Transfusion 1997;37 (Suppl 9S):35S

112. Daniels GL, Green CA, Mallinson G, et al. (abstract). Transf Med 1997;7 (Suppl 1):17

113. Lublin DM, Kompelli S, Reid ME. (abstract). Transfusion 1997;37 (Suppl 9S):102S

114. Daniels GL, Green CA, Powell R. (abstract). Transfusion 1997;37 (Suppl 9S):88S

115. Lublin DM, Thompson ES, Green AM, et al. J Clin Invest 1991;87:1945

116. Coyne KE, Hall SE, Thompson ES, et al. J Immunol 1992;149:2906

117. Petty AC, Daniels GL, Anstee DJ, et al. Vox Sang 1993;65:309

118. Lublin DM, Mallinson G, Poole J, et al. Blood 1994;84:1276

119. Telen MJ, Rao N, Udani M, et al. Blood 1994;84:3205

120. Telen MJ, Rao N, Lublin DM. (Letter). Transfusion 1995;35:278

121. Udani MN, Anderson N, Rao N, et al. Immunohematology 1995;11:1

122. Cash K, Strupp A, Uehlinger J, et al. (abstract). Transfusion 1997;37 (Suppl 9S):35S

123. Mudad R, Rao N, Issitt PD, et al. Transfusion 1995;35:925

124. Powell H, Moody S, Gooch A, et al. (abstract). Transf Med 1997;7 (Suppl 1):30

125. Anderson G, Donnelly S, Brady T, et al. (abstract). Transfusion 1993;33 (Suppl 9S):23S

126. Montgomery W, Nance S, Kavitsky D, et al. (abstract). Transfusion 1997;37 (Suppl 9S):41S

127. Thorpe SJ, Boult CE, Bailey SW, et al. Appl Immunochem 1996;4:190

128. Lubenko A, Rodi K, Williams M. (abstract). Transf Med 1997;7 (Suppl 1):32

129. Judd WJ, Steiner EA, Oberman HA, et al. Transfusion 1992;32:304

130. Alkhashan AA, Combs MR, Issitt PD. (abstract). Transfusion 1997;37 (Suppl 9S):28S

131. Rolih SD, Fisher FS, Figueroa D, et al. (abstract). Transfusion 1994;34 (Suppl 10S):19S

132. Alkhashan AA. MHS Thesis, Duke Univ 1996

133. Judd WJ, Fullen DR, Steiner EA, et al. (abstract). Transfusion 1997;37 (Suppl 9S):65S

134. Judd WJ, Steiner EA, Knafl PC. Immunohematology 1997;13:132

135. Issitt PD, Combs MR. Bradshaw T. (abstract). Transfusion 1997;37 (Suppl 9S):28S

136. Issitt, Combs MR, Booth K. (abstract). Transfusion 1997;37 (Suppl 9S):64S

137. Combs MR, Issitt PD, Malyska H. (abstract). Transfusion 1997;37 (Suppl 9S):31S

138. Combs MR, Issitt PD. (abstract). Transfusion 1997;37 (Suppl 9S):31S

139. Walker RH, Ed. Technical Manual, 11th Ed. Bethesda:Am Assoc Blood Banks, 1993:336 and 649

140. Vengelen-Tyler V. Ed. Technical Manual, 12th Ed. Bethesda:Am Assoc Blood Banks, 1993:354 and 643

141. Beattie K, Mallory DM, Eds. Immunohematology Methods and Procedures. Washington, D.C.:Am Red Cross Blood Program, 1993

142. Judd WJ. Methods in Immunohematology, 2nd Ed. Durham:Montgomery 1994:211

143. BCSH Blood Transfusion Task Force. Transf Med 1996;6:273

144. Kanter MH, Poole G, Garratty G. Transfusion 1997;37:816

145. Judd WJ, Davenport R. (Letter). Transfusion 1997;37:877

146. Case J. Editorial. Transfusion 1997;37:773

147. Kanter MH, Poole G, Garratty G. (Letter). Transfusion 1997;37:1221

148. Widmann FK. Transfusion 1997;37:665

149. Davenport RD, Kunkel SL. (abstract). Transfusion 1997;37 (Suppl 9S):1S

150. Davenport RD, Strieter RM, Standiford TJ, et al. Blood 1990;76:2439

151. Davenport RD, Streiter RM, Kunkel SL. Br J Haematol 1991;78:540

152. Davenport RD, Burdick M, Strieter RM, et al. Transfusion 1994;34:16

153. Udani M, Rao N, Telen MJ. Transfusion 1997;37:904

154. Barker RN, Casswell KM, Reid ME, et al. Br J Haematol 1992;82:126

155. Barker RN, Elson CJ. Eur J Immunol 1994;24:1578

156. Elson CJ, Barker RN, Thompson SJ, et al. Immunol Today 1995;16:71

157. Barker RN, Hall AM, Standen GR, et al. Blood 1997;90:2701

158. Arndt P, Garratty G, Borley R, et al. (abstract). Transfusion 1997;37 (Suppl 9S):34S

159. Madoz P, Muniz-Diaz E, Martinez C, et al. (abstract). Transfusion 1997;37 (Suppl 9S):36S

160. Boulton FE, Reynolds W. (abstract). Transf Med 1997;7 (Suppl 1):24

161. Boulton FE, Reynolds W, Brearley R, et al. (abstract). Transf Med 1997;7 (Suppl 1):24

162. Rankin A, Goodyear E, Boon S, et al. (abstract). Transf Med 1997;7 (Suppl 1):27

163. Yesus YW, Akhter JE. Am J Clin Pathol 1985;84:769

164. Shirey RS, Mirabella DC, Lumadue JA, et al. Transfusion 1997;37:493

165. Cash K, Brown T, Strupp A, et al. (abstract). Transfusion 1997;37 (Suppl 9S):34S

166. Hadley AG, Poole GD, Poole J, et al. Vox Sang 1996;71:108

167. Hadley A, Poole J, Poole G. (Letter). Transfusion 1997;37:985

168. Hall AR, Mason RP, Mallaband A. (abstract). Transf Med 1997;7 (Suppl 1):23

169. Armstrong-Fisher SS, Duncan JI, Urbaniak SJ, et al. (abstract). Transf Med 1997;7 (Suppl 1):24

170. Duncan JI. Reprod Fert Dev 1996;8:1547

171. Simpson MB, Pryzbylik JA, Denham JA, et al. Obstet

Gynecol 1978;52:616

172. Harrison KL, Popper EI. Transfusion 1981;21:90
173. Contreras M, Gordon H, Tidmarsh E. (Letter). Br J Haematol 1983;53:355
174. Barrie JV, Quinn MA. (Letter). Lancet 1985;1:1327
175. Pratt GA, Bowell PJ, MacKenzie IZ, et al. Clin Lab Haematol 1989;11:241
176. Todd A. BBTS Special Report No 6, May 1996:5
177. Viëtor HE, Kanhai HHH, Brand A. Transfusion 1994;34:970
178. Avent ND. Biotest Bull 1997;5:429
179. Aubin J-T, Le Van Kim C, Mouro I, et al. Br J Haematol 1997;98:356
180. Maaskant-van Wijk PA, Faas BHW, de Ruijter JAM, et al. (abstract). Transfusion 1997;37 (Suppl 9S):1S
181. Mueller TH, Gassner C, Gran S, et al. (abstract). Transfusion 1997;37 (Suppl 9S):19S
182. Faas BHW, Christiaens GCML, Maaskant PA, et al. (abstract). Transfusion 1997;37 (Suppl 9S):100S
183. Legler TJ, Blaschke V, Bustami N, et al. (abstract). Transfusion 1997;37 (Suppl 9S):100S
184. Gassner C, Mueller TH, Wagner FF, et al. (abstract). Transfusion 1997;37 (Suppl 9S):101S
185. Murphy MT, Fraser RH, Goddard JP. Transf Med 1996;6:133
186. Avent ND, Martin PG. Br J Haematol 1996;93:728
187. Lee S, Bennett PR, Overton T, et al. Am J Obstet Gynecol 1996;175:455
188. Hessner MJ, McFarland JG, Endean DJ. Transfusion 1996;36:495
189. Mifsud NA, Haddad AP, Sparrow RL, et al. (Letter). Blood 1997;89:4662
190. Kim DA, Kim TY, Choi TY. (abstract). Transfusion 1997;37 (Suppl 9S):33S
191. Rios M, Reid ME, Naime D, et al. (abstract). Transfusion 1997;37 (Suppl 9S):70S
192. Rios M, Reid ME, Naime D, et al. (abstract). Transfusion 1997;37 (Suppl 9S):101S
193. Olsson ML, Hansson C, Åkesson IE, et al. (abstract). Transfusion 1997;37 (Suppl 9S):102S
194. Arndt P, Hunt P, Garratty G, et al. (abstract). Transfusion 1997;37 (Suppl 9S):34S
195. Thorpe SJ. Biotest Bull 1997;5:523
196. Garratty G, Arndt P, Nance S. (abstract). Blood 1997;90 (Suppl 1, part 1):473a
197. Chu T, Reid ME, Øyen R, et al. (abstract). Blood 1997;90 (Suppl 1, part 1):435a
198. Yazdanbakhsh K, Øyen R, Reid ME. (abstract). Blood 1997;90 (Suppl 1, part 1):436a
199. Yazdanbakhsh K, Lee S, Reid ME. (abstract). Blood 1997;90 (Suppl 1, part 1):436a
200. Sandler SG, Mallory D, Nance ST. (abstract). Transfusion 1997;37 (Suppl 9S):95S
201. Zimmerman SA, Combs MR, Issitt PD, et al. (abstract). Blood 1997;90 (Suppl 1, part 1):458a
202. Win N, Logan RW, Cameron A. (Letter). Vox Sang 1997;73:56
203. BCSH Blood Transfusion Task Force. Transf Med 1996;6:261
204. Westgren M, Selbing A, Stangenberg M. Br Med J 1988;296:885
205. Galligan BR, Cairns R, Schifano JV, et al. Transfusion

206. Sesok-Pizzini D, Ratajczak M, Moore J, et al. (abstract). Blood 1997;90 (Suppl 1, part 1):472a
207. Palfi M, Hildén J-O. Vox Sang 1997;72:114
208. Garratty G, Arndt P, Domen R, et al. Vox Sang 1997;72:124
209. Rasamoelisolo M, Czerwinski M, Bruneau V, et al. Vox Sang 1997;72:185
210. Win N, Islam SIAM, Peterkin SA, et al. Vox Sang 1997;72:182
211. Gassner C, Schmarda A, Kilga-Nogler S, et al. Transfusion 1997;37:1020
212. Lee S, Naime DS, Reid ME, et al. Transfusion 1997;37:1117
213. Lee S. Unpublished observations cited in Reid ME, Lomas-Francis C. The Blood Group Antigen Facts Book. San Diego:Academic, 1997
214. King M-J, Kosanke J, Reid ME, et al. Transfusion 1997;37:1027
215. Thompson KM, Sutherland J, Barden G, et al. Scand J Immunol 1991;34:509
216. Borretzen M, Chapman C, Stevensen FK, et al. Scand J Immunol 1995;42:90
217. Silberstein LE, Jefferies LC, Goldman J, et al. Blood 1991;78:2372
218. Pascual V, Victor K, Spellerberg M, et al. J Immunol 1992;149:2337
219. Smith G, Spellergberg M, Boulton F, et al. Vox Sang 1995;68:231
220. Thorpe SJ, Boult CE, Stevenson FK, et al. Transfusion 1997;37:1111
221. Fukumori Y, Hori Y, Ohnoki S, et al. Transf Med 1997;7:227
222. Wallace M, Lomas-Francis C, Beckers E, et al. Transf Med 1997;7:233
223. Hunter CJ, Ziebol MD. Immunohematology 1997;13:136
224. Zago-Novaretti MC, Jorge CR, Jens E, et al. Immunohematology 1997;13:138
225. Øyen R, Halverson GR, Reid ME. Immunohematology 1997;13:75
226. Costamagna L, Barbarini M, Viarengo GL, et al. Immunohematology 1997;13:61
227. Mosley AL, Trich MB, Thomas NC, et al. Immunohematology 1997;37:58
228. Issitt LA. Immunohematology 1997;13:1
229. Kitchen KD. (Letter). Immunohematology 1997;13:145
230. Issitt, PD, personal communication to Issitt LA, and Issitt LA, personal communication to Issitt PD, 1997
231. Mendez MJ, Green LL, Corvalan JRF, et al. Nature Genet 1997;15:146
232. Griffiths M, Beaumont N, Yao SYN, et al. Nature Med 1997;3:89
233. Ogasawara K, Yabe R, Uchikawa M, et al. Blood 1996;88:2732
234. Suzuki K, Iwata M, Tsuji H, et al. Hum Genet 1997;99:454
235. Olsson ML, Guerreiro JF, Zago MA, et al. Biochem Biophys Res Comm 1997;234:779
236. Olsson ML, Chester MA, Santos SEB, et al. (abstract). Transfusion 1997;37 (Suppl 9S):103S
237. Marini A-M, Urrestarazu A, Beauwens R, et al. Trends Biochem Sci 1997;22:460

1989;29:179

In this index, most antigens but few antibodies are listed. Information about antibodies will be found on the pages indexed for the antigen defined. Numbers in bold face indicate that the information indexed is in Chapter 46, addenda. When the relationship to a blood group system is obvious, the antigen is included only in the listing for the blood group system. For example, Rh32, Rh33, et al. appear only in the Rh system listing. When the relationship is less obvious the antigen is included in the system listing but also has an independent entry. As examples, Wr^a and Wr^b are in the Diego system listing under D but also appear as Wr^a and Wr^b, under W. Some obsolete antigens are listed as a guide to where new names or information is given. Some of the smaller systems do not have system entries, as examples, the Scianna system antigens are listed individually as Sc1, Sc2, etc., those of the Indian system appear only under In^a and In^b. Finally, because the antigens are listed by system in Chapter 44, the antigen catalog, no index entries for pages 1145 to 1169 are given.